BRIEF CONTENTS

MATERNAL - NEWBORN NURSING

MATERNAL-NEWBORN NURSING

A FAMILY-CENTERED APPROACH

FIFTH EDITION

SALLY B. OLDS, RNC, MS
Associate Professor and Chair
Department of Holistic Nursing
Beth-El College of Nursing and Health Sciences
Colorado Springs, Colorado

MARCIA L. LONDON, RNC, MSN, NNP
Associate Professor and Director
Neonatal Nurse Practitioner Program
Beth-El College of Nursing and Health Sciences
Colorado Springs, Colorado

PATRICIA WIELAND LADEWIG, PhD, RNC, NP
Professor and Dean
School for Health Care Professions
Regis University
Denver, Colorado

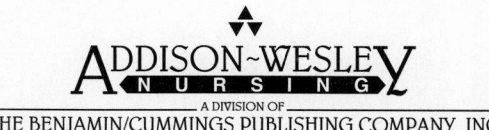

ADDISON~WESLEY NURSING
A DIVISION OF
THE BENJAMIN/CUMMINGS PUBLISHING COMPANY, INC.

Menlo Park, California • Reading, Massachusetts • New York • Don Mills, Ontario
Wokingham, U.K. • Amsterdam • Bonn • Paris • Milan • Madrid • Sydney
Singapore • Tokyo • Seoul • Taipei • Mexico City • San Juan, Puerto Rico

Executive Editor Patricia L. Cleary

Developmental Editor Elizabeth Maynard Schaefer

Managing Editor Wendy Earl

Production Editor David Rich

Editorial Assistant Marla Nowick

Text and Insert Designer Cloyce Wall

Cover Designer Yvo Riezebos Design

Page Designer Brenn Lea Pearson

Art Coordinator Bradley Burch

Photo Researcher Kathleen Cameron

Copy Editor Sylvia Stein Wright

Proofreader Kristin Barendsen

Indexer Karen Hollister

Senior Manufacturing Supervisor Merry Free Osborn

Compositor and Prepress Supplier GTS Graphics

Printer Von Hoffmann Press, Inc.

Cover Printer Color Dot, Inc.

Cover Quilt *I See the Moon* by Joy Baaklini

Library of Congress Cataloging-in-Publication Data

Olds, Sally B., 1940-
    Maternal-newborn nursing : a family centered approach /
Sally B. Olds, Marcia L. London, Patricia W. Ladewig. —
5th ed.
        p.   cm.
    Includes index.
    ISBN 0-8053-5612-6
    1. Maternity nursing.   I. London, Marcia L.   II.
Ladewig, Patricia W.   III. Title.
RG951.043   1995
810.73′878—dc20   95-38372
                                            CIP

ISBN 0-8053-5612-6
    2   3   4   5   6   7   8   9   10 - VH - 99   98   97   96

Photographic and art credits appear on page 1170.

Care has been taken to confirm the accuracy of information presented in this book. The authors, editors, and the publisher, however, cannot accept any responsibility for errors or omissions or for the consequences from application of the information in this book and make no warranty, expressed or implied, with respect to its contents.

The authors and publishers have exerted every effort to ensure that drug selections and dosages set forth in this text are in accord with current recommendations and practice at the time of publication. However, in view of ongoing research, changes in government regulations, and the constant flow of information relating to drug therapy and drug reactions, the reader is urged to check the package inserts of all drugs for any change in indications of dosage and for added warnings and precautions. This is particularly important when the recommended agent is a new and/or infrequently employed drug.

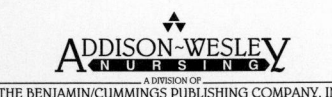
ADDISON-WESLEY NURSING
A DIVISION OF
THE BENJAMIN/CUMMINGS PUBLISHING COMPANY, INC.

2725 Sand Hill Road
Menlo Park, California 94025

DEDICATION

At this moment in time, when it seems that challenge and change are integral parts of every aspect of our personal and professional lives, we would like to pause to recognize some special women who have had and will continue to have tremendous impact upon our lives.

To Donna Johnson, my teacher and guide.
S B O

To my future colleagues, the neonatal nurses and neonatal nurse-practitioner students whose deep sense of caring for babies and their families provides an inspirational thread that is interwoven through my philosophy of teaching.
M L L

To Freda Ladewig, my mother-in law, who has taught me the meaning of courage.
P W L

We thank each of you for your gifts of love, friendship, guidance, and presence.

Tsulan Balka, RNC, MA, ACCE
Saint Joseph Hospital
Denver, Colorado

S Robin Barca, RNC, MS, CCE
Houston Valley Hospital and Medical Center
Kingsport, Tennessee

Emily Coogan Bennett, RNC, MS
Medical College of Virginia
Richmond, Virginia

Barbara E Carey, RNC, MN, NNP, CPNP
University of California, Los Angeles
Los Angeles, California

Nancy Kiernan Case, RN, PhD
Regis University
Denver, Colorado

Jane E Congleton, RN, BSN, MS, CGC
Memorial Hospital
Colorado Springs, Colorado

Mary English, RNC, MSN
Pennsylvania Reproductive Associates
Philadelphia, Pennsylvania

Vicky Flanagan, RN, BSN
Dartmouth-Hitchcock Medical Center
Lebanon, New Hampshire

Mary Hagedorn, RN, PhD, CPNP
Beth-El College of Nursing and Health Sciences
Colorado Springs, Colorado

Mary Ellen Honeyfield, RNC, MS, NNP
Innovative Health Care Incorporated
Denver, Colorado

Jeanne M Howell, RN, MS, CNM
Alexandria OB/GYN Associates
Alexandria, Minnesota

Sara L Jarrett, RN, MA, MS
Regis University
Denver, Colorado

Virginia Gramzow Kinnick, BSN, MSN, EdD, CNM
University of Northern Colorado
Greeley, Colorado

Cheryl Pope Kish, RN, MSN, EdD
Georgia College
Milledgeville, Georgia

Ruth Likler, RNC, BSN
Presbyterian/St Lukes Medical Center
Denver, Colorado

Marilyn Lowe, RNC, MSN
Nebraska Methodist Hospital
Omaha, Nebraska

Vicki A Lucas, RNC, PhD
Memorial Hospital Southwest
Houston, Texas

Kathy Marvel, RNC, MSN
Rose Medical Center
Denver, Colorado

Deborah Cooper McGee, RNC, MSN, PNNP
Presbyterian/St Lukes Medical Center
Denver, Colorado

Patricia Budd Moores, RN, PhD
Beth-El College of Nursing and Health Sciences
Colorado Springs, Colorado

Carol Myers, RNC, BSN
The Toledo Hosptial
Toledo, Ohio

Candace Layn Polzella, MSS, RD
Schwenksville, Pennsylvania

Diane Roth, RNC, BSN, RD, MS
HealthOne/Swedish Medical Center
Englewood, Colorado

Victoria Stetson, CNM, MS
Lovelace Medical Center
Albuquerque, New Mexico

Catherine E Theorell, RNC, MSN, NNP
Rush-Presbyterian St Lukes Medical Center
Chicago, Illinois

Candice J Tolve, RNC, MS
Regis University
Denver, Colorado

Susan Thompson Voss, RN, MSN
Blessing-Rieman College of Nursing
Quincy, Illinois

Helen B Walker, RNC, MSN, CNS
Mobile Infirmary Medical Center
Mobile, Alabama

REVIEWERS

Georgeanne Adamy, RN, MSW
DeAnza Community College
Cupertino, California

Bernadine Adams, RN, BSN, MN
Northeast Louisiana University
Monroe, Louisiana

Janet Azar, RN, BSN, MNEd
Tidewater Community College
Portsmouth, Virginia

Karen Bess, RN, MaEd, MSN
Jewish Hospital College of Nursing
  and Allied Health
St Louis, Missouri

Janet C Brookman, RN, BSN,
  MSN, DSN
The University of Alabama,
  Huntsville
Huntsville, Alabama

Judith Carveth, RN, BSN, MSN,
  PhD, CNM
University of North Carolina at
  Charlotte
Charlotte, North Carolina

Sandra K Cesario, RNC, BSN, MS
University of Oklahoma
Langston University
Tulsa, Oklahoma

Tom Coehlo, RN, BSN, MSN,
  C-FNP
Oregon Health Science University
  at Southern Oregon State College
Ashland, Oregon

José PC de Cangas, RN, MN
Lakehead University
Thunder Bay, Ontario, Canada

Dawn M Deford, RN, MS
Denton Community Hospital
Denton, Texas

Gretchen Stone Dimico, RNC,
  MN, PhD, IBCLC
Lewis-Clark State College, Coeur
  d'Alene Campus
Coeur d'Alene, Idaho

Sherry G Fader, BSN, MSN, RNC
Quincy College
Quincy, Massachusetts

Polly D Fehler, RN, AS, BSN,
  MSN
Tri-County Technical College
Pendleton, South Carolina

Sr Mary Jean Flaherty, PhD, RN,
  FAAN
The Catholic University of America
Washington, DC

Margaret Comerford Freda, EdD,
  RN, FAAN
Albert Einstein College of Medicine
Bronx, New York

Elizabeth Gualtieri, RN, BSN,
  MSN
Brookdale Community College
Lincroft, New Jersey

Margaret S Hamilton, RN, MNSc,
  DNS(C)
Purdue University
West Lafayette, Indiana

Mary Verweyst Kaufman, RN,
  MSN
Grand Rapids Community College
Grand Rapids, Michigan

Carol Kenner, RNC, DNS, FAAN
University of Cincinnati
Cincinnati, Ohio

Cheryl Pope Kish, RN, MSN, EdD
Georgia College
Milledgeville, Georgia

Mary M Lambert, RN, BS, MSEd
Western Oklahoma State College
Altus, Oklahoma

Jeanne Linhart, RN, C, BSN, MSN,
  FNP
Rockland Community College
Suffern, New York

Mary Maggio, RN, MN, CNP
Palo Alto Medical Foundation
Palo Alto, California

Myrtle Mayfield, RN, BSN, MEd
Watts School of Nursing
Durham, North Carolina

Alice Michaels, RN, BSCN, MSA
Central Queensland University
Rochapton, Queensland, Australia

Barbara S Migliore, RN, BSN
Los Angeles Pierce College
Woodland Hills, California

Laura R Romero, RN, MSN, CNM
East Los Angeles College
Monterey Park, California

Kathy J Schutler, RN, BSN, MSN
Belmont Technical College
St Clairsville, Ohio

Lynn C Tesh, RN, MSN
Randolph Community College
Asheboro, North Carolina

Louise F Timmer, RN, EdD
California State University,
  Sacramento
Sacramento, California

Leslie Young-Lewis, RN, BScN,
  MScN, PhD (c)
University of Toronto
Toronto, Ontario, Canada

Celesta L Warner, RN, MS
Wright State University
Dayton, Ohio

Judy E White, RN, BSN, MA, MSN
Rockland Community College
Suffern, New York

Susan Karn Wieczorek, RN, AAN,
  BSN, MSN
Health Education Consulting
  Institute
Columbus, Georgia

Norma N Wilkerson, RN, PhD
University of Wyoming
Laramie, Wyoming

Alex Wright, RN, RM, BA
The University of Sydney
Sydney, Australia

The wonder of childbirth remains unchanged. More than ever before, nurses play a central role in planning for and during the experience of birth, and in how families feel about the experience afterward. As women's choices about childbirth continue to expand, so do the responsibilities and commitment of the nurse. However, other forces are at work as well. The changes occurring in the health care delivery system have staggering implications for nurses everywhere, even nurses caring for childbearing families. Shortened length of stay, the trend toward greater use of home care options, the impact of HIV/AIDS, the increasing use of unlicensed assistive personnel, downsizing and mergers of large health care systems, the aging of the population—these and a myriad of other factors are altering the way we practice nursing today and in the future.

Now, more than ever, nurses must be flexible, creative, and open to change. They must be able to think critically and problem-solve effectively; they must be able to meet the teaching needs of their clients so that their clients can, in turn, better meet their own health care needs; they must be open to an increasingly multicultural population; they must understand and use the technology available in their chosen area of practice; and, most critically, they must never lose sight of the importance of excellent nursing care in improving the quality of people's lives.

The underlying philosophy of *Maternal-Newborn Nursing: A Family-Centered Approach* remains unchanged. We believe that pregnancy and birth are normal life processes and that family members are co-participants in care. However, we have also worked to provide a text that helps students develop the skills and abilities they will need in a changing health care environment.

NEW FEATURES

In this edition we have introduced several new features designed to enhance clinical skills and critical thinking abilities.

- **Critical Pathways** reflect a growing trend in the way nurses manage care. Four critical paths—intrapartal, newborn, postpartal, and cesarean birth—will help students plan and manage care within normally anticipated time frames. Students will become familiar with this approach to managing care so they are better prepared for clinical settings.

- **Critical Thinking in Practice** provides brief scenarios that ask students to determine the appropriate response to real-life clinical situations. Answers to the scenarios are provided in Appendix I to give students immediate feedback on their decision-making skills.

- **Essential Precautions in Practice** boxes appear throughout the text to help students apply appropriate blood and body fluid precautions in a variety of nursing care situations.

- **Teaching Moments** provide one of our favorite new features. These tips, or "pearls of wisdom," are gleaned from our own clinical practice or that of colleagues and are addressed directly to the students.

- A new chapter, **Client Teaching**, provides theoretical and practical information for students on approaches to client teaching. We devoted an entire chapter to this topic because of the role teaching plays in nursing today and because clients need accurate information presented in an understandable way if they are to problem-solve effectively.

- **Home care** is a growing trend in health care and it is called out by a colored heading in the chapters focusing on high-risk pregnancy and postpartal conditions.

- The **Research in Practice** boxes have been completely updated to reflect the latest research findings, and are redesigned to focus on the applicability of the findings for clinical practice. This helps students grasp the importance of clinical nursing research for effective practice.

- The new **full-color format** of the book provides an exciting and dramatic change. Color is used to highlight key features of the text for student readers. Full-color artwork is not only visually appealing, but clarifies anatomical structures and clinical procedures for easier understanding. The liberal use of new color photos brings students closer to the world of families and newborns.

Nursing Process and the Role of the Maternal-Newborn Nurse

While some books cover the role of the medical community in childbirth as a separate topic, our book gives an overview of *all* aspects of the childbearing process *with a specific emphasis on nursing care throughout pregnancy, labor and birth, and the postpartal period*. The nurse's role is clearly delineated and is presented within the framework of the nursing process. Chapters are organized around the five steps of the nursing process: assessment, diagnosis, planning, implementation, and evaluation. Numerous special features reinforce the nursing process as a framework for learning and for nursing care. The **Assessment Guides** incorporate expected findings, possible alterations, and causes, as well as guidelines for interventions. Revised and updated **Nursing Care Plans** are now easier to use and include a new section called *Essential Nursing Activities to Achieve Outcomes*. **Procedures,** such as those on pages 236 and 614, describe interventions specific to maternal-newborn nursing care in illustrated, step-by-step fashion.

Emphasis on Client/Family Teaching

Client and family teaching is a crucial responsibility of the maternal-newborn nurse, one we continue to strongly emphasize and highlight in this fifth edition. Again, our focus is on the teaching that nurses do at all stages of pregnancy and the childbearing process—including the important postpartal teaching that is done before and immediately after families are discharged. In several places a more detailed discussion of client/family teaching is summarized in the **Teaching Guides,** such as the one on *Sexual Activity During Pregnancy*, which starts on page 386. The tearout **Client/Family Teaching Cards** are also handy tools for the student to use while studying or for quick reference in the clinical setting. Furthermore, a fold-out, full-color **Fetal Development Chart** depicts maternal/fetal development month by month and provides specific teaching guidelines for each stage of pregnancy. Students can use this as another studying tool or as a quick clinical reference.

State-of-the-Art Teaching/Learning Tools

Instructors and students alike continue to praise the abundance of in-text learning aids included in our books. With this edition, we have once again created a book that is both easy to learn from and easy to use as a reference. Each chapter begins with behavioral **Objectives** and a list of **Key Terms,** and ends with a summary of **Key Con-**cepts as well as a list of **References.** Where appropriate, we have included **Drug Guides** for those medications commonly used in maternal-newborn nursing, to guide students in correctly administering medications. Additionally, photographs, quotes, and vignettes from nurses, clients, and students bring a personal perspective to the text by presenting real-life individuals. Finally, a **Glossary** of terms commonly used in the field of maternal-newborn nursing can be found at the back of the book.

Enhanced Visual Appeal

Because today's students are more visually oriented than ever, we have developed an exciting new full-color design and art program to command their interest and emphasize the key information they need to learn. Students are brought closer to the childbearing experience through the use of dramatic photographs of women and families from many cultures and backgrounds.

Commitment to Diversity

With this edition, we attempt to make our text even more inclusive through a commitment to diversity beyond multiculturalism. We realize such an approach is difficult at best, but feel its success cannot be measured simply in terms of specific photos, charts, or tables. Instead, we believe that with its subtle integration of a variety of issues and scenarios affecting maternal-newborn nursing care—beyond an emphasis on ethnicity alone—our approach is more accessible overall.

Complete Teaching/Learning Package

To help instructors make the best use of this new edition, we have developed a comprehensive package of new supplements with the following components:

- **Student Workbook**   This popular workbook has been revised and updated in keeping with the changes made in this revision. It incorporates strategies for students to increase synthesis of their knowledge.

- **1000-Item Test Bank**   Available in booklet form or as computer software for IBM or Apple, this updated and revised test bank helps faculty quickly and easily create numerous unique examinations. Test items are classified by cognitive level and nursing process step.

- **Clinical Handbook**   Written by the authors, this clinical handbook serves as a portable, succinct quick-reference to guide students in the clinical area.

- **Instructor's Manual** Written by Virginia Kinnick, CNM, EdD, this timesaving aid has been thoroughly revised and includes transparency masters.
- **Transparency Acetates** A set of full-color transparencies present enlarged versions of important text figures.

ACKNOWLEDGMENTS

Our goal with every revision is to incorporate the newest research and latest information from the literature of nursing and related fields to make our text as relevant and useful as possible. This would not be possible without the support and encouragement of our colleagues. The comments and suggestions we have received from nurse educators and practitioners around the country have helped us make the text accurate and up-to-date. Whenever a nurse takes the time to write or to speak to one of us at a professional gathering, we recognize again the intense commitment of nurses to excellence in practice. And so we thank our peers.

In publishing as in health care, quality assurance is an essential part of the process; that is the dimension our reviewers have added. Some reviewers assist us by validating the accuracy of the content, some by their attention to detail, and some by challenging us to examine our ways of thinking and to develop a new awareness. Thus we extend our sincere thanks to all those who reviewed the manuscript for this book; their names and affiliations are listed before this Preface.

We are also grateful to the contributors to the fifth edition of *Maternal-Newborn Nursing: A Family-Centered Approach.* Their knowledge of clinical practice and current literature in their areas of expertise helps make the chapters relevant and accurate. They, too, are listed just before this Preface.

During the process of revising this book, we often develop intense working relationships and long-term friendships. This is especially true of the two editors who worked with us—Peggy Adams and Patti Cleary. Peggy is warm, caring, and dedicated. She worked closely with us as the manuscript unfolded and sustained us during the rough times; she became a friend and confidante. Her life has taken a new, exciting turn and though we miss her, we wish her all the very best.

Patti Cleary is exceptional. We have known her for years, trust her implicitly, and value her guidance. She exemplifies all that is best about an editor and we are delighted to work with her again. She is a true friend.

Beth Schaefer, the developmental editor, brought a fresh eye to our book and helped us revise and update effectively. She is a woman of gentle speech and great patience, and we appreciate her commitment to our project.

The effort involved in coordinating the production phase of a book is mind-boggling. It requires an incredible eye for detail, the patience of a saint, and the ability to "crack a whip" judiciously. It also requires a high tolerance for crisis. Dave Rich, the production coordinator, is such a person. Even more amazing is the fact that, though we have never met him and he remains only a voice on the phone, we have absolute confidence in him. He has never let us down!

Bradley Burch of Wendy Earl Productions coordinated all the art for the manuscript. Each time we work with Brad we grow to appreciate even more his eye for detail, his commitment to the book, and his great patience. He knows what we want the book to convey and he helps us to achieve our goal.

Finally, we extend our warm thanks to the Marketing Manager at Addison-Wesley Nursing, John Harpster, and his wife, Barbara, for sharing with us their experiences of Barbara's pregnancy and their welcoming of their newborn son, Justin Christopher. The Harpsters are featured in the series of photos on the fold-out insert. Their experiences add a delightful personal touch to the book.

During these times of uncertainty in the health care environment, we are sustained by our passion for nursing and our vision of what childbirth means. Time and again we have seen the difference a skilled nurse can make in the lives of people in need. We, like you, are committed to helping all nurses recognize and take pride in that fact. Thank you for your letters, your comments, and your suggestions. We are renewed by your support.

DEAR STUDENTS:

We believe that working with childbearing families gives you the opportunity to experience the essence of nursing at its best. You can play a vital role in helping families learn what they need to know in order to be as independent as possible; you can improve and refine your assessment skills as you work with essentially healthy women and infants, and those with complications; and you can also use the other nursing skills you have learned in a variety of acute care settings.

We love this field and we know that many of you will as well. Some of you, on the other hand, may find that this area of nursing is not your first interest, and that's OK, too. We would have a real problem if every nurse loved the same area!

We do hope that you will use this opportunity to grow in professional ability and to appreciate the importance of all you do as nurses—not just the technical and organizational tasks, although they are undoubtedly crucial, but also the caring you bring to the role of nurse. When you hold the hand of a laboring woman or help an adolescent plan a way to tell her parents of her pregnancy; when you provide accepting care to a woman with AIDS or gently stroke the skin of a preterm infant; when you rejoice with a delighted father or console a grieving one; you are practicing the heart of nursing.

Caring in an optimal environment is not difficult, but caring in today's practice setting is more of a challenge. Finding a way to maintain a caring environment when you are overworked and stretched by fiscal constraints and a lack of adequate staffing requires great dedication, creativity, and personal resolve. We have attempted to help you translate caring into practice throughout this text through the tone of the book, the photos and art work, the personal quotes, and the content itself with its emphasis on holistic care.

As you work to translate what you learn into practice, please take care of yourselves as well. Providing excellent nursing care is infinitely rewarding and can be energizing, but it is also draining both physically and emotionally. Make time to play, rest, exercise, be with loved ones, and participate in things that rejuvenate you.

We think that nurses are very special people and we are proud to be counted among them. Good luck with your studies! We wish you well.

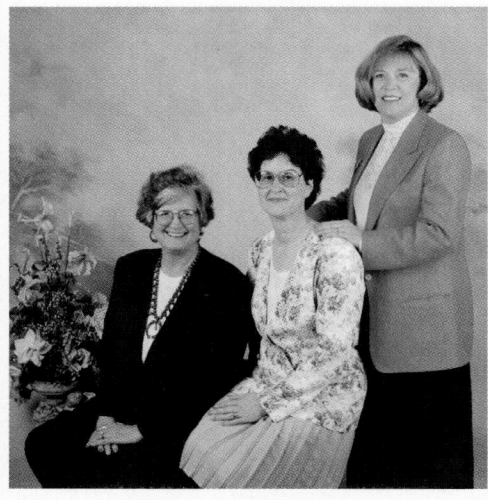

Left to right: Sally Olds; Marcia London; Pat Ladewig

SALLY B. OLDS
MARCIA L. LONDON
PAT W. LADEWIG

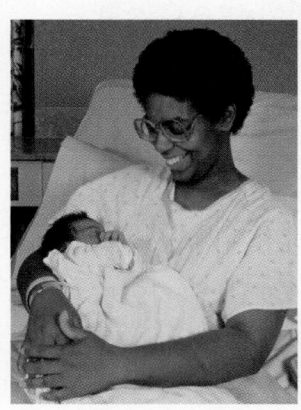

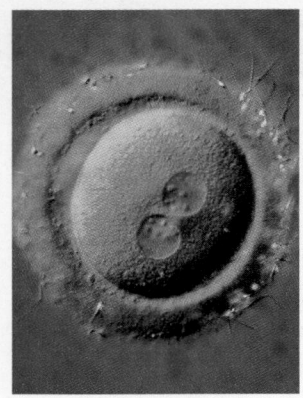

PART TWO
HUMAN REPRODUCTION

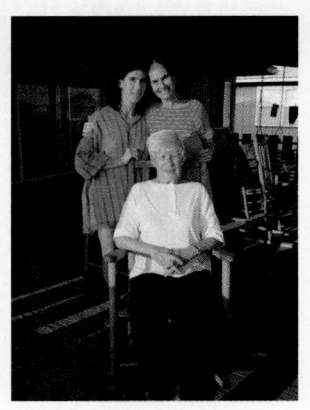

PART THREE
WOMEN'S HEALTH
THROUGHOUT THE
LIFESPAN

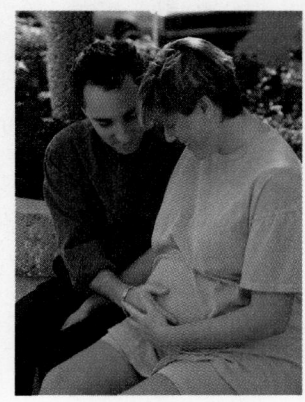

PART FOUR
PREGNANCY

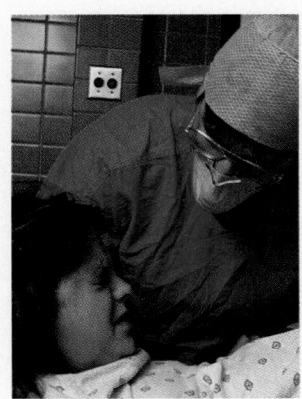

PART FIVE
BIRTH

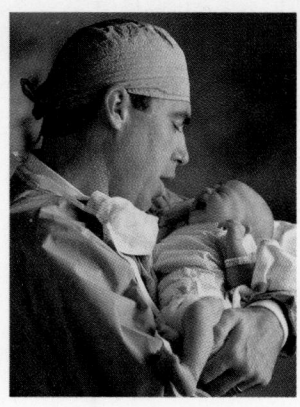

PART SIX
THE NEWBORN

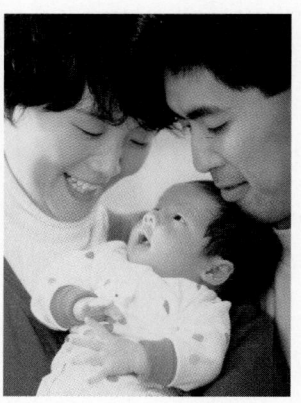

PART SEVEN
POSTPARTUM

TO THE STUDENT

*T*his textbook contains numerous learning tools to help increase your understanding of key concepts and guide you in applying maternal-newborn nursing care.

CRITICAL THINKING IN PRACTICE

A mother calls you to her room. She sounds frightened and says her baby can't breathe. You find the mother cradling her infant in her arms. The infant is mildly cyanotic, waving her arms, and has mucus coming from her nose and mouth. What would you do?

Answer (from Appendix I): Reassure mother that you will help her baby as you carry out the following activities:

- *Position the infant with her head lowered and to the side.*
- *Bulb suction the nares and mouth repeatedly until the airway is cleared.*
- *Hold and comfort the infant when normal respirations are restored.*
- *Reassure the mother, and review this procedure with her.*

NOTE: If bulb suctioning alone does not clear the airway, use DeLee wall suction and administer oxygen as needed to restore normal respirations.

CRITICAL THINKING IN PRACTICE boxes use a case study format to further develop effective problem-solving and decision-making skills. Responses are provided in the Appendix.

For additional examples, see pages 329, 381, and 1129.

Critical Thinking Question

What approaches might be effective in assessing medication use in a pregnant woman?

CRITICAL THINKING QUESTIONS are integrated throughout the text to encourage you to select appropriate strategies to support client needs.

For additional examples, see pages 197, 659, and 1096.

ESSENTIAL PRECAUTIONS IN PRACTICE

DURING PRENATAL EXAMINATIONS

Examples of times when gloves should be worn include the following:

- When drawing blood for lab work
- When handling urine specimens
- During pelvic examinations (sterile gloves)

In most instances in a clinic or office setting, gowns and goggles are not necessary because splashing of fluids is unlikely.

REMEMBER to wash your hands prior to putting the disposable gloves on and AGAIN immediately after you remove the gloves.

For further information consult OSHA and CDC guidelines.

ESSENTIAL PRECAUTIONS IN PRACTICE boxes, integrated throughout the text, show you how to apply appropriate infection control practices in a variety of situations.

For additional examples, see pages 761, 901, and 1118.

For additional examples, see pages 642, 860, and 1070.

CRITICAL PATHWAYS provide detailed, time-sequenced guides of anticipated care for women giving birth—whether vaginally or by cesarean section—for healthy newborns and for new mothers. In addition, numerous **nursing care plans** throughout the text help you structure your response to a wide range of situations you may encounter.

CESAREAN BIRTH CRITICAL PATHWAY

Category	Day of Surgery	Postoperative Day #1	Postoperative Day #2
Referral	Report from OR nurse	Lactation consultation if needed	Home nursing referral if indicated
Assessments	Assessments q15 min × 4, then q½ h × 2, then q4h if stable Vital signs: • BP WNL; no hypotension; no ↑ >30 mm systolic or 15 mm diastolic over baseline • Pulse: bradycardia normal; consistent with baseline • Respirations: 12–20/min; quiet, easy • Temperature 36.2–37.6 C (98–99.6 F); check initially; if WNL then q4h Pulse oxymetry: monitor first 2h; >90% Auscultate breath sounds: lungs clear, no adventitious sounds Breasts: soft, colostrum present Lochia: scant initially; rubra; no free flow or passage of clots Assess top of fundus (or sides depending on incision location) for firmness Dressings: clean & dry Comfort ≤5 on scale of 1 to 10 Auscultate for bowel sounds Check Homan's sign q shift: negative	Continue postpartum/postoperative assessments q4h until 24h postop, then q8h Vital signs assessment: all WNL; report temperature >38 C (100.4 F) Fundal height, location and firmness: normally firm, in the midline, at umbilicus Lochia—type, amount, odor; normally rubra, scant to moderate, earthy odor Lung sounds Bowel sounds checked until return of bowel sounds Assess abdomen for distention; should be soft, nondistended Dressings Homan's sign Breasts: Evaluate nipple status; should be no evidence of cracking or bruising Observe feeding technique with newborn Continue assessment of comfort level	Continue postpartum and postoperative assessments as described q8h Vital signs assessment q8h; all WNL; report temperature >38 C (100.4 F) Breasts: full; nipples should remain free of cracks, fissures, bruising Feeding technique with newborn: should be good or improving Incision: clean, dry; no redness, edema, drainage
Comfort	Institute comfort measures: position of comfort, adequate warmth Pain medication _____ by IV, PCA, or IM as ordered Epidural or intrathecal narcotic analgesia: follow analgesia orders from anesth. × 24h	Continue with pain management techniques Pain medication _____ as ordered PO once IV d/c'd Stool softener as ordered	Continue with pain management techniques
Teaching/ psychosocial	Orient to room if transferred from OR or delivery room Explain comfort measures, pain relief options Teach self-massage of fundus and expected findings If sufficiently alert, provide assistance with breastfeeding or bottle feeding Begin initial newborn teaching for woman or support person: bulb suctioning, positioning, diaper change, cord care Teach pericare	Provide information on early postpartum period Discuss postpartum psychologic changes Continue newborn teaching: soothing/comforting techniques, swaddling; return demonstrations indicate woman's understanding Provide opportunities for question and review; reinforce previous teaching Breastfeeding: nipple care; air-drying, lanolin, proper latch-on technique; tea bags Breast pumping if newborn in NICU Bottle feeding: supportive bra, ice bags, breast binder	Discuss incisional care Discuss involution, anticipated physical changes first two weeks postpartum, postpartum exercises, need to limit visitors Discuss postpartum nutrition: balanced diet, high protein and vitamin C to encourage wound healing Breastfeeding: • Increase calories by 500 kcal over nonpregnant state (200 kcal over pregnant intake) • Explain milk production, let-down reflex, use of supplements, breast pumping, and milk storage; answer questions Bottle feeding: • Return to normal caloric intake for nonpregnant state • Explain formula preparation and storage Discuss sibling rivalry: mother should have plan for supporting siblings at home Teaching evaluation completed

Category	Day of Surgery	Postoperative Day #1 *continued*	Postoperative Day #2 *continued*
	...ss if general ...d to questions ...ty and sensation ...thecal narcotics, ...: decreased ...ons < 11; ...tern; signs of ...int pupils; ...igns of sedation; ...ve nausea, ...tics: assess resp ...or 12 hours ...weigh pads if ...ad; presence of ...2h ...sary	If woman Rh⁻ and infant Rh⁺, RhoGAM work up; consent obtained; teaching completed, Administer RhoGAM if indicated Obtain consent for rubella vaccine if indicated; explain purpose, procedure, implications Obtain CBC D/C Foley	D/C buffalo cap Administer rubella vaccine if indicated Remove staples before discharge
Activity	Bed rest, position of comfort Siderails up for safety Maintain flat in bed if spinal anesthesia given May dangle p8h assistance (12p spinal)	Encourage leg exercises when in bed Progressive ambulation with assistance then independently as tolerated May shower with assistance p24h	Up ad lib as tolerated; encourage ambulation May shower independently
Nutrition	NPO until bowel sounds present, then begin clear liquids I&O q8h	Advance diet as tolerated once passing flatus Encourage fluids (2000 mL/day) D/C I&O when IV out and fluid intake adequate	Soft—regular if passing flatus Encourage fluid intake
Elimination	Foley catheter; catheter care q4–8h	D/C Foley Voiding large amt straw-colored urine Straight cath if bladder distended or unable to void	Same May have bowel movement; ask woman to report it to nurse
Medications	Continue pitocin infusion as ordered IV antibiotics as ordered Antiemetics prn as ordered If epidural or intrathecal narcotic analgesia used: • Naloxone 0.2 mg IV for respirations < 8/min or signs of resp distress • Diphenhydramine 25 mg IV or IM q2h prn itching	Buffalo cap IV when fluid intake adequate Heparin flush to BC per agency policy Antiflatulents PRN Stool softner _____	Continue medications May take own prenatal vitamins
Discharge planning/ home care	Evaluate knowledge of post cesarean recovery, newborn care	Discuss typical newborn schedule; stress need to plan for periods of rest Birth certificate paperwork completed Evaluate plans for transporting newborn; car seat available Arrangements made for baby pictures if desired	Review discharge instruction sheet and checklist Describe postpartum warning signs and when to call CNM/physician Provide prescriptions; gift pack to woman Newborn check schedule Postoperative/postpartum visit schedule
Family involvement	Evaluate support system Provide opportunities for woman and support persons to watch newborn assessments Recognize possible impact of culture on responses	Involve support persons in care, teaching; answer questions Evidence of parental bonding behaviors present Demonstrates culturally expected early parenting behaviors Contact social services if indicated	Plans made for care and support of mother following discharge Support person verbalizes understanding of need for woman to rest, eat nutritionally, recover, avoid overexertion Evidence of parental bonding behaviors clearly present

Teaching Guides help you understand how to assess common teaching needs in maternity care situations, create a particular teaching session, and evaluate the session's success.

For additional examples, see pages 376, 876, and 1112.

Assessment Guides summarize assessment findings, alterations and possible causes, and nursing responses to assessment data to help you make distinctions between normal and abnormal clinical findings.

For additional examples, see pages 341 and 357.

TEACHING GUIDE

Teaching Breast Self-Examination

Assessment: The nurse determines the woman's general knowledge about BSE, identifies previous experience with BSE, identifies risk factors for breast cancer (see Table 10–2), determines the woman's general knowledge about breast cancer, discusses the woman's feelings about her breasts and BSE, identifies barriers to BSE, and discusses her commitment to practice BSE.

Nursing Diagnosis: Knowledge deficit related to lack of information about breast self-examination

Nursing Plan and Implementation: The teaching plan will focus on assisting the woman to learn BSE so that she can use it effectively.

Client Goals: At completion of teaching, the woman will be able to:

1. Discuss her risk of breast cancer.
2. Describe the use of BSE in breast cancer detection.
3. Demonstrate the correct procedure for BSE.
4. List warning signs of breast cancer to be reported to the care giver.
5. Incorporate monthly BSE into her personal routine.

Teaching Plan

Content	Teaching Method
Content: Discuss the risk factors associated with breast cancer (see Table 10–2).	***Teaching Method:*** *This should be discussed in a private area free of interruptions. The room needs to have a mirror; bed, couch, or examining table; pillows; a patient gown; and a private area for the woman to disrobe.*
Stress the unique risk factors associated with the woman's personal history and life-style.	*The nurse should create a supportive, warm, and comfortable atmosphere by attitude and communication style—both verbal and nonverbal. A discussion of breast cancer may bring forth many emotions in the woman, including grief for previous breast cancer–related losses.*
Discuss the use of BSE in breast cancer detection.	*Focus on open discussion. A brochure with statistics and illustrations may be useful. Stress the positive outcomes of early detection to counterbalance fears.*
Describe and demonstrate the correct procedure for BSE. A. Instruct the woman to inspect her breasts by standing or sitting in front of a mirror. She needs to inspect her breasts in three positions: with both arms relaxed down at her side, both arms stretched straight over her head, and both hands placed on her hips while leaning forward (Figure 10–1).	*Learning is best accomplished when material is broken down into smaller steps and presented with multiple approaches. Prior to asking the woman to perform BSE, the nurse should use a model or a chart to demonstrate the procedure. Then the nurse should have the woman perform BSE. The nurse should be very supportive and give a lot of positive feedback because some women may be embarrassed. The nurse needs to demonstrate a nonjudgmental, accepting attitude.*

ontinued

Nursing Responses to Data†

Nursing Responses to Data

ovide opportunities for adequate rest; ovide nutritious meals and snacks that are nsistent with what the woman desires to eat d drink; provide opportunities to discuss th experience in nonjudgmental atmosere if the woman desires to do so.

plain postpartum blues; provide supportive nosphere; determine support available for other; consider referral for evidence of ofound depression.

ovide reinforcement and support for infant etaking behaviors; maintain nonjudgmen- approach and gather more information if etaking behaviors are not evident.

etermine whether woman understands glish and provide interpreter if needed; ovide reinforcement of information through nversation and through written material emember that some women and their milies may not be able to understand written aterials due to language difficulties or ability to read); provide information regard- infant care skills that are culturally con- stent; give woman opportunity to express r feelings; consider social service home erral for women who have no family or her support, are unable to take in informa- n about self-care and infant care, and monstrate no caretaking activities.

inued

Nursing Responses to Data†

to physician/certified nurse-midwife.

s size; apply ice glove or ice pack; to physician/certified nurse-midwife. rage sitz baths; review perineal care, riate wiping techniques. rage sitz baths, side-lying position; ads, anesthetic ointments, manual ement of hemorrhoids, stool softeners, sed fluid intake.

s for other symptoms of urinary tract n (UTI); obtain clean-catch urine; to physician/certified nurse-midwife.

to physician/certified nurse-midwife.

y nursing interventions to promote ; if not successful, obtain order for rization. symptoms of UTI to physician/certified midwife. rage fluids, ambulation, roughage in tz baths to promote healing of per- ; obtain order for stool softener.

Nursing Responses to Data†

e for specific request if possible. an is unable to provide specific infor- , the nurse may draw from general ation regarding cultural variation. an women may want food and fluids store hot-cold balance to the body. n of European background may ask for uids.

POSTPARTAL ASSESSMENT GUIDE

First Week After Birth

Physical Assessment/ Normal Findings	Alterations and Possible Causes*	Nursing Responses to Data†
Vital Signs		
Blood pressure (BP): Should remain consistent with baseline BP during pregnancy.	High BP (PIH, essential hypertension, renal disease, anxiety). Drop in BP (may be normal; uterine hemorrhage).	Evaluate history of preexisting disorders and check for other signs of PIH (edema, proteinuria). Assess for other signs of hemorrhage (↑ pulse, cool clammy skin).
Pulse: 50–90 beats/minute. May be bradycardia of 50–70 beats/minute.	Tachycardia (difficult labor and birth, hemorrhage).	Evaluate for other signs of hemorrhage (↓ BP, cool clammy skin).
Respirations: 16–24/minute.	Marked tachypnea (respiratory disease).	Assess for other signs of respiratory disease.
Temperature: 36.2–38 C (98–100.4 F).	After first 24 hours temperature of 38 C (100.4 F) or above suggests infection.	Assess for other signs of infection; notify physician/certified nurse-midwife.
Breasts		
General appearance: Smooth, even pigmentation, changes of pregnancy still apparent; one may appear larger.	Reddened area (mastitis).	Assess further for signs of infection.
Palpation: Depending on postpartal day, may be soft, filling, full, or engorged.	Palpable mass (caked breast, mastitis). Engorgement (venous stasis). Tenderness, heat, edema (engorgement, caked breast, mastitis).	Assess for other signs of infection: If blocked duct, consider heat, massage, position change for breastfeeding. Assess for further signs. Report mastitis to physician/certified nurse-midwife.
Nipples: Supple, pigmented, intact; become erect when stimulated.	Fissures, cracks, soreness (problems with breastfeeding), not erectile with stimulation (inverted nipples).	Reassess technique; recommend appropriate interventions.
Abdomen		
Musculature: Abdomen may be soft, have a "doughy" texture; rectus muscle intact.	Separation in musculature (diastasis recti abdominis).	Evaluate size of diastasis; teach appropriate exercises for decreasing the separation.
Fundus: Firm, midline; following expected schedule of involution.	Boggy (full bladder, uterine bleeding).	Massage until firm; assess bladder and have woman void if needed; attempt to express clots when firm. If bogginess remains or recurs, report to physician/certified nurse-midwife.
May be tender when palpated.	Constant tenderness (infection).	Assess for evidence of endometritis.
Lochia		
Scant to moderate amount, earthy odor; no clots.	Large amount, clots (hemorrhage). Foul-smelling lochia (infection).	Assess for firmness, express additional clots; begin peri-pad count. Assess for other signs of infection; report to physician/certified nurse-midwife.

*Possible causes of alterations are placed in parentheses.

†This column provides guidelines for further assessment and initial nursing actions.

➤

TEACHING MOMENT

When assessing blood pressure, have the pregnant woman sitting up with her arm resting on a table so that her arm is at the level of her heart.

Expect a decrease in her blood pressure from baseline during the second trimester because of normal physiologic changes. If this decrease doesn't occur, evaluate further for signs of pregnancy-induced hypertension (PIH).

Home Care

Because the mother with postpartum thromboembolic disease will depend on others for much of her initial home care, it is helpful for the father to be involved in preparations for discharge. Ample opportunities should be provided for questions to be answered and instructions clarified, verbally and in writing. The nurse will evaluate the extent to which both mother and father have understood instructions regarding the plan of care. It is especially important before discharge to assess the couple's plans in order to assure complete bed rest for the mother. They might explore ways for her to maintain bed rest and still spend quality time with her newborn and any other children. For example, young children can sit on the bed for storytelling or play quiet games, and the newborn's crib can be placed adjacent to the mother's bed.

Many concerns will not surface until the couple actually returns home and fully comprehends the reality of their situation. For that reason it is valuable to provide them with an accessible resource person and to plan telephone or home visit follow-up care.

The father may be assuming multiple roles in the circumstances—household manager, parent, worker, and care giver. Fatigue is inevitable. There may be financial concerns as a result of prolonged health care and/or his extended time away from work to care for the family. The couple must keep their communication lines open and spend quality time together. Referral to social services and assessment of the presence and use of a continued support system and coping strategies are necessary to avert potential crises.

Signs of postpartum thrombophlebitis may not occur until after discharge from the hospital. Consequently, all couples must be taught about the signs and symptoms and to appreciate the importance of reporting them immediately and of not massaging the affected leg. Should signs and symptoms occur after discharge from the postpartum unit, a short readmission might be required. Every effort is made in that case to allow mother, father, and newborn to remain together.

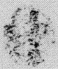

Teaching for Self-Care

The nurse instructs the woman to avoid prolonged standing or sitting because these positions contribute to venous stasis. She is also instructed to avoid crossing her legs because of the pressure it causes. The nurse also advises her to take frequent breaks such as when taking car trips or if she has a job where she sits most of the day. Walking is acceptable because it promotes venous return. The woman is reminded to identify her history of thrombosis/thrombophlebitis to her physician during subsequent pregnancies so that preventive measures may be instituted early.

Women who are discharged on warfarin must understand the purpose of the medication and be alert to signs of hemorrhage such as bleeding gums, epistaxis, petechiae or ecchymosis, or evidence of blood in the urine or stool. Because careful monitoring is important, the woman should clearly understand the need to keep scheduled appointments for prothrombin time assessment. Certain medications such as aspirin and non-steroidal anti-inflammatory drugs increase anticoagulant activity, so they should be avoided. In fact the woman should check for possible medication interaction before taking any medication while on warfarin. A woman may choose to carry a MedicAlert card in case of emergency and should inform all medical care providers, including dentists, that she is taking anticoagulants. She should also have vitamin K available in case bleeding occurs. Warfarin is excreted in the breast milk and thus may present problems for breastfeeding mothers. Women who wish to continue nursing may be maintained at home on low doses of subcutaneous heparin, because heparin is not excreted in breast milk.

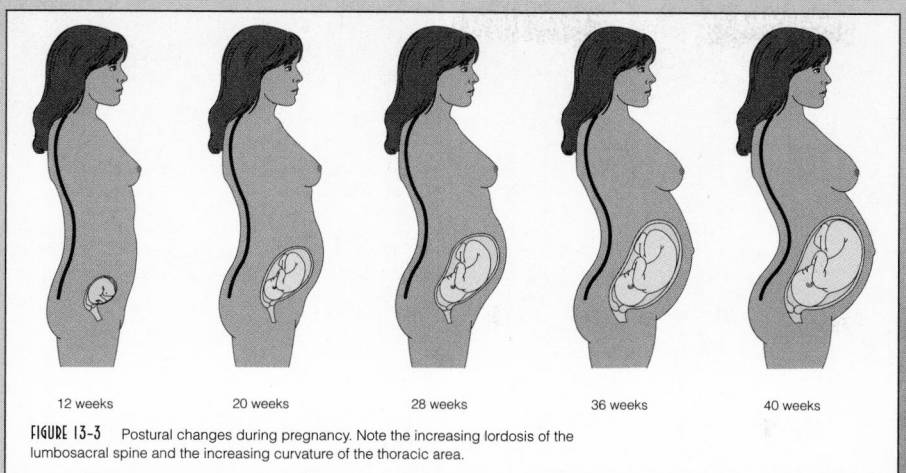

FIGURE 13-3   Postural changes during pregnancy. Note the increasing lordosis of the lumbosacral spine and the increasing curvature of the thoracic area.

| 12 weeks | 20 weeks | 28 weeks | 36 weeks | 40 weeks |

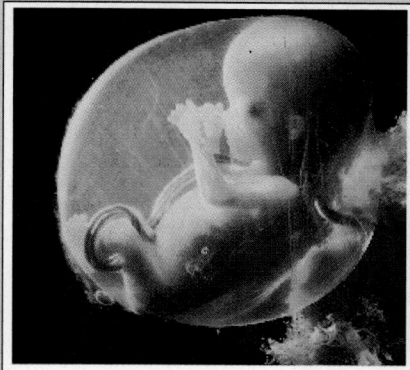

FIGURE 6-23   The fetus at 14 weeks. During this period of rapid growth the skin is so transparent that blood vessels are visible beneath it. More muscle tissue and body skeleton have developed, which holds the fetus more erect. SOURCE: Nilsson L: *A Child Is Born.* New York: Dell Publishing, 1990.

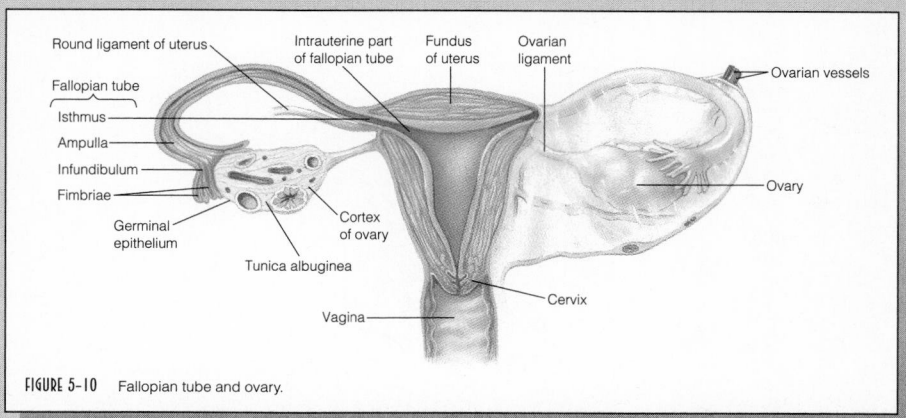

FIGURE 5-10   Fallopian tube and ovary.

FULL-COLOR FORMAT enhances visual learning of anatomy and physiologic processes and highlights key information. Dramatic photographs and personal reflections of childbearing women bring you closer to the childbearing experience.

Ideal for the Clinical Setting!

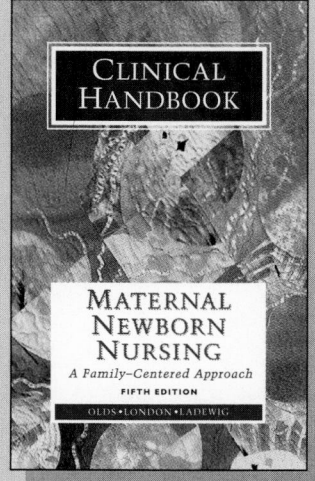

This portable quick-reference reviews vital maternity care information from pregnancy through the postpartal and newborn stages. Organized around the nursing process, this handy resource contains the information you need to provide safe, competent maternal-newborn nursing care, including:

- Special "Alert" signals for specific signs and symptoms

- Detailed Drug Guides and Procedures

- Common Abbreviations for Maternal-Newborn Terminology

- Normal Maternal and Neonatal Lab Values

- Projected Recommendations for Isolation Precautions (CDC 1995)

- Occupational Safety and Health Administration (OSHA) Blood-Borne Pathogens Standards

ISBN 0-8053-5614-2

PART ONE

CONTEMPORARY MATERNAL-NEWBORN NURSING

CHAPTER 1

CURRENT ISSUES IN MATERNAL-NEWBORN NURSING

*M*y daughter just told us that she is three months pregnant with our first grandchild. As a labor nurse for 25 years I've helped with hundreds of births, but it still seems magical to me, especially now. I'm excited for her and a little worried because I know all the risks as well as the joys. She is so happy, when I am with her I just want to laugh out loud. I already know I love being a grandmother, even though I really am too young!

KEY TERMS

Artificial insemination

Assisted reproductive technology (ART)

Certified nurse-midwife (CNM)

Client

Informed consent

Intrauterine fetal surgery

OBJECTIVES

Relate the concept of the expert nurse to nurses caring for childbearing families.

Discuss the impact of the self-care movement on contemporary childbirth.

Compare the nursing roles available to the maternal-newborn nurse.

Summarize the similarities and differences between certified nurse-midwives (CNMs) and lay midwives.

Describe significant legal and ethical issues for nurses caring for childbearing families.

Evaluate the potential impact of some of the special situations in contemporary maternity care.

The practice of most nurses is filled with special moments, shared experiences, times in which they know they have practiced the essence of nursing and, in doing so, have touched a life. What is the essence of nursing? Simply stated, nurses care *for* people, care *about* people, and use their expertise to help people help themselves.

I like working with students. I enjoy the enthusiasm they bring, the questions they ask, the ways they cause me to examine my practice. I love being a nurse. I am passionate about the importance of what I do, and I feel the need to seize every chance to influence those who will be practicing beside me some day. Last week was a perfect example. I had a junior nursing student working with me in one of our birthing rooms. It was her first day caring for a laboring woman, and she was scared and excited at the same time. We were taking care of a healthy woman who had two boys at home and really wanted a girl. As labor progressed, the student and I worked closely together monitoring contractions, teaching the woman and her husband, doing what we could to ease her discomfort. Sometimes the student would ask how I knew when to do something, a vaginal check, for example, and I'd have to think beyond "I just do" to give her some clues. At the birth the student stayed close to the mother, coaching and helping with breathing. The student was excited but felt she had an important role to play, and she handled it beautifully. At the moment of birth the student and the dad were leaning forward watching as the baby just slipped into the world. There wasn't a sound until the student said in a voice filled with awe, "Oh, it's a girl!" Then we all laughed and hugged each other. What a day—using my expertise to help others and helping a future nurse recognize the importance of what we do!

All nurses who provide care and support to childbearing women and their families can make a difference. But how does this happen? How do nurses develop expertise and become skilled, caring practitioners?

In her classic work Benner (1984) suggests that as nurses develop their skills in making clinical judgments and intervening appropriately, they progress through five levels of competence. Beginning as a novice, the new nurse progresses to advanced beginner and then to competent, proficient, and finally, expert nurse.

In the above situation, the student was clearly a novice. Lacking in experience, the novice relies on rules to guide actions. As nurses gain experience, they begin to draw on that experience to view situations more holistically, becoming increasingly aware of subtle cues that indicate physiologic and psychologic changes. Expert nurses, like the nurse in the preceding situation, have a clear vision of what is possible in a given situation. This holistic perspective is based on a wealth of knowledge bred of experience and enables nurses to act "intuitively" to provide effective care. In reality nurses' intuition reflects their internalization of information. When faced with a clinical situation, nurses draw almost subconsciously on their stored knowledge and judgment.

The use of intuitive perception is important to the "art of nursing," especially in areas such as maternal-newborn nursing, where change occurs quickly and families look to the nurse for help and guidance. Labor nurses become attuned to a woman's progress or lack of progress; nursery nurses detect subtle changes in their small charges; antepartal and postpartal nurses become adept at assessing and teaching. Similarly, nurses who are cross-trained as LDRP (labor, delivery, recovery, postpartum) nurses become skilled at caring for women and their newborns during all phases of childbirth. Thus skilled nursing practice depends on a solid base of knowledge and clinical expertise delivered in a caring, holistic manner. Benner and Wrubel (1989) emphasize the primacy of caring in nursing practice, as demonstrated in the following situation:

My first pregnancy ended in spontaneous abortion at 8 weeks, so this time I decided not to tell anyone I was pregnant until I was 3 months along. We had just told both families the news the preceding day when it happened again. I began bleeding heavily, and we rushed to the ER. Here I was, a maternal-newborn nursing instructor, and I couldn't seem to handle a pregnancy. I was in the bathroom when I passed the fetus into the johnny cap. My poor baby—so small, maybe 3 or 4 inches long. I began to sob uncontrollably as I rang for the nurse. I told her what happened, and she helped me to bed. My husband sat with his arm around me as I cried while the nurse took our baby out. A few minutes later she came back and said, "I saw on your record that you are Catholic. Would you like me to baptize your baby?" I said "Oh, yes, please," and she left. I've never forgotten how that made me feel. She saw me as a total person. I'm still teaching, and now I have two children. Whenever I teach high-risk pregnancy, I tell that story to the students. I want them to know what a difference a nurse can make.

We believe that many nurses who work with childbearing families are experts: They are sensitive, intuitive, and technically skilled. Such nurses do make a difference in the quality of care childbearing families receive.

CONTEMPORARY CHILDBIRTH

As anyone who has practiced in maternal or newborn nursing for several years will tell you, the field has changed dramatically. Today's maternal-newborn nurse has far broader responsibilities than the nurse of 25 years ago. Today nurses focus more on the specific goals of the individual childbearing woman and her family. The use of the nursing process has helped bring this about.

Not only has maternal-newborn nursing changed, so has the whole experience of childbirth. No longer do laboring women leave their partners and family at the labor room door while they work to give birth without the family's loving presence; no longer are newborns routinely whisked away for a prescribed period, to reappear magically for feedings every 4 hours and then return to the safe atmosphere of a central nursery; no longer are young siblings treated like walking sources of infection that threaten every infant. Today fathers are active participants in the birth experience. Families and friends are also often included. Siblings are encouraged to visit and meet their newest family member and may even attend the birth. Today the concept of "family-centered childbirth" is accepted and encouraged.

Childbearing women now have many choices. They can choose to give birth in hospital labor rooms, birthing rooms or birthing centers (attached to the hospital or free-standing), or even at home. The primary caregiver may be a physician, a nurse-midwife, or even a lay midwife. More choices are available with regard to use of analgesia, position for labor, and position for birth. Women may elect to give birth sitting, squatting, on hands and knees, sidelying, standing, or in the more traditional lithotomy position.

Unfortunately, some of the new choices open to educated consumers may also have a negative side. This is especially true with regard to the concept of early discharge. Until a few years ago even women with uncomplicated births were required to stay in the hospital for several days. However, many women who had supportive families were eager to return home as soon as possible following birth. They had the time and resources to return to the hospital or clinic for any necessary follow-up care and were well prepared to care for themselves and their newborns. In a somewhat unanticipated development, as hospitals have attempted to control costs, early discharge has become the norm, and women with little knowledge, experience, or support now find themselves discharged within 24 hours or less after giving birth. To compensate, nurses have been creative about devising effective strategies to do necessary teaching and discharge preparation while the woman is in the birthing facility. In this early postpartal period, however, women are often very tired and less ready emotionally to learn.

In some areas, follow-up care is provided to women who are discharged early. Nurses visit the women at home to assess their health and that of their infants and to do any necessary teaching. This trend toward home care is a positive one, and we hope that this method of meeting the needs of families becomes standard practice.

THE SELF-CARE MOVEMENT

At the end of the 19th century most individuals were self-reliant consumers. No standardization of medical education existed, and MD following the name gave no guarantee of the nature of the education, if any, or experience and background of the practitioner. Numerous syrups and nostrums were available for self-treatment, including many products that contained opium or morphine. Home "doctor books" were available and consulted widely by the general public. By the 1920s this situation had changed significantly. Medical education reform resulted in well-trained physicians with far more scientific knowledge than the average layperson. The more powerful medications were obtainable only through a physician. Thus the age of the physician-reliant consumer began. Increasing medical specialization and evolving technology also contributed to the trend toward consumer reliance on physicians. Phrases such as "whatever the doctor says" or "I just need to see the doctor and get a shot to fix it" characterized the prevailing attitude. The health care provider assumed the major portion of responsibility for health maintenance.

The self-care movement began to emerge in the late 1960s as new consumers sought to understand technology and take an interest in their own health and basic self-care skills. Toffler (1980) refers to these new consumers as "prosumers of medicine" because they are "people who are at the same time producers and consumers of health benefits." These prosumers exercise, control their diet, monitor their psychologic and physiologic status, and in some cases even do their own diagnostic tests. They thus assume many primary care functions. Furthermore, today's health care consumers are requiring greater information and accountability from their health care providers (Inlander 1990). These consumers recognize that information, indeed, is power.

In evaluating this trend toward self-care, Naisbitt (1982) refers to it as a move toward self-help and away from institutional help (medicine). He stresses the return to self-reliance, with a focus on holistic care, wellness, and preventive medicine.

Practicing self-care—assuming responsibility for one's own health—often requires assertiveness and taking an active role in seeking necessary information. Nurses can foster self-care by providing information readily and by acknowledging the right of individuals to ask questions and become actively involved in their own care.

Maternal-newborn care offers a special opportunity to promote active participation in health care because it is essentially health focused; in most cases clients are well when they enter the system; and the consumer movement that has already influenced childbirth encourages people to speak up for preferences in dealing with health care providers.

Self-care has gained an even broader appeal in recent years because literature suggests that it can significantly reduce health care costs. We believe that self-care will be a vital part of health care for years to come. Obviously, self-care is not always realistic or appropriate, especially in acute emergencies, but in many situations self-care is appropriate. With this in mind we have attempted throughout this book to suggest ways in which nurses might offer health education that would enable the childbearing woman or the parents of a newborn to meet their own health care needs. We see this as one of nursing's most important functions and one that nurses are especially well qualified to perform.

Because of our support of self-care, we have used the term **client** rather than patient when referring to the childbearing woman. The term client implies an active, rather than a passive, role. The client seeks assistance from individuals who have special skills and knowledge that the client does not. Information and suggestions for a plan of action regarding the client's particular situation are offered to the client by the health care professional. The client can choose not to accept the professional's advice. Furthermore, the health care professional cannot proceed with the plan of action without the client's consent. In this relationship clients assume responsibility for their decisions.

The nursing profession has been at the forefront in recognizing that people who are able should take an active role in their own health care, and the term client best fits this concept. Nurses in a maternity client–health care professional relationship must understand that it is their professional expertise and skill that is being sought. Any attempt to make decisions for the client is therefore inappropriate.

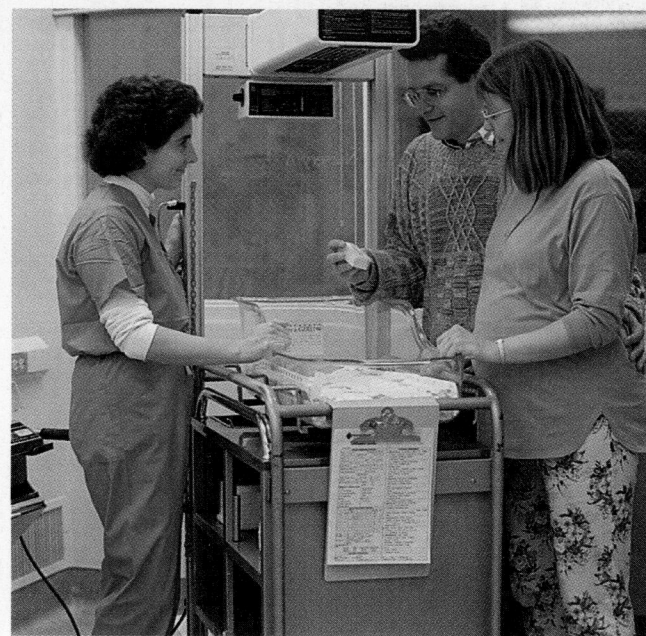

FIGURE 1-1 Individualized education for childbearing couples is one of the prime responsibilities of the maternal-newborn nurse.

NURSING ROLES

The contemporary maternal-newborn nurse has a variety of roles. In our opinion the most important roles are care giver, advocate, educator, researcher, change agent, and political activist.

Care Giver

The nurse uses professional expertise to help maintain and, when possible, maximize the health of the childbearing woman and her family. The nurse accomplishes this by making assessments, formulating nursing diagnoses, planning and providing care, and providing comfort and support when necessary. This may involve direct physical and emotional care of the childbearing woman or aid to the family caring for the mother.

Advocate

As a client *advocate*, the nurse supports clients' rights and assists them in making informed judgments. The maternity nurse advocate informs clients by clearly identifying the options available, as well as the risks of each one; by explaining simply but completely the nursing actions; and by answering questions with facts and not personal opinions. The maternity nurse advocate then supports the client's decision by adhering to it and ensuring that others do the same.

The nurse advocate can enhance the consumer–health care provider relationship both by providing complete information about desired services so that the consumer's expectations are realistic, and by helping individuals understand that having them participate in their health care is both desired and indeed necessary.

Educator

As discussed in the preceding section on self-care, the nurse has an important role as *educator*. The nurse assesses the need for education and information based on personal observation and input from the woman or her family. The nurse provides information at the client's level of understanding and confirms with the client that the information is understood. The nurse then provides any additional information necessary based on the individual's goals for learning. Nurses in maternity settings are especially active in client education. Nurses on many postpartum units, mother-baby units, and newborn nurseries have developed teaching checklists, a variety of handouts and literature, and teaching programs. However, individualized teaching between nurse and client is still the cornerstone of education for the maternal-newborn nurse (Figure 1–1).

Researcher

Nursing research is a process of systematic inquiry using scientific processes to solve a problem or answer a question. Well-done nursing research is vital to improving clinical practice. Fortunately, both the quality and quantity of nursing research have increased significantly over the past decade as more nurses become involved in research projects. To support these efforts, many clinical facilities now employ doctorally prepared nurses to work with staff nurses to develop and implement research proposals. Unfortunately, experts suggest that the results of nursing research are not being implemented effectively in clinical practice (Edwards-Beckett 1990) despite the evidence that research-based nursing interventions tend to result in more positive outcomes for clients (Heater et al 1990).

Professional nurses, whether involved directly in research or not, have a responsibility to be "critical consumers" of research findings. A major factor in helping nurses apply research results to clinical practice is the availability of methods to keep them informed about research findings. Evidence indicates that a monthly research newsletter is an effective approach to keeping nurses informed. Other useful approaches include research-focused meetings, continuing education offerings, computer networks, and interactive computer software (Pettengill et al 1994). We believe that the timely dissemination of research findings is an important area in which nurses in education and nurses in service can network and work together to improve the quality of care.

Because of our commitment to nursing research, we have incorporated research boxes into most of the chapters throughout this text. We have sought to select research that is well done and helpful in addressing specific aspects of care for women and childbearing families.

RESEARCH IN PRACTICE

The stories of women who repetitively contract sexually transmitted diseases (STDs), excluding AIDS, are characterized by feelings of powerlessness, stigma, victimization, and a sense of inevitability about these diseases. Nancy Redfern and Sally Hutchinson explored and described the experiences of eight women who had sought treatment for an STD at least twice in 2 years. Data included in-depth interviews as well as stories and anecdotes from the clinical practice of Redfern, a nurse practitioner. Data analysis consisted of line by line coding, collapsing codes into categories, and generation of themes.

This qualitative, descriptive study generated several themes relevant to the heterosexual relationships responsible for the women's multiple STDs. Monogamy surfaced as a state desired by all the women and was being practiced, at least by the women, at the time they contracted the STD. Several of the women wanted to feel "special" from their relationship. Sex emerged as an important component of the relationship, and companionship added a dimension to the sexual aspect. Some women indicated that they were searching for love and marriage. Lastly, many women discussed problems with the use of condoms, varying from lack of sensation to difficulty getting their partners to use them.

As noted, recurrent themes generated from this study include powerlessness and a sense of inevitability about STDs as part of life. Women in this study felt devalued by our culture and by their perceived need to accommodate men. The diagnosis of an STD made the women feel stigmatized and unclean. Four of the eight participants had experienced sexual molestation or rape. Models generated by the participants to explain and derive meaning from the experience of contracting STDs ranged from sexual behavior to weak immunity, to being able to get STDs from anything.

Clinical Application of the Study

As noted by the authors, nurses must recognize that the client's explanatory model may, and probably will, differ from that of the nurse. Failure to encourage the client to share her model may result in instructions and planned interventions that are not based on the client's view of the illness. The client's failure to follow instructions may result in subsequent exposure to STDs through unsafe sexual practice.

SOURCE: Redfern N, Hutchinson S: Women's experiences of repetitively contracting sexually transmitted diseases. *Health Care for Women International* 1994; 15:423.

Critical Thinking Question

Can you think of ways in which nurses might function as change agents? Do you know of any specific examples?

Change Agent

Today's nurse is a *change agent* who works within the health care setting to effect change that will ensure safe, satisfying childbirth experiences for families and promote competent care for women and their babies. Nurses accomplish this change in a variety of ways: by working on utilization, quality assurance, peer review, and protocols and procedures committees; by becoming active in professional organizations; and, informally, by sharing pertinent articles and workshop information with colleagues to help them become more aware and concerned.

Political Activist

Nurses must become more involved in the political arena. This involvement may begin simply with becoming active in one's professional organization and keeping abreast of political issues that affect nursing. Some nurses find a broader base for expressing concerns when they become members of their political party caucuses and are elected as delegates to their party conventions. Some nurses find that they can be most effective by writing logical, factual, and concerned letters to legislators about important health care issues. Nurses can also take action by contributing to the campaigns of candidates who are attuned to health care issues. The contributions should be accompanied by a letter specifying why the support was given.

Political representatives are always eager to know which of their actions gained them constituent support. Some nurses can best serve nursing by helping to develop public policy (by working in regulatory agencies or by running for political office). This level of involvement provides visibility and, more important, opportunities to make a difference through the laws of the country.

NURSE-PHYSICIAN RELATIONSHIPS

Today's professional nurse is being taught to function with physicians and other members of the health care team as a co-worker, not as the passive handmaiden of the past. Nursing students are learning to view their relationships as collegial rather than dependent. Relationships between nurses and physicians vary widely. In situations in which there is a high level of mutual confidence and respect, nurses find their work especially satisfying, and clients benefit from the high quality of the rapport (Figure 1–2).

A birthing area nurse recalls a situation in which she worked closely with a caring physician for the good of a childbearing woman and her family:

This happened several years ago before it was common to have families attend cesarean births. I was working evenings and was caring for a woman—I'll call her Mrs V. She was 39 weeks along, and her membranes had been ruptured for 26 hours. We tried to induce labor but it wasn't working. In those days the rule was that membranes should never be ruptured for more than 24 hours, so we were stretching it already. Finally her doctor decided her failure to progress made a cesarean necessary. He went in to discuss it with Mrs V and her husband and to get the permit signed. Dr Waters was a really caring doctor, and he spent a long time explaining, but she became terribly upset and just sobbed. He came out to the desk and said, "Mrs King, I can't seem to reach Mrs V. You have a good relationship with her. Will you please try?" I went in, let her cry for a while, and then talked to her about her feelings. She said that she had taken childbirth classes with her husband, and they had planned how they would share the birth of their baby. She couldn't stand the thought of facing surgery alone. I remembered reading that several hospitals throughout the country had started letting fathers attend nonemergency cesareans, but we had never done it at our hospital. I went out and told Dr Waters about her feelings and about the literature I had read on the subject. He had done some reading on it too and said, "I'm willing to try it if you are and if you feel you can support Mr V." The evening supervisor agreed to circulate so I could stay near Mr V. Dr Waters and I talked to the family together, explaining what would happen and giving them the choice. They were so excited; Mrs V was like a new woman. She had an epidural so she would be awake, and her husband sat at the head of the table near her. When their daughter was born, he held her for a while as he sat near his wife and then carried the baby to the nursery while Dr Waters finished the surgery. I'm not a big

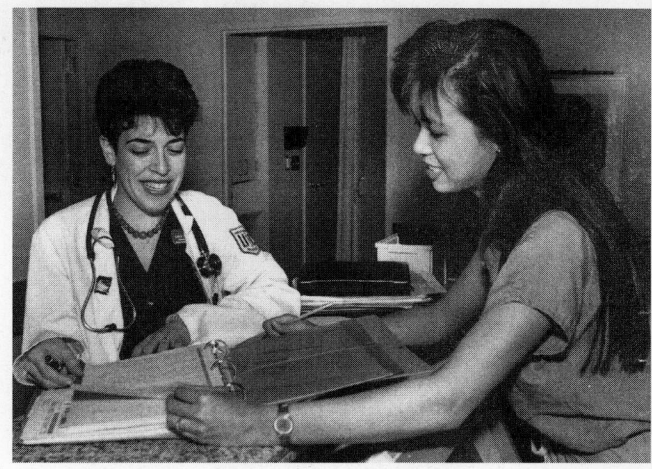

FIGURE 1-2   A collaborative nurse-physician relationship contributes to excellent client care.

trend setter or nursing leader, but that night Dr Waters and I took a risk together, and we made a difference. Afterward we sat in the nurses' station, had a cup of coffee, and just grinned at each other. I'll never forget it.

As the vignette shows, nurses and physicians working together as peers can have a tremendous positive impact on the quality of care provided. Moreover, one of the unexpected benefits of the current emphasis on health care reform is the realization it has brought to many health care providers and consumers of the vitally important role nurses play in providing excellent care to clients and families. As medicine becomes demystified, as consumers become active participants in their care, and as financial constraints demand cooperation, it is evident that a truly collegial relationship between nurses and physicians will benefit everyone.

PROFESSIONAL OPTIONS IN MATERNAL-NEWBORN NURSING PRACTICE

As a man, I don't always find it easy to be a labor and delivery nurse. I have three children of my own and attended all their births. It meant a lot to me to be there, and I like helping others to have good childbirth experiences, too. I don't fit some people's image of a nurse; so they refer to me as a "male nurse" as opposed to a real nurse, and they ask why I didn't go into medicine instead. Why can't they understand that I'm a nurse because it's what I really want to be—and I'm darned good at it, too. More men are choosing nursing now, and I think that will help. I hope to see the day when we don't have "female doctors" and "male nurses," but doctors and nurses, period!

Nursing is unique in its adaptability and flexibility in providing maternity care in various settings. Nurses are found in the maternity departments of acute care facilities, in physicians' offices, in public health department clinics, in college health services, in family planning clinics, in school nursing programs dealing with sex education or adolescent pregnancies, in volunteer community health services, in abortion clinics, and in any other setting where a client has a need for maternity care. The depth of nursing involvement in various settings is determined by the qualifications and the role or function of the nurse employed. Many different titles have evolved to describe the professional requirements of the nurse in various maternity care roles including the following:

- **Professional nurses** are graduates of an accredited basic program in nursing who have successfully completed the nursing examination (NCLEX) and are currently licensed as registered nurses. Professional nurses use the nursing process and employ their clinical skills in a variety of settings to provide basic nursing care. Today's nurse assumes a collaborative role with the physician and other members of the health care team and is competent, assertive, and willing to take risks in the role of client advocate.

- **Nurse practitioners (NPs)** are professional nurses who have received specialized education in either a master's degree program or a continuing education program. They function in a newer, expanded role, most often as providers of ambulatory care services, although some NPs do function in acute care settings. They focus on physical and psychosocial assessment, including health history, physical examination, and certain diagnostic tests and procedures. The nurse practitioner makes clinical judgments and begins appropriate treatments, seeking physician consultation when necessary. Within the scope of their clinical practice and expertise, nurse practitioners are well qualified to clinically manage a client whose illness has stabilized.

- **Clinical nurse specialists (CNSs)** are professional nurses with master's degrees who have additional specialized knowledge and competence in a specific clinical area. They assume a leadership role within their specialty and work to improve client care both directly and indirectly.

- **Certified nurse-midwives (CNMs)** are educated in the two disciplines of nursing and midwifery and possess evidence of certification according to the requirements of the American College of Nurse-Midwives (ACNM). Nurse-midwifery practice is the independent management of care of essentially normal women and newborns, antepartally, intrapartally, postpartally, and/or gynecologically. The certified nurse-midwife works within a health care system that provides for medical consultation, col-

laborative management, or referral in accord with the *Standards for the Practice of Nurse-Midwifery* as defined by the ACNM (1993).

The certified nurse-midwife practices within the framework of a medically directed health service. The CNM functions in private practice or as a member of the obstetric team in medical centers, institutions, universities, birth centers, and community health projects with active programs of nurse-midwifery.

The term *advanced practice nurse* is used to describe nurses who, by education and practice, function in an expanded nursing role. The term, often used in a legal sense in state nurse practice acts, most frequently applies to NPs, CNSs, CRNAs, and CNMs. As the importance of the nurse practitioner as a provider of care in a reformed health care system increases, the distinctions between the nurse practitioner role and the clinical nurse specialist role are beginning to blur, and these roles may ultimately merge.

CNMs and Lay Midwives

When nurse-midwifery began in the United States, it provided quality maternity care to those unable to afford physicians. Time and again CNMs demonstrated that the care they provided significantly lowered perinatal mortality. Today, as consumers of health care seek more involvement in decisions about their birth experience, an exciting trend is evolving: Women who can afford a choice of health care providers are choosing certified nurse-midwives. These women feel that CNMs recognize that the childbearing family wants to share an experience, to feel close and supported, and to control the birth experience (Figure 1–3).

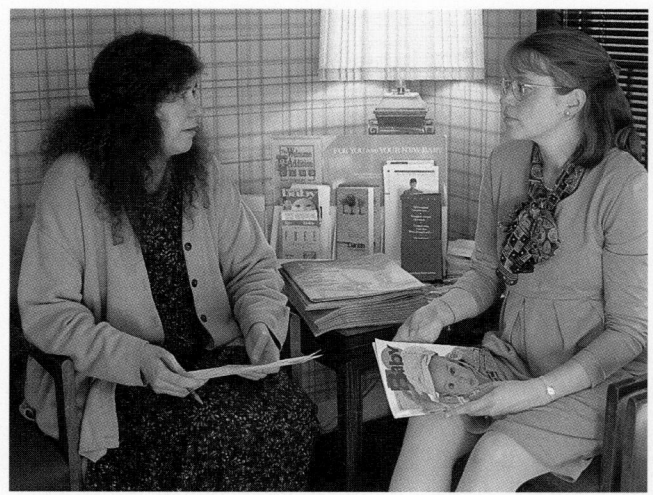

FIGURE 1-3   A certified nurse-midwife confers with her client.

The importance of certified nurse-midwives has been increasingly acknowledged. Certified nurse-midwives have prescription writing privileges in the District of Columbia and about one-half of the states and are receiving hospital privileges in many areas (Rooks 1990). This is due, in part, to a 1988 recommendation of the Institute of Medicine that physicians and state laws encourage hospital privileges for CNMs.

Lay midwives, or direct-entry midwives, usually are nonnurses who enter midwifery because of a desire to assist families to participate in home births. Lay midwives and certified nurse-midwives share many values: Both have a philosophy of nonintervention; both value a family-centered birth experience. However, certified nurse-midwives are concerned about the level of education of the lay midwife. Originally most lay midwives were experientially trained and unlicensed. Some states, such as Arizona, require that they must now be licensed. Lay midwives have begun efforts to improve their own standards and education, and a direct-entry midwifery school is now in existence in Seattle (Rooks 1990).

Many certified nurse-midwives believe that the education they received as nurses enhances their ability to function as midwives. Their nursing background helps CNMs function effectively in an emergency situation; it helps them deal with some of the broader health problems of the families they serve; it helps them understand how and when to collaborate with health professionals from other specialties; and it enables them to negotiate the health care system on behalf of their clients. Certification by the ACNM provides the public with some reassurance about the qualifications of a nurse-midwife.

Currently, the ACNM is working to develop more cordial relationships with the Midwives Alliance of North America (MANA), which is the association of lay midwives. Many CNMs support the idea of sharing continuing education course offerings with lay midwives because it is the childbearing woman who ultimately will benefit. Is there a place for a limited-focus care giver such as the lay midwife in this country? There has been in the past, and many states seem to be saying that a place exists today. Regardless of the outcome, there is a place for the CNM in today's process of childbirth. Midwifery helps provide balance, a recognition of the magic of a process that has become increasingly technical.

HEALTH CARE REFORM

Health care issues are at the top of the policy and legislative agendas of the nineties. Constant reminders of the American health care crisis can be found in the media and professional publications. Cost, access, and quality of health care have become the "bywords" of the times. However, cost of health care is the most compelling component driving policy change. Since 1965, this country's health care costs have increased from approximately 5%

of the gross national product to 15% currently. If system changes are not implemented, projections suggest this figure will escalate to 20% by the year 2000. Health care reform is in part a reaction to a cost problem out of control. The real question is whether the United States can develop solutions that are not simply reactive incremental changes, but solutions that truly address the cost issue and other fundamental problems in the system.

High cost and lack of access to appropriate health care services are two problems in the system. There are 37 million uninsured people in the United States and a debatable number underinsured. Many people who have insurance fear changing or losing jobs due to the structure of health care benefits and access to insurance. They may be denied insurance in the future due to preexisting conditions. The increase in illnesses such as AIDS and tuberculosis makes this problem of "job lock" and lack of transferability of insurance benefits even more significant. For some uninsured the only access to the health care system is an emergency room. This inappropriate use of expensive services for basic primary care is both an access and cost problem. Demographic and environmental changes are increasing the need for services. The number of elderly and chronically ill continues to rise. In this country 20% of children live in poverty. Homelessness, violence, AIDS, and substance abuse are on the increase.

Issues of cost and access overshadow most of the discussion and concern about quality of health care. Because the United States spends more per capita than any other country in the world on health care, can we assume that the quality of health care in America always receives a grade of A? Probably not. Outcomes of care in the US system usually are not determined. There has been little cost/benefit analysis to look at patient benefits and dollars spent. An outcome-based system is essential if there is to be comprehensive health care reform. Studies suggest that there is great variation in the level of care received in this country. Some procedures (as many as 30%) are unnecessary, inappropriate, or ineffective for a particular health care problem (Roberts 1993). The United States has some poor health outcomes that do not result in the world's best health. When the United States is measured by the World Health Organization health outcomes, it does not rank at the top. Coddington and colleagues (1990) identify characteristics to strive for in creating a viable and reasonable US health care system. They include universal access, reducing administrative costs, limiting inappropriate and unnecessary care, discouraging duplication of health services, increasing the number of primary care providers, reducing the need for cost shifting, developing a rationale for limiting care, reorganizing managed care, encouraging health care system mergers, and legal reform.

Changing the current system requires a new way of thinking and providing services. Primary health care services should be the base upon which all other secondary and tertiary services are built. Today in the United States the opposite is the case. The system emphasizes high-technology care; 75% of third-party payments are for hospital-based acute care. Further, 5% of the population spends 58% of the American health care resources (ANA 1993). To truly change the way the US health care system works, all segments of the population should have access to primary health care. This includes a focus on health promotion, prevention, and individual responsibility for one's own health. Secondary health care services would use a smaller amount of the health care dollar. Such services would include screening, diagnosis, and ongoing treatment of conditions. These services would be provided by clinics or long-term care facilities. Complex, highly technologic care would become the predominant type of service offered by hospitals. With this model the smallest proportion of the health care dollar and resources would be spent on high-tech tertiary care (ANA 1993).

The emerging shift in the US health care system presents a significant opportunity for the nursing profession. However, this opportunity for responding to and creating change in nursing and health care delivery requires a new way of thinking. Nursing as we now know it was designed with different "rules" and incentives. The nurse of the future will be shaped by the changing health care system. Nurses must clearly articulate our role in the changing environment. We must define and differentiate practice roles and the educational preparation required for those new roles, especially advanced practice roles such as nurse practitioners and CNMs. Roles of care giver and care manager must be delineated. Nurses will also have greater opportunities for roles in health promotion and disease prevention.

Nursing, if it is to survive, must change education, practice, and research. The uniqueness of nursing skills will become more visible if nursing develops firm partnerships with health professions other than medicine. Nurses should stress coalition building, discipline-specific skills, and collaborative advancement (Mundinger 1994). Essential characteristics and abilities of the nurse of the future include autonomy, risk taking, critical thinking, creativity, decision making, negotiation, conflict management, assessment, referral, teaching, and care management. Nurses must be prepared to assume new roles in new settings. Most future care will not be provided in the acute care (hospital-based) setting. Estimates suggest that by the turn of the century only 40% of nurses will work in the traditional hospital setting. Community-based health care providing primary care and some secondary care will be available in schools, workplaces, homes, churches, clinics, transitional care programs, and other ambulatory settings.

Nurses, through activities of the American Nurses Association (ANA), began to address issues related to health care reform as early as 1989. Then the ANA established a committee on cost, quality, and access for health care. At a 1991 Tricouncil meeting (composed of the ANA, NLN [National League for Nursing], AONE [American Organization of Nurse Executives], and AACN [American Association of Colleges of Nursing]) it was proposed to blend the work of the ANA and NLN into a *nursing* agenda for health reform. The result of that work led to the publication of *Nursing's Agenda for Health Care Reform.* That document is endorsed by more than 65 specialty nursing organizations and health care groups representing over a million nurses. When the document was published and distributed, it was viewed as a highly credible proposal by the American public. One poll ranked it second only to the American Association of Retired Persons' (AARP) proposal in credibility, believability, and potential for effectiveness.

Nurses suggest a new paradigm to define and describe US health care. The focus of health care must be on health, not illness; on behavioral aspects of care and technology and of care and cure; on the community, not just institutions; on systematic activities over time rather than episodic care; and on client choice rather than paternalism. Some basic elements of *Nursing's Agenda* include universal access to health care, definition of a standard benefit package available to all citizens and residents, a phase-in of the essential services to be financed (starting with coverage of pregnant women and young children), plans for long-term care that more appropriately meet the needs of the population, support for insurance reform, use of case management, assurance of direct access to a full range of primary health care providers, elimination of unnecessary administrative costs, and development of health care policies based on effectiveness and outcome research (ANA 1991). *Nursing's Agenda* offers solutions that will benefit the health care consumer. Nurses have a truly unique opportunity to be leaders in shaping the future of the US health care system.

Health care reform will have an impact on women's health and perinatal nursing. Klerman (1994) suggests that several factors, including demographic changes, the need to improve access to care, new research findings, and women's preferences for health care, will contribute to future changes in the field. Changes are predicted in clinical procedures, provider roles, the place where care is provided, and financing of care. As access to health care and the need to control costs increase, there will be a greater need for, and utilization of, nurses in advanced practice roles. It is estimated that 60% to 80% of primary and preventive care can be appropriately and cost effectively provided by advanced practice nurses (ANA 1992).

Nurses took a bold step with the *Agenda for Health Care Reform.* This position statement has allowed nurses to begin to participate as partners in shaping the future of the American health care delivery system. However, the work of the profession has only begun. Nursing must strive for unity in this process of change. Nurses must be willing to change and move into new roles. There must be a strong political presence to influence policymakers and consumers. Nurses must collaborate within nursing and with other providers. And last, for nursing to succeed in this era of dramatic change, nurses can no longer see their role as a job; it must be a professional career. If not now, when?

ETHICS, LAW, AND PROFESSIONAL PRACTICE

Professional nursing practice requires full understanding of practice standards, institutional or agency policies, and local, state, and federal laws. Professional practice also requires an understanding of the ethical implications of those standards, policies, and laws that impact care, care providers, and care recipients. Every professional nurse is responsible for obtaining and maintaining current information regarding ethics and laws related to nursing practice and health care.

Scope of Practice

State nurse practice acts protect the public by broadly defining the legal scope within which every nurse must practice and by excluding untrained or unlicensed individuals from practicing nursing. Although some state practice acts continue to limit nursing practice to the traditional responsibilities of providing client care related to health maintenance and disease prevention, most state practice acts cover expanded practice roles that include collaboration with other professionals in planning and providing care, physician-delegated diagnosis and prescriptive privilege, and the delegation of client care tasks to other specified licensed and unlicensed personnel. A few state practice acts specify nurses' ability to diagnose and treat health problems and incorporate definitions of nurse practitioner roles. Specified care activities for certified nurse-midwives and women's health, perinatal, or neonatal nurse practitioners may include diagnosis and prenatal management of uncomplicated pregnancies, management of births by certified nurse-midwives, and prescribing and dispensing medications using protocols in specified circumstances.

State practice acts also specify violations that may result in disciplinary action against a nurse. Correctly interpreting and understanding state practice acts enables the nurse to provide safe care within the limits of nursing practice. State boards of nursing may provide official interpretation of practice acts when the limits are not clear. On occasion hospital policy may conflict with a state's nurse practice act. It is important to recognize that *hospital or agency policy may restrict the scope of practice specified in a state practice act, but such policy cannot legally expand the scope of practice beyond the limits stated in the practice act.*

Nurse practice acts are subject to change. One component of professional nursing practice is the responsibility of each nurse to remain up-to-date regarding scope of practice and even to actively participate in promoting appropriate changes.

Standards of Nursing Care

Standards of care establish minimum criteria for competent, proficient delivery of nursing care. Such standards are designed to protect the public and are used to judge the quality of care provided. Legal interpretation of actions within standards of care is based on what a reasonably prudent nurse with similar education and experience would do in similar circumstances.

Written standards of care are provided by a number of different sources. The ANA has published standards of professional practice since 1950. In 1973 the ANA Congress for Nursing Practice began to write generic standards for all nurses in all settings. In addition the ANA Divisions of Practice have published standards that include nursing practice for maternal-child health. The Council of Perinatal Nurses has published standards for perinatal nursing. Other specialty organizations, such as the Association of Women's Health, Obstetrics, and Neonatal Nurses (AWHONN), the Association of Operating Room Nurses (AORN), and the National Association of Neonatal Nurses (NANN), have developed standards of specialty practice. Agency policies, procedures, and protocols also provide appropriate guidelines for care standards. The Joint Commission on Accreditation of Healthcare Organizations (JCAHO), a private, nongovernmental agency that audits the operation of hospitals and health care facilities, has also contributed to the development of nursing standards.

Some standards carry the force of law; others, although not legally based, still carry important legal significance. Any nurse who fails to meet appropriate standards of care invites allegations of negligence or malpractice. However, any nurse who practices within the guidelines established by agency, local, or national standards is assured that clients are provided with competent nursing care and therefore diminishes the potential for litigation.

Ethical Components of Care Standards

Standards of care are based on a legal model rather than on ethics. However, they incorporate important ethical components that extend the narrow legal interpretation of the term "standard." Although there is a great deal of interplay between the two disciplines, each has a different perspective.

Law is based primarily on a *rights model* that establishes rules of conduct to define our relationships with strangers and people we know. Law may also define our relationships to impersonal entities like formal organizations, agencies, or hospitals.

Ethics is based on a *responsibility* or *duty model* that considers a wider range of factors than the rights model of law. Ethics incorporates factors such as risks, benefits, other relationships, concerns, and the needs and abilities of persons affected by and affecting decisions.

Law and ethics are interrelated; they share a similar decision process and standards. Both disciplines incorporate fact finding, conflict negotiation, prioritization of related issues and values, and the application of resolutions of particular cases in decision making. Professional nurses must consider the ethical implications of legal decisions and the legal implications of ethical decisions.

Understanding the distinctions among medical or health care decisions, legal decisions, and ethical decisions is important. Consider the case in which parents from a culture unfamiliar to the nurse refuse surgery for their newborn based on a deeply held spiritual belief that intentional cutting of a body will result in spiritual death. Such a decision to forgo surgery may be viewed as negligent in the eyes of the law, unwise and inappropriate from a medical perspective, yet fully justifiable ethically. Similarly, legally sanctioned maintenance of life support for a severely damaged newborn with little hope for meaningful existence may remain a medically viable alternative, but to many is not ethically justifiable. Recognizing the type of decision to be made often helps measure the worth and outcome of a decision more appropriately.

Clients' Rights

Law and ethics impact all of nursing practice, and several topics have specific implications for maternal-child nursing practice. Consideration of clients' rights leads to the discussion of topics such as informed consent, privacy, and confidentiality.

Informed Consent

Informed consent as a concept is designed to allow clients to make intelligent decisions regarding their own health care. **Informed consent** means that a client, or designated decision maker, has granted permission for a specific treatment or procedure based on full information about that specific treatment or procedure as it relates to that client under the specific circumstances of the permission. Several elements must be addressed in order to be assured that informed consent has been given.

The information provided to the client must be clearly and concisely presented in a manner understandable to that individual and must include risks and benefits, the probability of success, and significant medical alternatives that exist. The client also needs to be told the consequences of receiving no treatment or procedure. Finally, the client must be told of the right to refuse a specific treatment or procedure. Each client should be told that refusal of the specified treatment or procedure does not mean that all support or care will be withdrawn as a result. Consent should always be freely given, without coercion. Even well-intentioned pressure to sway a client's

response to a request for permission is unethical and denies the client's fundamental right to informed consent.

To be sure to obtain informed consent, the nurse must ascertain client capacity and competence to decide. "Capacity" refers to a client's ability to understand information as presented. "Competence" refers to a client's ability to make a voluntary, rational, informed decision based on information provided and an understanding of the options and consequences of each option. Information should be provided by the individual who is ultimately responsible for the treatment or procedure. In most instances this is the physician. In such cases the nurse's role is to witness the client's signature giving consent. A nurse who knows the client and the procedure may certainly help the physician obtain the client's consent by clarifying the information the physician provides. It is also part of the nurse's role to determine that the client understands the information provided prior to making a decision.

Society grants to parents the authority and responsibility to give consent for their minor children. Parents are presumed to possess what a child lacks in maturity, experience, and capacity for judgment in life's difficult decisions. Although the age of majority is 18 years in most states, variations in certain states require that nurses be aware of the law in the state where they practice. Special problems can occur in maternity nursing when a minor gives birth. It is possible, depending upon state law, that a minor may consent to treatment for her infant but not for herself. In some states, however, a pregnant teenager is considered an emancipated minor and may therefore give consent for herself as well.

Additionally, some states require a married woman to obtain the consent of her spouse when a procedure involves sterilization or threatens the life of a fetus. Although childbearing women sign a general consent form on admission to an agency, separate informed consent is often required for surgery, cesarean birth, the administration of anesthesia, tubal ligation, or participation in research.

Refusal of a treatment, medication, or procedure after appropriate information also requires that a client sign a form to release the physician and agency from liability. Jehovah's Witnesses' refusal of blood transfusion or Rh_o (D) immune globulin is an example of such refusal.

Right to Privacy

The right to privacy is the right of a person to keep his or her person and property free from public scrutiny. Maternity nurses must remember that this includes unnecessary exposure of the childbearing woman's body. Only those responsible for her care should examine her or discuss her case. Although the United States Constitution does not explicitly sanction the right to privacy, the US Supreme Court has cited several constitutional amendments that imply the right to privacy (Loeb 1992). Most states have recognized the right to privacy through statutory or common law, and some states have written that right into their constitution. Professional standards protecting clients' privacy have been adopted by the ANA, NLN, and JCAHO. Health care agencies should also have written policies dealing with client privacy.

Laws regarding privacy specify that information about clients' treatment, condition, and prognosis can be shared only by the health professionals responsible for their care. Authorization for the release of any patient information should be obtained from competent patients or their surrogate decision maker. Although it may be legal to reveal vital statistics such as name, age, occupation, and prognosis, such information is often withheld because of ethical considerations. The client should be consulted regarding what information may be released and to whom. When a client is a celebrity or is considered newsworthy, inquiries may be best handled by the public relations department of the agency.

Confidentiality

Given the highly personal and intimate information requested of clients, the need for maintaining confidentiality is crucial for the development of trust in the client-provider relationship. Privileged communications exist between client and physician, client and attorney, husband and wife, clergy and those who seek their counsel. In some states nurses are also protected by laws of privilege. The wise nurse will become well informed regarding laws in the state of practice.

A client may waive the right to confidentiality of medical records by action or words. For example, if a childbearing woman sues a physician, hospital, or other care provider, she waives the right to confidentiality of the medical record because the record becomes a source of evidence. Clients commonly consent to disclose information to insurance companies or to employers. Computerization of records has created a greater concern for the integrity of records and the potential invasion of privacy. All information regarding a client belongs solely to that client. It is up to the client to authorize the release of that information. Liability becomes an issue if information about a client is released without prior approval from that client or the legally responsible guardian (Ellis & Hartley 1992).

In some instances the public good takes precedence over an individual's right to privacy. For example, state laws require that care providers report such things as gunshot wounds, child abuse, and some communicable diseases.

Basic Ethical Theories and Principles

An understanding of ethical theories and principles may help the nurse distinguish among the types of decisions often made in health care. Ethical decisions in health care are based primarily on one of two theoretical positions: *deontology*, which is duty-bound theory, and *utilitarianism* or *teleology*, which is consequence-bound theory. Although several ethical principles derive from these two theories, four principles impact current health care more than any others: autonomy, beneficence, nonmaleficence, and justice. (These are discussed in detail below.) Ethical principles and rules such as fidelity (promise keeping), veracity (truth telling), confidentiality, and privacy are other important considerations in reaching ethically justifiable health care decisions.

Deontology is the classical theory of ethics that suggests that the moral rightness or wrongness of human actions is determined according to the principle or motivation upon which the action is based rather than solely upon the consequences of the action. The determination of rightness or wrongness may be based, as in religious tradition, on an appeal to divine revelation or, as for some philosophers, on intuition and common sense (Beauchamps & Childress 1989). Deontology is based on the concept of moral duty or obligation (Ellis & Hartley 1992; Munson 1992).

Utilitarianism is based on the principle of utility or usefulness and is chiefly concerned with the consequences of actions to determine rightness and wrongness of human action. Utilitarianism seeks decisions that produce the greatest balance of good consequences over evil consequences in the world as a whole (Beauchamps & Walters 1989). Actions such as killing or lying, which are disallowed using deontology, may be justified under utilitarianism if the outcome produces greater good than evil consequences. If the consequence of an action is more positive than negative, the action is deemed good, and the means to achieve that end are justified (Ellis & Hartley 1992).

Ethical principles and rules that derive from these ethical theories often apply to nursing practice. Autonomy, beneficence, nonmaleficence, and justice are among those principles.

Autonomy

One of the most influential principles associated with health care ethics currently is autonomy. Autonomy is also referred to as the principle of respect for person. This principle of self-rule or self-determination refers to an individual's right to make free, uncoerced, informed decisions and to respect the decisions of others. The principle of autonomy also includes the acceptance of responsibility for one's choices. The principle of autonomy recognizes humans as unconditionally worthy agents. That is, humans are worthy regardless of any special circumstances or usefulness to others. Under this principle humans may not be treated as worthy only to serve one's own purposes (Beauchamps & Walters 1989). The concept of informed consent derives directly from the principle of autonomy.

Beneficence

Beneficence is the principle that invokes us to do good and to avoid harm. It requires nurses to abstain from injuring others and to help others promote their important and legitimate interests, primarily by preventing or removing possible harms (Beauchamps & Walters 1989; Mappes & Zembaty 1991). The client's welfare and best interests are at the heart of this principle. Promoting the client's welfare is inherent to the care provider role and therefore is central to the practice of maternal-child nursing.

Conflict often occurs between the principles of autonomy and beneficence. Consider the dilemma in which honoring the child's autonomy, the client's right to decide for self, conflicts with what is obviously in that client's best interest. This truly represents the conflict of one good with another (Davis 1990). This conflict between two goods is also evident in conflicts between maternal and fetal rights or maternal and paternal rights.

Nonmaleficence

Nonmaleficence is a corollary to beneficence that invokes us to do no harm. From the perspective of ethical theory, nonmaleficence carries greater moral weight than beneficence (Beauchamps & Walters 1989; Mappes & Zembaty 1991). What this means in nursing practice is that care providers must first be certain to honor their duty to do no harm before being free to promote the client's good. By this standard nurses must assure themselves that they will not hurt a client before being ethically justified in trying to help.

Justice

In the current environment of health care reform with the emphasis on the allocation of scarce health care resources, the principle of justice or fairness takes on great importance. Justice refers to the moral obligation to be fair to all according to what is due, owed, or deserved. What is fair, due, owed, or deserved may be either a benefit like political rights or economic goods or a burden such as taxes or military consignment. The principle of justice suggests that equals should be treated equally and unequals should be treated unequally. The determination of what is owed to an individual according to the principle of justice is very complex. It might be based on individual effort, merit, rights, need, societal contribution, or simple equal division (Beauchamps & Walters 1989).

Situations that create conflict among these ethical principles or among the rights of individuals occur in health care. Ethical decision making is based on the application of ethical principles and a consideration of the rights and values of the individuals involved. Conflicts are often heightened by the question of whose rights should prevail. Those of the individual and those of society are considered, and the risks and benefits are weighed. In many cases there are no clear-cut solutions.

Ethical Decisions

Health care and bioethical literature are filled with examples of ethical decision-making models and frameworks (Bandman & Bandman 1990; Benjamin & Curtis 1992; Ellis & Hartley 1992; Halloran 1982; Husted & Husted 1991; Silva 1990; Thompson & Thompson 1990). Decision-making models help guide nurses and other care providers through the decision-making process when they are confronted with seemingly unresolvable conflicts among the rights, duties, theories, principles, values, and individuals impacted by the ethical dilemmas of practice. Even without a formal decision-making framework, nurses are able to resolve ethical dilemmas by recognizing and utilizing the critical components of ethical decision-making models. There are six critical components of the ethical decision process that are very similar to the components of the nursing process.

When confronted by an ethical dilemma, one should first establish a means of determining who is involved in the dilemma, who is involved in the decision, and who will be affected by the outcome of the decision. This data-gathering step allows the nurse to identify and define the issue and determine who owns the problem, the information, the decision, and the consequences of it. A second data-gathering step is the establishment of the mechanism for obtaining all the information relevant to the conflict. Data related to diagnosis, prognosis, and treatment options should be collected in addition to information regarding available health care, psychosocial, spiritual, financial, and other appropriate resources.

The third step of any ethical decision-making process incorporates a plan to outline all potential options and the consequences of each. During this step the nurse should be sure that even opposing viewpoints are presented and considered. Setting individual values aside during this phase is important in order to encourage divergent views.

Fourth, the conflict resolution process must incorporate a review of driving and restraining forces, an assessment of risks and benefits, as well as the likelihood of a successful outcome with each option. At this stage the moral values of everyone involved need to be addressed. In addition, any more peripheral issues such as any impact on other individuals or systems related to the decision, changes in client condition, pertinent laws, or new information should be reviewed within the context of general and individual moral principles.

Fifth, there must be a plan to select and act on a resolution of the conflict. Determining, ahead of this step, who is ultimately responsible for the decision, who is most impacted by the outcome, and whether consensus is required may facilitate acting on the resolution.

Evaluation is the final step in the decision process. An evaluation of the resolution, its consequences, and the decision process itself is critically important if decisions in similar situations are not to be made in isolation.

Ethical decisions in maternal-child nursing are often complicated by moral obligations to more than one client. Straightforward solutions to the ethical dilemmas encountered in caring for childbearing families are often, quite simply, not available. Use of a formal decision structure may, however, increase the likelihood of addressing multiple needs in complex care situations in an ethically appropriate and legal manner.

Special Ethical Situations in Maternity Care

Ethical dilemmas confront nurses in all areas of practice. Dilemmas related to pregnancy, birth, and the newborn seem especially difficult to resolve. "New techniques for recognizing and responding to prenatal harms generate a variety of troubling issues which, in turn, pose fundamental challenges to the fields of medicine, biomedical ethics, law, and public policy" (Mathieu 1991, p 4). Social, cultural, and religious values and beliefs held by individuals are intricately interwoven with technological advances to compound the dilemmas in maternity care.

Maternal-Fetal Conflict

The status of the fetus as a person has long been debated. Until fairly recently the fetus was legally considered a nonperson. However, advances in technology have enabled physicians to monitor fetal development, to treat fetal problems, and even to provide pre-embryo diagnosis that may dramatically affect the outcome of the birth of a healthy baby. Increasingly, the fetus is viewed as a client separate from the mother, although treatment of the fetus necessarily involves the mother. Care providers may confront situations in which two clients assert "possibly contradictory moral claims on . . . [the] fundamental ethical obligation to do good and avoid harm" (J J Mitchell 1994, p 93).

In maternity care the moral assumption is made that the pregnant woman's decisions will be beneficial to both her life and well-being and that of her fetus (Mitchell 1994). In some cases, however, the pregnant woman refuses to consent to a medical intervention that is essential to the well-being of the fetus and of minimal risk to her. Situations also exist in which the pregnant woman engages in high-risk behaviors, such as substance abuse, that jeopardize the health of her fetus. In spite of care providers' noble intentions to protect the fetus, coercion of the pregnant woman, even through judicial intervention, is rarely justified. The pregnant woman remains the most appropriate evaluator of the benefits and risks of proposed treatments, interventions, or procedures in accordance with her values, goals, and philosophy. "Actions of coercion to obtain informed consent or force a course of action limiting maternal freedom of choice, threaten the doctor-patient relationship and violate the principles underlying the informed consent process" (ACOG 1987).

The American College of Obstetricians and Gynecologists (ACOG) Committee on Ethics 1987 position statement, *Patient Choices: Maternal-Fetal Conflict;* the American Academy of Pediatrics 1988 statement, *Fetal Therapy: Ethical Considerations;* and the American Medical Association Board of Trustees 1990 report, *Legal Interventions During Pregnancy,* all reaffirm the fundamental right of pregnant women to make informed, uncoerced decisions regarding medical interventions. All three major policy statements also recognize that cases of maternal-fetal conflict involve two clients, both of whom deserve respect and treatment. Further, all agree such cases "are best resolved through the use of internal hospital mechanisms including counseling, the intervention of specialists, and the utilization of ethics committees . . . and that a resort to judicial intervention is rarely, if ever, appropriate" (J J Mitchell 1994, p 94).

Abortion

Since the 1973 Supreme Court decision in *Roe v Wade,* abortion has been legal in the United States. It can be performed until the period of viability, after which abortion is permissible only when the life or health of the mother is threatened. Before viability the mother's rights are paramount; after viability the rights of the fetus take precedence. There are continuing efforts by individuals, organizations, and states to limit or abolish abortion by prohibiting Medicaid funding of abortions and putting other restrictions on the procedure. These efforts include restricting abortions to hospitals (which significantly increases the cost) and requiring agencies to provide graphic details of the procedure to the client, ostensibly to provide informed consent.

Efforts to restrict a woman's right to abortion gained momentum in 1989 when, in considering the case of *Webster v Reproductive Health Services,* the Supreme Court upheld a Missouri statute placing a variety of restrictions on abortion. In 1992 the Supreme Court upheld a US District Court decision in Pennsylvania that calls for restrictions on abortion that include providing information to the pregnant woman on the gestational age of the fetus, the risks of abortion, and the risks of pregnancy and childbirth. The Pennsylvania Abortion Council Act also requires 24-hours between informed consent and the abortion procedure and informed consent from one parent of a minor who wishes an abortion (Gill 1992).

In 1993, shortly after taking the oath of office, President Clinton signed executive orders that (1) lifted the gag rule prohibiting most health care providers at federally funded clinics from discussing abortion with pregnant women; (2) permitted the use of fetal tissue in federally funded research, even if the tissue was obtained from an abortion; and (3) permitted overseas US military personnel and their dependents to receive abortions at military hospitals at their own expense. Thus the controversy continues.

Techniques have been developed for the selective termination of pregnancy in instances of multiple pregnancy to reduce the number of fetuses in the uterus or to eliminate fetuses found, through prenatal testing, to be at risk for disease or disability. This relatively new technique raises serious concerns about its moral justification and the development of social policy delineating both access to and resource allocation for the procedure (Overall 1990).

The decision for abortion remains to be made by a woman and her physician. Care providers have the right to refuse to perform an abortion or to assist with the procedure if abortion is contrary to their moral and ethical beliefs. A nurse who refuses to participate in an abortion because of moral or ethical beliefs must be certain that someone with similar qualifications is able to provide appropriate care for the client. Clients may never be abandoned, regardless of the nurse's beliefs.

Fetal Research

Research with fetal tissue has been responsible for remarkable advances in the care and treatment of fetuses with health problems and advances in the treatment of progressive, debilitating adult diseases such as Parkinson's, Alzheimer's, and DiGeorge's syndromes. Although such research occurs in more than 13 countries worldwide, federally funded research using fetal tissue obtained from therapeutic abortions was not possible in the US from 1987 to 1993 due to a moratorium established during the presidency of George Bush and lifted by President Bill Clinton (Markowitz 1993). In 1994 a National Institutes of Health (NIH) expert advisory panel formulated rules to guide research using fetal tissue. The panel established strict, detailed guidelines for such research including, for example, the requirement that embryos to be used should not be allowed to develop for more than 14 days, which is consistent with the standard used worldwide. Sex selection of embryos is not permitted except in cases of sex-linked hereditary diseases such as hemophilia, nor are researchers permitted to implant human embryos in animals for gestation (Gorman 1994).

Therapeutic research with living fetuses has been instrumental in the treatment of Rh-sensitized infants, the evaluation of lung maturity using the lecithin/sphingomyelin ratio, and the treatment of pulmonary immaturity in the newborn. Because it is aimed at treating a fetal condition, therapeutic fetal research raises fewer ethical dilemmas than does nontherapeutic fetal research (Collins 1993). To be approved, nontherapeutic research requires that the risk to the fetus be minimal, that the knowledge to be gained be important, and that the information be unobtainable by any other means. Control over research standards and attention to state and federal regulations remain foci of debate regarding fetal research.

Intrauterine fetal surgery, which began in 1981 and developed through therapeutic research, is a therapy for anatomic lesions that can be corrected surgically and are incompatible with life if not treated. Bilateral hydronephrosis due to obstruction and congenital diaphragmatic hernia are examples of such lesions. In the early years of intrauterine fetal surgery prenatal approaches to correcting fetal hydrocephalus were attempted, but because of the poor natural history of the condition, this surgery is no longer done. Currently researchers are experimenting with intrauterine surgery to treat several conditions such as pleural effusion, obstructed cardiac valves, and sacrococcygeal teratoma, a rare tumor of the fetal buttocks (Contemporary OB/GYN 1994).

Intrauterine fetal surgery involves opening the uterus during the second trimester (prior to viability), treating the fetal lesion, and replacing the fetus in the uterus. The risks to the fetus are substantial, and the mother is committed to cesarean births for this and subsequent pregnancies because the upper, active segment of the uterus is incised during the surgery. Parents must, of course, be informed of the experimental nature of the treatment, the risks of the surgery, the commitment to cesarean birth, and alternatives to the treatment. As with other aspects of maternity care, the pregnant woman's autonomy must be respected. The procedure does involve health risks to the woman, and she retains the right to refuse any surgical procedure. Health care providers must be careful that their zeal for new technology does not lead them to focus unilaterally on the fetus at the expense of the mother (Contemporary OB/GYN 1994).

Reproductive Assistance

The number and sophistication of reproductive assistance techniques continue to grow. Infertile couples are now presented with reproductive options that include artificial insemination, in vitro fertilization, gamete intrafallopian transfer, embryo transfer, oocyte donation, and the possibility for surrogate childbearing.

Artificial insemination (AI) is accomplished by depositing into a woman sperm obtained from her husband, partner, or other donor. The sperm can be deposited into the vagina, the cervical canal, or the uterus. Homologous insemination (AIH) involves the husband's or partner's sperm; donor insemination (AID) involves a donor other than the husband or partner. No states prohibit AIH, so there is no question of the child's legitimacy. Legal problems may occur with AID, however. Because the child is the biologic child of the mother, legal concerns center around the donor. A donor must sign a form waiving all parental rights. The donor must also furnish accurate health information, particularly regarding genetic traits or diseases. Donor sperm must be tested for HIV. Husbands often are requested to sign a form to agree to the insemination and to assume parental responsibility for the child. Some men legally adopt the child so there is no question of parental rights and responsibilities. Several states have enacted legislation regarding paternity of the child conceived by insemination with donor sperm.

Assisted reproductive technology (ART) is the term used to describe the highly technologic approaches used to produce pregnancy. *In vitro fertilization and embryo transfer (IVF-ET)*, a therapy available to selected infertile couples, is perhaps the best known of ART techniques. In this process ovulation is induced; then one or more oocytes are retrieved by transvaginal ultrasound scanning in conjunction with transvaginal aspiration and fertilized with sperm from the husband, partner, or donor. Three to four embryos are transferred to the woman's uterus when they have developed to the four- to six-cell stage (Stillman & Gindoff 1994). *Zygote intrafallopian transfer (ZIFT)* is similar to IVF-ET, except that the developing embryo is implanted in the fallopian tube. The success rates of the procedures are low; clinical pregnancies result in approximately 16% of IVF-ET procedures and 22% of ZIFT procedures (Hurst & Schlaff 1994). Recently, researchers have begun to use natural cycle IVF (as opposed to the use of medications to stimulate ovulation). This approach eliminates the need to use fertility drugs to stimulate ovulation, with the associated risks of those medications, and results in the implantation of a single oocyte instead of multiple oocytes (Levy & Gindoff 1994). Legal and ethical issues associated with ART include questions of paternity if donor sperm is used, ownership and appropriate disposal of embryos that are not implanted, and the ethical ramifications of selective reduction when multiple pregnancy occurs.

Oocyte donation provides an alternative approach for women who lack oocytes (usually because of premature ovarian failure), women with genetic disorders who do not wish to use their own oocytes, and older women whose oocyte quality may be reduced. It is also used for women who have been unable to produce enough oocytes during IVF procedures (Goode & Hahn 1993). The oocyte donor may be known to the recipient or may be a stranger. Donor oocytes are fertilized with sperm from the recipient's partner in a way similar to that for IVF-ET. The recipient's endometrium is stimulated with hormones to prepare it to receive the fertilized oocytes, which are transferred using ET techniques.

Gamete intrafallopian transfer (GIFT) is used in women with at least one functioning tube whose infertility is due to unknown causes or male factors such as low sperm count. In GIFT multiple oocytes are retrieved by laparoscopy from the woman or a donor and transferred with sperm directly into the fallopian tubes. The resulting pregnancy is considered in vivo fertilization.

Surrogate childbearing occurs when a woman agrees to become pregnant for a childless couple. She is artificially inseminated with the male partner's sperm, a donor's sperm, or may even receive a gamete transfer, depending upon the infertile couple's needs. If the child is conceived by artificial insemination with sperm from the husband in the couple desiring the child, the child is the husband's biologic offspring. In this case the biologic mother agrees to relinquish the child at birth, the wife of the child's father agrees to adopt the child, and the biologic mother receives payment for expenses associated with the pregnancy and birth and usually a lump sum payment for her participation. Other agreements may be reached, depending on the source of the genetic material obtained to produce the embryo gestated by the surrogate mother. It is now possible to witness the birth of an infant with several parents—biologic or genetic parents, gestational parent, and adoptive parents. The complexity of ethical and legal issues surrounding such births seems obvious.

Surrogate childbearing remains controversial. Those in favor of it stress the surrogate mother's altruism in providing a couple who desperately want a child with the opportunity to be parents, the benefits and joys to the couple who receive the child, and the birth of a child who would otherwise not be born. Proponents suggest that the problems and risks are no different from other instances of artificial insemination by donor and note the emotional trauma of separating an infant from a birth mother for adoption.

Opponents of surrogacy cite the possibility of the birth of a defective newborn whom no one wants, a biologic mother who refuses to relinquish the newborn, the risks to the surrogate mother of a pregnancy without the benefits of motherhood, the appearance of buying a child (which is illegal in all states), and the identity problems of children who discover the complexities of their conceptions and gestations and wonder about relinquishment by their birth mothers. Others oppose surrogate childbearing on other moral, ethical, legal, or religious grounds.

Ethical and legal issues related to reproductive assistance continue to emerge. The questions of heritage and the legality of AID have not been resolved. The rights and responsibilities of donors are unclear. Other ethical questions include: What should be done with surplus fertilized oocytes? To whom do frozen embryos belong—parents together or separately? The hospital? Who is liable if a woman or her offspring contracts AIDS from donated sperm? Should children be told the method of their conception?

The Human Genome Project

The Human Genome Project, a multibillion dollar undertaking of NIH and the Department of Energy, was established to develop a human genetic map; formulate and improve techniques for DNA sequencing; create software to handle the information obtained; explore the ethical, social, and legal implications of genetic research (specifically as they relate to the project); establish research training programs for pre- and postdoctoral fellows; and explore ways to transfer the knowledge obtained to appropriate users in the medical and industrial communities (Raff & Eunpu 1994). As more genetic information becomes available as a result of the project, questions regarding use and protection of such information arise. Gene manipulation and gene therapy, once limited to science fiction novels, now present a reality that adds to the complex ethical questions of use and control of technology. Other emerging issues include the question of payment for genetic testing; appropriate counseling following testing; confidentiality; qualifications of individuals engaged in testing, counseling, and interventions; mandated testing; and the right to refuse genetic information.

Implications for Nursing Practice

New, complex issues and choices in maternal-newborn nursing continue to demand innovative nursing practice responses. Midwives at the Georgetown University School of Nursing in Washington, DC, for example, have, in anticipation of potential conflicts, initiated the use of advance directive birth plans to assist with the complex decisions surrounding the birthing experience. Prenatal birth plans are used to initiate discussions of treatment options, labor and birth preferences, and the family's goals throughout the birthing experience. "Having prenatal birth plans allows for a treatment decision to be known before the stress of labor itself . . . with the ultimate result being a bond of trust between health care provider and patient. The obligation of health care providers to respect maternal autonomy can be facilitated by the use of a birth plan that has been written by the pregnant woman or couple during a less stressful prenatal period" (Donohue 1994, p 43). Anticipation and planning cooperatively with clients may provide a proactive approach to conflict resolution.

The complex ethical issues facing maternal-newborn nurses have many social, cultural, legal, and professional ramifications. Nurses must learn to anticipate ethical dilemmas, clarify their own positions and values related to the issues, understand the legal implications of the issues, and develop appropriate strategies for ethical decision making.

KEY CONCEPTS

Many nurses working with childbearing families are expert practitioners who are able to serve as role models for nurses who have not yet attained the same level of competence.

Contemporary childbirth is family centered, offers choices about birth, and recognizes the needs of siblings and other family members.

The self-care movement, which emerged in the late 1960s, emphasizes personal health goals, a holistic approach, and an emphasis on preventive care.

Nurses function in a variety of roles, including care giver, advocate, educator, researcher, change agent, and political activist.

A nurse must practice within the scope of practice or be open to the accusation of practicing medicine without a license.

The standard of care is that of a reasonably prudent nurse.

The right to privacy is protected by state constitutions, statutes, and common law.

Informed consent—based on knowledge of a procedure and its benefits, risks, and alternatives—must be secured prior to providing treatment.

Intrauterine fetal surgery is a therapy for anatomic lesions that can be corrected surgically and are incompatible with life if left untreated.

Abortion can be performed until the age of viability. There are continuing efforts to restrict or abolish abortion. Care givers have the right to refuse to perform an abortion or assist with the procedure.

REFERENCES

American Academy of Pediatrics, Committee on Bioethics: Fetal therapy: Ethical considerations. *Pediatrics* 1988; 88:898.

American College of Obstetricians and Gynecologists, Committee on Ethics: *Opinion No. 55: Patient choices: Maternal-fetal conflict.* Washington, DC: ACOG, 1987.

American Medical Association, Board of Trustees: Legal interventions during pregnancy. *JAMA* 1990; 264:2663.

ANA: Advanced practice nursing: A new age in health care. In: *Nursing Facts.* Washington, DC: American Nurses Association, 1992.

ANA: *Nursing's Agenda for Health Care Reform.* Washington, DC: American Nurses Association, 1991.

ANA: Primary health care: The nurse solution. In: *Nursing Facts.* Washington, DC: American Nurses Association, 1993.

Bandman EL, Bandman B: *Nursing Ethics Through the Life Span,* 2nd ed. Norwalk, CT: Appleton & Lange, 1990.

Beauchamps TL, Childress JF: *Principles of Biomedical Ethics,* 3rd ed. New York: Oxford Univ Press, 1989.

Beauchamps TL, Walters LR: *Contemporary Issues in Bioethics,* 4th ed. Belmont, CA: Wadsworth, 1989.

Benjamin M, Curtis J: *Ethics in Nursing,* 3rd ed. New York: Oxford Univ Press, 1992.

Benner P: *From Novice to Expert.* Menlo Park, CA: Addison-Wesley, 1984.

Benner P, Wrubel J: *The Primacy of Caring.* Menlo Park, CA: Addison-Wesley, 1989.

Coddington DC et al: *The Crisis in Health Care.* San Francisco: Jossey-Bass, 1990.

Collins BA: Ethical issues in conducting clinical nursing research. *AWHONN Clin Issues Perinatal Women Health Nurs* 1993; 4(4):620.

Contemporary OB/GYN: Fetal surgery: Past, present, and future work in this frontier. April 15, 1994; 39(S):59. (Symposium.)

Davis AJ: Are there limits to caring? Conflict between autonomy and beneficence. In: *Ethical and Moral Dimensions of*

Care. Leininger MM (editor). Detroit, MI: Wayne State Univ Press, 1990.

Department of Health and Human Services, Secretary's Commission on Nursing: *Final Report*, vol 1. Washington, DC, 1988.

Donohue M: Midwives use advance directive birth plans to build trust. *Med Eth Advisor* 1994; 10(3): 43.

Edwards-Beckett J: Nursing research utilization techniques. *J Nurs Admin* 1990; 20(11):25.

Ellis JR, Hartley CL: *Nursing in Today's World: Challenges, Issues, and Trends*, 4th ed. Philadelphia: Lippincott, 1992.

Evans MI et al: Fetal therapy: The next generation. *Women's Health Issues* 1990; 1:31.

Fagin C, Lynaugh J: Reaping the rewards of radical change: A new agenda for nursing education. *Nurs Outlook* 1992; 40:213.

Gill S: The fate of Roe v Wade. *Hastings Center Report* 1992; 22(5):24.

Goode CJ, Hahn SJ: Oocyte donation and in vitro fertilization: The nurse's role with ethical and legal issues. *JOGNN* March/April 1993; 22(2):106.

Gorman C: Brave new embryos. *Time* August 29, 1994; 144(9):60.

Halloran MC: Rational ethical judgments utilizing a decision-making tool. *Heart Lung* 1982; 11(6):566.

Heater BS et al: Helping patients recover faster. *Am J Nurs* October 1990; 90:19.

Hurst BS, Schlaff WD: Assisted reproduction: What role for ZIFT? *Contemp OB/GYN* October 15, 1994; 39(S):9.

Husted GL, Husted JH: *Ethical Decision Making in Nursing*. St Louis, MO: Mosby-Year Book, 1991.

Inlander CB: Medicine and the consumer revolution. *The World and I* August 1990; 515.

Joint Commission on Accreditation of Healthcare Organizations: *The 1991 Joint Commission Accreditation Manual for Hospitals*, vol. 1, *Standards*. 1990.

Klerman L: Perinatal health care policy: How it will affect the family in the 21st century. *JOGNN* 1994; 23(2):124.

Levy MJ, Gindoff PR: Who benefits most from natural-cycle IVF? *Contemp OB/GYN* February 1994; 39(2):11.

Loeb S: *Nurses Handbook of Law and Ethics*. Springhouse, PA: Springhouse, 1992.

Mappes TA, Zembaty JS: *Biomedical Ethics*, 3rd ed. New York: McGraw-Hill, 1991.

Markowitz MS: Human fetal tissue: Ethical implications for use in research and treatment. *AWHONN Clin Issues Perinatal Women Health Nurs* 1993; 4(4):578.

Mathieu D: *Preventing Fetal Harm: Should the State Intervene?* Boston, MA: Kluwer Academic, 1991.

Mitchell C: Ethical dilemmas. *Crit Care Nurs Clin North Am* 1994; 2(3):427.

Mitchell JJ: Maternal-fetal conflict: A role for the healthcare ethics committee. *Healthcare Eth Comn Forum* 1994; 6(2):93.

Mundinger MO: Health care reform: Will nursing respond? *Nurs Health Care*. January 1994; 15(1):28.

Munson R: *Intervention and Reflection: Basic Issues in Medical Ethics*, 4th ed. Belmont, CA: Wadsworth, 1992.

Naisbitt J: *Megatrends*. New York: Warner Books, 1982.

Overall C: Selective termination of pregnancy and women's reproductive autonomy. *Hastings Center Report* 1990; 20(3):6.

Pettengill MM et al: Factors encouraging and discouraging the use of nursing research findings. *Image* Summer 1994; 26(2):143.

Raff BS, Eunpu D: The genome project. *JOGNN* July/August 1994; 23(6):488.

Roberts MJ, Clyde A: *Your Money or Your Life: The Health Care Crisis Explained*. New York: Doubleday, 1993.

Rooks JP: Nurse-midwifery: The window is wide open. *Am J Nurs* December 1990; 90:31.

Silva MC: *Ethical Decision Making in Nursing Administration*. Norwalk, CT: Appleton & Lange, 1990.

Stillman RJ, Gindoff PR: Assisted reproductive technology. In: *Danforth's Obstetrics and Gynecology*, 7th ed. Scott JR et al (editors). Philadelphia: Lippincott, 1994.

Thompson JE, Thompson HO: Ethical decision making: Process and models. *Neonatal Network* 1990; 9(1):69.

Toffler A: *The Third Wave*. New York: Morrow, 1980.

CHAPTER 2

TOOLS FOR CRITICAL THINKING IN MATERNAL-NEWBORN NURSING

*S*tatistics have never been so real for me as when I used them to prepare my speech to prospective legislators on "Meet the Candidates" night. I wanted them to acknowledge prevention of preterm birth as an important area that deserved funding. When I told them how many preterm babies were born in our state—and how much it cost taxpayers—the candidates listened and asked how they could help.

KEY TERMS

Birth rate

Critical thinking

Infant mortality rate

Maternal mortality rate

OBJECTIVES

Discuss critical thinking as it applies to the maternal-newborn nurse.

Describe the application of the nursing process in the maternal-newborn setting.

Contrast descriptive and inferential statistics.

Relate the availability of statistical data to the formulation of further research questions.

Discuss the application of nursing research in the maternal-newborn setting.

ost people are able to learn new information and consider factual data, but a more complex mental process is needed to use the facts learned and arrive at new insights and conclusions. This more complex process is critical thinking. **Critical thinking** involves separating fact from opinion, identifying prejudice and stereotypes that may influence information, exploring differing ideas and views, and coming to new conclusions or insights because of the thinking process.

Maternal-newborn nurses use critical thinking skills in all aspects of their nursing practice. Indeed, the hallmark of effective clinical nursing is the application of theory to practice in a logical, individualized way to analyze data and make decisions. In this text we have attempted to provide opportunities for nurses to enhance their critical thinking skills through several specially designed features, including *Critical Thinking Questions*, *Critical Thinking in Practice*, *Nursing Care Plans*, and *Research in Practice* boxes. This chapter begins with a brief discussion of critical thinking. It then focuses on several of the *tools for practice* that the nurse draws upon in providing thoughtful, effective nursing care.

The *nursing process* is a major tool for practice. It provides a logical, systematic approach to clinical decision making that aids the nurse in honing critical thinking skills. Some tools for practice, such as *communication skills*, help the nurse gather information; others, such as a *comprehensive knowledge base*, *standards of care*, *statistical data*, and *nursing research*, provide information for decision making.

CRITICAL THINKING

Today in nursing, as in all aspects of health care, the process of decision making has become more complex. Nurses have a myriad of data at their disposal and must be able to sort out the relevant information. In the current health care environment the nurse uses critical thinking to analyze the client's situation and to devise a plan or approach to care. The nurse analyzes information by mentally asking questions: What is important? Which data cluster together? What pieces of information are missing? Does the picture I see make sense intellectually? Does it "feel right"? What do I expect? What other experience have I had that I can draw on?

But what exactly is critical thinking? The National Council for Excellence in Critical Thinking Instruction (1992) has defined it as "the intellectually disciplined process of actively and skillfully conceptualizing, applying, analyzing, synthesizing, and evaluating information gathered from or generated by observation, experience,

reflection, reasoning, or communication, as a guide to belief and action" (p 2). Critical thinking skills enable the nurse to recognize and evaluate taken-for-granted assumptions that shape practice in order to identify valid information and seek out alternative courses of action when necessary (Brookfield 1993). It is a learned ability.

Experts stress that critical thinking has cognitive, psychomotor, and affective elements, which all must be addressed. Nurses learn the cognitive and psychomotor elements as they have opportunities to apply knowledge from classroom lectures, seminars, and readings to client situations in a variety of settings (Bowers & McCarthy 1993). The affective element, less easily taught but critically important, focuses on moral reasoning, awareness of self and personal beliefs, and the development of values and standards that guide activities and decisions (Woods 1993).

Each beginning professional nursing student gains experience in critical thinking as basic decisions are made regarding client care. To make these basic decisions, the student asks: Are the client's vital signs within normal limits? Should I expect them to be? If the vital signs are not "normal," what factors may be influencing them? As the student gains experience and faces additional challenges from more complex client care situations, the process of critical thinking becomes expanded and yet refined.

Consider the following: A 22-year-old woman named Isabella Johnson is in her third pregnancy and has been hospitalized for preterm labor. Her care involves remaining in bed at all times and lying on either her left or right side. Four times a day a monitor is used to assess whether she is having uterine contractions and to assess characteristics of the fetal heartbeat. Although the woman has smoked for the last 5 years and states that she smokes to relieve her stress, she has been forbidden to smoke in the hospital. She has been hospitalized for 4 weeks and has been told that she will need to remain in the hospital on bed rest for the remaining 7 weeks of her pregnancy. She has a 2-year-old and a 1-year-old at home. Her mother and a friend are sharing the responsibility of caring for her two children, although both women work full time. Isabella misses her children desperately and says that she has not been separated from them until this pregnancy.

In considering the nursing care for Isabella, a simplistic view would dictate that the nurse carry out the physician's orders and ensure that Isabella is compliant with the medical plan of care. However, the experienced nurse recognizes that the complex process of devising a plan of care involves considering the unique factors of Isabella's situation. As the plan of care is devised, the nurse will consider: What does the hospitalization mean for Isabella? Are the child care provisions working? Are other resources available? Are backup systems available for periodic relief or in the case of illness? How does the stress of worrying about her children and their care affect Isabella's course of treatment? What signs of stress are present now? What cultural and/or sociological values and beliefs does Isabella bring to the situation? How can her beliefs and values be incorporated into her plan of care? If smoking has been a part of the pregnancy to date, is there scientific evidence to support cessation now? If Isabella stops smoking now, will additional stress be added? Could other arrangements be made for Isabella to be monitored in the home if child care and help with cleaning and cooking could be arranged? Are there research studies that would support alternative arrangements for her care? Are my personal values and beliefs in any way influencing the nursing care I provide and my attitudes toward Isabella?

Once these questions are considered, the nurse pulls together the common threads of information; that which does not apply is discarded, and the relevant aspects are kept. For example, the nurse may be concerned about the child care arrangements; however, Isabella knows both care givers and is comfortable with the arrangements. Throughout the process the nurse has used critical thinking to explore different ideas and values, to differentiate between opinions and facts, and to consider the factors that are involved in Isabella Johnson's care.

Among the teaching strategies used to help individuals develop critical thinking skills, questioning, analyzing, and problem-solving tasks are used frequently because of their effectiveness. The *Critical Thinking Questions*, which have been incorporated throughout the text, are designed to assist readers in questioning and analyzing the subject being presented. Sometimes these questions require the reader to draw together information to analyze a cognitive problem; at other times they address an affective issue, often focusing on attitudes and beliefs. Because of the nature of the questions, we have not provided any answers.

The *Critical Thinking in Practice* scenarios provide clinical vignettes designed to challenge the reader to address a specific clinical situation by drawing on material presented in the chapter. Because this problem-solving approach is very specific, we have provided possible solutions in the back of the text.

THE NURSING PROCESS

The nursing process is an approach to problem solving that helps nurses collect and analyze data to identify and resolve client problems. Skillful, creative use of the nursing process enhances critical thinking abilities and provides a foundation for nursing practice. The nursing process, which consists of five steps—assessment, analysis/nursing diagnosis, planning, implementation, and evaluation—has its historical roots firmly based in the problem-solving process used by nurses since the time of Florence Nightingale.

Assessment

In the assessment phase of the nursing process the maternal-newborn nurse gathers both subjective and objective data about the health status of the childbearing woman. Subjective information may be obtained from the woman and family members and includes their perception of the health impairment or problem and its management. Objective data are measurable and include physical assessment findings and laboratory test results.

Analysis and Nursing Diagnosis

The second step in the nursing process is the analysis, assimilation, and clustering of assessment data into relevant categories from which nursing diagnoses are derived. Each nursing diagnosis describes a specific health problem, either actual or potential; its etiology; and the associated signs and symptoms. The formulation of a nursing diagnosis is the crucial step in the process, for the resulting plan of care is based on the problems as the nurse perceives them. In contrast to the medical diagnosis, which generally remains the same throughout the woman's health problem, the nursing diagnosis will reflect the changing response of the woman as her condition improves or worsens and as she and her family adjust to those changes (NAACOG 1989).

Consider the following nursing diagnosis: Ineffective breastfeeding related to sore nipples. The general problem, ineffective breastfeeding, is presented with the specific contributing factor, sore nipples. Ineffective breastfeeding is a client problem that is clearly in the realm of nursing care, not in that of medical diagnosis.

Once established, nursing diagnoses serve to direct the nursing plan of care. The nurse identifies expected outcomes (goals) and priorities of care as well as nursing interventions necessary to achieve the specified goals. Nursing interventions are directed at altering or eliminating the etiologic and/or contributing factors of the health problem, and the related signs and symptoms serve as a baseline for evaluation of the effectiveness of care.

Nursing diagnoses are incorporated in this text in various ways. In most chapters the nursing diagnosis appears clearly as a part of the nursing process. The chapters devoted to high-risk situations present examples of nursing diagnoses that may apply to specific problems being discussed. In addition, nursing diagnoses are emphasized in the *Nursing Care Plans* and in the *Critical Pathways*, which focus on selected conditions or situations. These nursing diagnoses are used as the basis for organizing and directing nursing care.

Planning

Once the analysis is completed and nursing diagnoses are formulated, the nurse establishes outcome goals. The nurse identifies interventions that will help the client meet the established goals and develops outcome criteria that will signify that the goals have been met. Lastly the nurse prioritizes the care needed. The beginning nurse usually works through this process step by step; the more experienced nurse frequently is able to develop an intricate plan of care covering all the steps simultaneously.

Implementation

In the fourth step of the nursing process the maternal-newborn nurse implements the identified plan of care and specific nursing interventions. The nurse uses many skills that are common to other areas of nursing, as well as many skills specific to the maternal-newborn setting. Common interventions include auscultating fetal heart rate, providing comfort measures for a laboring woman, changing maternal position to improve a fetal monitor tracing, using nursing techniques to help a postpartal woman void, and teaching a family about infant care.

Evaluation

The woman's progress or lack of progress toward the identified expected outcomes (goals) is evaluated by the woman and the nurse. The evaluation process includes asking questions: Have expected outcomes been met? Is reassessment needed? Are new problems present? Are changes in any part of the process necessary? Do new priorities need to be identified? Is revision of the plan of care required?

Evaluation is a logical end step, but it is also used continuously throughout the nursing process. The nurse continually evaluates the assessments that have been made, the priorities of care, and the effectiveness of the nursing interventions as nursing care is delivered. See Table 2–1 for an example illustrating application of the nursing process.

NURSING CARE PLAN AND CRITICAL PATHWAY

The outcome of the nursing process is the creation of a nursing care plan. In this text a nursing care plan with outcome-driven essential nursing activities has been developed for selected conditions or problems within various chapters. The nursing care plan begins with a section entitled "Client Assessment" that includes nursing history, physical examination, and diagnostic studies. The remainder of the nursing care plan includes sections in which nursing diagnoses, interventions, rationale for the interventions, and evaluation appear.

TABLE 2–1	Application of the Nursing Process

The following brief example illustrates the application of the nursing process.

Sarah, a 16-year-old, comes to the school nurse's office and asks why she seems to be having trouble with her pregnancy. She states she doesn't have any energy and can't keep her weight down. She is in her sixth month of pregnancy and has gained 3 lbs. She exercises every day for 1 hour, smokes one pack of cigarettes a day, and has trouble sleeping because of the pressure of homework and a part-time job each evening.

The nurse applies the nursing process as follows:

Assessment: Subjective data—Sarah states "I have trouble with my pregnancy; I have no energy, have trouble keeping my weight down, and lots of trouble sleeping." Objective data—3 lb weight gain in 6 months of pregnancy (below recommended rate). Sarah appears underweight for her height, pale with dark circles under her eyes.

Analysis/nursing diagnosis: The objective and subjective data support problems with adequate nutrition, and the statements regarding her weight suggest the need for information regarding nutritional needs during pregnancy. Sarah also needs to understand the need to obtain adequate rest and to clarify her perception of the role of exercise in pregnancy. The nurse ascertains that Sarah is going to the prenatal clinic on a fairly regular basis. The nurse decides the highest priority nursing diagnosis at this moment is Knowledge deficit related to lack of information about adequate nutritional intake during pregnancy. The nurse could also have identified a nursing diagnosis directed toward the sleep disturbance or the potential for alterations in nutrition related to inadequate intake for pregnancy needs. But overall she decided that giving Sarah information about her pregnancy would address a number of problems.

Planning: The goals of care include: Client will be able to verbalize the nutritional requirements in pregnancy and will begin gaining at least 3 lb per month.

Implementation: The nurse and Sarah plan sessions for the next few weeks during which there will be time for discussion and information to be shared. She gives Sarah some booklets designed for pregnant adolescents regarding nutritional and general care needs. The nurse obtains a current weight, and together they create a graph to record her weight each week. Sarah's interest in cartooning makes this a fun and creative project. The nurse asks her to keep a food intake record for 3 days and to drop it off at the end of the week.

Evaluation: As the relationship builds and they work together, the success of the interventions will be measured by Sarah's ability to verbalize nutritional needs and the objective data provided by her weight each week. The food intake record provides specific data to work with to encourage a diet to meet pregnancy needs.

In addition, *Critical Pathways* are provided in Chapter 23, The Family in Childbirth: Needs and Care; Chapter 29, The Normal Newborn: Needs and Care; and Chapter 34, The Postpartal Family: Needs and Care. These *Critical Pathways* apply the nursing process to caring for healthy individuals. The *Critical Pathways* are more specific than the care plans, however, because they provide basic guidelines as to expected outcomes at specified time intervals. This enables the reader to determine whether a client's responses meet general norms at any given time.

COMMUNICATION

The quality of information available for the nurse to use in decision making directly influences the success of the process. Thus communication is a major tool in effective

Technique	Example
Listening attentively	The nurse faces the woman, maintains eye contact, and positions herself or himself so that she or he is leaning slightly toward the client. The nurse concentrates attention on the interaction with the client.
Using open-ended questions	The nurse asks questions such as: "How do you feel about exercise during pregnancy?"
Clarifying	The nurse confirms the meaning of a comment. Client: "One person said to do exercises this way, and another person said I was not doing them right." Nurse: "So you feel you are getting conflicting instructions from us?" Client: "Yes, it's hard not knowing what to do."
Paraphrasing	The nurse restates the client's message in the nurse's own words. Client: "I can't exercise in the morning, and the evening seems so full, and. . ." Nurse: "You are having difficulty exercising."
Focusing	The nurse helps the woman focus on a particular aspect of the conversation. Client: "I am having strange feelings in my body, mostly in my abdomen." Nurse: "Describe the feeling."

critical thinking. This communication most often involves verbal and nonverbal interactions between the nurse and other health care providers or the nurse and client/family. The maternal-newborn nurse uses communication skills in all interactions with the childbearing woman and her family. The nurse begins by establishing rapport and a sense of trust with the client. Rapport and trust are enhanced when the client's individuality and beliefs are respected, when privacy is provided, and when the nurse is nonjudgmental.

The nurse uses therapeutic communication techniques (Table 2–2) during assessment, interventions, and all teaching activities. In order to ensure successful communication the nurse may need to use a variety of techniques.

Charting

Charting is an important means of communication within health care facilities. It enables health care providers to share pertinent information in a timely, lasting, and concise way. It also provides a legal record of the client's care. Changing practice has resulted in a variety of charting techniques: narrative charting, flow sheet charting, problem-oriented charting, charting by exception, and computerized charting. Whichever approach is used, nurses must clearly understand the process and ensure that their charting is accurate and well thought out.

Networking

Networking is a term that is used to describe the interaction of individuals. Networking may refer to the mechanism used by members of groups to exchange information or to establish new contacts. Although nurses have a long history of talking with each other, the process of creating a network of associates, acquaintances, and other professionals around a common goal is somewhat new. Currently, nurses are using networks to exchange information and ideas, to implement interventions suggested through research, and to collaborate on personal, professional, and client care issues.

Networking for professional nurses in the maternal-newborn setting include the following (Harter & Grossman 1989):

- Taking part in discussion groups through informal meetings or through a journal club

- Telephoning or writing to colleagues to share information

- Participating in opportunities to meet other nurses at professional meetings and conferences

- Getting involved with others in the community around a common cause

KNOWLEDGE BASE

Without sufficient, appropriate, and specific information effective decision making cannot take place. Critical thinking requires knowledge. Maternal-newborn nurses build their practice on a comprehensive knowledge base that includes information regarding pregnancy, labor and birth, the postpartal period, and the newborn period. Information includes normal anatomic, physiologic, and psychologic processes; factors that place the woman at risk; and complications that may occur in the childbearing period.

Nursing theories related to adaptation, stress, locus of control, human caring, and care of individuals may also be a part of the maternal-newborn nurse's knowledge base. In addition to the content/nursing theory knowledge base, the maternity nurse synthesizes knowledge from other disciplines. For example, knowledge of family development is obtained from sociology and psychology; anthropology provides insights into other cultural patterns, which increase understanding of the various women and their families who come into the childbearing health care setting.

Acquisition of knowledge is a lifelong process for today's professional nurse. New technology is being developed and implemented at a rapid rate; change and progress are inevitable. Maternal-newborn nurses, and nurses in other fields, find it a challenge to keep their knowledge base current with this information explosion; therefore specialization has become prevalent. Specialization provides a narrower focus and helps direct the learning process.

STANDARDS OF CARE

In the midst of a rapidly changing health care system and widely divergent approaches to basic nursing education, nursing standards provide direction and information for the practicing nurse. Standards of care identify the basic expectations and functions of a particular nursing role and therefore provide a framework for accountability in nursing practice. The standards of care also provide guidelines for ethical practice, as discussed in Chapter 1. In addition they provide a basis for identifying quality in specific health care settings.

The Association of Women's Health, Obstetric, and Neonatal Nurses (AWHONN) has assumed a leadership role in developing standards for nurses who care for childbearing families. These standards have played an integral part in providing direction for the development of high-quality maternity services in the United States. Because the health care setting may vary from one region to another, the standards are used as a basis for developing individualized policies and protocols.

Standards of Nursing Care: The AWHONN (Formerly NAACOG) Nursing Standard

Standard

Comprehensive obstetric, gynecologic, and neonatal (OGN) nursing care shall be provided to the client and her family and shall utilize all components of the nursing process, including assessment, nursing diagnosis, planning, implementation, and evaluation. It shall reflect informed consent and respect for the rights of the client and her family.

Interpretation

The nurse has the responsibility for collecting pertinent data and assessing the client's needs in order to determine the nursing intervention necessary to assist the client and her family. The care plan should take into consideration psychosocial as well as physical aspects of the client's history and should include active involvement of the client and her family.

The OGN nurse should support the client and family members' desire to participate in the nursing process as appropriate. In addition the client and her family should be supported throughout the nursing process by assessing the potential for individual or family crisis and evaluating their resources for coping, by use of supportive services, and by family interaction.

The OGN nurse should be familiar with the type of client records required and should share the responsibility for accurate and complete record keeping, maintaining appropriate confidentiality, to provide for continuity and coordination of nursing care, medical treatment, and client progress. The documentation of nursing care given should reflect the achievement or nonachievement of predetermined goals. Records should be retained for the appropriate interval of time as governed by law and local regulations (NAACOG 1991).

Application

Ms Gayle works in the mother-baby unit in a local hospital and has been participating on a committee to revise the chart forms. In reviewing the standards, the committee found the forms reflected the standards in using and documenting the nursing process and client care goals. The only areas not clearly reflected involved documentation of informed consent and client/family wishes for the birth experience. A place was added to the care plan, and each nurse was instructed to ask and record specific client/family wishes.

In addition to standards of care the AWHONN Committee on Practice develops OGN nursing practice resources as an aid to maternal-newborn nursing practice. The nursing practice resources do not define a standard of care; rather, they present techniques of practice that are currently accepted and recommended by leading authorities. For example, in December 1993 an AWHONN practice resource entitled *Cervical Ripening and Induction and Augmentation of Labor* became available. The resource guide provides information on indications and contraindications to inducing labor, as well as methods for cervical ripening and labor induction with an emphasis on nursing responsibilities. (See Chapter 26 for information regarding the incorporation of these guidelines into nursing care.)

STATISTICS

Evaluation of the health care system relies on *statistics*, the collection and analysis of pertinent numerical data. Health-related statistics provide an objective basis for projecting client needs, allocating resources, and analyzing new data for evaluation of treatment effectiveness.

There are two major types of statistics—descriptive and inferential. Descriptive statistics describe or summarize a set of data: They report facts—what *is*—in a concise and easily retrievable way. An example of a descriptive statistic is the birth rate in the United States. How the data are compiled and presented is determined by the question being asked. Although no conclusion about *why* some phenomenon has occurred may be drawn from these "vital" statistics, certain trends can be identified, high-risk "target groups" delineated, and research questions generated that will provoke further investigation using more sophisticated statistical testing.

Inferential statistics allow the investigator to draw conclusions or inferences about what is happening between two or more variables in a population and to establish or refute causal relationships between them. For example, descriptive statistics show that the infant mortality rate in the United States has declined over the past decade. Exactly *why* that trend has occurred cannot be answered by simply looking at these data, however. More data and inferential statistics, using smaller samples of the population of pregnant women, are needed to determine whether this finding is due to earlier prenatal care, improved maternal nutrition, use of electronic fetal monitoring during labor, and/or any number of factors potentially associated with maternal-fetal survival.

Descriptive statistics are the starting point that allows the formulation of research questions. Inferential statistics answer specific questions and generate theories to explain relationships between variables. Theory applied in nursing practice can help make changes in the specific variables that may be causing or contributing to certain health problems. The following section deals primarily with descriptive statistics, although inferential considerations are addressed through the use of possible research questions that may assist in identifying relevant variables.

Descriptive Statistics

Birth Rate

Birth rate refers to the number of live births per 1000 population. In the United States, after a peak in rate for all races of 25.0 in 1955, there has been a decline until the rate remained constant in 1975 and 1976—14.6 live births per 1000 population. This is the lowest recorded birth rate in the history of the United States. Beginning in 1975–1976 there was a small yearly increase through 1982 and then another decrease was recorded in 1983–1984. From 1985 to 1990 there was a steady yearly increase to 17.5 in June 1990. Since June 1990, the overall birth rate has decreased each year with 15.7 live births per 1000 total population in 1993 (National Center for Health Statistics 1994a). In 1992 there were 4,065,014 babies born in the United States, a decrease of 1% from 1991 and the second consecutive year of a decline in live births.

TABLE 2–3	Live Births and Birth Rates, Canada, 1980–1992	
Year	**Live Births***	**Birth Rate[†]**
1992[1] (preliminary)	398,642	14.0
1990	450,486	15.3
1980	370,709	15.5

*Live births = per 1000 population

[†]Live birth rate = per 1000 population

SOURCES: Modified from *Vital Statistics*. Vol. I. Births and deaths, 1985. Canada Health Division Vital Statistics and Disease Registry. Cat. 84-204. Minister of Supply and Services. November 1986. Table 1, p 2.
[1]Preliminary data. Personal contact. Statistics Canada, Publications Sales and Service. Ottawa, Ontario. March 20, 1995.

The number of live births and birth rate for Canada are presented in Table 2–3. The birth rate in Canada remains lower than in the United States.

Inferential considerations regarding birth rate may be identified by posing some of the following research questions:

- Is there an association with changing societal values?

- Is the difference in birth rate between various age groups reflective of education? Does it represent availability of contraceptive information?

- Women are averaging 1.8 children apiece, and the replacement rate is 2.1 per couple. What are the future implications of the declining rate?

Age of the Mother

In the United States in 1992 the highest birth rate was in women 25 to 29 years of age (117.4 per 1000 women in the specified age group), followed by a birth rate of 114.6 for women 20 to 24 years of age, 94.5 in 18- to 19-year-olds, and 80.2 in 30- to 34-year-olds (Table 2–4). An optimistic finding is that the birth rate among 15- to 17-year-olds declined 2% from 1991 (Figure 2–1). This is especially significant because the birth rate for this group of adolescents had increased 27% from 1986 to 1991. In considering births to 18- to 19-year-old adolescents, an interesting phenomenon is evident. The birth rate in this age group rose slightly in 1992, but the actual number of live births decreased by 4%. This is due to the 4% decrease in the number of women in this age group resulting from the fact that in 1973–74, when these young women were born, total births fell to historic low levels.

Birth rates for women age 35 to 39 (32.5 per 1000) increased 2% in 1992 and 3% overall from 1990 to 1992. This follows a 60% increase over the years from 1980 to

TABLE 2–4 Birth Rates by Age of Mother, Live Birth Order, and Race of Mother: United States, 1992
(Rates are live births per 1000 women in specified age and racial group. Live birth order refers to number of children born alive to mother)

| Live Birth Order and Race of Mother | 15–44 Years* | 10–14 Years | 15–19 Years | | | 20–24 Years | 25–29 Years | 30–34 Years | 35–39 Years | 40–44 Years | 45–49 Years |
			Total	15–17 Years	18–19 Years						
All races	68.9	1.4	60.7	37.8	94.5	114.6	117.4	80.2	32.5	5.9	0.3
First child	27.8	1.3	45.3	32.0	64.7	53.4	42.8	21.2	6.9	1.1	0.0
Second child	22.3	0.0	12.3	5.1	22.9	38.3	41.3	28.7	10.1	1.5	0.0
White	66.5	0.8	51.8	30.1	83.8	108.2	118.4	81.4	32.2	5.7	0.2
First child	27.3	0.7	40.5	26.5	61.1	53.4	44.7	22.0	7.1	1.1	0.0
Second child	22.0	0.0	9.5	3.3	18.6	36.7	42.7	29.7	10.2	1.5	0.0
Black	83.2	4.7	112.4	81.3	157.9	158.0	111.2	67.5	28.8	5.6	0.2
First child	30.6	4.5	74.3	63.8	89.6	56.5	28.7	13.2	4.4	0.8	0.0
Second child	24.3	0.2	27.7	14.8	46.6	51.0	35.0	20.1	7.4	1.1	0.0
American Indian†	75.4	1.6	84.4	53.8	132.6	145.5	109.4	63.0	28.0	6.1	*
First child	24.6	1.5	60.7	45.3	85.0	49.1	20.1	8.2	2.4	0.4	*
Second child	20.0	*	18.5	7.5	35.9	48.8	30.3	13.1	4.6	0.6	*
Asian or Pacific Islander	67.2	0.7	26.6	15.2	43.1	74.6	121.0	103.0	50.6	11.0	0.9
First child	29.4	0.7	19.8	12.6	30.2	41.5	60.4	36.0	12.4	2.3	0.1
Second child	21.8	*	4.9	2.1	9.1	20.5	37.6	39.7	18.2	2.9	0.1

* Rates computed by relating total births, regardless of age of mother, to women aged 15–44 years.
†Includes births to Aleuts and Eskimos.

SOURCE: National Center for Health Statistics: Advance report of final natality statistics, 1992. *Monthly Vital Statistics Report* vol 43, no 5, Suppl. Hyattsville, MD: National Center for Health Statistics, Public Health Service, 1994.

1990, the sharpest increase of any age group of women (National Center for Health Statistics 1994a).

Inferential considerations regarding birth rate may be identified by posing research questions such as the two that follow:

- Is there an association with changing societal values? With changing roles of women? With changing national economic conditions and financial status?

- Is there a correlation with years of education? With availability of contraceptive information for different age groups and races?

Weight at Birth

In 1992 the median weight at birth for all infants was 3360 g (approximately 7 lb, 7 oz). This is unchanged from 1991 and is the lowest reported median weight since 1981. The median birth weight was 3410 g (7 lb, 8 oz) for White babies and 3170 (7 lb) for Black babies.

The newborn posing the most concern to health professionals is the low-birth-weight (less than 2500 g) infant. From 1976 through 1988 low-birth-weight infants comprised about 6.9% of all births. Since 1988, there has been an increase, and in 1991 the incidence was 7.1%. As in previous years, a substantial racial difference in low-birth-weight infants persists, with 5.8% for White births,

13.3% for Black births, and 7.1% for all other races. The highest incidence of low birth weight tends to occur in the youngest and oldest mothers (National Center for Health Statistics 1994a).

Inferential considerations regarding weight at birth may be explored by posing various questions such as the following:

- Are there factors that affect different age and racial groups?

- Are there correlations with nutritional status before and during pregnancy?

- Educational level?

- Length of time between pregnancies?

- Availability of prenatal care?

- Desire and ability to seek prenatal care?

- Physical health of the mother?

- Presence of environmental factors such as high population levels or high altitude?

Infant Mortality

The **infant mortality rate** is the number of deaths of infants under 1 year of age per 1000 live births in a given population. *Neonatal mortality* is the number of deaths of infants less than 28 days of age per 1000 live births.

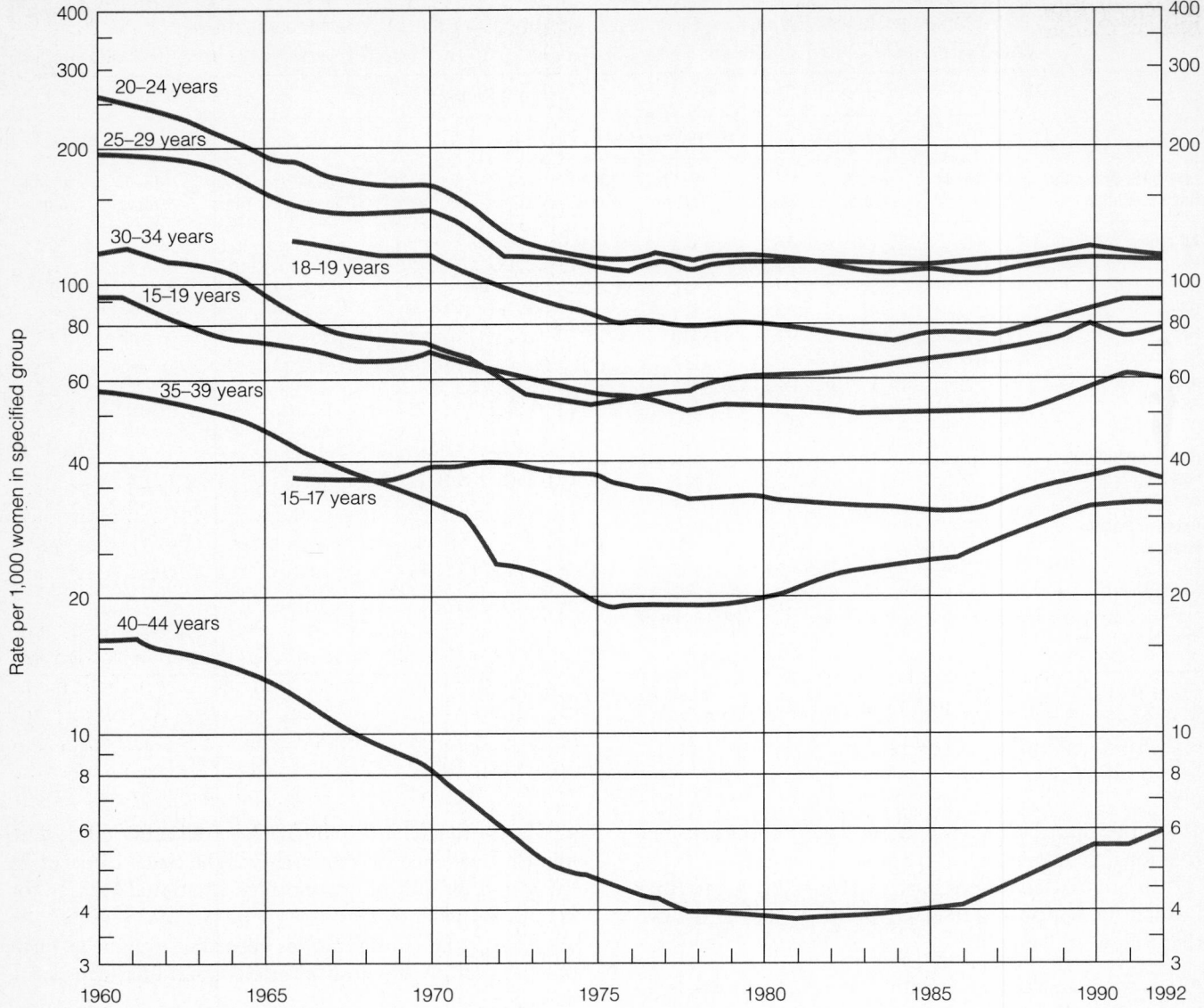

FIGURE 2-1   Birth rates by age of mother: United States, 1960–1992. SOURCE: National Center for Health Statistics: Advance report of final natality statistics, 1992. Monthly Vital Statistics Report vol 43, no 5, suppl, p 3. Hyattsville, MD: National Center for Health Statistics, Public Health Service, 1994.

Perinatal mortality encompasses both neonatal deaths and fetal deaths per 1000 live births. (Fetal death is death in utero at 20 weeks or more gestation.) For statistical purposes the period from 28 days to 11 months of age is designated the *postneonatal period.* Table 2–5 delineates infant mortality by age.

The infant mortality rate in 1993 was 8.3, which is the lowest rate ever recorded for the United States (National Center for Health Statistics 1994b). The infant mortality rate in Blacks has been approximately twice the rate in Whites since the early 1900s. In 1991 the mortality rate for White infants was 7.3, 17.6 for Blacks, and 7.6 for Hispanics (National Center for Health Statistics 1993).

Over half of infant deaths are caused by congenital anomalies, sudden infant death syndrome, respiratory distress syndrome, and disorders relating to short gestation and unspecified low birth weight (National Center for Health Statistics 1994b). Infant mortality for Canada is presented in Table 2–6. Comparison of Canadian and US infant mortality reveals a lower rate for Canada.

The US infant mortality rate has continued to be an area of concern, yet the United States has fallen to 22nd place among industrialized nations in infant mortality rankings. Health care professionals, policymakers, and the public have continued to stress the need in the United States for better prenatal care, coordination of health services, and the provision of comprehensive maternal-child

TABLE 2–5	Infant Mortality Rates by Age: United States. 1950–1994		
Year	Under 1 Year	Under 28 Days	28 days– 11 months
1994[1]	8.0 (provisional)		
1992[2]	8.5	5.4	3.1
1990[2]	9.2	5.8	3.4
1980[2]	12.6	8.5	4.1
1970[2]	20.0	15.1	4.9
1960[2]	26.0	18.7	7.3
1950[2]	29.2	20.5	8.7

SOURCES: [1]National Center for Health Statistics: Births, marriages, divorces, and deaths for August 1994. *Monthly Vital Statistics Report* vol 43, no 8. Hyattsville, MD: National Center for Health Statistics, Public Health Service, 1995.
[2]Kochanek KD, Hudson BL. Advance report of final mortality statistics, 1992. *Monthly Vital Statistics Report* Vol 43, No 6, Suppl. Hyattsville, MD: National Center for Health Statistics, Public Health Service. 1994.

TABLE 2–7	Maternal Mortality Rate per 100,000 Live Births: United States, 1950–1992
Year	Rate
1992[1]	7.8
1980[2]	9.2
1970[2]	21.5
1960[2]	37.1
1950[2]	83.3

SOURCES: [1]National Center for Health Statistics: Births, marriages, divorces, and deaths for August 1994. *Monthly Vital Statistics Report.* vol 42, no 8. Hyattsville, MD: National Center for Health Statistics, Public Health Service, 1995.
[2]National Center for Health Statistics: Advance report of final mortality statistics, 1984. *Monthly Vital Statistics Report.* vol 35, no 6, Suppl (2). DHHS Pub No (PHS) 86–1120. Public Health Service, Hyattsville, MD: September 26, 1986.

services. However, as many as one-fourth of pregnant women in some US communities do not receive prenatal care (Moore & Paul 1992), and our global ranking continues to fall.

Factors affecting the infant mortality rate may be identified by considering questions such as the following:

- Does infant mortality correlate with a specific maternal age?

- Is it associated with the time in pregnancy that the woman seeks prenatal care? With the number of prenatal visits?

- Is there a difference between racial groups? If so, is it associated with an educational level? With the availability of prenatal care?

Maternal Mortality

The **maternal mortality rate** for 1991 was 7.9 per 100,000 live births (323 women). The mortality rate for Black women at 18.3 was 3.2 times the rate of 5.8 for White women (National Center for Health Statistics

TABLE 2–6	Infant Mortality (Total Infant Death Rate per 1000 Live Births): Canada, 1980, 1985, and 1992
Year	Under 1 Year
1992[1]	6.4
1985	8.0
1980	10.4

SOURCES: Modified from *Vital Statistics, Vol. I. Births and deaths. 1985.* Canada Health Division Vital Statistics and Disease Registry. Cat. 84–204. Minister of Supply and Services. November 1986. Table 22, p 54.
[1]Preliminary data. Personal contact. Statistics Canada Publications, Sales and Services. Ottawa, Ontario. March 20, 1995.

1993). In the past the leading causes of death were hemorrhage, sepsis, and hypertensive disorders of pregnancy. Currently the leading causes are embolism, hypertensive disorders of pregnancy, hemorrhage, ectopic pregnancy, and infection (Scott et al 1994).

Factors influencing the decrease in maternal mortality include development of obstetrics as a recognized medical specialty, increased numbers of certified nurse-midwives, the establishment of high-risk centers for mother and newborn care, the prevention and control of infection with antibiotics and improved techniques, the availability of blood and blood products for transfusions, lowered rates of anesthesia-related deaths, and the application of research for the prevention of maternal deaths (Table 2–7).

Additional data affecting maternal mortality may be identified by asking the following:

- Is there a correlation with age? With availability of health care? With economic status? With access to health care?

- Is there adequate federal funding to reach women in need?

The maternal mortality rate in Canada was 3 in 1991 (Statistics Canada. Personal contact 3/20/1995).

Implications of Statistics for Nursing

The successful implementation of the nursing process depends on the appropriate application of statistics. Nurses can use statistics in a number of ways. For example, statistical data may be used to:

- Determine populations at risk

- Assess the relationship between specific factors

- Help establish a database for different client populations

- Determine the levels of care needed by particular client populations

- Evaluate the success of specific nursing interventions
- Determine priorities in caseloads
- Estimate staffing and equipment needs of hospital units and clinics

Statistical information is available through many sources, including professional literature; state and city health departments; vital statistics sections of private, county, state, and federal agencies; special programs or agencies (family-planning agencies); and demographic profiles of specific geographic areas. Nurses who make use of this information will find themselves well prepared to protect the health needs of maternity clients and their families.

NURSING RESEARCH

Research is a vital step in expanding the science of nursing. It is also a means of improving client care and continuing to advance the profession of nursing.

Once research is accomplished, it must be translated into the clinical practice setting, that is, made useful to nurses taking care of clients. Success in this effort ultimately depends on the willingness and ability of nurses to transfer research-generated knowledge into practical nursing interventions. This practical application can be accomplished by reading completed research studies of relevance to the specific health problem or client need and trying out the methods that worked for the investigator. Of course this example is an oversimplification, but we would like to emphasize that the process of applying research findings to improve client care can and should be made a relatively simple exercise in problem solving; otherwise the gap between research and action will remain wide. (See Research in Practice.)

Application of Research

The following two brief examples specific to maternal-newborn nursing help illustrate how the findings of a research study might be applied to improve client care and how clinical nurses and nursing faculty may collaborate on research studies.

Example 1: Clinical Implications

Assessment of fetal movement has been recognized as a method to provide some reassurance of fetal well-being and also to alert the expectant mother to possible fetal compromise. Some maternal-newborn health providers believe that assessment of fetal movement is appropriate for high-risk pregnancies but that it should not be recommended in low-risk pregnancies because it will increase maternal anxiety.

Gibby (1988) investigated whether the use of a fetal assessment method increased maternal anxiety. The study subjects were low-risk pregnant women who completed the State-Trait Anxiety Inventory at specified times during the pregnancy. The experimental group also completed daily fetal movement assessment. Gibby found that there was no significant difference between the two groups and that those in the group that completed daily fetal movement assessment did not indicate increased anxiety.

Although the study sample was small, the findings imply that fetal movement records may be used to provide information about the fetus without increasing maternal anxiety. The study results may be used to support the teaching of daily fetal movement assessment to low-risk women in many settings.

The clinical and/or research nurse may also identify future study questions such as: Does the time in pregnancy affect the findings? Is there a difference between various fetal movement assessment methods? What methods of teaching provide the most effective use of assessment tools? What other maternal factors might enhance the daily use of a fetal assessment method?

Example 2: Collaborative Research

Lyons et al (1990) report the results of a collaborative descriptive/correlational study designed to identify nursing diagnoses selected by postpartum mothers and their nurses. The investigators consisted of two hospital-based clinical nurse specialists, two nurse managers, and a university-based nursing professor. Working together, they submitted a proposal to Sigma Theta Tau, the national honor society for nursing, and each nurse pursued institutional approval. The study spanned approximately 1 year and provided a variety of benefits. The nursing staff identified an increased appreciation of nursing research, improved morale, and improvement of nursing care. Benefits for the institution included more effective uses of resources, visibility in research conferences and at conferences where data were reported, and enhanced recruitment opportunities. The researchers identified personal satisfaction and achievement and opportunities to work together as some of the benefits of the collaborative process.

The Lyons et al study may be used as an impetus to nurses in searching out other professionals who are interested in research. The collaborative process allows many investigators to share ideas, resources, talents, and the task of completing the study.

The examples just given are meant to illustrate how a practitioner might begin to think about using nursing research to improve maternal care. Of course, much time passes and much work will be required before an idea becomes an implemented practice. Change must be regarded in terms of costs and benefits before old ways are discarded for new ones.

Critical Thinking: An Example

Each of the tools of critical thinking—knowledge base, communication, nursing process, nursing standards, statistics, and nursing research—can exist separately, but in practice they overlap and build upon each other. An example of just one possible situation is presented in the following case study.

Two birthing unit nurses express concerns to each other about the seemingly high numbers of adolescents who have been giving birth in their unit.

At the next staff meeting they voice their concerns and raise questions about whether the number of teenage mothers seen in their unit is higher than normal. After discussion the nurses decide that they need to formulate a plan to gather more information. Each nurse volunteers to pursue a particular aspect of a plan of action. Their plan includes contacting the local public health department for local and national statistics on this age group; looking at the availability of health care for adolescents in their community; investigating the particular health problems of the pregnant teenager and risks to their infants; checking the availability of prenatal education groups for adolescents; finding out whether their community has school health programs and what the program content is; looking at national statistics regarding when adolescents seek prenatal care; talking with community nurse-midwives, physicians, and prenatal clinic personnel to see if the national statistics apply to their community; collecting information about current legislative issues affecting adolescent health care; seeking further information about the needs of adolescents during pregnancy and delivery by doing a library search; and looking for continuing education programs dealing with the pregnant adolescent client.

At subsequent staff meetings each nurse shares information, and other areas are investigated as the need is identified. How they evaluate the data and apply them will depend on the requirements of their maternity unit and the unique needs of their community.

Possible outcomes may include developing a research study, volunteering in local adolescent clinics, developing and teaching prenatal classes for adolescents, volunteering to teach in community school health programs, organizing a continuing education program on the adolescent mother for community hospitals, and forming a network within their professional nursing organization to stay informed about legislative issues pertaining to adolescents.

As the example illustrates, the application of the tools of critical thinking assists the nurse in analyzing data and planning a course of action.

KEY CONCEPTS

Today's nurse uses a variety of nursing skills in applying the critical thinking process in the setting of maternal-newborn nursing.

A comprehensive nursing knowledge base forms the foundation for nursing activities.

The nursing process, composed of assessment, analysis and nursing diagnosis, plan of care, implementation, and evaluation, provides a systematic method of approaching nursing practice.

Communication skills are important in obtaining client data and in providing nursing care.

Nursing standards provide information and guidelines for nurses in their own practice, in developing policies and protocols in health care settings, and in directing the development of quality nursing care.

Descriptive statistics describe or summarize a set of data. Inferential statistics allow the investigator to draw conclusions about what is happening between two or more variables in a population.

Nursing research is vital to add to the nursing knowledge base, expand clinical practice, and expand nursing theory.

REFERENCES

AWHONN: *Practice Resource: Cervical Ripening and Induction and Augmentation of Labor.* Washington, DC: AWHONN, 1993.

Bowers B and McCarthy D: Developing analytic thinking skills in early undergraduate education. *J Nurs Educ* March 1993; 32(3):107.

Brookfield S: On impostership, cultural suicide, and other dangers: How nurses learn critical thinking. *J Continuing Educ Nurs* September/October 1993; 24(5):197.

Gibby NW: Relationship between fetal movement charting and anxiety in low-risk pregnant women. *J Nurse-Midwifery* July/August 1988; 33(4):185.

Harter C, Grossman LK: Networking to implement effective health care. *MCN* November/December 1989; 14(6):387.

Lyons NB et al: Too busy for research? Collaboration: An answer. *MCN* March/April 1990; 15(2):67.

Moore ML, Paul NW: Improving access to prenatal care: Innovative responses to a national dilemma. White Plains, NY: March of Dimes Birth Defects Foundation. Birth Defects: Original article Series, vol 28, no 4, 1992.

NAACOG: *OGN Nursing Practice Resource: Nursing Diagnoses.* Washington, DC: NAACOG, 1989.

NAACOG: *Standards for the Nursing Care of Women and Newborns,* 4th ed. Washington, DC: NAACOG, 1991.

National Center for Health Statistics: Advance report of final mortality statistics, 1991. *Monthly Vital Stat Rep* 1993; 42(2S):1.

National Center for Health Statistics: Advance report of final natality statistics, 1992. *Monthly Vital Stat Rep* October 25, 1994a; 43(5S):1.

National Center for Health Statistics: Annual summary of births, marriages, divorces, and deaths: United States, 1993. *Monthly Vital Stat Rep* October 11, 1994b; 42(13):1.

National Council for Excellence in Critical Thinking. *Critical Thinking: Shaping the Mind of the 21st Century.* Rohnert Park, CA: Sonoma State University, Center for Critical Thinking and Moral Critique, 1992.

Scott JR et al (editors): *Danforth's Obstetrics and Gynecology,* 7th ed. Philadelphia: Lippincott, 1994.

Woods JH: Affective learning: One door to critical thinking. *Holistic Nurs Pract* 1993; 7(3):64.

CHAPTER 3

THE FAMILY IN CONTEMPORARY SOCIETY

*H*e didn't know what kind of father he'd make. He was so afraid our closeness and incredible happiness together would be cut into by a child—but of course he wanted us to have a baby more than anything in the world, he just would have to get used to the idea.

~ LAUREN BACALL, *BY MYSELF* ~

KEY TERMS

Blended or reconstituted family

Developmental framework

Family structure

Family systems framework

Interactional framework

Nuclear family

Structural-functional framework

OBJECTIVES

Summarize the status of the family in today's society.

Identify major variations in family structure and function.

List the social, psychologic, political, economic, and cultural factors that influence family structure and function.

Compare different approaches of conceptualizing family life as it relates to the childbearing family.

Develop an overview of instruments for assessing family functioning.

Explore the implications for nursing practice of treating the family as a unit of care.

Discuss the role of the nurse in assessing family dynamics and recommending possible interventions for the childbearing family.

*F*amily health, long the domain of public health professionals, is now becoming a primary concern of all health care providers. Consumer pressures, professional initiatives, and research on the family-illness relationship have increased the emphasis on family-centered health care. As people become more knowledgeable about their own health, they want to know more about the purpose and consequences of health care services for themselves and their families. Changing consumer needs and escalating health care costs have created consumer demand for alternative services and health care personnel. Growing awareness of the interdependence of stress and illness, as well as of physical fitness and health, has heightened interest in both individual and family self-care.

Family-centered care is also widely endorsed by health care professionals, who recognize the family as the primary source of physical and emotional support for individual members and as the primary influence on its children's development. Research on childbearing families has shown that family involvement during pregnancy and birth can enhance the birth experience, attachment between parents and infants, and parenting skills (Conner & Denson 1990; Fawcett 1989; Rempusheski 1990).

The recognition that effective health care of individuals requires the involvement of their support network has necessitated an expanded role for the nurse. The nurse now includes the family and/or significant others in health teaching, explanations of medical and surgical interventions, and coordination of health care activities. In addition, as the focus shifts from the parental unit to the entire family, nurses are incorporating siblings, grandparents, and other family members and significant others into the plan of care. The nurse can assist the entire family's adjustment to the arrival of a new infant by helping them to improve their communication patterns. For example, the family members can be encouraged to discuss their feelings and perceptions and identify potential role changes that may occur. When a family experiences a loss, such as the birth of a stillborn, disabled, or preterm infant, the maternal-newborn nurse can work with the entire family to assist them in coping with the event (Ross & Cobb 1990).

The ability to work effectively with a variety of families requires both understanding of how families function and willingness to consider the difficult issues inherent in achieving family-centered care. This chapter provides an introduction to varying family forms and functions, acquaints the reader with major conceptualizations of family life, and describes the instruments used to assess family functioning. It also focuses on understanding families and the major issues the nurse is likely to encounter in working with them.

THE CONTEMPORARY FAMILY

What is "the typical family"? In the 1950s and early 1960s (in the United States) that phrase evoked an image of a happily married, white, middle-class couple with two or three children, with the man as breadwinner and the woman as housewife. Divorce was infrequent because it was socially unacceptable. An aura of stability, contentment, and complacency surrounded the family.

Families responded to the political and social movements of the 1960s and 1970s in different ways. Some families remained virtually untouched by all that was going on around them; others responded by rethinking the values and assumptions underlying their views of family life. They questioned long-standing beliefs about what it meant to be a parent, a spouse, or a child and explored new forms of family grouping and ways of being a family.

Sweeping changes in the social, political, and economic profile of society have contributed to the changing structure of American families (Arnold & Brecht 1990). The family landscape has been altered by several factors, most notably the feminist movement, economic insecurity, increasing numbers of women in the work force, two-earner households, the rising rates of divorce resulting in single-parent households, and remarriages (Walsh 1993). Since the 1960s, the basic family unit of popular lore has all but vanished (Arnold & Brecht 1990). For many couples marriage and childbearing have been postponed until their late 20s or 30s. Other couples have chosen to cohabitate without marrying. Other individuals have chosen to have children through adoption or artificial insemination.

Contemporary family life is complex, with little room for complacency. What is typical about the typical family is that its members are faced with the difficult but gratifying task of coexisting with one another and their environment. In order to do this each family must maintain itself as a functioning unit in the face of an ever-changing situation. Hill (1974, p 374) captured the essence of the demands most families confront when he noted:

> The family is perhaps more subject to disturbance than any other organization because of its rapidly changing age composition and frequently changing plurality patterns. Its curious age and sex composition make it an inefficient work group, a poor planning committee, an unwieldy play group, and a group of uncertain congeniality. Its leadership is shared by two relatively inexperienced amateurs for most of their incumbency, new to the role of spouse and parent. They must work with a succession of disciples having few skills and lacking in judgment under conditions which never seem to remain stable long enough to bring about a settled organization.

A logical place to begin an exploration of this complex, changing entity called the family is with a definition. Not surprisingly, there is no single, generally accepted definition of family. Some authors focus on family structure or the configuration of actors and roles comprising the family. Others emphasize the activities or functions in which family members are engaged. The increase in nontraditional family forms has fostered a trend toward defining families in terms of the members' emotional ties to one another.

Stanhope and Lancaster (1988, p 353) define the family as "two or more individuals coming from the same or different kinship groups, who are involved in a continuous living arrangement, usually residing in the same household, experiencing common emotional bonds, and sharing certain obligations toward others."

Friedman (1992) defined the family as two or more persons joined by bonds of sharing and emotional closeness who identify themselves as being part of a family. This definition encompasses a variety of relationships formerly excluded by traditional definitions, including extended families living in two or more households, cohabitating couples, childless families, gay and lesbian families, bicoastal couples, and single-parent families. In many cases single parenting is the choice (Pakizegi 1990).

Regardless of the definition one chooses, a family has certain common characteristics. The members are joined emotionally and/or legally. Cultural values and beliefs are a part of every family, and these values and beliefs are transmitted by family members from generation to generation. The family unit is an interdependent group of individuals with definite role relationship and communication patterns that form a small social system. In addition the family serves as a buffer between the individual members and the larger society (Friedman 1992; Glick 1994). The concepts of family structure and function are discussed in more detail in the following section.

Family Structure

The term **family structure** refers to the organization of the family unit, the manner in which members are arranged, and how these members relate to each other (Friedman 1992). According to Friedman (1992) and Ross and Cobb (1990), most families belong to one of the following types of family configurations (Figure 3–1).

Nuclear Family

The traditional family structure in our society is the **nuclear family.** This configuration includes husband, wife, and all minor children living together in a single household, separate from the family of origin. Although the nuclear family remains the most prevalent family configuration in the United States today (US Bureau of the Census 1993), alternative family forms are increasing, and many families do not fit this pattern. Dissolution of a marriage results in dissolution of the nuclear family (Anderson et al 1994). Nuclear families today are often separated from their extended families because of career moves that have taken them thousands of miles from a close family and their roots.

Dual-Earner Family

Dual employment is often present in this family configuration. In the 90s the dual-earner family replaced the breadwinner/homemaker model as the statistical norm and is a trend likely to continue. In two-thirds of all two-parent households both parents hold a job (Walsh 1993). Many employed mothers now return to work before their infant is 1 year old due to limited maternity leave, a desire to be employed, or financial pressures (Tulman & Fawcett 1990). When both parents are employed, they often expect and seek assistance from each other to cope with the multiple roles they face (Tulman & Fawcett 1990). This type of family life-style is often associated with considerable stress due to the competing demands of the occupational structure and those associated with the family–child care, homemaking, and marital responsibilities. More stress is reported by the wife than the husband. Hall (1992) reported that employed mothers frequently indicated they had little time for themselves or their spousal relationships and felt exhausted. Employed fathers reported feeling less overwhelmed and maintained different views about the importance of household tasks.

Nuclear Dyad (Childless Family)

One variation of the nuclear family is the nuclear dyad. Frequently referred to as the *beginning family*, the nuclear dyad consists of a husband and wife, an unmarried heterosexual couple, or a homosexual couple living in a single-family residence. One or both partners are employed outside the home, and there are either no children or, in the case of an older couple, no children at home.

Single-Parent Family

One-parent families are becoming far more prevalent. Single-parent households, especially those headed by females, are on the rise (US Bureau of the Census 1993). This configuration of family life includes separated, divorced, or widowed parents; never married parents; single-parent adoptions; and single foster parents (Ross & Cobb 1990). Divorce is commonplace in today's society. Divorce rates, after climbing rapidly, have leveled off at around 50% (Glick 1994). In single-parent households one adult is left alone to raise minor children in a separate household with no other adults. Over one-third of all children can be expected to live in a single-parent household at some point in their development. Many single parents eventually marry for the first time or remarry, creating a need for additional role changes for both the former and the reconstituted family units.

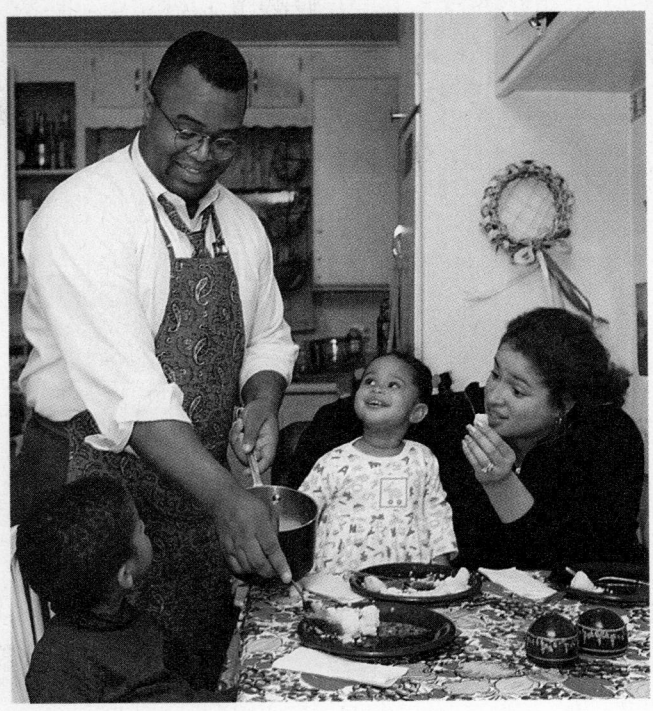

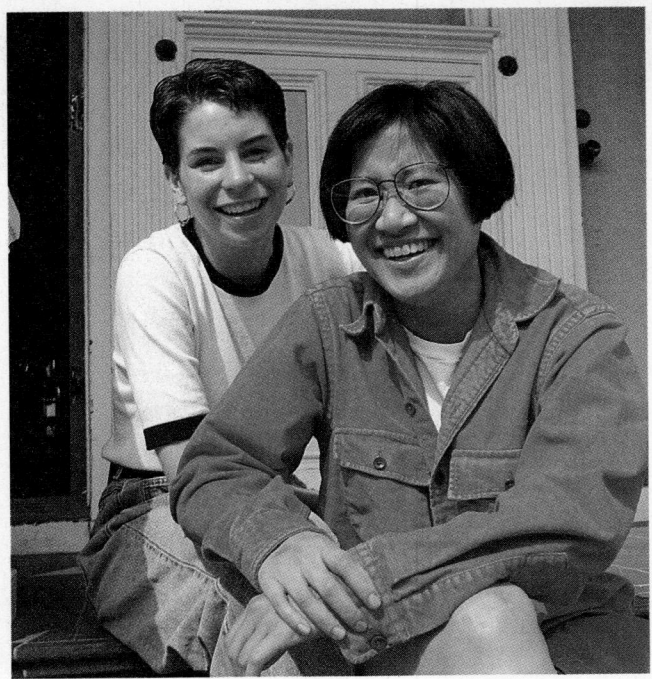

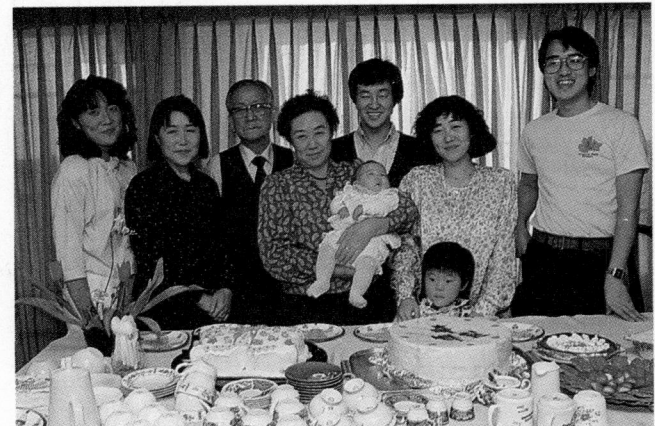

FIGURE 3-1   Different kinds of family configurations (clockwise from upper left): a nuclear family with two children, a nuclear dyad, a three-generation family, a single-parent family, a kin network

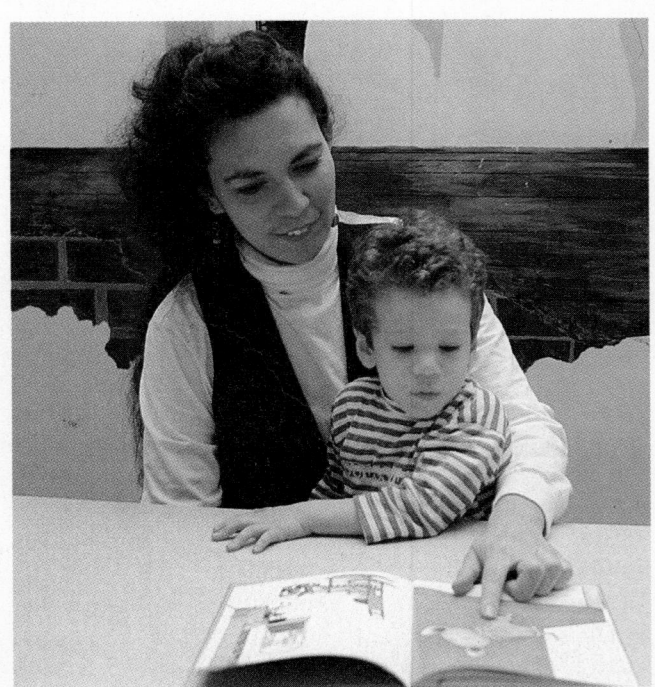

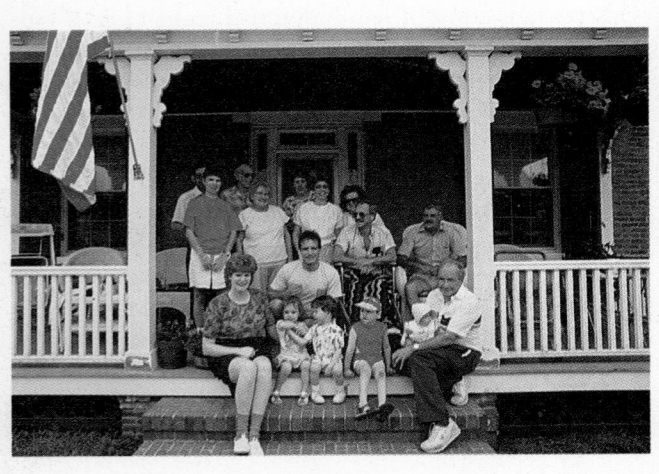

A majority of single-parent families are headed by women (US Bureau of the Census 1993). One of the major problems facing single-parent families is the economical burden of the configuration. Lack of adequate earning power, plus a lack of financial support from the fathers, continue to plague single-parent families headed by women. Women also continue to earn less in their positions than their male counterparts (Walsh 1993). Often the single-parent family is on government assistance because of lack of parental job skills or training or the expense of child care (Ross & Cobb 1990). In the past 20 years the number of unwed women bearing children has tripled (US Bureau of the Census 1993). Today one in four babies is born to an unwed mother (Walsh 1993). One in four adolescent girls becomes pregnant; over half of these births and over 90% of the births to Black teenagers are the result of a nonmarital relationship (Walsh 1993). Studies have documented the high risk of "children having children" as an entrance into a life of long-term poverty, poor quality parenting, and a cluster of health and psychosocial problems (Brooks-Gunn & Chase-Lansdale 1993; Chase-Lansdale & Brooks-Gunn 1991). Often these young mothers remain at home with parents and raise the child in an extended family situation (Ross & Cobb 1990).

Only 3% of single-parent families are headed by men. This number has increased only slightly over the past 20 years (US Bureau of the Census 1993) (Figure 3–2). Divorced fathers are often separated from their children, causing hardship and conflicts for all involved. Depending on the nature of the parents' relationship after divorce, collaborative parenting may or may not be possible. Father-child relationships are nearly always altered and contact is often infrequent. This may be due to the parent wanting to rid himself of financial responsibility ordered by the courts or the desire or need to move long distance from the child and the child's mother in order to make a living.

A variation of the single-parent family configuration that the maternal-newborn nurse may encounter is the *unmarried-parent* family, usually consisting of a mother and a child. With society's increasingly liberal attitudes toward sexuality, a large number of unmarried women are choosing to keep a child rather than giving it up for adoption or to conceive children through artificial insemination. An increasing number of single adults are adopting children.

Three-Generation Family

In the three-generation structure one or more grandparents live in a household with either a single-parent family or a nuclear family. Such a family can benefit from the grandparents' wisdom and experience; the grandmother's role may also include assisting with child care, freeing the mother to seek employment. This arrangement is a feature of many Asian, Hispanic, and African American families in the United States.

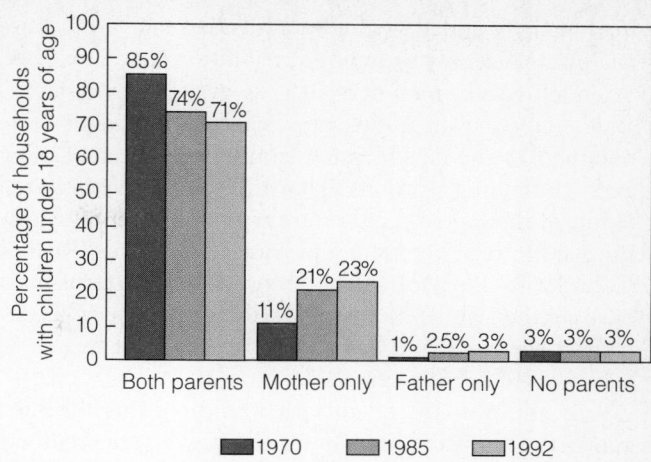

FIGURE 3-2 A comparison of family households with children under 18 years old: 1970, 1985, and 1992. SOURCE: Adapted from US Bureau of the Census: *Statistical Abstract of the United States.* Washington, DC: Government Printing Office, 1993.

Kin Network (Extended Family)

The *extended* family includes two or more nuclear or unmarried households or any of the previously described configurations living in proximity, exchanging goods, and looking to each other for interaction and support. There are ethnic communities in many large cities that have well-established kin networks (Ross & Cobb 1990). Although the parents have authority within their single households, the other adults are often consulted for advice, support, and authority in intrafamily affairs. A newly formed nuclear family may in fact be part of a *kin network* if relatives by blood or marriage are nearby and are part of the family's social group. For some families the trend for mothers to return to work has revived the need to depend on relatives living in separate households to care for children while parents are working (Ross & Cobb 1990). Many families are rediscovering the advantages of a well-maintained kinship system.

Blended (Reconstituted, Stepparent) Family

Recently, the nuclear family has been rocked by an increasing number of marital separations and divorces. Following divorce, about 75% of men and 65% of women remarry (Walsh 1993). Frequently these individuals bring children into the second marriage. When these families merge, the resulting union is termed a **blended family** or **reconstituted family** (Asmundsson 1981). A more recent term used to depict this configuration is the *stepfamily* (Walsh 1993). By the year 2000 this family configuration is predicted to be the dominant family form (Walsh 1993). The coming together of two families, often with very different histories, can be a challenge. Both of the parents and all of the children have functioned in a previous unit and now must develop methods of functioning in a new environment. Unlike nuclear families where members are added gradually, a blended family becomes an "instant" family grouping. In addition there are often extended family members such as grandparents, aunts, and uncles to which this new family must adapt. The members of the new blended family may be establishing and maintaining relationships with the newly constituted family at the same time they are trying to determine how to relate to relatives from a previous family unit (Ross & Cobb 1990). Both formal and informal role patterns must be examined and redefined. Childrearing decisions, financial concerns, and family functioning must be reconsidered, and conflict can arise.

In addition to the more common forms outlined above, the nurse may encounter clients who are members of other types of family structures.

Homosexual Unions

The social movement for gay and lesbian rights has led to advocacy for the normalization of homosexual orientation and families of choice (Walsh 1993). Increasingly, homosexual couples are demanding their rights in the legal system when they decide they wish to adopt children. Today many more lesbian couples are choosing to have biologic children through known or unknown donor insemination, and in some instances both women may choose to bear children (Goldner 1988; Pies 1990). These families face enormous challenges as they struggle with the day-to-day problems that all families face in addition to those imposed by society. Although gays and lesbians may "come out" to a much more tolerant society today, they clearly continue to face social stigma, isolation, and public humiliation. Homosexual relationships in most states lack legal sanction and are not afforded many of the social protections heterosexuals take for granted, their families face threats of dissolution through child removal, and their families of origin may disown them (Comstock 1991).

The estimates of how many children live with lesbian or gay parents fluctuate as widely as the estimates of gay and lesbian individuals (Laird 1993). Patterson (1992) reports that the estimates of lesbian mothers in the United States range from one to five million, whereas those of gay fathers fluctuate from one to three million. Although there have always been gay and lesbian parents, until recently, most children of gay and lesbian parents were born in the context of heterosexual marriages that later ended in divorce (Laird 1993).

Nonmarital Heterosexual Cohabiting Family

Some individuals choose to share living arrangements with other individuals for economic reasons or companionship or both. This family form is called *cohabitation* (Friedman 1992). These individuals are not legally married and often have no intentions of marrying. Other couples decide to live together as a trial or preliminary step to future marriage. Many young adults experience

this type of living arrangement, and larger numbers of older adults are beginning to choose it. Couples living within this arrangement are also choosing to have children.

Commune

When groups of individuals join together in one large household, farm, or community as a family unit, this is considered a *commune* (Ross & Cobb 1990). In communal situations the couples may maintain monogamous relationships, and childrearing becomes a jointly shared task. Other communes have all the individuals "married" to each other with offspring belonging to the entire group.

Although families are undergoing some important changes, we often lose sight of the fact that families have always been changing, just as they have struggled to maintain important continuities. In these new family arrangements many families find themselves in unfamiliar territory lacking a map or compass to guide their passage. The family is not only a locus of residence, but of meaning and relationship (Walsh 1993). As health care providers, we need to recognize the strengths and resilience provided by the traditional resources of kinship, culture, and religion.

Family Function

The concept of family function focuses on the family as a task performance group. By accomplishing certain goals, the family contributes to the survival of the wider social system of which it is a part, the family unit as a whole, and the individual members of that unit. In a broader sense *function* refers to the consequences or outcomes that a family's interrelated motives and subsequent behavior have for the family as a unit (Ritzer 1983), that is, what the family does. Although there is some variation among authors regarding specific family functions, the following are often cited as important goals that families must achieve to continue functioning.

Friedman (1992) has identified five major functions, plus an underlying mechanism by which these functions are achieved. These include (1) the *affective function*, which forms the primary basis for continuation of the family as a unit by meeting the family members' emotional needs; (2) the *reproductive function*, which provides for continuity within the family system and society; (3) the *socialization function*, which socializes children to their roles in society; (4) the *health care function* and provision of food, shelter, clothing, and warmth; and (5) the *economic function*, which provides the family with economic resources for survival (Table 3–1).

Family coping strategies provide the mechanism for carrying out these functions. Internal family coping strategies include (1) family group reliance, (2) humor, (3) greater family sharing, (4) reframing or controlling the meaning of a problem, (5) joint problem solving, and

TABLE 3-1   Guidelines for Functional Family Assessment

Affective Function

1. Do the family members display signs of affection for one another?
2. Do the family members appear to trust and respect one another?
3. Is the family supportive of its members?
4. What events or situations within the family could influence the parents' ability to provide nurturance of the children?
5. Do any of the children appear to be assuming adult or parenting roles that can influence how well their own emotional needs are being met?

Reproductive Function

1. Is the number of children within the family acceptable to both partners?
2. Are the family members comfortable with their own sexuality?
3. How is sexuality and reproductive information conveyed to the children?
4. Do members of the family use birth control? Are these methods satisfactory?
5. Do any of the family members have concerns related to sexuality and reproduction?

Socialization Function

1. Who in the family is primarily responsible for child care?
2. Who in the family is primarily responsible for discipline, rewards, or punishment?
3. What cultural influences affect the family's childrearing practices?
4. How does the family's socioeconomic class influence the family's childrearing practices?
5. What other variables influence the family's childrearing practices?
6. Does the family identify problem areas related to childrearing and discipline?

Health Care Function

1. Who in the family makes decisions related to the members' health care needs? Illness needs?
2. What health care facilities are available to the family?
3. What health care facilities are used by the family?
4. What is done when a family member becomes ill?

5. Does the family have adequate resources for health care needs? Does the family have health insurance?
6. Does the family have a private physician? Or do they visit a health clinic?
7. Are there specific health/illness practices related to the family's culture (ie, folk medicine practices)?
8. Is the "health practitioner" identified within the family's culture (ie, "granny," herbalist)?
9. What preventive health care practices are incorporated into the family's life-style?
10. What barriers to health care are perceived by the family?

Economic Function

1. What are the sources of the family income? Who in the family provides the economic resources?
2. Does the family have adequate income and/or resources to provide food, shelter, and clothing for the family members?
3. Does the family have health insurance or resources to pay for health care services?
4. What agencies need to be contacted to assist the family in the provision of adequate health care, food, clothing, or shelter?

Coping Function

1. What events or situations is the family experiencing that are potentially stressful? How does the family perceive these events or situations?
2. What resources or assets exist within the family to deal with the stressful events or situations?
3. Does the family have adequate support systems?
4. Does the family use humor? Is there joint problem solving?
5. Are the family roles flexible?
6. Is there family group reliance?
7. Is the family denying that a problem exists?
8. Does anyone in the family try to exploit the family members?
9. What is the family's level of adaptation?

SOURCE: Adapted from Friedman MM: *Family Nursing: Theory and Assessment*, 2nd ed. Norwalk, CT: Appleton-Century-Crofts, 1986.

(6) flexible roles. External family coping strategies include (1) seeking out information or knowledge about the stressor, (2) increasing linkages with community groups such as clubs and organizations, (3) using social support systems, (4) using self-help groups, and (5) seeking spiritual support. Without effective family coping strategies, the family's functions cannot be accomplished (Friedman 1992).

Given a particular configuration of members and a set of general tasks or goals that must be accomplished if the family is to survive, families develop rules and roles, usually informally communicated, that characterize their day-to-day functioning. This means that much of family life has a taken-for-granted quality about it. A *role* is a cluster of interpersonal behaviors, attitudes, and activities associated with an individual in a certain situation or position. The behaviors tend to be learned through interactions with parents and siblings. *Attitudes* are the expectations of the society in which the child is raised; they affect

and can be modified by the individuals' behaviors. Role activities are governed by expectations and behavior patterns of friends, relatives, and others outside the individual. Role behaviors, attitudes, and activities are learned to a large extent through the process of socialization.

Each family must define its role in the community and the roles of its individual members within the family unit. These roles are learned through interaction and imitation. Children learn the roles of their parents while learning their own roles and form their self-concepts on the basis of how well they execute their own roles. The roles that children assume affect their psychosocial development into adulthood.

Once the roles of family members are developed, family processes usually continue in a predictable pattern. When interruptions occur in the expected personal roles, family processes will also be interrupted. In most cases, one person will assume the other's role. For example, when the wage earner is disabled for a period, the spouse may need to find a job to replace the lost income, and the children may have to add more household duties and responsibilities to their roles.

THEORETICAL FRAMEWORKS FOR UNDERSTANDING THE FAMILY

By defining and interrelating concepts, theoretical frameworks provide a tool for understanding and analyzing families. Numerous frameworks are available for viewing family life, including the structural-functional, interactional, psychoanalytic, anthropologic, and developmental frameworks. The purpose of these various frameworks is to provide a nurse with a lens for viewing the family. Depending on which lens is selected, the nurse sees a somewhat different entity. Just as certain definitions of family focus attention on composition of the family, and others focus on function, theoretical frameworks provide a foundation for understanding family life, family assessment, and nursing care.

Overview of Frameworks

Four frameworks have been especially popular in nursing's study of the family: the *interactional framework*, the *structural-functional framework*, the *family systems framework*, and the *developmental framework*. The interactional framework looks at family members' subjective views of their situation, emphasizing internal family dynamics. The structural-functional framework focuses on the functional relationships between the family as a whole and other societal structures, as well as considering relationships within the family (Friedman 1992). The family systems framework, related to the structural-functional framework, focuses on the interaction of various family members rather than describing solely the functions of the members (Friedman 1992). This framework is also concerned with how families maintain stability in an ever-changing environment. The developmental framework emphasizes changing family structure and functions across the various stages of the family life cycle. Each stage has its own peculiar source of family conflict and solidarity. A brief discussion of each framework follows.

Interactional Framework

The **interactional framework** centers on understanding the family by discovering how individual members define their situation. The interactional perspective is broad and includes the perspectives of phenomenology, symbolic interaction, and role theory. Interactions focus on subjective meaning as indicated by the three basic premises on which the framework is grounded:

1. Human beings act toward things on the basis of the meaning these things have for them.

2. The meaning of such things is derived from or arises out of interactions one has with others.

3. Meanings are modified through an interpretive process people use in dealing with the things they encounter.

The concepts of self, interaction, communication processes, and role are central to the framework. The self is viewed as a constantly changing process that arises from interaction with others. Roles are seen as emergent rather than static entities. Interactionists focus on understanding how individuals define their roles and the implications of these definitions for how they enact them.

Knafl (1985) used an interactional perspective to study how families responded to a child's routine hospitalization. Hagedorn (1993), using an interactional perspective arising out of phenomenology, revealed the family's lived experience of childhood chronic illness. The data revealed seven "metathemes" about this experience, including embodiment of the illness, creating meaning and understanding of the illness, temporal changes, changing relationships, interacting with the environment, confronting death and affirming life, and a spiritual transcendence (faith, hope, and love). Key themes embedded within these metathemes included family members' struggle to maintain normalcy within their lives, the changing roles that emerge when family members become ill, and how time is experienced one day at a time.

The interactional framework is an appropriate lens for viewing families from the family's point of view. One can use data on these subjective views to identify common processes that family members use to define and manage various family situations. The framework is helpful in isolating specific potential sources of difficulties as family members relate to one another and to their community.

Structural-Functional Framework

The **structural-functional framework** defines the family as a social system. Using this approach, family analysis examines the family in terms of its relationship with other major social institutions such as health care, religion, education, government, and the economy. The primary goal is to determine how family patterns are related to other institutions and to consider the family in the overall structure of society. Emphasis is placed on the functions performed by the family. Artinian (1994) identified the following fundamental assumptions of the structural-functional perspective:

1. A family is a social system with functional requirements.

2. A family is a small group that has generic features common to all small groups.

3. Social systems such as the family accomplish functions that serve the individuals in addition to those that serve society.

4. Individuals act in accordance with a set of internalized norms and values that are learned primarily in the family through socialization.

Minuchin (1974) utilized the structural-functional framework in his research to conceptualize the family as an open sociocultural system that is continually faced with demands for change by its members as well as by inputs from the social systems within which the family is embedded. According to Minuchin, the family as a system has functional demands that organize how members of the family system interact. Through repeated transactions, patterns are established within the family concerning how, when, and to whom family members relate. These patterns become laws governing interactions and conduct of various family members. The family carries out its functions by differentiating into subsystems. Subsystems can consist of an individual, a pair, or a larger group and can be formed on the basis of sex, age, function, or mutual interest. Enduring subsystems in Minuchin's model include spouse subsystem (marital functions), parental subsystem (parental functions), and sibling subsystem (for peer socialization). Within this model boundaries ensure differentiation of the family subsystems. According to Minuchin, for a family to function adequately subsystem members must have contact with one another, but must not interfere with each other's functioning.

Family Systems Framework

The family is considered a system because it is a small group of interrelated and interdependent individuals (Artinian 1994). **Family systems framework** focuses on the interaction of various family members rather than solely describing their functions. The family systems framework emphasizes the concepts of structure, function, boundary maintenance, and change. Aldous (1978, p 26) identified four fundamental characteristics of the family as a social system:

1. The positions occupied by family members are interdependent.
2. The family maintains boundaries and therein constitutes an identifiable unit.
3. The family performs certain tasks both for the larger social system and for family members.
4. The family as a unit is capable of change.

Artinian (1994) identified the following three additional characteristics:

1. Family systems evolve to allow greater adaptability and tolerance to change.
2. Family systems change constantly in response to stresses and strains from within, as well as from the outside environment.
3. Family systems have homeostatic features to maintain stable patterns.

The family systems framework also considers what is called the energy level of the family. Energy may infuse into the family in the form of goods, services, and information. Energy may be released by the family in the form of motivation, skills, goods, or services. Families process energy through activities such as interacting, valuing, goal setting, decision making, and problem solving (Ross & Cobb 1990). In this framework all family systems are open. There is an open exchange of energy both inside and outside the family. The degree of openness varies, depending on the amount of interaction the family has with the environment.

Family structure is defined by the patterned interactions that develop over time among individuals occupying the various positions in the family. The positions (such as wife-mother and husband-father) that comprise the family are viewed as interdependent, although the degree of interdependence may vary both across families and within a single family over time. For example, children typically become less dependent on their parents as they grow older, but parents may become increasingly dependent on their children.

In the family systems framework family boundaries are phenomena such as attitudes, values, or rules that influence a family's exchange with its environment. Boundaries inhibit or facilitate human transactional processes between systems; thus they may be closed or diffuse (Artinian 1994). The family's ability to maintain control over its boundaries is linked to the previously described family functions. For example, if a family is unable to control a certain member's behavior, it may have to open its boundaries to law enforcement officials whether it wants to or not.

The family both initiates and reacts to change. In systems terminology these two processes are referred to as *positive* and *negative* feedback, respectively. Following a systems perspective, change is conceptualized in terms of goal attainment and information exchange. Families exchange information and receive feedback from their environment. Such feedback is processed by family members, who interpret it in terms of the family's goals and tasks. Depending on the "fit" between the feedback and the intended goal, the family may respond by altering either its behaviors or its goals. In a negative feedback situation the family takes a reactive stance and alters its behavior in response to outside input. For example, a couple changes their usual division of labor after their first child is born when they realize their former way of dividing household chores is no longer suitable. The change occurs only after a series of disruptive arguments in which each partner vehemently argues a different point of view. Such a change is reactive because it follows the birth of the baby and is made in the context of threatened family stability due to increased conflict between husband and wife. In a positive feedback situation the family takes a proactive stance and initiates change in response to an anticipated situation. In a proactive situation a couple anticipates that the birth of a baby will require a change in their established division of labor, and therefore they negotiate and try out several different arrangements before the baby is born.

The systems perspective is ideally suited to exploring family goal orientations, boundary maintenance, patterns of communication, and exchanges between the family and other social systems. It provides the nurse with a framework for understanding these aspects of family life.

Developmental Framework

The **developmental framework** looks at the family over time as it progresses through predictable stages of the life cycle. Duvall (1977) and Duvall and Miller (1985) view the family as having universal tasks as well as specific developmental tasks that must be accomplished at eight different stages (Table 3–2). Each stage is determined by the age and school placement of the oldest child. Each family member is involved in meeting his or her own individual tasks as well as contributing to the developmental tasks of the family as a unit. The first two stages, married couples/beginning families and childbearing families, are discussed in more detail.

The developmental approach has been criticized because of its lack of attention to diverse family forms, such as the childless family, and for what is described as its middle-class bias (Friedman 1992). Carter and McGoldrick (1989), for example, have developed a framework for studying families of varying forms. Dislocations of the family life cycle, such as divorce, require systematic changes in order for the family to proceed developmentally. However, the developmental framework can be useful for nurses and other health professionals because it allows the nurse to assess whether or not the developmental tasks are being accomplished and to anticipate change as the nuclear family progresses through the life cycle (Bradshaw 1988).

TABLE 3-2	The Eight-Stage Family Life Cycle

Stage 1	Beginning families (also referred to as married couples or the stage of marriage)
Stage 2	Childbearing families (the oldest child is an infant through 30 months)
Stage 3	Families with preschool children (oldest child is 2 1/2 to 6 years of age)
Stage 4	Families with schoolchildren (oldest child is 6 to 13 years of age)
Stage 5	Families with teenagers (oldest child is 13 to 20 years of age)
Stage 6	Families launching young adults (covering the first child who has left through the last child leaving home)
Stage 7	Middle-aged parents (empty nest through retirement)
Stage 8	Family in retirement and old age (also referred to as aging family members or retirement to death of both spouses)

SOURCE: The Eight Stage Family Life Cycle. In: *Marriage and Family Development,* 6th ed, by Duvall EM, Miller BC. Copyright © 1985 by Harper & Row, Publishers, Inc. Reprinted by permission of HarperCollins Publishers, Inc.

TABLE 3-3	Two-Parent Nuclear Family Life Cycle Stage 1 and Concomitant Family Developmental Tasks

Family Life Cycle Stage	Family Developmental Tasks
Beginning Families	1. Establishing mutually satisfying marriage
	2. Relating harmoniously to kin network
	3. Planning family (decisions about parenthood)

SOURCE: Two-Parent Nuclear Family Life Cycle Stages 1&2.... In: *Marriage and Family Development,* 6th ed, by Duvall EM, Miller BC. Copyright © 1985 by Harper & Row, Publishers, Inc. Reprinted by permission of HarperCollins Publishers, Inc.

Married Couple Stage

The first stage of Duvall's developmental family life cycle is the married couple/beginning family stage, which starts when the couple enters marriage and ends with the birth or adoption of the first child (Table 3–3).

The primary family tasks of the married couple/beginning family are establishing a mutually satisfying marriage relationship, forming a new household, and deciding whether to become parents. For the remarried an additional critical task is acceptance of the termination of the previous marriage in order to establish a healthy conjugal relationship with a new mate. In meeting the developmental tasks the newly formed couple must learn to live with and compromise with each other and to relate to each other's kin. Methods for resolving conflicts, as well as communication patterns and support of one another, must be developed. If the methods for resolving conflict and communicative patterns are healthy, the couple is more likely to achieve a satisfactory marital relationship. Unhealthy patterns may help short-term coping but will not aid long-term adaptation.

A couple may experience difficulty in sexual adjustment because of inaccurate or incomplete information resulting in unrealistic expectations of each other. The degree of sexual experience, particularly the amount of factual knowledge the partners bring to the marriage, affects their adaptation to the relationship. If a couple brings their own unresolved needs and desires into the relationship, it can have an adverse effect on the sexual relationship (Goldenberg & Goldenberg 1985). Marriage partners who recognize each other's varying needs and expectations are able to cooperate to achieve a mutually fulfilling sexual relationship.

One of the primary roles of the nurse working with families in this stage is that of health educator. The nurse can provide accurate information about family planning, pregnancy, sexuality concerns, role changes, and functional communication methods.

Couples who remain childless because of infertility will need support and education regarding their options. Infertility is often viewed as a crisis, and the nurse needs to be aware that the couple's relationship may be affected. The nurse can assist the couple by allowing them to verbalize their frustrations and concerns. The nurse can also provide the couple with information about various options, such as surgical or pharmacologic therapies. If these interventions are not successful, the nurse can discuss other options, such as in vitro fertilization, artificial insemination, and adoption, with the couple. Couples who choose to remain childless need to be supported in their decision. These couples must still work through the developmental tasks of establishing themselves as a unit.

Beginning Family Stage

In the latter part of the first stage in the family life cycle a couple's expectations of having their own child may be fulfilled. This marks the beginning family stage. Although this stage may cover the shortest time span in the cycle, this period is filled with many intense and diverse feelings. When the couple is told that conception has occurred, they may either accept or reject the pregnancy. Some pregnancies are unplanned, although either partner may subconsciously desire pregnancy. Others are planned and may even have been anticipated for months or years before conception actually takes place.

After their initial reactions to the fact that the wife is pregnant, the couple must accomplish certain tasks that are an offshoot of those from the earlier part of the married couple phase. For example, arrangements must be made for the physical care of the baby. These arrangements may mean drastic changes for the family if they have to move into larger quarters or to a place where children are accepted.

In the beginning family period the couple must make adjustments in *patterns of earning and spending*. Generally, the man is in the early phase of his career, and his salary may be low. The woman's salary, which may be a necessary part of the family income, may come to an end during the pregnancy. Many mothers choose to return to work after the baby is born, requiring that child care costs be added to the budget. Health care during the pregnancy and birth also requires large amounts of money, especially with rising medical costs.

Work loads and designation of authority in the household also change out of necessity during pregnancy. The man may assume more of the heavy household chores because it is difficult for the woman to bend and move about. At the same time, pregnant women do not find that their physical state prohibits them from pursuing many of the activities they enjoy, such as working, entertaining, or even participating in sports.

Sexual activities must also be altered to accommodate the physical and emotional changes of pregnancy. The pregnancy may have positive, negative, or no effects on the couple's sexual relationship. Husbands are as likely to feel changes in their sexual responses as their wives are. Because of changes in breast and abdominal size, the couple may need to alter their usual sexual activities.

As soon as the couple knows they are expecting a child, a new focus of interaction becomes evident, enlarging their need for and use of communication. Most couples feel a sense of fulfillment as they feel pride in their ability to conceive a child, as the wife begins to show signs of pregnancy, and as they make plans for the child's arrival. Husband and wife undergo changes in self-concepts in terms of masculinity, femininity, and parenthood. All of these tasks are accomplished with greater ease if the husband and wife develop communication patterns that help them cope with new responsibilities.

Communication with significant others also takes on a new perspective. Relatives and close friends may have a prominent role in helping the young couple with their baby after birth; they can give physical and emotional support to the wife as she undertakes the new tasks of child care. But significant others can interfere with the couple's adjustment to pregnancy and childbirth by telling "old wives' tales" and frightening myths. Reorienting relatives and friends to the kind of relationship that is most desirable for new parents and their child is a major task of the beginning expectant family.

Reorientation must also occur in *relationships with friends and in community activities*. Recreational and social activities can continue to be a major part of the couple's life, curtailed only to the extent that the pregnancy decreases the woman's ability to participate. The mother-to-be may be more sensitive about her partner's ability to continue his activities because his mobility is not affected. She may believe that he is seeking outside interests as she becomes more introspective about the birth of the child. The man may feel left out of many of the woman's activities as she visits the physician and attends groups to discuss the care and rearing of children. Planning joint activities while continuing to respect each other's needs for autonomy can help the couple make a comfortable transition to the complimentary relationship that will be needed in future years.

An expectant couple is open to and eager for knowledge about pregnancy, labor and delivery, and child care. Their background knowledge may be based more on hearsay than fact. They may have had little or no experience with infants and small children.

The couple must also resolve their questions about whether they are prepared to bring a child into their lives, how the baby will fit into their lives, and how they will alter their pattern of living for their child. As mentioned earlier, both partners feel emotions that are new to them and seek understanding from each other. The more one partner is able to meet the other's emotional needs, the more love each will be able to give to their child.

Childbearing Family Stage

The arrival of the first child marks a time of both crisis and great joy for the young family. Again the family faces a period of reorganization. Duvall and Miller (1985) explain that during the *childbearing family stage* (from the birth of the first child until that child is 30 months old) the baby and family become stabilized in their schedules

TABLE 3-4	Two-Parent Nuclear Family Life Cycle Stage 2 and Concomitant Family Developmental Tasks

Family Life Cycle Stage	Family Developmental Tasks
Childbearing families	1. Setting up the young family as a stable unit (integrating a new baby into family)
	2. Reconciling conflicting developmental tasks and needs of various family members
	3. Maintaining a satisfying marital relationship
	4. Expanding relationships with extended family by adding parenting and grandparenting roles

SOURCE: Two-Parent Nuclear Family Life Cycle Stages 1&2…. In: *Marriage and Family Development*, 6th ed, by Duvall EM, Miller BC. Copyright © 1985 by Harper & Row, Publishers, Inc. Reprinted by permission of HarperCollins Publishers, Inc.

and relationships with each other (Table 3–4). The parents feel great joy about the birth of their first child and share their joy with their family and friends; the new mother feels a sense of accomplishment and is ready to relax and let others care for her and her baby for a few days. At the same time the young couple has a feeling of great responsibility for their child's growth and development.

The first task of the childbearing family is *to arrange the home to meet the needs of the newborn infant*. The primary responsibility of the parents is to provide a safe, comfortable environment for the infant. A primary need of the newborn is a quiet, clean place to sleep. As children grow and become more mobile, their immediate environment enlarges even though they are still unable to protect themselves from many of its dangers.

Costs of raising a child are drastically increasing, creating additional problems for a couple already dealing with the increased costs of daily living. Even in the United States, where prosperity is relatively common, many families are below the poverty level, and children are raised with a minimum of economic expenditure.

The birth of the first child requires a *reworking of responsibility and accountability patterns*. A baby requires round-the-clock care, much of which is assumed by the mother, particularly if she is breast-feeding the child. The father may assume more of the household tasks, such as shopping and running errands outside the home. The partners share in seeking solutions to problems that arise during the day. The child also has accountability to parents as he or she grows older. The approval or disapproval of parents teaches the child what parents consider good and bad, and he or she recognizes good acts as pleasing ones.

Reestablishing a satisfying sexual relationship with one's partner is another task of the childbearing family stage. Sexual activity usually decreases or ceases during the postnatal period. The new mother becomes absorbed in her child, and her close physical relationship with the baby may decrease her sexual needs. The responsibilities of caring for a newborn may leave her physically exhausted. Her partner may feel rejected as the new mother focuses on the baby's needs instead of his. Much mutual patience and understanding are necessary as the couple strives to reunite to meet each other's needs.

Two stresses occur in the childbearing family period that can hinder or further the *development of effective communication:* the newborn's crying and the decreased sharing between the parents. Crying, the newborn's only means of communication, can be extremely disconcerting until the new parents are able to interpret what the various types of cries mean and until they learn to anticipate their infant's needs. When the parents believe they have met the needs of their child and the crying continues for no apparent reason, their frustration increases. However, as the parents attempt to meet the baby's needs lovingly, the baby's trust in them increases, and other methods of communication emerge such as smiling, cooing, and eventually talking.

The other strain on effective communication is decreased sharing between the parents. Their tasks may be more separately defined as the father works outside the home while the mother remains busy caring for their new baby and the house. They participate in different activities and have less time to be alone together. Instead of the one relationship of the couple, three relationships have developed to include the infant in the family circle. If the new mother returns to work soon after the baby is born, both parents may experience additional strain. However, even though the parents may have distinct tasks, they can share more as they watch their baby grow.

Relationships with relatives are also a facet of the development of the childbearing family. The new parents will receive much advice on how to care for the child. If they are mature and have successfully completed their previous developmental tasks, they are able to sift through this information and use what is most meaningful to them. The greater the difference between the two parental families, the greater the likelihood of conflicting advice, because each set of grandparents will want the child to be raised according to the traditions of their family. And, of course, the parental families can also supply a great deal of support and comfort to the new parents, who are trying to establish their own traditions.

The young family must participate in *community activities to establish relationships outside the home*. They are more involved in their home life than they were before their baby's birth and must find suitable babysitting arrangements if they desire to go out together. Their interests may change as they seek out congenial couples with young children who can share similar experiences.

A further responsibility of the childbearing family is to *decide whether or when to have more children* and to take appropriate measures. Having children in quick succession may prove to be a tremendous strain for both parents, although some couples prefer to have their children close together. If the first child has a defect or dies shortly after birth, the decision about whether or when to have another child becomes paramount.

Maintenance of motivation and morale in the childbearing family may become difficult. The repetitious tasks of everyday child care may overshadow the basic satisfactions of parenthood. Values placed on material objects may need to be changed, becoming dependent on what is good for the young child. The parents need to continue their independence as a couple while recognizing the child's dependence on them. The developmental needs of the child and those of the parents may be in conflict, so priorities must be set. The young family may need to accept assistance from relatives and friends at a time when they are still striving to be a separate unit.

The early childbearing and childrearing years have a significant influence on the ultimate strength of the family unit. Many crises occur that can either divide or unite the family. A division or conflict may not be evident while the children are still dependent but may manifest itself after the children have left home and there is little else to hold the parents together. Yet these same stresses can unite the family more solidly if they are faced as mutual problems and if individual needs and priorities are taken into account in family interrelationships.

The nurse can assist the family during this phase of family development by providing health teaching related to family planning, infant care, child development, and safety. The nurse can also give the couple support as they adjust to the physical and emotional demands of being parents. If other children are born during this phase, the nurse can assist the couple with problems related to sibling rivalry and time management. Drastic role changes accompany parenthood, and often the couple has little preparation. The nurse assists the family to communicate in an open manner about the various role changes that are occurring. Because wellness behaviors are learned at an early age, the nurse should provide the family with information related to stress management, nutrition, dental care, immunizations, exercise, and healthy life-style practices.

FACTORS AFFECTING FAMILY STRUCTURES AND FUNCTIONS

Regardless of its structure, the family does not function in isolation. The well-being of a family can be promoted or hindered by the acts or policies of other persons or institutions. Characteristics such as race, culture, ethnicity, and family configuration may affect the family's social status and standing, income level, and community acceptance. Religion often has a strong influence on the values, beliefs, and moral concepts of the family. Many religions also delineate behavioral codes, rituals, traditions of family life, cultural practices, societal traditions, and childrearing practices. The implications of these and other factors differ for each family. Members within each family can also be affected to varying degrees. The following sections explore the concepts of and factors affecting family life-style.

Family Life-Style

Families are characterized by diversity. As mentioned earlier, families come in widely varying sizes and behave in widely varying ways. Levin and Idler (1981, p 68) describe life-style as "this webbing material of values, beliefs, expectations, criteria of choice, problem solving, communication, and commitment that is unique to the family."

Traditionally, a family's socioeconomic status was determined by certain characteristics of the husband-father, including his occupation, education, and income. A more recent trend has been to include information from both parents in determining the family's socioeconomic status. (See Chapter 8 for discussion of the socioeconomic problems faced by single-parent families headed by women.) Social scientists consider education and occupational position to be the two main components of social class. Income is also a factor but is of less importance.

Family life across social classes has been shown to vary with regard to both structural and functional characteristics. There is an inverse relationship between social class and family size: The more affluent the family, the smaller it is. Differences have been noted as well in communication style and childbearing practices in families of differing social classes (Boyd-Franklin 1989).

Ethnic identity also influences family life. Ross and Cobb (1990) define ethnic identity as the way that an individual or family perceives themselves in relation to the larger society. Ethnic groups are subdivided into early ethnic minorities (such as Irish and German), recent and continuing ethnic minorities (such as Vietnamese and Cuban), historically subjugated ethnic minorities (such as Black and Native American), and socioreligious ethnic minorities (such as Mormon and Greek Orthodox). Structural and functional differences have often been associated with families of varying ethnic backgrounds. Members of a specific ethnic group share a distinct linguistic, social, and cultural background.

Nurse anthropologists and ethnographers such as Tripp-Reimer (1983) and Leininger (1985) have provided valuable insights into the family life and health care beliefs and practices of various ethnic groups. Speaking to the importance of understanding ethnomedical practices, Tripp-Reimer (1983, p 101) said: "While it is crucial to be sensitive to cultural beliefs and practices, it is just as essential not to overgeneralize and assume that all members of the subculture hold to a particular belief or practice." In a similar vein, Levin and Idler (1981, p 66) stressed the need for health care professionals to recognize the health care functions of the family in general.

> Many indigenous practices have emerged from historical test and may depend for their effectiveness on an

integrated, interacting set of values and beliefs. It may well be that their effective power lies in the family's commitment to them and their symbolic contribution to family identity.

Health care professionals need to be sensitive to clients' diverse needs and expectations. They must avoid attributing needs or expectations based on preconceived notions of what families in a given cultural, socioeconomic, or ethnic group's membership are like.

Societal Trends

Status of Women

The traditional role for a woman in society in the United States was once that of homemaker. Her role had value for the family; thus the home became the stronghold for women. Meanwhile, the man was traditionally considered the head of the household, and the status and life-style of those within the home depended to a large extent on him.

In reaction to the changing economic conditions within families women of childbearing age have entered the work force in record numbers in recent years. Previous generations of women had worked for noneconomic reasons, but today's families are increasingly dependent on the mother's income, be it primary or secondary. Women also continue to earn less than their male counterparts. The average full-time working wife contributes only 40% of the family's annual income (Walsh 1993). Currently about 58% of mothers with children under 1 year of age, 60% of mothers of preschool children, and 70% of mothers of school-age children are in the work force (Walsh 1993).

As women move into the work force, three areas of family life are likely to be influenced: division of labor within the home, marital adjustment, and parenting (Walsh 1993). For a more detailed discussion of women and societal issues see Chapter 8.

It is difficult to determine how the wife's employment affects marital satisfaction. Of the many variables likely to influence the relationship, two of the most important are the family's financial situation and each partner's values or beliefs regarding the woman's participation in the labor force. Dissatisfaction is most likely to occur when partners hold conflicting beliefs in this area.

Value of Children

The value of children varies greatly, depending on the meaning each culture and society attaches to children. In addition, the reaction of individual family members to a child is personalized and subjective (Figure 3–3). Historically, the motivations for having children have been religious, political, economic, and cultural. Some individuals want children for their own gratification—to have someone to guide and control, to reap economic gains, to improve one's status, to ensure one is cared for in old age, to

RESEARCH IN PRACTICE

Given that access to health care may be limited by language and cultural differences, Blanche Mikhail identified and assessed Hispanic American mothers' beliefs and practices concerning selected health problems of their children. Ms Mikhail recruited 105 Hispanic women with young children from a rural California clinic. A bilingual research assistant conducted interviews in the participant's language of choice, English or Spanish. Questions covered initial sources of advice; use of home remedies and folk healers; and perceived causes, seriousness, and management of health problems. The illnesses included fever, cough, diarrhea, vomiting, conjunctivitis, skin rash, minor wounds, and burns.

Data analysis included content and statistical analysis. Perceived causes of the illness varied. Some mothers believed that infections caused fever and cough while others stated the cause was an imbalance between hot and cold things. Diarrhea and vomiting were attributed to decomposed milk, something eaten not settling well in the stomach, or empacho (something believed to be stuck in the child's stomach). Perceived causes of conjunctivitis encompassed infections, allergies, pollution, or a draft.

Management of the problems included home remedies, using OTC drugs, seeking medical advice, or not knowing what to do. Common home remedies involved herbal teas for cough, rice water or suero (a liquid solution of water, sugar, lemon, or banana) for diarrhea, and chamomile or breast milk drops for conjunctivitis. Mothers also mentioned using aspirin for fever, Terramycin ointment for minor burns, and ophthalmic ointment for conjunctivitis. Many of the mothers obtained their drugs from Mexico, where they can be obtained without a prescription. Eleven percent of the mothers in the study admitted using azarcon (lead tetroxide) or greta (lead oxide) for treatment of stomach problems or empacho.

Clinical Application of the Study

In order to provide culturally sensitive health care, nurses must be aware of the belief systems and practices of their clients. As noted by the author, some of the home remedies used by the Hispanic mothers more than adequately treated the health problems. However, practices such as giving lead preparations to children with stomach ailments or giving aspirin for a fever create health risks.

SOURCE: Mikhail B: Hispanic mothers' beliefs and practices regarding selected children's health problems. *Western Journal of Nursing Research* 1994; 16(6):623.

satisfy cultural requirements, or to provide a means of personal immortality.

Many historical changes have influenced the importance of children in society. In agrarian societies children are valued for the economic gain they bring to their family and society. Industrialization and urbanization in North America have reduced the economic necessity of having children. As a result, children have become less "valuable" and more valued.

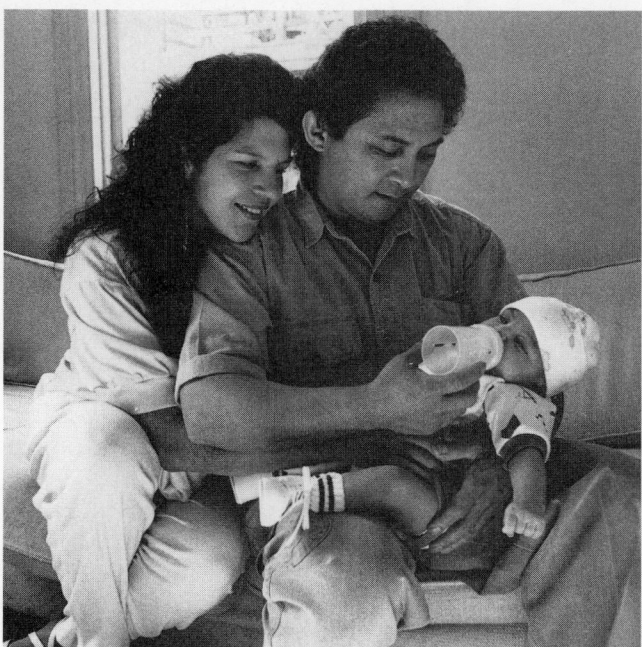

FIGURE 3-3 The value of a child to a family is personalized and depends on socioeconomic, religious, and cultural factors.

Environmental Factors

Environmental factors influencing the family are closely interrelated with the cultural and socioeconomic factors discussed previously. The environment includes outside forces that may alter the behaviors and activities of family members and the family group. Forces such as relatives, friends, and significant others; home, neighborhood, and community settings; and social, religious, and governmental institutions within the community all influence the family.

In childbearing families environmental factors are most significant in terms of their effects on parents. Parents, based on their experience and background, interpret the meaning of the interaction between environmental forces and the family for their children. If their explanations are positive, they transmit to their children feelings of security, stability, and well-being. However, if the parents feel negative toward or threatened by their surroundings, they may transmit feelings of danger, hostility, and anger. The way that the family interacts with its environment is likely to have a direct effect on the family's ability to meet members' needs individually and collectively.

The physical setting in which the family lives also affects family functioning. Poor housing may adversely influence family and member attitudes, behaviors, motivational levels, and self-esteem, which in turn increases stress and the risk of illness and accidents. The overcrowding of a home may interfere with privacy and result in inadequate childrearing and housekeeping practices. Chaotic, disorganized homes may contribute to a child's

developmental delay or deviances, which may be permanent. If family functioning continues to be impaired as the child's environment expands to settings outside the home, problems may become evident in the child's ability to communicate, solve problems, and form relationships.

Within the neighborhood and community, families tend to associate freely with community groups and other institutions to identify resources and receive services as needed. The family's ability to seek help through contact with others appears related in part to the family's perception of itself as a part of a whole and to its successful dealings with the larger community in meeting physical, psychologic, and social requirements.

NURSING IMPLICATIONS

Theories and research provide a basis for understanding families and suggest important areas of concern, typical patterns of behavior, and the range of variation surrounding the typical. Theories and research, however, do not prescribe what the nurse should do in a given situation. These decisions emanate from thoughtful interactions with family members in which nurses interpret the family's definition of the situation in light of their own knowledge. Nurses must be aware of their own cultural and value biases before making these decisions.

A major goal of family-centered maternity care is to help each member of an expectant family achieve optimal health by preventive, maintenance, and restorative measures. Nurses have the additional role of assisting families to accomplish appropriate developmental tasks at each family stage.

The success of the family depends on the achievement of these tasks. At times the family may find that success comes easily; at other times they must overcome delay or failure. Because failure tends to follow failure just as success follows success, the nurse may need to intervene to break a family's cycle of failures in performing tasks and to guide them toward success.

When giving care to a client, the nurse should keep in mind the long-term, intimate relationships among family members. The person receiving care has performed a unique role within the family group that must be acknowledged if the family is to function optimally. Thus families have the right to examine the kind of care and service a family member is receiving, to complain when the service is unsatisfactory, and to seek other sources of services when they are dissatisfied.

To ensure the provision of appropriate individualized care, the maternity nurse uses the nursing process as the framework for planning, implementing, and evaluating responsible health care.

The Family as Client

Because the individual develops as a member of a family unit, the nurse must understand the family in order to understand the individual. This is especially important in the maternity setting because the nurse is directly responsible for the well-being of the mother, father, and siblings, as well as the newborn.

The concept of the family as a client is one of the most important components of family-centered maternity nursing. Ideally, the family gives each member love and trust and responds consistently so that all may mature into individuals who are able to give these qualities to others.

Friedman (1992) identifies the family unit as being the critical resource for the delivery and success of health care services for the following reasons:

- In a family unit a dysfunction of one or more family members generally affects each individual as well as the family unit. If the nurse considers only the individual, the nursing assessment is fragmented rather than complete and holistic.

- Assessing the family helps the nurse understand the individuals functioning within their social context. With the expectant and childbearing family, the nurse is able to assist the prospective parents to prepare for the new family member.

- A strong interrelationship exists between the health status of a family as a unit and that of the individuals who constitute the family. By emphasizing health promotion and maintenance in the family, the nurse should have a positive effect not only on the individuals in the family, but also on the family unit.

- In considering the family as a whole the nurse identifies potential risk factors, thereby facilitating illness prevention.

- When illness occurs, the family is instrumental in seeking health care and in determining members' sick-role behaviors.

In family-centered maternity nursing the nurse generally focuses on health promotion and maintenance and prevention of illness, primarily with the beginning or childbearing family. To interact effectively with the wide variety of families they are likely to encounter, nurses need to do the following:

- Reevaluate personal cultural beliefs and values.

- Recognize personal biases and beliefs about a particular culture (stereotyping).

- Assess the individual/family carefully and openly, without judgment.

- Avoid generalizations and assumptions based on personal ideas and knowledge about a particular culture. There is diversity *within* every culture.

In view of these suggestions it is a good idea for the nurse to confirm any assumptions regarding the particular culture or group by speaking tactfully with the individual or family. The nurse's goal is to provide excellent care based on a complete biopsychologic assessment that includes a cultural component.

Through the assessment process discussed in the next section the nurse identifies risk factors that may lead to health problems. Planning with the family determines health goals that may require the involvement of other health team members. Assessment, intervention, and evaluation should be viewed as negotiative, interactive processes. Nurses and family members each bring unique knowledge and skills to a given health care situation. Ideally, they work together to achieve goals that are mutually acceptable.

APPLYING THE NURSING PROCESS

Most nurses in practice work simultaneously with individuals and family members. Use of the nursing process (assessment, diagnosis, planning, intervention, and evaluation) will often be more extensive and complex when working with families. Friedman (1992) introduced a two-level approach to assessing and carrying out family nursing care (Figure 3–4). The steps in this approach are interdependent, not strictly sequential or linear in organization. In practice steps or phases may overlap and take place simultaneously, with movement back and forth among the various steps.

Family Assessment

The process of nursing assessment is highlighted by continuous information gathering and professional judgments that attach meaning to the information gathered (Friedman 1992).

Assessment of the beginning or childbearing family's status is the first step in determining the family's level of functioning. Data may be gathered in a variety of settings, including the home, clinic, and birthing center. When assessing the family of a maternity client, the nurse should be comprehensive but focused on areas of particular relevance to the family. In-depth data collection is necessary in those areas that pose a problem for the family or are of concern to the nurse.

To collect valid, pertinent data, the nurse must establish a positive relationship with the client, a family member, and/or the family group. The use of empathy, positive regard, and active listening enables the nurse to gather complete, yet selective, information about the family. The nurse should obtain the following:

- Basic identifying information, including the names, ages, gender, and relationships of all family members

- Religious and cultural associations

- Type of family configuration

- Data about the members of the extended family who are closest to the nuclear family, especially if they reside nearby and form a strong support group for each other

- Individual and family perception of family functioning: communication patterns, division of labor

Health History

The nurse records a health history of the entire family because family health problems have potential effects on children. The nurse gathers information about the extended and nuclear family regarding past acute and chronic illnesses, congenital defects, mental health, obesity, or the occurrence of accidents. A family pedigree may be helpful in summarizing this information visually (see Chapter 7 on genetic counseling). With the beginning expectant family or the childbearing family, data about all pregnancies become significant. Knowledge of experiences of family members with health care delivery systems or hospitalization helps in deciding which approach to the family will be most helpful.

The nurse also needs to obtain data about the current health status of each family member. With the beginning and childbearing family, the nurse assesses the family's strengths and limitations in promoting and maintaining health by learning about the family's definitions of health and illness, their nutritional status, attitudes toward medicine use (prescription and nonprescription), recreational and exercise activities, exposure to environmental hazards, and sleep and rest practices. When a client is pregnant, prenatal assessment is essential (see Chapter 14). Other important information includes data on each family member's allergies, health problems requiring prescription medications, environmentally and genetically related illnesses, the family's knowledge about these disorders, and treatments that have been recommended and implemented.

Health Practices

Assessing the competency of the family to promote and maintain health, care for ill members, and carry out health care instructions is vital in determining the nurse's

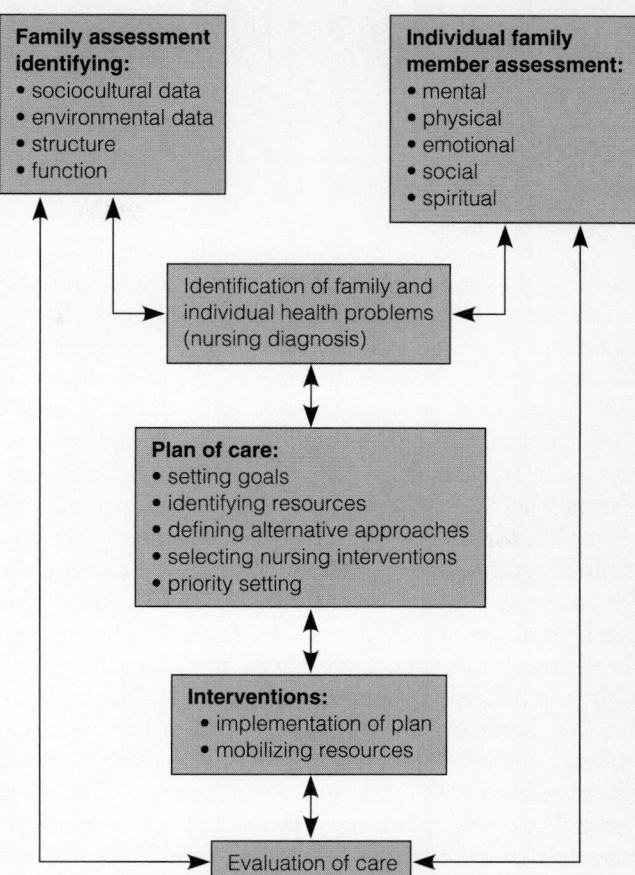

FIGURE 3-4 Steps in the individual and family nursing process. SOURCE: Adapted from Friedman MM: *Family Nursing Theory and Assessment,* 3rd ed. New York: Appleton-Century-Crofts, 1992, p 41.

interaction with the family. Many families use preventive health measures such as obtaining routine medical, dental, hearing, and ophthalmic examinations and immunizations and participating in other screening programs. If the family does not use such preventive measures, the nurse needs to assess the family's knowledge about or access to such measures. The nurse may find it necessary to identify health care facilities that are accessible to the family and to discuss how they are used.

Home Environment

A valid assessment of the family may require several home visits. Some families feel that a home visit by a nurse is an invasion of privacy, but most become more amenable as rapport is established. When assessing the characteristics of a home, the nurse must make objective observations; personal standards and values should not be allowed to distort evaluation of the living conditions. Living space that provides all family members with privacy and comfortable sleeping arrangements and permits each person to pursue interests and needs is important. If a new baby is expected, preparation for arrival should be evident. Adequate heat, light, cooking facilities, water, storage facilities, and hygienic equipment are necessary for maintaining the well-being of all family members. Age-appropriate toys, books, and other recreational and educational equipment should be available for any children in the home. Play areas should be away from safety hazards and should be adequately supervised. The distance of the home from health care facilities and the availability of transportation to them should also be investigated.

Appraisal of the home environment gives only some indication of the economic status of the family. Knowledge about the sources and amounts of family income and about the work skills of individual members aids in assessing health behavior and needs. Information about the allocation of income to shelter, clothing, food, savings, insurance, education, recreation, and health care reveals the family's economic priorities and its ability to meet the needs of all family members. However, at times nurses should not try to collect this information; social workers are the more appropriate professional.

The home assessment may also include observations of the population characteristics and resources of the neighborhood and the larger community in which the family lives, taking into account the family's associations and transactions within the community. How parents view their interaction with their neighborhood and community is significant because their children tend to relate in a similar fashion. Certain health problems can also have broad effects within a community. For example, diseases can be transmitted by children to other children in schools and from them to the rest of the family. After identifying such situations, a nurse can make recommendations to help families cope with such problems. With the greater emphasis on home health care today more maternal-newborn nurses will be making home visits because childbirth in-hospital stays have shortened to 24 hours in many cases.

Assessment Tools

In addition to the sources of information just described, several tools for objective data collection can be used to measure various aspects of family functioning. Some assessment tools concentrate on mother-infant interactions and needs for teaching and support. The Maternal Attachment Assessment Strategy provides a system of observing maternal-child behavior and establishing a profile of the mother's attachment behaviors (Avant 1982). The Mother-Infant Play Interaction Scale (MIPIS) is another tool that measures response reciprocity between mother and infant during unstructured play (Walker 1982).

The Feetman Family Functioning Scale (Roberts & Feetman 1982) assesses parents' views of relationships among family members and between the family and other social systems. It is a systematic method of assessing family functioning under stress. By identifying specific stressors, the maternal-newborn nurse can proceed to identify sources of support that will help diminish the stress. The Family APGAR test (Smilkstein 1984) assesses family functioning in the areas of adaptability, partnership, growth, affection, and resolve. The Family Environment Scale (Moos & Moos 1976) measures three components of family life: relationships, personal growth, and family system maintenance. The tool provides data that help the nurse compare parent and child perceptions and actual preferred family environment and to assess and facilitate change. The Family Assessment Device (FAD) is a self-reporting measure that identifies family strengths and limitations so that the nurse can reinforce family strengths or correct limitations (Epstein et al 1983).

Speer and Sachs (1985) provide an excellent overview and evaluation of nine family assessment tools. Their evaluation is based on the following criteria: understandable, easily administered and scored, reliable and valid, appropriate for all types of families, and clinically relevant. Such tools can facilitate the nurse's assessment of the family.

Analysis and Nursing Diagnosis

The family assessment culminates in an identification of family issues. In one approach the nurse describes the

---

TABLE 3-5	Family Assessment

Typology of 11 Functional Health Patterns

Health Perception/health management pattern: Describes family's perceived pattern of health and well-being and how health is managed

Nutritional/metabolic pattern: Describes pattern of food and fluid consumption relative to metabolic need and pattern indicators of local nutrient supply: family nutrition patterns

Elimination pattern: Describes patterns of excretory function (bowel, bladder, and skin); family waste disposal and hygiene practices

Activity/exercise pattern: Describes family's patterns of exercise, activity, leisure, and recreation

Cognitive/perceptual pattern: Describes sensory-perceptual and cognitive pattern; family decision making

Sleep/rest pattern: Describes patterns of sleep, rest, and relaxation of the family

Self-perception/self-concept pattern: Describes self-concept pattern and perceptions of self (eg, body comfort, body image, feeling state); family's perception of their image

Role/relationship pattern: Describes pattern of role engagement and relationships within the family

Sexuality-reproductive pattern: Describes family's patterns of satisfaction and dissatisfaction with sexual relationships, family planning, and reproduction

Coping/stress tolerance pattern: Describes general coping pattern and effectiveness of the pattern in terms of stress tolerance with the family; family's perceptions of events

Value/belief pattern: Describes patterns of values, beliefs (including spiritual), or goals that guide choices and decisions

SOURCE: Adapted from Gordon M: *Nursing Diagnosis: Process and Application,* 2nd ed. New York: McGraw-Hill, 1987, p 93.

TABLE 3-6	Possible Nursing Diagnoses for Family Nursing Practice

Functional Health Pattern	Possible Nursing Diagnoses
Health perception–health management pattern	Altered health management Health-seeking behaviors
Activity-exercise pattern	Impaired home maintenance management
Cognitive-perceptual pattern	Knowledge deficit Decisional conflict
Role-relationship pattern	Anticipatory grieving Dysfunctional grieving Parental role conflict Social isolation Alteration in family processes Altered role performance Altered parenting Violence, high risk: self-directed or directed at others
Coping–stress tolerance pattern	Family coping: potential for growth Ineffective family coping

SOURCE: Adapted from Gordon M: *Nursing Diagnosis: Process and Application,* 2nd ed. New York: McGraw-Hill, 1987; and 1992 NANDA Approved Nursing Diagnostic Categories.

functional health patterns of the family based on information gathered during the nursing history (Table 3–5). Family nursing diagnoses are extensions of family functional health patterns and are the outcomes of nursing assessment (Table 3–6). Ideally, the nurse gathers assessment data of families over a period of time. Data related to both previous and current patterns provide the nurse with information that leads to the development of nursing diagnoses.

Goals based on each nursing diagnosis are then established for the family. These are divided into short-range and long-range goals and should be a joint enterprise between the family and the nurse. Without this cooperative interaction the goals may not meet the needs that the family believes are important, may not be realistic for the family, or may not be accepted by the family as its responsibility.

The priority of these goals must then be determined. This is a highly individualized process; input from the family continues to have great importance. A severe illness, an unplanned child, and lack of funds for a needed purchase can all be crucial matters. The family may consider obtaining funds to be the most pressing goal, whereas the nurse may believe that accepting the child should receive immediate attention, and the physician may think that the treatment of the illness should be given top priority. Factors that affect priorities include the family's perceptions of its needs, the number of problems that require attention, the feasibility of goals set, the readiness of the family to meet the goals, and the amount of preparation or education necessary before the goals can be met. Working with the family, the nurse must validate the goals and their importance to gain the family's support in achieving them.

Planning

Planning interventions is the next step in the nursing process. The nursing care plan must be based on the goals set in consultation with the family. There are generally many approaches to every problem, and the nurse needs to identify the one that seems most likely to work in the family's particular framework of attitudes, beliefs, and values. Family participation in planning can be valuable because the family knows about its ability to deal with the situation. Therefore the nursing plan must be accepted by the family prior to putting it into action.

During the planning stage, decisions must be made about those health care workers, other professionals, and community agencies that will be of greatest value to the family. The nurse can explain the services available from these agencies. The family's needs may be best satisfied by several agencies, which will require interagency cooperation and coordination of efforts. The nurse may serve as the coordinator of these activities, assuring continuity of services to the family. One long-range goal for the family should be to strengthen its knowledge of community resources to meet its own health needs.

Implementation

In implementing a care plan the nurse must constantly keep in mind the short- and long-range goals that have been set for the family. Therapeutic interaction continues to be of primary importance. Changes in family needs often produce stress on some or all members. The recommendations and teaching of the nurse or other professionals may cause more stress because any change always causes some tension and anxiety. Family members may feel guilty about having certain needs and may be concerned about how these needs will be accepted by others. Any serious difficulties have probably already disrupted the family, and its members may have had to take on roles and responsibilities with which they are unfamiliar.

The nurse needs to be aware not only of the family's changing situation, but also of its members' changing views regarding their situation. In this sense assessment is ongoing and cuts across the intervention and assessment stages of the nursing process. Further resources may be needed to help the family cope in dealing with any problems.

When working with beginning and childbearing families, the nurse assumes many roles, including teacher, counselor, coordinator, researcher, and advocate. In these roles the nurse is careful to communicate in a manner that is understandable and meaningful to the family. Knowledge of the family's developmental level, internal processes, socioeconomic status, and cultural background helps in determining the most effective approach to use. A collaborative effort is necessary for learning to occur. The nurse assists the family to define strategies for change, and the family decides how to apply the learning primarily through their own resources. In some circumstances the nurse supports the family's position or initiates plans to foster further development, thus ensuring continued learning.

The nurse acts primarily as a teacher, counselor, and advocate in helping a couple determine their family-planning needs. The nurse offers information in a manner that the family can understand and use, demonstrating understanding and respect for needs and belief systems. Some families hesitate to use family-planning techniques because of fears or dislike of, or misunderstanding about, contraception; because of worries that they cannot afford family planning; or because of beliefs that others are trying to limit the size of their ethnic group.

The nurse's responsibilities to the beginning expectant family include preparing the couple for the woman's physical and emotional condition and needs and planning for the man's desires for involvement. Teaching expectant couples about pregnancy, labor, and birth and counseling them about child care and the parental role are important nursing responsibilities.

After the child is born, a primary concern of the nurse is to make sure that the family can meet the needs of the newborn infant. The nurse assumes the roles of teacher and counselor when discussing the needs of the infant and demonstrating infant care to the parents. In addition the nurse acts as the family advocate by giving emotional support to new parents and by providing guidance on effective use of health care professionals.

Evaluation

To interpret the success or failure of the nursing care plan, the nurse takes into account the goals set for the family and the effects produced. Again, the family should play an important part in this evaluation, as it has in other steps of the nursing process. Members need to be encouraged to respond freely and openly.

If a goal has been fully achieved, the nursing interventions have been successful. If a goal has not been attained, the nurse should explore the reasons for the failure and devise a new plan that might meet with greater success. If a goal has been partially achieved, the nurse and family determine whether the plan is realistic and simply needs more time or whether modifications are necessary. The nurse may find that changes in the family necessitate adjustments and adaptations in the nursing care plan at any point during its implementation. Even when all goals appear to have been attained, periodic reevaluation and encouragement are necessary for the family to continue to function at the best level.

REFERENCES

Aldous J: *Family Careers*. New York: Wiley, 1978.

Anderson KN, Anderson LE, Glanze WD (editors): *Mosby's Medical, Nursing, and Allied Health Dictionary*, 4th ed. St. Louis: Mosby, 1994.

Arnold L, Brecht M: Legislative issues affecting parenting: An overview of current policies. *J Perinatal Nurs* 1990; 4(2):24.

Artinian N: Selecting a model to guide family assessment. *Dimens Crit Care Nurs* 1994; 14(1):4.

Asmundsson R: Blended families: One plus one equals more than two. In: *Understanding the Family: Stress and Change in American Life*. Getty C, Humphreys W (editors). New York: Appleton-Century-Crofts, 1981.

Avant P: A maternal attachment assessment strategy. In: *Analysis of Current Assessment Strategies in the Health Care of Young Children and Childbearing Families*. Humenick S (editor). New York: Appleton-Century-Crofts, 1982.

Boyd-Franklin N: *Black Families in Therapy: A Multisystems Approach*. New York: Guilford Press, 1989.

Bradshaw MJ (editor): *Nursing of the Family in Health and Illness: A Developmental Approach*. Norwalk, CT: Appleton & Lange, 1988.

Brooks-Gunn J, Chase-Lansdale L: Correlates of adolescent pregnancy and parenthood. In: *Applied Developmental Psychology*. Fisher C, Lerner R (editors). Cambridge, MA: McGraw-Hill, 1993.

Carter B, McGoldrick M (editors): *The Changing Family Life Cycle: Framework for Family Therapy*. New York: Gardner, 1989.

Chase-Lansdale L, Brooks-Gunn J: Children having children: Effects on the family system. *Ped Ann* 1991; 20:467.

Comstock G: *Violence Against Lesbians and Gay Men*. New York: Columbia Univ Press, 1991.

Conner G, Denson V: Expectant father's response to pregnancy: Review of literature and implications for research in high risk pregnancy. *J Perinatal Nurs* 1990; 4(2):33.

Duvall EM: *Marriage and Family Development*, 5th ed. Philadelphia: Lippincott, 1977.

Duvall EM, Miller BC: *Marriage and Family Development*, 6th ed. New York: Harper & Row, 1985.

Epstein NB et al: The McMaster Family Assessment Device. *J Marital Fam Ther* 1983; 9:171.

Fawcett J: Spouses' experiences during pregnancy and the postpartum: A program of research and theory development. *Image* 1989; 21(3):149.

Friedman MM: *Family Nursing Theory and Assessment*, 3rd ed. New York: Appleton-Century-Crofts, 1992.

Glick P: American families: The way they are and were. In: *Families in Transition*, 8th ed. Scholnick A, Scholnick J (editors). New York: Harper Collins, 1994.

Goldenberg I and Goldenberg H: *Family Therapy, an Overview*, 2nd ed. Monterey, CA: Brooks/Cole, 1985.

Goldner V: Generation and gender: Normative and covert hierarchies. *Fam Process* 1988; 27:17.

Hagedorn M: *A Way of Life: A New Beginning Each Day. The Family's Lived Experience of Childhood Chronic Illness*. University Microfilms International, 1993.

Hall WA: A comparison of the experience of women and men in dual-earner families following the birth of their first infant. *Image* 1992; 24(1):33.

Hill RL: Modern systems theory and the family: A confrontation. In: *Sourcebook of Marriage and the Family*, 2nd ed. Sussman MB (editor). Boston: Houghton Mifflin, 1974.

Knafl KA: How families manage a pediatric hospitalization. *West J Nurs Res* 1985; 7:151.

Laird J: Lesbian and gay families. In: *Normal Family Processes*, 2nd ed. Walsh F (editor) New York: Guilford Press, 1993.

Leininger M: Transcultural care diversity and universality: A theory of nursing. *Nurs Health Care* 1985; 6:209.

Levin S, Idler E: *The Hidden Health Care System*. Cambridge, MA: Ballinger, 1981.

McCubbin H, Dahl B: *Marriage and Family: Individuals and Life Cycles*. New York: Wiley, 1985.

Minuchin S: *Families and Family Therapy*. Cambridge, MA: Harvard Univ Press, 1974.

Moos RW, Moos BS: A typology of family social environments. *Fam Process* 1976; 15:357.

Pakizegi B: Emerging family forms: Single mothers by choice—Demographic and psychosocial analysis. *Maternal-Child Nurs* 1990; 19(1):1.

Patterson C: Children of lesbian and gay parents. *Child Dev* 1992; 63:1025.

Pies C: Lesbians and the choice of parents. In: *Homosexuality and Family Relations*. Bozett F, Sussman M (editors). New York: Harrington Park Press, 1990.

Rempusheski V: Role of the extended family in parenting: A focus on grandparents of preterm infants. *J Perinatal Neonatal Nurs* 1990; 4(2):43.

Ritzer G: *Contemporary Sociological Theory*. New York: Knopf, 1983.

Roberts C, Feetman S: Assessing family functioning across three areas of relationships. *Nurs Res* April 1982; 231.

Ross B, Cobb KL: *Family Nursing: A Nursing Process Approach*. Redwood City, CA: Addison-Wesley, 1990.

Smilkstein G: The physician and family function assessment. *Fam Systems Med* Fall 1984; 263.

Speer J, Sachs B: Selecting the appropriate family assessment tool. *Ped Nurs* 1985; 11:349.

Stanhope M, Lancaster J: *Community Health Nursing: Process and Practice for Promoting Health*. St. Louis: Mosby, 1988.

Tripp-Reimer T: Retention of a folk health practice among four generations of urban Greek immigrants. *Nurs Res* 1983; 32:97.

Tulman L, Fawcett J: Maternal employment following childbirth. *Res Nurs Health* 1990; 13:181.

US Bureau of the Census: *Statistical Abstract of the United States*. Washington, DC: Government Printing Office, 1993.

Walker T: Mother-infant play. In: *Analysis of Current Assessment Strategies in the Health Care of Young Children and Childbearing Families*. Humenick S (editor). New York: Appleton-Century-Crofts, 1982.

Walsh F: Conceptualization of normal family process. In: *Normal Family Process*, 2nd ed. Walsh F (editor). New York: Guilford Press, 1993.

CHAPTER 4

CLIENT TEACHING

I can remember my nursing instructor stressing the need to use every opportunity available to do patient teaching. She told me that, no matter how I felt inside, I was an expert to the patients I cared for unless I acted otherwise. I was afraid to try teaching at first, but I soon realized that people did trust me and believed I knew what I was talking about. I felt good about that, but I felt a tremendous sense of responsibility, too. I had to be sure that I gave only accurate information. Even today, years later, when I don't know something or I'm not sure, I always make it my practice to say, "I don't know the answer, but I will find out for you." And then I do just that!

OBJECTIVES

Delineate the political, sociocultural, and technologic issues that influence client teaching.

Contrast the behavioral, cognitive field, perceptual-existential, and information-processing theories about learning.

Compare the key concepts that form the basis of selected theories about the "ways of knowing" or assimilating knowledge.

Describe the key concepts about adult learners that form the basis of the andragogical model developed by Knowles (1984).

Summarize the actions an educator needs to take to effectively implement the teaching/learning process.

lient education affords nurses the opportunity to profoundly influence the health and well-being of those for whom they care. The direct impact of this teaching can be realized when a nursing mother knows that her baby's refusal to suck results from sleepiness, not rejection of her or when a new father smiles and cuddles his infant after successfully completing his first "solo" bath at home. In this text, in keeping with our philosophy of a shared, mutually respectful relationship between health care provider and the individual, this teaching, commonly referred to as "patient teaching," will be referred to as "client teaching" or as "health teaching" because improvement in or maintenance of health status is the primary purpose of the teaching nurses do.

Nursing theorists and educators have long recognized the importance of client teaching and have written about this topic since the middle 1800s (Redman 1993b; Smith 1987). Nightingale spoke of the importance of health and implied that nurses could teach their homebound patients how to achieve efficient drainage and cleanliness and obtain pure air, light, and pure water in her *Notes on Nursing* (1969). In the 1920s, Lavinia Dock praised Margaret Sanger's efforts to provide information to underserved women of that era (Church 1990). Hildegard Peplau emphasized that client teaching should be developed around the individual's wants and ability to use the information (Peplau 1952).

In the 1970s a rebirth or reemphasis on client education occurred in response to several factors, including a new emphasis on health and self-care; a change in attitude toward physicians; and a trend toward long-term, outpatient, home management of chronic illnesses such as diabetes, hypertension, and sickle cell disease, which required that individuals with chronic illnesses be knowledgeable about their condition and its treatment (Redman 1993a). Today this trend toward home management has become a "given" in the health care system, with hospitalization indicated only during crisis periods or to stabilize newly diagnosed conditions.

Childbearing families have traditionally been viewed as important recipients of health teaching to prepare them for the challenges and responsibilities of childrearing. In the past, health teaching was a major part of the postpartal care provided during a hospitalization that typically lasted 72 hours for a vaginal birth and 4 to 5 days for a cesarean birth. Currently, women with vaginal births are discharged within 24 hours or less, and women with cesarean births remain for about 3 days. Thus the time for health teaching is extremely limited, and nurses have to use every opportunity to share information creatively with the new family. Concurrently, the teaching nurses provide during prenatal visits assumes new importance in preparing the pregnant woman for the pregnancy itself and the postpartum period.

Because the nurse is a primary provider of health teaching, we have attempted to assist readers to identify important areas of teaching and have used a variety of approaches to help nurses identify what to teach and how to do so. Teaching cards, which can be removed from the book and carried in a pocket, are provided. These cards contain information about teaching a variety of specific topics such as exercise during pregnancy, fetal heart monitoring, and breast-feeding. The text also contains a series of detailed teaching guides. Many of the chapters, especially those focusing on normal pregnancy and birth, contain the subheading "Teaching for Self-Care." These sections address areas of teaching about a specific topic. Finally, because we are teachers, too, we have created a special feature entitled "Teaching Moments." This is designed to help the nurse be more effective and contains tips we have learned through our own nursing practice or from our nurse colleagues.

This chapter addresses the topic of teaching from both theoretical and practical perspectives. It is designed to provide a framework for the health teaching that is an essential component of the nurse's role in working with the childbearing woman and her family.

ISSUES IMPACTING CLIENT TEACHING

Current political, sociocultural, and technologic issues can all impact client teaching. Each of these issues creates potential concerns for the client educator.

Political Issues

Political influences affecting client education include the trend toward self-care responsibility for health; the current educational climate of empowerment; the changing emphasis on women's health; health care reform; and the issue of jurisdiction over client education or who decides what, how, and when the client needs to be taught. The novice educator needs to be aware that education is inherently a political process and includes much more than just teaching a circumscribed set of content to specific individuals (Bevis & Watson 1989).

An increased emphasis on health, a trend toward less reliance on health care professionals, and general challenges to authority have all contributed to motivating people to take responsibility for themselves in matters of health (Redman 1993a; Stanhope & Lancaster 1992). Self-responsibility requires that the individual receive timely, correct health information, not only to practice a healthier life-style, but to manage and/or correct problems of chronic illness. Nurses play an important role in providing people with the necessary knowledge and skills to promote self-care (Loreno & Drick 1990).

Another client teaching factor with potential political impact involves the current educational movement toward empowerment. The empowered student, whether in a formal educational institution or in a health teaching situation, makes decisions based on knowledge and past experiences. Empowered students and empowered participants in health education seek equality in the educational process. Empowerment becomes a political process when an oppressed group seeks freedom from domination partially through the educational process (Shor & Freire 1987). As a result of the changing educational process, nurses who participate in health teaching will strive to facilitate informed, knowledgeable choices rather than compliant patient behavior. Teaching content will be negotiated between client and educator, and responsibility will be shared (Fleming 1992).

Women's issues have emerged as major factors in health care education. Recognition of the lack of information specific to women has resulted in more research and new publications (Belenky et al 1986; Gilligan 1982; Littlefield 1986; The Boston Women's Health Book Collective 1992). Knowledge of past and present attitudes toward women as well as current, accurate information based on research with and about women will assist anyone who plans health teaching involving mothers, babies, and families.

Even before the recent national movement toward health care reform, the health care industry had responded to political and legislative pressure to reduce costs. This response included shortened hospital stays and increased use of outpatient surgery and community-based facilities. Reduced interaction time with health care professionals intensifies the need for effective, interactive teaching/learning methods that enable the nurse to provide necessary information and ensure that the individual has learned the essential material.

The question of who becomes the gatekeeper of client education contains many political overtones because both nurses and physicians do client teaching. Many nurses suggest that because client education is a professional expectation and an independent nursing function, nurses have a legal obligation to provide health teaching to their clients (Ali 1993; Annand 1993). Physicians will also assume responsibility for client teaching, especially in areas of diagnosis and treatment of disease.

Sociocultural Issues

Sociocultural issues impact the nurse-educator and the client because both bring their own socioeconomic background, personal values, and cultural beliefs to the situation. If nurses do not recognize their own personal belief system, they will not be aware of how those beliefs impact their approach to client teaching and care.

Many societies are multicultural and contain both a dominant culture and other, smaller cultural groups. The increased frequency of international travel has led to greater mixing of peoples (Wilkins 1993). Nurses increasingly interact with clients of many ethnic backgrounds. Because of this, simply translating educational or health promotional materials from one language to another may create problems. Pictures or illustrations appropriate to individuals from the original culture may be offensive to the people from the receiving culture. Nevertheless, certain materials, such as informed consent or authorization for specific procedures, need to be translated into other languages. Any translated materials should be reviewed by bilingual health care providers for accuracy, ease of use, and cultural sensitivity (Poss et al 1993).

The nurse-educator must be aware of cultural norms that are different from the nurse's own belief system. Beliefs and values may vary in terms of time orientation, religious beliefs, folk remedies, cultural healers, and language and communication methods. Sociocultural influences may include folk beliefs about health and illness such as those found in Table 4–1 for people of Hispanic and African descent (Hautman 1979).

Hispanic folk healers or practitioners may include family members, a *curandero* or *curandera*, an *espiritualista*, a *yerbero*, or a *sabador* (Hautman 1979). Family members who do folk healing are those who possess knowledge of medicine learned from others or by studying. *Curanderos* or *curanderas* have knowledge about herbs, diet, massage, and rituals. They may have had training or received curative powers as a gift from God. An *espiritualista* or spiritualist is born with the ability to analyze dreams and foretell the future. A *yerbero* knows about growing and prescribing herbs. A *sabador* uses massage and manipulation of bones and muscles (Hautman 1979).

For people of African descent a folk practitioner may be a spiritualist, a voodoo priestess, or an "old lady." The spiritualist, usually associated with a fundamentalist Christian church, has been called by God to help others. A voodoo priestess establishes a therapeutic milieu, uses herbs, and can cure illnesses caused by voodoo. An "old lady" gives advice for common illness; her knowledge has been obtained through successful life experiences (Hautman 1979).

Beliefs about health and illness develop from world views, or how one sees the world. Most cultural groups believe in one of three major world views: magicoreligious, scientific, or holistic (Boyle & Andrews 1989).

In the magicoreligious world view supernatural forces control the world and the people in it. The supernatural forces may be a god, several gods, or other powers. Elements of this belief are found in African, Caribbean, and many Hispanic cultures. Some Western religious groups, such as Christian Scientists, believe in healing through the power of prayer alone (Boyle & Andrews 1989).

The scientific world view depends on objective, mechanistic thought processes. In this model health and health attributes have to be observable and measurable to

TABLE 4-1   Folk Illnesses in Hispanic and African American Cultures

Hispanic Culture

Folk Illness	Etiology	Symptoms	Practitioner	Treatment
Susto (fright)	An individual experiences a stressful event at some time prior to the onset of symptoms. The stressor may vary from the death of a significant person to a child's nightmare to the inability to adequately fulfill social role responsibility. Children are more susceptible to *susto* than adults. It is believed that the soul or spirit leaves the body.	Restlessness during sleep Anorexia Depression Listlessness Disinterest in personal appearance	*Curandero* *Espiritualista* *Espiritista*	A ceremony is performed using branches from a sweet pepper tree and a candle. Motions that form a cross are performed by the ill person and curer. Three Ave Marias or credos (Apostle's Creed) are said.
Empacho	Bolus of undigested food adheres to the stomach or wall of the intestine. The cause may be the food itself, or it may be due to eating when one is stressed or not hungry.	Stomach pain Diarrhea Anorexia	Family member *Sabador* *Curandero*	The stomach or back is massaged until a popping sound is heard. A laxative may be given.
Caida de la mollera (fallen fontanelle)	Trauma—a fall or blow to the head or the rapid dislodging of a nipple from an infant's mouth—causes the fontanelle to be sucked into the palate.	Inability to suckle Irritability Vomiting Diarrhea Sunken fontanelle	Family member *Curandero*	One or more of these practitioners insert a finger into the child's mouth and push the palate back into place. The child is held by the ankles with the top of the head just touching a pan of tepid water for a minute or two. A poultice of soap shavings is applied to the fontanelle. Herb tea is administered.
Mal de ojo (evil eye)	A disease of magical origin cast by a person who is jealous or envious of another person or something the person owns. The evil eye is cast by the envious person's vision upon the subject, thereby heating the subject's blood and producing symptoms. Usually a beautiful child is envied or admired but is not touched by the admirer, and the evil eye can be inflicted. The admirer may not be aware of the damage done. If the child is admired and then touched by that person, the evil eye is not inflicted.	Fever Diarrhea Vomiting Crying without apparent cause	*Curandero* *Brujo*	An unbroken egg is passed over the body or the body is rubbed with the egg to draw the heat (fever) from it. Prayers such as the Our Father or Hail Mary may be said simultaneously with the passing of the egg. The egg is then broken in a bowl, placed under the head of the bed, and left there all night. By morning if the egg is almost cooked from the heat of the body, this is a sign that the sick person had the *mal de ojo*.
Mal Puesto (evil)	Illness caused by a hex put on by a *brujo*, witch, *curandero*, or other person knowledgeable about witchcraft.	Vary considerably Strange behavioral changes Labile emotions Convulsions	*Curandero* *Brujo*	Varies, depending on the hex.

African Culture

Folk Illness	Etiology	Symptoms	Practitioner	Treatment
High blood (too much blood)	Diet very high in red meat and rich food. Belief that high blood causes stroke.	Weakness Paralysis Vertigo Other behaviors related to stroke	Family member Friend Spiritualist Self (after referring to a zodiac almanac)	Lemon juice, vinegar, epsom salts, or other astringent food is taken internally to sweat out the excess blood. Treatment varies, depending on what is appropriate for each person according to the zodiac almanac.
Low blood (not enough blood—anemia is conceptualized)	Too many astringent foods, too harsh a treatment for high blood. Remaining on high blood pressure medication for too long.	Fatigue Weakness	Same as for high blood	Rich red meat, raw beets are eaten. Treatment for high blood is stopped and the zodiac almanac is consulted.
Thin blood (predisposition to illness)	Occurs in women, children, or old people. Blood is very thin until puberty. It remains so until old age for women. May become thin in old men.	Greater susceptibility to illness	Individual	Individual should exercise caution in cold weather by wearing warm clothing or by staying indoors.
Rash appearing on a child after birth (no specific disease name —the concept is that of body defilement)	Impurities within the body coming out. The body is always being defiled and will therefore produce skin rashes.	Rash anywhere on the body; may be accompanied by fever	Family member	Catnip tea as a laxative or other commercial laxative is taken. The quality and kind depend on the age of the individual.
Diseases of witchcraft, "hex", or conjuring	Envy and sexual conflict are the most frequent causes of having someone hex another person.	Unusual behavior Sudden death Symptoms related to poisoning (ie, foul taste, falling off [weight loss], nausea, vomiting) A crawling sensation on the skin or in the stomach Psychotic behavior	Voodoo priest(ess) Spiritualist	*Conja* is the help given to the conjured person. Treatment varies, depending on the spell cast.

SOURCE: Adapted from Hautman MA: Folk health and illness beliefs. *Nurs Pract* 1979; 4(4):23.

TABLE 4-2 Cultural Beliefs About Activity and Pregnancy

Prescriptive Beliefs	Restrictive Beliefs	Taboo
Remain active during pregnancy to aid the baby's circulation. (Crow Indian)	Avoid cold air during pregnancy. (Mexican, Haitian, Asian)	Avoid lunar eclipses and moonlight, or the baby may be born with a deformity. (Mexican)
Remain happy to bring the baby joy and good fortune. (Pueblo and Navajo Indian)	Do not reach over your head, or the cord will wrap around the baby's neck. (African American, Hispanic, European American, Asian)	Don't walk on the streets at noon or five o'clock, or the spirits may become angry. (Vietnamese)
Sleep flat on your back to protect the baby. (Mexican)	Avoid weddings and funerals, or you will bring bad fortune to the baby. (Vietnamese)	Don't join in traditional ceremonies like Yei or Squaw dances, or spirits will harm the baby. (Navajo Indian)
Keep active during pregnancy to ensure a small baby and an easy labor. (Mexican)	Do not continue sexual intercourse, or harm will come to you and the baby. (Vietnamese, Filipino, Samoan)	Don't get involved with persons who cast spells, or the baby will be eaten in the womb. (Haitian)
Continue sexual intercourse to lubricate the birth canal and prevent dry labor. (Haitian, Mexican)	Do not tie knots or braid or allow the baby's father to do so, or you will have difficult labor. (Navajo Indian)	Don't say the baby's name before the naming ceremony, or harm might come to the baby. (Orthodox Jewish)
Continue daily baths and frequent shampoos during pregnancy to produce a clean baby. (Filipino)	Do not sew. (Pueblo Indian, Asian)	Don't have your picture taken because it might cause a stillbirth. (African decent)

SOURCE: Adapted from Boyle J and Andrews M: *Transcultural Concepts in Nursing Care.* Glenview, IL: Scott, Foresman/Little, Brown, 1989.

be real. This biomedical model, ascribed to by most of the dominant American cultural group, places greater importance on physical and chemical interventions than human relationships (Boyle & Andrews 1989).

The holistic health belief model stresses natural balance and harmony. "Everything in the universe has a place and a role to perform according to natural laws that maintain order. Disturbing these laws creates imbalance, chaos, and disease" (Boyle & Andrews 1989, p 29). Holistic world views are found in the American Indian and Asian cultures, for example. Two common metaphors for this belief system include the Chinese concept of yin and yang and the hot/cold theory of disease found in Asian, Hispanic, African, Arabic, Muslim, and Caribbean cultures. Yin, the feminine universal force, encompasses darkness, cold, the negative, inactivity, and emptiness. As an opposite, yang, the masculine force, is characterized by the positive, fullness, light, activity, and warmth (Babcock & Miller 1994; Boyle & Andrews 1989). Certain organs and health conditions are considered to be either yin or yang. Illness results from an imbalance between the two forces. Cancer, menstruation, and wasting are attributed to yin, for example; constipation, infection, and hangovers are characterized as yang conditions. The hot/cold theory of disease also includes the idea of balance, in this instance, between hot and cold humors (body fluids). Certain diseases, such as cancer, paralysis, and earache, are cold conditions and need hot medicine or food. Example of hot foods include gingerroot, cinnamon, and cod-liver oil (Giger & Davidhizar 1991).

In addition to health belief models and folk healing beliefs many cultures have specific beliefs about pregnancy, which may influence client teaching. Some of these beliefs are shown in Table 4–2.

In order to obtain pertinent client information, the nurse should always ask cultural assessment questions. Questions similar to those identified in Table 4–3 help both the nurse and the client identify important cultural issues that relate to health teaching. If nurses do not assess and honor cultural differences when teaching, the client will probably follow familiar practices and beliefs rather than attempt new approaches. A comprehensive coverage of cultural concepts is beyond the scope of this chapter; the reader is referred to several excellent texts listed in the References at the end of this chapter for more in-depth information.

Technologic Issues

In addition to political and sociocultural issues, technologic concerns also affect health teaching. Technologic aspects of client education involve issues of literacy as well as the explosion of knowledge and the transmission of information. Literacy pertains to the ability to read and write, but today can also be extended to basic knowledge of computers. Nurse-educators have the ability and technologic access to convey information through many different modalities. Therefore the educator should assess the client's literacy for the medium to be used.

TABLE 4-3	Suggested Cultural Questions for a Prenatal Assessment

Do you identify with either a particular ethnic group or a specific race?

Do you have beliefs and practices concerning pregnancy or birth that you learned while you were growing up?

Are there any practices or circumstances that you believe might harm you or your baby?

What foods do you believe to be important during your pregnancy (postpartum or during breastfeeding)?

Do you use or plan to use any type of cultural healers/practitioners or healing practices as part of your care?

Nurses also incorporate technology into their care on a daily basis and do not always consider how a piece of familiar equipment may appear to the individual for whom it is being used. In many cases the nurse's teaching about the technology being used puts the client at ease and enhances care.

One of every five adult Americans can be considered functionally illiterate, that is, reading at or below fifth grade level (Redman 1993b). Some strategies that can be used with these clients include presenting survival skills or essential information first; other information can be presented later. Each point should be made clearly, concisely, and vividly. Using simple language and examples can help the individual remember verbal information. Whenever possible, visuals such as line drawings are used. All written material should have large type and a simple format and be written at fifth grade level. Teaching is most effective if the nurse rehearses, demonstrates, and reviews all materials (Barnes 1992; Redman 1993b).

When using any type of technologic tool, such as a computer, to present information, the nurse must ascertain that the client has some comfort with the entire process and is not afraid, for example, of destroying the program or the computer by a keyboard stroke. Computer literacy is not necessary for the client to use the technology, but clear directions and a basic understanding of program usage are critical.

Technology has transformed health care, but many people are reluctant to reveal how frightening or incomprehensible they find a piece of machinery such as a fetal monitor. The nurse can create a teaching moment by showing the mother that her baby's heart rate varies from minute to minute and then reassuring her that this variability is desirable. Similarly, when the nurse shows the father how the monitor strip measures the contraction that he can feel when he places his hand on the mother's abdomen during labor, teaching takes place.

PRINCIPLES AND ASSUMPTIONS ABOUT TEACHING AND LEARNING

Learning implies change, or at least having the information to make a choice about whether or not to change one's thoughts or behavior. Daloz (1986) discusses the educational process as a transformative journey. Nurses can assist clients to learn the information needed to decide whether to transform a behavior, belief, or attitude. Most instructional practices are based on educational learning theories (Redman 1993b). Learning theory has evolved over time, and, as noted by Babcock and Miller (1994), theories help one make sense of observations and provide a way to examine observations and relationships. Theory-based teaching helps the nurse organize thinking and plan actions. Theoretical dimensions of learning include learning theories, ways of knowing, and assumptions about learners.

Theories About Learning

Current learning theories include behavioral, Gestalt or cognitive field, perceptual-existential, and information-processing theories.

Early learning theories, probably first conceptualized by Aristotle, focused on associating similar things and remembering them. This idea of associating similar things centuries later led to the school of thought entitled *behaviorism*. Through experimentation, Thorndike found that the learner remembered positive responses, acquired reinforced behaviors, and rejected behaviors that were not rewarded. Behaviorists believe that learning, or behavioral change, results from conditioning. Conditioning occurs when a stimulus and the resulting response lead to a certain pattern of behavior. For example, if a woman in early pregnancy learns that nausea (the stimulus) is reduced when she eats dry crackers before getting out of bed in the morning (response), she will probably remember to place crackers at her bedside before going to sleep.

Key terms in behaviorism include reinforcement, shaping, and extinction. "Reinforcement" involves giving a positive or negative reward in response to a behavior. A statement such as "You're doing great with your breathing" is positive reinforcement to the laboring mother. "Shaping" implies that the reinforcement becomes intermittent and then fades away as the desired behavior becomes established. Teaching the first-time mother to breastfeed uses shaping techniques with the nurse being initially involved with each step and reinforcing behavior, then gradually withdrawing as the mother gains confidence. "Extinction" occurs when no reinforcement occurs. When not rewarded, behavior tends to gradually decrease. Ignoring a child's temper tantrum, for example, may result in extinction of the behavior.

Gestalt or cognitive field theory is based on the premise that the learner is ready to perceive events in a new way. The term "Gestalt" means totality or the whole. This theory suggests that the whole is far more than simply the sum of its parts, so it is not possible to understand a given event or perception by reducing it into parts. This perspective incorporates both the learner and the learning context, which includes all the learner's perceptions and experiences (Babcock & Miller 1994). For example, parents who have never been in a hospital may consider a skin probe and a cardiac monitor taped to their preterm infant frightening, but the nurse caring for the infant sees them as simple and noninvasive tools. To Gestaltists and cognitive field theorists learning is a process in which the learner progresses in ability from simple recall to combining and synthesizing information to form new ideas. Learning eventually becomes the basis for problem solving (Whitman et al 1992).

A third type of learning theory, *humanistic or perceptual-existential*, integrates cognitive and behavioral concepts. It says that learning depends on the learner's actions, thoughts, and feelings. Behavioral change occurs when perceptions are modified. Learning necessitates total involvement by the learner—emotionally, intellectually, and physically. Learning should be self-directed; produce knowledgeable, caring learners; and be valued for its own sake (Babcock & Miller 1994).

The last learning theory under consideration, *information processing*, examines how information is encoded and remembered (Babcock & Miller 1994; Lesgold & Glaser 1989). There are short-term and long-term memory. Short-term memory consists of primary and working memory. As the first stage of the processing system, primary memory is transient because the contents are constantly displaced by incoming information. However, some information is moved to working memory. The working memory serves as an entry to the long-term memory and has a capacity for only a few items. Long-term memory may be of unlimited capacity and includes all the stored information the learner retains for more than a few seconds. This long-term memory provides the basis for learned skills and knowledge. Several subsystems are contained in long-term memory. For example, procedural memory stores routines that constitute skills and habits. Episodic memory contains temporal and situational contexts of events. Semantic or categorical memory includes meanings, facts, and rules independent of context. In a teaching situation the client's episodic memory might help her remember terms such as "placenta" and "fetal heart tones" from a prenatal class; semantic memory would provide more abstract information such as how nutrients get from the mother to the fetus (Lesgold & Glaser 1989).

Critical Thinking Question

Which of the learning theories just presented make the most sense to you? Why?

Ways of Knowing

Learning theories focus on intellectual functions and acquiring information, but several different "ways of knowing" or assimilating knowledge have also been described. Some of the most widely accepted models of how we use things such as experience and intuition to integrate what we know are described in this section.

Experiential Learning

Kolb (1984) described learning as a process in which knowledge is constructed from experience (Laschinger 1990). According to Kolb (1984), learners progress through four levels or learning modes. Stage one involves concrete experience, stage two incorporates the reflective phase of placing the experience in perspective, stage three consists of the abstraction of the experience to formulate concepts and generalizations, and stage four encompasses active experimental learning through formulating and testing hypotheses. Not all experiences call for the highest stage of learning, and exposure to different learning environments and other personal factors can help individuals develop a preferred learning style that incorporates more than one learning mode.

One type of learner, the *diverger*, combines concrete experiences and reflective observation to generate ideas and examine situations from several perspectives. The diverger often prefers discussion and group work. *Assimilators* develop meaningful conceptualizations of experience through reflective observation and abstract conceptualization; they like to study theoretical perspectives. A *converger* blends abstract conceptualizations with active experimentation to look for single solutions to problems. The converger tends to favor demonstrations and diagrams. The *accommodator*, using concrete experience and active experimentation, tends to rely on instinctual solutions, and enjoys demonstrations and question and answer sessions (Haggard 1989; Kolb 1984; Laschinger 1990).

Because individuals have different learning styles, they prefer to give and/or receive information in certain ways. Client educators need to be aware of the different ways individuals translate experience into knowledge because they will tend to use their favorite styles, which may or may not be the learner's preferred style.

Women's Ways of Knowing

To uncover women's ways of knowing, Belenky and her colleagues (1986) interviewed 135 women. They found that these learners progressed through five roles: the silent knower, the received knower, the subjective knower, the procedural knower, and the constructed knower.

Silent knowers perceive words as weapons to separate and diminish people. These women view themselves as seen but never heard and consider authority figures all-powerful. New nursing students sometimes feel like silent knowers before they can identify and define their abilities in nursing. *Received knowers* learn by listening and regard words as central to knowledge. They believe all knowledge originates outside of the self and listen to and repeat information from authority figures. The received knower can teach others, but only using the information provided by "experts." *Subjective knowers* have found an inner voice and have become their own authority. A pervasive theme of loss of trust in male authority due to sexual harassment and abuse exists in the stories of the subjective knower. Reliance on self has been established; truth and knowledge are viewed as personal, private, and intuitive. The subjective knower needs time to process new information and evaluate it against self-knowledge. *Procedural knowers*, usually college students or graduates, have incorporated the voice of reason. These women have acquired and applied procedures for obtaining and communicating knowledge. Method and objectivity have replaced intuition. Procedural knowers may be fascinated with proficient technique or correct sequencing for needed skills. *Constructed knowers* have integrated these methods. They construct their own reality by combining known procedure with knowledge they have generated. Constructed knowers have the capacity to empathize with others, regardless of their way of knowing.

Whatever their developmental level of knowing, women need confirmation of the self as knower. Whereas for men confirmation is important at the end of an educational process, for women "confirmation and community are prerequisites rather than consequences of development" (Belenky et al 1986, p 194). These authors point out that women do best with "connected teaching" in which the expert explores the learner's needs and abilities and constructs a message that is courteous to her.

Nurses' Ways of Knowing

Carper (1978) identified the patterns of knowing in nursing. These include empirics, ethics, personal knowing, and aesthetics.

Empiric knowledge describes or explains information through objective data. Many nurses use this pattern of knowing as the only method of conveying knowledge.

Ethical knowledge focuses on developing moral choices and value judgments, an area rarely addressed in client teaching, partially to avoid imposing value judgments on the client. However, nurses need to remember that unless learners are empowered to make their own decisions, they are vulnerable to implicit value statements of the right or wrong way to feel or behave contained in many teaching materials and presentations.

Personal knowing encompasses the capability of growth and realization of potential through self-knowledge. Authenticity and honesty enable the self to evaluate and change. Educators need to allow the client room to develop personal knowledge and grow as a result of the educational experience.

Aesthetic knowing embraces the art of nursing and is based on a "direct feeling of experience" (Carper 1978, p 17). Aesthetic knowing enables individuals to compare new knowledge with prior, personal experience. Nurses can integrate this pattern into their teaching by relating information to a client's previous experiences whenever possible. This form of knowing also involves intuition, an area addressed by both Benner and Noddings.

Noddings (Noddings & Glaser 1984) and Benner (1984) both recognize *intuition* as a way of knowing. Noddings indicates that once the urge to control and impose is put aside, one can become intentionally receptive to intuition. This intuitive mode of knowing is oriented toward understanding, as opposed to the analytic mode, which is goal oriented.

Benner (1984) describes the expert nurse as having intuitive knowledge about what actions to take in certain situations. This intuitive knowledge arises from years of experience. Intuitive judgment includes six aspects: pattern recognition, similarity recognition, commonsense understanding, skilled know-how, a sense of salience, and deliberative rationality (Leddy & Pepper 1989). A sense of salience refers to recognizing particularly significant situations, and deliberative rationality involves using analytic interpretation of past experiences to interpret findings. Expert nurses who rely on an intuitive way of knowing may have difficulty describing how they know something, but will often state "It just feels right."

> *I've worked in the high-risk nursery for 6 years now, and I really take pride in focusing on families and in helping them understand the purposes of the equipment we use and the procedures we do with the little ones. I want the families to feel that we are a team. Sometimes it is hard though. I remember trying to explain to one father, a physicist, why his prematurely born son needed to be under an oxygen hood. He kept interrupting me, asking me to tell him the partial pressure of oxygen. I tried to get him to laugh by joking that he probably knew more than I did about the partial pressure of oxygen and then asked him to just let me explain. Still he interrupted. Finally I realized that his reaction was the only way he knew to control what to him was an uncontrollable situation. Once I realized this, I quit trying to explain and turned the conversation to the shock of the preterm birth and the feelings people often have. I could see that talking about his feelings was very hard for him, but finally he did, at least a little.*

The nurse quoted above based much of her reaction to the father on aesthetic or intuitive knowing. In doing so she drew on internalized prior experiences. She did not rely on objective data; she sensed the problem.

Assumptions About Adult Learners

Knowles (1984) developed a theory of adult learning, which he termed *andragogy*, as opposed to pedagogy, the art and science of teaching as it applies to children. As part of his theory, he identified several assumptions about adult learners and how they best learn. Other theorists have expanded on his ideas. Recognizing and using these principles or assumptions will help nurses plan and use effective teaching designs.

Knowles (1984) described five areas in which adult learners differ from children: self-concept, experience, readiness to learn, orientation to learning, and motivation. The andragogic model assumes that adults have developed a *self-concept* of being responsible for their own decisions and their own lives. They need to be seen and treated by others as being capable of self-direction. The role of the learner's *experience* is important in that adults come to an educational activity with substantially more and very different experiences than a child. If their experiences are ignored or devalued, adults may perceive that not only have the experiences been rejected, but they have also been rejected as people. Adults become *ready to learn* when they see a need to know based on real-life situations, that is, when they need to be able to cope effectively. The *orientation to learning* for an adult is task centered or reality based, as opposed to subject centered. Adults are *motivated to learn* by external motivators such as the opportunity for a better job, but more compelling motivators come from internal pressures such as increased job satisfaction, self-esteem, or improved quality of life.

Other important assumptions about learning and learners relate to repetition, control, active participation, feedback, and organization (Babcock & Miller 1994; Van Hoozer et al 1987). *Repetition* and practice, especially when applied to tasks, help the learner remember. Having some *control* over the method and/or content facilitates learning for adults. *Active participation* enhances concept formation and improves learning. Immediate, positive *feedback* reinforces behavior. *Organization* of content can promote or hamper the learning process. Consideration of all these assumptions about the learner will enable a nurse to expedite the learning process.

TEACHING GUIDELINES

When an occasion for teaching arises, the nurse-educator needs to assess the situation, develop and present the teaching session, and examine the outcome to determine what changes, if any, need to be made. Each of these steps is important to the teaching/learning process.

Assessing the Situation

Several areas should be assessed prior to beginning a session. Essential categories include assessing the learner, evaluating oneself, and examining the setting. Even if the teaching session is spontaneous, the nurse will have a better outcome by assessing these three areas before beginning the session.

Assessment of the learner's readiness to learn consists of appraisal of the individual's health status, belief system including cultural background and values, developmental level, and past experiences (Whitman et al 1992). Evaluation of the learner's health status incorporates a perception of personal health, degree of physical comfort, extent of anxiety, energy level, and sensory abilities such as hearing and vision. An uncomfortable individual may have difficulty attending to new information. One's belief system encompasses health values, cultural influences, and presumed degree of control over one's own health. The learner's developmental level entails psychosocial development, ability to comprehend both verbal and written materials, and physical and cognitive maturity. Past experiences such as prior involvement with a health care environment or interactions with health care professionals may influence one's perceived need for education.

In addition to assessing learners, a nurse should also assess their personal abilities, knowledge, and values as they relate to the situation. After examining values and identifying potential strengths and limitations, the nurse-educator has a better idea of how to proceed with a teaching situation. Otherwise the nurse may either allow personal values to shade the presentation or attempt a teaching session without adequate knowledge.

The final step of assessing the situation includes examining the setting. Whether it is in a client's room or a more public area, the setting should afford privacy. The individual should be able to ask questions and receive information without feeling embarrassed. The immediate environment should be comfortable and quiet, so potential distractions are kept to a minimum. If a formal or group presentation is planned, everyone should be able to see both the presenter and any audiovisual aids. Prior to planning a group learning session, the educator should know what resources are available in the intended setting.

Creating the Teaching Session

Once the learner, self, and setting have been assessed, the nurse can develop the teaching session. Common elements include designing or planning the educational experience, developing the session through the selection of appropriate strategies, and evaluating the effectiveness of the session.

Designing the Educational Experience

Designing or planning a teaching session entails deciding about types of objectives or learning goals, determining subject content, and selecting the organizational pattern of the presentation. Even with a short teaching moment, nurses need to design or plan how to present the information.

The teaching session can be developed around behavioral objectives, teaching goals, or jointly developed teaching/learning outcomes (Bevis & Watson 1989; Redman 1993b). If behavioral objectives are used, they should be stated from the learner's perspective and focus, in measurable terms, on what the learner should be able to do, know, or feel after completion of instruction. Similarly, learning goals focus on identifying an outcome of the teaching/learning sessions from the learner's perspective. Jointly developed teaching/learning outcomes identify the outcome from the perspectives of both the teacher and the learner. Whichever option is selected—behavioral objectives, learning goals, or teaching/learning outcomes—they should be clearly identified by the teaching nurse.

Decisions about subject content or what to teach can be clarified by doing either a task description or a content analysis. A task description entails delineating how a task is performed step by step and can be used to determine that important information has not been left out. A content analysis examines specific subject material for fundamental underlying facts, concepts, and principles. By separating important from irrelevant information, the educator can determine essential content.

Preterm births account for 60% of perinatal morbidity and mortality. Because many women at risk for preterm birth are hospitalized and available for client education, Annette Gupton and Maureen Heaman designed a study to examine the learning priorities of these women. The convenience sample of 34 participants consisted of hospitalized women at risk for preterm birth. Reasons for hospitalization included spontaneous preterm rupture of membranes (12), twin pregnancy with dilation and/or contractions (6), antepartum hemorrhage (4), and other less frequent conditions.

The authors used a questionnaire developed for this study to collect data. The participants were asked to rate 18 categories of information commonly incorporated into educational programs designed for women at risk for preterm birth. Four open-ended questions asked the women about: (1) other information they needed, (2) their concerns, (3) information that they did not feel they needed, and (4) what they would tell a friend or relative to help her cope with being at risk for preterm birth. The questionnaire was evaluated for content validity but reliability scores were not reported.

Data analysis included both descriptive statistics and content analysis. The two most important categories of information for this group of women included: (1) wanting to know the consequences of prematurity for the baby, and (2) problems of the newborn associated with preterm birth. The open-ended questions elicited the women's expressions of the need to know the possible risks or complications for the baby, and the need to be reassured or receive assistance with coping. When asked what information was not needed, the women requested all available information. Several also requested complete honesty. They said they would tell a friend in this situation to rest and relax, to trust the health care system, and to keep herself informed.

Clinical Application of the Study

In order to meet client educational needs, nurses need to assess what information the client believes to be important and has the desire or motivation to learn. The authors note that many preterm birth prevention programs focus on defining preterm labor, risk factors, and how to palpate contractions. The women in this study voiced concern about the consequences of preterm birth for their babies and the need for reassurance. These concerns and anxieties need to be addressed before introducing other content.

SOURCE: Gupton A, Heaman M: Learning needs of hospitalized women at risk for preterm birth. *Appl Nurs Res* 1994; 7(3):118.

Learners need stability, order, pattern, and predictability in order to cope effectively with learning (Van Hoozer et al 1987). To develop a useful teaching session, nurses need to choose, organize, and present information in a way that helps learning to occur. Useful organizational methods include proceeding from beginning to end, familiar to unfamiliar, simple to complex, concrete to abstract, specific to general, or general to specific. The method used depends on the desired outcome, the identi-fied subject matter, and the assessed characteristics of the learner.

In a formal or group session the educator may wish to prepare an advanced organizer—a verbal summary, a written outline, a series of overhead transparencies, or a review and correlation of new content to previously learned material. For example, a review of previously learned material might consist of discussing how moss appears to be attached to a rock but can be peeled away with minimal damage to the moss. This concept is then related to the way the placenta peels away from the uterine wall and thus the mother's and baby's blood do not mix, but nutrients pass across the membrane. An advanced organizer is more abstract and general than the presentation but inclusive enough to help the learner organize content. Advanced organizers explicate and integrate the information to be presented. Whatever the organizational method, the session should be arranged to help the learner incorporate and retain new information.

Developing the Teaching Session

The development of the session partially depends on the objectives and organization of the content. Once these aspects of the session have been identified, the teacher can determine appropriate teaching strategies for delivering the information.

Teaching strategies are activities, materials, events, or techniques used to enable learners to attain knowledge or skills or develop or modify attitudes. They are used to motivate, stimulate critical thinking and problem solving, provoke a response, or evaluate the transfer of learning. The teaching strategy can be interactional, such as one-to-one instruction; it can be a method of conveying information, such as a video; or it can be an approach such as using an example to assist with learning. Strategies that can be used effectively for the identified purpose and that fit well with the teaching style of the instructor should be employed.

Teaching strategies can be either direct or indirect. A direct strategy involves face-to-face teacher interaction. Examples include lecture, demonstration, role playing, and discussion (Figure 4–1). Indirect strategies, such as the use of films, books, or games, provide vicarious or representative experiences, and the teacher's presence may not be required. Strategy selection is based on assessed learner needs, objectives or learning outcomes, teaching content, available resources, and teacher preference (Van Hoozer et al 1987). Table 4–4 identifies selected teaching strategies and their advantages and disadvantages.

Within a teaching session, comprehension is strongly affected by expectations. Regardless of the teaching strategy selected, a teacher should establish the "set" and accomplish closure within any teaching session. In a theater production the set develops atmosphere, establishes mood, and promotes viewer progression from scene to scene. In a teaching situation the set predisposes the

TABLE 4-4   Teaching Strategies: Advantages and Limitations

Strategy	Advantages	Limitations
Live, formal lecture with overhead transparencies or slides	Auditory and visual sensory input Same information delivered to large group of learners at one time Straightforward message delivery	Primarily one-way communication Immediate feedback and reinforcement limited or nonexistent
Discussion	Highly interactive Immediate feedback and reinforcement Flexible sequencing of information Branched organization of information	Lack of participation by some learners Message delivered to limited number of learners at one time Message not the same from one group or individual to another from time to time Primarily auditory input
Textbooks, readings	Same information conveyed to large group of learners at one time Flexible or fixed sequencing of information Highly portable Easy to repeat information	Visual input only Reading level may not be appropriate for all learners May lack immediate feedback and reinforcement
Live demonstration with return practice	Personalized role modeling Fixed or flexible sequencing of information Immediate feedback and reinforcement Active, overt, hands-on participation in learning	Not appropriate for large numbers of learners at one time Relatively expensive in terms of teaching time, equipment, and facility needs Scheduling problems
Computer assisted	Saves teaching and learning time Branched sequencing of information Immediate feedback and reinforcement Message easily repeated and manipulated Highly interactive Random access to information	Inadequate programming Scheduling problems Limited to one to three learners at a time Equipment expensive Backup needed in case of equipment failure
Video or 16 mm film of interview, lecture, or demonstration	Auditory, visual sensory input Fixed sequencing of information Saves teaching time Overcomes barriers of time, size, space, distance Conveys real action (motion) Message can be repeated Adaptable to group or individual	Learner dependent on equipment Rate and pace controlled by equipment Fixed sequencing of information Difficult to update and revise Equipment expensive; backup needed in case of malfunction Scheduling problems Usually lacks immediate feedback and reinforcement
Audioconferencing	Overcomes barriers of distance Flexible message delivery Highly interactive Immediate feedback and reinforcement Personalized Same information delivered to large group of learners at one time	Primarily auditory input Equipment malfunction Equipment and line time expensive Scheduling problems Message not easily repeated
2 × 2 slides	Easy to rearrange Fixed or flexible sequencing of information Adaptable to group or individual learning Multiple images can be displayed at one time Conveys realism Step-by-step disclosure of information	Still, visual input May lack immediate feedback and reinforcement Learner dependent on hardware May be lost or damaged by learners
Filmstrip	Fixed sequencing of information Step-by-step disclosure of information Adaptable to group or individual learning Message can be repeated Conveys realism	Still visual input Difficult and expensive to revise Learner dependent on hardware Easily damaged
Objects, models, mockups, simulators	Multisensory input Conveys realism Concrete, hands-on, overt participation in learning Immediate feedback and reinforcement	May oversimplify reality Damage, loss of parts Not suitable for large numbers of learners at same time
Teacher-directed clinical practicum	Real experiential learning Multisensory input Hands-on, overt participation in learning Immediate feedback and reinforcement Personalized	Limited to one-on-one or small groups of learners Facilities, scheduling problems Great amount of direct teaching time required

TABLE 4-4   continued

Strategy	Advantages	Limitations
Games, simulations, role play	Can be highly interactive or provide for independent participation in learning Consequences of actions realized Hands-on, overt participation in learning Immediate feedback and reinforcement Flexible sequencing of information Makes learning fun, rewarding Can simulate lifelike experiences	Some learners uncomfortable participating, especially in role playing. May oversimplify reality.
Modular instruction, learning activity packages	Multisensory input Can accommodate individual learning styles and preferences Facilitates mastery learning Step-by-step disclosure of information Highly organized Linear or branched organization of information Active, overt response Guided practice Easy to repeat information Learner can proceed at own rate and pace Objectives and procedures stated Immediate feedback and reinforcement	Instructor's management and record-keeping time great to track successful completion of modules or activities
Print programmed instruction (as in self-paced books)	Individualized Small, step-by-step disclosure of information Linear or branched organization of information Saves teaching and learning time Active, overt participation in learning Portable Easy to repeat Learner can proceed at own rate and pace Immediate feedback and reinforcement	Visual input only Readability may be a problem May foster boredom Allows learner procrastination

SOURCE: Adapted from Van Hoozer et al: *The Teaching Process: Theory and Practice in Nursing.* Norwalk, CT: Appleton-Century-Crofts, 1987.

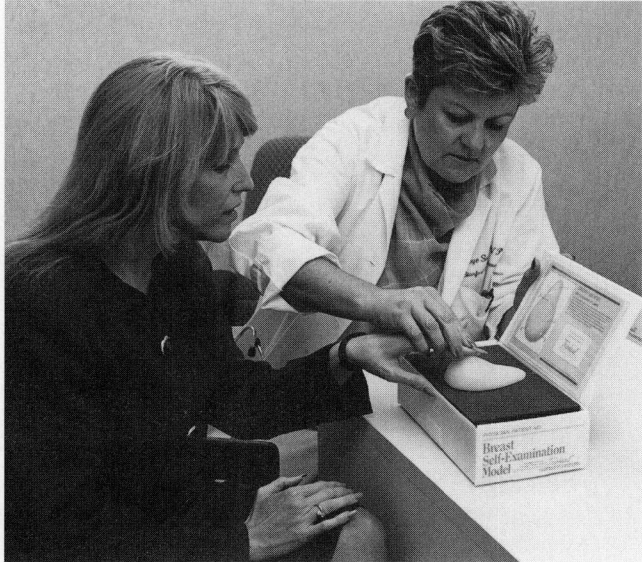

FIGURE 4-1   Teaching strategies that involve multiple forms of sensory input are most effective. In this case, the nurse explains breast self-examination and provides an opportunity for the woman to palpate a breast mass using a specially designed model.

learner to perceive information in a certain way. Establishing a set also helps learners achieve cognitive closure or make associations between old and new information (Van Hoozer et al 1987).

Set includes arousal, expectancy, and incentive. Arousal creates interest and focuses attention on the anticipated learning. Arousal requires capturing the audience's attention. Expectancy involves describing what the learner can anticipate with the learning experience. Incentive provides the motivation for attending to the session (de Tornyay & Thompson 1987). Set can be established through questions, such as asking a woman if she would like to know about specific information in a one-on-one teaching moment. In a group setting examples of set induction might include the use of short vignettes, role playing, or giving examples. Set "provides a common frame of reference, establishes a link between past and present messages, and facilitates transition to future messages" (Van Hoozer et al 1987, p 134).

Establishing set facilitates achieving closure. Closure means more than just a summary of what has been said. It involves combining old and new information, determining appropriateness, formulating associations, and transferring information to new learning experiences. Instructional closure occurs when the session is over and the instructor has linked new with old information. Cognitive closure results when the learner internally associates new with old knowledge. The teacher can achieve only instructional closure; cognitive closure happens within the individual learner.

Evaluating the Teaching Session

After assessing the situation and developing and presenting the teaching session, the nurse should evaluate the process. Evaluation consists of both formative and summative methods (Whitman et al 1992).

Formative evaluation assesses the process of the teaching session. It is continuous, allows for change, and provides ongoing feedback. Formative evaluation occurs when teachers ask themselves "How am I doing? Do they seem to be getting the information?" or checks with the participants about how they feel about the amount of information they have received. Peer evaluation or self-evaluation through the use of videotaping encompasses this type of evaluation because the entire process or session can be assessed. Any teaching session needs some preplanned, formative evaluation.

The second type of evaluation, summative evaluation, occurs after the teaching session. It can demonstrate behavioral change based on the teaching objectives or achievement of learning goals or outcomes. Summative evaluation can be accomplished by a variety of methods. Participants can be tested, although this is rarely practical in a clinical setting. Other effective methods include checklists to evaluate and document learning; interviews to discover knowledge; and observation of participants to ascertain development of psychomotor skills, alteration of health behaviors, or change in attitudes (Whitman et al 1992). All teaching sessions of more than momentary duration should have some type of summative evaluation.

KEY CONCEPTS

Although health-related teaching is commonly called "patient teaching," the term "client teaching" better reflects the notion of an equal partnership between the individual and the health care provider.

Political factors influencing client education include the trend toward self-care responsibility for health, the current educational climate of empowerment, the changing emphasis on women's health, the issue of jurisdiction over client education, and health care reform.

Sociocultural values profoundly influence clients' responses to health teaching.

Technologic tools such as computers can effectively enhance learning if the learner is comfortable with the process and not afraid of damaging the equipment.

Behavioral learning theory is based on concepts of positive responses, reinforced behavior, and rejected behavior, which work together to produce conditioning.

The information-processing learning theory is based on concepts regarding the ways information is remembered.

Different "ways of knowing" or assimilating knowledge have been described by theorists. Kolb called learning a process in which knowledge is developed from experience. Belenky addressed issues related to women's ways of knowing. Carper identified a framework based on types of knowledge used in nursing. Benner and Noddings addressed the concept of intuition as a way of knowing, especially as it relates to the expert nurse.

The andragogic model explores the characteristics of adult learners and the differences between them and younger learners. These differences involve self-concept, experience, readiness to learn, orientation to learning, and motivation.

When a teaching moment arises, the nurse-educator needs to assess the situation, develop and present the teaching situation, and examine or evaluate the outcome.

REFERENCES

Ali N: Preparing student nurses for patient education. *Nurse Educator* 1993; 18(2):27.

Annand F: A challenge for the 1990's: Patient education. *Today's OR Nurse* 1993; 15(1):31.

Babcock DE, Miller MA: *Client Education*. St. Louis: Mosby, 1994.

Barnes L: The illiterate client: Strategies in patient teaching. *MCN* 1992; 17(3):127.

Belenky M et al: *Women's Ways of Knowing: The Development of Self, Voice, and Mind*. New York: Basic Books, 1986.

Benner P: *From Novice to Expert*. Menlo Park, CA: Addison-Wesley, 1984.

Bevis E, Watson J: *Toward a Caring Curriculum: A New Pedagogy for Nursing*. New York: National League for Nursing, 1989.

Boyle J, Andrews M: *Transcultural Concepts in Nursing Care*. Glenview, IL: Scott, Foresman/Little, Brown, 1989.

Carper B: Fundamental patterns of knowing in nursing. *Advances Nurs Sci* 1978;1(1):13.

Church O: Nursing's history: What it was and what it was not. In: *The Nursing Profession: Turning Points*. Chaska N (editor). St. Louis: Mosby, 1990.

Daloz L: *Effective Teaching and Mentoring*. San Francisco: Jossey-Bass, 1986.

de Tornyay R, Thompson M: *Strategies for Teaching Nursing*. New York: Wiley, 1987.

Fleming V: Client education: A futuristic outlook. *J Adv Nurs* 1992; 17:158.

Giger J, Davidhizar R: *Transcultural Nursing*. St. Louis: Mosby-Year Book, 1991.

Gilligan C: *In a Different Voice*. Cambridge, MA: Harvard Univ Press, 1982.

Haggard A: *Handbook of Patient Education*. Rockville, MD: Aspen, 1989.

Hautman MA: Folk health and illness beliefs. *Nurse Pract* 1979; 4(4):23

Knowles D: *Andragogy in Action: Applying Modern Principles of Adult Learning.* San Francisco: Jossey-Bass, 1984.

Kolb D: *Experiential Learning.* Englewood Cliffs, NJ: Prentice Hall, 1984.

Laschinger H: Review of experiential learning theory research in the nursing profession. *J Adv Nurs* 1990;15:985.

Leddy S, Pepper JM: *Conceptual Bases of Professional Knowledge.* Philadelphia: Lippincott, 1989.

Lesgold A, Glaser R (editors): *Foundations for a Psychology of Education.* Hillsdale, NJ: Lawrence Erlbaum Associates, 1989.

Littlefield V: *Health Education for Women: A Guide for Nurses and Other Health Professionals.* Norwalk, CT: Appleton-Century-Crofts, 1986.

Loreno P, Drick C: Self-care identity formation: A nursing education perspective. *Holistic Nurs Pract* 1990; 4(2):79.

Nightingale F: *Notes on Nursing: What It Is, and What It Is Not.* New York: Dover, 1969.

Noddings N, Glaser R: *Awakening the Inner Eye: Intuition in Education.* New York: Teachers College Press, 1984.

Peplau H: *Interpersonal Relations in Nursing.* New York: Putnam's, 1952.

Poss R et al: Education literature for Hispanic patients. *Caring Magazine* February 1993; 104.

Rankin S, Stallings K: *Patient Education,* 2nd ed. Philadelphia: Lippincott, 1990.

Redman B: Patient education at 25 years. Where we have been and where we are going. *J Adv Nurs* 1993a; 18:725.

Redman B: *The Process of Patient Education,* 7th ed. St. Louis: Mosby-Year Book, 1993b.

Shor I, Freire P: *A Pedagogy for Liberation.* Granby, MA: Bergin & Garvey, 1987.

Smith C: *Patient Education: Nurses in Partnership with Other Health Professionals.* Orlando, FL: Grune & Stratton, 1987.

Stanhope M, Lancaster J: *Community Health Nursing: Process and Practice for Promoting Health.* St. Louis: Mosby-Year Book, 1992.

The Boston Women's Health Book Collective: *The New Our Bodies, Ourselves: A Book for and About Women.* New York: Touchstone, 1992.

Van Hoozer H et al: *The Teaching Process: Theory and Practice in Nursing.* Norwalk, CT: Appleton-Century-Crofts, 1987.

Whitman N et al: *Teaching in Nursing Practice.* Norwalk, CT: Appleton-Century-Crofts, 1992.

Wilkins H: Transcultural nursing: A selective review of the literature, 1985–1991. *J Adv Nurs* 1993; 18:602.

PART TWO

HUMAN REPRODUCTION

CHAPTER 5

THE REPRODUCTIVE SYSTEM

I always thought it was so boring to study anatomy and physiology. Who cares how many bones there are in the pelvis or the muscles involved. But now I'm with mothers having babies, and now it all makes sense.

~ A NURSING STUDENT ~

OBJECTIVES

Summarize the major changes in the reproductive system that occur during puberty.

Identify the structures and functions of the female and male reproductive systems.

Summarize the actions of the hormones that affect reproductive functioning.

Identify the two phases of the ovarian cycle and the changes that occur in each phase.

Describe the phases of the menstrual cycle, their dominant hormones, and the changes that occur in each phase.

Discuss the significance of specific female reproductive structures during childbirth.

*U*nderstanding childbearing requires more than understanding sexual intercourse or the process by which the female and male sex cells unite. One must also become familiar with the structures and functions that make childbearing possible and the phenomena that initiate it. This chapter considers the anatomic, physiologic, and sexual aspects of the female and male reproductive systems. Information regarding basic embryologic development is also presented in order to increase understanding of anatomy, physiology, and function. The psychosocial aspects of human sexuality are discussed in Chapter 9.

The female and male reproductive organs are *homologous*, that is, they are fundamentally similar in function and structure. The primary functions of both the female and male reproductive systems are to produce sex cells and to transport the sex cells to locations where their union can occur. The sex cells, called *gametes*, are produced by specialized organs called *gonads*. A series of ducts and glands within both the male and female reproductive systems contributes to the production and transport of the gametes.

EARLY DEVELOPMENT OF REPRODUCTIVE STRUCTURES AND PROCESSES

Although the genetic sex of an embryo is determined at fertilization, for about the first 8 weeks of gestation the male and female reproductive systems are undifferentiated. This undifferentiated period is followed by a period of rapid, dramatic changes as the reproductive organs differentiate into recognizable structures.

Ovaries and Testes

During the 5th week of gestation a primitive gonad arises from the intermediate mesoderm tissue known as gonadal ridges. The gonad develops a medulla (inner part of the organ) and cortex (outer part of the organ), which appear in the underlying mesenchyme (embryonic tissue from which connective and muscle tissue arises—Table 6–1). In genetic males during the 7th and 8th week the medulla develops into a testis, and the cortex regresses. In genetic females by about the 10th week the cortex develops into an ovary, and the medulla regresses.

Every egg available for maturation in a woman's reproductive life is present at her birth. During fetal life the ovary produces *oogonia*, cells that become primitive eggs called **oocytes,** by the process of **oogenesis** (see Chapter 6). No oocytes are formed after fetal development. About 150,000 oocytes are contained in the ovaries at birth

(Davies 1990). Each oocyte is contained in a small ovarian cavity called a *primitive follicle.*

Every month during a female's reproductive years one of the oocytes undergoes a process of cellular division and maturation that transforms it into a fertilizable egg, or **ovum.** At **ovulation** the ovum is released from its follicle. The remaining follicles and oocytes degenerate over time.

The testis produces the male gametes, called **spermatozoa** or *sperm*, by a process called **spermatogenesis.** This process will be described in Chapter 6. Spermatogenesis of mature sperm does not occur until the onset of puberty.

Figure 5–1 illustrates the embryologic development of the gonads and other internal reproductive organs.

Other Internal Structures

During the undifferentiated period—the first seven weeks—two pairs of genital ducts develop: the *mesonephric* and *paramesonephric* ducts.

In genetic females the fallopian tubes are formed from the unfused portions of the paramesonephric ducts, and the fused portions give rise to the epithelium and uterine glands. The endometrial stroma and the myometrium (thick layer of smooth muscle in the wall of the uterus) develop from the adjacent mesenchyme.

The vagina is derived from more than one embryologic structure. The vaginal epithelium develops from the endoderm of the urogenital sinus, and the musculature develops from the uterovaginal primordium.

The urethral and paraurethral glands develop from outgrowths of the urethra into the surrounding mesenchyme. Bartholin's glands arise from similar structures.

In genetic males the fetal testes secrete two hormones. The first, testosterone, stimulates the mesonephric ducts to develop into the male genital tract. The other hormone, müllerian regression factor, suppresses the development of the paramesonephric ducts, which would otherwise develop into the female genital tract.

From the mesonephric ducts comes development of the efferent ductule, vas deferens, epididymis, seminal vesicle, and ejaculatory duct. Both the prostate and the bulbourethral glands develop from endodermal outgrowths of the urethra.

External Structures

Genetic males and females possess the same external genitals until the end of the 9th week. By the 12th week differentiation of the external genitals is complete.

If fetal testosterone is not present, the indifferent external genitals are feminized. The phallus becomes the clitoris, and the urogenital folds remain open, forming

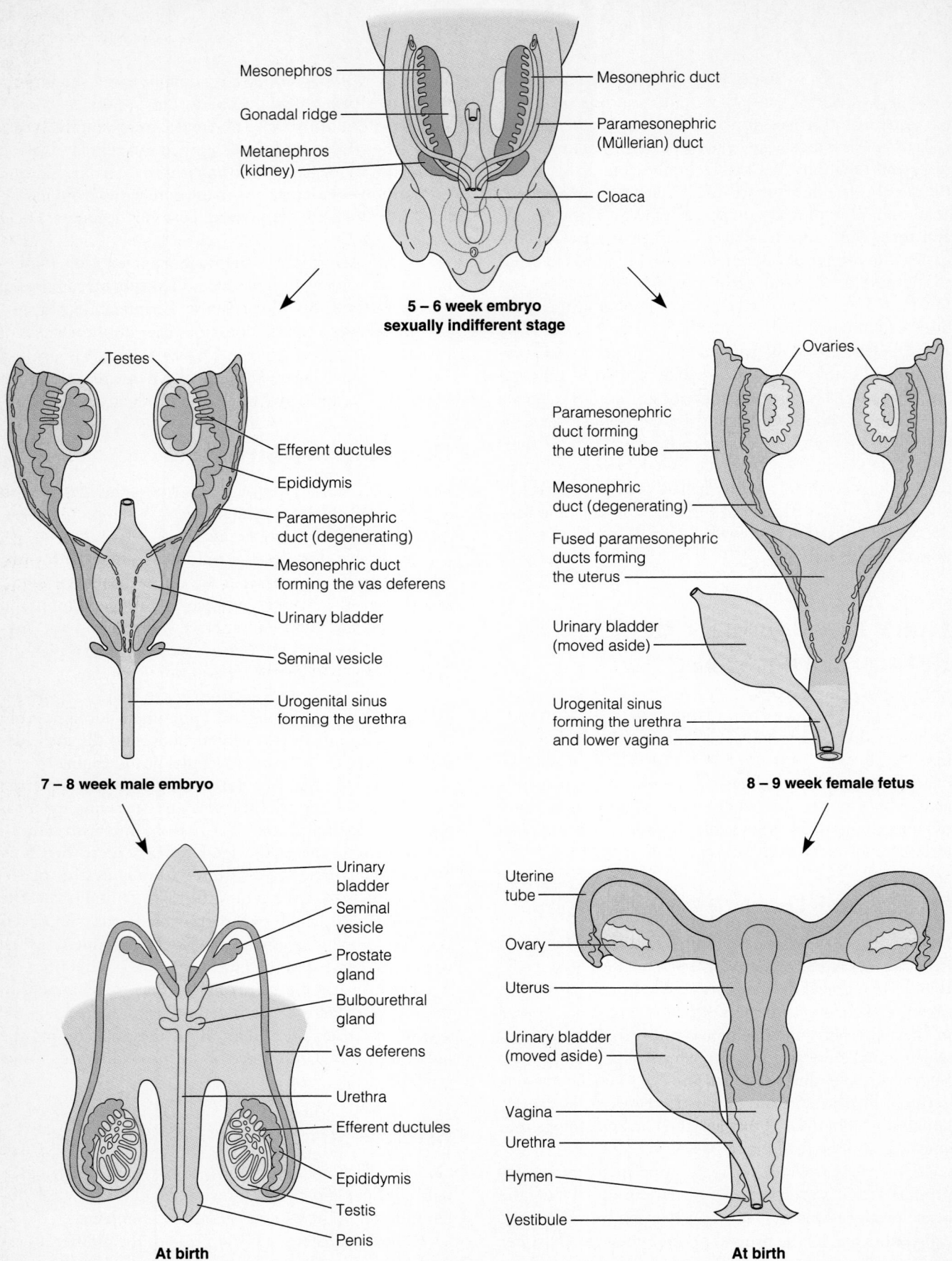

**5 – 6 week embryo
sexually indifferent stage**

Mesonephros

Gonadal ridge

Metanephros
(kidney)

Mesonephric duct

Paramesonephric
(Müllerian) duct

Cloaca

7 – 8 week male embryo

Testes

Efferent ductules

Epididymis

Paramesonephric
duct (degenerating)

Mesonephric duct
forming the vas deferens

Urinary bladder

Seminal vesicle

Urogenital sinus
forming the urethra

8 – 9 week female fetus

Ovaries

Paramesonephric
duct forming
the uterine tube

Mesonephric
duct (degenerating)

Fused paramesonephric
ducts forming
the uterus

Urinary bladder
(moved aside)

Urogenital sinus
forming the urethra
and lower vagina

At birth

Urinary
bladder

Seminal
vesicle

Prostate
gland

Bulbourethral
gland

Vas deferens

Urethra

Efferent ductules

Epididymis

Testis

Penis

At birth

Uterine
tube

Ovary

Uterus

Urinary bladder
(moved aside)

Vagina

Urethra

Hymen

Vestibule

FIGURE 5-1   Embryonic differentiation of male and female internal reproductive organs.

the labia minora. The labioscrotal folds form the labia majora.

If fetal testosterone is present, the indifferent external genitals become masculine. The phallus elongates, forming the penis. The fusion of the urogenital folds on the ventral surface of the penis forms the penile urethra, with the urethral meatus moving forward toward the glans penis.

PUBERTY

The term **puberty** refers to the developmental period between childhood and attainment of adult sexual characteristics and functioning. Its onset is never sudden, although it may appear so to parents or to the young person who is not prepared for the physical and emotional changes of puberty. Generally, boys mature physically about 2 years later than girls. In boys the age of onset of puberty ranges from 10 to 19 years; 14 years is the average age of onset. In girls the age of onset ranges from 9 to 17 years; 12 years is the average age of onset.

Puberty lasts from 1.5 to 5 years and involves profound physical, psychologic, and emotional changes. These changes include an altered body image, changing roles, and changing societal expectations and responses as the child matures to an adult.

Major Physical Changes

In both girls and boys, puberty is preceded by an accelerated growth rate called *adolescent spurt*. Widespread body system changes occur, including maturation of the reproductive organs.

Girls experience a broadening of the hips, then budding of the breasts, the appearance of pubic and axillary hair, and the onset of menstruation, called *menarche*. The average time between breast development and menarche is 2.3 years (Weiss & Goldsmith 1994).

Boys note such changes as an increase in the size of the external genitals; the appearance of pubic, axillary, and facial hair; the deepening of the voice; and nocturnal seminal emissions without sexual stimulation (mature sperm are not usually contained in these early emissions).

The physical changes of puberty present themselves differently in each person. The age at onset and progress of puberty vary widely, physical changes overlap, and the sequence of events can vary from person to person. This diversity results from people's different degrees of response to hormonal stimulation.

Physiology of Onset

Puberty is initiated by the maturation of the hypothalamic-pituitary-gonad complex (the *gonadostat*) and input from the central nervous system. The process, which begins during fetal life, is sequential and complex.

The central nervous system releases a neurotransmitter that stimulates the hypothalamus to synthesize and release **gonadotropin-releasing factor (GnRF)** (Tanner 1990). GnRF is transmitted to the anterior pituitary, where it causes the synthesis and secretion of the gonadotropins **follicle-stimulating hormone (FSH)** and **luteinizing hormone (LH)** (as seen in Figure 5–2).

Although the gonads do produce small amounts of **androgens** (male sex hormones) and **estrogens** (female sex hormones) before the onset of puberty, FSH and LH stimulate increased secretion of these hormones. Androgens and estrogens influence the development of secondary sex characteristics. FSH and LH stimulate the processes of spermatogenesis and maturation of ova.

Other hormones are involved in the onset of puberty. Although less direct, their action is essential. Abnormally high or low levels of adrenocorticotropic hormone (ACTH), thyroid hormone, or growth hormone (GH) can disrupt the onset of normal puberty (Tanner 1990).

FEMALE REPRODUCTIVE SYSTEM

The female reproductive system consists of the external and internal genitals and accessory organs of the breasts. The structure of the bony pelvis is also discussed in this section because of its importance in childbearing.

External Genitals

All the external reproductive organs, except the glandular structures, can be directly inspected. The size, color, and shape of these structures vary extensively among races and individuals.

The female external genitals, referred to as the **vulva** or *pudendum*, include the following structures (Figure 5–3):

- Mons pubis
- Labia majora
- Labia minora
- Clitoris
- Urethral meatus and opening of the paraurethral (Skene's) glands
- Vaginal vestibule (vaginal orifice, vulvovaginal glands, hymen, and fossa navicularis)
- Perineal body

Although they are not true parts of the female reproductive system, the urethral meatus and perineal body are considered here because of their proximity and relationship to the vulva.

The vulva has a generous supply of blood and nerves and is influenced by estrogenic hormones. As a woman ages, estrogen secretions decrease, causing the vulvar organs to atrophy and become subject to a variety of lesions.

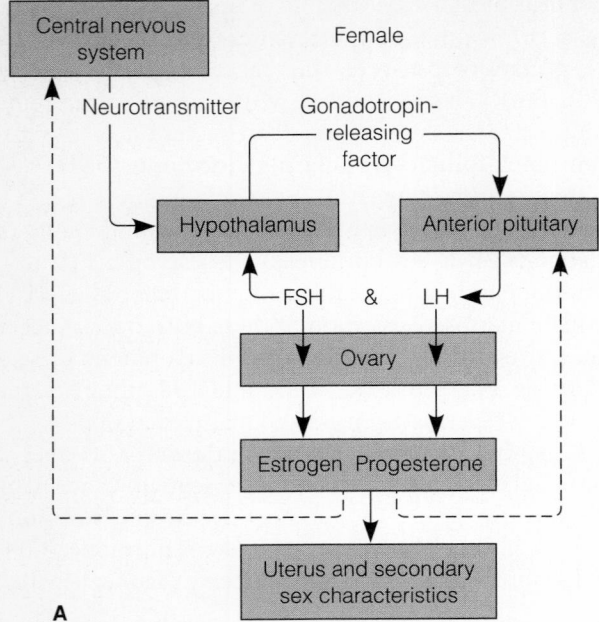

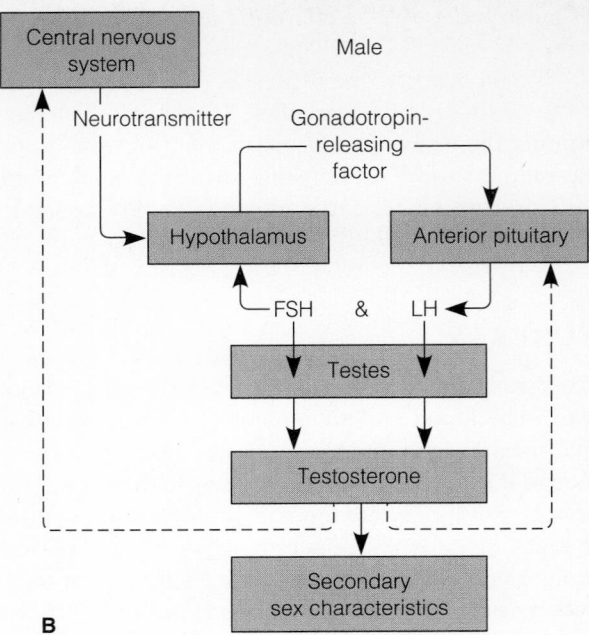

FIGURE 5-2 Physiologic changes leading to onset of puberty. *(A)* in females and *(B)* in males. Stimulation of hormone production is illustrated with solid lines, and inhibition is illustrated with broken lines. Through a neurotransmitter the CNS stimulates the hypothalamus, which in turn produces a gonadotropin-releasing factor that causes the anterior pituitary to produce gonadotropins (FSH or LH). These hormones stimulate specific structures in the gonads to secrete steroid hormones (estrogen, progesterone, or testosterone). The rise in pituitary hormone production increases hypothalamus activity. Elevated steroid hormone levels stimulate the CNS and pituitary gland to inhibit hormone production.

Mons Pubis

The *mons pubis* is a softly rounded mound of subcutaneous fatty tissue beginning at the lowest portion of the anterior abdominal wall. Also known as the mons veneris, this structure covers the anterior portion of the symphysis pubis. The mons pubis is covered with pubic hair, typically with the hairline forming a transverse line across the lower abdomen (Figure 5–3). The hair is short and varies from sparse and fine in the Asian woman to heavy, coarse, and curly in the Black woman. The mons pubis protects the pelvic bones, especially during coitus.

Labia Majora

The *labia majora* are longitudinal, raised folds of pigmented skin, one on either side of the vulvar cleft (Figure 5–3). As the pair descend, they narrow, enclosing the vulvar cleft, and merge to form the posterior junction of the perineal skin. Their chief function is protection of the structures lying between them. The labia majora are covered by stratified squamous epithelium containing hair follicles and sebaceous glands with underlying adipose and muscle tissue. Immediately under the skin is a sheet of dartos muscle, which is responsible for the wrinkled appearance of the labia majora as well as for their sensitivity to heat and cold.

The inner surface of the labia majora in women who have not had children is moist and looks like a mucous membrane, but after many births it is more skinlike (Cunningham et al 1993). With each pregnancy the labia majora becomes less prominent.

Arterial blood is supplied by the internal and external pudendal arteries. Because of the extensive venous network in the labia majora, varicosities may occur during

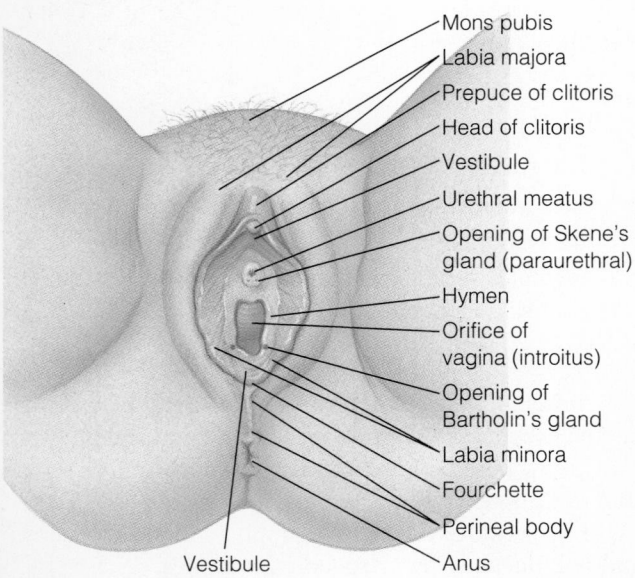

FIGURE 5-3 Female external genitals, longitudinal view.

pregnancy, and obstetric or sexual trauma may cause hematomas. The labia majora share an extensive lymphatic supply with the other structures of the vulva, which can facilitate the spread of cancer in the female reproductive organs. Because of the nerves supplying the labia majora (from the first lumbar and third sacral segment of the spinal cord), certain regional anesthesia blocks will affect them.

Labia Minora

The *labia minora* are soft folds of skin within the labia majora that converge near the anus, forming the *fourchette* (Figure 5–3). Each labium minora has the appearance of a shiny mucous membrane, moist and devoid of hair follicles. The labia minora are rich in sebaceous glands, which lubricate and waterproof the vulvar skin and provide bactericidal secretions. Because sebaceous glands do not open into hair follicles but directly onto the surface of the skin, sebaceous cysts commonly occur in this area. The labia minora are composed of erectile tissue containing loose connective tissue, blood vessels, numerous large venous spaces, and involuntary muscle tissue. Vulvovaginitis in this area is very irritating because of the many tactile nerve endings. The labia minora increase in size at puberty and decrease after menopause due to changes in estrogen levels.

Clitoris

The *clitoris* is the most erotically sensitive part of the female genital tract and is a common site of masturbation. The clitoris, located between the labia minora, is about 5 to 6 mm long and 6 to 8 mm across. Its tissue is essentially erectile. The clitoris consists primarily of the glans and the corpus or body (Figure 5–3). The glans is partially covered by a fold of skin called the *prepuce*. This area often looks like an opening to an orifice and may be confused with the urethral meatus. If an attempt is made to insert a catheter in this area, it will produce extreme discomfort. The clitoris has very rich blood and nerve supplies. Overall, it has a richer nerve supply than the penis.

The clitoris exists primarily for female sexual enjoyment. In addition it produces *smegma*, which along with other vulval secretions has a unique odor that may be sexually stimulating to the male.

Urethral Meatus and Paraurethral Glands

The *urethral meatus* is located 1 to 2.5 cm beneath the clitoris in the midline of the vestibule (Figure 5–3). At times the meatus is difficult to see because of the presence of blind dimples, small mucosal folds, or wide variance in location. Its appearance is often puckered and slitlike.

The *paraurethral glands*, or *Skene's glands*, open into the posterior wall of the urethra close to its orifice (Figure 5–3). Their secretions help lubricate the vaginal vestibule, facilitating sexual intercourse.

Vaginal Vestibule

The vaginal vestibule is a boat-shaped depression enclosed by the labia majora and visible when they are separated. The vestibule contains the vaginal opening, or *introitus*, which is the border between the external and internal genitals.

The *hymen* is a thin, elastic membrane that partially closes the vaginal opening. Its strength, shape, and size vary greatly among women. The hymen is essentially avascular. The belief that the intact hymen is a sign of virginity and that it is broken at first sexual intercourse with resultant bleeding is not valid. The hymen can be broken through strenuous physical activity, masturbation, menstruation, or the use of tampons. Once it is broken, the irregular tags of tissue that remain are called the myrtiform or hymenal carbuncles. Occasionally a woman about to give birth may still have an intact hymen.

External to the hymenal ring at the base of the vestibule are two small papular elevations containing the openings of the ducts of the *vulvovaginal (Bartholin's) glands*. They lie under the constrictor muscle of the vagina. The vulvovaginal glands are not generally palpable upon examination because they are placed deep in the perineal structures. These glands secrete a clear and thick mucus with an alkaline pH that enhances the viability and motility of sperm deposited in the vaginal vestibule.

These ducts of the vulvovaginal glands can harbor *Neisseria gonorrhoeae* and other bacteria, which can cause suppuration and Bartholin's gland abscesses (Davies 1990).

Innervation of the vestibular area is mainly by the perineal nerve from the sacral plexus. The area is not sensitive to touch generally; however, the hymen contains numerous free nerve endings as receptors to pain.

Perineal Body

The **perineal body** is a wedge-shaped mass of fibromuscular tissue measuring about $4 \times 4 \times 4$ cm, found between the lower part of the vagina and the anal canal (Figure 5–3). This area between the anus and the vagina is referred to as the *perineum*.

The muscles that meet at the perineal body are the external sphincter ani, both levator ani (the superficial and deep transverse perineal), and the bulbocavernosus. These muscles mingle with elastic fibers and connective tissue in an arrangement that allows a remarkable amount of stretching. The perineal body is much larger in the female than in the male. The perineal body is subject to lacerations and is the site of episiotomy during childbirth (see Chapter 26).

Female Internal Reproductive Organs

The female internal reproductive organs—the vagina, uterus, fallopian tubes, and ovaries—are target organs for estrogenic hormones. These organs play a unique part in

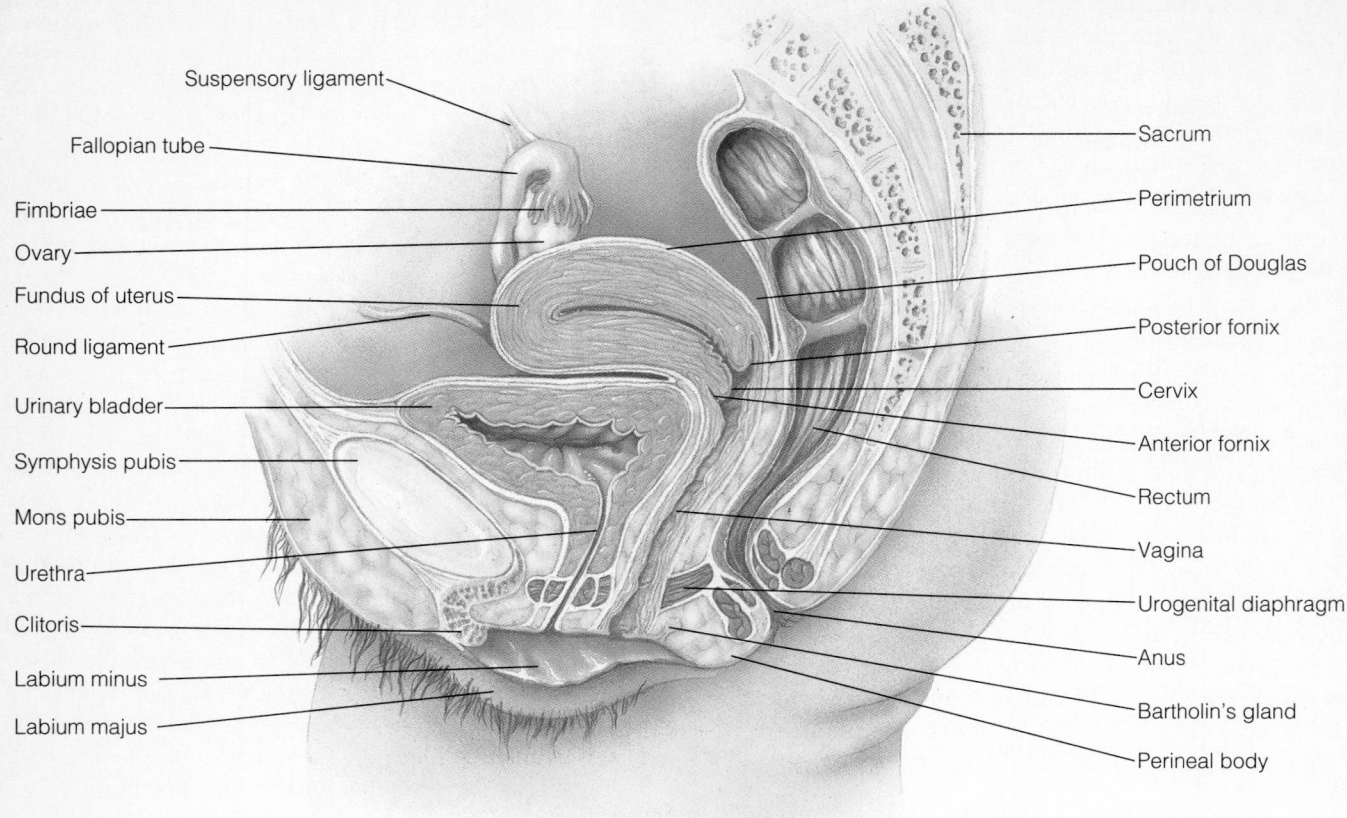

FIGURE 5-4 Female internal reproductive organs.

the reproductive cycle (Figure 5–4). The internal reproductive organs can be palpated during vaginal examination and assessed through use of various instruments.

Vagina

The **vagina** is a muscular and membranous tube that connects the external genitals with the *uterus* (Figure 5–4). It extends from the vulva to the uterus in a position nearly parallel to the plane of the pelvic brim. The vagina is often referred to as the *birth canal* because it forms the lower part of the axis through which the fetus must pass during birth.

Because the cervix of the uterus projects into the upper part of the anterior wall of the vagina, the anterior wall is approximately 2.5 cm shorter than the posterior wall. Measurements range from 6 to 8 cm for the anterior wall and 7 to 10 cm for the posterior wall.

In the upper part of the vagina, which is called the *vaginal vault,* there is a recess or hollow around the cervix. The area is referred to as the vaginal *fornix.* Because the

walls of the vaginal vault are very thin, various structures can be palpated through the walls and fornix of the vaginal vault, including the uterus, a distended bladder, the ovaries, the appendix, the cecum, the colon, and the ureters.

When a woman lies on her back after intercourse, the space in the fornix permits the pooling of semen. The collection of a large number of sperm near the cervix increases the chances of impregnation.

The walls of the vagina are covered with ridges, or *rugae,* crisscrossing each other. These rugae allow the vagina to stretch during the descent of the fetal head.

A rich blood supply is needed to maintain a high glycogen content in the epithelial cells as well as to nourish the underlying musculofascial layer, through which the vaginal vault has strong attachments to the cervix. These muscle layers are continuous with the superficial muscle fibers of the uterus. A thin band of striated muscle, the sphincter vaginae, is found at the lowest extremity of the vagina. However, the levator ani is the principal muscle that closes the vagina.

During a woman's reproductive life an acidic vaginal environment is normal (pH 4.0 to 5.0). Secretion from the vaginal epithelium provides a moist environment. The acidic environment is maintained by a symbiotic relationship between lactic acid–producing bacilli (Döderlein bacillus or lactobacillus) and the vaginal epithelial cells. These cells contain glycogen, which is broken down by the bacilli into lactic acid. The amount of glycogen is regulated by the ovarian hormones. Any interruption of this process can destroy the normal self-cleansing action of the vagina. Such interruption may be caused by antibiotic therapy, douching, or use of vaginal sprays or deodorants. For further discussion of comfort issues for women, see Chapter 9.

The acidic vaginal environment is normal only during the mature reproductive years and in the first days of life when maternal hormones are operating in the infant. A relatively neutral pH of 7.5 is normal from infancy until puberty and after menopause.

Each third of the vagina is supplied by a distinct vascular and lymphatic pattern. Venous drainage is accomplished by the venous plexus, which is also anastomosed to the vertebral venous plexus. This anastomosis makes it possible for a pelvic embolism or carcinoma to bypass the heart and lungs and lodge in the brain, spine, or other remote part of the body.

Lymphatic drainage in the upper third of the vagina drains into the external and internal iliac nodes; the middle third, into the hypogastric nodes; and the lower third, into the inguinal glands. The posterior wall drains into nodes lying in the rectovaginal septum. Any vaginal infection follows these routes.

The vagina has relatively little somatic innervation to its lower third by the pudendal nerve and virtually no special endings. Thus sensation during sexual excitement and coitus is minimal, as is vaginal pain during the second stage of labor. Nervous supply to the vagina is predominantly autonomic.

The vagina functions to:

- Serve as the passage for sperm and for the fetus during birth
- Provide passage for the menstrual products from the uterine endometrium to the outside of the body
- Protect against trauma from sexual intercourse and infection from pathogenic organisms

Uterus

As the core of reproduction and hence continuation of the human race, the uterus, or womb, has been endowed with a mystical aura. Numerous customs, taboos, mores, and values have evolved about women and their reproductive function. Although scientific knowledge has replaced much of this folklore, remnants of old ideas and superstitions persist. The nurse must be able to recognize

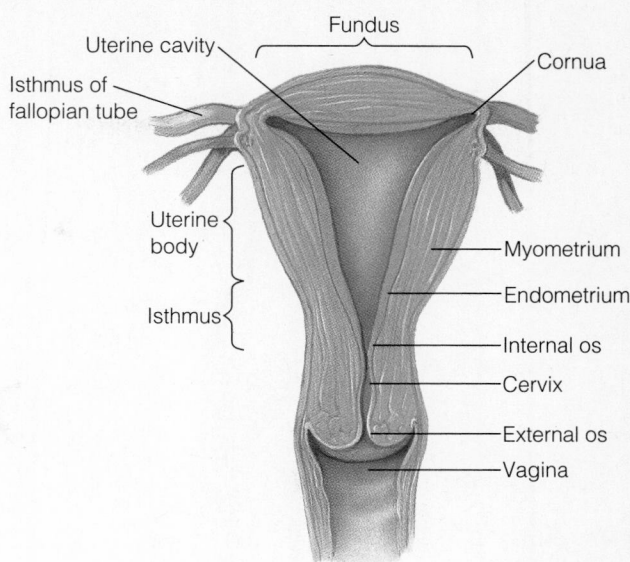

FIGURE 5-5   Structures of the uterus.

and deal with such attitudes and beliefs so that nursing care can be effective.

The **uterus** is a hollow, muscular, thick-walled, organ shaped like an upside-down pear. It lies in the center of the pelvic cavity between the base of the bladder and the rectum and above the vagina (Figure 5–5). It is level with or slightly below the brim of the pelvis, with the external opening of the cervix (the external os) about the level of the ischial spines. The mature organ weighs about 50 to 70 g and is approximately 7.5 cm long, 5 cm wide, and 1 to 2.5 cm thick (Resnick 1994).

Many uterine anomalies are thought to be congenital. Between the 6th and 9th week of embryonic development the paramesonephric ducts, which are adjacent to the mesonephric ducts, grow caudally (toward the head). Their ultimate fusion gives rise to the fallopian tubes, uterine fundus, cervix, and upper vagina. A normal uterus therefore requires two symmetric, parallel, equal-sized paramesonephric ducts to meet in the midline. Anomalies represent the absence of either one or both of the ducts, degrees of failure to fuse, or canalization defects. Uterine malformations such as the bicornuate ("two-horned") and didelphys ("double uterus") uterus are associated with habitual abortion. Because both the urinary and reproductive systems develop from the common urogenital fold in the embryo, anomalies in one system are frequently accompanied by anomalies in the other. Problems of infertility and premature labor and birth are common.

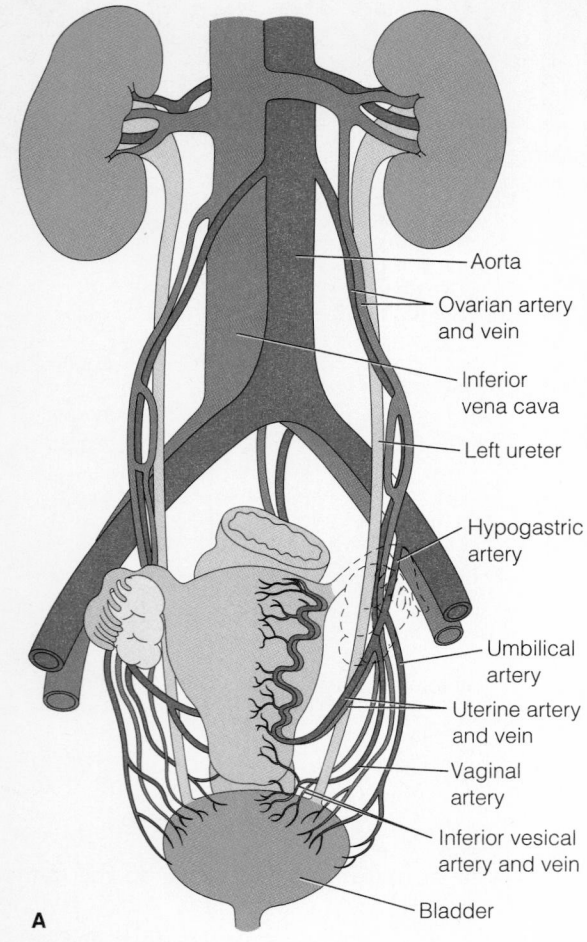

Aorta

Ovarian artery
and vein

Inferior
vena cava

Left ureter

Hypogastric
artery

Umbilical
artery

Uterine artery
and vein

Vaginal
artery

Inferior vesical
artery and vein

Bladder

A

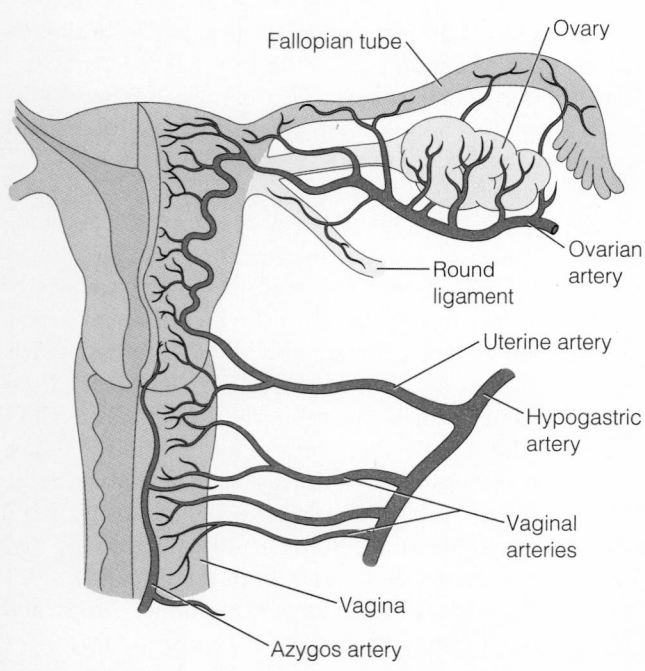

Fallopian tube

Ovary

Ovarian
artery

Round
ligament

Uterine artery

Hypogastric
artery

Vaginal
arteries

Vagina

Azygos artery

B

FIGURE 5-6 Blood supply to internal reproductive organs:
A Pelvic blood supply. *B* Blood supply to vagina, ovary,
uterus, and fallopian tube.

The uterus is kept in place by three sets of supports. The upper supports are the broad and round ligaments. The middle supports are the cardinal, pubocervical, and uterosacral ligaments. The lower supports are those structures considered to be the pelvic muscular floor.

The position of the uterus can vary, depending on a woman's posture, number of children borne, bladder and rectal fullness, and even normal respiratory patterns. Only the cervix is anchored laterally. The body of the uterus can move freely forward or backward. The axis also varies. Generally, the uterus bends forward, forming a sharp angle with the vagina. There is a bend in the area of the isthmus of the uterus, and from there the cervix points downward. The uterus is said to be *anteverted* when it is in this position. The anteverted position is considered normal.

The isthmus is a slight constriction in the uterus that divides it into two unequal parts. The upper two-thirds of the uterus is the **corpus,** or *body*, composed mainly of a smooth muscle layer (myometrium). The lower third is the **cervix,** or neck. The rounded uppermost portion of the corpus that extends above the points of attachment of the fallopian tubes is called the **fundus.** The elongated portion of the uterus where the fallopian tubes enter is called the **cornua.**

The **isthmus** joins the corpus and the cervix. It is located about 6 mm above the uterine opening of the cervix (the internal os), and it is in this area that the uterine lining changes into the mucous membrane of the cervix. The isthmus takes on importance in pregnancy because it becomes the lower uterine segment. With the cervix it is a passive segment and not part of the contractile uterus. At birth this thin lower segment, situated behind the bladder, is the site for lower-segment cesarean births (see Chapter 26).

The blood and lymphatic supplies to the uterus are extensive (Figure 5–6). Innervation of the uterus is entirely by the autonomic nervous system. Even without an intact nerve supply the uterus can contract adequately for birth. Thus, for example, hemiplegic women have adequate uterine contractions.

Pain of uterine contractions is carried to the central nervous system by the 11th and 12th thoracic nerve roots. Pain from the cervix and upper vagina passes through the ilioinguinal and pudendal nerves. The motor fibers to the uterus arise from the 7th and 8th thoracic vertebrae. Because the sensory and motor levels are separate, epidural anesthesia can be used during labor and birth.

The function of the uterus is to provide a safe environment for fetal development. The uterine lining is cyclically prepared by steroid hormones for implantation of the embryo **(nidation).** Once the embryo is implanted, the developing fetus is protected until it is expelled.

Both the body of the uterus and the cervix are changed permanently by pregnancy. The body never returns to its prepregnant size, and the external os changes from a circular opening of about 3 mm to a transverse slit with irregular edges.

The Corpus The uterine corpus is made up of three layers. The outermost layer is the *serosal layer* or **perimetrium,** which is composed of peritoneum. The middle layer is the *muscular uterine layer* or **myometrium.** This muscular uterine layer is continuous with the muscle layer of the fallopian tubes and with that of the vagina. This helps these organs present a unified reaction to various stimuli—ovulation, orgasm, or the deposit of sperm in the vagina. These muscle fibers also extend into the ovarian, round, and cardinal ligaments and minimally into the uterosacral ligaments, which helps explain the vague but disturbing pelvic "aches and pains" reported by many pregnant women.

The myometrium has three distinct layers of uterine (smooth) involuntary muscles (Figure 5–7). The outer layer, found mainly over the fundus, is made up of longitudinal muscles especially suited to expel the fetus during birth. The middle layer is thick and made up of interlacing muscle fibers in figure eight patterns. These muscle fibers surround large blood vessels, and their contraction produces a hemostatic action (a tourniquetlike action on blood vessels to stop bleeding after birth). The inner muscle layer is made up of circular fibers, which form sphincters at the fallopian tube attachment sites and at the internal os. The internal os sphincter inhibits the expulsion of the uterine contents during pregnancy but stretches in labor as cervical dilatation occurs. An incompetent cervical os can be caused by a torn, weak, or absent sphincter at the internal os. The sphincters at the fallopian tubes prevent menstrual blood from flowing backward into the fallopian tubes from the uterus.

Although each layer of muscle has been discussed as having a unique function, it must be remembered that the uterine musculature works as a whole. The uterine contractions of labor are responsible for the dilatation of the cervix and provide the major force for the passage of the fetus through the pelvic axis and vaginal canal at birth. The mucosal layer, or **endometrium,** of the uterine corpus is the innermost layer. It is composed of a single layer of columnar epithelium, glands, and stroma. From menarche to menopause, the endometrium undergoes monthly degeneration and renewal in the absence of pregnancy. As it responds to a governing hormonal cycle and prostaglandin influence as well, the endometrium varies in thickness from 0.5 to 5 mm.

The glands of the endometrium produce a thin, watery, alkaline secretion that keeps the uterine cavity moist. This *endometrial milk* not only assists the sperm as they travel to the fallopian tubes, but also nourishes the developing embryo before it lodges in the endometrium (Chapter 6).

The blood supply to the endometrium is unique. In the myometrium the radial arteries branch off from the arcuate arteries at right angles. Once inside the endometrium, they become the basal arteries supplying the zona basalis (a layer of the endometrium) and ultimately become the coiled arteries supplying the zona functionalis (also part of the endometrium). The straighter basal

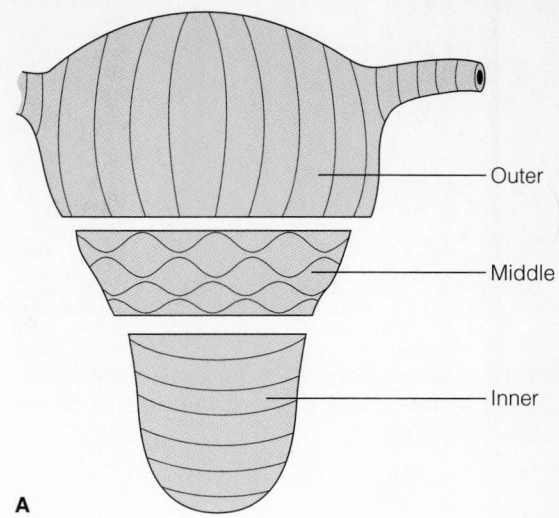

A

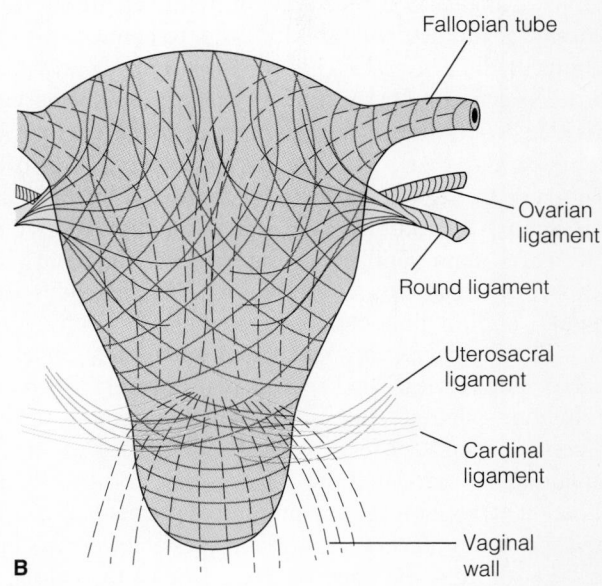

B

FIGURE 5-7 Uterine muscle layers: *A* Muscle fiber placement. *B* Interlacing of uterine muscle layers.

arteries are smaller than the coiled arteries and are not sensitive to cyclic hormonal control. Hence the zona basalis portion remains intact and is the site of new endometrial tissue generation. The coiled arteries are extremely sensitive to cyclic hormonal control. Their response is alternate relaxation and constriction during the ischemic or terminal phase of the menstrual cycle. This response allows for part of the endometrial tissue to remain intact while other endometrial tissue is shed during menstruation.

When pregnancy occurs and the endometrium is not shed, the reticular stromal cells surrounding the endometrial glands become the decidual cells of pregnancy. The stromal cells are highly vascular, channeling a rich blood supply to the endometrial surface.

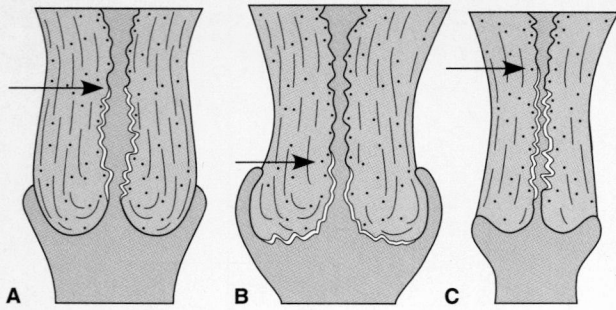

FIGURE 5-8   Changes in squamocolumnar junction (arrows) at various stages of life: *A* Childhood. *B* Reproductive years. *C* Postmenopausal years.

The Cervix   The narrow neck of the uterus is the cervix. Canal-like, it meets the body of the uterus at the *internal os* and descends about 2.5 cm to connect with the vagina at the *external os* (Figure 5–5). Thus it provides a protective portal for the body of the uterus. The cervix is divided by its line of attachment into the vaginal and supravaginal areas. The *vaginal cervix* projects into the vagina at an angle from 45 to 90 degrees. The *supravaginal cervix* is surrounded by the attachments that give the uterus its main support: the uterosacral ligaments, the transverse ligaments of the cervix (Mackenrodt's ligaments), and the pubocervical ligaments.

The vaginal cervix appears pink and ends at the external os. The cervical canal appears rosy red and is lined with columnar ciliated epithelium, which contains mucus-secreting glands. Most cervical cancer begins at this squamocolumnar junction. The specific location of the junction varies with age and number of pregnancies. Figure 5–8 shows this junction at various stages of a woman's life.

Elasticity is the chief characteristic of the cervix. Its ability to stretch is due to the high fibrous and collagenous content of the supportive tissues and also to the vast number of folds in the cervical lining.

The cervical mucosa has three functions:

- To provide lubrication for the vaginal canal
- To act as a bacteriostatic agent
- To provide an alkaline environment to shelter deposited sperm from the acidic vagina

At ovulation cervical mucus is clearer, thinner, and more alkaline than at other times.

Uterine Ligaments   The uterine ligaments support and stabilize the various reproductive organs. The ligaments shown in Figure 5–9 are described in this section.

- The **broad ligament** keeps the uterus centrally placed and provides stability within the pelvic cavity. It is a double layer that is continuous with the abdominal peritoneum. The broad ligament covers the uterus anteriorly and posteriorly and extends outward from the uterus to enfold and stabilize the fallopian tubes. The round and ovarian ligaments are at the upper border of the broad ligament. At its lower border it forms the cardinal ligaments. Between the folds of the broad ligament are connective tissue, involuntary muscle, blood and lymph vessels, and nerves.

- The **round ligaments** help the broad ligament keep the uterus in place. Each of the round ligaments arises from the sides of the uterus near the fallopian tube insertion. They extend outward between the folds of the broad ligament, passing through the inguinal ring and canals and eventually fusing with the connective tissue of the labia majora. The round ligaments are made up of longitudinal muscle and enlarge during pregnancy. During labor the round ligaments steady the uterus, pulling downward and forward, so that the presenting part of the fetus is forced into the cervix.

- The **ovarian ligaments** anchor the lower pole of the ovary to the cornua of the uterus. They are composed of muscle fibers, which allows the ligaments to contract. This contractile ability influences the position of the ovary to some extent, thus helping the fimbriae of the fallopian tubes to "catch" the ovum as it is released each month.

- The **cardinal ligaments** are the chief uterine supports, suspending the uterus from the side walls of the true pelvis. These ligaments, also known as *Mackenrodt's* or *transverse cervical ligaments*, arise from the sides of the pelvic walls and attach to the cervix in the upper vagina. These ligaments prevent uterine prolapse and also support the upper vagina.

- The **infundibulopelvic ligament** suspends and supports the ovaries. Arising from the outer third of the broad ligament, the infundibulopelvic ligament contains the ovarian vessels and nerves.

- The **uterosacral ligaments** provide support for the uterus and cervix at the level of the ischial spines. Arising on each side of the pelvis from the posterior wall of the uterus, the uterosacral ligaments sweep back around the rectum and insert on the sides of the first and second sacral vertebrae. The uterosacral ligaments contain smooth muscle fibers, connective tissue, blood and lymph vessels, and nerves. Providing support for the uterus and cervix at the level of the ischial spines, they also contain sensory nerve fibers that contribute to dysmenorrhea (painful menstruation; see Chapter 9).

Fallopian Tubes

The **fallopian tubes,** also known as *oviducts* or *uterine tubes* arise from each side of the uterus and reach almost to the side of the pelvis, where they turn toward the

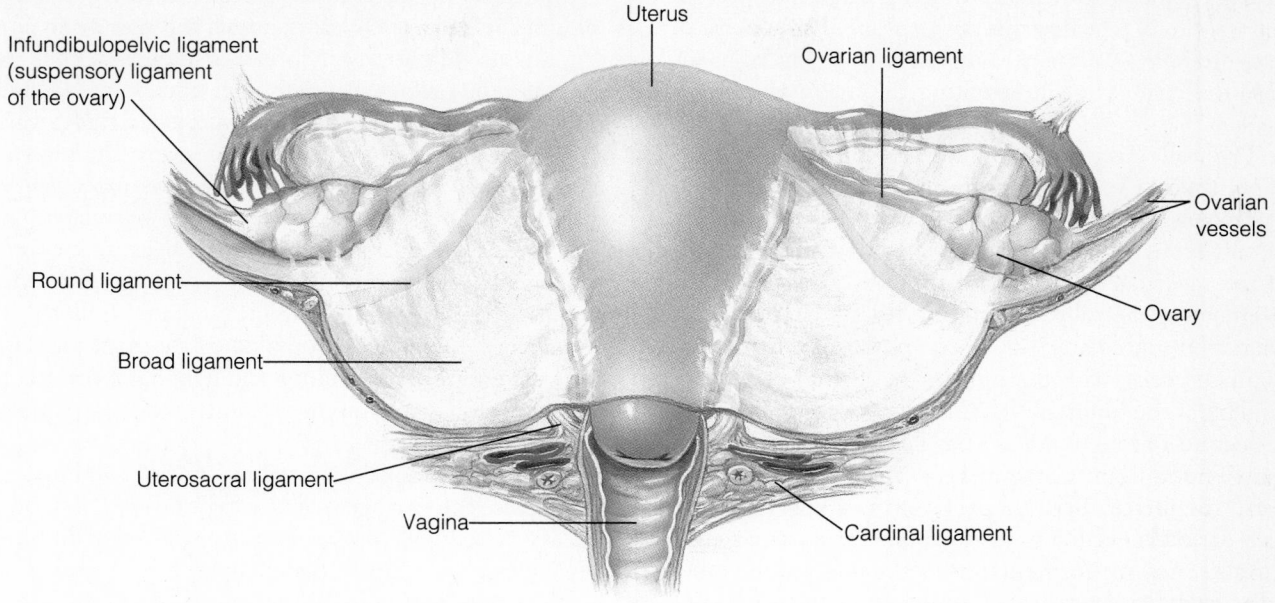

FIGURE 5-9   Uterine ligaments.

ovaries (Figure 5–10). Each tube is 8 to 13.5 cm long, lying in the superior border of the broad ligament (mesosalpinx). A short section of each fallopian tube is inside the uterus; its opening into the uterus is 1 mm in diameter. The fallopian tubes link the peritoneal cavity with the external environment through the uterus and vagina. This linkage increases a woman's vulnerability to disease processes.

Each fallopian tube may be divided into three parts: the isthmus, the ampulla, and the infundibulum or fimbria. The isthmus is straight and narrow, with a thick muscular wall and an opening (lumen) 2 to 3 mm in diameter. It is the site of tubal ligation (a surgical procedure to prevent pregnancy; see Chapter 9).

Next to the isthmus is the curved **ampulla,** which comprises the outer two-thirds of the tube. Fertilization

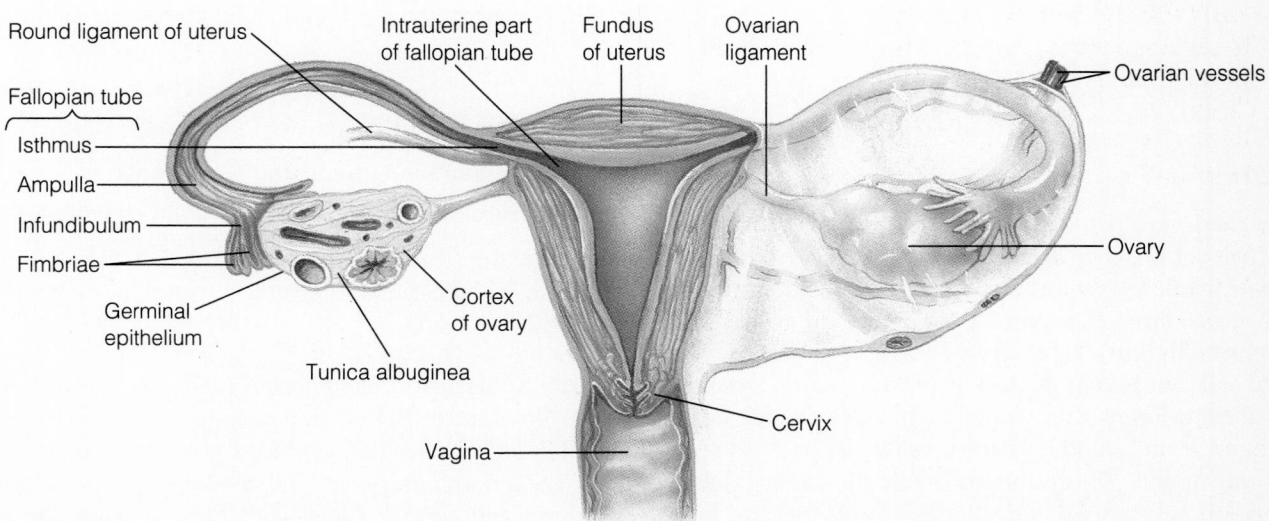

FIGURE 5-10   Fallopian tube and ovary.

of the secondary oocyte by a spermatozoon usually occurs here. The ampulla ends at the **fimbria,** which is a funnel-like enlargement with many moving fingerlike projections (fimbriae) reaching out to the ovary. The longest of these, the *fimbria ovarica*, is attached to the ovary to increase the chances of intercepting the ovum as it is released.

The wall of the fallopian tube is made up of four layers: peritoneal (serous), subserous (adventitial), muscular, and mucous tissues. The peritoneum covers the tubes. The subserous layer contains the blood and nerve supply, and the muscular layer is responsible for the peristaltic movement of the tube. The mucosal layer, immediately next to the muscular layer, is composed of ciliated and nonciliated cells, with the number of ciliated cells more abundant at the fimbria. Nonciliated cells are goblet cells that secrete a protein-rich, serous fluid that nourishes the ovum. The constantly moving tubal cilia propel the ovum toward the uterus. Because the ovum is a large cell, this ciliary action is needed to assist the tube's muscular layer peristalsis. Any malformation or malfunction of the tubes could result in infertility, ectopic pregnancy, or even sterility.

A well-functioning tubal transport system involves active fimbriae close to the ovary, peristalsis of the tube created by the muscular layer, ciliated currents beating toward the uterus, and the proximal contraction and distal relaxation of the tube caused by different types of prostaglandins.

Each fallopian tube is richly supplied with blood by the uterine and ovarian arteries. Thus the fallopian tubes have an unusual ability to recover from any inflammatory process. Lymphatic drainage occurs through the vessels close to the ureter into the lumbar nodes along the aorta. The functions of the fallopian tubes are as follows:

- To provide transport for the ovum from the ovary to the uterus (transport through the fallopian tubes varies from 3 to 4 days)
- To provide a site for fertilization
- To serve as a warm, moist, nourishing environment for the ovum or *zygote* (a fertilized egg). (See also Chapter 6.)

Ovaries

The *ovaries* are two almond-shaped glandular structures just below the pelvic brim. One ovary is located on each side of the pelvic cavity. Their size varies among women and according to the stage of the menstrual cycle. Each ovary weighs 6 to 10 g and is 1.5 to 3 cm wide, 2 to 5 cm long, and 1 to 1.5 cm thick. The ovaries of girls are small but become larger after puberty. They also change in appearance from smooth-surfaced, dull white organs to pitted gray organs. This pitting is caused by scarring due to ovulation. It is rare for both ovaries to be at the same level in the pelvic cavity. The ovary is held in place by the ovar-

ian, broad, and infundibulopelvic ligaments (Figure 5–9), which were discussed earlier in the chapter.

There is no peritoneal covering for the ovaries. Although this lack of covering assists the mature ovum to erupt, it also allows easier spread of malignant cells from cancer of the ovaries. A single layer of cuboidal epithelial cells, called the germinal epithelium, covers the ovaries. The ovaries are composed of three layers: the tunica albuginea, the cortex, and the medulla. The *tunica albuginea* is dense and dull white and serves as a protective layer. The *cortex* is the main functional part because it contains ova, graafian follicles, corpora lutea, degenerated corpora lutea (corpora albicantia), and degenerated follicles. The *medulla* is completely surrounded by the cortex and contains the nerves and the blood and lymphatic vessels. The ovaries are relatively insensitive unless they are squeezed or distended.

The ovaries are the primary source of two important hormones: the estrogens and progesterone. **Estrogens** are associated with those characteristics contributing to femaleness, including breast alveolar lobule growth and duct development. The ovaries secrete large amounts of estrogens; the adrenal cortex (extraglandular sites) produces minute amounts of estrogens in nonpregnant women.

Progesterone is often called the *hormone of pregnancy* because its effects on the uterus allow pregnancy to be maintained. The placenta is the primary source of progesterone during pregnancy. This hormone also inhibits the action of prolactin in α-lactalbumin synthesis, thereby preventing lactation during pregnancy (Cunningham et al 1993).

The interplay between the ovarian hormones and other hormones such as FSH and LH is responsible for the cyclic changes that allow pregnancy to occur. The hormonal and physical changes that occur during the female reproductive cycle will be discussed later in this chapter. Between the ages of 45 and 55 years the woman's ovaries secrete decreasing amounts of estrogen. Eventually, ovulatory activity ceases and menopause occurs.

Bony Pelvis

The female *bony pelvis* has two unique functions:

- To support and protect the pelvic contents
- To form the relatively fixed axis of the birth passage

Because the structural aspects of the pelvis are so important to childbearing, its structures must be understood clearly.

Bony Structure   The pelvis is made up of four bones: two innominate bones, the sacrum, and the coccyx (or tailbone). The pelvis resembles a bowl or basin; its sides are the innominate bones, and its back is composed of the sacrum and coccyx. Lined with fibrocartilage and held tightly together by ligaments, the four bones join at the

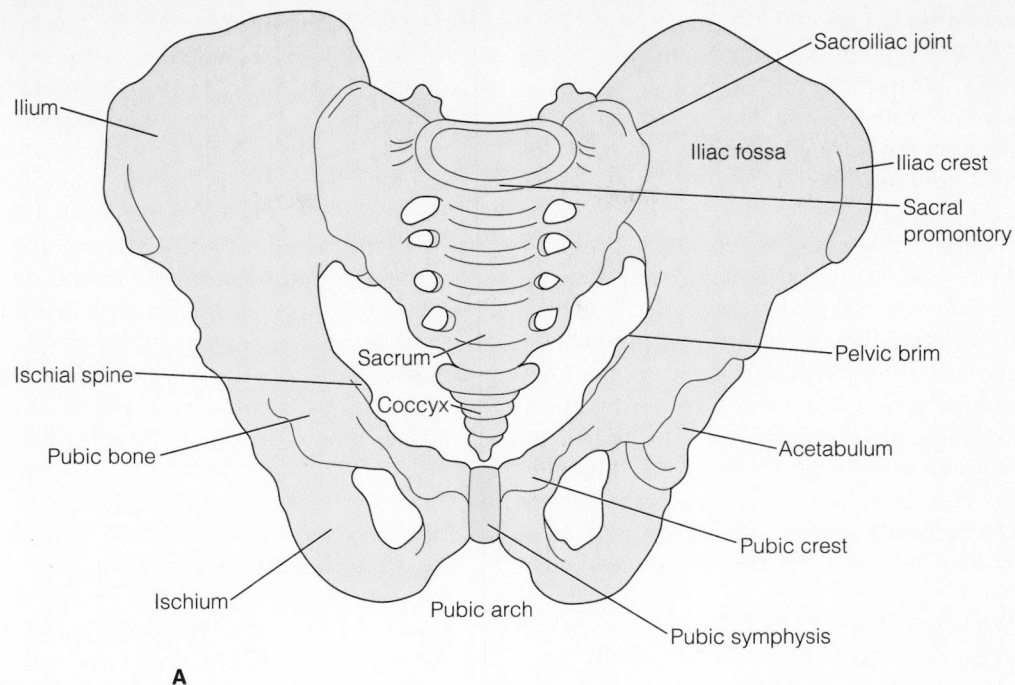

Ilium

Sacroiliac joint

Iliac fossa

Iliac crest

Sacral promontory

Pelvic brim

Acetabulum

Pubic crest

Pubic symphysis

Ischial spine

Sacrum

Coccyx

Pubic bone

Ischium

Pubic arch

A

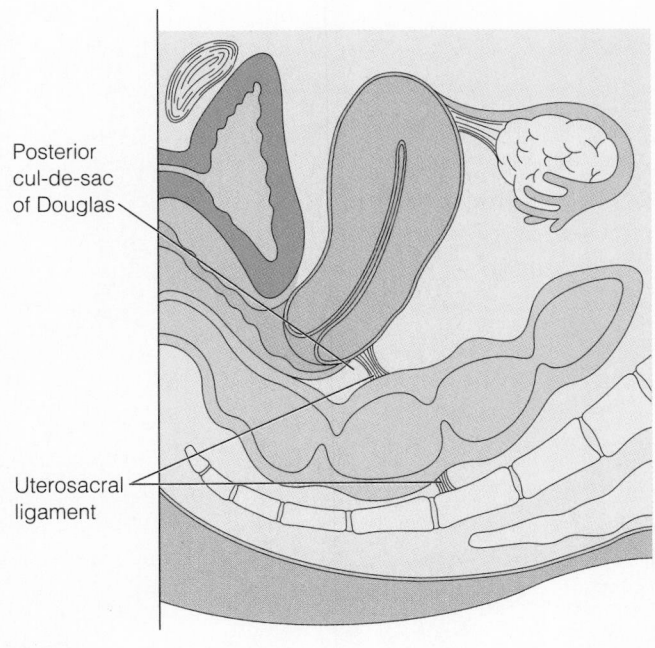

Posterior cul-de-sac of Douglas

Uterosacral ligament

B

FIGURE 5-11   Pelvis: *A* Pelvic bones. *B* Midsagittal view in supine position with some ligaments.

symphysis pubis, the two sacroiliac joints, and the sacro-coccygeal joints (Figure 5–11).

The **innominate bones,** also known as the *hip bones* or *os coxae,* are made up of three separate bones: the ilium, the ischium, and the pubis. These bones fuse to form a circular cavity, the *acetabulum,* which articulates with the femur.

The *ilium* is the broad, upper prominence of the hip. The *iliac crest* is the margin of the ilium. The *iliac spine,* the foremost projection nearest the groin, is the site of attachment for ligaments and muscles.

The *ischium,* the strongest bone, is under the ilium and below the acetabulum, the L-shaped ischium ends in a marked protuberance, the *ischial tuberosity,* on which the weight of a seated body rests. The **ischial spines** arise near the junction of the ilium and ischium and jut into the pelvic cavity. The shortest diameter of the pelvic cavity is located between the ischial spines. The ischial spines can serve as a reference point during labor to evaluate the descent of the fetal head into the birth canal. (See Chapter 21 and Figure 21–7.)

The *pubis* forms the slightly bowed front portion of the innominate bone. Extending medially from the acetabulum to the midpoint of the bony pelvis, the two pubic bones meet to form a joint, the **symphysis pubis.** The triangular space below this junction is known as the *pubic arch.* The fetal head passes under this arch during birth. The symphysis pubis is formed by heavy fibrocartilage and the superior and inferior pubic ligaments. The mobility of the inferior ligament, also known as the *arcuate pubic ligament,* increases during pregnancy and to a greater extent in subsequent pregnancies than in first pregnancies.

The sacroiliac joints also have a degree of mobility that increases near the end of pregnancy and results in an upward gliding movement. The pelvic outlet may be increased by 1.5 to 2 cm in the squatting, sitting, and dorsal lithotomy positions. These relaxations of the joints are induced by the hormones of pregnancy.

The *sacrum* is a wedge-shaped bone formed by the fusion of five vertebrae. On the anterior upper portion of the sacrum is a projection into the pelvic cavity known as the **sacral promontory.** This projection is another obstetric guide in determining pelvic measurements. (For discussion of pelvic measurements see Chapter 14.)

The small triangular bone last on the vertebral column is the *coccyx.* It articulates with the sacrum at the sacrococcygeal joint. The coccyx usually moves backward during labor to provide more room for the fetus.

Pelvic Floor   The muscular *pelvic floor* of the bony pelvis is designed to overcome the force of gravity exerted on the pelvic organs. It acts as a buttress to the irregularly shaped pelvic outlet, thereby providing stability and support for surrounding structures.

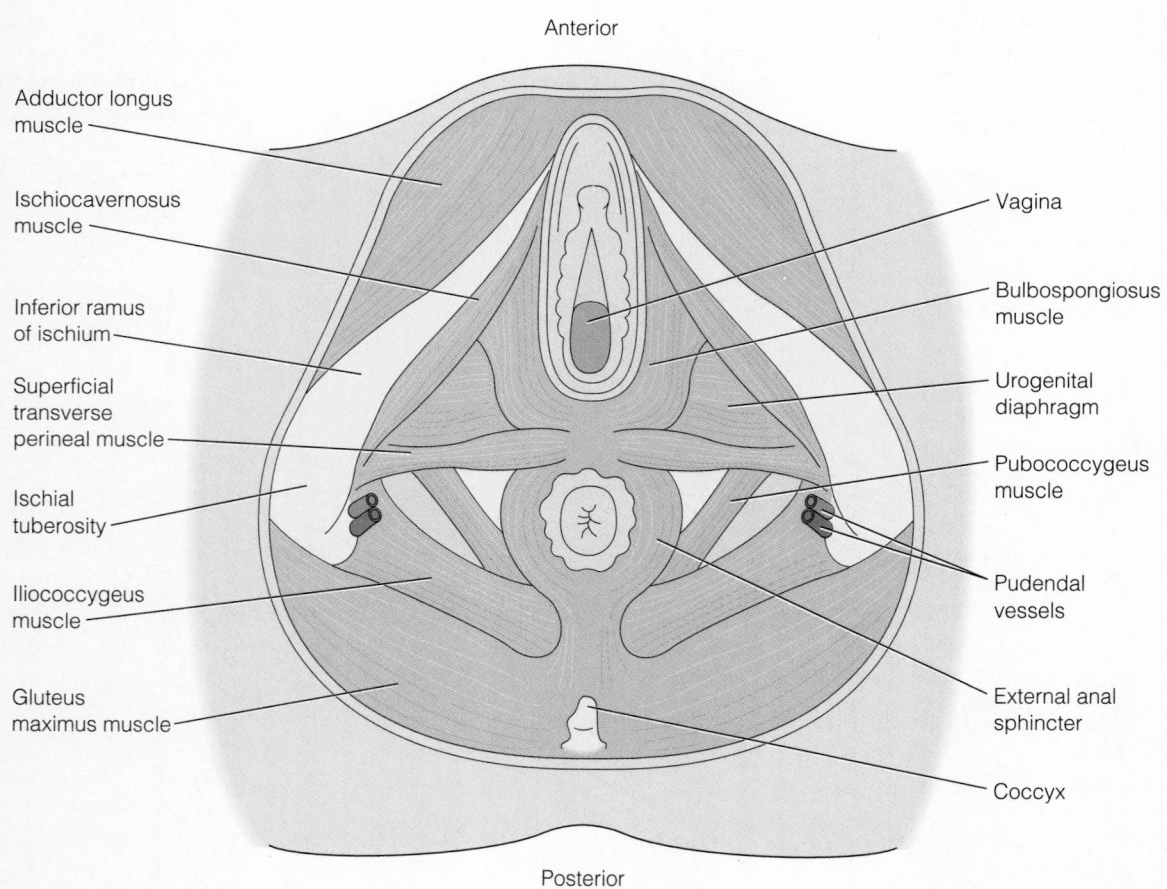

Anterior

Adductor longus muscle

Ischiocavernosus muscle

Inferior ramus of ischium

Superficial transverse perineal muscle

Ischial tuberosity

Iliococcygeus muscle

Gluteus maximus muscle

Vagina

Bulbospongiosus muscle

Urogenital diaphragm

Pubococcygeus muscle

Pudendal vessels

External anal sphincter

Coccyx

Posterior

FIGURE 5-12   Muscles of the pelvic floor. (The puborectalis, pubovaginalis, and coccygeal muscles cannot be seen from this view.)

Deep fascia and the levator ani and coccygeal muscles form the part of the pelvic floor known as the *pelvic diaphragm*. Above it is the pelvic cavity; below and behind it is the perineum. The sacrum is located posteriorly.

The *levator ani muscle* makes up the major portion of the pelvic diaphragm and consists of four muscles: ileococcygeus, pubococcygeus, puborectalis, and pubovaginalis. Forming a sling for the pelvic structures, the levator ani is interrupted by the urethra, vagina, and rectum. The ileococcygeal muscle, a thin muscular sheet underlying the sacrospinous ligament, helps the levator ani support the pelvic organs. Muscles of the pelvic floor are shown in Figure 5–12 and discussed in Table 5–1.

Endopelvic fascia covers the pelvic diaphragm. The components function as a whole, yet they are able to move over one another. This feature provides an exceptional capacity for dilatation during birth and return to prepregnant condition following birth.

The *urogenital triangle* (diaphragm) is external to the pelvic diaphragm, in the triangular area between the ischial tuberosities and the hollow of the pubic arch. It is made up of superficial and deep perineal membranes extending from the rami of the ischial and pubic bones. Most important in this region are the deep transverse perineal muscles, which are flat bands of muscle arising from the ischiopubic rami and intertwining in the midline to form a seam, or raphe. These muscles are modified to encircle both the urinary meatus and the vaginal orifice, forming the urethral and vaginal sphincters.

Pelvic Division   The pelvic cavity is divided into the false pelvis and the true pelvis (Figure 5–13).

The **false pelvis** is the portion above the pelvic brim, or linea terminalis, bounded by the lumbar vertebrae posteriorly, the iliac fossae laterally, and the lower abdominal wall anteriorly. Its primary function is to support the weight of the enlarged pregnant uterus and direct the presenting fetal part into the true pelvis below.

The **true pelvis** is the portion that lies below the pelvic brim. It is bounded above by the promontory of the sacrum and the upper margins of the pubic bones and below by the pelvic outlet. The true pelvis represents the bony limits of the birth canal. It measures about 5 cm at its anterior wall at the symphysis pubis and about 10 cm at its posterior wall. When a woman is standing upright, the upper portion of the pelvic cavity or canal is directed downward and backward and its lower portion, downward and forward. This forms an axis or curved canal through which the presenting part of the baby must pass during birth (Figure 5–13). The inclination of the pelvis is the angle formed by two planes, a horizontal plane passing through the tip of the coccyx and the superior border of the symphysis pubis and an inclined plane passing through the sacral promontory and the superior border of the symphysis pubis. This pelvic angle of inclination usually measures 50 to 60 degrees (Figure 5–14).

The bony circumference of the true pelvis is made up of the sacrum, coccyx, and innominate bones below the linea terminalis. This area is extremely important in obstetrics because its size and shape must be adequate for normal fetal passage during labor and at birth. The relationship of the fetal head to the true pelvic cavity is of critical importance.

TABLE 5-1	Muscles of the Pelvic Floor			
Muscle	**Origin**	**Insertion**	**Innervation**	**Action**
Levator ani	Pubis, lateral pelvic wall, and ischial spine	Blends with organs in pelvic cavity	Inferior rectal, second and third sacral nerves, plus anterior rami of third and fourth sacral nerves	Supports pelvic viscera; helps form pelvic diaphragm
Iliococcygeus	Pelvic surface of ischial spine and pelvic fascia	Central point of perineum, coccygeal raphe, and coccyx		Assists in supporting abdominal and pelvic viscera
Pubococcygeus	Pubis and pelvic fascia	Coccyx		
Puborectalis	Pubis	Blends with rectum; meets similar fibers from opposite side		Forms sling for rectum, just posterior to it; raises anus
Pubovaginalis	Pubis	Blends into vagina		Supports vagina
Coccygeus	Ischial spine and sacrospinous ligament	Lateral border of lower sacrum and upper coccyx	Third and fourth sacral nerves	Supports pelvic viscera; helps form pelvic diaphragm; flexes and abducts coccyx

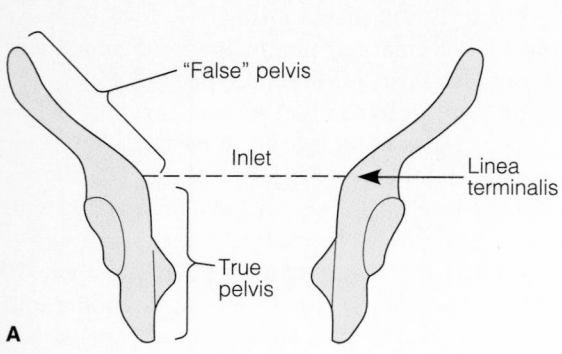

A

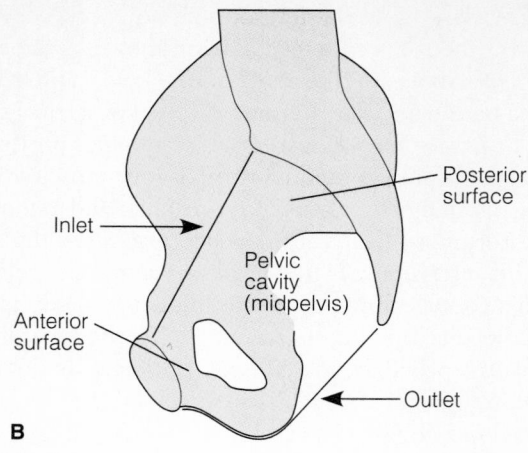

B

FIGURE 5-13   Female pelvis: *A* False pelvis is shallow cavity above inlet; true pelvis is deeper portion of the cavity below inlet. *B* True pelvis consists of inlet, cavity (midpelvis), and outlet.

The true pelvis consists of three parts: the inlet, the pelvic cavity, and the outlet. The pelvic planes are imaginary flat surfaces drawn across the three parts of the true pelvis at strategic levels (Figure 5–15). Associated with each part are distinct measurements that aid in evaluating the adequacy of the pelvis for childbirth.

The dimensions of the true pelvis and their obstetric implications are described here. Measurement techniques are discussed in Chapter 14. The effects of inadequate or abnormal pelvic diameters on labor and birth are further considered in Chapter 22.

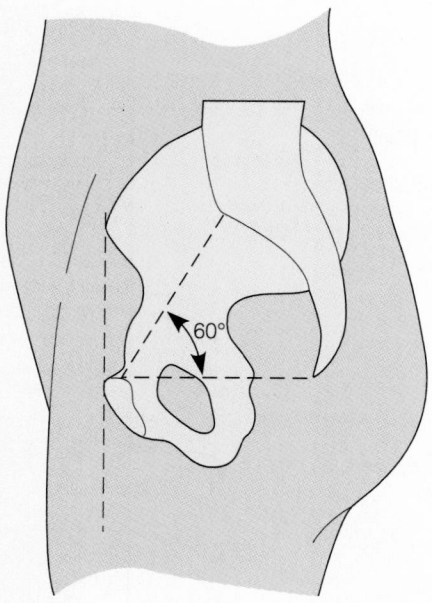

FIGURE 5-14   Pelvic angle of inclination while woman is standing.

The **pelvic inlet** is the upper border of the true pelvis and typically is round in the female. The size and shape of the pelvic inlet are determined by assessing three anteroposterior diameters: the diagonal conjugate, obstetric conjugate, and conjugate vera. (For an in-depth discussion see Chapter 14.) The **diagonal conjugate** extends from the subpubic angle to the middle of the sacral promontory and is typically 12.5 cm. The diagonal conjugate can be measured manually during a pelvic examination. The **obstetric conjugate** extends from the middle of the sacral promontory to an area approximately 1 cm below the pubic crest. Its length is estimated by subtracting 1.5 cm from the diagonal conjugate. The fetus passes through the obstetric conjugate, and the size of this diameter determines whether the fetus can move down into the birth canal in order for engagement to occur. The true (anatomic) conjugate, or **conjugate vera,** extends from the middle of the sacral promontory to the middle of the pubic crest (superior surface of the symphysis). One additional measurement, the **transverse diameter,** helps determine the shape of the inlet. The transverse diameter is the largest diameter of the inlet and is measured using the linea terminales as the points of reference.

The *pelvic cavity* (canal) has two planes with varying diameters. The largest part of the pelvis is called the *plane of the greatest dimensions* (Figure 5–15). It is a curved canal with a longer posterior than anterior wall. A change in the lumbar curve can increase or decrease the pelvic inclination and can influence the progress of labor because the fetus has to adjust itself to this curved path as well as to the different diameters of the true pelvis.

The smallest part of the pelvis is called the *plane of the least dimensions,* or the midpelvic plane (Figure 5–15). Arrest of labor occurs most frequently because of contracture (narrowing) in this plane, so its diameters are of great importance. The plane extends from the lower margin of

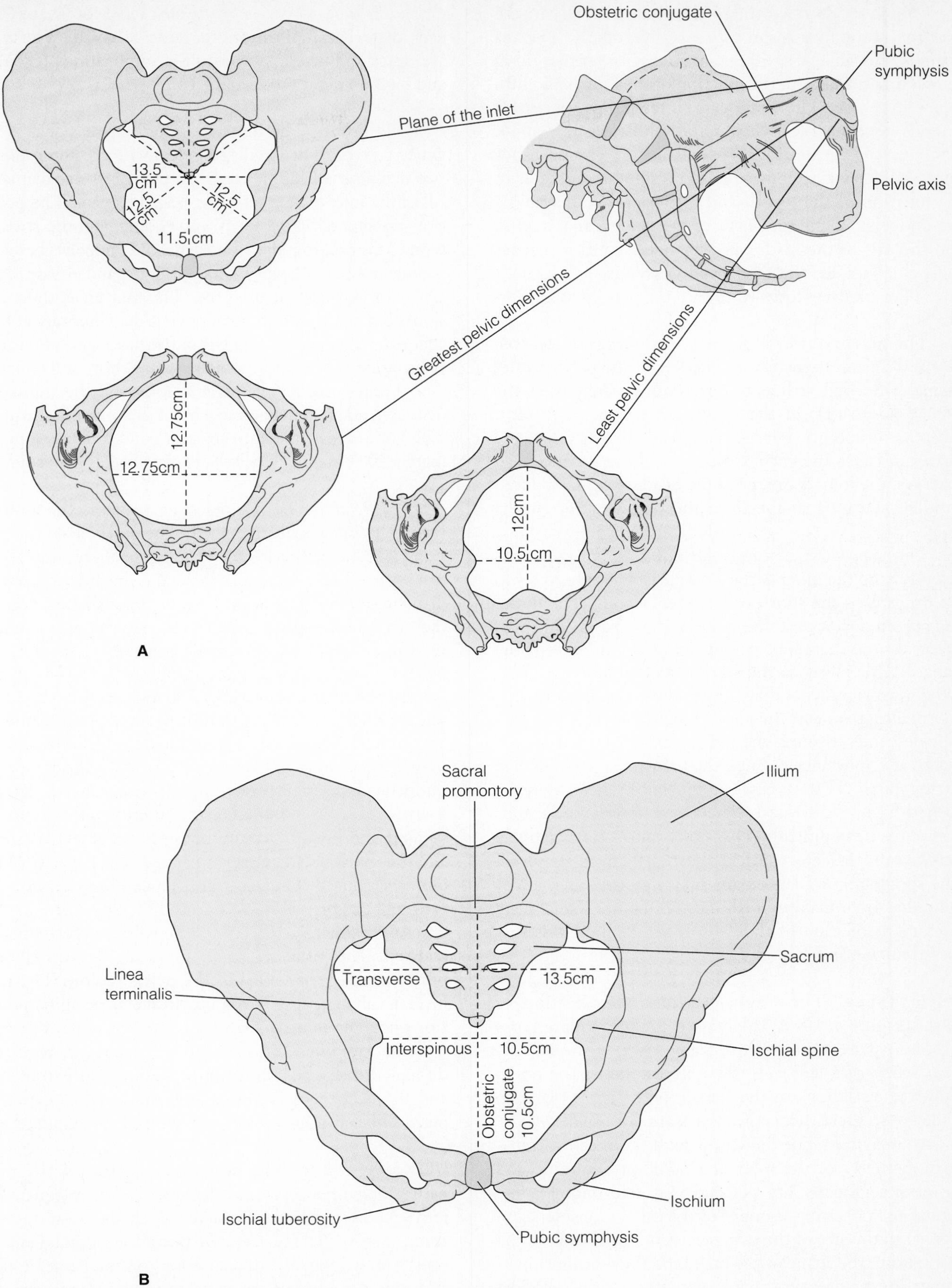

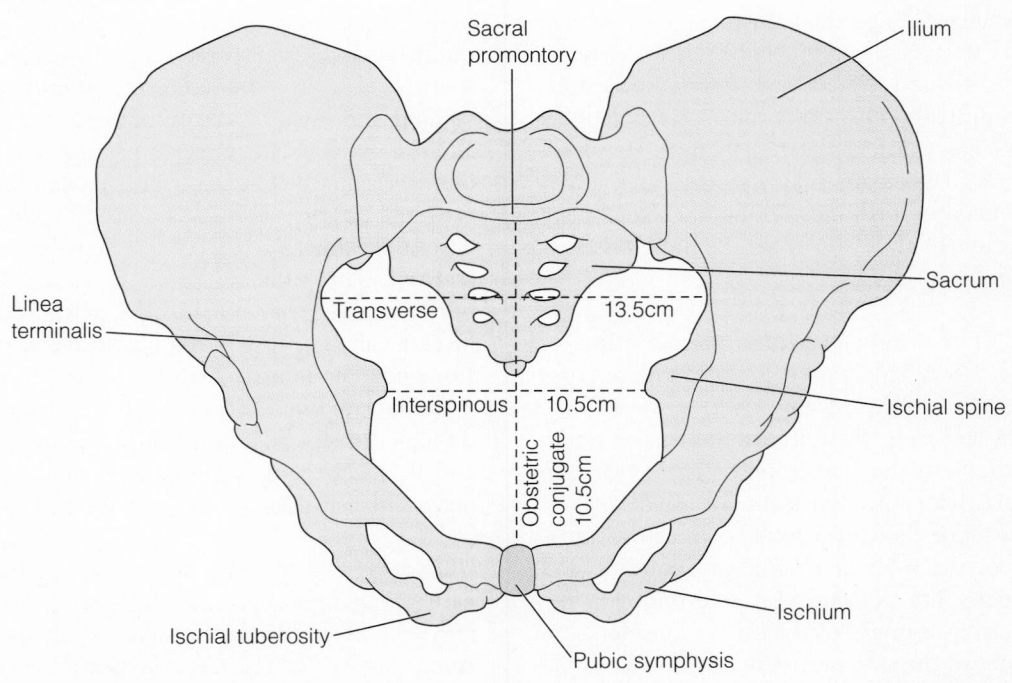

Obstetric conjugate

Pubic
symphysis

Plane of the inlet

13.5
cm
12.5
cm
12.5
cm

11.5 cm

Pelvic axis

Greatest pelvic dimensions

Least pelvic dimensions

12.75cm

12.75cm

12cm

10.5 cm

A

Sacral
promontory

Ilium

Linea
terminalis

Transverse   13.5cm

Sacrum

Interspinous   10.5cm

Ischial spine

Obstetric
conjugate
10.5cm

Ischial tuberosity

Ischium

Pubic symphysis

B

FIGURE 5-15   Pelvic planes: *A* Sagittal section of planes and diameters of the bony
pelvis. *B* Coronal section.

the symphysis pubis, through the ischial spines, to the junction of the fourth and fifth sacral vertebrae. The anteroposterior diameter extends from the lower margin of the symphysis pubis to the junction of the fourth and fifth sacral vertebrae. The transverse (interspinous) diameter extends between the ischial spines and measures about 10.5 cm; it is the shortest pelvic diameter. The posterior sagittal diameter extends from the bispinous diameter to the junction of the fourth and fifth sacral vertebrae. At the midpelvic plane the curve of the pelvic canal begins, and the axis of the birth canal changes. Until it reaches the ischial spines, the fetal head descends in a straight line. Then it curves forward toward the pelvic outlet (Figure 5–15).

The **pelvic outlet** is at the lower border of the true pelvis. The anteroposterior diameter of the pelvic outlet increases during birth as the presenting part pushes the coccyx posteriorly at the mobile sacrococcygeal joint. Decreased mobility, a large fetal head, and/or a forceful birth can cause the coccyx to snap. As the infant's head emerges, the long diameter of the head (occipital frontal) parallels the long diameter of the outlet (anteroposterior).

The transverse diameter (*bi-ischial* or *intertuberous*) extends from the inner surface of one ischial tuberosity to the other. It is the shortest diameter of the pelvic outlet and becomes shorter as the pubic arch narrows. The posterior sagittal diameter extends from the middle of the transverse diameter to the sacrococcygeal junction. This is the most significant diameter of the outlet because it is the smallest diameter through which the infant must pass as it descends through the pelvic canal. The pubic arch has great importance because the baby must pass under it during birth. If it is narrow, the baby's head may be pushed backward toward the coccyx, making the extension of the head difficult. This situation is known as *outlet dystocia*, and forceps (outlet) assisted birth is required. The shoulders of a large baby may also get stuck under the pubic arch, making birth more difficult. The clinical assessment of each of these obstetric diameters is discussed further in Chapter 14.

Pelvic Types The Caldwell-Moloy classification of pelves (Figure 5–16) is widely used to differentiate types of bony pelves (Caldwell & Moloy 1933). *Gynecoid, android, anthropoid,* and *platypelloid* are the four basic types. However, variations in the female pelvis from plane to plane are so great that classic types are not usual.

An imaginary line drawn through the greatest transverse diameter of the inlet divides it into anterior and posterior segments. The pelvis type is determined by assessing the posterior segment of the inlet. Consideration is given to the size of the sacrosciatic notch, flaring of the pelvic brim, the shape of the inlet, and the relationship of the greatest anteroposterior diameter to the greatest transverse diameter.

Each type of pelvis has a characteristic shape, and each shape has implications for labor and birth. The types are described briefly here and the implications for labor and birth in detail in Chapter 14.

Gynecoid Pelvis The most common female pelvis is the gynecoid type. The inlet is rounded, with the anteroposterior diameter a little shorter than the transverse diameter. All of the inlet diameters are at least adequate. The posterior segment is broad, deep, and roomy; and the anterior segment is well rounded. The gynecoid midpelvis has nonprominent ischial spines, straight and parallel side walls, and a wide, deep sacral curve. The sacrum is short and slopes backward. All of the midpelvic diameters are at least adequate. The gynecoid pelvic outlet has a wide and round pubic arch; the inferior pubic rami are short and concave. The anteroposterior diameter is long and the transverse diameter, adequate. The capacity of the outlet is adequate. The bones are of medium structure and weight. Approximately 50% of female pelves are classified as gynecoid.

Android Pelvis The normal male pelvis is the android type. The inlet is heart shaped. The anteroposterior and transverse diameters are adequate for birth, but the posterior sagittal diameter is too short, and the anterior sagittal diameter is long. The posterior segment is shallow because the sacral promontory is indented, resulting in a reduced capacity. The anterior segment is narrow, and the forepelvis is sharply angled. The android midpelvis has prominent ischial spines, convergent side walls, and a long, heavy sacrum inclining forward. All of the midpelvic diameters are reduced. The distance from the linea terminalis to the ischial tuberosities is long, yet the overall capacity of the midpelvis is reduced. The android outlet has a narrow, sharp, and deep pubic arch; the inferior pubic rami are straight and long. The anteroposterior diameter is short, and the transverse diameter is narrow. The capacity of the outlet is reduced. The bones are of medium to heavy structure and weight.

Approximately 20% of female pelves are classified as android. The influence of an android pelvis on labor is not favorable. Descent into the pelvis is slow. The fetal head usually engages in the transverse or occipital posterior diameter in asynclitism (oblique presentation) with extreme molding. Arrest of labor is frequent, requiring difficult forceps manipulation (rotation and extraction); and the deep, narrow pubic arch may lead to extensive perineal lacerations. Cesarean birth may be required.

Anthropoid Pelvis The anthropoid pelvis inlet is oval, with a long anteroposterior diameter and an adequate but rather short transverse diameter. Both the posterior and anterior segments are deep; the posterior sagittal diameter is extremely long, as is the anterior sagittal diameter. The anthropoid midpelvis has variable ischial spines, straight side walls, and a narrow and long sacrum that inclines

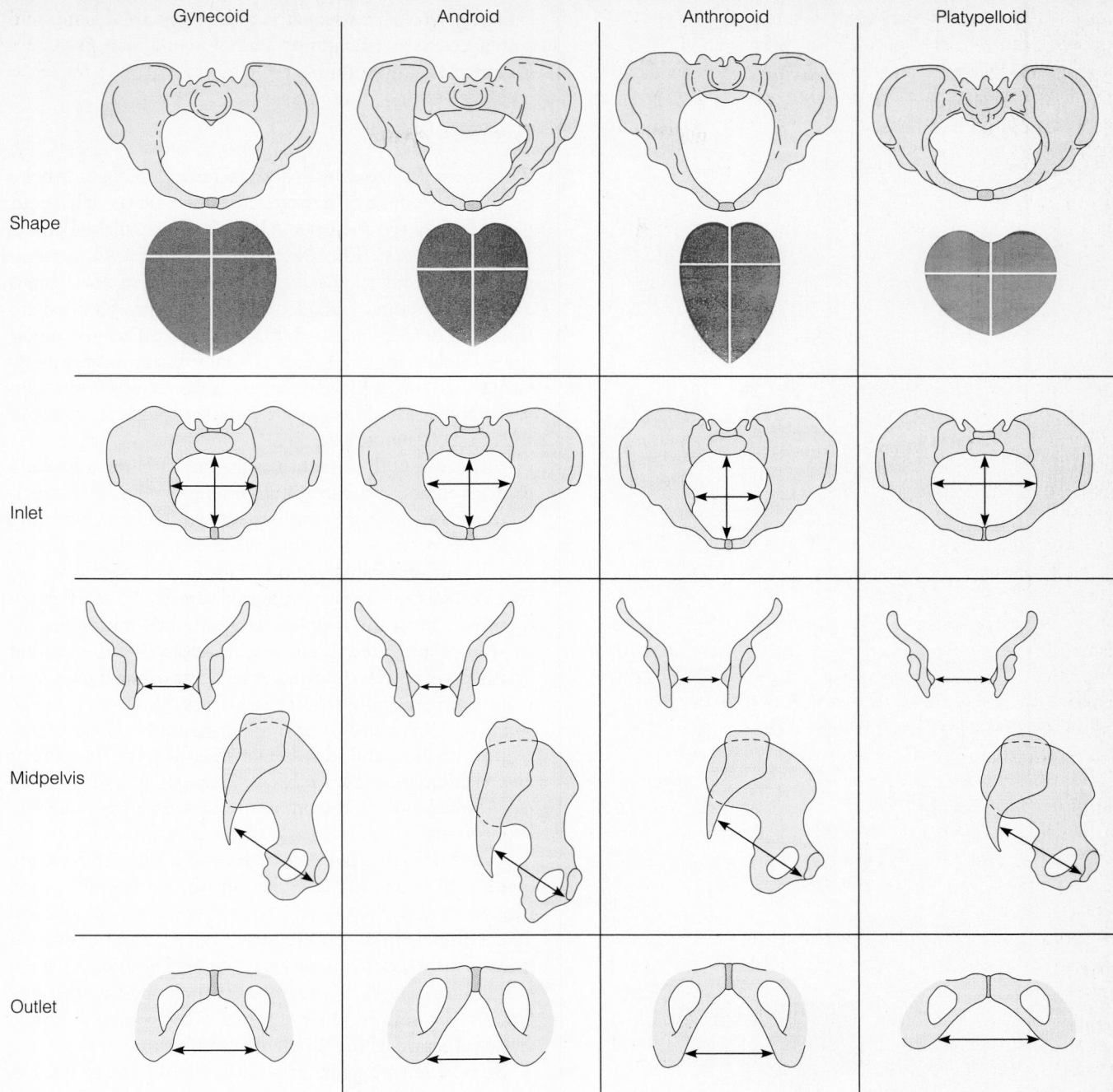

	Gynecoid	Android	Anthropoid	Platypelloid
Shape				
Inlet				
Midpelvis				
Outlet				

FIGURE 5-16   Comparison of Caldwell-Moloy pelvic types.

backward. The midpelvic diameters are at least adequate, making its capacity adequate. The anthropoid outlet has a normal or moderately narrow pubic arch; the interior pubic rami are long and narrow. The outlet capacity is adequate, and the bones are of medium weight and structure. Approximately 25% of female pelves are classified as anthropoid.

Platypelloid Pelvis   The platypelloid type refers to the flat female pelvis. The inlet is distinctly transverse oval, with a short anteroposterior and extremely short transverse diameter. The posterior sagittal and anterior sagittal diameters are short. Both the anterior and posterior segments are shallow. The platypelloid midpelvis has variable ischial spines, parallel side walls, and a wide sacrum with a deep curve inward. Only the transverse diameter is adequate; thus the midpelvic capacity is reduced. The platypelloid outlet has an extremely wide pubic arch; the inferior pubic rami are straight and short. The transverse diameter is wide, but the anteroposterior diameter is short. The outlet

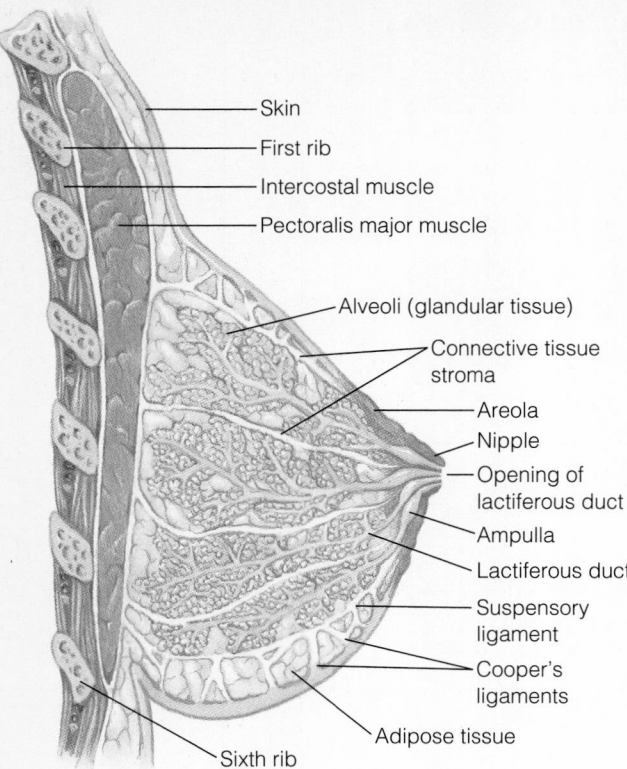

Skin
First rib
Intercostal muscle
Pectoralis major muscle

Alveoli (glandular tissue)

Connective tissue stroma

Areola
Nipple
Opening of lactiferous duct
Ampulla
Lactiferous duct
Suspensory ligament
Cooper's ligaments
Adipose tissue
Sixth rib

FIGURE 5-17 Anatomy of the breast: *A* Sagittal view of partially dissected left breast. *B* Sagittal view.

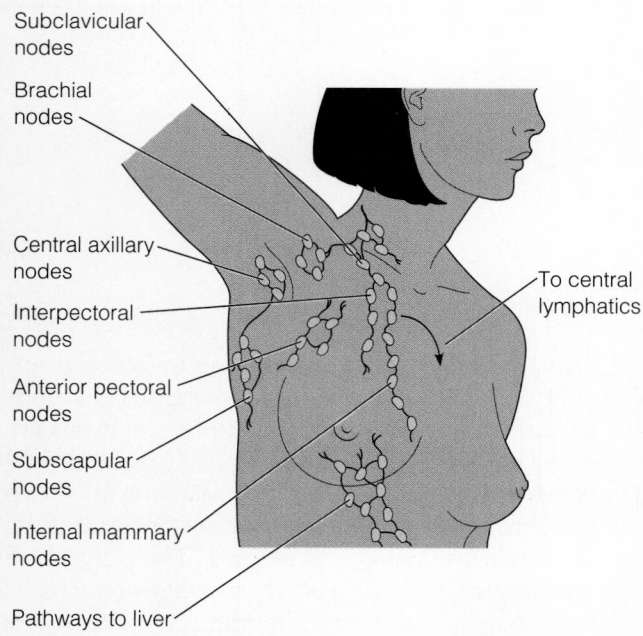

Subclavicular nodes
Brachial nodes
Central axillary nodes
Interpectoral nodes
Anterior pectoral nodes
Subscapular nodes
Internal mammary nodes
Pathways to liver
To central lymphatics

FIGURE 5-18 Lymphatic vessels draining the breast.

capacity may be inadequate. The platypelloid bones are similar to the gynecoid type. Only 5% of female pelves are classified as platypelloid.

Breasts

The *breasts*, or *mammary glands*, considered accessories of the reproductive system, are specialized sebaceous glands. They are conical and symmetrically placed on the sides of the chest. The greater pectoral and anterior seratus muscles underlie each breast. Suspending the breasts are fibrous tissues, called *Cooper's ligaments*, that extend from the deep fascia in the chest outward to just under the skin covering the breast. The left breast is frequently larger than the right. In different racial groups breasts develop at slightly different levels in the pectoral region of the chest (Rebar 1994).

In the center of each mature breast is the **nipple,** a protrusion about 0.5 to 1.3 cm in diameter. The nipple is composed mainly of erectile tissue, which becomes more rigid and prominent during the menstrual cycle, sexual excitement, pregnancy, and lactation. The nipple is surrounded by the heavily pigmented **areola,** 2.5 to 10 cm in diameter. Both the nipple and areola are roughened by small papillae called *Tubercles of Montgomery.* As an infant suckles, these tubercles secrete a fatty substance that helps lubricate and protect the breasts.

The breasts are composed of glandular, fibrous, and adipose tissue. The glandular tissue consists of acini or alveoli (Figure 5–17), which are arranged in a series of 15 to 24 lobes separated from each other by adipose and fibrous tissue.

Each lobe is made up of several lobules, which are comprised of many grapelike clusters of alveoli around tiny ducts. They are lined with a single layer of cuboidal epithelium, which secretes the various components of milk. The ducts from several lobules combine to form larger *lactiferous ducts,* or sinuses, which open on the surface of the nipple. The smooth muscle of the nipple causes erection of the nipple on contraction.

Cyclic hormonal control of the mature breast is complex. Essentially, estrogenic hormones stimulate the growth and development of the ductal epithelium. Progesterone, in association with estrogen, is responsible for the acinar and lobular development during the luteal phase of menstruation. Adrenal corticosteroids, prolactin, somatotropin (growth hormone), and thyroxine are also necessary for estrogen and progesterone to act.

The arterial, venous, and lymphatic systems communicate medially with the internal mammary vessels and laterally with the axillary vessels. Therefore in cancer of the breast metastasis follows the vascular supply both medially and laterally (Figure 5–18).

The biologic function of the breasts is to provide nourishment and protective maternal antibodies to infants through the lactation process. They are also a source of pleasurable sexual sensation.

FEMALE REPRODUCTIVE CYCLE

The monthly rhythmic changes in sexually mature females is usually called the menstrual cycle. A more accurate term is the **female reproductive cycle (FRC).** The FRC is composed of the *ovarian cycle*, during which ovulation occurs, and the *menstrual cycle*, during which menstruation occurs. These two cycles take place simultaneously (Figure 5–19).

Effects of Female Hormones

After menarche a female undergoes a cyclic pattern of ovulation and menstruation (if pregnancy does not occur) for a period of 30 to 40 years. This cycle is an orderly process under neurohormonal control: Each month one oocyte matures, ruptures from the ovary, and enters the fallopian tube. The ovary, vagina, uterus, and fallopian tubes are major target organs for female hormones. Each

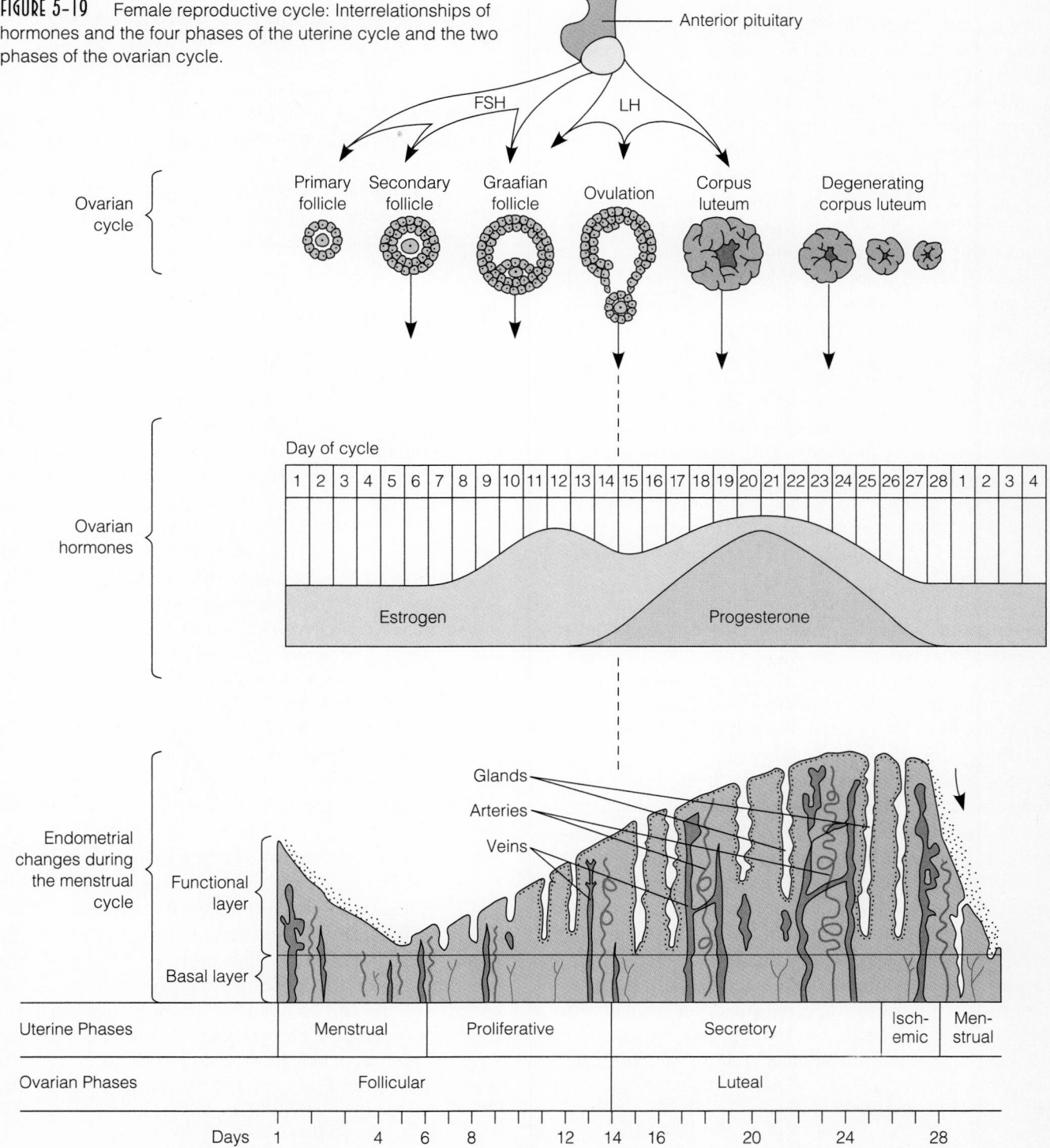

FIGURE 5-19 Female reproductive cycle: Interrelationships of hormones and the four phases of the uterine cycle and the two phases of the ovarian cycle.

organ undergoes changes indicative of the exact point in time of any menstrual cycle.

The ovaries not only produce mature gametes, but also secrete hormones. Ovarian hormones include the estrogens, progesterone, and testosterone. The ovary is sensitive to FSH and LH. The uterus is sensitive to estrogen and progesterone. The relative proportions of these hormones control the events of both ovarian and menstrual cycles.

Estrogens

Estrogens are associated with those characteristics contributing to "femaleness." The major estrogenic effects are due primarily to three classical estrogens: estrone, β-estradiol, and estriol. β-Estradiol is the major estrogen. Estrogens are secreted in large amounts by the ovaries in nonpregnant women.

Estrogens control the development of the female secondary sex characteristics: breast development, widening of the hips, and adipose deposits in the buttocks and mons pubis. The growth of body hair in females is also influenced by estrogen. In addition estrogens assist in the maturation of the ovarian follicles and cause the endometrial mucosa to proliferate following menstruation. The amount of estrogens is greatest during the proliferative (follicular or estrogenic) phase of the menstrual cycle. Estrogens also cause the uterus to increase in size and weight because of increased glycogen, amino acids, electrolytes, and water. Blood supply is expanded as well. Under the influence of estrogens myometrial contractility increases in both the uterus and the fallopian tubes, and there is increased uterine sensitivity to oxytocin. Estrogens inhibit FSH production and stimulate LH production.

Estrogens have effects on many hormones and other carrier proteins. This explains the increased amount of protein-bound iodine in pregnant women and in women who use oral contraceptives containing estrogen.

Estrogens may increase libidinal feelings in humans. They decrease the excitability of the hypothalamus, which may cause an increase in sexual desire.

For many years estrogens have been considered a preventive factor for coronary artery disease in women up to menopause, in the absence of diabetes or hypertension. Both lipoprotein and triglyceride metabolism are altered by estrogens. Although low estrogen levels do decrease serum cholesterol and β-lipoprotein levels and increase phospholipids and α-lipoprotein levels, numerous other factors must be considered in the development of coronary artery disease. Recent studies indicate that persistent high stress, coupled with specific types of personality patterns, diet (excessive calories, sodium, and saturated fats), smoking (especially in women taking oral contraceptives), obesity, and lack of exercise are influencing today's rise in incidence of coronary artery disease in women.

Progesterone

Progesterone is secreted by the corpus luteum and is found in greatest amounts during the secretory (luteal or progestational) phase of the menstrual cycle. It decreases the motility and contractility of the uterus caused by estrogens, thereby preparing the uterus for implantation after fertilization of the ovum. The endometrial mucosa is in a ready state as a result of estrogenic influence. Progesterone causes the uterine endometrium to further increase its supply of glycogen, arterial blood, secretory glands, amino acids, and water. This hormone is often called the *hormone of pregnancy* because its effects on the uterus allow pregnancy to be maintained.

Under the influence of progesterone the vaginal epithelium proliferates, and the cervix secretes thick, viscous mucus. Breast glandular tissue increases in size and complexity. Progesterone also prepares the breasts for lactation.

The temperature rise of about 0.35 C (0.5 F) that accompanies ovulation and persists throughout the secretory phase of the menstrual cycle is probably due to progesterone.

Prostaglandins (PGs)

Prostaglandins (oxygenated fatty acids), which are produced by the cells of the endometrium and are also classified as hormones, have varied actions in the body. The different types of PGs are indicated by Roman letters and either numbers (PGE_2) or Greek letters ($PGF_{2\alpha}$). Generally PGE relaxes smooth muscles and is a potent vasodilator; PGF is a potent vasoconstrictor and increases the contractility of muscles and arteries. Although their primary actions seem antagonistic, their basic regulatory functions in cells are achieved through an intricate pattern of reciprocal events. The discussion here will summarize their role in ovulation and menstruation.

Prostaglandin production increases during follicular maturation, is dependent on gonadotropins, and is essential to ovulation. Extrusion of the ovum, resulting from the increased contractility of the smooth muscle in the theca layer of the mature follicle, is thought to be caused by $PGF_{2\alpha}$ (Speroff et al 1994). Significant amounts of PGs are found in and around the follicle at the time of ovulation.

$PGF_{2\alpha}$ causes the corpus luteum to degenerate in the absence of pregnancy and induces luteolysis by blocking LH receptors in the corpus luteum (Speroff et al 1994).

During the late secretory phase the level of $PGF_{2\alpha}$ is higher than that of PGE. This event increases vasoconstriction and contractility of the myometrium, which contributes to the ischemia preceding menstruation. High concentration of PGs may also account for the vasoconstriction of the endometrium venous lacunae allowing for platelet aggregation at vascular rupture points, thereby preventing a rapid blood loss during menstruation. The menstrual flow's high concentration of PGs may also facilitate the process of tissue digestion, which allows for an orderly shedding of the endometrium during menstruation.

Neurohormonal Basis of the Female Reproductive Cycle

The FRC is controlled by complex interactions between the nervous and endocrine systems and their target tissues. These interactions involve the hypothalamus, anterior pituitary, and ovaries.

The hypothalamus secretes gonadotropin-releasing hormone (GnRH) to the pituitary gland in response to signals received from the central nervous system. This releasing hormone is often called luteinizing hormone–releasing hormone (LHRH) or follicle-stimulating hormone–releasing hormone (FSHRH).

In response to GnRH the anterior pituitary secretes the gonadotropic hormones FSH and LH. The ovaries contain specialized FSH and LH receptor cells. These receptor cells activate the production of adenylcyclase, causing increased cell growth and hormone secretion through the cyclic adenosine monophosphate (cAMP) mechanism. FSH is primarily responsible for the maturation of the ovarian follicle. As the follicle matures, it secretes increasing amounts of estrogen, which enhance the development of the follicle. (This estrogen also is responsible for the rebuilding/proliferation phase of the endometrium after it is shed during menstruation.)

Final maturation of the follicle will not come about without the action of LH. The anterior pituitary's production of LH increases sixfold to tenfold as the follicle matures. About 10 to 12 hours after the peak production of LH, ovulation occurs (Speroff et al 1994).

The LH is also responsible for the "luteinizing" of the theca and granulosa cells of the ruptured follicle (as described below). As a result, estrogen production is reduced and progesterone secretion continues. Thus estrogen levels fall a day before ovulation; tiny amounts of progesterone are in evidence. Ovulation takes place following the very rapid growth of the follicle as the sustained high level of estrogen diminishes and progesterone secretion begins.

The ruptured follicle undergoes rapid change and completes luteinization (the process of development of the corpus within a ruptured **graafian follicle**). The mass of lutein cells secretes large amounts of progesterone with smaller amounts of estrogen. (Concurrently, the excessive amounts of progesterone are responsible for the secretory phase of the uterine cycle.) Seven or 8 days following ovulation the corpus luteum begins to involute, losing its secretory function. The production of both progesterone and estrogen is severely diminished. The anterior pituitary responds with increasingly large amounts of FSH; a few days later LH production begins.

As a result new follicles become responsive to another ovarian cycle and begin maturing.

The Ovarian Cycle

The ovarian cycle has two phases: the follicular phase (days 1–14) and the luteal phase (days 15–28 in a 28-day cycle). Figure 5–20 depicts the changes that the follicle undergoes during the ovarian cycle. Usually only the length of the follicular phase varies in menstrual cycles of varying duration because the luteal phase is of fixed length. During the *follicular phase*, the immature follicle matures as a result of FSH. Within the follicle the oocyte grows. A mature graafian follicle appears about the 14th day under dual control of FSH and LH.

In the mature graafian follicle the cells surrounding the antral cavity are granulosa cells. The oocyte and follicular fluid are enclosed in the cumulus oophorus. The stromal elements of the ovary are condensed around the follicle in two layers: the *theca interna*, a vascular, hypertrophied layer; and the *theca externa*, an avascular layer of connective tissue. The theca interna cells resemble the luteal cells of the corpus luteum. In the mature graafian follicle the **zona pellucida** (oolemma), a thick, elastic capsule, develops around the oocyte. The fully mature graafian follicle is a large structure, measuring 5 to 10 mm. The mature follicle produces increasing amounts of estrogen.

Just before ovulation, the mature oocyte completes its first meiotic division (see Chapter 6 for a description of meiosis). As a result of this division, two cells are formed: a small cell called a *polar body* and a larger cell

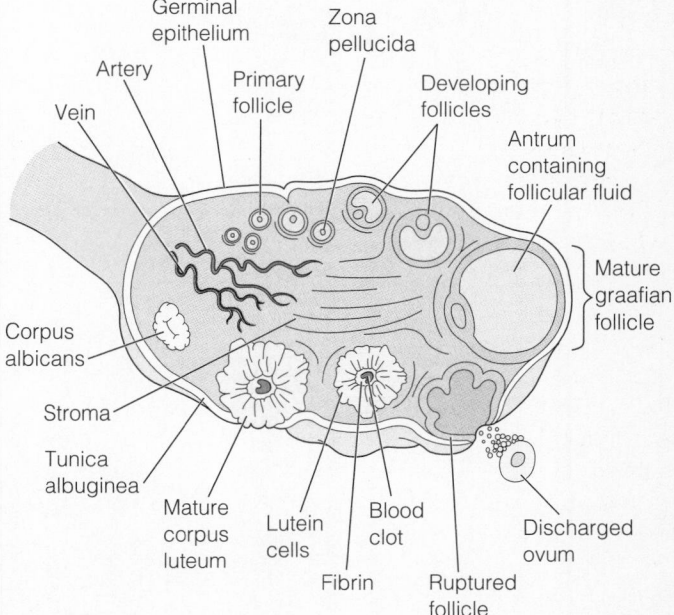

FIGURE 5-20 Various stages of development of the ovarian follicles.

called the *secondary oocyte*. The secondary oocyte matures into the ovum. (See Figure 6–4.)

As the graafian follicle matures and enlarges, it comes close to the surface of the ovary. The ovary surface has a blisterlike protrusion 10 to 15 mm in diameter, and the follicle's walls become thin. Extrusion of the ovum is aided by proteolytic enzyme formation by the theca externa and prostaglandin secretion into the follicular tissues. The secondary oocyte, polar body, and follicular fluid are pushed out. The ovum is discharged near the fimbria of the fallopian tube and is pulled into the tube to begin its journey toward the uterus.

Occasionally, ovulation is accompanied by midcycle pain, known as *mittelschmerz*. This pain may be caused by a thick tunica albuginea or by a local peritoneal reaction to the expelling of the follicular contents. Vaginal discharge may increase during ovulation, and a small amount of blood (midcycle spotting) may be discharged as well.

The body temperature increases about 0.3–0.6 C (0.5–1.0 F) 24 to 48 hours after the time of ovulation. It remains elevated until the day before menstruation begins. There may be an accompanying sharp basal body temperature drop just before the increase. These temperature changes are useful clinically to determine the approximate time ovulation occurs.

Generally, the ovum takes several minutes to travel through the ruptured follicle to the fallopian tube opening. The contractions of the tube's smooth muscle and its ciliary action propel the ovum through the tube. The ovum remains in the ampulla, where it may be fertilized and cleavage can begin. The ovum is thought to be fertile for only 6 to 24 hours. It reaches the uterus 72 to 96 hours after its release from the ovary.

The *luteal phase* begins when the ovum leaves its follicle. Under the influence of LH the **corpus luteum** develops from the ruptured follicle. Within 2 or 3 days the corpus luteum becomes yellowish and spherical and in-

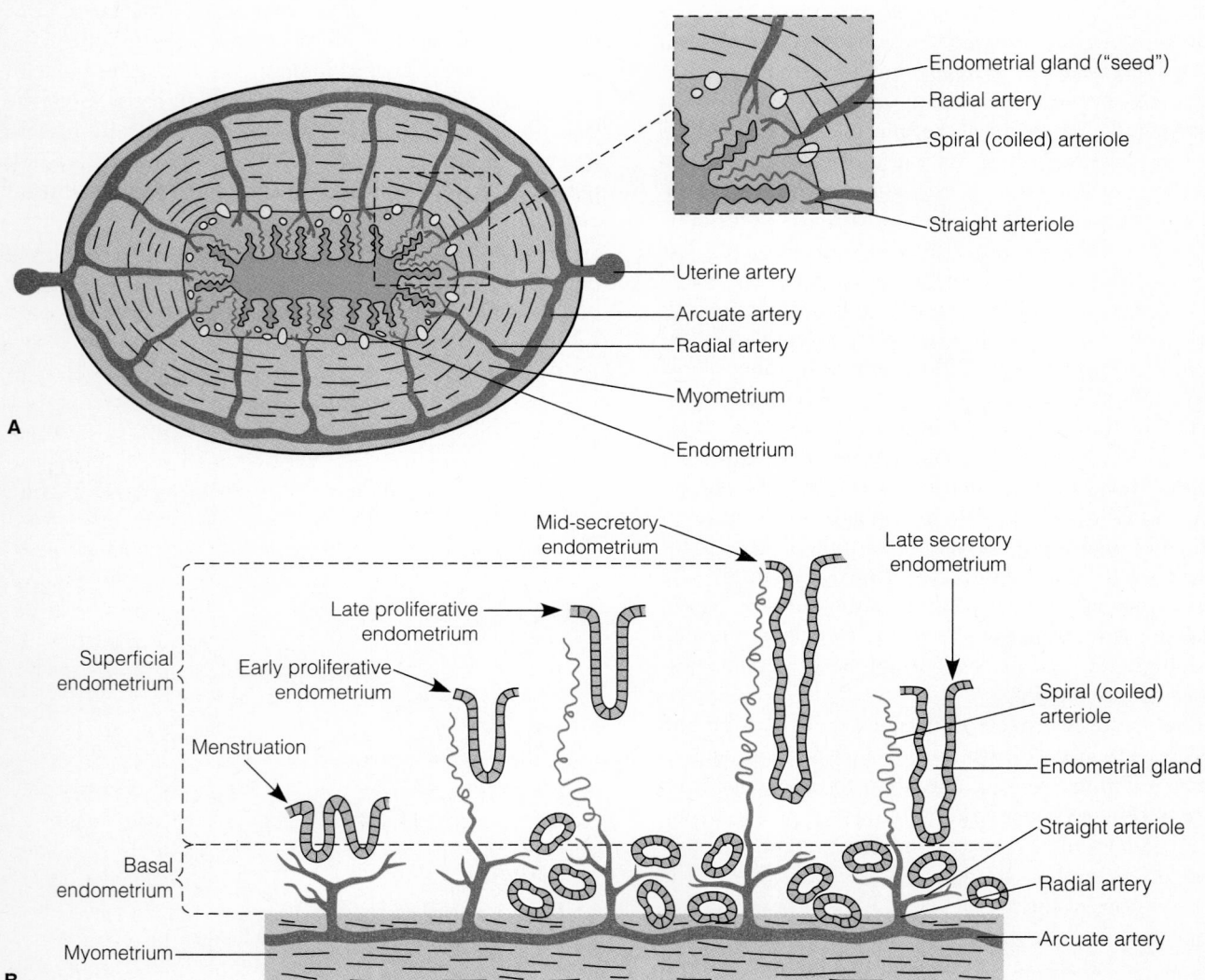

FIGURE 5–21   *A* Blood supply to the endometrium (cross-sectional view of the uterus).
B Schematic representation of blood supply during complete menstrual cycle.

creases in vascularity. If the ovum is fertilized and implants in the endometrium, the fertilized egg begins to secrete **human chorionic gonadotropin (hCG),** which is needed to maintain the corpus luteum. If fertilization does not occur, within about a week after ovulation the corpus luteum begins to degenerate, eventually becoming a connective tissue scar called the *corpus albicans*. With degeneration comes a decrease in estrogen and progesterone. This allows for an increase in LH and FSH, which triggers the hypothalamus. Approximately 14 days after ovulation (in a 28-day cycle), in the absence of pregnancy, menstruation begins.

The Menstrual Cycle

Menstruation is a physiologic event shared by all women, yet each woman's experience is unique. How a woman experiences menstruation depends on sociocultural factors and her attitudes about her body, sexuality, and reproductive function.

Menstruation is cyclic uterine bleeding in response to cyclic hormonal changes. Menstruation occurs when the ovum is not fertilized and begins about 14 days after ovulation in a 28-day cycle. The menstrual discharge, also referred to as the *menses* or *menstrual flow*, is composed of blood mixed with cervical and vaginal secretions, bacteria, mucus, leukocytes, and other cellular debris. The menstrual discharge is dark red and has a distinctive odor.

A review of the endometrium and its arterial blood supply will provide further understanding of the menstrual process. Blood flow from the spiral arterioles in the superficial endometrium is reduced, leading to a lack of blood and oxygen, which in turn produces tissue death (necrosis) and discharge of the superficial endometrium (menses). At the same time the straight arterioles provide the basal endometrium with sufficient blood flow to maintain this layer of the endometrium and the endometrial glands (or seeds) that are responsible for the generation of the endometrium in the next female reproductive or menstrual cycle (Figure 5–21). Bleeding is controlled by vasospasm of the straight basal arterioles, resulting in coagulative necrosis at the vessel tips.

Menarche—the onset of menstruation—usually occurs when a girl is about 12 to 13 years of age. Frequently, ovulation does not occur in early cycles; these are called anovulatory cycles. Early cycles also are often irregular in frequency, amount of flow, and duration. Within several months to 2 to 3 years a regular cycle becomes established.

Menstrual parameters vary greatly among individuals. Generally, menstruation occurs every 28 days, plus or minus 5 to 10 days. Emotional and physical factors such as illness, excessive fatigue, stress or anxiety, and rigorous exercise programs can alter the cycle interval. Certain environmental factors such as temperature and altitude may also affect the cycle.

TABLE 5-2	Characteristics of Menstrual Cycle and Ovulation
Menstrual phase (days 1–5)	Estrogen levels are low. Cervical mucus is scanty, viscous, and opaque. Endometrium is shed.
Proliferative phase (days 6–14)	Endometrium and myometrium thickness increases. Estrogen peaks just before ovulation. Cervical mucosa at ovulation: Is clear, thin, watery, and alkaline. Is more favorable to sperm. Has elasticity (*spinnbarkheit*) greater than 5 cm Shows ferning pattern on microscopic exam. Just prior to ovulation body temperature drops; then at ovulation basal body temperature increases 0.3 to 0.6C, and *mittelschmerz* and/or midcycle spotting may occur.
Secretory phase (days 15–26)	Estrogen drops sharply, and progesterone dominates. Vascularity of entire uterus increases. Tissue glycogen increases, and the uterus is made ready for implantation.
Ischemic phase (days 27–28)	Both estrogen and progesterone levels fall. Spiral arteries undergo vasoconstriction. Endometrium becomes pale. Blood vessels rupture. Blood escapes into uterine stromal cells.

The duration of menses is from 2 to 8 days, with the blood loss averaging 30 to 80 mL, and the loss of iron averaging 0.5 to 1 mg daily.

The menstrual cycle has four phases: menstrual phase, proliferative phase, secretory phase, and ischemic phase (Table 5–2). Menstruation occurs during the *menstrual phase*. Some endometrial areas are shed while others remain. Some of the remaining tips of the endometrial glands begin to regenerate. The endometrium is in a resting state following menstruation. Estrogen levels are low, and the endometrium is 1 to 2 mm deep. During this part of the cycle the cervical mucosa is scanty, viscous, and opaque.

The *proliferative phase* begins when the endometrial glands enlarge, becoming twisted and longer, in response to increasing amounts of estrogen. The blood vessels become prominent and dilated, and the endometrium increases in thickness sixfold to eightfold. This gradual process reaches its peak just before ovulation. The cervical mucosa becomes thin, clear, watery, and more alkaline, making the mucosa more favorable to spermatozoa. As ovulation nears, the cervical mucous shows increased elasticity, called *spinnbarkheit*. At ovulation the mucus will stretch more than 5 cm. The cervical mucosa pH increases from below 7.0 to 7.5 at the time of ovulation. On microscopic examination the mucosa shows a characteristic ferning pattern (Figure 7–4B). This ferning pattern is a useful aid in assessment of ovulation time (Table 5–3). For an in-depth discussion, see Chapter 7.

The *secretory phase* follows ovulation. The endometrium, under estrogenic influence, undergoes slight

| TABLE 5-3 | Signs of Ovulation |

The cervical mucosa changes in the following ways:

- The amount of mucus increases.
- It appears thin, watery, and clear.
- *Spinnbarkheit* greater than 5 cm is present.
- A ferning pattern appears on microscopic examination.

Basal body temperature increases 0.3 to 0.6 C 24 to 48 hours after ovulation.
Mittelschmerz may be present.
Midcycle spotting may occur.

---

cellular growth. Progesterone, however, causes such marked swelling and growth that the epithelium is warped into folds (Figure 5–22). The amount of tissue glycogen increases. The glandular epithelial cells begin to fill with cellular debris, and the glands become tortuous and dilate. The glands secrete small quantities of endometrial fluid in preparation for a fertilized ovum. The vascularity of the entire uterus increases greatly, providing a nourishing bed for implantation. If implantation occurs, the endometrium, under the influence of progesterone, continues to develop and become even thicker (Figure 5–23; see Chapter 6 for an in-depth discussion of implantation.)

If fertilization does not occur, the *ischemic phase* begins. The corpus luteum begins to degenerate, and as a result both estrogen and progesterone levels fall. Areas of necrosis appear under the epithelial lining. Extensive vascular changes also occur. Small blood vessels rupture, and the spiral arteries constrict and retract, causing a deficiency of blood in the endometrium, which becomes pale. This ischemic phase is characterized by the escape of blood into the stromal cells of the uterus. The menstrual flow begins, thus beginning the menstrual cycle again. After menstruation the basal layer remains so that the tips of the glands can regenerate the new functional endometrial layer. See Table 5–4 for a summary of the FRC.

MALE REPRODUCTIVE SYSTEM

The primary reproductive functions of the male genitals are to produce and transport the male sex cells (sperm) through and eventually out of the genital tract into the female genital tract. The male reproductive system consists of the external and internal genitals (Figure 5–24).

External Genitals

The two external reproductive organs are the penis and the scrotum.

Natural family planning entails knowing the fertile periods of the female partner and abstaining from sexual intercourse during those times to avoid a pregnancy, or having intercourse during those times to achieve a pregnancy. Determination of fertility is based on the presence or absence of cervical mucus. Richard Fehring, Donna Lawrence, and Connie Philpot determined the use effectiveness of the Creighton model of natural family planning. Two types of effectiveness apply to the use of natural planning to avoid pregnancy: Method effectiveness occurs when a method is taught and used correctly; use effectiveness refers to the actual use of the method and may include errors in both teaching and use.

The study sample included 242 couples who used the Creighton method for a combined total of 1,793 months. The method requires couples to attend an introductory teaching session and at least eight 1-hour follow-up sessions during the following year. Standardization of the session occurs through the use of a manual, extensive follow-up charting forms, a case management book, and a year-long program of training for the teachers.

At the 12th month of use for each couple the method was found to be 98.8% method-effective and 98.0% use-effective in avoiding pregnancy. The couples who were trying to conceive had a 24.4% use-effective rate in achieving pregnancy. Each pregnancy was evaluated and classified within the first 3 months. Classifications entailed achieving-related pregnancy with the method being used successfully, avoidance-related pregnancy with the method used to try to avoid a pregnancy that occurred anyway, or unresolved pregnancy in which the pregnancy cannot be classified as one of the first two categories. Avoidance-related pregnancy can be broken down into four sub-classifications: (1) method-related with the method being used correctly to avoid pregnancy, (2) use-related with the method being taught correctly but used incorrectly, (3) teaching-related with the method taught incorrectly but used correctly, and (4) using-teaching related with the method both taught and used incorrectly.

Clinical Application of Study

Natural family planning has the advantage of participation by both partners with a decision being made by each. Nurses should be conversant enough with all methods of family planning to recommend appropriate information to their clients based on client preference.

SOURCE: Fehring R, Lawrence D, Philpot C: Use effectiveness of the Creighton model ovulation method of natural family planning. *JOGNN* 1994; 23(4):303.

Penis

The *penis* is an elongated, cylindrical structure consisting of a body, termed the shaft, and a cone-shaped end called the glans. The penis lies in front of the scrotum.

The shaft of the penis is made up of three longitudinal columns of erectile tissue: the paired *corpora cavernosa* and a third, the *corpus spongiosum*. These columns are covered by a dense, fibrous connective tissue and then

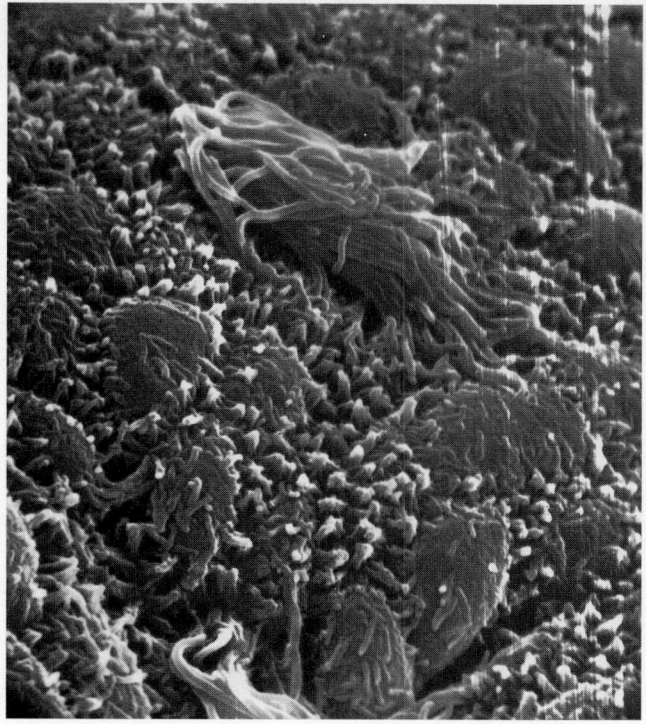

A

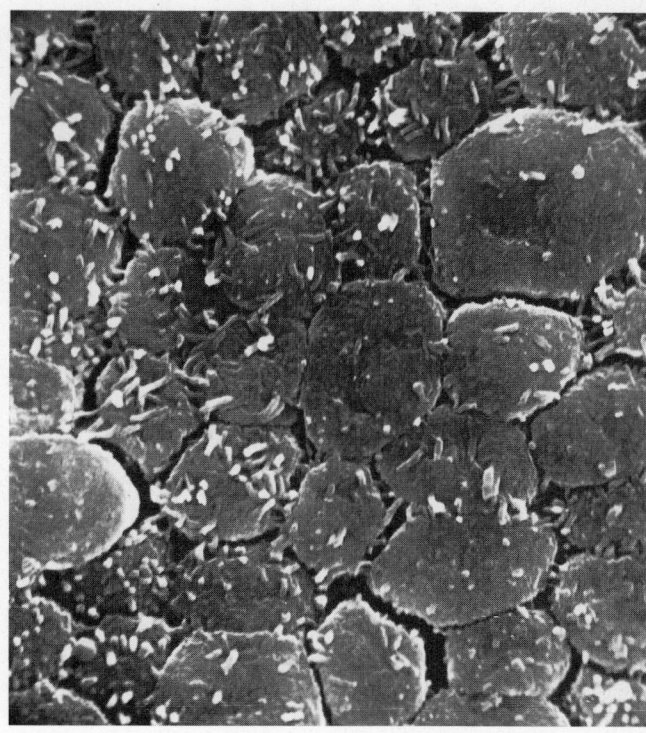

B

FIGURE 5-22 Scanning electron micrographs of the uterine lining during different phases of the uterine cycle. During the luteal phase *(A)* some of the cells have cilia, and some are secreting droplets. The secreting cells are covered with microvilli. In the secretory phase *(B)* microvilli are still present on the surface of the secreting cells, but the general surface of the lining has a lumpier appearance than during the proliferative phase, and the cilia appear shorter and less numerous. The named phases refer to the uterine condition at the time the photographs were taken.

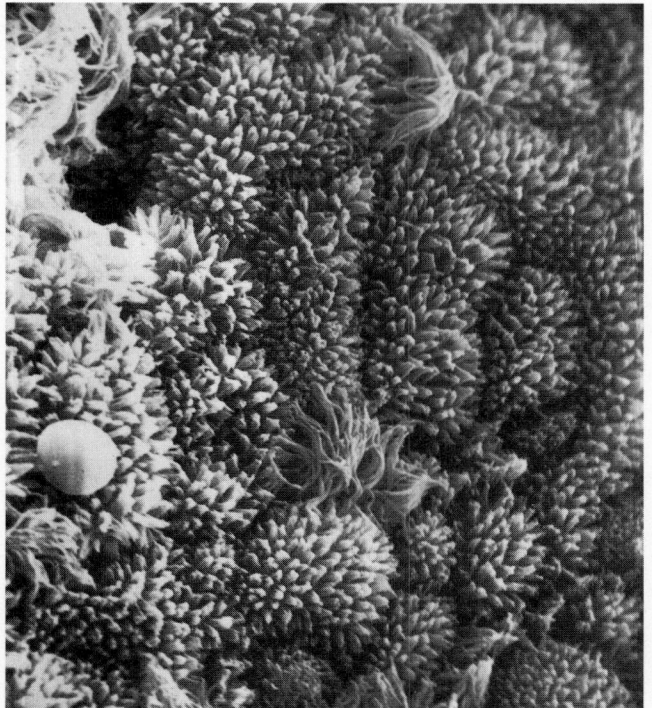

FIGURE 5-23 Scanning electron micrograph of the inner lining of the uterus at the time of blastocyst implantation. The blastocyst is an embryo at an early stage of development.

| **TABLE 5-4** | Summary of Female Reproductive Cycle |

Ovarian Cycle

Follicular phase (days 1–14): Primordial follicle matures under influence of FSH and LH up to the time of ovulation.

Luteal phase (days 15–28): Ovum leaves follicle; corpus luteum develops under LH influence and produces high levels of progesterone and low levels of estrogen.

Menstrual Cycle

Menstrual phase (days 1–5)

Proliferative phase (days 6–14): Estrogen peaks just prior to ovulation. Cervical mucus at ovulation is clear, thin, watery, alkaline, and more favorable to sperm; shows ferning pattern; and has *spinnbarkheit* greater than 5 cm. At ovulation body temperature drops, then rises sharply and remains elevated.

Secretory phase (days 15–26): Estrogen drops sharply and progesterone dominates.

Ischemic phase (days 27–28): Both estrogen and progesterone levels drop.

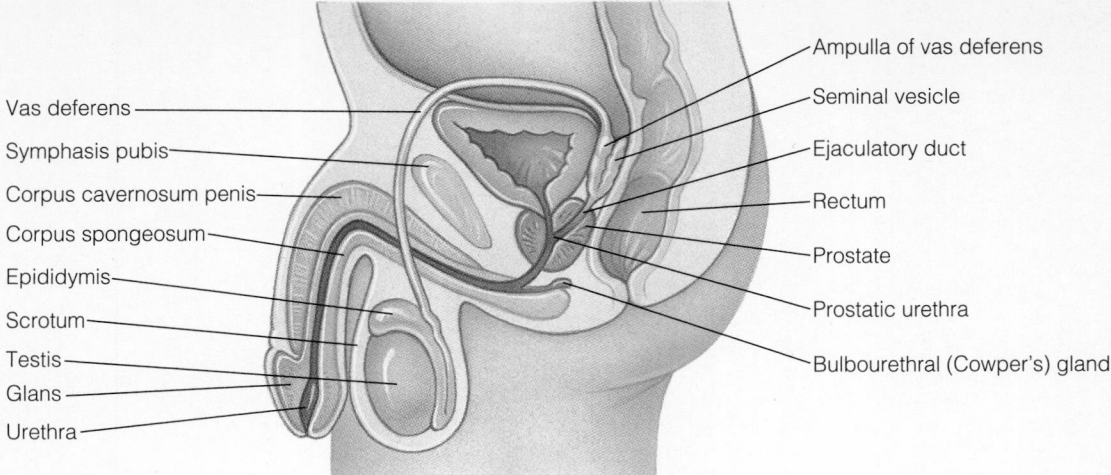

FIGURE 5-24   Male reproductive system, sagittal view.

enclosed by an elastic tissue. The penis is covered by a thin outer layer of skin.

The corpus spongiosum contains the urethra and extends beyond the corpora cavernosa to become the glans at the distal end of the penis. The urethra widens within the glans and ends in a slitlike orifice, located in the tip of the glans, called the *urethral meatus*. A circular fold of skin arises just behind the glans and covers it. Known as the *prepuce*, or *foreskin*, it is frequently removed by the surgical procedure of circumcision (Chapter 29). If the corpus spongiosum does not surround the urethra completely, the urethral meatus may occur on the ventral aspect of the penile shaft (hypospadias) or on the dorsal aspect (epispadias).

The penis is innervated by the pudendal nerve. Sympathetic fibers come from the hypogastric and pelvic plexuses; parasympathetic fibers from the third and fourth sacral nerves from the splanchnic nerves. During sexual stimulation the parasympathetic fibers are stimulated, and the ischiocavernous muscle contracts, preventing the return of venous blood from the cavernous sinuses. The blood vessels of the penis engorge, causing the penis to become erect. The penis elongates, thickens, and stiffens, a process called *erection*. If sexual stimulation is intense enough, the forceful and sudden expulsion of semen occurs through the rhythmic contractions of the penile muscles. This phenomenon is called *ejaculation*.

The penis serves both the urinary and reproductive systems. Urine is expelled through the urethral meatus. The primary function of the penis is to deposit sperm in the female vagina during sexual intercourse so that fertilization of the ovum can occur.

Scrotum

The *scrotum* is a pouchlike structure that hangs in front of the anus and behind the penis. Composed of skin and the *dartos* muscle, the scrotum shows increased pigmentation

and scattered hairs. The sebaceous glands open directly onto the scrotal surface; their secretion has a distinctive odor. Contraction of the dartos and cremasteric muscles shortens the scrotum and draws it closer to the body, thus wrinkling its outer surface. The degree of wrinkling is greatest in young men and at cold temperatures and is least in older men and at warm temperatures.

Inside the scrotum are two lateral compartments separated by a medial septum derived from the dartos muscle. Each compartment contains a testis with its related structures. Because the left spermatic cord grows longer, the left testis and its scrotal sac hang lower than the right.

TABLE 5-5	Summary of Male Reproductive Organ Functions

The testes house seminiferous tubules and gonads.

- Seminiferous tubules contain sperm cells in various stages of development and undergoing meiosis.
- Sertoli's cells nourish and protect spermatocytes (phase between spermatids and spermatozoa).
- Leydig's cells are the main source of testosterone.
- Epididymides provide an area for maturation of sperm and a reservoir for mature spermatozoa.
- The vas deferens connects the epididymis with the prostate gland, then connects with ducts from the seminal vesicle to become an ejaculatory duct.
- Ejaculatory ducts provide a passageway for semen and seminal fluid into the urethra.
- Seminal vesicles secrete yellowish fluid rich in fructose, prostaglandins, and fibrinogen. This provides nutrition that increases motility and fertilizing ability of sperm. Prostaglandins also aid fertilization by making the cervical mucus more receptive to sperm.
- The prostate gland secretes thin, alkaline fluid containing calcium, citric acid, and other substances. Alkalinity counteracts acidity of ductus and seminal vesicle secretions.
- Bulbourethral (Cowper's) glands secrete alkaline, viscous fluid into semen, aiding in neutralization of acidic vaginal secretions.

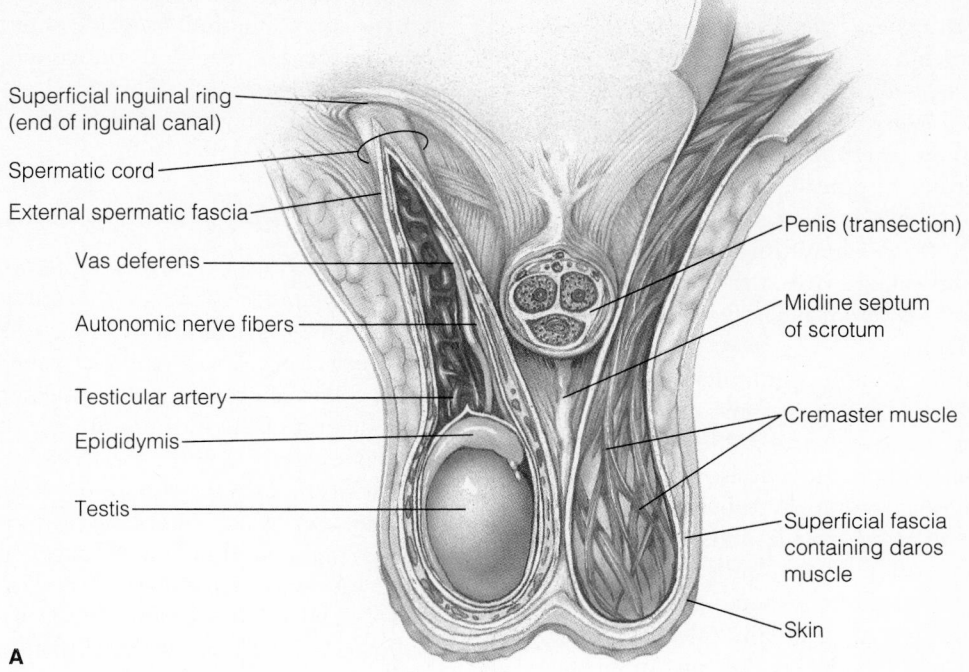

Superficial inguinal ring
(end of inguinal canal)

Spermatic cord

External spermatic fascia

Vas deferens

Autonomic nerve fibers

Testicular artery

Epididymis

Testis

Penis (transection)

Midline septum
of scrotum

Cremaster muscle

Superficial fascia
containing daros
muscle

Skin

A

A ridge (raphe) on the external scrotal surface marks the position of the medial septum and continues anteriorly on the urethral surface of the penis but disappears in the perineal area.

The function of the scrotum is to protect the testes and the sperm by maintaining a temperature lower than that of the body. Spermatogenesis will not occur if the testes fail to descend and thus remain at body temperature. Because it is sensitive to touch, pressure, temperature, and pain, the scrotum defends against potential harm to the testes.

Internal Reproductive Organs

The male internal reproductive organs include the gonads (testes or testicles), a system of ducts (epididymis, vas deferens, ejaculatory duct, and urethra), and accessory glands (seminal vesicles, prostate gland, bulbourethral glands, and urethral glands). See Table 5–5 for a summary of male reproductive organ functions.

Testes

The *testes* are a pair of oval, compound glandular organs contained in the scrotum (Figure 5–25). In the sexually mature male they are the site of spermatozoa production and the secretion of several male sex hormones.

Each testis is 4 to 6 cm long, 2 to 3 cm wide, and 3 to 4 cm deep. Each weighs 10 to 15 g. It is covered by a serous membrane and an inner capsule that is tough,

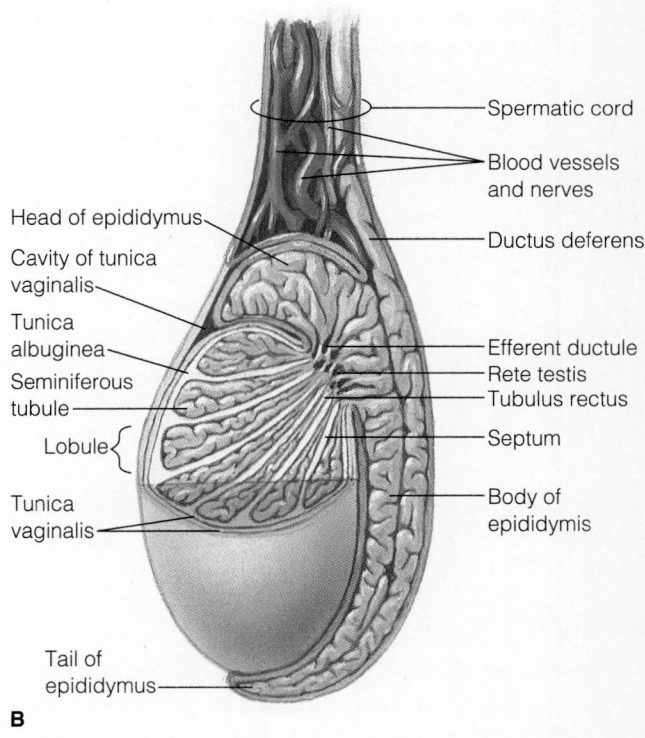

Spermatic cord

Blood vessels
and nerves

Head of epididymus

Cavity of tunica
vaginalis

Tunica
albuginea

Seminiferous
tubule

Lobule {

Tunica
vaginalis

Ductus deferens

Efferent ductule
Rete testis
Tubulus rectus

Septum

Body of
epididymis

Tail of
epididymus

B

FIGURE 5-25   The testes: *A* External view (at top of page). *B* Sagittal view showing interior anatomy.

white, and fibrous. The connective tissue sends projections inward to form septa, dividing the testis into 250 to 400 lobules. Each lobule contains one to three tightly packed *seminiferous tubules* containing sperm cells in all stages of development.

The seminiferous tubules are surrounded by loose connective tissue, which houses abundant blood and lymph vessels and the *interstitial (Leydig's) cells*. The cells produce testosterone, the primary male sex hormone. The seminiferous tubules come together to form the 20 or 30 straight tubules, which in turn form an anastomosing network of thin-walled spaces, the *rete testis*. The rete testis forms 10 to 15 efferent ducts that empty into the duct of the epididymis.

Most of the cells lining the seminiferous tubules undergo *spermatogenesis*, a process of maturation in which spermatocytes become spermatozoa. (See Chapter 6 for further discussion of spermatogenesis.) Sperm production varies among and within the tubules, with cells in different areas of the same tubule undergoing different stages of spermatogenesis. The seminiferous tubules also contain *Sertoli's cells*, which nourish and protect the spermatocytes. The sperm are eventually released from the tubules into the epididymis, where they mature further.

Like the female reproductive cycle, the process of spermatogenesis and other functions of the testes are the result of complex neural and hormonal controls. The hypothalamus secretes releasing factors, which stimulate the anterior pituitary to release the gonadotropins FSH and LH. These hormones cause the testes to produce *testosterone*, which maintains spermatogenesis, increases sperm production by the seminiferous tubules, and stimulates production of seminal fluid.

Testosterone is also responsible for the development of secondary male characteristics and certain behavioral patterns. The effects of testosterone include structural and functional development of the male genital tract, emission and ejaculation of seminal fluid, distribution of body hair, promotion of growth and strength of long bones, increased muscle mass, and enlargement of the vocal cords. The action of testosterone on the central nervous system is thought to produce aggressiveness and sexual drive. The action of testosterone is constant, not cyclic like that of the female hormones. Its production is not limited to a certain number of years, but is thought to decrease with age.

In summary, the primary functions of the testes are to serve as the site of spermatogenesis and to produce testosterone.

Epididymis

The epididymis (plural, *epididymides*) is a duct about 5.6 m long, although it is convoluted into a compact structure about 3.75 cm long. An epididymis lies behind each testis. It arises from the top of the testis, extends downward, and then passes upward, where it becomes the vas deferens.

The epididymis provides a reservoir where spermatozoa can survive for a long period. When discharged from the seminiferous tubules into the epididymis, the sperm are immobile and incapable of fertilizing an ovum. The spermatozoa remain in the epididymis for 2 to 10 days. As the sperm are transported along the tortuous course of the epididymis, they become both motile and fertile (Marieb & Mallatt 1992).

Vas Deferens and Ejaculatory Ducts

The *vas deferens*, also known as the *ductus deferens*, is about 40 cm long and connects the epididymis with the prostate. One vas deferens arises from the posterior border of each testis. It joins the spermatic cord and weaves over and between several pelvic structures until it meets the vas deferens from the opposite side. Each vas deferens terminus expands to form the *terminal ampulla*. It then unites with the seminal vesicle duct (a gland) to form the *ejaculatory duct*, which enters the prostate gland and ends in the prostatic urethra. The ejaculatory ducts serve as a passageway for semen and fluid secreted by the seminal vesicles. The main function of the vas deferens is to rapidly squeeze the sperm from their storage sites (the epididymis and distal part of the vas deferens) into the urethra.

Men who choose to take total responsibility for birth control may elect to have a vasectomy. In this procedure the scrotal portion of the vas deferens is surgically incised or cauterized. Although sperm continues to be produced for the next several years, they can no longer reach the outside of the body. Eventually, they deteriorate and are reabsorbed (Marieb & Mallatt 1992).

Urethra

The male urethra is a passageway for urine and semen. The urethra begins in the bladder and passes through the prostate gland, where it is called the *prostatic urethra*.

The urethra emerges from the prostate gland to become the *membranous urethra*. It terminates in the penis, where it is called the *penile urethra*. In the penile urethra goblet secretory cells are present, and smooth muscle is replaced by erectile tissue.

Accessory Glands

The male accessory glands are specialized structures under endocrine and neural control. Each secretes a unique and essential component of the total seminal fluid in an ordered sequence.

The *seminal vesicles* are two glands composed of many lobes. Each vesicle is about 7.5 cm long. They are situated between the bladder and rectum and immediately above the base of the prostate. The epithelium lining the seminal vesicles secretes an alkaline, viscous, clear fluid rich in high-energy fructose, prostaglandins, fibrinogen, and amino acids. During ejaculation this fluid mixes with

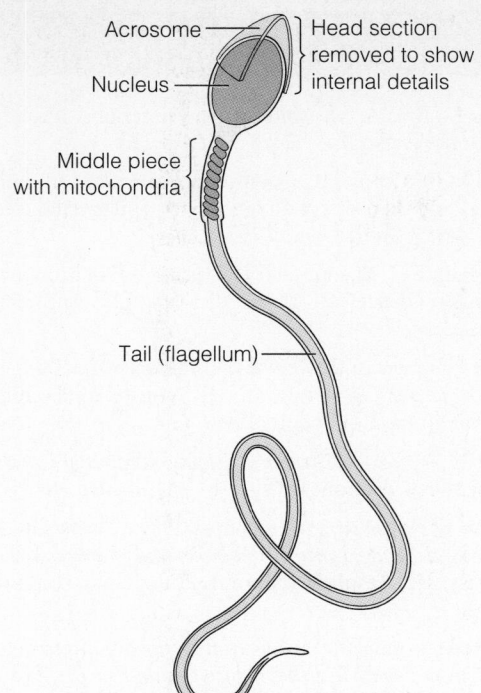

Acrosome
Nucleus
Head section removed to show internal details

Middle piece with mitochondria

Tail (flagellum)

FIGURE 5-26 Schematic representation of a mature spermatozoon.

sperm in the ejaculatory ducts. This fluid (about 70% of the semen fluid volume) helps provide an environment favorable to sperm motility and metabolism (Aumüller & Riva 1992).

The *prostate gland* encircles the upper part of the urethra and lies below the neck of the bladder. Made up of several lobes, it measures about 4 cm in diameter and weighs 20 to 30 g. The prostate is made up of both glandular and muscular tissue. It secretes a thin, milky, alkaline fluid containing high levels of zinc, calcium, citric acid, and acid phosphatase (Marieb & Mallatt 1992). This fluid protects the sperm from the acidic environment of the vagina and the male urethra, which could be spermicidal.

The *bulbourethral* or *Cowper's glands* are a pair of small round structures on either side of the membranous urethra. The glands secrete a clear, thick, alkaline fluid rich in mucoproteins that becomes part of the semen. This secretion also lubricates the penile urethra during sexual excitement and neutralizes the acid in the male urethra and the vagina, thereby enhancing sperm mobility.

The *urethral* or *Littre's glands* are tiny mucous-secreting glands found throughout the membranous lining of the penile urethra. Their secretions add to those of the bulbourethral glands.

Semen

The male ejaculate, *semen* or *seminal fluid*, is made up of spermatozoa and the secretions of all the accessory glands. The seminal fluid transports viable and motile

sperm to the female reproductive tract. Effective transportation of sperm requires adequate nutrients, an adequate pH (about 7.5), a specific concentration of sperm to fluid, and an optimal osmolarity.

A spermatozoon is made up of a *head* and a *tail* (Figure 5–26). The tail is divided into the middle piece and end piece. The head's main components are the *acrosome*, and the *nucleus*. The head carries the male's haploid number of chromosomes (23), and it is the part that enters the ovum at fertilization (Chapter 6). The tail, or *flagellum*, is specialized for motility.

Sperm may be stored in the male genital system up to 42 days, depending primarily on the frequency of ejaculations. The average volume of ejaculate following abstinence for several days is 2 to 5 mL but may vary from 1 to 10 mL. Repeated ejaculation results in decreased volume. Once ejaculated, sperm can live only 2 or 3 days in the female genital tract.

KEY CONCEPTS

Reproductive system events include developmental changes that lead to puberty, gametogenesis (spermatogenesis and oogenesis), sexual intercourse, development of sense of sexuality, pregnancy, embryo development, parturition, and lactation.

Reproductive activities require complex interactions between the reproductive structures, the central nervous system, and such endocrine glands as the pituitary, hypothalamus, testes, and ovaries.

At puberty an alteration in brain sensitivity leads to an increased release of GnRH, which stimulates LH and FSH, leading in the male to an increase in testosterone and in the female to an increase in estrogen and progesterone.

Estrogen is the principal cause of the events of puberty in females (maturation of ova, enlargement of the uterus and fallopian tubes, deposition of fat in the breasts and hips, and characteristic hair growth).

Puberty changes for the male (onset of spermatogenesis; enlargement of the penis, scrotum, and testes; voice changes; and characteristic hair growth) occur as a result of increased testosterone production by the testes.

The female reproductive system consists of the ovaries, where female germ cells and female sex hormones are formed; the fallopian tubes, which capture the ovum and allow transport to the uterus; the uterus, which is the implantation site for the fertilized ovum (blastocyst); the cervix, which is a protective portal for the body of the uterus and the connection between the vagina and the uterus; and the vagina, which is the passageway from the external genitals to the uterus and provides for discharge of menstrual products to the outside of the body.

The female reproductive cycle may be described in terms of the ovarian cycle, during which ovulation occurs, and the menstrual cycle, during which menstruation occurs. These two cycles take place simultaneously and are under neurohumoral control.

The ovarian cycle has two phases: the follicular phase and the luteal phase. During the follicular phase, the primordial follicle matures under the influence of FSH and LH until ovulation occurs. The luteal phase begins when the ovum leaves the follicle and the corpus luteum develops under the influence of LH. The corpus luteum produces high levels of progesterone and low levels of estrogen.

The menstrual cycle has four phases: menstrual, proliferative, secretory, and ischemic. Menstruation is the actual shedding of the endometrial lining, when estrogen levels are low. The proliferative phase begins when the endometrial glands begin to enlarge under the influence of estrogen and cervical mucosal changes occur; the changes peak at ovulation. The secretory phase follows ovulation, and, influenced primarily by progesterone, the uterus increases its vascularity to make ready for possible implantation. The ischemic phase is characterized by degeneration of the corpus luteum, decreases in both estrogen and progesterone levels, constriction of the spiral arteries, and escape of blood into the stromal cells of the endometrium.

The male reproductive system consists of the testes, where male germ cells and male sex hormones are formed; a series of continuous ducts through which spermatozoa are transported outside the body; accessory glands that produce secretions important to sperm nutrition, survival, and transport; and the penis, which serves as the reproductive organ of intercourse.

REFERENCES

Aumüller G, Riva A: Morphology and functions of the human seminal vesicle. *Andrologia* 1992; 24:183.

Caldwell WE, Moloy HC: Anatomical variations in the female pelvis and their effect on labor with a suggested classification. *Am J Obstet Gynecol* 1933; 26:479.

Cunningham FG, MacDonald PC, Gant NF (editors): *Williams Obstetrics*, 19th ed. Norwalk, CT: Appleton & Lange, 1993.

Davies J: Anatomy of the female genital tract. In: *Danforth's Obstetrics and Gynecology*, 6th ed. Scott JR et al (editors). Philadelphia: Lippincott, 1990.

Marieb EN, Mallatt J: *Human Anatomy*. Redwood City, CA: Benjamin/Cummings, 1992.

Rebar RW: The breast and the physiology of lactation. In: *Maternal-Fetal Medicine: Principles and Practice*, 3rd ed. Creasy RK, Resnik R (editors). Philadelphia: Saunders, 1994.

Resnik R: Anatomic alterations in the reproductive tract. In: *Maternal-Fetal Medicine: Principles and Practice*, 3rd ed. Creasy RK, Resnik R (editors). Philadelphia: Saunders, 1994.

Speroff L, Glass RH, Kase NG: *Clinical Gynecologic Endrocrinology and Infertility*, 5th ed. Baltimore: Williams & Wilkins, 1994.

Tanner JM: *Fetus into Man: Physical Growth from Conception to Maturity*, 2nd ed. Cambridge, MA: Harvard Univ Press, 1990.

Weiss G, Goldsmith LT: Puberty and pediatric and adolescent gynecology. In: *Danforth's Obstetrics and Gynecology*, 7th ed. Scott JR et al (editors). Philadelphia: Lippincott, 1994.

CONCEPTION AND FETAL DEVELOPMENT

*M*y friends tease me when I say this, but I *know* the moment my daughter was conceived. My husband and I had both been so busy at work, but we finally went away for a long weekend together. It was wonderful—we got back some of the magic as we took long walks and talked and talked. Until that weekend, whenever we discussed having children it was always "maybe someday."
On the second night we decided to skip the diaphragm for the first time ever. Our love-making seemed so special that evening, a true reflection of the emotional closeness we had recaptured. I never went back to using the diaphragm after that weekend, but I am convinced that Jennifer is the result of that night together!

OBJECTIVES

Explain the differences between mitotic cellular division and meiotic cellular division.

Compare the processes by which ova and sperm are produced.

Describe the process of fertilization.

Identify the differing processes by which fraternal (dizygotic) and identical (monozygotic) twins are formed.

Describe in order of increasing complexity the structures that form during the cellular multiplication and differentiation stages of intrauterine development.

Describe the development, structure, and functions of the placenta and umbilical cord during intrauterine life.

Summarize the significant changes in growth and development of the fetus in utero at 4, 6, 12, 16, 20, 24, 28, 32, 36, and 40 weeks' gestation.

Identify the vulnerable periods during which malformations of the various organ systems may occur, and describe the resulting congenital malformations.

Each person is unique. What is interesting about this uniqueness is that all of us have many if not all of the same "parts," and these parts usually function similarly. Even our chromosomes, those determinants of the structure and function of our organ systems and traits, are made of the same biochemical substances. How do we become unique, then? The answer lies in the physiologic mechanisms of heredity, the processes of cellular division, and the environmental factors that influence our development from the moment we are conceived. This chapter explores the processes involved in conception and fetal development—the basis of our uniqueness.

CHROMOSOMES

The body (somatic) cells of each individual contain within their nuclei threadlike bodies known as **chromosomes,** which are composed of strands of *deoxyribonucleic acid (DNA)* and protein. *Genes* are regions in the DNA strands that contain coded information used to determine the unique characteristics of the individual; they are arranged in linear order on the chromosomes.

The storage place for genetic information, DNA, does not leave the cell nucleus. The DNA strand splits and forms the template for a *ribonucleic acid (RNA)* molecule. The RNA passes out of the nucleus and carries coded information to the cytoplasm of the cell. An error in the "reading" of the code can cause a change that may have serious effects on the functioning of the organism.

Each chromosome contains two longitudinal halves called *chromatids*, which are joined together at a point called the centromere. Each animal species has a constant number of chromosomes in each of its body cells. Humans have 46 chromosomes divided into 23 pairs: 22 pairs of chromosomes are called autosomes and one pair (23rd pair) of sex chromosomes (designated either XX or XY). Each member of a pair carries either similar genes referred to as *homologous* (homozygous) or dissimilar genes referred to as *heterozygous* (Figure 6–1A).

The chromosomes are classified according to their length and to the position of their centromere. When the centromere is centrally located, the longitudinal halves are divided into one short arm region and one long arm region, and the chromosome resembles an X (Figure 6–1B).

CELLULAR DIVISION

All humans begin life as a single cell (fertilized ovum or zygote). This single cell reproduces itself, and in turn each new cell also reproduces itself in a continuing process. The new cells are similar to the cells from which they came.

Cells are reproduced by either mitosis or meiosis, two different but related processes. **Mitosis** results in the production of diploid body (somatic) cells, which are exact copies of the original cell. Mitosis makes growth and development possible, and in mature individuals it is the process by which our body cells continue to divide and replace themselves. **Meiosis** is the cell division process leading to the development of eggs and sperm needed to produce a new organism.

Mitosis

During mitosis the cell undergoes several changes, ending in cell division. Although mitosis is a continuous process, it is generally divided into five stages: interphase, prophase, metaphase, anaphase, and telophase (Figure 6–2).

During interphase, before cell division takes place, the DNA within the chromosomes replicates so that the genes will be doubled. Mitosis begins when the cell enters prophase. The chromosomes condense and form the shape we usually recognize as a chromosome. Next comes the appearance of a mitotic apparatus known as a spindle,

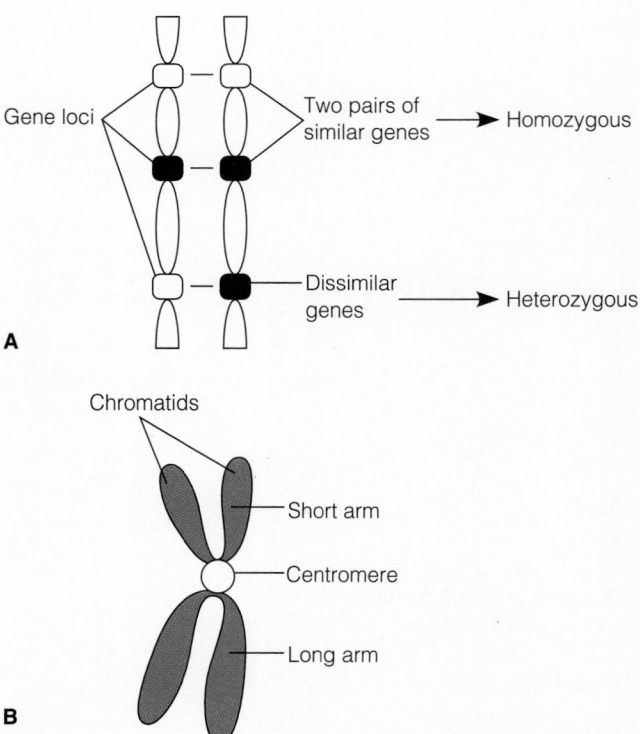

FIGURE 6-1   *A* One pair of homologous chromosomes with similar (homozygous) genes and dissimilar (heterozygous) genes. *B* Classification of chromosomal joining.

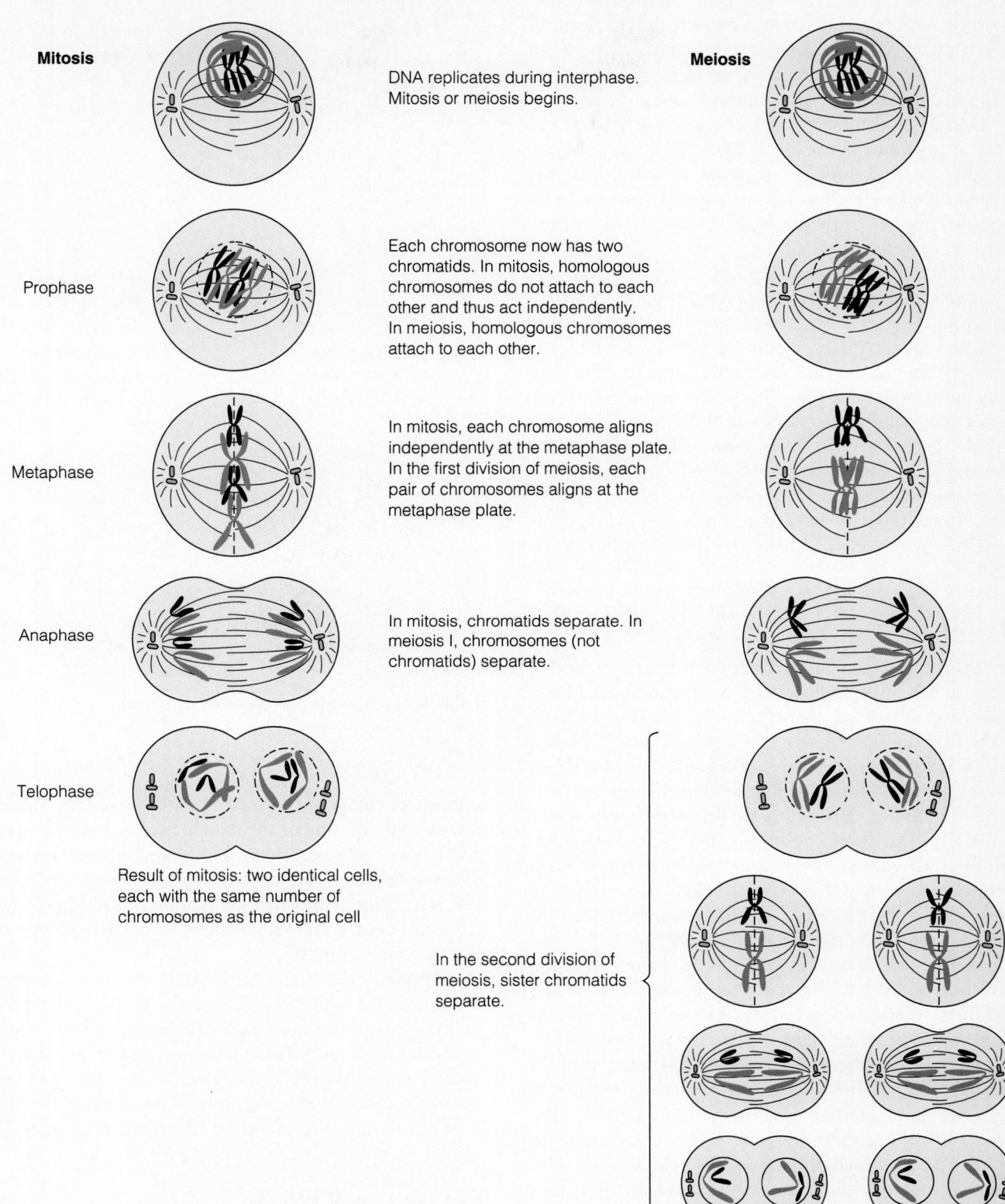

Mitosis

DNA replicates during interphase. Mitosis or meiosis begins.

Meiosis

Prophase

Each chromosome now has two chromatids. In mitosis, homologous chromosomes do not attach to each other and thus act independently. In meiosis, homologous chromosomes attach to each other.

Metaphase

In mitosis, each chromosome aligns independently at the metaphase plate. In the first division of meiosis, each pair of chromosomes aligns at the metaphase plate.

Anaphase

In mitosis, chromatids separate. In meiosis I, chromosomes (not chromatids) separate.

Telophase

Result of mitosis: two identical cells, each with the same number of chromosomes as the original cell

In the second division of meiosis, sister chromatids separate.

Result of meiosis: four haploid cells, each with half as many chromosomes as the original cell

FIGURE 6-2   Comparison of mitosis and meiosis.

in which fine threads extend from the top and bottom poles of the nucleus. At each pole of the spindle, a body known as the centriole is formed, so the threads of the spindle extend from one centriole to the other. Next the nuclear membrane, which separates the nucleus from the cytoplasm, disappears, the nucleus as a separate entity disappears, and the cell enters metaphase.

During metaphase the chromosomes line up at the equator (midway between the poles) of the spindle. Metaphase is followed by anaphase, in which the two chromatids of each chromosome separate and move to opposite ends of the spindle, where they cluster in masses near the two poles of the cell.

Telophase is essentially the opposite of prophase. A new nuclear membrane forms, separating each newly formed nucleus from the cytoplasm. The spindle disappears, and the centrioles relocate outside of each new nucleus. Within the nucleus the chromosomes lengthen and become threadlike. As telophase nears completion, a furrow develops in the cell cytoplasm and divides it into two daughter cells, each with its own nucleus. Daughter cells have the same **diploid number of chromosomes** (46) and the same genetic makeup as the cell from which they came. After a cell with 46 chromosomes goes through mitosis, two identical cells, each with 46 chromosomes, result.

Meiosis

Meiosis is a special type of cell division by which diploid cells give rise to haploid gametes (sperm and ova). Meiosis consists of two successive cell divisions (Figure 6–2). In the first division the chromosomes replicate. Next a pairing takes place between homologous chromosomes (Sadler 1990). Instead of separating immediately as in mitosis, the similar chromosomes become closely intertwined. At each point of contact, there is a physical exchange of genetic material between the chromatids (arms of the chromosomes). New combinations are provided by the newly formed chromosomes; these combinations account for the wide variation of traits, such as hair or eye color, in people. The chromosome pairs then separate, each member of a pair moving to opposite sides of the cell. (In contrast, during mitosis the chromatids of each chromosome separate and move to opposite poles.) The cell divides, forming two daughter cells, each with 23 doubled-structured chromosomes—the same amount of DNA as a normal somatic cell. In the second division the chromatids of each chromosome separate and move to opposite poles of each of the daughter cells. Cell division occurs, resulting in the formation of four cells, each containing 23 single chromosomes (the **haploid number of chromosomes**). These daughter cells contain only half the DNA of a normal somatic cell (Moore & Persaud 1993).

Mutations may occur during the second meiotic division if two of the chromatids do not move apart rapidly

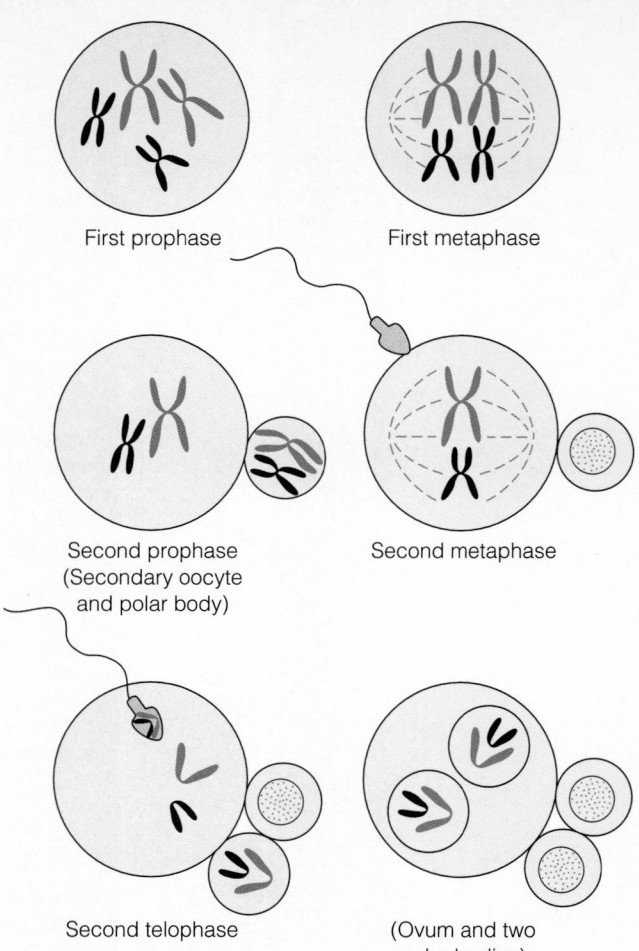

First prophase   First metaphase

Second prophase Second metaphase
(Secondary oocyte
and polar body)

Second telophase (Ovum and two
polar bodies)

FIGURE 6-3 Human oogenesis and fertilization.

enough when the cell divides. The still-paired chromatids are carried into one of the daughter cells and eventually form an extra chromosome. This condition is referred to as an *autosomal nondisjunction* (chromosomal mutation) and is harmful to the offspring that may result should fertilization occur. The implications of nondisjunction are discussed in Chapter 7.

Another type of chromosomal mutation can occur if chromosomes break during meiosis. If the broken segment is lost, the result is a shorter chromosome; this is known as a deletion. If the broken segment becomes attached to another chromosome, a harmful mutation called a translocation is the result (Thompson et al 1991). The effects of translocation are described in Chapter 7.

GAMETOGENESIS

Meiosis occurs during **gametogenesis,** the process by which germ cells, or **gametes** are produced. The gametes must have a haploid number of chromosomes (23) so that when the female gamete (the egg or ovum) and the male gamete (sperm or spermatozoon) unite to form the **zy-**

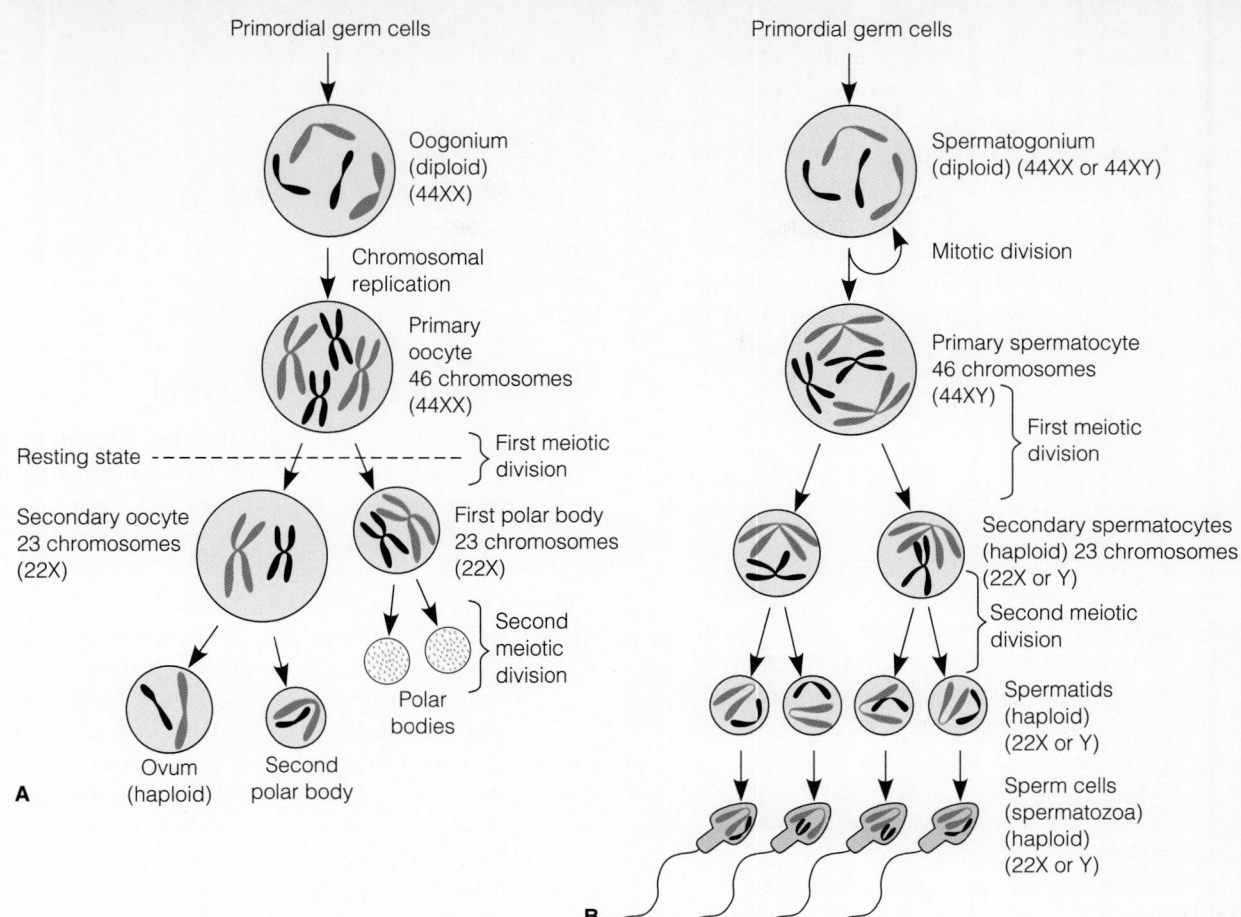

FIGURE 6-4   Gametogenesis involves meiosis within the ovary and testis. During meiosis each oogonium produces a single haploid ovum once some cytoplasm moves into the polar bodies *(A)*, whereas each spermatogonium produces four haploid spermatozoa *(B)*.

gote, the normal human diploid number of chromosomes (46) is reestablished.

Oogenesis

Oogenesis is the process by which female gametes or ova are produced. As discussed in Chapter 5, the ovaries begin to develop early in the fetal life of the female. All the ova that the female will produce in her lifetime are formed by the sixth month of fetal life. The ovary gives rise to oogonial cells, which develop into *oocytes*. Meiosis begins in all oocytes before the female infant is born but stops before the first division is complete and remains in this arrested phase until puberty. During puberty the mature primary oocyte continues through the first meiotic division in the graafian follicle of the ovary.

The first meiotic division produces two cells of unequal size with unequal amounts of cytoplasm, but the same number of chromosomes. These two cells are the *secondary oocyte* and a minute *polar body*. Both the secondary oocyte and the first polar body contain 22 double-structured autosomal chromosomes and one double-

structured sex chromosome (X). At the time of ovulation, the second meiotic division begins immediately and proceeds as the oocyte moves down the fallopian tube. Division is again not equal. The secondary oocyte proceeds to metaphase, where its meiotic division is arrested.

When the secondary oocyte completes the second meiotic division after fertilization, the result is a mature ovum with the haploid number of chromosomes and virtually all the cytoplasm. The second polar body (also haploid) is also formed at this time (Figure 6–3). The first polar body has now also divided, producing two additional polar bodies. Thus when meiosis is completed, four haploid cells have been produced: three small polar bodies, which eventually disintegrate, and one ovum (Sadler 1990) (Figure 6–4).

Spermatogenesis

During puberty the germinal epithelium in the seminiferous tubules of the testes begins the process of spermatogenesis, which produces the male gametes (sperm). As the (diploid number) spermatogonium enters the first meiotic division, it is called the *primary spermatocyte*. During this first meiotic division, the spermatogonium replicates and forms two haploid cells termed *secondary spermatocytes*, each of which contains 22 double-structured autosomal chromosomes and either a double-structured X sex chromosome or a double-structured Y sex chromosome. During the second meiotic division they divide to form four spermatids, each with the haploid number of chromosomes (Figure 6–4). The spermatids undergo a series of changes during which they lose most of their cytoplasm and become sperm (spermatozoa). The nucleus

becomes compacted into the head of the sperm, which is covered by a cap called an *acrosome*. A long tail is produced from one of the centrioles.

THE PROCESS OF FERTILIZATION

Fertilization is the process by which a sperm fuses with an ovum to form a new diploid cell, or zygote. Following are the events that lead to fertilization.

Preparation for Fertilization

The process of fertilization usually takes place in the ampulla (outer third) of the fallopian tube. During ovulation high estrogen levels increase peristalsis within the fallopian tubes, which helps move the ovum down the tube. The ovum has no inherent power of movement. The high estrogen levels also cause a thinning of the cervical mucus, facilitating movement of the sperm through the cervix, into the uterus, and up the fallopian tube.

The ovum's cell membrane is surrounded by two layers of tissue. The layer closest to the cell membrane is called the *zona pellucida*. It is a clear, noncellular layer whose function is not known. Surrounding the zona pellucida is a ring of elongated cells, called the *corona radiata* because they radiate from the ovum like the gaseous corona around the sun. These cells are held together by hyaluronic acid.

The mature ovum and spermatozoa have only a brief time to unite. Ova are considered fertile for about 24 hours after ovulation. Sperm can survive in the female reproductive tract for up to 72 hours but are believed to be healthy and highly fertile for only about 24 hours (Moore & Persaud 1993).

In a single ejaculation, the male deposits approximately 200 to 400 million spermatozoa in the vagina, of which fewer than 200 actually reach the ampulla (Moore & Persaud 1993). Fructose in the semen, secreted by the seminal vesicles, is the energy source for the sperm. The spermatozoa propel themselves up the female tract by the flagellar movement of their tails. Transit time from the cervix into the fallopian tube can be as short as 5 minutes but usually takes an average of 4–6 hours after ejaculation (Cunningham et al 1993). Prostaglandins in the semen may increase uterine smooth muscle contractions, which help transport the sperm. The fallopian tubes have a dual ciliary action that facilitates movement of the ovum toward the uterus and movement of the sperm from the uterus toward the ovary.

The sperm's nucleus, which contains its genetic material, is compacted into the head of the sperm and covered by a protective cap called an *acrosome*, which is in turn covered by a plasma membrane.

The sperm must undergo two processes before fertilization can happen: capacitation and the acrosomal reaction. **Capacitation** is the removal of the plasma membrane overlying the spermatozoa's acrosomal area and

RESEARCH IN PRACTICE

Approximately 8% of couples attempting pregnancy experience fertility problems. Jill Halman, Frank Andrews, and Antonia Abbey explored the differences between men and women in infertile couples regarding their perceptions and expectations about childbearing. The sample of 161 couples was representative of the majority of people seeking assistance for fertility issues in the United States—that is, they were white and middle class. Additional criteria for sample selection included being married, having no previous children, and having seen an infertility specialist but not yet having completed advanced treatments such as in vitro fertilization.

Individual 60-minute interviews with each member of the couple comprised the data collection. Areas assessed in the interview included fertility status as evaluated by length of time trying and difficulty having a baby, source of the fertility problem, acceptability of indicated treatment methods, importance of children, length of time by which the couple expected to have a child, ideal number of children, and expected number of children. An additional area of appraisal included measuring the stress experienced from tests and instrumentation for infertility. The authors used a combination of weighting the number of tests and the number of times performed with 12 questions of self-perceived stress from infertility tests and treatment. Reliability coefficients were given for this measure, but no validity issues were discussed in the article.

Data analysis using paired t-tests identified gender differences in several of the categories. Women endured more tests and treatments than the men and experienced more perceived stress from these tests. Women indicated more acceptance of possible treatments, placed more importance on having children, and desired a larger number of children than their male partners. No significant gender differences appeared in the estimation of the amount of time to have a child or in the expected number of children.

Clinical Application of Study

Even though a couple may go through the infertility work-up and treatment together, they bring different expectations and perceptions to the situation. Clinicians need to pay attention to possible gender differences in their interaction with each couple.

SOURCE: Halman J, Andrews F, Abbey A: Gender differences and perceptions about childbearing among infertile couples. *JOGNN* 1994; 23(7):593.

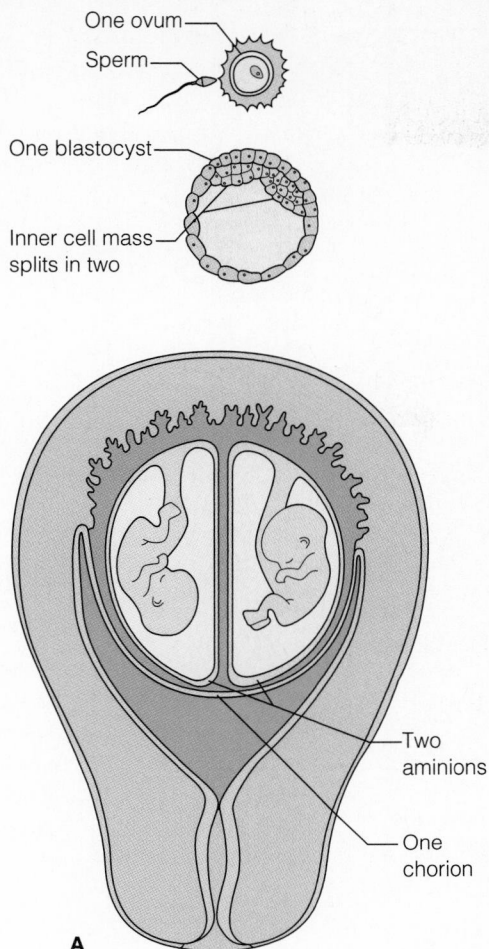

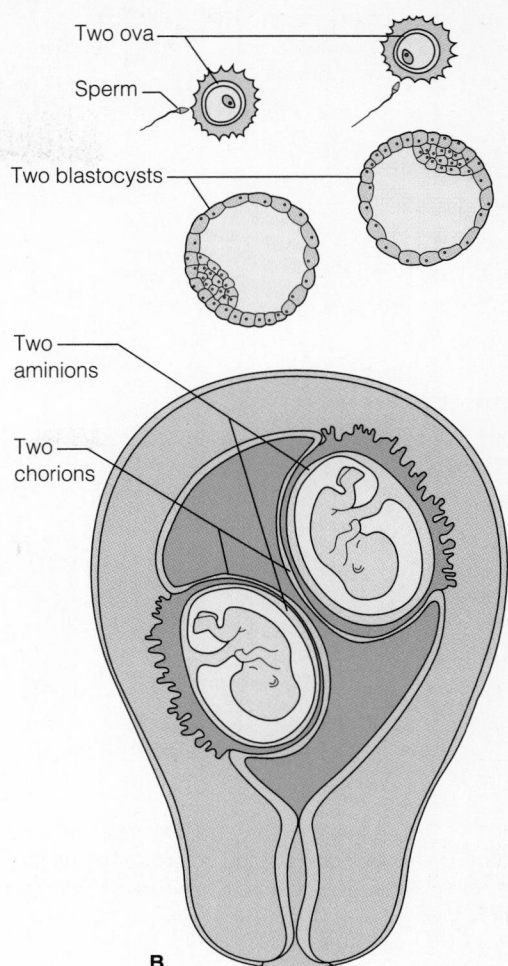

FIGURE 6-6 *A* Formation of identical twins. *B* Formation of fraternal twins.

The zygote now enters a period of rapid mitotic divisions called **cleavage,** during which it divides into two cells, four cells, eight cells, and so on. These cells, called *blastomeres,* are so small that the developing cell mass is only slightly larger than the original zygote. The blastomeres are held together by the zona pellucida, which is under the corona radiata. The blastomeres will eventually form a solid ball of 12 to 16 cells called the **morula.** As it enters the uterus, the intracellular fluid in the morula increases, and a central cavity forms within the cell mass.

The inner solid mass of cells is called the **blastocyst.** The outer layer of cells that surround the cavity and have replaced the zona pellucida is the **trophoblast.** Eventually, the trophoblast develops into one of the embryonic membranes, called the chorion. The blastocyst develops into a double layer of cells called the embryonic disk, from which the embryo will develop, and the other embryonic membrane called the amnion. The journey of the fertilized ovum to its destination in the uterus is illustrated in Figure 6–7.

Implantation (Nidation)

While floating in the uterine cavity, the blastocyst is nourished by the uterine glands, which secrete a mixture of lipids, mucopolysaccharides, and glycogen. The trophoblast attaches itself to the surface of the endometrium for further nourishment. The most frequent site of attachment is the upper part of the posterior uterine wall (Figure 6–7). Between days 7 and 9 after fertilization the zona pellucida disappears and the blastocyst implants itself by burrowing into the uterine lining and penetrating down toward the maternal capillaries until it is completely covered (Moore & Persaud 1993). The lining of the uterus thickens below the implanted blastocyst, and the cells of the trophoblast grow down into the thickened lining, forming processes called *villi.*

Under the influence of progesterone, the endometrium increases in thickness and vascularity in preparation for implantation and nourishment of the ovum. After implantation the endometrium is called the

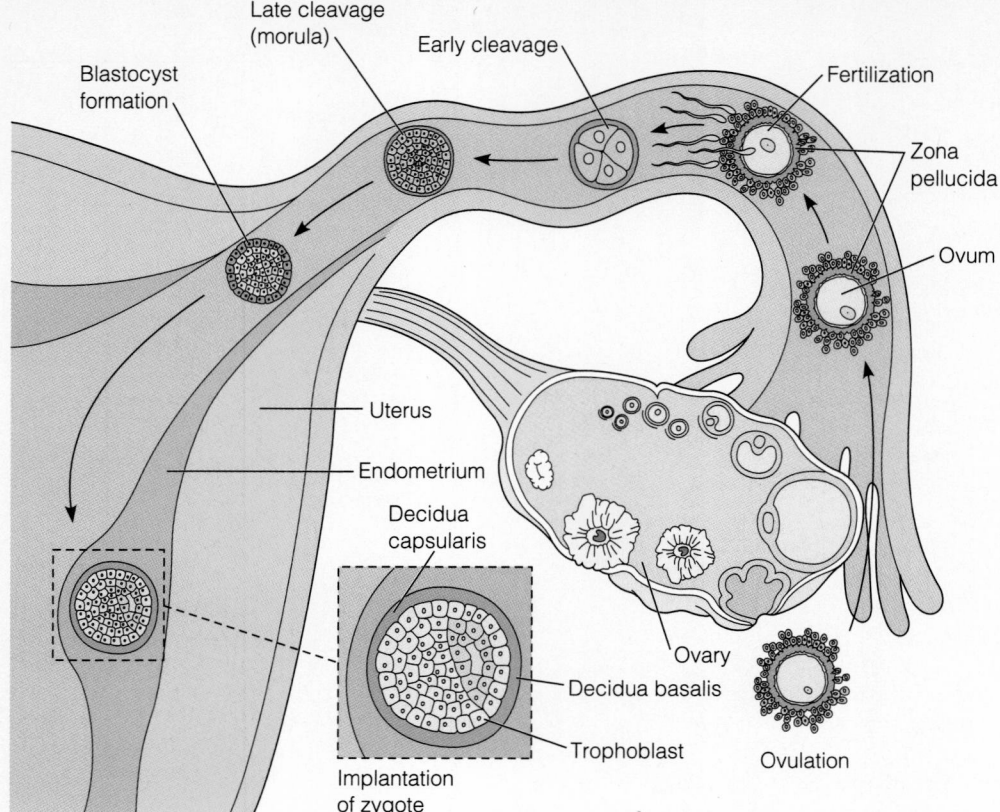

FIGURE 6-7 During ovulation the ovum leaves the ovary and enters the fallopian tube. Fertilization generally occurs in the outer third of the fallopian tube. Subsequent changes in the fertilized ovum from conception to implantation are depicted.

decidua. The portion of the decidua that covers the blastocyst is called the **decidua capsularis;** the portion directly under the implanted blastocyst is the **decidua basalis;** and the portion that lines the rest of the uterine cavity is the **decidua vera (parietalis)** (Figure 6–7 inset). The maternal part of the *placenta* develops from the decidua basalis, which contains large numbers of blood vessels. The chorionic villi (described below) in contact with the decidua basalis will form the fetal portion of the placenta.

Cellular Differentiation

Primary Germ Layers

About day 10 to 14 after conception, the homogenous mass of blastocyst cells differentiates into the primary germ layers. These layers, the **ectoderm, mesoderm,** and **endoderm** (Figure 6–8), are formed at the same time as the embryonic membranes. All tissues, organs, and organ systems will develop from these primary germ cell layers (Table 6–1 and Figure 6–9).

Embryonic Membranes

The **embryonic membranes** begin to form at the time of implantation (Figure 6–10). These membranes protect and support the embryo as it grows and develops inside the uterus. The first membrane to form is the **chorion,** the outermost embryonic membrane that encircles the amnion, embryo, and yolk sac. The chorion is a thick membrane that develops from the trophoblast and has many fingerlike projections, called *chorionic villi,* on its surface. These chorionic villi can be used for early genetic testing of the embryo at 8–10 weeks' gestation by chorionic villi sampling (see Chapter 20). As the pregnancy progresses, the villi begin to degenerate, except for those just under the embryo, which grow and branch into depressions in the uterine wall, forming the fetal portion of the placenta. By the fourth month of pregnancy, the

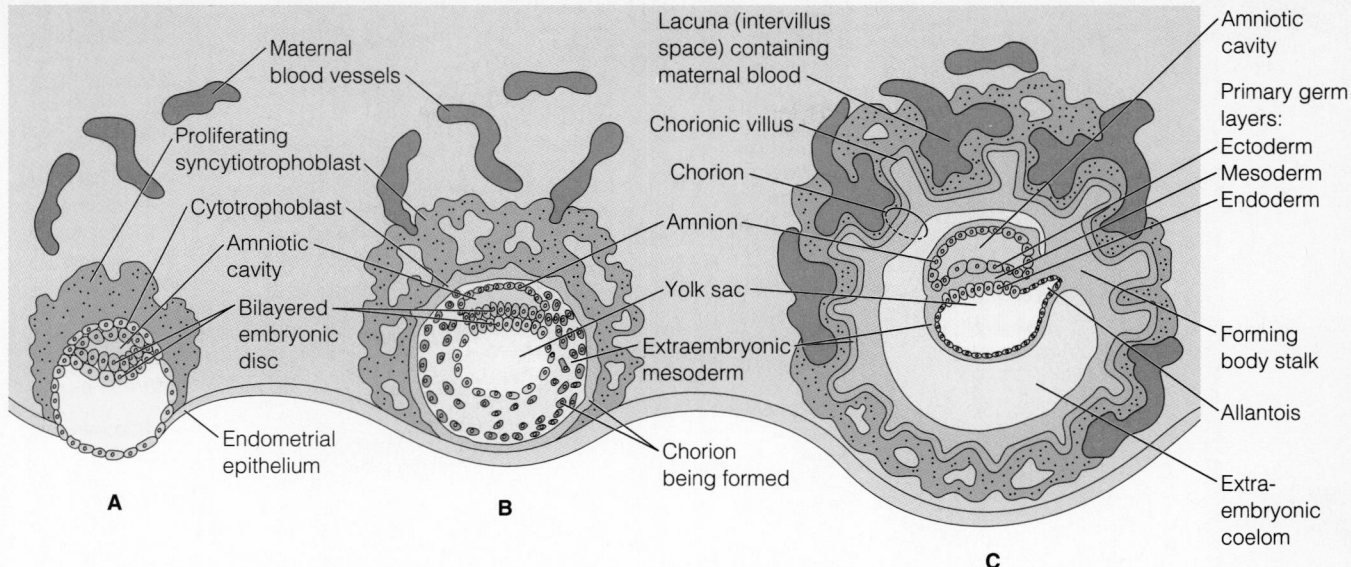

FIGURE 6-8 Formation of primary germ layers. *A* Implantation of a 7½-day blastocyst in which the cells of the embryonic disc are separated from the amnion by a fluid-filled space. The erosion of the endometrium by the syncytiotrophoblast is ongoing. *B* Implantation is completed by day 9 and extraembryonic mesoderm is beginning to form a discrete layer beneath the cytotrophoblast. *C* By day 16 the embryo shows all three germ layers, a yolk sac, and an allantois (an outpouching of the yolk sac that forms the structural basis of the body stalk, or umbilical cord). The cytotrophoblast and associated mesoderm has become the chorion, and chorionic villi are developing. SOURCE: Adapted from Marieb EN: *Human Anatomy and Physiology,* 3rd ed. Redwood City, CA: Benjamin/Cummings, 1995, p 1008.

surface of the chorion is smooth except at the place of attachment to the uterine wall.

The second membrane, the **amnion,** originates from the ectoderm, a primary germ layer, during the early stages of embryonic development. The amnion is a thin protective membrane that contains amniotic fluid. The space between the amniotic membrane and the embryo is the *amniotic cavity.* This cavity surrounds the embryo and yolk sac, except where the developing embryo (germ layer disk) attaches to the trophoblast via the umbilical cord. As the embryo grows, the amnion expands until it comes in contact with the chorion. These two slightly adherent membranes form the fluid-filled amniotic sac (or **bag of waters**) that protects the floating embryo.

TABLE 6-1	Derivation of Body Structures from Primary Cell Layers	
Ectoderm	**Mesoderm**	**Endoderm**
Epidermis	Dermis	Respiratory tract epithelium
Sweat glands	Wall of digestive tract	Epithelium (except nasal), including pharynx, tongue, tonsils, thyroid, parathyroid, thymus, tympanic cavity
Sebaceous glands	Kidneys and ureter (suprarenal cortex)	
Nails	Reproductive organs (gonads, genital ducts)	Lining of digestive tract
Hair follicles	Connective tissue (cartilage, bone, joint cavities)	Primary tissue of liver and pancreas
Lens of eye	Skeleton	Urethra and associated glands
Sensory epithelium of internal and external ear, nasal cavity, sinuses, mouth, anal canal	Muscles (all types)	Urinary bladder (except trigone)
Central and peripheral nervous systems	Cardiovascular system (heart, arteries, veins, blood, bone marrow)	Vagina (parts)
Nasal cavity	Pleura	
Oral glands and tooth enamel	Lymphatic tissue and cells	
Pituitary glands	Spleen	
Mammary glands		

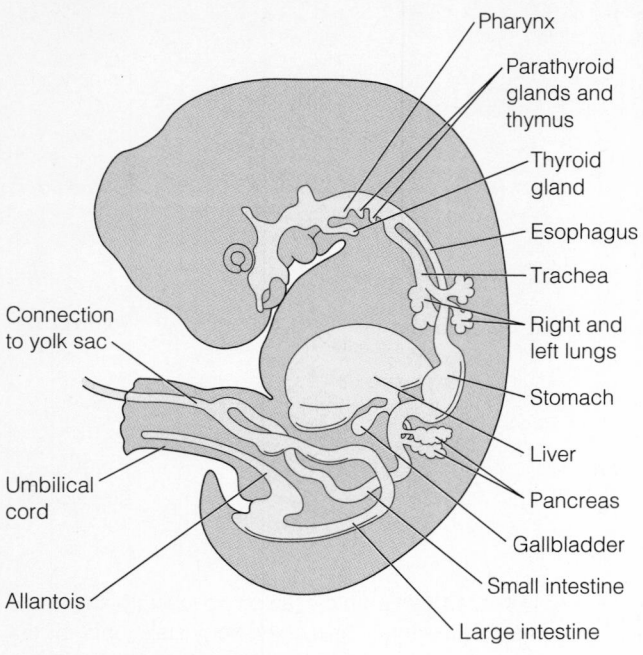

5-week embryo

FIGURE 6-9 Endoderm differentiates to form the epithelial lining of the digestive and respiratory tracts and associated glands. SOURCE: Adapted from Marieb EN: *Human Anatomy and Physiology,* 3rd ed. Redwood City, CA: Benjamin/Cummings, 1995, p 1013.

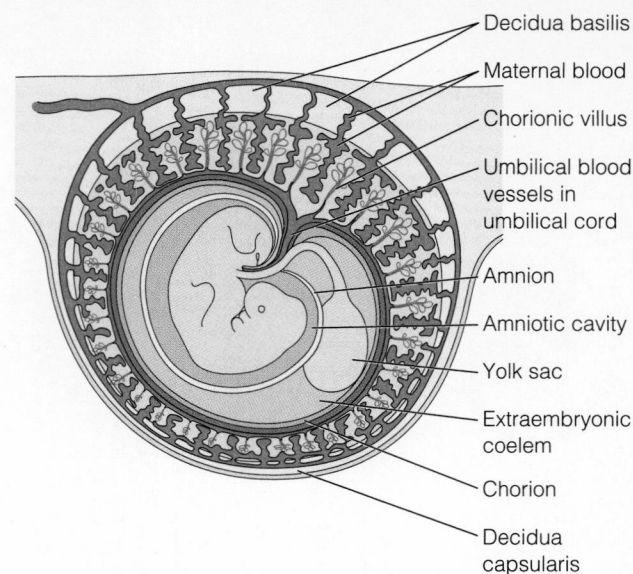

FIGURE 6-10 Early development of primary embryonic membranes. At 4½ weeks, the decidua capsularis (placental portion enclosing the embryo on the uterine surface) and decidua basalis (placental portion encompassing the elaborate chorionic villi and maternal endometrium) are well-formed. The chorionic villi lie in blood-filled intervillus spaces within the endometrium. The amnion and yolk sac are well-developed. SOURCE: Adapted from Marieb EN: *Human Anatomy and Physiology,* 3rd ed. Redwood City, CA: Benjamin/Cummings, 1995, p 1008.

Amniotic Fluid

Amniotic fluid functions as a cushion to protect against injury. It also helps control the embryo's temperature, permits symmetric external growth of the embryo, prevents adherence to the amnion, and allows freedom of movement so that the embryo-fetus can change position freely, thus aiding in musculoskeletal development.

The amount of amniotic fluid is about 30 mL at 10 weeks and increases to 350 mL at 20 weeks. After 20 weeks the volume ranges from 700 to 1000 mL (Moore & Persaud 1993). The amniotic fluid volume is constantly changing as the fluid moves back and forth across the placental membrane. As the pregnancy continues, the fetus contributes to the volume of amniotic fluid by excreting urine. The fetus also swallows up to 600 mL of the fluid every 24 hours. Approximately 400 mL of amniotic fluid flows out of the fetal lungs each day (Gilbert & Brace 1993). Amniotic fluid is slightly alkaline and contains albumin, urea, uric acid, creatinine, lecithin, sphingomyelin, bilirubin, fat, fructose, leukocytes, proteins, epithelial cells, enzymes, and fine hair called **lanugo.** Abnormal variations in amniotic fluid volume are oligohydramnios (less than normal amount of amniotic fluid)

and hydramnios (over 2000 mL of amniotic fluid). Hydramnios is also called polyhydramnios. Chapter 25 discusses alterations in amniotic fluid volume. Water and solutes must pass between the amniotic fluid and fetus. Figure 6–11 summarizes the major pathways of exchange.

Early in the first trimester of pregnancy, amniotic fluid is iso-osmolar with fetal and maternal plasma and is secreted from the developing trophoblast or embryo. Water and solutes move freely across the fetal skin before the time of skin keratinization. After 23–25 weeks thickening of the fetal skin inhibits this diffusion. During the rest of the pregnancy, the fetal kidneys are the major source of fluid that enters the amniotic sac. Abnormalities of fetal urine production can result in changes in amniotic fluid volume. For example, with obstruction of urine outflow, as in Potter's syndrome, oligohydramnios (less than 400 mL of amniotic fluid) develops. Conversely, Bartter's syndrome results in a fetal diuresis and hydramnios. Hydramnios is amniotic fluid volume of more than 2000 mL or amniotic fluid index (AFI) greater than the 97.5 percentile for the corresponding gestational age (Moise 1993). The fetal lungs are also significant contributors to amniotic fluid. Fetal breathing movements are associated with the bidirectional flow of fluid through the trachea.

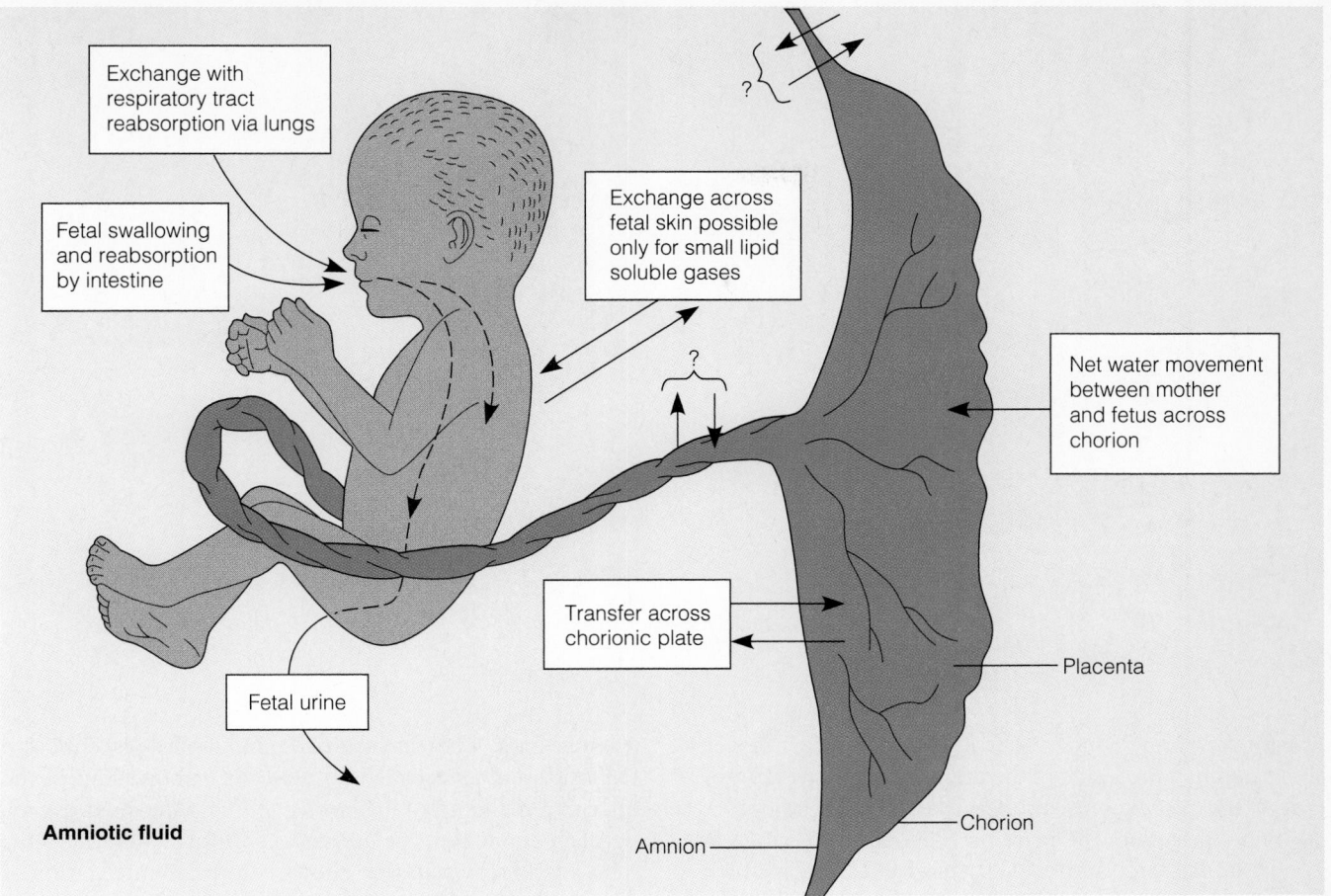

Exchange with
respiratory tract
reabsorption via lungs

Fetal swallowing
and reabsorption
by intestine

Exchange across
fetal skin possible
only for small lipid
soluble gases

Net water movement
between mother
and fetus across
chorion

Transfer across
chorionic plate

Fetal urine

Placenta

Amniotic fluid

Chorion

Amnion

FIGURE 6-11   Summary of the significant pathways of water and solute exchange
between the amniotic fluid and fetus. SOURCE: Seeds AE: Current concepts of amniotic
fluid dynamics. *Am J Obstet Gynecol* November 1980; 138:575.

Net outflow from the fetal lungs averages 4.3 mL/kg/
hour or 10% of body weight per day (Gilbert & Brace
1993). This outflow of lung and tracheal fluid is used as
the basis for amniotic fluid tests of fetal lung maturity.

The major mechanism by which amniotic fluid is removed in the last half of the pregnancy is fetal swallowing,
which occurs mostly during periods of fetal breathing
movements. In pregnancy when the fetus does not swallow normal amounts of amniotic fluid (as in esophageal
atresias and anencephalus), hydramnios will result. A potential route of amniotic fluid removal is by the trans-
membranous pathway, that is, the movement of fluid
across the amniochorion and into the maternal circulation
within the uterine wall. Another major regulator of amniotic fluid volume and composition is the intramembra-
nous pathway. This pathway causes amniotic water and/or
solutes to be absorbed by the fetal blood that perfuses the
fetal surface of the placenta (Gilbert & Brace 1993).

Yolk Sac

In humans the yolk sac is small and functions only in early
embryonic life. It develops as a second cavity in the blastocyst, about day 8 or 9 after conception, and forms primitive red blood cells during the first 6 weeks of development until the embryo's liver takes over the process. As
the embryo develops, the yolk sac is incorporated in the
umbilical cord, where it can be identified as a degenerate
structure after birth.

Placenta

The **placenta** is the means of metabolic and nutrient exchange between the embryonic and maternal circulations. Placental development and circulation does not begin until the third week of embryonic development. The
placenta develops at the site where the developing embryo attaches to the uterine wall. Expansion of the

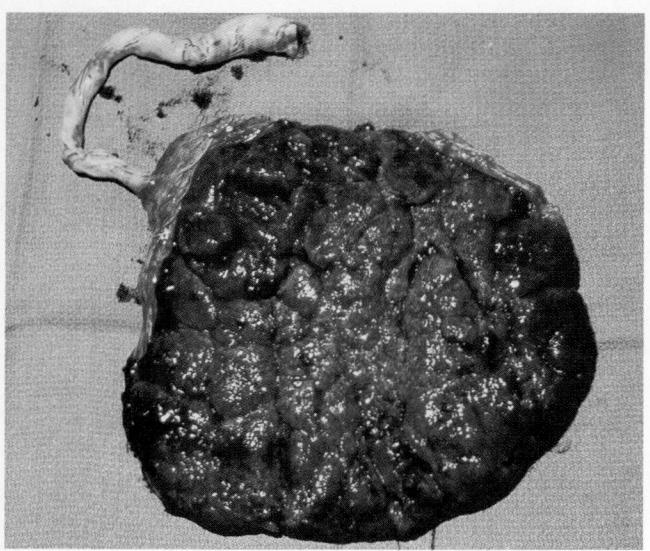

FIGURE 6-12   Maternal side of placenta.

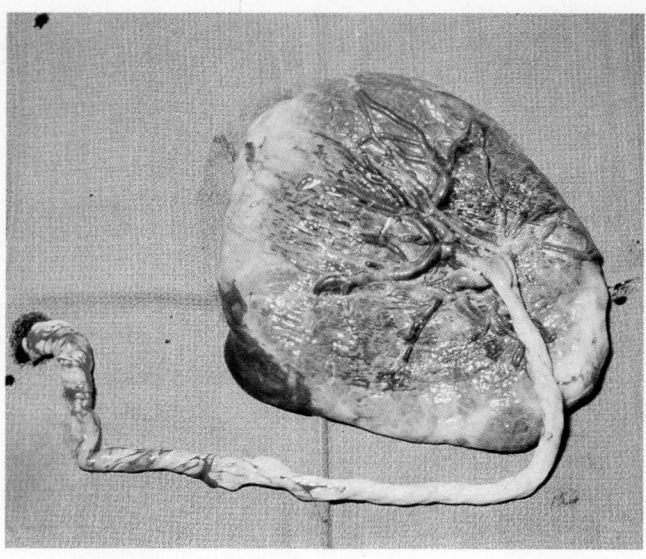

FIGURE 6-13   Fetal side of placenta.

placenta continues until about 20 weeks, when it covers about one-half the inside of the uterus. After 20 weeks' gestation, the placenta becomes thicker but not wider. At 40 weeks' gestation, the placenta is about 15–20 cm (5.9–7.9 in) in diameter and 2.5–3.0 cm (1.0–1.2 in) in thickness. At that time, it weighs approximately 400–600 g (14–21 oz).

The placenta has two parts: the maternal portion and the fetal portion. The maternal portion consists of the decidua basalis and its circulation. Its surface is red and fleshlike. The fetal portion consists of the chorionic villi and their circulation. The fetal surface of the placenta is covered by the amnion, which gives it a shiny, gray appearance (Figures 6–12 and 6–13).

Development of the placenta begins with the chorionic villi. The trophoblast cells of the chorionic villi form spaces in the tissue of the decidua basalis. These spaces fill with maternal blood, and the chorionic villi grow into these spaces. As the chorionic villi differentiate, two trophoblastic layers appear: an outer layer called the *syncytium* (consisting of syncytiotrophoblasts) and an inner layer known as the *cytotrophoblast* (Figure 6–14). The cytotrophoblast thins out and disappears about the fifth month, leaving only a single layer of syncytium covering the chorionic villi. The syncytium is in direct contact with the maternal blood in the intervillous spaces. It is the functional layer of the placenta and secretes the placental hormones of pregnancy.

A third, inner layer of connective mesoderm develops in the chorionic villi, forming *anchoring villi*. These anchoring villi eventually form the *septa* (partitions) of the placenta. These septa divide the mature placenta into 15 to 20 segments called **cotyledons** (subdivisions of the placenta made up of anchoring villi and decidual tissue). In each cotyledon, the *branching villi* form a highly complex vascular system that allows compartmentalization of the uteroplacental circulation. The exchange of gases and nutrients takes place across these vascular systems.

Exchange of substances across the placenta is minimal during the first 3 to 5 months of development because of limited permeability. The villous membrane is initially too thick. As the villous membrane thins, the placental permeability increases until about the last month of pregnancy, when permeability begins to decrease as the placenta ages. In the fully developed placenta fetal blood in the villi and maternal blood in the intervillous spaces are separated by three to four thin layers of tissue.

Placental Circulation   After implantation of the blastocyst, the cells differentiate into fetal cells and trophoblastic cells. The proliferating trophoblast successfully invades the decidua basalis of the endometrium, first opening the uterine capillaries and later opening the larger uterine vessels. The chorionic villi are an outgrowth of the blastocystic tissue. As these villi continue to grow and divide, the fetal vessels begin to form. The intervillous spaces in the decidua basalis develop as the endometrial spiral arteries are opened.

By the fourth week the placenta has begun to function as a means of metabolic exchange between embryo and mother. The completion of the maternal–placental–fetal circulation occurs about 17 days after conception

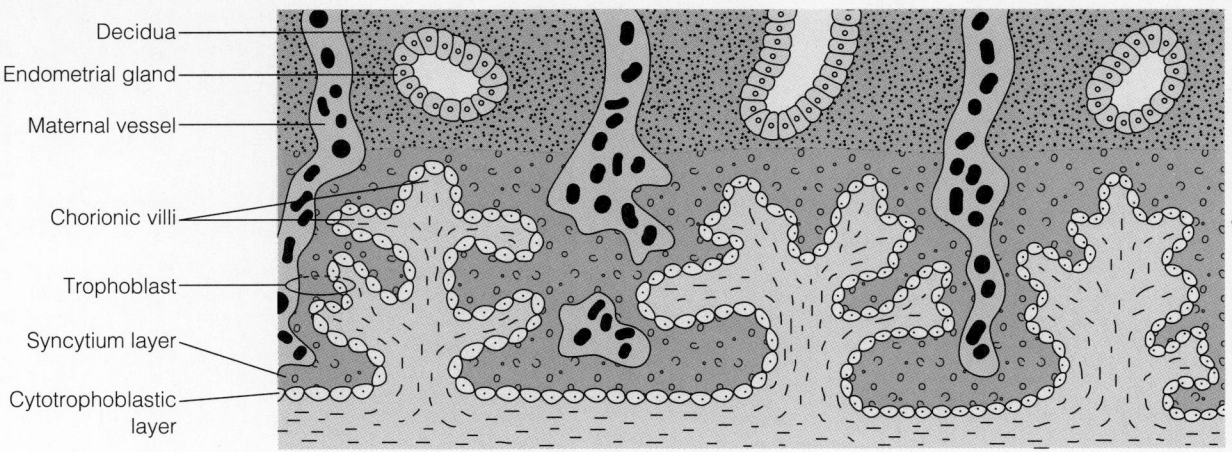

Decidua
Endometrial gland
Maternal vessel

Chorionic villi

Trophoblast

Syncytium layer

Cytotrophoblastic
layer

FIGURE 6-14 Longitudinal section of placental villus. Spaces formed in the maternal decidua are filled with maternal blood; chorionic villi proliferate into these maternal blood–filled spaces and differentiate into a syncytium layer and a cytotrophoblast layer.

when the embryonic heart begins functioning (Cunningham et al 1993).

By 14 weeks the placenta is a discrete organ. It has grown in thickness as a result of growth in the length and size of the chorionic villi and accompanying expansion of the intervillous space.

The *cotyledons* of the maternal surface contain branches of a single placental mainstream villus, allowing for some compartmentalization of the uteroplacental circulation. Each cotyledon is a vascular unit containing branching vessels that are distributed throughout a particular lobule and partially separated from other lobules by the cotyledon's thin septal partitions.

The capillaries of the villi are lined with an extremely thin endothelium and are surrounded by a layer of mesenchymal (connective) tissue. This connective tissue is covered by chorionic epithelium consisting of cytotrophoblast and syncytiotrophoblast (Figure 6–14). As previously discussed, the cytotrophoblast thins out and disappears after the fifth month.

In the fully developed placenta's umbilical cord, fetal blood flows through the two umbilical arteries to the capillaries of the villi, and oxygen-enriched blood flows back through the umbilical vein to the fetus (Figure 6–15). Late in pregnancy a soft blowing sound (*funic souffle)* can be heard over the area of the umbilical cord of the fetus. The sound is synchronous with the fetal heartbeat and the flow of fetal blood through the umbilical arteries.

Maternal blood, rich in oxygen and nutrients, spurts from the spiral uterine arteries into the intervillous spaces. These spurts are produced by the maternal blood pressure. The spurt of blood is directed toward the chorionic plate, and as the blood flow loses pressure, it becomes lateral (spreads out). Fresh blood continually enters and exerts pressure on the contents of the intervillous spaces, pushing blood toward the exits in the basal plate. Blood is then drained through the uterine and other pelvic veins. A *uterine souffle* is also heard in the later months of pregnancy. This uterine souffle, which is timed precisely with the mother's pulse and heard just above the mother's symphysis pubis, is caused by the augmented blood flow entering the dilated uterine arteries.

Circulation within the intervillous spaces depends on maternal blood pressure producing a gradient between arterial and venous channels. The lumen of the spiral uterine artery is narrow when it pierces the chorionic plate and enters the intervillous space, resulting in an increased blood pressure. The pressure in the arteries forces the blood into the intervillous spaces and bathes the numerous small villi in oxygenated blood. As the pressure decreases, the blood flows back from the chorionic plate toward the decidua, where it enters the endometrial veins.

Braxton Hicks contractions (Chapter 13) are believed to facilitate placental circulation by enhancing the movement of blood from the center of the cotyledon through the intervillous space. Placental blood flow is also enhanced when the woman is lying on her left side because the vena cava is not compromised.

Placental Functions Placental exchange functions occur only in those fetal vessels in intimate contact with the covering syncytial membrane. The syncytium villi have brush borders containing many microvilli, which greatly increase the exchange rate between maternal and fetal circulation (Sadler 1990).

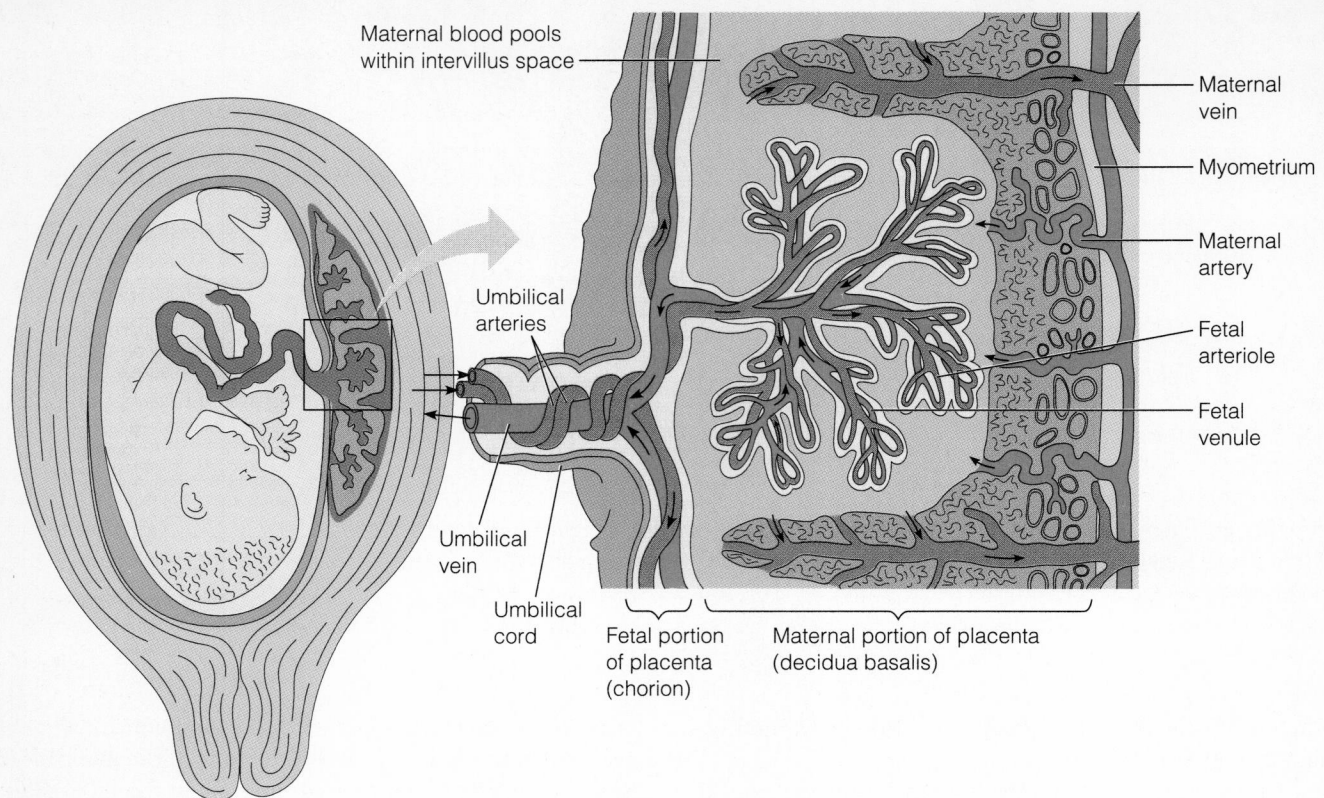

Maternal blood pools
within intervillus space

Maternal
vein

Myometrium

Maternal
artery

Fetal
arteriole

Fetal
venule

Umbilical
arteries

Umbilical
vein

Umbilical
cord

Fetal portion
of placenta
(chorion)

Maternal portion of placenta
(decidua basalis)

FIGURE 6-15   Vascular arrangement of the placenta. Arrows indicate the direction of
blood flow. Maternal blood flows through the uterine arteries to the intervillous spaces of
the placenta and returns through the uterine veins to maternal circulation. Fetal blood
flows through the umbilical arteries into the villous capillaries of the placenta and returns
through the umbilical vein to the fetal circulation.

The placental functions, many of which begin soon
after implantation, include fetal respiration, nutrition,
and excretion. To carry out these functions, the placenta
is involved in metabolic and transfer activities. It also has
endocrine functions and special immunologic properties.

Metabolic Activities   The placenta produces glycogen,
cholesterol, and fatty acids continuously for fetal use and
hormone production. The placenta also produces numerous enzymes required for fetoplacental transfer, and it
breaks down certain substances, such as epinephrine and
histamine. In addition it stores glycogen and iron.

Transport Functions   The placental membranes actively
control the transfer of a wide range of substances by five
major mechanisms:

1. *Simple diffusion* moves substances from an area of
    higher concentration to an area of lower concentra-
    tion. Substances that move across the placenta by
    simple diffusion include: water, oxygen, carbon
    dioxide, electrolytes (sodium and chloride), anes-
    thetic gases, and drugs. Insulin and steroid

hormones originating from the adrenals and thyroid
hormones also cross the placenta but at a very slow
rate. The rate of oxygen transfer across the placental
membrane is greater than that allowed by simple
diffusion, indicating that oxygen is also transferred
by facilitated diffusion of some type.

2. *Facilitated transport* involves a carrier system to move
    molecules from an area of greater concentration to
    an area of lower concentration. Molecules such as
    glucose, galactose, and some oxygen are transported
    by this method. The glucose level in the fetal blood
    ordinarily is approximately 20% to 30% lower than
    the glucose level in the maternal blood because glu-
    cose is being metabolized rapidly by the fetus. This
    in turn causes rapid transport of additional glucose
    from the maternal blood into the fetal blood.

3. *Active transport* can work against a concentration
    gradient, allowing molecules to move from areas of
    lower concentration to areas of higher concentra-
    tion. Amino acids, calcium, iron, iodine, water-
    soluble vitamins, and glucose are transferred across
    the placenta this way. The measured amino acid
    content of fetal blood is greater than that of mater-

nal blood, and calcium and inorganic phosphate occur in greater concentration in fetal blood than in maternal blood (Eden & Boehm 1990).

4. *Pinocytosis* is important for transferring large molecules, such as albumin and gamma-globulin. Materials are engulfed by amoebalike cells forming plasma droplets.

5. *Hydrostatic* and *osmotic pressures* allow the bulk flow of water and some solutes.

Other modes of transfer exist as well. For example, fetal red blood cells pass into the maternal circulation through breaks in the placental membrane, particularly during labor and birth. Certain cells, such as maternal leukocytes, and microorganisms, such as viruses (eg, the human immunodeficiency virus [HIV], which causes acquired immunodeficiency syndrome [AIDS]) and the bacterium *Treponema pallidum* (which causes syphilis), can also cross the placental membrane under their own power (Moore & Persaud 1993). Some bacteria and protozoa infect the placenta by causing lesions and then enter the fetal blood system.

Several factors, including the following, affect transfer rate:

* Molecular size
* Electrical charge
* Lipid solubility
* Placental area
* Diffusion distance
* Maternal–placental–fetal blood flow
* Blood saturation with gases and nutrients
* pK$_a$ of the substance
* Maternal–placental–fetal metabolism of the substance

Substances that have a molecular weight of 1000 daltons or more have difficulty crossing the placenta by simple diffusion. Therefore heparin, with a molecular weight above 6000, does not cross the placenta, but warfarin sodium (Coumadin), which has a molecular weight in the 300 to 400 range, crosses easily.

Electrically charged molecules cross the placenta more slowly. An example is the muscle relaxant, succinylcholine. A lipid-soluble substance moves quickly across the placenta into the fetal circulation. Reduction of the placental surface area, as with abruptio placentae (partial or complete premature separation of a normally implanted placenta) will lessen the area that is functional for exchange. Placental diffusion distance also affects exchange. In conditions such as diabetes and placental infection, edema of the villi increases the diffusion distance, thus increasing the distance the substance has to be transferred.

Changes in blood flow between the fetus and the maternal intervillous space can be influenced by the transfer rate of substances, the ratio of blood on each side of the placenta, and the binding and dissociation abilities of carrier molecules in the blood. Decreased intervillous space blood flow is seen during labor and with certain maternal disease conditions such as hypertension. Mild fetal hypoxia increases the umbilical blood flow, but severe hypoxia results in decreased blood flow.

As the maternal blood picks up fetal waste products and carbon dioxide, it drains back into the maternal circulation through the veins in the basal plate. Fetal blood is hypoxic by comparison; it therefore attracts oxygen from the mother's blood. Affinity for oxygen also increases as the fetal blood gives up its carbon dioxide, which decreases its acidity.

Endocrine Functions The placenta produces hormones that are vital to the survival of the fetus. These include human chorionic gonadotropin (hCG); human placental lactogen (hPL); and two steroid hormones, estrogen and progesterone.

The hormone *hCG* is similar to LH and prevents the normal involution of the corpus luteum at the end of the menstrual cycle (see Chapter 5). If the corpus luteum stops functioning before the 11th week of pregnancy, spontaneous abortion occurs. The hCG also causes the corpus luteum to secrete increased amounts of estrogen and progesterone.

After the 11th week the placenta produces enough progesterone and estrogen to maintain pregnancy. In the male fetus hCG also exerts an interstitial cell-stimulating effect on the testes, resulting in the production of testosterone. This small secretion of testosterone during embryonic development causes male sex organs to grow. Human chorionic gonadotropin may play a role in the trophoblast's immunologic capabilities (ability to exempt the placenta and embryo from rejection by the mother's system). This hormone is used as a basis for pregnancy tests (for discussion of pregnancy tests, see Chapter 13).

Human chorionic gonadotropin is present in maternal blood serum 8–10 days after fertilization, just as soon as implantation has occurred, and is detectable in maternal urine at the time of the missed menses. Chorionic gonadotropin reaches its maximum level at 50 to 70 days' gestation and then begins to decrease as placental hormone production increases.

Progesterone is a hormone essential for pregnancy. It increases the secretions of the fallopian tubes and uterus to provide appropriate nutritive matter for the developing morula and blastocyst. It also appears to aid in ovum transport through the fallopian tube (Moore & Persaud 1993). Progesterone causes decidual cells to develop in the uterine endometrium, and it must be present in high levels for implantation to occur. Progesterone also decreases the contractility of the uterus, thus preventing uterine contractions from causing spontaneous abortion.

Prior to hCG stimulation the production of progesterone by the corpus luteum reaches a peak about 7–10 days after ovulation. Implantation occurs at about the same time as this peak. At 16 days after ovulation, the production of progesterone reaches a level between 25 and 50 mg per day and continues to rise slowly in subsequent weeks (Cunningham et al 1993). After 10 weeks the placenta (specifically, the syncytiotrophoblast) takes over the production of progesterone and secretes it in tremendous quantities, reaching levels of more than 250 mg per day late in pregnancy.

By 7 weeks the placenta produces more than 50% of the *estrogens* in the maternal circulation. Estrogens serve mainly a proliferative function, causing enlargement of the uterus, breasts, and breast glandular tissue. Estrogens also have a significant role in increasing vascularity and vasodilation, particularly in the villous capillaries near the end of pregnancy. Placental estrogens increase markedly toward the end of pregnancy, to as much as 30 times the daily production in the middle of a normal monthly menstrual cycle. The primary estrogen secreted by the placenta is different from that secreted by the ovaries. The placenta secretes mainly *estriol*, whereas the ovaries secrete primarily *estradiol*. The placenta by itself cannot synthesize estriol. Essential precursors are provided by the adrenal glands of the fetus and are transported to the placenta for the final conversion to estriol.

The hormone *hPL* (human placental lactogen; sometimes referred to as human chorionic somatomammotropin or hCS) is similar to human pituitary growth hormone; hPL stimulates certain changes in the mother's metabolic processes. These changes ensure that more protein, glucose, and minerals are available for the fetus. Secretion of hPL can be detected by about 4 weeks. New placental proteins have been identified that may have clinical uses. These include SP 1 (Schwangerschaft's protein) and PP 5 (placental protein 5) and others (Eden & Boehm 1990).

Immunologic Properties The placenta and embryo are transplants of living tissue within the same species and are therefore considered *homografts*. Unlike other homografts, the placenta and embryo appear exempt from immunologic reaction by the host. Most recent data suggest that there is a suppression of cellular immunity by the placental hormones (progesterone and hCG) during pregnancy. One theory used to explain this phenomenon suggests that trophoblastic tissue is immunologically inert. It may contain a cell coating that masks transplantation antigens, repels sensitized lymphocytes, and protects against antibody formation.

Umbilical Cord

As the placenta is developing, the **umbilical cord** is also being formed from the amnion. The **body stalk,** which attaches the embryo to the yolk sac, contains blood vessels that extend into the chorionic villi. The body stalk fuses with the embryonic portion of the placenta to provide a circulatory pathway from the chorionic villi to the embryo. (See Figure 6–13.) As the body stalk elongates to become the umbilical cord, the vessels in the cord decrease to one large vein and two smaller arteries. About 1% of umbilical cords have only two vessels, an artery and a vein; this condition may be associated with congenital malformations, primarily of the cardiac and gastrointestinal systems. A specialized connective tissue known as **Wharton's jelly** surrounds the blood vessels in the umbilical cord. This tissue, plus the high blood volume pulsating through the vessels, prevents compression of the umbilical cord in utero. At term, the average cord is 2 cm (0.8 in) across and about 55 cm (22 in) long. The cord can attach itself to the placenta at various sites. Central insertion into the placenta is considered normal. (Chapter 19 discusses the various attachment sites.)

Umbilical cords appear twisted or spiraled. This is most likely caused by fetal movement. A true knot in the umbilical cord rarely occurs; if it does, the cord is usually long. More common are so-called false knots caused by the folding of cord vessels. A *nuchal cord* is said to exist when the umbilical cord encircles the fetal neck.

Fetal Circulatory System Development

The circulatory system of the fetus has several unique features that, by maintaining the blood flow to the placenta provide the fetus with oxygen and nutrients while removing carbon dioxide and other waste products.

Most of the blood supply bypasses the fetal lungs because they do not carry out respiratory gas exchange. The placenta assumes the function of the fetal lungs by supplying oxygen and allowing the fetus to excrete carbon dioxide into the maternal bloodstream. Figure 6–16 shows the fetal circulatory system. The blood from the placenta flows through the umbilical vein, which penetrates the abdominal wall of the fetus at the site that, after birth, is the umbilicus (belly button). It divides into two branches, one of which circulates a small amount of blood through the fetal liver and empties into the inferior vena cava through the hepatic vein. The second and larger branch, called the **ductus venosus,** empties directly into the fetal vena cava. This blood then enters the right atrium, passes through the **foramen ovale** into the left atrium, and pours into the left ventricle, which pumps it into the aorta. Some blood returning from the head and upper extremities by way of the superior vena cava is emptied into the right atrium and passes through the tricuspid valve into the right ventricle. This blood is pumped into the pulmonary artery, and a small amount passes to the lungs and provides nourishment only. The larger portion of blood passes from the pulmonary artery through the **ductus arteriosus** into the descending aorta, bypassing the lungs. Finally, blood returns to the placenta through the two umbilical arteries, and the process is repeated.

The fetus receives oxygen via diffusion from the maternal circulation because of the gradient difference of PO_2, of 50 mm Hg in maternal blood in the placenta to a

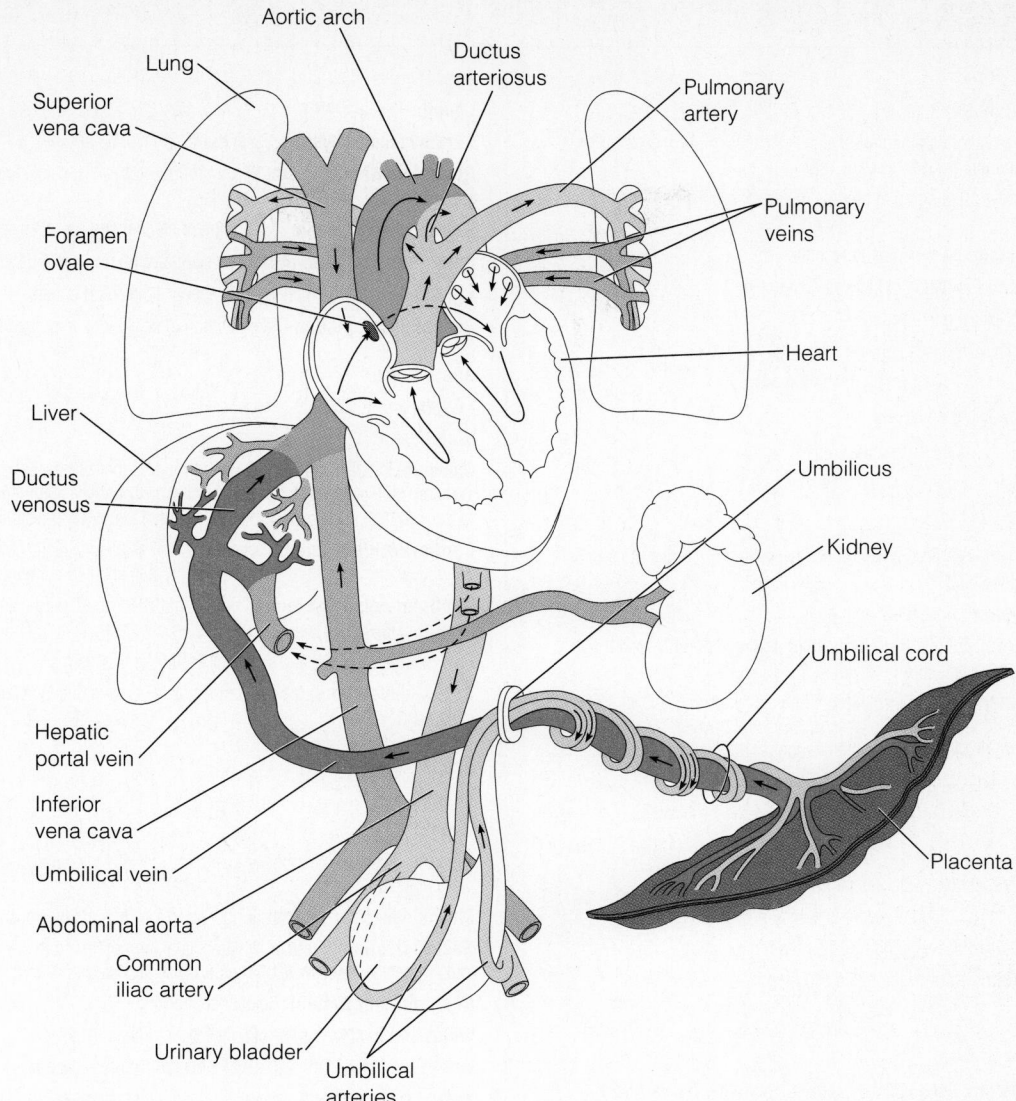

Aortic arch
Ductus
arteriosus
Lung
Pulmonary
artery
Superior
vena cava
Pulmonary
veins
Foramen
ovale
Heart
Liver
Umbilicus
Ductus
venosus
Kidney
Umbilical cord
Hepatic
portal vein
Inferior
vena cava
Placenta
Umbilical vein
Abdominal aorta
Common
iliac artery
Urinary bladder
Umbilical
arteries

High oxygenation

Moderate oxygenation

Low oxygenation

Very low oxygenation

FIGURE 6-16   Fetal circulation. Blood leaves the placenta and enters the fetus through the umbilical vein. After circulating through the fetus the blood returns to the placenta through the umbilical arteries. The ductus venosus, the foramen ovale, and the ductus arteriosus allow the blood to bypass the fetal liver and lungs.

30 mm Hg Po$_2$ in the fetus. At term the fetus receives oxygen from the mother's circulation at a rate of 20–30 mL/min (Sadler 1990). Fetal hemoglobin facilitates obtaining oxygen from the maternal circulation, since it carries as much as 20% to 30% more oxygen than adult hemoglobin. For further discussion see Chapter 27.

Fetal circulation delivers the highest available oxygen concentration to the head, neck, brain, and heart (coronary circulation) and a lesser amount of oxygenated blood to the abdominal organs and the lower body. This circulatory pattern leads to *cephalocaudal* (head-to-tail) development in the fetus.

Fetal Heart

The heart of the fetus, as in the adult, is under the control of its own pacemaker. The sinoatrial (S-A) node sets the rate and is supplied by the vagus nerve. Bridging the atrium and the ventricle is the atrioventricular (A-V) node. It is also supplied by the vagus nerve. Baseline changes in the fetal heartbeat have been shown to be under the influence of this nerve. Atropine will block this effect.

When the fetus is stressed, the sympathetic nervous system causes the release of norepinephrine, which in-

TABLE 6-2   Summary of Organ System Development

Age: 2–3 weeks

Length: 2 mm C–R (Crown-to-Rump)

Nervous system: Groove forms along middle back as cells thicken; neural tube forms from closure of neural groove.

Cardiovascular system: Beginning of blood circulation; tubular heart begins to form during third week.

Gastrointestinal system: Liver begins to function.

Genitourinary system: Formation of kidneys beginning.

Respiratory system: Nasal pits forming.

Endocrine system: Thyroid tissue appears.

Eyes: Optic cup and lens pit have formed; pigment in eyes.

Ear: Auditory pit is now enclosed structure.

Age: 4 weeks

Length: 4–6 mm C–R

Weight: 0.4 g

Nervous system: Anterior portion of neural tube closes to form brain; closure of posterior end forms spinal cord.

Musculoskeletal system: Noticeable limb buds.

Cardiovascular system: Tubular heart beats at 28 days and primitive red blood cells circulate through fetus and chorionic villi.

Gastrointestinal system: Mouth: formation of oral cavity; primitive jaws present; esophagotracheal septum begins division of esophagus and trachea. Digestive tract: stomach forms; esophagus and intestine become tubular; ducts of pancreas and liver forming.

Age: 5 weeks

Length: 8 mm C–R

Weight: Only 0.5% of total body weight is fat (to 20 weeks).

Nervous system: Brain has differentiated and cranial nerves are present.

Musculoskeletal system: Developing muscles have innervation.

Cardiovascular system: Atrial division has occurred.

Age: 6 weeks

Length: 12 mm C–R

Musculoskeletal system: Bone rudiments present; primitive skeletal shape forming; muscle mass begins to develop; ossification of skull and jaws begins.

Cardiovascular system: Chambers present in heart; groups of blood cells can be identified.

Gastrointestinal system: Oral and nasal cavities and upper lip formed; liver begins to form red blood cells.

Respiratory system: Trachea, bronchi, and lung buds present.

Ear: Formation of external, middle, and inner ear continues.

Sexual development: Embryonic sex glands appear.

Age: 7 weeks

Length: 18 mm C–R

Cardiovascular system: Fetal heartbeats can be detected.

Gastrointestinal system: Mouth: tongue separates; palate folds. Digestive tract: stomach attains final form.

Genitourinary system: Separation of bladder and urethra from rectum.

Respiratory system: Diaphragm separates abdominal and thoracic cavities.

Eyes: Optic nerve formed; eyelids appear, thickening of lens.

Sexual development: Differentiation of sex glands into ovaries and testes begins.

Age: 8 weeks

Length: 2.5–3 cm C–R

Weight: 2 g

Musculoskeletal system: Digits formed; further differentiation of cells in primitive skeleton; cartilaginous bones show first signs of ossification; development of muscles in trunk, limbs, and head; some movement of fetus now possible.

Cardiovascular system: Development of heart essentially complete; fetal circulation follows two circuits—four extraembryonic and two intraembryonic.

Gastrointestinal system: Mouth: completion of lip fusion. Digestive tract: rotation in midgut; anal membrane has perforated.

Ear: External, middle, and inner ear assuming final forms.

Sexual development: Male and female external genitals appear similar until end of ninth week.

Age: 10 weeks

Length: 5–6 cm C–H (Crown-to-Heel)

Weight: 14 g

Nervous system: Neurons appear at caudal end of spinal cord; basic divisions of brain present.

Musculoskeletal system: Fingers and toes begin nail growth.

Gastrointestinal system: Mouth: separation of lips from jaw; fusion of palate folds. Digestive tract: developing intestines enclosed in abdomen.

Genitourinary system: Bladder sac formed.

Endocrine system: Islets of Langerhans differentiated.

Eyes: Eyelids fused closed; development of lacrimal duct.

Sexual development: Males: production of testosterone and physical characteristics between 8 and 12 weeks.

Age: 12 weeks

Length: 8 cm C–R; 11.5 cm C–H

Weight: 45 g

Musculoskeletal system: Clear outlining of miniature bones (12–20 weeks); process of ossification is established throughout fetal body; appearance of involuntary muscles in viscera.

Note: Age refers to gestational age of fetus/conceptus; fertilization age.

---

creases the fetal heart rate. To counteract the increase in blood pressure, baroreceptors, which respond to stretch, are present in the vessel walls at the junction of the internal and external carotid arteries. When stimulated, these receptors, under the influence of the vagus and glossopharyngeal nerves, cause the heart rate to slow.

Chemoreceptors in the fetal peripheral and central nervous systems respond to decreased oxygen tensions and to increased carbon dioxide tensions, leading to fetal tachycardia and an increase in blood pressure. The central nervous system (CNS) also has control over heart rate. Increased activity of the fetus in a wakeful period is exhibited in an *increase in the beat-to-beat variability* of the fetal heart baseline. Sleep patterns demonstrate a *decrease in the beat-to-beat baseline variability*. In cases of severe hypoxia, increased levels of epinephrine and norepinephrine act on the fetal heart to produce a faster and stronger rate.

TABLE 6-2 continued

Gastrointestinal system: Mouth: completion of palate. Digestive tract: appearance of muscles in gut; bile secretion begins; liver is major producer of red blood cells.

Respiratory system: Lungs acquire definitive shape.

Skin: Pink and delicate.

Endocrine system: Hormonal secretion from thyroid; insulin present in pancreas.

Immunologic system: Appearance of lymphoid tissue in fetal thymus gland.

Age: 16 weeks

Length: 13.5 cm C–R; 15 cm C–H

Weight: 200 g

Musculoskeletal system: Teeth beginning to form hard tissue that will become central incisors.

Gastrointestinal system: Mouth: differentiation of hard and soft palate. Digestive tract: development of gastric and intestinal glands; intestines begin to collect meconium.

Genitourinary system: Kidneys assume typical shape and organization.

Skin: Appearance of scalp hair; lanugo present on body; transparent skin with visible blood vessels; sweat glands developing.

Eye, ear, and nose: Formed.

Sexual development: Sex determination possible.

Age: 18 weeks

Musculoskeletal system: Teeth beginning to form hard tissue (enamel and dentine) that will become lateral incisors.

Cardiovascular system: Fetal heart tones audible with fetoscope at 16–20 weeks.

Age: 20 weeks

Length: 19 cm C–R; 25 cm C–H

Weight: 435 g (6% of total body weight is fat)

Nervous system: Myelination of spinal cord begins.

Musculoskeletal system: Teeth beginning to form hard tissue that will become canine and first molar. Lower limbs are of final relative proportions.

Gastrointestinal system: Fetus actively sucks and swallows amniotic fluid; peristaltic movements begin.

Skin: Lanugo covers entire body; brown fat begins to form; vernix caseosa begins to form.

Immunologic system: Detectable levels of fetal antibodies (IgG type).

Blood formation: Iron is stored and bone marrow is increasingly important.

Age: 24 weeks

Length: 23 cm C–R; 28 cm C–H

Weight: 780 g

Nervous system: Brain looks like mature brain.

Musculoskeletal system: Teeth are beginning to form hard tissue that will become the second molar.

Respiratory system: Respiratory movements may occur (24–40 weeks). Nostrils reopen. Alveoli appear in lungs and begin production of surfactant; gas exchange possible.

Skin: Reddish and wrinkled, vernix caseosa present.

Immunologic system: IgG levels reach maternal levels.

Eyes: Structurally complete.

Age: 28 weeks

Length: 27 cm C–R; 35 cm C–H

Weight: 1200–1250 g

Nervous system: Begins regulation of some body functions.

Skin: Adipose tissue accumulates rapidly; nails appear; eyebrows and eyelashes present.

Eyes: Eyelids open (28–32 weeks).

Sexual development: Males: testes descend into inguinal canal and upper scrotum.

Age: 32 weeks

Length: 31 cm C–R; 38–43 cm C–H

Weight: 2000 g

Nervous system: More reflexes present.

Age: 36 weeks

Length: 35 cm C–R; 42–48 cm C–H

Weight: 2500–2750 g

Musculoskeletal system: Distal femoral ossification centers present.

Skin: Pale; body rounded, lanugo disappearing, hair fuzzy or woolly; few sole creases; sebaceous glands active and helping to produce vernix caseosa (36–40 weeks).

Ears: Ear lobes soft with little cartilage.

Sexual development: Males: scrotum small and few rugae present; descent of testes into upper scrotum to stay (36–40 weeks). Females: labia majora and minora equally prominent.

Age: 40 weeks

Length: 40 cm C–R; 48–52 cm C–H

Weight: 3200+ g (16% of total body weight is fat)

Respiratory system: At 38 weeks, lecithin-spingomyelin (L/S) ratio approaches 2:1 (indicates decreased risk of respiratory distress from inadequate surfactant production if born now).

Skin: Smooth and pink; vernix present in skinfolds; moderate to profuse silky hair; lanugo hair on shoulders and upper back; nails extend over tips or digits; creases cover sole.

Ears: Ear lobes firmer due to increased cartilage.

Sexual development: Males: rugous scrotum. Females: labia majora well developed and minora small or completely covered.

SOURCES: Sadler TW: *Langman's Medical Embryology,* 6th ed. Baltimore: Williams & Wilkins, 1990; and Moore KL, Persaud TVN: *The Developing Human: Clinically Oriented Embryology,* 5th ed. Philadelphia: Saunders, 1993.

EMBRYONIC AND FETAL DEVELOPMENT AND ORGAN FORMATION

Pregnancy is calculated to last an average of 10 lunar months: 40 weeks, or 280 days. This period of 280 days is calculated from the beginning of the last menstrual period to the time of birth. Estimated date of birth (EDB) is usually calculated by this method. The fertilization age or post-conception age of the fetus is calculated to be about 2 weeks less, or 266 days (38 weeks). The latter measurement is more accurate because it measures time from the fertilization of the ovum, or conception. The basic events of organ development in the embryo and fetus are outlined in Table 6-2. The time periods used are **postconception age periods.** For detailed discussion of each body system's development, see Chapter 27.

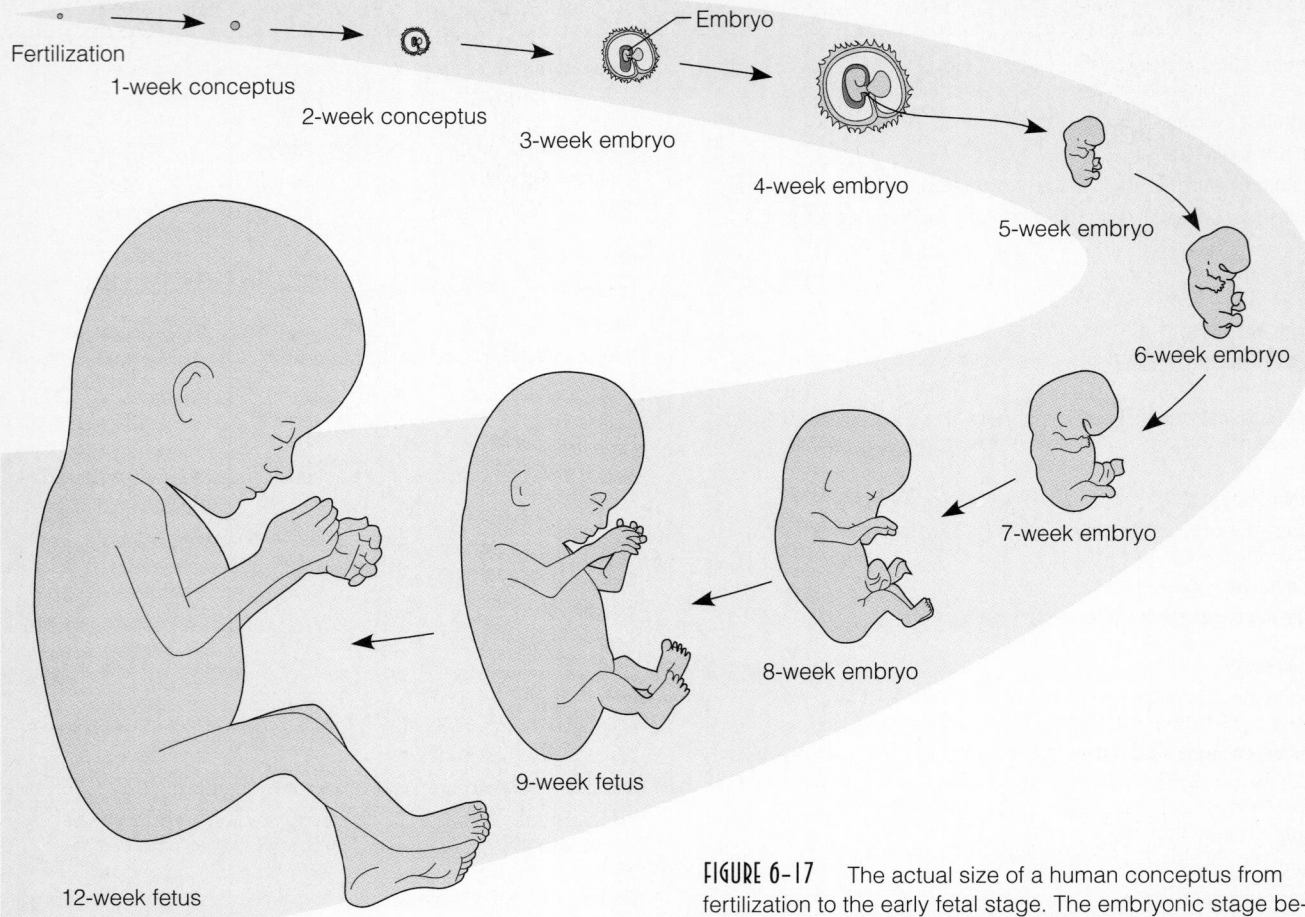

Fertilization

1-week conceptus

2-week conceptus

3-week embryo

Embryo

4-week embryo

5-week embryo

6-week embryo

7-week embryo

8-week embryo

9-week fetus

12-week fetus

FIGURE 6-17 The actual size of a human conceptus from fertilization to the early fetal stage. The embryonic stage begins in the third week after fertilization; the fetal stage begins in the ninth week. SOURCE: Adapted from Marieb EN: *Human Anatomy and Physiology,* 3rd ed. Redwood City, CA: Benjamin/Cummings, 1995, p 1000.

Human development follows three stages. The preembryonic stage consists of the first 14 days of development after the ovum is fertilized; the embryonic stage covers the period from day 15 until approximately the eighth week; and the fetal stage extends from the end of the eighth week until birth.

Preembryonic Stage

The first 14 days of human development, starting on the day the ovum is fertilized (conception), are referred to as the *preembryonic stage* or the *stage of the ovum.* This period is characterized by rapid cellular multiplication and differentiation and the establishment of the embryonic membranes and primary germ layers, discussed earlier.

Embryonic Stage

The stage of the **embryo** starts on day 14 or 15 (begins the third week after conception or fertilization) and continues until approximately 8 weeks or until the embryo reaches a *crown-to-rump* (C–R) length of 3 cm (1.2 in). This length is usually reached about 56 days after fertil-

ization (the end of the eighth gestational week). The embryonic stage is a period of differentiation of tissues into essential organs and development of the main external features (Figure 6–17). The embryo is most vulnerable to teratogens during this period.

Three Weeks

In the third week the embryonic disk becomes elongated and pear-shaped, with a broad cephalic end and a narrow caudal end. The ectoderm has formed a long cylindrical tube called the notochord for brain and spinal cord development. The gastrointestinal tract, created from the endoderm, appears as another tubelike structure communicating with the yolk sac. The most advanced organ is the heart. At 3 weeks a single tubular heart forms just outside the body cavity of the embryo.

Four to Five Weeks

During days 21 to 32, *somites,* a series of mesodermal blocks, form on either side of the embryo's midline. The vertebrae that form the spinal column will develop from these somites. Prior to 28 days, arm and leg buds are not

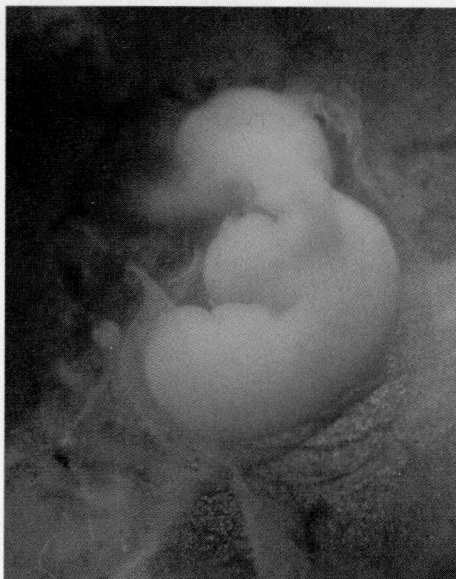

FIGURE 6-18   The embryo at 4 weeks. Pharyngeal arches, pharyngeal pouches, and primordia of the ear and eye are present.

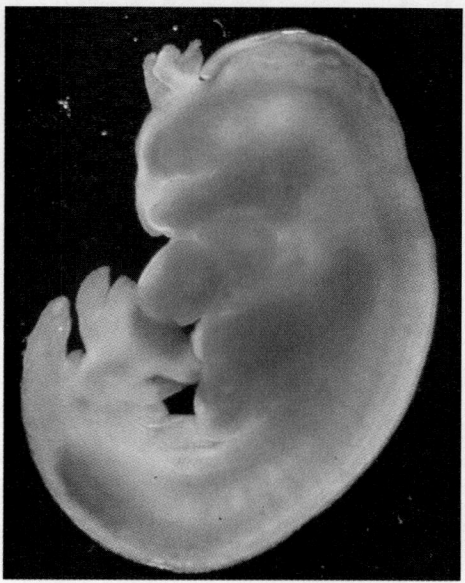

FIGURE 6-19   The embryo at 5 weeks. The embryo has a marked C-shaped body and a rudimentary tail.

visible, but the tail bud is present. The pharyngeal arches—which will form the lower jaw (mandibular arch), hyoid bone, and cartilage of the larynx—develop at this time. The pharyngeal pouches appear now; these pouches will form the eustachian tube and cavity of the middle ear, the tonsils, and the parathyroid and thymus glands. The primordia of the ear and eye are also present (Figure 6–18). By the end of 28 days, the tubular heart is beating at a regular rhythm and pushing its own primitive blood cells through the main blood vessels.

During the fifth week the optic cups and lens vesicles of the eye form and the nasal pits develop. Partitioning in the heart occurs with the dividing of the atrium. The embryo has a marked C-shaped body, accentuated by the rudimentary tail and the large head folded over a protuberant trunk (Figure 6–19). By day 35, the arm and leg buds are well developed, with paddle-shaped hand and foot plates. The heart, circulatory system, and brain show the most advanced development. The brain has differentiated into five areas, and ten pairs of cranial nerves are recognizable.

Six Weeks

At 6 weeks the head structures are more highly developed, and the trunk is straighter than in earlier stages. The upper and lower jaws are recognizable, and the external nares are well formed. The trachea has developed, and its caudal end is bifurcated for beginning lung formation. The upper lip has formed, and the palate is developing. The ears are developing rapidly. The arms have begun to extend ventrally across the chest, and both arms and legs have digits, although they may still be webbed. There is a slight elbow bend in the arm, which is more advanced in

development than the leg. Beginning at this stage the prominent tail will recede. The heart now has most of its definitive characteristics, and fetal circulation begins to be established. The liver begins to produce blood cells.

Seven Weeks

At 7 weeks the head of the embryo is rounded and nearly erect (Figure 6–20). The eyes have shifted from their original lateral position to a forward location, where they are closer together, and the eyelids are beginning to form. The palate is nearing completion, and the tongue is developing in the formed mouth. The gastrointestinal and genitourinary tracts undergo significant changes during

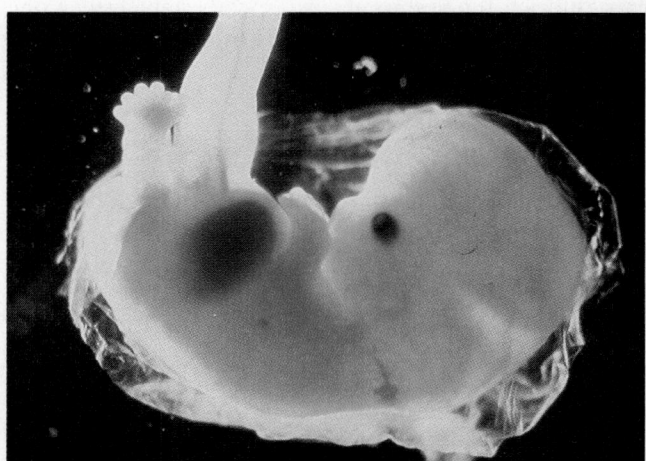

FIGURE 6-20   The embryo at 7 weeks. The head is rounded and nearly erect. The eyes have shifted forward and are closer together, and the eyelids begin to form.

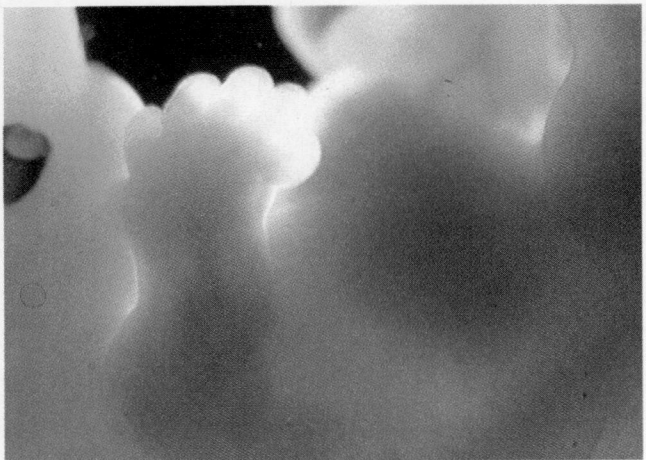

FIGURE 6-21　The embryo at 8 weeks. Although only 3 cm in C–R length, the embryo clearly resembles a human being. Facial features continue to develop.

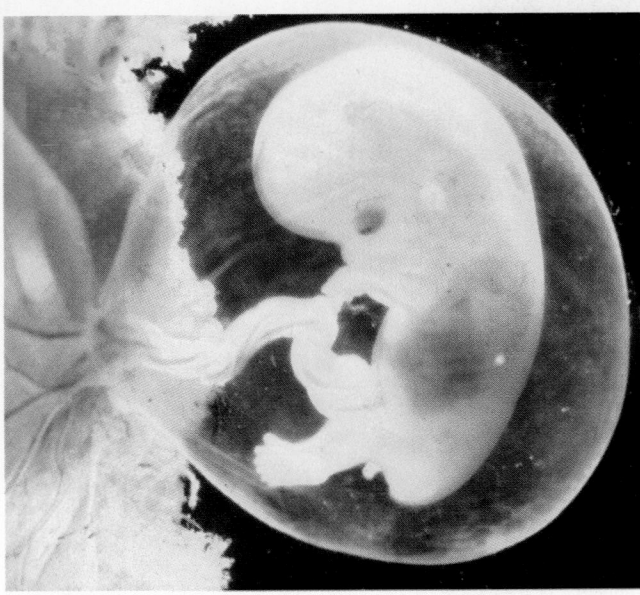

FIGURE 6-22　The fetus at 9 weeks. Every organ system and external structure is present. SOURCE: Nilsson L: *A Child Is Born.* New York: Dell Publishing, 1990.

the seventh week. Prior to this time the rectal and urogenital passages formed one tube that ended in a blind pouch; they now separate into two tubular structures. The intestines enter the extraembryonic coelom in the area of the umbilical cord (called umbilical herniation) (Moore & Persaud 1993). At this point the beginnings of all essential external and internal structures are present.

Eight Weeks

At 8 weeks the embryo is approximately 3 cm (1.2 in) C–R and clearly resembles a human being (Figure 6–21). Facial features continue to develop. The eyelids begin to fuse. Auricles of the external ears begin to assume their final shape, but they are still set low (Moore & Persaud 1993). External genitals appear, but the embryo's sex is not clearly identifiable. The rectal passage opens with the perforation of the anal membrane. The circulatory system through the umbilical cord is well established. Long bones are beginning to form, and the large muscles are now capable of contracting.

Fetal Stage

By the end of the eighth week the embryo is sufficiently developed to be called a **fetus.** Every organ system and external structure that will be found in the full-term newborn is present. The remainder of gestation is devoted to refining structures and perfecting function.

Nine to Twelve Weeks

By 10 weeks the fetus reaches a C–R length of 5 cm (2 in) and weighs about 14 g. The head is large and comprises almost half of the fetus's entire size (Figure 6–22). The neck is distinct from the head and body, and both the head and neck are straighter than in previous stages of development.

By 12 weeks the fetus reaches an 8-cm (3.2-in) C–R length and weighs about 45 g (1.6 oz). The face is well formed, with the nose protruding, the chin small and receding, and the ear acquiring a more adult shape. The eyelids close at about the tenth week and will not reopen until about 28 weeks. Some reflex movements of the lips suggestive of the sucking reflex have been observed at 3 months. Tooth buds now appear for all 20 of the child's first teeth (baby teeth). The limbs are long and slender, with well-formed digits. The fetus can curl the fingers toward the palm and make a tiny fist. The legs are still shorter and less developed than the arms. The urogenital tract completes its development, well-differentiated genitals appear, and the kidneys begin to produce urine. Red blood cells are produced primarily by the liver. Spontaneous movements of the fetus now occur. Fetal heart tones can be ascertained by electronic devices between 8 and 12 weeks. The heart rate is 120–160 beats per minute.

Thirteen to Sixteen Weeks

This is a period of rapid growth. At 13 weeks the fetus weighs 55–60 g and is about 9 cm (3.6 in) in C–R length. *Lanugo*, or fine hair, begins to develop, especially on the head. The skin is so transparent that blood vessels are clearly visible beneath it. More muscle tissue and body skeleton have developed, which hold the fetus more erect (Figure 6–23). Active movements are present—the fetus stretches and exercises its arms and legs. It makes sucking motions, swallows amniotic fluid, and produces meconium in the intestinal tract. Bronchial tubes are branching out in the primitive lungs, and sweat glands are devel-

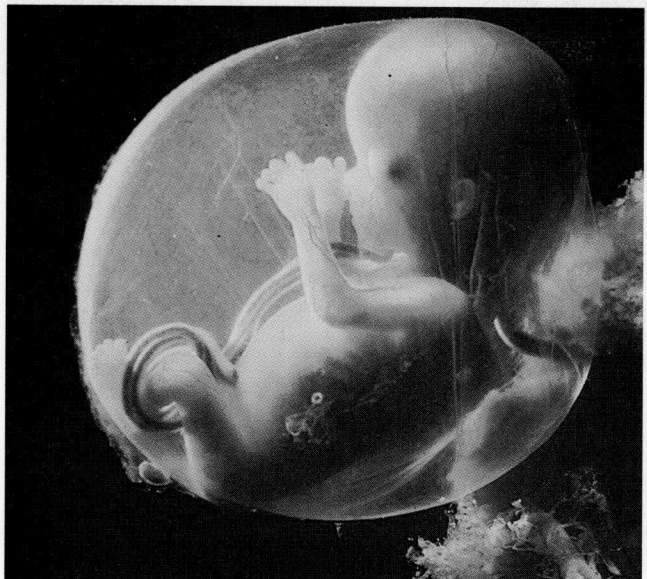

FIGURE 6-23   The fetus at 14 weeks. During this period of rapid growth the skin is so transparent that blood vessels are visible beneath it. More muscle tissue and body skeleton have developed, which holds the fetus more erect. SOURCE: Nilsson L: *A Child Is Born*. New York: Dell Publishing, 1990.

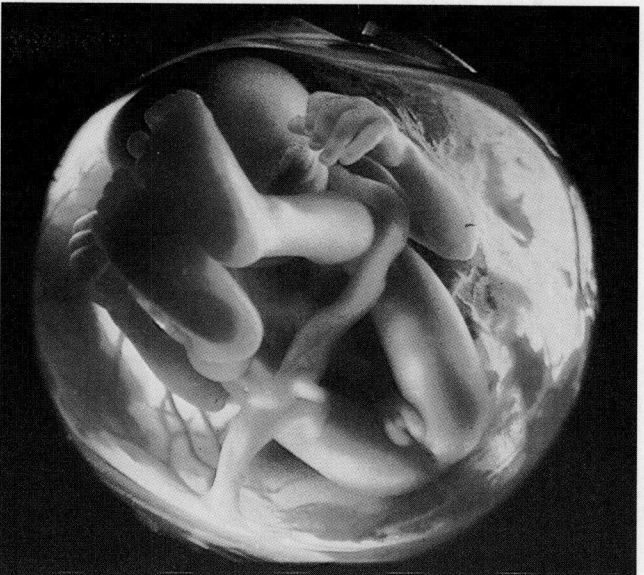

FIGURE 6-24   The fetus at 20 weeks. The fetus now weighs approximately 435–465 g and measures about 19 cm. Subcutaneous deposits of brown fat make the skin a little less transparent. "Woolly" hair covers the head, and nails have developed on the fingers and toes. SOURCE: Nilsson L: *A Child Is Born*. New York: Dell Publishing, 1990.

oping. The liver and pancreas now begin production of their appropriate secretions. By the beginning of week 16, skeletal ossification is clearly identifiable.

Twenty Weeks

The fetus doubles its C–R length and now measures about 19 cm (8 in). Fetal weight is between 435 and 465 g (15.2 to 16.3 oz). Lanugo covers the entire body and is especially prominent on the shoulders. Subcutaneous deposits of brown fat, which has a rich blood supply, makes the skin a little less transparent. Nipples now appear over the mammary glands. The head is covered with fine, "woolly" hair, and the eyebrows and eyelashes are beginning to form. The fetus has nails on both fingers and toes (Figure 6–24). Muscles are well developed, and the fetus is active. Fetal movement, known as *quickening*, is felt by the mother. The heartbeat is audible through the fetoscope. Quickening and fetal heartbeat can help in validating the estimated date of birth.

Twenty-four Weeks

The fetus at 24 weeks reaches a *crown-to-heel (C–H)* length of 28 cm (11.2 in). It weighs about 780 g (1 lb, 10 oz). The hair on the head is growing long, and eyebrows and eyelashes have formed. The eye is structurally complete and will soon open. The fetus has a reflex hand grip (grasp reflex) and, by the end of 6 months, a startle reflex. Skin covering the body is reddish and wrinkled, with little subcutaneous fat. Skin on the hands and feet has thickened, with skin ridges on palms and soles forming distinct footprints and fingerprints. The skin over the entire body

is covered with a protective cheeselike fatty substance secreted by the sebaceous glands called **vernix caseosa.** The alveoli in the lungs are just beginning to form.

Twenty-five to Twenty-eight Weeks

At 6 calendar months the fetal skin is still red, wrinkled, and covered with vernix caseosa. During this time the brain is developing rapidly, and the nervous system is complete enough to provide some degree of regulation of body functions. The eyelids open and close under neural control. If the fetus is a male, the testes begin to descend into the scrotal sac. Even though the lungs are still physiologically immature, they are sufficiently developed to provide gas exchange. A fetus born at this time will require immediate and prolonged intensive care in order to survive and to decrease the risk of major handicap. The fetus at 28 weeks is about 35–38 cm (14–15 in) long C–H and weighs 1200–1250 g (2 lb, 10.5 oz to 2 lb, 12 oz).

Twenty-nine to Thirty-two Weeks

At 30 weeks the pupillary light reflex is present (Moore & Persaud 1993). The fetus is gaining weight from an increase in body muscle and fat and weighs about 2000 g (4 lb, 6.5 oz) with a length of about 38–43 cm (15–17 in) by 32 weeks of age. The CNS has matured enough to direct rhythmic breathing movements and partially control body temperature. However, the lungs are not yet fully mature. Bones are now fully developed but are soft and flexible. The fetus begins storing iron, calcium, and phosphorus. In males the testicles may be located in the scrotal sac but are often still high in the inguinal canal.

Thirty-six Weeks

The fetus is beginning to get plump with less-wrinkled skin covering the deposits of subcutaneous fat. Lanugo hair is beginning to disappear, and the nails reach the edge of the fingertips. By 35 weeks the fetus has a firm grasp and exhibits spontaneous orientation to light. By 36 weeks of age the weight is usually 2500–2750 g (5 lb, 12 oz to 6 lb, 11.5 oz), and the C–H length of the fetus is about 42–48 cm (16–19 in). An infant born at this time has a good chance of surviving but may require some special care, especially if there is intrauterine growth retardation.

Thirty-eight to Forty Weeks

The fetus is considered full term at 38 weeks after conception. The C–H length varies from 48 to 52 cm (19 to 21 in) with males usually longer than females. Males also usually weigh more than females. The weight at term is about 3000–3600 g (6 lb, 10 oz to 7 lb, 15 oz). The skin is pink and has a smooth polished look. The only lanugo left is on the upper arms and shoulders. The hair on the head is no longer woolly but coarse and about an inch long. Vernix caseosa is present, with heavier deposits remaining in creases and folds of the skin. The body and extremities are plump, with good skin turgor, and the fingernails extend beyond the fingertips. The chest is prominent but still a little smaller than the head, and mammary glands protrude in both sexes. The testes are in the scrotum or are palpable in the inguinal canals. As the fetus enlarges, amniotic fluid diminishes to about 500 mL or less, and the fetal body mass fills the uterine cavity. The fetus assumes what is referred to as its *position of comfort*, or lie. The head is generally pointed downward, following the shape of the uterus (and also possibly because the head is heavier than the feet). The extremities and often the head are well flexed. After 5 months, feeding patterns, sleeping patterns, and activity patterns become established, so the fetus at term has its own body rhythms and individual style of response.

Table 6–3 lists some important developmental milestones.

Critical Thinking Question

How can knowing the gestational age of the fetus help us determine the potential effects of a teratogen?

FACTORS INFLUENCING EMBRYONIC AND FETAL DEVELOPMENT

Among factors that may affect embryonic development are the quality of the sperm or ovum from which the zygote was formed and the genetic code established at fer-

TABLE 6-3	Fetal Development: What Parents Want to Know
4 weeks:	The fetal heart begins to beat.
8 weeks:	All body organs are formed.
8–12 weeks:	Fetal heart tones can be heard by Doppler device.
16 weeks:	Baby's sex can be seen. Although thin, the fetus looks like a baby.
20 weeks:	Heartbeat can be heard with fetoscope. Mother feels movement (quickening). Baby develops a regular schedule of sleeping, sucking, and kicking. Hands can grasp. Baby assumes a favorite position in utero. Vernix (lanolinlike covering) protects the body and lanugo (fine hair) keeps oil on skin. Head hair, eyebrows, and eyelashes present.
24 weeks:	Weighs 1 lb 10 oz. Activity is increasing. Fetal respiratory movements begin.
28 weeks:	Eyes begin to open and close. Baby can breathe at this time. Surfactant needed for breathing at birth is formed. Baby is two-thirds its final size.
32 weeks:	Baby has fingernails and toenails. Subcutaneous fat is being laid down. Baby appears less red and wrinkled.
38–40 weeks:	Baby fills total uterus. Baby gets antibodies from mother.

tilization. In addition, the adequacy of the intrauterine environment is important for optimal growth. If the environment is unsuitable before cellular differentiation occurs, all the cells of the zygote are affected. The cells may die, which causes spontaneous abortion, or growth may be slowed, depending on the severity of the situation. When differentiation is complete and the fetal membranes have formed, an injurious agent has the greatest effect on those cells undergoing the most rapid growth. Thus the time of injury is critical in the development of anomalies.

Because organs are formed primarily during embryonic development, the growing organism is considered most vulnerable to hazardous agents during the first months of pregnancy. Table 6–4 lists potential malformations related to the time of insult. Any agent, such as a drug, virus, or radiation, that can cause development of abnormal structures in an embryo is referred to as a **teratogen.** Chapter 13 discusses the effects of specific teratogenic agents on the developing fetus.

Adequacy of the maternal environment is also important during the periods of rapid embryonic and fetal development. Maternal nutrition can affect brain development. The period of maximum brain growth and myelination begins with the fifth lunar month before birth and continues during the first 6 months after birth. During the first 6 months after birth there is a twofold increase in myelination; in the second 6 months to 2 years of age there is a 50% further increase (Volpe 1995). Amino acids, glucose, and fatty acids are considered to be

TABLE 6-4	Developmental Vulnerability Timetable
Weeks Since Conception	**Potential Teratogen-Induced Malformation**
3	Ectromelia (congenital absence of one or more limbs)
	Ectopia cordis (heart lies outside thoracic cavity)
4	Omphalocele (herniation of abdominal viscera into the umbilical cord)
	Tracheoesophageal fistula (abnormal connection between trachea and esophagus) (4–5 weeks)
	Hemivertebra (4–5* weeks)
5	Nuclear cataract
	Microphthalmia (abnormally small eyeballs) (5–6* weeks)
	Facial clefts
	Carpal or pedal ablation (5–6* weeks)
6	Gross septal or aortic abnormalities
	Cleft lip, agnathia (absence of the lower jaw)
7	Interventricular septal defects
	Pulmonary stenosis
	Cleft palate, micrognathia (smallness of the jaw)
	Epicanthus
	Brachycephalism (shortness of the head) (7–8* weeks)
	Mixed sexual characteristics
8	Persistent ostium primum (persistent opening in atrial septum)
	Digital stunting (shortening of fingers and toes)

*May occur in several time periods after conception.

SOURCE: Modified from Danforth DN, Scott JR: *Obstetrics and Gynecology*, 5th ed. Philadelphia: Lippincott, 1986, p 319.

the primary dietary factors in brain growth. A subtle type of damage that affects the associative capacity of the brain, possibly leading to learning disabilities, may be caused by nutritional deficiency at this stage. (Maternal nutrition is discussed in depth in Chapter 17.)

Another prenatal influence on the intrauterine environment is maternal hyperthermia associated with sauna baths or hot tub use (Milunsky et al 1992). Studies of the effects of maternal hyperthermia during the first trimester have raised concern about possible central nervous system defects and failure of neural tube closure. The effects of maternal substance abuse on fetal development are discussed in Chapters 18 and 31.

KEY CONCEPTS

Humans have 46 chromosomes, which are divided into 23 pairs—22 pairs of autosomes and one pair of sex chromosomes.

Mitosis is the process by which additional somatic (body) cells are formed. It provides growth and development of the organisms and replacement of body cells.

Meiosis is the process by which gametes are formed. It occurs during gametogenesis (oogenesis and spermatogenesis)

and consists of two successive cell divisions (reduction division), which produce a gamete with 23 chromosomes (22 chromosomes and 1 sex chromosome)—the haploid number of chromosomes.

Gametes must have a haploid number (23) of chromosomes so that, when the female gamete (ovum) and the male gamete (spermatozoon) unite (fertilization) to form the zygote, the normal human diploid number of chromosomes (46) is reestablished.

An ovum is considered fertile for about 24 hours after ovulation, and the sperm is capable of fertilizing the ovum for only about 24 hours after it is deposited in the female reproductive tract.

Fertilization usually takes place in the ampulla (outer third) of the fallopian tube.

Both capacitation and the acrosomal reaction must occur for the sperm to fertilize the ovum. Capacitation is the removal of the plasma membrane, which exposes the acrosomal covering of the sperm head. The acrosomal reaction is the deposit of hyaluronidase in the corona radiata, which allows the sperm head to penetrate the ovum.

Sex chromosomes are referred to as X and Y. Females have two X chromosomes and males have an X and a Y chromosome. Y chromosomes are carried only by the sperm. To produce a male child, the mother contributes an X chromosome and the father contributes a Y chromosome.

Twins are either monozygotic (identical) or dizygotic (fraternal). Dizygotic twins arise from two separate ova fertilized by two separate spermatozoa. Monozygotic twins develop from a single ovum fertilized by a single spermatozoon.

Intrauterine development first proceeds via cellular multiplication in which the zygote undergoes rapid mitotic division called cleavage. As a result of cleavage, the zygote divides and multiplies into cell groupings called blastomeres, which are held together by the zona pellucida. The blastomeres will eventually become a solid ball of cells called the morula. When a cavity forms in the morula cell mass, the inner solid cell mass is called the blastocyst.

Implantation usually occurs in the upper part of the posterior uterine wall when the blastocyst burrows into the uterine lining.

After implantation the endometrium is called the decidua. Decidua capsularis is the portion that covers the blastocyst. Decidua basalis is the portion that is directly under the blastocyst. Decidua vera is the portion that lines the rest of the uterine cavity.

Embryonic membranes are called the amnion and the chorion. The amnion is formed from the ectoderm and is a thin protective membrane that contains the amniotic fluid and the embryo. The chorion is a thick membrane that develops from the trophoblast and encloses the amnion, embryo, and yolk sac.

Amniotic fluid cushions the fetus against mechanical injury, controls the embryo's temperature, allows symmetrical external growth, prevents adherence to the amnion, and permits freedom of movement.

Primary germ layers will give rise to all tissues, organs, and organ systems. The three primary germ cell layers are ectoderm, endoderm, and mesoderm.

The placenta, which develops from the chorionic villi and the decidua basalis, has two parts: The maternal portion, consisting of the decidua basalis, is red and fresh-looking; the fetal portion, consisting of chorionic villi, is covered by the amnion and appears shiny and gray. The placenta is made up of 15–20 segments called cotyledons.

The placenta serves endocrine (production of hPL, hCG, estrogen, and progesterone), metabolic, and immunologic functions. It acts as the fetus's respiratory organ, is an organ of excretion, and aids in the exchange of nutrients.

The umbilical cord contains two umbilical arteries, which carry deoxygenated blood from the fetus to the placenta, and one umbilical vein, which carries oxygenated blood from the placenta to the fetus. The umbilical cord has a central insertion into the placenta. Wharton's jelly, a specialized connective tissue, prevents compression of the umbilical cord in utero.

Fetal circulation is a specially designed circulatory system that provides for oxygenation of the fetus while bypassing the fetal lungs.

Stages of fetal development include the preembryonic stage (the first 14 days of human development starting at fertilization), the embryonic stage (from day 15 after fertilization, or the beginning of the third week, until approximately 8 weeks after conception), and the fetal stage (from 8 weeks until birth at approximately 40 weeks postconception).

Significant events that occur during the embryonic stage are that at 4 weeks the fetal heart begins to beat and at 6 weeks fetal circulation is established.

The fetal stage is devoted to refining structures and perfecting function. The following are some significant developments during the fetal stage:

At 8–12 weeks all organ systems are formed and now require maturation.

At 16 weeks sex can be determined visually.

At 20 weeks fetal heartbeat can be auscultated by a fetoscope, and the mother can feel movement (quickening).

At 24 weeks vernix caseosa covers the entire body.

At 26–28 weeks the eyes reopen.

At 32 weeks skin appears less wrinkled and red, because subcutaneous fat has been laid down.

At 36 weeks fingernails reach the ends of fingers.

At 40 weeks vernix caseosa is apparent only in creases and folds of skin, and lanugo remains on upper arms and shoulders only.

The embryo is particularly vulnerable to teratogenesis during the first 8 weeks of cell differentiation and organ system development.

REFERENCES

Benirschke K: Normal development. In: Creasy RK, Resnik R (editors). *Maternal-Fetal Medicine: Principles and Practice*, 3rd ed. Philadelphia: Saunders, 1994.

Cunningham FG, MacDonald PC, Gant NG: *Williams Obstetrics*, 19th ed. Norwalk, CT: Appleton & Lange, 1993.

Eden RD, Boehm FH (editors). *Assessment and Care of the Fetus: Physiological, Clinical, and Medicolegal Principles.* Norwalk, CT: Appleton & Lange, 1990.

Gilbert WM, Brace RA: Amniotic fluid volume and normal flows to and from the amniotic cavity. *Semin Perinatol* 1993; 17(3):150.

Marieb EN, Mallatt J: *Human Anatomy.* Redwood City, CA: Benjamin/Cummings, 1992.

Milunsky A, Ulciclas M, Rothman KJ, et al: Maternal heat exposure and neural tube defects. *JAMA* 1992; 268(4):882.

Moise KJ: Polyhydramnios: Problems and treatment. *Semin Perinatol* 1993; 17(3):197.

Moore KL, Persaud TVN: *The Developing Human: Clinically Oriented Embryology*, 5th ed. Philadelphia: Saunders, 1993.

Revenis ME, Johnson LA: Multiple gestations. In: Avery GB, Fletcher M, MacDonald MG: *Neonatalogy: Pathophysiology and Management of the Newborn*, 4th ed. Philadelphia: Lippincott, 1994.

Sadler TW: *Langman's Medical Embryology*, 6th ed. Baltimore: Williams & Wilkins, 1990.

Speroff L, Glass RH, Kase NG: *Clinical Gynecologic Endocrinology and Infertility*, 5th ed. Baltimore: Williams & Wilkins, 1994.

Thompson MW, McInnes RR, Willard HF: *Thompson & Thompson's Genetics in Medicine*, 5th ed. Philadelphia: Saunders, 1991.

Volpe JJ: *Neurology of the Newborn*, 3rd ed. Philadelphia: Saunders, 1995.

SPECIAL REPRODUCTIVE CONCERNS

*A*s my husband and I sat in the waiting room at the in vitro clinic, I felt great apprehension. For 4 years we had been unable to conceive a child. I'd been through two surgeries, dozens of blood tests, hormone drugs that made me irrational and emotional, and many difficult times of blaming myself, feeling out of control, and having surprisingly painful reactions to seeing mothers with newborns. After many long discussions we had decided that, if in vitro didn't work for us, we would adopt a child. Still, we both felt that we wanted to experience childbirth together.

We were on the brink of the most expensive treatment in the infertility process—the last resort for most infertile couples. Each month's treatment would involve nearly $10,000 of uninsured costs; numerous injections, many of which I would have to administer to myself; egg retrieval; four or five ultrasounds; a dozen blood tests; and only a 30% chance of conceiving a child. Was I doing the right thing? Was this the right clinic for us? After so many disappointments did I dare to get my hopes up once again?

A young nurse burst into the office, tremendously excited and out of breath. She'd just come from the lab, having done a blood test, and had discovered that a patient, Judy, was pregnant. Watching the thrill and caring of these nurses' faces helped me to decide. Yes, I was in the right place. Yes, it was worth hoping again. Even if in vitro didn't work for us, we had to try.

OBJECTIVES

Describe how alterations in the normal male and female reproductive systems can contribute to a couple's infertility.

Identify indications for tests done in an infertility workup and associated treatments including assisted reproductive technologies.

Summarize the physiologic and psychologic effects of infertility on a couple.

Describe the nurse's roles as counselor, educator, and advocate for couples during infertility evaluation/treatment.

Discuss the indications for preconceptual chromosomal analysis and prenatal testing.

Identify the general characteristics of autosomal dominant, autosomal recessive, and X-linked recessive disorders.

Compare prenatal and postnatal diagnostic procedures used to determine the presence of genetic disorders.

Explore the emotional impact on a couple undergoing genetic testing or coping with the birth of a baby with a genetic disorder and explain the nurse's role in genetic counseling.

M ost couples who want children conceive with little difficulty. Pregnancy and childbirth usually take their normal course, and a healthy baby is born. But some less fortunate couples are unable to fulfill their dream of having a healthy baby because of infertility or genetic problems.

This chapter explores two particularly troubling reproductive problems facing some couples: the inability to conceive and the risk of bearing babies with genetic abnormalities.

INFERTILITY

Infertility is defined as lack of conception despite unprotected sexual intercourse for at least 12 months (Hatcher et al 1994). It can further be defined as a disease of the male or female reproductive system (American Fertility Society 1990). Approximately 10–15% of couples in their reproductive years are infertile (Speroff et al 1994). **Sterility** is a term applied when there is an absolute factor preventing reproduction. **Subfertility** is used to describe a couple having difficulty conceiving because both partners have reduced fecundity. Subfertility may be used interchangeably with the term *subfecundity* (Hatcher et al 1994).

Primary infertility identifies those women who have never conceived, whereas *secondary infertility* indicates those who have been pregnant in the past but have not conceived during 1 or more years of unprotected intercourse (Speroff et al 1994).

There is a public perception that infertility is on the rise and reaching epidemic proportions. But in fact the 1988 National Survey of Family Growth revealed that the incidence of infertility is unchanged from the last survey, which was conducted in 1982. Other sources even suggest it is on the decline (Mosher & Pratt 1993). What has changed is the composition of the infertile population; the infertility diagnosis has increased in the age group 25–44 because of delayed childbearing and the entry of the baby-boom cohort into this age range.

The following factors, gleaned from data revealed in the 1988 survey, may account for the perception that infertility is on the rise:

- The increase in open discussion about reproductive issues
- The increase in assisted reproduction techniques
- The increase in availability and use of infertility services
- The increase in public awareness of infertility due to media and popular literature
- The increase in insurance coverage of diagnosis of and treatment for infertility

- The increased number of childless women in the older age groups
- The increased number of childless women over 35 seeking medical attention for infertility (Speroff et al 1994)
- Increased incidence of sexually transmitted diseases (Wilcox & Mosher 1993)
- The decreasing population of adoptable babies

Essential Components of Fertility

Understanding the elements essential for normal fertility can help the nurse identify the many factors that may cause infertility. The following essential components must be presented for normal fertility:

Female partner:

1. The cervical mucus must be favorable to the survival of spermatozoa and allow passage to the upper genital tract.
2. There must be clear passage between the cervix and the fallopian tubes.
3. The fallopian tubes must be patent and have normal fimbria with peristaltic movements toward the uterus to facilitate normal transport and interaction of ovum and sperm.
4. The ovaries must produce and release normal ova in a timely manner.
5. There must be no obstruction between the ovaries and fallopian tubes.
6. The endometrium must be in a normal physiologic state to allow implantation of the blastocyst and to sustain normal growth and development.

Male partner:

1. The testes must produce adequate numbers of morphologically normal, motile sperm.
2. The male genital tract must not be obstructed.
3. The male genital tract secretions must be normal.
4. Ejaculated spermatozoa must be deposited in the female genital tract in such a manner that they reach the cervix.

These normal findings are correlated with possible causes of deviation in Table 7–1. In addition to these necessary elements, certain general physiologic and psychologic conditions must be present to support conception.

Considering the intricacies of the normal male and female reproductive cycle, it is an impressive phenomenon that approximately 92% of the couples in the United States are able to conceive. The remaining 8% suffer from either a male factor (40%) or a female factor (40%), or the cause of infertility cannot be identified, or prob-

TABLE 7-1   Possible Causes of Infertility

Necessary Norms	Deviations from Normal
Female	
Favorable cervical mucus	Cervicitis, cervical stenosis, use of coital lubricants, antisperm antibodies (immunologic response)
Clear passage between cervix and tubes	Myomas, adhesions, adenomyosis, polyps, endometritis, cervical stenosis, endometriosis, congenital anomalies (eg, septate uterus, DES exposure)
Patent tubes with normal motility	Pelvic inflammatory disease, peritubal adhesions, endometriosis, IUD, salpingitis (eg, chlamydia, recurrent STDs), neoplasm, ectopic pregnancy, tubal ligation
Ovulation and release of ova	Primary ovarian failure, polycystic ovarian disease, hypothyroidism, pituitary tumor, lactation, periovarian adhesions, endometriosis, premature ovarian failure, hyperprolactinemia, Turner syndrome
No obstruction between ovary and tubes	Adhesions, endometriosis, pelvic inflammatory disease
Endometrial preparation	Anovulation, luteal phase defect, malformation, uterine infection, Asherman's syndrome
Male	
Normal semen analysis	Abnormalities of sperm or semen, polyspermia, congenital defect in testicular development, mumps after adolescence, cryptorchidism, infections, gonadal exposure to x rays, chemotherapy, smoking, alcohol abuse, malnutrition, chronic or acute metabolic disease, medications (eg, morphine, ASA, ibuprofen), cocaine, marijuana use, constrictive underclothing, heat
Unobstructed genital tract	Infections, tumors, congenital anomalies, vasectomy, strictures, trauma, varicocele
Normal genital tract secretions	Infections, autoimmunity to semen, tumors
Ejaculate deposited at the cervix	Premature ejaculation, impotence, hypospadias, retrograde ejaculation (eg, diabetic), neurologic cord lesions, obesity (inhibiting adequate penetration)

lems exist with both partners (10–20%) (Speroff et al 1994). In 35% of the infertile couples there are multiple etiologies; with appropriate evaluation and therapy approximately half of these couples will become pregnant (Hill 1992).

Couples should be referred for infertility evaluation if they have been unable to conceive after at least 1 year of attempting to achieve pregnancy. If the woman is over 35 years old, it may be appropriate to refer the couple after only 6 to 9 months of unprotected intercourse without conception. At 25 years of age, the age at which couples are the most fertile, the average length of time needed to achieve conception is 5.3 months. The average 20- to 30-year-old American couple has intercourse one to three times a week, a frequency that should be sufficient to achieve pregnancy if all other factors are satisfactory. In about 20% of cases conception occurs within the first month of unprotected intercourse, in 72% by 6 months, in 85% by 12 months, and 95% within 24 months (Speroff et al 1994). There continues to be an increase in the number of women who give birth to their first child after the age of 30. Delaying parenthood appears to increase the possibility that one or more of the physiologic processes necessary for conception will be adversely affected (Speroff et al 1994).

Care of the Couple that Is Unable to Conceive

The easiest and least intrusive infertility testing approach is used first. Extensive testing is avoided until data confirm that the timing of intercourse and the length of coital exposure have been adequate. The couple should be informed of the most fertile times to have intercourse during the menstrual cycle. Teaching the couple the signs and timing of ovulation and the most effective times for intercourse within the cycle may solve the problem before extensive testing needs to be initiated. Primary assessment, including a comprehensive history (with a discussion of genetic conditions) and physical examination for any obvious causes of infertility, is done before a costly, time-consuming, and emotionally trying investigation is initiated. During the first visit for the preliminary investigation, the basic infertility workup is explained. The basic investigation for the couple depends on the individuals' history and usually includes assessment of ovarian function, cervical mucus adequacy and receptivity to sperm, sperm adequacy, tubal patency, and the general condition of the pelvic organs. Because approximately 40% of infertility is related to a male factor, a semen analysis should be one of the first diagnostic tests prior to moving on to the more invasive diagnostic procedures involving the woman.

It is never easy to discuss one's sexual activity, especially when potentially irreversible problems with fertility may exist. The mutual desire to have children is central to many marriages. Infertility has been described as a life crisis that may immobilize immediate life plans; strain existing emotional, financial, and physical resources; threaten long-term life goals; and awaken key issues from the couple's history (Morse & Van Hall 1986). The self-esteem of one or both partners may be threatened if the inability to conceive is seen as a lack of virility or femininity. The nurse can provide comfort to couples by

The indignities and invasion of privacy that occur with an infertility work-up and treatment program create problems even for those familiar with Western biomedicine. When the couple comes from another culture, these problems may be compounded because the couple may have to participate in behavior they deem culturally unacceptable. For these men and women, a culturally sensitive health care provider can make the difference between successful completion of the process and total failure. Janet Blenner used a qualitative methodology to explore health care providers' perceptions, approaches, and responses to infertile clients from culturally different backgrounds.

The sample included 28 health care providers who had been involved in infertility treatment for at least a year. Data collected by interviews were analyzed through a constant comparative technique, resulting in the generation of codes and clustering into categories.

Analysis resulted in the development of three major provider paths in the perception and response to culturally diverse clients. Path A included physicians, nurses, sonographic technicians, and radiologic technicians. These culturally unaware providers demonstrated a lack of awareness of cultural diversity, rigid approaches to treatment, and a perceived lack of commitment or noncompliance when their culturally diverse clients did not follow treatment programs. Path B providers

included only physicians; they were found to be culturally intolerant. Path C participants were physicians, nurses, sonographic technicians, and social workers; this group was culturally sensitive. Both the culturally intolerant (Path B) and culturally sensitive (Path C) providers recognized cultural diversity and identified conflicts and cultural barriers to treatment. Path B providers, however, described an unwillingness to tolerate the conflicts and barriers that affected treatment and would terminate the relationship or refer the clients to a more tolerant provider. Path C participants tolerated the necessary adjustments to the treatment protocols. These providers recognized gaps in their knowledge of culture and searched for information they lacked. They demonstrated a willingness to work within cultural limitations, and they adapted protocols and interventions to be more culturally sensitive.

Clinical Application of Study

This study contains invaluable information for anyone involved with culturally diverse clients, especially in situations where sexual practices or taboos impact client care.

SOURCE: Blenner J: Health care providers' treatment approaches to culturally diverse infertile clients. *J Transcultural Nurs* 1991; 2(2):24.

TABLE 7-2	Initial Infertility Physical Workup and Laboratory Evaluations

Female	Male

Physical examination
  Assessment of height, weight, blood pressure, temperature, and general health status
  Endocrine evaluation of thyroid for exophthalmos, lid lag, tremor, or palpable gland
  Optic fundi evaluation for presence of increased intracranial pressure, especially in oligomenorrheal or amenorrheal women (possible pituitary tumor)
  Reproductive features (including breast and external genital area)
  Physical ability to tolerate pregnancy
	Physical examination
	  General health (assessment of height, weight, blood pressure)
	  Endocrine evaluation (eg, presence of gyneco-mastia)
	  Visual fields evaluation for bitemporal hemianopia
	  Abnormal hair patterns

Pelvic examination
  Papanicolaou smear
  Culture for gonorrhea if indicated and possibly chlamydia or mycoplasma culture (opinions vary)
  Signs of vaginal infections (Chapter 10)
  Shape of escutcheon (eg, Does pubic hair distribution resemble that of a male?)
  Size of clitoris (enlargement caused by endocrine disorders)
  Evaluation of cervix: old lacerations, tears, erosion, polyps, condition and shape of os, signs of infections, cervical mucus (evaluate for estrogen effect of spinnbarkheit and cervical ferning)
	Urologic examination (includes presence or absence of phimosis; location of urethral meatus; size and consistency of each testis, vas deferens, and epididymis; presence of varicocele)

Bimanual examination
  Size, shape, position, and motility of uterus
  Presence of congenital anomalies
  Presence of endometriosis
  Evaluation of adnexa: ovarian size, cysts, fixations, or tumors
	Rectal examination
	  Size and consistency of the prostate with microscopic evaluation of prostate fluid for signs of infection
	  Size and consistency of seminal vesicles

Rectovaginal examination
  Presence of retroflexed or retroverted uterus
  Presence of rectouterine pouch masses
  Presence of possible endometriosis
	Laboratory examination
	  Complete blood count
	  Sedimentation rate if indicated
	  Serology
	  Urinalysis
	  Rh factor and blood grouping
	  Semen analysis
	  If indicated, testicular biopsy, buccal smear

Laboratory examination
  Complete blood count
  Sedimentation rate if indicated
  Serology
  Urinalysis
  Rh factor and blood grouping
  If indicated, thyroid function tests, prolactin levels, glucose tolerance test, 17-ketosteroid assay, 17-hydrocorticoid assay, testosterone or dehydroepiandrosterone levels	

offering a sympathetic ear, a nonjudgmental approach, and appropriate information and instructions throughout the diagnostic and therapeutic process.

Because infertility is a couple's issue, it is important for both partners to be present for the initial consultation. The first interview should include a comprehensive history of both partners and a physical and pelvic exam of the female. Table 7–2 outlines what is entailed in a complete infertility physical workup and laboratory evaluation for both partners. The historical data base, diagnostic tests usually performed, and health care interventions in cases of infertility are outlined in Figure 7–1.

Tests for Infertility

The infertility evaluation is based on information gleaned from a thorough history and physical examination. It is important to assess both partners due to the high incidence of multifactorial infertility. A thorough female evaluation includes assessment of the hypothalamic/pituitary axis in terms of ovulatory function, as well as structure and function of the cervix, uterus, fallopian tubes, and ovaries. See Chapter 5 for an in-depth discussion of the fertility cycle. Evaluation of the male may include at least two semen analyses to confirm or rule out a seminal

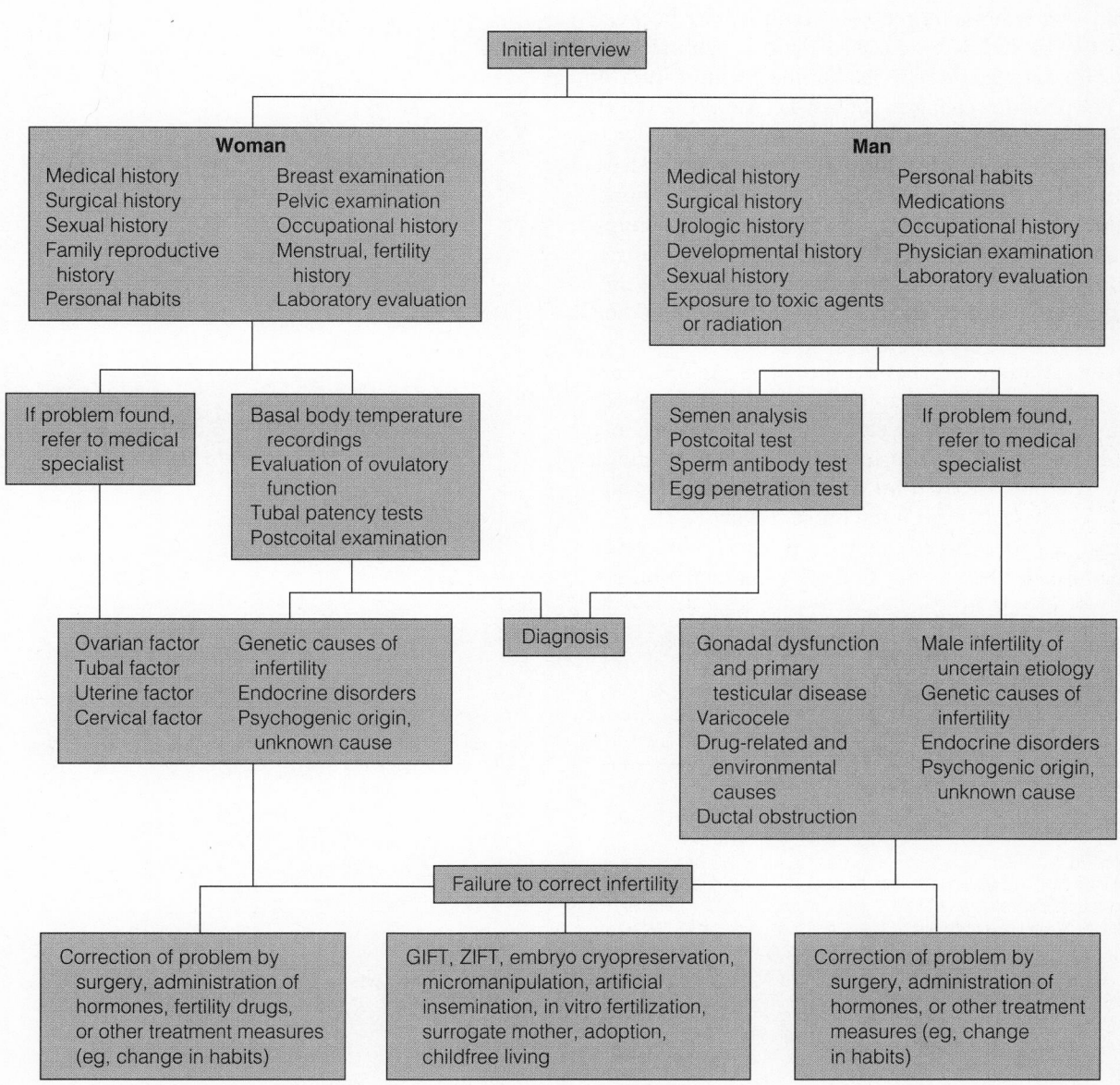

FIGURE 7–1   Flow chart for management of the infertile couple.

deficiency. Functional tests such as the hamster sperm penetration assay (SPA) or serum and semen immunobead testing for the presence of antisperm antibodies (immunologic infertility) may be performed. The female fertility assessments will be discussed first. For review of female reproductive cycle characteristics, see Table 7–3 and Figure 7–2.

Female Assessment

Evaluation of Ovulatory Factors Ovulation problems account for approximately 15% of couples' infertility (Speroff et al 1994). One basic test of ovulatory function is the **basal body temperature (BBT)** recording, which aids in identifying follicular, ovulatory, and luteal phase abnormalities. At the initial visit the woman is instructed in the technique of recording basal body temperature, which must be taken with a BBT thermometer. This special kind of thermometer measures temperature between 35.6 C (96 F) and 37.8 C (100 F) and is calibrated by tenths of a degree, thereby facilitating identification of slight temperature changes. The BBT should be taken every morning before getting out of bed (after at least 3 hours of sleep) (Hatcher et al 1994). Recent studies have demonstrated that, in addition to the traditional glass/mercury BBT thermometer, tympanic thermometry is a valid method to obtain basal body temperatures. Tympanic thermometry has the advantages of being simple and taking less than 2 seconds to get a reading (Wolf & Baker 1993).

Daily variations should be recorded on a temperature graph. The temperature graph typically shows a biphasic pattern during ovulatory cycles, whereas in anovulatory cycles it remains monophasic. The temperature graph and the readings are used for detecting timing of ovulation and the best time for intercourse (Figure 7–3).

Basal temperature for females in the preovulatory phase is usually below 36.7 C (98 F). As ovulation approaches, production of estrogen increases and at its peak may cause a slight drop, then rise, in the basal temperature. When ovulation occurs, there is a surge of luteinizing hormone (LH), and progesterone is produced by the corpus luteum, causing a 0.3 C to 0.6 C (0.5 F to 1.0 F) rise in basal temperature. These changes in the basal temperatures create the typical biphasic pattern. Figure 7–3B shows a biphasic ovulatory BBT chart. Progesterone is thermogenic (it produces heat), thereby maintaining the temperature increase during the second half of the menstrual cycle. Temperature elevation does not predict the day of ovulation but provides supportive evidence of ovulation about a day after it has occurred. Actual release of

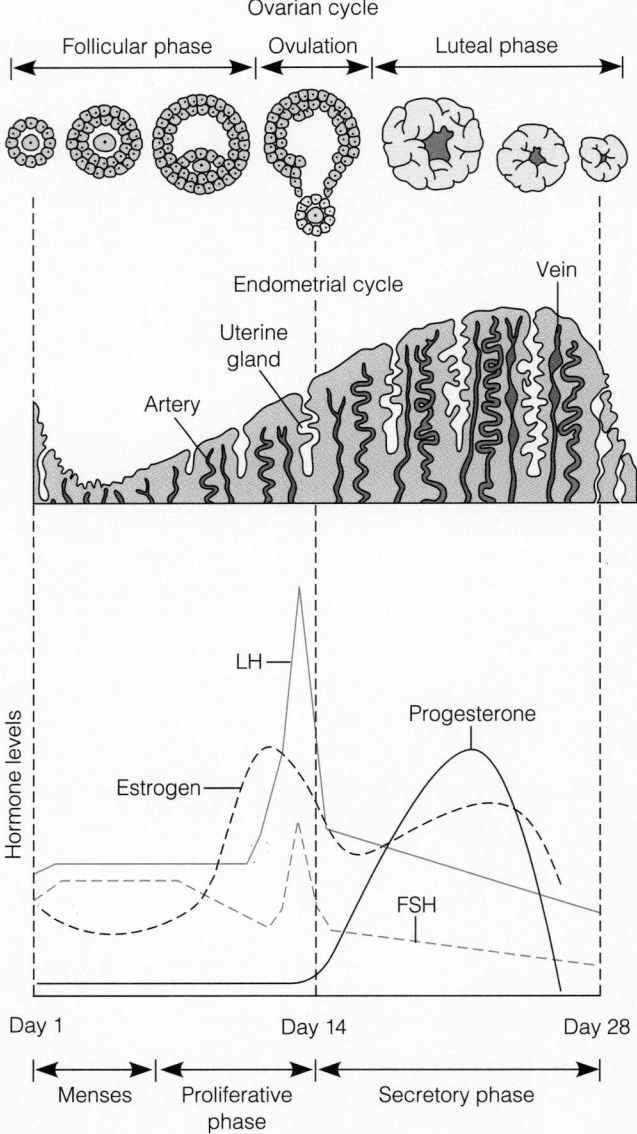

FIGURE 7-2 Sequence of events in a normal reproductive cycle showing the relationship of hormone levels to events in the ovarian and endometrial cycles.

TABLE 7–3	Female Reproductive Cycle
Ovarian Cycle	**Menstrual Cycle**
Follicular phase (days 1–14): Primordial follicle matures under influence of FSH and LH up to the time of ovulation.	*Menstrual phase* (days 1–5)
	Proliferative phase (days 6–14): Estrogen peaks just prior to ovulation. Cervical mucus at ovulation is clear, thin, watery, alkaline, and more favorable to sperm; shows ferning pattern; and has spinnbarkheit greater than 8 cm. At ovulation body temperature drops, then rises sharply and remains elevated.
Luteal phase (days 15–28): Ovum leaves follicle, corpus luteum develops under LH influence and produces high levels of progesterone and low levels of estrogen.	*Secretory phase* (days 15–26): Estrogen drops sharply and progesterone dominates.
	Ischemic phase (days 27–28): Both estrogen and progesterone levels drop.

the ovum probably occurs 24 to 36 hours prior to the first temperature elevation (Speroff et al 1994).

With the additional documentation of coitus, serial BBT charts can be used to indicate retrospectively if, and approximately when, the woman is ovulating and if intercourse is occurring at the proper time to achieve conception. A proposed schedule for intercourse based on serial BBT charts might be to recommend sexual intercourse *every other day* in the period of time beginning 3 to 4 days prior to and continuing for 2 to 3 days following the expected time of ovulation.

Hormonal assessments of ovulatory function fall into the following categories:

1. *Gonadotropin levels (FSH, LH).* Baseline hormonal assessment of FSH and LH provides valuable information concerning normal ovulatory function. Low levels may indicate hypothalamic/pituitary dysfunction, and high levels are indicative of poor ovarian function or failure. Measured on cycle day 3, basal FSH is the single most valuable test in assessing ovarian reserve and function and should always be measured, particularly in women over 35, to predict the potential for successful treatment with ovulation induction treatment cycles. High levels predict a very poor outcome for conception and pregnancy. LH levels may be measured early in the cycle to rule out disorders associated with androgen excess, causing a disruption in normal follicular development and oocyte maturation. Serial serum LH may also be measured at midcycle to document the LH surge, which is believed to be the time of maximum fertility. Urinary LH ovulation prediction kits are also available for home use and are used to better time postcoital testing, insemination, and coitus. Finally, an abnormal ratio of FSH to LH on cycle day 3 (with LH being elevated and FSH being low to normal) is indicative of polycystic ovarian disease.

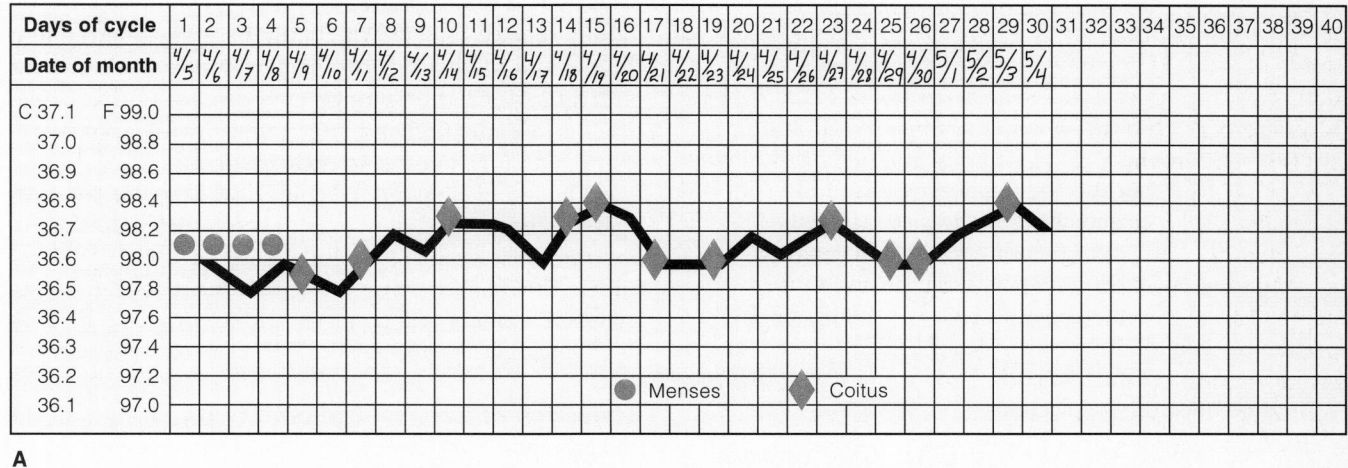

A

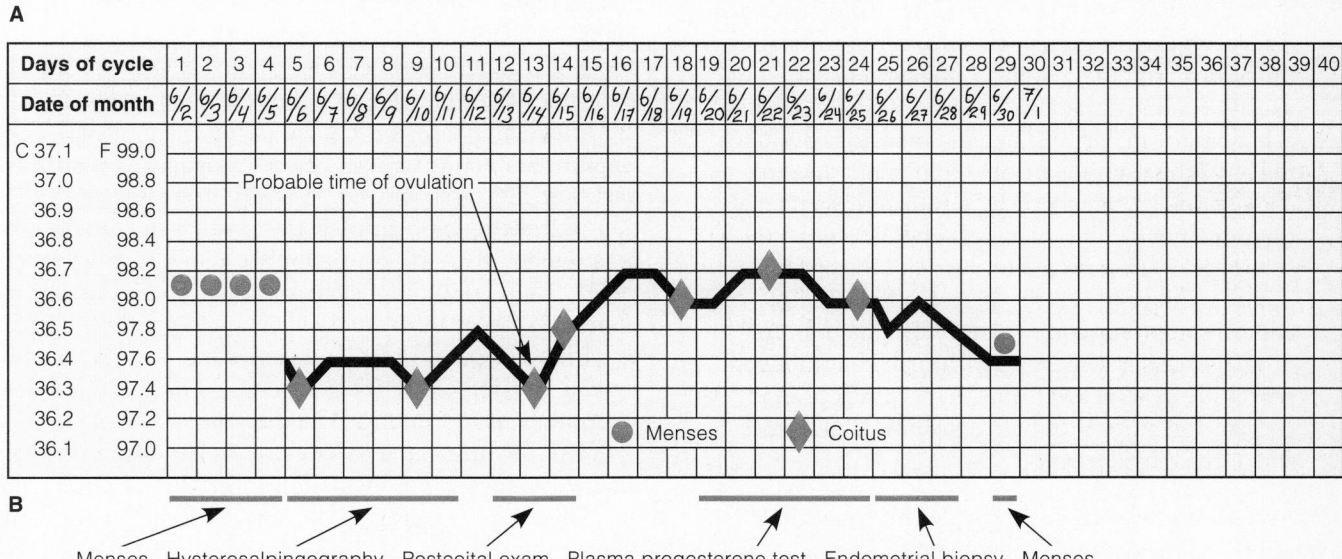

B

FIGURE 7-3   *A* A monophasic, anovulatory basal body temperature (BBT) chart.
B A biphasic BBT chart illustrating probable time of ovulation, the different types of testing, and the time in the cycle that each would be performed.

2. *Steroid hormones (estrogen, progesterone)*. Estrogen and progesterone levels measured by radioimmunoassay (RIA) are also valuable indicators of menstrual cycle function. Estradiol, the principal form of estrogen secreted from the ovary, provides an indirect measurement of oocyte development and maturation. Progesterone levels furnish the best evidence of ovulation and corpus luteum function. Serum levels begin to rise with the LH surge and peak about 8 days later. A level of 3 ng/mL 3 days after the LH surge confirms ovulation. Levels on day 21 (7 days postovulation) of 10 ng/mL or higher indicate an adequate luteal phase.

3. *Prolactin*. Elevated prolactin levels are a frequent cause of ovulatory dysfunction, which may range from a luteal phase defect to anovulation to amenorrhea. Prolactin levels also measured by RIA are generally considered normal if less than 20 ng/mL. High levels are associated with pituitary adenomas, and in such cases a CT scan is indicated. In the absence of thyroid dysfunction and pituitary adenomas, prolactin excess can be easily treated with bromocriptine (Parlodel) and normal ovulatory function restored in most cases.

4. *Thyroid stimulating hormone (TSH)*. Thyroid hormone is necessary for most body functions, not only metabolism, but specific tissue activities. TSH stimulates prolactin secretion by the pituitary gland (Speroff et al 1994). Hypothyroidism may have a dramatic effect on ovulatory function and cause menstrual irregularities and bleeding problems. It can be diagnosed by measuring TSH. Treatment is easily accomplished in cases of deficiency with thyroxine hormonal replacement.

5. *Androgen levels (testosterone, DHEAS, androstendione)*. Androgen excess can originate from the adrenal, ovary, or peripheral tissue. Despite the origin, it usually results in specific clinical symptoms such as acne, hirsutism, virilization, and ovulatory dysfunction—which can range from oligomenorrhea to anovulation to amenorrhea. Serum androgen levels can document androgen excess and determine the site of excess (ie, adrenal or ovarian). Successful treatment depends on the source and degree of clinical symptoms and ovulatory dysfunction. Androgen excess is associated with such conditions as polycystic ovarian syndrome, hyperprolactiremia, ovarian and adrenal tumors, Cushing's syndrome, and adrenal hyperplasia.

An **endometrial biopsy** provides information about ovulation by assessing the adequacy of corpus luteum function and endometrial receptivity. The biopsy is performed not earlier than 10–12 days postovulation using a paracervical block and is easily accomplished by removing a small sample of endometrium with a small pipette attached to suction. It is easy to perform and requires little cervical dilatation (3 mm diameter) (Speroff et al 1994). The patient should be informed that some pelvic discomfort, cramping, and vaginal spotting is normal during and following the procedure. The onset of menses following biopsy should be reported for accurate interpretation of the biopsy report. Contrary to popular belief, the risk of disruption to an early pregnancy is minimal (Corson 1990), but use of a urinary pregnancy test immediately prior to biopsy can further reduce the risk of biopsy after conception (Herbert et al 1990).

The pathologist evaluates the histologic development of the endometrium based on the day of the menstrual cycle to gauge the effect of progesterone on the endometrium. A dysfunction may exist if the endometrial lining does not show the expected amount of secretory tissue for that day of the woman's cycle. A repeat biopsy is indicated to confirm luteal phase dysfunction. Serum progesterone levels may also be indicated to confirm adequate luteal phase function.

Ultrasound is now an invaluable adjunct in infertility diagnosis and treatment. Transvaginal ultrasound has rapidly replaced the use of abdominal ultrasounds and is the method of choice for follicular monitoring of clients undergoing ovulation induction cycles, for timing ovulation for insemination and intercourse, for IVF oocyte retrieval, and for monitoring early pregnancy.

The use of transvaginal color flow Doppler to investigate uterine blood flow may in the future help the endocrinologist evaluate the adequacy of the developing follicle, further assessing oocyte maturity and endometrial development and patterns, and improve the diagnosis of luteal phase defect (Hill 1992).

Evaluation of Cervical Factors Cyclic changes in the presence and consistency of cervical mucus occur in response to changing estrogen and progesterone levels. Endocervical mucus cells consist predominantly of water, and under the influence of rising estrogen levels during the follicular phase the mucus changes significantly in amount and consistency. Mucus elasticity or **spinnbarkheit** increases and the viscosity decreases at ovulation. Excellent spinnbarkheit exists when the mucus can be stretched 8 to 10 cm or longer (Jaffe & Jewelewicz 1991). This is accomplished by using two glass slides (Figure 7–4A) or by grasping some mucus at the external os with a grasping forcep and stretching it in the vagina toward the introitus. (See Teaching Guide: Self-Care Methods of Determining Ovulation on pp 140–141.)

The **ferning capacity** (Figure 7–4B) of the cervical mucus also increases as ovulation approaches. Ferning, or crystallization, is caused by decreased levels of salt and water interacting with the glycoproteins in the mucus during the ovulatory period and is thus an indirect indication of estrogen production. To test for ferning, obtain mucus from the cervical os, spread it on a glass slide, allow it to air dry, and examine it under the microscope.

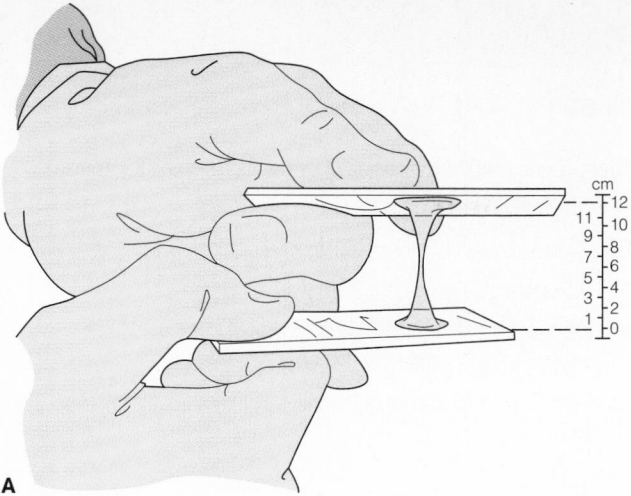

A

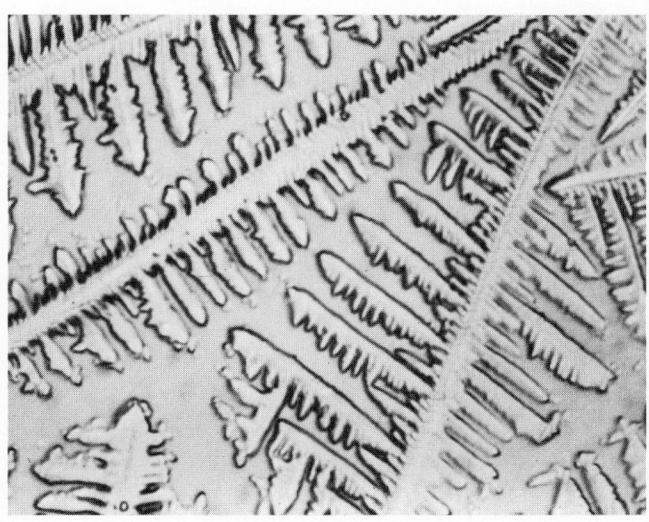

B

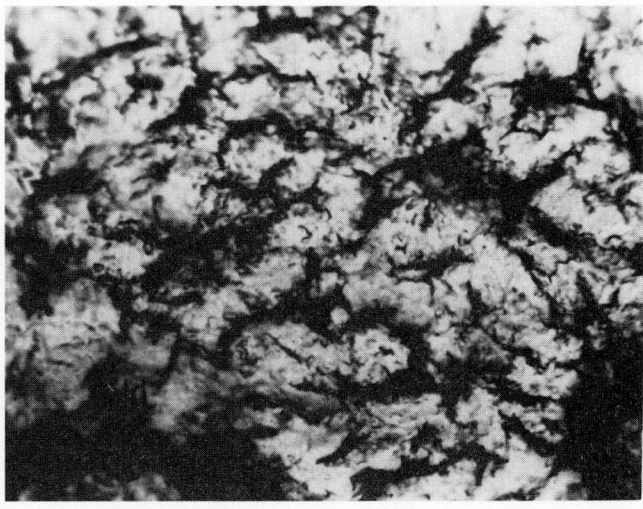

C

FIGURE 7-4 *A* Spinnbarkheit (elasticity). *B* Ferning pattern. *C* Lack of ferning pattern. SOURCE: Speroff L et al: *Clinical Gyneclogic Endocrinology and Infertility,* 5th ed. Baltimore: Williams & Wilkins, 1994, p 818.

Within 24–48 hours postovulation rising levels of progesterone cause a marked decrease in the quantity of cervical mucus and increase in viscosity and cellularity, resulting in absence of spinnbarkheit and ferning capacity and consequently sperm survival.

To be receptive to sperm, cervical mucus must be thin, clear, watery, profuse, alkaline, and acellular. As shown in Figure 7–5, the mazelike microscopic mucoid strands align in a parallel manner to allow for easy sperm passage. The mucus is termed inhospitable if these changes do not occur.

Cervical mucus inhospitable to sperm survival can have several causes, some of which are treatable. For example, estrogen secretion may be inadequate for the development of receptive mucus. Therapy with supplemental estrogen for approximately 6 days before expected ovulation encourages the formation of suitable spinnbarkheit (Speroff et al 1994). Cervical infection, another cause of mucosal hostility to sperm, can be treated, depending on the type of infection. Cone biopsy, electrocautery, or cryosurgery of the cervix may remove large numbers of mucus-producing glands, creating a "dry cervix" that decreases sperm survival (Hammond & Talbert 1985).

The cervix can also be the site of secretory immunologic reactions in which antisperm antibodies are produced, causing agglutination or immobilization of sperm. The most widely used serum sperm bioassay to detect specific classes of antibodies in serum and seminal fluid is immunobead testing by RIA. Treatment may include intrauterine insemination to bypass the cervical factor.

The postcoital test (Huhner's test) is a useful screening device to assess abnormalities in cervical mucus, sperm motility, sperm-mucus interaction, and the sperm's ability to negotiate the cervical mucus barrier. It is performed 1 to 2 days before ovulation as determined by

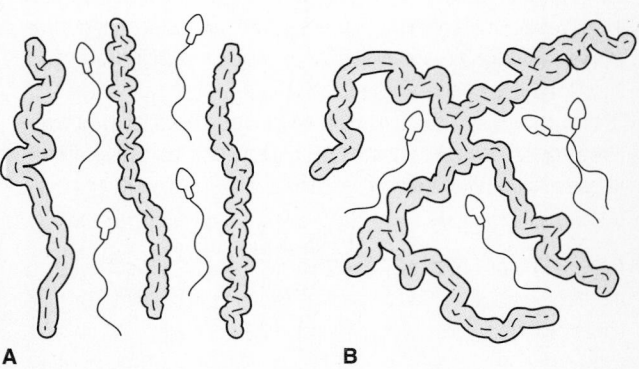

A   B

FIGURE 7-5 Sperm passage through cervical mucus. *A* Appearance at the time of ovulation with channels favoring efficient sperm penetration and migration upward. *B* Unfavorable mazelike configuration found at other times during the menstrual cycle. SOURCE: Corson S: *Conquering Infertility.* New York: Prentice Hall, 1990, p 16.

SELF-CARE METHODS OF DETERMINING OVULATION

Assessment   The nurse focuses on the woman's knowledge of her own body functions, mucus secretions, and menstrual cycle.

Nursing Diagnosis   The key nursing diagnosis will probably be: Knowledge deficit related to lack of information about normal body changes occurring with menstruation and ovulation.

Nursing Plan and Implementation   The teaching plan will include information on expected changes in cervical mucus and body temperature related to menstrual cycle, how to recognize that ovulation has occurred, and self-care methods for determining fertility days.

Client Goals   At the completion of the teaching session the woman will be able to:

1. Accurately identify cervical mucus changes
2. Accurately take and record BBT
3. Discuss the changes in BBT and cervical mucus that indicate ovulation has occurred
4. Summarize physical symptoms that may indicate ovulation has occurred.

Teaching Plan

Content

Basal Body Temperature (BBT)   Expected findings: The BBT can sometimes drop 12 to 24 hours before ovulation, but a sustained rise *almost always* follows for several days. Or a biphasic pattern with temperature elevation for 12 to 14 days prior to menstruation can be seen. At ovulation, temperature will rise 0.4–0.8 F above baseline preovulatory level. Some women notice a drop in temperature 24 hours prior to ovulation. Once a 0.4–0.8 F rise has occurred for 3 consecutive days, a woman who does not desire pregnancy can safely have intercourse because her fertile days have passed. All 3 days should have higher temperature readings than any of the previous days in the cycle. A woman needs to take her BBT for 3 to 4 months to develop a consistent pattern. Procedure: For accurate results the woman should take her temperature for 5 minutes every morning before she gets out of bed (needs at least 3 hours of sleep) and before starting any activity (including smoking). She should choose one site (oral, vaginal, rectal) and use same site each time. A BBT thermometer is preferable. After 5 minutes she should record her temperature on special BBT chart (with 0.1 markings). She connects the temperature dots for each day to see baseline temperature readings. After taking her temperature, the woman must shake down the thermometer to prepare for the next day. This is important because even the activity of shaking the thermometer before use can cause a small increase in basal temperature.
Special considerations include situations that can disturb body temperature: large alcohol intake, sleeplessness, gastrointestinal or other febrile illness, immunization, warm or hot climate, jet lag, shift work, or use of electric blanket.

Cervical Mucus Method   Expected findings: Pre- and postovulatory mucus is yellow, thick, and dry; absent; or white and cloudy. Close to or during ovulation mucus is clear, slippery (like egg whites), and elastic (can be stretched between two fingers—*spinnbarkheit*). Ovulation most likely occurs about 24 hours after the last day of abundant, slippery discharge (Hatcher et al 1994). Four days after peak mucus or when it is again dry, thick, and cloudy, the woman has passed her fertile days and may resume intercourse.

Teaching Method

Discuss BBT changes.
Demonstrate BBT thermometer and chart.
Provide pictures of anovulation cycle and biphasic cycle.

Show woman posters of mucus changes, spinnbarkheit of different elasticity.
Discuss feelings about actual procedure.

Mucus changes: During menstruation blood covers up sensation of wetness or mucus. For a few days after menstruation the vagina feels moist but is not distinctly wet (called "dry" days). The next mucus stage is thick, cloudy, whitish or yellowish, and sticky mucus. Vagina still doesn't feel wet, and this lasts for several days. As ovulation nears, mucus usually becomes more abundant, accompanied by an increasingly wet sensation. Next the clear slippery mucus decreases until it is no longer detectable, and either the thick, cloudy, sticky mucus returns or there is no mucus at all until the next menstrual period.

Procedure: The woman should check her vagina each day when she uses the bathroom, either by dabbing the vaginal opening with toilet paper or by putting a finger inside the opening. She should note the wetness (presence of mucus), collect mucus, and look at its color and consistency. Findings are recorded on chart each day. Several cycles of mucus changes are recorded to become familiar with the pattern before relying on this method.

Special considerations: Presence and consistency of mucus is altered by vaginal infection, vaginal medications such as creams or suppositories, spermicides, lubricants, douching, sexual arousal, or semen.

When pregnancy is not desired, some advise complete abstinence throughout the *first* cycle a woman charts her mucus changes to help her avoid confusing mucus with semen and normal sexual lubrication.

Other   Additional physical findings that may indicate ovulation include slight vaginal spotting, *mittelschmertz,* increased libido.

Discuss rationale for physical changes. Answer questions.

Evaluation   Teaching has been effective if the nurse discussed BBT and cervical mucus changes associated with ovulation, demonstrated BBT procedure and charting of BBT and cervical mucus changes. The woman feels comfortable with BBT and cervical mucus procedure and completion of charting. The woman is able to describe her body functions, how they change, and how they can be used to identify fertile periods and the time at which ovulation may occur.

previous BBT charts, the length of prior cycles, or a urinary LH kit.

The couple is asked to have intercourse 8–12 hours before examination. Mucus is aspirated from the endocervical canal, measured, and examined microscopically for signs of infection, spinnbarkheit, ferning, number of active spermatozoa per high-power field (HPF), and number of sperm with poor or no motility.

Normal findings in a postcoital test are acellular cervical mucus with 8–10 cm spinnbarkheit and ferning with 15–20 actively motile sperm cells per HPF. If fewer than five active sperm cells are seen, fertility may be severely compromised. When results are poor, it must be determined if it is due to a seminal problem, poor cervical mucus, or inappropriate timing.

Male Assessment

The semen analysis is the single most important diagnostic study of the male and should be done early in the couple's evaluation and prior to invasive testing of the female. Although a postcoital test can provide information about sperm viability, it does not provide sufficient information concerning normal seminal parameters.

To obtain accurate results, the specimen is collected after 2 to 3 days of abstinence and usually by masturbation to avoid contamination or loss of any ejaculate. If the male has difficulty producing sperm by masturbation, special condoms are available to collect the sperm through intercourse. Regular condoms should not be used because they contain spermicidal agents, and sperm

TABLE 7-4	Normal Semen Analysis

Factor	Value
Volume	2 to 6 mL
pH	7.0 to 8.0
Total sperm count	20 million
Liquefaction	Complete in 1 hour
Motility	50% or greater
Normal forms	60% or greater

SOURCE: Speroff L, Glass RH, Kase NG: *Clinical Gynecologic Endocrinology and Infertility,* 4th ed. Baltimore: Williams & Wilkins, 1989.

can be lost in the condom. The specimen should be placed in a sterile container and brought to the laboratory within an hour of collection if possible (2 to 3 hours maximum). It should be marked with the time of collection and date of previous ejaculation and maintained at body temperature. Repeated semen analysis may be required to assess the male's fertility potential adequately; a minimum of two separate analyses is recommended for confirmation. Because the cycle of spermatogenesis is 72 days, semen collections should be repeated at least 74 days apart to allow for new sperm maturation (Speroff et al 1994).

Semen analysis provides information about sperm motility and morphology as well as a determination of the absolute number of spermatozoa present (Table 7–4). Debate exists over the absolute number of sperm required for fertility. An infertile specimen is one that reveals fewer than 20 million sperm per mL, less than 50% motility, or less than 50% normal sperm forms (WHO 1992).

When a seminal deficiency has been identified, further investigation by an immunologist is warranted to look for an underlying cause such as an anatomic abnormality, GI infections including mycoplasma and chlamydia, a varicocele (dilatation of the spermatic cord veins in the scrotum), or an endocrine disorder such as elevated FSH levels in germ cell aplasia or decreased testosterone levels in hypogonadotropy. Some studies have indicated that the quality of sperm decreases with increased age. Infants born to 50- to 60-year-old fathers are at risk for trisomy 21 (Speroff et al 1994).

Treatment is directed toward correcting anatomic or endocrine problems with medical or surgical intervention. In many cases this is not possible, and treatment is directed toward compensating for the seminal deficiency. Treatment options depend on the severity of the seminal problem and may include intrauterine insemination with washed sperm collected from the partner, artificial insemination with donor sperm, or utilization of the assisted reproductive technologies (ARTs).

A variety of environmental factors can affect male fertility. Causes of increased scrotal heat such as jockey shorts, hot tubs, or occupations requiring long hours of sitting are thought to decrease fertility potential, but there are no clinical studies to substantiate this. Heavy use of marijuana, alcohol, or cocaine within 2 years of testing can depress sperm count and testosterone levels; cigarette smoking may depress sperm motility. Neurologic ejaculatory dysfunction can be caused by alpha blockers, phentolamine, methyldopa, quanethidine, and reserpine (Speroff et al 1994). Lead and pesticide exposure can also reduce sperm count (Hatcher et al 1994).

Spermatozoa have been shown to possess intrinsic antigens that can provoke male immunologic infertility. This is especially apparent following vasectomy reversals or genital trauma such as testicular torsion in which autoimmunity to sperm develops (the male produces antibodies to his own sperm) (Haas 1994). Research now indicates that it is the actual presence of antibodies on the spermatozoal surface (not just the presence of antibodies in the serum) that affects sperm function and thus leads to subfertility. Treatment for the presence of sperm antibodies in the male may include immunosuppression and sperm washing/dilution insemination techniques. Donor insemination is a treatment alternative for antibodies in the male and possibly in the female if she reacts only to her partner's sperm (Speroff et al 1994).

Evaluation of Uterine Structures and Tubal Patency

Tubal patency tests are usually done after BBT evaluation, semen analysis, and the other less invasive tests have been done and results evaluated. Tubal patency and uterine structure are usually evaluated by hysterosalpingography. Other invasive tests of the tubes' function are laparoscopy and hysteroscopy. Hysteroscopy may be performed earlier in the evaluation if the woman's history suggests possible tubal damage or uterine abnormalities.

Hysterosalpingography (HSG) or *hysterogram* involves an instillation of a radiopaque substance into the uterine cavity. As the substance fills the uterus and fallopian tubes and spills into the peritoneal cavity, it is viewed with x-ray techniques. This procedure can reveal tubal patency and any distortions of the uterine cavity. In addition the oil-based dye used in HSG may have a therapeutic effect. This effect may be caused by the flushing of debris, breaking of peritoneal adhesions, stimulation of cilia by the instillation, or improvement of cervical mucus because the iodine may exert a bacterostatic effect on the mucous membranes and decrease phagocytosis of sperm (Speroff et al 1994).

The hysterosalpingogram should be performed in the proliferative phase of the cycle to avoid interrupting an early pregnancy. This timing also avoids the lush secretory changes in the endometrium that occur after ovulation, which may prevent the passage of the dye through the tubes and present a false picture of cornual obstruction. Hysterosalpingography causes moderate discomfort. Women can take an OTC prostaglandin synthesis inhibitor 30 minutes prior to the procedure to decrease the pain. HSG can also cause serious recurrence of pelvic inflammatory disease, so prophylactic antibiotics are recommended (Hatcher et al 1994). A possible complication of oil dye intravasation is embolism. Venous or lymphatic intravasation can be detected immediately by fluoroscopy and injection of dye stopped (Speroff et al 1994).

Hysteroscopy allows the physician to further evaluate any areas of suspicion within the uterine cavity revealed by HSG. It is often done in conjunction with a laparoscopy but can be done independently in the office and does not require general anesthesia. A fiberoptic instrument is placed into the uterus for further evaluation of polyps, myomata, or structural variations (Speroff et al 1994).

Laparoscopy enables direct visualization of the pelvic organs and is usually done 6 to 8 months after HSG unless symptoms suggest the need for earlier evaluation. The woman usually is given a general anesthetic for this procedure. Entry is generally made through an incision in the umbilical area, although it is occasionally done suprapubically. The peritoneal cavity is distended with carbon dioxide gas, and the pelvic organs can be directly visualized with a fiberoptic instrument. Tube patency can be assessed by instilling dye into the uterine cavity through the cervix. The pelvis is evaluated for endometriosis, adhesions, organ fixations, pelvic inflammatory disease, tumors, and cysts. The intraperitoneal gas is usually manually expressed at the end of the procedure. Routine preanesthesia instructions should be given. The woman is told she may have some discomfort from organ displacement and shoulder to chest pain caused by gas in the abdomen lasting 24 to 48 hours after the procedure. She should be informed that she can resume normal activities after resting for about 2 days. Using postoperative pain medication and assuming a "knee-chest" position may help relieve discomfort.

Methods of Infertility Management

Pharmacologic Methods

If an ovulatory defect has been identified during fertility testing, the treatment depends on the specific cause of the problem. In the presence of normal ovaries, a normal prolactin level, and an intact pituitary gland, *clomiphene citrate* (Clomid, Serophene) is often used. See Drug Guide: Clomiphene Citrate. Clomiphene citrate acts by competing with estrogen receptor sites at the level of the hypothalamus, the pituitary, and the ovary, thus causing an increased secretion of FSH and LH, which stimulates follicular growth. Ovulation will occur in approximately 80% of properly selected patients, and conception rates approach 40%. The risk for multiple gestation with clomiphene is 5% and is almost exclusively twins (Speroff et al 1994).

The woman is instructed to take clomiphene beginning with 50 mg from cycle day 5 to 9. Ovulation can generally be expected to occur 5 to 10 days following the last dose. The presence of ovulation and evaluation of the response to therapy is assessed by BBT or urinary LH kit monitoring for in-home use, ultrasound evaluation, and possible luteal phase progesterone assays in conjunction

---

DRUG GUIDE

CLOMIPHENE CITRATE (CLOMID, SEROPHENE)

Overview of Action

Clomid stimulates follicular growth by increasing secretion of FSH and LH. Ovulation is expected to occur 5 to 10 days after last dose. Used when anovulation is caused by hypothalamic dysfunction, luteal phase dysfunction, or oligo-ovulation, and for in vitro fertilization.

Route, Dosage, Frequency

Administered orally. Fifty mg/day to 250 mg/day from day 5 to day 9 (total of 5 days) of the menstrual cycle. Usually start with 50 mg/day and increase dose 50 mg if no response, to a maximum of 250 mg (Mishell 1991). May need to give estrogen simultaneously if decrease in cervical mucus occurs.

Contraindications

Presence of ovarian enlargement, ovarian cysts, hyperstimulation syndrome, liver disease, visual problems, pregnancy.

Side Effects

Antiestrogenic effects may cause decrease in cervical mucus production and endometrial lining development. Other side effects include vasomotor flushes; abdominal distention and ovarian enlargement secondary to follicular growth and development and multiple corpus luteum formation; bloating, pain, soreness, breast discomfort; nausea and vomiting; visual symptoms (spots, flashes); headaches; dryness or loss of hair; multiple pregnancies.

Nursing Considerations

Determine if couple has been advised to have sexual intercourse every other day for 1 week beginning 5 days after the last day of medications.
Instruct couple on use of BBT chart to assess whether ovulation has occurred, or instruct on the use of urinary LH kits to predict the onset of LH surge. Also inform couple that plasma progesterone, cervical mucus, and postcoital test may be done. Remind couples that if the woman doesn't have a period, she must be checked for the possibility of pregnancy before another trial of Clomid is started.

with an endometrial biopsy. If ovulation is not achieved in the first cycle of therapy, the dosage may be increased in 50 mg increments to a maximum of 200 to 250 mg daily for 5 days. Additional use of human chorionic gonadotropin (hCG) may be used to induce ovulation in cases where the maximum dose is adequate for follicular development but not to stimulate ovulation or when a luteal phase defect is apparent. The hCG mimics the midcycle endogenous LH surge, induces final oocyte maturation, and stimulates progesterone production by the corpus luteum.

After the first treatment cycle a pelvic exam should be done to rule out ovarian enlargement or hyperstimulation. Ovarian enlargement and abdominal discomfort may result from follicular growth and the formation of multiple corpus lutea. Persistence of ovarian cysts is a contraindication for further clomiphene administration. Other side effects include hot flashes, abdominal distension, bloating, breast discomfort, nausea and vomiting, vision problems, headache, and dryness or loss of hair. Some women experience severe mood swings (Bambi-Hitler syndrome) (Blenner 1991).

Due to the antiestrogen effects of clomiphene citrate, high toxic levels of LH may exist during drug administration. It is important to instruct patients not to begin urinary LH kit home testing until at least 2 days after the last dose of clomiphene to avoid false positive results. Other antiestrogenic effects of Clomid include inhibition of mucus production and decreased development of endometrial lining. The occurrence of these effects can be determined by assessing preovulatory mucus in a postcoital test and measuring the endometrial lining by ultrasound. Supplemental low-dose estrogen may be given to ensure appropriate quality and quantity of cervical mucus.

Home-Care Measures

Women can assess the presence of ovulation and possible response to clomiphene therapy by doing BBT and urinary LH tests. The woman should be knowledgeable about side effects and call her health care provider if they occur. When visual disturbances (flashes, blurring, spots) occur, the woman should avoid brightly lit rooms. This side effect disappears within a few days or weeks after discontinuation of therapy (Speroff et al 1994). The occurrence of hot flashes may be due to the antiestrogenic properties of Clomid. Some relief can be obtained through increased intake of fluids and use of fans. Table 7–5 lists some of the drugs commonly used to treat infertility.

Human menopausal gonadotropin (hMG) therapy, also referred to as menotropins (Pergonal) and urofollitropin (Metrodin), is indicated as a first line of therapy for the anovulatory infertile woman with low to normal levels of gonadotropins (FSH and LH) and as a second line of

therapy in women who fail to ovulate or conceive with clomiphene citrate therapy. Menotropins is a mixture of FSH and LH in a 1:1 ratio, and urofollitropin is further purified and contains only FSH. Both are natural hormones extracted from the urine of postmenopausal women, purified, and freeze-dried into a powder. Immediately before intramuscular injection the powder is reconstituted with diluent.

Normal functioning of the pituitary is not necessary with menotropins or urofollitropin because their mechanisms of action are direct stimulation of follicular development in the ovary, thus totally bypassing the hypothalamic/pituitary axis. However, normal ovarian reserve and functioning are necessary to ensure that follicles can be stimulated by FSH and LH.

Menotropins is the primary preparation used for therapy. Urofollitropin is indicated for women who have excessive androgen production such as with polycystic ovary disease (PCO). Clients with PCO have high endogenous LH levels, and urofollitropin, which is predominantly FSH, is used to equalize the hormonal ratio and induce ovulation.

Menotropins and urofollitropin both require close observation with serum estradiol and ultrasound. Monitoring of follicle development is necessary to minimize the risk of multiple pregnancy and to avoid ovarian hyperstimulation syndrome. The daily dose of medication given is titrated based on serum estradiol and ultrasound findings. When follicle maturation has occurred, hCG may be administered by intramuscular injection to stimulate ovulation. The couple is advised to have intercourse on the day the hCG is administered and for the next 2 days. The multiple birth rate is reported to be about 20% with less than 1% resulting in multiples greater than triplets. Women who elect to have hMG medication usually have passed through all other forms of management without conceiving. Strong emotional support and thorough education are needed because of the numerous office visits and injections. Often the male partner is instructed, with return demonstration, to administer the daily injections.

When hyperprolactinemia accompanies anovulation, the infertility may be treated with *bromocriptine*. This medication acts directly on the prolactin-secreting cells in the anterior pituitary. It inhibits the pituitary's secretion of prolactin—thus preventing suppression of the pulsatile secretion of FSH and LH. This restores normal menstrual cycles—and induces ovulation by allowing FSH and LH production. High prolactin levels may impair production of FSH and LH and/or block their action on the ovaries. If treatment is successful, the tests of ovulatory function will indicate that ovulation is occurring with a normal luteal phase. Bromocriptine should be discontinued if pregnancy is suspected or at the anticipated time of ovulation because of its possible teratogenic ef-

| TABLE 7-5 | Drugs Commonly Used To Treat Infertility |

	Indications	
Drugs	**Women**	**Men**
Clomiphene citrate (Clomid, Serophene)	Polycystic ovarian disease (3 days, beginning day 5 of bleeding) Hyperandrogenemia (with no neoplasia) Premature follicular rupture	Low levels of gonadotropins Hypothalamic hypogonadism
Bromocriptine mesylate (Parlodel)	Hyperprolactinemia (functional or pituitary adenoma)	Hyperprolactinemia (functional or pituitary adenoma)
Progesterone	Luteal phase dysfunction	
hMG, menotropins (FSH and LH) (Pergonal) with hCG	Hypothalamic ovulatory dysfunction (after failure of clomiphene) Hypopituitarism Polycystic ovarian disease (rarely) Luteinized unruptured follicle syndrome (after failure of hCG alone) Inadequate cervical mucus In vitro fertilization, GIFT, ZIFT Controlled superovulation	Hypothalamic-pituitary failure due to Kallmann's syndrome or delayed puberty Hypogonadotropic hypogonadism (deficiency of FSH and LH)
hCG	Luteinized unruptured follicle syndrome Induction of ovulation	
FSH, urofollitropin (Metrodin) with hCG	Polycystic ovarian disease In vitro fertilization, GIFT, ZIFT	
GnRH (Factrel)	Hypothalamic ovulatory dysfunction (pulsed infusion)	Hypothalamic-pituitary failure due to Kallmann's syndrome or delayed puberty (pulsed infusion)
GnRH agonist Leuoprolide acetate (Lupron) Nafarelin acetate (Synarel)	Endometriosis Premature follicular rupture In vitro fertilization, GIFT, ZIFT	Hypogonadotropic gonadism

SOURCE: Adapted from Shane J: Evaluation and treatment of infertility. *Clin Symp* 1993; 45:2.

fects. Other side effects include nausea, diarrhea, dizziness, headache, and fatigue.

When endometriosis is determined to be the cause of the infertility, *danazol* (Danocrine) may be given to suppress ovulation and menstruation and to effect atrophy of the ectopic endometrial tissue. Other pharmologic treatments involve use of oral contraceptives or oral medroxyprogesterone acetate, and GnRH agonists (Haney 1994). For in-depth discussion of the management and care needed for endometriosis see Chapter 10.

Gonadotropin-releasing hormone (GnRH) is a therapeutic tool for ovulation stimulation. It is used for women who have insufficient endogenous release of GnRH. Administration is usually by continuous intravenous infusion accomplished by a portable infusion pump with a pulsatile mechanism worn on a belt around the waist. The length of treatment varies from 2 to 4 weeks, and hCG is also given to stimulate ovulation. The risk of multiple gestation and hyperstimulation is less than with hMG therapy, and the treatment is also less expensive (Speroff et al 1994). Significant client education and support are necessary for effective use of the pump. Some women find the pump cumbersome.

Treatment of luteal phase defects may include the use of progesterone to augment luteal phase progesterone levels or the use of ovulation induction agents such as clomiphene citrate or menotropins, which will augment proliferative phase FSH production of the developing follicle. Women with luteal phase defects have been found to have decreased FSH production in the proliferative phase. This is associated with a decline in luteal phase progesterone and estrogen production and is manifested by an out-of-phase endometrial biopsy. It is also common to use progesterone supplementation in conjunction with these ovulation induction agents if the drug alone does not correct the luteal phase. Occasionally, hCG therapy may be used in the luteal phase to stimulate corpus luteum production of progesterone.

Artificial Insemination

Artificial insemination with either the husband's semen (AIH) or the semen of a donor (AID) involves depositing sperm at the cervical os or in the uterus by mechanical means. Some people use the term therapeutic donor insemination (TDI) in place of AID (Speroff et al 1994).

AIH is generally indicated for such seminal deficiencies as oligospermia (low sperm count), asthenospermia (decreased motility), and teratospermia (low percentage, abnormal morphology), or anatomic defects that are accompanied by inadequate deposition of sperm, such as hypospadias (a congenital abnormal male urethral opening on the underside of the penis), and ejaculatory dysfunction such as retrograde ejaculation (Corson 1990). It is also indicated in unexplained infertility and some cases of female factor infertility, specifically with cervical factors such as scant or inhospitable mucus, persistent cervicitis, or cervical stenosis. In this case the insemination would be intrauterine (IUI) so as to bypass the cervical factor. Sperm preparation for IUI involves washing sperm from the seminal plasma.

IUI is an option for many couples with or without ovulation induction therapy before more aggressive treatments such in vitro fertilization (IVF) and gamete intrafallopian transfer (GIFT) are employed. Success rates vary from 10% to 25%, depending on indication for use and the woman's age.

Donor insemination is considered in cases of azoospermia (absence of sperm), severe oligo- or asthenospermia, inherited male sex-linked disorders, and autosomal dominant disorders (Speroff et al 1994). In the past several years indications for donor insemination have expanded to include single women or lesbians desirous of pregnancy (Daglish 1991). Some states have specified the parental rights of the single woman and the donor, but most are silent on this issue (Speroff et al 1994).

Donor insemination has become more complicated and expensive in the last decade because of the need for strict screening and processing procedures to prevent transmission of a genetic defect or sexually transmitted disease to the offspring or recipient. Guidelines established by the American Fertility Society (1990) include mandatory medical and infectious disease screening of both donor and recipient, the need for informed consent from all parties, the need to limit the number of pregnancies per donor, and the need to establish an accurate means of record keeping. Finally, because of the risk of infectious disease transmission, donated sperm must be frozen and quarantined for 6 months from the time of acquisition and the donor retested at this time before sperm can be released for use. Before AIDS was discovered, fresh semen was used.

Pregnancy rates with donor insemination are somewhat decreased per cycle with the use of frozen sperm because of the loss of motility in 15%–20% of the sperm caused by the freezing process. The usual number of cycles required to initiate pregnancy in a couple with a male factor only is approximately six. Couples who fail to conceive after six to eight cycles of well-timed inseminations require further evaluation and/or aggressive therapy such as the ARTs.

Numerous factors must be evaluated before AID is performed. Has every possible effort been made to diagnose and treat the cause of the male infertility? Do tests indicate normal ovulation and sperm/ovum transport in the woman? Has the couple had an opportunity to discuss this option with an infertility counselor to explore the issues of secrecy, disclosure, and potential feelings of loss the couple (particularly the male partner) may feel surrounding not having a genetic child (Townsend 1992). After making the decision, the couple should allow themselves time to further assess their concerns and explore their feelings individually and together to ensure that this option is acceptable to both. Couples need to consider how they will feel if the child is born with a congenital anomaly. Irrespective of natural intercourse or therapeutic insemination, congenital anomalies occur in 4–5% of all pregnancies (Amuzu et al 1990).

In Vitro Fertilization

Of all couples seeking infertility therapy, 85–90% are treated with conventional medical and surgical therapy. Of couples that are unable to conceive, 10–15% may resort to various methods of assisted reproduction such as **in vitro fertilization (IVF)** and gamete intrafallopian transfer (GIFT) (Office of Technology Assessment 1988).

In IVF a woman's eggs are collected from her ovaries, fertilized in the laboratory, and placed into her uterus after normal embryo development has begun. If the procedure is successful, the embryo continues to develop in the uterus, and pregnancy proceeds naturally.

The birth of the first child conceived through IVF occurred in Great Britain in 1978. IVF has now gone from an experimental procedure to an accepted treatment modality for infertile couples. Initially, the indication for IVF was absence, blockage, or irreparable damage of the fallopian tubes. Indications have expanded to include other conditions, such as male infertility, endometriosis, unexplained infertility, male and female immunologic infertility, and cervical factors.

The potential for a successful pregnancy with IVF is maximized when three to four embryos are replaced. For this reason ovulation is induced using fertility drugs. Follicular development and oocyte maturity are monitored frequently with ultrasound and hormonal assays. Monitoring usually begins around cycle day 7, and medications are titrated according to individual response. When the follicles appear mature, hCG is given to stimulate final egg maturation and control the induction of ovulation. Egg retrieval is performed approximately 35 hours later.

In the majority of cases egg retrieval is performed by a transvaginal approach under ultrasound guidance. It is an outpatient procedure performed with intravenous sedation and a cervical block for anesthesia. A needle guide that helps direct the aspirating needle through the posterior vaginal wall into the follicle is attached to the vaginal ultrasound probe. Many follicles can be aspirated with only one puncture, and the procedure generally lasts no more than 30 minutes. The client usually tolerates the procedure well and is discharged to home within 2 hours with instructions for limited activity for 24 hours.

Once identified, the oocytes are evaluated for maturity and incubated for a period of time prior to insemination. The gametes are incubated in a specially prepared culture medium supplemented with serum to provide nutrients. Fertilization should occur within 18 to 24 hours. Once it is documented, the fertilized eggs are transferred to growth medium and incubated for another 24 hours, at which time embryo development is assessed.

Embryo replacement is procedurally much like an IUI. Post–embryo replacement instructions include bed rest with minimal activity for 24 to 48 hours.

Success with IVF depends on many factors, the two most important being the woman's age and the indication. Women with three to six cycles of IVF have a good chance of achieving pregnancy. Many couples find the emotional, physical, and financial costs of going beyond three to six cycles too difficult (Speroff et al 1994). Clinical delivery rates reported by the Society of Assisted Reproductive Technology (SART) in 1992 were 19% per embryo replacement for women under the age of 40 when no male factor was present (SART 1993).

Other Assisted Reproductive Techniques

GIFT and ZIFT **Gamete intrafallopian transfer (GIFT),** developed in 1984, involves the retrieval of oocytes by laparoscopy; immediate placement of the oocytes in a catheter with washed, motile sperm; and placement of the gametes into the fimbriated end of the fallopian tube. Fertilization occurs in the fallopian tube as with normal conception (in vivo), rather than in the laboratory (in vitro), and is acceptable to the Catholic church (Mastroyannis 1993). The fertilized egg then travels through the fallopian tube to the uterus for implantation as in normal reproduction.

GIFT has proven to be a very effective therapy for couples whose infertility results from various seminal deficiencies, unexplained infertility, cervical factors, immunologic factors, and endometriosis when less aggressive means of therapy have failed. In cases of male factor infertility, GIFT offers an opportunity for the egg and an adequate concentration of sperm to meet in the fallopian tube, whereas with coitus sperm with low count or motility may never reach the tube.

The major prerequisite for GIFT is the presence of at least one normal fallopian tube. It is not an appropriate therapy for any woman with a history of PID, tubal disease, or ectopic gestation, due to the increased chance of sustaining an ectopic tubal pregnancy because the passage of the fertilized ova to the uterus is slowed.

From the GIFT technology evolved procedures such as **zygote intrafallopian transfer (ZIFT)** and tubal embryo transfer (TET). These procedures involve oocyte retrieval under ultrasound guidance, followed by in vitro fertilization and laparoscopic replacement of the fertilized eggs into the fimbriated end of the fallopian tube. In ZIFT, replacement of fertilized oocytes occurs at the zygote (just fertilized) stage. In TET this is done at the embryo stage. These procedures allow fertilization to be documented, which is not possible with GIFT, and the pregnancy rate is theoretically increased when the conceptus is placed in the fallopian tube so that normal fertilization and implantation are better mimicked than when replacement is in the uterus, as with IVF.

GIFT and ZIFT success rates reported by the SART registry in 1992 were 26.5% and 28.8% per procedure, respectively. Both gamete and embryo donation raise many questions for the couple as well as the possible child, such as what is the effect of secrecy, genetic discontinuance, and genealogic bewilderment on the child's development and on family dynamics (Goode & Hahn 1993; Townsend 1992).

Embryo Cryopreservation Research has shown that the replacement of three to four embryos in a treatment cycle offers the best chances for pregnancy. Replacing more than four increases only the chance for a multiple pregnancy (Schenker & Ezra 1994). To minimize this risk, excess embryos may be stored using freezing or cryopreservation. Should a pregnancy not ensue, frozen embryos can be thawed. After they are maintained in culture for a short time to confirm resumption of growth, they are replaced in the woman's uterus at the appropriate time in her menstrual cycle. Thus freezing affords the couple another attempt at pregnancy without having to undergo stimulation and egg retrieval.

Ethical issues to consider in this situation include: Who has legal custody of the embryos? How many is too many? When is selective reduction appropriate (Townsend 1992)? Perinatal nurses need to be involved in establishing standards and guidelines for assisted reproduction technologies (Jones 1994). Clinically, the perinatal nurse is instrumental in providing support, education, and counseling to couples considering assisted reproductive methods. The nurse assesses the couple for personal, marital, and parenting difficulties and initiates interventions that help establish family roles and bonds. Follow-up care mechanisms can be set, thereby aiding in individual growth, marital stability, and family development.

In Vitro Fertilization Utilizing Donor Oocytes The use of donor eggs, a natural extension of IVF, is reserved for women who do not produce viable eggs but have a functional uterus due to premature ovarian failure, surgical removal of the ovaries, advanced maternal age, or inherent oocyte defects. Women with normal ovarian function may also benefit from egg donation if they have an autosomal dominant or sex-linked genetic disorder such as hemophilia or Duchenne's muscular dystrophy.

Oocyte donors may be either known or anonymous. In either case both donors and recipients undergo exten-

ETHICAL CONSIDERATIONS AND THE ASSISTED REPRODUCTIVE TECHNOLOGIES

In vitro fertilization has been a welcome solution for many couples who have been unable to conceive. Recently, advances in the application of IVF technology have spurred the emergence of even more new avenues of achieving pregnancy and parenting. With hormonal replacement therapy and donor eggs or embryos women past menopause can achieve pregnancy. Other options include cryopreservation, fertilization of donor gametes (donor eggs, sperm, or both), IVF with the use of a gestational carrier, embryo adoption, and the use of surrogacy. All these options may be complicated by the introduction of a third party into the reproductive process, and for many this introduces a multitude of moral, legal, and ethical concerns. Some of the issues raised by these techniques include the following:

1. Is it a constitutional right for individuals or couples to be able to utilize donor gametes or to contract with a woman to carry their embryo in order to treat their infertility?

2. With a multiple pregnancy rate approaching 20% in couples undergoing IVF procedures, the potential (<3%) of having a grand multiple gestation (more than four fetuses) forces some couples to consider embryo reduction in order to avoid an adverse obstetrical and/or fetal outcome.

3. If excess embryos are frozen and kept, how long can and should they be stored? What should be done in cases of death of one or both of the partners, divorce, or when couples choose not to claim their embryos?

4. Do providers have the right to decide who can participate in using donor gametes, embryos, gestational carriers, and surrogates? What about single women, lesbian couples, or crossing generational lines (daughter being a donor for mother)?

5. Do the assisted reproductive technologies consider the best interests of the parties involved, including those of the resulting offspring? For example, what are the effects on a child of knowing or not knowing the identity of the donor in AID?

6. How can the potential for consanguinity (having an ancestor in common) be controlled in the case of gamete and/or embryo donation?

7. Does the existence of new technologies make it more difficult to accept childlessness by increasing pressure on women to follow every avenue in an attempt to conceive?

8. To what extent should health insurance policies cover these modes of treating infertility at a time of growing health care costs?

sive psychologic evaluation and counseling to ensure that all potential issues have been explored and discussed and that all parties involved are comfortable with the process (Lessor et al 1993). The nurse functions as a case manager by coordinating the many tests, procedures, and educational and counseling sessions that are involved for the donor and recipient couple.

Once donor eggs are available, they are inseminated with the sperm of the recipient's partner. After fertilization has occurred and embryo development has begun, the embryos are replaced in the recipient's uterus. Pregnancies can be achieved and maintained in these women with an estrogen/progesterone replacement protocol. When pregnancy occurs, hormonal support is continued until the placenta is capable of supporting the pregnancy—usually at 10 to 12 weeks. Some suggest loss of corpus luteum before 16 weeks may result in spontaneous abortion because the placenta may not really be fully functional.

Micromanipulation and Blastomere Analysis Micromanipulation allows individual eggs and sperm to be handled through the use of very fine, specialized instruments. Efforts are directed toward achieving fertilization in cases of severely compromised seminal problems that have not been successfully overcome with standard IVF procedures. Micromanipulation procedures involve introducing the sperm directly into the egg or carefully making very fine "slices" or perforations in the zona pellucida that facilitate sperm entry.

Recent advances in micromanipulation allow a single cell to be removed from the embryo for genetic study. Couples at risk for having a detectable single gene or chromosomal anomaly may wish to undergo such preimplantation genetic testing (blastomere analysis) (Pickler & Munro 1994). The single cell is obtained from a 6- to 8-cell embryo (blastomere biopsy) (Speroff et al 1994). The genetic content of the cell is examined using the polymerase chain reaction (PCR) technique. The cell's DNA is amplified 1,000,000 times and examined so that embryos affected with genetic disease are not replaced in the mother. Results of genetic testing on the preimplantation embryos are available in 4 to 24 hours, so unaffected embryos may still be replaced during the required biologic window of time without the need for cryopreservation (Cohen et al 1992).

The diagnosis of genetic disorders before implantation provides couples with the option of forgoing the attempt to establish a pregnancy and thereby avoiding a difficult decision about terminating an affected pregnancy. This technology also raises several issues, including the following:

• Identification of couples at risk. There is a need for criteria that identify couples at risk for diseases that constitute significant hardship and suffering so that "wrongful birth" cases can be avoided.

- Availability of and access to centers providing blastomere analysis. Should society provide access for those at risk for genetic transfer of disease but without the financial resources to pay for the services?

- The use of blastomere analysis for sex gene testing. In X-linked diseases the only way to prevent the disorder is to select against the Y chromosome.

* Identification of late onset diseases. The Human Genome Project has aided in the identification of genetic markers for late onset disease (Guyer & Collins 1993). Couples may wish to choose, for implantation, blastomeres that do not carry these markers.

In Vitro Fertilization Using a Gestational Carrier

The option of IVF utilizing a gestational carrier is appropriate for the infertile woman who is genetically sound but unable to carry a pregnancy due to (1) congenital absence or surgical removal of her uterus; (2) a reproductively impaired uterus, myomas, uterine synechiae (adhesion of uterus), or any other congenital abnormalities; or (3) a medical condition that might be life threatening during pregnancy, such as diabetes, immunological problems, or a severe heart, kidney, or liver disease (English 1991).

Use of the gestational carrier option allows a couple with any of these conditions to exercise the option of having their own biologic pregnancy. The couple undergoes the IVF procedure, and the resulting embryos are placed in a woman who has contracted with the infertile woman or couple to carry the child. This must be distinguished from surrogate motherhood, wherein the gestational surrogate mother makes a genetic contribution to the child (Snowdon 1994). In the carrier relationship the carrier has no genetic investment in the child. All participants are required to have medical and psychologic screening as well as legal counsel prior to acceptance into the program.

Critical Thinking Question

What makes a mother? Does motherhood require genetic, gestational, and social contributions to the child?

Adoption

The adoption of an infant can be a difficult and/or frustrating experience for all persons involved (Arms 1990). It is not uncommon for a couple to have to wait for several years before beginning the adoption process. The number of available infants has decreased because many infants are reared by their single mothers instead of being relinquished for adoption, as was customary in the past. In addition many unwanted pregnancies are being terminated by elective abortion. Some couples seek international adoptions or consider adopting older children, children with handicaps, or children of mixed parentage because the adoption process in such cases is quicker and more children are available. The nurse can assist couples considering adoption by providing information on community resources for adoption as well as by providing support through the adoption process. Couples also need support if they choose to remain childless (Menning 1988).

The Nurse's Role

Approximately 8% of the childbearing population in the United States (1 out of 12 couples) is unable to conceive or unable to carry a pregnancy to term. Infertility therapy taxes the financial, physical, and emotional resources of the couple. Treatment can cost over $20,000 a year, and insurance coverage may be limited. Years of effort and numerous evaluations and examinations may take place before a conception occurs, if one occurs at all. In a society that values children and considers them to be the natural result of marriage, infertile couples may face a myriad of tensions and discrimination.

The nurse needs to be constantly aware of the emotional needs of the couple confronting infertility evaluation and treatment. Often an intact marriage will become stressed with the intrusive but necessary infertility procedures and treatments. Constant attention to temperature charts and instructions about their sex life from a person outside the relationship naturally affect the spontaneity of a couple's interactions. Tests and treatments may heighten feelings of frustration or anger between the couple. The need to share this intimate area of a relationship, especially when one or the other is identified as "the cause" of infertility, may precipitate feelings of guilt or shame.

The nurse's role can be summarized as that of counselor, educator, and advocate. Tasks of the infertile couple and appropriate nursing interventions are summarized in Table 7–6. Throughout the evaluation process nurses can play a key role in lessening the stress these couples must endure by providing them with appropriate resources and

---

| TABLE 7-6 | Tasks of the Infertile Couple |

Tasks	Nursing Interventions
Recognize how infertility affects their lives and express feelings (may be negative toward self or mate)	Supportive: help to understand and facilitate free expression of feelings
Grieve the loss of potential offspring	Help to recognize feelings
Evaluate reasons for wanting a child	Help to understand motives
Decide about management	Identify alternatives; facilitate partner communication

SOURCE: Sawatzky M: Tasks of the infertile couple. *JOGNN* 1981; 10:132.

TABLE 7-7 Infertility Questionnaire

Self-Image

1. I feel bad about my body because of our inability to have a child.
2. Since our infertility, I feel I can do anything as well as I used to.
3. I feel as attractive as before our infertility.
4. I feel less masculine/feminine because of our inability to have a child.
5. Compared with others, I feel I am a worthwhile person.
6. Lately, I feel I am sexually attractive to my wife/husband.
7. I feel I will be incomplete as a man/woman if we cannot have a child.
8. Having an infertility problem makes me feel physically incompetent.

Guilt/Blame

1. I feel guilty about somehow causing our infertility.
2. I wonder if our infertility problem is due to something I did in the past.
3. My spouse makes me feel guilty about our problem.
4. There are times when I blame my spouse for our infertility.
5. I feel I am being punished because of our infertility.

Sexuality

1. Lately I feel I am able to respond to my spouse sexually.
2. I feel sex is a duty, not a pleasure.
3. Since our infertility problem, I enjoy sexual relations with my spouse.
4. We have sexual relations for the purpose of trying to conceive.
5. Sometimes I feel like a "sex machine," programmed to have sex during the fertile period.
6. Impaired fertility has helped our sexual relationship.
7. Our inability to have a child has increased my desire for sexual relations.
8. Our inability to have a child has decreased my desire for sexual relations.

Note: The questionnaire is scored on a Likert scale with responses ranging from "strongly agree" to "strongly disagree." Each question is scored separately, and the mean score is determined for each section (Self-Image, Guilt/Blame, Sexuality). The total mean score is then divided by 3. A final mean score of greater than 3 indicates distress.

SOURCE: Bernstein J: Assessment of psychological dysfunction associated with infertility. *JOGNN* 1985; 14(Suppl):63.

accurate information about what is entailed in treatment and what physical, emotional, and financial demands they can anticipate throughout the process. The nurse's ability to assess and respond to emotional and educational needs is essential to give infertile couples control. An assessment tool such as the infertility questionnaire (Table 7–7) may be helpful. Extensive and repeated explanations and written instruction may be necessary because the couple's anxiety often overwhelms their ability to retain all the information given.

Infertility may be perceived as a loss by one or both partners. The losses experienced have been described as loss of relationship with spouse, family, or friends; health; status or prestige; self-esteem; self-confidence; security; and fertility and potential child. Only one of these losses may precipitate a depression in adult life, and in many cases the crisis of infertility touches on them all (Mahlstedt 1985). Each couple passes through several stages of feelings, not unlike those identified by Kubler-Ross: sur-

prise, denial, anger, isolation, guilt, grief, and resolution (Menning 1988). The impact of these feelings on the couple and how fast they move into resolution, if ever, may depend on the cause and duration of treatment. Each partner may progress through the stages at different rates (Sandelowski 1994). Nonjudgmental acceptance and a professional, caring attitude on the nurse's part can go far to dissipate the negative emotions the couple may experience while going through this process.

This is also a time when the nurse may assess the quality of the couple's relationship: Are they able and willing to communicate verbally and share feelings? Are they mutually supportive? The answers to these questions may help the nurse identify areas of strength and weakness and construct an appropriate plan of care. Availability of mental health professionals for referral is helpful when the emotional issues become too disruptive in the couple's relationship or life. Couples should be made aware of infertility support and education organizations such as RESOLVE, which may help meet some of these needs and validate their feelings. Finally, individual or group counseling with other infertile couples may help the couple resolve feelings brought about by their own difficult situation.

Pregnancy After Infertility

The feeling of being infertile does not necessarily disappear with pregnancy. Although there may be initial ecstasy, the couple may also face a whole new arena of fear and anxieties, and the parents-to-be often do not know where they "fit in." They may feel a great sense of loss and isolation because those who have had no trouble conceiving cannot relate to the physical and emotional pain they endured to achieve the pregnancy. Contact with their past "infertile" support system may vanish when peers learn the couple has resolved their infertility (Braverman & English 1992).

Although the desperation to become pregnant may have superseded the couple's ability to acknowledge their concerns about undergoing various treatments or procedures, questions about the repeated cycle of fertility drugs or the achievement of pregnancy through IVF technology or cryopreservation may now arise. The expectant couple may be very concerned about the potential of these treatments for adverse effects on the fetus. Couples may need much reassurance throughout the pregnancy to allay these anxieties.

The nurse can assist couples who experience pregnancy after infertility by acknowledging their past experience of infertility treatment; validating their fears and anxieties as they face childbirth classes, birth, and parenting issues; and providing education and support regarding what to anticipate physically and emotionally throughout the pregnancy. These interventions will go a long way toward normalizing the experience for them.

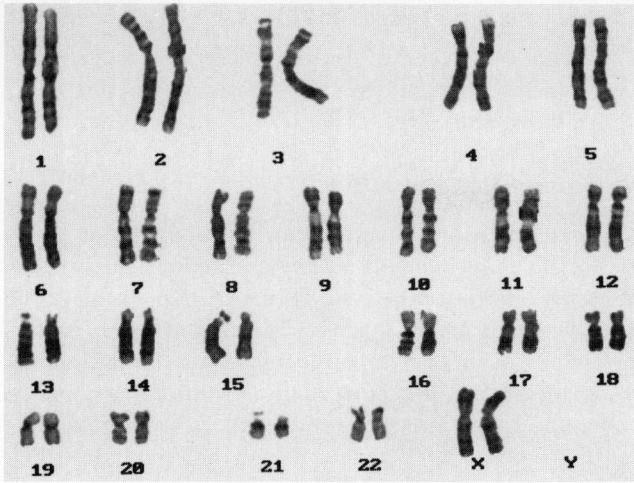

FIGURE 7-6 Normal female karotype. SOURCE: Courtesy David Peakman, Reproductive Genetics Center, Denver, CO.

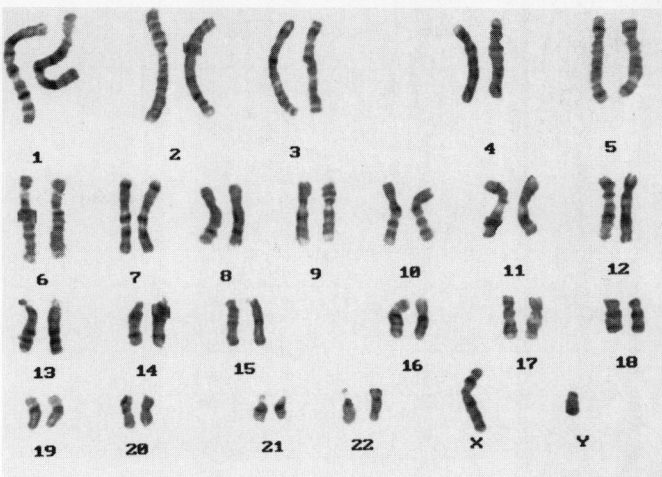

FIGURE 7-7 Normal male karotype. SOURCE: Courtesy David Peakman, Reproductive Genetics Center, Denver, CO.

GENETIC DISORDERS

Even when conception has been achieved, families can have special reproductive concerns. The desired and expected outcome of any pregnancy is the birth of a healthy, "perfect" baby. Parents experience grief, fear, and anger when they discover that their baby has been born with a defect or a genetic disease. Such an abnormality may be evident at birth or may not appear for some time. The baby may have inherited a disease from one parent, creating guilt and strife within the family.

Regardless of the type or scope of the problem, parents will have many questions: "What did I do?" "What caused it?" "Will it happen again?" The nurse must anticipate the parents' questions and concerns and guide, direct, and support the family (Olsen 1994). To do so, the nurse must have a basic knowledge of genetics and genetic counseling. Many congenital anomalies and diseases are genetic or have a strong genetic component. Others are not genetic at all. The genetic counselor attempts to categorize the problem and answer the family's questions. Professional nurses can help expedite this process if they understand the principles involved and are able to direct the family to the appropriate resources.

Chromosomes and Chromosomal Analysis

All hereditary material is carried on tightly coiled strands of DNA known as **chromosomes.** The chromosomes carry the genes, the smallest unit of inheritance, as discussed in greater detail in Chapter 6.

All *somatic* (body) cells contain 46 chromosomes, which is the *diploid number*; the sperm and egg contain half as many (23) chromosomes, or the *haploid number*

(see Chapter 6). There are 23 pairs of *homologous* chromosomes (a matched pair of chromosomes, one inherited from each parent). Twenty-two of the pairs are known as **autosomes** (nonsex chromosomes), and one pair is the **sex chromosomes,** X or Y. A normal female has a 46,XX chromosomes constitution, the normal male, 46,XY (Figures 7–6 and 7–7).

The **karyotype,** or pictorial analysis of an individual's chromosomes, is usually obtained from specially treated and stained peripheral blood lymphocytes. Once obtained, the cells are stimulated to undergo mitosis. The mitotic process is stopped during metaphase, the preparation is then stained, and the chromosomes become visible (Figure 7–8). Although the use of peripheral blood is

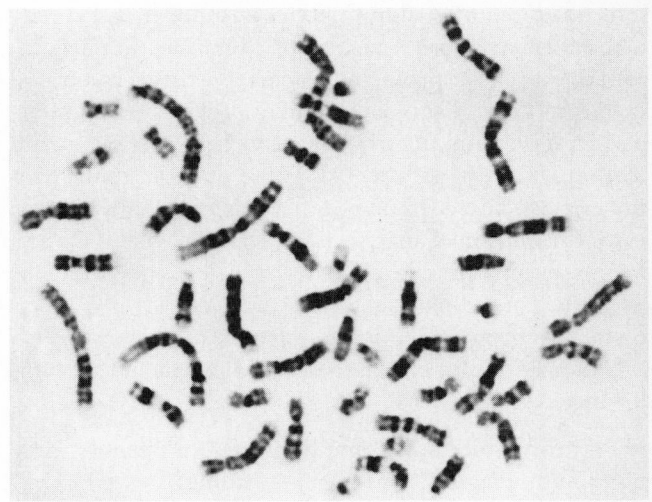

FIGURE 7-8 Chromosomes in metaphase spread. SOURCE: Courtesy Dr Arthur Robinson, National Jewish Hospital and Research Center, Denver, CO.

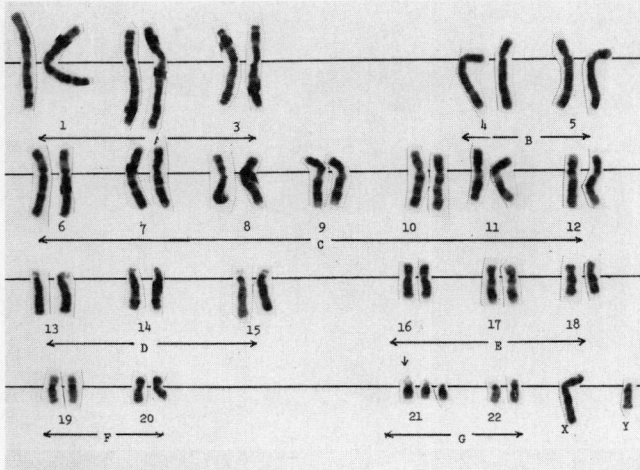

FIGURE 7-9   Karotype of a male who has trisomy 21, Down syndrome. Note the extra chromosome 21. SOURCE: Courtesy Dr Arthur Robinson, National Jewish Hospital and Research Center, Denver, CO.

- Multiple miscarriages
- Possible balanced translocation carrier (see discussion of abnormalities of chromosome structure in this chapter)

Autosomal Abnormalities

Abnormalities of Chromosome Number   Abnormalities of chromosome number are most commonly seen as trisomies, monosomies, and as mosaicism. In all three cases the abnormality is most often caused by *nondisjunction*, which occurs when paired chromosomes fail to separate during cell division. If nondisjunction occurs in either the sperm or the egg before fertilization, the resulting zygote (fertilized egg) will have an abnormal chromosome makeup in all of the cells (trisomy or monosomy). If nondisjunction occurs after fertilization, the developing zygote will have cells with two or more different chromosome makeups, evolving into two or more different cell lines (mosaicism).

Trisomies are the product of the union of a normal gamete (egg or sperm) with a gamete that contains an extra chromosome. The individual will have 47 chromosomes and be trisomic (have three copies of the same chromosome) for whichever chromosome is extra. Down syndrome (formerly called mongolism) is the most common trisomy abnormality seen in children (Figure 7–9). The presence of the extra chromosome 21 produces distinctive clinical features (see Table 7–8 and Figure 7–10). With the advent of modern surgical techniques and antibiotics children with Down syndrome are now living into their fifth or sixth decade of life.

Trisomies can occur among other autosomes; the two most common are trisomy 18 and trisomy 13 (Table 7–8 and Figures 7–11 and 7–12). The prognosis for children

an easy, convenient method of obtaining chromosomes, almost any tissue can be examined to get this information. In the case of a stillbirth or perinatal death in which there are multiple congenital abnormalities and there is a question of diagnosis or cause, karyotypes of cells in the child's internal organs (such as kidney, gonad, or thymus), rib, or skin can be examined if the tissues have not been fixed in formalin. In addition a piece (1 mm × 1 mm) of placenta taken from near the insertion of the cord and deep enough to include chorion may be sent for karyotyping. In the case of fetal death, obtaining placental tissue may yield results when fetal tissue does not.

Chromosome abnormalities can occur in either the autosomes or the sex chromosomes and can be divided into two categories: abnormalities of number and abnormalities of structure. Even small alterations in chromosomes can cause problems, especially those associated with slow growth and development or with mental retardation. The child does not need to have obvious major malformations to be affected. Some of these abnormalities can also be passed on to other offspring, thus in some cases chromosomal analysis is appropriate even if clinical manifestations are mild. Whatever the case, too much or too little genetic material usually produces adverse effects on normal growth and development.

Indications for chromosomal analysis include the following:

- Chromosome syndrome suspected (or clients with a clinical diagnosis of Down syndrome)
- Mental retardation and congenital malformations
- Abnormal sexual development (primary amenorrhea, lack of secondary sex characteristics
- Ambiguous genitalia

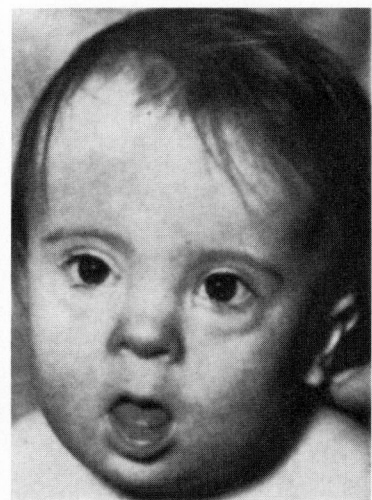

FIGURE 7-10   A child with Down syndrome. SOURCE: Jones KL: *Smith's Recognizable Patterns of Human Malformations,* 4th ed. Philadephia: WB Saunders, 1988.

with trisomy 13 or 18 is extremely poor. Most children (70%) die within the first 3 months of life due to complications related to respiratory and cardiac abnormalities. However, 10% survive the first year of life; therefore plans need to include the possibility of long-term care of a severely affected infant and family support.

Monosomies occur when a normal gamete unites with a gamete that is missing a chromosome. In this case the individual will have only 45 chromosomes and is said to be monosomic.

Mosaicism occurs after fertilization and results in an individual with two different cell lines, each with a

---

TABLE 7-8   Chromosomal Syndromes

Altered chromosome: 21 Genetic defect: trisomy 21 (Down syndrome) (secondary nondisjunction or 14/21 unbalanced translocation) Incidence: 1 in 700 live births **(Figure 7–10)**	**Characteristics:** CNS: mental retardation; hypotonia at birth Head: flattened occiput; depressed nasal bridge; mongoloid slant of eyes; epicanthal folds; white specking of the iris (Brushfield spots); protrusion of the tongue; high, arched palate; low-set ears Hands: broad, short fingers; abnormalities of finger and foot; dermal ridge patterns (dermatoglyphics); transverse palmar crease (simian line) Other: congenital heart disease
Altered chromosome: 18 Genetic defect: trisomy 18 Incidence: 1 in 3000 live births **(Figure 7–11)**	**Characteristics:** CNS: mental retardation; severe hypotonia Head: prominent occiput; low-set ears; corneal opacities; ptosis (drooping of eyelids) Hands: third and fourth fingers overlapped by second and fifth fingers; abnormal dermatoglyphics; syndactyly (webbing of fingers) Other: congenital heart defects; renal abnormalities; single umbilical artery; gastrointestinal tract abnormalities; rocker-bottom feet; cryptorchidism; various malformations of other organs
Altered chromosome: 18 Genetic defect: deletion of long arm of chromosome 18	**Characteristics:** CNS: severe psychomotor retardation Head: microcephaly; stenotic ear canals with conductive hearing loss Other: various other organ malformations
Altered chromosome: 13 Genetic defect: trisomy 13 Incidence: 1 in 5000 live births **(Figure 7–12)**	**Characteristics:** CNS: mental retardation; severe hypotonia; seizures Head: microcephaly; microphthalmia and/or coloboma (keyhole-shaped pupil); malformed ears; aplasia of external auditory canal; micrognathia (abnormally small lower jaw); cleft lip and palate Hands: polydactly (extra digits); abnormal posturing of fingers; abnormal dermatoglyphics Other: congenital heart defects; hemangiomas; gastrointestinal tract defects; various malformations of other organs
Altered chromosome: 5p Genetic defect: deletion of short arm of chromosome 5 (cri du chat, or cat cry, syndrome) Incidence: 1 in 20,000 live births **(Figure 7–14)**	**Characteristics:** CNS: severe mental retardation; a catlike cry in infancy Head: microcephaly; hypertelorism (widely spaced eyes); epicanthal folds; low-set ears Other: failure to thrive; various organ malformations
Altered chromosome: XO (sex chromosome) Genetic defect: only one X chromosome in female (Turner syndrome) Incidence: 1 in 300–7000 live female births **(Figure 7–15)**	**Characteristics:** CNS: no intellectual impairment; some perceptual difficulties Head: low hairline; webbed neck Trunk: short stature; cubitus valgus (increased carrying angle of arm); excessive nevi (congenital discoloration of skin due to pigmentation); broad shieldlike chest with widely spaced nipples; puffy feet; no toenails Other: fibrous streaks in ovaries; underdeveloped secondary sex characteristics; primary amenorrhea; usually infertile; renal anomalies; coarctation of the aorta
Altered chromosome: XXY (sex chromosome) Genetic defect: extra X chromosome in male (Klinefelter syndrome) Incidence: 1 in 1000 live male births, approximately 1–2% of institutionalized males	**Characteristics:** CNS: mild mental retardation Trunk: occasional gynecomastia (abnormally large male breasts); eunuchoid body proportions (lack of male muscular and sexual development) Other: small, soft testes; underdeveloped secondary sex characteristics; usually sterile

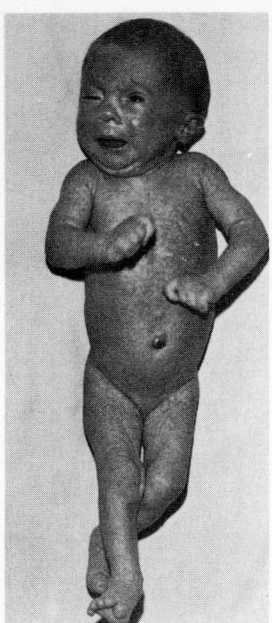

FIGURE 7-11 Infant with trisomy 18. SOURCE: Jones KL: *Smith's Recognizable Patterns of Human Malformations,* 4th ed. Philadelphia: Saunders, 1988.

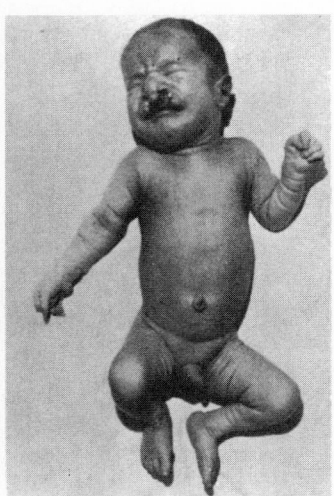

FIGURE 7-12 Infant with trisomy 13. SOURCE: Jones KL: *Smith's Recognizable Patterns of Human Malformations,* 4th ed. Philadelphia: Saunders, 1988

different chromosomal number. Mosaicism tends to be more common in the sex chromosomes, but when it does occur in the autosomes, it is most common in Down syndrome.

Clinical signs and symptoms may vary if mosaicism is present. In Down syndrome the clinical signs may be classic, minimal, or not apparent, depending on the number and location of the abnormal cells. An individual with many of the classic signs of Down syndrome but with normal intelligence should be investigated for the possibility of mosaicism. In such cases more than one tissue

may have to be examined to make the diagnosis. The peripheral blood may contain 46 chromosomes while the skin fibroblasts contain 47, +21.

Abnormalities of Chromosome Structure Abnormalities of chromosome structure involving only parts of the chromosome generally occur in two forms: translocation and deletions and/or additions. As the technology improves, more of these chromosomal structural abnormalities can be detected.

Not all children born with Down syndrome have trisomy 21. Instead, they may have an abnormal rearrangement of chromosomal material known as *translocation.* Clinically, the two types of Down syndrome are indistinguishable. What is of major importance to the family is that the two different types have significantly different risks of recurrence. The only way to distinguish between the two is to do a chromosome analysis. Risk of trisomy is 1 in 800 live births, in contrast with 1 in 1500 live births with a balanced translocation (Simpson 1990).

The translocation occurs when the carrier parent has 45 chromosomes, usually with one chromosome fused to another. A common translocation is one in which a particle of chromosome 14 breaks and fuses to chromosome 21. The parent has one normal 14, one normal 21, and one 14/21 chromosome. Because all the chromosomal material is present and functioning normally, the parent is clinically normal. This individual is known as a *balanced translocation carrier.*

When a person who is a balanced translocation carrier has a child with a person who has a structurally normal chromosome constitution, there are several possible outcomes (Figure 7–13). The offspring can receive the carrier parent's normal number 21 and the normal number 14 chromosomes in combination with the noncarrier parent's normal chromosomes 21 and 14. In this case the offspring is chromosomally normal. Alternatively, the child may receive one of the balanced translocations, thus becoming a carrier like the carrier parent—chromosomally abnormal genotype but clinically normal phenotype. If, however, the offspring receives the carrier parent's normal number 21 chromosome and the 14/21 chromosome and the noncarrier parent's normal chromosomes, the offspring receives two functioning number 14 chromosomes and three functioning number 21 chromosomes. At first glance the child seems to have 46 chromosomes but actually has an extra chromosome 21. Thus the child has an *unbalanced translocation* and has Down syndrome. Other types of translocations can occur. But regardless of the chromosome involved, any person having a balanced chromosome rearrangement (translocation) has the potential of having a child with an unbalanced chromosome constitution. This usually means a substantial negative effect on normal growth and development.

The other type of structural abnormality seen is caused by *additions or deletions* of chromosomal material.

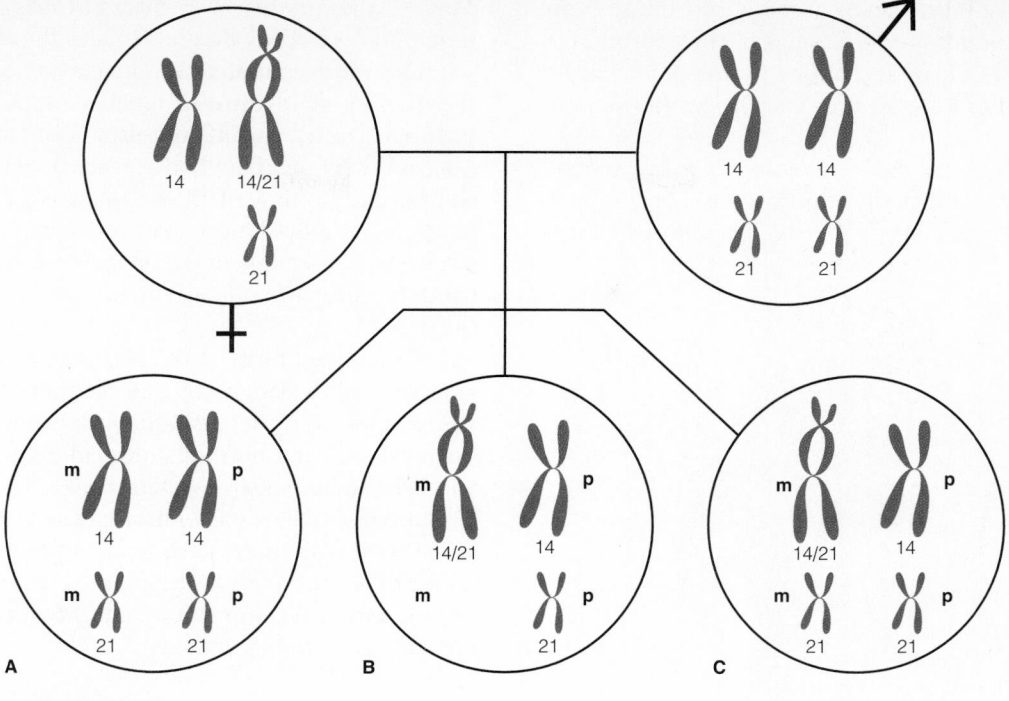

m = maternal origin
p = paternal origin

FIGURE 7-13   Diagram of various types of offspring when mother has a balanced translocation between chromosomes 14 and 21 and father has a normal arrangement of chromosomal material. *A* Normal offspring. *B* Balanced translocation carrier. *C* Unbalanced translocation. Child has Down syndrome.

Any portion of a chromosome may be lost or added, generally leading to some adverse effect. Depending on how much chromosomal material is involved, the clinical effects may be mild or severe. Many types of additions and deletions have been described, such as a deletion of the short arm of chromosome 5 (cri du chat, or cat cry, syndrome; Figure 7–14) or the deletion of the long arm of chromosome 18 (Edwards' syndrome). Table 7–8 lists other chromosomal syndromes.

Sex Chromosome Abnormalities   To better understand normal X chromosome function and thus abnormalities of the sex chromosomes, the nurse should know that in females, at an early embryonic stage, one of the two normal X chromosomes becomes inactive. The inactive X chromosome forms a dark staining area known as the *Barr body* or sex *chromatin body.*

The Barr body may be seen by examining the cells scraped from the inside of a woman's mouth. This procedure, the *buccal smear,* will show the number of inactive X chromosomes or Barr bodies present. The normal female has one Barr body because one of her two X chromosomes has been inactivated. The number of Barr bodies seen on the buccal smear is *always* one less than the number of X chromosomes present in the woman's cells. Chromosome analysis is preferred because the buccal

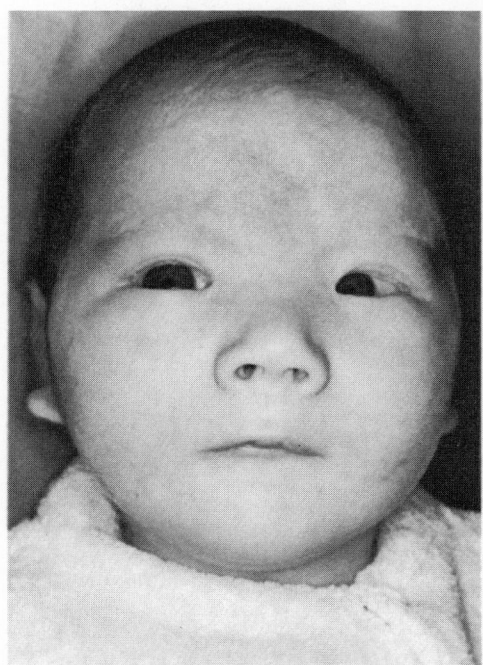

FIGURE 7-14   Infant with cri du chat syndrome resulting from deletion of part of the short arm of chromosome 5. Note characteristic facies with hypertelorism, epicanthus, and retrognathia. SOURCE: Thompson JS, Thompson MW: *Genetics in Medicine,* 5th ed. Philadelphia: Saunders, 1991.

smear is not diagnostic and has poor reliability. Now technology can target specific strands of chromosomes to determine the sex of the fetus. The normal male has no Barr bodies because he has only one X chromosome to begin with.

When Y chromosome–containing cells are stained and viewed, the Y chromosome appears as a bright body within the nucleus. The number of Y bodies present is equal to the number of Y chromosomes present. Males should have one Y body, and females should have none.

The most common sex chromosome abnormalities are **Turner syndrome** in females (45,X with no Barr bodies present) and **Klinefelter syndrome** in males (47,XXY with one Barr body present). See Table 7–8 for clinical descriptions of these abnormalities. During the newborn period, clinical signs and symptoms of Turner syndrome are lymphedema of the back (dorsum) of the hands (Figure 7–15) and of the feet, and excessive skin on the neck.

The mosaic form of the XO chromosome is associated with DES daughters, and fertility may not be impaired. However, there is a higher percentage of uterine malformation and hormonal difficulty associated with it, and hence a high degree of fetal wastage.

Other sex chromosome abnormalities may occur. Whether it is an increased number of X chromosomes or Y chromosomes or both, the affected individual generally has an increased number of abnormalities and severe mental retardation.

Modes of Inheritance

Many inherited diseases are produced by an abnormality in a single gene or pair of genes. In such instances the chromosomes are grossly normal. The defect is at the gene level. Some of these gene defects can be detected by new technologies, including DNA and other biochemical assays. The pattern of inheritance for a particular disease or defect is often determined by two methods: (1) close examination of the family in which the disease appears and (2) knowledge of how the disease has been previously inherited, when no laboratory methods of detection are available.

There are two major categories of inheritance: **Mendelian** or **single-gene inheritance** and **non-Mendelian** or **multifactorial inheritance**. Each single-gene trait is determined by a pair of genes working together. These genes are responsible for the observable expression of the traits (eg, brown eyes, dark skin), referred to as the **phenotype**. The total genetic makeup of an individual is referred to as the **genotype** (pattern of the genes on the chromosomes). One of the genes for a trait is inherited from the mother, the other, from the father. Individuals who have two identical genes at a given locus are considered to be **homozygous** for that trait. Individuals are considered to be **heterozygous** for a particular trait when they have two different *alleles* (alternate forms of the same gene) at a given locus on a pair of homologous chromosomes.

The well-known modes of single-gene inheritance are autosomal dominant, autosomal recessive, and X-linked (sex-linked) recessive. There is also a less common, X-linked dominant mode of inheritance and a newly identified mode of inheritance, the fragile X syndrome (discussed later in this chapter).

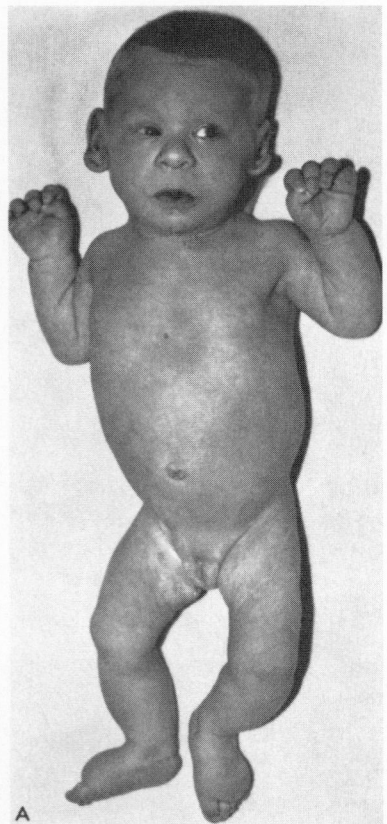

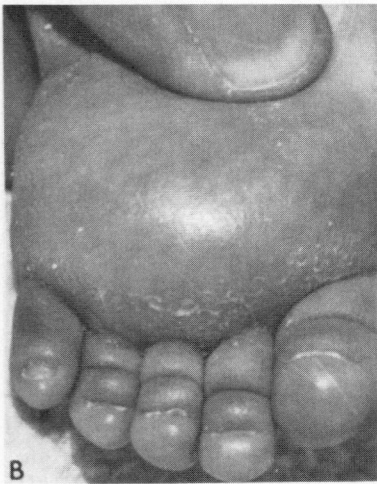

FIGURE 7-15 Infant with Turner syndrome at 1 month of age. Note: *A* Prominent ears. *B* Lymphedema. SOURCE: Lemli L, Smith DW: The XO syndrome: A study of the differential phenotype in 25 patients. *J Pediatr* 1963; 63:577.

Autosomal Dominant Inheritance

An individual is said to have an autosomal dominantly inherited disorder if the disease trait is heterozygous. That is, the abnormal gene overshadows the normal gene of the pair to produce the trait. The following occurs in autosomal dominant inheritance:

- An affected individual generally has an affected parent. The family pedigree (graphic representation of a family tree) usually shows multiple generations having the disorder.

- Affected individuals have a 50% chance of passing on the abnormal gene to each of their children (Figure 7–16).

- Both males and females are equally affected, and a father can pass the abnormal gene on to his son. This is an important principle when distinguishing autosomal dominant disorders from X-linked disorders.

- Unaffected individuals in most cases cannot transmit the disorder to their children.

- A mutation or a change of a normal gene into a dominant abnormal gene is possible. In this case this is the first time the disorder is seen in the family; an affected child is born to parents who are unaffected. In such instances there is not an increased risk of future children of the same parents being affected. The child, however, now has a 50% chance of passing the abnormal gene on to each offspring.

- Autosomal dominant inherited disorders have varying degrees of presentation. This is an important factor when counseling families concerning autosomal dominant disorders. Although a parent may have a mild form of the disease, the child may have a more severe form. Unfortunately, there is no method for predicting whether a child will be only mildly affected or more severely affected. The geneticist or health care provider must be thorough in the examination of family members to discern whether any of those individuals are indeed affected. They may express the disease in such a mild form that a cursory examination misses clinical signs of the disease.

Some common autosomal dominantly inherited disorders are Huntington's chorea, polycystic kidney disease, neurofibromatosis (von Recklinghausen's disease), and achondroplastic dwarfism.

Autosomal Recessive Inheritance

An individual has an autosomal recessively inherited disorder if the disease manifests itself only as a homozygous trait. That is, because the normal gene overshadows the abnormal one, the individual must have two abnormal genes to be affected. The notion of a *carrier state* is appropriate here. An individual who is heterozygous for the

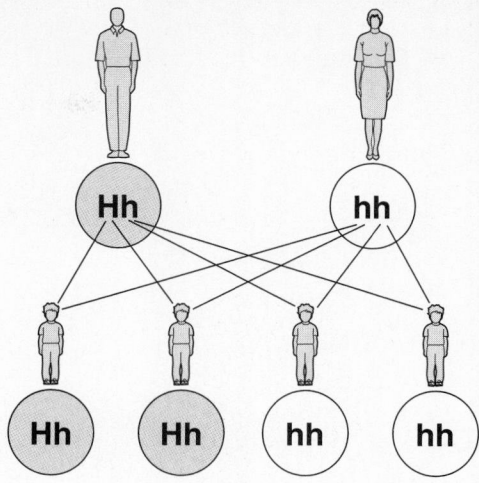

H = Gene for Huntington's chorea

h = Normal allele

(Hh) = Affected individual

(hh) = Nonaffected individual

A

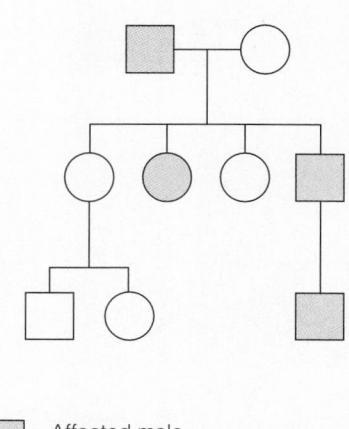

□ = Affected male

○ = Affected female

B

FIGURE 7-16 *A* Autosomal dominant inheritance. One parent is affected. Statistically, 50% of offspring will be affected, regardless of sex. *B* Autosomal dominant pedigree.

abnormal gene is clinically normal. It is not until two individuals mate and pass on the same abnormal gene that affected offspring may appear. The following occurs in autosomal recessive inheritance:

- An affected individual has clinically normal parents, but both are carriers of the abnormal gene (Figure 7–17).

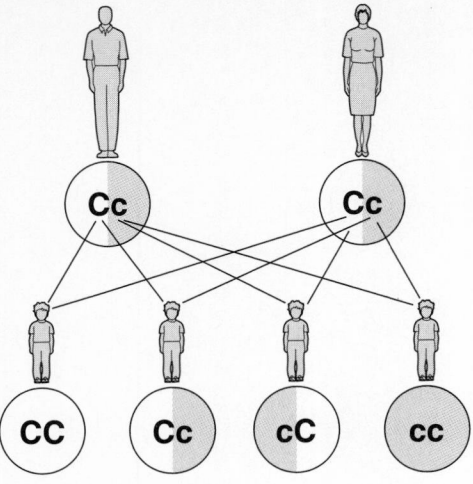

C = Normal allele

c = Gene for cystic fibrosis

(Cc) = Carrier, nonaffected individual

(cc) = Affected individual

A

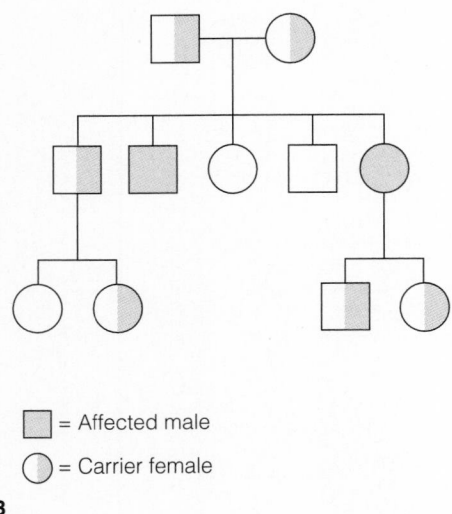

☐ = Affected male

◐ = Carrier female

B

FIGURE 7-17   *A* Autosomal recessive inheritance. Both parents are carriers. Statistically, 25% of offspring will be affected, regardless of sex. *B* Autosomal recessive pedigree.

- Parents who are both carriers of the same abnormal gene have a 25% chance of both passing the abnormal gene on to *any* of their children (Figure 7–17). Each pregnancy has a 25% chance of having an affected child.

- If the child of two carrier parents is clinically normal, there is a 50% chance that the child is a carrier of the gene (Figure 7–17).

- Both males and females are equally affected.

- The family pedigree usually shows siblings affected in a horizontal fashion (Figure 7–17). Future generations are not affected unless both parents carry the same abnormal gene.

- There is an increased history of consanguineous matings. Parents who are closely related are more likely to have the same genes in common than two parents who are unrelated.

- Recessively inherited disorders tend to be more severe in their clinical manifestations. Clinically normal carrier parents pass on the disorder, and the affected offspring will often not reproduce. If an affected individual does reproduce, all the children will be carriers of the disorder.

- The presence of the abnormal gene for some autosomal recessively inherited disorders can be detected in a normal carrier parent. For instance, Tay Sachs disease is caused by an inborn error of metabolism—that is, a deficiency of the enzyme hexosaminidase A. An affected individual has little or no enzyme activity present, whereas a carrier parent usually has 50% normal enzyme activity present. The carrier is biochemically abnormal but phenotypically normal. The heterozygous state can be detected even though it is asymptomatic.

Some other common autosomal recessive inherited disorders are cystic fibrosis, phenylketonuria (PKU), galactosemia, sickle-cell anemia, and most metabolic disorders.

X-Linked Recessive Inheritance

X-linked, or sex-linked, disorders are those for which the abnormal gene is carried on the X chromosome. A female may be heterozygous or homozygous for a trait carried on the X chromosome because she has two X chromosomes. A male, however, has only one X chromosome. The male in this case is considered to be *hemizygous*, having only one alternative form of the gene instead of a pair for a given trait or disorder. Thus an X-linked disorder is manifested in a male who carries the abnormal gene on his X chromosome. His mother is considered to be a carrier when the normal gene on one X chromosome overshadows the abnormal gene on the other X chromosome. The following occurs in X-linked recessive inheritance:

- There is no male-to-male transmission. Fathers pass only their Y chromosomes to their sons and their X chromosomes to their daughters. Daughters receive one X chromosome from the mother and one from the father.

- Affected males are related through the female line (Figure 7–18B).

- There is a 50% chance that a carrier mother will pass the abnormal gene to each of her sons, who will thus be affected. There is a 50% chance that a carrier mother will pass the normal gene to each of her sons, who will thus be unaffected. There is a 50% chance that a carrier mother will pass the abnormal gene to each of her daughters, who become carriers like their mother (Figure 7–18). There is also a 50% chance that a carrier mother will pass on her normal gene to her daughter, who will thus not be a carrier.

- Fathers affected with an X-linked disorder cannot pass the disorder to their sons, but *all* their daughters become carriers of the disorder.

- Occasionally, a female carrier may show some symptoms of an X-linked disorder. This situation is probably due to random inactivation of the X chromosome carrying the normal allele. Thus a heterozygous female may show some manifestation of an X-linked disorder.

Common X-linked recessive disorders are hemophilia, Duchenne muscular dystrophy, and some forms of color blindness.

X-Linked Dominant Inheritance

X-linked dominant disorders are extremely rare, the most common being vitamin D–resistant rickets. When X-linked dominance does occur, the pattern is similar to X-linked recessive inheritance except that heterozygous females are affected. The following occurs in X-linked dominant inheritance:

- The abnormal gene is dominant and overshadows the normal gene on the female's other X chromosome.

- There is no male-to-male transmission. An affected father will have affected daughters but no affected sons.

Fragile X Syndrome

Fragile X syndrome is a genetic disorder in which the abnormal gene is located on the X chromosome in a region that the chromatin failed to condense during mitosis. It is characterized in males by moderate retardation, large protuberant ears, and large testes after puberty. Females who carry the gene have more variable mentation—normal intelligence to moderate retardation.

The gene for this condition can be detected reliably with a DNA test called FMR-1. This gene appears to have repeated DNA sequences. Fifty to 200 repeats are considered a permutation with little phenotypic effect. When more than 200 repeats are present, a more severe phenotype is predicted. Prenatal diagnosis of carrier females, nonexpressing but transmitting males (men who carry the abnormal gene but have no symptoms), and fetuses can be carried out reliably (Nelson 1993; Oostra et al 1993).

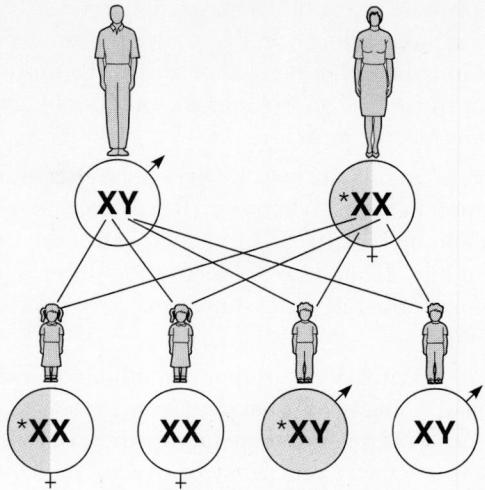

X = Chromosome carrying normal allele

***X** = Chromosome carrying gene for hemophilia

(XY)↗ = Affected male

(XX)• = Carrier female, nonaffected

A

= Affected male

(•) = Carrier female

B

FIGURE 7-18   *A* X-linked recessive inheritance. The mother is the carrier. Statistically, 50% of male offspring will be affected, and 50% of female offspring will be carriers. *B* X-linked pedigree.

Multifactorial Inheritance

Many common congenital malformations, such as cleft palate, heart defects, spina bifida, dislocated hips, clubfoot, and pyloric stenosis, are caused by an interaction of many genes and environmental factors. They are therefore multifactorial in origin. The following occur in multifactorial inheritance:

- The malformations may vary from mild to severe. For example, spina bifida may range in severity from mild, as spina bifida occulta, to more severe, as a myelomeningocele. It is believed that the more severe the defect, the greater the number of genes present for that defect.

- There is often a sex bias. Pyloric stenosis is more common in males, whereas cleft palate is more common among females. When a member of the less commonly affected sex shows the condition, a greater number of genes must usually be present to cause it.

- In the presence of environmental influence (such as seasonal changes, altitude, radiation exposure, chemicals in the environment, or exposure to toxic substances) fewer genes may be needed to manifest the disease in the offspring.

- In contrast to single-gene disorders, there is an additive effect in multifactorial inheritance. The more family members who have the defect, the greater the risk that the next pregnancy will also be affected.

- Risk factors are determined by the distribution of cases found in the general population. The risk of recurrence is usually 3% to 5% for all first-degree relatives (ie, parents, siblings, and children) if one family member is affected. The recurrence figure decreases with second-degree relatives (ie, grand-parents, grandchildren, aunts, and uncles) and so forth. Generally the recurrence risks increase the more family members who are affected (King & Schimke 1994).

Although most congenital malformations are multi-factorial tracts, a careful family history should always be taken because occasionally cleft lip and palate, certain congenital heart defects, and other malformations can also be inherited as autosomal dominant or recessive traits. Other disorders thought to be within the multifactorial inheritance group are diabetes, hypertension, some heart diseases, and mental illness.

Nongenetic Conditions

Not all disorders or congenital malformations are inherited or have an inherited component. Malformations present at birth may be caused by an environmental insult during pregnancy, such as exposure to a drug or an infectious agent (see Chapter 15). Some malformations, however, cannot be explained by genetic mechanisms or teratogens. These disorders are considered to have a developmental cause. A couple who has a child with phocomelia (abnormality of the limbs) in the absence of any other problems or family history may be reassured that the problem is developmental in etiology and the risk for future pregnancies is low. Such reassurance is also appropriate for families concerned about a child's seizures or developmental delays if they can be attributed to an acquired problem. Nurses should be very careful. A referral to a genetic center is warranted with any birth defect. Autosomal dominant conditions such as phocomelia can have very minimal expression in a parent but severe effects in a child. False reassurance or information can put any health care professional in jeopardy.

Prenatal Diagnosis

Parent-child and family planning counseling have become a major responsibility of professional nurses. To be effective counselors, nurses need to have the *most* current knowledge available concerning prenatal diagnosis (Wright 1994).

It is essential that the couple be completely informed as to the known and potential risks of each of the genetic diagnostic procedures. The nurse needs to recognize the emotional impact on the family of a decision to have or not to have a genetic diagnostic procedure.

The ability to diagnose certain genetic diseases by various diagnostic tools has enormous implications for the practice of preventive health care. Several methods are available for prenatal diagnosis, although some are still being used on an experimental basis.

Genetic Ultrasound

Ultrasound may be used to assess the fetus for genetic and/or congenital problems. With ultrasound one can visualize the fetal head for abnormalities in size, shape, and structure. Neural tube and cranial defects (anencephaly, microcephaly, hydrocephalus), gastrointestinal malformations (omphalocele, gastroschisis), renal malformations (dysplasia or obstruction), and skeletal malformations (caudal regression, conjoined twins) are only some of the disorders that have been diagnosed in utero by ultrasound.

Screening by ultrasound for congenital anomalies is best done at 18 to 20 weeks, when fetal structures have completed development (Chervenak et al 1993; Simpson & Elias 1993). There is no information documenting harm to the fetus or long-term effects with exposure to ultrasound. However, there is no guarantee of complete safety; therefore the practitioner and the parents must evaluate the risks against the benefits on an individual basis (Chervenak et al 1993).

Genetic Amniocentesis

A major method of prenatal diagnosis is genetic amniocentesis (Figure 7–19). The procedure is described in Chapter 20. The indications for genetic amniocentesis include the following:

- Advanced maternal age. Any woman 35 or older is at greater risk for having children with chromosome

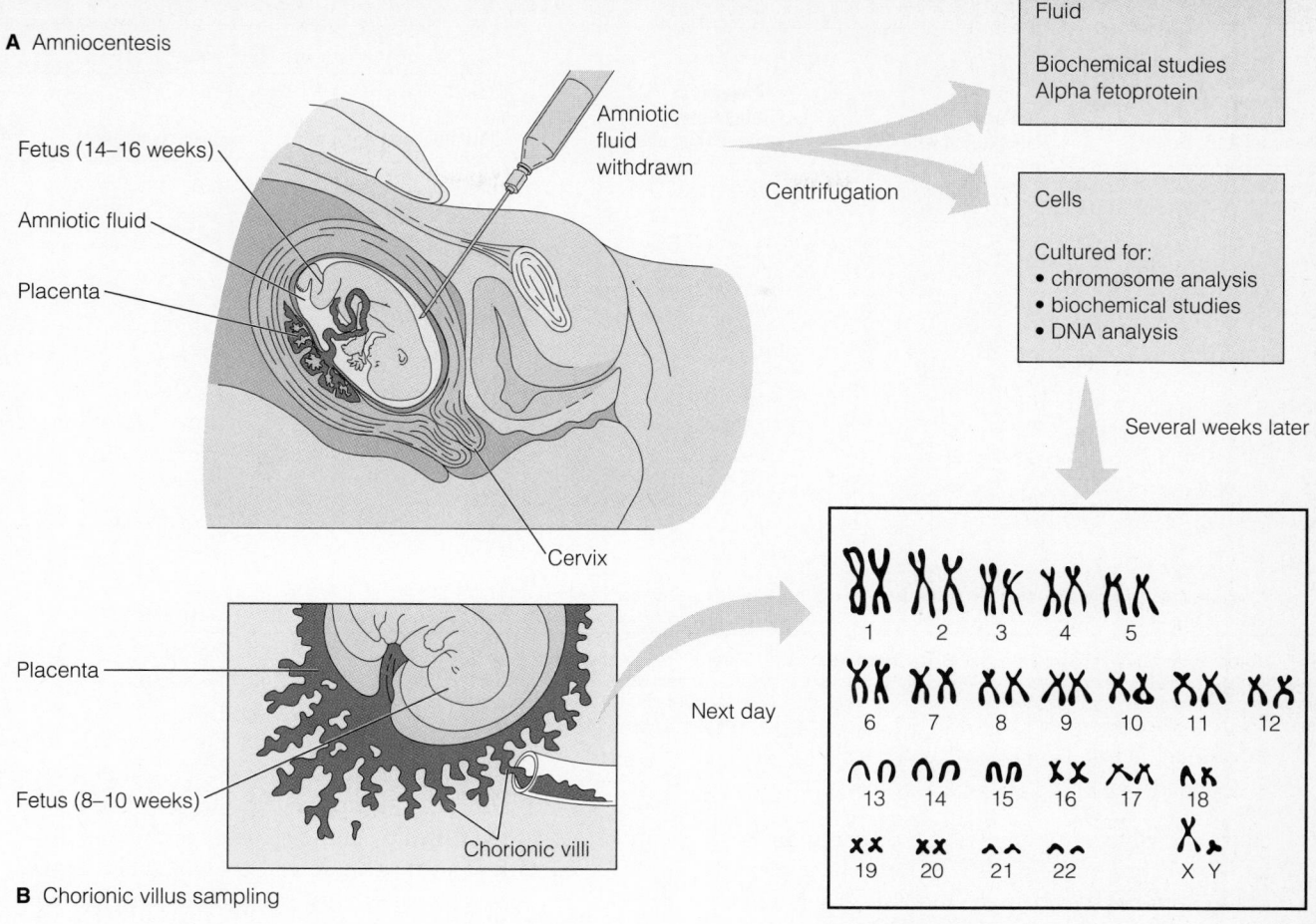

A Amniocentesis

Fetus (14–16 weeks)

Amniotic fluid

Placenta

Amniotic fluid withdrawn

Cervix

Fluid

Biochemical studies
Alpha fetoprotein

Centrifugation

Cells

Cultured for:
• chromosome analysis
• biochemical studies
• DNA analysis

Several weeks later

Placenta

Fetus (8–10 weeks)

Chorionic villi

B Chorionic villus sampling

Next day

Human karyotype

FIGURE 7-19   *A* Genetic amniocentesis for prenatal diagnosis is done at 14–16 weeks' gestation. *B* Chorionic villus sampling is done at 8–10 weeks, and the cells are karotyped within 48–72 hours. SOURCE: Adapted from Marieb EN: *Human Anatomy and Physiology,* 3rd ed. Redwood City, CA: Benjamin/Cummings, 1995, p 1037.

abnormalities. Approximately 95% of trisomy 21 cases occur because of advanced maternal age (Simpson & Elias 1993). See Chapter 20 for further discussion. Half of the chromosomal abnormalities due to maternal age are trisomy 21, and half are other abnormalities of chromosome number, such as trisomy 13, 18, XXX, or XXY. The risk of having a live born infant with a chromosome problem is 1 in 200 for a 35-year-old woman; the risk for trisomy 21 is 1 in 400. At age 45 the risks are 1 in 20 and 1 in 40, respectively (Hook et al 1988). Table 7–9 presents maternal age–related risks at different gestational ages.

• Previous child born with a chromosomal abnormality. Young couples who have had a child with trisomy 21, 18, or 13 have approximately a 1% to 2% risk of a future child having a chromosome abnormality. Genetic amniocentesis is made available to any couple who has already had a child with a chromosome abnormality.

• Parent carrying a chromosomal abnormality (balanced translocation). Any couple in which one of the partners is a carrier of a balanced translocation should be considered for prenatal diagnosis. Although the person with the chromosome rearrangement is clinically normal, he or she has the potential for conceiving a child with an unbalanced chromosome constitution, which usually has substantial adverse effects on normal development. For example, a woman who carries a balanced 14/21 translocation has a risk of approximately 10% to 15% that her children will be affected with the unbalanced translocation of Down syndrome; if the father is a carrier, there is a 2% to 5% risk. Translocation errors occur more often during maternal meiosis than paternal meiosis.

• Mother carrying an X-linked disease. In families in which the woman is a known or possible carrier of an X-linked disorder, such as Duchenne's muscular dystrophy or hemophilia, genetic amniocentesis,

Maternal Age (Years)	10 Weeks Rates Noted with CVS	17 Weeks Rates Noted with Amniocentesis	Birth	
			Chromosomal Anomalies	Down Syndrome*
33		1/200	1/300	1/600
34		1/170	1/250	1/500
35	1/110	1/130	1/200	1/400
36	1/80	1/100	1/170	1/340
37	1/65	1/80	1/130	1/260
38	1/50	1/65	1/100	1/200
39	1/35	1/50	1/80	1/160
40	1/30	1/40	1/65	1/130
41	1/20	1/30	1/50	1/100
42	1/15	1/25	1/40	1/80
43	1/13	1/20	1/30	1/60
44	1/10	1/15	1/25	1/50
45	1/7	1/12	1/20	1/40
46	1/6	1/10	1/16	1/32
47	1/4	1/8	1/12	1/24
48	1/3	1/6	1/10	1/20

*Risk for Down syndrome is approximately half of each number listed above (eg, age 33 risk for live born Down syndrome is 1 in 600).

SOURCES: Approximate (rounded) estimates from Hook EB et al: Maternal age-specific rates of 47, +21 and other cytogenetic abnormalities diagnosed in the first trimester of pregnancy in chorionic villus biopsy specimens: Comparison with rates expected from observations at amniocentesis. *Am J Hum Genet* 1988; 42:797; and Hook EB, Cross PK and Schreimachers DM: Chromosomal abnormality rates at amniocentesis and in live-born infants. *JAMA* 1983; 249:2034. Rates for maternal ages >45 years are based on very small numbers.

chorionic villus sampling (CVS), or percutaneous umbilical cord sampling (PUBS) may be appropriate options. Increasingly, these disorders can be diagnosed in utero. For a known female carrier the risk of an affected male fetus is 50%. With new technologies such as DNA testing it may be possible to differentiate between affected and nonaffected males in some disorders. In disorders where female carriers can be distinguished from noncarriers, only the carrier females would be offered prenatal diagnosis.

- Parents carrying an inborn error of metabolism that can be diagnosed in utero. The number of inherited metabolic disorders that can be diagnosed in utero is increasing at a rapid rate. Metabolic disorders detectable in utero include argininosuccinicaciduria, cystinosis, fabry disease, galactosemia, Gaucher disease, homocystinuria, Hunter syndrome, Hurler disease, Krabbe disease, Lesch-Nyhan syndrome, maple syrup urine disease, metachromatic leukodystrophy, methylmalonic aciduria, Niemann-Pick disease, Pompe disease, Sanfilippo syndrome, and Tay Sachs disease.

- Both parents carrying an autosomal recessive disease. When both parents are carriers of an autosomal recessive disease, there is a 25% risk for each pregnancy that the fetus will be affected. Diagnosis is made by testing the cultured amniotic fluid cells (enzyme level, substrate level, product level, or DNA) or the fluid itself. Autosomal recessive dis-

eases identified by amniocentesis are hemoglobinopathies such as sickle-cell anemia, thalassemia, and cystic fibrosis. Most research to date has been in the prenatal diagnosis of hemoglobinopathies. Both sickle-cell anemia and β-thalassemia once were diagnosed using fetal blood samples obtained by amnioscopy, which has a 3% to 5% risk of fetal demise and spontaneous abortion. Prenatal diagnosis of these conditions can be accomplished on uncultured amniotic fluid from an amniocentesis using various DNA analyses (D'Alton 1994). With the detection of the deletion that causes 70% of the cases of cystic fibrosis, carrier testing and prenatal diagnosis are available for some families. It is theorized that the other 30% of the cases of cystic fibrosis are caused by numerous different deletions (Simpson & Elias 1993). For those families without a known deletion but with a living affected relative, carrier detection and prenatal diagnosis may be possible with DNA testing and/or biochemical analysis of amniotic fluid with the microvillar enzyme activity (Simpson & Elias 1993).

- Family history of neural tube defects. Genetic amniocentesis is available to those couples who have had a child with neural tube defects or who have a family history of these conditions, which include anencephaly, spina bifida, and myelomeningocele. Neural tube defects are usually multifactorial traits. Regardless of the statistical risk for a given family, whether for an isolated neural tube defect or a dis-

TABLE 7-10 — Couples To Be Offered Prenatal Diagnosis

Women 35 or over at time of birth

Couples having a balanced translocation (chromosomal abnormality)

Mother carrying X-linked disease (eg, hemophilia)

Couples having a previous child with chromosomal abnormality

Couples in which either partner or a previous child is affected with a diagnosable metabolic disorder

Couples in which both partners are carriers for a diagnosable metabolic or autosomal recessive disorder

Family or personal history of neural tube defects

Ethnic groups at increased risk for specific disorders (Table 7–11)

Couples with history of two or more first trimester spontaneous abortions

Women with an abnormal maternal serum alpha fetoprotein (MSAFP or AFP3) test

---

order in which a neural tube defect is a constant feature, the risk of recurrence can be reduced (possibly by as much as 90%) through α-fetoprotein (AFP) determination of the amniotic fluid (Simpson & Elias 1993). In pregnancies in which the fetus has an open neural tube defect, α-fetoprotein leaks into the amniotic fluid, and levels are elevated (Filly et al 1993; Simpson & Elias 1993). Thus genetic amniocentesis allows those families for whom the risk of a neural tube defect is increased the opportunity to choose whether to have a child with such a disorder (Table 7–10 and 7–11). For those who would not terminate a pregnancy, cesarean section is generally advised prior to the onset of labor (Luthy et al 1992).

Chorionic Villus Sampling (CVS)

Chorionic villus sampling is a technique used in selected regional centers. Its diagnostic capability is similar to amniocentesis. Its advantages are that diagnostic information is available at 8 to 10 weeks' gestation and that products of conception are tested directly. (For further discussion see Chapter 20.)

Percutaneous Umbilical Blood Sampling

Percutaneous umbilical blood sampling (PUBS) is a technique used for obtaining blood that allows for more rapid chromosome diagnosis, for genetic studies, or for transfusion for Rh isoimmunization or hydrops (Shulman et al 1993). For more in-depth discussion see Chapter 20.

Alpha Fetoprotein (AFP and AFP3)

AFP is a substance produced by the fetal liver, kidney, and gastrointestinal tract. This fetal protein is normally found in small amounts in maternal circulation. In addition to the infant with open neural tube defect, infants with anencephaly, omphalocele, gastroschisis, or multiple gestation have elevated maternal serum AFP (MSAFP). Low MSAFP has been associated with Down syndrome. Ultrasound and amniocentesis are offered with low or high MSAFP. Inaccurate dating is the most common cause for abnormal AFP; therefore ultrasound dating is very important. Amniocentesis will reveal what the AFP level is in the amniotic fluid. With high MSAFP, normal amniotic fluid AFP, and normal ultrasound, there is an increased risk for preterm labor, perinatal death, and intrauterine growth restriction (Filly et al 1993).

AFP3 is a test on maternal blood with AFP, unconjugated estriol, and hCG (Wright 1994). AFP3, in addition

---

TABLE 7-11 — Genetic Screening Recommendations for Various Ethnic and Age Groups

Background of Population at Risk	Disorder	Screening Test	Definitive Test
Ashkenazic Jewish	Tay Sachs disease	Decreased serum hexosaminidase-A	CVS* or amniocentesis for hexosaminidase-A assay
African; Hispanic from Caribbean, Central America, South America (*Journal of Black Nurses* 1992)	Sickle-cell anemia	Presence of sickle-cell hemoglobin; confirmatory hemoglobin electrophoresis	CVS or amniocentesis for genotype determination; direct molecular studies
Greek, Italian	β-thalassemia	Mean corpuscular volume <80%; confirmatory hemoglobin electrophoresis	CVS or amniocentesis for genotype determination (direct molecular studies or indirect RFLP[†] analysis)
Southeast Asian (Vietnamese, Laotian, Cambodian), Philippine	α-thalassemia	Mean corpuscular volume <80%; confirmatory hemoglobin electrophoresis	CVS or amniocentesis for genotype determination (direct molecular studies)
Women over age 35 (EDB) (all ethnic groups)	Chromosomal trisomies	None	CVS or amniocentesis for cytogenetic analysis
Women of any age (all ethnic groups; particularly suggested for women from British Isles, Ireland)	Neural tube defects and selected other anomalies	Maternal serum α-fetoprotein (MSAFP)	Amniocentesis for amniotic fluid, α-fetoprotein, and acetylcholinesterase assays

*Chorionic villus sampling

[†]Restriction fragment length polymorphism

to testing for open spine or ventral wall defects, will detect 60% of Down syndrome and about 50% of trisomy 18, compared with MSAFP alone, which detects, for example, just 30% of Down syndrome (D'Alton 1994). Folic acid supplements (0.4 mg/day) are recommended beginning preconceptually for an individual with no family history of neural tube defects because the neural tube begins to form 16 days after conception and is completely closed by 28 days, often before a woman knows she is pregnant. Women with a family history of neural tube defects should consult their prenatal care provider for higher doses of folic acid (CDC 1993; King & Schimke 1994).

Implications of Prenatal Diagnostic Testing

It is imperative that counseling precede any procedure for prenatal diagnosis. Many questions and points must be considered if the family is to reach a satisfactory decision.

With the advent of diagnostic techniques such as amniocentesis, couples at risk, who would not otherwise have additional children, can decide to conceive. Alternatively, after prenatal diagnosis a couple can decide not to have a child with a genetic disease. However, the percentage of therapeutic abortions after amniocentesis is small. For many couples prenatal diagnosis is not a solution because they choose not to prevent the genetic disease by aborting the fetus. The decision whether or not to use prenatal diagnosis can be made only by the family.

Families with a baby having a lethal anomaly, such as trisomy 13 or 18, may wish to consider nonaggressive intervention. This may include no tocolytic therapy for preterm labor, no monitoring during labor, no cesarean section, and no resuscitation or intensive care after birth. These alternatives must be discussed with the delivering health care professional and in some cases taken before the hospital ethics committee for approval. By having prenatal diagnosis, even when termination is not an option, parents can prepare for the birth of a child with special needs, contact other families with a child with a similar problem, or contact support services before the birth (Chervenak & McCullough 1989).

Genetic counselors give nondirective information and discuss with the family all available options if an abnormal fetus is discovered or suspected. Every pregnancy has a 3% to 5% risk for an infant to be born with a birth defect, some of which can be diagnosed before birth. When an abnormality is detected or suspected, an attempt is made to determine the diagnosis by assessing the family health history (via the pedigree) and the pregnancy history and by evaluating the fetal anomaly or anomalies. The parents are then presented with options.

Prenatal diagnosis cannot guarantee the birth of a normal child. It can only determine the presence or absence of specific disorders (within the limits of laboratory error). Many disorders can be prenatally diagnosed; the list has grown and continues to grow almost daily. Ex-

perts on a specific disorder should be consulted before information is given to couples and before options regarding prenatal diagnosis are discussed.

Treatment of prenatally diagnosed disorders may begin during the pregnancy, thus possibly preventing irreversible damage. For example, a galactose-free diet may be given to a mother carrying a fetus with galactosemia. In light of the philosophy of preventive health care, information on what data can be obtained prenatally should be made available to all couples who are expecting a baby or who are contemplating pregnancy.

Critical Thinking Question

What implications does the human genome project have for families with genetic conditions?

Postnatal Diagnosis

Questions concerning genetic disorders, cause, treatment, and prognosis are most often first discussed in the newborn nursery or during the infant's first few months of life. When a child is born with anomalies, has a stormy neonatal period, or does not progress as expected, a genetic evaluation may well be warranted.

Accurate diagnosis and an optimal treatment plan incorporate the following:

- Complete and detailed histories to determine if the problem is prenatal (congenital), postnatal, or familial in origin
- Thorough physical examination, including dermatoglyphic analysis
- Laboratory analysis, which includes chromosome analysis; enzyme assay for inborn errors of metabolism (see Chapter 29 for further discussion on these specific tests); and antibody titers for infectious teratogens, such as toxoplasmosis, rubella, cytomegalovirus, and herpes virus **(TORCH)** (see Chapter 19).

To make an accurate diagnosis, the geneticist consults with other specialists and reviews the current literature. This permits the geneticist to evaluate all the available information before arriving at a diagnosis and plan of action.

Physical Examination

The physical examination is essential in helping to establish the diagnosis. The geneticist must attend to minute details and look for specific patterns of abnormalities. Two major questions should be kept in mind: Is just one organ system involved, or are multiple systems involved? Does the abnormality have a prenatal or postnatal onset? If only a single malformation is present (cleft palate) or only one organ system is involved (the skin), the geneticist tends to think in terms of multifactorial, single-gene disorders or developmental causes. If multiple malformations are present, chromosomal and teratogenic causes are often the first possibilities to consider. Many chromosomal abnormalities and single-gene disorders are associated with a specific pattern of malformations. Thus one must have expertise in syndrome recognition to be able to arrive at an accurate diagnosis. Also, minor anomalies such as skin tags, open sinus tracts in ear lobes, or a single umbilical artery are often signs of internal defects.

Dermatoglyphic Analysis

Dermatoglyphics are the patterns of the ridged skin found on the fingers, palms, toes, and soles (Thompson et al 1991). Although each individual has a unique ridge pattern, specific types of patterns that can be systematically classified exist. Because differentiation of dermal ridges is complete by the end of the fourth month of gestation, many genetic disorders that affect multiple systems also affect the dermatoglyphics. Thus a child with a chromosomal abnormality often exhibits certain characteristic dermatoglyphics. For example, palmar creases are associated with trisomy 21.

Pattern combinations and frequencies considered together are more significant than pattern types alone. In Down syndrome or any other abnormality any one of the particular specified patterns seen can also be found in normal individuals. It is when these patterns are in *combination* that they are associated with a specific disorder, such as Down syndrome.

Children with Down syndrome often have a single flexion crease (single transverse palmar crease) on the palms, an increased number of ulnar loops on the fingertips (often on all ten fingers) (Figure 7–20), and also a characteristic pattern on the soles of the feet (the hallucal pattern), known as an arch tibial. Children with trisomy 13 have an increased number of arch patterns on the fingertips and single flexion creases of the palms (Thompson et al 1991). Chromosome abnormalities are only one area in which unusual dermatoglyphics have been described; they can also be associated with other single-gene or multifactorial disorders.

Laboratory Analysis

Laboratory studies include chromosome analysis (discussed previously), enzyme assays, DNA studies (both direct and by linkage), and serologic and microscopic studies. Enzyme assays are performed to diagnose inherited metabolic diseases. These usually are done if the result on newborn screening is abnormal or if the child has any combination of the following: nausea and vomiting, enlarged viscera, poor feeding, lethargy, and seizures. Metabolic abnormalities should also be considered in any child who does well during the neonatal period with normal developmental milestones but then deteriorates, particularly in CNS functioning. The major tests assay amino

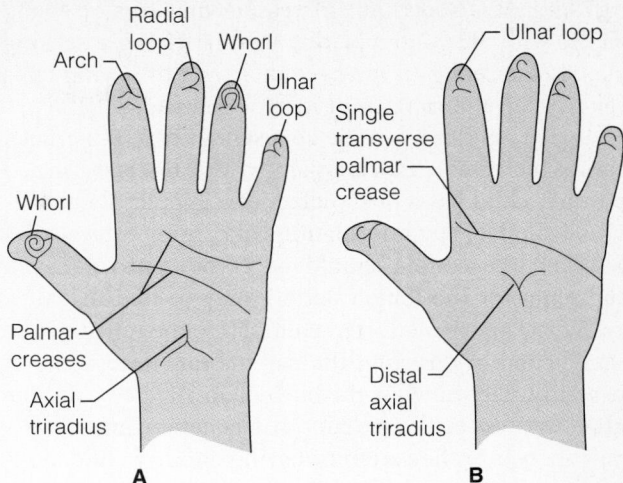

FIGURE 7-20 Dermatoglyphic patterns of the hands in (A) a normal individual and (B) a child with Down syndrome. Note the single transverse palmar crease, distally placed axial triradius, and increased number of ulnar loops.

and organic acids. Other specific enzyme assays are performed only if the clinical picture warrants them.

As mentioned, some genetic disorders are identified on newborn screening. The major purpose of screening programs is to identify affected newborns as soon as possible after birth so that corrective treatment can be instituted before irreversible damage is done. Many institutions now screen for six inborn errors of metabolism: PKU, galactosemia, hypothyroidism, sickle-cell anemia, maple syrup urine disease, and homocystinuria. (See Chapter 32 for further discussion of these conditions.)

The Family, the Nurse, and the Genetic Counseling Process

Genetic counseling is a communication process in which the genetic counselor tries to provide a family with the most complete and accurate information on the occurrence or the risk of recurrence of a genetic disease in that family (Inati et al 1994). The goals inherent in this definition are threefold:

1. Genetic counseling allows families to make informed decisions about reproduction.

2. It helps families assess the available treatments, consider appropriate alternatives to decrease the risk, learn about the usual course and outcome of the genetic disease or abnormality, and deal with other psychologic and social implications that often accompany such problems.

3. Genetic counseling may help decrease the incidence and impact of genetic disease.

Timing is an important aspect of the counseling, process. Preferably, counseling should be *prospective*—before the birth of an affected child. Increasing numbers of young couples who are contemplating childbearing are seeking genetic counseling to discover their risk of having children with an abnormality or genetic disease.

In retrospective genetic counseling, time is a crucial factor. One cannot expect a family who has just learned that their child has a birth defect or a genetic abnormality to assimilate any information concerning future risks. However, the couple should never be "put off" from counseling for too long a period, only to find that they have borne another affected child. Here the nurse can be instrumental in directing the parents into counseling at the appropriate time. At the birth of an affected child the nurse can inform the parents that genetic counseling is available before they attempt having another child. Asking one or two members of a genetics team to introduce themselves to the family is often enough to bring up the subject of genetic counseling. When the parents have begun to recover from the initial shock of bearing a child with an abnormality, or when they begin to contemplate having more children, the nurse can encourage the couple to seek counseling.

Referring Couples for Counseling

Nurses who are aware of families at an increased risk for having a child with a genetic disorder are in an ideal position to make referrals. Genetic counseling is an appropriate course of action for any family wondering, "Will it happen again?" The nursery nurse frequently has the first contact with the family that has a newborn with a congenital abnormality. The family nurse practitioner or family-planning nurse is in an excellent position to reach at-risk families before the birth of another baby with a congenital problem. Genetic counseling referral is advised for any of the following categories:

- *Congenital abnormalities, including mental retardation.* Any couple who has a child or a relative with a congenital malformation may be at an increased risk and should be so informed. If mental retardation of unidentified cause has occurred in a family, there may be an increased risk of recurrence.

  In many cases the genetic counselor will identify the cause of a malformation as a teratogen (see Chapter 15). The family should be aware of teratogenic substances so they can avoid exposure during any subsequent pregnancy.

- *Familial disorders.* Families should be told that certain diseases may have a genetic component and that the risk of their occurrence in a particular family may be higher than that for the general population. Such disorders as diabetes, heart disease, cancer, and mental illness fall into this category.

- *Known inherited diseases.* Families may know that a disease is inherited but not know the mechanism or the specific risk for them. An important point to

remember is that family members who are not at risk for passing on a disorder should be as well informed as family members who are at increased risk.

- *Metabolic disorders.* Any families at risk for having a child with a metabolic disorder or biochemical defect should be referred. Because most inborn errors of metabolism are autosomal recessively inherited ones, a family may not be identified as at risk until the birth of an affected child.

  Carriers of the sickle-cell trait can be identified before pregnancy is begun, and the risk of having an affected child can be determined. Prenatal diagnosis of an affected fetus is available.

- *Chromosomal abnormalities.* As discussed previously, any couple who has had a child with a chromosomal abnormality may be at an increased risk of having another child similarly affected. This group includes families in which there is concern for a possible translocation.

The process of genetic counseling usually begins after the birth of a child diagnosed as having a congenital problem or genetic disease. After the parents have been referred to the genetic clinic, they are sent a form requesting information on the health status of various family members. At this time the nurse can help by discussing the form with the family or clarifying the information needed to complete it.

A **pedigree** (graphic representation of a family tree) and family health history facilitate identification of other family members who might also be at risk for the same disorder. The family being counseled may wish to notify those relatives at risk so that they, too, can be given genetic counseling. When done correctly, the family history and pedigree become one of the most powerful and useful tools for determining a family risk.

A screening pedigree generally includes the affected individual, siblings, parents, aunts, uncles, and grandparents (Figure 7–21). If the family does not have all the necessary information at hand, the nurse can urge them to obtain the information in time for their first genetic counseling session, when a more complete pedigree will be taken.

The pedigree is a fairly easy and productive method for screening families. The nurse can obtain the necessary information and draw a screening pedigree in approximately 15 minutes. Information that should be obtained when drawing the family pedigree includes names (maiden names if appropriate) and birth dates of members of the immediate family; names and ages of the remainder of the family (including deceased members), with a description of their health status; causes of death of family members; and any other information the family feels is significant. In discussing the affected individual the nurse should obtain information on the pregnancy history of the mother (including miscarriages), medica-

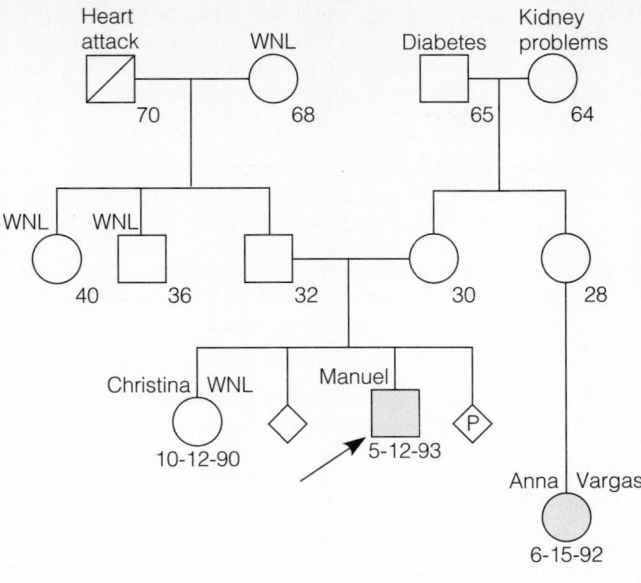

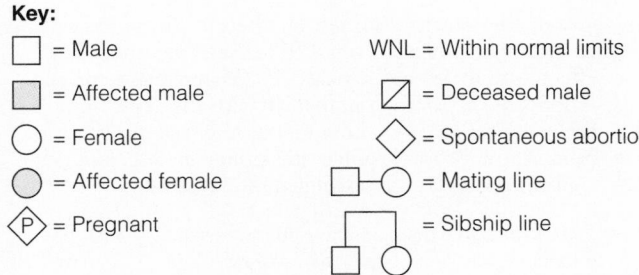

Key:

- ☐ = Male
- ▨ = Affected male
- ○ = Female
- ▨ = Affected female
- ⬦P = Pregnant

- WNL = Within normal limits
- ⬕ = Deceased male
- ◇ = Spontaneous abortion
- ☐○ = Mating line
- = Sibship line

FIGURE 7-21 Screening pedigree. Arrow indicates the nearest family member affected with the disorder being investigated. Basic data have been recorded. Numbers refer to the ages of family members.

tions and drugs taken during pregnancy, x-ray exposure, infections or illness during pregnancy, type of birth control used prior to pregnancy, and the method used to diagnose the pregnancy. A complete childbirth history should be taken, including a description of any complications. It is also appropriate for the nurse to ask the family when the problem was evident to them or was diagnosed.

The nurse should inquire about the affected child's growth and development. The information obtained should include developmental milestones, growth in comparison to siblings or other children the same age, symptoms of a problem, school records, and any previous testing.

Finally, information concerning ethnic background, family origin, and/or religion should be elicited. Many genetic disorders are more common among certain ethnic groups or in particular geographic areas. For example, families from the British Isles are at higher risk of having children with neural tube defects; the Ashkenazi Jews are at higher risk of Tay Sachs disease; Blacks are at risk for sickle-cell anemia; and people of Mediterranean heritage have a higher risk of thalassemias.

Follow-Up Counseling

When all the data have been carefully examined and analyzed, the family returns for a follow-up visit. At this time the parents are given all the information available, including the medical facts, diagnosis, probable course of the disorder, and any available management; the inheritance pattern for this particular family and their risk of recurrence; and the options or alternatives for dealing with the risk of recurrence. The remainder of the counseling session is spent discussing the course of action that seems appropriate to the family in view of their risk and family goals.

Among those options or alternatives are prenatal diagnosis and early detection and treatment and in some cases adoption, artificial insemination, or delayed childbearing.

The family may consider *artificial insemination by donor (AID)*, discussed earlier in this chapter. This alternative is appropriate in several instances; for example, if the male partner has an autosomal dominant disease, AID would decrease to zero the risk of having an affected child (if the sperm donor is not at risk) because the child would not inherit any genes from the affected parent. If the man is affected with an X-linked disorder and does not wish to continue the gene in the family (all his daughters will be carriers), AID would be an alternative to terminating all pregnancies with a female fetus. If the man is a carrier for a balanced translocation and if termination of pregnancy is against family ethics, AID is the most appropriate alternative. AID is also appropriate if both parents are carriers of an autosomal recessive disease. AID lowers the risk to a very low level or to zero if a carrier test is available. Finally, AID may be appropriate if the family is at high risk for a multifactorial disorder.

Couples who are young and at risk may decide to delay childbearing for a few years. Medical science and medical genetics are continually making breakthroughs in early detection and treatment. These couples may find in a few years that prenatal diagnosis will be available or that a disease can be detected and treated early to prevent irreversible damage.

The family may return to the genetic counselor a number of times to air their questions and concerns. It is desirable for the nurse working with the family to attend many or all of these counseling sessions. Because the nurse has already established a rapport with the family, the nurse can act as a liaison between the family and the genetic counselor. Hearing directly what the genetic counselor says helps the nurse clarify issues for the family, which in turn helps them formulate questions.

When the parents have completed the counseling sessions, the counselor sends them and their physician a letter detailing the contents of the sessions. The family keeps this document for reference. See Table 7–12.

Perhaps one of the most important and crucial aspects of genetic counseling in which the nurse is involved

TABLE 7-12	Nursing Responsibilities in Genetic Counseling

Identify families at risk for genetic problems.

Assist families in acquiring accurate information about the specific problem.

Act as liaison between family and genetic counselor.

Assist the family in understanding/dealing with information received.

Provide information on support groups.

Aid families in coping with this crisis.

Provide information about known genetic factors.

Assure continuity of nursing care to the family.

is follow-up counseling. The nurse with the appropriate knowledge of genetics is in an ideal position to help families review what has been discussed during the counseling sessions and to answer any additional questions they might have. As the family returns to the daily aspects of living, the nurse can provide helpful information on the day-to-day aspects of caring for the child, answer questions as they arise, support parents in their decisions, and refer the family to other health and community agencies (Mackta & Weiss 1994).

If the couple is considering having more children or if siblings want information concerning their affected brother or sister, the nurse should recommend that the family return for another follow-up visit with the genetic counselor. Appropriate options can again be defined and discussed, and any new information available can be given to the family. Many genetic centers have found the public health nurse to be the ideal health professional to provide such follow-up care.

Care must be taken not to assume a diagnosis, determine carrier status or recurrence risks, or provide genetic counseling without adequate information and training. Inadequate, inappropriate, or inaccurate information may be misleading or harmful. Health care professionals need to learn the appropriate referral systems and options for care in their region.

KEY CONCEPTS

A couple is considered infertile when they do not conceive after 1 year of unprotected coitus.

At least 10–15% of couples in the United States are infertile.

A thorough history and physical of both partners is essential as a basis for infertility investigation.

General fertility investigations include evaluation of ovarian function, cervical mucus adequacy and receptivity to sperm, sperm number and function, tubal patency, general condition of the pelvic organs, and certain laboratory tests.

Among cases of infertility, 40% involve male factors, 40% involve female factors, 10–20% have no identifiable cause, and 35% have multifactorial etiologies.

Medications may be prescribed to induce ovulation, facilitate cervical mucus formation, reduce antibody concentration, increase sperm count and motility, and suppress endometriosis.

The emotional aspect of infertility may be more difficult for the couple than the testing and therapy.

The nurse needs to be prepared to provide accurate information about infertility and dispel myths.

The nurse assesses coping responses and initiates counseling referrals as indicated.

In autosomal dominant disorders an affected parent has a 50% chance of having an affected child. Such disorders equally affect both males and females. The characteristic presentation will vary in each individual with the gene. Some of the common autosomal dominant inherited disorders are Huntington's chorea, polycystic kidney disease, and neurofibromatosis (von Recklinghausen's disease).

Autosomal recessive disorders are characterized by both parents being carriers; each offspring having a 25% chance of having the disease, a 25% chance of not being affected, and a 50% chance of being a carrier; and males and females being equally affected. Some common autosomal recessive inheritance disorders are cystic fibrosis, phenylketonuria (PKU), galactosemia, sickle-cell anemia, Tay Sachs disease, and most metabolic disorders.

X-linked recessive disorders are characterized by no male-to-male transmission; effects limited to males; a 50% chance that a carrier mother will pass the abnormal gene to her son; a 50% chance that her daughter will be a carrier; and a 100% chance that daughters of affected fathers will be carriers. Common X-linked recessive disorders are hemophilia, some forms of color blindness, and Duchenne muscular dystrophy.

Multifactorial inheritance disorders include cleft lip and palate, spina bifida, dislocated hips, clubfoot, and pyloric stenosis.

Some genetic conditions that can currently be diagnosed prenatally are neurotube and cranial defects, renal malformations, hemophilia, fragile X syndrome, thalassemia, cystic fibrosis, many inborn errors of metabolism such as Tay Sachs disease, and neural tube defects. This list expands daily as new technology allows more conditions to be detected.

The chief tools of prenatal diagnosis are ultrasound, maternal serum alpha fetoprotein testing, amniocentesis, chorionic villus sampling, and percutaneous umbilical blood sampling.

Based on sound knowledge about common genetic problems, the nurse should prepare the family for counseling and act as a resource person during and after the counseling sessions.

REFERENCES

American Fertility Society: New guidelines for the use of semen donor insemination. *Fertil Steril* 1990; 53(3):1s.

Amuzu B, Laxova R, Shapiro SS: Pregnancy outcome, health of children, and family adjustment after donor insemination. *Obstet Gynecol* 1990; 75:899.

Arms S: *Adoption: A Handful of Hope.* Berkeley, CA: Celestial Arts, 1990.

Blenner JL: Clomiphene-induced mood swings. *JOGNN* 1991; 20(4):321.

Braverman A, English M: Creating brave new families with advanced reproductive technologies. *NAACOG Clin Issues Perinat Women Health Nurs* 1992; 3(2):353.

CDC: Recommendations for use of folic acid to reduce number of spina bifida cases and other neural tube defects. *JAMA* 1993; 269(10):1233.

Chervenak FA, Issaacson GC, Campbell S: *Ultrasounds in Obstetrics and Gynecology.* Boston: Little, Brown, 1993.

Chervenak FA, McCullough LB: Nonaggressive obstetric management: An option for some fetal anomalies during the third trimester. *JAMA* 1989; 261(23):3439.

Cohen J, Malter HE, Talansky BE, Brifo J: *Micromanipulation of Human Gametes and Embryos,* New York: Raven Press, 1992.

Corson S: *Conquering Infertility.* New York: Prentice Hall, 1990.

Daglish CS: Therapeutic donor insemination. In: *Principles of Infertility Nursing.* Garner C (editor). Boston: CRC Press, 1991.

D'Alton ME: Prenatal diagnostic procedures. *Semin Perinatol* 1994; 18(3):140.

English M: Frontiers of reproductive technology: A review of assisted methods of reproduction. In: *Principles of Infertility Nursing.* Garner C (editor). Boston: CRC Press, 1991.

Filly RA, Callen PW, Goldstein RB: Alpha-fetoprotein screening programs: What every obstetric sonologist should know. *Radiology* 1993; 188(1):1.

Goode CJ, Hahn SJ: Oocyte donation and in vitro fertilization: The nurse's role with ethical and legal issues. *JOGNN* 1993; 22(2):106.

Guyer MS, Collins FS: The human genome project and the future of medicine. *AJDC* 1993; 147:1145.

Haas G: Antisperm antibodies. In: *Progress in Infertility.* Behrman S, Patton G, Holtz G (editors). Boston: Little, Brown, 1994.

Hammond M, Talbert L: *Infertility.* Oradell, NJ: Medical Economics Books, 1985.

Haney A: Treatment of endometriosis. In: *Progress in Infertility.* Behrman S, Patton G, Holtz G (editors). Boston: Little, Brown, 1994.

Hatcher RA et al: *Contraceptive Technology,* 16th ed. New York: Irvington, 1994.

Herbert C et al: Use of a sensitive pregnancy test before endometrial biopsies taken in the late luteal phase. *Fertil Steril* 1990; 53(1):162.

Hill L: Infertility and reproductive assistance. In: *Transvaginal Ultrasound.* Nyberg D et al (editors). St Louis: Mosby, 1992.

Hook EB et al: Maternal age-specific rates of 47,+21 and other cytogenetic abnormalities diagnosed in the first trimester of pregnancy in chorionic villus biopsy specimens: Comparison with rates expected from observations at amniocentesis. *Am J Hum Genet* 1988; 42:797.

Inati MN, Lazar EC, Haskin-Leahy L: The role of the genetic counselor in a perinatal unit. *Semin Perinatol* 1994; 18(3):133.

Jaffe SB, Jewelewicz R: The basic infertility investigation. *Fertil Steril* 1991; 56(4):599.

Jones SL: Assisted reproductive technologies: Genetic and nursing implications. *JOGNN* 1994; 23(6):492.

Journal of Black Nurses: A lay educator's approach to sickle cell disease education. 1992.

King CR, Schimke RN: Multifactorial inheritance. In: *Gynecology and Obstetrics* Vol. 5. Sciarra JJ (editor). Philadelphia: Harper & Row, 1994.

King RA, Rotter JI, Motulsky AG: *The Genetics of Common Diseases.* New York: Oxford Univ Press, 1992.

Lessor R et al: An analysis of social and psychological characteristics of women volunteering to become oocyte donors. *Fertil Steril* 1993; 59(1):65.

Luthy DA et al: Cesarean section before the onset of labor and subsequent motor function in infants with meningomyelocele diagnosed antenatally. *NEJM* 1992; 324(10):662.

Mackta J, Weiss JO: The role of genetic support groups. *JOGNN* 1994; 23(6):519.

Mahlstedt PP: The psychological components of infertility. *Fertil Steril* 1985; 43:335.

Mastroyannis C: Gamete intrafallopian transfer: Ethical considerations, historical development of the procedure, and comparison with other advanced reproductive technologies. *Fertil Steril* 1993; 60(3):389.

Menning E: *Infertility: A Guide for the Childless Couple,* 2nd ed. New York: Prentice Hall, 1988.

Mishell DR, Davajan V, Lobo RA: *Infertility, Contraception and Reproductive Endocrinology.* Boston: Blackwell Scientific Publications, 1991.

Morse C, Van Hall E: Psychosocial aspects of infertility: A review of current concepts. *J Psychosom Obstet & Gynecol* 1986; 6:157.

Mosher WD, Pratt WF: The demography of infertility in the United States. In: *Annual Progress in Reproductive Medicine.* Asch RH, Studd JW (editors). Pearl River, NY: Parthenon Publishing Group, 1993.

Nelson DL: Fragile X syndrome: Review and current status. *Growth—Genet & Hor* 1993; 9(2):1.

Office of Technology Assessment: Infertility: Medical and social consequences. Washington, DC: US Government Printing Office, 1988.

Olsen DG: Parental adjustment to a child with genetic disease: One parent's reflections. *JOGNN* 1994; 23(6):516.

Oostra BA et al: Guidelines for the diagnosis of fragile X syndrome. *J Med Genet* 1993; 30(5):410.

Pickler RH, Munro CL: Blastomere analysis: Issues for discussion. *JOGNN* 1994; 23(5):379.

Sandelowski M: On infertility. *JOGNN* 1994; 23(9):749.

Sawatzky M: Tasks of the infertile couple. *JOGNN* 1981; 10:132.

Schenker JG, Ezra Y: Complications of assisted reproductive techniques. *Fertil Steril* 1994; 61(3):411.

Shane J: Evaluation and treatment of infertility. *Clin Symp* 1993; 45:2.

Shulman LP et al: Mode of ascertainment is critical in assessing safety of percutaneous umbilical blood sampling. *Am J Perinatol* 1993; 10(1):27.

Simpson JL: Genetic factors in obstetrics and gynecology. In: *Danforth's Obstetrics and Gynecology*, 6th ed. Scott JR et al (editors). Philadelphia: Lippincott, 1990.

Simpson JL, Elias S: *Essentials of Prenatal Diagnosis*. New York: Churchill Livingstone, 1993.

Snowdon C: What makes a mother? Interviews with women involved in egg donation and surrogacy. *Birth* 1994; 21(2):77.

Society for Assisted Reproductive Technology, The American Fertility Society: Assisted reproductive technology in the United States and Canada: 1991 results from the Society for Assisted Reproductive Technology generated from the American Fertility Society Registry. *Fertil Steril* 1993; 59(5):956.

Speroff L, Glass RH, Kase NG: *Clinical Gynecologic Endocrinology and Infertility*, 5th ed. Baltimore: Williams & Wilkins, 1994.

Thompson MW, McInnes RR, Willard HF: *Thompson & Thompson's Genetics in Medicine*, 5th ed. Philadelphia: Saunders, 1991.

Townsend AB: Ethical issues of gamete and embryo donation: Implications for nursing. *J Perinatol* 1992; 12(4):359.

Wilcox LS, Mosher WD: Use of infertility services in the United States. *Obstet Gynecol* 1993; 82:122.

Wilcox LS et al: Defining and interpreting pregnancy success rates for in vitro fertilization. *Fertil Steril* 1993; 60(1):18.

Wolf GC, Baker CA: Tympanic thermometry for recording basal body temperatures. *Fertil Steril* 1993; 60(5):922.

World Health Organization: *WHO Manual for the Examination of Human Semen and Sperm–Cervical Mucus Interaction*. Cambridge, England: Cambridge Univ Press, 1992.

Wright L: Prenatal diagnosis in the 1990s. *JOGNN* 1994; 23(6):506.

PART THREE

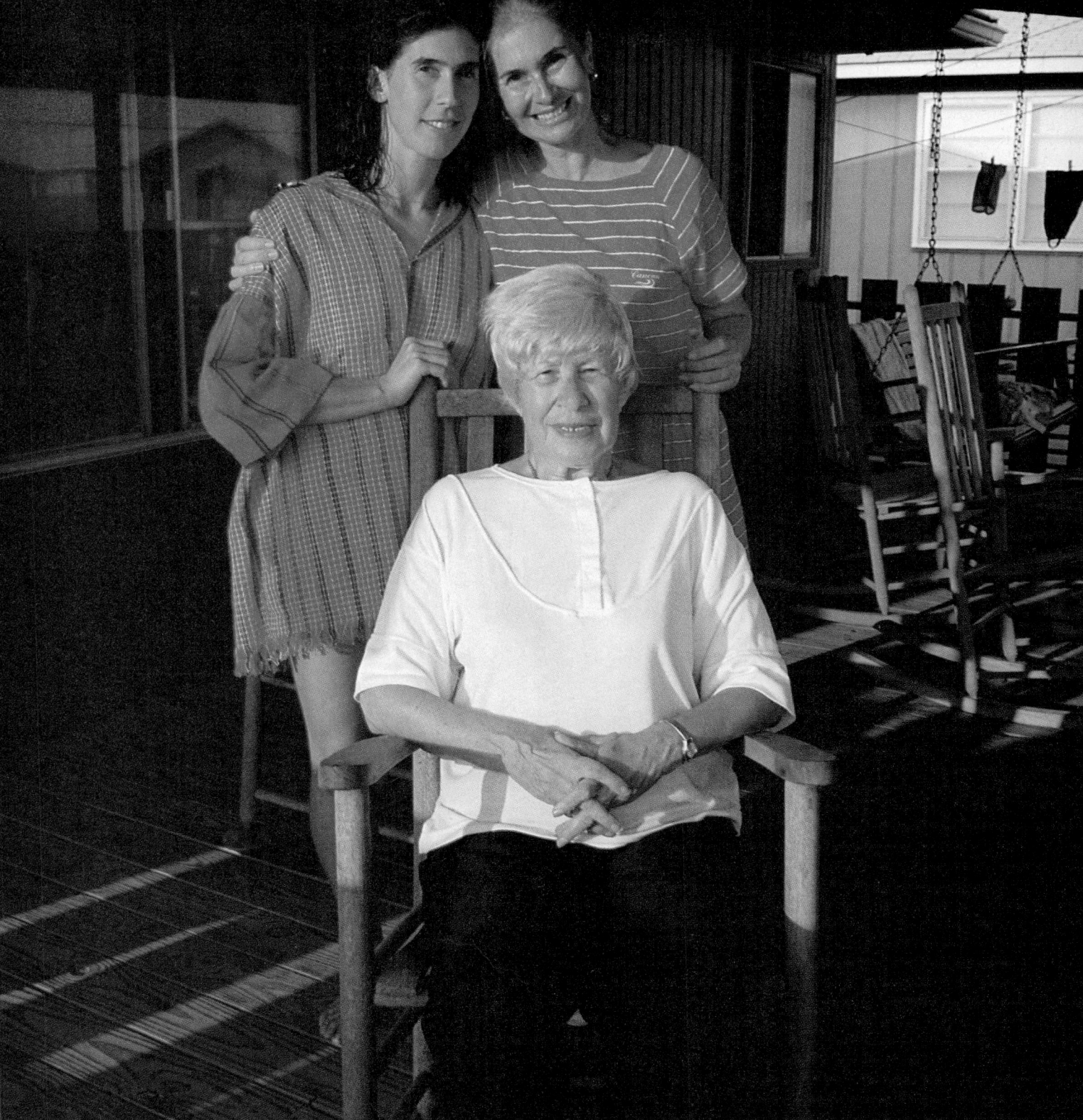

WOMEN'S HEALTH THROUGHOUT THE LIFESPAN

CHAPTER 8

WOMEN'S CARE: SOCIAL ISSUES

I don't think there has ever been a more exciting time for women. There are many challenges that face us: work, wage and role issues, safety in pregnancy and childbearing, and conflict over women's rights. On the other hand, women have never been more active and involved in the issues that affect them. The 1990's hold much promise for our future.

KEY TERMS

Child abuse

Child neglect

OBJECTIVES

Describe the concept of feminization of poverty.

Discuss the current work environment and the factors that affect women's wages.

Discuss work benefits that affect the childbearing woman.

Describe environmental hazards present in a childbearing woman's work setting.

Summarize the philosophical differences in the question of abortion.

Identify the factors that place parents at risk for child abuse.

Delineate the short- and long-term effects of child abuse on the child and other members of the family.

Identify the responsibilities of the nurse who suspects child abuse.

Cite the community resources available to violence-prone parents.

*W*omen of today have the opportunity to be dynamic, challenging, and challenged individuals. They have opportunities for personal and professional growth that did not exist 25 years ago. Because of political and social changes that have occurred in this country since the early 1970s, women's options have expanded dramatically. Although many women still choose the traditional "women's" careers and become nurses, teachers, and "at-home" mothers, others are entering occupations that until recently were filled almost exclusively by men. More women than ever have joined the ranks of lawyers and judges, managers and corporate heads, scientists, journalists, legislators, construction workers, plumbers, and other laborers. Women can be found in almost all occupations and thus are sharing in many of the benefits that come with these positions.

Progress has its costs, however. For example, the woman with a career and a family may have difficulty maintaining both. The woman who would like nothing more than to be an "at-home" wife and mother may be forced by the high cost of living to work outside the home and entrust the care of her children to others. The woman who has devoted her prime childbearing years to establishing a career rather than a family may find herself feeling pressure to find a partner and have children before it is too late.

Nurses must deal with many of the issues facing women, if not personally, then in their dealings with women as they come into the health care setting for maternal-newborn care. To help nurses better understand their clients' concerns and problems, this chapter addresses a few of the more serious issues facing women today.

WOMEN AND POVERTY

The harsh economic plight of many women is dramatically reflected in the growing phenomenon referred to as the *feminization of poverty*, a term suggested by Diana Pearce (1993). Simply stated, an increasing number of women live on incomes that fall below the poverty level, which in 1992 was $14,335 for a family of four (Bureau of the Census 1994).

The extent of this problem is enormous and increasing at a rapid rate. In 1991, 7% of two-parent households fell below the poverty level, and a staggering 46% of households headed by single mothers lived in poverty. Currently, about 20% of families with children are maintained by a woman alone, but that number is expected to increase dramatically in the coming decade. With a divorce rate approaching 50% and an out-of-wedlock birth rate of about 25%, the reality is that many children will spend at least a portion of their lives in a single-parent family. One researcher suggests that 50% of White children and 90% of children of African descent will be affected by this trend (Pearce 1993).

Even more disturbing is the portion of children in this country living in poverty. No other age group, not even the elderly, has a higher rate of poverty. Almost a quarter (23%) of children in the United States live below the poverty level. Two risk factors are especially significant in documenting poverty in children: female-headed family and race (Devine & Wright 1993). Approximately 59% of children living in female-headed homes fall below the poverty level. For children from minority groups who live in female-headed households the percentage falling below the poverty level is even more disturbing: 69.2% of African American children and 68.6% of Hispanic children (Bureau of the Census 1993). Currently, two-thirds of all poor people in this country are women and children; it is projected that by the year 2000 they will account for most of the people living in poverty (Figure 8–1).

The feminization of poverty extends beyond the United States. Females make up over half of the approximately 23.4% of people living in absolute poverty worldwide (Brown et al 1990), and women are expected to continue to be the majority of the over 50% worldwide

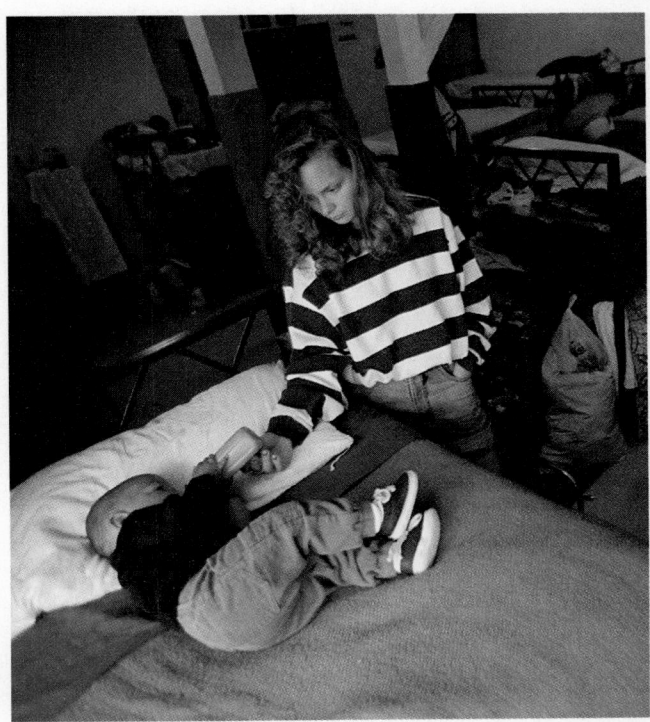

FIGURE 8–1 Two-thirds of all those Americans living in poverty are women and children.

poverty rate in 2050–2075 (Brown et al 1990). Considered globally, women must cope with some special problems: they live with the burden of working more than men but are being paid less for the same work; they are often expected to bear, raise, and feed many (preferably male) children; they are frequently abused and beaten in their own home; often they have few legal rights. The literacy rate for females is lower than that for males, and education—when available—is more frequently provided for men (Brown et al 1990).

Although the statistics on poverty may be shocking, they reveal little about what living with poverty is like. It is a day-by-day experience fraught with struggle and hardship.

I never thought this would happen to me. Things were so good for us and our daughter that I thought we would not be another one of those divorced families. Two months after I became pregnant with our second child, it was over. My husband left us. Suddenly, I am the sole support of myself and my children. It's like I'm dreaming, like a nightmare. I'm a teacher, and I've always had a good job, but I have taken time off to stay with our first child and haven't worked for the last two years. I thought it was important to stay at home and take care of our baby, and Jim felt that way too. Since he left I haven't been able to get a teaching position or any job. So now I don't have medical insurance or any benefits to help with this pregnancy. Applying for Medicaid has to be one of the most humiliating experiences I have ever had. I'm an intelligent woman with a college degree, and I couldn't figure out the forms. I'm smart really, surely I am, but I felt so dumb. The lines and the impersonal treatment that I had heard about but never believed in were there. I was a number and felt shuttled from one place to the next. You know, they don't do it on purpose. I know they have heard so many awful stories, but you know it hurt. It will take six weeks to qualify, and that means I will be more than halfway through the pregnancy. I've called and no one will accept me now, without paying money I don't have. I feel really caught. I know I should be getting prenatal care. I had problems with the last pregnancy, and I know care is important. I'm caught. I can't get care without money, and I'm afraid when I start care, they will be angry with me because I waited so long. It seems there is no way to win. There are only two doctors in our town who will accept Medicaid, and they are clear across town. It's all right. I'm thankful that I can get some help now when I need it, but it is so hard. I never dreamed I'd be in this position. I just never dreamed.

Contributing Factors

The feminization of poverty has occurred as a result of three major factors:

- The increase of families headed by females and the fact that these women bear almost all the economic burden of raising the children

- A labor market characterized by several factors that are not advantageous for women: women's lower wages; occupational gender segregation; and the disproportionately large number of women employed in temporary, part-time, or dead-end jobs (Matteo 1993)

- The welfare system

RESEARCH IN PRACTICE

Urban dwelling, socially disadvantaged women may be at increased risk for contracting and dying from AIDS. When these women become pregnant, a substantial number of them seek prenatal care, and thus the health care system may be able to interrupt the horizontal or vertical spread of AIDS. However, limited understanding of the knowledge and experiences of these clients may handicap health professionals in their efforts to design effective intervention programs. Katherine Kinsey developed a study to describe and explore the HIV/AIDS knowledge, attitudes, and beliefs of urban childbearing women.

The sample of 105 women came from an urban area classified as "distressed" with a high incidence of HIV/AIDS cases and 75% of the residents receiving some form of public assistance. At least 40% of the women described having one or more previous pregnancies fathered by different men and reported a history of one or more sexually transmitted diseases. All participants had received state mandated HIV/AIDS counseling and 71% had completed the HIV screening test.

Data collection included interviews, focus group discussions, and record reviews. Seventy percent of the women stated that they had no current risk of having HIV/AIDS, and 63% believed that they were not at risk for getting HIV/AIDS. The participants typically asserted that they were not at risk because they "knew their man." The rationale for their risk appraisals included commitment to their present monogamous relationships, results of negative prenatal screening for HIV, and personal strategies used to distance themselves from the possibility of contracting HIV and AIDS. During the focus groups the women reinforced each other's belief system and reassured the interviewer about the validity of their risk appraisals.

Clinical Application of Study

The author recommends abandoning the one-time counseling and HIV testing for this group of women in order to reduce their reliance on one test to apprise risk. With ongoing HIV/AIDS counseling and discussion during the entire prenatal period, the women might better understand HIV/AIDS testing and be more able to accurately assess their risk. The author further asserts that this population needs specific information about the actual meaning of HIV testing, partner responsibility, condom use and efficacy, and the effects of sexually transmitted diseases on themselves and their children.

SOURCE: Kinsey K: "But I know my man!" HIV/AIDS risk appraisals and heuristical reasoning patterns among childbearing women. *Holistic Nursing Practice* 1994; 8(2):79.

Increase in Female-Headed Households

The increase in the number of female-headed families is closely associated with divorce. Almost one out of every two marriages ends in divorce. As a result of divorce the woman's standard of living generally decreases significantly while the male's increases. This dramatic change in the standard of living is usually associated with the lower earning capacity of women and the fact that the children typically remain with the mother. Women receive custody of the children in over 75% of cases (Clarke 1995), but the economic assistance provided by the father often is minimal. Only about a third of divorced women receive child support from their former husbands (Devine & Wright 1993), and these legally awarded payments are frequently inadequate. Moreover, until recently, society has not really held men accountable for these payments. It fell to the woman to initiate the process of support enforcement through the courts, an emotionally draining and time-consuming effort that placed a further burden on her. Current trends are focusing on requiring recalcitrant divorced fathers to make their child support payments, and states are cooperating to help identify these men. A few states are testing programs in which unemployed men who owe child support are assigned to work programs so they can earn the money necessary to make their child support payments (Mead 1992).

Labor Market

Women have steadily increased their participation in the labor force. In 1970, 43.3% of females were employed; by 1992 that number had increased to 57.8%; and it is predicted that by the year 2005, 63% of females over age 16 will be part of the labor force (Bureau of the Census 1993). Unfortunately, the average woman employed year-round and full time makes only 71 cents for every dollar earned by a man (Pearce 1993). This occurs for a variety of reasons. About a third of women work in a cluster of occupations including cashier, child care worker, waitress, nurse, retail sales clerk, elementary school teacher, and secretary, which tend to be poorly paid when compared to male-dominated positions requiring comparable levels of responsibility, skill, and education. Although more women are entering professional fields such as medicine and law, the number of women in professions such as engineering and the hard sciences has not increased. Proportionately, the number of women in nontraditional occupations remains at 9%, unchanged over the past decade (Pearce 1993). Equally significant two-thirds of part-time workers are women; as such, their wages typically are lower, and they often have no fringe benefits, such as sick leave and health insurance.

For working divorced or single women with children the issue of child care is especially difficult. Child care is expensive and may place a burden on the household budget. Moreover, the responsibilities women face for ensuring the safety and well-being of their children may cause them to be viewed as unreliable or uncommitted to employers if they miss work because their children become sick. Currently, more enlightened employers are beginning to recognize and accommodate the needs of a female work force. Like other areas of reform, however, this trend tends to benefit women in better paying, more secure positions far more than it benefits women who are poor and in low-paying positions.

Welfare System

The welfare system provides much needed assistance to many women. Unfortunately, the amount of support provided is not sufficient even to raise the family income to the identified poverty level. Furthermore, the welfare system as it is currently designed provides disincentives to women to work. For example, a woman who works may need to use a large portion of her income to pay for child care. She may find that her income is significantly less when she works in a low-paying job and pays child care than when she stays home with her children and receives support, including food stamps and Aid to Families with Dependent Children (AFDC). In addition AFDC typically qualifies a woman for Medicaid payments. Because so many of the jobs available to women are low paying and without benefits, the value of the health care coverage Medicaid provides is often greater than the salary the woman would receive (Devine & Wright 1993).

Obviously, the welfare system provides disincentives to work, but, as Devine and Wright (1993, p 60) point out, "When the welfare system is more attractive than work, the solution is not to make work less attractive but rather to *make work more attractive.* . . . When the critics demand that people get off the welfare rolls and into jobs, they should understand that under current conditions they are asking poor people to make an economically irrational decision." To address this problem, an obvious first step is to supply ample opportunities for jobs with normal fringe benefits (especially health care), sufficient hours, and reasonable wages.

Other industrialized countries have avoided creating this subculture of impoverished women and children. Countries such as Germany, France, Austria, Denmark, Israel, Sweden, and the Netherlands view the support of female-headed households as a public responsibility. In these cases, a government agency first gives child support to the custodial parent and then seeks to collect the support money from the absent parent. Moreover, these countries also have reasonable family workplace policies, including child care, job protection, extended maternity leave, and health care for all (Couture 1991).

Homelessness

For many individuals the thought of a homeless person conjures up a vision of an older man curled in a doorway or making a home under a bridge. However, this vision is less accurate today than in the past; today's homeless have very different characteristics. Women and children now comprise approximately 33–40% of the homeless population (Kline & Saperstein 1992). Indeed, of the total homeless population, families with children are the fastest growing group (Whitman et al 1990).

A major factor contributing to the incidence of homelessness is the high cost of housing. During the past 20 years the costs of housing have increased far more than wages or other income sources, especially for women. Single-parent, female-headed households have seen their rent burden increase from an average of 35% of their income in 1974 to over 58% (Wolch & Dear 1993). The incidence of homelessness is also related to the extent of a woman's social support system. Because middle-class women typically have relatives and friends with more space and resources, they are able to avoid becoming homeless to a greater extent than poorer women. As Dornbusch (1993, p 162) states, "The women who typically head homeless families are desperately trying to avoid homelessness, but they can no longer count on their social-support network."

Health risks and problems of the homeless are greater than in the general population. Malnutrition predisposes the homeless to a variety of respiratory and nutritional disorders. A study of a group of homeless children revealed that half had current or recurrent health problems of which more than 80% were classified as acute (Eddins 1993). A disproportionately high number of homeless children have not received preventive health care services such as immunizations.

Effects on Health Care

The effects of poverty on health care are extensive. Since 1981, many funding cuts have directly affected programs that benefited those living in poverty. Funding cuts to Aid to Families with Dependent Children resulted in the discontinuation of support to over half the working families that had received AFDC prior to 1981. Equally significant, the value of AFDC payments dropped so that by 1990 the median AFDC monthly benefit for a family of three was $364, which is less than half the current poverty level (Wolch & Dear 1993). The Food Stamp Program has stopped assisting a million people due to decreased funding, and the Women, Infants, and Children (WIC) Program is currently able to provide assistance to less than half those who are eligible (Dutton 1993). These cuts come at a time when the benefits of adequate nutrition and prenatal care have been documented to have significant health care dollars for every dollar spent.

Lack of health insurance is also a major problem for the poor. Thirty-seven million Americans have no health insurance, and another seven to ten million have inadequate coverage. In 1990 over half with incomes less than $20,000 were without medical coverage. Medicaid cur-

rently serves only 40% of the poor and near poor, which is a decrease from the 65% served in 1976 (Dutton 1993). Decreases in health insurance have led to declines in preventive health care that are costing American dollars and even lives. For example, children's immunization rates have fallen significantly in recent years, especially among non-Whites; so a resurgence of childhood illnesses is occurring, especially in urban areas. For example, the incidence of measles in the US increased from 1497 in 1983 to over 30,000 in 1990, with over 60 reported deaths. This is especially important in light of the fact that immunizations are a very effective preventive health care approach estimated to save $10 for every $1 spent (Dutton 1993).

The issue of universal health care coverage is a significant one, especially for women living in poverty. Statistical data already are beginning to reflect the change in health insurance coverage and funding cuts. Women who do not receive prenatal care are three times more likely to have low-birth-weight babies, and the incidence of low-birth-weight babies is increasing. Overall, infant mortality has decreased fairly rapidly throughout this century until 1980. At that time the infant mortality rate continued to decline but at a much slower rate. In the late 1980s there was no further decline, and the overall rate even showed some trend toward a slight increase. In poor areas the increase in infant mortality has been marked.

Suggestions for Nursing Action

The issue of women and poverty is critical, and the implications for childbearing care are very real. A pregnant woman who is suffering economically may also suffer physically and psychologically. The physical and psychologic states of the woman depend on her access to health care and her financial ability to act on her health care providers' recommendations. In the end it is often the children who suffer the most, bearing the physical and psychologic scars of their mothers' struggles.

Nurses should be concerned about the issue of women and poverty for two primary reasons. One is related to the nurse's professional role. The health care system and thus nursing are intricately woven into the political and social structures of society. Nurses often work with women on welfare; they *see* the effects of poverty on childbearing families and the pain and struggles of these families. The limited resources of these women often stymie nurses' efforts to provide quality care.

The other reason for concern is largely personal. The majority of nurses are women, and like the teacher quoted earlier, some nurses may find themselves in financial difficulty, frequently due to circumstances beyond their control.

What can nurses do about the growing problem of female poverty? The following sections include suggestions for action that nurses can take to ease this crisis.

Personal Action

Be aware of your own beliefs about poverty and the women who need public assistance.

Explore your feelings regarding poverty.

Remain knowledgeable about the impact of poverty on the childbearing woman and her family.

Speak out to inform others of the facts; correct misconceptions.

Client Action

Be sensitive in assessing a woman's economic status during intake interviews. Use the knowledge of the current extent of this problem to try to identify other women who may be at risk.

Provide supportive counseling, and determine the woman's ability to follow a treatment plan or accomplish self-care measures, especially when extra expenditure of funds is required.

Stay knowledgeable about community resources to assist the woman with financial need and be prepared to offer suggestions and counseling regarding possible resources. It is much more helpful to give a group name and a phone number than to send the woman out to search on her own.

Community Action

When possible, work with community organizations and planners to identify financial needs of childbearing women in the community.

Offer your nursing expertise to community groups to help them meet the financial and health needs of childbearing women and their families.

Political Action

Know your legislators and their views. Be available to discuss issues and act as a resource for them as they become more knowledgeable about issues that affect childbearing women.

Make your opinions and ideas known to your legislators.

Support programs that benefit childbearing women and help identify areas that need to be addressed.

Educate the legislators about the alarming increase in poverty among women.

Research Action

Investigate the impact of poverty on the health and welfare of childbearing women and their families.

When women are unable to obtain adequate care, document it so this information will be available for future use.

Conduct research projects to dispel myths associated with poverty.

WOMEN IN THE WORKPLACE

The discrepancy between men's and women's wages is caused by many factors. From the beginning women's wages were purposely set lower than men's simply because it was a woman doing the job. The work of men and women was not valued equally. Unfortunately, this belief still affects women in the workplace.

Young women traditionally have been socialized in ways that affect their opportunities and expectations, and this may ultimately contribute to wage discrepancy. Boys are encouraged to develop a competitive spirit first in sports and then in other areas of their lives. They learn that "being a winner" and "knowing how to play the game" are valued qualities. Girls are usually not encouraged to develop a competitive spirit; many cultures do not view competitiveness as an important or desirable trait for a girl to have. Girls learn from parents, the media, their peers, and others that physical attractiveness is the key to success because it is more likely to earn popularity than being smart.

Education is also a significant factor in the socializing of women. The AAUW (American Association of University Women) report, *How Schools Shortchange Girls* (1992), identifies stereotypes and addresses issues influencing the education girls receive, including:

- Historically, girls have been seen as stronger in verbal areas than boys, but recent research suggests that these differences have decreased significantly.

- Differences between boys and girls in mathematics achievement are small and decreasing. The differences that exist are related to sample age, academic selectivity, and cognitive level being tested. No differences exist at age 9, the differences are minimal at age 13, but by age 17 a large difference, favoring males, exists.

- Girls tend to doubt their competence in math more than boys do.

- Gender differences in science may be increasing.

- More boys choose careers in science and engineering. Girls who choose careers in these fields report that the encouragement of teachers played an important role in their decision.

- Despite some progress, textbooks continue to show subtle language bias, absence of women from accounts of technological advances, neglect of information on women as shapers of history, and a scarcity of scholarship on women.

- Girls' self-esteem decreases as they go through school, although the exact reason has not been identified. Researchers have suggested that the continuous curricular message that the lives of women count for less than those of men may play a role in this decrease.

- Males typically receive more teacher attention than females as well as more specific, helpful evaluative comments about the quality of their work.

- Evidence indicates that boys do not treat girls well. Reports of sexual harassment in junior high and high school are increasing. These episodes reflect attitudes about power as much as about sexuality and can be very demoralizing to girls if not controlled by school officials.

The information in the AAUW report has sparked important discussions among parents and educators. If it leads to improved experiences for girls in academic settings, these will in turn contribute to more women seeking higher education and higher paying jobs and to a decrease in wage discrepancy.

Fortunately, there are also several factors exerting a positive force on the issue of wage discrimination.

- The number of women obtaining a college education continues to increase, and these women influence the work environment as they enter the work force.

- Many working women are holding their jobs for extended periods and are not as likely to work for short periods. They are gaining more experience in performing their jobs, and this has a positive effect on their productivity. As productivity rises, wages generally rise.

- Women have become more involved in the political arena and are raising the issue of *comparable worth*.

The basic premise of comparable worth is that the same wages should be paid for work that requires comparable skills, responsibility, education, and experience. This issue is quite controversial. Opponents suggest that, to the extent that job reevaluation results in major increases in women's salaries, comparable worth will increase unemployment and inefficiency, encourage women to remain in female-dominated jobs, decrease US ability to compete with foreign manufacturers, and reallocate limited salary resources away from lower-class, minority men to White, middle-class women (Rhode 1993). Research does suggest, however, that the costs of pay equity adjustments have been overestimated and could be accommodated if phased in gradually and logically (Rhode 1993). Moreover, in some companies comparable worth is a reality. Major companies such as IBM, AT&T, and Bank of America have instituted some forms of comparable

worth. At least 20 states have comparable worth legislation pending or have commissions studying the issue.

Nurses' Pay

Nurses as a group experience many of the same problems that confront women in the general work force. The average starting salary of a staff nurse in 1990 was $24,768, and the average maximum salary was $37,168. Nurses' salaries are still below what other professionals with similar education and responsibilities are paid. There is a variety of reasons for the continuing low wages for nurses, including the following:

- 96% of nurses are women, and as with other professions or job categories that are held mainly by women, wages stay in the low range.

- The majority of nurses are employed in hospitals, and in many communities there is only one hospital. Because of this lack of competition, the hospitals are in a position to keep wages low.

- There are only a few organized collective-bargaining groups for nurses.

- The recent federal, state, and local efforts to cut and contain health care costs have created a climate in which jobs are eliminated and pay increases are delayed.

Suggestions for Nursing Action

What can nurses do about wage discrimination in the health care system? What can nurses do to help clients who are suffering financially because of wage discrimination? The following sections include suggestions for actions nurses can take.

Personal Action

Seek information regarding the wages for nurses in your community.

Share wage information with other nurses so more people will be informed. When wages are kept secret, disparities are more likely to exist.

Validate what it is that you do as a nurse and why you are cost-efficient so you will know your own worth and will be better able to discuss wages.

Help other nurses maintain their self-esteem and feelings of worth.

Client Action

Encourage women to push for wage equity.

Encourage women to talk together about wages so inequities can be identified.

Community Action

Work with community leaders and groups to identify the lack of adequate jobs and wage inequity in your community.

Political Action

Educate legislators about the status of womens' wages and the impact low wages have on health care for the childbearing woman and her family.

Support programs that enhance employment opportunities for fair wages for women.

Research Action

Investigate variables affecting the variations in pay across the country, by sex of the nurse and position.

Investigate salary negotiating skills and characteristics of nurses who are able to negotiate.

MATERNITY LEAVES AND CHILD CARE BENEFITS

Maternity Leaves

Combining a career with childbearing can be a challenging task. Moreover, leaving a job to have a child may result at the very least in lost experience, most commonly in lost benefits, perhaps a lost opportunity for promotion, and sometimes loss of the job completely.

Family options improved somewhat in 1993 when the Family and Medical Leave Act was signed into law by President Bill Clinton. This law permits employees to take up to 12 weeks of unpaid leave from work following the birth or adoption of a child. Employees may also take leave if faced with a personal serious illness or the illness of a spouse, child, or parent. During the leave, health insurance benefits must be continued, and employees are entitled to return to their former position or one considered comparable. Coverage is not mandated for employees who work less than 25 hours per week or who have been employed less than 1 year. Under the law eligible employees are required to provide 30 days' notice when possible and must furnish a physician's statement verifying the need.

Because the Family and Medical Leave Act applies only to companies with 50 or more employees, the vast majority of companies and about 25 million employees are not covered by the law (O'Brien et al 1993). Those employees still must rely on the policies, if any, that their employers have established. Over 30 states currently have legislation related to maternity or medical leave, and the 1993 act does not automatically supersede the legislation previously passed by these states. Companies are required to follow the statute that offers employees greater protection (Karsten 1994).

Discrimination against pregnant women remains an issue in some areas, so women need to be aware of their rights, which were established by the Pregnancy Discrimination Act of 1978. This act guarantees the following:

- A pregnant woman cannot be denied a job if she is able to perform major job functions.

- The same procedure for using sick-leave pay or disability benefits must be used for the pregnant woman as for other employees.

- Employee medical coverage must include pregnancy benefits.

- The mother can use all her maternity benefits without penalty.

When a woman is planning a pregnancy, she should acquire information regarding pregnancy benefits in her work setting. The state in which she lives will also have guidelines or regulations regarding pregnancy. Questions that the woman may need to address include the following:

- Can I be forced to go on leave because I am pregnant?

- What are my rights to sick leave or disability leave with my pregnancy?

- Can I lose my job for taking disability leave associated with pregnancy?

- Do I have any rights concerning infant care?

- Is my employer required to provide maternity benefits and insurance coverage?

Child Care Benefits

Child care has been a working woman's problem for years. Although some fathers are actively involved in meshing work and family responsibilities, the high percentage of single-parent households headed by a woman results in child care remaining a significant concern for women. Access to safe, reliable child care varies. In some areas there is a surplus of child care slots, but in major metropolitan areas such as New York and San Francisco actual availability is an issue (Ellis 1993). The biggest problem, however, is affordability. In the United States working women commonly spend 25% of their take-home pay for child care. Typically, a parent pays approximately $3000 annually, although this cost can reach $6000 or more in certain areas of the Northeast (Ellis 1993). This means that, on an average, a woman working full time must earn an extra $1.50/hour just to cover the cost of day care, more if she works only part time (Pearce 1993).

Currently, about 5400 employers provide some form of support for employees' child care needs through referral programs, on-site or near-site centers, or financial assistance (Friedman 1994). Other creative approaches to handling child care are also gaining in popularity. These include flextime scheduling, part-time work, job sharing, and telecommuting (working at home). For many women, however, child care is the most challenging of all the issues they face. Given increased attention from citizens, legislators, and business, a uniform child care policy may not be far away.

Critical Thinking Question

What benefits will be important for you as you enter your professional career?

Suggestions for Nursing Action

Personal Action

Examine the maternity and child care benefits in your own work environment. When questions arise or unmet needs are identified, follow the guidelines in your facility to suggest changes or additions in benefit policies.

Be knowledgeable about the current status of wage inequity and its effect on the childbearing woman's ability to afford adequate child care.

Once prepared with accurate knowledge, speak out when needed to provide information and correct inaccurate information about women's wages.

Client Action

Talk with women to identify whether their benefit packages are useful.

Encourage women to investigate the benefits in their own work setting.

Provide resources that can be used to learn about regulations regarding benefits on the community, state, and national levels.

Encourage women to pursue their questions regarding benefits until they are answered satisfactorily.

Community Action

Provide community leaders with information about the need for comprehensive maternal and child care benefits for childbearing women and their families.

Work within the community to identify benefits for the nursing profession.

Work with community and professional nursing groups to enhance the status of nursing.

Work with your professional nursing organizations to improve benefits for nursing.

Political Action

Write your legislators and support legislation that addresses and corrects wage inequities. Let your legislators know if you do not support legislation and why. Educate legislators about the importance of a national policy on parental leaves and child care.

Research Action

Investigate factors currently affecting public view of comparable pay.

ENVIRONMENTAL HAZARDS IN THE WORKPLACE

As more women enter the work force, they are exposed to an ever-increasing number of chemicals and environmental pollutants. Of the approximately 50,000 chemicals used today in industry, about 500 have been implicated as having potentially hazardous effects on reproduction (Bernhardt 1990). These include the following:

1. *Hazards of the microelectronic industry.* Study of the microelectronic industry has indicated that there is a link between various substances used in this field and birth defects, spontaneous abortions, and other reproductive problems. Among the "high-tech" hazards are glycol ethers, arsenic, lead, and radiation (Hembree 1986).

2. *Lead.* Lead was one of the first agents found to have adverse effects on reproduction. Lead contamination causes an increased rate of spontaneous abortions, stillbirths, and prematurity; surviving children are more likely to have impaired growth and neurologic damage (Bang et al 1983). A study of 35,000 female factory workers in Finland (Hembree 1986) demonstrated an increased spontaneous abortion rate in women who worked in electronics and with lead soldering.

   Changes related to the reproductive system have also been reported in male workers who are exposed to lead. Several studies have indicated decreased libido, decreased sperm count, and abnormal sperm morphology. There is also an increased number of spontaneous abortions or stillbirths in pregnancies fathered by male workers exposed to lead (Winder 1989). The effects on the male reproductive system have been observed with high-level exposure and also with exposure that is within current recommendations of regulatory authorities for the workplace (Winder 1989).

Although research suggests that lead has adverse effects on the reproductive function of both female and male workers, only women are now excluded from exposure to lead in the workplace. This is based on a fetal protection policy stating that a woman in her reproductive years may be excluded from working with lead (Scialli 1989). The policy developed from the belief that a woman's exposure to lead can directly intoxicate the fetus.

3. *Vinyl chloride.* Vinyl chloride is used in the manufacture of plastics and resin (Bernhardt 1990). There is an increased incidence of spontaneous abortion and stillbirth in partners of male workers exposed to vinyl chloride. Studies indicate that the fetal death may be caused by chromosomal changes in the sperm (Schnorr 1988).

4. *Halogenated hydrocarbons.* Polychlorinated biphenyls (PCBs) are the most widely known halogenated hydrocarbons. They are used in the manufacture of plastics and as heat-exchange fluids in the electrical industry (Lione 1988). High-level exposure to PCBs has been associated with an increased spontaneous abortion rate, low birth weight, hyperpigmentation of Caucasian infants at birth (cola-colored skin), gingival hyperplasia, and tooth eruption at birth. Low-level exposure, which may occur from eating fish caught from PCB-contaminated waterways, may also cause low birth weight and reduced infant head size. PCBs may also be transferred to newborns through breast milk (Lione 1988).

5. *Antineoplastic drugs.* Female nurses who administer antineoplastic drugs may be at increased risk of menstrual irregularities, giving birth to infants with congenital anomalies, and fetal loss (Hewitt et al 1993). The Occupational Safety and Health Administration (OSHA) has outlined preventive measures nurses can employ to decrease the risk of exposure. These include using vertical laminar air flow (VLAF) hoods to reconstitute the medications and wearing disposable, impermeable gowns and latex gloves to prevent skin contact when handling the medication. In addition pregnant or lactating health care workers should be able to choose not to work with these medications or the individuals receiving them (Hewitt et al 1993).

6. *Video display terminals (VDTs).* Questions regarding the safety of exposure to video display terminals have arisen in recent years, and various studies have produced contradictory results. However, a well-designed, comprehensive study by Schnorr and colleagues (1991) at NIOSH (National Institute for Occupational Safety and Health) found no increased risk of spontaneous abortion or overall fetal loss in women whose work exposed them regularly to VDTs. Until more is known about the possibility of other biologic effects of chronic exposure to the low-frequency electromagnetic fields found with VDTs, women should avoid chronic exposure. Because the strength of the field decreases significantly with distance, this can be accomplished by sitting at least 50 cm (20 in) from the screen and at least 1 m (3.25 feet) from the sides or back of adjacent machines (because electromagnetic field strength is typically higher from the back and sides). Exposure is also decreased by turning off VDTs, printers, and other electrical devices when they are not in use (Paul 1993).

7. *Anesthetics.* Exposure to anesthetic agents such as nitrous oxide has been associated with increased spontaneous abortion rates and increased numbers of congenital anomalies (Schumann 1990). Anesthetists, exposed daily to anesthetic gases, have an increased risk of infertility as well as statistically significant higher rates of spontaneous abortion or children born with congenital anomalies (Collins 1990).

8. *Ionizing radiation.* Exposure to ionizing radiation for diagnosis or treatment has long been recognized as a significant risk during pregnancy. Radiation exposure has been associated with spontaneous abortions, stillbirths, congenital anomalies, developmental delays, mental retardation, seizures, and leukemia in the child exposed in utero (McAbee et al 1993). Workplace exposure is regulated primarily by three agencies: OSHA, the Nuclear Regulatory Commission (NRC), and the Mine Safety and Health Administration. Specific exposure limitations have been established. Workers who are anticipating pregnancy should be given accurate information about exposure levels, including dosage, frequency, and timing of exposure (Paul 1993).

9. Nurses have an occupational hazard in the exposure inherent in providing care for sick people. Exposure to toxoplasmosis, rubella, cytomegalovirus, herpes simplex, and hepatitis B may affect pregnancy and fetal outcome (Hewitt et al 1993). Exposure to HIV infection has also been a concern to health care professionals.

Environmental hazards are increasing with the discovery and development of new products, and they exert their effect on everyone in their environment. Women are at particular risk while they are in the childbearing years. Because no work environment is without risks, it is becoming more important for each woman to become knowledgeable about her own workplace. Information can be obtained from libraries, the public health department, and special agencies that collect data regarding environmental hazards.

Suggestions for Nursing Action

Environmental hazards are an area of particular interest and importance to maternal-newborn nurses. Not only does the health care environment carry some risk to each nurse, but also the nurse needs to be knowledgeable about the possible risks to which childbearing women are exposed. Nurses can be influential in encouraging more investigation of chemical substances and environmental hazards so that work environments will be safer for all.

Personal Action

Be knowledgeable about hazards in your own work environment.

Collect information regarding the effects of various environmental hazards on the childbearing woman and her family.

Follow guidelines and procedures in the work setting to decrease your risk.

Client Action

Obtain information about environmental hazards in the woman's work environment.

Suggest resources to the woman to enhance her knowledge.

Recommend resource groups to obtain more information.

Community Action

Work with community leaders and groups to identify environmental hazards in your community.

Provide education regarding the hazards to childbearing women.

Political Action

Provide information about environmental hazards in your community to your legislators.

Educate your legislators regarding the special effects of environmental hazards on the childbearing woman and her family.

Support legislation that addresses and solves problems involving environmental hazards.

Research Action

Document problems that are observed during your care of clients.

ABORTION

Abortion is a highly charged issue, and people for and against legalized abortion are known for their heated confrontations. Even the terms used to refer to those with differing philosophic opinions about abortion are cause for argument. The antiabortion philosophy is dubbed "pro-life," and the proabortion philosophy is called "pro-choice." This seems to suggest that the pro-choice philosophy would not be in favor of life. It is partly this politicizing terminology that works to polarize opposing viewpoints.

The abortion issue is one that different factions have dealt with in one way or another for centuries. For the past 200 years the policies and philosophies in the United States have been directed primarily by the medical community. Through the first half of this century, abortion was a topic not to be discussed; it was a private matter. An important result of this privacy was that even though people held many divergent opinions about abortion, those adhering to each philosophic position believed their opinions were those of the majority. In the 1960s an effort to clarify laws and philosophies made the issue of abortion an open one; it was no longer a private issue that one could quietly hope others would solve in the "right way." More importantly, people discovered that their opinion was not necessarily that of the majority.

There are many different opinions and many issues associated with abortion. Four major arguments that are the basis of differing feelings about the rightness or wrongness of abortion are often presented. These include the following:

1. The moral status of the embryo. Historically, the status of the embryo has been ambiguous from philosophic, religious, and moral viewpoints. Questions of the legal status of the fetus, the use of medical technology, and the value of children are central to this argument.

2. The moment that life begins. The fact that the heartbeat of a developing embryo can be observed by the end of the first month of gestation is accepted by both sides. However, there is no agreement on what this fact means. A heartbeat is necessary for life, but the ability to breathe is also critical to maintain life. Does the fact that there is a heartbeat prove that life exists, or does life require a heartbeat and the ability to breathe?

3. The personhood of the embryo. Personhood carries with it inalienable rights to due process in our society. The question, then, is whether the embryo is a person.

4. The woman's role in our society. The ability to have an abortion gives the woman control over her reproductive life. In establishing this control, however, the role of motherhood becomes just one role that women might choose. Some opponents fear that legal abortion devalues motherhood and the decision to remain in the home to raise children.

The abortion issue is clearly a complex one involving many philosophic points, values, and opinions. Debate regarding abortion continues in the 1990s as groups speak out and protest publicly against those with perceived opposing views. The Supreme Court continues to consider cases that challenge the 1973 *Roe v Wade* decision, such as *Webster v Reproductive Health Services* (1989). Individual states are also striving to enact abortion policies that address at what point an abortion may be done and under what circumstances, where it may be done, and if spousal or parental permission is required. Some states are adding a required informational session that precedes the abortion decision and a waiting period between the informational session and the abortion procedure. The debate extends into the development of new contraceptive techniques and has focused on the testing of RU 486 (a French drug that has been used to cause abortion) at selected sites in the United States.

One of the questions that concerns both proabortion and antiabortion groups is the possible psychologic impact of having an abortion or of carrying an unwanted pregnancy to term. Clearly, on the public scene, in the legislative arena, and in people's private beliefs, the abortion issue is one that continues to raise many questions (Annas 1989; Ashley & O'Rourke 1994).

The implications of abortion for maternal-newborn nurses are also complex. All nurses will have many opportunities over the course of a professional nursing career to examine their personal feelings and opinions, and there is a good chance that these opinions will change over time as they have new experiences and insights.

The philosophies of nurses mirror those of the society at large and it may be difficult to provide care for an individual who is participating in a procedure with which the nurse disagrees. If a client is having an abortion, the nurse who does not support abortion may be faced with a decision about whether to provide care. In some settings nurses do not have to provide care for women having an abortion if it is against their own personal philosophy and if another nurse is available to provide care. The nurse with a pro-choice philosophy may have difficulty understanding how a professional colleague could possibly choose not to care for a client based on the client's personal beliefs. If a nurse can choose not to care for a woman having an abortion, can the nurse also choose not to provide care for an alcoholic? A drug addict? A person of another race or religion? The questions facing nurses about the abortion issue have implications for other areas of nursing.

Suggestions for Nursing Action

Personal Action

Explore your own feelings and beliefs regarding abortion.

Talk with others and gather information about abortion.

Be knowledgeable about the issues involved.

Client Action

If your beliefs allow you to care for women considering abortion, provide counseling and support to women as they seek information. If your beliefs do not allow you to care for women who choose abortion, avoid imposing your opinions on them. Provide factual information.

Be nonjudgmental when working with women who have abortions.

Community Action

Work with community groups that support your views.

Support adequate health care for women regardless of the option that the woman choose (to seek an abortion or to continue with the pregnancy).

Political Action

Provide education, support, and assistance to legislators in order to attain legislation that promotes your philosophy and ensures safe care for women.

FAMILY VIOLENCE

Family violence is a major health issue for women worldwide. Violence against women in the form of female partner abuse or sexual assault is covered in detail in Chapter 11. Violence against children is discussed in this chapter.

Child Abuse

My daughter looks at me, her eyes brimming with tears and her face strained. We sit across from each other clutching ceramic cups of hot chocolate—something to try to bring comfort. She has heard me spill out part of the memories of childhood sexual abuse that I have been reliving and has seen part of the pain that is my insides. She has listened, and with each word it looks like I have struck her, that the words reach out and lash at her. She is hearing and feeling my pain, and I think maybe I shouldn't do this, maybe she shouldn't know, maybe I should protect her, maybe my tormentors were right, I shouldn't tell. But I need her to know. I need her to be able to share this life-changing process with me and mostly to know that her mother is alright.

The pain is there, swirling on the red formica tabletop. It is in her eyes. It is in my fingers that clench the cup. It is in the napkin that I twist. It is in my shoulders that I no longer seem to be able to hold up. It is in my downward gaze as I consider whether it is alright to look up at her and in that instant that our eyes meet to fear that this is the moment I will see doubt and disgust in her eyes. It is in my heart and soul and in every cell of my body. And she looks at me. There is no doubt, no disgust. She says, "I know this happens to people, but, oh no, not you . . . not my mom." And inside I say, "Thank you my daughter, thank you for believing me."

One of the most disastrous results of dysfunctional parenting is child abuse. Child abuse arises in part from the cultural sanctioning of physical discipline of children by their parents. Among the many serious effects of child abuse are physical handicaps, poor self-image, inability to love others, antisocial or violent behavior in later life, and death. Over 2.9 million reports of suspected physical or sexual child abuse or neglect are filed annually in the United States. Abuse or neglect results in the deaths of more than 1000 children each year (Devlin & Reynolds 1994). The problem is far more pervasive than these numbers indicate, however, because of the untold number of cases of abuse or neglect that are never reported.

A small number of abusing parents are mentally ill, but most have less serious problems that respond to intervention. Parents at risk for abusive behavior may manifest one or more of the risk factors identified in Table 8–1.

TABLE 8–1	Parental Risk Factors for Child Maltreatment
Risk Factor	**Assessment Finding**
Lack of nurturing experience	Inadequate experience with parenting (eg, multiple foster homes)
	Parent neglected or abused as a child
	Parent expected to meet high demands of own parents as a child
Lack of knowledge of normal growth and development	Inability to read "cues" of child
	Impatience when child does not respond as expected; unreasonable discipline
	Unrealistically high expectations for the child
Isolation	Inadequate use of supports
	Inability to identify resources
	Unknown to others in community
Low self-esteem	Lack of trust, particularly of authority figures
	Expects rejection
High vulnerability to criticism	History of family violence in family of origin or in current family system (eg, female partner abuse)
	Impulsive
Many unmet needs	Feelings of being unloved or having unresponsive partner, unstable marriage, or no relationship at all
	Youthful marriage, forced marriage, unwanted pregnancy
Multiple stressors	Poverty, unemployment, substandard housing, lack of job opportunities
	Inadequate clothing and insufficient food
Substance abuse	Abuse of alcohol or drugs
Role reversal	Emotional immaturity, lack of patience, inability to make judgments
	Preoccupied with self
	Depression
	Dependent on others

SOURCE: Adapted from Mott SR et al: *Nursing Care of Children and Families,* 2nd ed. Redwood City, CA: Addison-Wesley Nursing, 1990, p 589.

Child abusers are found among all socioeconomic, religious, and ethnic groups. Some child abusers are irrational or even psychotic, but most are ordinary people who feel trapped in stressful life situations with which they cannot cope satisfactorily. Many abusive parents are simply confused and overwhelmed by parenthood or by life in general and vent their frustrations on their children. Because all parents have negative feelings about their children at one time or another, the difference between parents who abuse and those who do not is often only a matter of degree. All parents are at risk occasionally, but most are able to channel their frustration and anger appropriately.

The parent with a potential for abuse is one who feels isolated, is unable to trust others, is too passive to be able to give, or has very unrealistic expectations for children. Parents at risk for abuse tend to expect their children to perform for their gratification, and they tend to use severe physical punishment to ensure a child's proper behavior. Parents who abuse their children are likely to have been abused as children. This multigenerational pattern of child abuse, although disturbing, does help in identifying families in need of prevention.

Many abusive parents also have unrealistic expectations for themselves and unknowingly contribute to their problems. For example, one parent waxed the kitchen floor during a snowstorm and then abused the child who tracked mud into the house. The parent's behavior and their expectations for the child clearly contributed to the problem.

Parents with a potential for abuse often expect their children to meet their needs and therefore are most likely to abuse a child who is viewed as "different."

Children at risk for abuse may be the result of difficult pregnancies or births or those born at inconvenient times, born out of wedlock, the "wrong" sex, or too active or too passive. Some children are abused because they are the result of a forced pregnancy with an unloved partner or the result of rape or incest. Others have characteristics, such as looks and mannerisms, that evoke negative associations in the abusing parent. Children who have been separated from their families because of prematurity or neonatal disease are more likely to be at risk for abuse. Children with congenital anomalies, mental retardation, hyperactivity, or chronic illness are also at risk. Children with abnormal sleep-wake patterns or feeding difficulties and those who are unresponsive to care giving might also be at risk if they are living in a family with other risk factors (Mott et al 1990). Only a small percentage of premature or difficult children, however, are abused, and for all abused children it is the combination of parental deficiencies and characteristics of the child that create the problems leading to abuse.

Child abuse is most likely to occur during times of crisis. The parent's loss of a job, for example, might be just enough to make the crying of a fretful infant unbearable. Some families hover on the brink of perpetual crisis, living with constant changes that contribute to feelings of inadequacy. The magnitude of the crisis is not always in proportion to the abuse. A relatively minor crisis might be viewed as the "last straw" in an unhappy situation.

Solving a crisis for troubled families is not enough if new crises and stressors merely reestablish dysfunctional patterns. Instead, the nurse teaches parents to develop their own coping strategies and to identify when and how to seek help. Parents who learn the problems inherent in isolation, for example, will then seek assistance when under stress and will avoid the patterns of behavior that cause them to abuse their children.

Types of Abuse

Child abuse or maltreatment may be physical, emotional, or sexual. The nurse needs to assess for all forms of abuse (Figure 8–2). The consequences of emotional and sexual abuse are not as obvious as those of physical abuse, but the effects of these types of abuse may last longer and be more damaging to the personal development of the child. Munchausen syndrome by proxy (MSP) is an unusual type of child abuse in which the parent invents or directly induces the child's illness or injury symptoms and then seeks medical assistance, which results in the child undergoing unnecessary, expensive, potentially harmful medical tests and procedures. Approximately 10% of children who are victims of MSP die each year; 25–33% of cases involve more than one child in a given family (Smith & Killam 1994). Although the perpetrator of this abuse may be the father or another caretaker, it is most often the mother. The reasons for the perpetrator's need to have the child be ill are not well understood, and MSP remains a difficult problem to diagnose and treat. Care of these families requires a multidisciplinary approach and long-term therapy.

Documentation

Child *neglect* can be defined as failure by parents or other custodian to meet the medical, emotional, physical, or supervisory needs of a child, whereas **child** *abuse* is nonaccidental physical or threatened harm and includes mental and emotional injury, sexual abuse, and sexual exploitation (Allen & Hollowell 1990). In situations of child abuse and neglect, documentation of evidence is vital.

Records provide the legal basis for intervening on behalf of the child. Nursing history and daily notes need to be accurate, timely, and objective. The goal of documentation is to provide a written account of each visit or contact. If the nursing records become part of a court proceeding, they need to portray a family by specifying behaviors that indicate progress or failure in providing a safe, nurturing environment for the child. In some neglect cases much of the evidence is intangible and difficult to prove; therefore input from many professionals is necessary to convince the court that a child is actually at risk for abuse or neglect. Evidence of risk might include the

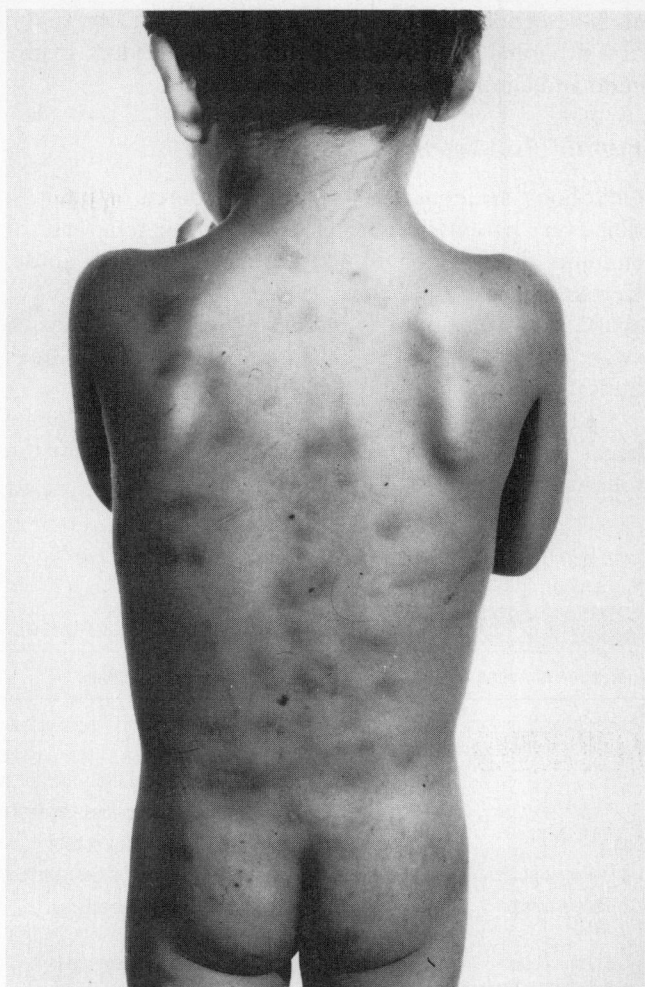

FIGURE 8-2 An abused child may display numerous bruises and scars. SOURCE: Mott SR et al: *Nursing Care of Children and Families,* 2nd ed. Redwood City, CA: Addison-Wesley Nursing, 1990, p 603.

doctor's and nurse's notes on the child, the school nurse's report, and the social worker's impressions during a home visit regarding the child's physical appearance; interactions with parents, peers, and other adults; ability to respond to questions; and general development. Evidence of neglect might include developmental delays, substance abuse, poor medical care, poor school attendance, or lack of supervision. Careful documentation and recorded evidence are essential when presenting a case to the judicial system.

Child Abuse and the Role of the Nurse

By the nature of their work, nurses in a variety of settings are involved in the identification, treatment, and prevention of child abuse and neglect. In most states nurses and other health care providers are legally obligated to report any case of suspected child abuse or neglect. The nurse's early detection of child abuse and neglect may lead to the first attempts to intervene and provide services to the child and family.

Family Assessment

Childhood accidents are a common source of injuries; thus every parent who brings a child in for treatment of an injury should not automatically be suspected of abuse. Certain physical and behavioral findings are indicative of abuse, however, and it is important for the nurse to be aware of these clues. Tables 8–2 and 8–3 list the findings indicative of physical and sexual abuse.

In all cases of suspected abuse or neglect the nurse needs to ask the child and family members present the following questions:

1. How did the accident (or incident) happen?
2. When did the accident happen?
3. Where were the child and other family members at the time?
4. Who was caring for the child at the time?
5. Who saw the accident?
6. What did the child do after the accident?
7. What measures were taken by the parent?

Questions to the parents should be phrased in a nonjudgmental way to decrease the likelihood of hostile or defensive responses. For example, it is more effective to ask "How did this burn occur?" than to ask "How did you do this?" Similarly, open-ended questioning of the child in

---

TABLE 8-2   Signs and Symptoms of Physical Abuse

Indication of Abuse	Assessment Findings
Bruises or welts on ears, eyes, mouth, lips, torso, buttocks, genital areas, calves	Injuries may be in shape of object used to produce them (eg, sticks, belts, hairbrushes, buckles)
	Injuries located on parts of body not usually injured, such as bruising behind the ear, bleeding into the conjunctiva or retina, pinch marks on genitals (normal bruises commonly appear on forehead, shins, knees, elbows)
	Injuries often in various stages of healing
Burns	Shape suggests type of burn
Immersion burns	Immersion burns on feet have "socklike," on hands "glovelike," on buttocks or genitals "donutlike" appearance
Pattern burns	Pattern suggests object used (eg, iron, stove grate, electric burner, heater); small, circular burns on feet, face, hands, chest, or buttocks suggest cigar or cigarette
Friction burns	Friction burns on legs, arms, neck, or torso may be caused by child having been tied up with rope
Scald burns	Caused by hot liquid poured over trunk or extremities; multiple splash marks may appear on body; depth of burn varies with temperature of liquid, length of contact, and presence of clothing
Fractures of skull, face, nose, orbit, long bones, ribs	Multiple or spiral fractures caused by twisting motion
	Evidence of epiphyseal separations and periosteal shearing
	Shaft fractures from direct blows
	Fractures may be in various stages of healing if earlier fractures went untreated
Lacerations or abrasions on mouth, lips, gums, eyes, genitals	Human bite marks, especially those of adult size, may be evident
	Torn frenulum in infant from forcing object into mouth
	Puncture wounds or deep scratch marks from fingernails around face or genital area
Head trauma	Evidence of increased intracranial pressure in infant (eg, bulging fontanelle)
	Subdural hematomas from being dropped on the head or from receiving blows to the head; if abuse is repetitive, separation of cranial sutures may be evident due to chronic subdural hematoma
	Areas of baldness and swelling from hair being pulled out when dragging the child by the hair
Neck trauma	Limited range of motion from whiplash injury due to being shaken
	Dislocation or subluxation of neck
Somatic	Persistent vomiting or abdominal pain
	Rigid abdomen due to internal bleeding
	Shock
Child's behaviors	Extreme aggressiveness or withdrawal; wariness of adults; fear of going home; apprehension when other children cry
	Appears disinterested or frightened of parents, shows no emotion when parents leave or return
	Indiscriminate friendliness and immediate affection shown toward anyone providing attention
	Vacant stare; no eye contact
	Surveys environment but remains motionless
	Stiffens when approached as if expecting punishment of a physical nature
	Inappropriate response to painful procedures

SOURCE: Adapted from Mott SR et al: *Nursing Care of Children and Families,* 2nd ed. Redwood City, CA: Addison-Wesley Nursing,1990, p 593.

private ("Would you tell me more about this?") will elicit more information than questions requiring a "yes" or "no" response. To protect the child, do not reveal to the parents information given by the child (Devlin & Reynolds 1994). After recording answers to these questions, the nurse proceeds with the physical assessment, noting the location, color, and characteristics of all cutaneous lesions. Photographs might be needed as legal evidence.

Orthopedic, surgical, ophthalmologic, and gynecologic examinations also might be needed, depending on the type of injuries. Gynecologic examination includes cultures for gonorrhea and other sexually transmitted infections, microscopic examination for blood and sperm, pregnancy testing, and clothing examination for semen, blood, or pubic hairs. Strict procedures must be followed in collecting evidence and specimens to provide data the courts will accept.

The most important determination to make during the assessment is the risk of reinjury to the victim or injury to other children in the household. Assessment of family functioning, coping strategies, and current state of crisis provides valuable data for such determination. Sometimes, even when the injuries are not severe, hospitalization or foster home placement is necessary. Protection of the child (or children) is always the priority.

In assessing neglected or abused children and their families, the nurse considers the long-term consequences of neglect and their possible effects on family cooperation in meeting goals. Assessment of neglected or abused children and their families include the following:

- The parents' emotional ability to accept services
- Communication patterns within the family
- The range and availability of services
- The family's use of services
- Supportive counseling for all family members
- The children's growth and developmental patterns
- The parents' attempts to diminish isolation
- The parents' responses to expectations to change behaviors
- The quality of nurturance within the family
- Family dynamics and other risk factors such as substance abuse or spouse abuse
- Environmental stressors such as inadequate housing, hygiene, or nutrition

Support for Dysfunctional Parents

Providing parental supports to marginally functioning parents is preferable to removing the child from the home. Removing children is traumatic, and most communities lack adequate foster care homes. Foster care is more expensive than maintaining the family system. Dysfunctional parents also tend to continue the cycle of dysfunctional parenting with other children in the family.

TABLE 8-3	Signs of Sexual Abuse
Physical Signs	**Behavioral Signs**
Laceration of labia, vagina, or perineum	Advanced knowledge of adult sexual behavior
Irritation, pain, or injury to genital area	Discussion of or implied involvement in sexual activity
Hematomas in genital area	Expression of severe emotional conflict at home with fear of intervention
Vaginal or penile discharge	Reluctance to participate in sports, showers, changing of clothes
Dysuria or urinary frequency	Excessive bathing
Sexually transmitted infection in young child (on eyes, mouth, anus, or genitals)	Sitting carefully because of injuries
Pregnancy	Unusual interest in genital area (eg, fondling of genitals, excessive masturbation, etc)
Itching, bruises, or bleeding in genital area	Sexual acting out with peers
Unexplained vaginal or rectal bleeding	Sleep disturbances (eg, nightmares, fear of sleeping alone)
Enlarged vaginal or rectal orifice	Reluctance to participate in activities with a particular person or at a particular place
Foreign objects in vagina or rectum	Increased number of new fears
Increased rectal pigmentation	Fear of being alone
Gait disturbance	Poor peer relations
	Depression
	Change in performance at school
	Eating disorders
	Vague somatic complaints
	Extreme shyness
	Increased aggressive or hostile behavior
	Encopresis
	Enuresis
	Self-destructive or suicidal behaviors
	Substance abuse
	Runaway behaviors

SOURCE: Adapted from Mott SR et al: *Nursing Care of Children and Families,* 2nd ed. Redwood City, CA: Addison-Wesley Nursing, 1990, p 597.

Although both professionals and nonprofessionals acknowledge intense feelings concerning child abuse and neglect, they often have little concern for the abusive parents. However, parents as well as children need support in these situations.

Working with neglectful and abusive parents is emotionally draining and disturbing for all people involved. Seeing a child victimized calls forth strong emotions, particularly among nurses, who might be required to provide nursing care during the time of the acute injury. The tendency is to protect the victim, the innocent child, and to punish the parent, who after all is the offender. But the nurse who perceives the family as a system understands that both child and parent are victims (Wissow 1990). The etiology of abuse is complex and multifaceted.

A major task for the nurse is helping dysfunctional parents understand the impact of stress and crises in their lives and the appropriate responses to these crises. In a family that is providing only marginal child care any

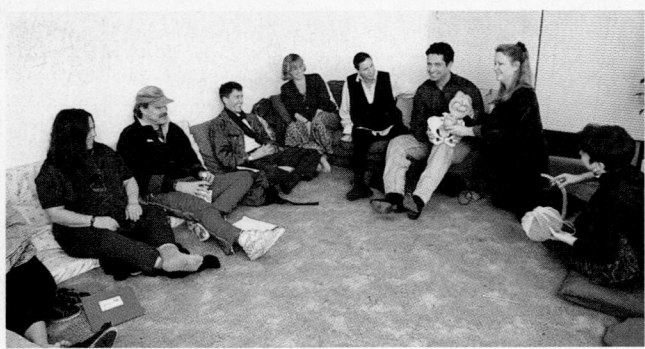

FIGURE 8-3 Parents explore ideas and ways to cope with stress in parenting classes and group therapy sessions.

stress, however small, might create a crisis. The nurse who identifies stress in dysfunctional families therefore needs to assess coping strategies. Successful coping patterns suggest growth and motivation. The nurse may need to teach appropriate ways to cope with stress. A family's reaction to stress is often a measure of the family's strength as a system.

Most parents need support services as they learn to develop new coping techniques. Group therapy, which provides peer support, might assist abusive parents because finding others with similar problems minimizes isolation (Figure 8–3). Nurse-therapists can address and help parents verbalize common fears and misconceptions about parenting.

Nurses and other professionals often need to make contracts and establish realistic deadlines in working with families. This in turn is good role modeling. Dysfunctional families need to be informed that their pattern of child care is inadequate and not acceptable to the community or school system. Facts of legal consequence, including removal of the children, need to be both verbalized and written out. These measures might seem drastic, but if they are handled in too gentle a manner and the family misinterprets the message, valuable time may be lost in mixed messages and conflicts.

Some parents appear to be docile, cooperative, and open but have merely learned responses that please. The nurse therefore is careful to identify concrete changes that indicate progress. Otherwise the therapeutic contact might end too early for a family that appears to have changed. Periodic evaluation of family dynamics and interagency accomplishments and conflicts should ensure that the family does not manipulate workers or agencies and decrease the effectiveness of the plan. In some instances a child protective worker is needed to function as coordinator.

Intervention is more effective when multiple resources are available and the family can help choose which resources to use. Most families need to draw on a variety of resources to break the cycle of a dysfunctional life-style. Nurses and other health professionals therefore need to be aware of the services available within their communities. They need to help families find those programs most geared to their needs and then coordinate the program goals and the family's progress.

Parents Anonymous, a self-help group for abusive parents, is often an excellent source of information and support for abusive parents seeking to change their behavior. Formerly abusive parents often report increased self-esteem as they assist other parents in distress. Some continue to attend Parents Anonymous meetings long after their initial needs are met, and many parents report pleasurable relationships with their children for the first time in their lives.

Support for the Child

If significant changes in the family are unavoidable, the child needs assistance in working through feelings of having caused the changes. Siblings also need to be included in the treatment plan of an abused or neglected child. If the child is hospitalized, fears of pain or violence are intensified by the unfamiliar surroundings and people. If a parent does visit, the parent is often unsupportive and may be angry with the child. The child is often confused, hurt, and frightened. Nurses and other hospital staff can identify pain, fear, and confusion and help the child discuss those feelings. The child needs to be told what will happen in developmentally appropriate terms and be reassured, as much as possible, that the parent will be back. The fewer the number of care givers, the more likely it is that the child will establish trusting relationships.

Some children have never heard their names spoken in a gentle voice, and a slow, gentle approach is essential to build any degree of trust. Children who withdraw from human contact must be allowed a reasonable period of time in which to grieve and appraise new people. If the child regresses, the regressive behavior needs to be accepted until the child can ease into a more appropriate developmental stage.

Younger children are likely to need nurturing in the form of rocking, cuddling, and soothing. The child initially might appear to reject any comforting, however, or become aggressive in response to overwhelming anxiety. The aggressive behaviors are learned responses to chaotic living and can become a problem if the child manages to manipulate many people. Team members need to set consistent limits in a firm but kindly manner and help the child learn more acceptable behaviors. Aggressive children usually have feelings of deprivation, sadness, and loneliness and may believe themselves to be unworthy and bad. Such children have little faith in their ability to inspire approval and affection.

Individual therapy may help aggressive children to discuss family dynamics and expectations their parents have for them. The therapeutic approach is to face reality honestly and not to arouse expectations in the child that the parent cannot or will not fulfill. Children who have been severely abused or have witnessed severe abuse of a sibling also need support in developing future relationships that are free of fears, guilt, and anxieties. Children facing loss or separation from their parents need therapeutic assistance to handle the loss and time to mourn.

Long-term follow-up of dysfunctional families has no set time for completion. In some instances services are required until the children reach adulthood. Periodic evaluation of parental progress and family growth includes monitoring the behaviors of the children, who might exhibit anger, anxiety, intense loneliness, or apathy. The children's progress in school must also be assessed, together with their response to authority figures. Dysfunctional behaviors suggest that the child needs individual attention.

Suggestions for Nursing Action

Personal Action

Avoid "rescuer fantasies," which can blind you to the real needs of the child and family.

Spend time working through your own thoughts and beliefs about child abuse. Identify any stereotypical ideas you may have about abuse and abusers.

Always bear in mind that the child with whom you are interacting, regardless of the setting, may be in an abusive family environment. Develop skill in identifying these children and in working as a member of an interdisciplinary team.

Client Action

When possible, advocate for two-nurse teams—one to care for the child and the other to work with the parent. This approach often helps channel negative feelings and maintain lines of communication.

Be nonjudgmental in working with abusive families.

Be aware of resources in your community that might assist abusive parents and their children.

Community Action

Support community programs designed to assist abused children and their parents.

Be an advocate for educational programs designed to help community members understand the complex factors contributing to child abuse and for effective programs for intervening to break the cycle of abuse.

Political Action

Provide education, support, and assistance to legislators in enacting laws designed to help abused children and their families break the cycle of violence and dysfunction in which they are caught.

REFERENCES

Allen JM, Hollowell EE: Nurses and child abuse/neglect reporting: Duties, responsibilities, and issues. *J Pract Nurs* June 1990; 40(2):56.

American Association of University Women: *The AAUW Report: How Schools Shortchange Girls.* Washington, DC: AAUW, 1992.

Annas GJ: Webster and the politics of abortion. *Hastings Center Report* March/April 1989; 1936.

Ashley BM, O'Rourke KD: *Ethics of Health Care: An Introductory Textbook.* Washington, DC: Georgetown Univ Press, 1994.

Bang KM et al: Reproductive hazards in the work place. *Fam Commun Health* May 1983; 6:44.

Bernhardt JH: Potential workplace hazards to reproductive health: Information for primary prevention. *JOGNN* January/February 1990; 19:53.

Brown LR et al: *State of the World 1990: A Worldwatch Institute Report on Progress Toward a Sustainable Society.* New York: Norton, 1990.

Bureau of the Census: *Statistical Abstract of the United States, 1994,* 114th ed. Washington, DC, 1994.

Clarke SC: Advance report on final divorce statistics, 1989 and 1990. *Monthly Vital Statistics Report,* vol 43 no 8, suppl. Hyattsville, MD: National Center for Health Statistics, 1995.

Collins J: Health care of women in the workplace. *Health Care Women Int* 1990; 11:21.

Couture PD: *Blessed Are the Poor?* Nashville: Abingdon Press, 1991.

Devine JA, Wright JD: *The Greatest of Evils.* New York: Aldine de Gruyter, 1993.

Devlin BK, Reynolds E: Child abuse: How to recognize it, how to intervene. *AJN* March 1994; 94(3):26.

Dornbusch, SM: Some political implications of the Stanford studies of homeless families. In: *American Women in the Nineties.* Matteo S (editor). Boston: Northeastern Univ Press, 1993.

Dutton DB: Poorer and sicker: Legacies of the 1980s, lessons for the 1990s. In: *American Women in the Nineties.* Matteo S (editor). Boston: Northeastern Univ Press, 1993.

Eddins E: Characteristics, health status and service needs of sheltered homeless families. *ABNFJ* Spring 1993; 4(2):40.

Ellis JE: What price child care? *Business Week* February 8, 1993; p 64.

Friedman DE: Work and family: The new strategic plan. In: *Management and Gender.* Karsten MF. Westport, CT: Quorum Books, 1994.

Hembree D: High-tech hazards. *Ms* March 1986; 14:79.

Hermelin FG: Legislating Fair Pay. *Working Woman* January 1995; p 34.

Hewitt JB et al: Health hazards of nursing: Identifying workplace hazards and reducing risks. *AWHONN Clin Issues Perinatal Women Health Nurs* 1993; 4(2):320.

Karsten MF: *Management and Gender.* Westport, CT: Quorum Books, 1994.

Kline EN, Saperstein AB: Homeless women. *Nurs Clin North Am* December 1992; 27(4):885.

Lione A: Polychlorinated biphenyls and reproduction. *Reprod Toxicol* 1988; 2(2):83.

Matteo S: *American Women in the Nineties: Today's Critical Issues.* Boston: Northeastern Univ Press, 1993.

McAbee RR et al: Adverse reproductive outcomes and occupational exposures among nurses. *AAOHNJ* March 1993; 41(3):110.

Mead LM: *The New Politics of Poverty.* New York: Basic Books, 1992.

Mott SR et al: *Nursing Care of Children and Families,* 2nd ed. Redwood City, CA: Addison-Wesley Nursing, 1990.

O'Brien T et al: Most small businesses appear prepared to cope with new family-leave rules. *Wall Street Journal* February 8, 1993; p B1.

Paul ME: Physical agents in the workplace. *Sem Perinatol* February 1993; 17(1):5.

Pearce DM: Something old, something new: Women's poverty in the 1990s. In: *American Women in the Nineties.* Matteo S (editor). Boston: Northeastern Univ Press, 1993.

Rhode DL: Gender equality and employment policy. In: *American Women in the Nineties.* Matteo S (editor). Boston: Northeastern Univ Press, 1993.

Schnorr TM: NIOSH epidemiologic studies of pregnancy outcomes. *Reprod Toxicol* 1990; 4:61.

Schnorr TM et al: Video display terminals and the risk of spontaneous abortion. *N Engl J Med* 1991; 324:727.

Schumann D: Nitrous oxide anesthetic: Risks to healthy personnel. *Int Nurs Rev* January/February 1990; 37:214.

Scialli AR: Who should paint the nursery? *Reprod Toxicol* 1989; 3(3):159.

Smith K and Killam P: Munchausen syndrome by proxy. *MCN* July/August 1994; 19(4):214.

Whitman D et al: The return of skid row. *US News and World Reports* January 15, 1990, p 27.

Winder C: Reproductive and chromosomal effects of occupational exposure to lead in the male. *Reprod Toxicol* 1989; 3:221.

Wissow L: *Child Advocacy for the Clinician.* Baltimore: Williams & Wilkins, 1990.

Wolch J and Dear M: *Malign Neglect.* San Francisco: Jossey-Bass, 1993.

CHAPTER 9

WOMEN'S SEXUALITY

*O*ur daughter and her family were visiting us from out of town for the holidays, and we had our four children and their families for a festive family dinner. I found myself sitting back and enjoying their good-natured ribbing and camaraderie and could sense the love and closeness among them. It was interesting noting the similarities and also differences in each offspring's personality. I remembered each of their births vividly. Oh yes, there is a great emotional risk having a family, and I learned I must cope with the sorrows as well as the great joy. In rearing my family I ran the gamut of emotions. There were times of intense pride; times of impatience and aggravation when my perfect little angels weren't so perfect; times of guilt when Mother wasn't so perfect either; times I felt fiercely protective but had to let them go so they could become self-sufficient, independent people. As I watched and studied my family I suddenly realized I not only love them all completely but I LIKE THEM as people in their own right because they are good and caring as well as wonderful parents to our grandchildren. I experienced such a feeling of thankfulness because my husband and I were truly blessed. Would I be willing to do it again? Yes! Yes! Yes!

KEY TERMS

Amenorrhea

Cervical cap

Climacteric

Coitus

Coitus interruptus

Condoms

Contraceptive sponge

Depo-Provera

Diaphragm

Dysmenorrhea

Female condom

Fertility awareness methods

Hormone replacement therapy (HRT)

Hot flashes

Intrauterine device (IUD)

Menarche

Menopause

Mifepristone (RU 486)

Norplant

Oral contraceptives (OC)

Orgasm

Premenstrual syndrome (PMS)

Spermicides

Subdermal implants

Tubal ligation

Vasectomy

OBJECTIVES

Summarize the factors that influence the development of attitudes about sexuality.

Compare the sexual responses of males and females as identified by Masters and Johnson.

Describe techniques a nurse can use to be more effective when taking a sexual history.

Identify information nurses should provide to young women about menstruation and self-care.

Summarize current findings about the causes and treatment of premenstrual syndrome (PMS).

Discuss methods of alleviating dysmenorrhea.

Compare the various methods of fertility control with regard to advantages, disadvantages, and effectiveness.

Develop a teaching plan that could be used to instruct a client about a specific method of contraception.

Delineate the physical and psychologic aspects of menopause.

Discuss hormone replacement therapy in menopausal women with regard to purpose, procedures, benefits, and risks.

People are sexual beings. Men and women develop sexual identities, make sexual choices, and establish personal standards of appropriate sexual behavior. Human sexuality begins developing at conception and evolves throughout an individual's life. The sexual experimentation and exploration of children gives way to the more urgent activities of the adolescent. With maturity, sexual contact becomes part of a broader and usually more meaningful relationship.

This chapter focuses on the concept of sexuality particularly as it relates to women through their lifespan. It provides information on preconception planning for women or couples who choose to become parents. The chapter also focuses on available methods of contraception and on the needs of the menopausal woman.

DEVELOPMENT OF SEXUALITY

Sexual development begins at conception, when biologic sex is determined: XX chromosomes, a female; XY, a male. As the embryo becomes a fetus and development continues, sexual differentiation takes place (see Figure 5–1), and the sex organs begin functioning. Even as the sex organs are developing, other senses and systems are developing that enable the infant to react to sexual stimuli at birth. The sense of touch, for example, which is fundamental in the development of sexuality, is highly developed by 8 weeks' gestation.

The stimuli, experiences, and relationships that are essential to the development of sexuality come into play at birth. The infant learns to find satisfaction through oral stimuli, through contact with another, and through cuddling and holding. Young infants learn to touch their genitals and seem to be capable of sexual arousal.

Toddlers facing toilet training become even more aware of their bodies and may more consciously practice masturbation, although their parents often discourage it. By age 3 most children are aware of their sexual identity as a result of consistent parental and social reinforcement. During the childhood years, from 5 through 12, sexual activity and interest may be less apparent, but it has not disappeared. Games such as "playing house" or "playing doctor" help children learn sex roles and more about the differences between the sexes. Children show a preference for playmates of the same sex, although they may begin to show some romantic interest in members of the opposite sex as the preteen years approach.

Puberty and adolescence are a time of transition from childhood to adulthood. Adolescence finds physically and sexually mature young people trying to cope with new situations and sensations while they are still psychologically immature. Sexual experimentation begins, and masturbation accompanied by fantasy is common. Homosexual experiences may occur, and mutual masturbation for boys is not uncommon. Heterosexual contacts progress over 4 or 5 years from initial kissing and fondling, to mutual body exploration and masturbation, to sexual intercourse.

With adulthood comes responsibility and choice. Because sexual expression in marriage has the most widespread legitimacy in our society, many adults choose to marry. However, new life-styles, recognition of a variety of views of morality, and increasing numbers of contraceptive choices have made more commonplace other situations in which sexuality can be expressed.

Sexual Orientation

The exact origins of sexual orientation, especially homosexuality, have been studied extensively over the years, but no definitive theory has yet been developed. Early research focused on psychosocial theories related to parenting patterns, life events, or the psychologic makeup of the individual. Homosexuality was considered a poor second choice for people who lacked satisfactory heterosexual experiences (Crooks & Baur 1993). However, a classic study by Bell and associates (1981) of the development of sexual orientation found that no specific phenomenon of family life could be identified as especially significant for either heterosexual or homosexual development. They stated, "[A] boy or a girl is predisposed to be homosexual or heterosexual, and during childhood and adolescence this basic sexual orientation begins to become evident" (p 187).

Current research focuses on biologic theories of sexual orientation. For example, a study of three groups of men (identical twins, fraternal twins, and adoptive brothers) found that, if one brother was homosexual, so were 11% of the adoptive brothers, 22% of the fraternal twins, and 52% of the identical twins. Although environment may play a role, a genetic component seems indicated by the differences between the identical twins and the other groups (Bailey & Pillard 1991). Other studies have focused on differences in the brains of homosexual and heterosexual individuals.

A biologic cause for homosexuality might influence the attitudes of society. A recent study found that people who believed homosexuals were born with their sexual orientation were more accepting and positive about homosexuality than those who believed that people learned or chose to be homosexual (Gelman et al 1992).

At present research suggests a biologic predisposition to exclusive homosexuality, but the exact causes of sexual orientation remain uncertain. Sexual orientation may be best viewed as a continuum influenced by the interaction of biologic and psychologic factors, which may be unique for each individual (Crooks & Baur 1993).

Sexual Attitudes and Beliefs

Attitudes about sex are influenced by a variety of factors. The home environment is one of the greatest influences. Children raised by parents who are comfortable with and open about sexuality will probably be more comfortable with their sexuality than children raised in more restrictive environments. The following anecdote from a young mother provides an example.

When I was growing up, my parents always showed affection for each other and for us. Hugs, kisses, and pats on the shoulder were common. In discussing sexual issues with me, my mother was very direct and always used correct terminology. She never seemed embarrassed to answer questions. My closest girlfriend couldn't talk to her mother about anything. She told me once that she had never seen her parents show any physical affection for each other. They never kissed or hugged her either. She had an older sister, but they weren't close, so I ended up telling her what my mother told me. When we started high school and had so many questions, it was harder. One day a neat thing happened. My mom made some cocoa, and the three of us sat and talked all afternoon. Mom answered our questions about sex and got us thinking about more abstract aspects of sexuality like ethics and choices. It was one of the most special times I ever shared with my mother. I hope I can do the same for my children.

Even if parents are not openly demonstrative, they can convey to children that sexuality is a natural, acceptable, and satisfying part of life by creating a positive home atmosphere.

Cultural background can profoundly influence the home and environment and thereby have a major impact on the child's socialization. Individuals raised in a male-dominated or strongly moralistic culture will usually have very different attitudes from those of individuals raised in a culture that views sexual expression as a shared experience between equals. People can reject cultural norms as adults, but doing so is often difficult and may cause stress.

Similarly, religious teachings can profoundly influence attitudes about sexuality. The concept of reproduction as the only legitimate purpose for sexual activity has its roots in Judeo-Christian teachings and may devalue other forms of noncoital sexual expression such as sexual fantasy, masturbation, or oral or anal sex, which many researchers view as alternative sexual options for those who select them (Crooks & Baur 1993). Comfort with various forms of sexual expression; attitudes about fertility control, abortion, and homosexuality; beliefs about the roles of women and men in society; and childrearing practices all may be influenced by an individual's religious beliefs.

Attitudes about sex are influenced by education and socioeconomic level. People with more income and education tend to be more comfortable with a wider variety of sexual activities. Sexual attitudes can be profoundly af-

RESEARCH IN PRACTICE

Using grounded theory methodology, Shirley Bruenjes generated a theory of health for middle-aged women. Health, for these women, becomes a process lived daily rather than a static end product to be achieved. The women in the study orchestrated their health by balancing physical, emotional, spiritual, and personal factors to achieve a sense of harmony.

The sample consisted of 7 women ranging in age from 45 to 65 years. All of the women were married, employed full time, considered themselves to be in good health, and had at least a bachelor's degree. Data collection involved in-depth interviews that were transcribed and analyzed using a constant comparative method. Substantive codes were merged into theoretical categories.

The theoretial categories generated from this study included environment, health, feedback, personal factors, emotional health, physical health, spiritual health, relationships, and conducting. Personal factors included genetics, aging, and disease. The conducting category incorporated prioritizing, choices, balance, moderation, interaction, and responsibility. The core category, orchestrating health, explained the development of the theoretical categories as well as organized the entire study. For example, physical health, a theoretical category, contained substantive codes of nutrition, exercise, sleep, and self care. These components could be compared to the individual musical instruments of an orchestra section that must be balanced both within the section and with the other sections by the conductor. The study indicated that the woman, as conductor, remained in control of her own health and directed the interplay of physical, spiritual, and emotional health against the background of her environment. Personal factors played a part of being "in tune," and the interactive audience incorporated the women's relationships.

Clinical Application of Study

These women controlled their own health; they did not want to give up their "conducting" to someone else. They saw the balance and tuning of their health as their responsibility. In nurse-client relationships that promote the client's continued orchestration of her health, the nurse can act as a participating member of the audience to give feedback and critique, but cannot wrestle away the baton.

SOURCE: Bruenjes S: Orchestrating health: Middle-aged women's process of living health. *Holistic Nursing Practice* 1994; 8(4): 22.

fected by previous sexual experiences, especially very intense experiences such as incest, sexual abuse, rape, or severe punishment for sexual experimentation.

Personal characteristics are influential in the development of sexual attitudes. Although it is difficult to negate the influence of environment, people are born with different personality characteristics: Some are shy, others more adventuresome, and so forth. There are also variations in sex drive or libido that significantly influence an individual's view of sexuality.

Sexuality must be considered within the context of a person's life and life choices. Sex is a major focus to some and a minor consideration to others. Some feel sex is only appropriate in a close and loving relationship; others feel that love and sex are separate and do not necessarily have to occur together.

Opinions also vary about the purpose of sexual intercourse. More traditional views hold that the sole purpose of sex is procreation. Pleasure may be experienced, but it is not essential. For those who view sex as only for procreation, it is necessary for the male to achieve an orgasm so that sperm are ejaculated; however, a woman may or may not achieve one. Some believe that any sexual activities engaged in for pleasure only are selfish and immoral. Others believe that the purpose of sex is pleasure: If an action brings pleasure, it is good. Nothing is unacceptable as long as it provides pleasure and release. Sex is only "bad" if it does not bring satisfaction to either or both parties. Sexual expression can also be viewed as a means of expression, a sharing of feelings, a union of two individuals seeking to communicate. This communication may involve demonstration of a variety of messages: tenderness, domination, passion, or even anger.

Although the basic patterns of psychosexual development are established by the end of adolescence, a person continues to develop and modify beliefs and attitudes throughout life. Many adults broaden their attitudes about sexual activities and experiment with different sexual life-styles. During adulthood an individual usually resolves any psychosexual conflicts and develops a set of sexual values.

Sexual Response Cycle

People obtain sexual satisfaction in a variety of ways. A person alone may find sexual pleasure in a book, a film, or a stirring musical piece; fantasy; or masturbation. Couples may experience sexual pleasure through a shared experience; through physical closeness such as holding each other or cuddling together; through touching, kissing, and stroking each other; through mutual masturbation; or through sexual intercourse.

Many terms are used to describe the sexual mating of a sexually mature male and female. These include coitus, sexual intercourse, copulation, making love, and the sex act. **Coitus** is defined as the insertion of the erect penis into the vagina. After repeated thrusting movements of the penis, the man experiences ejaculation of semen concurrent with orgasm. **Orgasm** is the involuntary climax of the sexual experience, involving a series of muscular contractions, profound physiologic bodily response, and intense sensual pleasure. Orgasm may be achieved by other methods of sexual stimulation besides sexual intercourse, such as masturbation and oral stimulation. Although the basic events of coitus are the same for all heterosexual couples, wide variation exists in sexual positions, technique, duration, intent, meaning, and reactions among individuals.

Coitus is a personal act between two consenting individuals. It can signify a variety of feelings, beliefs, and at-

TABLE 9-1   Anatomic and Physiologic Summary of Female Sexual Response

Organ	Excitement (foreplay)	Plateau (entry and coital movements)	Orgasm (climax)	Resolution (relaxation)
Clitoris	Size of glans increases; engorgement of dorsal vein occurs; shaft elongates	Glans retracts under hood after erection	Rhythmic muscular contractions occur, ranging from mild to intense	Returns to normal; no refractory period; multiple orgasms possible
Labia majora	Vasocongestion and swelling occur; nulliparous: flatten and widen; multiparous: widen by movement from vaginal introitus	Increase		Return to normal size and color
Labia minora	Vasocongestion of erectile tissue occurs; color darkens; extension of tissue	Increase		Return to normal size and color
Vagina	Vaginal lubrication appears; in 10–30 seconds widens and lengthens 1 cm; walls become purplish; progressive distention occurs; upper portion "tents"; rugae become smooth	Engorgement occurs; outer third of vagina swells; "orgasmic platform" develops; interior lumen decreases to "grasp" penis	Outer third has spasm, then rhythmic contractions; perivaginal muscles contract	Outer third relaxes after clitoris returns to normal, remaining portion returns to normal
Cervix	Moves upward and backward posteriorly	Cervical os opens slightly	Rhythmic contractions from fundus to cervix occur	Returns to normal position; os closes in 20–30 minutes
Uterus	Moves upward and backward	Increases in size	Sex flush most pronounced	Returns to precoital size slowly
Breasts	Areolae increase in size; nipples become erect and size increases; sex flush may appear			Slow return to normal; sex flush disappears

TABLE 9–2 — Anatomic and Physiologic Summary of Male Sexual Response

Organ	Excitement (foreplay)	Plateau (entry and coital movements)	Orgasm (climax)	Resolution (relaxation)
Scrotum	Skin thickens; scrotal sac elevates and flattens against body (spermatic cord contracts)	Remains tense and close to body		
Testes	Elevate with scrotum	May increase in size by 50%; remain elevated		
Penis	Engorgement and erection is rapid; size increases; position changes; angle of protrusion created	Coronal ridge size increases; glans becomes purplish	Contracts	Becomes flaccid; refractory period: erection may not be experienced
Urethra	Moistened with mucus	Mucus increases; becomes distended with semen just before orgasm	Semen ejected with force as bulb contracts	Minor contractions persist even after semen is ejected
Seminal vesicles			Semen is discharged into urethral bulb	
Prostate			Contracts, expelling fluid into urethral bulb	
Bulbourethral glands		Few drops of fluid may be discharged (contain sperm)		
Breasts	Nipples may become erect; sex flush may appear		Sex flush most pronounced	Slow return to normal; sex flush fades slowly

titudes. It may reflect their mutual commitment and caring, or it may be a more immediate interaction for the purpose of personal pleasure or merely temporary companionship.

Physiology of Sexual Response

In their classic study of human sexuality Masters and Johnson (Masters et al 1986) identified and described the physiology of the sexual response in both males and females. All the responses can be classified as either vasocongestive or myotonic. *Vasocongestion* involves the congestion or engorgement of blood vessels and is the most common physiologic response to sexual arousal. *Myotonia*, a secondary physiologic response, is increased muscular tone or tension.

Human sexual response occurs in four separate phases: excitement, plateau, orgasm, and resolution. Female (Table 9–1) and male (Table 9–2) anatomic and physiologic reactions are similar. Wide variations occur, however, in duration and intensity of response.

Female sexual response varies considerably. Not all women experience orgasm consistently; they are influenced by their psychologic state, health, current sexual motivation, and environmental distractions. A woman may not experience orgasm during a particular act of coitus, or she may experience one or multiple orgasms of varying intensity (Figure 9–1A). Such variation is common.

The male physical response is relatively constant, resulting in orgasm if erection and sexual stimulation are maintained (Figure 9–1B).

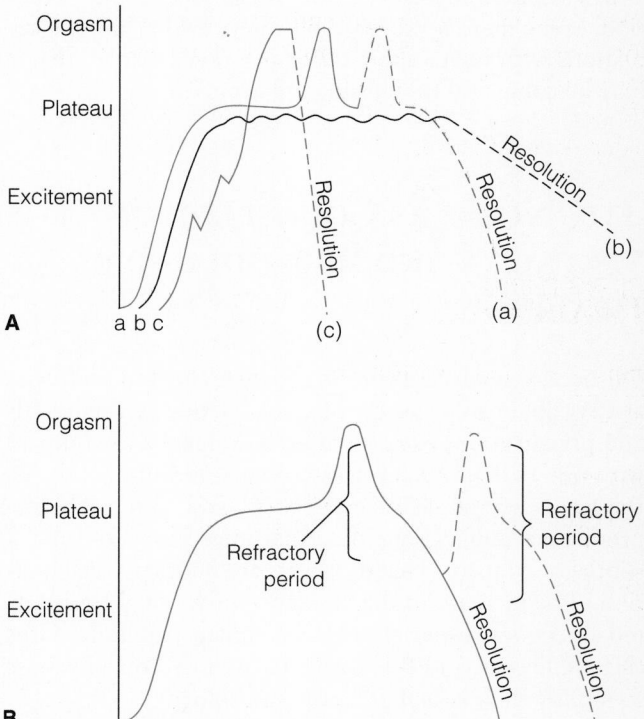

FIGURE 9–1   *A* Three variations of the female sexual response: (a) reaction pattern with single or multiple orgasms, (b) reaction pattern that reaches plateau but not orgasm, (c) reaction pattern without distinct plateau. *B* Reaction pattern of most typical male sexual response. The dotted line indicates another possible pattern involving a second orgasm occurring after the refractory period. SOURCE: Masters WH et al: *Masters and Johnson on Sex and Human Loving.* Boston: Little, Brown, 1986.

Women and men exhibit several identical responses. The *sex flush* is a maculopapular rash that usually begins in the epigastric area and spreads quickly to the breasts. More than half of women experience sex flush, whereas less than half of men do. Heart rate and blood pressure increase in proportion to the degree of sexual excitement. Muscles tense beginning in the excitement phase. This tension increases during the plateau phase. Hyperventilation occurs just before and during orgasm. At orgasm muscle tension is extreme. The face may contort while muscles of the neck, extremities, abdomen, and buttocks contract tightly. Individuals may moan, murmur, or cry out and will experience a brief total surrender to bodily responses, accompanied by acute pleasure and relief.

During resolution the body returns to the unaroused state. Muscular tension is dramatically reduced, and blood is released from the engorged tissues. If orgasm did not occur, the lingering vasocongestion may cause feelings of pelvic fullness and pressure that take a longer time to resolve.

Although women are capable of achieving multiple orgasms, men are more limited in that respect. Practically all men experience a *refractory period* as part of their resolution phase. During this period, which may last from a few minutes in young men to several hours in older men, a man is physiologically unable to achieve another erection. Some men, however, can achieve two or more ejaculations with such a short refractory time between that it may be compared to multiple orgasm.

THE NURSE AS COUNSELOR ON SEXUALITY AND REPRODUCTIVE HEALTH

On occasion most people experience concern and even anxiety about some aspect of sexuality. Societal standards and pressures can cause people to evaluate and compare with others their sexual attractiveness, technical abilities, the frequency of sexual interaction, and so on. The reproductive implications of sexual intercourse are also a source of concern. Health factors are another consideration. The increase in the incidence of sexually transmitted infections, especially AIDS, human papilloma virus (HPV), herpes, and chlamydia, have caused many people to modify their sexual practices and activities.

Because sexuality and its reproductive implications are such an intrinsic and emotion-laden part of life, people have many concerns, problems, and questions about sex roles, sexual behaviors, sex education, family planning, sexual inhibitions, sexual values, and related areas.

To be effective in providing sexual health care, nurses must develop an awareness of their own feelings, values, and attitudes about sexuality. Often people believe that their own sexual values and patterns of sexual behavior are the best ones, the "right" ones. This of course implies that all other attitudes and practices are not as good or are "wrong." Nurses must recognize their own beliefs and attitudes so that they can be more sensitive and objective when confronted with the beliefs of others. Nurses who recognize that they are not comfortable dealing with issues related to sexuality should avoid situations that require sexual counseling and should refer clients to nurses who are more at ease in this area.

Many nurses who care for childbearing families will be faced with questions about sexuality, sexual practices, and so forth. These nurses need to have accurate, up-to-date knowledge about these topics. They should also know about the structure and functions of the male and female reproductive systems.

Continuing education for practicing nurses and appropriate courses in undergraduate and graduate nursing education programs can provide opportunities for nurses to learn about sexual values, attitudes, alternative lifestyles, cultural factors, and misconceptions and myths about sex and reproduction. Nurses can then update this knowledge by regular reading so that they are familiar with current literature on the subject.

Self-awareness and a sound knowledge base are not, by themselves, sufficient to make the nurse an effective counselor. The nurse also needs to develop skills in listening, communicating, interviewing, assessing, and intervening. Nurses today are often responsible for taking a woman's initial history. Opening the discussion with a brief explanation of the purpose of such questions is often helpful. For example, the nurse might say,

> As your nurse I'm interested in all aspects of your well-being. Often women have concerns or questions about sexual matters, especially when they are pregnant (starting to be sexually active). I will be asking you some questions about your sexual history as part of your general health history.

The nurse may find the following additional suggestions useful when taking a sexual history:

- Provide a quiet, private place, free of distractions.

- Approach the situation in a relaxed, unhurried way and with an attitude of honesty and acceptance.

- Use direct eye contact as much as possible unless you know that this is culturally unacceptable to the woman.

- Fit the taking of the sexual history into the gynecologic and obstetric history rather than isolating it.

- Do little if any writing during the discussion, especially if the woman seems ill at ease or is discussing very personal issues.

- Avoid sitting across a desk. Sit as close to the woman as seems comfortable to you both.

- Pay attention to nonverbal cues and body language.

- Ask open-ended questions. Often nurses develop the habit of asking questions that require a "yes" or "no" response. Open-ended questions often elicit far more information. For example, "What, if anything, would you change about your current sex life?" will produce more information than "Are you happy with your sex life now?"

- If the woman has no questions or concerns, it is not necessary to press for a lengthy discussion. It may be that she is satisfied, or that your relationship has not reached the point where she is comfortable with such a discussion.

- Clarify terminology. If the woman uses a slang term, find out what she means by it. If the word she uses is not comfortable for you, use one that is comfortable without being too clinical.

- Proceed from easier topics to those that are more difficult to discuss. Often it is easier to discuss the menstrual history, for example, before considering sexually transmitted infections or unusual sexual practices.

- Before asking direct questions, it is often useful to make a generality or normalcy statement such as "Many women worry about . . . " or "Often women have questions about . . . . "

- Try to determine whether the woman has already identified specific concerns or if she attributes problems to something specific. For example, you might ask, "Do you feel that anything is affecting your sexual health or happiness in any way?"

- The phrase "How do you feel about that?" is used so often that it has become trite. Instead try "What would you like to change about that situation?" or "You seem uncomfortable. What are you thinking about now?"

- Self-disclosure can occasionally help the woman be more at ease. Before making any self-disclosure statement, however, the nurse should internally question whose needs will be met by the disclosure and whether there is any sense of being in competition with the client.

- Violence against women is a major health risk. When taking a history, provide opportunities for the woman to discuss sexual abuse (see Chapter 11).

A complete sexual history may not be necessary in every situation, and the depth of the information obtained will vary with the client's situation. It may take several encounters to complete a sexual history. Clients may not share such personal information until they have developed a trusting relationship with the care giver.

Applying the Nursing Process

After completing the sexual history, the nurse assesses the information obtained. If the nurse identifies a problem that requires further assessment, referral to a nurse practitioner, nurse-midwife, physician, or counselor may be

necessary. In many instances the nurse will be able to develop a nursing diagnosis and then plan and implement interventions. For example, if the nurse determines that a woman who is interested in conceiving a child does not have a clear understanding of when she ovulates, the nurse may formulate the following nursing diagnosis: Knowledge deficit related to lack of information about the timing of ovulation. The nurse could then evaluate the woman's knowledge through discussion and work with the woman to provide necessary knowledge. The nurse might also suggest that the woman keep a menstrual calendar and monitor basal body temperatures and cervical mucus to identify the time of ovulation.

It is important for the nurse to be realistic in making assessments and planning interventions. It requires insight and skill to recognize when a woman's problem requires interventions that are beyond a nurse's preparation and ability. In such situations appropriate referrals should be made.

SOCIOCULTURAL ASPECTS OF MENSTRUATION

The consistent and somewhat mysterious recurrence of menstruation has engendered menstrual belief systems over the millennia that remain with us and become the social reality. Cultural, religious, and personal attitudes about menstruation are part of the menstrual experience and, unfortunately, often reflect negative attitudes toward women.

Critical Thinking Question

How have you been influenced by attitudes and customs about menstruation?

Some cultures have isolated women entirely (in menstrual huts, for example) or restricted them to the company of other women during menstruation because they believed that menstrual blood was "unclean" and dangerous. Some beliefs emanating from this myth are that menstruating women have the ability to harm growing crops, wither flowers, and cause bread not to rise. A common belief is that menstruating women are able to contaminate their husbands, so sexual intercourse is contraindicated (the Talmud, and Leviticus 15:19 of the Bible). Menstruating women have been accused of having supernatural powers (because of the association of bleeding with death), which are sometimes good but more often destructive.

Although many of these myths have disappeared, there is a tendency to regard the menstruating woman as vulnerable or less capable. Current customs include refraining from exercise, showers, and sexual intercourse and hiding the fact of menstruation entirely.

Some people have used these myths to deny jobs to women and treat them as inferior. The belief that women lose a lot of time from work is largely unsupported. Women still work where they are needed at home, in factories, or in offices with no concessions in schedules or routines to take account of individual differences in cycles. It is interesting to note that men, who are more prone to incapacitating and unpredictable diseases such as heart problems, are encouraged to continue in highly responsible positions.

Fortunately, the 1990s have afforded a more enlightened view of menstruating women in the United States. As they have appeared in increasing numbers in the work force, women have shown their competence in a male-dominated world. Women have worked hard to gain equal treatment and have proven conclusively that the menstrual cycle is a normal event, rarely a reason to avoid work or responsibility.

Male Attitudes and Sexual Activity

Most women have been socialized to refrain from discussing menstruation with men. This cultural taboo is usually supported by the tendency to separate into gender groups for school discussions of growth and development. As a result, many men, even male physicians, lack information about menstruation. It is important to be open and tell both daughters and sons about the many events of the life cycle so that they can be comfortable and open about these changes and the maturational processes.

Cultural taboos against coitus during menses are of long duration, but the health reasons for such taboos have been found to be invalid. Nurses discussing this area with clients may want to confirm that sexual activity during menses is common practice and is not contraindicated; however, not all couples desire it.

THE ROLE OF THE NURSE IN MENSTRUAL COUNSELING

Girls today begin to learn about puberty and menstruation at a surprisingly young age. Unfortunately, the source of their "information" is sometimes their peers, and thus the information may be incomplete, inaccurate, and sensationalized. Nurses who work with young girls and adolescents recognize this and are working hard to provide accurate health teaching and to correct misinformation about **menarche** (the onset of menses) and the menstrual cycle.

The nurse provides information about what is normal and expected during menstruation. Some of the objective data needed to assess individual women and determine normalcy include:

- *Length of the average cycle.* Early in a female's menstrual life the median cycle length is 29 days; this will decrease slightly to a median of 25 + days prior to menopause. Cycle length that varies from 21 to 35 days is considered normal. Cycle length is calculated by counting the number of days from the onset of one menses to the onset of the next menses. There is a wide variation among women.

- *Individual variability.* The typical month-to-month variation in an individual's cycle is plus or minus 2 days, although greater normal variations are frequently noted. No woman's cycle is exactly the same length every month.

- *Amount of flow.* The average flow is approximately 30 mL in a period; users of IUDs may double this amount. The average woman can characterize the amount of flow by the number of pads or tampons used. Increase or decrease in the number of pads or tampons used is a good subjective indicator of changes in menstrual flow.

- *Length of menses.* The length of the menses is usually from 2 to 8 days. Here again there is wide variability. The number of days is another indicator of amount of flow.

Information of a subjective nature may be elicited by general questions such as, "How do you feel?" "Has there been any change?" "Do you have any problems with your menstrual period?" Skilled interviewing will yield information about the social, environmental, and biophysical impacts of the individual's menstrual cycle.

Promotion of Successful Adaptation to Menarche

Many young women find it embarrassing or stressful to discuss the menstrual experience, both because of the many taboos associated with the subject and because of their immaturity. The young woman who physically matures earlier than her peers is especially likely to be at a disadvantage; because the event has not been expected to occur so soon, she is less likely to have an adequate knowledge base for coping with her experience. A girl 10 or 11 years of age is also limited by her cognitive immaturity; the "magical thinking" typical of her developmental stage may lead to such thoughts as "everyone will know I have my period."

The most critical factor in successful adaptation to menarche is the adolescent's level of preparedness. A direct relationship exists between adequacy of preparation and the degree to which the menarcheal experience is positive. The nurse should make it clear that, within limits, variations in age at menarche, length of cycle, and duration of menses are normal because girls are likely to become concerned if they are not "on time" as compared with their peers. It is helpful to acknowledge the negative aspects of menstruation (messiness, embarrassment) as well as its positive role as a symbol of maturity and womanhood.

Rita Cooper is a 16-year-old, vivacious teenager who comes to the clinic because of irregular menses. She is captain of the cheerleading squad at the local high school and believes that her periods are "really messed up" and interfering with her cheering activities. She wants to get her periods regulated and asks for birth control pills.

As you take Rita's menstrual history, you find that her menarche was at age 12 and that her periods occur every 24–34 days. She usually has cramps, and the flow, which she describes as heavy, lasts 4–5 days. She uses an average of five tampons per day. What should you advise Rita about her menstrual cycle?

Answers can be found in Appendix I.

Teaching About Comfort Measures and Issues During Menstruation

Menstrual fluid contains blood; cervical mucus; vaginal secretions, mucus, and cells; and degenerated endometrial particles. It usually does not have an odor until it makes contact with bacteria on the skin or in the air.

Tampons and Pads

Women in different cultures have handled their menstrual flow in many ways. Since early times, women have made tampons and pads from cloths or rags, which required washing but were reusable. Commercial tampons were introduced in the 1930s.

Today's adhesive stripped mini- and maxipads and flushable tampons have made life easier. Unfortunately, in their zeal to perfect a comfortable, convenient, leak- and odorproof product, manufacturers have added deodorants to both sanitary napkins and tampons and have increased their absorbency. Both these "improvements" may prove harmful. The chemical used to deodorize can create a rash on the vulva and can do worse damage to the tender mucous lining of the vagina itself. Excessive or inappropriate use of superabsorbent tampons can produce dryness and even small sores or ulcers in the vagina.

Superabsorbent tampons are to be used only for exceptionally heavy menstrual flow, not during the whole period. In the absence of a heavy menstrual flow these tampons will absorb all moisture, leaving the vaginal walls dry and subject to injury. The absorbency of even regular tampons can vary. If the tampon is hard to pull out or shreds when removed or if the vagina becomes dry, the tampon is probably too absorbent. If a woman is worried about accidental spotting, she should check the diagrams on the packages of regular tampons. Those that expand in width are better able to prevent leakage without being too absorbent.

A woman may want to use tampons only during the day and switch to pads at night to avoid vaginal irritation. Tampons should be avoided on the last spotty days of the period. If a woman experiences vaginal irritation, itching, soreness, or unusual odor while using tampons, she should stop using them or change brands or absorbencies to see if that helps.

Toxic shock syndrome (TSS) has been linked to menstruation and tampon use. Warning signs of TSS include the following:

- Fever (temperature of 38.9 C [102 F] or more)
- Diarrhea
- Vomiting
- Muscle aches (myalgia)
- Sunburnlike diffuse rash
- Inflamed mucous membranes

A woman should be advised to seek *immediate* medical attention if these symptoms occur during a menstrual cycle or when using a barrier method of contraception such as a diaphragm, cervical cap, or contraceptive sponge. For further discussion of TSS, see Chapter 10.

The choice of sanitary protection must meet the individual's needs, and she should feel comfortable using it whether it be pads or tampons.

Vaginal Sprays and Douches

Another comfort issue is the use of douches and vaginal sprays. Many women have been led to believe that regular douching is as fundamental as a morning shower and that use of hygiene spray deodorant is as essential as use of underarm deodorants. In fact these douches and deodorants are not only unnecessary, but they also can be harmful. Vaginal sprays can cause infections, itching, burning, irritation, vaginal discharge, rashes, and other problems.

Women who choose to use female deodorant sprays should carefully follow the directions for proper use. These sprays should not be used with sanitary napkins or applied to broken, irritated, or itching skin. The two circumstances in which women may be most concerned with vaginal odor are during menstruation and during intercourse, and these are times when use of feminine deodorant spray is clearly contraindicated.

Douching is unnecessary because the vagina cleanses itself; simply wiping the labia is sufficient for cleanliness. Douching washes away the natural mucus and upsets the vaginal ecology, which can make the vagina more susceptible to infection. Douching with one of the perfumed or flavored douches can cause allergic reactions, and too frequent use of an undiluted or strong douche solution can induce severe irritation and even tissue damage. Propelling water up the vagina may also erode the antibacterial cervical plug and force microorganisms from the vagina into the uterus. Women should not douche during menstruation because the cervix is slightly dilated to permit the downward flow of menstrual fluid from the uterine lining. It may be easier to introduce infection at this time, resulting in endometritis (infection of the lining [endometrium] of the uterus).

The mucous secretions that continually bathe the vagina are completely odorfree while they are in the vagina; only when they mingle with perspiration and hit the air does odor develop. Keeping one's skin clean and free of bacteria with plain soap and water is the most effective method of controlling odor. A soapy finger or soft washcloth should be used to wash gently between the vulvar folds. Bathing is as important (if not more so) during the menstrual period as at any other time. There is no evidence that bathing will bring on cramps or interrupt blood flow. On the contrary, a long, leisurely soak in a warm tub will promote menstrual blood flow and relieve cramps by relaxing the muscles.

Keeping the vaginal area fresh throughout the day means keeping it dry and clean. After bathing or showering and patting herself dry a woman should wear cotton panties. She should make sure that her clothes are loose enough to permit the vaginal area to breathe. After using the toilet, a woman should always wipe herself from front to back and, if necessary, follow up with a moistened paper towel or toilet paper. If an unusual odor persists despite these efforts, it may be a sign that something is awry. Certain conditions such as vaginitis produce a foul-smelling discharge.

Relief of Discomfort

Cramping and general discomfort may be alleviated by instituting certain nutritional practices, exercise, the use of heat and massage, and mild analgesics (see discussion of dysmenorrhea that follows).

Nutritional Self-Care   The B-complex vitamins, especially vitamin B_6, play a role in neutralizing the excessive amounts of estrogen produced by the ovaries during the course of a normal menstrual cycle and therefore may prevent the bloating and irritability that sometimes occur premenstrually. Vitamin E, a mild prostaglandin inhibitor, may help decrease menstrual discomfort. Vitamin E is also able to improve circulation, which reduces muscular spasms and pain by reducing the uterus's need for oxygen. Supplements may be taken, but these vitamins are also available in a well-balanced diet. Women should avoid excess salt because it can contribute to fluid retention. The methylxanthines in caffeine may contribute to breast tenderness during menses, so women may find it helpful to avoid coffee, teas, colas, and chocolate.

Exercise   Exercise, if performed daily, can relieve existing discomfort and help prevent menstrual cramps and associated complaints. It relieves constipation by increasing intestinal activity and curbs bloating by increasing

perspiration. The deep breathing required during exercise brings more oxygen to the blood, which relaxes the uterus and helps ease discomfort. Exercise helps alleviate anxiety and tension. Helpful exercises include jogging, swimming, fast-paced walking, and bicycling.

Heat and Massage   Heat is soothing and promotes increased blood flow. Any type of warmth, from sipping herbal tea to soaking in a hot tub or using a heating pad, may be helpful during painful periods. Massage can also soothe aching back muscles and promote relaxation and blood flow.

ASSOCIATED MENSTRUAL CONDITIONS

Premenstrual Syndrome

Premenstrual syndrome (PMS) refers to a symptom complex associated with the luteal phase of the menstrual cycle. The symptoms must, by definition, occur between the time of ovulation and the onset of menses. They are repetitive in each menstrual cycle during the same time frame. Symptoms that last beyond the second day of menses generally are not considered premenstrual, and alternative causes should be pursued.

The exact cause of PMS is unknown, but a multitude of theories have been postulated to explain it. These range from hormone imbalance to nutritional deficiency and include prostaglandin deficiency, prostaglandin excess, vitamin B_6 deficiency, β-endorphin deficiency, serotonin deficiency, and hypothalmic-pituitary-adrenal dysregulation. A great deal of research is currently being done on PMS, and it is likely that our understanding of the condition will increase in the future.

Women over age 30 are more likely to develop PMS than those under 30. Five percent to 10% of ovulating women report severe symptoms of PMS at some time in their lives (Copeland 1993). Symptoms include:

- *Psychologic:* irritability, lethargy, depression, low morale, anxiety, sleep disorders, crying spells, and hostility
- *Neurologic:* classic migraine, vertigo, syncope
- *Respiratory:* nasal congestion, hoarseness, asthma
- *Gastrointestinal:* nausea, vomiting, constipation, abdominal bloating, diarrhea, craving for sweets, chocolate, or salt
- *Urinary:* retention and oliguria
- *Dermatologic:* acne
- *Mammary:* swelling and tenderness

Most women experience only some of these symptoms. The most disconcerting symptoms, and the ones that many women seek treatment for, are the psychologic ones. The symptoms usually are most pronounced 2 to 3 days before the onset of menstruation (although they may be present for up to 2 weeks before the onset of menstruation) and subside as menstrual flow begins, with or without treatment.

Nursing Care

The nurse can help the woman identify specific premenstrual symptoms and develop healthy behavior. After assessment, counseling for PMS may include restriction of foods containing methylxanthines (eg, chocolate and coffee), fat, salt, and sugar; increased intake of complex carbohydrates and protein; and increased frequency of meals. Supplementation with B complex vitamins, especially B_6, may reduce anxiety and depression. A dose of 25 to 50 mg twice daily is recommended. Megadoses should be avoided because of the risk of B_6 toxicity (Rayburn 1992). Vitamin E supplementation may reduce breast tenderness. A program of regular aerobic exercise such as fast walking, jogging, or aerobic dancing is often helpful in alleviating PMS.

Pharmacologic treatments for PMS have varied greatly. In addition to vitamin supplements the more widely known remedies include progesterone suppositories, diuretics, and prostaglandin inhibitors. Bromocriptine (Parlodel) reduces breast symptoms, and danazol decreases breast symptoms and other general symptoms as well (Chuong et al 1994) but has more associated serious side effects. All have been effective in some women and not in others. Antianxiety drugs and antidepressants have been used with some effectiveness in women who have psychologic symptoms as their major problem. They must be used with caution and in the lowest possible therapeutic dose (Rayburn 1992).

An empathetic relationship with a health care professional to whom the woman feels free to voice her concerns is highly beneficial. Encouragement to keep a diary may help the woman identify life events associated with PMS. Self-care groups and self-help literature may help women gain control over their bodies and reduce stress. Group members share helpful therapies, including nutrition information and exercise and relaxation techniques. Biofeedback techniques can be learned and used to treat specific symptoms such as headache.

Dysmenorrhea

Dysmenorrhea, or painful menses, usually occurs a day or two prior to the onset of menstruation and subsides by the end of menses. Multiple studies report that 45% to 50% of women experience painful periods. Cramps may be accompanied by headache, dizziness, backache, leg pain, nausea, vomiting, or diarrhea. Typically, a young girl's menstrual cycle is irregular and painless until regular ovulation is established. At that time dysmenorrhea may occur in a cyclic fashion until a woman reaches her late 20s or until after a full-term pregnancy, when menstrual cramps often subside.

Primary dysmenorrhea is defined as cramps without underlying disease. Prostaglandin hormones (F_2 and $F_{2\alpha}$), which are produced by the uterus in higher concentrations during menstruation, are the cause of primary dysmenorrhea. Prostaglandins increase uterine contractions and decrease uterine artery blood flow, causing ischemia. The end result is the painful sensation of cramps.

Secondary dysmenorrhea is associated with an underlying pathologic condition of the reproductive tract and usually appears after menstruation has been established. Conditions that most frequently cause secondary dysmenorrhea include the presence of an IUD, endometriosis, pelvic inflammatory disease, anatomic anomalies such as cervical stenosis or imperforate hymen, uterine displacement, or ovarian cysts. Because primary and secondary dysmenorrhea may coexist, accurate differential diagnosis is essential for appropriate treatment.

Effective treatment for primary dysmenorrhea includes prostaglandin inhibitors and oral contraceptives. Prostaglandin inhibitors work by reducing the amount of local uterine release of prostaglandins, thereby reducing cramping. A variety of prostaglandin inhibitors are available. These include aspirin, ibuprofen, mefenamic acid, and naproxen. Some are over-the-counter medications and others require a prescription. Oral contraceptives work primarily by blocking ovulation. Oral contraceptives, too, are numerous, and a physical examination of the client is required before they can be prescribed. Women should consult their health care provider for advice about the best therapy for them.

Nursing Care

The nurse can assist women by becoming informed about self-care measures for dysmenorrhea. Self-care measures include starting an exercise program; using the pelvic rock exercise, which can decrease the pain; using heat in the form of baths, showers, or heating pads to relieve discomfort by increasing blood flow and decreasing muscle spasms; and getting more rest during menstruation. Hot drinks such as soups or spiced or herbal teas are soothing and relaxing and can help break the pain-tension cycle. Good nutrition can also promote a sense of well-being.

Menstrual Cycle Variations

Amenorrhea, the absence of menses, is classified as primary or secondary. *Primary amenorrhea* is said to occur if menstruation has not been established by age 18 years. *Secondary amenorrhea* is said to occur when an established menses (of longer than 3 months) ceases. Any of the functional causes of delayed menarche may also cause secondary amenorrhea.

Primary amenorrhea necessitates a thorough assessment of the young woman to determine its cause. The identified causes include congenital obstructions, congenital absence of the uterus, testicular feminization, or absence or imbalance of hormones. Successful treatment is determined by causative factors. Many causes are not correctable, and infertility will result.

Secondary amenorrhea is caused most frequently by pregnancy. Additional causes include lactation, hormonal imbalances, poor nutrition (anorexia nervosa, obesity, fad dieting), ovarian lesions, strenuous exercise (associated with long-distance runners with low body fat ratios), debilitating systemic diseases, stress of high intensity and/or long duration, stressful life events, a change in season or climate, use of oral contraceptives, the phenothiazine and chlorpromazine group of tranquilizers, and syndromes such as Cushing and Sheehan. Treatment is dictated by causative factors. If the cause is related to such conditions, the nurse can explain that once the underlying condition has been corrected—for example, when sufficient body weight is gained—menses will resume. Women who participate in strenuous exercise routines may be advised to increase their caloric intake or reduce their exercise levels for a month or two to see whether a normal cycle ensues. If it does not, medical referral is indicated.

An abnormally short menstrual cycle is termed *hypomenorrhea*; an abnormally long one is called *hypermenorrhea*. Excessive, profuse flow is called *menorrhagia*, and bleeding between periods is known as *metrorrhagia*. Infrequent and too frequent menses are termed *oligomenorrhea* and *polymenorrhea*, respectively. Such irregularities should be investigated to rule out any disease process.

Anovulatory Cycle

An anovulatory cycle is a cycle in which ovulation does not occur, even though the woman is not taking oral contraceptives. These cycles are noted for their irregularity, the absence of any symptoms of menstrual distress, and (often) heavy bleeding. The bleeding, if severe, is termed *dysfunctional uterine bleeding (DUB)*. In anovulatory DUB, estrogen excess results in the proliferation of endometrial growth because the secretory changes stimulated by progesterone fail to occur.

Anovulatory cycles are common in young adolescents for up to 2 years after menarche as the hypothalmic-pituitary-ovarian axis matures and begins producing normal levels of estrogen and the luteinizing hormone surge, which are necessary for normal ovulation and menstruation. Anovulatory cycles in mature females are most commonly caused by polycystic ovary disease, regular strenuous exercise, extreme weight changes, stress, or chronic substance abuse.

In women taking oral contraceptives, an ovulation-suppressed cycle occurs. Although administration of the birth control pill is interrupted each month so that cyclic withdrawal bleeding can occur, these episodes of bleeding are unlike normal menses in some respects. Typically, the flow is light to scant, and the woman experiences no dysmenorrhea.

CONTRACEPTIVE METHODS

A couple's decision to use a method of contraception is often motivated by a desire to gain control over the number of children they will conceive, if any, and/or to determine the spacing of future children. In choosing a specific method, consistency of use is more important than the absolute reliability of a given method. Other factors to be considered are the side effects and contraindications for use of a particular contraceptive method.

The nurse often assists the couple in selecting a contraceptive method. To be able to suggest a method that has practical application and is compatible with the couple's health and physical needs, the nurse must assess the couple to gather relevant data. The woman's past medical, surgical, menstrual, and obstetric history, including former contraceptive use, should be reviewed. The history should include immediate family incidences of diabetes, bleeding or clotting problems, heart problems or high blood pressure, migraine headaches or seizure disorders, kidney or liver disease, anemia, tuberculosis, stroke, cancer, or mental problems. This information provides a baseline of risk factors that could influence or contraindicate the prescription of oral contraceptives.

A physical examination should include, at a minimum, thyroid, breast, and pelvic examinations. Weight, age, and blood pressure can indicate risk factors that may preclude prescribing certain forms of birth control. Minimal laboratory testing includes a hemoglobin/hematocrit analysis; dipstick urine for sugar and protein; Pap smear; endocervical culture for *Neisseria gonorrhoeae* and chlamydia; serologic test for syphillis; and any other test identified during the history or physical exam as being appropriate. Women seeking contraception should be offered HIV testing, especially if they consider themselves in a risk group. Pre- and post-test counseling for HIV should be provided.

The couple's decisions about contraception should be made voluntarily, with full knowledge of options, advantages, disadvantages, effectiveness, side effects, and long-term effects; with access to alternatives; without pressure by health professionals; and with the strictest confidentiality. Many outside factors influence a couple's choice, including cultural influences, religious beliefs, personality, cost, effectiveness, misinformation, practicability of method, and self-esteem. Different methods of contraception may be appropriate at different times in a couple's life.

Following is a review of the major contraceptive methods available, with an examination of their advantages and disadvantages. Figure 9–2 identifies first-year failure rates for the various birth control methods.

Fertility Awareness Methods

Fertility awareness methods, also referred to as natural family planning, are based on an understanding of the changes that occur throughout a woman's ovulatory cy-

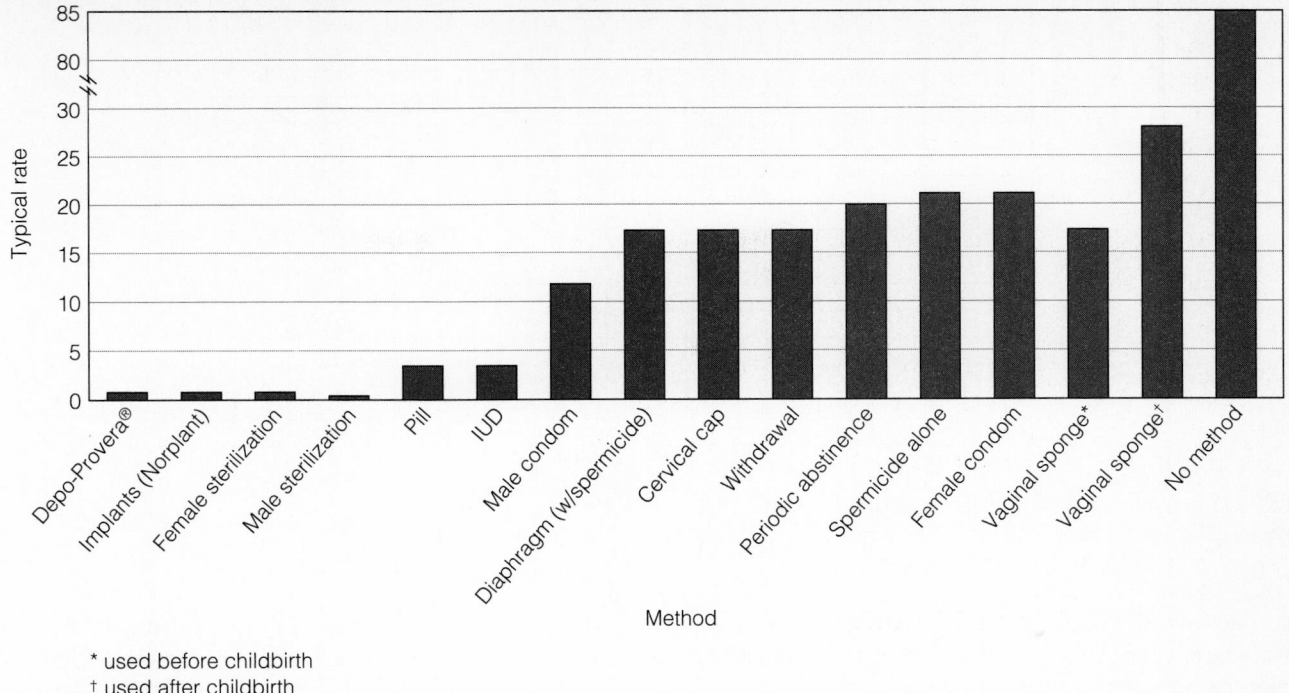

* used before childbirth
† used after childbirth

FIGURE 9-2 Percent of women experiencing accidental pregnancy in the first year of continuous use of various contraceptives.

cle. All these methods require periods of abstinence and recording of certain events throughout the cycle; hence cooperation of the partner is important.

Advantages of fertility awareness methods include the following: The methods are free, safe, acceptable to many whose religious beliefs prohibit other methods, provide an increased awareness of the body, involve no artificial substances or devices, encourage a couple to communicate about sexual activity and family planning, and are also useful in helping a couple plan a pregnancy.

Disadvantages include the following: They require extensive initial counseling to use effectively; they may interfere with sexual spontaneity; they require extensive maintenance of records for several cycles prior to beginning to use them; they may be difficult or impossible for women with irregular cycles to use; and, although theoretically they should be very reliable, in actual practice they may not be as reliable in preventing pregnancy as other methods.

The *basal body temperature (BBT) method* to detect ovulation requires that a woman take her BBT every morning upon awakening (before any activity such as drinking, smoking, or going to the bathroom) and record the readings on a temperature graph. For best results the woman should use a BBT thermometer, which records in tenths of a degree rather than two-tenths, as found in standard thermometers. After 3 to 4 months of recording temperatures, the woman with regular cycles should be able to predict when ovulation will occur. The method is based on the fact that the temperature sometimes drops

just prior to ovulation and almost always rises and remains elevated for several days after. The temperature rise occurs in response to the increased progesterone levels that occur in the second half of the cycle. Figure 9–3 shows a sample BBT chart. To avoid conception, the couple must avoid intercourse on the day of the temperature rise and for 3 days after. Because the temperature rise does not occur until after ovulation, a woman who had intercourse just prior to the rise is at risk of pregnancy. To decrease this risk, some couples abstain from intercourse for several days before the *anticipated* time of ovulation and then for 3 days after.

The *calendar method*, also referred to as the rhythm method, is based on the assumptions that ovulation tends to occur 14 days (plus or minus 2 days) before the start of the next menstrual period, sperm are viable for 48 to 72 hours, and the ovum is viable for 24 hours (Hatcher et al 1994). To use this method, the woman must record her menstrual cycles for 6 to 8 months so that the shortest and longest cycles can be identified. The first day of menstruation is the first day of the cycle. The fertile phase is calculated from 18 days before the end of the shortest recorded cycle through 11 days from the end of the longest recorded cycle (Hatcher et al 1994). For example, if a woman's cycle lasts from 24 to 28 days, the fertile phase would be calculated as day 6 through day 17. Once this information is obtained, the woman can identify the fertile and infertile phases of her cycle. For effective use of this method, she must abstain from intercourse during the fertile phase.

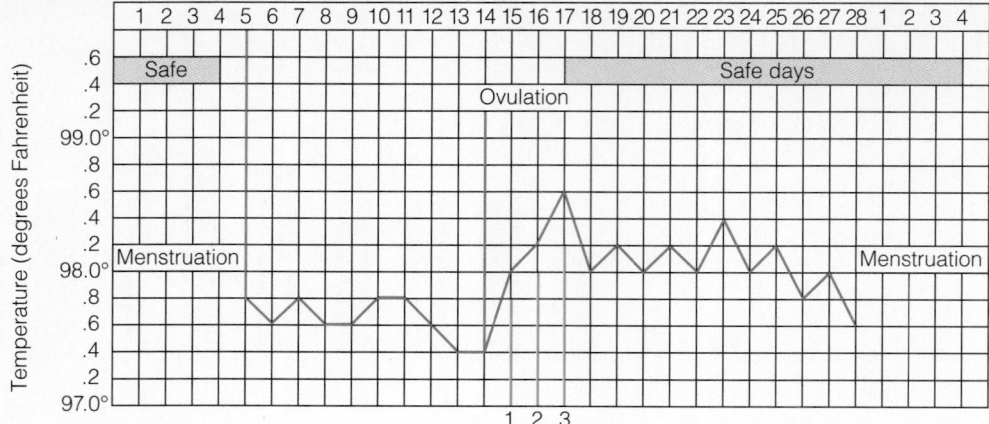

FIGURE 9-3 Sample basal body temperature chart. SOURCE: Crooks R, Baur K: *Our Sexuality,* 5th ed. Redwood City, CA: Benjamin/Cummings, 1993.

The calendar method is the least reliable of the fertility awareness methods and has largely been replaced by the other, more scientific approaches.

The *cervical mucus method*, sometimes called the *ovulation method* or the *Billings method*, involves the assessment of cervical mucus changes that occur during the menstrual cycle. The amount and character of cervical mucus change as a result of the influence of estrogen and progesterone on the mucous secretory glands present in the cervix.

At ovulation, estrogen-dominant mucus is greatest in amount and stretchability. The woman notices a feeling of wetness around the vagina. This mucus shows a ferning pattern that becomes apparent when the mucus is placed on a glass slide and allowed to dry (Figure 7–4). The stretchability (spinnbarkheit) of the cervical mucus is greatest at the time of ovulation and may vary from 5 to 20 cm. This type of mucus allows increased permeability to sperm.

During the luteal phase the characteristics of the cervical mucus change. Progesterone-dominant mucus becomes thick and sticky and forms a network in the cervical canal that traps the sperm and makes their passage more difficult.

To use the ovulation method, the woman should abstain from intercourse for the first menstrual cycle. Cervical mucus should be assessed on a daily basis for the woman to become more familiar with varying characteristics. After a pattern has been established, abstinence from intercourse is necessary when estrogen-dominant mucus predominates and for 4 days following ovulation.

The *symptothermal method* consists of various assessments that are made and recorded by the couple. They use a chart to record information regarding cycle days, coitus, cervical mucus changes, and secondary signs such as increased libido, abdominal bloating, mittelschmerz, and basal body temperature. Through the various assessments the couple learns to recognize signs of ovulation.

This combined approach tends to improve the effectiveness of fertility awareness contraception methods.

Coitus interruptus, or the withdrawal method of birth control, allows couples to have sexual intercourse until ejaculation is imminent. At that time the man withdraws his penis and ejaculates completely away from the external genitalia of his female partner. The method is available in any situation, costs nothing, and requires no medication or devices. Because of its high failure rate, which among typical couples is 19%, it is not a recommended method of contraception. It is, however, considerably better than no method at all (Hatcher et al 1994).

Failure tends to occur for two reasons: First, this method demands great self-control on the part of the man, who must withdraw just as he feels the urge for deeper penetration with impending orgasm. Second, some preejaculatory fluid, which can contain sperm, may escape from the penis during the excitement phase prior to ejaculation. Because the quantity of sperm in this preejaculatory fluid is increased after a recent ejaculation, this is especially significant for couples who engage in repeated episodes of orgasm within a short period of time. To use the method correctly, the man should void and wipe the tip of his penis before intercourse. This removes any sperm that may have remained in the urethra from a previous ejaculation. When the man senses that he is about to ejaculate, he should withdraw his penis completely and ejaculate away from his partner's genitalia. Withdrawal is not effective in men who cannot sense when ejaculation is imminent. Couples who use this method should be aware of postcoital contraceptive options should the man fail to withdraw in time.

Abstinence can also be considered a situational contraceptive and, because of changing values and the increased risk of infection with intercourse, is gaining increased acceptance as a viable alternative to intercourse.

Douching after intercourse is an ineffective method of contraception and is not recommended. It may actually

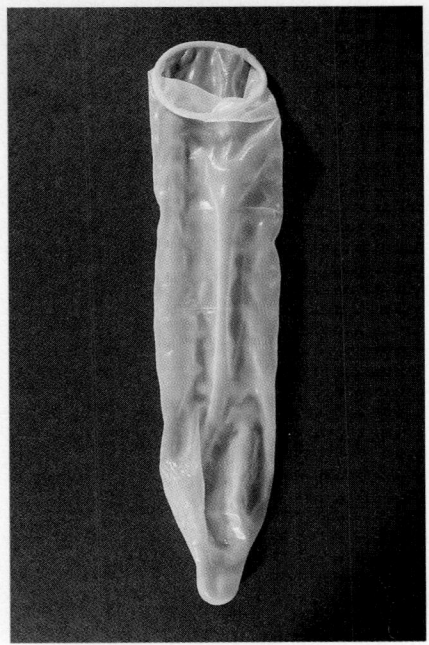

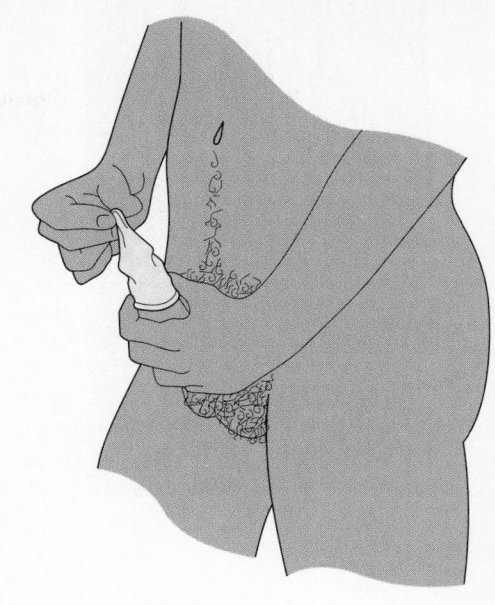

FIGURE 9-4 *A* Unrolled condom with reservoir tip. *B* Correct use of a condom.

facilitate conception by pushing the sperm farther up the birth canal. Furthermore, sperm have been identified in the fallopian tubes as soon as 90 seconds after ejaculation.

Barrier Contraceptives

Mechanical contraceptive methods act as barriers preventing either the transport of sperm to the ovum or the implantation of the ovum/zygote.

Male Condom

Condoms are an effective means of contraception when used consistently and properly (Figure 9–4). Acceptance has been increasing as a growing number of men assumes responsibility for regulation of fertility. Another reason for the increased use of condoms is the protection they afford against many sexually transmitted infections, especially HIV.

Condoms are applied to the erect penis, rolled from the tip to the end of the shaft, before vulvar or vaginal contact is made. A small space must be left at the end of the condom to allow for collection of the ejaculate so that the condom will not break at the time of ejaculation. Water-soluble lubricants, such as K-Y Jelly, should be used if the condom and/or vagina are dry, to prevent irritation and possible condom breakage. For optimum effectiveness the penis should be withdrawn from the vagina while still erect and the condom rim held to prevent spillage. If after ejaculation the penis becomes flaccid while still in the vagina, the male should hold onto the edge of the condom while withdrawing from the vagina to avoid

spilling the semen and to prevent the condom from slipping off.

The effectiveness of condoms is largely determined by their use. The condom is small, lightweight, disposable, and inexpensive; has no side effects; requires no medical examination or supervision; offers visual evidence of effectiveness; and protects against many sexually transmitted infections. Many women now insist that their sexual partners use condoms, and many women carry condoms with them.

With their increasing popularity comes increased choice. Condoms are now available with ribbed sides or smooth sides, tapered or straight-sided, lubricated or unlubricated, with spermicide and without. Condoms called "skin condoms" made from lamb's intestines are also available and are preferred by some men, especially those who have difficulty tolerating latex. They are *not* considered effective in preventing the spread of infection; in fact viruses such as HIV, hepatitis B, and herpes simplex can pass through them. Latex condoms are superior in that regard. Spermicidal condoms or concurrent use of a vaginal spermicide increases overall effectiveness.

Breakage, displacement, possible perineal or vaginal irritation, and dulled sensation are cited as disadvantages of the condom.

Female Condom

The Reality **female condom** (Figure 9–5) is a thin polyurethane sheath with a flexible ring at each end. The inner ring, at the closed end of the condom, serves as the means of insertion and covers the cervix like a diaphragm.

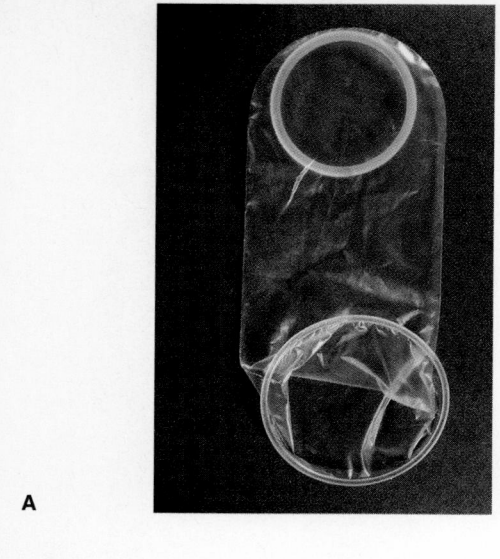

A

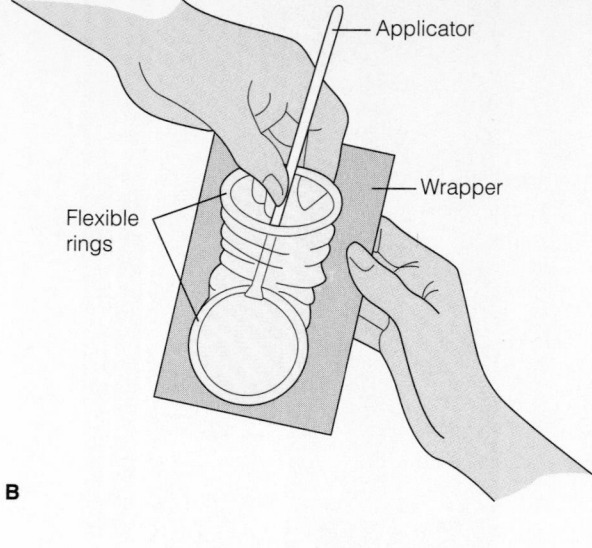

B

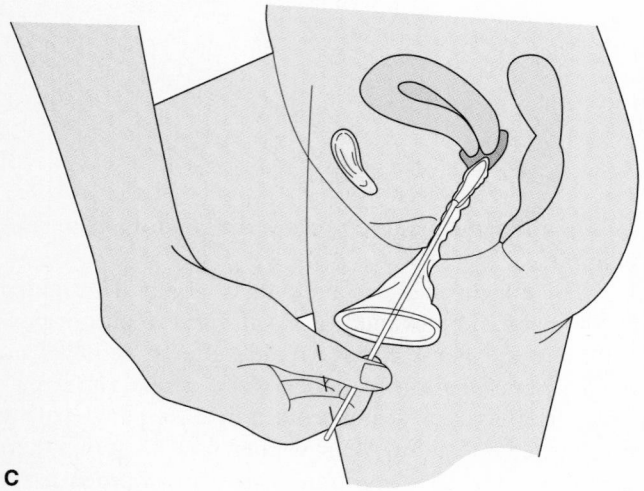

C

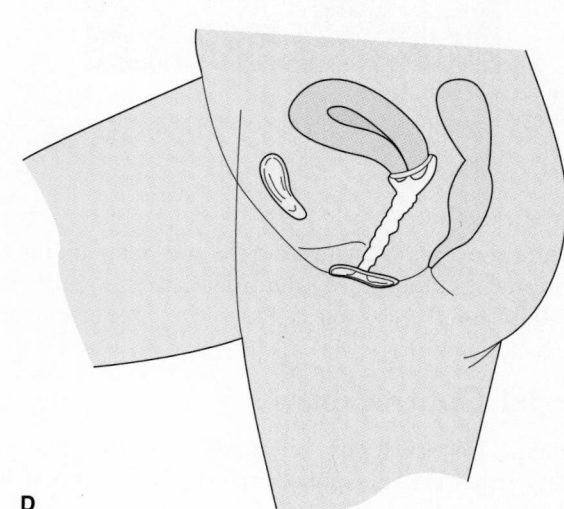

D

FIGURE 9-5 *A* The female condom. To insert the condom: *B* Remove condom and applicator from wrapper by pulling up on the ring. *C* Insert condom slowly by gently pushing the applicator toward the small of the back. *D* When properly inserted, the outer ring should rest on the folds of skin around the vaginal opening, and the inner ring (closed end) should fit loosely against the cervix. SOURCE: Crooks R, Baur K: *Our Sexuality,* 5th ed. Monterey, CA: Brooks Cole, 1993.

The second ring remains outside the vagina and covers a portion of the woman's perineum. It also covers the base of the man's penis during intercourse. Available over the counter and designed for one-time use, it may be inserted just prior to or up to 8 hours before intercourse. The inner sheath is prelubricated but does not contain spermicide and is not designed to be used with a male condom. Data on its effectiveness against pregnancy are still limited, although the female condom has been compared to other barrier methods. It probably provides better protection against pathogens than some other methods because it lines the entire vagina. The female condom is re-garded positively because it is the first woman-controlled barrier contraceptive that provides some protection against sexually transmitted infections. Its cost (about $2.25) may be a factor for some couples. The ultimate acceptance and usage of the female condom by women and their partners has yet to be determined (Connell 1994).

Diaphragm

The **diaphragm** (Figure 9–6) is used with spermicidal cream or jelly and offers a good level of protection from conception. The woman must be fitted with a diaphragm

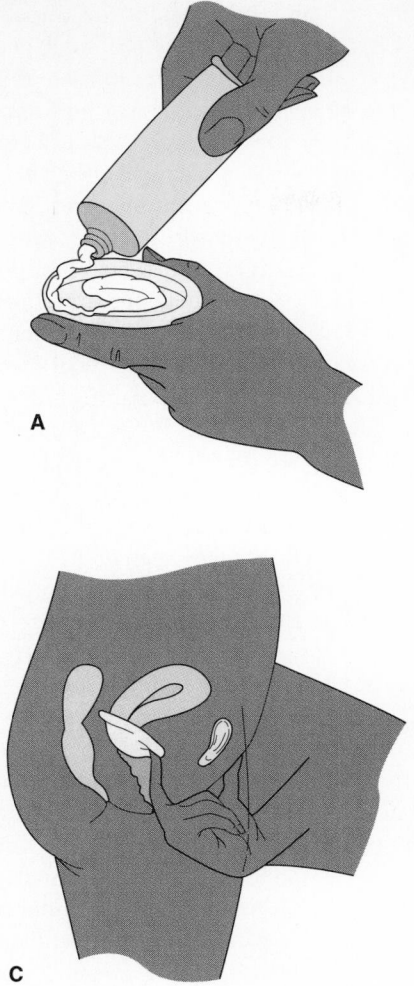

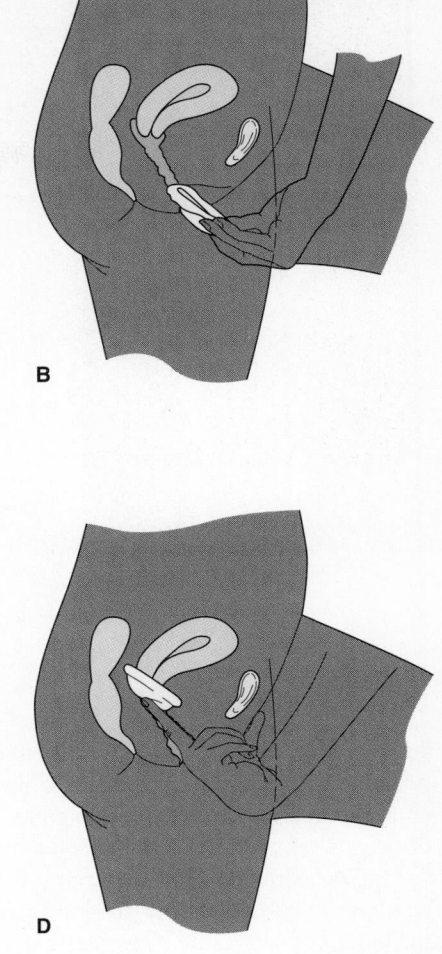

FIGURE 9-6   *A* Apply jelly to the rim and center of the diaphragm. *B* Insert the diaphragm. *C* Push the rim of the diaphragm under the symphysis pubis. *D* Check placement of the diaphragm. Cervix should be felt through the diaphragm.

and given instructions by trained personnel. It should be rechecked for correct size after each childbirth and if a woman has gained or lost 15 pounds or more.

The diaphragm must be inserted prior to intercourse, with approximately 1 teaspoonful (or 1½ inches from the tube) of spermicidal jelly placed around its rim and in the cup. This serves as a chemical barrier to supplement the mechanical barrier of the diaphragm. The diaphragm is inserted into the vagina and covers the cervix. The last step is to push the edge of the diaphragm under the symphysis pubis, which may result in a "popping" sensation. When fitted properly and correctly in place, the diaphragm should not cause discomfort to the woman or her partner. Correct placement of the diaphragm can be checked by touching the cervix with a fingertip through the cup. The cervix feels like a small rounded structure and has a consistency similar to that of the tip of the nose. The center of the diaphragm should be over the cervix. If more than 4 hours elapse between insertion of the diaphragm and intercourse, additional spermicidal cream should be used. It is necessary to leave

the diaphragm in place for at least 6 to 8 hours after coitus. If intercourse is desired again within the 6 hours, another type of contraception must be used or additional spermicidal jelly placed in the vagina with an applicator, taking care not to disturb the placement of the diaphragm. The diaphragm should be held up to the light periodically and carefully inspected for tears or holes.

Some couples feel that the use of a diaphragm interferes with the spontaneity of intercourse. The nurse can suggest that the partner insert the diaphragm as part of foreplay.

Diaphragms are an excellent contraceptive method for women who are lactating, who cannot or do not wish to use the pill (oral contraceptives), or who wish to avoid the increased risk of pelvic inflammatory disease associated with intrauterine devices. They are also a good choice for older women who smoke but don't wish to be sterilized.

Women who object to manipulating their genitals to insert the diaphragm, check its placement, and remove it may find this method unsatisfactory. Also, it is not

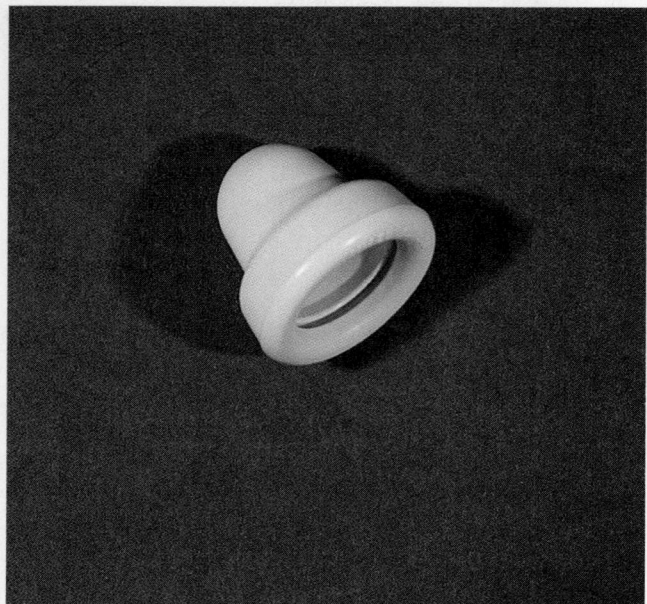

FIGURE 9-7   Cervical cap.

recommended for women with a history of urinary tract infection (UTI) because pressure from the diaphragm on the urethra may interfere with complete bladder emptying and lead to recurrent UTI. Women with a history of toxic shock syndrome should not use diaphragms or any of the barrier methods because they are left in place for prolonged periods. For the same reason the diaphragm should not be used during a menstrual period or if a woman has abnormal vaginal discharge.

Cervical Cap

The **cervical cap** (Figure 9–7) is a cup-shaped device, used with spermicidal cream or jelly, that fits snugly over the cervix and is held in place by suction. Effectiveness rates are similar to those for the diaphragm. Widely used in Europe, it is beginning to gain popularity in the United States. Use of the cervical cap is similar to that of the diaphragm. Unlike the diaphragm, however, the cap may be left in place for up to 48 hours, and it does not require additional spermicide for repeated intercourse. The cervical cap may be more difficult to fit because of limited size options. It also tends to be more difficult for women to insert and remove (Hatcher et al 1994).

Intrauterine Device

An **intrauterine device (IUD)** is designed to be inserted into the uterus and left in place for prolonged periods of time, providing continuous contraceptive protection. The exact mechanism of IUD action is not clearly understood. Traditionally, the IUD was believed to act by preventing implantation of a fertilized ovum. Thus the IUD

was considered an abortifacient or abortion-causing method. Current evidence on the new generation of IUDs suggests that they truly are contraceptives; they act by immobilizing sperm in some way and impeding their progress from the cervix through the uterus to the fallopian tubes (Chez & Mishell 1994). Other evidence indicates that they may also prevent fertilization by speeding the movement of the ovum through the fallopian tubes to the uterus. The IUD is also known to have local inflammatory effects on the endometrium as well as other biochemical and enzymatic processes, but their impact on IUD action is not yet clear (Hatcher et al 1994).

Two IUDs are currently available, and a third is being tested. The two available IUDs are medicated, containing either copper (Cu380T—ParaGard) or progesterone (Progestasert) (Figure 9–8). The Progestasert must be changed every year and should therefore be used only in special circumstances such as in women with an allergy to copper. The ParaGard was originally approved by the FDA to be changed every 4 years; recently, however, it was approved for 8 years' use. If approved, the Levonorgestrel IUD (LNg IUD), which releases levonorgestrel, will probably be changed every 5 years.

Advantages of IUDs include high rate of effectiveness, continuous contraceptive protection, no need for coitus-related activity, and relative inexpensiveness over time. The possible adverse effects of IUDs limit their use somewhat. These include pelvic inflammatory disease, severe dysmenorrhea, irregular menses, increased bleeding during menses, uterine perforation, and expulsion. In addition, if the IUD fails and a pregnancy results, there is an increased incidence of ectopic pregnancy (Hatcher et al 1994).

IUDs are best suited to women who are multiparous and in a stable monogamous relationship. They are not recommended for women who have multiple sexual partners and are thus at risk for STDs because they provide no protection against STDs.

The IUD is inserted into the uterus with its string or tail protruding through the cervix into the vagina. It may be inserted during a menstrual period or during the 4- to

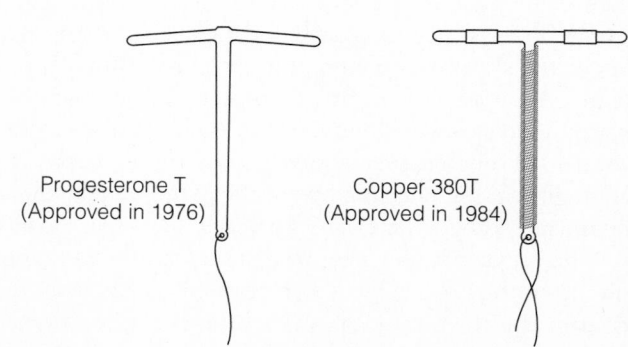

Progesterone T
(Approved in 1976)

Copper 380T
(Approved in 1984)

FIGURE 9-8   Two types of IUDs.

6-week postpartum check. After insertion, the woman should be instructed to check for the presence of the string once a week for the first month and then after each menses. She is told that she may have some cramping and/or bleeding intermittently for 2 to 6 weeks and that her first few menses may be irregular. Follow-up examination is suggested 4 to 8 weeks after insertion.

Women with IUDs should be advised to contact their health care provider immediately if they experience any of the following warning signs, which can be remembered by thinking of the acronym "PAINS" (Hatcher et al 1994, p 375):

P   Period late (pregnancy), abnormal spotting or bleeding
A   Abdominal pain, pain with intercourse
I   Infection exposure (any STD), abnormal discharge
N   Not feeling well, fever, chills
S   String missing, shorter, or longer

Oral Contraceptives

The use of hormones, specifically the combination of estrogen and progesterone, is a very successful birth control method. **Oral contraceptives (OC)** work by inhibiting the release of an ovum and by maintaining cervical mucus that is inhibitory to sperm passage. Numerous oral contraceptives are available. The "pill" is taken daily for 21 days beginning on the Sunday after the first day of the menstrual cycle. In most cases menses will occur 1 to 4 days after the last pill is taken. Seven days after completing her last pill, the woman restarts the pill. Thus the woman always begins the pill on the same day of the week. Companies also offer a 28-day pack with seven "blank" pills so that the woman never stops taking a pill. The pill should be taken at approximately the same time each day for optimum effectiveness—usually upon arising or before retiring in the evening. Certain medications such as dilantin or tetracycline may decrease the effectiveness of oral contraceptives. The woman should discuss all medication use with her health care provider. It may be necessary to increase the strength of her OC or advise that she use a backup method of contraception in some cases.

Although they are highly effective, oral contraceptives may produce side effects ranging from breakthrough bleeding to thrombus formation. Side effects from oral contraceptives may be either progesterone or estrogen related (Table 9–3). The use of low-dose (35 μg or less estrogen) preparations has reduced many of the side effects, but the threat of potential risk is sufficient to deter some women from using oral contraceptives.

Another oral contraceptive is the seldom used progesterone-only pill, also called the *minipill*. It is used primarily by women who have a contraindication to the estrogen component of the combination preparation, such as history of thrombophlebitis, but are strongly motivated toward this form of contraception. The major problems with this preparation are amenorrhea or irregular spotting and bleeding patterns.

Contraindications to the use of oral contraceptives include pregnancy, previous history of thrombophlebitis or thrombolic disease, acute or chronic liver disease of cholestatic type with abnormal function, presence of estrogen-dependent carcinomas, undiagnosed uterine bleeding, heavy smoking, hypertension, diabetes, and hyperlipidemia. Women with any of the following conditions who use oral contraceptives should be examined every 3 months: migraine headaches, epilepsy, depression, oligomenorrhea, and amenorrhea. Women who choose this method of contraception should be fully advised of potential side effects.

Oral contraceptives also have some important noncontraceptive benefits. Many women experience relief of uncomfortable menstrual symptoms. Cramps are lessened, flow is decreased, and cycle regularity is increased. Mittelschmerz is eliminated, and the incidence of functional ovarian cysts is decreased. More importantly, there is a substantial reduction in the incidence of ectopic pregnancy, ovarian cancer, endometrial cancer, iron-deficiency anemia, and benign breast disease. The FDA recently revised the oral contraceptive labeling material to state that for healthy, nonsmoking women over age 40, the benefits of oral contraceptives may outweigh possible risks (Hatcher et al 1994).

The woman using oral contraceptives should be advised to contact her health care provider if she becomes depressed, develops a breast lump, becomes jaundiced, or experiences any of the following warning signs, which can

TABLE 9-3	Side Effects Associated with Oral Contraceptives
Estrogen Effects	**Progestin Effects**
Alterations in lipid metabolism	Acne, oily skin
Breast tenderness, engorgement; increased breast size	Breast tenderness; increased breast size
Cerebrovascular accident	Decreased libido
Changes in carbohydrate metabolism	Decreased high-density lipoprotein (HDL) cholesterol levels
Chloasma	Depression
Fluid retention; cyclic weight gain	Fatigue
Headache	Hirsutism
Hepatic adenomas	Increased appetite; weight gain
Hypertension	Increased low-density lipoprotein (LDL) cholesterol levels
Leukorrhea, cervical erosion, ectopia	Oligomenorrhea, amenorrhea
Nausea	Pruritus
Nervousness, irritability	Sebaceous cysts
Telangiectasia	
Thromboembolic complications – thrombophlebitis, pulmonary embolism	

be remembered using the acronym "ACHES" (Hatcher et al 1994, p 276):

A Abdominal pain (severe)
C Chest pain (severe), cough, shortness of breath
H Headache (severe), dizziness, weakness, or numbness
E Eye problems (vision loss or blurring), speech problems
S Severe leg pain (calf or thigh)

Spermicides

Spermicides, available as creams, jellies, foam, vaginal film, and suppositories, are inserted into the vagina prior to intercourse. They destroy sperm or neutralize vaginal secretions and thereby immobilize sperm. Spermicides that effervesce in a moist environment offer more rapid protection, and coitus may take place immediately after they are inserted. Suppositories may require up to 30 minutes to dissolve and will *not* offer protection until they do so. The woman should be instructed to insert these spermicide preparations high in the vagina and maintain a supine position.

Spermicides are minimally effective when used alone, but their effectiveness increases in conjunction with a condom. They provide a significant protection against gonorrhea and chlamydia and some protection against trichomonas and herpes (Hatcher et al 1994). Unfortunately, the effectiveness of spermicides against HIV has been called into question. Nonoxynol-9, the active ingredient in spermicides, is lethal to HIV in laboratory tests. However, spermicides are known to be irritating to vaginal and cervical epithelium, especially with frequent use. Evidence suggests that microscopic lesions of the vaginal tissue can facilitate the transmission of HIV. Researchers question whether frequent use of spermicide with its resulting irritation to the vaginal epithelium actually enhances the transmission of HIV (Pollack & Moore, 1994). Because the impact of spermicides on vaginal tissue does seem to be dose related, women who have frequent intercourse and who are at high risk for HIV should be counseled about the possible implications of spermicide use.

The major advantages of spermicides are their wide availability and low toxicity. Although some studies have suggested that the use of spermicides at the time of conception or early in pregnancy may be associated with an increased risk of congenital anomalies, recent studies show no increased incidence.

Long-Acting Progestin Contraceptives

Subdermal Implants (Norplant)

Subdermal implants (Norplant) consist of six silastic capsules containing levonorgestrel, a progestin, which are

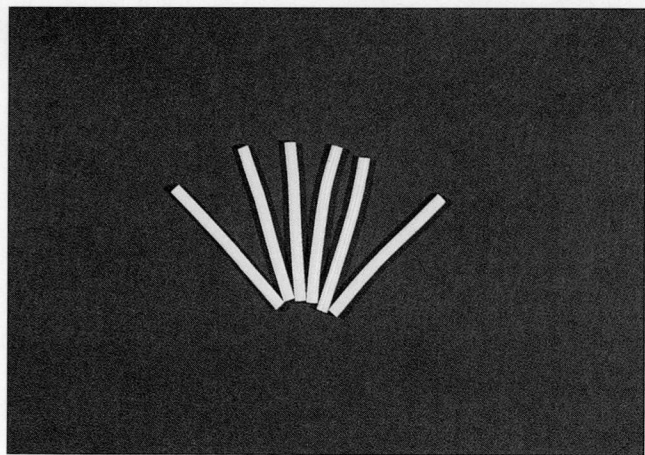

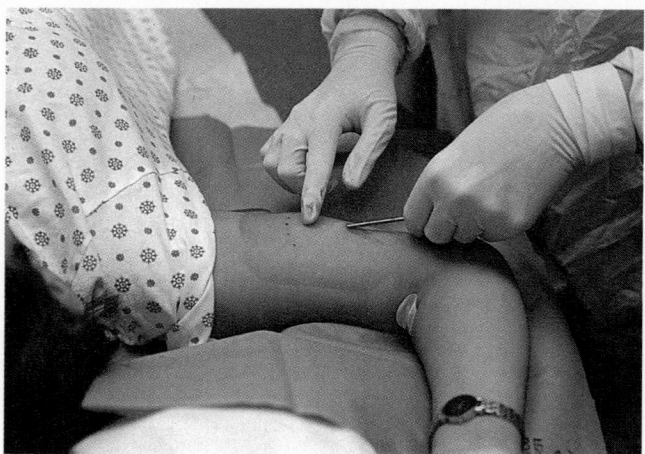

FIGURE 9-9   Norplant, a long-acting progestin contraceptive, is implanted in a woman's upper arm.

implanted in a woman's arm. They are effective for up to 5 years (Figure 9–9).

Norplant acts by preventing ovulation in most women. It also stimulates the production of thick cervical mucus, which inhibits sperm penetration. Norplant provides effective continuous contraception that is removed from the act of coitus. Possible side effects include spotting, irregular bleeding or amenorrhea, an increased incidence of ovarian cysts, weight gain, headaches, acne, hirsutism, and depression (Hinkle 1994). Women should be advised that the implants may be visible, especially in very slender users, and a minor surgical procedure is required to insert and remove the implants.

Injectable Progestin (Depo-Provera)

Medroxyprogesterone acetate suspension (**Depo-Provera**), a long-acting, injectable progestin, has been approved for contraceptive use in the United States. A single intramuscular injection of 150 mg Depo-Provera provides highly effective birth control for 3 months. This method, which acts primarily by suppressing ovulation, is safe, convenient, private, and relatively inexpensive. It also separates birth control from the act of coitus. It can safely be given to nursing mothers because it contains no estrogen. Common side effects include menstrual irregularities, amenorrhea, weight gain, and headache. Return of fertility may be delayed for up to 12 to 18 months after injections are stopped.

Emergency Postcoital Contraception

Emergency postcoital contraception is indicated when a woman is worried about pregnancy because of unprotected intercourse or a possible contraceptive failure (eg, a broken condom, slipped diaphragm, or too long between Depo-Provera injections). Postcoital contraceptive regimens are most effective when taken within 72 hours of coitus.

The most commonly prescribed postcoital emergency contraceptive is Ovral, a combination OC containing 50 μg estrogen. This is occasionally referred to as "the morning-after pill," but the woman actually takes two pills as soon as possible after unprotected intercourse and two more 12 hours later. Unfortunately, a common side effect is vomiting, especially after the second two pills. Some care givers prescribe an antiemetic to help prevent the vomiting.

Other currently used regimens for emergency contraception include larger than normal doses of certain other combination contraceptives, conjugated estrogens, or danazol, or the insertion of a copper IUD (Contemporary OB/GYN 1994).

Male Contraception

The vasectomy and the condom are currently the only forms of male contraception available in the United States. Hormonal contraception for men has yet to be developed, although studies are under way.

Future Trends

A wide variety of contraception methods are currently being investigated for use in the United States. Many are already available in other countries, but the FDA requires extensive study to determine efficacy and safety prior to marketing in this country.

Potential future contraceptive options include **mifepristone (RU 486),** which has gained widespread recognition as an abortifacient in Europe and China. A progesterone antagonist, it may be most appropriately used as a safe, effective postcoital contraceptive. By blocking progesterone, mifepristone alters the endometrium, making it unsuitable for implantation. Research indicates that it has excellent efficacy with minimal side effects when given within 72 hours of unprotected intercourse (Hatcher et al 1994). It currently is being tested at selected US clinics.

Research continues on the use of contraceptive vaccinations for men and women and male hormonal methods

such as long-acting testosterone injections and progestin-androgen combination injections. Other products currently being tested include disposable, spermicide-containing diaphragms; a new contraceptive sponge; Lea's shield, which is similar to a cervical cap but with a valve to allow cervical secretions to flow out; transdermal contraceptives; and progesterone-containing vaginal rings (Mastroianni 1994).

Operative Sterilization

Before sterilization is performed on either partner, a thorough explanation of the procedure should be given to both. Each should understand that sterilization is not a decision to be taken lightly or entered into when psychologic stresses, such as separation or divorce, exist. Even though male and female procedures are theoretically reversible, the permanency of the procedure should be stressed and understood. All forms of reversible contraception should be explained and discussed in detail to assist the client in making an informed decision.

Male sterilization is achieved by a relatively minor procedure called a **vasectomy.** Under local anesthesia a 2 to 3 cm incision is made over the vas deferens on each side of the scrotum. The ducts are isolated; severed; and occluded by ligation of the ends, by coagulation of the lumen, by burial of the cut ends, or by use of clips or polyethylene tubing with a stopcock for potentially reversible procedures. Absorbable sutures are used to close the skin. The man is instructed to apply ice when pain or swelling occurs and to use a scrotal support for a week. It takes about 4 to 6 weeks and 6 to 36 ejaculations to clear remaining sperm from the vas deferens. During that period the couple is advised to use another method of birth control and to bring in two or three semen samples for a sperm count. The man is rechecked at 6 and 12 months to ensure that fertility has not been restored by recanalization. Side effects of a vasectomy are uncommon, but they include hematoma, sperm granulomas, and spontaneous reanastomosis.

Vasectomies can be reversed with the use of microsurgery techniques. Restored fertility, as measured by subsequent pregnancy, ranges from 30–85% (Hatcher et al 1994).

Female sterilization **(tubal ligation)** can be accomplished by several abdominal and vaginal procedures. The fallopian tubes are transected or occluded by electrocautery. Postpartal laparotomy is done 1 to 3 days after childbirth, under general anesthesia and usually with a small subumbilical incision. The tubes are isolated and may then be crushed, ligated, electrocoagulated, banded, or plugged (in the newer reversible procedures). The interval minilaparotomy uses a suprapubic incision with similar techniques for interrupting tubal patency.

Laparoscopic sterilization may be done at any time. One or two incisions are made in the subumbilical area. The abdomen is distended with carbon dioxide gas, the laparoscope is introduced through a trocar, and the fallopian tube is visualized. The isthmic portion of the tube is grasped and coagulated, transected, clipped, or banded. The procedure is repeated on the other tube.

Complications of female sterilization procedures include coagulation burns on the bowels, bowel perforation, infection, hemorrhage, and adverse anesthesia effects. Reversal of a tubal ligation depends on many factors, including the portion of the tube excised, the presence or absence of the fimbriae, and the length of the tube remaining. Microsurgical techniques are now the standard reversal approach, with successful pregnancy rates of 40% to 75%.

No reversible form of sterilization holds promise of widespread use at the present time. However, a reversible form of sterilization is currently being investigated. It incorporates the use of a hysteroscope for direct visualization of the tubal openings into the uterus. The openings are injected with a silicone substance that hardens and occludes the cornual section of the fallopian tube. Hysterosalpingography confirms the success of the procedure, and a thread is left in the uterine cavity for future removal.

I think I'm like a lot of women. During my life I've used a variety of contraceptive methods. I took the pill back when the doses were higher, I used foam alone and had a baby, then used spermicidal cream and condoms more successfully. I never wanted a tubal, and my husband refuses to consider vasectomy, so the IUD was a perfect alternative. I'm 41 and I like something I don't have to think about every time we want to make love. Women my age need choices, too.

Nursing Care

In most cases the nurse who provides information and guidance about contraceptive methods works with a woman because most contraceptive methods are female oriented. Because a man can purchase condoms without seeing a health care provider, only in the case of vasectomy does a man require counseling and interaction with a nurse. The nurse can play an important role in helping a woman choose a method of contraception that is acceptable to her and to her partner (Table 9–4).

In addition to the assessments described on page 202 the nurse can spend time with the woman learning about her life-style, personal attitudes toward particular contraceptive methods, and plans for future childbearing. If a woman has multiple sexual partners and a high rate of sexual activity, for example, a spermicide alone offers only limited protection against pregnancy, and an IUD greatly increases her chances of developing pelvic inflammatory disease. Birth control pills may provide the greatest protection for this woman if future childbearing ability is important to her.

Religious beliefs are often important in selecting a method of fertility control, and the nurse counseling women about contraception should be sensitive to them.

TABLE 9-4	Factors to Consider in Choosing a Method of Contraception

Effectiveness of method in preventing pregnancy
Safety of the method:
    Are there inherent risks?
    Does it offer protection against STDs or other conditions?
Client's age and future childbearing plans
Any contraindications in client's health history
Religious or moral factors influencing choice
Personal preferences, biases
Life-style:
    How frequently does client have intercourse?
    Does she have multiple partners?
    Does she have ready access to medical care in the event of complications?
    Is cost a factor?
Partner's support and willingness to cooperate
Personal motivation to use method

Some women accept only fertility awareness methods of contraception. The nurse working with these women can help by providing them with the information and support they need to follow this method effectively.

Personal bias also plays a role in selection of method. Some women are reluctant to take birth control pills because they fear the associated risk factors. If the woman remains fearful even after careful explanation and reassurance that the risks of the pill are limited in women who are good candidates for the pill, the nurse should recommend another method. By the same token, if a woman is uncomfortable with touching her genitals and thus finds many of the barrier methods distasteful, she should choose another method.

Personal bias can also influence the nurse unless care is taken. Nurses tend to recommend the methods they prefer and have confidence in. Although this is understandable, it could also interfere with the effectiveness of the counseling the nurse provides. Nurses should examine their own feelings, attitudes, and biases about contraceptive choices.

Once a method is chosen, the nurse can help the woman learn to use it effectively (see Teaching Guide: Using a Method of Contraception). Often it is the nurse who is available to answer questions about a particular method.

If a woman is considering a tubal ligation or her partner is considering a vasectomy, careful preoperative preparation and explanation are essential. The couple should clearly understand the risks and the surgical techniques used and should accept the idea that the method is essentially irreversible. Although the physician does much of the counseling for these procedures, nurses are often responsible for reinforcing the information and answering questions.

USING A METHOD OF CONTRACEPTION

Assessment   The nurse determines the woman's general knowledge about contraceptive methods, identifies the methods the woman has used previously (if any), identifies contraindications or risk factors for any methods, discusses the woman's personal preferences and biases about various methods, and discusses her commitment (and her partner's commitment if appropriate) to a chosen method.

Nursing Diagnosis   Knowledge deficit related to lack of information about the correct use of chosen method of contraception.

Nursing Plan and Implementation   The teaching plan will focus on confirming that a chosen method of contraception is a good choice for the woman. The nurse will then help the woman learn the method so that she can use it effectively.

Client Goals   At the completion of teaching, the woman will be able to:

1.   Confirm for herself that the chosen method of contraception is appropriate for her.

2.   List the advantages, disadvantages, and risks of the chosen method.

3.   Describe (or demonstrate) the correct procedure for using the chosen method.

4.   Cite warning signs that should be reported to the care giver.

Teaching Plan

Content   Discuss the factors that a woman should consider in choosing a method of contraception (Table 9–4). Stress that the different methods may be appropriate at different times in the woman's life. Review the woman's reasons for selecting a particular method and confirm any contraindications to specific methods.

Discuss the advantages, disadvantages, and risks of the chosen method.

Describe the correct procedure for using a method. Go through step-by-step. Periodically stop and have the woman review the information for you. If a technique is to be learned (as with inserting a diaphragm or charting BBT), demonstrate and then have the woman do a return demonstration as appropriate. (Note: If certain aspects are beyond the nurse's level of expertise, the nurse can review the content and confirm that a woman has the opportunity to do a return demonstration. For example, an office nurse who does not do cervical cap fittings may cover information on its use, have the woman try inserting the cap herself, and then have the placement checked by the nurse practitioner or physician.)

Provide information on what the woman should do if unusual circumstances arise (she forgets a pill or misses a morning temperature).

Stress warning signs that require immediate action on the part of the woman, and explain why these signs indicate a risk. Carefully delineate the actions the woman should take: Should she contact her care giver? Stop the method?

Arrange to talk with the woman again soon, either on the phone or at a return visit, to determine if she has any questions about the method and to ensure that no problems have arisen.

Teaching Method   *Contraception is a personal decision, so the discussion should take place in a private area free of interruptions.*

The nurse should create a supportive, warm, and comfortable atmosphere by her or his attitude and communication style—both verbal and nonverbal.

The nurse needs to consciously recognize that her or his personal preferences about contraception may be very different from those of the woman being counseled. The nurse has the responsibility to provide accurate information in an open, nonjudgmental way.

Focus on open discussion. It may help to have written information about the method chosen. If a signed permit is required (as with sterilization or IUD insertion), the physician should also discuss the advantages, disadvantages, and risks.

Learning is best accomplished when material is broken down into smaller steps.

People learn best when multiple approaches are used, so it is helpful to have a model or chart to enable the woman to visualize what is being described. The nurse can also have a sample of the chosen method available: a package of oral contraceptives, an open IUD, or a symptothermal chart.

Provide a written handout identifying the warning signs and listing the actions a woman should take. The handout should also cover actions the woman should take if an unusual situation develops. For example, what should she do if she vomits or has diarrhea while taking oral contraceptives? What action should she take if she and her partner are using a condom and it breaks?

The woman should know that she is free to call if she has questions or concerns once she starts using the method. This increases her comfort level and enables the nurse to detect potential problems early.

The nurse also reviews any possible side effects and warning signs of the method chosen and counsels the woman about what action to take if she suspects she is pregnant. In many cases the nurse may become involved in telephone counseling for women who call with questions and concerns. Thus the nurse must be knowledgeable about this topic and have resources available to find answers to less common questions.

Menopause

Menopause, the cessation of menses, marks a developmental transition in a woman's life. It signals the end of reproductive potential and implies aging, if not old age. The current approximate age of menopause in the United States is 51 years. Approximately one-third of the entire female population of the Western world is postmenopausal (Hammond 1994). **Climacteric,** or change of life, a word often used synonymously with menopause, refers to the host of psychologic and physical alterations that occur around the time of menopause.

Health Promotion and Aging

As women's life expectancy has lengthened, our knowledge and attitudes about aging have changed. Increased awareness of health and factors that promote it at all ages has become part of the American culture. For example, many women are engaged in exercise and fitness activities to promote cardiovascular health. The harmful effects of smoking have been thoroughly documented, and many women are quitting smoking. Nutrition for a healthy life with an emphasis on a low-fat, high-fiber diet is now taught in school, through the mass media, and even in supermarkets. All these factors have helped contribute to a significantly healthier female population at all ages. In addition women have spoken out to demand better, more comprehensive research on health issues affecting them and have begun to take more active roles in their own health care.

Menopause, too, has become a subject of increasing interest to both the lay public and researchers. This has occurred in part because in the 1990s nearly 50 million women in the United States will be 50 years of age or over (the median age for menopause) and can expect to live another 30 years because life expectancy for women now exceeds 80 years (McKeon 1994). Traditional views held that menopause was a time of crisis, emotional struggle, depression, anxiety, and loss of self-esteem. Thankfully, this is no longer true. As the number of women reaching menopause increases, the negative emotional connotations society attaches to menopause are diminishing, enabling menopausal women to cope more effectively with the changes they are experiencing and even enabling them to view menopause as a time of personal growth. Fortunately, at the same time many of the physiologic changes of menopause are being moderated by the widespread use of hormone replacement therapy.

Physical and Psychologic Aspects

Physical characteristics of menopause are linked to the shift from a cyclic to a noncyclic hormone pattern. The age of onset may be influenced by nutritional, cultural, or genetic factors. The exact physiologic mechanisms initiating its onset are not known. Onset occurs when ovarian function ceases, resulting in estrogen levels diminishing to the point that menstruation stops.

Generally, ovulation ceases prior to menopause. Individual variations exist, and as much as 6 to 8 years of transition prior to menopause has been noted. The change is usually gradual, and normal menstrual irregularities do not include menorrhagia or metrorrhagia. Atrophy of the ovaries occurs gradually; FSH levels rise and less estrogen is produced. Menopausal symptoms include atrophic changes in the vagina, vulva, and urethra and in the trigonal area of the bladder.

Menopausal women often experience certain vasomotor disturbances that are clearly related to hormonal changes and the cessation of menstruation. Fifty percent of women report symptoms of heat arising on the chest and spreading to the neck and face (caused by vasodilation), sweating (mild to drenching), sleep disturbances, and occasional chills. This cluster of symptoms is often called **hot flashes.** There may be 20 to 30 of these a day, lasting 3 to 5 minutes. Dizzy spells, palpitations, and weakness are also reported by some women. Increased perspiration may occur at night as well as during the hot flash. Vasomotor symptoms in menopausal women vary widely. Some women have severe hot flashes as described; others experience few, if any.

Many women experience no emotional difficulties during menopause. Approximately 30–40%, however, report affective symptoms such as insomnia, fatigue, decreased concentration, memory loss, irritability, depression, and dissatisfaction with personal performance and achievement (McKeon 1994).

Vulvar atrophy occurs late, and the pubic hair thins, turns gray or white, and may ultimately disappear. The labia lose substance and their heightened pigmentation. Pelvic fascia and muscles atrophy, resulting in decreased pelvic support. The breasts become pendulous and decrease in size and firmness.

The uterine endometrium and myometrium atrophy, as do the cervical glands. The uterine cavity becomes stenosed. The fallopian tubes atrophy extensively. The vaginal mucosa becomes smooth and thin, and the rugae disappear, leading to loss of elasticity. As a result intercourse may be painful. Dryness of the mucous membrane can lead to burning and itching. The vaginal pH level increases as the number of Döderlein's bacilli decreases.

Menopausal women remain orgasmic, although the excitement phase of the female sexual response cycle may be prolonged. For some, sexual interest and activity may improve as the need for contraception disappears and personal growth and awareness increase. Others may experience a decrease in libido due to lowered levels of testosterone.

The estrogen deprivation that occurs in menopausal women may significantly increase their risk of coronary heart disease. Estrogens improve the lipid profile by increasing high-density lipoprotein (HDL) and triglycerides and decreasing low-density lipoprotein (LDL) and total cholesterol. Furthermore, researchers speculate that estrogens may act directly on coronary arteries in a way not understood (Bowman 1990).

Menopause is also associated with the onset of osteoporosis, a condition characterized by loss of bone mass, which puts an individual at risk for nontraumatic fractures. Osteoporosis is more common in women who are middle-aged or older. The following risk factors are also associated with osteoporosis: White or Asian, small-boned and thin, family history of osteoporosis, lack of regular exercise, nulliparous, early onset of menopause, consistently low intake of calcium, cigarette smoking, and moderate to heavy alcohol intake.

Hormone Replacement Therapy (HRT)

Hormone replacement therapy (HRT), usually involving estrogen with or without a progestin, for menopausal women has been controversial for many years, but currently the American College of Obstetricians and Gynecologists recommends HRT in menopause. Estrogen replacement is helpful in stopping hot flashes and night sweats and in reversing atrophic vaginal changes. It also decreases the psychologic changes for many women. Perhaps most significantly, HRT may reduce the incidence of cardiovascular heart disease and is effective in retarding bone loss and decreasing the fractures associated with osteoporosis.

Pre- or postmenopausal women with four or more risk factors for osteoporosis should have bone mass measurements done. The woman's height should be measured at each visit because a loss of height is often an early sign that vertebrae are being compressed because of reduced bone mass (Kase 1993). A variety of conditions, including malabsorption syndrome, cancer, cirrhosis of the liver, chronic use of cortisone, and rheumatoid arthritis, can cause secondary arthritis, which resembles osteoporosis. If these secondary causes have been eliminated, treatment for osteoporosis is instituted.

Prevention of osteoporosis is a primary goal of care. Women are advised to maintain an adequate calcium intake. Approximately 1200 mg of elemental calcium is recommended for premenopausal women and 1500 mg for postmenopausal women. To achieve this level, most women require supplements. Vitamin D supplements are sometimes also recommended because vitamin D increases the absorption of calcium from the stomach.

Women are advised to participate regularly in exercise, to consume only modest quantities of alcohol and caffeine, and to stop smoking. This is especially important because alcohol and smoking have a negative effect on the rate of bone resorption. Women with no contraindications to estrogen who are showing evidence of bone loss are good candidates for HRT.

When estrogen is given alone, it can produce endometrial hyperplasia and increase the risk of endometrial cancer. Thus, in women who still have a uterus, estrogen is opposed by giving a progestin for a portion of the cycle. Currently, opinion varies as to the number of days that progesterone (Provera) should be included. Typically, estrogen is given the first 25 days of the month with 10 mg Provera added during the last 12 days of the estrogen administration (Schnare 1993). (Some care givers still prefer to add the Provera for the last 10 days instead.) An alternative approach involves the daily administration of 0.625 mg estrogen with 2.5 mg Provera. This regimen is associated with less vaginal bleeding, is sufficient to prevent endometrial hyperplasia and osteoporosis, and also retains most of the cardiovascular protective effects of the estrogen (Sitruk-Ware 1991; Whitehead et al 1992).

Although most women take estrogen in tablet form, some prefer the transdermal estrogen skin patch, which is applied twice a week to an area of skin free of hair. For women experiencing decreased libido, combination estrogen-testosterone preparations are available.

A thorough history, physical examination including Pap smear, and baseline mammogram are indicated before starting HRT. An initial endometrial biopsy is no longer recommended for all woman beginning HRT but is indicated for women with an increased risk of endometrial cancer. It is also indicated if excessive, unexpected, or prolonged bleeding occurs (McKeon 1994).

Women taking estrogen should be advised to stop immediately if they develop headaches, visual changes, signs of thrombophlebitis, or chest pain.

Etidonate diphosphate is a new treatment that is administered in an intermittent, cyclic fashion. It acts by inhibiting bone resorption and increasing bone mass. The drug, currently approved in the United States for the treatment of Paget's disease, is useful for menopausal women with osteoporosis who cannot take estrogen.

Nursing Care

Menopausal women may need assistance in the form of counseling to adjust successfully to this developmental phase of life. Reaction to menopause is determined to a large extent by the kind of life the woman has lived, by the security she has in her feminine identity, and by her feelings of self-worth and self-esteem.

Nurses or other health professionals can help the menopausal woman achieve high-level functioning at this time in her life. Of paramount importance is the nurse's ability to understand and provide support for the woman's views and feelings. Whether the woman expresses "relief and delight" or "tearfulness and fear," the nurse needs to use an empathetic approach in counseling, health teaching, or providing physical care.

Nurses should explore the question of comfort during sexual intercourse. In counseling the woman the nurse may say, for example, "After menopause many women notice that their vagina seems dryer, and intercourse can be uncomfortable. Have you noticed any changes?" This gives the woman information and may open discussion. The nurse can then go on to suggest that lubrication with a water-soluble jelly may help provide relief. Use of estrogen, orally or in vaginal creams, may also be indicated. Increased frequency of intercourse will maintain some elasticity in the vagina. When assessing the menopausal woman, the nurse should address the question of sexual activity openly but tactfully because many women in this age group may have been socialized to be reticent in discussing sex.

The crucial need of women in the perimenopausal period of life is adequate information about the changes taking place in their bodies and their lives. Supplying that information provides both a challenge and an opportunity for nurses.

KEY CONCEPTS

Sexual development begins at conception. The development of sexuality continues throughout an individual's lifetime.

Attitudes about sex are influenced by a variety of factors, including family and home environment, culture, education, socioeconomic level, previous sexual experiences, and individual personality characteristics.

Masters and Johnson identified four phases in the human sexual response cycle: excitement, plateau, orgasm, and resolution.

To be effective as a counselor on sexual matters, nurses must be aware of and comfortable with their feelings and attitudes, have accurate up-to-date knowledge, be skilled in communicating, and be insightful enough to recognize those occasions when a woman's problem requires more specialized intervention so that appropriate referral can be made.

Girls and women should be provided with clear information about comfort measures and issues during menstruation such as tampons (deodorant and absorbency); vaginal spray and douching practices; and self-care comfort measures, such as nutrition, exercise, and use of heat and massage.

Premenstrual syndrome occurs most often in women over 30. Symptoms occur 2 to 3 days before onset of menstruation and subside as menstruation starts with or without treatment. Medical management includes progesterone agonists and prostaglandin inhibitors. Self-care measures include improved nutrition (vitamin B complex and E supplementation and avoidance of methylxanthines, such

as in chocolate and caffeine), a program of aerobic exercise, and participation in self-care support groups.

Dysmenorrhea usually begins at, or a day before, onset of menses and disappears by the end of menstruation. Therapy with hormones, such as oral contraceptives, or with nonsteroidal anti-inflammatory drugs or prostaglandin inhibitors is useful. Self-care measures include improved nutrition, exercise, applications of heat, and extra rest.

Fertility awareness methods are "natural," noninvasive techniques often used by people whose religious beliefs keep them from using other methods of contraception.

Barrier contraceptives such as the diaphragm, cervical cap, contraceptive sponge, male condom, and female condom act as barriers to prevent the transport of sperm. These methods are used in conjunction with a spermicide.

The IUD is a mechanical contraceptive that works primarily by preventing fertilization and implantation.

Oral contraceptives (the "pill") are combinations of estrogen and progesterone. When taken correctly, they are one of the most effective of the reversible methods of fertility control.

Spermicides are less effective in preventing pregnancy when they are not used with a barrier method.

Permanent sterilization is accomplished by tubal ligation for women and vasectomy for men. Clients are advised that the method should be considered irreversible.

Menopause is a physiologic maturational change in a woman's life that may be associated with emotional attributes. Physiologic changes include the cessation of menses and decrease in circulating hormones. The more common symptoms are "hot flashes," palpitations, dyspareunia, dizziness, insomnia, mood changes, depression, memory loss, and increased perspiration at night. The woman's anatomy also undergoes changes such as atrophy of the vagina, reduction in size and pigmentation of the labia, and myometrial atrophy. The risk of developing osteoporosis or coronary heart disease increases.

Current management of menopause still centers around hormone replacement and calcium supplementation therapy.

REFERENCES

Bailey JM, Pillard R: A genetic study of male sexual orientation. *Arch Gen Psychiatry* 1991; 48:1089.

Bell A et al: *Sexual Preference: Its Development in Men and Women.* Bloomington, IN: Indiana Univ Press, 1981.

Bowman M: Hormone replacement therapy: A new look at the combination regimen. *Female Patient* September 1990; 15:63.

Chez RA, Mishell DR: Control of human reproduction: Contraception, sterilization, and pregnancy termination. In: *Danforth's Obstetrics and Gynecology*, 7th ed. Scott JR et al (editors). Philadelphia: Lippincott, 1994.

Chuong CJ et al: Revising treatments for premenstrual syndrome. *Contemp OB/GYN* January 1994; 39(1):66.

Connell EB: The female condom—a new contraception option. *Contemp OB/GYN* October 15, 1994; 39:20.

Contemporary OB/GYN. Emergency postcoital contraception. January 1994; 39(1):78.

Cook MJ: Perimenopause: An opportunity for health promotion. *JOGNN* May/June 1993; 22(3):223.

Copeland L: *Textbook of Gynecology*. Philadelphia: Saunders, 1993.

Crooks R, Baur K: *Our Sexuality*, 5th ed. Monterey, CA: Brooks Cole, 1993.

Dan A: The law and women's bodies: Menstruation leave in Japan. Presented at Socio-Cultural Issues in Menstrual Cycle Research, an Inter-Disciplinary Conference, University of California, San Francisco, May 20–21, 1983.

Edge V et al: *Women's Health Care*. St. Louis: Mosby, 1994.

Gelman D et al: Born or bred? *Newsweek* February 24, 1992; 24:46.

Hammond CB: Climacteric. In: *Danforth's Obstetrics and Gynecology*, 7th ed. Scott JR et al (editors). Philadelphia: Lippincott, 1994.

Hatcher RA et al: *Contraceptive Technology*, 16th ed. New York: Irvington, 1994.

Hinkle LT: Education and counseling for Norplant users. *JOGNN* June 1994; 23(5):387.

Kase NG et al: *Principles and Practices of Clinical Gynecology*. New York: Wiley, 1993.

Lobo RA: *Treatment of the Postmenopausal Woman*. New York: Raven Press, 1994.

Masters WH et al: *Masters and Johnson on Sex and Human Loving*. Boston: Little, Brown, 1986.

Mastroianni L: Future contraceptive methods. *Contracep Rep* September 1994; 5(4):4.

McKeon VA: Hormone replacement therapy: Evaluating the risks and benefits. *JOGNN* October 1994; 23(8):647.

Pollack AE, Moore C: New issues in spermicide use. *Contemp OB/GYN* April 15, 1994; 39:29.

Rayburn W: *Drug Therapy in Obstetrics and Gynecology*, 3rd ed. St Louis: Mosby-Year Book, 1992.

Schnare S: Hormone therapy. *Contemp OB/GYN* September 1993; 1(3):3.

Siegel SJ: The effect of culture on the way women experience menstruation: Jewish women and mikvah. Presented at Socio-Cultural Issues in Menstrual Cycle Research, an Inter-Disciplinary Conference, University of California, San Francisco, May 20–21, 1983.

Sitruk-Ware R et al: *The Menopause and Hormonal Replacement Therapy*. New York: Marcel Dekker, 1991.

Whitehead M et al: *Hormone Replacement Therapy*. Edinburgh, Scotland: Churchill-Livingstone, 1992.

CHAPTER 10

WOMEN'S HEALTH PROBLEMS

I was 35 when my husband divorced me for another woman. During the following year I had sex with only two men, but one of them gave me herpes. I was devastated when my nurse practitioner diagnosed it. I felt embarrassed, ashamed, dirty. My self-esteem had never been lower. My nurse practitioner was wonderful. She explained the disease and how it was spread and helped me find ways to relieve the symptoms. More than that, though, I always knew she cared about me personally. She helped me realize I was still a worthwhile person. Knowing she still liked and respected me helped me start feeling good about myself again. When I met a man I really cared about, she helped me figure a way to tell him about my herpes. He was able to accept it and still love me. We are married now and I've never been happier. We've followed my practitioner's advice about ways to avoid infecting my husband, and he hasn't had any sign of infection. When I think about all the changes and stress in my life, I can't imagine how I would have coped without my practitioner. She gave me support when I needed it and encouraged me to stand alone when I was ready. She's a special woman.

KEY TERMS

Breast self-examination (BSE)

Colposcopy

Dilation and curettage (D&C)

Endometriosis

Fibrocystic breast disease (FBD)

Galactorrhea

Hysterectomy

Mammogram

Pelvic inflammatory disease (PID)

Sexually transmitted disease (STD)

Sexually transmitted infection

Toxic shock syndrome (TSS)

Vulvovaginal candidiasis (VVC)

OBJECTIVES

Differentiate the common benign breast disorders.

Identify the nursing needs of a woman with cancer of the breast.

Discuss the signs, symptoms, and treatment of endometriosis.

Describe toxic shock syndrome with regard to diagnosis, treatment, and health teaching.

Compare the common sexually transmitted infections with regard to causative organism, signs and symptoms, treatment, and long-term implications.

Summarize health teaching the nurse should provide to a woman with a sexually transmitted infection.

Relate the development and progression of pelvic inflammatory disease to the possible development of infertility.

Identify measures that should be employed to establish a diagnosis when a woman has an abnormal finding during a pelvic examination.

Compare lower urinary tract infections with upper urinary tract infections.

Discuss the issues and concerns surrounding gynecologic surgery.

Describe the most common gynecologic surgical procedures.

Discuss the nursing care of women during gynecologic surgery.

*W*omen's health refers to a holistic view of women and their health-related needs within the context of their everyday lives. It is based on the awareness that a woman's physical, mental, and social status are interdependent and determine her state of health or illness. The woman's view of her situation, her assessment of her needs, her values, and her beliefs are valid and important factors to be incorporated into any health care intervention.

The contemporary woman is likely to encounter various gynecologic or urinary problems during her lifetime. Nurses can assist women by providing them with accurate, sensitive, and supportive health education and counseling. This chapter provides basic information about a variety of gynecologic health problems. To simplify learning, information is presented according to specific disease processes and female body parts. It is essential to remember, however, that women are multidimensional, complex beings who are entitled to holistic health care.

THE FEMALE BREAST

The female breast has for centuries assumed an importance far out of proportion to its natural purpose—the nourishment of an infant. Sexual interest in breasts is peculiar to humans and is a long-standing cultural phenomenon, as can be seen in the paintings and sculpture displayed in museums throughout the world and in the idealized images of "perfect" breasts that are often used by the media to sell a variety of products and services. These attitudes have perpetuated the belief among some women that breasts are their "badge of femininity."

A complex interaction of cultural and psychosocial factors determines the significance of the breasts for each woman. Because people develop their body images in part via external feedback, the disproportionate glorification of the breasts may have profound effects on a woman's body image. Some women are willing to subject themselves to potentially disfiguring surgeries in order to alter the appearance of their breasts. Some women even choose the loss of life over the loss of a breast in their delay or refusal to seek medical care for a breast lump.

Breasts develop as a secondary sex characteristic during puberty. For the developing adolescent, breasts are a visible symbol of her feminine identity and an important part of her body image and self-esteem. Because a woman's primary sexual organs cannot be observed, breast development provides visual confirmation that the adolescent is becoming a woman. Breasts are a source of erotic stimulation for many women, and they play a role in the expression of women's sexuality.

Normal Cyclic Changes in the Nonlactating Breast

Like the uterus, the breast functions dynamically in a cyclic process that is regulated by the nervous and hormonal systems. Each month, in rhythm with the cycle of ovulation and under the direct influence of the hormone estrogen, the breasts become engorged with fluid in anticipation of pregnancy. The contours of the breasts' lobular structure become apparent, producing the sensations of lumpiness, tenderness, and perhaps pain. *Mastodynia* (premenstrual swelling and tenderness of the breasts) is common. It usually lasts for 3 to 4 days prior to the onset of menstruation, but the symptoms may persist throughout the month.

Such symptoms may be diagnosed erroneously as fibrocystic breast disease but are more accurately identified as increased physiologic nodularity, an exaggerated response to normal cyclic changes. If conception does not occur, the accumulated fluid drains away via the lymphatic network.

After menopause, adipose breast tissue atrophies and is replaced by connective tissue. Elasticity is diminished, and breasts tend to hang more loosely from the chest wall because of these tissue changes and relaxation of the suspensory ligaments. The nipples become smaller, flatter, and lose some erectile ability. The skin over the breasts may take on a relatively dry, thin texture. Cyclic engorgement of the breast tissue does not occur after menopause. However, the engorgement may resume with estrogen replacement therapy.

CARE OF THE WOMAN WITH FIBROCYSTIC BREAST DISEASE

Fibrocystic breast disease (FBD), the most common of the benign breast disorders, is characterized by a thickening of normal breast tissue and the formation of cysts. *Mammary dysplasia* or *chronic cystic mastitis* are also terms used to describe this benign condition. It is estimated that 50% of women of childbearing age will have palpable evidence of cystic disease sometime during their reproductive years (Mansel 1992). There are two types of FBD: proliferative breast disease (PD) and nonproliferative breast disease (NPD). Fibrosis and/or cyst formation are associated with NPD, and epithelial hyperplasia is associated with PD (Hughes 1992). Epithelial hyperplasia may be classified as atypical hyperplasia (AH) as determined by a histologic evaluation. Women with PD and AH have 4.3 times the breast cancer risk of women without PD. In women with PD but without AH, the relative risk for developing breast cancer is 1.3. A family history of breast cancer increases breast cancer risk 2.4 times. The joint occurrence of family history and atypical hyperplasia has been shown to have a strong synergistic effect on breast cancer risk (Worrell et al 1993). NPD is not considered to be a risk factor for breast cancer.

FBD appears to improve during pregnancy and lactation and resolve with menopause. Early cystic changes have been found in teenagers and women in their twenties; however, the occurrence of breast cysts is most prevalent in women 30 to 50 years of age (Mansel 1992).

Fibrosis is a thickening of normal breast tissue. The breast may become multinodular with a periodic mass. Cyst formation that may accompany fibrosis is considered a later change in fibrocystic disease. Cyst formation may result when normal secretions within the ductal network are unable to drain away. Their accumulation can then create a fluid-filled sac or cyst.

FBD is probably caused by an imbalance in estrogen and progesterone, which distorts the normal breast changes of the menstrual cycle. Current theories suggest that unopposed estrogen in the luteal phase related to progesterone deficiency may be the cause of fibrocystic breast disease. Because the condition responds to the changes of the menstrual cycle, a woman may actually observe a lessening in the size of a lump with the onset of her menstrual cycle related to a decrease in the estrogen level. The symptoms often increase as the woman approaches menopause; the condition generally improves following menopause. However, if a postmenopausal woman is treated with hormone replacement therapy, the cyclic breast changes may resume (Mansel 1992).

Medical Therapy

The woman often reports pain, tenderness, and swelling that occurs cyclically and is most pronounced just before her menses begins. Physical examination may reveal only mild signs of irregularity, or the breasts may feel dense, with areas of irregularity and nodularity. Women often refer to this as "lumpiness." Some women may also have clear, milky, straw-colored, or greenish nipple discharge. Nipple discharge is called **galactorrhea,** which means inappropriate lactation. Galactorrhea may be physiologic, which is the case with FBD, drug induced, idiopathic, or pathologic. Clear, milky, straw-colored, or greenish nipple discharge is usually associated with benign conditions, whereas bloody or serosanguineous discharge is usually associated with malignant conditions. Regardless of its character, all breast discharge should have a cytologic evaluation (Edge & Segatore 1993).

If the woman has a large, fluid-filled cyst, she may experience a localized painful area as the capsule containing the accumulated fluid distends coincident with her cycle. However, if small cyst formation occurs, the woman may experience not a solitary tender lump but a diffuse tenderness.

Mammography, sonography, palpation, and fine-needle aspiration are used to confirm fibrocystic breast disease. Often, fine-needle aspiration is the treatment as well, affording relief from the tenderness or the pain (De-Freitar et al 1992).

Diagnostic criteria for fibrocystic breast disease are as follows:

- A palpable, fluid-filled mass is felt.
- The mass can be aspirated.
- Histologic examination confirms cystic disease.
- Mammography indicates cystic formation.

Physical examination reveals that cysts are round, movable, and well delineated in appearance. Specific characteristics that differentiate a cyst from a malignant neoplasm are mobility, tenderness, and the absence of skin retraction (or pulling) in surrounding tissue. Well-circumscribed lesions have a 98% benign rate and generally do not require a biopsy.

Fine-needle aspiration, an office procedure, is used in conjunction with physical examination for diagnosis. Fluid withdrawal confirms the presence of a cyst. The fluid aspirated is sent for cytologic examination. If aspiration is incomplete, yielding no fluid, or yields bloody fluid, a biopsy is necessary. If the physical findings remain unclear, a mammogram is ordered to clarify the diagnosis. A mammogram revealing an unexplained or suspicious area warrants surgical exploration or biopsy (Olson 1993).

Treatment of palpable cysts is conservative; invasive procedures such as biopsy are used only if the diagnosis is questionable. If a question persists, surgical exploration of the tissue and removal of the affected area are scheduled as an outpatient procedure. The mass or affected area is reexamined after 4 weeks to determine if the cyst has refilled.

Women with mild symptoms may benefit from restricting sodium intake and taking a mild diuretic during the week before the onset of menses. This counteracts fluid retention, relieves pressure in the breast, and helps decrease the pain. In other cases a mild analgesic might be necessary.

Controversy surrounds the practice of limiting caffeine to relieve symptoms. Some studies have found a positive correlation between intake of methylxanthines (found in caffeine products such as coffee, tea, cola, chocolate, and some medications) and breast pain in women with FBD (Bullough et al 1990). Other studies reported no change when methylxanthines were limited, and one study reported that symptoms worsened when caffeine was eliminated (Norwood 1990).

In severe cases of FBD the hormone inhibitor tamoxifen has been used. It produces marked regression of fibrocystic changes, including precancerous ones.

Additional medical therapies that have been found beneficial in varying degrees include oral contraceptives, progestins, and bromocriptine (Herbst & Berek 1993). These all work on the principle of estrogen suppression and progesterone stimulation or augmentation.

Nursing Assessment

The nurse assesses the woman's understanding of fibrocystic breast disease and the importance of regular breast self-examination. Some specially trained nurses perform breast examinations of healthy women. The nurse reviews the woman's history for close relatives with fibrocystic breast disease or cancer of the breast. The nurse also obtains information on relief measures that have been effective for the woman.

Nursing Diagnosis

Nursing diagnoses that may apply to a woman with fibrocystic breast disease include the following:

- Knowledge deficit related to lack of understanding of self-care measures

- Pain related to the cyclic breast changes that occur premenstrually

Critical Thinking Question

Why do you suppose so many women are unwilling to do monthly breast self-examination despite its value in detecting cancer early?

Nursing Plan and Implementation

Breast Self-Examination

Monthly **breast self-examination (BSE)** is the best method for detecting breast masses early. Women need to be taught to practice monthly BSE from the time that they develop breast tissue during puberty. A woman who knows the texture and feel of her own breasts is far more likely to detect changes that develop. All health professionals need to include breast examination and the teaching of routine BSE in regular checkups. Often the nurse, particularly in a clinic, office, or community health setting, assumes responsibility for teaching BSE to women. Nurses also have the opportunity to teach BSE in hospital settings. See Teaching Guide: Teaching Breast Self-Examination on page 222.

All premenopausal women should perform BSE monthly approximately 1 week after their menses. Pregnant women, women who have had a hysterectomy, and postmenopausal women should pick a certain day of the month—perhaps the first day or the date of their birth—as their regular day to do BSE. Postmenopausal women who are on cyclic hormone replacement therapy should perform BSE at the end of the time period when they do not take hormones.

The American Cancer Society has a pamphlet, "How to Examine Your Breasts," that can be obtained free of charge for distribution to clients.

Teaching for Self-Care

In addition to teaching BSE, the nurse suggests measures the woman can employ to help alleviate her discomfort. These include the following:

- Wearing a well-fitting, supportive bra, at night as well as during the day when symptoms are severe

- Applying ice packs to tender areas of the breasts

- Using nonprescription salicylates or anti-inflammatory medication

- Limiting caffeine and salt intake

Provision of Psychologic Support

By carefully explaining FBD and its relationship to the monthly cycle, the nurse can alleviate the woman's anxiety while reinforcing the importance of having any suspected abnormality investigated promptly. The major concern is that, because of the lumpiness of the breasts, small malignant neoplasms will be missed. In reality, women with FBD make up a minority of breast cancer cases, and the breast cancer risk is not uniform in all women with FBD. As mentioned previously, breast cancer tends to be concentrated in those women with proliferative lesions, especially with atypia, and a contributory family history (Worrell et al 1993).

The nurse can also point out that frequent professional breast examination and regular mammograms are tools that help detect any abnormalities, and that the woman who practices monthly BSE, follows her care giver's advice, and is examined regularly has taken positive action to protect her health.

Evaluation

Anticipated outcomes of nursing care include:

- The woman incorporates monthly BSE into her personal routine.

- The woman implements measures to help alleviate her discomfort.

- The woman understands fibrocystic breast disease, deals with her anxiety over the potential complications, and takes positive action to protect her health.

Text continues on page 224

TEACHING BREAST SELF-EXAMINATION

Assessment: The nurse determines the woman's general knowledge about BSE, identifies previous experience with BSE, identifies risk factors for breast cancer (see Table 10–2), determines the woman's general knowledge about breast cancer, discusses the woman's feelings about her breasts and BSE, identifies barriers to BSE, and discusses her commitment to practice BSE.

Nursing Diagnosis: Knowledge deficit related to lack of information about breast self-examination

Nursing Plan and Implementation: The teaching plan will focus on assisting the woman to learn BSE so that she can use it effectively.

Client Goals: At completion of teaching, the woman will be able to:

1. Discuss her risk of breast cancer.
2. Describe the use of BSE in breast cancer detection.
3. Demonstrate the correct procedure for BSE.
4. List warning signs of breast cancer to be reported to the care giver.
5. Incorporate monthly BSE into her personal routine.

Teaching Plan

Content: Discuss the risk factors associated with breast cancer (see Table 10–2).

Teaching Method: *This should be discussed in a private area free of interruptions. The room needs to have a mirror; bed, couch, or examining table; pillows; a patient gown; and a private area for the woman to disrobe.*

Stress the unique risk factors associated with the woman's personal history and life-style.

The nurse should create a supportive, warm, and comfortable atmosphere by attitude and communication style—both verbal and nonverbal. A discussion of breast cancer may bring forth many emotions in the woman, including grief for previous breast cancer–related losses.

Discuss the use of BSE in breast cancer detection.

Focus on open discussion. A brochure with statistics and illustrations may be useful. Stress the positive outcomes of early detection to counterbalance fears.

Describe and demonstrate the correct procedure for BSE.
A. Instruct the woman to inspect her breasts by standing or sitting in front of a mirror. She needs to inspect her breasts in three positions: with both arms relaxed down at her side, both arms stretched straight over her head, and both hands placed on her hips while leaning forward (Figure 10–1).

Learning is best accomplished when material is broken down into smaller steps and presented with multiple approaches. Prior to asking the woman to perform BSE, the nurse should use a model or a chart to demonstrate the procedure. Then the nurse should have the woman perform BSE. The nurse should be very supportive and give a lot of positive feedback because some women may be embarrassed. The nurse needs to demonstrate a nonjudgmental, accepting attitude.

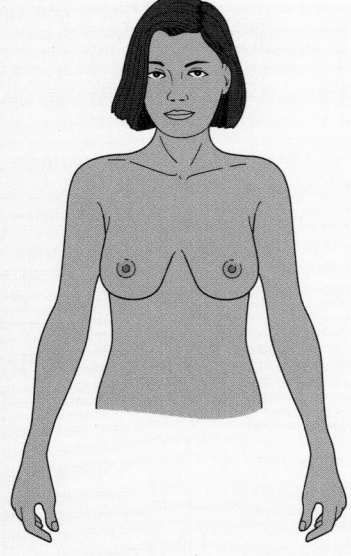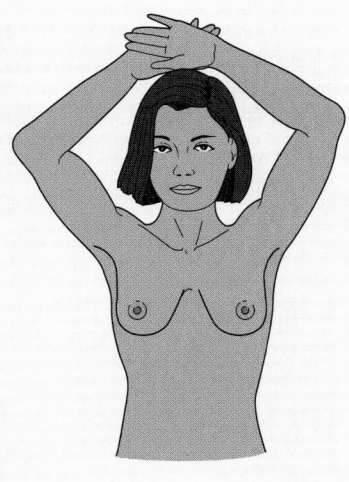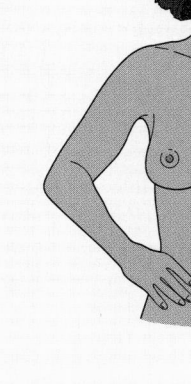

FIGURE 10-1   Positions for inspection.

B. Advise the woman to look at her breasts individually and in comparison with one another. Note and record the following characteristics for each position:

Size and Symmetry of the Breasts

1. Breasts may vary, but the variations should remain constant during rest or movement—note abnormal contours.

2. Some size difference between the breasts is normal.

Shape and Direction of the Breasts

1. The shape of the breasts can be rounded or pendulous with some variation between breasts.

2. The breasts should be pointing slightly laterally.

Color, Thickening, Edema, and Venous Patterns

1. Check for redness or inflammation.

2. A blue hue with a marked venous pattern that is focal or unilateral may indicate an area of increased blood supply due to tumor. Symmetric venous patterns are normal.

3. Skin edema observed as thickened skin with enlarged pores ("orange peel") may indicate blocked lymphatic drainage due to tumor.

Surface of the Breasts

1. Skin dimpling, puckering, or retraction (pulling) when the woman presses her hands together or against her hips suggests malignancy.

2. Striae (stretch marks) red at onset and whitish with age are normal.

Nipple Size and Shape, Direction, Rashes, Ulcerations, and Discharge

1. Long-standing nipple inversion is normal, but an inverted nipple previously capable of erection is suspicious. Note any deviation, flattening, or broadening of the nipples.

2. Check for rashes, ulcerations, or discharge.

C. Instruct the woman to palpate (feel) her breasts as follows:

1. Lie down. Put one hand behind your head. With the other hand, fingers flattened, gently feel your breast. Press lightly (Figure 10–2A). Now examine the breast.

2. Figure 10–2B shows you how to check each breast. Begin as you see in B and follow the arrows, feeling gently for a lump or thickening. Remember to feel all parts of each breast.

3. Now repeat the same procedure sitting up, with the hand still behind your head (Figure 10–2C).

4. Squeeze the nipple between your thumb and forefinger. Look for any discharge—clear or bloody (Figure 10–2D).

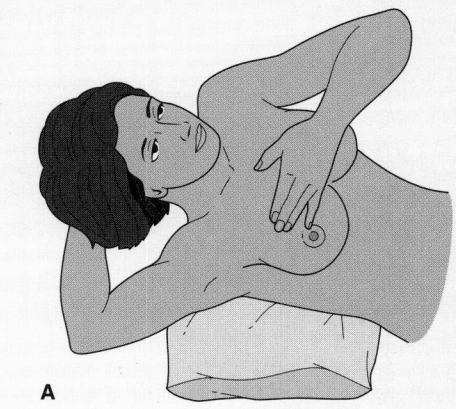

A

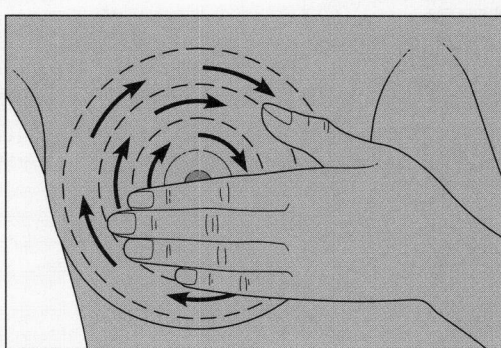

B

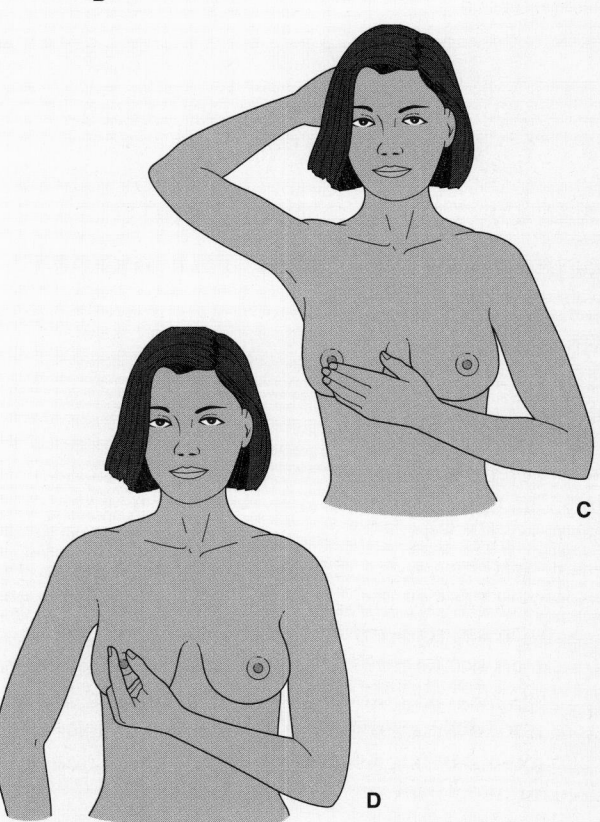

C

D

FIGURE 10-2   Breast self-examination

TEACHING BREAST SELF-EXAMINATION *continued*

D. Take the woman's hand and help her to identify her "normal lumps" (eg, mammary ridge, ribs and nodularity in the upper outer quadrants).

Demonstrate "normal lumps" on the woman herself while guiding her hand and identifying the area.

E. After she examines her breasts and identifies her normal lumps, instruct her to palpate her breasts once more to identify any areas that she may have questions about. If questions arise, the nurse should palpate the area and attempt to identify if it is normal.

Allowing the woman to differentiate normal from abnormal lumps on herself and a model will increase confidence that she will recognize an abnormal finding. Having the nurse check her immediately afterwards will positively reinforce her and diminish the fear associated with BSE.

F. If a breast model is available, instruct the woman to palpate it and identify the lumps.

G. Provide information on the warning signs of breast cancer and what she should do if she identifies any of these signs during BSE.

Provide a written handout on the warning signs of breast cancer. The handout should also cover actions that she should take if a warning sign is discovered. Stress the positive effects of early detection.

Timing: Instruct the woman to perform BSE on a monthly basis. Be specific based on whether she is premenopausal, pregnant, postmenopausal, or postmenopausal receiving hormone replacement therapy.

Teaching Method: *Provide the woman with a reminder symbol for monthly BSE. The American Cancer Society provides such items to hang in the shower, place on a refrigerator, and so forth. Ask her when she plans to do BSE each month. This will serve as a method of evaluation and reinforcement. Praise her commitment to do monthly BSE. Give the woman a follow-up telephone number (eg, American Cancer Society) to use if she needs additional information or has questions. This will increase her comfort level with BSE and enable her to detect potential problems early.*

SOURCE: American Cancer Society: *Breast Self-Examination and the Nurse*, No. 3408 PE. New York, 1973.

CARE OF THE WOMAN WITH A BENIGN DISORDER OF THE BREAST

Table 10–1 summarizes common benign breast disorders. Mastitis is discussed in Chapter 36.

Fibroadenoma

The *fibroadenoma* is a common benign tumor seen in women in their teens and early twenties. It is the third most common tumor of the breast; its incidence is exceeded only by carcinoma and fibrocystic disease. Fibroadenomas found in adolescent breasts appear closely linked to breast hypertrophy, which may occur during the pubertal growth spurt. Fibroadenomas will respond to hormonal influence and are known to increase in size and secrete milk during pregnancy. Unlike cystic disease, fibroadenoma has not been significantly associated with malignant neoplasms.

Fibroadenomas are solid tumors that are well defined, sharply delineated, and rounded, with a rubbery firmness. These tumors can be moved freely within the breast tissue and are not associated with any fibroblastic response in surrounding tissue. A solitary nodule is common, but multiple tumors have been observed in about 15% of cases (Mansel 1992). The size of a fibroadenoma ranges from 1 to 5 cm, with the nodule commonly occurring around the nipple or in the upper quadrant of the breast along the lateral side. Fibroadenomas are asymptomatic and nontender. They are usually discovered by accident.

Medical Therapy

Fibroadenomas are characterized by their appearance on physical examination. They are well outlined, rounded, lobulated in appearance, rubbery, and relatively movable.

If there are any disquieting features to the appearance of the lump, fine-needle biopsy and/or excision of the mass may be indicated. Caution is exercised when deciding upon biopsy because excision of the mass in a young girl may interfere with normal breast development. Watchful observation and possible surgical excision are the only treatments for fibroadenomas. Mammography is not useful in young women due to their

TABLE 10-1　Summary of Benign Breast Disorders

Condition	Age	Pain	Cancer Risk	Nipple Discharge	Location	Consistency and Mobility	Diagnosis and Treatment
Fibrocystic breast disease	30–50	Yes	Yes with proliferative disease and atypical hyperplasia	Varies: none at all or may be clear, milky, straw-colored, or green	Upper outer quadrant	Multiple lumps occurring bilaterally, influenced by menstrual cycle, nodular	Needle aspiration, Pap smear of nipple discharge, observation, biopsy if unresolved mass exists or mammographic changes, sonography
Fibroadenoma	15–25, median age 20	No	No	No, but milky discharge in pregnancy	Nipple or upper outer quadrant along the lateral side	Solid, well defined, sharply delineated, rounded, rubbery, mobile	Mammography, observation, surgical excision
Intraductal papilloma	Menopausal 50–60	Yes on palpation	Yes with multiple papillomas	Yes: serous, bloody, or brownish-green	No specific location	Nonpalpable or small, ball-like, poorly delineated	Pap smear of nipple discharge, mammography, ductogram, surgical excision
Duct ectasia	45–55	Yes: burning and itching around the nipple	No	Yes in perimenopausal women: thick, sticky, green, greenish-brown, or bloodstained	Mass behind or around the nipple	Poorly circumscribed, inflammation, nipple retraction, axillary lymph adenopathy	Pap smear of breast discharge, mammography, drug therapy for symptoms, surgical excision, observation

dense breast tissue. Surgery is often deferred, but if surgery is indicated, it is performed under local anesthesia on an outpatient basis. Surgical removal of a fibroadenoma concludes its treatment.

Intraductal Papilloma

Although *intraductal papillomas* are relatively uncommon, they constitute the primary cause of nipple discharge in women who are not pregnant or lactating. Intraductal papillomas are primarily a disease of the menopausal years, although they may be found in women of any age.

Papillomas are fragile, fingerlike projections into the duct lumen that result from proliferation of the duct epithelium. Minimal trauma will cause blood or serum to collect in the involved duct and will result in spontaneous serous or bloody nipple discharge. No evidence currently exists linking a solitary intraductal papilloma with breast cancer. Multiple intraductal papillomas, however, have been associated with malignant transformation (Morrow 1992).

Medical Therapy

The majority of papillomas present as solitary nodules. These small, ball-like lesions may be detected on mammography but are most often nonpalpable, although palpation may elicit some tenderness. The presence of a pa-

pilloma is often frightening to the woman because her primary symptom is a discharge from the nipple that may be serosanguinous or brownish-green due to the presence of old blood.

If the woman reports a nipple discharge, the breast should be milked to obtain fluid. The fluid obtained is sent for a Papanicolaou (Pap) smear. The diagnosis is confirmed if papilloma cells are present. The diagnosis may also be confirmed by a ductogram, which involves injecting radiopaque dye into the duct followed by a mammogram. The lesion may be excised and histologically examined to differentiate between a benign papilloma and a papillary carcinoma.

Treatment for benign papilloma is excision. Medical follow-up visits may be more frequent because of the possibility of recurrence and the similarity of papillary carcinoma to the benign condition (Mansel 1992).

Duct Ectasia (Comedomastitis or Plasma Cell Mastitis)

Mammary *duct ectasia* is a benign condition that involves inflammation of the ducts behind the nipple, duct enlargement, and collection of cellular debris and fluid in the involved ducts. The disease is most commonly seen in women ages 45 to 55, although it can be found in younger women.

Breast pain and a palpable mass are common symptoms in premenopausal women; nipple discharge predominates in perimenopausal women; and nipple retraction is more often noted in postmenopausal women. This disease is not associated with cancer (Mansel 1992).

Medical Therapy

The woman often reports a thick, sticky nipple discharge with burning pain, pruritus, and inflammation. The drainage may be green, greenish-brown, or blood stained. Masses associated with duct ectasia may be poorly circumscribed. Nipple retraction, bloody nipple discharge, and axillary lymphadenopathy accompanying inflammation further complicate accurate differentiation of the disease from breast cancer. Treatment is conservative, with drug therapy aimed at symptomatic relief. The major central ducts of the breast occasionally have to be excised. Local excision of the involved ducts has been effective in controlling symptoms. Treatment plans are dependent upon the severity of the problem. The vast majority of women will require nothing more than routine follow-up with physical examination. In the early stages of inflammation women should be advised to keep their nipples clean to minimize the risk of infection. The symptoms may be frightening, and the woman may need emotional support in addition to reassurance that this disorder is not associated with cancer.

APPLYING THE NURSING PROCESS

Nursing Assessment

During the period of diagnosis the woman may be anxious about a possible change in body image or a diagnosis of cancer. The nurse can use therapeutic communication to assess the significance the woman places on her breasts; her current emotional status and coping mechanisms used during periods of stress; knowledge and beliefs about cancer; and other variables that may influence her coping and adjustment.

Nursing Diagnosis

Nursing diagnoses that may apply to a woman with a benign disorder of the breast include the following:

- Knowledge deficit related to a lack of understanding of diagnostic procedures
- Anxiety related to threat to body image

Nursing Plan and Implementation

During the prediagnosis period the woman should be encouraged to express her anxiety. Misconceptions need to be clarified. The woman may find herself considering the implications for her personal life, her family, and the future if the diagnosis is cancer. This "what next" concern helps the woman consider the implications of cancer and enables her to begin planning. It is tempting to disregard these concerns by simply responding, "Oh, don't think like that. Everything will be fine." Such an approach, however, invalidates the woman's concerns and denies her the opportunity to begin considering the future. The sensitive nurse avoids unnecessary pessimism while recognizing that the woman's concerns are valid, and provides accurate information about diagnosis and treatment options.

Evaluation

Anticipated outcomes of nursing care include:

- The woman feels comfortable discussing her fears, concerns, and questions during the period of diagnosis.
- The diagnosis is made accurately and quickly.

CARE OF THE WOMAN WITH CARCINOMA OF THE BREAST

An estimated one in nine women will be diagnosed with breast cancer, which is second only to lung cancer as a cause of cancer deaths in women. Major advances in breast cancer therapies include the widespread use of screening mammography, resulting in mortality reduction; the evolution of multimodality treatment planning, resulting in more coordinated care; and the use of adjuvant therapies such as radiation, chemotherapy, and hormones, which result in prolonged survival (Coleman 1993). Early detection seems to influence the outcome of breast cancer more than the particular type or combination of treatment used. A woman's chances of survival are directly linked to the stage of the disease at diagnosis (Mahon 1993).

Risk Factors for Breast Cancer

Factors placing women at risk for breast cancer have been studied extensively by epidemiologists and other clinical researchers. The risk factors associated with carcinoma of the breast are summarized in Table 10–2. The most significant risk factors are female gender, older age, and positive family history in a first-degree relative. However, only 20% of women who have breast cancer have sisters or mothers with a history of breast cancer. A woman's age is the most important risk factor in determining when to begin mammography screening. Women aged 40 or older have 90% of breast cancers. Women over age 65 are

TABLE 10-2	Summary of Risk Factors for Breast Cancer		
Factor	**Higher risk**	**Lower risk**
Age	≥ 40	< 40
History of cancer in one breast	Yes	No
Family history of premenopausal bilateral breast cancer	Yes	No
Country of residence	North America, Northern Europe	Asia, Africa
Any first-degree relative with breast cancer	Yes	No
History of fibrocystic condition with atypical hyperplasia	Yes	No
Alcohol consumption	> 9 drinks/week	< 9 drinks/week
History of primary cancer in ovary or endometrium	Yes	No
Radiation to chest	Large doses	Minimal exposure
Socioeconomic class	Upper	Lower
Age at first full-term pregnancy	> 30	< 20
Oophorectomy	Yes	No
Postmenopausal body build	Obese	Thin
Race	White	Black
Marital status	Never married	Never married
Age at menarche	Early	Late
Age at menopause	Late	Early
US place of residence	Urban Northern	Rural Southern

twice as likely to develop or die from breast cancer as those aged 40 to 64. Women who have had cancer in one breast have an increased risk of developing it in the other breast (National Cancer Institute 1993).

Other risk factors that have been implicated include early age of menarche (before 12 years) and nulliparity or first pregnancy resulting in the birth of a child after the age of 30. Fibrocystic disease with hyperplasia has also been implicated. Several life-style aspects have been identified as suspected risk factors including being overweight, particularly in the upper body; using alcohol; and eating a high-fat diet. Caffeine has not been shown to increase risk for breast cancer.

Studies have not shown that oral contraceptives increase breast cancer risk. There is no increased risk with postmenopausal hormone replacement therapy that includes both estrogen and progesterone. There is some controversy over the use of hormone replacement therapy in postmenopausal women with a history of breast cancer. Each woman must be counseled as to her relative risk of breast cancer recurrence versus her risk of osteoporosis and cardiovascular disease (DiSaia 1993).

Nurses need to help women assess their risk for breast cancer and teach them about risk reduction through life-style modifications and screening techniques such as BSE. Although a majority of breast lumps are discovered by women themselves, they may delay seeking further evaluation. The earlier the detection, the greater the chance of cure. Women delay or avoid seeking health care when they detect a lump for a variety of reasons: denial, maintaining control over their life, threats to body image, and the fear of cancer and ultimately death (Ellerhorst-Ryan & Goeldner 1992).

Pathophysiology of Breast Cancer

Theories about the causes of breast cancer include genetic alterations and trace genes (Black & Soloman 1993; Walker & Varley 1993), hormonal mechanisms, and immunologic processes. Because breast cancer does not occur in the prepubertal female, it is thought that prior conditioning of the breast tissue by endogenous steroids may be essential for its development.

A malignant breast neoplasm may originate either in a duct or in the epithelium of the breast lobes. The size and location of the tumor cell at diagnosis is of major importance in the treatment options available to the woman. In situ cancers are found within the basement membrane of the duct or lobule. In situ cancer of the duct is often identified on mammography as microcalcifications clustered in one area of the breast. Among the most common reasons for biopsies, microcalcifications constitute 20% of cancers found by mammography. They cannot be felt by breast physical exam. Lobule in situ cancer is often discovered in premenopausal women who have a biopsy for minimal thickening or other unexplained abnormality. If lobule in situ cancer is found in one breast, it may occur in the other breast as well.

Infiltrating or invasive cancer cells that have passed through the basement membrane of the duct into the fatty tissue will eventually form a fibrous lump that can be felt on examination. Infiltrating ductal carcinoma is the most common type of cancer. Infiltrating cancer of the lobules occurs when the cells break through the basement membrane in single file and invade the surrounding tissue. It is estimated that 15% of breast cancer is of the infiltrating lobular type. This type is more difficult to see on mammograms and is usually felt as a soft thickening in the breast (Hirshaut & Pressman 1993).

Other less common types of malignant breast disease may also be found by physical examination and mammography. About 50% of all breast cancers originate in the upper outer quadrant and spread or metastasize to the auxiliary lymph nodes. Approximately 25% of all breast cancers arise in the central portion of the breast and metastasize to the mammary lymph node chain and bloodstream. Common sites of distant metastasis are the lymph nodes, lungs, liver, brain, and bone.

During the early stage of development a lump in the breast is usually isolated, movable, and painless. A hard distinct mass that is not freely movable suggests cancer. More advanced signs, such as fixation to the skin, skin edema, deep fixation, nipple retraction, or bloody nipple discharge, are further evidence of malignancy.

Classification of tumors has been developed around size and degree of spreading by local invasion, lymph, or bloodstream. Small tumors that have not metastasized and are under 2 cm (about ¾ in) in diameter have the best prognosis following treatment.

Screening, Detection, and Diagnosis

The purpose of breast screening programs is to identify women with breast cancer who have no clinical signs. The primary screening tools currently available include monthly BSE, annual examination by a health professional, and mammography. Advanced radiologic exams such as ultrasonography, thermography, and diaphanography are used occasionally. Fine-needle aspiration may be requested for women with cysts. However, a surgical biopsy is necessary for definitive diagnosis. Prior to the collection of objective data, a thorough history of risk factors, breast self-examination findings, and relevant health history data should be completed (Drugay 1993).

Monthly Breast Self-Examination

Monthly BSE has been shown to be the most effective method for early detection of breast cancer (Ludwick 1992). Approximately 75% of breast lumps are found by women themselves (Hirshaut & Pressman 1993). Refer to Teaching Guide: Teaching Breast Self-Examination on page 222.

Breast Examination by a Health Care Provider

The American Cancer Society and the American College of Obstetricians and Gynecologists recommend that all women have their breasts examined annually, or more often if the woman is at increased risk, by a trained health care provider. Nurses can be certified in performing breast examinations (Ludwick 1992). If the health care provider finds a suspicious lump during the breast examination, a mammogram will be ordered. Additional testing may be ordered, and a referral to a breast specialist, surgeon, or oncologist may be made.

> The physician also felt the lump and thickening, and now I'm waiting for my mammogram. In these few days my thoughts and feelings have been a roller coaster. I'm 46, and I'm wondering if this is it. Am I dying? Now? I'm afraid as I have not been afraid since one of our children was very ill. Try as I may to fill my head with other thoughts, it keeps slipping back to this.

Mammogram

A film screen **mammogram** is a soft-tissue x-ray image of the compressed breast taken without injecting a contrast medium. Able to detect many lesions in the breast before they can be felt, a mammogram also serves as a diagnostic tool in making a differential diagnosis.

Currently, the American Cancer Society, the AMA Council on Scientific Affairs, and the American College of Radiology suggest the following mammogram screening guidelines:

- Baseline mammogram between ages 35 and 40
- Mammogram every 1 to 2 years between ages 40 and 49
- Mammogram annually for all women over age 50

Mammography is less effective for diagnosing abnormalities in younger, denser breast tissue (Clark 1992). In light of the low incidence of breast cancer in women under age 30, it is suggested that sonography and aspiration are of benefit in evaluating breast masses in these women. A screening mammogram should be used only for women in this age group with a strong clinical suggestion of cancer. Controversy exists about the benefit of a screening mammogram in young women who have undergone augmentation mammoplasty (Douglas et al 1991). In this case the concern is that, because 22–83% of breast tissue is obscured by the implants, a lump may not be felt, even during professional examination.

Mammography is a useful tool, but it cannot replace BSE or physical examination. Up to 15% of early-stage breast cancers are detected by physical examination and not detected by mammogram (Ellerhorst-Ryan & Goeldner 1992).

Needle Biopsy

A fine-needle aspiration (biopsy) is accomplished by inserting a needle into the mass to withdraw cells or cystic fluid for microscopic examination. A fine needle on a hypodermic syringe is typically used to aspirate cystic fluid. A wider needle may be used when removing a biopsy sample of cells from a solid mass. Needle biopsy is not always a definitive diagnostic procedure, and a surgical (open) biopsy may still be necessary. Needle biopsies cannot conclusively rule out the presence of cancerous cells. Hence practitioners view aspiration biopsy as only a supplemental diagnostic technique.

Needle localizations are done for nonpalpable, mammographically suspicious breast lesions. The radiologist places the needle marker in the breast tissue under the guidance of mammography or ultrasound. The surgeon uses this marker to locate the area to be biopsied. The most recent advances have involved a technique for stereotactic biopsy called the Mammotest. This procedure is done in the radiology department under local anesthesia. Core biopsies of the suspicious lesion are taken by the computer-guided insertion of a large-gauge needle into the compressed breast tissue (Miller et al 1992).

Surgical (Open) Biopsy

Biopsy is the primary diagnostic technique for confirming the presence of cancer. There are two types of biopsy. An *incisional biopsy* is used if the lump is large. A small section of the tumor is removed for examination by a pathologist, and further treatment is initiated in a second step. An *excisional biopsy*, used for smaller lesions, removes the suspicious area or small lump in its entirety, as well as an additional margin of surrounding tissue. Skin is not removed during an excisional biopsy. The excised tissue and preoperative mammograms (if needle localization was used) are sent to pathology for microscopic evaluation by immediate frozen section and permanent section. Immediate diagnosis and confirmation of "clean margins" around the tumor can be obtained. This is effectively a lumpectomy for very small tumors and is basic surgical treatment for early breast cancer; radiation therapy is also strongly recommended (National Cancer Institute 1993).

Surgical biopsy is usually performed on an outpatient basis with local anesthesia. If the pathologist examines the excised tissue by frozen section, the physician may be immediately able to share a preliminary diagnosis and will then offer more detailed information at a follow-up visit in the office. A staging or classification system for breast cancer has been developed by the American Joint Committee on Cancer. This system correlates combinations of characteristics of the tumor (T), the nodes (N), and the metastasis (M). Staging is carried out following biopsy of the tumor and, if necessary, the lymph nodes (Hirshaut & Pressman 1993).

In this two-step approach to diagnosis the woman and her physician then have an opportunity to discuss future treatment alternatives. The woman meanwhile can also increase her knowledge and well-being by seeking a second opinion, talking with her family and support systems, seeking counseling, and arranging her schedule to enhance her sense of well-being. This approach to breast cancer diagnosis has gained support from women and health care professionals alike. A decision made in this fashion is less likely to be regretted later (Neufeld et al 1993).

Treatment of Breast Cancer

Controversy regarding treatment alternatives for breast cancer persists within the medical profession. The woman may not want the treatment her physician recommends for a newly diagnosed breast cancer. The physician's major concern may be a cure, which may include more radical surgical treatments, whereas the woman may feel the threatened loss of a valued body part is equally important.

Treatment options are determined by the extent of disease and the type of breast cancer. Treatments include surgery, radiation, chemotherapy, and hormone therapy. At times some or all of these are used either in combination or sequentially. Newer experimental therapies also show promise. Breast cancer is a slow growing disease and, if detected early, is curable. However once the disease has spread beyond the breast and regional lymph nodes, it is not generally curable (Palmer 1993). Thus early breast cancer is difficult to diagnose but easy to cure. Late breast cancer is easy to diagnose but difficult to cure.

If a woman is diagnosed with breast cancer during pregnancy, much more conservative treatment modalities are used. Treatment depends on the stage of the disease at the time of diagnosis. If possible, treatment is delayed until after childbirth. If waiting until then is not possible, the surgical treatment modality is initiated with special attention to anesthesia. Radiation therapy, chemotherapy, and hormone therapy should be avoided during pregnancy, if at all possible, due to potential danger to the fetus.

Surgical Treatment Alternatives

Radical mastectomy used to be the surgery of choice for breast cancer. The unfortunate aspect of this option is the mutilation it causes. Breast cancer treatment has a significant emotional impact on the woman's integrity, body image, self-concept, and sexual identity. Because of the possibility of residual cancer cells after surgical intervention, many surgeons believe it is logical to remove the greatest amount of tissue in the hope of curative treatment. However, recent studies have proved that conservative breast surgery in early disease combined with radiation or adjuvant chemotherapy gives 5-year survival results that are as satisfactory. Of course, the earlier the detection, the more conservative the surgery can be. It is important for the nurse to realize that the aim of surgical breast cancer treatment is threefold:

1. To preserve the woman's life
2. To minimize recurrence
3. To provide the best cosmetic results possible

Currently available surgical approaches include excisional biopsy (discussed previously), lumpectomy, partial mastectomy, total (simple) mastectomy, radical mastectomy, and breast reconstruction.

Lumpectomy involves removing the tumor mass and a narrow margin of normal tissue surrounding it.
Partial mastectomy involves removing the tumor and 2–3 cm of surrounding tissue.
Total (simple) mastectomy refers to the surgical removal of the breast but not the pectoral muscle.
Radical mastectomy is the surgical removal of the entire breast, skin, pectoralis major and minor muscles, lymph nodes of the axilla, and surrounding fat tissue.

Treating breast cancer with immediate breast reconstruction using a variety of implants and surgical approaches is becoming increasingly common. This has the advantages of lower cost, reduced anesthesia exposure, and a strong psychologic boost. Studies have shown that immediate reconstruction does not increase the risk of cancer recurrence or metastasis. Women who have undergone a radical mastectomy are not good candidates for reconstruction because they lack sufficient amounts of skin and muscle.

Radiation Therapy

Radiation therapy is used for breast cancer either to reduce tumor size prior to surgery or to kill any lingering malignant cells following surgery. It is particularly useful following conservative surgical techniques.

Chemotherapy

Adjuvant chemotherapy is recommended to cure microscopic metastatic disease by destroying malignant cells in women with positive lymph nodes. The standard chemotherapeutic approach is CMF (ie, *c*yclophosphamide [Cytoxon], *m*ethotrexate, and 5-*f*luorouracil), although other regimens are also used. Opinion varies as to the value of using chemotherapy or tamoxifen in women with negative lymph nodes. The use of adjuvant chemotherapy in treating all breast cancer is becoming increasingly common because of the close proximity of the breasts to the lymphatic circulation, which results in rapid metastasis of the disease.

Hormone Therapy

Tumors are tested to determine if they are estrogen-receptor–positive or –negative. An estrogen-receptor–positive tumor is one that is stimulated by estrogen. Therefore the goal of hormone therapy is to suppress estrogen stimulation, which will result in tumor regression. Antiestrogen therapy has produced positive results in 70% of women with estrogen-receptor–positive tumors. Tamoxifen, the most common antiestrogen used, is the most prescribed anticancer medication in the world. Tamoxifen is presently being studied in the prophylaxis of breast cancer in high-risk postmenopausal women. In premenopausal women with estrogen-receptor–positive tumors, a bilateral oophorectomy can provide a 65% chance of tumor remission (Leis 1993).

Other hormone therapies include treatment with androgen, progestin, or large doses of estrogen in postmenopausal women. High doses of these hormones cause tumor regression, although the exact mechanism of action is unknown.

Metastatic Disease

Metastatic breast cancer is characterized by the presence of cancer cells in distant parts of the body. Four common sites of metastasis are the lungs, liver, brain, and bone. The woman with breast cancer metastasis has a shortened life expectancy, and her survival is frequently contingent on the organ systems involved in the metastasis and her response to therapy. In metastatic disease endocrine manipulation and chemotherapy are used to interrupt the cellular growth and spread of the cancer cells. Radiation therapy directed at a specific area and surgery are used palliatively to relieve the pain or obstruction associated with metastatic tumor spread. Metastatic disease is considered to be advanced or terminal when the cancer spread cannot be controlled by any of the therapeutic interventions previously discussed.

Psychosocial issues related to metastatic breast cancer range from those related to cure and restoration of body image to those related to the achievement of quality survival and symptom control. In the presence of a disease that is not yet curable hope takes on new meaning. Hope for cure is replaced by hope for continuing availability of therapeutic options, treatment responsiveness, long-term survival, freedom from symptoms, and hope that life-style patterns and interpersonal relationships will remain intact.

Psychosocial Concerns of the Woman with Breast Cancer

When a woman is confronted with a breast mass, she initiates a decision-making process about her diagnostic and treatment options and her approach to her condition. The woman is the only person who can decide what benefits of surgery are worth what personal risks. Despite the seriousness of the diagnosis, the time constraints, and the expense involved, the woman should be encouraged to seek a second opinion, which is now paid for by many third-party payment plans.

In the early phases of treatment an emotional dichotomy often prevails: The woman experiencing a mastectomy deals with both the potential loss of life due to cancer and the loss of a breast or a portion of it. Yet in the period immediately preceding and following mastectomy, health professionals tend to emphasize treatment of the cancer so that the woman will comply with her therapeutic regimen. The issue of breast loss is postponed. In the early postoperative phase the woman may experience strong pressure from her partner, family, friends, and health care team to "do well" by adjusting quickly and easily to the surgery. Most American women have been socialized to be "good" by pleasing others. To please her mate or her physician, a woman may begin to deny some of her feelings, particularly about the loss of the breast. She may hold back her questions and refrain from talking about her feelings to make a good impression. By providing information, resources, and support, nurses can help women with breast cancer increase their self-esteem and improve interpersonal relationships, body image, and identity, thereby enabling them to manage their illness more effectively (Kahane 1993). Nurses need to encourage women to discuss breast loss and body disfigurement. Otherwise the natural grieving associated with this loss may be delayed.

The course of adjustment confronting the woman with breast cancer has been described as four phases: shock, reaction, recovery, and reorientation. In the shock phase women make statements like "Everything is unreal" or "I can't understand what is happening to me."

Shock extends from the discovery of the lump through the process of diagnosis.

Reaction occurs in conjunction with the initiation of treatment. As treatment begins, the woman is compelled to face what has occurred and begins to take in what has happened. Coping mechanisms become evident during this phase. Reaction coincides with the length of treatment, and for many women radiation treatment or chemotherapy prolongs this period to months. During the phases of shock and reaction the woman is completely absorbed with what has caused the problem. Treatment reinforces the diagnosis of cancer and the immediate consequences of the disease. Denial of breast loss and the reality of the illness is common during the periods of diagnosis and treatment. Denial protects the woman, making therapy tolerable.

Recovery begins during convalescence following the completion of medical treatment. Anxiety about her illness diminishes, and the woman looks to the future once more. She turns outward and gradually resumes her former activities. Conversely, depression and social isolation occur if the woman is unable to negotiate the recovery phase successfully.

A woman's family and friends significantly influence her recovery. Women often perceive their partners as their primary source of support. Both members of a couple must adjust to her condition and its implications as well as to the effect of therapy on their sexual intimacy. Difficulties with psychosocial adjustment to breast cancer tend to be similar for women and their partners except in the area of role adjustments, where women have more difficulty. The American Cancer Society sponsors numerous support groups for cancer survivors and their families. They also have a highly successful program, Reach to Recovery, for women following surgery.

Friends and relatives may be reluctant to initiate social interaction during the recovery period. The woman's own uncertainty about resuming previous activities coupled with friends' reticence about "pushing her" may result in a more withdrawn life-style.

Reorientation follows recovery and is unending. It is accomplished when the woman can acknowledge that breast cancer is a part of her life, yet living, for her, has returned to or perhaps exceeded its former fullness and meaning.

Nursing Care of the Woman with Breast Cancer

Nursing care of the woman with breast cancer is multidimensional. It involves meeting the educational, psychosocial, psychosexual, and physical needs of the woman and to a certain extent those of her family. In meeting these needs the nurse functions as care giver, counselor, educator, liaison, and advocate. Nurses need to support women in their efforts to provide self-care. This increases

their self-esteem and their sense of control. The nursing care changes as the woman progresses from the period of diagnosis to the recovery period.

Nursing Care During the Diagnostic Period

Nursing care begins before a woman faces a diagnosis of breast cancer. Indeed, the nurse can significantly affect the woman's prognosis by encouraging early detection of malignant tumors. Health teaching can assist the woman in understanding breast cancer treatment alternatives. Awareness of possible choices enables a woman to select the treatment regimen she perceives is best for her individual needs.

APPLYING THE NURSING PROCESS

Nursing Assessment

The woman seeking health care following discovery of a lump is likely to be apprehensive. She may hold unfounded beliefs about breast cancer. Holistic health assessment should be conducted in an understanding, unhurried, emotionally supportive atmosphere. Such an assessment has therapeutic value in itself. It should include the following:

- A systems review emphasizing the reproductive system, particularly the breast
- The significance the woman attributes to her breasts
- The woman's knowledge and beliefs about breast cancer
- Identification of social support (family, friends, clergy)
- The woman's emotional status and coping mechanisms she has used during periods of stress
- Environmental factors that may influence coping and adjustment

Assessment of the woman facing a diagnosis of breast cancer must be an ongoing process. Sufficient data must be obtained to provide the nurse and other health team members with increasing insight into the client's biophysical, mental, emotional, and social situation.

Nursing Diagnosis

Nursing diagnoses that may apply during the diagnostic period include the following:

- Knowledge deficit related to lack of information about the diagnostic procedures

- Fear related to the possibility of a diagnosis of cancer

Nursing Plan and Implementation

The nurse should assure the woman that she will be able to participate in decision making about her treatment once the biopsy results are known. Nursing advocacy involves supporting the woman's right to make the best decision for her. With the assistance of the nurse the woman can explore her fears, clarify her values, and identify the treatment options that would be personally acceptable. Once the woman has made an informed decision, the nurse's role becomes one of support. The woman and her partner or support person should discuss the treatment alternatives together with the health care provider once the results of the biopsy are known. At the time of the discovery of a suspicious lump and certainly after the diagnosis of breast cancer the woman should be referred to a team of cancer specialists.

Evaluation

Anticipated outcomes of nursing care include:

- The woman is able to discuss her diagnosis, treatment options, and long-term prognosis.
- After assessing her alternatives the woman chooses the treatment that seems most appropriate to her.

CARE OF THE WOMAN WITH ENDOMETRIOSIS

Endometriosis is a condition characterized by the presence of endometrial tissue outside the endometrial cavity. This tissue responds to the hormonal changes of the menstrual cycle and bleeds in a cyclic fashion. This bleeding results in inflammation, fibrosis, and formation of adhesions. The most common symptoms include progressive dysmenorrhea, dyspareunia (painful intercourse), and infertility.

Endometriosis may occur at any age after puberty, although it is most common in women between 30 and 40 and is rare in postmenopausal women. A familial tendency does seem to exist.

The exact cause of endometriosis is unknown. Proposed theories of etiology include retrograde menstrual flow and inflammation of endometrium, hereditary tendency, and, most recently, an immunologic defect (Kauppila 1993).

The pelvic pain associated with endometriosis is cyclic in nature due to the normal monthly fluctuations in hormones. It is postulated that estrogen and progesterone stimulate endometrial-like tissue growth, like that which occurs in the uterus during the menstrual cycle. The bleeding that occurs leads to pressure and inflammation in the adjacent tissues, causing pain. The character of the pain has limited value in predicting the stage of endometriosis. It is associated with the volume of implants and the presence of the disease in the cul-de-sac and the uterosacral ligaments (Ripps & Martin 1992).

The most common sites of endometriosis are the ovaries, the uterosacral ligaments, and the cul-de-sac. However, endometriosis can involve many body organs remote from the pelvis (such as the lungs) and can thus produce a host of complications. For example, intrathoracic endometriosis can result in pneumothorax.

Women with certain menstrual characteristics are more at risk for developing endometriosis. A woman with a menstrual cycle length of 27 days or less and a menstrual flow lasting a week or more has twice the risk of a woman with longer cycle length and shorter flow duration. Women with heavy flow and those who have used tampons for longer than 14 years are also at increased risk (Darrow et al 1993). Moreover research indicates that severe dysmenorrhea is the only symptom predictive of endometriosis (Forman et al 1993).

The long-term sequelae of endometriosis are many and range from minor complications to the most serious complication, infertility. This is caused by interference with ovum release and tubal movement secondary to tubal adhesions.

Medical Therapy

The most common symptom of endometriosis is pelvic pain, which is often a dull ache or cramping sensation. It is often related to menstruation and generally ceases following the completion of the woman's menses. Dyspareunia, another common symptom, occurs most frequently if the uterus is retroverted and lesions are present in the area of the posterior vaginal fornix or the uterosacral ligaments. Another frequently cited symptom is abnormal uterine bleeding. No specific pattern exists, although it may be frequent, prolonged, and excessive.

Endometriosis is often diagnosed when a woman seeks treatment or evaluation for infertility. Bimanual examination may reveal a fixed, tender, retroverted uterus and palpable nodules in the cul-de-sac. The diagnosis of endometriosis can be confirmed by laparoscopy or laparotomy.

Treatment may be medical, surgical, or a combination of the two. The surgical treatment of endometriosis is shifting from laparotomy toward laparoscopy. Various lasers as well as sharp dissection and bipolar cautery are used through the laparoscope in the surgical treatment of endometriosis (Younger 1993).

The medical treatment of endometriosis revolves around hormone repressive therapies. Because endome-

DANAZOL (DANOCRINE)

Overview of Action

Danazol is a testosterone derivative with a mild androgenic effect. The drug has an antigonadotropic effect that results in the suppression of both follicle-stimulating hormone (FSH) and luteinizing hormone (LH). As a consequence ovulation is suppressed and amenorrhea develops. Danazol also reduces levels of sex steroids by inhibiting the enzymes responsible for their production and binds steroid hormone receptors on endometrial tissue implants. This results in atrophy of endometrial tissue implants and endometrium within the uterus. Dose-related menstrual changes have been associated with this drug. At lower dosages (50–100 mg) menstrual bleeding may be regular or irregular. With dosages of 200–400 mg, 40% to 90% of women experience amenorrhea. Progress of endometriosis is stopped, and the woman's pain is relieved. The drug may also be used to treat fibrocystic breast disease.

Route, Dosage, Frequency

Endometriosis: 200–400 mg orally two times per day for 3–6 months. Therapy is begun if pregnancy test is negative or during woman's menstrual period. Treatment may be extended for 9 months or restarted if symptoms recur.

Breast disease: 100–400 mg/day orally two times per day for 3–6 months. Long-term effects of treatment not known.

Contraindications

Pregnancy
Breastfeeding women
Impaired kidney, heart, or liver function
Undiagnosed abnormal vaginal bleeding
Porphyria

Side Effects

Vaginal bleeding	Acne
Vasomotor instability	Oily skin and hair
Hirsutism	Weight gain
Reduced libido	Decreased breast size
Voice changes, hoarseness	Irritability, depression
Edema	Sleep disorders, fatigue
Muscle cramps	Gastroenteritis
Headaches	Signs of atrophic vaginitis
Nausea	Alopecia
Clitoral enlargement	Amenorrhea

Changed lab values, including reduced high-density lipoprotein (HDL); increased low-density lipoprotein (LDL); increased liver enzyme levels (serum glutamic-oxaloacetic transaminase [SGOT], serum glutamic-pyruvic transaminase [SGPT], creatinine phosphokinase [CPK], lactic dehydrogenase [LDH])

Nursing Considerations

1. Inform woman about potential side effects; stress that menses and ovulation usually resume within 2 to 3 months after discontinuing therapy.

2. Continue routine breast examinations and report any enlarged or hardened breast nodules.

3. Obtain baseline and other liver function tests as ordered.

4. Voice changes should be reported immediately and the medication stopped to avoid permanent damage.

5. Observe woman for signs of virilization.

6. Because ovulation may not be suppressed, a backup, nonhormonal form of birth control should be used if the woman wishes to avoid conception.

triosis is perpetuated by menstrual cycle hormone changes, the goal of the therapy is to suppress the menstrual cycle. This can be accomplished by various medications. The two most commonly used are danazol and a gonadotropin-releasing hormone (GnRH) agonist. Danazol (see Drug Guide: Danazol [Danocrine]) suppresses the menstrual cycle through its androgenic action. This may result in the side effects of acne or weight gain. The GnRH agonists suppress the menstrual cycle through estrogen antagonism; this may result in the hypoestrogen side effects of hot flashes, vaginal dryness, and loss of bone density. Recent studies have indicated that these side effects may be modified when the GnRH agonists are combined with a progestin (Kauppila 1993). If the woman does not desire pregnancy at the present time, she may be started on oral contraceptives. Low-dose oral contraceptives have been effective in treating pelvic pain and dysmenorrhea in these women (Vercellini et al 1993).

In women with minimal disease and symptoms treatment includes observation, analgesics, and nonsteroidal anti-inflammatory drugs (NSAIDs). The woman who desires pregnancy and has been unsuccessful in her attempts to conceive is treated with a 3- to 6-month course of danazol or a GnRH agonist such as leuprolide (Lupron) or nafarelin. After she has completed the course of therapy, she will attempt to conceive, probably with the aid of ovulation stimulation medications. The chances of a woman achieving a pregnancy following the surgical and medical treatment for endometriosis are increased with active ovulation management (Kemmann et al 1993).

Women treated with medical therapies only are likely to experience recurrence of their endometriosis after the therapy is discontinued, particularly if their disease is severe at the outset. Women who have only surgical treatment experience a 25% recurrence rate. This is why most women are treated with a combination of medical and surgical therapies. These therapies appear to be equally effective in the subsequent pregnancy rates of infertile women (Walker & Shaw 1993).

In more advanced cases a laparotomy may be done to remove implants and break up adhesions. If severe dyspareunia or dysmenorrhea are symptoms, the surgeon may perform a presacral neurectomy, or severing of the presacral nerve, which relieves pain to the central pelvis. In advanced cases in which childbearing is not an issue a hysterectomy with bilateral salpingo-oophorectomy may be done.

APPLYING THE NURSING PROCESS

Nursing Assessment

The nurse should be aware of the common symptoms of endometriosis and elicit an accurate history if a woman mentions these symptoms. If a woman is being treated for endometriosis, the nurse should assess the woman's understanding of the condition, its implications, and the treatment alternatives.

Nursing Diagnosis

Nursing diagnoses that may apply to a woman with endometriosis include the following:

- Pain related to peritoneal irritation secondary to endometriosis.

- Ineffective individual coping related to depression secondary to infertility.

Nursing Plan and Implementation

The nurse can be available to explain the condition, its symptoms, treatment alternatives, and prognosis. The nurse can help the woman evaluate treatment options and make choices that are appropriate for her. If medication is begun, the nurse can review the dosage, schedule, possible side effects, and any warning signs. Women are often advised to avoid delaying pregnancy because of the risk of infertility. The woman may wish to discuss the implications of this decision on her life choices, relationship with her partner, and personal preferences. The nurse can be a nonjudgmental listener and help the woman consider her options.

Evaluation

Anticipated outcomes of nursing care include:

- The woman clearly understands her condition, its implications for fertility, and her treatment options.

- The woman successfully copes with the discomfort and long-term implications of her diagnosis.

- After considering her options, the woman chooses appropriate treatment options and therapy.

CARE OF THE WOMAN WITH TOXIC SHOCK SYNDROME

Toxic shock syndrome (TSS) was first described in children, but soon afterward the association between TSS and menstruation was identified (Colbry 1992). Although TSS has been reported in children, postmenopausal women, and men, it is primarily a disease of women of reproductive age, especially at or near menses or during the postpartum period. The causative organism is a strain of *Staphylococcus aureus* that produces a specific toxin called TSST-1. Although the vast majority of women have antibodies to *S aureus*, only a few ever develop signs of the disease. Research indicates a possible link between high levels of estradiol and inhibition of toxin production. If this is the case, it would explain the higher incidence of TSS during menstruation and the postpartal period when estradiol levels are low.

The use of high-absorbency tampons has been widely publicized as being related to an increased incidence of TSS. However, occluding the cervical os with a contraceptive device such as a cervical cap, diaphragm, or contraceptive sponge, especially if they are left in place for more than 24 hours, may also increase the risk of TSS.

A nonmenstrual form of toxic shock syndrome may also occur. It is found in men, women, and children following burns or surgery. It has a 65% rate of nosocomial acquisition (Kain et al 1993).

Medical Therapy

Early diagnosis and treatment are important in preventing a fatal outcome. The case-to-fatality ratio has decreased from 15% to 3% (Eschenbach 1994).

The most common signs of TSS include fever (often greater than 38.9 C [102 F]); desquamation of the skin, especially the palms and soles, which usually occurs 1 to 2 weeks after the onset of symptoms; a sunburnlike rash; hypotension; and dizziness. Systemic symptoms often include vomiting, diarrhea, severe myalgia, and inflamed mucous membranes (oropharyngeal, conjunctival, or vaginal). In addition, disorders of the central nervous system, including alterations in consciousness, disorientation, and coma, may occur.

Laboratory findings reveal elevated BUN, creatinine, SGOT, SGPT, and total bilirubin; platelets are often less than $100,000/mm^3$. Blood, throat, and CSF cultures are negative, as are tests for Rocky Mountain spotted fever (Colbry 1992).

Women with TSS are generally hospitalized and given supportive therapy, including intravenous fluids to maintain blood pressure. If a tampon is in place, it should be removed. Severe cases may require dialysis, administration of vasopressors, and intubation. Penicillinase-resistant antibiotics, although of only limited value during the acute phase, do help reduce the risk of recurrence (Eschenbach 1994).

Nursing Care

Nurses play a major role in helping educate women about ways of preventing the development of TSS. Women should understand the importance of avoiding prolonged use of tampons. Tampons should be changed every 3 to 6 hours, and super-absorbency tampons should be avoided. Some women may choose to use other products, such as sanitary napkins or minipads. The woman who chooses to continue using tampons may reduce her risk by alternating them with napkins and by avoiding overnight use of tampons.

Postpartal women are advised to avoid the use of tampons for 6 to 8 weeks after childbirth. Women with a history of TSS should totally refrain from using tampons (Schuchat & Broome 1991).

Women who use barrier contraceptives such as diaphragms, cervical caps, or contraceptive sponges should avoid leaving them in place for prolonged periods. These devices should not be used during the postpartum period or when the woman is menstruating.

Nurses can also help make women aware of the signs and symptoms of TSS so that women will seek treatment promptly if signs occur.

CARE OF THE WOMAN DURING A PELVIC EXAMINATION

Women have a pelvic examination performed for a variety of reasons ranging from health maintenance to disease diagnosis. The pelvic exam is often perceived by women as an uncomfortable and embarrassing procedure. The negative feelings may cause women to delay having yearly gynecologic examinations, and this avoidance may pose a threat to life and health.

To make the pelvic examination less threatening, and thus improve health-seeking behavior, it is important to create a trusting environment and incorporate practices that help the woman maintain a sense of control. Some health care providers are performing what is called an educational pelvic examination. During this type of exam the woman becomes an active participant and has an opportunity to learn about her body, voice her concerns, and share decisions regarding her care.

The educational exam includes offering the woman a mirror to watch the procedure, pointing out anatomic parts to her, and positioning and draping her to allow eye-to-eye contact with the practitioner. The woman is encouraged to participate by asking questions and giving feedback.

Nurse practitioners, certified nurse-midwives, and physicians all perform pelvic examinations. Nurses assist the practitioner and the woman during the examination. Procedure 10–1, on page 236, provides information on assisting with a pelvic examination.

Vulvar Self-Examination

During the pelvic examination many care givers also provide education about self-examination of the vulva. This procedure, like the self-examination of the breasts, permits early detection of abnormalities, thereby maximizing the possibility of cure and the use of conservative treatment approaches.

Self-examination of the vulva is simple to perform. The woman is advised to assume a sitting position on a bed or chair. In good light she holds a mirror in one hand and uses her other hand to expose the tissue of her perineum while she carefully inspects and palpates the area. Pregnant or obese women may find it easier to inspect the area while standing with one foot placed on a low stool. Figure 10–3 demonstrates the correct procedure for vulvar self-examination. Any abnormalities or changes should be reported to the woman's health care provider.

The examination should be performed monthly at the same time as the BSE in all sexually active asymptomatic women or women over age 18. Women with a history of vulvar lesions or women with symptoms should inspect their vulva more frequently.

CARE OF THE WOMAN WITH A VAGINAL INFECTION

Vulvovaginal Candidiasis (VVC)

Vulvovaginal candidiasis (often called "yeast infection") is the most common form of vaginitis affecting the vagina and vulva. An estimated 75% of women will

Nursing Action	Rationale

Objective: Assemble and prepare equipment.

Prepare and arrange following equipment so that it is easily accessible:

1. Various sized vaginal specula, warmed with water or on a heating pad prior to insertion

   Examination is facilitated.

   Warmed speculum assists in lubrication and facilitates initial insertion when culture and smears are to be taken. Do not use lubricant on speculum prior to insertion. This may alter findings or cultures.

2. Gloves

3. Water-soluble lubricant

4. Materials for Pap smear and cultures

5. Good light source

Objective: Prepare woman.

Explain procedure.

Explanation of procedure decreases anxiety.

Instruct woman to empty her bladder and to remove clothing below waist. She may be encouraged to keep her shoes on and will be given a disposable drape or sheet to place on her lap. Encourage her to sit on the end of the examining table with the drape across her lap prior to examination. Provide a warm environment either through overhead heat lights or through central heat. If a woman has never had a pelvic examination before, show her the equipment and explain the procedure prior to examination.

Comfort is promoted during internal examination. She may feel more comfortable with shoes on rather than supporting her weight with bare heels against cold stirrups.

Position woman in lithotomy position with thighs flexed and adducted. Place her feet in stirrups. Buttocks should extend slightly beyond end of examining table.

Drape woman with a sheet, leaving flap so perineum can be exposed.

Objective: Provide support to woman as physician or nurse practitioner carries out examination.

Explain each part of examination as it is performed: inspection of external genitals, vagina, and cervix; bimanual examination of internal organs. Instruct woman to relax and breathe slowly.

Relaxation is promoted.

Advise woman when speculum is to be inserted and ask her to bear down.

When speculum is inserted, woman may feel intravaginal pressure. Bearing down helps open vaginal orifice and relax perineal muscles.

Lubricate examiner's fingers well prior to bimanual examination.

Lubrication decreases friction and eases insertion.

Objective: Provide for woman's comfort at end of examination.

Move to the end of the examining table and face woman's perineum. Cover the woman with the drape. Apply gentle pressure to the woman's knees and encourage her to move toward the head of the table. Offer your hand to the woman, remove her heels from the stirrups, and assist the woman to a sitting position. Be sure that she is not dizzy and that she is sitting or standing safely before you leave the room.

Supine position may create postural hypotension.

Provide tissues to wipe lubricant from perineum.

Upon assuming sitting position, vaginal secretions along with lubricant may be discharged.

Provide privacy for woman to dress.

Comfort and sense of privacy is promoted.

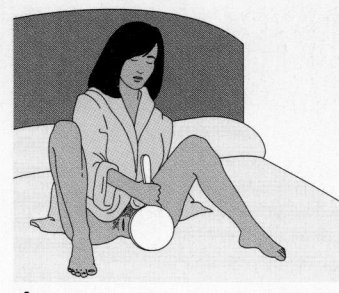

A

Choose a position that is comfortable and exposes the labia. To make viewing easier, use a mirror with a handle.

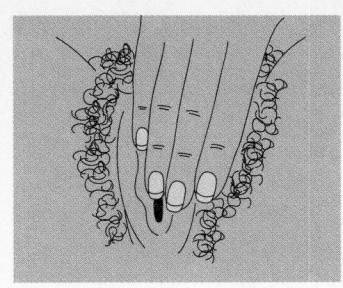

E

Press all areas of the vulva with the flat part of the fingers.

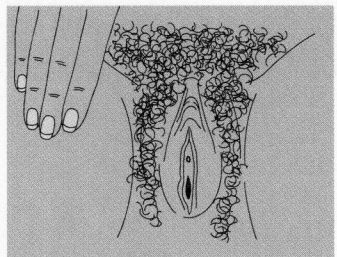

B

Observe the entire vulva and determine whether one side resembles the other.

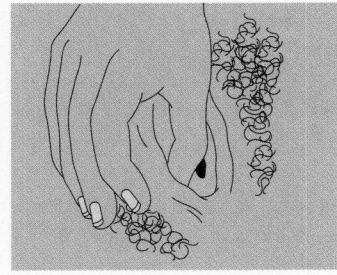

F

Insert the thumb inside the labia and palpate the area between the thumb and the index finger.

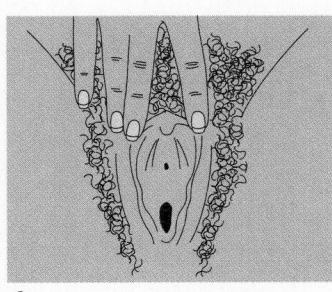

C

Gently push back the covering, or the hood, of the clitoris to inspect the area.

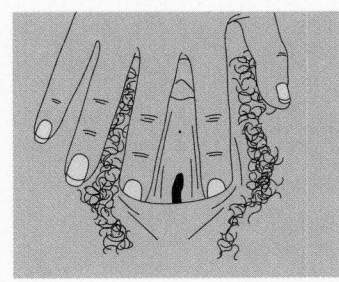

G

Encircle the vaginal opening with index and middle fingers and compress the tissue. The tissue should be soft, moist, elastic, and non-tender.

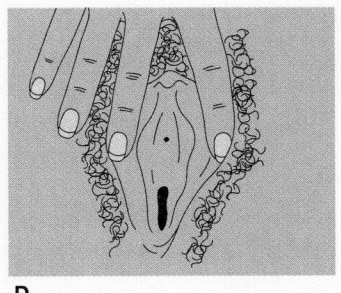
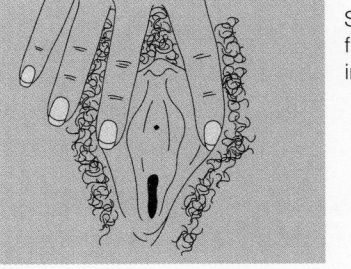

D

Separate the labia with the fingers and examine the inner parts.

FIGURE 10-3   Steps to follow to perform vulvar self-examination.

experience at least one episode of VVC during their lifetime, and 40–45% will experience two or more episodes (CDC 1993). Recurrences are frequent for some women. Factors that contribute to the occurrence of this infection are use of oral contraceptives, use of antibiotics, pregnancy, immunosuppression, diabetes mellitus, presence of human immunodeficiency virus (HIV), use of feminine hygiene products, and other premenstrual factors that are unclear. A gram-positive fungus (*Candida albicans*) is the causative organism. *Candida* is a resident of the mouth,

intestines, and vagina in 25–50% of healthy women. Infection seems to occur when there is overgrowth of this organism.

Medical Therapy

The goal of medical therapy is to diagnose the infection and treat it effectively. The woman will often complain of thick, white, curdy vaginal discharge; severe itching, dysuria; and dyspareunia. A male sexual partner may develop a rash or excoriation of the skin of the penis and possibly pruritus.

On physical examination the woman's labia may be swollen and excoriated if the pruritus has been severe. A speculum examination reveals thick, white, tenacious, cheeselike patches adhering to the vaginal mucosa. Diagnosis is confirmed by microscopic examination of the vaginal discharge; hyphae and spores will usually be seen on a potassium hydroxide (KOH) wet mount preparation (Figure 10–4).

Medical treatment of monilial vaginitis includes intravaginal insertion of miconazole, tioconazole, butaconazole, teraconazole, or clotrimazole suppositories, tablets, or cream at bedtime for 3 days to 1 week. Recently, these medications have become available over the counter. Because a prescription is no longer needed, it is important to counsel women to have VVC diagnosed by a health care provider at least once prior to self-treatment with over-the-counter medications.

If the vulva is also infected, the cream form is prescribed and may be applied topically. Nystatin and single-dose therapies are less effective than recommended therapies. Pregnant women are treated the same as nonpregnant women (CDC 1993). Infection at the time of childbirth may cause thrush in the newborn.

Topical miconazole usually eliminates the yeast infection from the male. However, the CDC states that treatment of the sex partner is not necessary unless candidal balanitis (inflammation of the glans penis) is present or chronicity is a problem. Women with frequent unexplained infections should be evaluated for predisposing conditions and the diagnosis confirmed with a culture. The optimal treatment for recurrent VVC is ketoconazole 100 mg orally, daily for up to 6 months (CDC 1993).

If miconazole cream is being used by both partners, sexual intercourse is permitted and may assure the spread of the cream throughout the vagina. With other methods of treatment abstinence is recommended until both partners are cured.

APPLYING THE NURSING PROCESS

Nursing Assessment

The nurse caring for the woman should suspect monilial vaginitis if the woman complains of intense vulvar itching and a curdy, white discharge. Because the woman with diabetes mellitus during pregnancy is especially susceptible to this infection, the nurse should be alert for symptoms in these women. In some areas nurses are trained to do speculum examinations and wet mount preparations and can therefore confirm the diagnosis themselves. In most cases, however, the nurse who suspects a vaginal infection

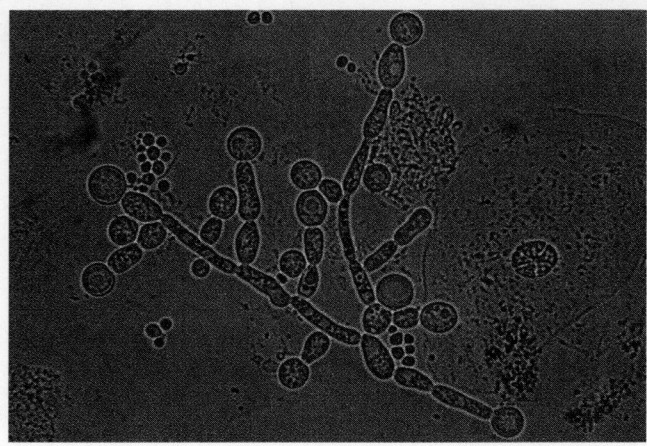

FIGURE 10-4   The hyphae and spores of *Candida albicans.*
SOURCE: Courtesy Centers for Disease Control and Prevention.

reports this to the woman's physician, nurse practitioner, or certified nurse-midwife.

Nursing Diagnosis

Nursing diagnoses that might apply to the woman with VVC include the following:

- Risk for impaired skin integrity related to scratching secondary to the effects of the infection
- Knowledge deficit related to lack of information about ways of preventing the development of VVC

Nursing Plan and Implementation

If the woman is experiencing discomfort due to the pruritus, the nurse can recommend gentle bathing of the vulva with a weak sodium bicarbonate solution. If a topical treatment is being used, the woman should bathe the area before applying the medication.

The nurse also discusses with the woman the factors that contribute to the development of VVC and can suggest ways to prevent recurrences. Some women report that the addition of yogurt to the diet or the use of activated culture of plain yogurt as a vaginal douche helps prevent recurrences by maintaining high levels of lactobacillus.

Evaluation

Anticipated outcomes of nursing care include:

- The woman's symptoms are relieved, and the infection is cured.
- The woman is able to identify self-care measures to prevent further episodes of VVC.

Bacterial Vaginosis (*Gardnerella vaginalis* Vaginitis) (BV)

Many flora normally inhabit the vagina of the healthy woman. Some of these organisms are potentially pathogenic. In some women these bacteria begin to "overgrow," causing a vaginitis. The cause of this overgrowth is not clear, although tissue trauma and sexual intercourse are sometimes identified as contributing factors. The *Gardnerella vaginalis* organism (formerly referred to as *Hemophilus vaginalis*) has been found in the vast majority of cases, along with an increased concentration of anaerobic bacteria. *G vaginalis* can be isolated from vaginal cultures from half of healthy women (CDC 1993). The infected woman often notices an excessive amount of thin, watery, white vaginal discharge with a foul odor described as "fishy." The vaginal discharge is noninflammatory. The characteristic "clue" cell is seen on a wet mount preparation (Figure 10–5). There is also a positive amine "whiff" test. When the discharge is mixed with the potassium hydroxide on a wet mount, a "fishy odor" is emitted. Bacterial vaginitis can also be diagnosed with a Gram stain or a pH of vaginal fluid >4.5.

The nonpregnant woman is generally treated with metronidazole (Flagyl). (See Drug Guide: Metronidazole on page 240.) Because of its potential teratogenic effects, metronidazole is avoided during the first trimester of pregnancy. During the second and third trimesters oral metronidazole can be used, although vaginal metronidazole gel or clindamycin cream may be preferable. During the first trimester of pregnancy one full applicator (5 g) of 2% clindamycin cream is inserted intravaginally at bedtime for 7 days (CDC 1993). Studies suggest that BV in pregnancy may be a factor in premature rupture of the membranes and preterm birth (CDC 1993).

Asymptomatic infections are common in nonpregnant women and generally are not treated. No clinical counterpart of bacterial vaginosis exists in males, and treatment of male sex partners has not shown to be beneficial for the woman or the male partner (CDC 1993).

CARE OF THE WOMAN WITH A SEXUALLY TRANSMITTED INFECTION

The occurrence of **sexually transmitted infection** (also called a **sexually transmitted disease [STD]**) has increased over the past few decades. The terms *venereal disease* and *VD* are being used less frequently; they appear outdated and carry value-laden, negative connotations. No matter how these infections are classified, women often feel anxious, guilty, embarrassed, or fearful when they have or suspect they have vaginitis or a sexually transmitted infection. Vaginitis and sexually transmitted infections are the most common reasons for outpatient treatment of women.

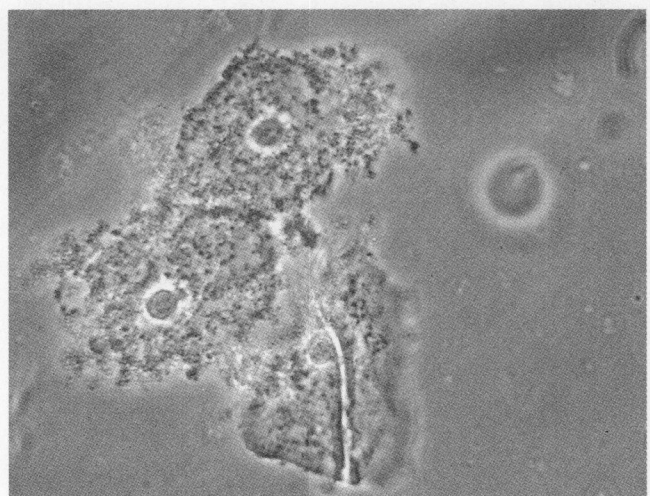

FIGURE 10–5 Depiction of the clue cells characteristically seen in bacterial vaginosis. (*Gardnerella vaginalis*).

Table 10–3 provides a summary of sexually transmitted infections and their treatment. Precautions specific to a particular sexually transmitted infection are noted with discussion of that infection.

Trichomoniasis

Between 15% and 20% of all women are infected with trichomoniasis at some time. This infection is most frequently seen in females 16 to 35 years of age. Women are usually symptomatic, although some women who are carriers have no noticeable discomfort. Between 60% and 90% of the male partners may be asymptomatic. Worldwide, trichomoniasis infects an estimated 180 million people annually.

T vaginalis is a microscopic motile protozoan that thrives in an alkaline environment. Most infections are acquired through sexual intimacy. Transmission by shared bath facilities, wet towels, or wet swimsuits may be possible (CDC 1993). In women this parasite lives only in the genitourinary tract—on squamous epithelial cells lining the vagina, Skene's glands, and urethra. In men it lives in the urethra, prostate gland, and—in uncircumcised males—under the foreskin.

Medical Therapy

Symptoms of trichomoniasis include a yellow-green, frothy, odorous discharge frequently accompanied by inflammation of the vagina and cervix, dysuria, and dyspareunia. Visualization of *T vaginalis* under the microscope on a wet mount preparation of vaginal discharge confirms the diagnosis (Figure 10–6).

Prescriptive treatment for trichomoniasis is oral metronidazole administered over 7 days or in a single 2-g dose for both male and female sexual partners. Intercourse should be avoided until both partners are cured.

The woman should be informed that metronidazole is contraindicated in the first trimester of pregnancy because of possible teratogenic effects on the fetus. However, no other adequate therapy exists. For women with severe symptoms *after the first trimester*, treatment with 2 g of metronidazole in a single dose may be considered (CDC 1993). Vaginal trichomoniasis has been associated with premature rupture of membranes and preterm birth (CDC 1993). The woman and her partner should be cautioned to avoid alcohol while taking metronidazole; the combination has an effect similar to that of alcohol and Antabuse—abdominal pain, flushing, or tremors.

Various vaginal creams, suppositories, or douches may decrease symptoms without clearing up the infection. The only treatment proven effective is metronidazole. Therefore other methods are not recommended.

Chlamydial Infection

Chlamydial infection, caused by *Chlamydia trachomatis*, is the most common sexually transmitted infection in the United States. The organism is an intracellular bacterium with several different immunotypes. Immunotypes of *Chlamydia* are responsible for lymphogranuloma venereum and trachoma, which is the world's leading cause of preventable blindness.

DRUG GUIDE

METRONIDAZOLE (FLAGYL)

Overview of Action

Metronidazole is an antiprotozoal and antibacterial agent. It possesses direct trichomonacidal and amebicidal activity against *T vaginalis* and *E histolytica*. Metronidazole is active in vitro against most obligate anaerobes but does not appear to possess any clinically relevant activity against facultative anaerobes or obligate aerobes. It is used in the treatment of various infections caused by organisms that are sensitive to this drug. It is used predominantly to treat the following infections in women: *T vaginalis,* bacterial vaginosis, endometritis, endomyometritis, tuboovarian abscess, and postsurgical vaginal cuff infection.

Route, Dosage, Frequency

Trichomoniasis—1-day treatment: 2 g orally in a single dose or two divided doses of 1 g each given in the same day; 7-day treatment: 250 mg orally three times a day for 7 consecutive days.
Amebiasis—Adults: 750 mg orally three times a day for 5–10 days; children: 35–50 mg/kg/24 hours orally divided into three doses for 10 days.
Anaerobic bacterial infection—7.5 mg/kg orally every 6 hours, not to exceed 4 g in a 24-hour period, for 7–10 days. In the treatment of serious anaerobic infections the IV form of the drug is used initially.

Contraindications

First trimester of pregnancy
Breastfeeding women (drug secreted in breast milk)
Impaired kidney or liver function

Side Effects

Convulsive seizures	Weakness
Peripheral neuropathy	Insomnia
Nausea/Vomiting	Cystitis

Headache	Dysuria
Anorexia	Reversible neutropenia and thrombocytopenia
Diarrhea	
Epigastric distress	Flattening of the T-wave on EKG
Abdominal cramping	Polyuria
Constipation	Incontinence
Metallic taste in mouth	Pelvic pressure
Dizziness	Proliferation of *Candida* in the vagina and mouth
Vertigo	
Uncoordination	Joint pains
Ataxia	Decreased libido
Confusion	Dryness in the mouth, vulva, and vagina
Irritability	
Depression	Dyspareunia

Nursing Considerations

1. Inform woman about potential side effects.

2. Rule out first trimester pregnancy, and stress the importance of contraceptive compliance during course of treatment.

3. Obtain baseline renal, liver, and hepatic function tests as ordered.

4. Teach woman about the signs, symptoms, and treatment of vulvovaginal candidiasis.

5. Counsel woman to avoid alcoholic beverages while taking the medication.

6. If the woman is taking oral contraceptives, a backup nonhormonal contraceptive method is recommended during treatment.

7. Take thorough history to rule out the woman's exposure to this medication within the last 6 weeks.

8. Teach woman to monitor the signs and symptoms of her infection.

9. Encourage cooperation with the entire course of treatment.

TABLE 10-3   Summary of Sexually Transmitted Infections

Disease	Organism	Diagnosis	Treatment Nonpregnant	Treatment Pregnant
Vulvovaginal candidiasis	*Candida albicans*	Wet mount hyphae	Topically applied azole drugs	Topically applied azole drugs
Bacterial vaginosis	*G vaginalis* and *Mycoplasma hominis*	Wet mount clue cells	Metronidazole	Clindamycin cream
Trichomoniasis	*T Vaginalis*	Wet mount trichomonads	Metronidazole	Metronidazole after 1st trimester
Syphilis	*Treponema pallidum*	Dark-field examination VDRL, RPR, or MHA-TP	Benzathine Penicillin G	Benzathine Penicillin G
Herpes genitalis	Herpes simplex virus	Herpes culture or titre	Acyclovir	None
Chlamydia	*Chlamydia trachomatis*	Chlamydia culture	Doxycycline	Erythromycin base
Gonorrhea	*Neisseria gonorrhoeae*	Gonorrhea culture	Ceftriaxone and Doxycycline	Ceftriaxone and Erythromycin
Acquired immunodeficiency syndrome	Human immunodeficiency virus	ELISA test and Western blot	Varies	Varies
Genital warts	Human papilloma virus	Virapap, biopsy, Pap smear, colposcopy	Cryotherapy Podophyllum, podofilox	Cryotherapy Trichloracectic acid
Pediculosis pubis	*Phthirus*	Microscopic identification of lice or nits	Permethrin 1% cream rinse or Lindane 1% shampoo	Permethrin 1% cream rinse
Scabies	*Sarcoptes scabiei*	Confirmation of symptoms or scraping of furrows	Lindane 1% lotion or permethrin 5% cream	Crotamiton 10% lotion or permethrin 5% cream

Chlamydia is a major cause of nongonococcal urethritis (NGU) in men. In women it can cause infections similar to those that occur with gonorrhea. It can infect the fallopian tubes, cervix, urethra, and Bartholin's glands. Pelvic inflammatory disease, infertility, and ectopic pregnancy are also associated with chlamydia (CDC 1993).

The infant of a woman with untreated chlamydia is at risk of developing ophthalmia neonatorum, which, although responsive to erythromycin ophthalmic ointment, does not respond to silver nitrate eye prophylaxis.

The newborn may also develop chlamydial pneumonia. In fact approximately 30,000 cases of pneumonia in infants 6 months old or less are traceable to chlamydial infections. Pregnant women with asymptomatic cases of chlamydia have a 40% to 70% incidence of neonatal chlamydial infection. Chlamydia may also be responsible for premature labor and fetal death.

Symptoms of chlamydia include a thin or purulent discharge, burning and frequency of urination, and lower abdominal pain. Women, however, are often asymptomatic. Diagnosis is frequently made after treatment of a male partner for NGU or in a symptomatic woman with a negative gonorrhea culture. Moreover, 25% to 60% of heterosexual women with gonorrheal infections also have chlamydia (CDC 1993). Laboratory detection is now simpler due to the availability of a test to detect monoclonal antibodies specific for *Chlamydia*. However, as is the case with syphilis and gonorrhea, women are not routinely screened for chlamydia due to the added expense of the test. The CDC (1993) has identified priority groups for chlamydia screening, including high-risk pregnant women, adolescents, and women 20–24 years of age with multiple sexual partners, new sexual partners, and those who do not consistently use condoms.

The usual prescribed treatment for chlamydia is azithromycin or doxycycline. Doxycycline has a longer history of extensive use, safety, efficacy, and low cost; azithromycin has the advantage of single-dose administration. Any woman diagnosed with gonorrhea should also be treated with one of these medications because of the high risk of co-infection with chlamydia. The male

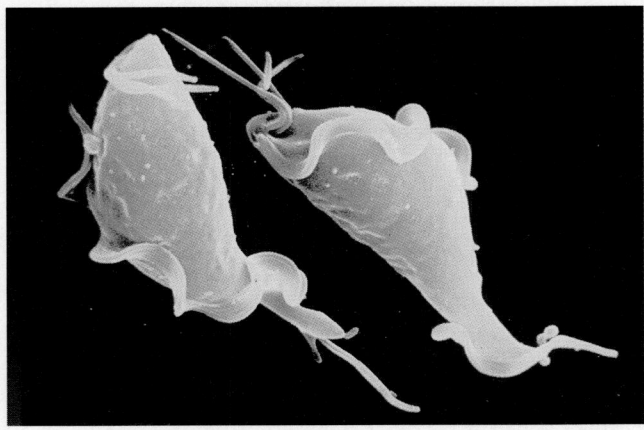

FIGURE 10-6   Microscopic appearance of *Trichomonas vaginalis.*

sexual partner should also be tested and treated. Pregnant women should be treated with erythromycin (CDC 1993). Many authorities recommend routine treatment of newborns with tetracycline or erythromycin eye ointment to avoid the possibility of ophthalmia neonatorum or conjunctivitis. Barrier contraceptives, especially spermicidally treated condoms, offer some protection against chlamydia.

Herpes Genitalis (Herpes Simplex Virus)

Estimates suggest that 30 million people in the United States have genital herpes and that 500,000 new cases occur each year (CDC 1993). The herpes simplex virus is the causative organism. There are two types of herpes:

- Type 1—usually noted to be present above the waist and not usually sexually transmitted. The "cold sore" is the most common herpes type 1 lesion. This type may occur in the genital area, usually as a result of oral-genital sexual contact.

- Type 2—usually associated with genital infections. This type can occur as oral lesions after oral-genital sexual contact if genital lesions are present.

The clinical symptoms and treatment of type 1 and type 2 herpes are the same when they occur in the genital area.

Primary Episode

Multiple blisterlike vesicles appear, usually in the genital area and sometimes affecting the vaginal walls, cervix, urethra, and anus. The vesicles may appear within a few hours to 20 days after exposure and rupture spontaneously to form extremely painful, open, ulcerated lesions. Inflammation and pain secondary to the presence of herpes lesions can cause difficult urination and urinary retention. Inguinal lymph node enlargement may be present. Flulike symptoms and genital pruritus or tingling also may be noticed. A severe primary episode does not necessarily indicate that a woman will be predisposed to frequent or severe recurrences. Primary episodes usually last the longest and are the most severe. Lesions heal spontaneously in 2 to 4 weeks.

Recurrent Episodes

After the lesions heal the virus enters a dormant phase, residing in the nerve ganglia of the affected area. Some individuals never have a recurrence, whereas others have regular recurrences. Recurrent lesions usually occur at the site of the primary episode. Recurrences are usually less severe than the initial episode and seem to be triggered by emotional stress, menstruation, ovulation, pregnancy, frequent or vigorous intercourse, poor health status or a generally rundown physical condition, tight

clothing, or overheating. Some genital herpes infections may be asymptomatic. It has been reported that 14% to 43% of women with cytologically detected herpes simplex virus may have asymptomatic viral shedding. It is assumed that asymptomatic viral shedding may transmit the herpes infection; this could explain the acquisition of the disease from individuals with no history of genital lesions. Diagnosis is made on the basis of the appearance of the lesions, Pap smear, or culture of the lesions, and blood testing for antibodies.

Medical Therapy

There is no known cure for herpes. Prescriptive treatment is available to provide relief from pain and prevent complications from secondary infection. For treatment of the first clinical episode of genital herpes oral acyclovir, 200 mg five times a day for 7 to 10 days or until clinical resolution, is recommended. For treatment of recurrent episodes oral acyclovir, 200–800 mg two to five times a day for 5 days, is recommended. Treatment for recurrent episodes should be instituted during the prodrome or within 2 days of the onset of the lesion. Frequent recurrences are defined as six or more per year. Daily suppressive therapy, oral acyclovir 400 mg twice daily, reduces the frequency of recurrences by at least 75% among women with frequent recurrences. Topical therapy with acyclovir is substantially less effective than the oral drug, and its use is discouraged. Acyclovir should not be used for pregnant women because its safety has not been established for that group (CDC 1993).

Self-help suggestions include cleansing with povidone-iodine (Betadine) solution to prevent secondary infection and Burow's solution to relieve discomfort. Use of vitamin C or lysine is frequently suggested to prevent recurrence, although studies have not documented the effectiveness of these supplements. Keeping the genital area clean and dry, wearing loose clothing, and wearing cotton underwear or none at all will promote healing. Primary and recurrent lesions will heal without prescriptive therapies.

Women should be advised to abstain from sexual activity during the prodrome and while lesions are present. Genital herpes and other diseases causing genital ulcers have been associated with an increased risk of acquiring HIV infection; therefore condoms should be used during all sexual contact (CDC 1993).

Syphilis

Syphilis is a chronic infection caused by a spirochete, *Treponema pallidum*. Syphilis can be acquired congenitally, through transplacental inoculation, and can result from maternal exposure to infected exudate during sexual contact or from contact with open wounds or infected blood. The incubation period varies from 10 to 90 days, and even though no symptoms or lesions are noted during this time, the woman's blood contains spirochetes and is infectious. The infection is divided into early (primary and secondary stages) and late (tertiary) syphilis. During primary syphilis a painless chancre appears at the site where the *Treponema pallidum* organism entered the body. Symptoms include slight fever, loss of weight, and malaise. The chancre persists for about 4 weeks and then disappears. In 6 weeks to 6 months secondary symptoms appear. Skin eruptions called condylomata lata, which resemble wartlike plaques, may appear on the vulva. Other secondary symptoms are acute arthritis, other skin lesions, adenopathy, enlargement of the liver and spleen, iritis, and a chronic sore throat with hoarseness. Signs of secondary syphilis tend to disappear in 3 to 12 weeks; then the disease may lie dormant for a short period or for as long as 15 years or more before signs of tertiary syphilis appear. Late syphilis may affect the heart, central nervous system, eyes, ears, bone, or any other body organ. It is often fatal. When infected in utero, the newborn will exhibit secondary stage symptoms of syphilis. Transplacentally transmitted syphilis, if not treated, can result in stillbirth, preterm birth, and neonatal death (CDC 1993).

The incidence of syphilis declined after the discovery of penicillin, but since 1958, the incidence has been increasing. As a result of the increased incidence and the disease's impact on the fetus in utero, serologic testing of every pregnant woman is recommended; testing is required by some state laws. Testing is done at the initial prenatal screening and repeated in the third trimester. With adequate early treatment congenital syphilis is preventable. The clinical manifestations and treatment of the syphilitic newborn are discussed in Chapter 32.

Medical Therapy

The goal of medical therapy is to identify women with syphilis and begin antibiotic treatment. Definitive diagnosis is made by dark-field examination and direct fluorescent antibody tests of lesion exudate or tissue for spirochetes. Blood tests such as VDRL (Venereal Disease Research Laboratories), RPR (Rapid Plasma Reagin), or the more specific FTA-ABS (fluorescent treponemal antibody absorption test) and microhemagglutination assay for antibodies to *T pallidum* (MHA-TP) are commonly done for presumptive diagnosis. Blood studies may be negative if blood is drawn too early.

For women with syphilis of less than a year's duration the CDC recommend 2.4 million units of benzathine penicillin G intramuscularly. If syphilis is of long (more than a year) duration, 2.4 million units of benzathine penicillin G is given intramuscularly once a week for 3 weeks. If a nonpregnant woman is allergic to penicillin, doxycycline, 100 mg by mouth twice daily for 2 weeks, can be given. Maternal serologic testing may remain positive for 8 months, and the newborn may have a positive test for 3 months.

In the pregnant woman treatment with penicillin should begin after the first positive test rather than waiting for further testing. Pregnant women who are allergic to penicillin should not be treated with doxycycline or tetracycline. Erythromycin has not been found to be effective in treating pregnant women. Therefore it is recommended that allergic women be skin-tested to validate their allergy to penicillin and be desensitized in order to be treated with penicillin. Parenteral penicillin G is the only therapy with documented efficacy for syphilis during pregnancy (CDC 1993). All sex partners need to be screened and tested.

Gonorrhea

Gonorrhea (often called "clap," "GC," "drip," or "dose") is an infection caused by the bacterium *Neisseria gonorrhoeae*. An estimated one million new infections with *N gonorrhoeae* occur in the United States each year (CDC 1993). If a nonpregnant woman contracts the disease, she is at risk of developing pelvic inflammatory disease, which can lead to tubal scarring, infertility, and ectopic pregnancy. If a woman becomes infected after the third month of pregnancy, the mucus plug in the cervix will prevent the infection from ascending, and it will remain localized in the urethra, cervix, and Bartholin's glands until the membranes rupture. Then the disease can spread upward.

Medical Therapy

The majority of women with gonorrhea are asymptomatic. Thus it is accepted practice to screen for this infection by doing a cervical culture during the initial prenatal examination and during well woman examinations in high-risk populations. Cultures of the urethra, throat, and rectum may also be required for diagnosis, depending on the body orifices used for intercourse.

The most common symptoms of gonorrheal infection include a purulent, greenish-yellow vaginal discharge; dysuria; and urinary frequency. Some women also develop inflammation and swelling of the vulva. The cervix may appear swollen and eroded and may secrete a foul-smelling discharge in which gonococci are present.

Treatment consists of antibiotic therapy with 125 mg ceftriaxone intramuscularly once plus 100 mg doxycycline by mouth twice a day for 7 days. If the woman is allergic to ceftriaxone, spectinomycin is given followed by the doxycycline. Additional treatment may be required if the cultures remain positive 7 to 14 days after completion of treatment. All sexual partners must also be treated, or the woman may become reinfected. Pregnant women should be treated with 125 mg ceftriaxone intramuscularly once plus 500 mg erythromycin by mouth twice a day for 7 days (CDC 1993).

Women should be informed of the need for reculture to verify cure and the need for abstinence or condom use until cure is confirmed. Both sexual partners should be

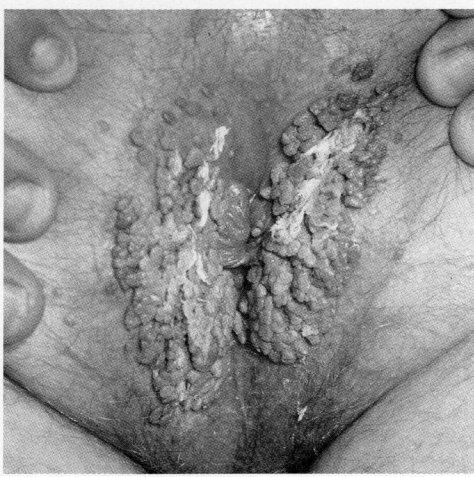

FIGURE 10-7 Condylomata acuminata on the vulva.

treated if either has a positive test for gonorrhea. It is important to explain why treatment is necessary even if the client has a negative culture or is asymptomatic. For example, false-negative reports are possible. Gonorrhea may be asymptomatic. Untreated infections are associated with the following risks:

- Pelvic inflammatory disease and secondary infertility are possible.

- Disseminated gonorrhea can involve joints or cause septicemia.

- Infection present at the time of birth causes ophthalmia neonatorum in the infant (Zenilman 1993).

Acquired Immunodeficiency Syndrome (AIDS)

Acquired immunodeficiency syndrome (AIDS) is a fatal disorder caused by the human immunodeficiency virus (HIV), which may be transmitted sexually. The care of a person with AIDS is primarily supportive, although some medications that seem to prolong life and reduce symptoms are being developed. The reader is referred to a medical-surgical nursing text for a complete description of this care.

However, because the diagnosis of AIDS or the presence of the AIDS antibody has profound implications for a fetus if the woman is pregnant, AIDS is discussed in greater detail in Chapter 18.

Condyloma Acuminata (Venereal Warts)

Venereal warts occur in all age groups and develop in more than 50% to 70% of sexual partners of infected individuals. They are relatively common, with an incidence of 50 per 100,000 population. The causative organism is human papilloma virus (HPV). These benign warts are most commonly caused by HPV types 6 or 11. A woman often seeks medical care after noting "bumps" in the genital area. Single or multiple soft, grayish-pink, cauliflowerlike lesions may be observed (Figure 10–7).

The moist warmth of the genital area is conducive to the growth of condyloma, which may be present on the vulva, vagina, cervix, and anus. The virus is transmitted through sexual contact. The incubation period following exposure is 3 weeks to 3 years.

Approximately 50 HPV types have been identified so far, and a number of these (types 16, 18, 31, 33, and 35) are associated with malignant transformation resulting in cancer of the anogenital tract. In women with abnormal Pap smears the prevalence of HPV is 80% to 96%. HPV proliferates during pregnancy due to immunosuppression, increased hormonal activity, and increased vascularity. HPV in pregnancy has been associated with laryngeal papilloma in the newborn.

Medical Therapy

Because condyloma sometimes resembles other lesions and malignant transformation is possible, all atypical, pigmented, and persistent warts should be treated promptly. Diagnosis is made by clinical examination, Pap smear, Virapap, colposcopy, or a biopsy. The treatment of choice for pregnant and nonpregnant women is cryotherapy with liquid nitrogen to destroy the lesions (CDC 1993). An alternative therapy is topically applied podophyllin or podofilox, which the woman is instructed to wash off 4 hours after application. Podofilox is used for self-treatment; the woman applies this to the warts twice daily for 3 days, followed by 4 days of no therapy. This cycle may be repeated as necessary for a total of four cycles. Podophyllin is applied to the warts by a health care provider and may be repeated once weekly for 6 weeks. These drugs are not used during pregnancy because they are thought to be teratogenic and in large doses have been associated with fetal death. If the woman is pregnant or if the lesions do not respond to podophyllin, trichloroacetic acid (TCA) may be used. Carbon dioxide laser therapy, performed under colposcopy, has a good success rate. This is probably because use of the colposcope aids in detecting tiny "satellite" lesions.

Generally, HPV is asymptomatic, although recently it has been associated with monilialike symptoms. Women with chronic yeast infections with a negative monilia culture should be screened for HPV with colposcopy. HPV is most commonly detected by Pap smear and the visualization of external lesions. The type of HPV virus may be identified using the recently developed Virapap test.

Medical literature has indicated a link between the occurrence of condyloma and abnormal cell changes of the cervix or possibly cervical cancer. Women with ab-

normal Pap smears, especially if condyloma is identified, should be screened for HPV with a colposcopic examination. During the colposcopy biopsies are taken to confirm the diagnosis. If the cellular atypia is due to HPV, treatment is initiated promptly with cryotherapy or laser therapy. Screening sex partners is not necessary because of the high incidence of subclinical lesions. Pregnant women are treated with cryotherapy, laser therapy, or TCA. A cesarean birth is not necessary because the perinatal rate of transmission is low (CDC 1993).

Pediculosis Pubis (Pubic or Crab Louse)

Pubic lice occur more commonly in adults than in children. Pediculosis pubis is cased by *Phthirus*, a grayish, parasitic "crab" louse that lays eggs that attach to the hair shaft. Transmission is primarily by sexual contact, although shared towels and bed linens are also possible sources.

Medical Therapy

Symptoms include intense pruritus in areas covered by pubic hair. Occasionally, lice are present in chest hair, armpits, eyelashes, and eyebrows. "Crabs" or brown-red spots may be noted in the underwear. Diagnosis is made by clinical and microscopic identification of adult lice or nits (eggs). Pediculosis is treated with 1% Permethrin creme rinse applied to the affected area for 10 minutes, plus combing of the pubic hair with a fine-tooth comb. Over-the-counter medications are safe but less effective. All contaminated linens or clothing should be laundered or dry cleaned. All sexual partners or members of the household should be treated. The woman should be warned of possible toxicity with overuse of the medication. Women should be cautioned not to use medication in or around their eyes. Pediculosis of the eyelashes should be treated by the application of occlusive ophthalmic ointment to the eyelid margins, two times a day for 10 days, to smother lice (CDC 1993).

Clients should be reevaluated in 1 week if symptoms persist. Retreatment may be necessary if lice are found or eggs are observed at the hair-stem junction. Alternative treatment is with pyrethrins and piperonyl butoxide applied to the affected area and washed off after 10 minutes or lindane 1% (Kwell) shampoo applied for 4 minutes and thoroughly washed off. Lindane is not recommended in pregnant or lactating women (CDC 1993).

Scabies

Sarcoptes scabiei is an ectoparasitic itch mite. The female mite burrows under the skin to deposit her eggs. Transmission is by intimate sexual contact and contact with household members.

Medical Therapy

Symptoms include pruritus that worsens at night or when the individual is warm. Noticeable erythematous, papular lesions, or furrows may be present. Diagnosis is made by confirmation of the symptoms or scraping of the furrows to obtain mites. Prescriptive therapy is 1% lindane (Kwell) lotion applied from the neck down after taking a bath and thoroughly washed off after 8 hours. This treatment is not recommended in pregnant or lactating women. In the pregnant woman, permethrin 5% cream should be applied from the neck down and washed off after 8 to 14 hours. Clothing and bed linen should be washed and dried in a hot dryer or dry cleaned (CDC 1993).

The woman should be advised that sexual partners and other household members should also be treated. Persistent pruritus often occurs after treatment; the woman should be aware that pruritus does not signify that the treatment is ineffective. She should be cautioned that overuse of lotion can cause toxicity.

APPLYING THE NURSING PROCESS

Nursing Assessment

The nurse working with women must become adept at taking a thorough history and identifying women at risk for sexually transmitted infections. Factors that place a woman at risk for STDs are multiple sexual partners, partners with high-risk behaviors, a partner's involvement with other sexual partners, use of feminine hygiene products, high-risk sexual activities such as intercourse without barrier contraception or anal intercourse, treatment with antibiotics while taking oral contraceptives, and young age at onset of sexual activity. The nurse should be alert for signs and symptoms of sexually transmitted infections and familiar with diagnostic procedures if infection is suspected.

Although each STD has certain distinctive characteristics, the following complaints suggest the possibility of infection and warrant further investigation.

- Presence of a "sore" or lesion on the vulva
- Increased vaginal discharge or malodorous vaginal discharge
- Burning with urination
- Dyspareunia
- Bleeding after intercourse
- Pelvic pain

In many instances the woman is asymptomatic but may report symptoms in her partner, especially painful urination or urethral discharge. It is often helpful to ask the woman whether her partner is experiencing any symptoms.

Nursing Diagnosis

Nursing diagnoses that may apply when a woman has a sexually transmitted infection include the following:

- Altered family processes related to the effects of a diagnosis of STD on the couple's relationship
- Knowledge deficit related to lack of information about the long-term effects of the diagnosis on childbearing status
- Self-esteem disturbance related to difficulty in accepting the knowledge that the condition is sexually transmitted

Nursing Plan and Implementation

Teaching for Self-Care

Nurses can play a vital role in preventing sexually transmitted infections. They can educate women as to how to protect themselves with safer sexual practices and with various contraceptive methods that guard against sexually transmitted infections as well as pregnancy. Spermicides have been reported to kill a wide range of bacteria and viruses, including HIV, gonorrhea, and chlamydia. Condoms and diaphragms give some protection from bacterial and viral infections of the genital tract. Hormonal contraception and tubal ligation safeguard the upper genital tract but not the cervix. Women who use IUDs are at increased risk for pelvic inflammatory disease (Kirkman & Chantler 1993).

In a supportive and nonjudgmental way the nurse provides the woman who has a sexually transmitted infection with information about the disease, methods of transmission, implications for pregnancy or future fertility, and importance of thorough treatment. If treatment of her partner is indicated, the woman must understand that it is important to prevent a continuous cycle of reinfection. She should also understand the need to abstain from sexual activity, if necessary, during treatment.

The woman should be instructed about the correct procedure for taking her medication and should clearly understand the importance of any follow-up assessments. Prevention of STDs should be stressed with all women. Women in a monogamous relationship with a low-risk partner are at least risk for STD. Multiple sexual partners, history of STD, and IV drug use are associated with higher risk, as are high-risk activities such as anal intercourse and exchange of body fluids. Women should be encouraged to require partners, especially new partners, to use a condom.

If a woman suspects she has an infection, she should abstain from intercourse and seek testing. Disappearance

CRITICAL THINKING IN PRACTICE

CW is a 21-year-old, single woman, G0P0, who comes to the office today complaining of excessive, odorous vaginal discharge. She uses an IUD for contraception and has several sex partners. She states that she douches with a medicated douche after intercourse. What should you tell CW about feminine hygiene? What would you tell CW about the relationship between contraceptives and sexually transmitted infections?

Answers can be found in Appendix I.

of symptoms does not mean the infection is cured. If medication is prescribed, it is important to complete the full prescription. Treatment of sexual partners is an important part of therapy to prevent recurrence or spread. Informing her sex partner may be very difficult for her, and she could be faced with accusations of infidelity on her or her partner's part. The nurse must make a special effort to provide the woman with correct information and support during this time. It is often helpful for the couple to discuss an STD together with the health care provider.

Provision of Psychologic Support

Some sexually transmitted infections such as trichomoniasis or chlamydia may cause a woman concern but once diagnosed are rather simply treated. Other STDs may also be fairly simple to treat medically but may carry a stigma and be emotionally devastating for the woman. Diseases such as pediculosis pubis may cause a woman to feel "unclean"; syphilis, because it is reportable, may leave the woman feeling exposed and vulnerable. Herpes can be especially difficult to deal with emotionally because it causes discomfort and is not presently curable.

The sensitive nurse can be especially helpful in encouraging the woman to explore her feelings about the diagnosis. She may experience anger or feel "betrayed" by a partner; she may feel guilt or see her diagnosis as a form of "punishment"; or she may feel concern about the long-term implications for future childbearing or ongoing intimate relationships. She may experience a myriad of differing emotions that she never expected. Opportunities to discuss her feelings in a nonjudgmental environment can be especially helpful. The nurse can offer suggestions about support groups if indicated and assist the woman in planning for her future with regard to sexual activity.

More subtly, the nurse's attitude of acceptance and matter-of-factness conveys to the woman that she is still an acceptable person who happens to have an infection.

Evaluation

Anticipated outcomes of nursing care include:

- The infection is identified and cured if possible. If not, supportive therapy is provided.
- The woman and her partner understand the infection, its method of transmission, its implications, and the therapy.
- The woman copes successfully with the impact of the diagnosis on her self-concept.

CARE OF THE WOMAN WITH PELVIC INFLAMMATORY DISEASE

Pelvic inflammatory disease (PID) occurs in approximately 1% of women between 15 and 39, although sexually active young women between 15 and 24 have the highest infection rate. Fifteen percent to 40% of all infertility is attributed to PID. The disease is more common in women who have had multiple sexual partners, a history of PID, early onset of sexual activity, a recent gynecologic procedure, or an intrauterine device. It usually produces a tubal infection (salpingitis) that may or may not be accompanied by a pelvic abscess. It also may produce endometritis or pelvic peritonitis. However, perhaps the greatest problem of PID is that postinfection tubal damage is associated with a high incidence of infertility and ectopic pregnancy (Hillis et al 1993).

The organisms most frequently identified with PID include *Chlamydia trachomatis* and *Neisseria gonorrhoeae*, although other aerobic and anaerobic organisms that are often part of the normal vaginal flora have also been found in women with PID (CDC 1993).

Medical Therapy

Symptoms of PID include bilateral sharp, cramping pain in the lower quadrants, fever, chills, purulent vaginal discharge, irregular bleeding, malaise, dysuria, nausea, dyspareunia, and vomiting. However, it is possible to be asymptomatic and have normal laboratory findings.

Women with chlamydia-associated PID are young (75% are younger than 25 years of age), asymptomatic, experience only low-grade pelvic pain, rarely have an elevated temperature, and frequently have irregular bleeding. Women with gonorrhea-associated PID have a more pronounced clinical picture (fever, initial pain at menstrual bleeding, and palpable adnexal swelling) (Jossens & Sweet 1993). Cervical motion tenderness (Chandelier

sign) and adnexal swelling are also common with PID, but these signs also occur in appendicitis and ectopic pregnancy, which must be ruled out (CDC 1993).

Diagnosis consists of a clinical examination to define symptoms plus blood tests and a gonorrhea culture and test for chlamydia. Other diagnostic procedures that may help confirm the diagnosis include the following:

- Elevated erythrocyte sedimentation rate
- Wet prep of vaginal secretions that reveals the presence of numerous inflammatory white blood cells, and coccoid bacteria
- Elevated C-reactive protein
- Ultrasound to detect the presence of a pelvic abscess
- Laparoscopy to confirm the diagnosis and enable the examiner to obtain cultures from the fimbriated ends of the fallopian tubes
- Endometrial biopsy that reveals histopathologic evidence of endometritis (Romanowski 1993).

Diagnosing PID is difficult because many women are asymptomatic or have only mild or nonspecific signs and symptoms. The following signs and symptoms are consistent with the diagnosis of PID: lower abdominal tenderness, adnexal tenderness, cervical motion tenderness, and an oral temperature higher than 38.3 C. The CDC recommends that providers maintain a low threshold for the diagnosis of PID and immediately initiate empiric antimicrobial therapy. These recommendations are based on the fact that diagnosis and management of other common causes of lower abdominal pain (such as ectopic pregnancy, acute appendicitis, and functional pain) are unlikely to be impaired by initiating antimicrobial therapy for PID.

PID therapy regimes must provide broad-spectrum antibiotic coverage of likely pathogens. Inpatient treatment is recommended when the following criteria are met:

- The diagnosis is uncertain, and surgical emergencies such as appendicitis and ectopic pregnancy cannot be excluded
- Pelvic abscess is suspected
- The woman is pregnant
- The woman is an adolescent (cooperation is unpredictable)
- The woman has HIV infection
- Severe illness or nausea and vomiting preclude outpatient management
- The woman is unable to follow or tolerate an outpatient regimen
- The woman has failed to respond clinically to outpatient therapy
- Clinical follow-up within 72 hours of starting antibiotic treatment cannot be arranged

Intravenous administration of cefoxitan sodium, cefotetan disodium, or clindamycin plus gentamicin provides effective inpatient therapy. Outpatient therapy usually includes antibiotics such as cefoxitin, ceftriaxone, doxycycline, ofloxacin, and clindamycin used singly or in combination.

Women being treated with inpatient regimes should show substantial clinical improvement within 3 to 5 days of therapy. Women being treated with outpatient regimes must be examined within 72 hours of the initiation of therapy. Because of the risk of persistent infection, clients should have a microbiologic reexamination 7 to 10 days after completing therapy and have a test of cure 4 to 6 weeks after completing therapy (CDC 1993).

The sexual partner should also be treated. If the woman has an IUD, it is generally removed 24 to 48 hours after antibiotic therapy is started. After the infection is treated, microsurgical techniques are sometimes used to release any adhesions and repair tubal damage if the woman desires to bear children (Ault & Faro 1993).

APPLYING THE NURSING PROCESS

Nursing Assessment

The nurse is alert to factors in a woman's history that put her at risk for PID. Even though fewer types of IUDs are available now, many women still have them, and the nurse should question the woman about possible symptoms, such as aching pain in the lower abdomen, foul-smelling discharge, malaise, and the like. The woman who is acutely ill will have obvious symptoms, but a low-grade infection is more difficult to detect.

Nursing Diagnosis

Nursing diagnoses that may apply to a woman with PID include the following:

- Pain related to peritoneal irritation
- Knowledge deficit related to a lack of information about possible effects of PID on fertility

Nursing Plan and Implementation

The nurse plays a vital role in helping to prevent or detect PID and should discuss related risk factors with clients. The woman who uses an IUD for contraception and has multiple sexual partners should clearly understand the risk she faces. The nurse should discuss signs and symptoms of PID and stress the importance of early detection should the woman develop symptoms.

The woman who develops PID should understand the importance of completing her antibiotic treatment and of returning for follow-up evaluation. She should also understand the possibility of decreased fertility following the infection. If appropriate, the nurse can answer the woman's questions about microsurgical techniques (Jossens & Sweet 1993).

The care of the woman who is acutely ill with pelvic abscess following childbirth is discussed in Chapter 36.

Evaluation

Anticipated outcomes of nursing care include:

- The woman clearly understands her condition, her therapy, and the possible long-term implications of PID on her fertility.
- The woman completes her course of therapy, and the PID is cured.

CARE OF THE WOMAN WITH VULVITIS

Genital pruritus and soreness may be secondary to a non-pathogenic process. Common causes are:

- Frequent douching or use of over-the-counter douches
- Feminine deodorant spray
- Detergents or harsh soaps
- Colored or perfumed toilet paper
- Contraceptive creams, foams, or suppositories
- Dye (as in new clothing)
- Synthetic clothing that traps moisture, such as nylon underwear, polyester slacks
- Intercourse without proper lubrication
- Deodorant menstrual pads or tampons
- Estrogen deprivation after menopause

Teaching for Self-Care

Although women are often told that the practices listed above contribute to vaginitis, this is not necessarily so. In many cases the woman may be experiencing vulvitis without vaginitis.

The nurse can inform women of the possible factors contributing to local irritation and encourage them to avoid practices that contribute to symptoms. Suggestions for good genital hygiene are advisable. The nurse should encourage medical evaluation if symptoms persist. Specifically, a medical evaluation is warranted in post-menopausal women with symptoms because they are at increased risk for vulvar cancer. The nurse should discourage women from treating themselves with over-the-counter anti-inflammatory creams and douches (Secor & Fertitta 1992).

CARE OF THE WOMAN WITH CERVICITIS

Cervicitis is an inflammation of the cervix. It may be caused by an infective process such as gonorrhea, herpes, *Trichomonas*, *Candida*, or *Gardnerella*. Chemical or hygienic products used in the vagina or the presence of foreign bodies may cause cervicitis.

Medical Therapy

Symptoms of cervicitis include yellow discharge with odor, dyspareunia, postcoital bleeding, and irregular bleeding. A woman may be asymptomatic. Diagnosis consists of a clinical examination and appropriate wet mount smear, cultures, or Pap smear. Appropriate treatment is antibiotic therapy, cryotherapy, or removal of any foreign object (IUD, contraceptive sponge, or tampon).

Teaching for Self-Care

The woman should be advised to avoid possible vaginal irritants such as douches or tampons. Medical care should be sought if the woman is symptomatic. If an abnormal reading occurs on a Pap smear report, the nurse should clarify the report for the woman. If the inflammatory finding or Pap smear indicates HPV or condylomata, a colposcopy is performed for further evaluation. It may be reassuring to inform women that an infectious process and cervical irritants can result in an abnormal Pap smear reading. The Pap smear should be repeated after these problems are eliminated.

CARE OF THE WOMAN WITH AN ABNORMAL FINDING DURING PELVIC EXAMINATION

The Pap Smear

A Papanicolaou (Pap) smear is used to screen for cervical cancer, but it can also provide information on hormonal status and identify sexually transmitted organisms such as HPV. The Pap test is the cytologic examination of cells taken from the endocervix, the area of greatest cellular change and thus the area at greatest risk for cellular ab-

---

RESEARCH IN PRACTICE

Women experience perimenstrual symptoms varying from scarcely perceptible to exceedingly distressful. Ellen Mitchell, Nancy Woods, and Martha Lentz differentiated among three symptom patterns of perimenstrual severity: premenstrual magnification (PMM), premenstrual syndrome (PMS), and low symptoms (LS). From literature on the subject, the authors proposed that social demands, personal resources, socialization, parity, age, personal health practices, and psychologic distress could be used to distinguish among the three groups.

In order to obtain an appropriate sample of healthy women, the authors chose an epidemiological approach in which they first selected census block groups based on age, income, and ethnicity. Telephone contact with 5755 households identified 1135 women between the ages of 18 and 45. Of these, 656 women met the study criteria. Of the 343 women who had a home interview and returned the 3-month long, daily diary, 142 fell into one of the three symptom patterns considered in this study.

The authors used a variety of preexisting tools to determine the subjects' social demands based on stressful life events in the past year, their menstrual socialization and mothers' premenstrual symptoms, feminine socialization, self-reported parity, personal health habits such as cigarette smoking and caffeine ingestion, and psychologic distress in the form of depression. Psychometric properties of each tool were reported.

Discriminant analysis showed that, compared to the LS group, women with PMS tended to have more education, more psychologic distress, and a mother who had more premenstrual symptoms. Women with PMM had more life stress events and were younger than the LS group. Women with PMS differed from the PMM group by being older, having more education, engaging in healthier lifestyles, and having more non-traditional views about women.

Clinical Application of Study

This study increases awareness that symptoms of PMS can be classified according to severity and that these classifications are associated with a wide variety of factors. According to this study, if a woman suffers from PMS or PMM she may be experiencing psychologic distress, a problem that may be amenable to treatment. Also, the authors suggest that if menstrual socialization plays a part in PMS, then non-judgmental presentation of information at menarche might affect future perimenstrual symptoms.

SOURCE: Mitchell E, Woods N, Lentz M: Differentiation of women with three perimenstrual symptom patterns. *Nurs Res* 1994; 43(1):25.

---

normalities, as well as the exocervix and the vaginal walls. The squamocolumnar junction (also known as the transition [T] zone), is located in the endocervix in adult women. It is the area where, through a process of squamous metaplasia, the squamous epithelium grows over the columnar epithelium of the cervix.

TABLE 10–4 The 1991 Bethesda System (TBS) for Classifying Pap Smears

Adequacy of the Specimen

Satisfactory for evaluation
Satisfactory for evaluation but limited by. . .(specify reason)
Unsatisfactory for evaluation

General Categorization (optional)

Within normal limits
Benign cellular changes (See descriptive diagnoses.)
Epithelial cell abnormality (See descriptive diagnoses.)

Descriptive Diagnoses

Benign cellular changes
  Infection
    Trichomonas vaginalis
    Fungal organisms morphologically consistent with *Candide* spp
    Predominance of coccobacilli consistent with shift in vaginal flora
    Bacteria morphologically consistent with *Actinomyces* spp
    Cellular changes associated with herpes simplex virus
    Other
  Reactive changes
    Reactive cellular changes associated with:
      Inflammation (includes typical repair)
      Atrophy with inflammation ("atrophic vaginitis")
      Radiation
      Intrauterine contraceptive device (IUD)
      Other

Reactive changes *(continued)*
  Epithelial cell abnormalities
    Squamous cell
    Atypical squamous cells of undetermined significance (ASCUS): Qualify*
    Low-grade squamous intraepithelial lesion (SIL) encompassing HPV[†] mild dysplasia/CIN 1
    High-grade squamous intraepithelial lesion encompassing: Moderate and severe dysplasia, CIS/CIN 2 and CIN 3
    Squamous cell carcinoma
  Glandular cell
    Endometrial cells, cytologically benign, in a postmenopausal woman
    Atypical glandular cells of undetermined significance: Qualify*
    Endocervical adenocarcinoma
    Endometrial adenocarcinoma
    Extrauterine adenocarcinoma
    Adenocarcinoma, not otherwise specified
  Other malignant neoplasms: Specify
    Hormonal evaluation (applies to vaginal smears only)
    Hormonal pattern compatible with age and history
    Hormonal pattern incompatible with age and history: Specify
    Hormonal evaluation not possible due to: Specify

*Atypical squamous or glandular cells of undetermined significance should be further qualified as to whether a reactive or a premalignant/malignant process is favored.

†Cellular changes of human papillomavirus (HPV)—previously termed koilocytosis, koilocytotic atypia, or condylomatous atypia—are included in the category of low-grade squamous intraepithelial lesion.

Women should be advised to avoid douching, intercourse, feminine hygiene products, and spermicidal agents immediately prior to a Pap smear. Pap smears should not be obtained during menstruation or when visible cervicitis exists. Women should also be instructed to tell their health care provider if they are taking any hormones.

To obtain a Pap smear, a water-lubricated speculum is inserted into the vagina to permit visualization of the cervix. Cells of the exocervix are obtained using a wooden or plastic spatula. The endocervix is sampled using a cotton swab or cytobrush. The cytobrush has been shown to produce the most accurate results. A sample of cells from the vaginal walls is also obtained. The cells are placed on a labeled glass slide (or slides), sprayed with fixative, and sent to a cytology lab for microscopic examination.

Various laboratories use different Pap smear classification systems. All systems range from a normal result to invasive cancer. The 1991 Bethesda system is recognized by the CDC as the most appropriate system to use in reporting findings (CDC 1993) (Table 10–4).

Recommendations for Pap smear screening vary widely and are based upon the woman's risk for developing cervical cancer. Factors that place a woman at high risk for cervical cancer include the following:

- Coitus at an early age
- History of multiple sex partners
- Sex partner with a history of multiple sex partners
- Exposure to sexually transmitted infections
- History of immunosuppressive therapy
- Antenatal exposure to diethylstilbestrol (DES)
- History of dysplasia

Abnormal Pap Smear Results

Cervical cancer is the seventh most common cancer in women in the United States today, but it was number one 50 years ago. This decline occurred in large part because of the effectiveness of screening for early cervical cancer. Worldwide, however, it remains the most common cancer affecting women, with approximately 500,000 new cases each year (DiSaia 1994a). Cervical cancer is considered a preventable disease because it is slow growing, has a lengthy preinvasive state, has inexpensive and available screening programs, and has effective treatment approaches for preinvasive lesions (Yoder & Rubin 1992).

Because cervical neoplasia (and its precursor cervical dysplasia) is almost never encountered in virgins, it is considered a form of sexually transmitted infection. The role of HPV in the development of cervical dysplasia is not totally understood, but evidence suggests that HPV DNA is present in 80–90% of dysplasias (DiSaia 1994a). Increased sexual activity among teenagers has resulted in increased rates of HPV infection and abnormal Pap smears in that age group. Thus annual Pap smears and the use of barrier contraceptives should be stressed in all sexually active women (Yoder & Rubin 1992).

Women tend to expect a normal report when a Pap smear is done, but various abnormal findings are common. Early detection of abnormalities allows infections or early changes to be treated before cells reach a precancerous or cancerous stage.

Medical Therapy

A Pap smear report based on the Bethesda system provides three types of information: adequacy of the sample, general categorization, and descriptive diagnosis. General categorization is listed as within normal limits, benign cellular changes, or epithelial cell abnormality. The benign cellular changes are related to an inflammatory or infectious process that is not related to malignant transformation (Herbst et al 1993). The recommended followup for this classification is to treat the underlying cause and repeat the Pap smear within 3 months (CDC 1993).

Epithelial cell abnormalities are classified as atypical squamous cells of undetermined significance (ASCUS), low-grade squamous intraepithelial lesion (SIL), or highgrace SIL. A woman with ASCUS or low-grade SIL should either have a repeat Pap smear to confirm the results or be referred for colposcopy and biopsy. A woman with high-grade SIL should *always* be referred for colposcopy and directed biopsies (CDC 1993).

Colposcopy has evolved as an appropriate "second step" in many cases when a Pap smear is abnormal. The examination, typically done in an office or clinic, permits more detailed visualization of the cervix in bright light using a microscope with 6 to 40 times magnification. The cervix can be visualized directly and again following application of 3% acetic acid, which causes abnormal epithelium to assume a characteristic white appearance. The colposcope allows a lesion to be localized to obtain a "directed biopsy."

If a pregnant woman has an abnormal Pap smear, a colposcopy and biopsies are done to evaluate the disease further. If the biopsy shows anything less than invasive cancer, treatment is postponed until after birth. However, continued evaluation during pregnancy is recommended with Pap smears and colposcopic exams every 3 to 6 months.

Specific nursing care includes the following (Barsevick & Lauver 1990):

- Providing concrete, objective information about the examination and self-care instruction

- Anticipating the need for information about the cause and meaning of abnormalities

- Answering general questions about treatment options and procedures

- Assisting and encouraging slow breathing or other relaxation techniques during the procedure

Surgical Interventions for Abnormal Cytology

Although malignant lesions may be treated with radical surgical techniques as well as chemotherapy and radiation, surgical interventions are also important for the diagnosis and treatment of premalignant lesions. The goal of a biopsy is to obtain a tissue sample of the lesion in order to base a diagnosis on a pathology evaluation. A diagnosis of cancer can be made only after a pathology evaluation of tissue. The goal of the four other surgical interventions is to destroy and/or remove the abnormal tissue.

The treatment of cervical cancer depends on the stage of the disease, which is determined by the extent of its spread. Table 10–5 describes the staging of cervical cancer. The surgical treatment of cervical cancer may include a total abdominal hysterectomy (TAH) and bilateral lymphadenectomy. It will also include radiation therapy and possibly chemotherapy.

Biopsy A cervical biopsy is performed to investigate suspicious cervical tissue to diagnose or rule out cancer of the cervix at its earliest stages. Occasionally, the biopsy can be therapeutic as well as diagnostic if the entire lesion is removed. An endometrial biopsy is used to diagnose several functional menstruation disorders, infertility

TABLE 10-5	Staging of Cervical Cancer
Stage 0:	Carcinoma in situ, intraepithelial carcinoma
Stage I:	Carcinoma is strictly confined to the cervix. Extension to the corpus should be disregarded.
Stage II:	Carcinoma extends beyond the cervix but has not extended to the pelvic wall. The vagina is involved, but not as far as the lower third.
Stage III:	Carcinoma extends to the pelvic wall. On rectal examination, there is no cancer-free space between the tumor and the pelvic wall. The tumor involves the lower third of the vagina. All cases with hydronephrosis or nonfunctioning kidney are included.
IIIa:	No extension to the pelvic wall.
IIIb:	Extension to the pelvic wall and/or hydronephrosis or nonfunctioning kidney
Stage IV:	Carcinoma extends beyond the true pelvis or clinically involves the mucosa of the bladder or rectum. Bullous edema alone does not permit a case to be allotted to stage IV.
IVa:	Spread of the growth to adjacent organs
IVb:	Spread to distant organs

SOURCE: DiSaia P: Disorders of the uterine cervix. In: *Danforth's Obstetrics and Gynecology*, 7th ed. Scott JR et al (editors). Philadelphia: Lippincott, 1994, pp 910–911.

problems related to ovulation, and benign or malignant lesions.

The woman may experience moderate to severe cramplike pains during the procedure and afterward. A small amount of bleeding also may occur after the biopsy and may continue for up to 2 weeks. Bleeding as heavy as a menstrual period should be reported to the physician or clinic.

An endocervical curettage is performed prior to biopsies to confirm the presence or absence of disease in the endocervix. The endocervical canal is scraped from the internal to external os. The woman needs to be prepared for some cramping and pain during the procedure.

Laser Therapy The laser is used to treat cervical, vaginal, and vulvar intraepithelial neoplasia. It is reported to be safer, less mutilating, and less costly than conization and hysterectomy. The laser is used when all boundaries of the lesion are visible on colposcopy and the endocervical curettage is negative. The invisible, highly concentrated beam is absorbed by water in the tissues, and the energy is converted to heat, causing evaporation of the cellular water and cellular death. Normal tissue remains intact (Gilbride 1992; Rubin & Curtin 1992).

The laser can be used in outpatient settings. No anesthesia is needed for cervical lesions, and bleeding is minimal. The woman may experience minor cramping and a slight discharge for 5–7 days. She should avoid the use of tampons, douching, and sexual intercourse for 2 weeks. Healing may take 6–12 weeks. Laser therapy is specific to the lesion and should not affect fertility.

Conization A conization is generally performed when the entire lesion cannot be visualized by colposcopic examination. In this procedure a cone of tissue, the size and length of which are determined by the extent of the lesion, is surgically removed. A large amount of normal tissue is removed along with the abnormal tissue. Conization can be performed as an inpatient or outpatient procedure and under local or general anesthesia. There is a risk of postoperative infection and hemorrhage, and premature labor and abortion may be experienced in future pregnancies. A prolonged or profuse menstrual period can occur with the next two or three cycles.

Loop Electrosurgical Excision Procedure (LEEP)
LEEP can be used to treat cervical, vaginal, and vulvar intraepithelial neoplasia. After an abnormal Pap smear and a colposcopic evaluation that indicates a premalignant lesion, a small wire loop is used to excise the entire lesion, squamocolumnar junction, and transformation zone. This can all be performed in an outpatient setting under local anesthesia and is virtually bloodless and painless. With the advent of LEEP many physicians have stopped performing cryosurgery and laser surgery for almost all intraepithelial neoplasia of the female genital tract.

LEEP can also be used to treat external lesions such as genital warts (Baggish et al 1992).

Cryosurgery Cervical dysplasia, endocervicitis, and nabothian cysts may be treated by cryosurgery. The procedure uses freezing to cause tissue necrosis. A double freeze method is advocated, with nitrous oxide or carbon dioxide as the refrigerant. The freezing also can destroy normal tissue.

The procedure is usually performed a week after the menstrual period. Cryosurgery can be performed in the physician's office or clinic without anesthesia. It is not a painful procedure, although the woman may experience some cramping.

The woman should be told to expect a heavy, persistent, watery discharge for several weeks. She should not use tampons and should avoid sexual intercourse while the discharge is present because the cervix can be easily damaged.

Ovarian Masses

Between 70% and 80% of ovarian masses are benign. More than 50% are functional cysts occurring most commonly in women 20 to 40 years of age. Functional cysts are rare in women who take oral contraceptives.

Ovarian cysts usually represent physiologic variations in the menstrual cycle. Dermoid cysts (cystic teratomas) comprise 10% of all benign ovarian masses. Cartilage, bone, teeth, skin, or hair can be observed in these cysts. Endometriomas, or "chocolate cysts," are another common type of ovarian mass (Perricone et al 1992).

No relationship exists between ovarian cysts and ovarian cancer. However, ovarian cancer is the most fatal of all cancers in women because it is very difficult to diagnose and often has spread throughout the pelvis before it is detected. Ovarian cancer occurs most commonly in perimenopausal and menopausal women, with an average client age of 50 to 59 years, although the incidence does increase with age. It is more common in industrialized countries, in women with a personal history of breast cancer or a family history of ovarian cancer in a first-degree relative, and in women who are nulliparous or had their first pregnancy at an older age. Asbestos and talc exposure have been suggested as causative agents, but that link has not been confirmed (DiSaia 1994b).

Currently no adequate screening techniques for ovarian cancer exist. Elevated levels of CA 125, a circulating tumor marker, are found in ovarian cancer, but similar elevations are found in a variety of benign diseases, so the test is not especially useful as a screening technique. Unfortunately, pelvic examination detects only tumors that are large enough to palpate. The symptoms of ovarian cancer are vague and nonspecific. They include abdominal swelling and heaviness, pelvic pressure, mild constipation, and increased abdominal girth.

Medical Therapy

A woman with an ovarian mass may be asymptomatic; the mass may be noted on a routine pelvic examination. She may experience a sensation of fullness or cramping in the lower abdomen (often unilateral), dyspareunia, irregular bleeding, or delayed menstruation.

Diagnosis is made on the basis of a palpable mass with or without tenderness and other related symptoms. Radiography or ultrasonography may be used to assist or confirm the diagnosis. Transvaginal ultrasonography has been found to provide a sharper image of the ovaries than abdominal ultrasonography. The diagnosis may be confirmed using laparoscopy or laparotomy (Kramer et al 1993).

The woman is frequently kept under observation for 1 or 2 months because most cysts will resolve on their own and are harmless. Alternatively, oral contraceptives may be prescribed for 1 or 2 months to suppress ovarian function. If this regimen has been effective, a repeat pelvic examination should be normal. If the mass is still present after 60 days of observation and oral contraceptive therapy, a diagnostic laparoscopy or laparotomy may be considered. Tubal or ovarian lesions, ectopic pregnancy, cancer, infection, or appendicitis also must be ruled out before a diagnosis can be confirmed.

Surgery is not always necessary but will be considered if the mass is larger than 6 to 7 cm in circumference; if the woman is over 40 years of age with an adnexal mass, a persistent mass, or continuous pain; and if the woman is taking oral contraceptives. Surgical exploration is also indicated when a palpable mass is found in an infant or young girl or in a postmenopausal woman.

Women who are taking oral contraceptives should be informed of their preventive effect against ovarian masses. Women may need clear explanations about why the initial therapy is observation. A discussion of the origin and resolution of ovarian cysts may clarify this treatment plan. If surgery should involve removal or impaired function of one ovary, the woman should be assured that the remaining ovary should take over ovarian functioning and that pregnancy is still possible.

All stages of diagnosed ovarian cancer are treated with a TAH and bilateral salpingo-oophorectomy (BSO). Radiation and chemotherapy are often used following surgery.

Uterine Masses

Uterine masses may be benign or malignant. Fibroid tumors, also called leiomyomas, are among the most common benign disease entities in women and are the most common reason for gynecologic surgery. Between 20% and 50% of women develop leiomyomas by 40 years of age. The potential for cancer is minimal. Leiomyomas are more common in women of African descent.

Endometrial cancer is most commonly a disease of postmenopausal women. It has a high rate of cure if detected early. The key to early detection lies in educating women to recognize symptoms and seek care. The hallmark sign is vaginal bleeding in postmenopausal women not treated with hormone replacement therapy. Risk factors associated with endometrial cancer include early menarche (before age 12); late menopause (after age 50); low parity; obesity; unopposed estrogen replacement therapy; family history of endometrial, breast, or colon cancer; and personal history of diabetes, hypertension, endometrial hyperplasia, or liver disease.

Medical Therapy

Fibroid tumors develop when smooth muscle cells are present in whorls and arise from uterine muscles and connective tissue. The size varies from 1 to 2 cm to the size of a 10-week fetus. Frequently, the woman is asymptomatic. Lower abdominal pain, fullness or pressure, menorrhagia, metrorrhagia, or increased dysmenorrhea may occur, particularly with large leiomyomas. Ultrasonography, especially transvaginal ultrasonography, can reveal masses or nodules and assist in and confirm the diagnosis. Leiomyoma is also considered as a possible diagnosis when masses or nodules involving the uterus are palpated on a pelvic examination.

The majority of these masses require no treatment and will shrink after menopause. Close observation for symptoms or an increase in size of the uterus or the masses may be the only management most women will require. Routine repeat pelvic examinations every 3 to 6 months are commonly recommended unless there are other symptoms. Of particular concern is a mass that does not shrink postmenopausally or that develops postmenopausally and is associated with postmenopausal bleeding. These symptoms are associated with endometrial cancer. This concern does not apply to postmenopausal women on hormone replacement therapy.

If a woman notices symptoms or if pelvic examination reveals that the mass is increasing in size, surgery (myomectomy, dilation and curettage, endometrial ablation, or hysterectomy) will be recommended. The choice of surgery depends on the age and reproductive status of the woman and/or the significance of the noted changes. There are no medications or therapies to prevent fibroids. However, fibroids are estrogen-dependent tumors; estrogen supplementation (premarin) can stimulate their growth, and antiestrogen medications (danazol) can prevent their growth.

The diagnosis of endometrial cancer is made by an endometrial biopsy or by the posthysterectomy pathology examination of the uterus. The treatment of endometrial cancer depends on the stage of the disease. Table 10–6 delineates the staging of endometrial cancer. All stages of endometrial cancer are treated surgically

TABLE 10-6	Staging of Endometrial Cancer

Stage Ia G123:	Tumor limited to endometrium
Ib G123:	Invasion to less than one-half the myometrium
Ic G123:	Invasion to more than one-half the myometrium
Stage IIa G123:	Endocervical glandular involvement only
IIb G123:	Cervical stromal invasion
Stage IIIa G123:	Tumor invades serosa and/or adnexa, and/or positive peritoneal cytology
IIIb G123:	Vaginal metastases
IIIc G123:	Metastases to pelvic and/or para-aortic lymph nodes
Stage IVa G123:	Tumor invasion of bladder and/or bowel mucosa
IV b:	Distant metastases including intra-abdominal and/or inguinal lymph nodes

Graded according to the degree of histologic differentiation:

G1: 5% or less of a nonsquamous or nonmorular solid growth pattern
G2: 6% to 50% of a nonsquamous or nonmorular solid growth pattern
G3: More than 50% of a nonsquamous or nonmorular solid growth pattern

SOURCE: Creasman WT: New gynecologic cancer staging. *Obstet Gynecol* February 1990; 75:287. Reprinted with permission from the American College of Obstetricians and Gynecologists.

with a TAH and BSO. Stage II tumors are treated with lymph node dissection and radiation therapy. Stage III and IV tumors are treated with external and/or intracavity irradiation.

Vulvar and Vaginal Lesions

Vulvar and vaginal lesions are rare. Vulvar lesions are most commonly associated with vulvitis or vulvar cancer. Atrophic vaginitis is a benign condition caused by a lack of estrogen stimulation to the vulva and vagina (both are estrogen-dependent tissues).

Vulvar cancer is most common in women between 70 and 80 years of age who have chronic vulvitis. The following risk factors are associated with vulvar cancer: chronic vulvitis, vulvar demotoses, STDs, and cancer of the cervix. The most common forms of vulvar cancer are Paget's disease, squamous cell carcinoma, and vulvar intraepithelial neoplasia (VIN).

A common vulvovaginal lesion is Bartholin's gland cyst. This is a benign lesion caused by an infection in the Bartholin's glands. The infection can be caused by a number of organisms, the most common being gonorrhea or staphylococcus. Women who have multiple sex partners or who use non-water-soluble lubricants are at risk for this infection.

Vaginal cancer is extremely rare; the only risk factors are cancer of the cervix and diethystilbestereol (DES) exposure of the female fetus in utero.

Medical Therapy

The symptoms of all vulvar lesions are the same—itching and burning. The diagnostic tests used to establish a specific diagnosis are wet mount with potassium hydroxide, culture, and biopsy. The treatment is based upon the specific diagnosis. Atrophic vaginitis is treated with oral or topical estrogen. Vulvar cancer is treated with a vulvectomy and removal of the superficial inguinal lymph nodes.

A Bartholin's gland cyst is characterized by unilateral, hard, painful swelling of the vulva in the area of the Bartholin's glands. The treatment for this is incision and drainage of the abscess with follow-up antibiotic therapy based upon the culture and sensitivity.

Women with vaginal cancer are usually asymptomatic, although occasionally they have progressive vaginal discharge or painless, intermittent vaginal bleeding. Examination may reveal an exophytic or ulcerative lesion. Diagnosis is by a Pap smear and biopsy of the lesions. Treatment is the surgical removal of affected tissue and possibly adjacent tissue.

General Principles of Nursing Intervention

Except for those nurses specially trained to do pelvic examinations and Pap smears, these procedures are not routinely done by nurses. In most cases nursing assessment is directed toward an evaluation of the woman's understanding of the findings, their implications, and her psychosocial response.

Research indicates that women undergoing colposcopy have questions about the procedure (such as timing of events), the sensations they will experience, the meaning of the results, and treatment options (Barsevick & Lauver 1990). Nurses are able to provide information about colposcopy and other diagnostic procedures the woman will undergo. In addition the woman needs accurate information on etiology, symptomatology, and treatment options. She should be encouraged to report symptoms and keep appointments for follow-up examination and evaluation. The woman needs realistic reassurance if her condition is benign; she may require counseling and effective emotional support if a malignancy is likely. If the management plan includes surgery, she may need the nurse's support in obtaining a second opinion and making her decision.

CARE OF THE WOMAN DURING GYNECOLOGIC SURGERY

Before I was faced with cancer, I thought that doctors were the people with all the information. But it was the nurse who explained the test results and the diagnosis the doctor had given me. Because of my nurse, I know just what to expect and how to take care of myself. I think nurses should speak up more so people know all the wonderful things they do.

The women's health movement has increased public and professional awareness of issues related to gynecologic problems and treatments. Information on new, improved diagnostic and surgical techniques that may be used as alternatives to major surgery is being disseminated to consumers and nurses by various groups. The field of reproductive surgery has changed considerably since the late nineteenth century. Continuing increases in the number of reproductive surgical procedures being performed, particularly hysterectomies, remain a cause for concern, however. Hysterectomy is still the most common surgical procedure in the United States (Bachmann 1990).

There are many components to an informed decision to undergo reproductive surgery. The first question that should be addressed is: What are the indications for having the surgery? An explanation of the surgical procedure and the reasons it was selected over other available alternative procedures should be given to the woman. Effects on childbearing ability and/or sexual performance should be explained, as well as effects on the general functioning of the body. An explanation of the risks of the surgery should include the common risks, the nonserious risks, the rare or unusual complications, and the risk of death.

The question whether a second opinion on the necessity for surgery should be sought is somewhat controversial. In the case of elective surgery different physicians may have different opinions. A woman should be encouraged to consult other physicians when there is controversy about a treatment (such as, for example, treatment of early cervical cancers) or when the surgeon is unknown to the woman. A specialist in gynecology is the preferred source for a second opinion. Some third-party payment plans require second opinions. The woman can analyze the information and discuss her concerns with the nurse or physician before she signs a written consent that acknowledges the information given and the authorization for the surgery.

Other concerns that may influence the decision to have reproductive surgery may be categorized as general concerns about surgery and specific concerns related to gynecologic surgery. General concerns include:

- Anesthesia: fear of general anesthesia because of loss of control; fear of regional anesthesia because of possible postoperative problems and concern about being awake during surgery

- Anticipation of postoperative pain

- Fear of death or disability

- Concerns about limitation of normal functioning and dependency during recovery

- Financial coverage for hospitalization

- Family members: welfare of family members while the woman is undergoing surgery (eg, child care, loss of wages, help for household chores)

Specific concerns related to gynecologic surgery are related to the significance of the reproductive organs for the woman. Surgery to alter or remove a reproductive organ may be perceived as a threat to self-concept.

Body image is affected whenever a body part is lost. The degree of mourning for that loss is related to the significance attached to it. Even though there is no outwardly apparent change with a hysterectomy, the loss may be felt strongly. Many women fear postoperative changes such as masculinization, weight gain, and loss of sexuality. Reproductive surgery may also be seen as a threat to femininity in our society, which emphasizes childbearing and motherhood.

Hysterectomy

A **hysterectomy** involves the removal of the uterus through an abdominal incision or through the vagina. When the fallopian tubes and both ovaries are also removed, the procedure is called a total abdominal hysterectomy with bilateral salpingo-oophorectomy (TAH-BSO) or total vaginal hysterectomy (TVH-BSO).

The most recent advance in hysterectomy surgery is the laparoscopy-assisted vaginal hysterectomy (LAVH). In this technique, the laparoscope is inserted into the umbilicus and used to assist with visualization and dissection to facilitate the vaginal removal of the uterus. The advantage of this method is that the surgeon is able to produce results similar to a TAH but without a large abdominal scar. Theoretically, women should recover more quickly from this surgery than from a TAH. This technique is somewhat controversial because of the added expense resulting from increased time in the operating room and the risks of prolonged anesthesia exposure.

Indications

Hysterectomy is the usual treatment for several conditions, although there is no medical consensus about absolute indications. Abdominal hysterectomies are generally performed for cancer of the cervix, endometrium, and ovary; fibroids; endometriosis; chronic pelvic inflammatory disease (PID); and adenomyosis.

TVH is usually performed for pelvic relaxation (see discussion later in this chapter) and abnormal uterine bleeding. Some current techniques can be used to manage abnormal uterine bleeding, thus avoiding a hysterectomy. Hysteroscopy allows the physician to look inside the uterus and perform minor surgical procedures. Endometrial ablation is used to cauterize the entire endometrium, thus preventing it from regenerating and bleeding. Women who still wish to have children are not candidates for endometrial ablation and would most likely be treated with dilation and curettage (described later in this chapter).

Surgical Procedures

Abdominal procedures are usually performed in women who have had previous pelvic surgery with resulting adhesions, scarring, or endometriosis and in nulliparous women whose fallopian tubes and ovaries are also to be removed. Abdominal hysterectomy is preferred when malignancy is suspected or confirmed because the procedure allows exploration of the abdomen and pelvis to determine the degree of tumor extension. Disadvantages of the abdominal procedure over the vaginal approach include scarring, more postoperative pain, slower recovery, and more problems with bowel function.

Vaginal hysterectomy is usually the preferred treatment for uterine prolapse and pelvic relaxation. An anterior and/or posterior repair of the vaginal walls may also be performed with vaginal hysterectomy. This surgical repair is done when weakened pelvic supports have displaced one or more of the pelvic organs (urethra, bladder, rectum), causing urinary incontinence, constipation, or defecation problems. The advantages of vaginal hysterectomy include earlier ambulation, less postoperative pain, less anesthesia and operative time, less blood loss, no visible scar, and a shorter hospital stay. The vaginal route is preferred for the elderly, obese, or debilitated woman who is a poor risk for abdominal surgery. The major disadvantage of a vaginal hysterectomy is the increased risk of trauma to the bladder.

Removal of the ovaries with the uterus remains controversial. Some surgeons recommend that the ovaries never be removed in premenopausal women because bilateral oophorectomy results in surgical castration and menopause. Other physicians recommend removal of the ovaries in all hysterectomy patients over 40 years of age because of the risk of ovarian cancer. Still other recommend removal of ovaries at the time of a hysterectomy if the woman has a family history of ovarian cancer. In any case oophorectomy should not be considered routine with hysterectomy. The woman should be informed about the alternatives so that she can decide which option she prefers. If the ovaries are removed in a premenopausal woman, estrogen replacement therapy needs to be initiated.

Preoperative preparation for the hysterectomy generally includes the following:

- Laboratory work (complete blood count, hemoglobin, hematocrit, type and cross-match of blood, urinalysis, chest radiographs, electrocardiogram)

- Vaginal examination and/or complete physical examination

- Surgical preparation (enema, douche, abdominal-pubic or perineal shave)

- Maintaining NPO status for 8 hours prior to surgery

- Emptying of bladder just prior to surgery

- Preoperative medication and intravenous fluids

Nursing Assessment

Nursing assessment of the woman undergoing a hysterectomy will include psychosocial aspects and determination of the learning needs of the woman.

It is important for the nurse to thoroughly assess the physiologic, psychosocial, and sexual needs of the woman. Factors known to affect psychologic adjustment after surgery include the age of the woman, her cultural background and educational level, the attitude of her partner, her family situation, her preoperative preparation, and whether or not cancer is involved. The significance of the uterus in the woman's self-image will be reflected in her attitudes about menstruation, childbearing, body image, and sexuality. If the woman equates her uterus with femininity, she may feel an acute loss. She may feel that she will become an "empty shell." If she sees childbearing as a major role in life, loss of reproductive ability can cause distress. The loss of menses is viewed with relief if there have been dysmenorrhea or other menstrual problems but with sadness if menses is seen as a cleansing process or a sign of youth. The woman may feel that sexual ability and desire depend on the presence of the uterus and that hysterectomy will affect satisfaction and ability (Haslett 1993).

Misconceptions and fears about the effects of hysterectomy need to be identified preoperatively so that correct information is provided to the woman and reassurances are given that assist her in making a positive emotional adjustment to surgery.

Nursing Diagnosis

Examples of nursing diagnoses that may apply to the woman having a hysterectomy include the following:

- Knowledge deficit related to lack of information about preoperative routines, postoperative exercises/activity and/or postoperative alterations/sensations

- Fear related to unknown outcome of surgery

Nursing Plan and Implementation

Provision of Preoperative Teaching

Preoperative information and teaching can be done individually or in groups. Being informed about hysterectomy prior to surgery can decrease anxiety and prepare the woman for the procedure and the postoperative period. The preoperative information given should include the consequences of the surgery (what is removed, effect on reproductive ability, and so on), the type of anesthesia used, possible risks and complications, postoperative care routines, convalescence, and when various activities can be resumed.

Promotion of Physical Well-Being in the Postoperative Period

Routine postoperative care includes monitoring vital signs, temperature, and fluid intake and output; checking the amount of bleeding by assessing the abdominal dressing and/or perineal pads; assessing the need for pain relief; and encouraging early ambulation, leg exercises, turning, coughing, and deep breathing. In addition to these routine interventions, the diet will be advanced from clear liquids to a regular diet when bowel sounds are present. Sitz baths, heat lamps, and ice packs may be used to relieve perineal discomfort, decrease swelling, and promote healing (for vaginal hysterectomy). Foley catheters are usually discontinued 8 to 10 hours after surgery unless anterior repairs were done with vaginal hysterectomy, in which case the Foley or suprapubic catheter may remain in place for up to 7 days even though the woman returns home 24 to 48 hours after surgery.

Postoperative complications can occur with both abdominal and vaginal hysterectomies. Hemorrhage, urinary tract complications, and wound infections occur more frequently with the vaginal procedure. Complications associated more frequently with abdominal procedures include intestinal obstruction (paralytic ileus), thromboembolism, pulmonary embolism, atelectasis, pneumonia, and wound dehiscence. Emotional complications can occur with both procedures (see the following section on psychosexual reactions). A complication unique to an LAVH is severe chest and shoulder pain due to the injection of CO_2 during the use of the laparoscope.

Discharge planning begins prior to admission. The nurse and other members of the health care team should discuss and reinforce information concerning physical and emotional recovery. Topics to be covered include physical changes the woman can expect, physical limitations or restrictions during convalescence, anticipatory guidance, and emotional reactions that can occur.

Anticipated physical changes include weakness and fatigue, cessation of menses, inability to become pregnant, possibility of painful intercourse after vaginal hysterectomy with repair (until vaginal walls are stretched), possible bowel irregularity, possible lack of appetite, possible phantom pain (uterine cramps), and possible temporary loss of vaginal sensation after vaginal hysterectomy. Restrictions after surgery may include avoidance of heavy lifting, strenuous work, or active sports for at least 1 month; avoidance of tub baths, douches, and sexual intercourse for 3 to 6 weeks; and avoidance of sitting for long periods of time to prevent pelvic congestion. Anticipatory guidance is given to stress the need for the postoperative

checkup in 4 to 6 weeks. The woman also should be taught the signs of infection, hemorrhage, and bladder problems because these complications can occur after she leaves the hospital. Discussions about possible emotional responses should clear up any misconceptions about hysterectomy causing masculinization, detrimental effects on sexual responses, or mental illness.

Addressing Psychosexual Concerns

A variety of feelings may be associated with a hysterectomy. The woman may feel fear, anxiety, lowered self-esteem, and depression. Depression is more frequently seen in women who have had a hysterectomy for treatment of cancer—because these clients must also face the possibility of death from the disease—and in women who have an abdominal hysterectomy rather than a vaginal procedure (Haslett 1993).

Wide variations in sexual adjustment occur after a hysterectomy. Specific information that may assist with sexual adjustment after surgery includes the following:

- The vagina shrinks temporarily postoperatively and coitus will help stretch it.

- Using water-soluble lubricants may make coitus more comfortable.

- Clitoral orgasm may be encouraged.

- The goal is overall sensual enjoyment.

- Orgasm will feel different because of the loss of uterine contractions.

Nurses who are not comfortable with or knowledgeable about sexual counseling should either seek more education in human sexuality or refer the client to someone who is more comfortable discussing it.

Evaluation

Anticipated outcomes of nursing care include:

- The woman can discuss the reason for the hysterectomy, the alternatives, the expected outcome of surgery, the risks, and aspects of self-care after surgery.

- The woman has an uneventful recovery without complications.

- The woman feels she is able to ask questions and obtain support.

- The woman participates in decision making about her care.

Dilation and Curettage

Dilation and curettage (D & C) is the most frequently performed minor gynecologic surgical procedure. Indications for D & C can be diagnostic or therapeutic. Diagnostic indications include checking for uterine malignancy, evaluating infertility causes, and investigating dysfunctional uterine bleeding. Therapeutic indications include therapeutic abortion; treatment of heavy bleeding, incomplete abortion, or dysmenorrhea; and removal of polyps. A D & C is generally performed under general anesthesia but can be done in outpatient surgery.

Salpingectomy

Salpingectomy is the unilateral or bilateral removal of the fallopian tubes. Indications include diseases of the tubes, sepsis, malignancy, and tubal pregnancy. Salpingectomy for tubal pregnancy is generally an emergency procedure because the placenta erodes the fallopian tube and can cause hemorrhage once the fallopian tube is completely eroded.

Tubal Reconstruction

Microsurgery has significantly affected gynecologic surgery, primarily in the treatment of infertility and reversal of sterilization. The tubal reconstruction procedure involves "unblocking" the tubes and reconnecting the remaining portions (tubal reanastomosis), using magnification and microsurgical techniques to obtain proper alignment and accurate approximation of the tubes. The success rate in reversal of sterilization surgery is 60% (Fischer 1991).

Oophorectomy

Oophorectomy is unilateral or bilateral removal of the entire ovary. Indications include severe pelvic inflammatory disease, malignancy, ectopic pregnancy, and ovarian cysts. Ovaries may be removed when a hysterectomy is performed if the woman is menopausal but are often not removed in premenopausal women, depending on the indication for the hysterectomy.

When both ovaries are removed in premenopausal women, abrupt surgical menopause occurs. This may cause decreased libido, decreased vaginal lubrication, and decreased sensations in the lower vaginal tract. Symptoms of menopause—such as hot flashes and atrophy of the vaginal epithelium—may be treated with hormone replacement therapy. Women at risk of developing osteoporosis or who have a strong family history of cardiovascular disease are prime candidates for hormone replacement therapy. There is no consensus on the risk factors, benefits, or side effects of estrogen replacement in women who have had hysterectomies. Some clinicians advocate administration of progesterone for a portion of each cycle to oppose the estrogen effects. Whether or not a woman who does not have a uterus should receive progestin is controversial. There is a need for further research on this issue.

Vulvectomy

A simple vulvectomy is performed for leukoplakia and intractible pruritus, whereas a radical procedure is done for malignant disease. A simple vulvectomy is the removal of the labia majora and minora and the clitoris. Radical vulvectomy is the removal of the whole vulva, the skin and fat of the femoral triangle, and the pelvic lymph nodes. Skin grafts may be necessary.

This disfiguring procedure is associated with marked psychosexual disturbances. Most women report decreased sexual arousal levels and low self-image. The woman may express grief over her loss by crying, withdrawing, or becoming depressed or angry.

Sexual activity can be resumed within 3 months, but adjustments are necessary owing to the loss of sensory perception for foreplay. Stimulation of breasts, thighs, buttocks, or anterior abdominal wall can be suggested.

Pelvic Exenteration

A pelvic exenteration is performed for recurrence of cervical cancer. Only about 5% of women with recurrence are candidates for the procedure, which is not performed if there is any evidence of tumor outside the pelvis, if the cancer has metastasized to the lymph nodes, or if all of the tumor cannot be removed.

Exenteration can be of the anterior or posterior pelvis or of the total pelvis. *Anterior exenteration* is the removal of the uterus, ovaries, fallopian tubes, vagina, bladder, urethra, and pelvic lymph nodes. Urine is diverted through an ileal conduit. *Posterior exenteration* is the removal of the uterus, fallopian tubes, ovaries, descending colon, rectum, and anal canal. A colostomy is created. A *total exenteration* is a combination of the anterior and posterior procedures. A vagina can be reconstructed from split-thickness skin grafts or a segment of small bowel.

Complications associated with exenteration include intestinal and urinary obstruction, thrombophlebitis, pulmonary embolism, pyelonephritis, hypovolemia, peritonitis, pneumonia, and wound infection.

Nursing Care

Postoperative care for vulvectomy includes urinary drainage via an indwelling catheter to prevent wound contamination and meticulous wound care to debride and promote healing. Wound care usually consists of debriding with a solution of half-strength peroxide followed by normal saline. The wound is then dried with either a heat lamp or a hair dryer (cold air).

Postoperative care for the woman with pelvic exenteration usually begins with three or four days in the intensive care unit because of the risk of shock, cardiac changes, and kidney failure. Once the woman returns to the regular postoperative unit, care includes the usual postoperative interventions, as well as care for the ileal conduit or colostomy. The nurse needs to continue to assess the woman for a grief reaction to the drastic changes in her body and should expect emotional fluctuations.

SURGICAL INTERRUPTION OF PREGNANCY

Although for centuries abortion was banned by both church and public law, many women still sought to terminate their pregnancies. Because of the illegal status of abortion, however, the procedure was always dangerous. Illegal abortions became the single highest cause of maternal death in this country. Since 1973, when induced abortion became a legal option in the United States, the maternal mortality rate has declined steadily.

Although legalized abortion has been in effect for more than two decades, the controversy over the moral and legal issues continues. This controversy is, of course, readily apparent in the medical and nursing professions. See Chapter 8 for further discussion of the belief system and social issues surrounding abortion.

Factors Influencing the Decision to Seek Abortion

A number of physical and psychosocial factors influence a woman's decision to seek an abortion. The presence of a disease or health state that jeopardizes the mother's life and serious, life-threatening fetal problems are frequently suggested as indications for abortion. In other instances the timing or circumstance of the pregnancy creates an inordinate stress on the woman, and she chooses an abortion. Some of these situations may involve contraceptive failure, rape, or incest. In all cases the decision is best made by the woman or couple involved because they will bear the impact of the continuance or termination of the pregnancy.

Methods

The method of abortion differs depending on the length of gestation. See Table 10–7 for summaries of various techniques.

Nursing Assessment

The nurse must assess the woman's knowledge base regarding the abortion and her emotional status in order to devise a teaching plan and provide emotional support.

Nursing Diagnosis

Examples of nursing diagnoses that may apply to the woman having an abortion include the following:

- Knowledge deficit related to lack of information about the abortion procedure, alternatives, risks, and associated self-care
- Pain related to the procedure and uterine cramping

Nursing Plan and Implementation

As the woman makes her decision about having an abortion, she will need information about the types of abortion and the associated risks. The woman needs to understand the available alternatives and the possible problems. The debate about abortion is frequently impassioned, which makes it very difficult to obtain accurate, unbiased facts on which to base a decision. The nurse helps provide valuable information so that the woman can make an informed choice.

Important aspects of care include allowance for verbalization by the woman; support before, during, and after the procedure; monitoring of vital signs, intake, and output; providing for physical comfort and privacy throughout the procedure; and health teaching regarding self-care, the importance of the postabortion checkup, and contraception review.

Evaluation

Anticipated outcomes of nursing care include:

- The woman understands the procedure, the alternatives, and the associated risks.
- The woman has been able to participate in informed decision making.
- The woman has not suffered any complications of the procedure.
- The woman has a support base and is aware of resources in her community that she may use if needed.

TABLE 10-7 Methods Used in Termination of Pregnancy

First-Trimester Abortion	Complications
Dilation and Curettage (D & C) Dilation and curettage is the oldest method. It involves the use of a metal curette to scrape out the inside of the uterus. This procedure is performed under general anesthesia. It is not done frequently now because other methods are deemed safer and less traumatic.	Perforation of the uterus, laceration of the cervix, systemic reaction to the anesthetic agent, hemorrhage
Minisuction A minisuction is accomplished with a small-bore cannula and a 50 mL syringe as a vacuum source. This technique is also called menstrual regulation or menstrual extraction.	Perforation of the uterus, laceration of the cervix, systemic reaction to the anesthetic agent, hemorrhage
Vacuum Curettage After a paracervical block, the cervix is dilated, and a vacuum suction cannula is inserted to remove the contents of the uterus. Laminaria or magnesium sulfate sponges may be inserted into the cervix for several hours or overnight to dilate the cervix.	Perforation of the uterus, laceration of the cervix, systemic reaction to the anesthetic agent, hemorrhage

Second Trimester (mid-trimester)	Complications
Hypertonic Saline Hypertonic saline is still a method used after 20 weeks. A laminaria is inserted the day before. Hypertonic saline is injected or infused into the amniotic cavity. The procedure takes an average of 33 to 35 hours to completion. Some clinicians begin intravenous oxytocin a few hours after the instillation of hypertonic saline. In this case the procedure takes an average of 25 hours. The addition of oxytocin increases the risk to the woman.	Cervical laceration, uterine rupture, cardiovascular collapse, pulmonary and/or cerebral edema, renal failure, failed abortion, hemorrhage, infection, embolism
Dilation and Extraction (D & E) Laminaria are inserted 1 or 2 days before the procedure. During the D & E an IV is started for the administration of analgesia and other medications, a paracervical block is administered, and the contents are removed with a combination of suction and forceps. The procedure usually takes 10 to 20 minutes.	Perforation of the uterus with bladder or intestinal injury, amniotic fluid embolism, disseminated intravascular coagulation
Systemic Prostaglandins Prostaglandin E_2 vaginal suppositories or 15-methyl $PGF_{2\alpha}$ (Prostin 15M) may be used. The average time for either of these procedures is 13 to 15 hours.	Nausea, vomiting, fever
Intrauterine Prostaglandins Insertion of laminaria is done the night before. Prostaglandin $F_{2\alpha}$ is injected into the amniotic sac. The abortion procedure usually averages about 14 hours after the $PGF_{2\alpha}$ is instilled. In some instances urea is also instilled.	Vomiting, diarrhea, fever, cervical rupture, hemorrhage, infection

CARE OF THE WOMAN WITH A URINARY TRACT INFECTION

A urinary tract infection (UTI) may be a mere inconvenience or may reach life-threatening severity. Bacteria usually enter the urinary tract at its distal end, that is, by way of the urethra. The organisms are capable of migrating against the downward flow of urine. The shortness of the female urethra facilitates the passage of bacteria into the bladder. Other conditions that are associated with bacterial entry are relative incompetence of the urinary sphincter, frequent enuresis (bedwetting) prior to adolescence, and urinary catheterization. A habit of wiping from the back to front after urination may transfer bacteria from the anorectal area to the urethra.

About 5% of women have at least one UTI before becoming sexually active. The prevalence increases 1% per decade of life. Voluntarily suppressing the desire to urinate is a predisposing factor. Elderly women who have more difficulty in the awareness of the urge to void and the ability to hold urine have a significantly higher incidence of UTI than younger women. Retention overdistends the bladder and can lead to an infection. For reasons that are unclear there seems to be a relationship between recurring UTI and sexual intercourse. Women may be at increased risk for a UTI with a new sex partner and a sudden increase in sexual activity. This is commonly called "honeymoon cystitis." General poor health or lowered resistance to infection can also increase a woman's susceptibility to urinary tract infections. Stasis of urine, compression of ureters (especially the right ureter), decreased bactericidal capabilities of leukocytes in the urine, and vesicoureteral reflux (backward urine flow) make the pregnant woman even more susceptible to urinary tract infections.

The highest prevalence of UTI is among women of high parity in the low socioeconomic level, women with a history of UTI, and women with sickle cell disease or sickle cell trait.

Asymptomatic bacteriuria (ASB) (bacteria in the urine actively multiplying without accompanying clinical symptoms) constitutes about 6% to 8% of cases of UTI. This becomes especially significant if the woman is pregnant. Between 25% and 30% of pregnant women with untreated ASB will go on to develop pyelonephritis, which can result in preterm labor (Kiningham 1993). Asymptomatic bacteriuria is almost always caused by a single organism. If more than one type of bacteria is cultured, the possibility of urine culture contamination must be considered. The most common cause of ASB is *Escherichia coli*. Other commonly found causative organisms include *Klebsiella* and *Proteus*.

If a pregnant woman develops an acute UTI, especially with high temperature, amniotic fluid infection may develop and retard the growth of the placenta.

Lower Urinary Tract Infection (Cystitis)

Because urinary tract infections are ascending, it is important to recognize and diagnose a lower UTI early to avoid the sequelae associated with upper UTI.

Interstitial cystitis is a chronic inflammatory condition of unknown etiology involving the bladder wall. It is a relatively uncommon type of cystitis that is frequently misdiagnosed as either bacterial, urologic, or gynecologic in origin. Women between the ages of 20 and 70 are most often affected. Clients complain of bladder pain, urgency, frequency, genital pain, dyspareunia, and sleep disturbances. The urine culture is negative, and the only physical finding may be some urethral or vaginal tenderness. Interstitial cystitis does not respond to antibiotic therapy, and no effective treatment regimen has been found (Fihn 1992).

Medical Therapy

Symptoms of frequency, pyuria, and dysuria without bacteriuria may indicate urethritis caused by *Chlamydia trachomatis*. It has become a common pathogen in the genitourinary system.

When cystitis develops, the initial symptom is often dysuria, specifically at the end of urination. Urgency and frequency also occur. Cystitis is usually accompanied by a low-grade fever (38.3 C [101 F] or lower), and hematuria is seen occasionally. Urine specimens usually contain an abnormal number of leukocytes and bacteria.

Oral sulfonamides, particularly sulfisoxazole, are generally effective against lower UTI. If the woman is pregnant, these should be used only in early pregnancy because they interfere with protein binding of bilirubin in the fetus. Use of sulfonamides in the last few weeks of pregnancy can lead to neonatal hyperbilirubinemia and kernicterus. Other drugs that are usually effective (and apparently safe for a fetus) are ampicillin and nitrofurantoin (Furadantin). Nitrofurantoin crosses the placenta, but no harm to the fetus has been demonstrated (Tan & File 1992).

Phenazopyridine (Pyridium), a bladder analgesic, may also be prescribed to treat the dysuria.

Nursing Assessment

During each visit the nurse notes any complaints from the woman of pain on urination or other urinary difficulties. If any concerns arise, the nurse obtains a clean-catch urine specimen from the woman.

Nursing Diagnosis

Nursing diagnoses that may apply to a woman with a lower UTI include the following:

- Pain related to dysuria secondary to the urinary tract infection
- Knowledge deficit related to a lack of understanding of self-care measures to help prevent recurrence of UTI

Nursing Plan and Implementation

Teaching for Self-Care

The nurse should make sure the woman is aware of good hygiene practices because most bacteria enter through the urethra after having spread from the anal area. Table 10–8 identifies measures for preventing cystitis. The nurse should also reinforce instructions or answer questions regarding the prescribed antibiotic, the amount of liquids to take, and the reasons for these treatments.

TABLE 10-8 Measures for Preventing Cystitis

If you use a diaphragm for contraception, try changing methods or using another size of diaphragm.

Avoid bladder irritants such as alcohol, caffeine products, and carbonated beverages.

Increase fluid intake, especially water, to a minimum of six to eight glasses per day.

Make regular urination a habit; avoid long waits.

Practice good genital hygiene, including wiping from front to back after urination and bowel movements.

Be aware that vigorous or frequent sexual activity may contribute to urinary tract infection.

Urinate before and after intercourse to empty the bladder and cleanse the urethra.

Complete medication regimens even if symptoms decrease.

Do not use medication left over from previous infections.

Drink cranberry juice to acidify the urine. This has been found to relieve symptoms in some cases.

Cystitis usually responds rapidly to treatment, but follow-up urinary cultures are important.

Evaluation

Anticipated outcomes of nursing care include:

- The woman implements self-care measures to help prevent cystitis as part of her personal routine.
- The woman can identify the signs, symptoms, therapy, and possible complications of cystitis.
- The woman's infection is cured.

Upper Urinary Tract Infection (Pyelonephritis)

Pyelonephritis (inflammatory disease of the kidneys) is less common but more serious than cystitis and is often preceded by lower UTI. It is more common during the latter part of pregnancy or early postpartum and poses a serious threat to maternal and fetal well-being. Women with symptomatic pyelonephritis during pregnancy have an increased risk of premature births as well as intrauterine growth retardation.

Medical Therapy

The goal of medical intervention is to diagnose acute pyelonephritis and begin treatment as soon as possible. Acute pyelonephritis has a sudden onset with chills, high fever of 39.6–40.6 C (103–105 F), and flank pain (either unilateral or bilateral). The right side is almost always in-

volved if the woman is pregnant because the large bulk of intestines to the left pushes the uterus to the right, putting pressure on the right ureter and kidney. Nausea, vomiting, and general malaise may ensue. With accompanying cystitis, frequency, urgency, and burning with urination may be experienced.

Edema of the renal parenchyma or ureteritis with blockage and swelling of the ureter may lead to temporary suppression of urinary output. This is accompanied by severe colicky pain, vomiting, dehydration, and ileus of the large bowel. The woman with acute pyelonephritis will generally have increased diastolic blood pressure, positive fluorescent antibody titer (FA-test), low creatinine clearance, significant bacteremia in urine culture, pyuria, and presence of white blood cell casts.

During pregnancy, acute pyelonephritis can lead to maternal sepsis and is life threatening to both the woman and her unborn child. Consequently, the woman is hospitalized and started on intravenous antibiotic therapy as soon as an acute upper UTI is diagnosed by symptoms and urine culture. In the case of obstructed pyelonephritis a blood culture is necessary. The woman is kept in bed. After a sensitivity report the antibiotic may be changed to one more specific for the infecting organism. Ampicillin, nitrofurantoin, or one of these in combination with a sulfonamide is commonly prescribed. Other antibiotics considered safe during pregnancy include cephalexin, sulfisoxazole, and methenamine (Elder 1992).

If signs of urinary obstruction occur or continue, the ureter may need to be catheterized to establish adequate drainage.

With appropriate drug therapy the woman's temperature should return to normal. The pain subsides, and the urine shows no bacteria within 2 to 3 days. Follow-up urinary cultures are needed to ensure that the infection has been eliminated completely.

Nursing Assessment

During the woman's visit the nurse obtains a sexual and medical history to identify the woman at risk for UTI. A clean-catch urine specimen is evaluated for evidence of ASB.

Teaching for Self-Care

The nurse provides the woman with information to help her recognize the signs of UTI so she can contact her care giver as soon as possible when needed. The nurse also discusses hygiene practices, the advantages of wearing cotton underwear, and the need to void frequently to prevent urinary stasis.

The nurse stresses the importance of maintaining a good fluid intake. Drinking cranberry juice daily and taking 500 mg vitamin C both help acidify the urine and may help prevent recurrence of infection. Women with a history of UTI find it helpful to drink a glass of fluid prior to sexual intercourse and void before and afterward.

Pelvic Relaxation

There are several forms of pelvic relaxation. A cystocele is the downward displacement of the bladder, which appears as a bulge in the anterior vaginal wall. A rectocele is the downward displacement of the rectum, which appears as a bulge in the posterior vaginal wall. An enterocele is the downward displacement of the intestines into the vagina. Uterine prolapse occurs when the ligaments that suspend the uterus become relaxed and the uterus bulges down into the vagina. Arbitrary classifications of mild to severe are frequently given. Genetic predisposition, vaginal childbearing, obesity, lifting, standing for long periods, and increased age are factors that may contribute to pelvic relaxation (Hanzal et al 1993).

Medical Therapy

Symptoms of stress incontinence, including loss of urine with coughing, sneezing, laughing, or sudden exertion, are most common with a cystocele. Constipation is a common symptom with a rectocele or an enterocele. Dyspareunia and increased vaginal discharge may be associated with uterine prolapse. Vaginal fullness, a bulging out of the vaginal wall, or a dragging sensation may also be noticeable with all forms of pelvic relaxation.

If pelvic relaxation is mild, Kegel exercises are helpful in restoring tone. The exercises involve contraction and relaxation of the pubococcygeal muscle. Women have found these exercises helpful before and after childbirth in maintaining vaginal muscle tone. Estrogen may improve the condition of vaginal mucous membranes—especially in menopausal women (see Chapter 9). Vaginal pessaries or rings may be used if surgery is undesirable or impossible or until surgery can be scheduled (Kaminski et al 1993). An anterior repair and/or a bladder suspension are surgical procedures that may be used to correct a cystocele. A posterior repair may be used to correct a rectocele. In women who have ceased childbearing, a TVH may be the surgical treatment of choice.

Teaching for Self-Care

The nurse may instruct the woman in the use of Kegel exercises. Information on the causes and contributing factors and discussion of possible alternative therapies will greatly assist the woman.

KEY CONCEPTS

The breasts function in a cyclic process that is regulated by nervous and hormonal systems. Thus many women experience breast tenderness and swelling premenstrually.

In fibrocystic breast disease the cysts tend to be round, mobile, and well delineated. The woman generally experiences increased discomfort premenstrually. Because of the increased risk of developing breast cancer, women with FBD should understand the importance of monthly BSE.

Factors that increase a woman's risk of developing breast cancer include advancing age (most occur after age 40), family history (especially mother or sister) of breast cancer, early menarche, late menopause, personal history of cancer in one breast, high levels of dietary fat, and high-protein and low-selenium diet.

Recommendations for frequency of screening mammograms are as follows:

- Baseline mammogram between ages 35 and 40
- Mammogram every 1 to 2 years between ages 40 and 50
- Mammogram annually for all women after age 50

Diagnosis of suspicious breast mass is made by fine-needle biopsy.

A variety of surgical treatment alternatives now exist for women with breast cancer, including radical mastectomy, modified radical mastectomy, simple mastectomy, subcutaneous mastectomy, partial mastectomy, and lumpectomy. Breast reconstruction following surgery is becoming a more common alternative. Other treatment modalities for breast cancer include radiation therapy, chemotherapy, and endocrine therapy.

A woman with breast cancer faces many psychologic concerns, including fear of the diagnosis, altered body image, and the response of family and friends. She must also deal with the long-term prognosis and her physical response to the treatment she receives. Nurses play a vital role in providing information and psychologic support.

Endometriosis is a condition in which endometrial tissue occurs outside the endometrial cavity. This tissue bleeds in a cyclic fashion in response to the menstrual cycle. The bleeding leads to inflammation, scarring, and adhesions. The prime symptoms include dysmenorrhea, dyspareunia, and infertility.

Treatment of endometriosis may be medical, surgical, or a combination. For the woman not desiring pregnancy at present oral contraceptives are used. Women desiring pregnancy are treated with a course of danazol.

Toxic shock syndrome, caused by a toxin of *Staphylococcus aureus*, is most common in women of childbearing age. There is an increased incidence in women who use tampons or barrier methods of contraception.

Moniliasis, a vaginal infection caused by *Candida albicans*, is most common in women who use oral contraceptives, are on antibiotics, are currently pregnant, or have diabetes mellitus. It is generally treated with intravaginal miconazole or clotrimazole suppositories.

Chlamydial infection is difficult to detect in a woman but may result in PID and infertility. It is treated with doxycycline.

Herpes genitalis, caused by the herpes simplex virus, is a recurrent infection with no known cure. Acyclovir (Zovirax) may provide a reduction in symptoms.

Syphilis, caused by *Treponema pallidum*, is a sexually transmitted infection that is treatable if diagnosed. The characteristic lesion is the chancre. Syphilis can also be transmitted in utero to the fetus of an infected woman. The treatment of choice is penicillin.

Gonorrhea, a common sexually transmitted infection, may be asymptomatic in women initially but may cause PID if not diagnosed early. The treatment of choice is ceftriaxone and doxycycline.

Condyloma accuminata (venereal warts) is transmitted by a virus. Treatment is indicated because research suggests a possible link with cervical cancer. The treatment chosen depends on the size and location of the warts.

Nurses caring for women with an STD should discuss methods of prevention, signs and symptoms, and treatment alternatives in a supportive, nonjudgmental way.

Women with an abnormal finding on a pelvic examination will need careful explanation of the finding and techniques of diagnosis and emotional support during the diagnostic period.

When abnormal Pap smear results are discovered, associated procedures may include colposcopy, biopsy, laser surgery, conization, or cryosurgery.

Gynecologic cancer involves carcinoma of the cervix, ovaries, uterus, endometrium, and/or vulva.

Components of an informed decision regarding reproductive surgery include an explanation of the indications for the surgery, the surgical procedure, the treatment and alternatives, the risks, and the effects on the woman.

The nurse focuses on the information the woman needs to make an informed decision and on the assessment of data and implementation of nursing care.

A hysterectomy involves the removal of the uterus. It may be done abdominally or vaginally.

Dilation and curettage is the most frequently performed minor gynecologic surgical procedure. It is done for heavy bleeding, incomplete abortion, therapeutic abortion, dysmenorrhea, or removal of a polyp.

A number of physical and psychologic factors influence a woman's decision to seek an abortion.

The classic symptoms of a lower UTI are dysuria, urgency, frequency, and sometimes hematuria. Oral sulfonamides are the treatment of choice.

An upper UTI is a serious infection that can permanently damage the kidneys if untreated. Generally, the woman is acutely ill and may require supportive therapy as well as antibiotics.

Pelvic relaxation is a downward displacement of the pelvic organs into the vagina. Often it is accompanied by stress incontinence and constipation. Kegel exercises may help restore tone in mild cases.

REFERENCES

Ault KA, Faro S: Pelvic inflammatory disease: Current diagnostic criteria and treatment guidelines. *Postgrad Med* February 1993; 93(2):85.

Bachmann GA: Hysterectomy: A critical review. *J Reprod Med* September 1990; 35(9):839.

Baggish MS et al: Ways of using LEEP for external lesions. *Contemp OB/GYN* May 1992; 138.

Barsevick AM, Lauver D: Women's informational needs about colposcopy. *Image* Spring 1990; 22(1):23.

Bassett LW, Kimme-Smith C: Breast sonography. *Am J Roentgen* March 1991; 156(3):449.

Black DM, Solomon E: The search for the familial breast/ovarian cancer gene. *Trends Genet* January 1993; 9(1):22.

Bullough B et al: Methylxanthines and fibrocystic breast disease: A study of correlations. *Nurse Pract* 1990; 15(3):36.

Centers for Disease Control and Prevention: 1993 Sexually transmitted diseases treatment guidelines. *MMWR* 1993; 42(RR-14):4.

Clark RM: Benign and malignant breast pathology. *Cur Op Obstet Gynecol* August 1992; 4(4):601.

Colbry SL: A review of toxic shock syndrome: The need for education still exists. *Nurse Pract* September 1992; 17(9):39.

Coleman C: The role of the comprehensive breast center. *Nurse Pract Forum* June 1993; 4(2):110.

Darrow SL et al: Menstrual cycle characteristics and the risk of endometriosis. *Epidemiology* March 1993; 4(2):135.

De-Freitas R et al: Fine needle aspiration cytology of palpable breast lesions. *Br J Clin Practice* Autumn 1992; 46(3):187.

DiSaia PJ: Disorders of the uterine cervix. In: *Danforth's Obstetrics and Gynecology*, 7th ed. Scott JR et al (editors). Philadelphia: Lippincott, 1994a.

DiSaia PJ: Hormone-replacement therapy in patients with breast cancer: A reappraisal. *Cancer* February 1993; 71(4 suppl):1490.

DiSaia PJ: Ovarian neoplasms. In: *Danforth's Obstetrics and Gynecology*, 7th ed. Scott JR et al (editors). Philadelphia: Lippincott, 1994b.

Douglas KP et al: Roentgenographic evaluation of the augmented breast. *Southern Med J* January 1991; 84(1):49.

Drugay M: Focus on breast cancer screening. *J Gerontol Nurs* August 1993; 19(8):43.

Edge DS, Segatore M: Assessment and management of galactorrhea. *Nurs Pract* June 1993; 18(6):35.

Elder NC: Acute urinary tract infection in women: What kind of antibiotic therapy is optimal? *Postgrad Med* November 1, 1992; 92(6):159.

Ellerhorst-Ryan JM, Goeldner J: Breast cancer. *Nurs Clin North Am* December 1992; 27(4):821.

Eschenbach DA: Pelvic infections and sexually transmitted disease. In: *Danforth's Obstetrics and Gynecology*, 7th ed. Scott JR et al (editors). Philadelphia: Lippincott, 1994.

Fihn SD: Lower urinary tract infection in women. *Cur Op Obstet Gynecol* August 1992; 4(4):571.

Fischer CK: Microtuboplasty as an outpatient procedure. *J Reprod Med* January 1991; 36(1):74.

Forman RG et al: Patient history as a simple predictor of pelvic pathology in subfertile women. *Human Reprod* January 1993; 8(1):53.

Gilbride M: What is the mechanism of action for lasers that are being used to treat gynecologic conditions? *NAACOG Newsletter* October 1992; 19(10):9.

Hanzal et al: Levator ani muscle morphology and recurrent genuine stress incontinence. *Obstet Gynecol* March 1993; 81(3):426.

Haslett S: Hysterectomy (continuing education credit). *Nurs Standard* January 27–February 2, 1993; 7(19):31.

Herbst AL, Berek JS: Impact of contraception on gynecologic cancers. *Am J Obstet Gynecol* June 1993; 168(PT2):1980.

Herbst AL et al: Interpreting the new Bethesda classification system. *Contemp OB/GYN* August 1993; 86.

Hillis SD et al: Delayed care of pelvic inflammatory disease as a risk factor for impaired fertility. *Am J Obstet Gynecol* May 1993; 168(5):1503.

Hirshaut Y, Pressman P: *Breast Cancer: The Complete Guide.* New York: Bantam Books, 1993.

Hughes KK: Psychosocial and functional status of breast cancer patients: The influence of diagnosis and treatment choice. *Cancer Nurs* June 1993; 16(3):222.

Hughes LE: Benign breast disorders: The clinician's view. *Cancer Det Prev* 1992; 16(1):1.

Jossens MO, Sweet RL: Pelvic inflammatory disease: Risk factors and microbial etiologies. *JOGNN* March/April 1993; 22(2):169.

Judd HL: Gonadotropin-releasing hormone agonists: Strategies for managing the hypoestragenic effects of therapy. *Am J Obstet Gynecol* February 1992; 146(2):752.

Kahane DH: The management of the psychosocial impact of breast cancer. *Nurse Pract Forum* June 1993; 4(2):105.

Kain KC et al: Clinical spectrum of nonmenstrual toxic shock syndrome (TSS): Comparison with menstrual TSS by multivariate discriminant analyses. *Clin Infect Dis* January 1993; 16(1):100.

Kaminski PF et al: Correction of massive vaginal prolapse in an older population: A four-year experience at a rural tertiary care center. *J Am Ger Soc* January 1993; 41(1):42.

Kauppila A: Changing concepts of medical treatment of endometriosis. *Acta Obstet Gynecol Scand* July 1993; 72(5):324.

Kelly PT: Breast cancer risk: The role of the nurse practitioner. *Nurse Pract Forum* June 1993; 4(2):91.

Kemmann E et al: Does ovulation stimulation improve fertility in women with minimal/mild endometriosis after laser laparoscopy? *Internat J Fertil Menopausal Studies* January/February 1993; 38(1):16.

Kiningham RB: Asymptomatic bacteriuria in pregnancy. *Am Fam Phys* April 1993; 47(5):1232.

Kirkman R, Chantler E: Contraception and the prevention of sexually transmitted diseases. *Brit Med Bul* January 1993; 49(1):171.

Kramer BS et al: A National Cancer Institute sponsored screening trial for prostatic, lung, colorectal, and ovarian cancers. *Cancer* January 15, 1993; 71(2 suppl):589.

Krebs HB, Helmkamp BF: Assuring successful cone biopsy. *Contemp OB/GYN* March 1991; 131.

Leis HP Jr: The role of tamoxifen in the prevention and treatment of benign and malignant breast lesions: A chemopreventive. *Internat Surgery* April/June 1993; 78(2):176.

Ludwick R: Registered nurses' knowledge and practices of teaching and performing breast exams among elderly women. *Cancer Nurs* February 1992; 15(1):68.

Mahon SM: Early detection of breast cancer: Implications for nurses. *Missouri Nurse* July/August 1993; 62(4):14.

Mansel R: Benign breast disease. *Practitioner* September 1992; 236(1518):830.

McGonigle KF, Huggins ER: Oral contraceptives and breast disease. *Fertil Steril* November 1991; 56(5):799.

Miller RS et al: The early detection of nonpalpable breast carcinoma with needle localization: Experience with 500 patients in a community hospital. *Am Surgeon* March 1992; 58(3):193.

Morrow M: Pre-cancerous breast lesions: Implications for breast cancer prevention trials. *Internat J Radiol Oncol Biol Physiol* 1992; 23(5):1071.

Muscatello R et al: Multiple serum marker assay in the diagnosis of endometriosis. *Gynecol Endocrin* December 1992; 6(4):265.

Nagamani M et al: Calas levels in menitamy therapy for endometriosis and in prediction of recurrence. *Internat J Fertil Menopausal Studies* July/August 1992; 37(4):227.

National Cancer Institute: *What You Need to Know About Breast Cancer.* Washington DC: NIH Publication No. 94-1556, 1993.

Neufeld KR et al: A nursing intervention strategy to foster patient involvement in treatment decisions. *Oncol Nurs Forum* May 1993; 20(4):631.

Norwood SL: Fibrocystic breast disease: An update and review. *JOGNN* 1990; 19(2):116.

Olson LK: Interpreting the mammogram report. *Am Fam Phys* February 1, 1993; 47(2):396.

Palmer GA: Breast cancer: Diagnosis and treatment. *Nurs Pract Forum* June 1993; 4(2):100.

Perricone R et al: Cystic ovaries in women affected with hereditary angioedema. *Clin Exper Immunol* December 1992; 90(3):401.

Petitti DB, Reingold AL: Recent trends in the incidence of toxic shock syndrome in Northern California. *Am J Pub Health* September 1991; 81(9):1209.

Podczaski E et al: Detection and patterns of treatment failure in 300 consecutive cases of "early" endometrial cancer after primary surgery. *Gynecol Oncol* December 1992; 47(3):323.

Ripps BA, Martin DC: Correlation of focal pelvic tenderness with implant dimension and stage of endometriosis. *J Reprod Med* July 1992; 37(7):620.

Romanowski B: Pelvic inflammatory disease: Current approaches. *Can Fam Phys* February 1993; 39:346.

Rosenberg MJ, Phillips RS: Does douching promote ascending infection? *J Reprod Med* November 1992; 37(11):930.

Rubin MM, Lauver D: Assessment and management of cervical intraepithelial neoplasia. *Nurs Pract* October 1990; 15(10):23.

Rubin SC, Curtin JP: Surgery for gynecologic malignances. *Cur Op Oncol* October 1992; 4(5):923.

Sammarco MJ et al: Local anesthesia for cryosurgery on the cervix. *J Reprod Med* March 1993; 38(3):170.

Schuchat A, Broome CV: Toxic shock syndrome and tampons. *Epidemiol Rev* 1991; 13:99.

Secor RM, Fertitta L: Vulvar vestibulitis syndrome. *Nurs Pract Forum* September 1992; 3(3):161.

Suginura K et al: Endometriosis detection and diagnosis with chemical shift MR imaging. *Radiology* August 1993; 188(2):435.

Tan JS, File TM Jr: Treatment of bacteriuria in pregnancy. *Drugs* December 1992; 44(6):972.

Vercellini P et al: A gonadotropin-releasing hormone agonist versus a low-dose oral contraceptive for pelvic pain associated with endometriosis. *Fert Steril* July 1993; 60(1):75.

Walker KG, Shaw RW: Gonadotropin-releasing hormone analogues for the treatment of endometriosis: Long term follow-up. *Fertil Steril* March 1993; 59(3):511.

Walker RA, Varley JM: The molecular pathology of human breast cancer. *Cancer Surveys* 1993; 16:31.

Worrell JA et al: Breast cancer risk associated with proliferative breast disease and atypical hyperplasia. *Cancer* February 15, 1993; 71(4):1258.

Yoder L, Rubin M: The epidemiology of cervical cancer and its precursors. *Oncol Nurs Forum* 1992; 19(3):485.

Younger JB: Endometriosis. *Curr Op Obstet Gynecol* June 1993; 5(3):333.

Zenilman JM: Gonorrhea: Clinical and public health issues. *Hosp Prac* (office ed.) February 28, 1993; 28(2A):29.

CHAPTER 11

VIOLENCE AGAINST WOMEN

To my friends I'm living the American dream. My husband is a successful broker; we have a lovely house; we take exotic vacations. Even if I told them about the occasional slap, the shove, the sex when I really didn't want it, they would think it was probably worth putting up with it. Sometimes I do think about leaving, but it would mean admitting I failed. Even as I tell you this, I know it doesn't make sense—he does the hitting, but I feel ashamed. I'm not a battered wife; I can't be. My husband just has a quick temper.

KEY TERMS

Cycle of violence

Date rape

Female partner abuse

Rape

Rape trauma syndrome

OBJECTIVES

List the social, psychologic, political, and cultural factors that contribute to the occurrence of female partner abuse and rape.

Identify the phases of the "cycle of violence."

Describe the myths and facts about female partner abuse.

Delineate the role of the nurse who cares for battered women.

Contrast the nonsexual and sexual aspects of rape.

Compare the types of rape.

Identify the phases of the rape trauma syndrome.

Explain the reasons why nurses who care for rape survivors should first explore their personal values and beliefs about rape.

Discuss the nurse's role as client advocate and counselor with rape survivors.

Summarize the procedures for collecting and preserving physical evidence of sexual assault.

Discuss the preventive and legal responsibilities of the community.

*V*iolence against women has reached epidemic proportions in society today. Experts suggest that as many as one in three women will be the victim of abuse at some time in her life. Violence affects women of all ages, races, and ethnic backgrounds, from all socioeconomic levels, all educational levels, and all walks of life. Two of the most common forms of violence are partner abuse and rape. Society not only accepts these forms of violence against women; it subtly, and sometimes not so subtly, shifts the blame for the violence to the woman herself by asking questions such as "What did she do to make him so mad?" "Why does she stay?" "What was she doing out so late?"

Violence against women is a major health concern. It costs the health care system millions of dollars and thousands of lives each year (Campbell 1993). In response to this epidemic a number of health-related organizations have begun to address the issue. *Healthy People 2000* (1992), a national health promotion and disease prevention project, includes in its summary report objectives to decrease the violence experienced by women. The Joint Commission on the Accreditation of Healthcare Organizations (JCAHO) has mandated that emergency departments have in place protocols for caring for battered women. The American Nurses Association (1991) advocates education for all nurses on the identification and prevention of violence against women as well as routine assessment for abuse in all women.

HISTORICAL AND SOCIETAL FACTORS CONTRIBUTING TO VIOLENCE AGAINST WOMEN

Violence against women is not new. Throughout history, for thousands of years in patriarchal societies, women have been victims of violence. Wives, concubines, sisters, daughters, mothers—none was immune. Female partner abuse (wife battering) is as old as the institution of marriage. Wives were considered the "property" of husbands, subject to their wishes and demands. A husband had the right—even the duty—to "keep her in line," even to kill her. The phrase "rule of thumb" comes from the judicial restriction that when a man beat his wife, the stick he used could be no larger around than the width of his thumb. Outsiders were expected to "keep out of it"; battering was a family matter.

The legal status of women has improved over the years in many cultures. However, many people still hold to the traditional views of male dominance in marriage or any intimate relationship, which can contribute to the occurrence of female partner abuse (Bohn 1990). Traditionally, rape was viewed not as an act of a man against a woman, but as an act of aggression against another man—the woman's husband or father, that is, her "owner." To rape a man's daughter or wife was the ultimate insult, an act of power. On conclusion of a battle, rape of the wives and daughters of the losers symbolized the triumph of the conquerors and the humiliation of the vanquished.

Violence against women is viewed as a means of control by society. Men are generally physically stronger than women and, in a patriarchal society, have greater power and influence. Many women grow up knowing a vague sense of fear that limits their choices and activities because they feel the need always to be on guard. Thus they look to males to serve in the role of "protector," keeping women safe from harm. Unfortunately, these protectors are the very ones who may perpetrate the acts of violence. But because society often fails to hold men accountable, the violence continues.

FEMALE PARTNER ABUSE

A variety of terms has been used to describe violence occurring between partners in an ongoing relationship: domestic violence, partner abuse, spouse abuse. These terms suggest a neutrality, a balance of abuse that is totally inaccurate because approximately 95% of the victims of this form of violence are women (Furniss et al 1993). Consequently, the term **female partner abuse** will be used in this text.

Typically, the batterer is a male, although there are reports of abuse in lesbian relationships. The woman may or may not be married to her abuser. She may be living with, dating, or divorced from him.

Female partner abuse is the most common form of violence in the United States but the least reported serious crime. Estimates suggest that a battering incident occurs every 15 seconds in the United States. In 1990, 30% of all female murder victims were killed by a husband or boyfriend (Federal Bureau of Investigation 1992). At least two-thirds of the women who lose their lives at the hands of a partner or ex-partner were experiencing physical abuse by the man before the murder (Campbell 1993).

The women's movement and heightened public sensitivity to violence against women have stimulated recognition of the extent of this problem.

Female partner abuse may take many forms, including the following:

- Verbal attacks and insults
- Intimidation and threats
- Emotional deprivation and aggravation
- Social isolation and economic deprivation
- Intellectual derision and ridicule

- Sexual demands or deprivation
- Physical pain and injury

According to Walker (1984) and Helton and Snodgrass (1987), a battered woman is one who has suffered one or more episodes of battery from her male partner or ex-partners. Battering involves coercing a woman with physical, social, and/or psychologic behaviors. Physical battering includes slapping, kicking, shoving, punching, forms of torture, use of objects or weapons, and sexual assault. Women who are physically abused can also suffer psychologic and emotional abuse.

Studies have found that battering is more prevalent among lower-income groups, urban families, blue-collar workers, minority racial groups, people who have not completed high school, families in which the husband is unemployed, families with more than three children, and individuals with no religious affiliation. It is more likely that the problem of battering is simply better hidden among the middle- and higher-income groups, where women have access to private health care providers, psychiatrists, and attorneys.

Contributing Factors

Female partner abuse is a result of the complex and dynamic interaction of social, cultural, political, and psychologic factors.

- *Childhood experiences.* Children who witness or experience abuse and battering are more likely to become batterers (males) or to be abused (females) in their own relationships. Perhaps they view this as normal behavior in intimate relationships.

- *Sex role conditioning.* Traditionally, females have been socialized to believe they are inferior, inadequate, and dependent on males for approval. Women are often expected to seek male approval by being nurturing and submissive. Males have traditionally been socialized to expect these behaviors of females and to expect to be financially successful, aggressive, and independent.

- *Economic insecurity of women.* Women typically receive less education and less pay and learn fewer job skills than men. Those with children are often financially dependent on their partners because their own earning power is limited. When they leave the relationship, they frequently fall into poverty.

- *Fear of humiliation.* Family members, friends, and neighbors may think the woman brought abuse on herself or may not understand why she does not leave the batterer. These personal supports may desert the battered woman in fear of their own safety.

- *Ages of children.* Families with young children are subject to more stress and demands; mothers may be more dependent on their husbands for economic and emotional support for themselves and their children.

- *Institutional indifference.* Law enforcement personnel, social service agencies, and the judicial system often do not understand. They feel frustrated and impotent when battered women repeatedly return to their partners.

- *Belief that violence among family members is a private matter.* Belief in the sacredness and privacy of the family has contributed to lack of intervention by legal, social, and medical agencies (King 1993).

- *Perception of inequity of power.* Men who perceive they lack power or resources in their homes or jobs may feel the need to prove themselves and resort to violence against those they perceive as less powerful to assert their superiority (King & Ryan 1989).

- *Religious traditions.* Most religions support the inferiority of women and believe that women should be dependent on their husbands. Laws and statutes based on these doctrines protect battering husbands from prosecution. Religion supports patriarchy, which is written into the laws and economic system to enforce the order of society.

Common Myths About Battering and Battered Women

Numerous myths about battering and battered women are believed by both professionals and the public. These myths often reinforce misunderstanding of battering and perpetuate the problem by keeping battered women silent. Myths range from the belief that the battered woman is a passive, innocent victim to the belief that she asked for and desires the beating. Professionals who provide services for battered women need to recognize and counteract these myths. Some commonly accepted myths are discussed here.

Battering occurs in a small percentage of the population. The statistics on reported cases underrepresent the true incidence. As indicated earlier, as many as one in three women will be the victim of assault by her partner in her lifetime. Battering is a seriously underreported crime: It generally occurs at night, in the home, and without witnesses. It is estimated that only one in ten women reports battering assaults.

Battering is a lower-class problem. It is true that lower-class families have a higher incidence of reported battering and are more likely to have contact with community agencies concerning this problem, but female partner abuse also occurs in middle- and upper-income families. Lower-class families have more unemployment and less education and may have a tradition of expressing anger physically rather than verbally. Middle- and upper-class women are also abused. They may stay in an abusive relationship because they have no financial resources of their own or to avoid exposing the abuse so as to protect their professional lives or those of their partners (Kennedy 1993).

Battered women provoke males to beat them; women push men beyond the breaking point and incite physical violence. Women are often socialized to feel responsible for the state of their relationship. It is important to recognize that people are individually responsible for their behavior: Batterers become violent because of their own internal inadequacies and not because of what the women did or did not do.

Alcohol and drug abuse cause battering. Studies do show a relationship between battering incidents and alcohol use by batterers. In many cases alcohol is viewed as the primary trigger precipitating the battering. However, alcohol use may be an underlying problem in the relationship. King and Ryan (1989) proposed that batterers use alcohol as an excuse to carry out a violent act and shift the blame from themselves to the alcohol. Others suggest that alcohol reduces the batterers' inhibitions, increasing the likelihood of violent acts. Battered women often blame the violence on the batterer's drunkenness and think that the abuse will stop if their partners stop drinking. Unfortunately, this usually does not happen.

Battered women were battered children. This myth holds true in only a few cases; the majority did not grow up in violent homes (Bohn 1990). Most women report that their partners were the first person to beat them. Many battered women, however, were exposed to sex-role stereotyping that reinforces their own belief in their inability to take care of themselves. Consequently, they assume a dependent role with men.

Battered women can easily leave the situation. Leaving is easier said than done. Women assume they are responsible for their marriages and children; they may still love their husbands, rely on them for financial support, and feel their children need a father. Usually battered women have been psychologically abused and have come to believe that family problems are their fault. They often have isolated themselves from family, friends, and agencies that could assist them. Many women with children have no place to go, and shelters have long waiting lists. Most importantly, battered women are at the greatest risk for severe battering or murder when they leave the batterer.

Batterers and battered women cannot change. If psychosocial learning theory is accurate, both batterers and battered women can be resocialized and can learn more effective ways of relating and interacting. Batterers can learn to verbalize their feelings, rechannel their aggressions, and accept the fact that women are not their property to punish or beat. Batterers must also learn not to psychologically abuse their partners. Battered women can be resocialized to recognize their self-worth and develop assertive skills. They can learn to relate with men in more productive ways.

Battered women will be safer when they are pregnant. Battering may occur for the first time during pregnancy or may escalate in intensity if the woman is already being abused. The abuse is frequently aimed at the breasts, abdomen, or vagina. One theory as to why this occurs relates to the husband's or partner's low self-esteem. He already views his partner as his personal property and may feel that the fetus is an intruder. He may also resent the extra attention his partner receives from family, friends, and health care givers (Chez 1994).

The police can protect battered women. Women have been severely beaten and killed by partners against whom they had restraining orders. To adequately safeguard a battered woman, 24-hour protection would be necessary; police are not able to provide this level of protection.

Cycle of Violence

Walker (1984), in an effort to better explain the experience of battered women, developed the theory of the **cycle of violence.** Battering takes place in a cyclic fashion through three phases.

The first, the tension-building phase, is manifested by the batterer demonstrating power and control. Tension builds for both the batterer and the woman. This phase is characterized by anger, arguing, blaming the woman for external problems, and possibly minor battering incidents. Often the woman is in a stage of denial or blames herself for the battering. The woman believes she can prevent the escalation of the batterer's anger by her own action (Walker 1984).

The second phase is termed the acute battering incident. This is manifested when the tension has reached its peak. This battering is distinguished by a lack of control, lack of predictability, and the major destructiveness of the incident. Some external event or internal state of the batterer usually triggers the acute incident. This is generally the briefest of the three phases. The cycle of violence can be interrupted before the acute battering incident if proper interventions take place (Walker 1984).

The third phase, the tranquil, loving phase, is sometimes called the honeymoon period. This phase may be characterized by extremely loving, kind, and contrite behaviors by the batterer as he tries to make up with the woman. This phase is not always present. Instead there could be simply an absence of tension and violence. Without intervention this phase will end at some point, and the cycle of violence will repeat (Walker 1984). Researchers have shown that over time the cycle of violence increases in severity and frequency (Walker 1984).

Characteristics of Battered Women

Battered women often hold traditional views of sex roles. Many were raised to be submissive, passive, and dependent and to seek approval from male figures. Whereas some battered women were exposed to domestic violence between their parents, others first experience it from their partners. Battered women are likely to accept the traditional female role in their marriage or relationship and believe their husbands/partners will love and protect them. As traditionalists, they believe in family unity and accept prescribed female sex-role stereotypes, believing it is a woman's responsibility to keep her man happy. They believe that they are responsible for the relationship; they have an investment in it and want to make it work. If the relationship fails, they think they have failed as women, that it is their fault, and that their "punishment" is justified.

Battered women typically attribute their beatings to some personal shortcoming or inadequacy. Battered women report that they believed their partners' insults and accusations of being bad wives/partners and negligent mothers. As these women become more isolated, it becomes harder for them to judge who is right. Convinced that they are to blame, they find it easier to admit their guilt than to confront their partners/husbands. For years the men they love and trust have been telling them how bad or incompetent they are. Eventually they fully believe in their inadequacy; they are psychologically destroyed. Their low self-esteem reinforces their belief that they deserve to be beaten.

Many battered women do not work outside the home. They are isolated from their families, friends, and neighbors and totally dependent on their partners/husbands for financial and emotional needs. Their extreme dependency sets the stage for the partner/husband to exert almost complete control of their environment and finances. The woman does not believe that she can be independent or self-sufficient.

After repeated beatings, a woman's self-esteem is virtually nonexistent. She feels depressed and guilty about a situation over which she has no control. Her sense of hopelessness and helplessness reduces her problem-solving ability. Ignorance of available resources and personal despondency further contribute to their sense of powerlessness. Some women develop a pattern of behavior termed "learned helplessness." Because experience has taught her that she often cannot predict the effect her actions will have, she is likely to choose behaviors and responses that have the greatest likelihood of triggering a known response. The unknown is terrifying. Learned helplessness often plays a role in a woman's decision to stay in a known situation, even though abusive, rather than face the unknown by leaving.

Battered women often feel a pervasive, undefined guilt. They may internalize their anger at their partners/husbands and the situation into depression or may express it indirectly with severe stress reactions and psychophysiologic symptoms. Fear becomes part of daily life because they know that the slightest provocation, suspicion, or jealousy may incite another attack. Caught between their terror of remaining in the home and fear of the unknown if they leave, trapped by psychologic paralysis and complete dependence on their partners/husbands, some women attempt suicide. Bohn (1990) reported that 20% to 50% of battered women attempt suicide.

Characteristics of Batterers

Batterers come from all racial, ethnic, and religious groups and all professions, occupations, and socioeconomic groups. Physical abuse may be seen in the batterer's history and is only one of the many power tactics abusers may use to control their partner (Bohn 1990). Battering is also more common in families where the husband or partner is experiencing difficulty at work or is unemployed.

Many of the frustrations that abusive men cannot handle are related to their jobs, their perceptions of themselves and their partners/wives, and their inability to achieve their goals. Their feelings of insecurity, socioeconomic inferiority, powerlessness, and helplessness conflict with their assumptions of male supremacy. Emotionally immature or aggressive men may have a tendency to express these overwhelming feelings of inadequacy through violence.

Many batterers feel undeserving of their partners, yet they blame and punish the very person they value. Extreme jealousy and possessiveness are the hallmarks of abusers. They characteristically express their ambivalence by alternating episodes of unmerciful beatings with periods of remorse and loving attention. Extremes in behavior and overreacting are typical patterns.

Battered women often describe their husbands/partners as lacking respect toward women in general, having come from homes where they have witnessed abuse of their mothers or were themselves abused as children, and having a hidden rage that erupts occasionally. Batterers accept conventional "macho" values, yet when they are not angry or aggressive, they appear childlike, dependent, seductive, manipulative, and in need of nurturing. They may be well respected in the community. This dual personality of batterers reflects the conflict between their belief that they must live up to their macho image and their feelings of inadequacy and insecurity in the role of husband or provider. Combined with low frustration tolerance and poor impulse control, their pervasive sense of powerlessness leads them to strike out at life's inequities by abusing women.

RESEARCH IN PRACTICE

Carol Ann Mitchell and Carole Smyth used a case study approach to examine elder abuse. Domestic violence toward elders encompasses five categories of abuse: passive neglect, active neglect, psychologic abuse, financial abuse, and physical abuse. Neglect occurs when a care giver fails to meet an elder's needs, such as requirements for food or health care. Passive neglect results from a lack of understanding about the elder's needs, while active neglect involves a conscious decision not to meet known needs. Psychologic abuse may occur when a poor relationship exists between the abused and the abuser. Financial abuse usually results from greed. Physical abuse such as hitting, slapping, or sexual molestation is the most discussed, least believed, and most difficult to validate of these problems, because the victim usually gives a potentially valid reason for the injury.

The victim of elder abuse typically presents as a white, elderly, single or widowed female with a physical impairment or treatable health problem. The abuser usually is a relative, such as a spouse, child, or grandchild. Detection of abuse requires taking a careful history and performing a physical and mental examination to assess the elder's cognitive, physical, functional, and other capabilities. The suspected victim should be completely examined for possible injury in the absence of the care giver.

In the case presented, the victim, a 70-year-old woman, experienced emotional and sexual abuse from her husband, also in his 70s. On admission, the woman exhibited multiple bruises, pain with range of motion, and vaginal bleeding, which she attributed to prior chemotherapy. The authors use the case to exemplify elder abuse and describe a decision-making model to apply in suspected cases.

Clinical Application of Study

With identification of a suspicious injury in an elderly woman, the nurse should assess for potential risk factors associated with elder abuse including a history of physician hopping, unexplained delays in treatment, bizarrely or inconsistently explained injuries, family history of violence, isolation, or dependency. Once an abusive situation has been identified, necessary interventions may include referral, couseling for both victim and abuser, family education, and continuous monitoring by a health care professional. In the case study presented, the team instituted home health care for the victim because typically less abuse and neglect occur when a third party is present in the home.

SOURCE: Mitchell CA, Smyth C: A case study of an abused older woman. *Health Care for Women International* 1994; 15:521.

The Battered Woman and the Role of the Nurse

Increased publicity and public sensitivity and heightened awareness of women's rights are encouraging battered women to leave their homes and seek shelter and community assistance. In the past decade many communities have developed domestic violence programs, shelters, and resources for battered women. However, the needs of battered women and their children are still insufficiently met. Beds in shelters are often full. The National Domestic Violence Hotline was discontinued due to lack of funds. Very few services exist for battered women and their children in rural areas (Fishwick 1993).

Battered women enter the health care system in many different settings. Nurses may see them in the physician's office with minor trauma or in the emergency room with multiple severe injuries. Battered women are frequently seen in obstetric services because battering often begins and occurs more frequently during pregnancy. Nurses in psychiatric–mental health services frequently counsel women who have been battered, and community health nurses may find battered women during home visits. Unfortunately, emergency rooms, hospitals, and social service agencies do not routinely recognize and report battering cases to the legal authorities for action and followup, although some states are initiating this policy.

Female partner abuse is a major social problem that ignorance and lack of resources allow to continue. Former Surgeon General C. Everett Koop (1989) stated that domestic violence is "an overwhelming moral, economic, and public health burden that our society can no longer bear." Society and health professionals now need to move beyond mere recognition of the problem to develop a better understanding of the dynamics of battering. Nurses can intervene in the cycle of violence by helping battered women recognize their options and take appropriate action.

The Nurse's Attitudes and Characteristics

Nurses in many different health care settings often come in contact with battered and abused women but fail to recognize them, especially if their bruises are not visible. Nurses who wish to help battered women need advanced knowledge of the dynamics of battered women, assessment skills for recognizing subtle cues of battering, and appropriate intervention skills in counseling and referral. Nurses need to be sensitive to battered women's problems and able to tolerate their own empathic feelings of fear and terror as battered women describe their violent experiences and abusive situations. Other skills required by the nurse include compassion, a sense of reality, and a sense of humor, along with the ability to set limits in decision making.

Working with battered women is often frustrating, and many health care providers feel impotent when these women repeatedly return to their abusive situations without developing sufficient ego strength or coping abilities. Many health care workers are reluctant to become involved, knowing that battered women require long-term assistance and counseling, often for many years, before they are able to change or leave the situation. Nurses must realize that they cannot rescue battered women; these women must decide on their own how to handle the situation. The effective nurse provides battered women with information that empowers them in decision making and supports their decisions knowing that incremental assistance over the years may be the only alternative until they are ready to explore other options.

Critical Thinking Question

Imagine that you have just arrived at a shelter for battered women. You have two children, ages 6 and 8, no cash or credit cards. Because you have been isolated for 10 years, you have no close friends; your parents are living in a nursing home. You haven't held a job since you got married. You will be able to remain at the shelter for 3 weeks. The shelter personnel have helped you find a job as a checker for which you will be paid $5.25/hour. Calculate a budget for 1 month. What problems do you foresee?

APPLYING THE NURSING PROCESS

Nursing Assessment

Victims of family violence may be clients in any setting, yet they are difficult to identify because they rarely disclose their problems. Women who are at high risk of battering often have a history of alcohol or drug abuse, child abuse, or abuse in the previous or present marriage. Other signs of possible abuse include the following:

- Expressions of helplessness and powerlessness: an attitude that the woman lacks control over her life

- Low self-esteem, as seen in the woman's dress, her appearance, and the way she relates to health care providers

- Signs of depression in remarks about fatigue, hopelessness, and somatic problems such as headache, insomnia, choking sensations, or chest, back, or pelvic pain; possible suicide attempts

During the assessment of female clients, the nurse should be alert to the following cues of abuse:

- *Hesitancy in providing detailed information about the injury and how it occurred.* The woman may appear timid and evasive and may avoid eye contact; she may seem embarrassed about having been injured.

- *Inappropriate affect for the situation.* The woman may appear overly frightened, disoriented, or depressed over minor injuries. She may display extremes in behavior by minimizing the importance of significant injuries or appearing fragile with minor injuries.

- *Delayed reporting of symptoms.* Considerable time may elapse between the injury and the woman's seeking treatment. She may have waited until the batterer left home to come in for treatment, or she may have hoped that her symptoms would disappear.

- *Types and sites of injuries.* The usual injuries are bruises, abrasions, or contusions to the head (eyes and back of neck), throat, chest, breast, abdomen, or genitals. Usually there are multiple injury sites. Nonbattered women's injuries are usually located at one or two sites and on the extremities such as sprains and strains. There may be scars and evidence of old injuries that have healed.

- *Inappropriate explanation.* The woman's account of the cause does not fit the type and location of the injuries. She may state she fell down the stairs or walked into a door, although she has abrasions and contusions around her eyes and throat. She (or her partner) may describe her as "accident prone."

- *Increased anxiety in the presence of the possible batterer.* The woman may look to her partner for approval before answering questions about her injury and its cause. He may remain close, appear reluctant to leave her alone for fear she will talk, or demand to be present during the examination.

- *History of missed appointments or frequently changed appointments.* She may have been unable to come in because she had obvious signs of abuse or because her partner wouldn't permit it.

Because battering is now so prevalent, it is important to include questions about domestic violence in all primary care encounters. Furniss and associates (1993) recommend asking the following screening questions:

1. Has your partner ever emotionally or physically abused you?

2. During the past year, have you been hurt physically by anyone?

3. (For pregnant women) Since you became pregnant, has anyone hurt you physically?

The assessment interview should be conducted in a quiet, private place in which the woman can feel safe. When culturally appropriate, it is important to maintain eye contact and avoid excessive note taking. The nurse should assure the woman that her privacy will be respected. It is essential that the nurse remain nonjudgmental, create a warm, caring climate conducive to sharing, and demonstrate a willingness to talk about violence.

A battered woman will often interpret the nurse's willingness to discuss violence as permission for her to discuss it as well (Hoff 1992).

The assessment of the woman should include information about her strengths and her support system. Strengths may include education, employment history, activities in the home, community involvement, and her ability to cope or handle past problems. The woman's support system may include her family, friends, neighbors, and community agencies or organizations.

During the assessment phase, the nurse begins building a relationship with the woman based on trust, understanding, and advocacy. A woman may feel ashamed and embarrassed about her injuries and situation. It is important to assure her that all information she provides will be kept confidential. Trust begins as the nurse conveys an attitude of unconditional acceptance, empathy, and positive regard for the woman's worth and dignity. The woman may need to be asked or given permission to discuss her problems before she shares them. Asking questions with sensitivity is better than avoiding the issues. A gentle, firm approach is useful. Nurses should show that they recognize the woman's feelings and that they accept her right to feel as she does. If and when a woman reveals that she has been beaten, she may begin crying and pouring out details of her years of abuse. Empathic listening and support are essential. See the Nursing Care Plan: The Battered Woman.

Nursing Diagnosis

Analysis of the woman's history and physical examination reveals patterns that may lead the nurse to suspect abuse and battering. If the woman's story of how she received her injuries is inconsistent with her symptoms, the nurse should record the woman's statements and the evidence,

CRITICAL THINKING IN PRACTICE

Marsha Martin, age 23, has come to the emergency room for an injury to her upper left shoulder. She is accompanied by her boyfriend with whom she lives, Fred Schultz. The nurse asks Marsha to tell her the details surrounding the injury to her shoulder. Marsha relates that she is very clumsy and was walking through the house in a hurry when she ran into the door jamb. She said the incident happened 2 hours ago. She complains of discomfort in the shoulder. While relating her story, she often looks at Fred. Fred nods his head in agreement with Marsha's statements. Upon assessment the nurse discovers that Marsha's shoulder is very edematous and bruised. The amount of edema and bruising is not consistent with an injury that happened 2 hours ago. What would you as the nurse do next?

Answers can be found in Appendix I.

noting that the inconsistency suggests possible abuse and that further follow-up is recommended. The nurse can write in the chart, "injuries are inconsistent with her account of the accident" or "injuries are consistent with assault" if that is the case or "She denies being beaten" if the woman was asked directly and so responded.

In cases where the woman states she has been beaten, kicked, punched, or attacked but does not identify the assailant, the nurse should record the extent of injuries, note the woman's exact words, and describe the incident with a diagnosis of probable battering. Those cases in which the woman states she was beaten by a husband or partner may be diagnosed as battering with all evidence recorded, including the woman's statements.

When abuse or battering is suspected or determined, the nurse should formulate nursing diagnoses based on the assessment findings. Nursing diagnoses related to nonphysical components of abuse or battering may include the following:

- Self-esteem disturbance related to feelings of worthlessness and powerlessness
- Knowledge deficit related to lack of information about community resources to assist her

Nursing Plan and Implementation

Provision of Psychologic and Emotional Support

When a battered woman comes in for treatment, she needs to feel safe physically and safe in talking about her injuries and problems. If a man is with her, the nurse should ask or tell him to wait in the waiting room while the woman is examined. This may reduce her fear, help establish trust, and facilitate her expressions of guilt, shame, and embarrassment, along with pent-up anger, rage, and terror about her battering situation. Anger may be directed toward herself, the batterer, or health professionals.

A battered woman also needs to reestablish a feeling of control over her world. She needs to regain a sense of predictability by knowing what to expect and how she can interact. The nurse should provide sufficient information about what to expect in terms the woman can understand. Simple explanations about how long she will stay, whom she will see, and what will be done are important. Some women ask no questions, whereas others produce a barrage of questions. Giving the woman control can be accomplished by asking her permission to do simple tasks and providing her with choices whenever possible. She should be informed that her record will be kept confidential and not released or seen by anyone outside the hospital or agency without her permission.

The nurse encourages the woman to talk about her injuries and home situation by asking, "How did this happen to you?" or saying, "We often see injuries like yours when a woman has been beaten. Has this happened to

NURSING CARE PLAN

THE BATTERED WOMAN

Nursing Assessment

Nursing History

History of delay between time of injury and time when treatment sought

Vague or evasive accounts of the cause of injuries

Inappropriate affect for situation

History of drug or child abuse

Type and sites of injuries

History of emotional complaints

Increased anxiety in presence of possible batterer

History of missed or changed appointments

Physical Examination

Complete physical examination

Injuries at multiple sites, especially in area of head, face, neck, chest, abdomen, and upper extremities

Evidence of old, healed injuries

NURSING DIAGNOSIS: Ineffective individual coping related to low self-esteem secondary to ongoing abusive relationship

EXPECTED OUTCOME: Woman can identify her strengths and her need for self-determination.

Nursing Interventions	Rationale
Provide supportive counseling and reassurance. Accept and acknowledge woman's state of confusion. Encourage woman to express her feelings and concerns. Assist woman to identify her strengths and reestablish her feelings of control.	Women often come to believe that they are to blame for abuse or are dependent on abuser. Battered women can be assisted in recognizing their self-worth and developing assertiveness skills.

OUTCOME MET IF:

- Woman verbalizes her feelings, strengths, and needs.
- Woman verbalizes belief that she is a worthwhile person.
- Woman verbalizes realization that no one deserves to be battered, that the problem lies in the batterer, not the victim.

NURSING DIAGNOSIS: Knowledge deficit related to the lack of information about available community resources and support services

EXPECTED OUTCOME: Woman discusses resources and support services available to her.

Nursing Interventions	Rationale
Identify the woman's support systems.	Women's support system may include her family, friends, or neighbors.
Discuss the woman's options with her.	Woman may feel she is trapped in the relationship and has no options.
Identify available community resources such as shelters, financial aid, child care, job training, or employment counseling.	Women are often unaware of available resources for support or assistance.
Explain the purpose of an exit plan. Assist woman to develop one appropriate for her situation.	An exit plan is a plan, thought out in advance, that helps the woman escape if her life is threatened. Because an abused woman is often isolated, this advance preparation can enable her to cope with the tasks of living without her partner.

OUTCOME MET IF:

- Woman discusses resources and services available to her.
- Woman keeps resource phone numbers available if she chooses to return to the abusive situation.
- Woman has an exit plan so that she can leave when necessary.

you?" Directly confronting the injuries and possible battering may provide an opening for the woman who is trying to cope in private; she may feel less ashamed and frightened when offered this lead in a relaxed, supportive, and nonjudgmental manner. A woman may continue to deny her battering. The nurse should encourage her to talk but should avoid badgering her.

Supportive counseling and reassurance are professional skills nurses use throughout each phase of the nursing process with a battered woman. The nurse should do the following:

- Let the woman work through her story, problems, and situation at her own pace.

- Let the woman know that she is believed and not considered crazy.

- Anticipate her ambivalence in the love-hate relationship with the batterer. She knows he may be loving and contrite after the incident if she has been through the cycle of violence before.

- Respect the woman's capacity to change and grow when she is ready.

- Assist her in identifying specific problems, and support realistic ideas for reducing or eliminating those problems.

- Help clarify the woman's beliefs and myths, and provide information to change her false beliefs.

- Stress that no one should be abused and that the abuse is *not her fault*.

For example, if the woman feels she is responsible for or deserves the beating, the nurse assures her that her husband or partner is totally responsible for his own actions and that she cannot be held responsible for another person's behavior. If the woman thinks that all men beat women and that there is no way to avoid this problem, the nurse explains that this is not so and that both people in a relationship can change. If the woman thinks she is the only one who is beaten, the nurse tells her that many women are battered and that until recently their problems were ignored, but that now various community agencies are available to assist battered women. If, having been through the cycle of violence, a woman thinks her partner will change, the nurse tells her that the abuse and beatings usually continue to get worse over time until the woman takes the initiative and changes the situation with the help of community resources. If a woman continues to see the positive side of the family situation, such as that the marriage is still intact; the children have a father, home, and food; and she loves the man, she needs to examine the benefits and consequences of remaining in the situation. The appropriate intervention is not to tell her what to do, but to help her recognize her options and resources and make her own decisions. Advising or encouraging a woman to leave an abusive situation is not always

in the woman's best interest; leaving the home is a major decision with long-lasting consequences. The woman may be economically unable to leave the situation, especially if she has young children. If the woman leaves and then later returns home, both husband and wife may become more frustrated, increasing the possibility of further beatings and even homicide. The most acceptable course of action is one that the woman freely chooses.

If the woman returns to an abusive situation, the nurse should encourage her to develop an exit plan for herself and her children, if she has any. As part of the plan, she should pack a change of clothes for herself and the children, including toilet articles and an extra set of car and house keys. She should store these away from the house with a friend or neighbor. If possible, she should have money, identification papers (driver's license, social security card), checkbook, savings account information, other financial records (such as mortgage papers, automobile title), and information about the children to help her enroll them in school. She should also plan where she will go, regardless of the day or time. The nurse should ensure that the woman has a planned escape route and emergency telephone numbers she can call, including the local police, a phone hotline, and a women's shelter if one is available in the community.

Provision of Information About Community Resources

Besides offering emotional support, medical treatment, and counseling, the nurse should inform any woman she suspects may be in an abusive situation of the services available in the hospital, agency, and community. Battered women have many needs that require the assistance and coordination of different community agencies. Unfortunately, many battered women are unaware of community agencies that can assist them. Battered women may need the following:

- Medical treatment for injuries

- Temporary shelter to provide a safe environment for themselves and their children

- Counseling to raise their self-esteem and help them understand the dynamics of family violence

- Legal assistance for protection and/or prosecution

- Financial assistance to provide shelter, food, and clothing

- Job training or employment counseling

- An ongoing support group with counseling on relationships with males and children

A network of community agencies can meet these numerous, varied needs of women, children, and batterers. It is important that employees in these agencies understand the complex dynamics of family violence and female partner abuse as well as how their services and those of other agencies can assist these families. Services that are available to the battered woman are discussed in the following sections.

Emergency Room Services   Many battered women are first seen and diagnosed in the emergency rooms of their neighborhood hospitals. Approximately 20% to 50% of all female emergency room clients are battered women (Campbell & Sheridan 1989).

Emergency room nurses and personnel need to be alert to symptoms of battering, recognize these cues, and encourage women to seek assistance from community agencies. Some states require that suspected cases of abuse and battering be reported to the legal authorities or social service agencies.

Shelter and Housing   Since family violence has been recognized as a major social problem, many community agencies have sought federal and state funds to provide needed services and shelters.

Shelters differ in the services they provide, depending on the governing body, financial resources and funding agencies, organizational structure, staff qualifications, and range of available community services. Typical shelters provide battered women and their children with a room, beds, food, clothing, and other basic necessities. If professional staff is available, the shelter may offer crisis counseling, individual and group counseling, and information about community agencies such as legal aid, welfare, job training, financial and employment agencies, and women's counseling or support groups.

For safety reasons the location of most shelters is undisclosed, but they can be contacted through a community crisis line. Unfortunately, admission requirements usually state that the woman must have been beaten in the past; this eliminates those women in potentially violent situations until they have been beaten.

Legal Services and Options   During incidents of domestic violence, the police are frequently called by the victim or neighbors. Family violence typically occurs on the weekend or in late evening when most social service agencies are closed; therefore the police department is often the first major agency involved. Approximately 25 states have laws requiring that arrest occur if a domestic disturbance report is marked by violence. The arrest is considered a "cooling down" period for the man. Unfortunately, in states with no such laws, or if the woman refuses to press charges, the police may still simply issue a warning and leave. Some states have passed tough laws aimed at protecting the victims. In Colorado, for example, police are required to take into custody abusers who have committed a violent act; New York has a similar law in place (Smolowe 1994).

Legal options for battered women vary according to state laws and services. In some states a woman may seek a restraining order from the family court or a domestic relations court to protect herself from the batterer. This restraining order specifies that the man may not physically abuse any family members but does not give him a criminal record. Unfortunately, many abusive men violate the restraining order and continue to stalk, harass, intimidate, and abuse their female partner. As part of Colorado's law, police are required to arrest the batterer if he violates the restraining order once. If he violates it again, he faces mandatory jail time (Smolowe 1994). Other states are considering similar legislation. If the battered woman decides to prosecute, the case is usually heard in criminal court, which handles crimes of assault, harassment, and battery. Criminal court hearings may result in a fine, probation, and/or a jail sentence if the batterer is convicted; in this case the man would have a criminal record. The prosecution process is often lengthy and may last more than a year. Some state judicial systems are introducing more lenient options such as mandatory counseling for batterers in lieu of prosecution. Divorce is another legal recourse a woman may choose, but divorce may take several months to a year.

Most battered women are unaware of their legal options. They fear further beatings if they prosecute the batterer. Limited financial resources may also keep them from seeking legal assistance. Some women do not understand the complex judicial process and their options within it. Therefore few battered women press charges against the batterer, so their fear and vulnerability to repeated beatings continue, with minimal assistance from the police and legal system. Some communities provide legal advocacy services to help battered women understand the judicial process and its consequences to the woman, children, and batterer.

Financial Services   Once battered women leave their homes or seek legal assistance, they usually receive no financial support from the batterer. Without funds battered women and their children are at the mercy of community social service agencies, and it usually takes weeks for papers to be processed before any money is forthcoming. Agencies that may provide financial assistance to battered women include their county welfare department, Aid to Families with Dependent Children, The United Way, women's support groups, religious organizations, and possibly the Salvation Army. There may be other local groups to assist these women in various ways such as providing food or clothing.

Employment Training or Placement   Many battered women are full-time mothers who lack advanced education, training, and job experience. High unemployment rates, minimal skills, and inadequate transportation make it difficult for these women to obtain employment with an adequate salary. Women who have children must consider where to place them during working hours as well as the added cost of child care. Often the woman's choice is restricted to accepting welfare or taking a low-paying job. Either choice usually means lowering the standard of living to subsistence. Avoiding beatings at such a cost may not seem like a viable option.

Some women do seek job training if the opportunities are available, but training provides no guarantee of future job placement. A woman may still have to arrange for financial support and child care while obtaining advanced employment skills or an education.

Counseling   Battered women may need a variety of counseling services, such as crisis intervention, short-term individual therapy, group therapy, or peer support groups, over an extended period. Counseling and therapy may be provided by nurses, social workers, psychologists, mental health specialists, or clergy with special training.

Evaluation

After interacting with a battered woman, nurses may wonder how to judge the effectiveness of their actions. It is helpful to remember that the average battered woman endures the situation for years before seeking meaningful assistance. The nurse may see the woman at the beginning of this long process when she is not yet ready to change her situation. Most women return home in resignation after each battering. Some seek temporary shelter several times before taking final steps to change their situation.

It may take a long time for a woman to concede that life may be better outside the battering situation and that there are effective ways to change the situation. Each woman needs to plan her own life when she has sufficient strength and knowledge of her options and consequences. The nurse should remember that if the woman decides to return home, it is the woman's decision and not the nurse's problem. Having recognized the battered woman, provided counsel, and properly referred her, the nurse has planted the seed for release from the cycle of violence. The seed may lie dormant for years; at a critical moment it may sprout and change the woman's life.

RAPE

If you really want to help her, the first thing you must do is believe her—even if no weapons were used, she knew the single assailant, she didn't make a police report, and/or there is no evidence of harm. It is not necessary for you to decide if she was

"really raped." She says she was raped, and that's enough. She feels raped, and she needs your support.
    ~ LINDA E. LEDRAY, *RECOVERING FROM RAPE* ~

As rape is being recognized as one of today's most serious violent crimes, rape crisis counseling centers are emerging to meet the needs of rape survivors. Nevertheless, society continues to harbor many myths and misconceptions about rape and rape survivors. Fear related to these myths may discourage the rape survivor from reporting the assault and may deprive her of the care she needs.

In its broadest sense **rape** is involuntary sexual contact with another person. However, the legal definition varies according to state. In some states rape involves vaginal penetration by a penis. In other states all types of forced sex, including oral or anal sex or vaginal penetration by a hand or object, are included in the definition. The term *sexual assault* is also used to label such acts. Legally, three elements are necessary for a charge of rape: nonconsent of the victim, the use of force, threat, or deception; and vaginal penetration, however slight.

In a personal sense rape is about violation: violation of an individual's autonomy "at the level of basic bodily integrity. The body is invaded, injured, defiled" (Herman 1992, p 53). Survivors of rape report feelings of shame, which result from the profound sense of helplessness, violation, and indignity. They also identify feelings of guilt and inferiority that they were unable to protect themselves, unable to ward off attack (Herman 1992).

The rapist may be an acquaintance, a husband, an employer, or a stranger. Rape is *an act of violence expressed sexually*. The act is not motivated by sexual desire but by issues of power, anger, or control. It is a male's aggression and rage acted out against a female.

Rape has been reported against females from age 6 months to 93 years, but it remains one of the most underreported violent crimes in the United States. Official statistics reveal only a portion of the actual incidence of rape. For example, in 1991 the FBI's Uniform Crime Report (UCR) recorded 106,593 rapes or 12 rapes per hour, 1 rape every 5 minutes. Figures issued by the Crime Victims Research and Treatment Center in the National Women's Study (NWS) (1992) reveal a far more serious picture. Only about 1 out of 6 rapes (16%) was ever reported to the police. Consequently, the actual number of rapes in the United States each year is probably closer to 639,500, or 1 rape every 1.2 minutes (Buchwald et al 1993). Rape by an assailant known to the woman occurs approximately 78% of the time, although it is especially unlikely to be reported (NWS 1992). Even more disturbing, only 1% of rapists are arrested and convicted (Herman 1992).

The National Center for the Prevention and Control of Rape estimates that one out of every three women will be raped at some time in her life. The incidence of rape in the United States is 4 times the rate in Germany, 13 times that of England, and 20 times that of Japan (*Newsweek* 1990).

Rape is more common during the summer months (especially the month of August) and in large metropolitan areas, although the rate of rape is increasing more rapidly in midsize cities than in large metropolitan areas. Younger women are more likely to be victims, as are women of African descent, but no group is immune (Gordon & Riger 1989).

Myths About Rape

Many people believe the myths that rape commonly occurs at night to provocatively clothed, promiscuous women by unknown assailants. They believe that rapists are sex-starved lunatics who were provoked by the clothing or appearance of the woman. Furthermore, it is a common misconception that no truly virtuous woman can be raped against her will, so that if rape occurs, the woman must have "asked for it." Conversely, the myth continues, because there is nothing a woman can do about rape, she should just relax and enjoy it.

The belief in some or all of these myths has shaped people's response to the rape survivor. Research indicates that Blacks, males, and people with traditional views of women's roles tend to believe more that women are responsible for causing rape and are less desirable after the rape; they consider rapists as madmen driven by passion and favor harsh punishment for rapists (Gordon & Riger 1989). Culture plays an important role in people's response to rape. "In cultures in which virginity is viewed as a prized possession of single women, rape victims are blamed and punished for losing their family honor" (Mollica & Son 1989, p 375). Fortunately, education does seem to be changing societal views about these myths to some extent.

Societal Views of Rape

Recently, rape survivors have been accused of provoking the assault by their appearance or behavior or merely by being present in a secluded area. This neomedieval concept of rape portrays a woman as a temptress preying on men's susceptibility to passion, destroying their always tenuous control, until she "gets what she is asking for."

Rape has also been portrayed as a universal female fantasy—the secret dream of every American girl. Sudden attack, physical abuse, and the threat to her life were believed to "turn her on." Actually, rape appears to be the fantasy of some men. Malamuth (1981) asked male students at the University of California whether they would rape a woman if they knew they would not be caught and punished. Approximately 35% of the men interviewed said they might.

Who Commits Rape—and Why

Characteristics of Rapists

Like their victims, rapists come from all ethnic backgrounds and walks of life. More than half are under 25 years of age, and three out of five are married and leading "normal" sex lives. Why do these men rape? Of the many theories proposed in answer to this question none provides a concrete explanation.

Unfortunately, so few rapists are actually caught and convicted that a clear characterization of the assailant has not been developed. Far from being lusty, overly amorous, or perverted, the rapist tends to be emotionally weak and insecure and may have difficulty maintaining interpersonal relationships. Many rapists also have trouble dealing with the stresses of daily life. "A man of low self-esteem with recurrent failures in social relationships buffeted by daily stresses becomes angry and feels powerless. He then performs a sexual act as an expression of anger or power" (Dupre et al 1993, pp 642–643).

Types of Rape

Rape has been categorized in different ways. One method considers whether the rapist was known to the survivor. In *blitz rape* the assailant and victim are strangers, and the rape is sudden and unexpected. In blitz rape the rapist is more likely to use a weapon and threaten violence or murder.

Confidence rape (also called *acquaintance rape*) involves an assailant with whom the victim had previous nonviolent interaction. The attacker uses deception and trust to gain access to the victim and then betrays that trust. **Date rape** is a type of confidence rape. This type of rape is commonly found on college campuses and occurs between a dating couple. Research suggests that the incidence of date rape on campuses is as high as 15–25% of females (DeKeseredy et al 1993). In date rape situations the male has usually planned to have sex and will do what he feels necessary if denied. Thus in this case the primary motivation of the rapist is sexual gratification (Crooks & Baur 1993). Research suggests that men tend to justify rape more when the woman initiated the date, when the man paid the expenses, and when they went to the man's residence (Muehlenhard 1988). In confidence rape the victim is more likely to have consumed drugs or alcohol prior to the attack and tends to delay in reporting the attack (Silverman et al 1988).

Critical Thinking Question

Why do you think the incidence of date rape is increasing? What can women do to protect themselves from acquaintance rape?

Rape has also been categorized as *power rape, anger rape,* or *sadistic rape.* The purpose of power rape is control or mastery. The male uses sexual intercourse to place a woman in a powerless position so that he can feel dominant, potent, and strong. He often believes his victim enjoys the assault, and he exerts only the amount of force necessary to subdue his victim (Dupre et al 1993). Often power rape is a planned blitz attack, but most acquaintance rapes are also power rapes.

Anger rape is the use of a sexual act to express feelings of rage. Typically, the assailant feels abused and mistreated by significant women in his life, and the rape becomes a symbolic act of revenge. Often the act is characterized by considerable brutality and degradation. Attacks on older women often are a form of anger rape.

The sadistic rapist has an antisocial personality, and sadism usually characterizes all his relationships. He delights in torture and mutilation and is aroused by his victim's struggles and pain. In this type of rape the victim and assailant are generally strangers, and the assault is planned. This type of rape, while fortunately rare, usually receives media attention. Most rape homicides are sadistic rapes.

Gang rape is more common in younger men who are responding to peer pressure. Typically, only one or two of the men may have a rapist mentality, but they are able to incite the others to commit acts they would not do individually. Often gang rape can escalate to severe violence and sadistic behavior as the young men seek to outdo each other.

The foregoing classifications are not mutually exclusive; they categorize the dominant motive in a given rape. Regardless of the style of attack, anger, power, and sadism are components of any rape, which is essentially the use of sexual behavior to meet nonsexual needs.

Rape Trauma Syndrome

Rape is viewed as a situational crisis, that is, an unanticipated traumatic event that the victim generally is unprepared to handle because it is unforeseen. Following rape, the survivor may experience a cluster of symptoms described by Burgess and Holmstrom (1979) as **rape trauma syndrome.** Burgess and Holmstrom originally described this syndrome as having two phases: the acute phase and the adjustment or reorganization phase. Sutherland and Scherl proposed an intermediate "outward adjustment" phase (Golan 1978). These phases are summarized in Table 11–1. Other authors have described an alternative "silent reaction." Survivors also suffer long-term effects.

Although the phases of response are discussed individually in the following sections, they often overlap. Individual responses and their duration vary greatly.

TABLE 11–1	Phases of the Rape Trauma Syndrome
Phase	**Response**
Acute phase	Fear, shock, disbelief, desire for revenge, anger, denial, anxiety, guilt, embarrassment, humiliation, helplessness, dependency; survivor may seek help or may remain silent.
Outward adjustment phase	Survivor appears outwardly composed, denying and repressing feelings; for example, she returns to work, buys a weapon, adds security measures to her residence, and denies need for counseling.
Reorganizational phase	Survivor experiences sexual dysfunction, phobias, sleep disorders, anxiety, and a strong urge to talk about or resolve feelings; survivor may seek counseling or may remain silent.

Acute Phase

The acute phase of rape trauma syndrome begins during the rape and may last for a few days or up to 3 weeks (Gordon & Riger 1989). The woman may experience fear, shock, and disbelief and sometimes denial. The woman may feel embarrassed, humiliated, guilty, and unclean; her wish to cleanse herself by bathing or douching may be overpowering, even if she knows that by doing so she is destroying evidence. She may feel angry or anxious, powerless or helpless. Some women blame themselves and feel guilty or feel compelled to "play the scene over and over in their minds."

The rape survivor may suppress her emotions or may reveal them by crying, sobbing, or acting tense and restless. Survivors who control or mask their emotions may appear calm, composed, or subdued. Physical manifestations of rape trauma syndrome include (Burgess & Holmstrom 1979, p 234):

- *Circulatory:* flushing, perspiration, feeling hot or cold
- *Respiratory:* sighing respirations, hyperventilation, dizziness
- *Gastrointestinal:* abdominal pain, nausea, anorexia, diarrhea, constipation
- *Genitourinary:* urinary frequency, interference with sexual function
- *Mental:* impaired attention, poor concentration, poor memory, changes in outlook and planning

Many rape survivors also experience alterations in sleep patterns such as insomnia, nightmares, or crying out at night.

Outward Adjustment Phase

Once the acute stage has passed, the survivor may appear adjusted. She returns to work or school and resumes her usual roles. But although she appears composed, she is actually coping by denial and suppression. The survivor needs the outward adjustment phase to cope with the experience of rape; it is a means of regaining control of her life. During this time, she may move to a different residence or may institute security measures such as installing extra locks or requesting an unlisted telephone number. She may buy a weapon or take a course in self-defense. These activities do not resolve her emotional trauma; they simply push it further into her subconscious. In addition she may get less support from others who perceive her as being "over it."

Reorganizational Phase

Because the rape experience had not been resolved, denial and suppression cannot sustain the survivor for long. These coping mechanisms deteriorate; she becomes depressed and anxious and feels a strong urge to talk about the rape. At this point the woman enters the reorganizational phase of the rape trauma syndrome. She must alter her self-concept and resolve her feelings about the rape.

During this phase, the rape survivor experiences numerous difficulties. Survivors frequently report prolonged menstrual and/or gynecologic disorders. The woman may develop phobias. Fears of being indoors or outdoors or of being attacked from behind—depending on how the attack took place—are common. Because of these fears, the woman may alter her life-style. If she is afraid of crowds, of being out after dark, or of returning to an empty house, she may become a virtual recluse.

Rape survivors frequently report sexual dysfunction. Some women become totally averse to sexual activity. Those who do try to engage in sex often report a decrease in vaginal lubrication, inability to be aroused, unusual sensations in the genital area, and inability to achieve orgasm.

Sleep disorders persist. Survivors report repeated nightmares in which they either relive the rape or thwart the rapist's attempt. In either case the dream contains disturbing violence. The woman repeatedly replays the role of victim until she comes to terms with the experience.

The Silent Reaction

Women who do not report the rape go through the phases of the rape trauma syndrome without using available support systems. Their reasons for keeping silent vary; a woman may be embarrassed, she may accept society's "temptress view" and blame herself, or she may fear retaliation. Her experience may be discovered much later, perhaps when she seeks professional help in resolving a different crisis.

Some women seek medical help for their physical injuries without disclosing that a rape was the cause. The nurse who suspects that a woman has been raped should seek validation through sympathetic questioning.

Rape as a Cause of Post-Traumatic Stress Disorder

Recent research has demonstrated that rape survivors exhibit high levels of post-traumatic stress disorder, the same disorder that developed in many of the veterans of the Vietnam War. Although there are many common characteristics of post-traumatic stress disorder, there is no one set of predictable behaviors; each individual's symptom pattern tends to reflect his or her childhood experiences, adaptive style, and emotional conflicts (Herman 1992). For example, some individuals will develop symptoms of depression, and others will develop symptoms of anger and irritability.

Post-traumatic stress disorder is marked by varying degrees of intensity. One mitigating factor is individual resiliency. Women who remained calm during a rape attack, used a variety of active strategies, and did their best to thwart the attack tend to fare better and have fewer symptoms of distress afterward than women who were rendered helpless and unable to function because of their terror (Herman 1992). Not surprisingly, the intensity of the post-traumatic disorder is often greatest for women who had psychiatric disorders prior to their assault.

The stages of post-traumatic stress disorder include hyperarousal, intrusion, and constriction (Herman 1992).

Hyperarousal is best described as a state of permanent alertness, a readiness for the return of the danger. In this stage the individual takes longer to fall asleep, sleeps poorly, startles easily, and reacts with great intensity to any stimulus associated with the traumatic event.

The *intrusion* stage is one of continuously reliving the traumatic event as flashbacks while awake and traumatic nightmares during sleep. Intense memories can also be triggered by insignificant events. Most importantly, reliving carries the same emotional intensity as the original trauma, and the affected individual will typically go to great lengths to avoid that experience.

The third stage, *constriction*, is a form of dissociation characterized by a sense of numbing, of distorted perceptions, an altered consciousness, and a detached calm. This narrowing may also apply to an individual's life choices so that, for example, a rape survivor may be afraid to leave her home alone or interact with people.

The stages of the post-traumatic stress syndrome are difficult to treat. Because they keep an individual from addressing the problem, she cannot integrate the event into her life, and healing is blocked. Recovery depends on empowering the woman to seek control of her life within the context of healing relationships.

Physical Care of the Rape Survivor

Traditionally, the health care system has met the physical needs of the rape survivor (often to the detriment of emotional needs). Repair of tissue damage and prevention of complications are primary concerns. Because rape is a crime as well as a traumatic emergency, however, some aspects of medical care are governed by the need to collect and preserve legal evidence for use in prosecuting the assailant. In so doing, health care providers must respect the rights of the rape survivor. To better meet women's needs, many emergency departments use multidisciplinary teams to provide effective care to rape survivors and their families.

Detailed History

Obtaining a detailed history is an essential first step in acquiring necessary medical and forensic data, but it can also be a therapeutic tool if done in a sensitive, caring way. Because rape survivors may appear relaxed and normal when first seen, care givers may underestimate the woman's needs, but it is essential that rape survivors receive immediate attention (Robinson 1990). An explicit sexual history is usually taken immediately after the woman has received any necessary emergency care. Because care givers often lack experience in obtaining the necessary information in enough depth and detail, many agencies use a standardized history flow sheet to record information.

The care giver should use a nonjudgmental approach and avoid leading or coaching the woman. Once the sheet is completed, the woman can be given her own copy to take home.

Collection of Evidence

The collection of evidence may, in itself, be traumatic for the woman. It is valuable to have someone available to provide support and act as an advocate during these procedures. This person may be a family member or close friend, but often it is a nurse. An interpreter should also be provided as necessary.

The woman should receive a thorough explanation of the procedures to be carried out and should sign a consent form. An important legal concept when dealing with rape survivors is the need to preserve the *chain of evidence*, meaning that all physical evidence and specimens should remain in the hands of a professional until they are turned over to a police officer. The chain of evidence is preserved to prevent confusion and the possibility of tampering with evidence (Dupre et al 1993). Most agencies have special sexual assault kits that contain all necessary supplies for collecting and labeling evidence.

Vaginal and rectal examinations are performed, along with a complete physical examination for trauma. Any lacerations of the vaginal wall are repaired and noted. A colposcope with photographic capability can be used to document injuries to the genitalia.

Clothing   The woman is asked to remove her clothing while standing on a clean sheet. The sheet and clothing are then placed in a paper bag, sealed, and labeled appropriately.

Swabs of Stains and Secretions   Swabs of body stains are analyzed for semen or sperm. Because victims are often forced to commit fellatio, oral swabs are examined for semen. Gonorrhea and chlamydia cultures also are taken from vaginal, rectal, and oral cavities. Specimens of the woman's saliva are examined to determine whether she is a secretor or nonsecretor of certain blood-group antigens. If she is a nonsecretor—that is, if these antigens are not present in her saliva—the presence of antigens in her mouth and/or vagina may be evidence of semen from the assailant.

Vaginal and rectal swabs are necessary to document the presence of sperm. Because sperm are sensitive to air and do not survive for long periods, a screen for vaginal sperm is performed as soon as possible. A vaginal smear is placed on a wet mount and stained; any sperm that are present will appear light blue. The absence of sperm, however, does not signify that no rape has occurred. Many rapists suffer from sexual dysfunction during the rape and do not ejaculate.

Hair and Scrapings   Clippings or scrapings of the woman's fingernails are examined for blood or tissue from the assailant. Approximately 15 hairs are pulled from her head to analyze the root structure and identify foreign hairs. Her pubic hair is combed to check for loose pubic hair that may have been transferred from the rapist, and 15 to 20 of her pubic hairs are closely clipped to provide a comparison for forensics.

Blood Samples   Blood is drawn to test for syphilis and to determine the woman's blood type.

Photographs   The procedure for taking photographs, if any, is determined by institutional policy.

Prevention of Sexually Transmitted Infections

The survivor is offered prophylactic treatment for sexually transmitted diseases (STDs). Usually 250 mg ceftriaxone is given intramuscularly, followed by 100 mg doxycycline orally, twice daily for 7 days (Dupre et al 1993). In addition any identified STDs are treated. The woman should be offered human immunodeficiency virus (HIV) testing and hepatitis B testing at the time she seeks care and again in 3 to 6 months. If she tests positive, she should be referred to a center specializing in the treatment of AIDS. Some agencies advocate treating the woman with a vaginal application of nonoxynol-9 as a possible anti-HIV (anti-AIDS) treatment (Foster & Bartlett 1989). If the survivor chooses not to receive prophylactic treatment, the nurse should instruct her to return in 2 weeks to be tested for gonorrhea and again in 4 to 6 weeks to be tested for syphilis.

Prevention of Pregnancy

The woman is questioned about her menstrual cycle and contraceptive practices. If she could become pregnant as a result of the rape, postcoital therapy is offered. Treatment involves 5 mg ethinyl estradiol orally, twice daily for 5 days with 10 mg prochlorperazine (Compazine) orally or by suppository every 8 hours to control nausea (Beckmann & Groetzinger 1989). Other side effects include vomiting, headache, breast tenderness, and menstrual irregularities. Estrogen therapy should begin within 72 hours and ideally within 24 hours of intercourse to be effective. Because the estrogen may be teratogenic, a pregnancy test should be performed first. The woman should be advised that if she becomes pregnant despite the therapy, one of her options is a therapeutic abortion.

The Rape Survivor and the Role of the Nurse

Rape survivors frequently enter the health care system by way of the emergency room; nurses are often the first to counsel them. It is essential to remember that the rape survivor is not sick; she is in a crisis state.

The values, attitudes, and beliefs of a caregiver will necessarily affect the competency and focus of the care that person gives. Interaction with a rape survivor may provoke anxiety, ambivalence, or feelings of personal vulnerability to rape. The nurse may feel overwhelmed by sympathetic feelings or by a sense of inadequacy. Conversely, the nurse may consciously or subconsciously accept the view that a woman was "asking for it." Such feelings interfere with the nurse's ability to give empathic, advocative assistance. Moreover, the nurse may silently convey these feelings to the woman, thus increasing her distress.

Nurses who work with rape survivors must understand their own attitudes and beliefs about rape. With the aid of a skilled facilitator, nurses can discuss their feelings about rape and rape survivors and resolve any conflicts.

APPLYING THE NURSING PROCESS

Nursing Assessment

Policies for admitting and examining rape survivors vary among institutions. A woman who has been raped is under great stress and needs the sensitive care of professionals who are aware of her special needs. The manner in which she is treated at this crucial time will strongly affect her ability to function in the future.

CONTEMPORARY ISSUE

SHOULD INVOLUNTARY HIV TESTING OF AN ACCUSED RAPIST BE PERMITTED?

One of the ongoing fears a woman faces after surviving rape is the possibility of developing HIV infection if the rapist was HIV positive. This fear may be especially pronounced when the assailant is a stranger. The risk of developing HIV varies with the type of sexual exposure (vaginal, oral, or anal), the number of sexual penetrations, the associated trauma the woman experiences (the presence of blood, lesions, or tissue trauma increases the risk), and the infectiousness of the rapist (infectiousness is highest in recently infected individuals and those in the late stages of the disease). Infectiousness is also increased in the presence of other sexually transmitted infections (Gostin et al 1994).

Unfortunately, in many cases the assailant is not apprehended by the police, or he is apprehended but state laws prohibit HIV testing before conviction. Thus the woman often must live with uncertainty for a prolonged period because seroconversion to positive HIV may take 6 to 12 months. In addition to the ongoing worry the woman must make conscious life-style choices, including the decision whether to immediately begin costly prophylaxis with zidovudine. She may also decide to alter life plans, such as delaying marriage, sexual relationships, or pregnancy. Risks extend to others as well. If the survivor was pregnant at the time of the rape, worry about the HIV status of the fetus may be intense. If the woman chooses to have a sexual relationship during the months following the assault, improper use of condoms (if her assailant infected her) could put her partner at risk of infection as well.

Consequently, some states are moving toward mandatory testing of accused rapists. Currently, over 30 states authorize mandatory testing, but fewer than half of those authorize preconviction testing (Gostin et al 1994). Opponents of preconviction involuntary testing believe that such testing violates the accused's rights to privacy, autonomy, and procedural fairness, especially because the US legal system is based on the principle that an individual is presumed innocent until proven guilty.

The issue raises several questions:

- Do the benefits the rape survivor would receive from such information outweigh the rights of the accused to autonomy and privacy?

- Should the right of the accused *not* to know the results, should he so choose, be upheld if mandatory testing is permitted?

- Can sufficient safeguards be built into any mandatory testing law to ensure that the information gained would not lead to the wrongful conviction of an innocent person?

- Should a warrant be required before mandatory testing of the accused is done?

- If the survivor subsequently becomes HIV positive, what would be required to prove that seroconversion occurred as a result of the assault and not due to her own risk-taking behaviors?

The first priority is creating a safe, secure milieu. Admission information should be gathered in a quiet, private room. The woman should be reassured that she is not alone and will not be abandoned and that she is safe from a second attack. During this time, the nurse can develop a relationship so that the rape survivor has a person to whom she can relate consistently throughout her hospital experience.

The survivor's level of emotional distress must as assessed, both for the purpose of planning care and as possible courtroom evidence. Scrupulous documentation is essential because the survivor's medical record is often used in the courtroom to verify her testimony if the rapist is prosecuted. The mental status examination includes the following:

- *General appearance and behavior.* What is the woman's attitude? Her posture? What mannerisms does she display?
- *Consciousness/awareness.* Is the woman oriented to time, place, and identity? Is she able to focus on a subject, theme, or event?
- *Affectivity and mood.* Is the woman depressed? Anxious? Displaying elation anxiety? Is she fearful or apathetic? Is she expressing her feelings or controlling them?
- *Motor behavior.* Is the woman inactive, hyperactive, or underactive?
- *Thought control.* How logical is the woman's flow of ideas and associations?
- *Intellectual functioning.* How intelligent does the woman appear? What is her level of general knowledge? How well does she remember events? How sound is her judgment?

Nursing Diagnosis

Examples of nursing diagnoses that may apply to the rape survivor include the following:

- Fear related to invasion of personal space secondary to rape
- Powerlessness related to inability to regain sense of control secondary to rape

Nursing Plan and Implementation

Table 11–2 outlines the general nursing actions that are appropriate during each of the phases of the rape trauma syndrome.

Provision of Support

It is imperative that control be returned to the woman as quickly as possible. She has suffered trauma in which all control was taken from her. The nurse can return control

TABLE 11–2	Nursing Actions Appropriate to Phases of the Rape Trauma Syndrome
Phase	**Nursing Action**
Acute phase	Create a safe milieu.
	Explain the sequence of events in the health care facility.
	Allow the woman to grieve and express her feelings.
	Provide care for significant others.
Outward adjustment phase	Provide advocacy and support at the level requested by the woman.
	Provide assistance to significant others.
Reorganizational phase	Establish a trusting relationship.
	Assist the woman to understand her role in the assault.
	Clarify and enhance the woman's feelings.
	Assist the woman in planning for her future.

by encouraging the woman to make contact. When feasible, the woman should decide on the sequence of hospital events. In this way the nurse helps her deal with her crisis in small, manageable increments.

The woman should be encouraged to express her feelings and reassured that anger and fear are normal, appropriate responses. The nurse can also address expressed or unexpressed guilt by assuring the woman that the rape was not her fault.

By explaining the medical examination and the sequence of events in the emergency department, the nurse alleviates anxiety related to fear of the unknown. The woman should know what is going to happen and why and how she can assist in each phase of the examination.

Throughout the experience the nurse acts as the survivor's advocate, providing support without usurping decision making. The nurse need not agree with all the survivor's decisions but should respect and defend her right to make them.

The family members or friends on whom the survivor calls also need nursing care. Like those of the survivor, the reactions of the family will depend on the values to which they ascribe. Sonstegard et al (1982) reported that the most common reaction is to regard rape as a sexual act rather than an act of violence. Many families or mates blame the survivor for the rape and feel angry with her for not having been more careful. They may feel personally wronged or attacked and see the survivor as being devalued or unclean. These reactions compound the survivor's crisis.

By spending some time with family members before their first interaction with the survivor, the nurse can reduce their anxiety and absorb their frustrations, sparing the woman further trauma.

A survivor who is in the outward adjustment phase may deny any need for counseling. The nurse, respecting the woman's wishes, does not force counseling on her. The family, however, may still need assistance in coping with anger or guilt. The survivor's behavior may confuse them. By providing information and support, the nurse can help them examine and reconcile their feelings.

As the woman enters the reorganizational phase, she usually feels a strong urge to discuss and resolve her feelings about herself and her assailant. During this phase, the survivor may benefit from counseling.

Provision of Effective Rape Counseling

Rape counseling is an extended process of supporting the rape survivor as she comes to terms with her assault and its impact on her life. In many instances counselors who work with women who have been raped are nurses with additional education, but other health professionals also provide this counseling. (In this section the terms "counselor" and "nurse" are used interchangeably.)

Initially, the counselor and survivor explore the survivor's feelings and establish rapport. Feelings that have been denied and suppressed are brought into the woman's awareness. She should be encouraged to express those feelings openly, identify their source, and understand that they belong to her. Acceptance of the woman and respect for her are essential. The woman must feel that she can come to the nurse in a safe, stable, nonjudgmental environment to express her feelings fully and get in touch with them.

Having identified her feelings, the survivor and the nurse go on to clarify them and understand their source. Understanding the reasons for her feelings enables the woman to decide on actions that will resolve her problems. The nurse can assist her in understanding the larger context of the rape. It is important for the nurse to avoid reinforcing the prevalent myth that rape is the survivor's "fault." Rather, the nurse can use questions and discussion to encourage the woman to conclude that the blame lies with the rapist. Similarly, the nurse assists the individual in formulating strategies for returning to her pre-rape level of functioning.

In the final phase of counseling the survivor makes specific plans for overcoming her problems and tests them with the nurse's support. With the nurse, the woman explores her thoughts and feelings about self-care, celebrates her victories, and evaluates her defeats. It is important to emphasize that the loss of control that occurred during the rape was temporary and that the woman does have control over other aspects of her life.

Evaluation

Nurses working in an area such as an emergency department where survivors of rape are seen for evaluation and treatment are usually not able to learn of the woman's ultimate adjustment following sexual abuse. In evaluating the effectiveness of care, however, certain factors are important. Care has been effective if, when the woman leaves the area, she has developed a measure of trust in the staff and feels that she has been treated with courtesy and respect and has not been blamed *in any way* for her rape.

Her physical care should have been done efficiently and carefully, and the chain of evidence should have been maintained. The woman should have a list of community resources for rape survivors and should have information on the follow-up care and testing she requires. This information should include a referral to someone skilled in counseling the survivors of rape. Her friends and family, if present, should feel that they have been treated courteously and had their questions answered and their concerns addressed.

Rape as a Community Responsibility

Preventive education, funding of rape crisis counseling centers, and prosecution of the rapist are community responsibilities.

Preventive Education

Community colleges or local rape awareness groups may offer courses in preventive strategies. Some classes focus on increasing women's awareness of situations in which they are at risk. Others are concerned with changing societal attitudes about rape and rape survivors. Because rape is a considerable risk for any woman, courses in what to do during and after a rape may also be helpful. Nurses are well qualified to initiate or participate in preventive instruction.

Rape Crisis Counseling

Most rape crisis counseling centers operate 24 hours a day, 7 days a week. Their services are invaluable. Properly trained telephone counselors can help the woman regain control early in the crisis. Early crisis intervention often encourages the woman to seek professional treatment and assistance. Many rape crisis centers offer free counseling to rape survivors or can refer them to qualified counselors. Information on sexually transmitted infections and pregnancy alternatives may also be obtained from these centers.

Prosecution of the Rapist

Legally, rape, like any criminal action, is considered a crime against the state rather than against the victim. Therefore, prosecution of the assailant is a community responsibility in which the district attorney will act on the victim's behalf. The victim, however, must initiate the process by reporting the crime and pressing charges against her assailant. Once authorities have apprehended the alleged rapist, the judicial system is set into motion.

Procedures vary from state to state. A judge or magistrate generally conducts a hearing to determine whether there is sufficient evidence that a crime has in fact been committed and that the accused has committed it. If so, the alleged assailant will be bound over for the grand jury. The grand jury will hear the state's evidence (not the defense), again to determine whether the evidence is sufficient for trial. If so, the defendant is indicted; if not, he is acquitted. Once indicted, a defendant must stand trial unless he waives this right. He may elect to have his case heard by a judge rather than a jury. Either a judge or a jury will find the defendant guilty or not guilty, and he will be retained or set free accordingly.

Many rape survivors who have gone through the judicial process refer to it as a second rape—and sometimes a more damaging one. The survivor will be repeatedly asked to identify the assailant and describe the rape in intimate detail. Throughout the pretrial period the defense attorney may use delaying tactics, obtaining continuances or postponements, further frustrating the survivor and her support system. Publicity may intensify her feelings of humiliation, and if the assailant is released on bail, she may fear retaliation.

During the trial itself, cross-examination by the defense attorney can be a severely degrading experience in which the "victim as temptress" myth is continually evoked. Although some states have altered their laws so that the survivor's sexual history may not be made public, others have not. The defense attorney will try to discredit her testimony, causing her to feel victimized a second time.

The nurse acting as a counselor needs to be aware of the judicial sequence to anticipate rising tension and frustration in the survivor and her support system. They will need consistent, effective support at this crucial time.

KEY CONCEPTS

Female partner battering is a common occurrence, but it is the least reported serious crime in the United States.

Battering occurs in a cyclic pattern called the "cycle of violence," which increases in frequency and severity over time.

Nurses are in an excellent position to intervene and assist battered women by recognizing their cues, diagnosing their problems appropriately, and understanding the complex dynamics of the battering family. The nurse provides information about available community resources, medical attention, and emotional support.

The FBI's Uniform Crime Report indicates that a rape occurs every 5 minutes in the United States, yet a majority of rapes are unreported. The assailant is known to the woman 78% of the time. Estimates suggest that one out of every three women will be raped at some time in her life.

Why men rape remains a mystery, although it has been established that rape is an act of violence acted out sexually. Most rapes are expressions of anger or power.

Following rape, the survivor will usually experience an assortment of symptoms known as the rape trauma syndrome. Recent research also links the effects of rape to the post-traumatic stress disorder experienced by many veterans following the Vietnam War.

The nursing actions to assist rape survivors are encompassed in the roles of advocate, educator, and counselor.

Nurses inform the woman of the sequence of events involved in providing her care and developing the chain of evidence and support the survivor's decisions.

The counseling process used by the nurse follows the crisis intervention model because the survivor is in a situational crisis rather than being ill.

Widespread education is needed to abolish societal myths surrounding rape.

REFERENCES

American Nurses Association: Position Statement on Physical Violence Against Women. Washington DC: ANA, 1991.

Beckmann CRB, Groetzinger LL: Treating sexual assault victims: A protocol for health professionals. *Female Patient* May 1989; 14:78.

Bohn DK: Domestic violence and pregnancy: Implications for practice. *J Nurse-Midwifery* February 1990; 35(2):86.

Buchwald E et al: *Transforming a Rape Culture*. Minneapolis, MN: Milkweed Editions, 1993.

Bullock LFC et al: Breaking the cycle of abuse: How nurses can intervene. *J Psychosoc Nurs* 1989; 27(8):1113.

Burge SK: Violence against women as a health care issue. *Fam Med* September/October 1989; 21:368.

Burgess AW, Holmstrom LL: *Rape: Crisis and Recovery*. Englewood Cliffs, NJ: Prentice Hall, 1979.

Campbell JC: Woman abuse and public policy: Potential for nursing action. *AWHONN Clin Issues Perinatal Women Health Nurs* 1993; 4(3):503.

Campbell JC, Sheridan DJ: Emergency nursing interventions with battered women. *J Emerg Nurs* 1989; 15(1):12.

Chez N: Helping the victim of domestic violence. *AJN* July 1994; 94(7):32.

Crooks R, Baur K: *Our Sexuality*, 5th ed. Monterey, CA: Brooks Cole, 1993.

DeKeseredy WS et al: Sexual assault and stranger aggression on a Canadian university campus. *Sex Roles* 1993; 28(5/6):263.

Dennis LI: Adolescent rape: The role of nursing. *Issues Comprehensive Pediat Nurs* 1988; 11:59.

Department of Health & Human Services, Public Health Services: *Healthy People 2000*. Washington DC: Publication No. PHS 91-50213, 1990.

Dupre AR et al: Sexual assault. *Obstet Gynecol Survey* 1993; 48(9):640.

Federal Bureau of Investigation, US Department of Justice: *Crime in the United States, 1991*. August 30, 1992; 14.

Fishwick N: Nursing care of rural battered women. *AWHONN Clin Issues Perinatal Women Health Nurs* 1993; 4(3):441.

Foster IM, Bartlett J: Anti-HIV substances for rape victims (letter). *JAMA* 1989; 261(23):3407

Furniss K et al: What you can do to stop domestic violence. *Contemp OB/GYN* November 1993; 1(4):5.

Golan N: *Treatment in Crisis Situations*. New York: Free Press, 1978.

Gordon MT, Riger S: *The Female Fear*. New York: Free Press, 1989.

Gostin LO et al: HIV testing, counseling, and prophylaxis after sexual assault. *JAMA* May 11, 1994; 271(18):1436.

Helton AS, Snodgrass FG: Battering during pregnancy: Intervention strategies. *Birth* 1987; 14(3):142.

Herman JL: *Trauma and Recovery*. New York: Basic Books, 1992.

Hoff LA: Battered women: Understanding, identification, and assessment. *J Am Acad Nurs Pract* October/December 1992; 4(4):148.

Kennedy PH: Sexual abuse within adult intimate relationships. *AWHONN Clin Issues Perinatal Women Health Nurs* 1993; 4(3):391.

King MC: Changing women's lives: The primary prevention of violence against women. *AWHONN Clin Issues Perinatal Women Health Nurs* 1993; 4(3):449.

King MC, Ryan J: Abused women: Dispelling myths and encouraging intervention. *Nurse Pract* 1989; 14(5):47.

Koop CE: Doctors announce campaign to combat domestic violence. ACOG news release, January 3, 1989.

Malamuth N: Rape proclivity among males. *J Soc Issues* 1981; 37:138.

Mollica RF, Son L: Cultural dimensions in the evaluation and treatment of sexual trauma. *Psych Clin North Am* June 1989; 12:363.

Muehlenhard CL: Misinterpreted dating behaviors and the risk of date rape. *J Soc Clin Psychol* 1988; 6(1):20.

National Victim Center and the Crime Victim's Research and Treatment Center: *Rape in America: A Report to the Nation*. April 23, 1992.

Renshaw DC: Treatment of sexual exploitation: Rape and incest. *Psych Clin North Am* June 1989; 12:257.

Robinson JC: Rape—A crime with health consequences. *Female Patient* March 1990; 15:25.

Silverman DC et al: Blitz rape and confidence rape: A typology applied to 1,000 consecutive cases. *Am J Psychiatry* November 1988; 145:1438.

Smolowe J: When violence hits home. *Time* July 4, 1994, p 19.

Sonstegard LJ et al: *Women's Health Ambulatory Care*, vol. 1. New York: Grune & Stratton, 1982.

Stenchever MA, Stenchever DH: Abuse of women: An overview. *Women's Health Issues* Fall 1991; 1(4):187.

The mind of the rapist. *Newsweek*, July 23, 1990, p 46.

Walker L: *The Battered Woman Syndrome*. New York: Springer, 1984.

PART FOUR

PREGNANCY

CHAPTER 12

PREPARATION FOR CHILDBIRTH

*C*hoices are important. They determine how you experience giving birth and how your baby enters the world. They must be made in the present and lived with in the future.

~ PREGNANT FEELINGS ~

KEY TERMS

Birth plan

Disassociation relaxation

Doula

Effleurage

Prenatal education

Progressive relaxation

Psychoprophylactic (Lamaze) method

Touch relaxation

OBJECTIVES

Apply the nursing process in assisting couples to prepare for childbirth.

Identify the various issues related to pregnancy, labor, and birth that require decision making by parents.

Discuss the basic goals of childbirth education.

Summarize the role of the doula/labor companion during labor and birth.

Describe the types of prenatal education programs available to expectant families.

Delineate the childbirth educator's role in decreasing anxiety for pregnant women.

Compare methods of childbirth preparation.

*P*reparation for parenthood begins with one's own birth into a family. Attitudes, feelings, and fears about parenthood are molded by relationships with one's own parents and the relationships observed in others' families.

A person's experiences with parenting or children may have been pleasant or uncomfortable. The information an individual has about parenthood and related areas may or may not be accurate. Because people bring their beliefs and fears with them to the childbearing period, the nurse can do much to correct misconceptions and calm fears regarding pregnancy, childbirth, and early parenting. One way that a couple can cope with feelings about impending parenthood is to assume an active, participatory role during the preconception, prenatal, intrapartal, and postpartal periods. This involvement enables them to take part in many of the decisions regarding the conduct of the birth. It offers them a degree of control over what could be an overwhelming experience.

Some of the decisions that the childbearing family must consider are presented in this chapter. The chapter addresses issues such as the decision to have a baby, choice of care provider, type of childbirth preparation, place of birth, activities during the birth, method of infant feeding, and choices surrounding treatment of the newborn. It also considers the role of the nurse, who provides information that enables the family to make informed decisions.

Throughout this chapter the term "childbearing family" is used. In today's society the childbearing family may be composed of a man and a woman joined by marriage or simply by mutual personal commitment, a single woman living alone or with another partner or a family member, or a lesbian couple. No matter what the family structure and configuration, the expectant woman and her support person have similar concerns and educational needs during this time. In this chapter the term "childbearing family" includes all family types.

Today's professional nurse has many opportunities to help the childbearing family make the decisions that are part of pregnancy and birth. The nurse can help families select a health care provider, find prenatal classes that meet their needs, and make informed choices. Even more important, as the family works through these decisions, the nurse is able to affirm their decision-making abilities and their ability to take on parenting roles. For first-time parents in particular the decisions may seem numerous and complicated. The nurse has a unique opportunity to help these families establish a pattern of decision making that will serve them well in their years as parents (Figure 12–1).

PRECONCEPTION COUNSELING

One of the first questions a couple should ask prior to conception is whether they wish to have children. This involves consideration of each person's personal goals, expectations of their relationship, and desire to be a parent. Often one individual wishes to have a child while the other does not. In such situations, an open discussion is

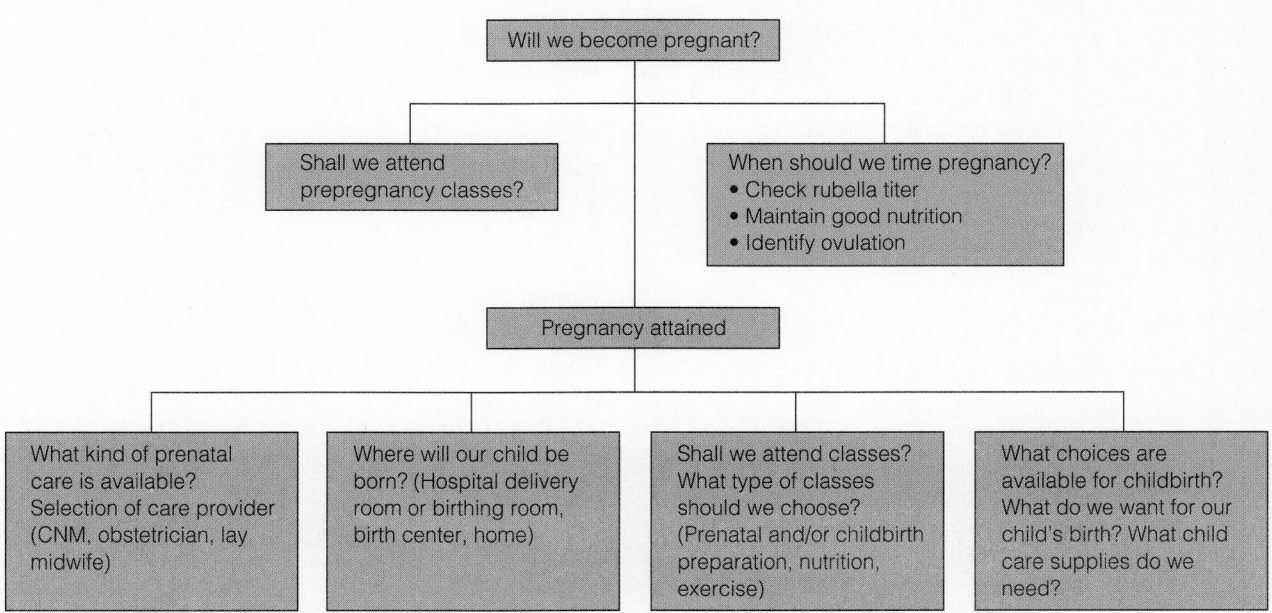

FIGURE 12-1   Pregnancy decision tree.

essential to reach a mutually acceptable decision. In some cases this may require couple's counseling.

Couples who wish to have children face a decision about the timing of pregnancy. At what point in their lives do they believe it would be best to become parents? Pregnancy comes as a surprise even when the decision about timing is made, but at least the couple has some control over it.

RESEARCH IN PRACTICE

A woman's psychologic well-being during the developmental stage of pregnancy may significantly moderate her transition to motherhood and her relationship with her child. The woman's attachments with her mother and with her husband are two influential factors in the woman's psychologic well-being during pregnancy. These attachments provide an important portion of the pregnant woman's social support. Theories hold that mother-daughter relationships lay the foundation for the daughter's future attachments and impact her adaptation to the maternal role. A positive husband-wife relationship correlates with maternal warmth and positive attitudes about childbirth.

Rachel Zachariah used this conceptual framework to test a model hypothesizing that both attachment with her husband and attachment with her mother would correlate with a pregnant woman's psychologic well-being. Zachariah further hypothesized that, after controlling for sociodemographic variables, these two attachments combined would contribute significantly to the woman's psychologic well-being. The sample included 115 pregnant Canadian women reared by their mothers, living with their husbands, expecting their first child, and at least 18 years of age. The author used established tools to measure husband-wife attachment, mother-daughter attachment, social support, and psychologic well-being. Reliability and validity issues were addressed for each tool.

Both mother-daughter and husband-wife attachment correlated with psychologic well-being. In addition, emotional support, socioeconomic status, and age of the woman all correlated positively with psychologic well-being. Multiple regression analysis showed that the husband-wife attachment, age of wife, and mother-daughter attachment explained 36% of the variability for the pregnant woman's psychologic well-being. Of these factors, the husband-wife attachment made the most significant contribution (beta = 0.42, $p < 0.001$).

Clinical Application of Study

In any pregnancy, the nurse needs to assess the support system available to the pregnant woman. Because the woman's relationship with her husband and with her mother relate to her psychologic well-being, health care professionals should assess and support these relationships in particular. If either or both of these supportive participants is not available, the nurse can assist the woman in strengthening other important relationships.

SOURCE: Zachariah R: Mother-daughter and husband-wife attachment as predictors of psychological well-being during pregnancy. *Clin Nurs Res* 1994; 3(4): 371.

For couples who have religious beliefs that do not support contraception or who feel that fertility planning is unnatural and wrong, planning the timing of pregnancy is unacceptable and irrelevant. These couples can still take steps to ensure that they are in the best possible physical and mental health when pregnancy occurs.

Preconception Health Measures

If a couple has decided to have a child or if the couple does not find planning acceptable, they may make an effort to maximize the quality of their health. This effort should include making life-style changes to avoid known or potential health risks such as alcohol.

Because there is no definite safe level for alcohol consumption during pregnancy and because the woman is often pregnant before she realizes it, a woman planning to become pregnant should be advised to stop drinking totally if possible. Because the effects on the embryo of heavy drinking by the father are not as well understood, less emphasis has been placed on male drinking. However, studies suggest that heavy alcohol consumption may decrease a man's fertility. Furthermore, the woman may find it more difficult to avoid alcohol if her partner continues to drink. Thus it is helpful if her partner also restricts his alcohol intake.

Smoking during pregnancy has been associated with decreased weight gain of the fetus and preterm labor (Kochenour 1994).

The effects of caffeine are less clearly understood. Because it poses a potential risk, women are advised to stop drinking beverages containing caffeine completely if possible or at least limit them to two drinks per day. In addition to coffee, tea, colas, and chocolate, caffeine is found in medications such as Excedrin, Anacin, and many appetite suppressants.

Many of the social (cocaine, marijuana, LSD) and street (heroin, crack) drugs pose a very serious threat to a fetus. Prescription drugs can also be hazardous. A woman who uses any drugs or medications should discuss the implications of their use with her health care provider. In most cases it is best to avoid the use of medication whenever possible.

Certain jobs result in exposure to agents that can reduce a man's or woman's fertility or that might cause harm to the fetus if the woman becomes pregnant. This is especially true of exposure to radiation, photographic chemicals, and anesthetic agents. When a couple is contemplating pregnancy, they should carefully consider whether they are exposed to any environmental hazards at work or in their community. (See Chapter 8.)

Physical Examination

It is advisable for both partners to have a physical examination to identify any health problems so that they can be corrected if possible. These might include medical conditions such as high blood pressure or obesity; problems that pose a threat to fertility, such as certain sexually transmitted diseases; or conditions that keep the individual from achieving optimal health, such as anemia or colitis. If the family history indicates previous genetic disorders or if the couple is planning pregnancy when the woman is over age 35, the health care provider may suggest that the couple consider genetic counseling (see Chapter 7 for additional discussion). In addition to the history and physical exam the woman may have the following laboratory tests: urinalysis, complete blood count, Rh factor, Venereal Disease Research Laboratory (VDRL) test, Pap smear, gonorrhea culture, and rubella and hepatitis screens (Rosen 1990).

Prior to conception the woman is also advised to have a dental examination and any necessary dental work to avoid exposure to x-rays and the risk of infection.

Nutrition

Prior to conception it is advisable for the woman to be at an average weight for her body build and height. She should follow a nutritious diet that contains ample quantities of all the essential nutrients. Some nutritionists advocate emphasizing the following nutrients: calcium, protein, iron, B complex vitamins, vitamin C, folic acid, and magnesium. Excessive vitamin intake can cause severe fetal problems and should be avoided.

Exercise

A woman is advised to establish a regular exercise plan beginning at least 3 months before she plans to attempt to become pregnant. The exercise chosen should be one she enjoys and will continue. It should provide some aerobic conditioning and some general toning. Exercise improves the woman's circulation and general health and tones her muscles. Once an exercise program is well established, the woman is generally encouraged to continue it during pregnancy. For a discussion of exercise during pregnancy see Chapter 15.

Contraception

Women who wish to conceive and who take birth control pills are advised to stop the pill and have two or three normal menses before attempting pregnancy. This allows the natural hormonal cycle to return and facilitates dating the subsequent pregnancy. Women using an intrauterine device are advised to have it removed and wait 1 month before attempting to conceive. This allows the endometrium to be resterilized. During the waiting period barrier methods of contraception (condoms, diaphragm, cervical cap, or spermicides) are recommended.

Conception

Most preconception recommendations focus on helping the couple attain their best possible health state so that they do not enter pregnancy with unnecessary risks. Conception is a personal and emotional experience, and even if a couple is prepared, they may feel some ambivalence. This is a normal response, but they may require reassurance that the ambivalence will pass. A couple may get so caught up in preparation and in their efforts to "do things right" that they lose sight of the pleasure they derive from each other and their lives together and cease to value the joy of spontaneity in their relationship. It is often helpful for the health care provider to remind an overly zealous couple that moderation is always appropriate and that there is value in taking "time to smell the roses."

CHILDBEARING DECISIONS

When a couple discovers that the woman is pregnant, they are faced with many decisions. For instance they must make decisions about who will provide health care, where their child will be born, who will attend the birth, and whether to attend prepregnancy or prenatal classes. The woman must also make decisions about whether to have analgesia, perineal preparation, an enema, or the use of stirrups; what position to use during labor and birth; and whether to breastfeed her child.

Some parents deal with the numerous decisions regarding childbirth by devising a **birth plan.** In this plan they identify aspects of the childbearing experience that are most important to them. The birth plan helps identify options that may be available, and it becomes a tool for communication between the couple, the health care providers, and the personnel at the birth setting (Kitzinger 1992). The plan helps the couple set priorities for activities that they want. A sample birth plan is presented in Figure 12–2.

The birth plan identifies many factors associated with childbirth. One of the first decisions that the woman or couple needs to make is the type of care provider to use and how to choose that health care provider. The choice and the place of birth frequently go hand in hand.

As the couple seeks information, nurses can assist in the decision-making process. The nurse can discuss various types of care providers so that the couple knows what to expect from each type. The couple needs to know the differences between the educational preparation, skill level, and general philosophy of certified nurse-midwives, obstetricians, family practice physicians, and lay midwives. The nurse also provides information about different types of birth settings and assists the couple in obtaining further information through tours of facilities and reading. Questions regarding the care provider's credentials, basic and special education and training, fee schedule, the health insurance plans that are accepted, and availability for new patients can be answered by telephoning a receptionist in the office. As the couple prepares to interview different care providers, they may want to develop a list of questions so that they will learn the desired information during the interview process. Sample questions may include:

Choice	I would like to have		Available	
	Yes	No	Yes	No
Care provider:				
Certified nurse-midwife				
Obstetrician				
Lay midwife				
Birth setting				
Hospital:				
Birthing room				
Delivery room				
Birth center				
Home				
Partner present				
During labor				
During birth				
During cesarean				
During whole postpartum period				
During labor:				
Ambulate as desired				
Shower if desired				
Wear own clothes				
Use hot tub				
Use own rocking chair				
Have perineal prep				
Have enema				
Water birth				
Electronic fetal monitor				
Membranes:				
Rupture naturally				
Amniotomy if needed				
Labor stimulation if needed				
Medication:				
Identify type desired				
Fluids or ice as desired				
Music during labor and birth				
Position during birth:				
On side				
Hands and knees				
Kneeling				
Squatting				
Birthing chair				
Birthing bed				
Other:				
Family present (sibs)				
Filming of birth				
Leboyer				
Episiotomy				
No sterile drapes				
Partner to cut umbilical cord				
Hold baby immediately after birth				
Breastfeed immediately after birth				
No separation after birth				
Save the placenta				
Newborn care:				
Eye treatment for the baby				
Vitamin K injection				
Breastfeeding				
Formula feeding				
Glucose water				
Circumcision				
Postpartum care:				
Rooming-in				
Short stay				
Sibling visitation				
Infant care classes				
Self-care classes				
Other:				

- Who is in practice with you, or who covers for you when you are off?
- How do your partners' philosophies compare to yours?
- What are your feelings about my partner (or other children) coming to the prenatal visits?
- What weight gain do you recommend and why?
- How many of your parents attend prenatal and/or childbirth preparation classes, and what type do they choose?
- What are your feelings about (add in special desires for the birth event, such as ambulation and different positions during labor, analgesics and regional blocks, episiotomy, induction of labor, electronic fetal monitoring, other people being present during birth, breastfeeding immediately after birth, no separation of infant and parents following birth, and so on)?
- If a cesarean is necessary, could my partner be present?
- What birthing facilities do you usually use?

The couple will also need to discuss the qualities that they want in a care provider for their newborn. They will probably want to visit with care providers prior to birth in order to select one who meets their needs.

Choosing a care provider is just one of the myriad of choices and decisions with which the couple is faced (see Table 12–1). Another area of decision making is demonstrated in the following situation:

Mr and Mrs Cline were discussing newborn care with Ms Gayle, the clinic nurse, during one of their prenatal appointments. The Clines had been gathering information about the clothes needed for a newborn and about infant feeding, but had not yet considered whether to use reuseable (cloth) or single-use (disposable) diapers. They wanted some help in getting information. Ms Gayle helped them devise a plan to collect information from a variety of sources regarding cost, convenience, and any implications for their baby. The Clines called a number of stores to determine the prices for cloth and single-use diapers. They investigated the cost of a diaper service, as well as the cost of laundering their own diapers. They found that laundering their own diapers was the least expensive, but having a diaper

FIGURE 12-2 Birth plan for childbirth choices. The column on the left lists various choices that the couple may consider during their childbirth experience. Once the couple has considered each of the choices, they may mark the "yes" or "no" space in the middle columns. The right columns are used to note the availability of some of the choices. For instance the couple may want to use a hot tub during labor, but the birthing settings in their community do not have hot tubs available. All choices need to be made in the context of what is available in the couple's community.

Issue	Benefits	Risks
Breastfeeding	No additional expense Contains maternal antibodies Decreases incidence of infant otitis media, vomiting, and diarrhea Easier to digest than formula Immediately after birth promotes uterine contractions and decreases incidence of postpartum hemorrhage	Transmission of pollutants that mother is exposed to such as pesticides to newborn Irregular ovulation and menses can cause false sense of security and nonuse of contraceptives Increased nutritional requirement in mother
Perineal prep	May decrease risk of infection Facilitates episiotomy repair	Nicks can be portal for bacteria Discomfort as hair grows back
Ambulation during labor	Comfort for laboring woman May assist in labor progression by stimulating contractions, allowing gravity to help descent of fetus, and giving sense of independence and control	Cord prolapse with ruptured membranes unless engagement has occurred Birth of infant in undesirable situations
Electronic fetal monitoring	Helps evaluate fetal well-being Helps identify fetal stress Useful in diagnostic testing Helps evaluate labor progress	Supine postural hypotension Intrauterine perforation (with internal uterine pressure device) Infection (with internal monitoring) Decreases personal interaction with mother because of attention paid to the machine Mother unable to ambulate or change her position freely
Whirlpool (jet hydrotherapy)	Increased relaxation Decreased anxiety Stimulation of labor Nonmedicated pain relief Slight decrease in B/P Increased diuresis	May slow contractions if used before active labor is established Possible risk of infection if membranes are ruptured Slight increase in maternal temperature and heart rate and fetal heart rate during whirlpool and/or in first 30 minutes after being in tub (Aderhold & Perry 1991)
Analgesia	Maternal relaxation facilitates labor	All drugs reach the fetus in varying degrees and with varying effects
Episiotomy	Decreased irregular tearing of perineum	Increased pain after birth and for 3 months following birth Infection Increased frequency of third- and fourth-degree lacerations (Mynaugh 1991)

service was only about a dollar more per week, and convenience was important to them because of their work schedules. Single-use diapers were the most expensive—approximately 50% higher than for a diaper service and 60% higher than laundering their own reuseable diapers (Lehrburger et al 1991). They had seen coupons for single-use and knew that would affect the price, but the Clines anticipated a storage problem if they purchased too many at once.

The Clines then turned to a consideration of ecologic issues and the implications of using a natural product (cotton cloth diapers) versus the use of natural resources (trees) to create the single-use diapers and the problems associated with disposal of the diapers. Currently in the United States single-use diapers make up 2% of landfills (Holaday et al 1995; Korte 1993). Although this seems a small amount, it translates into more than 2.6 million tons of disposable diapers that are thrown into landfills every year. Once in the landfill, it takes about 500 years (approximately 20 generations of one family) for the single-use diapers to decompose (Brink 1990). The Clines also discovered that over 100 types of viruses can be left in single-use diapers. Once the diapers are in the landfill, viruses can be carried into the ground water. That is why it is illegal in many communities to dump human or animal waste in landfills.

After a thorough study the Clines decided to use a diaper service. They shared their information with Ms Gayle and put

together a packet for other parents to use. The Clines felt they had investigated the questions thoroughly and made an informed decision.

Communication is the key to decision making. A discussion of childbirth expectations between the couple and the health care provider will create a foundation on which to build. This process represents one of many life skills inherent in preparation for birth.

Although most birth experiences are very close to the desired experience, at times the expectations cannot be met. This may be due to unavailability of some choices in the couple's community or the presence of unexpected problems during pregnancy or birth. It is important for nurses to help expectant parents keep sight of what is realistic and possible and to help them understand that when choices are made, alternatives may be necessary.

Birthing Environments: Choices

Until recently, the most prevalent setting for labor and birth was a hospital labor unit, composed of separate labor rooms, birthing rooms, and recovery area, and a different unit for the remaining hospital stay. This type of unit is still available in some hospitals. However, many hospitals have changed their labor and birth units to reflect the philosophy of family-centered care. In the newer units the woman is not moved from room to room during labor and birth.

Couples in some communities also have the option of using a free-standing birth center. These facilities have been created in answer to consumer demand for a more homelike, natural setting for their childbearing experience. The childbearing consumer wants to know what is happening, to maintain a sense of dignity, and to maintain control over the childbearing experience.

For the small number of couples who feel that even the family-centered hospital setting or a free-standing birth center do not offer them enough control, home birth is another option (Figure 12–3).

The Hospital Setting

In hospitals offering the more traditional maternity service with a separate labor and birth area, newborn nursery, and postpartum area the nursing staff remains constant in one area, and a certified nurse-midwife or physician may be involved with the birth. This type of birth setting tends to be a large metropolitan hospital with many births per year.

In many other hospitals the "birth center" room is usually decorated in a homelike manner with drapes, wall paper, and wooden furniture. The laboring woman is admitted into the birthing room and remains there during labor, birth, and the recovery period, and the newborn remains in the room with the mother. In many centers she also remains in this room throughout the postpartum stay. The nursing community calls these rooms "single purpose" and may refer to them as LDR (labor, delivery, and recovery room), LDB (labor, delivery, and birth room), or LDRP (labor, delivery, recovery, and postpartum room).

In contrast with the traditional labor and delivery unit, in which health care professionals wear sterile gowns and masks for the birth and the woman is not encouraged to choose alternative birth positions, the birthing center of a less traditional hospital is much more relaxed. The personnel may wear bright-colored scrub suits, the individual choices of the birthing couple are encouraged, the woman may assume a variety of positions for labor and birth, and the couple is permitted to invite whoever they wish for the birth. The newborn remains with the mother for a time after birth, and breastfeeding is encouraged immediately after birth. The emphasis is placed on family unity and family desires. The expectant couple may choose this environment because it offers the more homelike setting while also offering high-risk care and the availability of emergency assistance.

Free-Standing Birth Centers

Care in free-standing birth centers is given by certified nurse-midwives, labor and birth nurses, nurse practitioners, physicians, nonmedical assistants, public health nurses, families themselves, or any combination of these. *Birth centers* require families to take more responsibility for the birth experience than usual while providing a more flexible and less costly way to give birth.

Birth centers strive for a warm, homelike atmosphere, with birthing rooms similar to typical bedrooms. The room is generally furnished with a bed, in which the woman labors and gives birth, comfortable chairs for the father and other relatives or friends, a cradle, and private bath and/or shower. Some free-standing centers also have play rooms for siblings, kitchens where families may keep food or beverages, and other amenities. Most free-standing centers encourage children to participate to whatever extent they choose. Some hospital-based centers are somewhat more reluctant to allow total participation in childbirth by siblings.

Birth centers meet criteria for maintaining safety in out-of-hospital births. These criteria include attendance by qualified health care professionals, screening and transfer criteria, a transport system immediately available, and a readily accessible backup physician and hospital facility.

In keeping with the concept of birth as a normal event most birth centers are set up for nurse-midwife management of labor and birth rather than for obstetric technology and treatment. Therefore these centers are not appropriate for high-risk birth. Couples intending to use the centers are screened during pregnancy for high-risk factors (see Chapters 18 and 19). The presence of any one factor does not automatically exclude the woman from giving birth in a birth center, but it does mean that careful and continuous assessment is vital.

> *What I've seen time and again is that the technology of the hospital overwhelms patients' natural instincts; they are intimidated, afraid of appearing stupid or clumsy or sentimental in a surrounding that seems too efficient and immaculate and intelligent.*
> ~ A MIDWIFE'S STORY ~

Each center also has policies about various circumstances that would require the woman to be transferred to a hospital birth setting. These may include, but are not limited to, the following:

- An increase in maternal temperature to over 37.8 C (100.4 F)
- A significant change in blood pressure
- Meconium-stained amniotic fluid
- Prolonged true labor
- Significant vaginal bleeding
- Prolonged second stage of labor (more than 2 hours for a nullipara and more than 1 hour for a multipara)
- Indications of fetal stress or distress

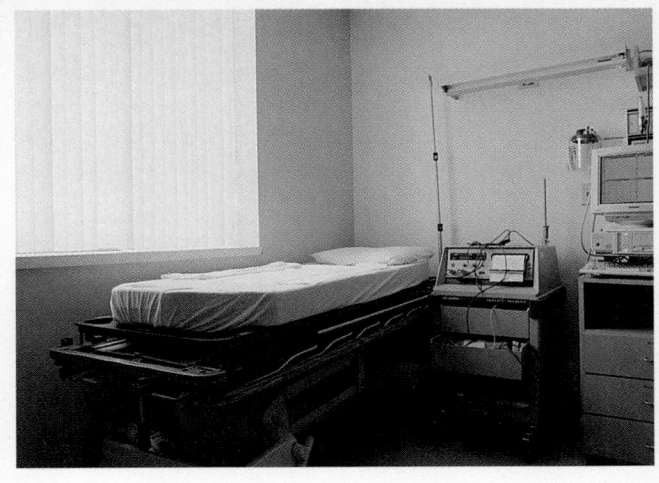

A

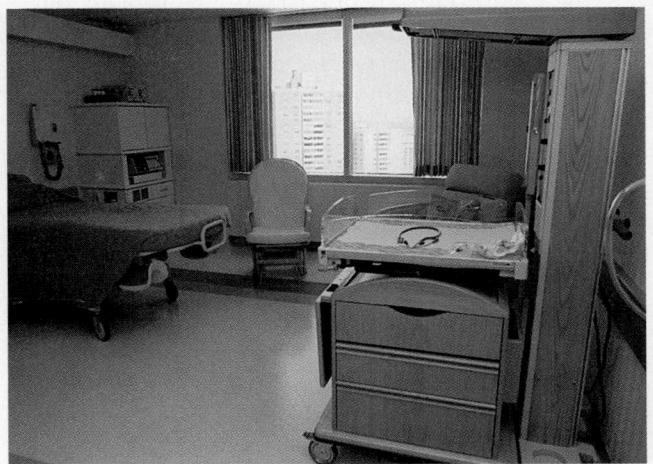

B

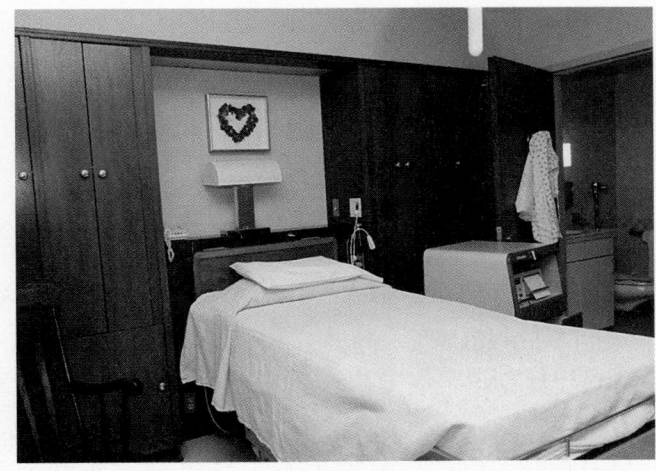

C

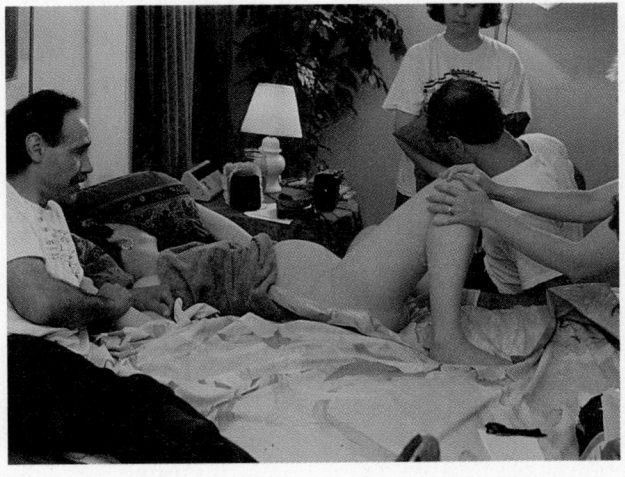

D

FIGURE 12-3 Birth settings. *A* In-hospital maternity unit. *B* In-hospital birthing room.
C Free-standing birth center. *D* Home birth.

The couple is encouraged to attend prenatal classes to prepare for childbirth. They are also encouraged to meet birthing center personnel and to discuss their desires and preferences.

Traditional obstetric procedures are generally omitted. Episiotomies are not routine, forceps are not used, and in many centers the woman may give birth in the position of her choice. After the birth physical contact between the parents and newborn is encouraged. The mother may breastfeed immediately. Siblings and accompanying support persons are also encouraged to interact with the newborn as they choose.

If rooming-in is immediate, healthy newborns and their families are not separated. The initial pediatric examination is frequently conducted in the presence of the family. The mother and newborn are monitored for 2 to 24 hours after birth and then discharged.

Birth center personnel usually perform a home visit after discharge. The home visit provides an opportunity to see the family in their home setting, to make assessments of the mother and newborn, to answer questions, and to provide information and support.

Home Births

Another alternative to the traditional hospital birth is home birth. Couples who choose home birth generally have strong beliefs about their rights to make their own birth choices. Couples choosing home births believe that the responsibility for the birth outcome is theirs. Furthermore, they do not believe the hospital is necessarily the safest place to give birth, and they see standard medical practice as frequently involving unnecessary trauma and intervention. Some women may feel that hospital routines and expectations will not allow them to conform to their cultural norms for childbearing behavior.

In making the choice between home and hospital birth medical risk is only one issue. The effect on the family unit is another issue. Parents who take responsibility for a home birth feel that it is a warm, close, loving experience under their control. The newborn is immediately incorporated into the family, and the continuous contact between the newborn and the family helps to bond the family as a unit. Siblings present during the birth are able to welcome the newborn into the family and are participants in an exciting and beautiful experience.

The safety of any home birth is maximized by thorough planning, careful prenatal care and screening, skilled physicians or nurse-midwives, and an organized and tested transport system to a facility where accepting care givers are available. However, adequate medical backup care is frequently unobtainable. Obstetricians as a group are particularly vocal opponents of home birth. Their opposition is often based on memories of serious emergencies they have witnessed at the time of birth. Therefore they usually view home birth as a backward step in maternal-child care.

Choosing the Birth Setting

Information regarding the birth setting can be obtained from tours of the facilities and from talking with nurses and recent parents. Expectant couples may ask recent parents the following questions:

- What kind of support did you receive during labor? Was it what you wanted?
- If the setting has both labor and delivery rooms and birthing rooms, was the type of room you wanted available when you wanted it?
- Were you encouraged to be mobile during labor or to do what you wanted to do (walking, sitting in a rocking chair, remaining in bed, sitting in a hot tub, standing in a shower, and so on)?
- Was your labor partner or coach treated well?
- Was your birth plan respected? Did you share it with the facility before the birth? If something did not work, why do you think there were problems?
- How were medications handled during labor? Were you comfortable with it?
- Were siblings welcomed in the birth setting? After the birth?
- Was the nursing staff helpful after the baby was born? Did you receive self-care and infant care information? Was it in a usable form? Did you have a choice about what information you got? Did they let you decide what information you needed?

The Labor Support Person

Some of the first formal childbirth preparation classes were patterned after a book entitled *Husband Coached Childbirth* by Dr Robert Bradley, published in 1965. Since that time, husbands and other partners of the expectant woman have been very involved in acting as "coaches" during childbirth classes, labor, and birth. Recently, however, there has been recognition of the facts that some partners do not want to play an active role during labor and birth, and some pregnant women are not finding the kind of support they desire. Chapman (1991) studied fathers during childbirth and found that they usually take on one of three roles: (1) In the "coach" role the father actively assists the woman in comfort and breathing techniques and seems to assume responsibility for helping direct the course of her responses during labor. (2) The "teammate" is very willing to help, but waits for direction from the nurse or physician. (3) The "witness" is willing to hold the woman's hand, but for the most part does not seek further involvement and is comfortable to simply observe the process. Chapman's study and other information about partners' comfort levels and their personal and cultural expectations of their role have created awareness that some women need support from another source.

When the partner is not actively involved in supportive, attentive care, most women look to another woman for empathy and help (Simkin 1992). Out of this need for companionship and special support in the birthing journey the role of the **doula** has evolved. "Doula" is a Greek word that means "woman's servant." In the birthing environment doula refers to a companion who provides support but does not perform any clinical tasks. The doula provides emotional, physical, and informational support and acts as an advocate for the woman and her family by verbalizing their wishes to the nurses and physicians or certified nurse-midwives. A doula may also be trained to provide support and care during the postpartum period (Simkin 1992). The doula may accompany the childbearing couple on a volunteer basis or may be paid a fee by the family. Synonyms for doula are labor support person, birth assistant, and labor assistant (Simkin 1992). Another support person who has been involved in labor and birthing is a *monitrice*. "Monitrice" is a French word that refers to a specially trained nurse who provides assessment, nursing care, and support (Simkin 1992). The role of monitrice is not common in the United States.

Currently, many women and physicians favor the use of an epidural to provide more comfort for the woman during labor, and therefore the need for a doula is perceived as less vital (Klaus et al 1993). But because birthing practices change over time, the use of epidural regional blocks is predicted to decrease as women once again want less intervention and a more natural, unmedicated approach to labor.

Siblings at Birth

The couple may decide to have their other children present at the birth. Children who will attend a birth can be prepared through books, audiovisual materials, models, discussion, and sibling classes. Nurses can assist parents with sibling preparation by helping them understand the stresses a child may experience. For example, the child may feel left out when there is a new child to love or disappointed if a brother is born when a sister is expected.

It is highly recommended that the child have his or her own support person or coach whose sole responsibility is tending to the needs of the child. The support person should be well known to the child, warm, sensitive, flexible, knowledgeable about the birth process, and comfortable with sexuality and birth. This person must be prepared to interpret what is happening to the child and to intervene when necessary. The support person should not be one who would be hesitant to leave (such as a maternal grandmother). Instead, the person responsible for the child must be amenable to the child's desire to leave the birthing room.

The child should be given the option of relating to the birth in whatever manner she or he chooses as long as it is not disruptive. Children should understand that it is their own choice to be there and that they may stay or leave the room as they choose. To help the child meet his or her goal, the nurse may wish to elicit exactly what the child expects from the experience. The child needs to feel free to ask questions and express feelings.

In general siblings' presence at birth engenders feelings of interest and the desire to nurture "our" baby, as opposed to jealousy and rivalry directed at "Mom's" baby. The mother does not disappear mysteriously to the hospital and return with a demanding outsider. Instead the family attending the birth together finds a new opportunity for closeness and growth by sharing in the birth of a new member.

CLASSES FOR FAMILY MEMBERS DURING PREGNANCY

Prenatal Education

Programs of **prenatal education** vary in their goals, content, leadership techniques, and method of teaching. The content of a class is generally dictated by its goals (Fleming 1992). For example, if the goal of a class is to prepare the couple for childbirth, it may not address the discomforts of pregnancy and the care of the newborn. Other classes may focus only on pregnancy, not labor and birth. Special classes are also available for couples who know that the woman will be having a cesarean birth. Nurses should be aware of couples' goals before directing them to specific classes.

Class Content

Childbirth preparation classes usually contain information regarding changes in the woman and the developing baby (Table 12–2).

From the expectant parents' point of view class content is best presented in chronology with the pregnancy. Although both parents expect to learn breathing and relaxation techniques and infant care, fathers usually expect facts, and mothers expect coping strategies. It is important that the classes begin by finding out what each parent wants to learn (Shearer 1990).

At times prenatal classes are divided into early and late classes.

Early Classes: First Trimester

Early prenatal classes should include both couples in early pregnancy and preconception couples. The classes contain information regarding early gestational changes, self-care during pregnancy, fetal development and environmental dangers for the fetus, sexuality in pregnancy, birth settings and types of care providers, nutrition, rest and exercise suggestions, common discomforts of pregnancy and relief measures, psychologic changes in pregnancy for the woman and man, and information needed to get the pregnancy off to a good start. Early classes should provide information about factors that place the woman at risk for preterm labor and about recognition of

TABLE 12-2   Possible Content for Childbirth Preparation Classes

Early classes (first trimester)
    Early gestational changes
    Self-care during pregnancy
    Fetal development, environmental dangers for the fetus (teratogens)
    Sexuality in pregnancy
    Birth settings and types of care providers
    Nutrition, rest, and exercise suggestions
    Relief measures for common discomforts of pregnancy
    Psychologic changes in pregnancy
    Information for getting pregnancy off to a good start

Later classes (second and third trimesters)
    Preparation for birth process
    Role of partner, doula, labor companion
    Birth choices (episiotomy, medications, fetal monitoring, perineal prep, enema)
    Postpartum self-care
    Newborn safety issues (ie, car seats)
    Transition to early parenting

Adolescent preparation classes
    How to be a good parent
    Newborn care
    Health dangers for the baby
    Healthy diet during pregnancy
    How to recognize when baby is ill
    Baby care: physical and emotional

Breastfeeding programs
    Advantages and disadvantages
    Techniques of breastfeeding
    Methods of breast preparation
    Involvement of fathers in feeding process

Sibling preparation

Grandparents' classes

Preparation for cesarean birth

Preparation for vaginal birth after cesarean birth (VBAC)

---

possible signs and symptoms of preterm labor. Early classes should also include information on infant feeding to lay the groundwork for decision making.

Later Classes: Second and Third Trimesters

The later classes focus on preparation for the birth, infant care and feeding, postpartum self-care, birth choices (episiotomy, medications, fetal monitoring, perineal prep, enema, and so forth), and newborn safety issues. Because many parents purchase a car seat prior to birth, later classes should include information regarding how car seats work, the importance of car seats, and how to select an approved car seat (Baer 1992).

Broussard and Rich (1990) suggest that infant stimulation concepts that can be used later with the new baby be incorporated into childbirth preparation classes. This will aid in the development of parenting skills and enhance prenatal and newborn bonding. Infant stimulation that could be used include tactile, vestibular, auditory, and visual stimulation. Information regarding tactile stimulation can be presented while discussing maternal anatomy and physiology. As the uterine wall thins during the pregnancy the mother and father are better able to feel the baby, and the fetus can sense the parents' stroking and patting through the abdominal wall. Abdominal effleurage (a light stroking movement made over the abdominal wall with the fingertips) can also be used to provide tactile stimulation to the fetus.

Vestibular stimulation through movement of the fetus is provided while the expectant woman does the pelvic-tilt exercise. Rocking in a rocking chair is also a comfortable way to provide relaxation for the expectant woman and vestibular stimulation for the fetus. Auditory stimulation can be provided by playing music. Classical music (such as Vivaldi, Mozart, Beethoven, and Bach) is found to be pleasing to the fetus. In the prenatal period actual visual stimulation for the fetus is not possible because of the intrauterine environment. However, the parents can be encouraged to participate by visualizing the fetus "as lying calmly inside, all flexed, sucking its thumb, swallowing amniotic fluid, and opening its eyes to look toward the sunlight filtering through the abdominal wall" (Broussard & Rich 1990, p 384).

Adolescent Parenting Classes

Adolescents have special content learning needs during pregnancy. Bachman (1993) reported that teens in school-based health classes wanted to learn about infant illnesses and about complications of pregnancy, labor, and birth. In a study by Causby, Nixon, and Bright (1991) teens involved in schools with specialized educational programs for pregnant adolescents and new teenage parents were more prepared for parenthood and interacted more with their children, including talking more with them, having more structured play periods, and consciously encouraging the child's development.

Breastfeeding Programs

Programs offering prenatal and postpartal information on breastfeeding are increasing. Women who attend these classes are more likely to breastfeed and to start their infants on semisolid foods at the appropriate time (Shoham-Yakubovich et al 1993). The most important aspects of motivation to breastfeed are information, education, and contact with other breastfeeding women (Bergh 1993). Content of these classes includes advantages and disadvantages of breastfeeding techniques and methods of breast preparation.

The father is being included in educational programs more frequently because his support and encouragement are vital (Matich & Sims 1992), and it is important to include him in decision making. Some fathers feel that the act of feeding the newborn enhances the baby's relationship with the parent and therefore that breastfeeding means fathers and mothers will have inherently different relationships with their newborn (Gamble & Morse 1993). Breastfeeding classes provide fathers with opportunities for sharing information and discussion of their feelings about breastfeeding (Gamble & Morse 1993).

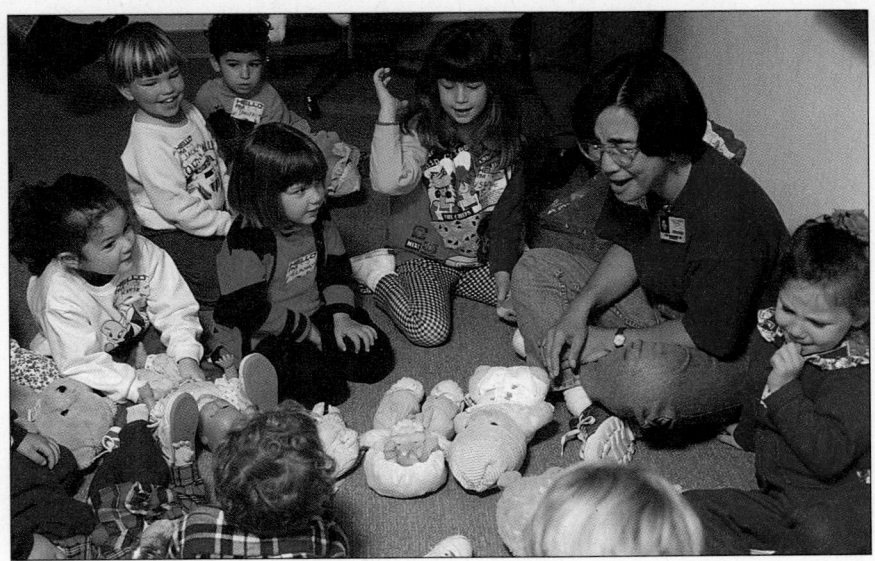

FIGURE 12-4   It is especially important that siblings be well prepared when they are going to be present for the birth. However, all siblings can benefit from information about birth and the new baby ahead of time.

Prepared Sibling Programs

The birth of a new sibling is a significant event in a child's life. It may be associated with negative behavior toward the newborn, withdrawal, and sleep problems. More positively, the older siblings tend to exhibit fewer anxieties, and the mothers feel more able to cope with their older child when the new baby arrives (Spero 1993). With increased emphasis on family-centered birth, siblings are now being included more often in the birthing process. Their involvement may include visiting during labor, being present at birth, and/or visiting in the postpartal period.

Sibling preparation classes usually involve a tour of the birthing unit where the children will visit their mothers. Children generally show interest in such items as television sets, electric beds, and telephones the mothers will use to call them. The youngsters can climb on footstools at the nursery window to see the new babies. Most tours involve a visit to a birthing room. After the tour the children have an opportunity to see and hear more about what happens to the parents and newborn in the hospital, how babies are born, and what babies are like. This teaching may involve a combination of books, audiovisual materials, models, play experiences, making a birthday care package, packing a bag, and making foot and hand prints (Figure 12–4). They also have the opportunity to express their feelings about having a new baby in the family (Spero 1993). Discussion sessions may be divided into two age groups if the ages of the children attending vary greatly.

After the class parents usually receive additional resources that tell how to prepare children for a baby in the family. Some programs award certificates to the children who attend, offer refreshments to the children and their parents, and give gift packets with articles similar to those new mothers receive (lotion, diapers for the new baby).

Classes that prepare children for attendance at birth vary. It is important that the children be at least familiar with what to expect during labor and birth: how the parents will act, especially the sounds and faces the mother will make; what they will see, including the messiness, blood, and equipment; and how the baby will look and act at birth. In addition parents are encouraged to involve the child early in the pregnancy, including taking the child on a prenatal visit to see the CNM/physician and listen to the fetal heart beat. Most advocates feel the child also needs to be comfortable with seeing the mother without clothes prior to seeing her during labor and birth.

Classes for Grandparents

Grandparents are an important source of support and information for prospective and new parents. They are now being included in the birthing process more frequently. Prenatal programs for grandparents can be an important source of information regarding current beliefs and practices in childbearing. The most useful content may include changes in birthing and parenting practices and helpful tips for being a supportive grandparent.

EDUCATION OF THE FAMILY HAVING CESAREAN BIRTH

Preparation for Cesarean Birth

Cesarean birth is an alternative method of childbirth. Because one out of every four births is a cesarean, preparation for this possibility should be an integral part of every childbirth education curriculum. The instructor should treat cesarean birth as a normal event and present factual information that will allow a couple to make choices and participate in their birth experience. The instructor can emphasize the similarities between cesarean and vaginal births to minimize undertones of "normal" versus "abnormal" birth. This will diminish feelings of anger, loss, and grief that often accompany cesarean births.

Cesarean birth classes should cover what happens during a cesarean birth, what the parents will feel, and what the parents can do.

All couples should be encouraged to discuss with their physician or nurse-midwife what the approach would be in the event of a cesarean. They can also discuss their needs and desires. Their preferences may include the following:

• Participating in the choice of anesthetic

• Father (or significant other) being present during the procedures and/or birth

• Type of anesthesia: epidural, spinal, or general

Preparation for Repeat Cesarean Birth

When a couple is anticipating a repeat cesarean birth, they have time to analyze the experience, synthesize information, and prepare for some of the specifics. Some hospitals or local groups (such as C-Sec, Inc) provide preparation classes for cesarean birth. Couples who have had previous negative experiences need an opportunity to discuss issues that contributed to their negative feelings. They should be encouraged to identify what they would like to change and to list interventions that would make the experience more positive. Those who have had positive experiences need reassurance that their needs and desires will be met in the same manner. In addition an opportunity should be given to discuss any fears or anxieties.

A specific concern of the woman facing a repeat cesarean is anticipation of the pain. She needs reassurance that subsequent cesareans are often less painful than the first. If her first cesarean was preceded by a long or strenuous labor, she will not experience the same fatigue. Giving this information will help her cope more effectively with stressful stimuli, including pain. The nurse can remind the client that she has already had experience with how to prevent, cope with, and alleviate painful stimuli.

Preparation for Couples Desiring Vaginal Birth After Cesarean Birth (VBAC)

Couples who have had a cesarean birth and are now anticipating a vaginal birth have different needs from other couples. Because they may have unresolved questions and concerns about the last birth, it is helpful to begin the series of classes with an informational session. During this session couples can ask questions, share experiences, and begin to form bonds with each other. The nurse can supply information regarding the criteria necessary to attempt a trial of labor and identify decisions regarding the birth experience. Some childbirth educators find it is

helpful to have the couples prepare two birth plans: one for vaginal birth and one for cesarean birth. The preparation of the birth plans seems to assist the couple in taking more control of the birth experience and tends to increase the positive aspects of the experience (Austin 1986).

After an informational session the classes may be divided, depending on the needs of the couples. Those with recent coached childbirth experiences may need only refresher classes; other couples may need complete training. Some couples may choose to attend regular classes after obtaining the beginning information in the informational session.

SELECTED METHODS OF CHILDBIRTH PREPARATION

Various methods of childbirth preparation are taught in North America. Some prenatal classes are more specifically oriented to preparation for labor and birth, have a name indicating a theory of pain reduction in childbirth, and teach specific exercises to reduce pain. The most common methods of this type are the Read (natural childbirth), the Lamaze (psychoprophylactic), the Kitzinger (sensory-memory method), and the Bradley (partner-coached childbirth) methods. Hypnosis is also discussed here because it is sometimes used to help the expectant mother reduce or even eliminate pain in labor and birth. See Table 12–3 for differentiating characteristics of each method. This chapter focuses on the Lamaze method because it is the most widely used in the United States today. Each of these methods is designed to provide the woman with understanding and coping measures so that her pregnancy and birth are healthy and happy events in which she participates.

Childbirth education effectively helps parents make positive life-style choices and can reduce risks associated with poor outcomes (Jeffers 1993). Expectant parents are taught that childbirth exercises and preparation for childbirth do not exclude the use of analgesics but that they often reduce the amount necessary. Some women will not require medication. Unfortunately, some groups teach that childbirth without pain relief medication is the desired goal. This feeling can be extremely destructive to the woman's self-concept at a time when she needs positive reinforcement in her abilities to achieve and perform competently. Fortunately, current thinking recognizes that individuals vary in their responses to stress, that the character of individual labors differs, and that pain medication used judiciously may enhance the woman's ability to use relaxation techniques (Crowe 1990).

The programs in prepared childbirth have some similarities. All have an educational component to help eliminate fear. The classes vary in the amount of coverage of various subjects related to the maternity cycle, but they all teach relaxation techniques, and they all prepare the

TABLE 12-3	Summary of Selected Childbirth Preparation Methods	
Method	**Characteristics**	**Breathing Technique**
Lamaze	See narrative discussion.	
Read	First of the "natural" childbirth methods. Method utilizes information on progressive relaxation techniques and on abdominal breathing.	Primarily abdominal. Woman concentrates on forcing the abdominal muscles to rise. Works on slowing number of respirations per minute so that she can take one breath/minute (30-second inhalation and 30-second exhalation). Slow abdominal breathing used during first stage. Rapid chest breathing used toward end of labor if abdominal breathing not sufficient; panting is used to prevent pushing until needed.
Bradley	Frequently referred to as partner- or husband-coached natural childbirth. The exercises used to accomplish relaxation and slow controlled breathing are basically those used in the Read method. Emphasis on abstaining from use of medication.	Primarily abdominal as in Read method.
Kitzinger	Uses sensory memory to help the woman understand and work with her body in preparation for birth. Incorporates the Stanislavsky method of acting as a way to teach relaxation.	Uses chest breathing in conjunction with abdominal relaxation.
Hypnosis	Basic technique of hypnosis used in obstetrics is called hypnoreflexogenous method and is a combination of hypnosis and conditioned reflexes.	Normal breathing pattern.

participants for what to expect during labor and birth. Except for hypnosis, these methods also feature exercises to condition muscles and breathing patterns used in labor. The greatest differences among the methods lie in the theories of why they work and in the relaxation techniques and breathing patterns they teach.

The advantages of these methods of childbirth preparation are several. The most important is that the baby may be healthier because of the reduced need for analgesics and anesthetics. Another advantage is the satisfaction of the couples for whom childbirth becomes a shared and profound emotional experience. In addition proponents of each method claim that they shorten the labor process, a claim that has been clinically validated.

All maternal-newborn nurses need to know how these methods differ so that they can support each couple in their chosen method. It is important for nurses to assess the couple's emotional resources and their expectations so they can help them achieve their goals more effectively.

The maternal-newborn nurse may also assist the expectant couple in locating a childbirth education class that best meets their needs. Expectant parents need to know that the qualifications of childbirth educators vary. The oldest nationally accredited certification program in Lamaze childbirth is offered through the American Society for Psychoprophylaxis in Obstetrics, Inc (ASPO). Lamaze childbirth educators participate in rigorous training and maintain ongoing continuing education. Other educators have a variety of preparation and requirements. In choosing a childbirth education class that will best meet their needs, the expectant family may want to ask the following:

- What is the expected course content?

- What is the class size, and what are the major teaching-learning techniques?

- What is the education and experience of the class leader?

- Is the childbirth educator open to adding content that the class participants want?

Psychoprophylactic (Lamaze) Method

The terms **psychoprophylactic** and *Lamaze* are used interchangeably. Psychoprophylactic means "mind prevention," and Dr Fernand Lamaze, a French obstetrician, was the first person to introduce this method of childbirth preparation to the Western world. Psychoprophylaxis actually originated in Russia and is based on Pavlov's research with conditioned reflexes. Pavlov found that the cortical centers of the brain can respond to only one set of signals at a time and that they accept only the strongest signal; the weaker signals are inhibited. Therefore the Lamaze method seeks to focus on specific relaxation and breathing exercises as a distraction from the discomforts of labor. As a result of practicing breathing exercises, when true labor is occurring, the conditioned response (the exercises) will be able to be used.

The two components of Lamaze classes are education and training. In addition to relaxation techniques and breathing exercises class content includes information on prenatal nutrition, sexuality, exercise, labor and usual variations of labor, vaginal and cesarean birth, infant feeding, early parenting, and coping skills for the postpartum period.

The fear-tension-pain cycle serves as a framework for the Lamaze method. The woman without prenatal childbirth education is more likely to be afraid. This fear

TABLE 12-4   Touch Relaxation

Practice is vital to the following exercises, which require that the pregnant woman and her partner work very closely together. Tell the woman, "With practice you will train yourself to release not only in response to your partner's touch but also to the touch of doctors or nurses as they examine you. This technique will also help you to be more comfortable with your own body."

Goals:

(For her) To recognize and release tension in response to partner's touch; to be able to do this automatically and spontaneously.
(For partner) To recognize her tension in its very early stages; to learn how to touch in a firm yet sensitive way; to concentrate on her problem areas.

Tools:

(For her) Conscious relaxation, comfortable positioning, and trust.
(For partner) Sensitivity, patience, and warm hands!

Procedure:

She tenses.
Partner touches.
She immediately releases toward touch.
Partner strokes, "drawing" tension from her.
She releases all residual tensions.

Sequence:

- Contract muscles of the scalp and raise eyebrows. Partner cups hands on either side of the scalp. Immediately release tension in response to the pressure of your partner's touch. Then release any residual tension as your partner strokes your head.

- Frown, wrinkle nose, and squeeze eyes shut. Partner rests hands on brow and then strokes down over temples. Release.

- Grit teeth and clench jaw. Partner rests hands on either side of jaw. Release.

- Press shoulder blades back. Partner rests hands on front of shoulders. Release.

- Pull abdominal wall toward spine. Partner rests hands on sides of abdomen and then strokes down over hips. Partner might also stroke the lower curve of abdomen across pubic symphysis. Release.

- Press thighs together. Partner touches outside of each leg. Relax and let legs move apart. Partner strokes firmly down outside of leg with light strokes up on inner thigh.

- Press legs outward, still flexed but forcing thighs apart. Partner rests hands with fingers pointing downward on inner thighs. Firmly stroke down to knees, then lightly stroke upward on outside of leg. Release.

- Tense arm muscles. Partner places hands on the upper arm and shoulder area, one on the inside and one on the outside of the arm. Stroke down to the elbow and then down forearm to wrist and over fingertips. Release. Repeat with other arm.

- Tighten leg muscles, being careful not to cramp them. Partner touches foot around the instep, firmly without tickling. Release whole leg. Partner moves hands up, placing one on either side of the thigh, stroking down to the knee then down the calf to the foot and over the toes. Release. Repeat with other leg.

- Change to the Sims lateral or side-lying position. Raise chin, contracting the muscles at the back of the neck. Partner rests hand on nape of neck and massages. Release.

- Curl into fetal position, drawing shoulders forward. Partner applies pressure to back of shoulders. Stroke upper back. Release.

- Hollow the small of back by arching back. Partner rests hands against either side of spine and follows with stroking down over buttocks. Release.

- Press buttocks together. Partner rests one hand on each buttock. After initial release, stroke down toward thighs.

SOURCE: O'Halloran S: *Pregnant and Prepared: A Guide to Preparing for Childbirth*. Wayne, NJ: Avery, 1984, pp 43–44. Courtesy of NACE: The Nashua Association for Childbirth Education.

produces tension in the muscles of her body, and the tense muscles lead to more pain. Lamaze education seeks to break this cycle. Educational intervention decreases uncertainty and fear of the unknown. The resultant relaxation decreases muscle tension. Specific breathing patterns are also used to distract attention away from the pain. In addition to causing tension fear causes the release of adrenaline, which counteracts the effects of oxytocin, making uterine contractions less effective. Thus the labor for a prepared woman may be shorter than that for an unprepared woman.

Instructors teaching the method in this country have modified many of the original exercises, but the basic theory of conditioned reflex remains the same. Women are taught to substitute favorable conditioned responses for unfavorable ones. Rather than restlessness and loss of control in labor, the woman learns to respond to contractions with conditioned relaxation of the uninvolved muscles and a learned respiratory pattern. Exercise taught in these classes include proper body mechanics and body conditioning.

Another integral part of the Lamaze method involves encouraging the childbearing family to explore, discuss, and develop a list of their wishes regarding their birth experience (see the discussion of the birth plan in "Childbearing Decisions"). The couple is encouraged to discuss their wishes with the certified nurse-midwife or physician prior to birth and with the maternal-newborn nursing personnel upon admission. The nursing staff that knows the couple's wishes is able to offer more effective support. Another movement in the Lamaze curriculum is toward applying selected life skills. Decision making, relaxation, and communication are skills learned in class that can then be applied throughout life.

Toning Exercises

Some of the body conditioning exercises, such as the pelvic tilt, pelvic rock, and Kegel's exercises, are taught in childbirth preparation classes. Other exercises strengthen the abdominal muscles for the expulsive phase of labor. (See Chapter 15 for a description of recommended exercises.)

Relaxation Exercises

Relaxation during labor allows the woman to conserve energy and allows the uterine muscles to work more efficiently. Without practice it is very difficult to relax the whole body in the midst of intense uterine contractions. Many people are familiar with **progressive relaxation** exercises such as those taught to aid relaxation and induce sleep. One example follows: Lie down on your back or side. (The left side position is best for pregnant women.)

TABLE 12-5	Disassociation Relaxation

The uterus, an involuntary muscle, will work most efficiently and effectively when the rest of your body is free from tension. The following exercises will give you further practice in conscious release. They will also give you and your partner a way to evaluate your progress.

Goals:

During pregnancy disassociation relaxation will teach you consciously to release certain sets of muscles while contracting others and to disassociate yourself from voluntary tension.
During labor this technique will release all voluntary muscles of your body at will while the uterus contracts. This conserves energy and fights fatigue.

Tools:

Body awareness, touch release, and concentration.

Procedure:

Partner gives consistent suggestions.
Partner checks relaxation using touching.

Example:

Partner: "Contraction begins."
Mother: Relaxation breath (following with a comfortable rate of breathing).
Partner: See suggested patterns below.
Mother: Relaxation breath.

Sequence:

"Contract right arm. Hold. Release."
"Contract left arm. Hold. Release."
"Contract right leg. Hold. Release."
"Contract left leg. Hold. Release."
"Contract both arms. Hold. Release."
"Contract both legs. Hold. Release."
"Contract right side (arm and leg). Hold. Release."
"Contract left side (arm and leg). Hold. Release."
"Contract right arm and left leg. Hold. Release."
"Contract left arm and right leg. Hold. Release."

For Variety:

Contract right arm and left leg.
Release left leg. Contract right leg. Release right arm. Contract left arm.
Release.

SOURCE: O'Halloran S: *Pregnant and Prepared: A Guide to Preparing for Childbirth.* Wayne, NJ: Avery, 1984, pp 45–46. Courtesy of NACE: The Nashua Association for Childbirth Education.

Tighten your muscles in both feet. Hold the tightness for a few seconds, and then relax the muscles completely, letting all the tension drain out. Tighten your lower legs, hold for a few seconds, and then relax the muscles, letting all the tension drain out. Continue tensing and relaxing parts of your body, moving up the body as you do so.

Another type of relaxation exercise called **touch relaxation** requires cooperation between the woman and her coach. It is particularly useful in learning how to work together during labor. See Table 12–4.

An additional exercise specific to Lamaze is **disassociation relaxation.** This pattern of active relaxation is in contrast to the Read method of passive relaxation. The woman is taught to become familiar with the sensation of contracting and relaxing the voluntary muscle groups throughout her body. She then learns to contract a specific muscle group and relax the rest of her body. This process of isolating the action of one group of voluntary muscles from the rest of the body is called *neuromuscular disassociation* and is basic to the psychoprophylaxis method of prepared childbirth. The exercise conditions the woman to relax uninvolved muscles while the uterus contracts. See Table 12–5.

In order to practice the relaxation exercises in a more realistic setting the coach may use two methods to induce some discomfort:

1. The coach places both hands in a grasping position firmly on the upper arm and turns them in opposite directions to create a burning sensation. This is begun slowly and gently and increased at the direction of the woman as she continues to practice relaxation and/or practices the breathing techniques (Figure 12–5).

2. The coach places a hand on the woman's inner thigh just above the knee and pinches the area.

While practicing, the coach checks the woman's neck, shoulders, arms, and legs for relaxation. As tense areas are found, the coach encourages the woman to relax that particular body part. The woman learns to respond to her own perceptions of tense muscles and also to the suggestion from others. The suggestion can come verbally or from touch. The exercises are usually practiced each day so that they become comfortable and easy to do.

A specific type of cutaneous stimulation used prior to the transitional phase of labor is known as abdominal **effleurage** (Figure 12–6). This light abdominal stroking is

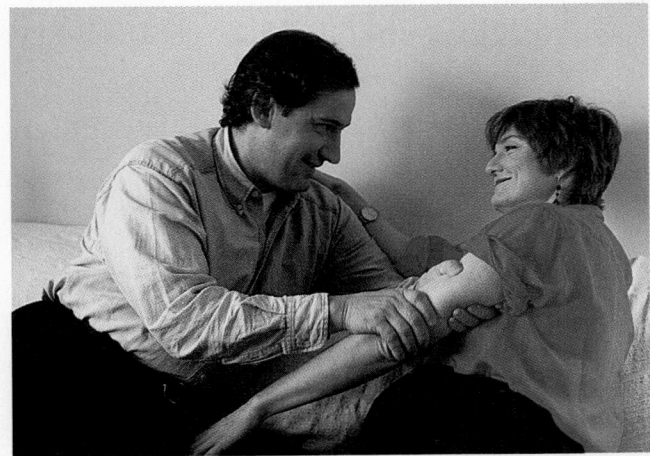

FIGURE 12-5   To help the woman practice relaxing in the presence of discomfort, the coach can induce discomfort by "twisting" the skin of her upper arm or by pinching her inner thigh.

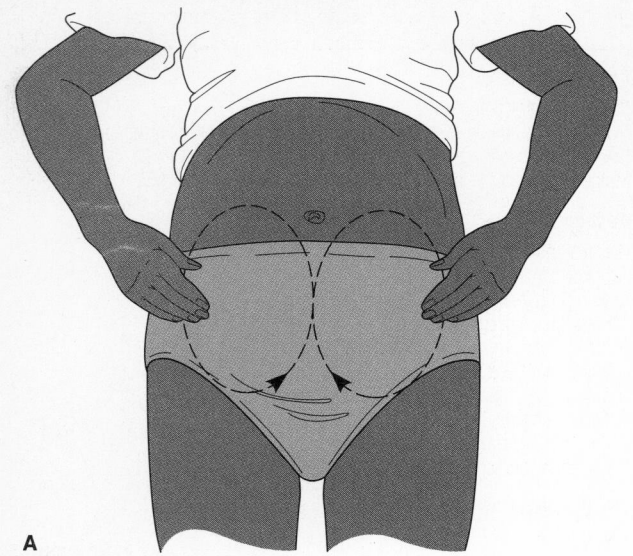

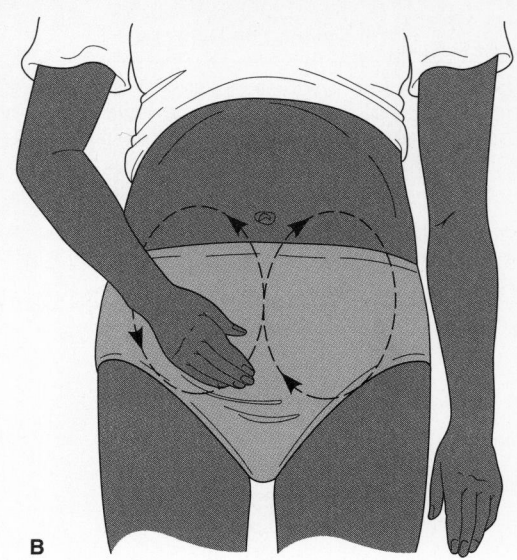

FIGURE 12-6 Effleurage is light stroking of the abdomen with the fingertips. *A* Starting at the symphysis, the woman lightly moves her fingertips up and around in a circular pattern.

B An alternative approach involves using one hand in a figure eight pattern. This light stroking can also be done by the support person.

used in the Lamaze method of childbirth preparation. It effectively relieves mild to moderate pain, but not intense pain. Deep pressure over the sacrum is more effective for relieving back pain. In addition to the measures just described the nurse can promote relaxation by encouraging and supporting the client's controlled breathing.

Other methods that may be used to enhance relaxation are guided imagery and meditation.

Breathing Techniques

Breathing techniques are a key element of most childbirth preparation programs. They help keep the mother and her unborn baby adequately oxygenated and help the mother relax and focus her attention appropriately. Lamaze breathing techniques are described in detail in Chapter 23.

KEY CONCEPTS

Many couples are choosing preconception counseling and classes as they begin to prepare for pregnancy. Preconception preparation includes reviewing life-style beliefs and habits, learning about nutrition and exercise, and preparing the body for pregnancy.

A variety of decisions regarding pregnancy and birth must be made. The childbearing family needs to choose the type of health care provider to use, the birth setting, and whether to use a labor support person such as a doula. In addition there will be many specific wishes that the couple may consider regarding the birth. A birth plan assists the

childbearing family as it directs them to some areas they may want to consider and helps them prioritize their choices.

Prenatal education programs vary in their goals, content, leadership techniques, and method of teaching.

Prenatal classes may be offered early and/or late in the gestational period. The class content varies depending on the type of class and the individual offering it. Expectant parents tend to want information in chronologic sequence with the pregnancy. Adolescents have special content learning needs.

Breastfeeding programs are offered in the prenatal period.

Siblings are now being included in the whole birthing process, and classes for them are available from many sources.

Grandparents have unique needs for information in grandparents' classes.

Information regarding cesarean birth is included in antepartal classes to help prepare parents.

The major types of childbirth preparation methods are Lamaze, Bradley, Read, Kitzinger, and hypnosis.

Lamaze is a type of psychoprophylactic method. The classes include information on toning exercises, relaxation exercises and techniques, and breathing methods for labor.

REFERENCES

Aderhold KJ, Perry L: Jet hydrotherapy for labor and postpartum pain relief. *MCN* 1991; 16:97.

Austin SEJ: Childbirth classes for couples desiring VBAC. *MCN* 1986; 11:250.

Bachman JA: Self-described learning needs of pregnant teen participants in an innovative university/community partnership. *Mat Child Nurs J* April/June 1993; 21(2):65.

Baer D: Buckle up! *Lamaze Par Mag* 1992; p 95.

Bergh AM: Obstacles to and motivation for successful breast-feeding. *Curationis* 1993; 16:24.

Bradley R: *Husband Coached Childbirth.* New York: Harper & Row 1965.

Brink S: Cloth diapers help hospital to soften the bottom line. *Boston Herald,* July 11, 1990.

Broussard AB, Rich SK: Incorporating infant stimulation concepts into prenatal classes. *JOGNN* September/October 1990; 19(5):381.

Causby V, Nixon C, Bright JM: Influences on adolescent mother-infant interactions. *Adolescence* 1991; 26:619.

Center for Policy Alternatives: Update on diapers. September 1990. (Available from 2000 Florida Avenue NW, Washington, DC 20009)

Chapman L: Co-laboring: Expectant fathers' experience during labor and birth. *J Mat Child Nurse* 1991; 5:92.

Crowe K, von Baeyer C: Predictors of a positive childbirth experience. *Birth* June 1990; 16:59.

Fortier JC et al: Adjustment to a newborn: Sibling preparation makes a difference. *JOGNN* January/February 1991; 20(1):73.

Fleming VM: Client education: A futuristic outlook. *J Advanced Nurs* 1992; 17:158.

Gamble D, Morse JM: Fathers of breastfed infants: Postponing and types of involvement. *JOGNN* 1993; 22:358.

Holaday B et al: Fecal contamination in child day care centers: Cloth vs paper diapers. *Am J Pub Health* 1995; 85:1.

Jeffers DF: Outreach childbirth education classes for low-income families: A strategy for program development. *AWHONN Clin Issues Perinatal Women Health Nurs* 1993; 4:95.

Jones ME, Bonte C: Conceptualizing community interventions in social service needs of pregnant adolescents. *J Ped Health Care* 1990; 4:193.

Kitzinger S: Sheila Kitzinger's letter from England: Birth plans. *Birth* 1992; 19(1):36.

Klaus MH, Kennel JH, Klaus PH: *Mothering the Mother.* Redwood City, CA: Addison-Wesley, 1993.

Kochenour NK: Normal pregnancy and prenatal care. In: *Danforth's Obstetrics and Gynecology,* 7th ed. Scott JR et al (editors). Philadelphia: Lippincott, 1994.

Korte D: *Bringing up Baby.* National Association of Diaper Services 1993.

Lehrburger C, Mullen J, Jones CV: Diapers: Environmental impacts and lifecycle analysis. Report to the National Association of Diaper Services. January 1991. (Available from Carl Lehrburger, PO Box 998, Great Barrington, MA 01230)

Matich JR, Sims LS: A comparison of social support variables between women who intend to breast or bottle feed. *Soc Sci Med* 1992; 34:919.

Mynaugh PA: A randomized study of two methods of teaching perineal massage: Effects of practice rates, episiotomy rates, and lacerations. *Birth* September 1991; 18(3):153.

Primono J et al: The high environmental cost of disposable diapers. *MCN* September/October 1990; 15:279.

Rosen MG: Preconception care: Why is it necessary? *Female Patient* May 1990; 15:73.

Shearer M: Effects of prenatal education depend on the attitudes and practices of obstetric caregivers. *Birth* June 1990; 17:73.

Shoham-Yakubovich I, Pliskin JS, Carr D: Infant feeding practices: An evaluation of the impact of a health education course. *Am J Pub Health* 1993; 4:122.

Simkin P: The labor support person. *ICEA Rev* 1992; 16:19.

Spero D: Sibling preparation classes. *AWHONN Clin Issues Perinatal Women Health Nurs* 1993; 4:122.

CHAPTER 13

PHYSICAL AND PSYCHOLOGIC CHANGES OF PREGNANCY

*T*he atmosphere of approval in which I was bathed—even by strangers on the street, it seemed—was like an aura I carried with me. . . . This is what women have always done.

~ ADRIENNE RICH, *OF WOMAN BORN* ~

KEY TERMS

Ballottement

Braxton Hicks contractions

Chadwick's sign

Chloasma

Colostrum

Couvade

Diastasis recti

Ethnocentrism

Goodell's sign

Hegar's sign

Linea nigra

McDonald's sign

Morning sickness

Physiologic anemia of pregnancy

Quickening

Striae

Supine hypotensive syndrome (vena caval syndrome; aortocaval compression)

OBJECTIVES

Identify the anatomic and physiologic changes that occur during pregnancy.

Relate the physiologic and anatomic changes that occur in the body systems during pregnancy to the signs and symptoms that develop in the woman.

Compare subjective (presumptive), objective (probable), and diagnostic (positive) changes of pregnancy.

Contrast the various types of pregnancy tests.

Discuss the emotional and psychologic changes that commonly occur in a woman, her partner, and her family during pregnancy.

Summarize cultural factors that may influence a family's response to pregnancy.

Through modern technology and highly evolved research methods we know a great deal about how pregnancy occurs and what happens to the fetus and the woman's body during gestation. Yet no matter how much we learn about this event, it never ceases to amaze us. First, it is nothing short of a miracle that the union of two microscopic entities—an ovum and a sperm—can produce a living being. Second, the woman's body must undergo extraordinary physical changes to sustain a pregnancy. A pregnant woman's body changes in size and shape, and all her organ systems modify their functions to create an environment that protects and nurtures the growing fetus.

Pregnancy is divided into three trimesters, each a 3-month period. Each trimester has its own predictable developments in both the fetus and the mother. This chapter describes both obvious and subtle physical and psychologic changes caused by pregnancy. It also discusses the various cultural factors that can affect a woman's well-being during pregnancy.

ANATOMY AND PHYSIOLOGY OF PREGNANCY

The changes that occur in the pregnant woman's body are caused by several factors. Many changes are the results of hormonal influences, some are caused by the growth of the fetus inside the uterus, and some are a result of the mother's physical adaptation to the changes that are occurring.

Reproductive System

The changes in the body during pregnancy are most obvious in the organs of the reproductive system.

Uterus

The changes in the uterus during pregnancy are phenomenal. Before pregnancy the uterus is a small, semisolid, pear-shaped organ measuring approximately 7.5 × 5 × 2.5 cm and weighing about 60 g (2 oz). At the end of pregnancy the dimensions are approximately 28 × 24 × 21 cm, with an organ weight of approximately 1000 g (2.2 lb). Its capacity increases from 10 mL to 5 L or more.

The enlargement of the uterus is primarily a result of an increase in size (*hypertrophy*) of the preexisting myometrial cells. There is only a limited increase in cell number (*hyperplasia*). The amount of fibrous tissue between the muscle bands increases markedly, which adds to the strength and elasticity of the muscle wall.

The uterine walls are considerably thicker during the first few months of pregnancy than during the nonpregnant state. The initial changes are stimulated by increased estrogen and progesterone levels and not by mechanical distention by the products of conception. After approximately the third month, intrauterine pressure begins to be exerted by the uterine contents. The myometrial hypertrophy continues during the first few months of pregnancy. Then the musculature begins to distend, resulting in a thinning of the muscle wall to a thickness of about 5 mm or less at term. The ease of palpating the fetus through the abdominal wall attests to this thinning.

The circulatory requirements of the uterus increase as the uterus enlarges and the fetus and placenta develop. The size and number of the blood vessels and lymphatics increase greatly. By the end of pregnancy one-sixth the total maternal blood volume is contained within the vascular system of the uterus.

Braxton Hicks contractions—irregular, generally painless contractions of the uterus—occur intermittently throughout pregnancy. They may be palpated bimanually beginning about the fourth month of pregnancy. These contractions help stimulate the movement of blood through the intervillous spaces of the placenta. In late pregnancy as these contractions increase in frequency, they can become uncomfortable and may be confused with true labor contractions.

Cervix

Estrogen stimulates the glandular tissue of the cervix, which increases in cell number and becomes hyperactive. The endocervical glands occupy about half the mass of the cervix at term, as compared to a small fraction in the nonpregnant state. They secrete a thick, tenacious mucus, which accumulates and thickens to form the mucus plug that seals the endocervical canal and prevents the ascent of bacteria or other substances into the uterus. This plug is expelled when cervical dilatation begins. The hyperactive glandular tissue also causes an increase in the normal physiologic mucorrhea, at times resulting in a profuse discharge. Increased vascularization causes both the softening of the cervix (**Goodell's sign**) and a blue-purple discoloration of the cervix (**Chadwick's sign**). Increased vascularization is a result of hypertrophy and engorgement of the vessels below the growing uterus.

Ovaries

The ovaries cease ovum production during pregnancy. Many follicles develop temporarily but never to the point of maturity. The cells lining these follicles, the thecal cells, become active in hormone production and have been called the *interstitial glands of pregnancy*.

During early pregnancy human chorionic gonadotrophin (hCG) maintains the corpus luteum, which persists and produces hormones until about week 10 to 12 of pregnancy. It engulfs approximately a third of the ovary at its peak of hypertrophy. By the middle of pregnancy it has regressed to almost complete obliteration. The progesterone it secretes maintains the endometrium until the placenta produces enough progesterone to maintain the pregnancy.

Vagina

The vaginal epithelium undergoes hypertrophy, increased vascularization, and hyperplasia during pregnancy. As with the cervical changes, these changes are estrogen induced and result in a thickening of mucosa, a loosening of connective tissue, and an increase in vaginal secretions. The secretions are thick, white, and acidic (pH 3.5–6.0). The acid pH plays a significant role in preventing infections. However, it also favors the growth of yeast organisms, resulting in moniliasis, a common vaginal infection during pregnancy.

As in the uterus, the smooth muscle cells of the vagina become hypertrophied, with an accompanying loosening of the supportive connective tissue. By the end of pregnancy the vaginal wall and perineal body have become sufficiently relaxed to permit distention of the tissues and passage of the infant.

Because the blood flow to the vagina is increased, it may show the same blue-purple color (Chadwick's sign) seen in the cervix.

Breasts

Soon after the first menstrual period is missed estrogen- and progesterone-induced changes are noted in the mammary glands. Increases in breast size and nodularity are the result of glandular hyperplasia and hypertrophy in preparation for lactation. By the end of the second month superficial veins are prominent, nipples are more erectile, and pigmentation of the areola is obvious. Pigmentation tends to be more pronounced in women with dark complexions. Hypertrophy of Montgomery's follicles is noted within the primary areola. **Striae** (stretch marks) may develop as the pregnancy progresses. Breast changes are often most noticeable in the woman who is pregnant for the first time.

Colostrum, an antibody-rich, yellow secretion, may be expressed manually by the 12th week and may leak from the breasts during the last trimester of pregnancy. Colostrum gradually converts to mature milk during the first few days following childbirth.

Respiratory System

Pulmonary function is modified throughout pregnancy. Pregnancy induces a small degree of hyperventilation as the tidal volume (amount of air breathed with ordinary respiration) increases steadily throughout pregnancy. There is a 30% to 40% rise from nonpregnant values in the volume of air breathed each minute. Between weeks 16 and 40 oxygen consumption increases approximately 15% to 20% to meet the increased needs of the mother as well as those of the fetus and placenta. The vital capacity (maximum amount of air that can be moved in and out of the lungs with forced respiration) increases slightly while lung compliance and pulmonary diffusion remain constant. Measurements of airway resistance show a marked decrease in pregnancy in response to elevated progesterone levels. This permits increases in oxygen consumption, in carbon dioxide production, and in the respiratory functional reserve.

The diaphragm is elevated and the subcostal angle is increased as a result of pressure from the enlarging uterus. This change causes the rib cage to flare, with a decrease in the vertical diameter and increases in the anteroposterior and transverse diameters. The circumference of the chest may increase by as much as 6 cm. The increase compensates for the elevated diaphragm, and there is no significant loss of intrathoracic volume. Breathing changes from abdominal to thoracic as pregnancy progresses, and descent of the diaphragm on inspiration becomes less possible.

Nasal "stuffiness" and epistaxis are not uncommon. They occur because of estrogen-induced edema and vascular congestion of the nasal mucosa.

Cardiovascular System

The growing uterus exerts pressure on the diaphragm, pushing the heart upward and to the left and rotating it forward. This lateral displacement makes the heart appear somewhat enlarged on x-ray examination.

Blood volume progressively increases throughout pregnancy, beginning in the first trimester and peaking in the middle of the third trimester at about 45% above nonpregnant levels. This increase is due to increases in both plasma and erythrocytes. No increase occurs in pulmonary capillary wedge pressure or in central venous pressure despite the increase in blood volume. This is due to decreases in both systemic vascular resistance (21%) and pulmonary vascular resistance (34%), which enable the circulation to adapt to higher blood volume while maintaining normal vessel pressures (Clark et al 1989). Cardiac output begins to increase early in pregnancy and peaks at 24–28 weeks' gestation at 30% to 50% above prepregnant levels. It then remains elevated for the duration of the pregnancy (Blackburn & Loper 1992).

During pregnancy, organ systems receive additional blood flow according to their increased work load. Thus blood flow to the uterus and kidneys increases while hepatic and cerebral flow remains unchanged.

The pulse rate frequently increases during pregnancy, although the amount varies from almost no increase to an increase of 10 to 15 beats per minute. The blood pressure decreases slightly during pregnancy, reaching its lowest point during the second trimester.

The blood pressure then gradually increases during the third trimester and is near prepregnant levels at term (when the baby is due).

The femoral venous pressure slowly rises as the uterus exerts increasing pressure on return blood flow. There is an increased tendency toward stagnation of blood in the lower extremities, with a resulting dependent edema and tendency toward varicose vein formation in the legs, vulva, and rectum late in pregnancy. In addition to the effects of increased femoral venous pressure, a reduction of plasma colloid osmotic pressure resulting from a reduction in plasma albumin further maintains the presence of fluid in the extravascular space. The pregnant woman becomes more prone to develop postural hypotension because of the increased blood volume in the lower extremities.

Researchers have long recognized that the enlarging uterus may put pressure on the vena cava when the woman is supine, resulting in **supine hypotensive syndrome** or **vena caval syndrome.** This pressure interferes with returning blood flow and produces a marked decrease in blood pressure with accompanying dizziness, pallor, and clamminess, which can be corrected by having the woman lie on her left side. Recent research indicates that the enlarging uterus may press on the aorta and its collateral circulation as well, which suggests that the term **aortocaval compression** is more accurate (Blackburn & Loper 1992) (Figure 13–1).

The total erythrocyte volume increases by about 30% in women who receive iron supplementation but increases only about 18% without iron supplements (Cruikshank & Hays 1991). This increase is necessary to transport the additional oxygen required during pregnancy. The increase in plasma volume averages about 50%. Because the plasma volume increase is greater than the erythrocyte increase, however, the hematocrit, which measures the portion of whole blood that is composed of erythrocytes, decreases by an average of about 7%. This decrease is referred to as the **physiologic anemia of pregnancy** (pseudoanemia).

Iron is necessary for hemoglobin formation, and hemoglobin is the oxygen-carrying component of erythrocytes. Thus the increase in erythrocyte levels results in an increased need for iron by the pregnant woman. Even though the gastrointestinal absorption of iron is moderately increased during pregnancy, it is usually necessary to add supplemental iron to the diet to meet the expanded red blood cell and fetal needs.

Leukocyte production equals or is slightly greater than the increase in blood volume. The average cell count is 5000 to 12,000/mm^3, with an occasional woman developing a physiologic leukocytosis of 15,000/mm^3. During labor and the early postpartum period these levels may reach 25,000/mm^3. The reason for this dramatic increase remains unknown, but similar leukocyte changes occur with physiologic stress such as vigorous exercise. It probably represents the return to the circulation of mature

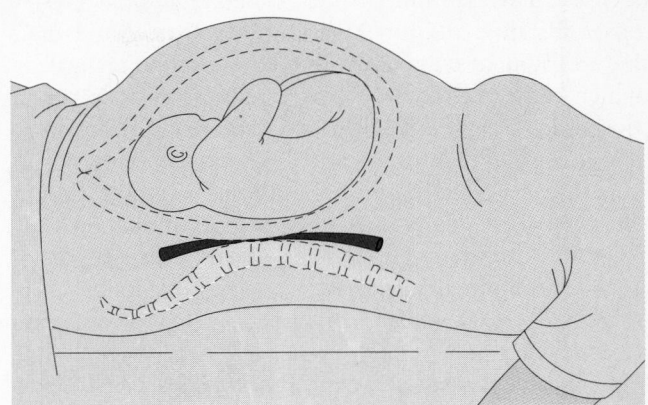

FIGURE 13-1 Vena caval syndrome. The gravid uterus compresses the vena cava when the woman is supine. This reduces the blood flow returning to the heart and may cause maternal hypotension.

leukocytes that had been shunted out of the circulatory system (Blackburn & Loper 1992).

The fibrin level in the blood is increased by as much as 40% at term, and the plasma fibrinogen has been known to increase by as much as 50%. The increased fibrinogen accounts for the nonpathologic rise of the sedimentation rate. Although the clotting time of the pregnant woman does not differ significantly from that of the nonpregnant woman, blood factors VII, VIII, IX, and X are increased so that pregnancy becomes a somewhat hypercoagulable state. These changes, coupled with venous stasis in late pregnancy, place the pregnant woman at increased risk of developing venous thrombosis.

Gastrointestinal System

Many of the discomforts of pregnancy are attributed to changes in the gastrointestinal system. Nausea and vomiting during the first trimester are associated with the hCG secreted by the implanted blastocyst and with a change in carbohydrate metabolism that occurs in early pregnancy. Peculiarities of taste and smell are common and can further aggravate gastrointestinal discomfort. Gum tissue may become hyperemic and softened and may bleed when only mildly traumatized. The secretion of saliva may increase or even become excessive (*ptyalism*). The gastric contents become more acidic as a result of elevated gastrin levels (produced by the placenta) (Camann & Ostheimer 1990).

During the second half of pregnancy, numerous gastrointestinal symptoms are attributable to the pressure of the growing uterus and smooth muscle relaxation due to elevated progesterone levels. The intestines are displaced laterally and posteriorly and the stomach superiorly. Heartburn (*pyrosis*) is caused by the reflux of acidic secretions from the stomach into the lower esophagus as a result of relaxation of the cardiac sphincter. Gastric emptying time and intestinal motility are delayed, leading to frequent complaints of bloating and constipation, which can be aggravated by the smooth muscle relaxation and increased electrolyte and water reabsorption in the large intestine. Hemorrhoids frequently develop if constipation is a problem or, in the second half of pregnancy, from pressure on vessels below the level of the uterus.

Only minor liver changes occur with pregnancy. Plasma albumin concentrations and serum cholinesterase activity decrease with normal pregnancy as with certain liver diseases.

The emptying time of the gallbladder is prolonged during pregnancy as a result of smooth muscle relaxation from progesterone. Hypercholesterolemia may follow, and it can predispose the woman to gallstone formation.

Urinary Tract

During the first trimester, the growing uterus puts pressure on the bladder, producing urinary frequency until the second trimester when the uterus becomes an abdominal organ. Near term, when the presenting part engages in the pelvis, pressure is again exerted on the bladder. This pressure can impair the drainage of blood and lymph from the hyperemic bladder, rendering it more susceptible to infection and trauma. The bladder, normally a convex organ, becomes concave from the external pressure, and its retention capacity is greatly reduced.

Dilation of the kidneys and ureter may occur, most frequently on the right side above the pelvic brim, due to the lie of the uterus. This dilation is accompanied by elongation and curvature of the ureter. There appears to be no single factor accounting for this anatomic variation; instead a combination of ureteral atonia and hypoperistalsis, possibly caused by the placental progesterone and by pressure from the enlarging fetus, seems to be involved. The presence of amino acids and glucose in the urine in conjunction with the tendency toward ureteral atonia and stasis of urine in the ureters may increase the risk of urinary tract infection (Blackburn & Loper 1992).

The glomerular filtration rate (GFR) and renal plasma flow (RPF) increase early in pregnancy. The GFR rises by as much as 50% by the beginning of the second trimester and remains elevated until birth. The increase in RPF is slightly less and decreases somewhat during the third trimester (Cunningham et al 1993). The mechanism for these rises remains unclear, but human placental lactogen (hPL) may play a part because it possesses properties similar to the pituitary growth hormone and has been shown experimentally to produce rises in GFR.

An increased renal tubular reabsorption rate compensates for the increased glomerular activity. Amino acids and water-soluble vitamins are excreted in greater amounts than in the nonpregnant woman. Glycosuria is not uncommon or necessarily pathogenic during pregnancy but is merely a reflection of the kidneys' inability to reabsorb all of the glucose filtered by the glomeruli. However, pregnancy can be diabetogenic, so the possibility of diabetes mellitus cannot be disregarded.

The increased renal function during pregnancy results in an increased clearance of urea and creatinine and in a lowering of the blood urea and nonprotein nitrogen values. Because of this, measurement of creatinine clearance provides an accurate test of renal functioning during pregnancy.

Skin and Hair

Changes in skin pigmentation commonly occur during pregnancy. These changes are thought to be stimulated by increased estrogen levels and perhaps by increased progesterone levels because these hormones are melanogenic stimulants (Blackburn & Loper 1992).

Pigmentation of the skin increases primarily in areas that are already hyperpigmented: the areola, the nipples, the vulva, the perianal area, and the linea alba. The *linea alba* refers to the midline of the abdomen from the pubic area to the umbilicus and above. During pregnancy increased pigmentation may cause this area to darken. It is then referred to as the **linea nigra** (Figure 13–2). Some women also develop facial **chloasma** or the "mask of pregnancy." This is an irregular pigmentation of the

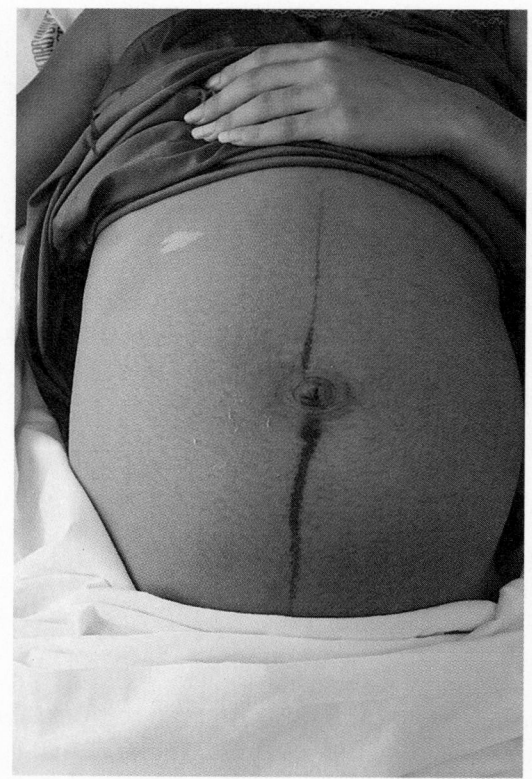

FIGURE 13-2   Linea nigra.

cheeks, forehead, and nose that occurs in many women during pregnancy and is accentuated by sun exposure. Similar changes may occur in women who are taking oral contraceptives. Facial chloasma is more prominent in dark-haired women and is occasionally disfiguring. Fortunately, it fades or at least regresses soon after birth when the hormonal influence of pregnancy has stopped. In addition the sweat and sebaceous glands are frequently hyperactive during pregnancy.

Striae, or stretch marks, are reddish, wavy, depressed streaks that may occur over the abdomen, breasts, and thighs as pregnancy progresses. They are caused by reduced connective tissue strength due to elevated adrenal steroid levels.

Vascular spider nevi may develop on the chest, neck, face, arms, and legs. They are small, bright-red elevations of the skin radiating from a central body. They may be caused by increased subcutaneous blood flow in response to increased estrogen levels. This condition is of no clinical significance and disappears after pregnancy ends.

The rate of hair growth may be decreased during pregnancy and the number of hair follicles in the resting or dormant phase is also decreased. After birth the number of hair follicles in the resting phase increases sharply, and the woman may notice increased shedding of hair for 1 to 4 months. Fortunately, this shedding is self-limiting, and normal hair growth is usually restored by 6 to 12 months (Cunningham et al 1993).

Musculoskeletal System

No demonstrable changes occur in the teeth of the pregnant woman. No demineralization takes place. The fairly common occurrence of dental caries during pregnancy has led to the myth "a tooth for every pregnancy." The dental caries that may accompany pregnancy are likely to be caused by inadequate oral hygiene and dental care.

The sacroiliac, sacrococcygeal, and pubic joints of the pelvis relax in the later part of the pregnancy, presumably as a result of relaxin and progesterone. This often causes a waddling gait. A slight separation of the symphysis pubis can often be demonstrated on radiologic examination.

As the pregnant woman's center of gravity gradually changes, the lumbodorsal spinal curve is accentuated, and the woman's posture changes (Figure 13–3). This posture change compensates for the increased weight of the uterus anteriorly and frequently results in low backache. Late in pregnancy, neck, shoulder, and upper extremity aching may occur because of shoulder slumping and anterior flexion of the neck accompanying the lumbodorsal lordosis. Paresthesias of the extremities may occur late in pregnancy as a result of pressure on peripheral nerves.

Often pressure of the enlarging uterus on the abdominal muscles causes the rectus abdominis muscle to separate, producing **diastasis recti.** If the separation is severe and muscle tone is not regained postpartally,

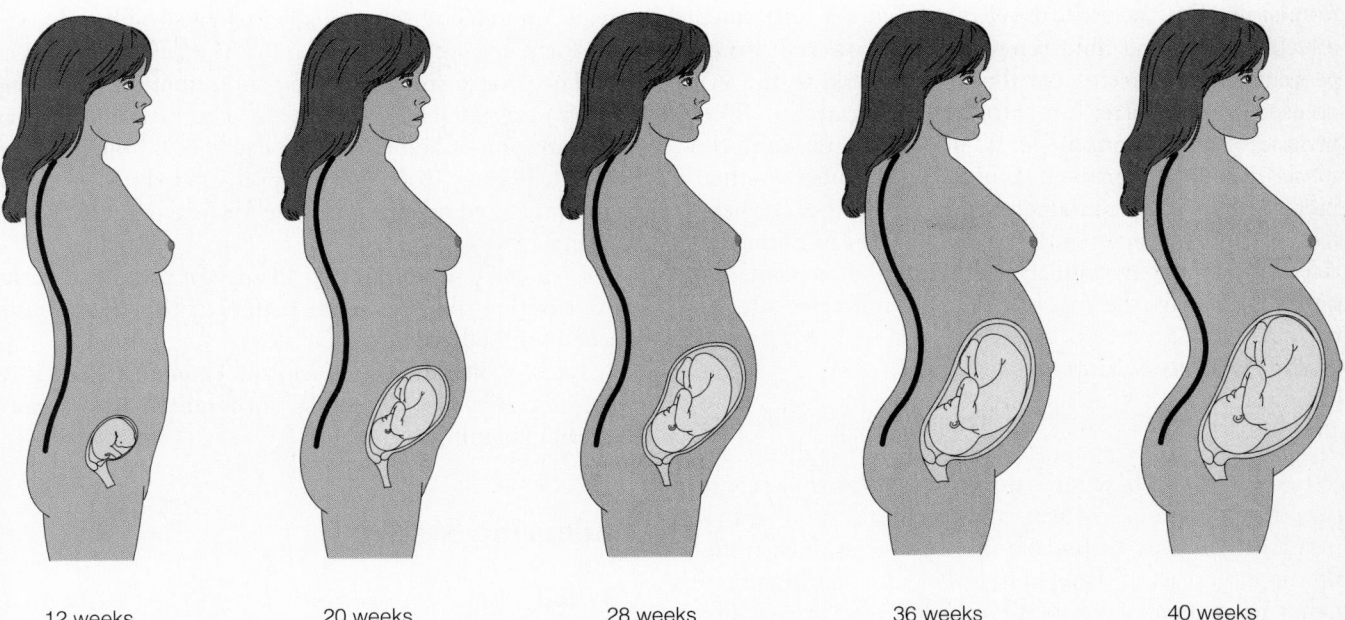

| 12 weeks | 20 weeks | 28 weeks | 36 weeks | 40 weeks |

FIGURE 13-3 Postural changes during pregnancy. Note the increasing lordosis of the lumbosacral spine and the increasing curvature of the thoracic area.

subsequent pregnancies will not have adequate support, and the woman's abdomen may appear pendulous.

Metabolism

Most metabolic functions accelerate during pregnancy to support the additional demands of the growing fetus and its support system. The expectant mother must meet her own tissue replacement needs, those of the fetus, and those preparatory for labor and lactation. No other event in life induces such profound metabolic changes.

Weight Gain

The recommended total weight gain during pregnancy for a woman of normal weight prior to pregnancy is 11.5–16 kg (25–35 lb); for women who were overweight the recommended gain is 7–11.5 kg (15–25 lb); and for underweight women, 12.5–18 kg (28–40 lb) (Institute of Medicine 1990). Weight may decrease slightly during the first trimester due to nausea, vomiting, and food intolerances of early pregnancy. The lost weight is soon regained, and an average increase of 1.4–2.3 kg (3–5 lb), 5.5–6.8 kg (12–15 lb), and 5.5–6.8 kg (12–15 lb) occurs in the first, second, and third trimesters, respectively. The average weight gain is distributed as follows: 11 lb, fetus, placenta, amniotic fluid; 2 lb, uterus; 4 lb, increased blood volume; 3 lb, breasts; 5–10 lb, maternal stores.

Adequate nutrition and weight gain are important during pregnancy. Maternal nutrition is discussed in detail in Chapter 17.

Water Metabolism

Increased water retention is a basic chemical alteration of pregnancy. Several interrelated factors cause this phenomenon. The increased level of steroid sex hormones affects sodium and fluid retention. The lowered serum protein also influences the fluid balance, as do the increased intracapillary pressure and permeability. The products of conception—fetus, placenta, and amniotic fluid—account for an average of 3.5 L of water. Another increase of 3.5 L is contained within the mother's hypertrophied organs, augmented blood volume, and interstitial fluids. The extracellular fluid is distributed primarily below the uterus, the area of elevated venous pressure.

Nutrient Metabolism

The fetus makes its greatest protein and fat demands during the last half of gestation, doubling in weight in the last 6 to 8 weeks. The increased nitrogen (protein) retention that begins in early pregnancy is initially used for hyperplasia and hypertrophy of maternal tissues, such as the uterus and breasts. Nitrogen must be stored during pregnancy to maintain a constant level within the breast milk and to avoid depletion of maternal tissues.

Fats are more completely absorbed during pregnancy, resulting in a marked increase in the serum lipids, lipoproteins, and cholesterol and decreased elimination through the bowel. Fat deposits in the fetus increase from about 2% at midpregnancy to almost 12% at term. The excess nitrogen and lipidemia are considered to be a preparation for lactation.

The demand for *carbohydrate* increases, especially during the last two trimesters. Ketosis can be a problem, especially with the diabetic woman, due to glycosuria, reduced alkaline reserves, and lipidemia. Intermittent glycosuria is not uncommon during pregnancy. When it is not accompanied by a rise in blood sugar levels, glycosuria is a physiologic entity secondary to the increased glomerular filtration rate. Fasting blood sugar levels tend to fall slightly, returning to more normal levels by the sixth postpartal month. The oral glucose tolerance test shows no change with pregnancy.

The possibility of diabetes must not be overlooked during pregnancy. Plasma levels of insulin are increased during pregnancy (probably due to hormonal changes), and rapid destruction of insulin takes place within the placenta. Insulin production must be increased by the mother, and any marginal pancreatic function quickly becomes apparent. The diabetic woman often experiences increased exogenous insulin demands during pregnancy.

The demand for *iron* during pregnancy is accelerated, and the pregnant woman needs to guard against anemia. Iron is necessary for the increase in erythrocytes, hemoglobin, and blood volume, as well as for the increased tissue demands of both woman and fetus.

Iron transfer takes place at the placenta in only one direction—toward the fetus. It has been demonstrated that approximately five-sixths of the iron stored in the fetal liver has been assimilated during the last trimester of pregnancy. This stored iron in the fetal liver compensates in the first 4 months of neonatal life for the normal inadequate amounts of iron available in breast milk and non-iron-fortified formulas.

The progressive absorption and retention of *calcium* during pregnancy has been noted. The maternal plasma concentration of bound calcium decreases as the levels of bindable plasma proteins fall. Approximately 30 g of calcium is retained in maternal bone for fetal deposition late in pregnancy.

Pregnancy produces little change in the metabolism of most other minerals other than retention of amounts needed for fetal growth.

Vitamin metabolism does not change appreciably with pregnancy (see Chapter 17 for requirements of minerals and vitamins).

Endocrine System

Thyroid

Pregnancy influences the thyroid gland's size and activity. Often a palpable change is noted, which represents an increase in vascularity and hyperplasia of glandular tissue.

Serum-free thyroxine (T_4) increases in early pregnancy and thyroid-stimulating hormone (TSH) decreases. The increased free T_4 and decreased TSH have been linked, with elevated hCG, to nausea and vomiting in early pregnancy (Blackburn & Loper 1992). The elevated T_4 levels continue until 6 to 12 weeks postpartum. Increased thyroxine-binding capacity is represented by the change in serum protein-bound iodine (PBI) from a nonpregnant level of 5–12 μg/dL to a pregnant level of 9–16 μg/dL, probably caused by the increase in the levels of circulating estrogens.

The basal metabolic rate (BMR) increases by as much as 20 to 25% during pregnancy, beginning at 4 months (Blackburn & Loper 1992). Most of the increase in oxygen consumption is a result of fetal metabolic activity.

Parathyroid

The concentration of the parathyroid hormone and the size of the parathyroid glands increase, paralleling the fetal calcium requirements. Parathyroid hormone concentration reaches its highest level of approximately twofold between 15 and 35 weeks of gestation, returning to a normal or even subnormal level before childbirth.

Pituitary

During pregnancy, the pituitary gland enlarges somewhat, but it returns to normal size after birth. There is no significant change in the posterior lobe of the gland, although the anterior lobe increases in weight with each successive pregnancy.

Pregnancy is made possible by the hypothalamic stimulation of the anterior pituitary hormones: FSH, which stimulates ovum growth, and LH, which effects ovulation. Pituitary stimulation prolongs the corpus luteal phase of the ovary, which maintains the secretory endometrium for development of the pregnancy. Two additional pituitary hormones, thyrotropin and adrenotropin, alter maternal metabolism to support the pregnancy. Prolactin, also an anterior pituitary secretion, is responsible for initial lactation. (Continued lactation depends on the suckling of the infant.)

The posterior pituitary contains the mechanism for the release of oxytocin and vasopressin, which exert oxytocic, vasopressor, and antidiuretic effects. The main effects of oxytocin are the promotion of uterine contractility and the stimulation of milk ejection from the breasts. Vasopressin causes vasoconstriction, which results in increased blood pressure; it also has an antidiuretic effect and plays an important role in the regulation of water balance. Vasopressin secretion is controlled by changes in plasma osmolarity and blood volume.

Adrenals

Little structural change occurs in the adrenal glands during a normal pregnancy. Estrogen-induced increases in the levels of circulating cortisol result primarily from lowered renal excretion. The circulating cortisol levels regulate carbohydrate and protein metabolism. A normal level resumes 1 to 6 weeks postpartum.

The adrenals secrete increased levels of aldosterone by the early part of the second trimester. The levels of secretion are even more elevated in the woman on a sodium-restricted diet. This increase in aldosterone in a normal pregnancy may be the body's protective response to the increased sodium excretion associated with progesterone (Cunningham et al 1993).

Pancreas

The pregnant woman has increased insulin needs. The islets of Langerhans are stressed to meet this increased demand, and a latent deficiency may become apparent during pregnancy, producing symptoms of gestational diabetes (Chapter 18).

Hormones in Pregnancy

Several hormones are required to maintain pregnancy. Most of these are produced initially by the corpus luteum; production is then assumed by the placenta. The hormones produced during pregnancy are human chorionic gonadotropin, human placental lactogen, estrogen, progesterone, and relaxin. (For an in-depth discussion of placental hormones see Chapter 6.)

Human Chorionic Gonadotropin (hCG)   The trophoblast secretes hCG in early pregnancy. This hormone stimulates progesterone and estrogen production by the corpus luteum to maintain the pregnancy until the placenta is developed sufficiently to assume that function.

Human Placental Lactogen (hPL)   Also called human chorionic somatomammotropin (hCS), hPL is produced by the syncytiotrophoblast. This hormone is an antagonist of insulin; it increases the amount of circulating free fatty acids for maternal metabolic needs and decreases maternal metabolism of glucose to favor fetal growth.

Estrogen   Secreted originally by the corpus luteum, estrogen is produced primarily by the placenta as early as the seventh week of pregnancy. Estrogen stimulates uterine development to provide a suitable environment for the fetus. It also helps to develop the ductal system of the breasts in preparation for lactation.

Progesterone   Progesterone, also produced initially by the corpus luteum and then by the placenta, plays the greatest role in maintaining pregnancy. It maintains the endometrium and inhibits spontaneous uterine contractility, thus preventing early spontaneous abortion due to uterine activity. Progesterone also helps develop the acini and lobules of the breasts in preparation for lactation.

Relaxin   Relaxin is detectable in the serum of a pregnant woman by the time of the first missed menstrual period. Relaxin inhibits uterine activity, diminishes the strength of uterine contractions, aids in the softening of the cervix, and has the long-term effect of remodeling collagen. Its primary source is the corpus luteum, but small amounts are believed to be produced by the uterine decidua throughout pregnancy (Cunningham et al 1993).

Prostaglandins in Pregnancy

Prostaglandins (PGs) are lipid substances that can arise from most body tissues but occur in high concentrations in the female reproductive tract and are present in the decidua during pregnancy. The exact functions of PGs during pregnancy are still unknown, although it has been proposed that they are responsible for maintaining reduced placental vascular resistance. Decreased prostaglandin levels may contribute to hypertension and pregnancy-induced hypertension (PIH). Prostaglandins are also believed to play a role in the complex biochemistry that initiates labor, although their specific functions are still being defined (Blackburn & Loper 1992).

SIGNS OF PREGNANCY

Many of the changes women experience during pregnancy are used to diagnose the pregnancy itself. They are called the subjective or presumptive changes, the objective or probable changes, and the diagnostic or positive changes of pregnancy.

Subjective (Presumptive) Changes

The subjective changes of pregnancy are the symptoms the woman experiences and reports. They can be caused by other conditions (Table 13–1) and therefore cannot be considered proof of pregnancy. The following can be diagnostic clues when other signs and symptoms of pregnancy are also present.

Amenorrhea is the earliest symptom of pregnancy. In a healthy woman whose menstrual cycles are regular, missing one or more menstrual periods leads to the consideration of pregnancy.

Nausea and vomiting are experienced by almost half of all pregnant women during the first 3 months of pregnancy and result from elevated hCG levels and changed carbohydrate metabolism. The woman may feel merely a distaste for food or may suffer extreme vomiting, which may be accompanied by dehydration and ketosis. These symptoms frequently occur in the early part of the day and disappear within a few hours and hence are commonly called **morning sickness.** Some women may complain of nausea or vomiting in late afternoon and evening, especially in association with fatigue. This gastrointestinal disturbance usually appears about 6 weeks after the first day of the last menstrual period and usually disappears spontaneously 6 to 12 weeks later, although it may be prolonged in some instances. Recent research suggests

TABLE 13-1	Differential Diagnosis of Pregnancy— Subjective Changes
Subjective Changes	**Possible Causes**
Amenorrhea	Endocrine factors: early menopause; lactation; thyroid, pituitary, adrenal, ovarian dysfunction Metabolic factors: malnutrition, anemia, climatic changes, diabetes mellitus, degenerative disorders, long-distance running Psychologic factors: emotional shock, fear of pregnancy or sexually transmitted infection, intense desire for pregnancy (pseudocyesis), stress Obliteration of endometrial cavity by infection or curettage Systemic disease (acute or chronic), such as tuberculosis or malignancy
Nausea and vomiting	Gastrointestinal disorders Acute infections such as encephalitis Emotional disorders such as pseudocyesis or anorexia nervosa
Urinary frequency	Urinary tract infection Cystocele Pelvic tumors Urethral diverticula Emotional tension
Breast tenderness	Premenstrual tension Chronic cystic mastitis Pseudocyesis Hyperestrinism
Quickening	Increased peristalsis Flatus ("gas") Abdominal muscle contractions Shifting of abdominal contents

that women who experience nausea and vomiting in pregnancy have decreased incidence of spontaneous abortion and perinatal mortality (Blackburn & Loper 1992).

Excessive fatigue may be noted within a few weeks after the first missed menstrual period and may persist throughout the first trimester.

Urinary frequency is experienced during the first trimester as the enlarging uterus exerts pressure on the bladder. The increased vascularization and pelvic congestion that occur in each pregnancy can also cause frequent voiding. This symptom decreases during the second trimester, when the uterus is an abdominal organ, but reappears during the third trimester, when the presenting part descends into the pelvis.

Changes in the breasts are frequently noted in early pregnancy. Some women report significant breast changes prior to missing their first menses. Engorgement of the breasts due to the hormone-induced growth of the secretory ductal system results in the subjective symptoms of tenderness and tingling, especially of the nipple area.

Quickening, or the mother's perception of fetal movement, occurs about 18 to 20 weeks after the *last menstrual period (LMP)* in a primigravida but may occur as early as 16 weeks in a multigravida (woman who has been pregnant more than once). Quickening is a fluttering sen-

TABLE 13-2   Differential Diagnosis of Pregnancy—Objective Changes

Objective Changes	Possible Causes
Changes in pelvic organs	Increased vascular congestion
Goodell's sign	Estrogen-progestin oral contraceptives
Chadwick's sign	Vulvar, vaginal, cervical hyperemia
Hegar's sign	Excessively soft walls of nonpregnant uterus
Uterine enlargement	Uterine tumors
Braun von Fernwald's sign	Uterine tumors
Piskacek's sign	Uterine tumors
Enlargement of abdomen	Obesity, ascites, pelvic tumors
Braxton Hicks contractions	Hematometra, pedunculated, submucous, and soft myomas
Uterine souffle	Large uterine myomas, large ovarian tumors, or any condition with greatly increased uterine blood flow
Pigmentation of skin	Estrogen-progestin oral contraceptives
Chloasma	Melanocyte hormonal stimulation
Linea nigra	
Nipples/areola	
Abdominal striae	Obesity, pelvic tumor
Ballottement	Uterine tumors/polyps, ascites
Pregnancy tests	Increased pituitary gonadotropins at menopause, choriocarcinoma, hydatidiform mole
Palpation for fetal outline	Uterine myomas

sation in the abdomen that gradually increases in intensity and frequency.

Objective (Probable) Changes

An examiner can perceive the objective changes that occur in pregnancy. They are more diagnostic than the subjective symptoms. However, their presence does not offer a definite diagnosis of pregnancy (Table 13–2).

Changes in the pelvic organs caused by increased vascular congestion are the only physical signs detectable within the first 3 months of pregnancy. These changes are noted on pelvic examination. There is a softening of the cervix, called Goodell's sign. Chadwick's sign is the deep red to purple or bluish coloration of the mucous membranes of the cervix, vagina, and vulva due to increased vasocongestion of the pelvic vessels. (Cunningham et al [1993] consider Chadwick's sign a subjective sign; Scott et al [1994] consider it an objective sign.) **Hegar's sign** is a softening of the isthmus of the uterus, the area between the cervix and the body of the uterus, which occurs at 6 to 8 weeks of pregnancy. This area may become so soft that on a bimanual exam there seems to be nothing between the cervix and the body of the uterus (Figure 13–4). *Ladin's sign* is a soft spot anteriorly in the middle of the uterus near the junction of the body of the uterus and cervix (Figure 13–5*A*). **McDonald's sign** is an ease in flexing the body of the uterus against the cervix.

The uterus assumes an irregular globular shape during the early months of pregnancy. Irregular softening and enlargement at the site of implantation, known as

Braun von Fernwald's sign, occurs about the fifth week (Figure 13–5*B*). Occasionally an almost tumorlike, asymmetric enlargement occurs, called *Piskacek's sign* (Figure 13–5*C*). Generalized enlargement and softening of the body of the uterus are present after the eighth week of pregnancy. The fundus of the uterus is palpable just above the symphysis pubis at approximately 10 to 12 weeks' gestation and at the level of the umbilicus at 20 to 22 weeks' gestation (Figure 13–6).

Enlargement of the abdomen during the childbearing years is usually regarded as evidence of pregnancy, especially if the enlargement is progressive and is accompanied by a continuing amenorrhea. It is generally more pronounced in a woman whose abdominal musculature has lost some of its tone because of previous childbirth.

As mentioned earlier, Braxton Hicks contractions are ordinarily painless contractions that occur at irregular intervals throughout pregnancy but are felt with abdominal palpation after week 28. As the woman approaches the end of the pregnancy, these contractions may become more uncomfortable and are often called "false labor."

Uterine souffle may be heard when auscultating the abdomen over the uterus. It is a soft blowing sound at the same rate as the maternal pulse and is due to the increased uterine vascularization and the blood pulsating through the placenta. It is sometimes confused with the *funic souffle*, which is a soft blowing sound of blood pulsating through the umbilical arteries. The funic souffle is at the same rate as the fetal heart rate.

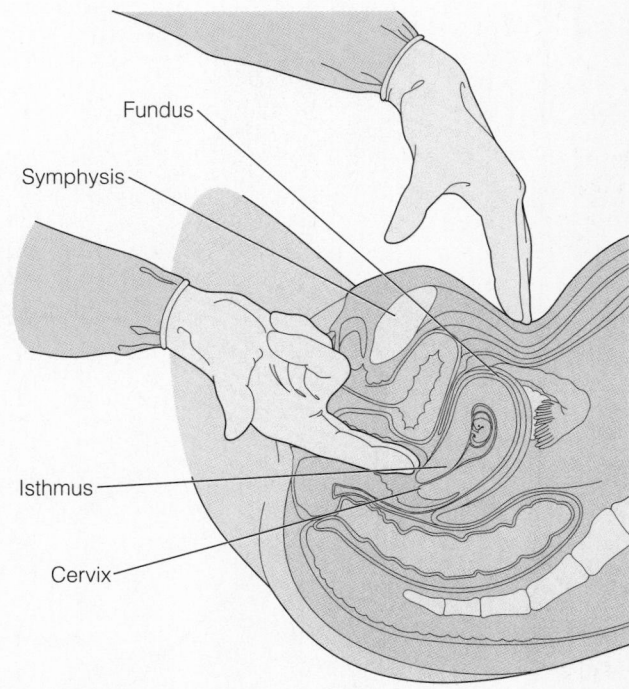

Fundus

Symphysis

Isthmus

Cervix

FIGURE 13-4   Hegar's sign, a softening of the isthmus of the uterus, can be determined by the examiner during a vaginal examination.

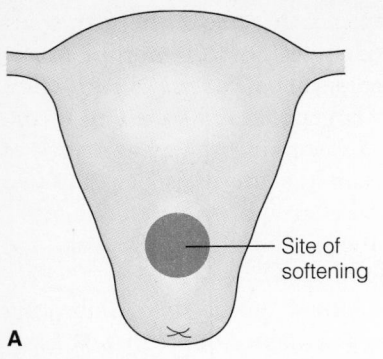 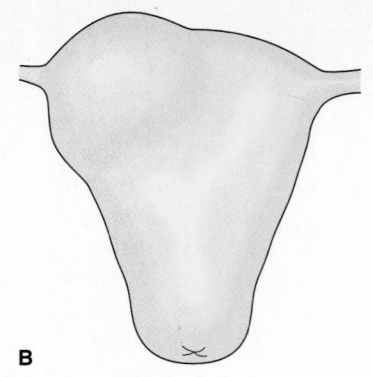 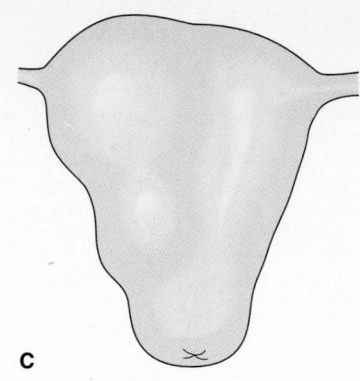

A   B   C

Site of softening

FIGURE 13-5   Early uterine changes of pregnancy. *A* Ladin's sign, a soft spot anteriorly in the middle of the uterus near the junction of the body of the uterus and the cervix. *B* Braun von Fernwald's sign, irregular softening and enlargement at the site of implantation. *C* Piskacek's sign, a tumorlike, asymmetric enlargement.

Changes in pigmentation of the skin and the *appearance of abdominal striae* are common manifestations in pregnancy. Facial chloasma occurs in varying degrees after week 16. The pigmentation of the nipple and areola may darken, especially in primigravidas and dark-haired women. The Montgomery glands of the areola may become enlarged. The skin in the midline of the abdomen may develop a pigmented line, the linea nigra. As pregnancy progresses striae appear on the abdomen and buttocks.

The *fetal outline* may be identified by palpation in many pregnant women after 24 weeks of gestation, becoming easier to distinguish as term approaches. **Ballottement** is the passive fetal movement elicited by pushing up against the cervix with two fingers. This pushes the fetal body up and, as it falls back, the examiner feels a rebound.

Pregnancy tests are based on analysis of maternal blood or urine for the detection of human chorionic gonadotropin, the hormone secreted by the trophoblast. These tests are not considered positive signs of pregnancy because the similarity of hCG and the pituitary-secreted LH occasionally results in cross-reactions. In addition certain conditions other than pregnancy can cause elevated levels of hCG.

Pregnancy Tests

Most pregnancy tests in the past were bioassays that used laboratory animals. These tests were time-consuming and subject to error. Consequently, they have been replaced by immunoassays and radioreceptor assay tests.

Immunoassay   The immunologic pregnancy tests are based on the antigenic property of hCG. There are four types of tests.

1. *Hemagglutination-inhibition test (Pregnosticon R)* is based on the fact that no clumping of cells occurs when the urine of a pregnant woman is added to the hCG-sensitized red blood cells of sheep.

2. *Latex agglutination tests (Gravindex and Pregnosticon slide test)* are based on the fact that latex particle agglutination is inhibited in the presence of urine containing hCG.

The hemagglutination-inhibition test and the latex agglutination tests are approximately 95% accurate in di-

FIGURE 13-6   Approximate height of the fundus at various weeks of pregnancy.

agnosing pregnancy and 98% accurate in determining the absence of pregnancy. The tests become positive approximately 10 to 14 days after the first missed menstrual period. The specimen used for the tests is the first early morning midstream urine because it is adequately concentrated for accuracy. The presence of protein substances (such as blood) in the specimen should be avoided because false-positive results may occur.

3. *β subunit radioimmunoassay or RIA* uses an antiserum with specificity for the β subunit of hCG in blood plasma. This is a very accurate pregnancy test that becomes positive a few days after presumed implantation, thereby permitting earlier diagnosis of pregnancy. This test is also used in the diagnosis of ectopic pregnancy or trophoblastic disease. However, because it requires several hours to perform and has only limited sensitivity, it is being replaced by other simpler tests (Buster & Carson 1991).

4. *Enzyme-Linked Immunosorbent Assay (ELISA)* is useful for detecting and quantifying small amounts of material. A blue color develops, the intensity of which is related to the amount of hCG present (Cunningham et al 1993). The test is sensitive, quick, and can detect hCG levels as early as 7–9 days after ovulation and conception, which is 5 days before the first missed period (Buster & Carson 1991).

5. *Radioreceptor Assay (RRA)* radioreceptor assay (Biocept-G) uses the principle of high-affinity receptors to detect pregnancy. It is a sensitive test and can be performed in 1 hour, but because it fails to distinguish between hCG and LH, cross-reactions may occur.

Over-the-Counter Pregnancy Tests   Home pregnancy tests are available over-the-counter at a reasonable cost. These enzyme immunoassay tests are quite sensitive and detect even low levels of hCG in urine. Best results are obtained with the first morning-voided urine, although some of the tests can be used at any time. To obtain the specimen, the woman generally voids on the absorbent end of a test stick for at least 5 seconds (a few kits still use drops of urine for testing). A color change in the test window (typically blue or purple, depending on the manufacturer) indicates a positive pregnancy test. Results appear in 3 to 5 minutes.

The false-positive rate of these tests is quite low, but the false-negative results are higher and should be followed up in the presence of pregnancy symptoms. Most of the kits available today can detect a pregnancy as early as the day of a missed period, although, to avoid false-negative results, women should be encouraged to wait 6 to 9 days after a missed menstrual period before completing the test. A false-negative result may lead to delays in beginning prenatal care or discontinuing drugs that may be harmful to the fetus (Contemporary OB/GYN 1993).

It is important that women using the home kits understand that a positive result merely indicates growing trophoblastic tissue and not necessarily a uterine pregnancy. If the woman delays seeking prenatal care after pregnancy is confirmed, an early ectopic pregnancy may be missed.

Critical Thinking Question

What factors might cause a woman to choose a home pregnancy test rather than have a pregnancy test done in a health care facility?

Diagnostic (Positive) Changes

The positive signs of pregnancy are completely objective, cannot be confused with pathologic states, and offer conclusive proof of pregnancy, but they are usually not present until after the fourth month of pregnancy.

The *fetal heartbeat* can be detected with a fetoscope by approximately week 17 to 20 of pregnancy. With the electronic Doppler device it is possible to detect the fetal heartbeat as early as week 10 to 12. The fetal heart rate is between 120 and 160 beats per minute and must be counted and compared with the maternal pulse for differentiation. Auscultation of the abdomen may reveal sounds other than that of the fetal heart. The maternal pulse, emanating from the abdominal aorta, may be unusually loud, or a uterine souffle may be heard.

Fetal movements are actively palpable by a trained examiner after about 20 weeks' gestation. They vary from a faint flutter in the early months to more vigorous movements late in pregnancy.

Ultrasound is a technique that can be used for a positive diagnosis as early as the fourth to fifth week of pregnancy. The gestational sac can be observed by 4 to 5 weeks' gestation (2 to 3 weeks after conception); fetal parts and fetal heart movement can be seen as early as 8 weeks (Cunningham et al 1993). Fetal movement can be detected with the real-time methods at approximately 12 weeks after the LMP (10 weeks after conception). (See Chapter 20 for further discussion.)

More recently ultrasound using a vaginal probe has been employed to detect a gestational sac as early as 10 days after implantation (Cunningham et al 1993).

PSYCHOLOGIC RESPONSE OF THE EXPECTANT FAMILY TO PREGNANCY

Pregnancy is a developmental challenge, a turning point, in a family's life and therefore is accompanied by stress and anxiety whether the pregnancy is desired or not. Pregnancy confirms one's biologic capabilities to reproduce. It is evidence of one's participation in sexual activity and as such is an affirmation of one's sexuality. For beginning families pregnancy is the transition period from childlessness to parenthood. If the pregnancy terminates in the birth of a child, the couple enters a new stage of their life together, one that is irreversible and characterized by awesome responsibilities.

The expectant couple may be unaware of the physical, emotional, and cognitive states peculiar to pregnancy. The couple may anticipate no problem from such a normal event as pregnancy and therefore may be confused and distressed by the feelings and behaviors commonly associated with childbearing.

If the expectant woman is married or has a stable partner, she no longer is only a mate but also must assume the role of mother. Her partner will soon be a father. Career goals and mobility may be altered or thwarted for one or both partners. Each partner begins to see the other in a different light. Their relationship takes on a different meaning to them and within the larger family and community. Their life-style changes. Role reorientation and re-identification are inevitable with each additional pregnancy and child. The set routines, family dynamics, and interactions are altered again with each pregnancy and require readjustment and realignment.

If a pregnant woman is without a stable partner, by design or circumstance, she will still experience changes in role identity and psychobiologic maturation. She must deal alone with the role changes, fears, and adjustments of pregnancy or seek support from family and friends. She also faces the reality of planning for the future as a single parent.

Decisions about financial matters need to be made at this time. Will the woman work during the pregnancy and return to work after the baby is born? If she chooses to return to work, how soon after the birth of the child will she return? Decisions may also need to be made about the division of tasks within the home. If the woman expects to share household and child care tasks with the man, but he believes that women take care of home and children and men provide the income, conflicts will inevitably arise. Similarly, problems may also arise if a father wishes to assume an active parenting role, but the mother feels she has the "final say" about parenting issues. When these differences are discussed openly, needs are identified, and solutions developed mutually, the newly forming family moves toward meeting the needs of its members.

The couple must face the realities of labor and birth before parenthood can be realized. Many nonparents have little idea what labor entails. Their information is frequently based on experiences related to them by family members or friends, and these tales are often fraught with myths and exaggerations. Classes in prepared childbirth can help them overcome much of this lack of information or misinformation.

Labor is threatening in many respects. Pain, disfigurement, disruption of bodily function, and even death are potential threats for the woman. The man faces the potential disfigurement of his wife, impairment of her health, or her death. Both fear that the baby may be ill or disfigured. The expectant couple is subject to anxiety during this period, and no one can reassure them about the outcome.

For some couples pregnancy is more than a developmental stage; it is a crisis. *Crisis* can be defined as a disturbance or conflict in which the individual cannot maintain a state of equilibrium. Pregnancy can be considered a *maturational crisis* since it is a common event in the normal growth and development of the family. During such a crisis the individual or family is in disequilibrium. Egos weaken, usual defense mechanisms lose their effectiveness, unresolved material from the past reappears, and relationships shift. The period of disequilibrium and disorganization is characterized by abortive attempts to solve the perceived problems. If the crisis is unresolved, it will result in maladaptive behaviors in one or more family members and possible disintegration of the family. Families who are able to resolve a maturational crisis successfully will return to normal functioning and can even strengthen the bonds in the family relationship.

Pregnancy as a Developmental Stage

Pregnancy can be viewed as a developmental stage with its own distinct developmental tasks. Pregnancy can be a time of support or conflict for a couple, depending on the amount of adjustment each is willing to make to maintain the family's equilibrium. Family dynamics are an important factor in adjusting to pregnancy. Family strengths include the ability of the couple to talk about issues that are important to them, to resolve conflicts and make compromises, and to seek and receive assistance and support from loved ones (Tomlinson et al 1990).

During pregnancy the couple plans together for the first child's arrival, collecting information on how to be parents. At the same time each continues to participate in some separate activities with friends or family members. The availability of social support is an important factor in psychosocial well-being during pregnancy. The social network often is a major source of advice for the pregnant woman. Research suggests that both folk beliefs and sound information are given. The most commonly reported myth for women is that reaching above the head will cause the umbilical cord to wrap around the baby's neck (St Clair & Anderson 1989).

Although individual activities are important, some conflict may arise if the couple's activities become too divergent. Thus they may find it necessary to limit their outside associations.

During pregnancy the expectant mother and father both face significant changes and must deal with major psychosocial adjustments (Table 13–3). Other family members, especially the couple's other children and the grandparents-to-be, must also adjust to the pregnancy.

TABLE 13-3   Parental Reactions to Pregnancy

First Trimester	Second Trimester	Third Trimester
Mother's Reactions	**Mother's Reactions**	**Mother's Reactions**
Informs father secretively or openly	Remains regressive and introspective, projects all problems with authority figures onto partner, may become angry as if lack of interest is sign of weakness in him	Experiences more anxiety and tension, with physical awkwardness
Feels ambivalent toward pregnancy, anxious about labor and responsibility of child	Continues to deal with feelings as a mother and looks for furniture as something concrete	Feels much discomfort and insomnia from physical condition
Is aware of physical changes, daydreams of possible miscarriage	May have other extreme of anxiety and wait until ninth month to look for furniture and clothes for baby	Prepares for birth, assembles layette, picks out names
Develops special feelings for, renewed interest in her own mother, with formation of a personal identity	Feels movement and is aware of fetus and incorporates it into herself	Dreams often about misplacing baby or not being able to give birth, fears birth of deformed baby
	Dreams that partner will be killed, telephones him often for reassurance	Feels ecstasy and excitement, has spurt of energy during last month
	Experiences more distinct physical changes, sexual desires may increase or decrease	
Father's Reactions	**Father's Reactions**	**Father's Reactions**
Differ according to age, parity, desire for child, economic stability	If he can cope, will give her extra attention she needs; if he cannot cope, will develop a new time-consuming interest outside of home	Adapts to alternative methods of sexual contact
Acceptance of pregnant woman's attitude or complete rejection and lack of communication	May develop a creative feeling and a "closeness to nature"	Becomes concerned over financial responsibility
Is aware of his own sexual feelings, may develop more or less sexual arousal	May become involved in pregnancy and buy or make furniture	May show new sense of tenderness and concern, treats partner like doll
Accepts, rejects, or resents mother-in-law	Feels for movement of baby, listens to heartbeat, or remains aloof, with no physical contact	Daydreams about child as if older and not newborn, dreams of losing partner
May develop new hobby outside of family as sign of stress	May have fears and fantasies about himself being pregnant, may become uneasy with this feminine aspect in himself	Renewed sexual attraction to partner
	May react negatively if partner is too demanding, may become jealous of physician and of his/her importance to partner and her pregnancy	Feels he is ultimately responsible for whatever happens

The Mother

Pregnancy is a condition that alters body image and also necessitates a reordering of social relationships and changes in roles of family members. The way a particular woman meets the stresses of pregnancy is influenced by her emotional makeup, her sociologic and cultural background, and her acceptance or rejection of the pregnancy. Many women manifest similar psychologic and emotional responses during pregnancy, including ambivalence, acceptance, introversion, mood swings, and changes in body image.

Ambivalence

Initially, even if the pregnancy is planned, there is an element of surprise that conception has occurred. This feeling is generally coupled with a feeling that the timing is wrong, that pregnancy is desirable "some day" but "not now." The reasons women cite may vary widely—long-term plans, job commitments, financial stress, the needs of an existing child—but the general feeling is that one is not ready to have a child at this time. This feeling accounts for much of the ambivalence commonly experienced by women during early pregnancy. Ambivalence may also be related to the need to modify personal relationships or career plans, to fear coupled with excitement about assuming a new role, to unresolved emotional conflicts with one's own mother, and to fears about pregnancy, labor, and birth. Such feelings may be even more pronounced in the event of an unplanned or unwanted pregnancy. Indirect evidence of ambivalence includes complaints about depression, physical discomfort, and feeling "ugly" and unattractive (Lederman 1984).

During the early months the pregnant woman may seriously consider the possibility of an abortion if the pregnancy is unwanted. In the event of religious conflicts about induced abortion the woman may experience guilt feelings about her thoughts or may tend to focus on the possibility of spontaneous abortion (miscarriage). Even when the pregnancy is consciously planned and desired, thoughts of abortion and miscarriage arise. The idea that the baby might be lost has a certain emotional appeal because it represents the possible relief of fears and ambivalence. Concurrently, the pregnant woman may feel guilty for having such negative thoughts and may worry that in some way these thoughts will harm the baby (Robinson & Stewart 1990).

RESEARCH IN PRACTICE

Stillbirths contribute substantially to perinatal mortality worldwide, and the rate of late intrauterine death has remained relatively constant over the past decade. Despite this, prospective mothers are not routinely taught fetal movement counting, a technique that potentially identifies reduced fetal activity. Obstetric literature suggests that self-monitoring may create psychologic stress for the pregnant woman by increasing her attention to fetal movements. Robert Liston, Kathleen Bloom, and Pamela Zimmer asked whether state/trait anxiety, locus of control, or maternal attitude toward pregnancy changed between the 27th and 37th week of gestation as a result of fetal movement counting.

The sample consisted of 590 consenting low-risk primigravidas with no preexisting medical or psychologic problems who were referred by family physicians. Pretesting was carried out in the 27th week using established psychologic inventories. Participants were randomly assigned to one of three groups. The first group, fetal movement counters, received instruction on counting and recording fetal movement. A protocol established for ethical reasons required a woman who had not felt at least 10 fetal movements by noon on any day to immediately notify her physician for a biophysical profile of non-stress testing and ultrasound. The second group of women served as a control for possible Hawthorne effects and received instructions to record their periods of sleeping and wakefulness including any nighttime sleep interruptions. The third group, non-recording women, was only told that they would complete the psychologic testing again at 37 weeks' gestation.

Statistical analysis showed significant changes in the psychologic parameters of the women but were unrelated to group. The fetal counting group did not differ from the other two groups according to repeated measures analysis of variance. Overall the sample of 590 women demonstrated a slight rise in state anxiety, a decrease in trait anxiety, a slightly increased sense of internal control, a slight decrease in sense of well being, and a slight increase in positive attitudes toward the infant.

Clinical Application of Study

Although the results of two previous large studies differ on the question of whether fetal movement counting reduces late intrauterine death, this study identified no change in pregnant women's psychologic distress as a result of monitoring fetal movement. With explicit instructions and clear, careful response protocols, self-monitoring might reduce stillbirth risk.

SOURCE: Liston R, Bloom K, Zimmer P: The psychological effects of counting fetal movements. *Birth* 1994; 21(3):135.

Acceptance

Acceptance of pregnancy is influenced by many factors. Lower acceptance tends to be related to an unplanned pregnancy and greater evidence of fear and conflict. The woman carrying an unplanned pregnancy tends to experience more physical discomfort and depression. When a pregnancy is well accepted, the woman demonstrates feelings of happiness and pleasure in the pregnancy. She experiences less physical discomfort and shows a high degree of tolerance for the discomforts associated with the third trimester (Lederman 1984).

During the *first trimester*, evidence of pregnancy is limited to amenorrhea and to the word of the care giver that the pregnancy test was positive. In an effort to verify her condition a woman may become minutely conscious of changes in her body that could validate the pregnancy. During the first trimester the woman's baby does not seem real to her, and she focuses on herself and her pregnancy (Rubin 1984).

The *second trimester* is relatively tranquil. Morning sickness generally passes, the threat of spontaneous abortion diminishes, and the woman begins to accept the reality of her pregnancy. It is not unusual for an enthusiastic primagravida to don maternity clothes at the beginning of this trimester even when it is not truly necessary. The clothing serves as a verification of her pregnant state.

The highlight of the second trimester is quickening, which generally occurs about week 20—midway through the pregnancy. Actual perception of fetal movement frequently produces dramatic changes in the woman. She now perceives her baby as a real person and generally becomes excited about the pregnancy even if she hasn't been prior to this time.

As quickening and her altered physical appearance confirm her pregnant state, the woman adjusts to the idea of change and begins to prepare for her new role and her new set of relationships—with her partner and family, the child-to-be and other children, friends, and loved ones. When the pregnancy is well accepted, the woman takes pleasure in the sensations of pregnancy and attempts to picture her baby in order to know him or her better. The woman may avidly delve into folklore regarding the child's sex and may carefully study photos of herself and her partner to gain some clues about her child's appearance. She may ask her friends about childbirth and seek out other women who are pregnant or have recently given birth. She feels well, is excited, and may exhibit the "glow" so often attributed to pregnant women.

The *third trimester* combines a sense of pride with anxiety about what is to come in order for the child to be born. During this time the special prerogatives of pregnancy may be most marked. As her protruding abdomen proclaims her advanced pregnancy, the woman may find that others become more solicitous, that a chair may be offered in a crowded room, that others may carry her parcels. The woman may actually need this help, she may simply enjoy the attention as a privilege of pregnancy, or she may reject it if she fears that such gestures indicate she is helpless.

During the final trimester physical discomforts again increase, and adequate rest becomes a necessity. The woman, eager for the pregnancy to end, wonders if her baby's expected date of birth is accurate. She makes final preparation for the baby and may spend long periods considering names for the child. During this time the woman worries more about the health and safety of her unborn child and may have concerns that she will not behave well during childbirth (Robinson & Stewart 1990).

The woman may feel vulnerable to rejection, loss, or insult. She may worry about a variety of things and hesitate to go out unless accompanied by someone she is certain cares about her. She may withdraw into the security and quiet of her home. Toward the end of this period there is often a burst of energy as the woman prepares the "nest" for her expected infant. Many women report bursts of energy in which they vigorously clean and organize their homes.

Introversion

Introversion, or turning in on oneself, is a common occurrence in pregnancy. An active, outgoing woman may become less interested in previous activities and more concerned with needs for rest and time alone. This concentration of attention permits the woman to plan, adjust, adapt, build, and draw strength in preparation for her child's birth (Rubin 1975). As she becomes more aware of herself, her partner may feel she is being overly sensitive. He may perceive her introversion and passivity as exclusion of him and may in turn become unable to interact with her, either verbally or physically, or to provide the affection, support, and consideration she requires. This change may result in disequilibrium and stress for the entire family. It is essential that the couple work together to establish new, mutually acceptable patterns of response in order to overcome these blocks to communication.

> I don't know if this is really considered a problem or not, but at times it seems like a problem. I'm really subject to drastic mood changes. That, or I'll be extremely emotional. For no reason at all I'll start crying or just laughing until I can hardly breathe. I don't know why; and if I can't understand it, it's twice as hard for John, especially if I'm bummed out or crying. It doesn't seem normal for a person to cry for no reason and I never did it before.
>
> ~ QUOTED IN RP LEDERMAN ~
> ~ PSYCHOSOCIAL ADAPTATION IN PREGNANCY ~

Mood Swings

Throughout pregnancy the emotions of many women are characterized by mood swings, from great joy to deep despair. Frequently, the woman will become tearful with little apparent cause. When asked why she is crying, she may find it difficult or impossible to give a reason. The situation is extremely unsettling for the partner, causing him to feel confused and inadequate. Because the man may feel unable to handle the woman's tears, he often reacts by withdrawing and ignoring the problem. Because the pregnant woman needs increased love and affection, she may perceive his reaction as unloving and nonsupportive. Once the couple understands that this behavior is characteristic of pregnancy, it becomes easier for them to deal with it more effectively—although it will be a source of stress to some extent throughout pregnancy.

Changes in Body Image

Pregnancy produces marked changes in a woman's body within a relatively short period of time. Women perceive that they require more body space as pregnancy progresses (Fawcett et al 1986). They also experience changes in body image. The degree of this change is related to a certain extent to personality factors, social network responses, and attitudes toward pregnancy.

Body boundary is another aspect of body image. It is the boundary that defines self, "containing and demarcating self as an entity separate from the surroundings" (Rubin 1984, p 17). When the body boundary is definite, the body is seen as firm, strong, and distinct from its environment. Body boundary vulnerability occurs when the body boundary is perceived as delicate, capable of being penetrated, and not readily distinguishable from its environment. The pregnant woman may feel both increased body boundary definitions and body boundary vulnerability, which suggests that the woman may perceive her body as vulnerable and yet as a protective container (Fawcett 1978).

Changes in body image are normal but can be very stressful for the pregnant woman. Explanation of the changes and discussion of the alterations in body image may help both the woman and her partner deal with the stress associated with this aspect of pregnancy.

Psychologic Tasks of the Mother

Rubin (1984) has identified four major tasks that the pregnant woman undertakes to maintain her intactness and that of her family and at the same time incorporate her new child into the family system. These tasks form the foundation for a mutually gratifying relationship with her infant:

1. *Ensuring safe passage through pregnancy, labor, and birth.* The pregnant woman feels concern for both her unborn child and herself. She seeks competent maternity care to provide a sense of control and wishes to establish a relationship with her nurse-midwife or physician so that they "know" her and her needs. The woman also seeks knowledge from literature, observation of other pregnant women and new mothers, and discussion with others who have borne children. The pregnant woman also seeks to

ensure safe passage by engaging in self-care activities related to diet, exercise, alcohol consumption, and so forth (Patterson et al 1990). In the third trimester, as her movements slow and her body mass increases, she becomes aware of external threats in the environment—a toy on a stair, the awkwardness of an escalator—that pose a threat to her intactness and represent hazards to be overcome. External threats become more significant, and the woman worries if her partner is late or she is home alone. Sleep becomes difficult, and she begins to long for the baby's birth, even though it, too, is frightening.

2. *Seeking of acceptance of this child by others.* The birth of a child alters a woman's primary support group, her family, and her secondary affiliative groups. During the first trimester the woman may feel sorrow at the anticipated changes, but in most cases the transition from existing social groupings to newer groupings occurs smoothly. The family generally makes the transition, and the woman slowly and subtly alters her secondary network to meet the needs of her pregnancy. In this adjustment the woman's partner is the most important figure. His support and acceptance influence her completion of her maternal tasks, the formation of her maternal identity, indeed the entire course of her pregnancy. If there are other children in the home, the mother also works to ensure their acceptance of the coming child. Accepting the coming change in exclusive relationships—woman and partner or mother and first child— is sometimes stressful, and the woman will often work to maintain some special time with her partner or older child. Achieving social acceptance of the child and herself as mother may be more difficult for the adolescent mother or single woman. The child to come is not always wanted, and the woman often must direct her energies to changing this situation.

3. *Seeking of commitment and acceptance of self as mother to the infant (binding-in).* During the first trimester the child remains a rather abstract concept. With quickening, however, the child begins to become a real person, and the mother begins to develop bonds of attachment. The mother experiences the movement of the child within her in an intimate, exclusive way, and out of this experience bonds of love form. The mother develops a fantasy image of her ideal child. This possessive love increases her maternal commitment to protect her fetus now and her child after he or she is born.

4. *Learning to give of oneself on behalf of one's child.* Childbirth involves many acts of giving. The man "gives" a child to a woman; she in turn "gives" a child to the man. Life is given to an infant; a sibling is given to older children of the family. The woman begins to develop a capacity for self-denial and learns to delay immediate personal gratification to meet the needs of another. Baby showers and baby gifts are acts of giving that help the mother's self-esteem while also helping her acknowledge the separateness and needs of the coming baby.

Accomplishment of these tasks helps the expectant woman develop her self-concept as mother. Often the expectant mother turns to her own mother during pregnancy because her mother is a source of information and can serve as a role model (Lederman 1984). A woman's self-concept as mother expands with actual experience and continues to grow through subsequent childbearing and child rearing. Occasionally, a woman never accepts the mother role but plays the role of babysitter or older sister.

The Father

Until fairly recently the expectant father was often viewed as a "bystander" or observer of his partner's pregnancy. He was necessary for conception, for bill paying, and for providing male guidance as his child matured. This view has changed, and the father of today is expected to fulfill the role of provider as well as nurturing, caring, involved parent (Henderson & Brouse 1991). Previously, little attention was given to his needs, responses, and adjustments during pregnancy. Research suggests, however, that the father's stresses, adaptive behaviors, and developmental processes are as complex as those of his mate (Longobucco & Freston 1989).

In response to societal pressures, the influence of the woman's movement, and the economic pressures that result in more women employed outside the home, shared parenting and breadwinning have become more commonplace. Then, too, many men have actively sought to be more involved in the experience of childbirth and parenting.

Thus the expectant father must first deal with the reality of the pregnancy and then struggle to gain recognition as a parent from his partner, family, friends, co-workers, society—and from his baby as well. The expectant mother can help her partner be a participant and not merely a helpmate to her if she has a definite sense of the experience as *their* pregnancy and *their* infant and not *her* pregnancy and *her* infant (Jordan 1990).

The expectant father faces psychologic stress as he makes the transition from nonparent to parent or from parent of one or more to parent of two or more. The stressor most frequently identified by expectant fathers has often been financial concern. Research suggests that major sources of stress include concern that the baby will not be healthy and normal and worry about the pain the partner will experience in childbirth, about unexpected events during pregnancy, and about the baby's condition at birth (Glazer 1989). Other sources of stress for expectant fathers include concern over the changing relationship with their partner, diminished sexual responsiveness in their partner or in themselves, change in relationships with their family or male friends, their role during labor and birth, and their ability to parent.

Expectant fathers experience many of the same feelings and conflicts experienced by expectant mothers when the pregnancy has been confirmed. Feelings of ambivalence are prevalent. The extent of ambivalence depends on many factors, such as whether the pregnancy was planned, the man's relationship with his partner, his previous experiences with pregnancy, his age, and his economic stability.

The expectant father must establish a fatherhood role just as the woman develops a concept of herself as mother. Fathers who are most successful at this generally like children, are excited about the prospect of fatherhood, are eager to nurture a child, have confidence in their ability to be a parent, and share the experiences of pregnancy and childbirth with their partners (Lederman 1984).

First Trimester

After the initial excitement of the announcement of the pregnancy to friends and relatives and their congratulations, an expectant father may begin to feel left out of the pregnancy. He is also often confused by his partner's mood changes and perhaps bewildered by his responses to her changing body. He may resent the attention given to the woman and the need to change their relationship as she experiences fatigue and a decreased interest in sex.

During this time his child is a "potential baby." Fathers often picture interacting with a child of 5 or 6 rather than a newborn. Even the pregnancy itself may seem unreal until the woman shows more physical signs (Jordan 1990).

Second Trimester

The father's role in the pregnancy is still vague in the second trimester, but his involvement can be increased by his watching and feeling fetal movement. Many women report that their partner kisses them on the abdomen more in pregnancy than at any other time. Both may find this sexually arousing, and, during the second trimester especially, it can be a facilitator to increasing sexual activity.

It is helpful if the father, as well as the mother, has the opportunity to hear the fetal heartbeat. That requires a visit to the nurse-midwife's or physician's office. Involvement of fathers in antepartal care is increasing as fathers become more comfortable with this new role. For many men seeing the infant on ultrasound is an important experience in accepting the reality of the pregnancy.

The expectant father needs to confront and resolve some of his own conflicts about the fathering he experienced. He will need to sort out those behaviors in his own fathering that he wants and does not want to imitate. This process usually occurs gradually as the pregnancy progresses. Because a more active involvement in childbirth and parenting by fathers is somewhat new, men may have few role models available to them. Fishbein (1984) suggests that the actual role a father assumes is less important than the process of negotiating between partners to reach agreement on the father's role. Fishbein found that agreement was more important than the actual degree of paternal involvement. Agreement between partners tended to increase with age and combined family income.

The woman's appearance begins to alter at this time too, and men react differently to the physical change. For some it decreases sexual interest; for others it may have the opposite effect. A multitude of emotions are experienced by both partners, and it continues to be important for them to communicate and accept each other's feelings and concerns. In situations in which the expectant mother's demands dominate the relationship, the expectant father's resentment may increase to the point that he is spending more time at work, involved in a hobby, or with his friends. The behavior is even more likely if the expectant father did not want the pregnancy and/or if the relationship was not a good one prior to the pregnancy.

Third Trimester

If the couple have communicated their concerns and feelings to one another and grown in their relationship, the third trimester is a special and rewarding time. A more clearly defined role evolves at this time for the expectant father, and it becomes more obvious how the couple can prepare together for the coming event. They may become involved in childbirth education classes, and more concrete preparations for the arrival of the baby begin, such as shopping for a crib, car seat, and other equipment. If the expectant father has developed a detached attitude about the pregnancy prior to this time, however, it is unlikely that he will become a willing participant even though his role becomes more obvious.

Concerns and fears may recur. Many men are afraid of hurting the unborn baby during intercourse. The father may also begin to have anxiety and fantasies about what could happen to his partner and the unborn baby during labor and birth and feels a great sense of responsibility. The questions asked earlier in pregnancy emerge again. What kind of parents will he and his partner be? Will he really be able to help his partner in labor? Can they afford to have a baby?

Couvade

The term **couvade** traditionally has referred to the observance of certain rituals and taboos by the male to signify the transition to fatherhood. In non-Western society these taboos may have taken specific form—for example, the man may have been forbidden to eat certain foods or carry certain weapons. More recently, the term has been used to describe the unintentional development of physical symptoms by the partner of a pregnant woman. The incidence of couvade has been cited as ranging from 11% to 97% (Conner & Denson 1990).

The most commonly occurring symptoms include gastrointestinal disturbances, upper respiratory disturbances, aches and pains, and behavioral manifestations (Conner & Denson 1990). Research suggests that those men who demonstrate couvade syndrome tend to have a higher degree of paternal role preparation and be involved in more activities related to this preparation (Longobucco & Freston 1989).

Siblings

The introduction of a new baby into the family is often the beginning of sibling rivalry. Sibling rivalry results from children's fear of change in the security of their relationships with their parents. Some of the behaviors demonstrating feelings of sibling rivalry may even be directed toward the mother during the pregnancy as she experiences more fatigue and less patience with her toddler. Parents who recognize the situation early in pregnancy and begin constructive actions can help minimize the problems of sibling rivalry.

Preparation for the young child begins several weeks prior to the anticipated birth and is designed according to the age and experience of the child. Because they do not have a clear concept of time, young children should not be told too early about the pregnancy. From the toddler's point of view "several weeks" is an extremely long time. The mother may let the child feel the baby moving in her uterus, explaining that this is "a special place where babies grow." The child can help the parents put the baby clothes in drawers or prepare the nursery. The child will probably be interested in trying on the clothes, lying in the crib, and trying out other baby items.

The concept of consistency is important in dealing with young children. They need reassurance that certain people, special things, and familiar places will continue to exist after the new baby arrives. The crib is an important though transient object in a child's life. If it is to be given to the new baby, the parents should thoughtfully help the child adjust to this change (Honig 1986). Any move from crib to bed or from one room to another should precede the baby's birth.

If the child is ready for toilet training, it is most effectively done several months before or after the baby's arrival. Parents should know that the older, toilet-trained child may regress to wetting or soiling because he or she sees the new baby getting attention for such behavior. The older, weaned child may want to drink from a bottle again after the new baby comes. Lack of knowledge of these common occurrences can be frustrating to the new mother and can compound the stress that she feels during the early postpartum days.

During the pregnancy older children should be introduced to a new baby for short periods to get an idea of what a new baby is like. This introduction dispels fantasies that the new arrival will be big enough to be a playmate. Pregnant women may also find it helpful to bring their children to a prenatal visit after they have been told about the expected baby. The children are encouraged to become involved in prenatal care and to ask any questions they may have. They are also given the opportunity to hear the baby's heartbeat, either with a stethoscope or with the Doppler. This helps make the baby more real to them.

The school-age child should be involved in the pregnancy. If the pregnancy is viewed as a family affair, the child is not excluded from the experience. Teaching about the pregnancy should be based on the child's level of understanding and interest. Overeager parents may go into lengthier and more in-depth responses than the child is interested in. Some children are more curious than others. Books at their level of understanding can be made available in the home. Involvement in family discussions, attendance at sibling preparation classes, encouragement to feel fetal movement, and an opportunity to listen to the fetal heart supplement the learning process and help make the school-age child feel part of the pregnancy. Studies have demonstrated that sibling preparation classes assist in the transition process for both parents and children. After attending the classes, children exhibit less anxiety and increased ability to express their feelings. Parents are often better able to cope with the older child after birth.

The older child may appear to have a sophisticated knowledge base, but it may be intermingled with many misconceptions. Thus opportunities for discussion and participation should be provided.

Even after the birth siblings need to feel that they are part of a family affair. Changes in hospital regulations allowing siblings to be present at the birth or to visit their mother and the new baby facilitate this process. On arrival at home, siblings can share in "showing off" the new baby.

Preparation of siblings for the arrival of a new baby is essential, but other factors are equally important. These include the amount of parental attention focused on the new arrival, amount of parental attention given the older child after the birth of the new arrival, and parental reinforcement of regressive and/or aggressive behavior.

Grandparents

The first relatives told about a pregnancy are usually the grandparents. Although relationships with parents can be very complex, this period in a family's life most often promotes a closer relationship between the expectant couple and their parents. Usually the expectant grandparents become increasingly supportive of the expectant couple, even if disapproval of the couple's marriage and/or other conflicts were previously present.

Grandparents may be unsure about the amount of involvement they are "allowed" during the pregnancy and childbearing process. Most want to be helpful; some may bestow advice and/or gifts unsparingly. Because grandparenting can occur over a wide span of years, people's response to this role can vary considerably. For some this new role may occur at a relatively young age, and the connotation of aging that accompanies the role may affect their response to the pregnancy. The younger grandparent may also be involved in work and other activities and may not demonstrate as much interest as the young couple would like.

It can be difficult for even sensitive grandparents to know how much involvement the couple wants. Expectant couples want to feel in control of their new situation, which may be initially difficult in their changing roles. Grandparents find that this factor, as well as changing roles in their own life (eg, retirement, financial concerns, menopause of the expectant grandmother, death of a friend), may contribute to conflicts in the changing family structure. Some parents of expectant couples may already be grandparents and have already developed their own style of grandparenting, which will be an important factor in how they respond to the pregnancy.

Childbearing and childrearing practices are very different for today's childbearing couple. It helps family cohesiveness for young couples to share with interested grandparents what today's practices are and why they feel they are effective. For example, Biasella (1993) describes a comprehensive perinatal education program for families that includes grandparents in one to two classes that discuss current obstetrical and childrearing practices. Some couples may even choose to have grandparents attend the birth. At the same time it is important for young couples to listen to any differences expectant grandparents want to explain. When grandparents give advice, it helps to remember that they care. When their recommendations seem effective, it is significant to grandparents that young couples do listen and follow advice.

Occasionally young couples feel they are receiving more advice than they can tolerate. Too often they perceive parents' suggestions as criticizing their ability to prepare adequately for the childbearing process—and later as criticizing their care of the newborn. It is helpful for the young couple to discuss the problem and agree on a plan of action. The role of the helping grandparents when the new baby is brought home needs to be clarified before the event to ensure a comfortable situation for all.

CULTURAL DIVERSITY AND PREGNANCY

Critical Thinking Question

How might nurses learn more about the cultural beliefs and practices of the ethnic groups that live in their area?

A universal tendency exists to create ceremonial rituals and rites around important life events. Thus pregnancy, childbirth, marriage, and death are often tied to ritual. Many of these rituals have their origins in the practices of ancient human beings (Spector 1991). For example, pregnancy rituals described in the Korean culture include Tae Mong and Tae Kyo. After the Korean woman has a dream about conception, Tae Mong, she follows the Tae Kyo ritual for pregnancy. Tae Kyo is a set of rules for safe and easy childbirth that the woman follows to protect the infant from disease and retardation and to protect the family from misfortune (Pritham & Sammons 1993).

The rituals, customs, and practices of a group are a reflection of the group's values. Thus the identification of cultural values is useful in planning and providing culturally sensitive care. An understanding of male and female roles, family life-styles, or the meaning of children in a culture may explain reactions of joy or shame. Pregnancy is a joyful event in a culture that values children. In some cultures, however, pregnancy is a shameful event if it occurs outside of marriage.

Health values and beliefs are also important in understanding reactions and behavior. Certain behaviors can be expected if a culture views pregnancy as a sickness, whereas other behaviors can be expected if pregnancy is viewed as a natural occurrence. Prenatal care may not be a priority for women who view pregnancy as a natural occurrence. For example, in the Southeast Asian culture pregnancy is not considered an illness, so seeking prenatal care may not be important to this group (Mattson & Lew 1992). Health care in Southeast Asia is crisis oriented, with symptom relief as the goal (D'Avanzo 1992).

Generalizations about cultural characteristics or cultural values are difficult since these characteristics may not be exhibited by every individual within a culture. Just as variations are seen *between* cultures, variations are also seen *within* cultures. These variations are often related to social and economic factors such as class, income, and education. For example, a third-generation Chinese American family might have very different values and beliefs than a traditional Chinese family because of their exposure to the American culture. For this reason the nurse needs to supplement a general knowledge of cultural values and practices with a complete assessment of the individual's values and practices.

Attitudes about pregnancy may vary somewhat among cultures. Americans of African descent, for example, usually consider pregnancy as a state of wellness. Mexican Americans generally view pregnancy as a natural and desirable condition, and most Native American groups consider pregnancy a normal process. In all these cultures children are desired. Children ensure continuation of the family and cultural values. A woman who gives birth to a child, especially a son, often achieves higher status. This is true in traditional Chinese families, for example. Similarly, in the western United States culture of Mormonism, motherhood is thought to be the most important aspect of a woman's life and equated with the male role of priesthood (Conley 1990). In Mexican American society and among many Hispanic groups having children is evidence of the male's virility and is a sign of manliness or *machismo*, a desired trait.

Health Beliefs

Although pregnancy is perceived as a natural occurrence in many cultures, it may also be viewed as a time of increased vulnerability. In groups that adhere to beliefs in evil spirits certain protective precautions are often followed. For example, pregnant Vietnamese women are warned to avoid funerals, places of worship, and streets at noon and five o'clock in the afternoon because spirits are present at these times (Stringfellow 1978). Traditional beliefs often guide the Southeast Asian individual in the prenatal period, such as the belief that raising the arms over the head pulls on the placenta and may cause it to break (D'Avanzo 1992). In the Mexican American culture the concept of *mal aire* or bad air is sometimes related to evil spirits. It is thought that air, especially night air, may enter the body and cause harm. Preventive measures, such as keeping the windows closed or covering the head, are used. For many Southeast Asians, "wind" represents a bad external influence that may enter a person when the body is vulnerable, such as during and after childbirth or during surgery (Lee et al 1988).

Most of the taboos stemming from the belief in evil spirits exist for fear of injuring the unborn child. Taboos also emanate from the fear that a pregnant woman has evil powers. For this reason pregnant women are sometimes prohibited from taking part in certain activities. For example, the pregnant Vietnamese woman cannot attend a wedding for fear of bringing bad luck to the newlyweds (Hollingsworth et al 1980).

The equilibrium model of health is based on the concept of balance between light and dark, heat and cold. Asian belief focuses on the notion of *yin* and *yang*. Yin represents the female, passive principle—darkness, cold, wetness—and yang is the masculine, active part—light, heat, and dryness. When the two are combined, they are all that can be. The hot-cold classification is seen in cultures in Latin America, the Near East, and Asia. The dimensions and meanings of this classification vary, however, and require further investigation.

Mexican Americans often consider illness to be an excess of either hot or cold. To restore health, imbalances are often corrected by the proper use of foods, medications, or herbs. These substances are also classified as hot or cold. For example, an illness attributed to an excess of coldness will be treated only with hot foods or medications. The classification of foods is not always consistent, but it does conform to a general structure of traditional knowledge. Certain foods, spices, herbs, and medications are perceived to cool or heat the body. These perceptions do not necessarily correspond to the actual temperature; some hot dishes are said to have a cooling quality.

Southeast Asians believe it is important to keep the woman "warm" after the birth because blood, which is considered "hot," has been lost, and the woman is at risk of becoming "cold." Therefore they avoid cold drinks and foods following birth (Mattson & Lew 1992). Hindu women, on the other hand, consider pregnancy a "hot" period and eat "cool" foods to counterbalance the hot state (Wollett & Dosanjh-Matwala 1990).

The concepts of hot and cold are not as important in Native American or African American beliefs. There are some similarities, however, in all of these groups because of the emphasis on a balance in nature.

Health Practices

Health care practices during pregnancy are influenced by numerous factors, such as the prevalence of traditional home remedies and folk beliefs, the importance of indigenous healers, and the influence of professional health care workers. In an urban setting the age, length of time in the city, marital status, and strength of the family may affect these patterns. Socioeconomic status is also important because modern medical services are more accessible to those who can afford it. The social network is an important source of information for a pregnant woman. Often the advice is sound, but sometimes the rationale is incorrect or the advice, if followed, could be harmful (St. Clair & Anderson 1989).

An awareness of alternative health sources is crucial for health professionals because these practices affect health outcomes. For example, many members of the Mexican American community utilize the *partera*, a lay midwife, as a healer who gives advice and treats illnesses during pregnancy as well as being in attendance during labor and birth (Spector 1991).

Indigenous healers are also important in some cultures. In the Mexican American culture the healer is called a *curandero*. In some Native American tribes the medicine man may fulfill the healing role. Herbalists are often found in Asian cultures; and faith healers, root doctors, and spiritualists are sometimes consulted in the African American culture.

Cultural Factors and Nursing Care

In recent years people from a variety of cultures have immigrated to North America. This influx of people has had a significant impact on the health care system. Numerous differences exist in beliefs, values, health care practices and expectations, language, world views, and etiquette between these newly arrived people and the majority of health care providers.

Health care providers are often unaware of the cultural characteristics they themselves demonstrate. Without cultural awareness care givers tend to project their own cultural responses onto foreign-born clients and assume that the clients are demonstrating a specific behavior for the same reason that they would. For example, health care providers sometimes label a pregnant or post-partum Filipino woman as "lazy" because of her rather sedentary life-style. In reality this style results from the cultural belief that inactivity is necessary to protect the mother and child (Stern et al 1985). Thiederman (1986) suggests that if health care providers fail to understand the reasons for a person's behavior, it is impossible for them to intervene appropriately and ensure cooperation.

To a certain extent most of us are guilty of ethnocentrism, at least some of the time. **Ethnocentrism** "refers to an individual's belief that his or her own cultural group's beliefs and values are the best or the only acceptable beliefs. It includes an inability to understand the worldview or beliefs of another culture" (Eliason 1993). Thus the nurse who values stoicism during labor may be uncomfortable with the more vocal response of a Latin American woman. Another nurse may be disconcerted by the Southeast Asian woman who believes that pain is something to be endured rather than alleviated and is very intent on maintaining self-control in labor (Mattson & Lew 1992).

Health care providers sometimes believe that if members of other cultures do not share Western values, they should adopt them. This is especially difficult for some nurses caring for childbearing families if the nurse is a firm believer in the equality of the sexes and women's liberation. The nurse may find it difficult to remain silent if a woman from a Middle Eastern culture defers to her husband in decision making. It is important to remember that pressure to defy cultural values and beliefs can be stressful and anxiety provoking for these women (Thiederman 1986).

Members of minority culture groups are often found living in a certain area of a community. The nurse can begin developing cultural sensitivity by becoming knowledgeable about the cultural practices of local groups. For example, is it considered courteous to avoid eye contact? Should last names be used in conversation as a sign of respect? Is a female health care provider necessary?

Cultural assessment is an important aspect of prenatal care. Health care professionals are becoming increasingly aware of the importance of addressing cultural, physiologic, and psychologic needs in the prenatal assessment in order to provide culture-specific health care during pregnancy (Pritham & Sammons 1993). The nurse should identify the main beliefs, values, and behaviors that relate to pregnancy and childbearing. This includes information about ethnic background, amount of affiliation with the ethnic group, patterns of decision making, religious preferences, language, communication style, and common etiquette practices (Tripp-Reimer et al 1984). The nurse can also explore the woman's (or family's) expectations of the health care system.

In planning care the nurse considers the extent to which the woman's personal values, beliefs, and customs are in accord with those of the woman's identified cultural group, the nurse providing care, and the health care agency. If discrepancies exist, the nurse then considers

CRITICAL THINKING IN PRACTICE

Mr and Mrs Nguyen have recently immigrated to the United States from Southeast Asia after spending 1 year in a refugee camp. Mr Nguyen speaks only a few phrases of English, and Mrs Nguyen speaks no English. They present to the prenatal clinic where you are working as the triage nurse. Mr Nguyen explains that his wife is expecting her third child and has not received any prenatal care. He states that this is their first time utilizing a health care facility in the United States. The language barrier renders you unable to obtain any further information. You examine Mrs Nguyen and find her vital signs and brief physical examination to be within normal range. Her fundal height measures 28 cm, the fetal heart rate is 132 beats per minute. What would you do?

Answers can be found in Appendix I.

whether the woman's system is supportive, neutral, or harmful in relation to possible interventions (Tripp-Reimer et al 1984). If the woman's system is supportive or neutral, it can be incorporated into the plan. For example, individual food practices or methods of pain expression may differ from those of the nurse or agency but would not necessarily interfere with the nursing plan. However, certain cultural practices might pose a threat to the health of the childbearing woman. For example, some Filipino women will not take any medication during pregnancy. The health care provider may consider a certain medication essential to the woman's well-being. In

TABLE 13-4	Providing Effective Prenatal Care to Families of Different Cultures

Nurses who are **interacting** with expectant families from a different culture or ethnic group can provide more effective, culturally sensitive nursing care by:

- Critically examining their own cultural beliefs
- Identifying personal biases, attitudes, stereotypes, and prejudices
- Making a conscious commitment to respect the values and beliefs of others
- Using sensitive, current language when describing their culture
- Learning the rituals, customs, and practices of the major cultural and ethnic groups with whom they have contact
- Including cultural assessment and assessment of the family's expectations of the health care system as a routine part of prenatal nursing care
- Incorporating the family's cultural practices into prenatal care as much as possible
- Fostering an attitude of respect for and cooperating with alternative healers and care givers whenever possible
- Providing for the services of an interpreter if language barriers exist
- Learning the language (or at least several key phrases) of at least one of the cultural groups with whom they interact
- Recognizing that ultimately it is the woman's right to make her own health care choices
- Evaluating whether client's health care beliefs have any potential negative consequences for the client's health

this case the woman's cultural belief may be detrimental to her own health. The nurse then faces two alternatives:

1. Identifying ways of persuading the woman to accept the proposed therapy

2. Accepting the woman's rationale for refusing therapy if she is not willing to adapt her belief system (Tripp-Reimer et al 1984)

Table 13–4 on page 329 summarizes the key actions a nurse can take to become more culturally aware.

Siblings of all ages require assistance in dealing with the birth of a new baby.

Cultural values, beliefs, and behaviors influence a couple's response to childbearing and the health care system.

Ethnocentrism is the belief that one's own cultural beliefs, values, and practices are the best ones, indeed the only ones worth considering.

A cultural assessment should focus on factors that will influence the practices of the childbearing family with regard to their health needs.

KEY CONCEPTS

Virtually all systems of a woman's body are altered in some way during pregnancy.

Blood pressure decreases slightly during pregnancy. It reaches its lowest point in the second trimester and gradually increases to near normal levels in the third trimester.

The enlarging uterus may exert pressure on the vena cava when the woman lies supine. This is called the vena caval syndrome.

A physiologic anemia may occur during pregnancy because the total plasma volume increases more than the total number of erythrocytes. This produces a drop in the hematocrit.

The glomerular filtration rate increases during pregnancy. Glycosuria may be caused by the body's inability to reabsorb all the glucose filtered by the glomeruli.

Changes in the skin include the development of chloasma; linea nigra; darkened nipples, areola, and vulva; striae; spider nevi; and palmar erythema.

Insulin needs are increased during pregnancy. A woman with a latent deficiency state may respond to the increased stress on the islets of Langerhans by developing gestational diabetes.

The subjective (presumptive) signs of pregnancy are those symptoms experienced and reported by the woman, such as amenorrhea, nausea and vomiting, fatigue, urinary frequency, breast changes, and quickening.

The objective (probable) signs of pregnancy can be perceived by the examiner but may be caused by conditions other than pregnancy.

The diagnostic (positive) signs of pregnancy can be perceived by the examiner and can be caused only by pregnancy.

During pregnancy the expectant woman may experience ambivalence, acceptance, introversion, emotional lability, and changes in body image.

Rubin (1984) has identified four developmental tasks for the pregnant woman: (1) ensuring safe passage through pregnancy, labor, and birth; (2) seeking acceptance of this child by others; (3) seeking commitment and acceptance of self as mother to the infant; and (4) learning to give of oneself on behalf of one's child.

Fathers also face a series of adjustments as they accept their new role.

REFERENCES

Biasella S: A comprehensive perinatal education class. *AWHONN Clin Issues Perinatal Women Health Nurs* 1993; 4(1):5.

Blackburn ST, Loper DL: *Maternal, Fetal, and Neonatal Physiology: A Clinical Perspective.* Philadelphia: WB Saunders, 1992.

Buster JE, Carson SA: Placental endocrinology and diagnosis of pregnancy. In: *Obstetrics: Normal and Problem Pregnancies,* 2nd ed. Gabbe SG et al (editors). New York: Churchill-Livingstone, 1991.

Camann WR, Ostheimer GW: Physiological adaptations during pregnancy. *Internat Anesthesiol Clin* Winter 1990; 28(1):2.

Clark SL et al: Central hemodynamic assessment of normal term pregnancy. *Am J Obstet Gynecol* December 1989; 161:1439.

Conley LJ: Childbearing and childrearing practices in Mormonism. *Neonatal Network* October 1990; 9(3):41.

Conner GK, Denson V: Expectant fathers' response to pregnancy: Review of literature and implications for research in high risk pregnancy. *J Perinatal Neonatal Nurs* September 1990; 4(2):33.

Contemporary OB/GYN: Demystifying ovulation and pregnancy hits for your patients. April 15, 1993; 38S:67.

Cruikshank DP, Hays PM: Maternal physiology in pregnancy. In: *Obstetrics: Normal and Problem Pregnancies.* Gabbe SG et al (editors). New York: Churchill-Livingstone, 1991.

Cunningham FG et al: *Williams Obstetrics,* 19th ed. Norwalk, CT: Appleton & Lange, 1993.

D'Avanzo CE: Bridging the cultural gap with Southeast Asians. *MCN* July/August 1992; 17:204.

Eliason MJ: Ethics and transcultural nursing care. *Nurs Outlook* September/October 1993; 41(5):225.

Fawcett J: Body image and the expectant couple. *MCN* July/August 1978; 3:227.

Fawcett J et al: Spouses' body image changes during and after pregnancy: A replication and extension. *Nurs Res* July/August 1986; 35:220.

Fishbein EG: Expectant father's stress—Due to mother's expectations? *JOGNN* September/October 1984; 13:325.

Glazer G: Anxiety and stressors of expectant fathers. *West J Nurs Res* 1989; 11(1):47.

Henderson AD, Brouse AJ: The experiences of new fathers during the first 3 weeks of life. *J Adv Nurs* 1991; 16:293.

Hofmeyr CJ, Marcos EF, Butchart AM: Pregnant women's perceptions of themselves: A survey. *Birth* December 1990; 17(4):205.

Hollingsworth AO et al: The refugees and childbearing. What to expect. *RN* November 1980; 43:45.

Honig JC: Preparing preschool-aged children to be siblings. *MCN* January/February 1986; 11:37.

Hytten FE: Weight gain in pregnancy. In: *Clinical Physiology in Obstetrics*, 2nd ed. Hytten FE, Chamberlain G (editors) Oxford, England: Blackwell, 1991.

Institute of Medicine: Nutrition during pregnancy: I Weight gain. Washington, DC: National Academy Press, 1990.

Jordan PL: Laboring for relevance: Expectant and new fatherhood. *Nurs Res* January/February 1990; 39:11.

Khanobdee C, Sukratanachaiyakul V, Templeton GJ: Couvade syndrome in expectant Thai fathers. *Internat J Nurs Studies* 1993; 30(2):125.

Kimura M et al: Physiologic thyroid activation in normal early pregnancy is induced by circulating hCG. *Obstet Gynecol* May 1990; 75:775.

Lederman RP: *Psychosocial Adaptation in Pregnancy*. Englewood Cliffs, NJ: Prentice Hall, 1984.

Lee RV et al: Southeast Asian folklore about pregnancy and parturition. *Obstet Gynecol* April 1988; 71:643.

Longobucco DC, Freston MS: Relation of somatic symptoms to degree of paternal-role preparation of first-time expectant fathers. *JOGNN* November/December 1989; 18:482.

Mattson S, Lew L: Culturally sensitive prenatal care for Southeast Asians. *JOGNN* January/February 1992; 21(1):48.

Oakley A, Rajan L, Gant A: Social support and pregnancy outcome. *Brit J Obstet Gynecol* February 1990; 97:155.

Patterson ET et al: Seeking safe passage: Utilizing health care during pregnancy. *Image* Spring 1990; 22(1):27.

Pritham UA, Sammons LN: Korean women's attitudes toward pregnancy and prenatal care. *Health Care Women Int* 1993; 14:145.

Robinson GE, Stewart DE: Motivation for motherhood and the experience of pregnancy. *Can J Psych* December 1990; 34:861.

Rubin R: *Maternal Identity and the Maternal Experience*. New York: Springer, 1984.

Rubin R: Maternal tasks in pregnancy. *Mat Child Nurs J* Fall 1975; 4:143.

Scott JR et al: *Danforth's Obstetrics and Gynecology*, 7th ed. Philadelphia: Lippincott, 1994.

Spector RE: *Cultural Diversity in Health and Illness*. Norwalk, CT: Appleton & Lange, 1991.

Spero D: Sibling preparation classes. *AWHONN Clin Issues Perinatal Women Health Nurs* 1993; 4(1):122.

St Clair PA, Anderson NA: Social network advice during pregnancy: Myths, misinformation, and sound counsel. *Birth* September 1989; 16:103.

Stern PN et al: Culturally induced stress during childbearing: The Philippine-American experience. *Health Care Women Int* 1985; 6:105.

Stringfellow L: The Vietnamese. In: *Culture, Childbearing, Health Professionals*. Clark AL (editor). Philadelphia: Davis, 1978.

Thiederman SB: Ethnocentrism: A barrier to effective health care. *Nurs Pract* August 1986; 11:52.

Tomlinson B et al: Family dynamics during pregnancy. *J Adv Nurs* 1990; 15:683.

Tripp-Reimer T et al: Cultural assessment: Content and process. *Nurs Outlook* March/April 1984; 32:78.

Wollett A, Dosanjh-Matwala N: Pregnancy and antenatal care: The attitudes and experiences of Asian women. *Child Care Health Dev* 1990; 16:63.

CHAPTER 14

ANTEPARTAL NURSING ASSESSMENT

*O*ur daughter, one of the authors of this book, invited me to write a few paragraphs. What would I write about? How about comparing the father's role at childbirth when she was born to the role of today's father. The father of the 1940s. . . . Main objective: Get your wife to the hospital on time. No delays. Don't wait too long. You're not schooled in delivering babies. Next, check her in and find the father's waiting lounge. You won't be needed until the baby is born. Fathers are really useless at this time. Try not to be nervous. Smoking is in fashion so you're well equipped with a fresh pack. Coffee is available. Lots and lots of coffee. This hospital is very considerate. The delivery may take a long time. It's always at night. It seems babies are never born in the daytime. You're tired. Maybe you can pace. It's hard to pace in a room ten foot square. Delivery may take anywhere from twenty minutes to twenty hours. Hope it's not twenty hours.

More coffee, more cigarettes, no sleep. What a drain on the father. . . . The baby finally comes. Two hours later the doctor remembers the father is waiting. "It's a beautiful, healthy baby girl. Mother and baby are doing fine. You can see them now, but only for five minutes." What a relief. The pressure is finally off. Isn't nature wonderful?. . . Today's father, my son. Schooled in Lamaze. Drives his wife to the hospital. Coaches her through her labor. Helps her find a comfortable position to birth their baby. His camera is ready. The baby is born. He cuts the cord. What a relief. The pressure is finally off. Isn't nature wonderful?

KEY TERMS

Abortion

Antepartum

Diagonal conjugate

Estimated date of birth (EDB)

Gestation

Gravida

Intrapartum

Multigravida

Multipara

Nägele's rule

Nulligravida

Nullipara

Obstetric conjugate

Para

Postpartum

Postterm labor

Preterm or premature labor

Primigravida

Primipara

Risk factors

Stillbirth

Term

OBJECTIVES

Summarize the essential components of a prenatal history.

Explain common obstetric terminology found in the history of maternity clients.

Identify factors related to the father's health that should be recorded on the prenatal record.

Describe the normal physiologic changes one would expect to find when performing a physical assessment on a pregnant woman.

Explain the use of Nägele's rule to determine the estimated date of birth.

Develop an outline of the essential measurements that can be determined by clinical pelvimetry.

Describe areas that should be evaluated as part of the initial assessment of psychosocial factors related to a woman's pregnancy.

Relate the danger signs of pregnancy to their possible causes.

Today nurses are assuming a more important role in prenatal care, particularly in the area of assessment. The certified nurse-midwife has the education and skill to perform in-depth prenatal assessments. The nurse practitioner may share the assessment responsibilities with a physician. An office nurse, whose primary role may be to counsel and meet the psychologic needs of the expectant family, performs assessments in those areas.

An environment of comfort and open communication should be established with each antepartal visit. The nurse should convey concern for the woman as an individual and availability to listen and discuss the woman's concerns and desires. A supportive atmosphere coupled with the information found in the prenatal assessment guides in this chapter will enable the nurse to identify needed areas of education and counseling.

INITIAL CLIENT HISTORY

The course of a pregnancy depends on a number of factors, including the prepregnancy health of the woman, presence of disease states, emotional status, and past health care. Ideally, health care before the advent of pregnancy has been adequate, and antenatal care will be a continuation of that established care. One important method of determining the adequacy of a woman's prepregnancy care is a thorough history.

Definition of Terms

The following terms are used in the obstetric history of maternity clients:

Gestation: The number of weeks since the first day of the last menstrual period (LMP)

Abortion: Birth that occurs prior to the end of 20 weeks' gestation

Term: The normal duration of pregnancy

Preterm or premature labor: Labor that occurs after 20 weeks but before the completion of 37 weeks of gestation

Postterm labor: Labor that occurs after 42 weeks of gestation

Antepartum: Time between conception and onset of labor; usually used to describe the period during which a woman is pregnant; used interchangeably with "prenatal"

Intrapartum: Time from onset of labor until the birth of the infant and placenta

Postpartum: Time from birth until the woman's body returns to an essentially prepregnant condition

Gravida: Any pregnancy, regardless of duration, including present pregnancy

Nulligravida: A woman who has never been pregnant

Primigravida: A woman who is pregnant for the first time

Multigravida: A woman who is in her second or any subsequent pregnancy

Para: Birth after 20 weeks' gestation regardless of whether the infant is born alive or dead

Nullipara: A woman who has not given birth at more than 20 weeks' gestation

Primipara: A woman who has had one birth at more than 20 weeks' gestation, regardless of whether the infant is born alive or dead

Multipara: A woman who has had two or more births at more than 20 weeks' gestation

Stillbirth: A fetus born dead after 20 weeks of gestation

The terms *gravida* and *para* refer to pregnancies/births, not to the fetus. Thus twins, triplets, and so forth count as one pregnancy and one birth.

The following examples illustrate how these terms are applied in clinical situations:

1. Jean Smith has one child born at 38 weeks and is pregnant for the second time. At Jean's initial prenatal visit the nurse indicates her obstetric history as "gravida 2 para 1 ab 0." Jean Smith's present pregnancy terminates at 16 weeks' gestation. She is now "gravida 2 para 1 ab 1."

2. Liz Alexander is pregnant for the fourth time. She has a child born at 35 weeks at home. She lost one pregnancy at 10 weeks' gestation and gave birth to another infant stillborn at term. At her prenatal assessment the nurse records Liz Alexander's obstetric history as "gravida 4 para 2 ab 1."

To provide more comprehensive data, a more detailed approach is used in some settings. Using the detailed system, gravida keeps the same meaning, but that of para is altered somewhat to focus on the number of infants born rather than the number of deliveries. A useful acronym for remembering the system is TPAL.

First digit, T: number of *term* infants, that is, the number of infants born at the completion of 37 weeks' gestation or beyond

Second digit, P: number of *preterm* infants born, that is, the number of infants born before the completion of 37 weeks' gestation

Third digit, A: number of pregnancies ending in either spontaneous or therapeutic *abortion*

Fourth digit, L: number of currently *living* children to whom the woman has given birth

Using this approach, the nurse would have initially classified Jean Smith (described in the first example) as "gravida 2 para 1001." Following her spontaneous abortion, she would be "gravida 2 para 1011." Liz Alexander would be described as "gravida 4 para 1111" (Figure 14–1).

Name	Gravida	Term	Preterm	Abort	Living Child
Jean Smith	2	1	0	0	1
Liz Alexander	4	1	1	1	1

FIGURE 14-1   The TPAL approach provides more detailed information about the woman's pregnancy history.

Client Profile

The history is essentially a screening tool that identifies the factors that may detrimentally affect the course of a pregnancy. For optimal prenatal care the following information should be obtained for each maternity client at the first prenatal assessment:

1. Current pregnancy
   - First day of last normal menstrual period (LMP)
   - Presence of cramping, bleeding, or spotting since LMP
   - Woman's opinion about when conception occurred and when infant is due
   - Woman's attitude toward pregnancy (Is pregnancy planned? Wanted?)
   - Results of pregnancy test, if completed
   - Any discomforts since LMP: nausea, vomiting, urinary frequency, fatigue, breast tenderness, etc

2. Past pregnancies
   - Number of pregnancies
   - Number of abortions, spontaneous or induced
   - Number of living children
   - History of previous pregnancies: length of pregnancy, length of labor and birth, type of birth (vaginal, forceps or silastic cup, cesarean), type of anesthesia used, if any, woman's perception of the experience, complications (antepartal, intrapartal, postpartal)
   - Perinatal status of previous children: Apgar scores, birth weights, general development, complications, feeding patterns (breast/bottle)
   - Blood type and Rh factor (if negative—medication after birth to prevent sensitization)
   - Prenatal education classes, resources (books)

3. Gynecologic history
   - Previous infections: vaginal, cervical, tubal, sexually transmitted
   - Previous surgery
   - Age of menarche
   - Regularity, frequency, and duration of menstrual flow
   - History of dysmenorrhea
   - Sexual history
   - Contraceptive history (If birth control pills were used, did pregnancy immediately follow cessation of pills? If not how long after?)
   - Date of last Pap smear, any history of abnormal Pap smear

4. Current medical history
   - Weight
   - Blood type and Rh factor, if known
   - General health, including nutrition, regular exercise program (type, frequency, duration)
   - Any medications presently being taken (including nonprescription medications) or taken since the onset of pregnancy
   - Previous or present use of alcohol, tobacco, or caffeine (Ask specifically about the amounts of alcohol, cigarettes, and caffeine [specify coffee, tea, colas, chocolate] consumed each day.)
   - Illicit drug use and/or abuse (Ask about specific drugs such as cocaine, crack, marijuana.)
   - Drug and other allergies
   - Potential teratogenic insults to this pregnancy, such as viral infections, medications, x-ray examinations, surgery, cats in home (possible source of toxoplasmosis)
   - Presence of disease conditions, such as diabetes, hypertension, cardiovascular disease, renal problems
   - Record of immunizations (especially rubella)
   - Presence of any abnormal symptoms

5. Past medical history
   - Childhood diseases
   - Past treatment for any disease condition: Any hospitalizations? History of hepatitis? Rheumatic fever? Pyelonephritis?
   - Surgical procedures
   - Presence of bleeding disorders or tendencies (Has she received blood transfusions?)

6. Family medical history
   - Presence of diabetes, cardiovascular disease, hypertension, hematologic disorders, tuberculosis, preeclampsia-eclampsia (pregnancy-induced hypertension [PIH])
   - Occurrence of multiple births
   - History of congenital diseases or deformities

- History of mental illness
- Occurrence of cesarean births
- Cause of death of deceased parents or siblings

7. Religious/cultural history
   - Does the woman wish to specify a religious preference on her chart? Does she have any religious beliefs or practices that might influence her health care or that of her child, such as prohibition against receiving blood products, dietary considerations, circumcision rites, etc?
   - Are there practices in her culture or that of her partner that might influence her care or that of her child?

8. Occupational history
   - Occupation
   - Does she stand all day, or are there opportunities to sit and elevate her legs? Does she do any heavy lifting?
   - Exposure to chemicals or other harmful substances
   - Opportunity for regular lunch, breaks for nutritious snacks
   - Provision for maternity leave

9. Partner's history
   - Presence of genetic conditions or diseases
   - Age
   - Significant health problems
   - Previous or present alcohol intake, drug use, tobacco use
   - Blood type and Rh factor
   - Occupation
   - Educational level
   - Attitude toward the pregnancy

10. Personal information
    - Age
    - Educational level
    - Race or ethnic group (to identify need for prenatal genetic screening or counseling)
    - Stability of living conditions
    - Economic level
    - Housing
    - Any history of emotional or physical deprivation or abuse (herself or children)
    - History of emotional problems
    - Support systems
    - Overuse or underuse of health care system
    - Acceptance of pregnancy

- Personal preferences about the birth (expectations of both the woman and her partner, presence of others, and so on).
- Plans for care of child following birth

Obtaining Data

A questionnaire like the one shown in Figure 14–2 is used in many instances to obtain information. The woman should complete the questionnaire in a quiet place with a minimum of distractions.

The nurse can obtain further information in a direct interview, which allows the pregnant woman to expand or clarify her responses to questions and gives the nurse and client the opportunity to begin developing a good relationship.

The expectant father should be encouraged to attend the initial and subsequent prenatal assessments. He is often able to contribute information to the history and may use the opportunity to ask questions and express concerns that may be of particular importance to him.

Prenatal High-Risk Screening

A highly significant part of the prenatal assessment is the screening for high-risk factors. **Risk factors** are any findings that have been shown to have a negative effect on pregnancy outcome, either for the woman or her unborn child. Many risk factors can be identified during the initial prenatal assessment; others may be detected during subsequent prenatal visits. It is important that high-risk pregnancies be identified early so that appropriate interventions can be instituted immediately.

All risk factors do not threaten the pregnancy to the same degree. Thus many agencies use a risk-scoring sheet to determine the degree of risk. The sheet is initiated at the first visit and becomes a permanent part of the woman's record. Information may be updated throughout the pregnancy as necessary. It is always possible that a pregnancy may begin as low risk and change to high risk because of complications. Risk is also assessed intrapartally and postpartally.

Table 14–1 is an example of one risk-scoring protocol that evaluates the woman for factors that increase her risk of spontaneous preterm birth. Table 14–2 identifies the major risk factors currently recognized. The table describes maternal and fetal/neonatal implications should the risk be present in the pregnancy. In addition to the factors listed, the perinatal health team also needs to evaluate such psychosocial factors as ethnic background; occupation and education; financial status; environment, including living arrangements and location; and the woman's and her family's or significant other's concept of health, which might influence her attitude toward seeking health care.

INITIAL ANTEPARTAL ASSESSMENT

Critical Thinking Question

What approaches might the nurse use to effectively assess the woman's psychosocial status at the initial visit? What behavioral cues in the woman might be helpful?

The antepartal assessment focuses on the woman holistically by considering physical, cultural, and psychosocial factors that influence her health. At the initial visit the woman may be concerned with the diagnosis of pregnancy. However, during this visit she and her primary support person are also evaluating the health team that she has chosen. The establishment of the nurse-client relationship will help the woman evaluate the health team

---

Name _____ Age _____

Address _____ Home Phone _____

What was the last year of schooling completed? _____

How old were you when your menstrual periods started? _____

How many days does a normal period last? _____

How many days are there between periods? _____

Do you have cramping with your periods? yes ____ no ____

Is the pain: minimal _____

moderate _____

severe _____

What was the date of your last normal menstrual period? _____

Have you had bleeding or spotting

since your last menstrual period? yes ____ no ____

Have you been on birth control pills? yes ____ no ____

If yes, when did you stop taking them? _____

How many previous pregnancies have you had? _____

How many living children do you have? _____

Have you had any abortions or stillbirths? yes ____ no ____

If yes, how many? _____

Were any of your previous babies born prematurely?

yes ____ no ____

List the birth weight of all previous children.

1. _____   3. _____

2. _____   4. _____

Did any of your children have problems immediately after birth?

yes ____ no ____

If yes, check the problems that occurred:

____ Respiratory   ____ Feeding

____ Jaundice   ____ Heart

____ Bleeding

Did you have any problems with:

previous pregnancies? yes ____ no ____

If yes, what was the problem? _____

previous labors? yes ____ no ____

If yes, what was the problem? _____

previous postpartal periods: yes ____ no ____

if yes, what was the problem? _____

Are you Rh negative: yes ____ no ____

Did you receive RhoGAM after each pregnancy? yes ____ no ____

What is your present weight? _____

Are you presently taking any prescription or nonprescription drugs?

yes ____ no ____

If yes, please list the medications:

1. _____   3. _____

2. _____   4. _____

Do you smoke? yes ____ no ____

If yes, how many cigarettes per day? _____

How much alcohol do you consume each day? _____

each week? _____

How much caffeine do you consume each day? _____

If you have had any of the following diseases, place a check beside it.

____ Chickenpox	____ High blood pressure
____ Mumps	____ Heart disease
____ Measles (3 day)	____ Respiratory disease
____ Measles (2 week)	____ Kidney disease
____ Asthma	____ Frequent bladder
____ Hepatitis	infections

If any of the following diseases is present in your family, place a check beside the item.

____ Diabetes	____ Preeclampsia-eclampsia
____ Cardiovascular disease	____ Multiple pregnancies
____ High blood pressure	____ Congenital disorder
____ Breast cancer	

The following questions pertain to the father of this child.

What is the father's age? _____

Does he take prescription or nonprescription drugs?

yes ____ no ____

If yes, please list the medications:

1. _____   3. _____

2. _____   4. _____

What is his alcohol intake each day? _____

each week? _____

FIGURE 14-2   Sample prenatal questionnaire.

TABLE 14-1 System for Determining Risk of Spontaneous Preterm Birth

Points Assigned	Socioeconomic Factors	Previous Medical History	Daily Habits	Aspects of Current Pregnancy
1	Two children at home Low socioeconomic status	Abortion × 1 Less than 1 year since last birth	Works outside home	Unusual fatigue
2	Maternal age 18–20 years or > 40 years Single parent	Abortion × 2	Smokes more than 10 cigarettes per day	Gain of less than 5 kg by 32 weeks
3	Very low socioeconomic status Height < 150 cm Weight < 45 kg	Abortion × 3	Heavy or stressful work Long, tiring trip	Breech at 32 weeks Weight loss of 2 kg Head engaged at 32 weeks Febrile illness
4	Maternal age < 18 years	Pyelonephritis		Bleeding after 12 weeks Effacement Dilation Uterine irritability
5		Uterine anomaly Second trimester abortion DES exposure Cone biopsy		Placenta previa Hydramnios
10		Preterm birth Repeated second trimester abortion		Twins Abdominal surgery

NOTE: The score is computed by adding the number of points given any item. The score is computed at the first visit and again at 22 to 26 weeks' gestation. A total score of 10 or more places the woman at high risk of spontaneous preterm birth.

SOURCE: Adapted from Creasy RK, Gummer BA, and Liggins GC: A system for predicting spontaneous preterm birth. *Obstet Gynecol* 1980; 55:692.

TABLE 14-2 Prenatal High-Risk Factors

Factor	Maternal Implication	Fetal/Neonatal Implication
Social-Personal		
Low income level and/or low educational level	Poor antenatal care Poor nutrition ↑ risk of preeclampsia	Low birth weight Intrauterine growth retardation (IUGR)
Poor diet	Inadequate nutrition ↑ risk anemia ↑ risk preeclampsia	Fetal malnutrition Prematurity
Living at high altitude	↑ hemoglobin	Prematurity IUGR
Multiparity > 3	↑ risk antepartum/postpartum hemorrhage	Anemia Fetal death
Weight < 45.5 kg (100 lb)	Poor nutrition Cephalopelvic disproportion Prolonged labor	IUGR Hypoxia associated with difficult labor and birth
Weight > 91 kg (200 lb)	↑ risk hypertension ↑ risk cephalopelvic disproportion	↓ fetal nutrition
Age < 16	Poor nutrition Poor antenatal care ↑ risk preeclampsia ↑ risk cephalopelvic disproportion	Low birth weight ↑ fetal demise
Age > 35	↑ risk preeclampsia ↑ risk cesarean birth	↑ risk congenital anomalies ↑ chromosomal aberrations
Smoking one pack/day or more	↑ risk hypertension ↑ risk cancer	↓ placental perfusion → ↓ O_2 and nutrients available Low birth weight IUGR Preterm birth
Use of addicting drugs	↑ risk poor nutrition ↑ risk of infection with IV drugs	↑ risk congenital anomalies ↑ risk low birth weight Neonatal withdrawal Lower serum bilirubin
Excessive alcohol consumption	↑ risk poor nutrition Possible hepatic effects with long-term consumption	↑ risk fetal alcohol syndrome

TABLE 14-2   Prenatal High-Risk Factors *continued*

Factor	Maternal Implication	Fetal/Neonatal Implication
Preexisting Medical Disorders		
Diabetes mellitus	↑ risk preeclampsia, hypertension Episodes of hypoglycemia and hyperglycemia ↑ risk cesarean birth	Low birth weight Macrosomia Neonatal hypoglycemia ↑ risk congenital anomalies ↑ risk respiratory distress syndrome
Cardiac disease	Cardiac decompensation Further strain on mother's body ↑ maternal death rate	↑ risk fetal demise ↑ perinatal mortality
Anemia: hemoglobin < 9 g/dL (White) < 29% hematocrit (White) < 8.2 g/dL hemoglobin (Black) < 26% hematocrit (Black)	Iron deficiency anemia Low energy level Decreased oxygen-carrying capacity	Fetal death Prematurity Low birth weight
Hypertension	↑ vasospasm ↑ risk CNS irritability → convulsions ↑ risk CVA ↑ risk renal damage	↓ placental perfusion → low birth weight Preterm birth
Thyroid disorder Hypothyroidism	↑ infertility ↓ BMR, goiter, myxedema	↑ spontaneous abortion ↑ risk congenital goiter Mental retardation → cretinism ↑ incidence congenital anomalies
Hyperthyroidism	↑ risk postpartum hemorrhage ↑ risk preeclampsia Danger of thyroid storm	↑ incidence preterm birth ↑ tendency to thyrotoxicosis
Renal disease (moderate to severe)	↑ risk renal failure	↑ risk IUGR ↑ risk preterm birth
DES exposure	↑ infertility, spontaneous abortion ↑ cervical incompetence	↑ spontaneous abortion ↑ risk preterm birth
Obstetric Considerations		
Previous Pregnancy		
Stillborn	↑ emotional/psychologic distress	↑ risk IUGR ↑ risk preterm birth
Habitual abortion	↑ emotional/psychologic distress ↑ possibility diagnostic workup	↑ risk abortion
Cesarean birth	↑ possibility repeat cesarean birth	↑ risk preterm birth ↑ risk respiratory distress
Rh or blood group sensitization	↑ financial expenditure for testing	Hydrops fetalis Icterus gravis Neonatal anemia Kernicterus Hypoglycemia
Large baby	↑ risk cesarean birth ↑ risk gestational diabetes	Birth injury Hypoglycemia

and also provide the nurse with a basis for developing an atmosphere that is conducive to interviewing, support, and education. Because many women are excited and anxious at the first antepartal visit, the initial psychosocial-cultural assessment is general.

As part of the initial psychosocial-cultural assessment the nurse discusses with the woman any religious, cultural, or socioeconomic factors that influence the woman's expectations of the childbearing experience. It is especially helpful if the nurse is familiar with common practices of various religious and cultural groups who re-

side in the community. If the nurse gathers this data in a tactful, caring way, it can help make the childbearing woman's experience a positive one.

After the history is obtained, the woman is prepared for the physical examination. The physical examination begins with assessment of vital signs; then the woman's body is examined. The pelvic examination is performed last.

Before the examination the woman should provide a clean urine specimen. When the bladder is empty, the woman is more comfortable during the pelvic examina-

TABLE 14-2   *continued*

Factor	Maternal Implication	Fetal/Neonatal Implication
Current Pregnancy		
Rubella (first trimester)		Congenital heart disease
		Cataracts
		Nerve deafness
		Bone lesions
		Prolonged virus shedding
Rubella (second trimester)		Hepatitis
		Thrombocytopenia
Cytomegalovirus		IUGR
		Encephalopathy
Herpesvirus type 2	Severe discomfort	Neonatal herpesvirus type 2
	Concern about possibility of cesarean birth, fetal infection	2° hepatitis with jaundice
		Neurologic abnormalities
Syphilis	↑ incidence abortion	↑ fetal demise
		Congenital syphilis
Abruptio placenta and placenta previa	↑ risk hemorrhage	Fetal/neonatal anemia
	Bed rest	Intrauterine hemorrhage
	Extended hospitalization	↑ fetal demise
Preeclampsia/eclampsia (PIH)	See hypertension	↓ placental perfusion
		→ low birth weight
Multiple gestation	↑ risk postpartum hemorrhage	↑ risk preterm birth
		↑ risk fetal demise
Elevated hematocrit	Increased viscosity of blood	Fetal death rate 5 times normal rate
> 41% (White)		
> 38% (Black)		
Spontaneous premature rupture of membranes	↑ uterine infection	↑ risk preterm birth
		↑ fetal demise

tion, and the examiner can palpate the pelvic organs more easily. After emptying her bladder, the woman is asked to disrobe and is given a sheet or some other protective covering.

Increasing numbers of nurses, such as certified nurse-midwives and other nurses in advanced practice, are prepared to perform physical examinations. The nurse who has not yet fully developed specific assessment skills assesses the woman's vital signs, explains the procedures to allay apprehension, positions her for examination, and assists the examiner as necessary.

Each nurse is responsible for operating at the expected standard for someone with that individual nurse's skill and knowledge base.

Thoroughness and a systematic procedure are the most important considerations when performing the physical portion of an antepartal examination (see the Initial Prenatal Assessment Guide on page 341). To promote completeness, the Initial Prenatal Assessment Guide is organized into three columns that address the areas to be assessed, the variations or alterations that may be observed, and nursing responses to the data. The nurse should be aware that certain organs and systems are assessed concurrently with other systems during the physi-

CRITICAL THINKING IN PRACTICE

Karen Blade, a 23-year-old, G1P0, is 10 weeks pregnant when she sees the certified nurse-midwife (CNM) for her first prenatal exam. She has been experiencing some mild nausea and fatigue but otherwise is feeling well. She asks the CNM about continuing with her routine exercises (walking 3 miles a day and lifting light weights). She also asks about using the heated pool and a hot tub. What should she be told?

Answers can be found in Appendix I.

cal portion of the examination. Essential Precautions in Practice: During Prenatal Examinations provides basic information on appropriate body fluid precautions.

Nursing interventions based on assessment of the normal physical and psychosocial changes, as well as the cultural influences associated with pregnancy and client teaching and counseling needs that have been mutually defined, are discussed further in Chapter 15.

When assessing blood pressure, have the pregnant woman sitting up with her arm resting on a table so that her arm is at the level of her heart.

Expect a decrease in her blood pressure from baseline during the second trimester because of normal physiologic changes. If this decrease doesn't occur, evaluate further for signs of pregnancy-induced hypertension (PIH).

DETERMINATION OF DUE DATE

Childbearing families generally want to know the "due date," or the date around which childbirth will occur. Historically, the due date has been called the estimated date of confinement (EDC). The concept of confinement is, however, rather negative, and there is a trend in the literature to avoid it by referring to the birth date as the EDD or *estimated date of delivery*. Childbirth educators often stress that babies are not "delivered" like a package; they are *born*. In keeping with a view that emphasizes the normality of the process, we have chosen to refer to the due date as the **EDB (estimated date of birth)** throughout this text.

To calculate the EDB, it is helpful to know the first day of the woman's last menstrual period (LMP). However, some women have episodes of irregular bleeding or fail to keep track of menstrual cycles. Thus other techniques also help determine how far along a woman is in her pregnancy, that is, at how many weeks' gestation she is. Other techniques that can be used include evaluating uterine size, determining when quickening occurs, and auscultating fetal heart rate with a doppler and later a fetoscope.

DURING PRENATAL EXAMINATIONS

Examples of times when gloves should be worn include the following:

- When drawing blood for lab work
- When handling urine specimens
- During pelvic examinations (sterile gloves)

In most instances in a clinic or office setting, gowns and goggles are not necessary because splashing of fluids is unlikely.

REMEMBER to wash your hands prior to putting the disposable gloves on and AGAIN immediately after you remove the gloves.

For further information consult OSHA and CDC guidelines.

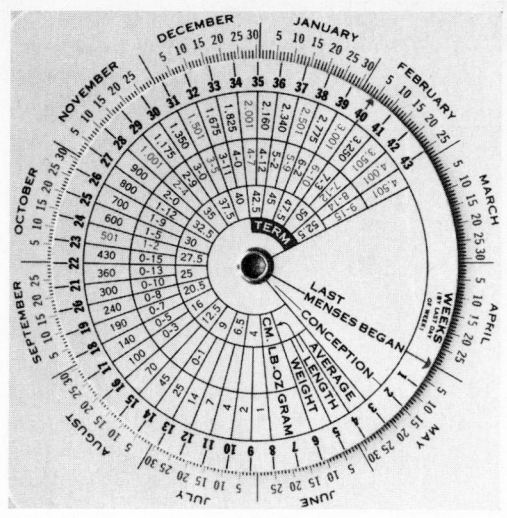

FIGURE 14-3   The EDB wheel can be used to calculate the due date. To use it, place the *last menses began* arrow on the date of the woman's LMP. Then read the EDB at the arrow labeled *40*. In this case the LMP is April 30 and the EDB is February 4.

Nägele's Rule

The most common method of determining the EDB is **Nägele's rule.** To use this method, begin with the first day of the last menstrual period, subtract 3 months, and add 7 days. For example,

First day of LMP	November 21
Subtract 3 months	− 3 months
	August 21
Add 7 days	+ 7 days
EDB	August 28

It is simpler to change the months to numeric terms:

November 21 becomes	11–21
Subtract 3 months	− 3
	8–21
Add 7 days	+ 7
EDB	August 28

If a woman with a history of menses every 28 days remembers her LMP and was not taking oral contraceptives prior to becoming pregnant, Nägele's rule may be a fairly accurate determiner of her predicted birth date. However, if her cycle is irregular or 35 to 40 days in length, the time of ovulation may be delayed by several days. If she has been on oral contraceptives, ovulation may be delayed several weeks following her last menses. *Ovulation usually occurs 14 days before the onset of the next menses, not 14 days after the previous menses.* Thus Nägele's rule, while helpful, is not foolproof. Mittendorf et al (1990) found that the average length of gestation in uncomplicated pregnancies is longer than Nägele's rule suggests, especially for White primiparas (+7 days). A gestation calculator or "wheel" permits the care giver to calculate the EDB even more quickly (Figure 14–3).

Text continues on page 349

Physical Assessment/ Normal Findings	Alterations and Possible Causes*	Nursing Responses to Data†

Vital Signs

Blood pressure (BP): 90–140/60–90	High BP (essential hypertension; renal disease; pregestational hypertension; apprehension or anxiety associated with pregnancy diagnosis, exam, or other crises; PIH if initial assessment not done until after 20 weeks' gestation)	BP > 140/90 requires immediate consideration; establish woman's BP; refer to physician if necessary. Assess woman's knowledge about high BP; counsel on self-care and medical management.
Pulse: 60–90 beats/min. Rate may increase 10 beats/min during pregnancy	Increased pulse rate (excitement or anxiety, cardiac disorders)	Count for 1 full minute; note irregularities.
Respiration: 16–24 breaths/min (or pulse rate divided by four). Pregnancy may induce a degree of hyperventilation; thoracic breathing predominant	Marked tachypnea or abnormal patterns	Assess for respiratory disease.
Temperature: 36.2–37.6 C (98–99.6 F)	Elevated temperature (infection)	Assess for infection process or disease state if temperature is elevated; refer to physician/CNM.

Weight

Depends on body build	Weight < 45 kg (100 lb) or > 91 kg (200 lb); rapid, sudden weight gain (PIH)	Evaluate need for nutritional counseling; obtain information on eating habits, cooking practices, foods regularly eaten, income limitations, need for food supplements, pica and other abnormal food habits. Note initial weight to establish baseline for weight gain throughout pregnancy.

Skin

Color: Consistent with racial background; pink nail beds	Pallor (anemia); bronze, yellow (hepatic disease, other causes of jaundice)	The following tests should be performed: complete blood count (CBC), bilirubin level, urinalysis, and blood urea nitrogen (BUN).
	Bluish, reddish, mottled; dusky appearance or pallor of palms and nail beds in dark-skinned women (anemia)	If abnormal, refer to physician.
Condition: Absence of edema (slight edema of lower extremities is normal during pregnancy)	Edema (PIH); rashes, dermatitis (allergic response)	Counsel on relief measures for slight edema. Initiate PIH assessment; refer to physician.
Lesions: Absence of lesions	Ulceration (varicose veins, decreased circulation)	Further assess circulatory status; refer to physician if lesion severe.
Spider nevi common in pregnancy	Petechiae, multiple bruises, ecchymosis (hemorrhagic disorders; abuse)	Evaluate for bleeding or clotting disorder. Provide oportunities to discuss abuse if suspected.
Moles	Change in size or color (carcinoma)	Refer to physician.

*Possible causes of alterations are placed in parentheses.

†This column provides guidelines for further assessment and initial nursing intervention.

Physical Assessment/ Normal Findings	Alterations and Possible Causes*	Nursing Responses to Data†
Pigmentation: Pigmentation changes of pregnancy include linea nigra, striae gravidarum, chloasma		Assure woman that these are normal manifestations of pregnancy and explain the physiologic basis for the changes.
Café-au-lait spots	Six or more (Albright's syndrome or neurofibromatosis)	Consult with physician.
Nose		
Character of mucosa: Redder than oral mucosa; in pregnancy nasal mucosa is edematous in response to increased estrogen, resulting in nasal stuffiness and nosebleeds	Olfactory loss (first cranial nerve deficit)	Counsel woman about possible relief measures for nasal stuffiness and nosebleeds (epistaxis); refer to physician for olfactory loss.
Mouth		
May note hypertrophy of gingival tissue because of estrogen	Edema, inflammation (infection); pale in color (anemia)	Assess hematocrit for anemia; counsel regarding dental hygiene habits. Refer to physician or dentist if necessary. Routine dental care appropriate during pregnancy (no x-rays, no gas).
Neck		
Nodes: Small, mobile, nontender nodes	Tender, hard, fixed or prominent nodes (infection, carcinoma)	Examine for local infection; refer to physician.
Thyroid: Small, smooth, lateral lobes palpable on either side of trachea; slight hyperplasia by third month of pregnancy	Enlargement or nodule tenderness (hyperthyroidism)	Listen over thyroid for bruits, which may indicate hyperthyroidism. Question woman about dietary habits (iodine intake). Ascertain history of thyroid problems; refer to physician.
Chest and Lungs		
Chest: Symmetric, elliptical, smaller anteroposterior (A-P) than transverse diameter	Increased A-P diameter, funnel chest, pigeon chest (emphysema, asthma, chronic obstructive pulmonary disease [COPD])	Evaluate for emphysema, asthma, pulmonary disease (COPD).
Ribs: Slope downward from nipple line	More horizontal (COPD) Angular bumps Rachitic rosary (vitamin C deficiency)	Evaluate for COPD. Evaluate for fractures. Consult physician. Consult nutritionist.
Inspection and palpation: No retraction or bulging of intercostal spaces (ICS) during inspiration or expiration; symmetrical expansion	ICS retractions with inspiration, bulging with expiration; unequal expansion (respiratory disease)	Do thorough initial assessment. Refer to physician.
Tactile fremitus	Tachypnea, hyperpnea, Cheyne-Stokes respirations (respiratory disease)	Refer to physician.
Percussion: Bilateral symmetry in tone	Flatness of percussion, which may be affected by chest wall thickness	Evaluate for pleural effusions, consolidations, or tumor.

*Possible causes of alterations are placed in parentheses.

†This column provides guidelines for further assessment and initial nursing intervention.

Physical Assessment/ Normal Findings	Alterations and Possible Causes*	Nursing Responses to Data†
Low-pitched resonance of moderate intensity	High diaphragm (atelectasis or paralysis), pleural effusion	Refer to physician.
Auscultation: Upper lobes: bronchovesicular sounds above sternum and scapulas; equal expiratory and inspiratory phases	Abnormal if heard over any other area of chest	Refer to physician.
Remainder of chest: vesicular breath sounds heard; inspiratory phase longer (3:1)	Rales, rhonchi, wheezes; pleural friction rub; absence of breath sounds; bronchophony, egophony, whispered pectoriloquy	Refer to physician.

Breasts

Physical Assessment/ Normal Findings	Alterations and Possible Causes*	Nursing Responses to Data†
Supple; symmetric in size and contour; darker pigmentation of nipple and areola; may have supernumerary nipples, usually 5–6 cm below normal nipple line	"Pigskin" or orange-peel appearance, nipple retractions, swelling, hardness (carcinoma); redness, heat, tenderness, cracked or fissured nipple (infection)	Encourage monthly self-breast checks; instruct woman how to examine own breasts.
Axillary nodes unpalpable or pellet sized	Tenderness, enlargement, hard node (carcinoma); may be visible bump (infection)	Refer to physician if evidence of inflammation.

Pregnancy changes:

1. Size increase noted primarily in first 20 weeks.
2. Become nodular.
3. Tingling sensation may be felt during first and third trimester; woman may report feeling of heaviness.
4. Pigmentation of nipples and areolas darkens.
5. Superficial veins dilate and become more prominent.
6. Striae seen in multiparas.
7. Tubercles of Montgomery enlarge.
8. Colostrum may be present after 12th week.
9. Secondary areola appears at 20 weeks, characterized by series of washed-out spots surrounding primary areola.
10. Breasts less firm, old striae may be present in multiparas.

Discuss normalcy of changes and their meaning with the woman.
Teach and/or institute appropriate relief measures.
Encourage use of supportive, well-fitting brassiere.

Heart

Physical Assessment/ Normal Findings	Alterations and Possible Causes*	Nursing Responses to Data†
Normal rate, rhythm, and heart sounds	Enlargement, thrills, thrusts, gross irregularity or skipped beats, gallop rhythm or extra sounds (cardiac disease)	Complete an initial assessment. Explain normalcy of pregnancy-induced changes. Refer to physician if indicated.

Pregnancy changes:

1. Palpitations may occur due to sympathetic nervous system disturbance.

*Possible causes of alterations are placed in parentheses.

†This column provides guidelines for further assessment and initial nursing intervention.

Physical Assessment/ Normal Findings	Alterations and Possible Causes*	Nursing Responses to Data†
2. Short systolic murmurs that ↑ in held expiration are normal due to increased volume.		

Abdomen

Physical Assessment/ Normal Findings	Alterations and Possible Causes*	Nursing Responses to Data†
Normal appearance, skin texture, and hair distribution; liver nonpalpable; abdomen nontender	Muscle guarding (anxiety, acute tenderness); tenderness, mass (ectopic pregnancy, inflammation, carcinoma)	Assure client of normalcy of diastasis. Provide initial information about appropriate postpartum exercises. Evaluate client anxiety level. Refer to physician if indicated.

Pregnancy changes:

1. Purple striae may be present (or silver striae on a multipara) as well as linea nigra.
2. Diastasis of the rectus muscles late in pregnancy.

3. Size: Flat or rotund abdomen; progressive enlargement of uterus due to pregnancy. 10–12 weeks: Fundus slightly above symphysis pubis. 16 weeks: Fundus halfway between symphysis and umbilicus.	Size of uterus inconsistent with length of gestation (intrauterine growth retardation [IUGR] multiple pregnancy, fetal demise, hydatidiform mole)	Reassess menstrual history regarding pregnancy dating. Evaluate increase in size using McDonald's method. Use ultrasound to establish diagnosis.

20–22 weeks: Fundus at umbilicus.

28 weeks: Fundus three finger breadths above umbilicus.

36 weeks: Fundus just below ensiform cartilage.

4. Fetal heartbeats: 120–160 beats/min may be heard with Doppler at 10–12 weeks' gestation; may be heard with fetoscope at 17–20 weeks.	Failure to hear fetal heartbeat with stethoscope after 17–20 weeks (fetal demise, hydatidiform mole)	Refer to physician. Administer pregnancy tests. Use ultrasound to establish diagnosis.
5. Fetal movement palpable by a trained examiner after the 18th week.	Failure to feel fetal movements after 20 weeks' gestation (fetal demise, hydatidiform mole)	Refer to physician for evaluation of fetal status.
6. Ballottement: During fourth to fifth month fetus rises and then rebounds to original position when uterus is tapped sharply.	No ballottement (oligohydramnios)	Refer to physician for evaluation of fetal status.

Extremities

Physical Assessment/ Normal Findings	Alterations and Possible Causes*	Nursing Responses to Data†
Skin warm, pulses palpable, full range of motion; may be some edema of hands and ankles in late pregnancy; varicose veins may become more pronounced; palmar erythema may be present	Unpalpable or diminished pulses (arterial insufficiency); marked edema (PIH)	Evaluate for other symptoms of heart disease; initiate follow-up if woman mentions that her rings feel tight. Discuss prevention and self-treatment measures for varicose veins; refer to physician if indicated.

*Possible causes of alterations are placed in parentheses.

†This column provides guidelines for further assessment and initial nursing intervention.

Physical Assessment/ Normal Findings	Alterations and Possible Causes*	Nursing Responses to Data†
Spine		
Normal spinal curves: Concave cervical, convex thoracic, concave lumbar	Abnormal spinal curves: flatness, kyphosis, lordosis	Refer to physician for assessment of cephalopelvic disproportion (CPD).
In pregnancy lumbar spinal curve may be accentuated	Backache	May have implications for administration of spinal anesthetics; see Chapter 15 for relief measures.
Shoulders and iliac crests should be even	Uneven shoulders and iliac crests (scoliosis)	Refer very young women to a physician; discuss back-stretching exercises with older women.
Reflexes		
Normal and symmetrical	Hyperactivity, clonus (PIH)	Evaluate for other symptoms of PIH.
Pelvic Area		
External female genitals: Normally formed with female hair distribution; in multiparas, labia majora loose and pigmented; urinary and vaginal orifices visible and appropriately located	Lesions, hematomas, varicosities, inflammation of Bartholin's glands; clitoral hypertrophy (masculinization)	Exp lain pelvic examination procedure (Procedure 10–1). Encourage woman to minimize her discomfort by relaxing her hips. Provide privacy.
Vagina: Pink or dark pink; vaginal discharge odorless, nonirritating; in multiparas, vaginal folds smooth and flattened; may have episiotomy scar	Abnormal discharge associated with vaginal infections	Obtain vaginal smear. Provide understandable verbal and written instructions about treatment for woman and partner, if indicated.
Cervix: Pink color; os closed except in multiparas, in whom os admits fingertip	Eversion, reddish erosion, Nabothian or retention cysts, cervical polyp; granular area that bleeds (carcinoma of cervix); lesions (herpes, human papilloma virus [HPV]) Presence of string or plastic tip from cervix (intrauterine device [IUD] in uterus)	Provide woman with a hand mirror and identify genital structures for her; encourage her to view her cervix if she wishes. Refer to physician if indicated. Advise woman of potential serious risks of leaving an IUD in place during pregnancy; refer to physician for removal.
Pregnancy changes: 1–4 weeks' gestation: Enlargement in antero-posterior diameter	Absence of Goodell's sign (inflammatory conditions, carcinoma)	Refer to physician.
4–6 weeks' gestation: Softening of cervix (Goodell's sign), softening of isthmus of uterus (Hegar's sign); cervix takes on bluish coloring (Chadwick's sign)		
8–12 weeks' gestation: Vagina and cervix appear bluish-violet in color (Chadwick's sign)		
Uterus: Pear-shaped, mobile; smooth surface	Fixed (pelvic inflammatory disease [PID]); nodular surface (fibromas)	Refer to physician.
Ovaries: Small, walnut-shaped, nontender (ovaries and fallopian tubes are located in the adnexal areas)	Pain on movement of cervix (PID); enlarged or nodular ovaries (cyst, tumor, tubal pregnancy, corpus luteum of pregnancy)	Evaluate adnexal areas; refer to physician.

*Possible causes of alterations are placed in parentheses.

†This column provides guidelines for further assessment and initial nursing intervention.

Physical Assessment/ Normal Findings	Alterations and Possible Causes*	Nursing Responses to Data†
Pelvic Measurements		
Internal measurements:	Measurement below normal	Vaginal birth may not be possible if deviations are present.
1. Diagonal conjugate at least 11.5 cm (Figure 14–7)		
2. Obstetric conjugate estimated by subtracting 1.5–2 cm from diagonal conjugate	Disproportion of pubic arch	
3. Inclination of sacrum	Abnormal curvature of sacrum	
4. Motility of coccyx; external intertuberosity diameter > 8 cm	Fixed or malposition of coccyx	
Anus and Rectum		
No lumps, rashes, excoriation, tenderness; cervix may be felt through rectal wall	Hemorrhoids, rectal prolapse; nodular lesion (carcinoma)	Counsel about appropriate prevention and relief measures; refer to physician for further evaluation.
Laboratory Evaluation		
Hemoglobin: 12–16 g/dL; women residing in high altitudes may have higher levels of hemoglobin	< 12 g/dL (anemia)	Note: Wear gloves when drawing blood. Hemoglobin < 12 g/dL requires nutritional counseling. < 11 g/dL requires iron supplementation.
ABO and Rh typing: Normal distribution of blood types	Rh negative	If Rh negative, check for presence of anti-Rh antibodies.
		Check partner's blood type; if partner is Rh positive, discuss with woman the need for antibody titers during pregnancy, management during the intrapartal period, and possible candidacy for RhIgG.
Complete blood count (CBC)		
Hematocrit: 38%–47%; physiologic anemia (pseudoanemia) may occur	Marked anemia or blood dyscrasias	Perform CBC and Schilling differential cell count.
Red blood cells (RBC): 4.2–5.4 million/μL		
White blood cells (WBC): 4500–11,000/μL	Presence of infection; may be elevated in pregnancy and with labor	Evaluate for other signs of infection.
Differential		
Neutrophils: 40%–60%		
Bands: up to 5%		
Eosinophils: 1%–3%		
Basophils: up to 1%		
Lymphocytes: 20%–40%		
Monocytes: 4%–8%		

*Possible causes of alterations are placed in parentheses.

†This column provides guidelines for further assessment and initial nursing intervention.

Physical Assessment/ Normal Findings	Alterations and Possible Causes*	Nursing Responses to Data†
Syphilis tests—serologic test for syphilis (STS), complement fixation test, Venereal Disease Research Laboratory (VDRL) test—nonreactive	Positive reaction STS—tests may have 25%–45% incidence of biologic false-positive results; false results may occur in individuals who have acute viral or bacterial infections, hypersensitivity reactions, recent vaccinations, collagen disease, malaria, or tuberculosis.	Positive results may be confirmed with the fluorescent treponemal antibody absorption (FTA-ABS) tests; all tests for syphilis give positive results in the secondary stage of the disease; antibiotic tests may cause negative test results.
Gonorrhea culture: Negative	Positive	Refer for treatment.
Urinalysis (u/a): Normal color, specific gravity; pH 4.6–8.0	Abnormal color (porphyria, hemoglobinuria, bilirubinemia); alkaline urine (metabolic alkalemia, *Proteus* infection, old specimen)	Repeat u/a; refer to physician.
Negative for protein, red blood cells, white blood cells, casts	Positive findings (contaminated specimen, kidney disease)	Repeat u/a; refer to physician.
Glucose: Negative (small degree of glycosuria may occur in pregnancy)	Glycosuria (low renal threshold for glucose, diabetes mellitus)	Assess blood glucose; test urine for ketones.
Rubella titer: Hemagglutination-inhibition test (HAI) > 1:10 indicates woman is immune	HAI titer < 1:10	Immunization will be given on postpartum or within 6 weeks after childbirth. Instruct woman whose titers are < 1:10 to avoid children who have rubella.
HIV screen: Offered to all women; encouraged for those at risk; negative	Positive	Refer to physician.
Illicit drug screen: Offered to all women; negative	Positive	Refer to physician.
Sickle cell screen for clients of African descent: Negative	Positive; test results would include a description of cells	Refer to physician.
Pap test: Negative	Test results that show atypical cells	Refer to physician. Discuss the meaning of the findings with the woman and importance of follow-up.

Cultural Assessment	Variations to Consider	Nursing Responses to Data†
Determine the woman's fluency in English	Woman may be fluent in a language other than English.	Work with a knowledgeable translator to provide information and answer questions.
Ask the woman how she prefers to be addressed.	Some women prefer informality; others prefer to use titles.	Address the woman according to her preference. Maintain formality in introducing oneself if that seems preferred.
Determine customs and practices regarding prenatal care:	Practices are influenced by individual preference, cultural expectations, or religious beliefs.	Honor a woman's practices and provide for specific preferences unless they are contraindicated because of safety.

*Possible causes of alterations are placed in parentheses.

†This column provides guidelines for further assessment and initial nursing intervention.

Cultural Assessment	Variations to Consider	Nursing Responses to Data[†]
• Ask the woman if there are certain practices she expects to follow when she is pregnant.	Some women believe that they should perform certain acts related to sleep, activity, or clothing.	Have information printed in the language of different cultural groups that live in the area.
• Ask the woman if there are any activities she cannot do while she is pregnant.	Some women have restrictions or taboos they follow related to work, activity, sexual, environmental, or emotional factors (Boyle & Andrews 1989).	
• Ask the woman whether there are certain foods she is expected to eat or avoid while she is pregnant. Determine whether she has lactose intolerance.	Foods are an important cultural factor. Some women may have certain foods they must eat or avoid; many women have lactose intolerance and have difficulty consuming sufficient calcium.	Respect the woman's food preferences, help her plan an adequate prenatal diet within the framework of her preferences, and refer to a dietician if necessary.
• Ask the woman whether the gender of her care giver is of concern.	Some women are comfortable only with a female care giver.	Arrange for a female care giver if it is the woman's preference.
• Ask the woman about the degree of involvement in her pregnancy that she expects or wants from her support person, mother, and other significant people.	If the woman does have a partner, she may not want this person involved in the pregnancy. For some the role falls to the woman's mother or a female relative or friend.	Respect the woman's preferences about her partner/husband's involvement; avoid imposing personal values or expectations.
• Ask the woman about her sources of support/counseling during pregnancy	Some women seek advice from a family member, *curandera,* tribal healer, and so forth.	Respect and honor the woman's sources of support.

Psychosocial Assessment	Variations to Consider*	Nursing Responses to Data[†]
Psychologic Status		
Excitement and/or apprehension; ambivalence	Marked anxiety (fear of pregnancy diagnosis, fear of medical facility)	Establish lines of communication. Active listening is useful. Establish trusting relationship. Encourage woman to take active part in her care.
	Apathy Display of anger with pregnancy diagnosis	Establish communication and begin counseling. Use active listening techniques.
Educational Needs		
May have questions about pregnancy or may need time to adjust to reality of pregnancy		Establish educational, supporting environment that can be expanded throughout pregnancy.
Support Systems		
Can identify at least two or three individuals with whom woman is emotionally intimate (partner, parent, sibling, friend)	Isolated (no telephone, unlisted number); cannot name a neighbor or friend whom she can call upon in an emergency; does not perceive parents as part of her support system	Institute support system through community groups. Help woman to develop trusting relationship with health care professionals.

*Possible causes of alterations are placed in parentheses.

[†]This column provides guidelines for further assessment and initial nursing intervention.

Psychosocial Assessment	Variations to Consider*	Nursing Responses to Data[†]
Family Functioning		
Emotionally supportive Communications adequate Mutually satisfying Cohesiveness in times of trouble	Long-term problems or specific problems related to this pregnancy, potential stressors within the family, pessimistic attitudes, unilateral decision making, unrealistic expectations of this pregnancy and/or child	Help identify the problems and stressors, encourage communication, discuss role changes and adaptations.
Economic Status		
Source of income is stable and sufficient to meet basic needs of daily living and medical needs	Limited prenatal care Poor physical health Limited use of health care system Unstable economic status	Discuss available resources for health maintenance and the birth. Institute appropriate referral for meeting expanding family's needs—food stamps and so forth.
Stability of Living Conditions		
Adequate, stable housing for expanding family's needs	Crowded living conditions Questionable supportive environment for newborn	Refer to appropriate community agency. Work with family on self-help ways to improve situation.

*Possible causes of alterations are placed in parentheses.

[†]This column provides guidelines for further assessment and initial nursing intervention.

Uterine Assessment

Physical Examination

When a woman is examined in the first 10 to 12 weeks of her pregnancy and the nurse practitioner, certified nurse-midwife, or physician thinks that her uterine size is compatible with her menstrual history, uterine size may be the single most important clinical method for dating her pregnancy. In many cases, however, women do not seek obstetric care until well into their second trimester, when it becomes much more difficult to evaluate specific uterine size. In the case of the obese woman it is most difficult to determine uterine size early in pregnancy.

Fundal Height

Fundal height may be used as an indicator of uterine size, although this cannot be used late in pregnancy. A centimeter tape measure is used to measure the distance from the top of the symphysis pubis over the curve of the abdomen to the top of the uterine fundus (McDonald's method) (Figure 14–4). Fundal height in centimeters correlates well with weeks of gestation between 22–24 weeks and 34 weeks. At 26 weeks' gestation, for example, fundal height is probably about 26 cm. To be most accurate, fundal height should be measured by the same examiner each time. The bladder must be emptied before making the measurement (Cunningham et al 1993). Maternal position (trunk elevation, knee flexion) also influences fundal height measurement (Engstrom et al 1993). If the woman is very tall or very short, fundal height will differ. In the third trimester, variations in fetal weight decrease the accuracy of fundal height measurements.

Measurements of fundal height from month to month and week to week may give indications of intrauterine growth retardation (IUGR) if there is a lag in progression or indications of the presence of twins or hydramnios if there is a sudden increase in height. Unfortunately, this method of dating a pregnancy can be quite inaccurate in obese women, in women with uterine fibroids, and in mothers who develop hydramnios.

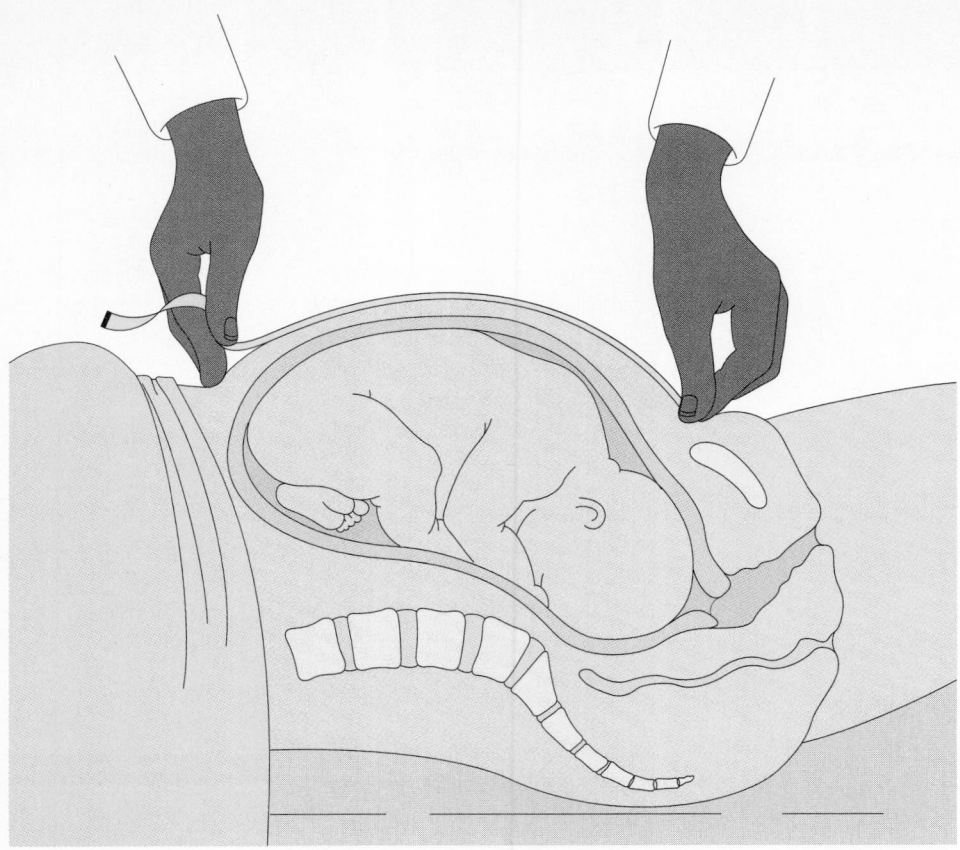

FIGURE 14-4   A cross-sectional view of fetal position when McDonald's method is used to assess fundal height.

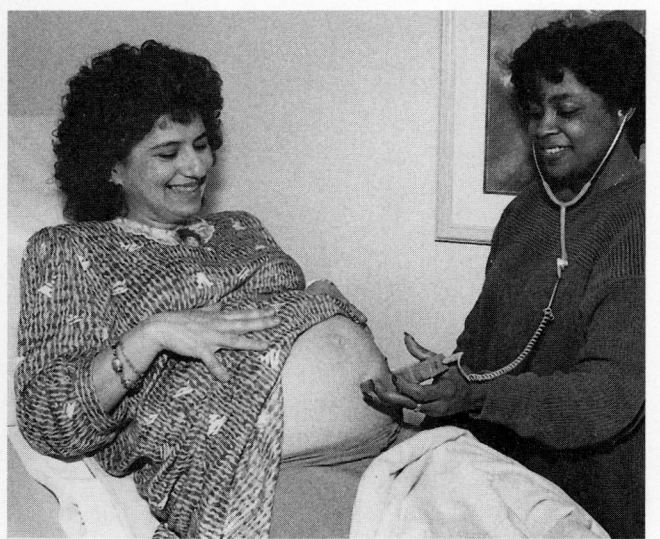

FIGURE 14-5   Listening to the fetal heartbeat with a Doppler device.

Fetal Development

Quickening

Fetal movements felt by the mother may give some indications that the fetus is nearing 20 weeks' gestation. However, quickening may be experienced between 16 and 22 weeks' gestation, so this is not a completely accurate method. Because multiparous women have experienced quickening before, they often report it earlier than a primigravida does.

Fetal Heartbeat

The fetal heartbeat can be detected as early as week 16 and almost always by 19 or 20 weeks of gestation with an ordinary fetoscope. In the case of twins or the obese woman it may be later than this before the fetal heartbeat can be detected. Fetal heartbeat may be detected with the ultrasonic Doppler device (Figure 14–5) at about 10 to 12 weeks' gestation.

Ultrasound

In the first trimester, ultrasound scanning can detect a gestational sac as early as 5 to 6 weeks after the LMP, fetal heart activity by 9 to 10 weeks and occasionally earlier, and fetal breathing movement by 11 weeks of pregnancy. Crown-to-rump measurements can be made for assessment of fetal age until the fetal head can be defined. Biparietal diameter measurements can be made by approximately 12 to 13 weeks and are most accurate between 20 and 30 weeks, when rapid growth in biparietal diameter occurs. (See Chapter 20 for an in-depth discussion of ultrasound scanning of the fetus.)

ASSESSMENT OF PELVIC ADEQUACY

The pelvis is assessed vaginally to determine whether its size is adequate for a vaginal birth. Nurses with special preparation may perform the vaginal assessment and interpret pelvimetry findings. This is sometimes referred to as clinical pelvimetry.

Pelvic Inlet

The important anteroposterior diameters of the inlet for childbearing are the diagonal conjugate, the obstetric conjugate, and the conjugata vera or true conjugate (Figure 14–6). Other diameters are the transverse (approximately 13.5 cm) and the oblique (averages 12.75 cm).

The anteroposterior diameters of the pelvic inlet may be assessed by attempting to reach from the lower border of the symphysis pubis to the sacral promontory with the middle finger. The clinician should determine the length of the finger before attempting this. The **diagonal conjugate** can then be measured by marking the place where the proximal part of the hand makes contact with the pubis (Figure 14–7). Then the distance is measured (normally measures at least 11.5 cm or more). The **obstetric conjugate** is the smallest and thus the most important anteroposterior diameter through which the fetus must pass. It extends from the sacral promontory to the upper inner point on the symphysis. Because it cannot be measured manually (but only by x-ray examination), it is estimated by subtracting 1.5–2 cm from the length of the diagonal conjugate. It should measure 10 cm or more in order for an average size baby (7.5–8 lb) to pass through without difficulty. The true conjugate extends from the upper border of the symphysis pubis to the middle of the sacral promontory. It can be determined by subtracting 1 cm from the diagonal conjugate.

Pelvic Cavity (Midpelvis)

Important midpelvic measurements include the plane of least dimension, or midplane (anteroposterior diameter, normally 11.5–12 cm; posterior sagittal diameter, 4.5–5

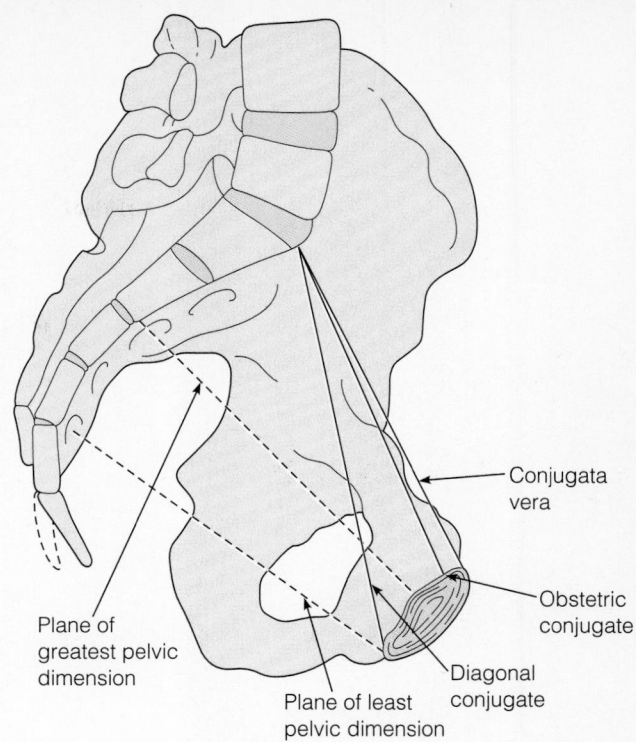

FIGURE 14-6 Anteroposterior diameters of the pelvic inlet and their relationship to the pelvic planes.

cm; and transverse diameter [interspinous], 10 cm). The planes of the midpelvis cannot be accurately measured by clinical examination. An evaluation of adequacy is made based on the prominence of the ischial spines and degree of convergence of the side walls.

Location of the sacrospinous ligament, a firm ridge of tissue, makes location of the ischial spines easier. When this ligament is located, the examiner should run the fingers along it laterally toward the anterior portion of the pelvis. The spines may range from a small firm bump like the knuckle of a finger (termed *not encroaching*) to a very prominent bone (called *encroaching*).

The sacrosciatic notch should admit two fingers. A wide notch means that the sacrum curves posteriorly, giving the anteroposterior diameter of the midpelvis a greater length. A narrow notch indicates a decreased diameter. The width of the sacrosciatic notch is more accurately evaluated through x-ray examination but can be estimated through vaginal examination.

The length of the sacrospinous ligament is measured by tracing the ligament from its origin on the ischial spines to its insertion on the sacrum. It is usually 4 cm or two to three finger breadths long.

The capacity of the cavity can be assessed by sweeping the fingers down the side walls bilaterally to evaluate

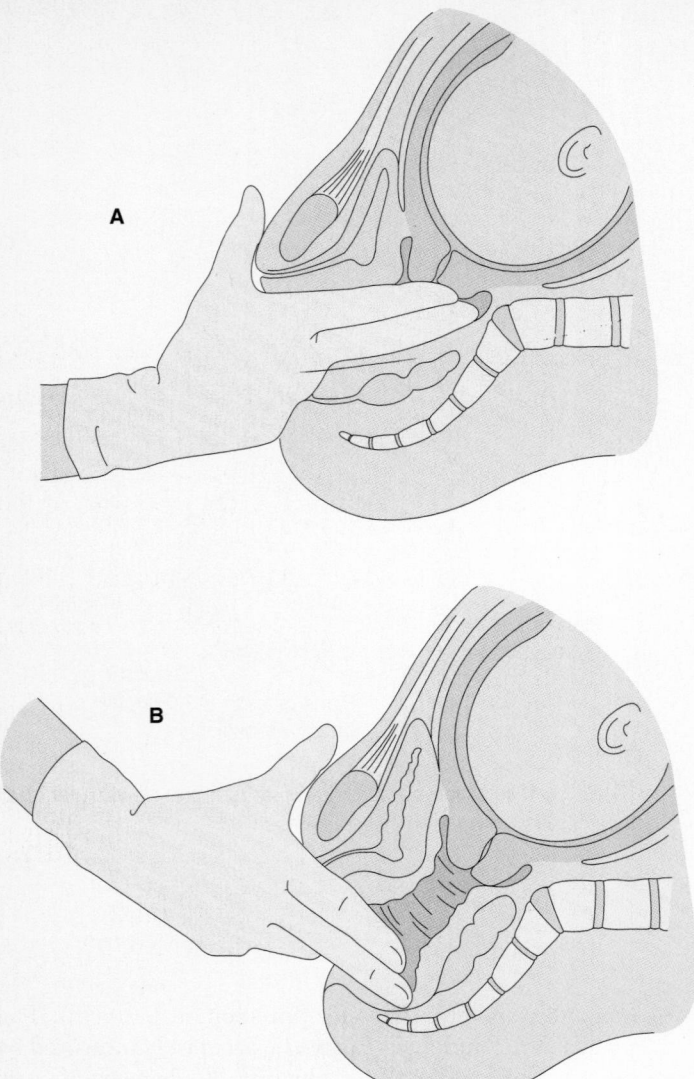

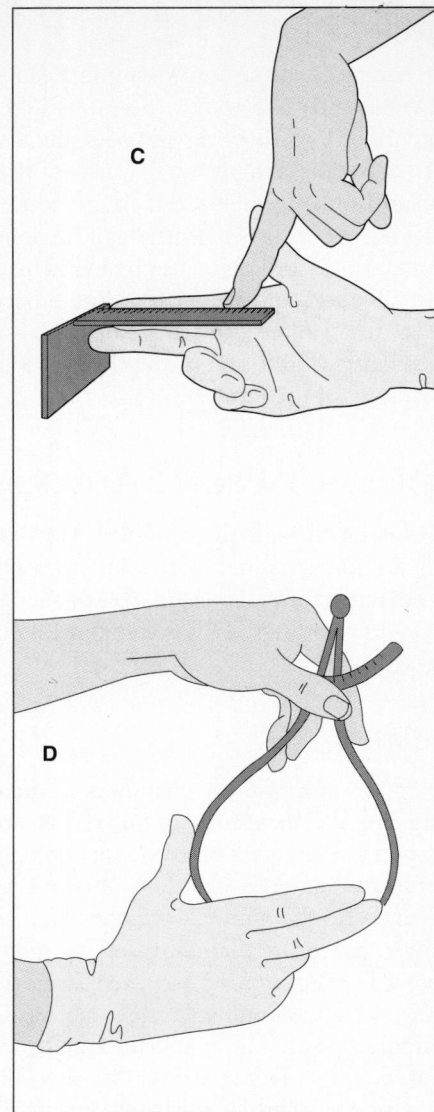

FIGURE 14-7   Manual measurement of inlet and outlet. *A* Estimation of the diagonal conjugate, which extends from the lower border of the symphysis pubis to the sacral promontory. *B* Estimation of the anteroposterior diameter of the outlet, which extends from the lower border of the symphysis pubis to the tip of the sacrum. *C and D* Methods that may be used to check the manual estimation of anteroposterior measurements.

the shape of the pelvic side walls. They may be termed *convergent* (closer together at the outlet than the inlet, like a funnel), *divergent* (side walls farther apart at the outlet, which typically means the pubic arch will have a wide angle), or *straight* (normal finding). The curvature, inclination, and hollowness of the sacrum help indicate the capacity of the posterior pelvis. It is estimated digitally by palpating the sacrococcygeal junction and by inching up toward the promontory. The examiner then estimates the hollowness of the sacrum. A flat or shallow sacrum has less room; a hollow sacrum is considered normal.

The plane of greatest pelvic dimensions represents the largest portion of the pelvic cavity and has no obstetric significance.

Pelvic Outlet

The anteroposterior diameter of the pelvic outlet (9.5–11.5 cm), which extends from the lower border of the symphysis pubis to the tip of the sacrum, can be measured digitally (Figure 14–7). The transverse diameter of the outlet is measured by placing the fist between the ischial tuberosities. It usually measures 8 to 10 cm (Figure 14–8). The posterior sagittal diameter, the third important outlet diameter, normally measures at least 7.5 cm.

The mobility of the coccyx is determined by pressing down on it with the forefinger and middle finger during the initial vaginal examination. An immobile coccyx can decrease the diameter of the outlet.

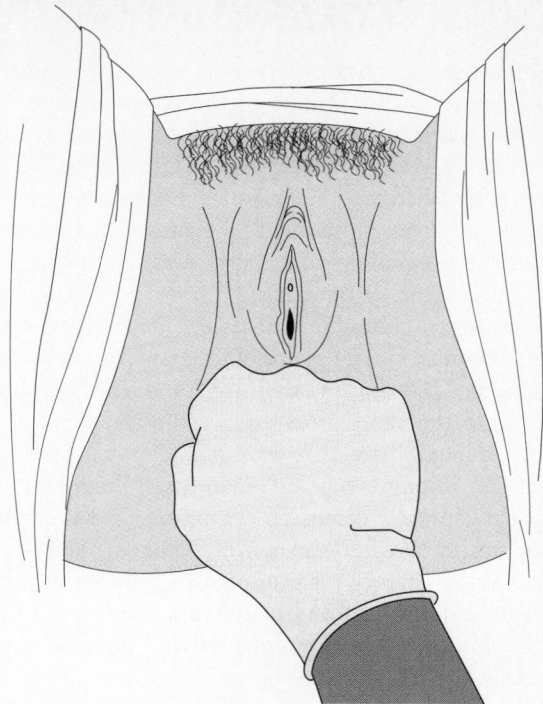

FIGURE 14-8   Use of a closed fist to measure the outlet. Most examiners know the distance between their first and last proximal knuckles. If they don't, they can use a measuring device.

The subpubic angle is estimated by palpating the bony structure externally. It should be 85 to 90 degrees. The subpubic angle is estimated by placing two fingers side by side at the border of the symphysis (Figure 14–9). It is probably reduced if the examiner cannot separate his or her fingers.

The length and shape of the pubic rami affect the transverse diameter of the outlet. The pubic ramus is expected to be short and concave inward, as opposed to straight and long.

The height and inclination of the symphysis pubis are measured, and the contour of the pubic arch is estimated. Excessively long or angulated bone structure shortens the diameter of the obstetric conjugate. Height can be determined by placing the index finger of the gloved hand up to the superior border of the symphysis. The examiner should measure the length of the first phalanx of the index finger (normally about 2.5 cm). Inclination can be determined by externally placing one finger on the top of the symphysis while the internal finger palpates the internal margin. An imaginary line is drawn between the fingers, and the angle is estimated.

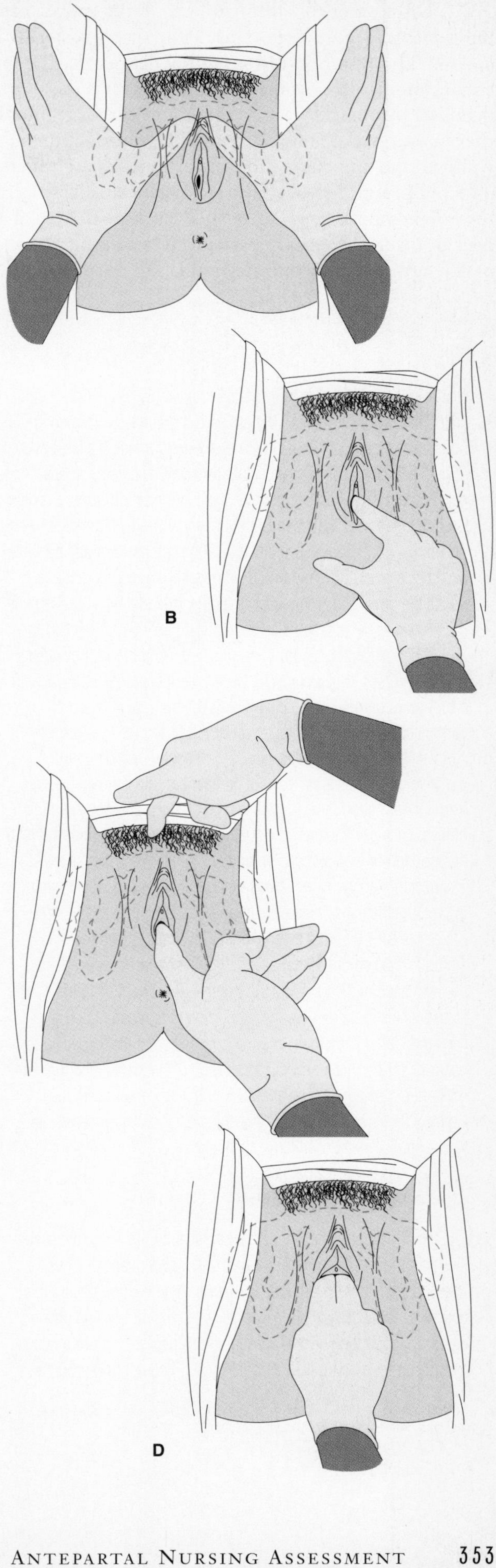

FIGURE 14-9   Evaluation of the outlet. *A* Estimation of the subpubic angle. *B* Estimation of the length of the pubic ramus. *C* Estimation of the depth and inclination of the pubis. *D* Estimation of the contour of the subpubic angle.

A

B

C

D

A posterior inclination with the lower border of the pubis slanting inward decreases the anteroposterior diameter. The anteroposterior sagittal diameter is the most significant diameter of the outlet because it is the shortest diameter through which the infant must pass. Estimating the contour of the pubic arch provides information on the width of the angle at which these bones come together. The pubic arch has obstetric importance; if it is narrow, the infant's head may be pushed backward toward the coccyx, making extension of the fetal head difficult, which may lengthen the second stage of labor.

RESEARCH IN PRACTICE

Health professionals use biophysical profiles (BPPs) to assess fetal status in the third trimester of high-risk pregnancies. BPPs combine non-stress testing and real-time ultrasound to image the fetus and assess fetal behavior. In many fetal assessment centers, nurses perform non-stress tests and physicians interpret the BPPs. Carolyn Gregor, Lisa Paine, Kathleen Costigan, and Timothy Johnson proposed that nurses with specialty education can perform and evaluate all aspects of the BPP and report nonreassuring results to the responsible physician. Their study hypothesized that fetal assessment nurses would be as reliable as obstetricians in interpreting BPPs.

The interpreters or study sample consisted of four physicians and four nurses. The physicians were experienced obstetricians with 1 to 5 years of ultrasound experience. The nurses, who had all completed a 40-hour practicum on BPPs during the year prior to the study, either staffed the fetal assessment center or were certified nurse-midwives. The standard of comparison for evaluation came from interpretation by a physician expert in fetal assessment techniques. Each participant individually evaluated 23 videotapes of fetal ultrasound imaging and copies of these fetuses' non-stress tests. The gestational age of the fetus ranged from 29 to 42 weeks excluding multiple fetuses and severe anomalies. Each participant interpreted the BPP in terms of fetal tone, movement, breathing, and amniotic fluid volume. After calculating the degree of agreement between each participant and the expert, the authors used the Kappa statistical test to determine the proportion of agreement between each individual participant and the expert beyond that expected to occur by chance. The physicians showed 5% substantial agreement, 55% moderate agreement, and 40% slight agreement with the expert. The nurses exhibited 10% substantial, 70% moderate, and 10% slight agreement with the expert.

Clinical Application for Study

This study demonstrates that expert clinical nurses with advanced skill training can interpret BPPs of high-risk pregnancies, thus freeing physicians for other tasks. The authors caution that a high degree of collaboration must exist between the nurses and physicians working together, and appropriate standards and protocols must be utilized along with a rigorous, certified training program.

SOURCE: Gregor C, Paine L, Costigan K, Johnson T: Interpretation of biophysical profiles by nurses and physicians. *JOGNN* 1994; 23(5):405.

SUBSEQUENT CLIENT HISTORY

At subsequent prenatal visits the nurse continues to gather data about the course of the pregnancy to date. The nurse asks specifically whether the woman has experienced any discomfort, especially the kinds of discomfort that are often seen at specific times during a pregnancy. The nurse inquires about physical changes that relate directly to the pregnancy, such as the woman's perception of fetal movement. Other pertinent information includes any exposure to contagious illnesses, medical treatment and therapy prescribed for nonpregnancy problems since the last visit, and any prescription or over-the-counter medications that were not prescribed as part of the woman's prenatal care.

The danger signs that a woman should report immediately are generally discussed during the initial prenatal visit and reviewed when she comes for her second prenatal visit. Many care givers also provide printed information on the subject written in lay terms. Table 14–3 identifies the danger signs of pregnancy and possible causes for each.

Periodic prenatal examinations offer the nurse an opportunity to assess the childbearing woman's psychologic needs and emotional status. If the woman's partner attends the prenatal visits, his needs and concerns can also be identified.

The interchange between the nurse and woman will be facilitated if it takes place in a friendly, trusting environment. The woman should be given sufficient time to ask questions and to air concerns. If the nurse provides the time and demonstrates genuine interest, the woman

TABLE 14-3	Danger Signs in Pregnancy
Danger Sign	**Possible Cause**
Sudden gush of fluid from vagina	Premature rupture of membranes
Vaginal bleeding	Abruptio placentae, placenta previa Lesions of cervix or vagina "Bloody show"
Abdominal pain	Preterm labor, abruptio placentae
Temperature above 38.3 C (101 F) and chills	Infection
Dizziness, blurring of vision, double vision, spots before eyes	Hypertension, preeclampsia
Persistent vomiting	Hyperemesis gravidarum
Severe headache	Hypertension, preeclampsia
Edema of hands, face, legs, and feet	Preeclampsia
Muscular irritability, convulsions	Preeclampsia, eclampsia
Epigastric pain	Preeclampsia—ischemia in major abdominal vessels
Oliguria	Renal impairment, decreased fluid intake
Dysuria	Urinary tract infection
Absence of fetal movement	Maternal medication, obesity, fetal death

will feel more at ease bringing up questions that she may believe are silly or concerns that she has been afraid to verbalize. The nurse who has an accurate understanding of all the changes of pregnancy is most able to answer questions and provide information. See the foldout color chart, "Maternal-Fetal Development," for vivid illustrations of some of this information.

The nurse should be sensitive to religious, cultural, and socioeconomic factors that may influence a family's response to pregnancy, as well as to their expectations of the health care system. The nurse can avoid stereotyping clients simply by asking each woman about her expectations for the antepartal period. Although many women's responses may reflect traditional norms, other women will have decidedly different views or may have expectations that represent a blending of beliefs or cultures.

During the prenatal period, it is essential to begin assessing the ability of the woman (and her partner, if possible) to successfully assume their responsibilities as parents. Table 14–4 identifies areas for assessment and provides some sample questions the nurse might use to obtain necessary information. If the woman's responses are primarily negative, interventions can be planned for the prenatal and postpartal periods.

SUBSEQUENT ANTEPARTAL ASSESSMENT

The Subsequent Prenatal Assessment Guide, which begins on page 357, provides a systematic approach to the regular physical examinations the pregnant woman

Text continues on page 360

TABLE 14-4	Prenatal Assessment of Parenting Guide	

Areas Assessed	Sample Questions
I. Perception of complexities of mothering	
A. Desires baby for itself	1. Did you plan on getting pregnant?
Positive:	2. How do you feel about being pregnant?
1. Feels positive about pregnancy	3. Why do you want this baby?
Negative:	
1. Wants baby to meet own needs such as someone to love her, someone to get her out of unhappy home	
B. Expresses concern about impact of mothering role on other roles (wife, career, school)	1. What do you think it will be like to take care of a baby?
Positive:	2. How do you think your life will be different after you have your baby?
1. Realistic expectations of how baby will affect job, career, school, and personal goals	3. How do you feel this baby will affect your job, career, school, and personal goals?
2. Interested in learning about child care	4. How will the baby affect your relationship with your boyfriend or husband?
Negative:	5. Have you done any reading, babysitting, or made any things for a baby?
1. Feels pregnancy and baby will make no emotional, physical, or social demands on self	
2. Has no insight that mothering role will affect other roles or life-style	
C. Gives up routine habits because "not good for baby" (eg, quits smoking, adjusts time schedule)	
Positive:	
1. Gives up routines not good for baby (quits smoking, adjusts eating habits)	
II. Attachment	
A. Strong feelings regarding sex of baby. Why?	1. Why do you prefer a certain sex? (Is reason inappropriate for a baby?)
Positive:	2. Note comments client makes about baby not being normal and why client feels this way.
1. Verbalizes positive thoughts about the baby	
Negative:	
1. Baby will be like negative aspects of self and partner	
B. Interested in data regarding fetus (eg, growth and development, heart tones)	
Positive:	
1. As above	
Negative:	
1. Shows no interest in fetal growth and development, quickening, and fetal heart tones	
2. Expresses negative feelings about fetus by rejecting counseling regarding nutrition, rest, hygiene	

TABLE 14-4 Prenatal Assessment of Parenting *continued*

Areas Assessed	Sample Questions
C. Fantasies about baby	1. What did you think or feel when you first felt the baby move?
Positive:	2. Have you started preparing for the baby?
1. Follows cultural norms regarding preparation	3. What do you think your baby will look like—what age do you see your baby at?
2. Time of attachment behaviors appropriate to her history of pregnancy loss	4. How would you like your new baby to look?
Negative:	
1. Bonding conditional depending on sex, age of baby, and/or labor and birth experience	
2. Woman considers only own needs when making plans for baby	
3. Exhibits no attachment behaviors after critical period of previous pregnancy	
4. Failure to follow cultural norms regarding preparation	
III. Acceptance of child by significant others	
A. Acknowledges acceptance by significant other of the new responsibility inherent in child	1. How does your partner feel about this pregnancy?
Positive:	2. How do your parents feel?
	3. What do your friends think?
1. Acknowledges unconditional acceptance of pregnancy and baby by significant others	4. Does your partner have a preference regarding the baby's sex? Why?
2. Partner accepts new responsibility inherent with child	5. How does your partner feel about being a father?
3. Timely sharing of experience of pregnancy with significant others	6. What do you think he'll be like as a father?
Negative:	7. What do you think he'll do to help you with child care?
1. Significant others not supportively involved with pregnancy	8. Have you and your partner talked about how the baby might change your lives?
2. Conditional acceptance of pregnancy depending on sex, race, age of baby	9. Who have you told about your pregnancy?
3. Decision making does not take in needs of fetus (eg, spends food money on new car)	
4. Takes no/little responsibility for needs of pregnancy, woman/fetus	
B. Concrete demonstration of acceptance of pregnancy/baby by significant others (eg, baby shower, significant other involved in prenatal education)	1. Note if partner attends clinic with client (degree of interest; eg, listens to heart tones). Significant other plans to be with client during labor and birth.
Positive:	2. Is your partner contributing financially?
1. Baby shower	
2. Significant other attends prenatal class with client	
IV. Ensures physical well-being	
A. Concerns about having normal pregnancy, labor and birth, and baby	1. What have you heard about labor and birth?
Positive:	2. Note data about client's reaction to prenatal class.
1. Preparing for labor and birth, attends prenatal classes, interested in labor and birth	
2. Aware of danger signs of pregnancy	
3. Seeks and uses appropriate health care (eg, time of initial visit, keeps appointments, follows through on recommendations)	
Negative:	
1. Denies signs and symptoms that might suggest complications of pregnancy	
2. Verbalizes extreme fear of labor and birth—refuses to talk about labor and birth	
3. Fails appointments, fails to follow instructions, refuses to attend prenatal classes	
B. Family/client decisions reflect concern for health of mother and baby (eg, use of finances, time)	
Positive:	
1. As above	

NOTE: When "Negative" is not listed in a section, the reader may assume that negative is the absence of positive responses.

SOURCE: Modified and used with permission of the Minneapolis Health Dept, Minneapolis, MN.

Physical Assessment/ Normal Findings	Alterations and Possible Causes*	Nursing Responses to Data†
Vital Signs		
Temperature: 36.2–37.6 C (98–99.6 F)	Elevated temperature (infection)	Evaluate for signs of infection. Refer to physician.
Pulse: 60–90/min Rate may increase 10 beats/min during pregnancy	Increased pulse rate (anxiety, cardiac disorders)	Note irregularities. Assess for anxiety and stress.
Respiration: 16–24/min	Marked tachypnea or abnormal patterns (respiratory disease)	Refer to physician.
Blood pressure: 90–140/60–90 (falls in second trimester)	> 140/90 or increase of 30 mm systolic and 15 mm diastolic (PIH)	Assess for edema, proteinuria, hyperreflexia. Refer to physician. Schedule appointments more frequently.
Weight Gain		
First trimester: 1.4–2.3 kg (3–5 lb) *Second trimester:* 5.5–6.8 kg (12–15 lb) *Third trimester:* 5.5–6.8 kg (12–15 lb)	Inadequate weight gain (poor nutrition, nausea, IUGR) Excessive weight gain (excessive caloric intake, edema, PIH)	Discuss appropriate weight gain. Provide nutritional counseling. Assess for presence of edema or anemia.
Edema		
Small amount of dependent edema, especially in last weeks of pregnancy	Edema in hands, face, legs, feet (PIH)	Identify any correlation between edema and activities, blood pressure, or proteinuria. Refer to physician if indicated.
Uterine Size		
See Initial Prenatal Assessment Guide for normal changes during pregnancy	Unusually rapid growth (multiple gestation, hydatidiform mole, hydramnios, miscalculation of EDB)	Evaluate fetal status. Determine height of fundus (p 349). Use diagnostic ultrasound.
Fetal Heartbeat		
120–160/min Funic souffle	Absence of fetal heartbeat after 20 weeks' gestation (maternal obesity, fetal demise)	Evaluate fetal status.
Laboratory Evaluation		
Hemoglobin: 12–16 g/dL Pseudoanemia of pregnancy	< 12 g/dL (anemia)	Provide nutritional counseling. Hemoglobin is repeated at 7 months' gestation. Women of Mediterranean heritage need a close check on hemoglobin because of possibility of thalassemia.
Maternal serum α-fetoprotein (MSAFP): normal levels (done at 16–18 weeks' gestation)	Elevated (neural tube defect, underestimated gestational age, multiple gestation, fetal demise, Rh disease)	Refer to physician.

*Possible causes of alterations are placed in parentheses.

†This column provides guidelines for further assessment and initial nursing intervention.

Physical Assessment/ Normal Findings	Alterations and Possible Causes*	Nursing Responses to Data†
50 g, 1-hour glucose screen (done between 24 and 28 weeks' gestation)	Plasma glucose level > 140 mg/dL (gestational diabetes mellitus [GDM])	Discuss implications of GDM. Refer for a diagnostic glucose tolerance test.
Urinalysis: See Initial Prenatal Assessment Guide for normal findings	See Initial Prenatal Assessment Guide for deviations	Repeat urinalysis at 7 months' gestation. Dipstick test at each visit.
Protein: Negative	Proteinuria, albuminuria (contamination by vaginal discharge, urinary tract infection, PIH)	Obtain dipstick urine sample. Refer to physician if deviations are present.
Glucose: Negative	Persistent glycosuria (diabetes mellitus)	Refer to physician.
Note: Glycosuria may be present due to physiologic alterations in glomerular filtration rate and renal threshold		

Cultural Assessment	Variations to Consider	Nursing Responses to Data†
Determine the mother's (and family's) attitudes about the sex of the unborn child.	Some women have no preference about the sex of the child; others do. In many cultures boys are especially valued as firstborn children.	Provide opportunities to discuss preferences and expectations; avoid a judgmental attitude to the response.
Ask about the woman's expectations of childbirth. Will she want someone with her for the birth? Whom does she choose? What is the role of her partner?	Some women want their partner present for labor and birth; others prefer a female relative or friend. Some women expect to be separated from their partner once cervical dilatation has occurred (Boyle & Andrews 1989).	Provide information on birth options, but accept the woman's decision about who will attend.
Ask about preparations for the baby. Determine what is customary for the woman.	Some women may have a fully prepared nursery; others may not have a separate room for the baby.	Explore reasons for not preparing for the baby. Support the mother's preferences, and provide information about possible sources of assistance if the decision is related to a lack of resources.

Psychosocial Assessment	Variations to Consider*	Nursing Responses to Data†
Expectant Mother		
Psychologic status: *First trimester:* Incorporates idea of pregnancy; may feel ambivalent, especially if she must give up desired role; usually looks for signs of verification of pregnancy, such as increase in abdominal size or fetal movement *Second trimester:* Baby becomes more real to woman as abdominal size increases and she feels movement; she begins to turn inward, becoming more introspective	Increasing stress and anxiety Inability to establish communication; inability to accept pregnancy; inappropriate response or actions; denial of pregnancy; inability to cope	Encourage woman to take an active part in her care. Establish lines of communication. Establish a trusting relationship. Counsel as necessary. Refer to appropriate professional as needed.

*Possible causes of alterations are placed in parentheses.

†This column provides guidelines for further assessment and initial nursing intervention.

Psychosocial Assessment	Variations to Consider*	Nursing Responses to Data†
Third trimester: Begins to think of baby as separate being; may feel restless and may feel that time of labor will never come; remains self-centered and concentrates on preparing place for baby		
Educational needs: *Self-care measures and knowledge about following:*	Inadequate information	Teach and/or institute appropriate relief measures (Chapter 15).
Health promotion		
Breast care		
Hygiene		
Rest		
Exercise		
Nutrition		
Relief measures for common discomforts of pregnancy		
Danger signs in pregnancy (Table 14–3)		
Sexual activity: Woman knows how pregnancy affects sexual activity	Lack of information about effects of pregnancy and/or alternative positions during sexual intercourse	Provide counseling.
Preparation for parenting: Appropriate preparation (Table 14–4)	Lack of preparation (denial, failure to adjust to baby, unwanted child) See Table 14–4	Counsel. If lack of preparation is due to inadequacy of information, provide information (Chapter 15).
Preparation for childbirth: *Client aware of following:*		If couple chooses particular technique, refer to classes (see Chapter 12 for description of childbirth preparation techniques). Encourage prenatal class attendance. Educate woman during visits based on current physical status. Provide reading list for more specific information.
1. Prepared childbirth techniques		
2. Normal processes and changes during childbirth		
3. Problems that may occur as a result of drug and alcohol use and of smoking	Continued abuse of drugs and alcohol; denial of possible effect on self and baby	Review danger signs that were presented on initial visit.
Woman has met other physician and/or nurse-midwife who may be attending her birth in the absence of primary care giver	Introduction of new individual at birth may increase stress and anxiety for woman and partner	Introduce woman to all members of group practice.
Impending labor: *Client knows signs of impending labor:*	Lack of information	Provide appropriate teaching, stressing importance of seeking appropriate medical assistance.
1. Uterine contractions that increase in frequency, duration, intensity		
2. Bloody show		
3. Expulsion of mucous plug		
4. Rupture of membranes		

*Possible causes of alterations are placed in parentheses.

†This column provides guidelines for further assessment and initial nursing intervention.

Psychosocial Assessment	Variations to Consider*	Nursing Responses to Data†
Expectant Father		
Psychologic status:		
First trimester: May express excitement over confirmation of pregnancy and of his virility; concerns move toward providing for financial needs; energetic; may identify with some discomforts of pregnancy and may even exhibit symptoms	Increasing stress and anxiety Inability to establish communication Inability to accept pregnancy diagnosis Withdrawal of support Abandonment of the mother	Encourage expectant father to come to prenatal visits. Establish lines of communication. Establish trusting relationship.
Second trimester: May feel more confident and be less concerned with financial matters; may have concerns about wife's changing size and shape, her increasing introspection		Counsel. Let expectant father know that it is normal for him to experience these feelings.
Third trimester: May have feelings of rivalry with fetus, especially during sexual activity; may make changes in his physical appearance and exhibit more interest in himself; may become more energetic; fantasizes about child but usually imagines older child; fears of mutilation and death of woman and child		Include expectant father in pregnancy activities as he desires. Provide education, information, and support. Increasing numbers of expectant fathers are demonstrating desire to be involved in many or all aspects of prenatal care, education, and preparation.

*Possible causes of alterations are placed in parentheses.

†This column provides guidelines for further assessment and initial nursing intervention.

should undergo for optimal prenatal care, and a model for evaluating both the pregnant woman and the expectant father, if he is involved in the pregnancy.

The frequency of subsequent visits should be determined by the woman's individual needs and the assessment of her risks. Generally, the recommended frequency of prenatal visits is as follows:

- Every 4 weeks for the first 28 weeks of gestation
- Every 2 weeks until 36 weeks' gestation
- After week 36, every week until childbirth

During the subsequent antepartal assessments, a woman may exhibit psychologic problems such as the following:

- Increasing anxiety
- Inability to establish communication
- Inappropriate responses or actions
- Denial of pregnancy
- Inability to cope with stress
- Intense preoccupation with the sex of the baby

- Failure to acknowledge quickening
- Failure to plan and prepare for the baby (for example, living arrangements, clothing, feeding methods)
- Indications of substance abuse

If the woman appears to have these or other critical psychologic problems, the nurse should provide ongoing support and counseling and also refer her to appropriate professionals.

KEY CONCEPTS

A complete history forms the basis of prenatal care and is reevaluated and updated as necessary throughout the pregnancy.

The initial prenatal assessment is a careful and thorough physical examination and cultural and psychosocial assessment designed to identify variations and potential risk factors.

Laboratory tests completed at the initial visit, such as a complete blood count, ABO and Rh typing, urinalysis, Pap smear, gonorrhea culture, rubella titer, and various blood screens, provide information about the woman's health during early pregnancy and also help detect potential problems.

The estimated date of birth can be calculated using Nägele's rule. Using this approach, one begins with the first day of the last menstrual period, subtracts 3 months, and adds 7 days. A "wheel" may also be used to calculate the EDB.

Accuracy of the EDB may be evaluated by physical examination to assess uterine size, measurement of fundal height, and ultrasound. Perception of quickening and auscultation of fetal heartbeat are also useful tools in confirming the gestation of a pregnancy.

The diagonal conjugate is the distance from the lower posterior border of the symphysis pubis to the sacral promontory. The obstetric conjugate is estimated by subtracting 1.5 to 2.0 cm from the length of the diagonal conjugate.

As part of the assessment of the pelvic cavity (midpelvis), the prominence of the ischial spines is assessed, the sacrosciatic notch and the length of the sacrospinous ligament are measured, and the shape of the pelvic side walls is evaluated. Finally, the hollowness of the sacrum is determined.

The anteroposterior diameter of the pelvic outlet is determined, the mobility of the coccyx is assessed, the suprapubic angle is estimated, and the contour of the pubic arch is evaluated to assess the adequacy of the pelvic outlet.

The nurse begins evaluating the woman psychosocially during the initial prenatal assessment. This assessment continues and is modified throughout the pregnancy.

Cultural and ethnic beliefs may strongly influence the woman's attitudes and apparent cooperation with care during pregnancy.

REFERENCES

Boyle JS, Andrews MM: *Transcultural Concepts in Nursing Care.* Glenview, IL: Scott, Foresman/Little, Brown, 1989.

Cunningham FG et al: *Williams Obstetrics*, 19th ed. Norwalk, CT: Appleton & Lange, 1993.

Engstrom JL et al: Fundal height measurement. *J Nurse-Midwifery* January/February 1993; 38:26.

Milunsky A et al: Maternal heat exposure and neural tube defects. *JAMA* August 19, 1992; 268(7):882.

Mittendorf R et al: The length of uncomplicated human gestation. *Obstet Gynecol* June 1990; 75:929.

CHAPTER 15

THE EXPECTANT FAMILY: NEEDS AND CARE

I don't know how I timed it, but my nursing program OB rotation finishes up right about my due date. Watching all the births during my rotation has been really exciting. The labor and delivery nurses laugh and say my hormones should be hopping now, but I think this baby is subliminally telling me that we won't "hatch" until I take my last final exam!

KEY TERMS

Fetal activity diary (FAD)

Fetal alcohol syndrome (FAS)

Fetal movement records (FMR)

Kegel's exercises

Leukorrhea

Nipple preparation

Pelvic tilt

Ptyalism

Teratogens

OBJECTIVES

Summarize communication skills that nurses can use to enhance effectiveness in nursing assessments and implementation of care.

Explain the causes of the common discomforts of pregnancy and appropriate measures to alleviate these discomforts.

Develop a plan of care incorporating anticipatory guidance of the pregnant woman and her family to maintain and promote well-being for each trimester of pregnancy.

Discuss the significance of cultural considerations in managing nursing care during pregnancy and common practices of specific cultures.

Describe the significance of using the nursing process to promote health in the woman and her family during pregnancy.

Compare similarities and differences in the needs of expectant women in various age groups.

From the moment a woman finds out that she is pregnant she faces a future marked by dramatic changes. Her appearance will be altered. Her relationships will change. She will experience a variety of unique physical changes throughout the pregnancy. Even her psychologic state will be affected.

Her family must also adjust to the pregnancy. Roles and responsibilities of family members will be altered as the woman's ability to perform certain activities changes. They too must adapt psychologically to the situation.

The expectant woman and her family will probably have many questions about the pregnancy and its impact on her and the other members of the family. In addition the daily activities and health care practices of the woman become of concern when she and her family realize that the well-being of the unborn child can be affected by what she does.

Nurses caring for pregnant women need a clear understanding of pregnancy and the changes it brings if they are to be effective in implementing the nursing process to plan and provide care. With this in mind, Chapter 13 provided a data base for the nurse by presenting material related to the normal physical and psychologic, social, and cultural changes of pregnancy. Chapter 14 then used that data base to begin the nursing process by focusing on client assessment. This chapter continues the application of the nursing process to the expectant woman by discussing analysis and nursing diagnosis, planning, implementation, and evaluation. Planning and implementation are combined here to avoid redundancy.

NURSING DIAGNOSIS DURING PREGNANCY

The nurse may see a pregnant woman only once every 3–4 weeks during the first several months of her pregnancy. This is why a written care plan that incorporates the data base, nursing diagnoses, and client goals is essential to ensure continuity of care.

The nurse can anticipate that, for many women with a low-risk pregnancy, certain nursing diagnoses will be made more frequently than others. This will, of course, vary from woman to woman and according to the time in the pregnancy. Examples of common nursing diagnoses include the following:

- Knowledge deficit related to a lack of information about the use of medication during pregnancy

- Constipation related to the physiologic effects of pregnancy

- Altered sexuality patterns related to discomfort during late pregnancy

After formulating an appropriate diagnosis, the nurse establishes related goals to guide the nursing plan and interventions.

NURSING PLAN AND IMPLEMENTATION DURING PREGNANCY

Once nursing diagnoses have been identified, the next step is to establish priorities of nursing care. Sometimes priorities of care are based on the most immediate needs or concerns perceived by the woman. For example, during the first trimester, when a woman is experiencing nausea or is concerned about sexual intimacy with her partner, she is not likely to be ready to hear about labor and birth.

The woman's priorities may not always be the same as the nurse's. If the safety of the woman or her fetus is at issue, however, that takes priority over other concerns of the woman or her family. It is the responsibility of medical and nursing professionals to help the woman and her family understand the significance of a problem and to plan appropriate interventions to deal with it.

The intervention methods most used by nurses in caring for the expectant woman and her family are communication techniques and teaching-learning strategies. These intervention methods are most obvious when used in groups, such as early pregnancy classes and childbirth education classes, but the nurse in the prenatal setting often applies these techniques on an individual basis.

The value of providing a primary care nurse to coordinate care for each childbearing family is beginning to be recognized. The nurse in a clinic or HMO may be the only source of continuity for the woman, who may see a different physician or certified nurse-midwife at each visit. The nurse can be extremely effective in working with the expectant family by providing them with necessary and complete information about pregnancy, self-care measures, and community resources or referral agencies that may be of help to them. Such education allows the family to assume equal responsibility with health care providers in working toward their common goal of a positive childbearing experience.

Promotion of Family Wellness

Relieving the expectant woman's discomforts and maintaining her physical health are important parts of the nursing plan. The plan also anticipates the need for information and guidance (Table 15–1). Interventions are timed to coincide with the woman's (couple's) readiness and needs. In addition, because the woman's well-being is

TABLE 15-1	Topics for Client Teaching During Pregnancy

All Three Trimesters
Discomforts of pregnancy (see Table 15–3)
Nutrition and weight gain
Sexual activity
Sibling preparation

First Trimester
Attitude toward pregnancy
Exercise and rest
Smoking; use of alcohol and other drugs
Traveling
Fetal growth and development
Danger signals associated with spontaneous abortion
Employment
Early pregnancy classes

Second Trimester
Concerns related to changes in body
Fetal growth and development
Fetal movement
Clothing
Care of skin and breasts
Beginning preparation for care of the infant (equipment and room)
Decisions about infant feeding

Third Trimester
Exercise and rest
Traveling
Danger signals
Preparation for labor and birth
Completion of preparation in home for new baby
Decisions about the infant (circumcision, method of feeding, and so forth)
Decision making for the early postpartum period
Education about psychologic and physical expectations in the early postpartum period

directly related to the well-being of those to whom she is closest, the nurse helps meet the needs of the woman's family to better maintain the harmony and integrity of the family unit. The nurse does this by providing support and prenatal education. If the nurse is effective, family members may gain greater problem-solving ability, self-esteem, self-confidence, and ability to participate in health care.

Father

Although the father of the baby is present in most cases, his presence cannot be assumed. If he is not a part of the family structure, it is important to assess the woman's support system to determine what significant persons in her life will play a major role during this childbearing experience.

When the father is part of the family or support system, providing anticipatory guidance to him is a neces-

sary part of any plan of care. He may need information about the anatomic, physiologic, and emotional changes that occur during pregnancy and postpartum, the couple's sexuality and sexual response, and the reactions that he may experience. He may wish to express his feelings about breast- versus bottle-feeding, the sex of the child, and other topics. If it is culturally acceptable to the couple and personally acceptable to him, the nurse refers the couple to expectant parents' classes for further information and support from other couples.

The nurse assesses the father's intended degree of participation during labor and birth and his knowledge of what to expect. If the couple prefers that his participation be minimal or restricted, the nurse supports their decision. With this type of consideration and collaboration, the father is less apt to develop feelings of alienation, helplessness, and guilt during the intrapartal period. The relationship between the couple may be strengthened and his self-esteem raised. He is then better able to provide physical and emotional support to his partner during labor and birth.

Siblings

The nurse incorporates in the plan for prenatal care a discussion about the negative feelings that older children may have. Parents may be distressed to see an older child become aggressive toward the newborn. Parents who are unprepared for the older child's feeling of anger, jealousy, and rejection may respond inappropriately in their confusion and surprise. The nurse emphasizes that open communication between parents and children (or acting out feelings with a doll if the child is too young to verbalize) helps children master their feelings and may prevent them from hurting the baby when they are unsupervised. Children may feel less neglected and more secure if they know that their parents are willing to help with their anger and aggressiveness.

Parents may be encouraged to bring their children to antepartal visits. Seeing what is involved and listening to the fetal heartbeat may make the pregnancy more real to siblings. Many agencies also provide sibling classes geared to different ages and levels of understanding.

Prenatal Education

Throughout the prenatal period the nurse provides informal and formal education to the childbearing family. This education is designed to help the family carry out self-care when appropriate and to report changes that may indicate a possible health problem. The nurse also provides anticipatory guidance to help the family plan for changes that will occur following childbirth. Issues that could be possible sources of postpartal stress should be discussed by the expectant couple. Issues to be resolved beforehand may include the sharing of infant and household chores, help in the first few days, reapportionment of family finances, options for babysitting to allow the mother (and couple) some free time, the mother's return to work after the baby's birth, and sibling rivalry.

Relationship changes with in-laws should be addressed as well as the woman's or couple's expectations of the grandparents. Although some grandparents are eager to assist with child care by babysitting, others are not. The parents should also give some thought to the best ways of dealing with possible conflicts with the grandparents over childraising approaches. Couples resolve these issues in different ways; however, postpartal adjustment is easier for a couple who agrees on the issues beforehand than for a couple who does not confront and resolve these issues.

TEACHING MOMENT

At each prenatal visit focus your teaching on changes or possible discomforts the woman might encounter during the coming month and the next trimester. If the pregnancy is progressing normally, spend a few minutes describing her baby at this stage of development.

Cultural Considerations in Pregnancy

As discussed in Chapter 13, specific actions during pregnancy are often determined by cultural beliefs. Some beliefs, which have been passed down from generation to generation, may be called "old wives' tales." These beliefs certainly had some meaning at one time, but the meanings have often been lost with the passing of time. Other beliefs have definite meanings that are retained. Table 15–2 presents activities that are encouraged or forbidden by specific cultures. The table is not meant to be all-inclusive; it offers a few examples of cultural activities that may be important to some clients during the prenatal period.

In working with clients of another culture the health care professional should be as open as possible to other beliefs. If certain activities are not harmful, there is no need to impose one's beliefs and practices upon a person of another culture. If the activities are harmful, the nurse can consult or work with someone within the culture or someone aware of cultural beliefs and values to help modify a client's behavior or to determine alternatives (see Nursing Care Plan: Handling Language Barriers at First Prenatal Visit on page 366).

Text continues on page 368

| TABLE 15-2 | Cultural Beliefs and Activities During Pregnancy |

Here are a few examples of cultural beliefs and activities related to pregnancy. It is important not to make assumptions about a client's beliefs since cultural norms vary greatly within a culture and from generation to generation. The nurse should observe the client carefully and take the time to ask questions. The client will benefit greatly from this awareness of differences.

Belief or Activity	Nursing Considerations
Home Remedies	
People of European background may use nonprescription medications to relieve discomfort or ensure better health. People of Mexican background may use spearmint or sassafras tea to ease morning sickness and cathartics during the last month of pregnancy to ensure a healthy birth (Brown 1976). Clients of Chinese descent may drink ginseng tea for faintness after childbirth or as a sedative when mixed with bamboo leaves (Spector 1991).	Find out what medications and home remedies your client is using, and counsel your client regarding overall effects. It is common for individuals to avoid telling health care workers about home remedies—the client may feel this will be judged unfavorably. Phrase your questions in a sensitive, accepting way.
Some people of African heritage may use self-medication for pregnancy discomforts—for example, castor oil for constipation, herbs for nausea and vomiting, and vinegar and baking soda for heartburn (Carrington 1978).	In some cases you might want to suggest remedies that may be more effective—for example, eating high-fiber foods to reduce constipation. If the home remedy is not harmful, there is no reason to ask a client to discontinue this practice.
Clothing	
Women of Mexican background may wear certain clothing—for example, a muneco-cord worn beneath the breasts and knotted over the umbilicus to ensure a safe birth (Brown 1976).	Ask your client how she feels about hospital clothing. You may want to find out if certain styles of clothing or jewelry have special meaning for her. Respect these clothing choices, intervening only if the clothing could be harmful in any way.
Some women of European heritage may be concerned that they look fat while pregnant and may choose clothing based on self-image.	Discuss these concerns about self-image with your client.
Exercise	
Some people of African, European, and Mexican cultural heritage feel that reaching over the head can harm the baby. Some people of European background may fear that lifting heavy objects will cause the placenta to separate.	Ask your client if there are any activities she is afraid to do because of the pregnancy. Assure her that reaching over her head will not harm the baby, and evaluate other activities related to their effect on the pregnancy.
Spirituality	
Navajo Indians may meet with the medicine man 2 months prior to birth, feeling that the prayers will ensure a safe birth and healthy baby. Some people of European background may tend to pay more attention to spirituality in their life to alleviate fears and assure a safe birth.	Encourage the use of support systems and spiritual aids that provide comfort for the mother.

NURSING CARE PLAN

HANDLING LANGUAGE BARRIERS AT FIRST PRENATAL VISIT

Nursing Assessment

Nursing History
1. Degree of communication possible
2. Course of pregnancy
3. Estimated gestational age
4. Sensitivity to medications
5. Existing problems or concerns

Physical Examination
1. Vital signs, height, weight, general appearance
2. Signs of confusion, fear, or anxiety

Diagnostic Studies
1. Urinalysis
2. CBC
3. Rubella titer, hepatitis screen if indicated
4. Other lab work as appropriate

NURSING DIAGNOSIS: Impaired verbal communication related to lack of understanding of care giver's language

EXPECTED OUTCOME: Woman/family will have an opportunity to share and receive all needed information.

Nursing Interventions	Rationale
Arrange for an interpreter—family member, friend, or staff person—to be present at this visit and subsequent visits as needed. If interpreter not available, use pictures related to basic needs such as food, water, toileting, pain, and medication. Avoid rushing interview.	For effective ongoing communication a shared language is essential.

OUTCOME MET IF:
- Interpreter is present at all visits.
- Woman/family verbalize through interpreter understanding of all information and have no further questions.

NURSING DIAGNOSIS: Impaired social interaction related to differing cultural practices and expectations between client and nurse

EXPECTED OUTCOME: The woman will discuss her expectations.

Nursing Interventions	Rationale
Ask the woman to describe her expectations of the health care system.	To provide effective, culturally sensitive care, the nurse must gather information about acceptable and proscribed activities for the woman and her family.
Ask the woman about customs and culturally specific practices that are important to her.	
Ask the woman to describe any practices that are specifically forbidden in her culture.	
Describe procedures usually performed during a prenatal visit and discuss the woman's feelings about them.	
Postpone any nonessential procedures to a subsequent visit if the woman appears overwhelmed.	

OUTCOME MET IF:
- Woman's expectations and cultural beliefs are made known to the health care provider.
- Woman verbalizes understanding of needed prenatal procedures and voices acceptance of them.

HANDLING LANGUAGE BARRIERS AT FIRST PRENATAL VISIT *continued*

NURSING DIAGNOSIS: Impaired social interaction related to culturally specific expectations of the role of the partner in the pregnancy and birth

EXPECTED OUTCOME: The woman will have an opportunity to discuss her wishes regarding her partner's involvement

Nursing Interventions	Rationale
Ask the woman to identify her primary support person and discuss their expectations of this person's involvement in the pregnancy and birth.	The role of the primary support person is often culturally specific and may vary greatly. The nurse recognizes this and respects the family's wishes.

OUTCOME MET IF:
- Woman verbalizes expectations and preferences in regard to primary support person.

NURSING DIAGNOSIS: Knowledge deficit: related to lack of information about the changes associated with pregnancy and about prenatal care practices in the adopted country

EXPECTED OUTCOME: The woman will gain information regarding pregnancy changes and prenatal care.

Nursing Interventions	Rationale
Provide basic information about pregnancy and prenatal care. Plan additional sessions as needed so that the woman is not overwhelmed with information. Provide opportunities for questions and clarifications. If possible, provide printed information in the woman's language. Establish a mutually acceptable method for the woman to contact a care giver if she has questions or problems or in an emergency.	All pregnant women have the right to clear, accurate information in order to be active participants in their health care.

OUTCOME MET IF:
- Woman verbalizes understanding of information regarding pregnancy, prenatal care, methods and phone numbers for contacting health care providers, and available community resources.

Essential Nursing Activities To Achieve Outcomes

Initial Visit

1. Contact and have interpreter at this and every visit if possible.
2. Make prenatal appointments with both the woman and the interpreter, so same interpreter can be utilized for consistency and relationship building.
3. Provide as much printed information in the woman's language as possible.
4. Keep information basic.
5. Determine woman's expectations and cultural preferences in regard to prenatal care and labor/birth.
6. Make available phone numbers and contact methods for health care providers and community resources.

Following Visits

1. Have interpreter available.
2. Evaluate further need for information.
3. Continue to identify appropriate community resources.
4. Honor cultural customs and beliefs.

During periods of crisis such as the transition to parenthood, marital relationships may be stressed and marital satisfaction may decline. Satisfaction depends not only on the exchange of support but also on the confirmation of expected support. Childbirth education classes could address preparation for parenthood and marital relationship development rather than focusing solely on the labor and birth experience. Based on this conceptual framework, Sherrilyn Coffman, Mary Levitt, and Linda Brown hypothesized that parents who perceive greater confirmation of expected support will have a more positive emotional affect, higher relationship satisfaction scores, and more positive attitudes toward the baby. They further hypothesized that confirmation of support would impact relationship satisfaction even after support was accounted for, and that parents who participated in a childbirth education class that focused on expectations for support would perceive greater confirmation of expectations and more positive outcomes.

Married couples recruited from 18 childbirth education classes served as the sample. Each married participant, 282 total, completed instruments measuring relationship satisfaction, emotional affect, attitude toward the baby, received support index, and expectancy confirmation. After random assignment of each class into either the experimental or the control group, the instructor initiated a 1-hour study session. In the experimental group the focus was on expectations for mutual support after childbirth with time for the husband and wife to discuss the issues and for group discussion. The control group discussion focused on sex role behavior, a topic unrelated to support. The final study sample consisted of 204 participants who, between the third and sixth months postpartum, completed and returned the same prenatal questionnaire as that given in the class.

Study results supported the first hypothesis, that parents with greater confirmation of support had more positive outcomes. The second hypothesis, that confirmation of expected support was independent of actual support in its effect on relationship satisfaction, was validated for women but not for men. Hypothesis three was not validated, possibly because the treatment, a 1-hour class, was not strong enough to create an effect.

Clinical Application of Study

Interactions with nurses, such as in childbirth education classes, should provide opportunities to explore issues other than the actual birth. This study identifies one such issue.

SOURCE: Coffman S, Levitt M, Brown L: Effects of clarification of support expectations in prenatal couples. *Nurs Res* 1994; 43(2):111.

Relief of the Common Discomforts of Pregnancy

Common discomforts of pregnancy are often referred to as minor discomforts by health care professionals. These discomforts, however, are not minor to the pregnant woman.

Most of the discomforts of pregnancy are a result of physiologic and anatomic changes and are fairly specific to each of the three trimesters. Table 15–3 identifies the common discomforts of pregnancy, their possible causes, and the self-care measures that might relieve the discomfort.

First Trimester

Nausea and Vomiting   Nausea and vomiting are early symptoms in pregnancy. Some degree of nausea occurs in the majority of pregnant women. These symptoms appear sometime after the first missed menstrual period and usually cease by the fourth missed menstrual period. Approximately 50% to 88% of pregnant women experience some degree of nausea (Blackburn & Loper 1992). Some women develop an aversion only to specific foods, many experience nausea upon arising in the morning, and others experience nausea throughout the day or in the evening. Vomiting does not occur in the majority of these women.

The exact cause of nausea and vomiting of pregnancy is unknown but is believed to be multifactorial. Research has identified possible hormonal, metabolic, toxic, neurologic, and psychosomatic factors contributing to its development (Kousen 1993). Because hCG begins to be present in the body at about the time symptoms of morning sickness usually begin and hCG levels are subsiding when the discomfort of nausea and vomiting usually ends, hCG is often cited as a major factor. This is further supported by the fact that hCG levels tend to be significantly higher in molar pregnancy (characterized by an abnormal proliferation of trophoblastic tissue and changes in the chorionic villi of the placenta [Chapter 19, Gestational Trophoblastic Disease]), than in normal pregnancy, and nausea and vomiting are common symptoms of this disorder. Research has not yet confirmed this theory, however (Cunningham et al 1993). Changes in carbohydrate metabolism, fatigue, and emotional factors may also play a role in the development of nausea and vomiting of pregnancy.

Teaching for Self-Care   Treatment of nausea and vomiting is not always successful, but the symptoms can be reduced. The nurse must assess when the nausea and/or vomiting occurs to be helpful in suggesting methods of relief. For some women nausea may be relieved simply by avoiding the odor of certain foods or other conditions that precipitate the problem. If nausea occurs most frequently during early morning, the woman may find it helpful to eat dry

TABLE 15-3	Self-Care Measures for Common Discomforts of Pregnancy	

Discomfort	Influencing Factors	Self-Care Measures
First Trimester		
Nausea and vomiting	Increased levels of hCG Changes in carbohydrate metabolism Emotional factors Fatigue	Avoid odors or causative factors. Eat dry crackers or toast before arising in morning. Have small but frequent meals. Avoid greasy or highly seasoned foods. Take dry meals with fluids between meals. Drink carbonated beverages.
Urinary frequency	Pressure of uterus on bladder in both first and third trimesters	Void when urge is felt. Increase fluid intake during the day. Decrease fluid intake *only* in the evening to decrease nocturia.
Fatigue	Specific causative factors unknown May be aggravated by nocturia due to urinary frequency	Plan time for a nap or rest period daily. Go to bed earlier. Seek family support and assistance with responsibilities so that more time is available to rest.
Breast tenderness	Increased levels of estrogen and progesterone	Wear well-fitting, supportive bra.
Increased vaginal discharge	Hyperplasia of vaginal mucosa and increased production of mucus by the endocervical glands due to the increase in estrogen levels	Promote cleanliness by daily bathing. Avoid douching, nylon underpants, and pantyhose; cotton underpants are more absorbent; powder can be used to maintain dryness if not allowed to cake.
Nasal stuffiness and nosebleed (epistaxis)	Elevated estrogen levels	May be unresponsive, but cool air vaporizer may help; avoid use of nasal sprays and decongestants.
Ptyalism (excessive, often bitter salivation)	Specific causative factors unknown	Use astringent mouthwashes, chew gum, or suck hard candy.
Second and Third Trimesters		
Heartburn (pyrosis)	Increased production of progesterone, decreasing gastroin-testinal motility and increasing relaxation of cardiac sphincter, displacement of stomach by enlarging uterus, thus regurgitation of acidic gastric contents into esophagus	Eat small and more frequent meals. Use low-sodium antacids. Avoid overeating, fatty and fried foods, lying down after eating, and sodium bicarbonate.
Ankle edema	Prolonged standing or sitting Increased levels of sodium due to hormonal influences Circulatory congestion of lower extremities Increased capillary permeability Varicose veins	Practice frequent dorsiflexion of feet when prolonged sitting or standing is necessary. Elevate legs when sitting or resting. Avoid tight garters or restrictive bands around legs.
Varicose veins	Venous congestion in the lower veins that increases with pregnancy Hereditary factors (weakening of walls of veins, faulty valves) Increased age and weight gain	Elevate legs frequently. Wear supportive hose. Avoid crossing legs at the knees, standing for long periods, garters, and hosiery with constrictive bands.
Hemorrhoids	Constipation (see following discussion) Increased pressure from gravid uterus on hemorrhoidal veins	Avoid constipation. Apply ice packs, topical ointments, anesthetic agents, warm soaks, or sitz baths; gently reinsert into rectum as necessary.
Constipation	Increased levels of progesterone, which cause general bowel sluggishness Pressure of enlarging uterus on intestine Iron supplements Diet, lack of exercise, and decreased fluids	Increase fluid intake, fiber in the diet, and exercise. Develop regular bowel habits. Use stool softeners as recommended by physician.
Backache	Increased curvature of the lumbosacral vertebrae as the uterus enlarges Increased levels of hormones, which cause softening of cartilage in body joints Fatigue Poor body mechanics	Use proper body mechanics. Practice the pelvic tilt exercise. Avoid uncomfortable working heights, high-heeled shoes, lifting heavy loads, and fatigue.
Leg cramps	Imbalance of calcium/phosphorus ratio Increased pressure of uterus on nerves Fatigue Poor circulation to lower extremities Pointing the toes	Practice dorsiflexion of feet in order to stretch affected muscle. Evaluate diet. Apply heat to affected muscles.

TABLE 15-3   Self-Care Measures *continued*

Discomfort	Influencing Factors	Self-Care Measures
Second and Third Trimesters		
Faintness	Postural hypotension Sudden change of position causing venous pooling in dependent veins Standing for long periods in warm area Anemia	Arise slowly from resting position. Avoid prolonged standing in warm or stuffy environments. Evaluate hematocrit/hemoglobin.
Dyspnea	Decreased vital capacity from pressure of enlarging uterus on the diaphragm	Use proper posture when sitting and standing. Sleep propped up with pillows for relief if problem occurs at night.
Flatulence	Decreased gastrointestinal motility leading to delayed emptying time Pressure of growing uterus on large intestine Air swallowing	Avoid gas-forming foods. Chew food thoroughly. Get regular daily exercise. Maintain normal bowel habits.
Carpal tunnel syndrome	Compression of median nerve in carpal tunnel of wrist Aggravated by repetitive hand movements	Avoid aggravating hand movements. Use splint as prescribed. Elevate affected arm.

crackers or toast before arising slowly. Arising slowly and avoiding sudden position changes throughout the day may also help prevent nausea due to hypotensive episodes. The woman can also be advised to avoid brushing her teeth right after eating, as this, too, may trigger vomiting.

Generally, it is helpful to eat small meals every 2 to 3 hours during the day and to avoid greasy or highly seasoned foods. Food may be salted to taste. The salt increases the palatability of the food and replaces any chloride lost when the woman vomits hydrochloric acid from the stomach. Eating dry meals and taking all liquids, including soups, between meals may help some women by avoiding overdistention of the stomach. Sudden changes in blood sugar levels can be avoided if the small meals are high in low-fat protein or complex carbohydrates. Some women find that slowly sipping herbal tea (peppermint, chamomile, raspberry leaf, spearmint) or a carbonated beverage helps reduce nausea.

More recently, some women have obtained relief from acupressure wrist bands. As an alternative to the wrist bands women can be taught to use acupressure to the pressure point located proximal to the wrist crease. Research suggests that women who do this procedure for 10 minutes four times each day experience significantly less nausea (Belluomini et al 1994). Although health care providers are reluctant to prescribe any medication during pregnancy, some women find 25 mg pyridoxine (vitamin B₆) helpful when taken every 8 hours for several days (Newman et al 1993; Sahakian et al 1991).

Although some nausea is common, the woman who suffers from extreme nausea coupled with vomiting requires additional assessment. She should be advised to contact her health care provider if she vomits more than

once per day or shows signs of dehydration such as dry mouth, decreased amounts of highly concentrated urine, and the like. In such cases the physician/certified nurse-midwife may order antiemetics. However, antiemetics should be avoided if at all possible during the first trimester because of the danger of teratogenic effects on embryo development.

Nausea and vomiting generally cease by the fourth month of pregnancy. If they do not, hyperemesis gravidarum (a complication of pregnancy discussed in Chapter 19) may develop.

Nasal Stuffiness and Epistaxis   Once pregnancy is well established, elevated estrogen levels may produce edema of the nasal mucosa resulting in nasal stuffiness, nasal discharge, and obstruction. Epistaxis (nosebleed) may also result.

Teaching for Self-Care   Cool air vaporizers and normal saline nose drops may be helpful. However, the problem is often unresponsive to treatment. Women experiencing these problems find it difficult to sleep and may resort to nasal sprays and decongestants to relieve the problem. Such interventions can exaggerate the nasal stuffiness and create other discomforts. The use of any medication in pregnancy should be avoided if possible.

Fatigue   Marked fatigue, often out of proportion to the woman's normal pattern, is so common in early pregnancy that it is considered a presumptive sign of pregnancy. It is aggravated if the woman has to arise several times each night because of urinary frequency. Typically, it resolves soon after the end of the first trimester.

Teaching for Self-Care Scheduling activities to allow for napping is helpful. Women should be encouraged to use every opportunity available to rest, including going to bed earlier in the evening. The woman's partner, if he is involved in the pregnancy, needs to understand that the fatigue is normal and will subside. He can be encouraged to assume more home responsibilities to support the woman and enable her to rest.

Urinary Frequency Urinary frequency is a common discomfort of pregnancy. It occurs early in pregnancy because of the pressure of the enlarging uterus on the bladder. This condition subsides for a while when the uterus moves out of the pelvic area into the abdominal cavity around the 12th week. Although the glomerular filtration rate increases in pregnancy, it does not cause a significant increase in urine output. Frequency recurs in the last trimester as the enlarging uterus begins to press on the bladder again. Coughing or sneezing in the last month may even cause leakage of urine.

As long as other symptoms of urinary tract infection do not appear, frequency of urination is considered normal during the first and third trimesters.

Teaching for Self-Care There are no methods of decreasing the frequency of urination in pregnancy. Fluid intake should never be decreased to prevent frequency. The woman should be encouraged to maintain an adequate fluid intake: at least 2000 mL/day. She should also be encouraged to empty her bladder frequently (approximately every 2 hours while awake).

Frequent bladder emptying helps decrease the incidence of leakage of urine. Because frequency often results in several trips to the bathroom each night, it is important to remind the woman to consider safety factors in the home such as a clear path to the bathroom, the use of a night light, and the like. The woman who leaks urine may choose to wear pantyliners during the day. If she does, she should change them as soon as they become damp to avoid perineal excoriation and to avoid contamination of the perineum from the rectal area if the pads move back and forth as she walks. Tightening of the pubococcygeus muscle, which supports internal organs and controls voiding, can help maintain good perineal tone. This procedure, known as Kegel's exercise, is discussed in "Perineal Exercises" later in this chapter.

Although frequency is considered normal during the first and third trimesters, signs of bladder infection, such as pain, burning with voiding, or blood in the urine, should be reported to the woman's health care provider.

Breast Tenderness Sensitivity of the breasts occurs early and continues throughout the pregnancy. Increased levels of estrogen and progesterone play large roles in the soreness and tingling sensation felt in the breasts and in the increased sensitivity of the nipples.

Teaching for Self-Care A well-fitting, supportive brassiere gives the most relief for this discomfort. The qualities of a properly supportive brassiere are discussed in Breast Care later in this chapter.

Ptyalism Ptyalism is a rare discomfort of pregnancy in which excessive, often bitter saliva is produced. Causal theories are vague, and effective treatments are limited.

Teaching for Self-Care Using astringent mouthwashes, chewing gum, or sucking on hard candy may minimize the problem of ptyalism.

Increased Vaginal Discharge Increased vaginal discharge (**leukorrhea**) is common in pregnancy. The discharge is usually whitish and consists of mucus and exfoliated vaginal epithelial cells. It occurs as the result of hyperplasia of vaginal mucosa and increased production of mucus by the endocervical glands. In addition the increased acidity of the secretions encourages the growth of *Candida albicans*, and the woman is thus more susceptible to monilial vaginitis.

Teaching for Self-Care Cleanliness is important in preventing excoriation and vaginal infections. Daily bathing is adequate; douching should be avoided during pregnancy. Nylon underpants and pantyhose retain heat and moisture in the genital area; absorbent cotton underpants should be worn to help prevent problems. The pregnant woman should be encouraged to report any change in vaginal discharge, any irritation in the perineal area, and intense vaginal itching. These changes frequently indicate vaginal infections.

Second and Third Trimesters

It is difficult to classify discomforts as specifically occurring in the second or third trimester because many problems are due to individual variations in women such as number of previously existing conditions. The symptoms discussed in this section usually do not appear until the third trimester in primigravidas but occur earlier with each succeeding pregnancy.

Heartburn (Pyrosis) Heartburn is the regurgitation of acidic gastric contents into the esophagus. It creates a burning or irritating sensation in the esophagus and radiates upward, sometimes leaving a bad taste in the mouth. Heartburn appears to be primarily a result of the displacement of the stomach by the enlarging uterus. The increased production of progesterone in pregnancy, decreases in gastrointestinal motility, and relaxation of the cardiac sphincter also contribute to heartburn.

Teaching for Self-Care Heartburn is aggravated by overeating, ingesting fatty and fried foods, and lying down soon after eating. These situations should therefore be avoided. The woman should be encouraged to drink an adequate amount of fluid (6 to 8 glasses) each day and to eat smaller, more frequent meals to accommodate the decreased size of her stomach. Good posture is important because it allows more room for the stomach to function. The care giver may recommend a low-sodium antacid such as aluminum hydroxide (Amphojel) or a combination of aluminum hydroxide and magnesium hydroxide (Maalox). Because aluminum alone tends to cause constipation and magnesium alone is associated with diarrhea, the combined approach is more desirable. Sodium bicarbonate (baking soda) and Alka-Seltzer should be avoided because of the potential for electrolyte imbalance.

Ankle Edema Most women experience ankle edema in the last part of pregnancy because of the increasing difficulty of venous return from the lower extremities. Prolonged standing or sitting and warm weather increase the edema. It is also associated with varicose veins. Ankle edema becomes a concern only when accompanied by hypertension or proteinuria or when the edema is not postural in origin.

Teaching for Self-Care The aggravating conditions just mentioned should be avoided. If the woman has to sit or stand for long periods, frequent dorsiflexion of her feet will help contract muscles, thereby squeezing the fluid back into circulation. The pregnant woman should not wear tight garters or other restrictive bands around her legs. During rest periods the woman should elevate her legs and hips as described in the following section on varicose veins.

Varicose Veins Varicose veins are a result of weakening of the walls of veins or faulty functioning of the valves. Poor circulation in the lower extremities predisposes to varicose veins in the legs and thighs. With poor circulation stasis of the blood exerts pressure that gradually weakens the walls of the veins and causes varicosities. In other cases faulty functioning of the valves causes pooling of blood in the lower extremities with concomitant pressure on the vein walls.

The weight of the gravid uterus in the pelvis aggravates the development of varicosities in the legs and pelvic area by preventing good venous return. Increased maternal age, excessive weight gain, a large fetus, heredity, and multiple pregnancy can all contribute to the problem.

Women with leg varicosities experience aching and tiredness in the lower extremities, with the discomfort increasing throughout the day. Prevention or relief of the discomfort occurs when good venous return from the lower extremities is restored.

Vulvar varicosities may also be a problem in pregnancy, although they are less common. Varicosities in the vulva and perineum cause aching and a sense of heaviness. Support in these areas promotes relief.

Treatment of varicose veins by surgery or the injection method is not recommended during pregnancy. The woman should be aware that treatment may be needed after pregnancy because the problem will be aggravated by a succeeding pregnancy.

Phlebothrombosis and thrombophlebitis are possible complications of varicose veins, but they usually do not occur in a healthy pregnant woman. If these complications occur, the cause is often a local injury.

Teaching for Self-Care Regular exercise such as swimming, cycling, or walking promotes venous return, which helps prevent varicosities. Avoiding factors that contribute to venous stasis is also helpful. The pregnant woman should avoid standing or sitting for prolonged periods. She should also avoid crossing her legs at the knees because of the pressure on her veins. She should not wear garters or hosiery with constricting bands, such as knee-high hose. However, supportive hose or elastic stockings may be extremely helpful. Supportive hose should be put on in the morning and should be washed daily with soap and warm water to help retain its elasticity.

The pregnant woman should be encouraged to elevate her legs level with her hips when she sits. Comfort is enhanced if she supports the entire leg rather than simply propping her feet up on a stool, which may lead to hyperextension of the knees. The woman who sits or stands for long periods should walk around frequently to promote venous return to the heart. She can also be encouraged to dorsiflex her feet, hold the position for 3 seconds, then release, with 8 to 10 repetitions several times each day. Venous return is most effectively promoted if the woman lies down with her feet elevated several times a day. To avoid difficulty related to pressure of the uterus on the vena cava, the woman can lie with her legs elevated on pillows and a pillow placed under one hip to displace the uterus to one side (Figure 15–1).

Support for vulvar varicosities can be provided by wearing two sanitary pads inside the underpants. Elevation of only the legs aggravates vulvar varicosities by creating stasis of blood in the pelvic area. Therefore it is important that the pelvic area also be elevated to promote venous drainage into the trunk of the body. More than one firm pillow under the hips may be needed to accomplish this elevation. Near the end of pregnancy this position may be extremely awkward; the woman may best relieve uterine pressure on the pelvic veins by resting on her side. Blocks may also be placed under the foot of her bed to elevate it slightly.

Flatulence Flatulence results from decreased gastrointestinal motility, leading to delayed emptying, and from pressure upon the large intestine by the growing uterus. Air swallowing may also contribute to the problem.

Teaching for Self-Care The woman should be advised to avoid gas-forming foods and to chew her food thoroughly.

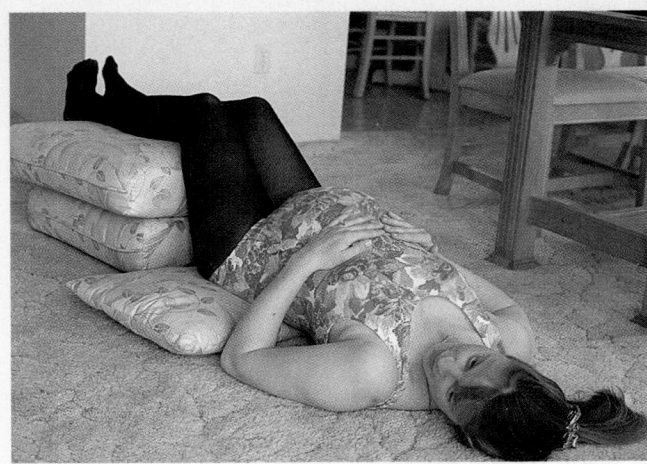

FIGURE 15-1   Swelling and discomfort from varicosities can be decreased by lying down with the legs and one hip elevated (to avoid compression of the vena cava).

Teaching for Self-Care   Relief can be achieved by gently reinserting the hemorrhoid. Reinsertion is aided by gravity; it is more successful if the woman lies on her side or in the knee to chest position. She places some lubricant on her finger and presses against the hemorrhoids, pushing them inside. She holds them in place for 1 to 2 minutes and then gently withdraws her finger. The anal sphincter should then hold them inside the rectum. The woman will find it especially helpful if she can then maintain a side-lying (Sims') position for a time, so this procedure is best done before bed or prior to a daily rest period.

Avoiding constipation is important in preventing and/or relieving the discomfort of hemorrhoids. Relief measures for existing hemorrhoid symptoms include ice packs, use of topical ointments and anesthetic agents, and warm soaks.

The woman should contact her health care provider if the hemorrhoids become hardened and noticeably tender to touch. Rectal bleeding that is more than spotting following defecation should also be reported.

Constipation   Conditions in pregnancy that predispose the woman to constipation include general bowel sluggishness caused by increased progesterone and steroid metabolism; displacement of the intestines, which increases with the growth of the fetus; and oral iron supplements, which may be needed by the pregnant woman.

Teaching for Self-Care   Increased fluid intake (at least 2000 mL/day), adequate roughage or bulk in the diet, regular bowel habits, and adequate daily exercise can often maintain good bowel function in women who have not had previous problems. Some women find it helpful to drink a warm beverage or glass of prune juice in the morning. Women should leave sufficient time following breakfast so that the natural action of the body will produce defecation. Some women, rushing to leave for work or school, ignore or suppress the urge to defecate.

Women who try to develop good bowel habits during pregnancy will be prepared to maintain good bowel function after birth; meanwhile they may need to use mild laxatives, stool softeners, and suppositories as recommended by their care giver. The nurse should help women with constipation to develop good daily bowel habits and to avoid becoming dependent on laxatives during pregnancy, a habit that may continue after birth.

Flatulence can be decreased by regular bowel habits and by exercise.

Hemorrhoids   Hemorrhoids are varicosities of the veins around the lower end of the rectum and anus. In the nonpregnant state, hemorrhoids are usually caused by the straining that occurs with constipation. When a woman becomes pregnant, the gravid uterus creates pressure on the veins and thus interferes with venous circulation. As the pregnancy progresses and the fetus grows, greater pressure on the veins and displacement of intestines occur, increasing the problem of constipation and often resulting in hemorrhoids.

Some women may not be bothered by hemorrhoids until the second stage of labor, when the hemorrhoids appear as they push just before birth. Hemorrhoids that occur in pregnancy or at birth usually become asymptomatic after the early postpartal period.

Women who have hemorrhoids prior to pregnancy probably experience more difficulties with them during pregnancy because of the aggravating conditions just discussed.

Symptoms of hemorrhoids include itching, swelling, and pain, as well as hemorrhoidal bleeding. Internal hemorrhoids are located above the anal sphincter and are responsible for bleeding, usually with defecation. They are not usually painful unless they protrude from the anus. External hemorrhoids are located outside the anal sphincter. They are not usually the source of bleeding or pain; however, thrombosis of the hemorrhoids can occur, and in that case they become extremely painful. The thrombosis may resolve itself in 24 hours, or it can be treated in the physician's office by incising and evacuating the blood clot.

Backache   Many pregnant women experience backache. As the uterus enlarges, increased curvature of the lumbosacral vertebrae occurs. Circulating steroid hormones cause a softening and relaxation of pelvic joints, the growing uterus stretches the abdominal muscles, and the increasing weight creates a gradual tilt of the anterior portion of the pelvis. As the anterior portion of the pelvis tilts downward, the spinal curvature increases. If the woman does not learn how to correct this curvature, the strain on the muscles and ligaments will cause backache.

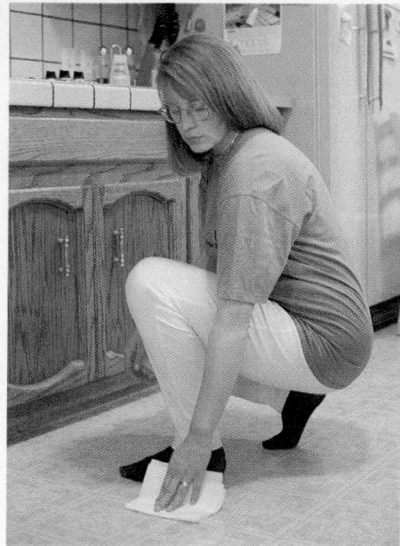

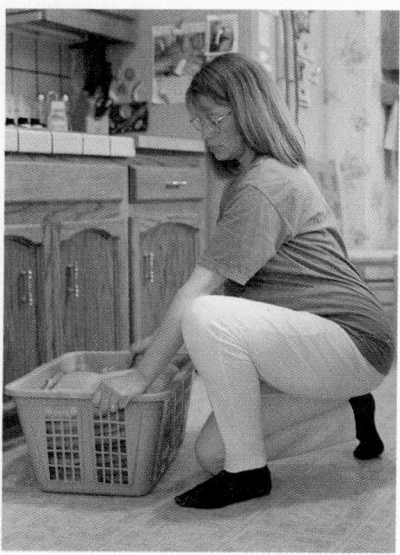

FIGURE 15-2   When picking up objects from floor level or lifting objects, the pregnant woman must use proper body mechanics.

Teaching for Self-Care   An exercise called the pelvic tilt can help restore proper body alignment. As the anterior pelvis is tilted upward, the curvature of the back is automatically decreased, relieving much of the discomfort. If proper body alignment is maintained throughout pregnancy, backaches can be relieved or even prevented. See "Exercises To Prepare for Childbirth" later in this chapter.

The use of proper posture and good body mechanics throughout pregnancy is important. The pregnant woman should not curve her back by bending over to lift or pick up items from the floor. The strain is felt in the muscles of the back. Leg muscles should be used to do the work instead. The woman can keep her back straight by bending her knees to lower her body into the squatting position (Figure 15–2). Her feet should be placed 12 to 18 inches apart to maintain body balance. When lifting a

heavy object such as a child, she should place one foot flat on the floor, slightly in front of the other foot, and lower herself to the other knee. The object is held close to her body for lifting. This same principle of keeping the back straight and bending the knees applies when the woman sits down or gets out of a chair.

Work heights that require constant bending can contribute to backache and should be adjusted as necessary. Women who do not experience backache in pregnancy may become aware of it later as they bend to change a newborn's diaper.

A pendulous abdomen contributes to backache by increasing the curvature of the spine. The use of a supportive maternity girdle is discussed in "Clothing" later in this chapter, as is the role of high-heeled shoes in increasing the lumbosacral curvature.

Leg Cramps   Leg cramps are painful muscle spasms in the gastrocnemius muscles. They occur most frequently at night after the woman has gone to bed but may occur at other times. Extension of the foot can often cause leg cramps. The nurse should warn the pregnant woman not to extend the foot during childbirth preparation exercises or during rest periods.

The exact cause of leg cramps is not known. Proposed contributing factors include an inadequate calcium intake, an imbalance in the calcium/phosphorus ratio, pressure of the enlarged uterus on the pelvic nerves leading to the legs, or pressure on the pelvic vessels causing impaired circulation.

Leg cramps are more common in the third trimester because of increased weight of the uterus on the nerves supplying the lower extremities. Fatigue and poor circulation in the lower extremities contribute to this problem.

Teaching for Self-Care   Immediate relief of the muscle spasm is achieved by stretching the muscle. This is most effectively done with the woman lying on her back and another person pressing the woman's knee down to straighten her leg while pushing her foot toward her leg. Foot flexion techniques, massage, and warm packs can be used to alleviate discomfort from leg cramps (Figure 15–3).

The physician may recommend that the woman drink no more than a pint of milk daily and take calcium lactate or may suggest a quart of milk daily and prescribe aluminum hydroxide gel. Aluminum hydroxide gel absorbs phosphorus and eliminates it directly through the intestinal tract. The treatment recommendations depend on the frequency of the leg cramps.

When planning a treatment regimen, one must be careful not to totally exclude milk from the woman's diet because it is an excellent source of several other essential nutrients.

Faintness   Many pregnant women occasionally feel faint, especially in warm, crowded areas. Faintness is caused by a combination of changes in the blood volume

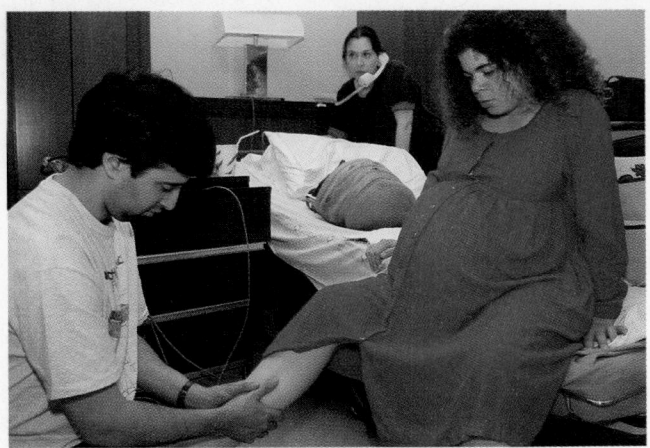

FIGURE 15-3 The expectant father can help relieve the woman's painful leg cramps by massaging her calf.

and postural hypotension due to venous pooling of blood in the dependent veins. Sudden change of position or standing for prolonged periods can cause this sensation, and fainting can occur.

Teaching for Self-Care The nurse should first be certain that the pregnant woman understands the symptoms of faintness. These include slight dizziness, a "swirling" or "floating" sensation, and a decreased ability to hear or focus attention. If faintness is experienced from prolonged standing or being in a warm, crowded room, the woman should sit down and lower her head between her legs. If this procedure does not help, the woman should be assisted to an area where she can lie down and get fresh air. When arising from a resting position, she should move slowly. Women whose jobs require standing in one place for long periods should march in place regularly to increase venous return from the legs.

Shortness of Breath Shortness of breath occurs as the uterus rises into the abdomen and causes pressure on the diaphragm. This problem worsens in the last trimester as the enlarged uterus presses directly on the diaphragm, decreasing vital capacity. The primigravida experiences considerable relief from shortness of breath in the last few weeks of pregnancy, when lightening occurs, and the fetus and uterus move down in the pelvis. Because the multigravida does not usually experience lightening until labor, shortness of breath will continue throughout her pregnancy.

Teaching for Self-Care During the day, sitting straight in a chair and using proper posture when standing help provide relief. If distress is great at night, the woman can sleep propped up in bed with several pillows behind her head and shoulders.

Difficulty Sleeping Although the pregnant woman may experience difficulty sleeping for many of the same psychologic reasons as the nonpregnant woman, many physical factors also contribute to this problem. The enlarged uterus may make it difficult to find a comfortable position for sleep, and an active fetus may aggravate the problem. The other discomforts of pregnancy such as urinary frequency, shortness of breath, and leg cramps may also be contributing factors.

Teaching for Self-Care The pregnant woman may find it helpful to drink a warm (caffeine-free) beverage before bed and may benefit from a soothing backrub given by her partner or a family member. Pillows may be used to provide support for her back, between her legs, or for her upper arm when she lies on her side. Relaxation techniques may also help. The woman should avoid caffeine products, stimulating activity, and sleeping medication.

Round Ligament Pain As the uterus enlarges during pregnancy, the round ligaments stretch, hypertrophy, and lengthen as the uterus rises up in the abdomen. Round ligament pain is attributed to this stretching.

Teaching for Self-Care The woman may feel concern when she first experiences round ligament pain because it is often intense and causes a "grabbing" sensation in the lower abdomen and inguinal area. The nurse should warn women of this possible discomfort. Few treatment measures really alleviate this discomfort, but understanding the cause will help decrease anxiety. Once the care giver has ascertained that the cause of the discomfort is not related to a medical complication such as appendicitis or gall bladder disease, the woman may find that a heating pad applied to the abdomen brings some relief. She may also benefit from bringing her knees up on her abdomen.

Carpal Tunnel Syndrome Carpal tunnel syndrome (CTS) results from compression of the median nerve in the carpal tunnel of the wrist. The syndrome is commonly bilateral but may be more pronounced in the dominant hand. Typically, the woman with CTS awakens with numbness, tingling, or burning in the fleshy part of the palm near the thumb. She may also experience numbness in her fingers and mild hand weakness. The syndrome is aggravated by repetitive hand movements such as typing. Symptoms often disappear following the birth. Treatment involves splinting, avoiding aggravating movements, and in some cases injecting steroids into the carpal tunnel. Surgery is indicated in severe cases.

Teaching for Self-Care Although the condition is not preventable, the woman should be advised to avoid aggravating activities and use her splint as directed.

Text continues on page 378

WHAT TO TELL THE PREGNANT WOMAN ABOUT ASSESSING FETAL ACTIVITY

Assessment: The nurse focuses on the woman's prior knowledge and former use of fetal movement assessment methods, the week of gestation, and her communication and ability to understand and process information.

Nursing Diagnosis: The essential nursing diagnosis will probably be knowledge deficit related to lack of information about fetal movement assessment methods.

Nursing Plan and Implementation: The goal of the teaching sessions is to provide general information regarding fetal movement and assessment methods.

Client Goals: At the completion of the teaching session the woman will:

- Discuss the types of fetal assessment methods, reasons for assessment, how to accomplish the assessment, and methods of record keeping.
- Demonstrate the use of a movement record.
- Identify resources to call if questions arise.
- Agree to bring the movement record to each prenatal visit.

Teaching Plan

Content: The expectant woman needs to know that fetal movements are first felt around 18 weeks' gestation. From that time the fetal movements get stronger and easier to detect. A slowing or stopping of fetal movement may be an indication that the fetus needs some attention and evaluation. The normal amount of movement varies considerably; however, most healthy fetuses move at least ten times in 3 hours.

Cardiff Count-to-Ten (Figure 15–4)

The woman begins these assessments in the 27th week of gestation. The woman chooses what time she will start each day but keeps the time relatively consistent. She can either place a mark for each fetal movement until ten have been recorded or place an X at the beginning of the counting period and then again at the time ten movements have been felt.

It will be advantageous for the woman to schedule the counting periods about 1 hour past eating and to combine the counting period with rest. A side-lying position provides optimal circulation to the uterus-placenta-fetus unit. In addition the fetus's movements are felt more readily while lying on the side. Later in the pregnancy some women may be bothered by indigestion after eating. In this case they can prop up the upper body but still maintain a side-lying position.

When to Contact the Care Provider

When there are questions or concerns.

If there are fewer than ten movements in 3 hours.

If overall the fetus's movements are slowing, and it takes much longer each day to note ten movements.

What Happens Next

The care provider will probably suggest a nonstress test (NST) to further evaluate the fetus. Additional testing may include a contraction stress test (CST), tests for pulmonary maturity, and ultrasound. (These tests are discussed in Chapter 20.)

Teaching Method: *Describe procedures and demonstrate how to assess fetal movement. Sit beside woman and show her how to place her hand on the fundus to feel fetal movement.*

Provide a written teaching sheet for the woman's use at home.

Demonstrate how to record movements on Cardiff Count-to-Ten scoring card.

Watch woman fill out record as examples are provided. Encourage her to complete the record each day and bring it with her to each prenatal visit. Assure her that the record will be discussed at each prenatal visit, and questions may be addressed at that time if desired.

Provide the woman with a name and phone number in case she has further questions.

Teaching Plan continued

Evaluation: The nurse may evaluate learning by having the woman explain the method to the nurse and by asking the woman to fill the card in using a fictitious situation. At each prenatal visit the expectant woman's record is reviewed, and this provides another opportunity for evaluation of learning. Asking about the record at each visit will demonstrate that it is an important part of the woman's care. Review of the record provides wonderful opportunities for questions and clarification.

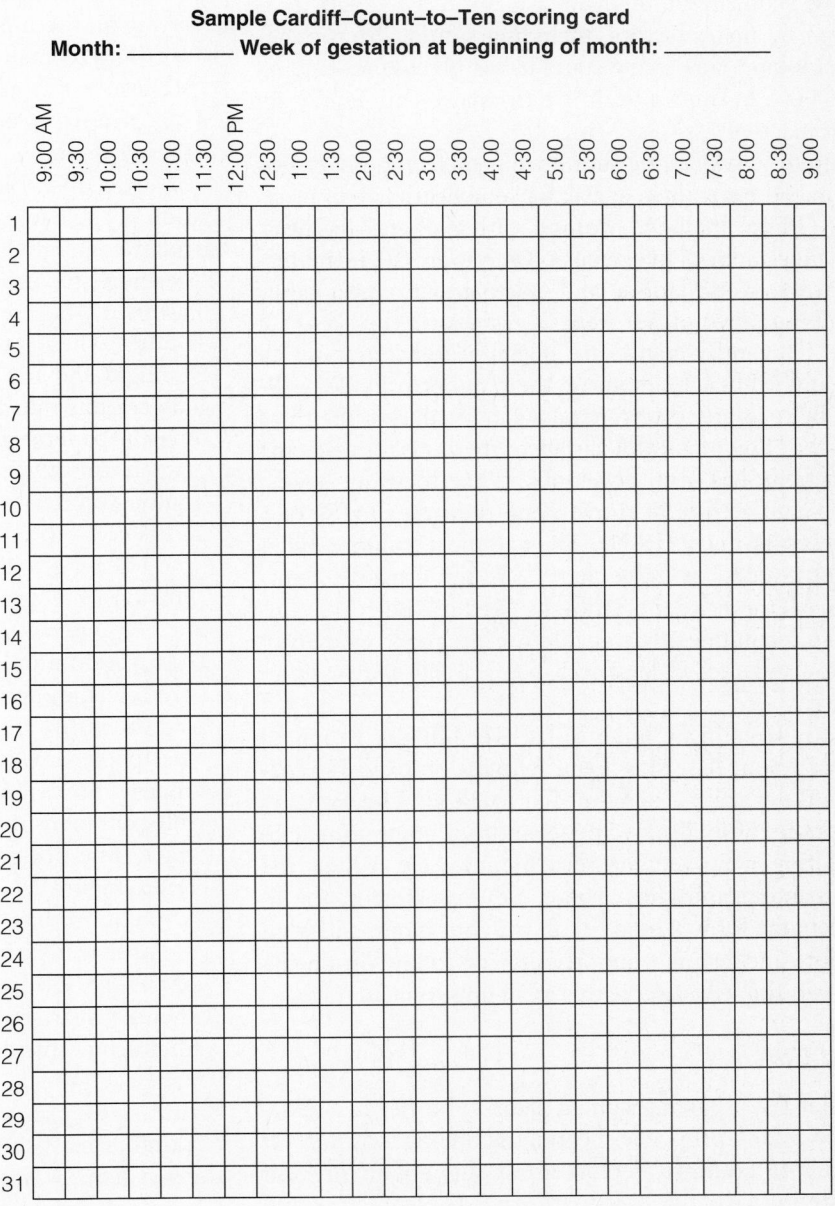

FIGURE 15-4 Fetal movement assessment method: the Cardiff Count-to-Ten scoring card (adaptation).

Promotion of Maternal and Fetal Well-Being During Pregnancy

The pregnant woman is faced with the important responsibility of maintaining her health not only for her sake but also for the sake of her fetus. Nurses can help promote maternal and fetal well-being by providing expectant couples with accurate and complete information about health behaviors that can affect pregnancy and childbirth.

Fetal Activity Monitoring

Since the early 1970s, researchers have recognized the value of assessing fetal activity as a measure of fetal well-being. Vigorous fetal activity generally provides reassurance of fetal well-being; a marked decrease in activity or cessation of movement may indicate possible fetal compromise requiring immediate evaluation. Fetal activity is affected by many factors, including sound, drugs, cigarette smoking, fetal sleep state, blood glucose levels, and time of day. At times a healthy fetus may be minimally active or inactive.

Initially, systematic monitoring of fetal activity was encouraged for women at risk for fetal death late in pregnancy. These included women with diabetes mellitus, pregnancy-induced hypertension (Chapter 19), intrauterine growth retardation, and postmaturity (pregnancy continuing beyond 42 weeks' gestation) (Freda et al 1993). Currently, many care givers are encouraging all pregnant women to monitor their unborn child's well-being by regularly assessing fetal activity during the third trimester of pregnancy. A variety of methods for assessing fetal activity has been developed. They focus on having the woman keep **fetal movement records (FMR)** or a **fetal activity diary (FAD)**. The two most common types of "kick counts" or "kick charts" are the Cardiff Count-to-Ten Method and the Sadovsky Method. Both are noninvasive techniques that enable the pregnant woman to monitor and record fetal well-being easily and without expense.

The Teaching Guide: What To Tell the Pregnant Woman About Assessing Fetal Activity, on page 376, describes the Cardiff Count-to-Ten Method. The woman's perceptions of fetal movements and her commitment to completing a movement record may vary. When the woman understands the purpose of the assessment, how to complete the form, whom to call with questions, and what to report and has the opportunity for follow-up during each visit, she will also see this as an important activity.

Breast Care

Whether the pregnant woman plans to bottle- or breast-feed her infant, proper support of the breasts is important to promote comfort, retain breast shape, and prevent back strain, particularly if the breasts become large and pendulous. The sensitivity of the breasts in pregnancy is also relieved by good support.

A well-fitting, supportive brassiere has the following qualities:

- The straps are wide and do not stretch (elastic straps soon lose their tautness due to the weight of the breasts and frequent washing).
- The cup holds all breast tissue comfortably.
- The brassiere has tucks or other devices that allow it to expand, thus accommodating the enlarging chest circumference.
- The brassiere supports the nipple line approximately midway between the elbow and shoulder. At the same time the brassiere is not pulled up in the back by the weight of the breasts.

Cleanliness of the breasts is important, especially as the woman begins producing colostrum. Colostrum that crusts on the nipples should be removed with warm water. The woman planning to breastfeed should not use soap on her nipples because of its drying effect.

Nipple preparation, begun during the third trimester, helps prevent soreness during the early days of breastfeeding. Nipple preparation promotes the distribution of the natural lubricants produced by Montgomery's tubercles, stimulates blood flow to the breast, and helps develop the protective layer of skin over the nipple. Women who are planning to nurse can begin by going braless when possible and by exposing their nipples to sunlight and air. Rubbing the nipples removes protective lubrication and should be avoided, but rolling the nipple may be beneficial. This is done by grasping the nipple between thumb and forefinger and gently rolling and pulling on it. A woman with a history of preterm labor is advised *not* to do this because nipple stimulation triggers the release of oxytocin. (See Chapter 19 for further discussion.)

Nipple rolling is more difficult for women with flat or inverted nipples, but it is still a useful preparation for breastfeeding. Nipple inversion is usually diagnosed during the initial antepartal assessment. Occasionally, a nipple appears inverted at all times. In other cases the nipple appears normal initially, but pressure on the alveoli with the examiner's thumb and finger causes the nipple to retract. The normal or flat nipple protrudes when this is done (Figure 15–5).

The woman with nipple inversion can increase nipple protractility by performing Hoffman's exercises (Figure 15–6) (Hoffman 1953). If the nipple is truly inverted, she can wear special breast shields (such as Woolrich or Eschmann shields) for the last 3 or 4 months of pregnancy (Figure 15–7). These shields tend to absorb moisture, so they should not be worn more than a few hours at a time. Breast shields appear to be the only measure that really helps women with inverted nipples.

Oral stimulation of the nipple by the woman's partner during sex play is also an excellent technique for toughening the nipple in preparation for breastfeeding.

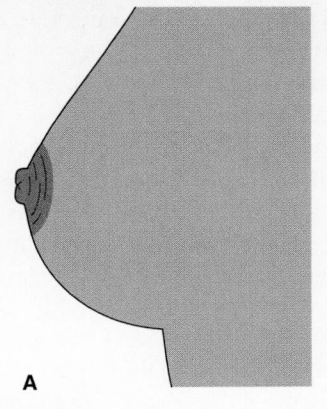
A

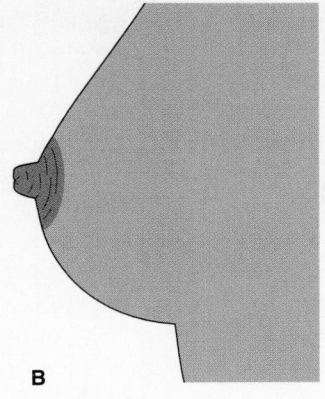
B

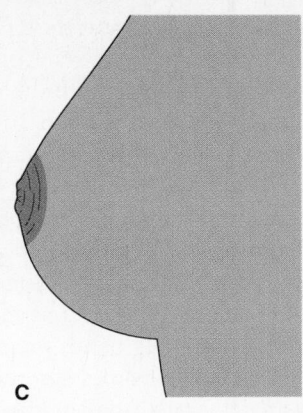
C

FIGURE 15-5   *A* When not stimulated, normal and inverted nipples often look alike. *B* When stimulated, the normal nipple protrudes. *C* When stimulated, the inverted nipple retracts.

However, great variation exists. In some women one or both nipples always appear inverted, even when not stimulated.

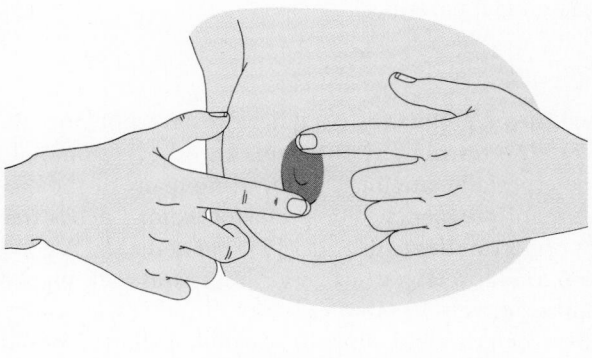

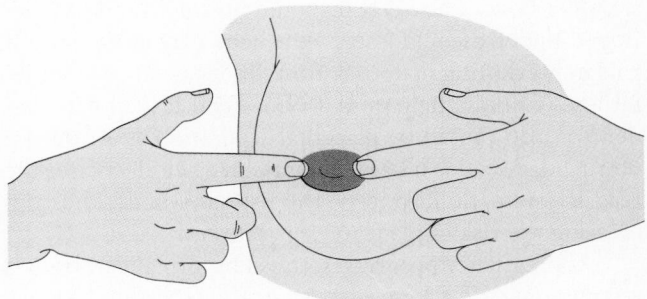

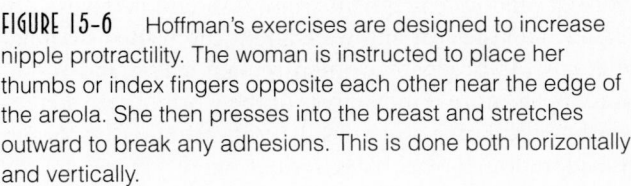

FIGURE 15-6   Hoffman's exercises are designed to increase nipple protractility. The woman is instructed to place her thumbs or index fingers opposite each other near the edge of the areola. She then presses into the breast and stretches outward to break any adhesions. This is done both horizontally and vertically.

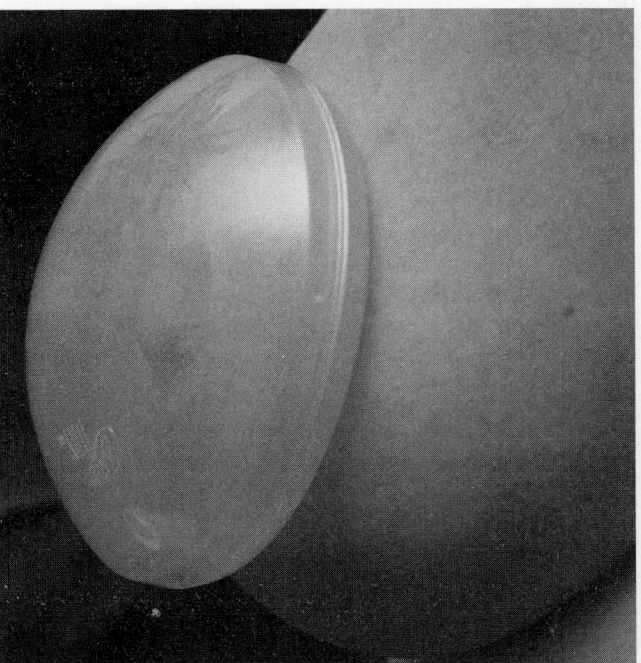

FIGURE 15-7   This breast shield is designed to increase the protractility of inverted nipples. Worn the last 3 to 4 months of pregnancy, they exert gentle pulling pressure at the edge of the areola, gradually forcing the nipple through the center of the shield. They may be used after birth if still necessary.

The couple who enjoy this stimulation should be encouraged to continue it throughout the pregnancy except when the woman has a history of preterm labor, as discussed earlier.

Clothing

Maternity clothes are constructed with fuller lines to allow for the increase in abdominal size during pregnancy. Skirts and slacks have soft elastic waistbands and a stretchable panel over the abdominal area. Maternity clothes keep pace with fashion trends, enabling the woman to feel stylish. However, maternity clothing is expensive and is worn for a relatively short time. Women can economize by sharing clothes with friends, sewing their own garments, or buying used maternity clothing.

Clothing should be loose and nonconstricting both for general comfort and to prevent some of the specific discomforts of pregnancy. For example, restricting bands such as garters can interfere with venous circulation and predispose to varicose veins or aggravate existing ones.

Maternity girdles are seldom worn today and are not necessary for most women. They are sometimes used by women athletes, such as runners, dancers, or gymnasts, who maintain a light workout schedule during pregnancy. Women with large, pendulous abdomens may also benefit from a well-fitting, supportive girdle. Without this support the pendulous abdomen increases the curvature of the back and is a source of backache and general discomfort. Tight leg bands on girdles should be avoided.

High-heeled shoes aggravate back discomfort by increasing the curvature of the back. They should not be worn if the woman experiences backache or problems with her balance. Shoes should fit properly and feel comfortable.

Bathing

Daily bathing is important because of the increased perspiration and mucoid vaginal discharge that occurs during pregnancy. The woman may take either a shower or a tub bath, according to her preference. Caution is needed during tub baths because balance becomes a problem as pregnancy advances. Rubber tub mats and hand grips are valuable safety devices. Moreover, vasodilation due to the warm water may cause the woman to experience some faintness when she attempts to get out of the tub. Thus she may require assistance, especially in the third trimester. *To avoid introducing infection, tub baths are contraindicated in the presence of vaginal bleeding or when the membranes are ruptured.* Women are advised to avoid hot tubs, saunas, or prolonged immersion in a very hot bath. Research suggests that maternal exposure to heat (hot tubs, sauna, or fever) in the first trimester is associated with an increased risk of neural tube defects in the fetus/newborn (Milunsky et al 1992).

Employment

Studies of women who are employed during pregnancy show distinct differences. Women who work in office jobs tend to have slightly lower odds of having a small-for-gestational-age (SGA) baby than unemployed women. This may be because of better access to health care or because these women tend to be healthier as a group. However, women who work in strenuous manual jobs have a higher incidence of preterm or SGA infants than either office workers or unemployed women. This difference may be related to decreased uteroplacental perfusion as blood is shunted to muscle tissue or may reflect the fact that women who are better off tend to work in less strenuous jobs (Launer et al 1990).

Although more recent research suggests no differences in perinatal outcomes between pregnant women who are employed and those who are not, these data may be influenced by the "healthy worker effect." This effect suggests that more healthy women continue to work during their pregnancies. Thus when these women are compared with nonworking pregnant women, the groups may not actually be comparable in terms of health, economic status, or educational level (DeJoseph 1993).

Major deterrents to employment during pregnancy include fetotoxic hazards in the environment, excessive physical strain, overfatigue, and medical or pregnancy-related complications. In the last half of pregnancy occupations involving balance should be adjusted to protect the mother.

Fetotoxic hazards in the environment are always a concern to the expectant couple. If the pregnant woman or the woman contemplating pregnancy is working in industry, she should contact her company physician or nurse about possible hazards in her work environment and should do her own reading and research on environmental hazards. (See also Chapter 8 for a discussion of environmental hazards.)

Travel

If medical or pregnancy complications are not present, there are no restrictions on travel. Travel by automobile can be especially fatiguing, aggravating many of the discomforts of pregnancy. The pregnant woman needs frequent opportunities to get out of the car and walk. A good pattern to follow is to stop every 2 hours and walk around for approximately 10 minutes.

Seat belts should be worn, including both lap and shoulder belts. The lap belt should fit snugly and be positioned under the abdomen. Seat belts play an important role in preventing maternal mortality with subsequent fetal loss (Cunningham et al 1993). Fetal loss in car accidents is also caused by placental separation as a result of uterine distortion. Use of the shoulder belt decreases the risk of traumatic flexion of the woman's body, thus decreasing the risk of placental separation.

As pregnancy progresses, travel by airplane or train is recommended for long distances. To avoid the development of phlebitis, pregnant women should be advised to request an aisle seat and walk about the plane at regular intervals. As pregnant women remain active and sometimes fly to more remote areas of the world, the availability of medical care at her destination is another important consideration for the near-term woman. Travel should usually be avoided if there is a history of bleeding or pregnancy-induced hypertension or if multiple births are anticipated.

Activity and Rest

Critical Thinking Question

What factors should be considered in advising a woman about exercise during pregnancy?

Exercise during pregnancy helps maintain maternal fitness and muscle tone, leads to improved self-image and sense of control, increases energy, improves sleep, relieves tension, helps control weight gain, promotes regular bowel function, and is associated with improved postpartum recovery. Normal participation in exercise can continue throughout an uncomplicated pregnancy. Furthermore, physically fit women who run or do aerobic exercise regularly during pregnancy have been found to have less fetal distress during labor, shorter active labors, fewer cesarean births, and less meconium-stained amniotic fluid (Cunningham et al 1993).

Certain conditions do contraindicate exercise. These include preterm rupture of the membranes, pregnancy-induced hypertension, incompetent cervix (cerclage), persistent second or third trimester bleeding, a history of preterm labor in the prior or current pregnancy, or intrauterine growth retardation. Women with other obstetric conditions or preexisting medical conditions such as chronic hypertension or cardiac or pulmonary disease should be evaluated carefully to determine whether any form of exercise is appropriate (ACOG 1994).

Research related to the effects of maternal exercise on the fetus is varied and contradictory. Exercise can lead to increased maternal core temperature and hyperthermia. However, research suggests that the incidence of neural tube defects or other birth defects is not increased in the pregnancies of women who continue to exercise, even vigorously, during early pregnancy (ACOG 1994; Artal Mittelmark et al 1991).

Uterine blood flow is reduced during exercise as blood is shunted from visceral organs to muscles. The fetus does seem able to withstand this stress, however, without developing hypoxia. Research indicates that, for most healthy pregnant women with no additional risk factors for preterm labor, exercise does not increase the incidence of preterm labor and birth or baseline uterine activity (ACOG 1994).

In most instances normal participation in regular exercise can continue and in fact is encouraged throughout an uncomplicated pregnancy. Before beginning an exercise program a pregnant woman should be examined by her certified nurse-midwife or physician. A pregnant woman who is already in an exercise program can discuss her degree of participation with her care giver. Women should also seek the opinion of their health care provider about taking part in strenuous sports such as skiing, diving, and horseback riding. In general the skilled sportswoman is no longer discouraged from participating in these activities if her pregnancy is uncomplicated. Pregnancy is not the time, however, to learn a new or strenuous sport.

The American College of Obstetricians and Gynecologists (ACOG) has formulated new guidelines about exercise during pregnancy (ACOG 1994). These include the following:

- Even mild to moderate exercise is beneficial during pregnancy. Regular exercise, which occurs at least three times a week, is preferred.

- After the first trimester women should avoid exercising in the supine position. In most pregnant women the supine position is associated with decreased cardiac output. Because uterine blood flow is reduced during exercise as blood is shunted from the visceral organs to the muscles, the remaining cardiac output is further decreased. Similarly, women should avoid standing motionless for prolonged periods.

- Because decreased oxygen is available for aerobic exercise during pregnancy, women should modify the intensity of their exercise based on their symptoms, should stop when they become fatigued, and should avoid exercising to the point of exhaustion. Non–weight-bearing exercises such as swimming or cycling are recommended because they decrease the risk of injury and provide fitness with comfort.

- As pregnancy progresses and the center of gravity changes, especially in the third trimester, exercises in which the loss of balance could pose a risk to mother or fetus should be avoided. Similarly, the woman should avoid any type of exercise that might result in even mild abdominal trauma.

- A normal pregnancy requires an additional 300 kcal per day. Women who exercise regularly during pregnancy should be careful to ensure that they consume an adequate diet.

- To augment heat dissipation, especially during the first trimester, pregnant women who exercise should

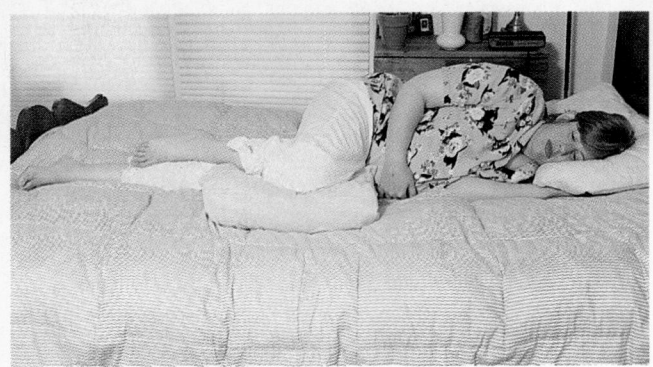

FIGURE 15-8   Position for relaxation and rest as pregnancy progresses.

wear appropriate clothing, ensure adequate hydration, and avoid the prolonged overheating associated with vigorous exercise in hot, humid weather.

In addition to the ACOG (1994) recommendations, the nurse may suggest that the woman wear a supportive bra and appropriate shoes when exercising. She should be advised to warm up and stretch to help prepare the joints for activity and cool down with a period of mild activity to help restore circulation and avoid pooling of blood. A moderate, rhythmic exercise routine involving large muscle groups such as swimming, cycling, walking, or cross-country skiing is best. Jogging or running is acceptable for women already conditioned to these activities. High-risk activities requiring balance and coordination such as sky diving, mountain climbing, scuba diving, ice skating, surfing, and racquetball should be avoided.

Warning signs of overexertion include the following: extreme fatigue, sudden sharp pain, difficulty in breathing, nausea or vomiting, dizziness or faintness, pain, or excessive muscle soreness. Exercise should be stopped and then the program modified if these occur. If the symptoms persist, the woman should contact her care giver (ACOG 1992).

Adequate rest in pregnancy is important for both physical and emotional health. Women need more sleep throughout pregnancy, particularly in the first and last trimesters, when they tire easily. Without adequate rest pregnant women have less resilience.

Finding time to rest during the day may be difficult for women who work or have small children. The nurse can help the expectant mother examine her daily schedule to develop a realistic plan for short periods of rest and relaxation.

Sleeping becomes more difficult during the last trimester because of the enlarged abdomen, increased frequency of urination, and greater activity of the fetus. Finding a comfortable position becomes difficult for the pregnant woman. Figure 15–8 shows a position most pregnant women find comfortable. Progressive relaxation

techniques similar to those taught in prepared childbirth classes can help prepare the woman for sleep (see Chapter 23).

Exercises To Prepare for Childbirth

Certain exercises help strengthen muscle tone in preparation for birth and promote more rapid restoration of muscle tone after birth. Some physical changes of pregnancy can be reduced considerably by faithfully practicing prescribed body-conditioning exercises. Many body-conditioning exercises for pregnancy are taught; a few of the more common ones are discussed here.

The **pelvic tilt,** or pelvic rocking, helps prevent or reduce back strain and strengthens abdominal muscle tone. To do the pelvic tilt, the pregnant woman lies on her back and puts her feet flat on the floor. This bent position of the knees helps prevent strain and discomfort (Figure 15–9). She decreases the curvature in her back by pressing her spine toward the floor. With her back pressed to the floor, the woman tightens her buttocks and abdominal muscles as she tucks in her buttocks. The pelvic tilt can also be performed on hands and knees, while sitting in a chair, or while standing with the back against a wall. The body alignment achieved when the pelvic tilt is correctly done should be maintained as much as possible throughout the day.

TEACHING MOMENT

Doing the pelvic rock on hands and knees may aggravate back strain. Teach women with a history of minor back problems to do the pelvic rock only in the standing position.

Abdominal Exercises   A basic exercise to increase abdominal muscle tone is tightening abdominal muscles in synchronization with respirations. It can be done in any position, but it is best learned while the woman lies supine. With knees flexed and feet flat on the floor the woman expands her abdomen and slowly takes a deep breath. As she slowly exhales, she gradually pulls in her abdominal muscles until they are fully contracted. She relaxes for a few seconds and then repeats the exercise.

Partial sit-ups strengthen abdominal muscle tone and are done according to individual comfort levels. When doing a partial sit-up, the woman lies on the floor as described above (Figure 15–10). This exercise is done with the knees bent and the feet flat on the floor to avoid undue strain on the lower back. She stretches her arms toward her knees as she slowly pulls her head and shoulders off the floor to a comfortable level. (If she has poor abdominal muscle tone, she may not be able to pull up very far.) She then slowly returns to the starting position, takes a deep breath, and repeats the exercise. To strengthen the

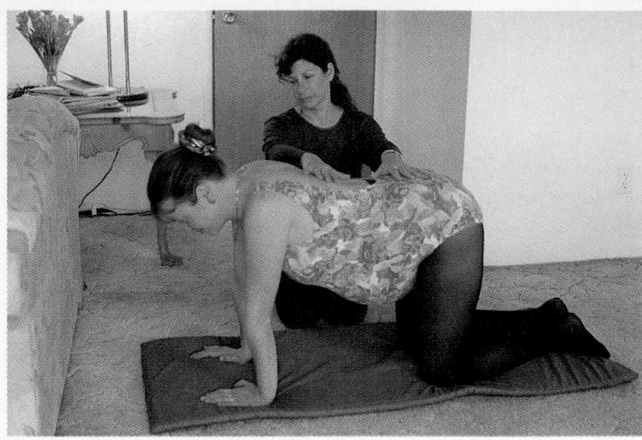

A

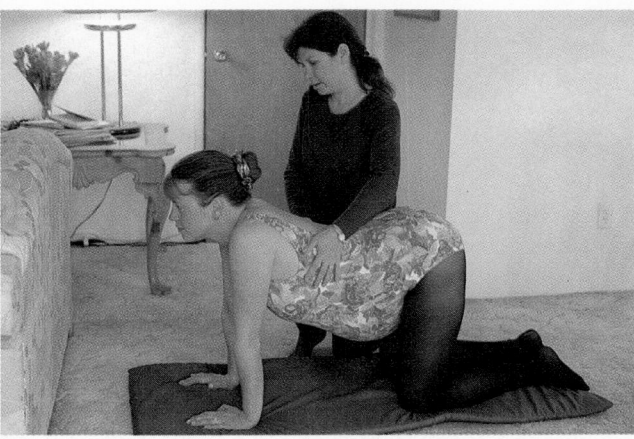

B

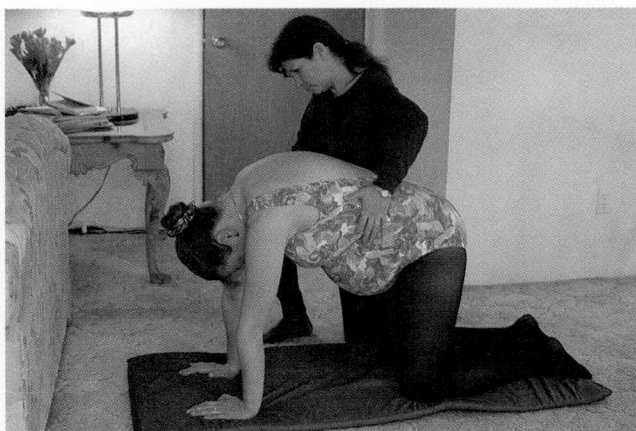

C

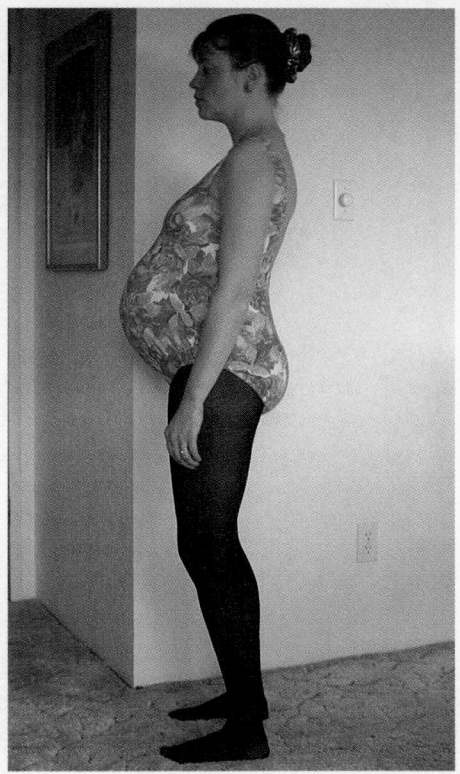

D

FIGURE 15-9 *A* Starting position when the pelvic tilt is done on hands and knees. The back is flat and parallel to the floor, the hands are under the head, and the knees are directly under the buttocks. *B* A prenatal yoga instructor offers pointers for proper positioning for the first part of the tilt: head up, neck long and separated from the shoulders, buttocks up, and pelvis thrust back, allowing the back to drop and release on an inhaled breath. *C* The instructor helps the woman assume the correct position for the next part of the tilt. It is done on a long exhalation, allowing the pregnant woman to arch her back, drop her head loosely, push away from her hands, and draw in the muscles of her abdomen to strengthen them. Note that in this position the pelvis and buttocks are tucked under, and the buttock muscles are tightened. *D* Proper posture. The knees are slightly bent but not locked, the pelvis and buttocks are tucked under, thereby lengthening the spine and helping support the weighty abdomen. With her chin tucked in, this woman's neck, shoulders, hips, knees, and feet are all in a straight line perpendicular to the floor. Her feet are parallel. This is also the starting position for doing the pelvic tilt while standing.

oblique abdominal muscles, she repeats the process, but stretches the left arm to the side of her right knee, returns to the floor, takes a deep breath, and then reaches with the right arm to the left knee.

These exercises can be done approximately five times in a sequence, and the sequence can be repeated several times during the day as desired. It is important to do the exercises slowly to prevent muscle strain and overtiring.

Perineal Exercises Perineal muscle tightening also referred to as **Kegel's exercises,** strengthen the pubococcygeus muscle and increases its elasticity (Figure 15–11). The woman can feel the specific muscle group to be exercised by stopping urination midstream. However, doing Kegel's exercises while urinating is discouraged because this practice has been associated with urinary stasis and urinary tract infection.

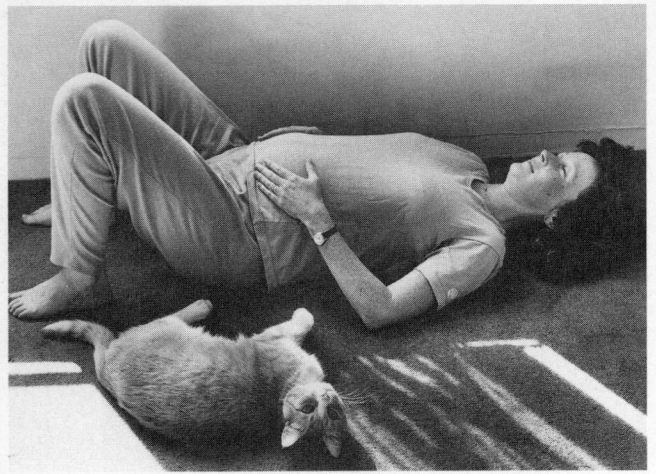

As a result of the physiologic, anatomic, and emotional changes of pregnancy, the couple usually have many questions and concerns about sexual activity during pregnancy. Often these questions are about possible injury to the baby or the woman during intercourse and about changes in the desire each partner feels for the other.

In the past couples were frequently warned to avoid sexual intercourse during the last 6 to 8 weeks of pregnancy to prevent complications such as infection or premature rupture of the membranes. However, these fears

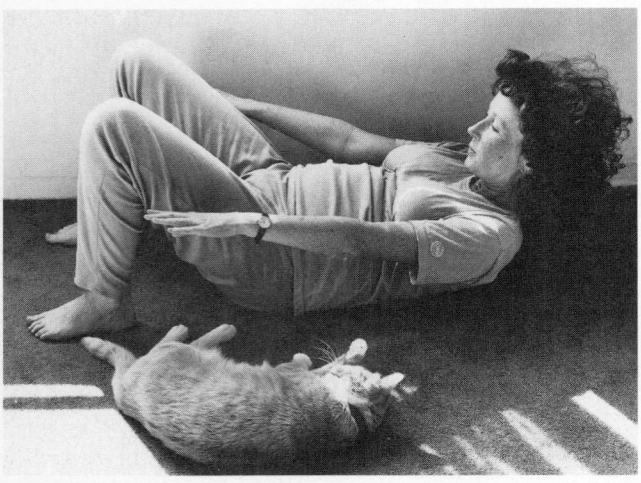

FIGURE 15-10   The pregnant woman can strengthen her abdominal muscles by doing partial sit-ups.

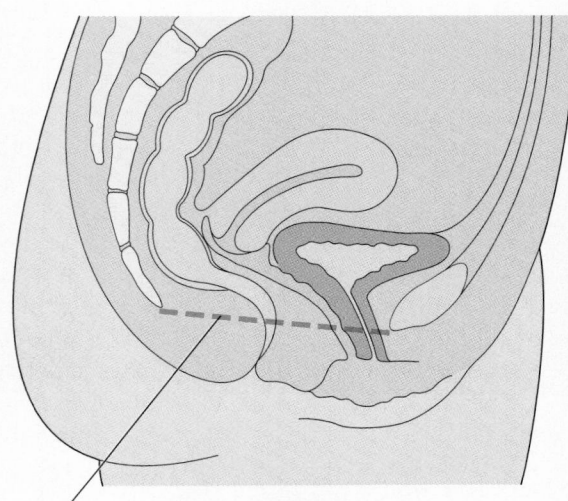

Pubococcygeus muscle with good tone

Childbirth educators sometimes use the following technique to teach Kegel's exercises. They tell the woman to think of her perineal muscles as an elevator. When she relaxes, the elevator is on the first floor. To do the exercises, she contracts, bringing the elevator to the second, third, and fourth floors. She keeps the elevator on the fourth floor for a few seconds, and then gradually relaxes the area. If the exercise is properly done, the woman does not contract the muscles of the buttocks and thighs.

Kegel's exercises can be done at almost any time. Some women use ordinary events—for instance, stopping at a red light—as a cue to remember to do the exercise. Others do Kegel's exercises while waiting in a checkout line, talking on the telephone, or watching television.

Inner Thigh Exercises   The pregnant woman should assume a cross-legged sitting position whenever possible. The *tailor sit* stretches the muscles of the inner thighs in preparation for labor and birth.

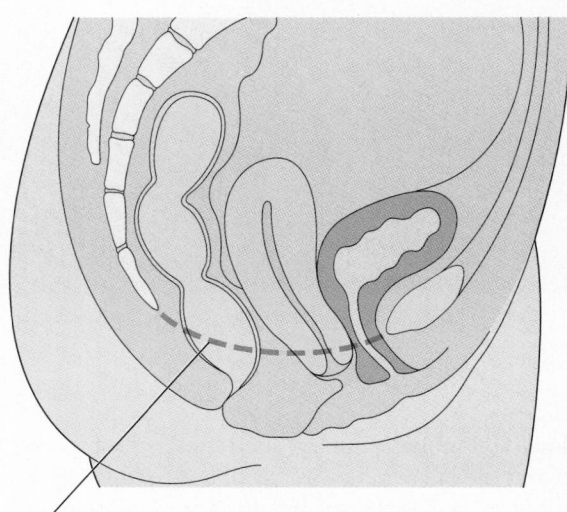

Pubococcygeus muscle with poor tone

FIGURE 15-11   Kegel's exercises. The woman learns to tighten the pubococcygeus muscle, which improves support to the pelvic organs.

seem to be unfounded. In a healthy pregnancy there is no valid reason to limit sexual activity. Intercourse is contraindicated when bleeding is present or the membranes are ruptured. Women with a history of preterm labor or premature rupture of the membranes and those who experience strong uterine contractions following orgasm should be advised of the possible risks of coitus after 32 weeks' gestation (Kochenour 1994).

The expectant mother may experience changes in sexual desire and response. Often these are related to the various discomforts that occur throughout pregnancy. For instance, during the first trimester, fatigue or nausea and vomiting may decrease desire, and breast tenderness may make the woman less responsive to fondling of her breasts. During the second trimester, many of the discomforts have lessened, and with the vascular congestion of the pelvis the woman may experience even greater sexual satisfaction than she experienced prior to pregnancy.

During the third trimester, interest in coitus may again decrease as the woman becomes more uncomfortable and fatigued. In addition, shortness of breath, painful pelvic ligaments, urinary frequency, and decreased mobility may lessen sexual desire and activity. If they are not already using them, the couple should consider coital positions other than male superior, such as side-by-side, female superior, and vaginal rear entry.

Sexual activity does not have to include intercourse. Many of the nurturing and sexual needs of the pregnant woman can be satisfied by cuddling, kissing, and being held. The warm, sensual feelings that accompany these activities can be an end in themselves. Her partner, however, may need to masturbate more frequently than before.

The sexual desires of men are also affected by many factors in pregnancy. These include the previous relationship with the partner, acceptance of the pregnancy, attitudes toward the partner's change of appearance, and concern about hurting the expectant mother or baby. Some men may withdraw from sexual contact because of a belief that sex with a pregnant woman is immoral. This may be especially true for the couple whose religious beliefs teach that sexual intercourse is only for procreation. Some men find it difficult to view their partners as sexually appealing while they are adjusting to the concept of her as a mother. Some men feel their partner's pregnancy arousing and experience feelings of increased happiness, intimacy, and closeness.

The expectant couple should be aware of their changing sexual desires, the normality of these changes, and the importance of communicating these changes to each other so that they can make nurturing adaptations. The nurse has an important role in helping the expecting couple adapt. The couple must feel free to express concerns about sexual activity, and the nurse must be able to respond and give anticipatory guidance in a comfortable manner (Teaching Guide: Sexual Activity During Pregnancy on page 386).

Dental Care

Ongoing dental hygiene is important in pregnancy. In spite of such discomforts as nausea and vomiting, gum hypertrophy and tenderness, possible ptyalism, and heartburn, regular oral hygiene must not be neglected.

The pregnant woman is encouraged to have a dental checkup early in her pregnancy. Women who neglect to obtain dental care prior to pregnancy become aware of dental problems during this time and thus may associate these problems with pregnancy. General dental repair and extractions can be done during pregnancy, preferably under local anesthetic. The woman should inform her dentist of her pregnancy so that she is not exposed to teratogenic substances. Dental x-ray examinations and extensive dental work should be delayed when possible until after birth. Extensive dental care during pregnancy requires consultation between the dentist and the maternal health care professional.

Immunizations

All women of childbearing age need to be fully aware of the risks of receiving specific immunizations if pregnancy is possible. Expectant women, especially those who intend to travel internationally, should be aware of the immunizations that are contraindicated during pregnancy. In addition it is important that expectant women clearly understand the recommendations that are made regarding other immunizations, such as those for influenza epidemics.

Immunizations with attenuated live viruses, such as rubella vaccine, should not be given in pregnancy because of the possible harmful effect of the live viruses on the developing embryo. Vaccinations using killed viruses can be used. Recommendations for immunizations during pregnancy are given in Table 15–4.

Teratogenic Substances

Substances that adversely affect the normal growth and development of the fetus are called **teratogens.** Many of these effects are readily apparent at birth, but others may not be identified for years. A well-known example is the development of cervical cancer in adolescent females whose mothers took diethylstilbestrol (DES) during pregnancy.

Many suspected teratogenic substances exist. The harmful effects of others, such as some pesticides and exposure to radiation (x rays, radioactive iodine, and atomic fallout) in the first trimester of pregnancy, have been documented.

Some environmental factors are also suspected to be teratogenic, but due to the complexities of the environment, causal relationships are difficult to demonstrate. For example, expectant women who live in high-altitude areas have been found to have an increased incidence of SGA babies.

SEXUAL ACTIVITY DURING PREGNANCY

Assessment: Occasionally, a woman indicates her beliefs about sexual activity during pregnancy by asking a direct question. This is most likely to occur if the woman and the nurse have a good rapport. Often, however, the nurse must ask some general questions to determine the woman's level of understanding. A general statement may trigger a discussion and help the nurse make a determination. In many cases teaching about this topic is coupled with ongoing assessment of the woman's understanding of sexual activity during pregnancy.

Nursing Diagnosis: The key nursing diagnosis will probably be: knowledge deficit related to lack of information about changes in sexuality and sexual activity during pregnancy.

Nursing Plan and Implementation: The teaching plan will generally focus on discussion or use of a "question and answer" format. The presence of both partners may be beneficial in fostering communication between them and is acceptable unless personal or cultural factors indicate otherwise.

Client Goals: At the completion of the teaching the woman will:

1. Relate the changes in sexuality and sexual response that may occur during pregnancy to changes in technique, frequency, and response that may be indicated.

2. Explore personal attitudes, beliefs, and expectations about sexual activity during pregnancy.

3. Cite maternal factors that would contraindicate sexual intercourse.

Teaching Plan

Content: Begin by explaining that the pregnant woman may experience changes in desire during the course of pregnancy. During the first trimester, discomforts such as nausea, fatigue, and breast tenderness may make intercourse less desirable for many women.

Other women may have fewer discomforts and may find that their sexual desire is unchanged. In the second trimester, as symptoms decrease, desire may increase. In the third trimester, discomfort and fatigue may lead to decreased desire in the woman.

Men may notice changes in their level of desire, too. Among other things, this may be related to feelings about their partner's changing appearance, their belief about the acceptability of sexual activity with a pregnant woman, or concern about hurting the woman or fetus. Some men find the changes of pregnancy erotic; others must adjust to the notion of their partner as a mother.

Explain that the woman may notice that orgasms are much more intense during the last weeks of pregnancy and may be followed by cramping. Because of the presence of the enlarging uterus on the vena cava, the woman should not lie flat on her back for intercourse after about the fourth month. If the couple prefer that position, a pillow should be placed under her right hip to displace the uterus. Alternate positions such as side-lying, female superior, or vaginal rear entry may become necessary as her uterus enlarges.

Stress that sexual activities that both partners enjoy are generally acceptable. It is not advisable for couples who favor anal sex to go from anal penetration to vaginal penetration because of the risk of introducing *E coli* into the vagina.

Alternative methods of expressing intimacy and affection such as cuddling, holding and stroking each other, and kissing may help maintain the couple's feelings of warmth and closeness.

Teaching Method: *Universal statements that give permission, such as "Many couples experience changes in sexual desire during pregnancy. What kind of changes have you experienced?" are often effective in starting discussion. Depending on the woman's (or couple's) level of knowledge and sophistication, part or all of this discussion may be necessary.*

If the partner is present, approach him in the same nonjudgmental way used above. If not, ask the woman if she has noticed any changes in her partner or if he has expressed any concerns.

Deal with any specific questions about the physical and psychologic changes that the couple may have.

Discussion about various sexual activities requires that nurses be comfortable with their sexuality and be tactful. Often the nurse may find it advisable to volunteer such information to show that discussion of sexual variations is acceptable.

The couple may be content with these approaches to meeting their sexual needs, or they may require assurance that such approaches are indeed "normal."

If the man feels desire for further sexual release, his partner may help him masturbate to ejaculation, or he may prefer to masturbate in private.

The woman who is interested in masturbation as a form of gratification should be advised that the orgasmic contractions may be especially intense in later pregnancy.

Stress that sexual intercourse is contraindicated once the membranes are ruptured or if bleeding is present. Women with a history of preterm labor may be advised to avoid intercourse because the oxytocin that is released with orgasm stimulates uterine contractions and may trigger preterm labor. Because oxytocin is also released with nipple stimulation, fondling the breasts may also be contraindicated in those cases.

An explanation of the contraindications accompanied by their rationale provides specific guidelines that most couples find helpful.

A discussion of sexuality and sexual activity should stress the importance of open communication so that the couple feel comfortable expressing their feelings, preferences, and concerns.

Some couples are skilled at expressing their feelings about sexual activity. Others find it difficult and can benefit from specific suggestions. The nurse should provide opportunities for discussion throughout the talk.

Specific handouts on sexual activity are also helpful for couples and may address topics that were not discussed.

Evaluation: The nurse determines the effectiveness of teaching by evaluating the woman's (or couple's) response to information throughout the discussion. The nurse may also ask the woman to express information such as the contraindications to intercourse in her own words. Follow-up sessions and questions from the woman also provide information about teaching effectiveness.

Medications are perhaps the most likely documented teratogens, but other factors can also harm the fetus, including certain infections such as rubella, syphilis, herpesvirus type 2, toxoplasmosis, and cytomegalovirus (CMV). Hyperthermia (temperature greater than 39 C [102.9 F]), especially if it occurs in the critical period of organ development, may account for the increased incidence of congenital anomalies that has been associated with the use of hot tubs early in pregnancy (Milunsky et al 1992).

During pregnancy women need to have adequate information available and a realistic perspective on

---

TABLE 15-4	Summary of Recommendations for Immunization During Pregnancy

Live Virus Vaccines

Measles—contraindicated
Mumps—contraindicated
Poliomyelitis—not routine; increased risk exposure
Rubella—contraindicated
Yellow fever—travel to high-risk areas only

Inactive Virus Vaccines

Influenza—serious underlying diseases
Rabies—same as nonpregnant
Hepatitis B—at high risk and negative for B antigen

Inactivated Bacterial Vaccines

Cholera—to meet international travel requirements
Pneumococcus—same as nonpregnant
Plague—selective vaccination of exposed persons
Typhoid—travel to endemic areas

Toxoids

Tetanus-diphtheria—same as nonpregnant

Hyperimmune Globulins

Hepatitis B—postexposure prophylaxis: given along with hepatitis B vaccine initially, then vaccine alone at 1 and 6 months
Rabies—postexposure prophylaxis
Tetanus—postexposure prophylaxis
Varicella—consider for postexposure (within 96 hours)

Pooled Immune Serum Globulins

Hepatitis A—postexposure prophylaxis
Measles—postexposure prophylaxis

SOURCE: Cunningham FG et al: *Williams Obstetrics*, 19th ed. Norwalk, CT: Appleton & Lange, 1993, p 264.

potential environmental hazards. Factors that are suspected to be hazardous to the general population should obviously be avoided if possible. The expectant woman must remember that factors present in the environment for lengthy periods of time, such as pollution, have not resulted in epidemics of newborn defects.

Much research is being conducted on medications, alcohol, and cigarettes and their roles as teratogenic substances. This information is discussed in the following sections.

Medications

Critical Thinking Question

What approaches might be effective in assessing medication use in a pregnant woman?

The prevalent use of medication in pregnancy is of great concern. Studies have demonstrated that the average pregnant woman takes many more medications than commonly believed, including over-the-counter (OTC) drugs as well as prescription drugs. Medications sold over the counter can be as dangerous as prescription drugs. For example, aspirin is known to inhibit prostaglandin synthesis. This may result in prolonged pregnancy or labor if the woman has used aspirin regularly. Aspirin also interferes with platelet functioning, which may increase the risk of bleeding antepartally or at birth (Niebyl 1994).

Many pregnant women need medication for therapeutic purposes, such as the treatment of infections, allergies, or other pathologic processes. In these situations the problem can be extremely complex. Known teratogenic agents are not prescribed and usually can be replaced by medications considered safe. Even when a woman is highly motivated to avoid taking any medications, she may have taken potentially teratogenic medications before her pregnancy was diagnosed, especially if she had an irregular menstrual cycle.

The greatest potential for gross abnormalities in the fetus occurs during the first trimester of pregnancy, when fetal organs are first developing. The classic period of teratogenesis in a woman with a 28-day cycle extends from day 31 after the LMP (17 days after fertilization) to day 71 (54 days after fertilization) (Niebyl 1994). Many factors influence teratogenic effects, including timing and duration of exposure to the medication as correlated with specific organ development; route of administration; individual metabolic and circulatory factors in the mother, placenta, and fetus; concurrent exposure to other agents; and species susceptibility to the effects (Kochenour 1992). For example, the commonly prescribed acne medication isotretinoin (Accutane) is associated with a high incidence of spontaneous abortion and congenital malformations if taken early in pregnancy. Valproic acid, an anticonvulsant, is associated with an increased risk of

spina bifida. Table 15–5 identifies the possible effects of selected drugs on the fetus and newborn.

To provide information for care givers and clients, the Food and Drug Administration has developed the following classification system for medications administered during pregnancy:

Category A: Controlled studies in women have demonstrated no associated fetal risk. Few drugs fall into this category.

Category B: Animal studies show no risk, but there are no controlled studies in women, or animal studies indicate a risk, but controlled human studies fail to demonstrate a risk. Heparin and the penicillins fall into this category.

Category C: No adequate studies, either in animals or women, are available, or animal studies show teratogenic effects, but no controlled studies in women are available. Many drugs fall into this category, which, because of the lack of information, is a problematic one for care givers. Epinephrine, β-blockers, and acyclovir fall into this category.

Category D: Evidence of human fetal risk does exist, but the benefits of the drug in certain situations are thought to outweigh the risks. Examples of drugs in this category include tetracycline, vincristine, lithium, and hydrochlorothiazide.

Category X: The demonstrated fetal risks clearly outweigh any possible benefit. Examples of drugs in this category include isotretinoin (Accutane), estrogens, and clomiphene.

If a woman has taken a drug in category D or X, she should be informed of the risks associated with that drug and of her alternatives. Similarly, a woman who has taken a drug in the safer categories can be reassured (Cunningham et al 1993).

Although the first trimester is the critical period for teratogenesis, some medications are known to have teratogenic effect when taken in the second and third trimesters. For example, tetracycline taken in late pregnancy is commonly associated with staining of teeth in children and has been shown to depress skeletal growth, especially in premature infants. Sulfonamides taken in the last few weeks of pregnancy are known to compete with bilirubin attachment of protein-binding sites, increasing the risk of jaundice in the newborn (Niebyl 1994). Warfarin (Coumadin), a commonly prescribed anticoagulant, is associated with CNS defects following fetal exposure during the second and third trimesters (Kochenour 1992).

Other medications affect the fetus in much the same way that an adult is affected by an overdose. For example, the use of anticoagulants to treat thromboembolism in the mother can interfere with clotting factors in the fetus. However, this risk is lessened by frequent monitoring of prothrombin time in the mother, accompanied by appropriate changes in dosages of the anticoagulants. Because heparin does not cross the placenta, it is safer for the fetus than warfarin and other anticoagulants.

All medication should be avoided if possible. If no alternative exists, it is wisest to select a well-known medication rather than a newer drug whose potential teratogenic effects may not be known. When possible, the oral form of the drug should be used, and it should be prescribed in the lowest possible therapeutic dose for the shortest time possible. Finally, the care giver should carefully consider the multiple components of the medication.

Consumers today are more aware of the potential risk of taking medications during pregnancy. They are asking for information, and physicians are being held accountable to provide it.

A woman clearly has a right to the most comprehensive information available concerning medications. The nurse can assist her by suggesting appropriate references and helping her research information. Some fine reference books on drugs and pregnancy are currently available and should be part of the library of every office and clinic that provides prenatal care.

The nurse should also remind the woman of the importance of checking with her certified nurse-midwife or physician about medications she was taking when pregnancy occurred and about any nonprescription drugs she is contemplating using. A good rule to follow is that the advantage of using a particular medication must outweigh the risks. Any medication with possible teratogenic effects must be avoided.

Smoking Smoking has been linked to higher infertility rates in both men and women. In women smoking has been identified as a factor in ovulatory, tubal function, and implantation disorders, as well as oocyte depletion and early pregnancy loss. In men smoking has been linked to impaired sperm concentration and changes in sperm motility and morphology (ACOG 1993).

Infants of mothers who smoke tend to have a lower birth weight and a higher incidence of perinatal deaths than infants of mothers who do not smoke (Cunningham et al 1993). These findings increase significantly as maternal age increases. This may be related to the fact that older women have probably been smoking longer and may have some chronic vascular disease; they may consume more cigarettes daily, thus increasing their dose; or they may be more sensitive to the vasoconstrictive effects of cigarettes (Wen et al 1990). In addition mothers who smoke have an increased risk of spontaneous abortion, preterm birth, placenta previa, abruptio placentae, and premature rupture of the membranes. This risk is related to the number of cigarettes smoked (ACOG 1993). Research also links maternal smoking, both during pregnancy and afterward, with an increased risk of sudden infant death syndrome (SIDS), as well as with pneumonia and other respiratory infections (Petersen et al 1992).

TABLE 15–5	Possible Effects of Selected Drugs on the Fetus and Neonate
Maternal Drug	**Effects on Fetus and Neonate**
Risk outweighs benefits if the following drugs are given in the first trimester:	
Thalidomide	Limb, auricle, eye, and visceral malformations
Tolbutamide (Orinase)	Increase of anomalies
Streptomycin	Eighth nerve damage; multiple skeletal anomalies
Tetracycline	Inhibition of bone growth; syndactyly; discoloration of teeth
Iodide	Congenital goiter; hypothyroidism; mental retardation
Methotrexate	Multiple anomalies
Diethylstilbestrol	Clear-cell adenocarcinoma of the vagina and cervix; genital tract anomalies
Warfarin (Coumadin)	Skeletal and facial anomalies; mental retardation
Risk vs. benefits uncertain in the first trimester:	
Gentamicin	Eighth cranial nerve damage
Kanamycin	Eighth cranial nerve damage
Lithium	Goiter; eye anomalies; cleft palate
Barbiturates	Increase of anomalies
Quinine	Increase of anomalies
Septra or Bactrim	Cleft palate
Cytotoxic drugs	Increase of anomalies
Benefit outweighs risk in the first trimester:	
Clomiphene (Clomid)	Increase of anomalies; neural tube defects; Down syndrome
Glucocorticoids	Cleft palate; cardiac defects
General anesthesia	Increase of anomalies
Tricyclic antidepressants	CNS and limb malformations
Sulfonamides	Cleft palate; facial and skeletal defects
Antacids	Increase of anomalies
Salicylates	Central nervous system, visceral, and skeletal malformations
Acetaminophen	None
Heparin	None
Terbutaline	None
Phenothiazines	None
Insulin	Skeletal malformations
Penicillins	None
Chloramphenicol	None
Isoniazid (INH)	Increase of anomalies

SOURCE: Adapted from Howard FM, Hill JM: *Obstet Gynecol Survey* 1979; 34:643.

The specific mechanism by which smoking affects the fetus is not known. Smoking appears to decrease placental blood flow and plasma volume. In addition changes found in the placentas of smokers suggest toxicity related to elements in tobacco smoke and ischemia caused by the vasoconstrictive effects of nicotine on uterine vessels. Smoking may also interfere with maternal absorption or metabolism of calcium, vitamin C, vitamin B_{12}, and perhaps vitamins A, B_6, and B_1 (Aaronson & MacNee 1989).

Fewer women smoke today than 20 years ago. Although approximately 25% of women continue to smoke during pregnancy (Floyd et al 1991), many stop smoking or at least reduce their intake once pregnancy is confirmed. Unfortunately, a majority of women who quit smoking during pregnancy resume after birth; this percentage is lower for women who quit early in pregnancy. This finding suggests that although women are aware of the potential impact of smoking on the fetus, they may be less knowledgeable about the effects of passive smoke on the baby (Fingerhut et al 1990).

Studies demonstrate that any decrease in smoking during pregnancy improves fetal outcome, and researchers continue to explore approaches designed to help women quit smoking (O'Connor et al 1992; Petersen et al 1992). Pregnancy may be a difficult time for a woman to stop smoking, but the nurse should encourage her to reduce the number of cigarettes she smokes daily. The need to protect her unborn child may dramatically increase her motivation.

Alcohol   Alcohol is now considered one of the primary teratogens in the Western world. Fetuses of women who are heavy drinkers are at increased risk for developing **fetal alcohol syndrome (FAS)** (Chapter 31).

The effects of moderate consumption of alcohol during pregnancy are not clearly known, but research suggests there is an increased incidence of lower birth weight and of some neurologic effects, such as attention-deficit disorder. Evidence suggests that the risk of teratogenic effects increases proportionately with increased average daily intake of alcohol. Although studies of light drinkers (women who consumed fewer than seven drinks per week) demonstrate a degree of risk for adverse pregnancy effects similar to that of nondrinkers, no safe level of drinking during pregnancy has been identified, and care givers recommend that pregnant women be advised to *abstain from all alcohol during pregnancy* (Bruce et al 1993).

Alcohol passes the placental barrier within minutes after consumption, with fetal blood alcohol levels becoming equivalent to maternal blood alcohol levels. The effects of alcohol consumption vary according to the stage of fetal development. During the first trimester, alcohol probably alters embryonic development; throughout pregnancy alcohol may interfere with cell division and growth; in the third trimester, the time of most rapid brain growth, alcohol may alter CNS development and contribute to growth retardation (Bruce et al 1993). The risk of neurologic damage is lessened if heavy drinking ceases in the third trimester. Decreased consumption of alcohol in midpregnancy is associated with a lower incidence of growth retardation. Malnutrition, common in heavy drinkers, and alcohol-induced maternal hypoglycemia may also contribute to fetal problems (Niebyl 1994).

Assessment of a woman's alcohol intake should be a chief part of each woman's medical history, with questions asked in a direct and nonjudgmental manner. All women should be counseled about the role of alcohol in pregnancy. When pregnant women become aware of the risk of alcohol to the fetus, most usually attempt to modify their alcohol consumption. If heavy consumption is involved, these women should be referred early to an alcoholic treatment program. Because the drug disulfiram (Antabuse)—often used in the treatment of alcoholism—is suspected as a teratogenic agent, a woman in such a program should inform her counselor if she becomes pregnant.

Counseling about the effects of alcohol during pregnancy has been effective and should, of course, continue. Because the most profound impact of alcohol occurs in the first weeks after conception, nurses and other health care providers will see the most dramatic decrease in the effects of alcohol during pregnancy by increasing their teaching efforts in the period prior to conception.

Caffeine   Current research reveals no evidence that caffeine increases reproductive or teratogenic risk in humans (Cunningham et al 1993). However, maternal coffee consumption does decrease iron absorption and may increase the risk of anemia (Niebyl 1994). Until more definitive data are available, nurses should advise women of common sources of caffeine, including coffee, tea, colas, and chocolate, and suggest they use good judgment in moderating their caffeine intake.

Marijuana   The prevalence of marijuana use in our society raises many concerns about its effect on the fetus, but to date no teratogenic effects of marijuana use during pregnancy have been documented (Cunningham et al 1993). Doing research on marijuana use in pregnancy is difficult, however, because it is an illegal drug. Unreliability of reporting, lack of a representative population, inability to determine strength or composition of the marijuana used, presence of herbicides, and use of other drugs at the same time are major factors complicating the research being done.

Cocaine   A woman who uses cocaine is at increased risk for acute myocardial infarction, cardiac arrhythmias, ruptured ascending aorta, seizures, cerebrovascular accidents, hyperthermia, bowel ischemia, and sudden death (AAP and ACOG 1992). During pregnancy, cocaine use has been related to abruptio placentae, preterm birth, fetal distress, low birth weight, neonatal withdrawal, and SIDS (Blume et al 1993). Several congenital anomalies in the neonate have also been linked to maternal cocaine use, including genitourinary anomalies, congenital heart defects, limb reduction defects, CNS anomalies, prune belly syndrome, and segmental intestinal atresia (Cunningham et al 1993). (See also Chapter 18.)

As cocaine becomes more widely used by women of childbearing age, health care providers must become alert to early signs of cocaine use. It is often difficult for a nurse or physician to face the fact that a woman with whom they have a relationship may be using cocaine, but ongoing alertness and an open, nonjudgmental approach are important in early detection. Urine screening for cocaine is valuable, but because cocaine is metabolized rapidly, the drug screen is negative within 24 to 48 hours after cocaine use. Thus it is probable that many abusers are missed. It is possible to use radioimmunoassays (RIA) of neonatal meconium to detect cocaine. This tool is valuable in detecting newborns of cocaine-abusing women (Dombrowski & Sokol 1990).

EVALUATION

Throughout the antepartal period evaluation is an essential part of effective nursing care. As nurses ask questions of the pregnant woman and her family or make observations of physical changes, they are evaluating the results of previous interventions. In evaluating the effectiveness of the interventions the nurse should not be afraid to try creative solutions if they are logical and carefully thought out. This is especially important in dealing with families from other cultures. If a practice is important to a woman and not harmful, the culturally sensitive nurse will not discourage it.

In completing an evaluation the nurse must also recognize situations that require referral for further evaluation. For example, a woman who has gained 4 lb in 1 week probably does not require counseling about nutrition; she needs further assessment for pregnancy-induced hypertension. The nurse who has a sound knowledge of theory will recognize this and act immediately.

The ongoing and cyclic nature of the nursing process is especially evident in the prenatal setting. However, throughout the course of pregnancy certain criteria can be used to determine the quality of care provided. In essence nursing care has been effective if:

- The common discomforts of pregnancy are quickly identified and are relieved or lessened effectively.
- The woman is able to discuss the physiologic and psychologic changes of pregnancy.
- The woman implements appropriate self-care measures if they are indicated during pregnancy.
- The woman avoids substances and situations that pose a risk to her well-being or that of her child.
- The woman seeks regular prenatal care.

KEY CONCEPTS

Provision of anticipatory guidance about childbirth, the postpartum period, and childrearing is a primary responsibility of the nurse caring for women in an antepartal setting.

The nurse assesses the expectant father's knowledge level and intended degree of participation and then works with the couple to help ensure a satisfying experience.

Culturally based practices and proscribed activities may have a major impact on the childbearing family.

The common discomforts of pregnancy occur as a result of physiologic and anatomic changes. The nurse provides the woman with information about self-care activities aimed at reducing or relieving discomfort.

To make appropriate self-care choices and ensure healthful habits, a pregnant woman requires accurate information about a range of subjects from exercise to sexual activity, from bathing to immunization.

Teratogenic substances are substances that adversely affect the normal growth and development of the fetus.

A pregnant woman should avoid taking medications or using over-the-counter preparations during pregnancy.

Evidence exists that smoking, consuming alcohol, or using social drugs during pregnancy may be harmful to the fetus.

Maternal assessment of fetal activity keeps the woman "in touch" with her fetus and provides ongoing assessment of fetal status.

REFERENCES

Aaronson LS, MacNee CL: Tobacco, alcohol, and caffeine use during pregnancy. *JOGNN* 1989; 18(4):279.

American Academy of Pediatrics (AAP) and American College of Obstetricians and Gynecologists (ACOG): *Guidelines for Perinatal Care*, 3rd ed. Elk Grove Village, IL: AAP, 1992.

American College of Obstetricians and Gynecologists (ACOG): Exercise during pregnancy and the postpartum period. *ACOG Technical Bulletin 189*. Washington, DC: ACOG, February 1994.

American College of Obstetricians and Gynecologists (ACOG): Smoking and reproductive health. *ACOG Technical Bulletin 180*. Washington, DC: ACOG, May 1993.

American College of Obstetricians and Gynecologists (ACOG): Women and exercise. *ACOG Technical Bulletin 173*. Washington, DC: ACOG, October 1992.

Artal Mittelmark R et al: *Exercise in Pregnancy*, 2nd ed. Baltimore: Williams & Wilkins, 1991.

Barry M, Bia F: Pregnancy and travel. *JAMA* February 1989; 261:728.

Belluomini J et al: Acupressure for nausea and vomiting of pregnancy: A randomized, blinded study. *Obstet Gynecol* August 1994; 84(2):245.

Blackburn ST, Loper DL: *Maternal, Fetal, and Neonatal Physiology: A Clinical Perspective*. Philadelphia: Saunders, 1992.

Blume SB et al: When you first suspect substance abuse. *Contemp OB/GYN* March 1993; 38(3):74.

Brown MS: A cross-cultural look at pregnancy, labor, and delivery. *JOGNN* September/October 1976; 5:35.

Bruce FC et al: Alcohol use before and during pregnancy. *Am J Prev Med* 1993; 9(5):267.

Carrington BW: The Afro American. In: *Culture, Childbearing, Health Professionals.* Clark AL (editor). Philadelphia: Davis, 1978.

Cunningham FG et al: *Williams Obstetrics,* 19th ed. Norwalk, CT: Appleton & Lange, 1993.

DeJoseph JF: Redefining women's work during pregnancy: Toward a more comprehensive approach. *Birth* June 1993; 20(2):86.

Dombrowski MP, Sokol RJ: Cocaine and abruption. *Contemp OB/GYN* April 1990; 35:13.

Fingerhut LA et al: Smoking before, during, and after pregnancy. *Am J Public Health* May 1990; 80(5):541.

Floyd RL et al: Smoking during pregnancy: Prevalence, effects, and intervention strategies. *Birth* March 1991; 18(1):48.

Freda MC et al: Fetal movement counting: Which method? *MCN* November/December 1993; 18:314.

Hoffman JB: A suggested treatment for inverted nipples. *Am J Obstet Gynecol* 1953; 66:346.

Kochenour NK: Medication in pregnancy: Minimize the risks. *Contemp OB/GYN* February 1992; 37(2):59.

Kochenour NK: Normal pregnancy and prenatal care. In: *Danforth's Obstetrics and Gynecology,* 7th ed. Scott JR et al (editors). Philadelphia: Lippincott, 1994.

Kousen M: Treatment of nausea and vomiting in pregnancy. *Am Fam Phys* November 15, 1993; 48(7):1279.

Launer LJ et al: The effect of maternal work on fetal growth and duration of pregnancy: A prospective study. *Brit J Obstet Gynecol* January 1990; 97:62.

Masters WH, Johnson VE: *Human Sexual Response.* Boston: Little, Brown, 1966.

Milunsky A et al: Maternal heat exposure and neural tube defects. *JAMA* August 19, 1992; 268(7):882.

Newman V et al: Clinical advances in the management of severe nausea and vomiting during pregnancy. *JOGNN* November/December 1993; 22(6):483.

Niebyl JR: Teratology and drug use during pregnancy and lactation. In: *Danforth's Obstetrics and Gynecology,* 7th ed. Scott JR et al (editors). Philadelphia: Lippincott, 1994.

O'Connor AM et al: Effectiveness of a pregnancy smoking cessation program. *JOGNN* September/October 1992; 21(5):385.

Petersen L et al: Smoking reduction during pregnancy by a program of self-help and clinical support. *Obstet Gynecol* June 1992; 79(6):924.

Sahakian V et al: Vitamin B_6 is effective therapy for nausea and vomiting of pregnancy: A randomized, double-blind placebo-controlled study. *Obstet Gynecol* 1991; 78:33.

Spector RE: *Cultural Diversity in Health and Illness,* 3rd ed. Norwalk, CT: Appleton & Lange, 1991.

Wakefield M et al: Characteristics associated with smoking cessation during pregnancy among working class women. *Addiction* October 1993; 88:1423.

Wen SW et al: Smoking, maternal age, fetal growth, and gestational age at delivery. *Am J Obstet Gynecol* 1990; 162:53.

CHAPTER 16

THE EXPECTANT FAMILY: AGE-RELATED CONSIDERATIONS

I am a freshman in college and so is my daughter. I had her when I was 15 and that forced me to grow up in a hurry. For years I've thought about being a nurse, and now is my chance. Please understand, my daughter is very precious to me, but a part of me knows that if I had it to do over, I would change so much of my life—if only I had known!

KEY TERMS

Blended family

Early adolescence

Emancipated minors

Late adolescence

Middle adolescence

OBJECTIVES

Describe different reasons for teenage pregnancy and their implications for nursing care.

Summarize the physical, psychologic, and sociologic risks faced by an adolescent who is pregnant.

Describe the reactions and needs of the adolescent father.

Discuss the reactions of the adolescent's family to her pregnancy.

Formulate a plan of care to meet the needs of a pregnant adolescent.

Identify the medical risks faced by an older expectant couple.

Relate the concerns of older expectant couples to their adaptation to pregnancy.

$\mathcal{P}$regnancy is a challenging time for all women as they adjust to the changes they experience and prepare to assume a new role as mother of one or more children. Even if a woman chooses to terminate her pregnancy, the very fact that she has been pregnant has a lasting effect on her. Age at the time of pregnancy may be a factor in a woman's adjustment, both physically and psychologically. This chapter explores the special needs and concerns of pregnant adolescents and of women who become pregnant over age 35 years.

CARE OF THE PREGNANT ADOLESCENT

In the United States each year over one million teenage girls become pregnant, and most of these pregnancies are unplanned (Adolescent unintended pregnancy, 1994). Regardless of race, teenage girls in the lowest socioeconomic quartile are four times as likely to have a baby as those in the highest socioeconomic quartile (Rosenheim & Testa 1992). Although some choose to believe that welfare policies are to blame for this problem, data tend to indicate that this is not the case (Rosenheim & Testa 1992; Williams 1991).

Teenage pregnancy is a multifaceted problem with no single cause or cure. For a teen, pregnancy comes at a time when her physical development is incomplete and available support systems may be limited. Pregnancy interrupts her education and makes it tremendously difficult for her to complete the developmental tasks of adolescence as well as those related to pregnancy and parenthood (Table 16–1).

Significantly, adolescents are engaging in sexual intercourse at an earlier age than seen previously (Adolescent unintended pregnancy 1994). This is especially true for white, nonpoor teenage females (Children's Defense Fund 1991) because sexual activity among African American female adolescents remains unchanged, and a slight decline in sexual activity has occurred among Hispanic adolescents (Rosenheim & Testa 1992). However, birth rates for nonwhite teens remain twice as high as those for white teenagers (National Center for Health Statistics 1991). The total public cost for teen births is approximately $25.1 billion. Estimates suggest that simply delaying these births until the mother is age 20 could result in an annual savings of $10 billion primarily because of the improvements in both educational and occupational status these young women could experience by delaying motherhood (Burnhill 1994).

The incidence of teenage sexual activity in the United States is similar to that in industrialized European nations and Canada, but the incidence of teen pregnancy, induced abortion, and births among adolescents is signif-

icantly higher in the United States (Teens and contraception 1992). Researchers suggest that these countries may have lower adolescent pregnancy rates because of family influences, a greater openness about sexuality, better accessibility to contraceptives, and a more comprehensive approach to sex education (Crooks & Baur 1993; Peckham 1993).

Authorities believe that many factors contribute to the increased incidence of adolescent pregnancy in the United States. Cohabitation and premarital sexual activity are commonplace. Sexual innuendo permeates every aspect of the popular media, including music, music videos, television, and movies, but issues of sexual responsibility are commonly ignored. As a result of these trends sexual activity is occurring at a younger age and is encouraged by peer pressure in the adolescent population. In fact the statistics lead many to believe that sexual activity is the normative experience of high school teenagers today (Steinberg 1993).

Pregnancy risk taking (sexual activity without use of pregnancy prevention measures) is believed to stem from a variety of factors. Many teenage girls feel that they are not vulnerable to pregnancy, that because of their uniqueness, they are immune (Humenick et al 1991). Others, because of confusion or misinformation about conception, do not understand the risk ("I thought I was too young. . . " or "I don't make love that frequently. . . "). Still others fail to anticipate intercourse.

Reports of contraception use with the first experience of intercourse vary tremendously. However, as many as one-half to two-thirds of teenagers do not use contraception with their first experience. If contraception is used, condoms are most likely to be employed, followed by the pill (Kahn et al 1990; Mosher & McNally 1991). Those under the age of 15 are less likely to use contraception than the older teenager (Mosher & McNally 1991). Errors in contraception use among teenagers are probably common, thus decreasing their protective effects.

Not surprisingly, adolescents who have a future orientation to educational goals are more likely to use contraception than those who do not have access to middle-class opportunities (Humenick et al 1991; Ravoira & Cherry 1992). Other factors affecting the use of contraception include access or availability, cost of supplies, and concern regarding confidentiality. Results of a large study conducted with high school students indicated that many are unaware of their rights to confidentiality for certain health problems (Cheng et al 1993).

A woman's intrapsychic conflict about becoming pregnant is also cited as a factor in pregnancy risk taking (Flanigan et al 1990). The adolescent girl may use pregnancy for various subconscious or conscious reasons: to punish her father and/or mother, to escape from an undesirable home situation, to gain attention, or to feel that

| | TABLE 16-1 | Developmental Tasks of Adolescence |

Tasks	Description of Successful Resolution	High-Risk Factors for Teen Pregnancy
Developing an identity	As individuals enter puberty, their physical appearance begins to change, and others begin to respond differently to them. The media present idealized images of the teenage female. Fluctuation in self-esteem may occur, and hormonal changes create awareness of sexual desire. Adolescents experience confusion about their self-image. This is a time of experimentation until they become comfortable with who they are.	If the young adolescent feels she cannot live up to parents' expectations or is in a dysfunctional family situation, she may adopt a negative identity. She may become rebellious and actively involved in risk-taking behaviors such as substance abuse and early sexual activity.
Gaining independence	Adolescents gradually move away from parental control and are influenced by peers. Eventually, they develop values that help govern their behavior responsibly without extrinsic control of peers or parents.	Peer pressure is highest during early and middle adolescence. If peers are involved in antisocial behavior, this influences their behavior and all other developmental tasks. Substance abuse and sexual activity are common in these groups.
Developing emotional intimacy in relationships	Adolescents begin to develop a close emotional attachment with another individual. They can share innermost feelings and have empathy for the other. This usually begins with a friend of the same sex and eventually develops into a trusting and loving relationship with someone of the opposite sex.	Research conducted with a group of pregnant teenage girls and teenage mothers reported that their needs for intimacy were not being met by their peers or families. Sexual activity was an attempt to meet these needs (Ravoira & Cherry 1992). This is a problem for victims of neglect or abuse. Although sexual intercourse has become a common adolescent experience, emotional intimacy as described is not associated with the majority of dating relationships, and most teenage marriages end in divorce.
Developing comfort with their sexuality	Puberty causes a new awareness of sexual desire and new meaning about physical contact with others. Adolescents learn to express sexual feelings appropriately and comfortably in a relationship.	Many young adolescent females who become sexually involved at an early age do so for a variety of reasons that do not lead to comfort with their own sexuality: peer pressure, pressure from an older male partner, rebellion against parents, sexual abuse and its consequences.
Gaining a sense of achievement	Adolescents begin to look toward the future and compare talents, work skills, and/or academic achievement with reality in preparing for adult working roles.	Approximately one-fourth of American adolescents drop out of high school. Those who drop out of school prematurely tend to be from economically disadvantaged backgrounds. Data show that early sexual experimentation by adolescents correlates with poor school performance whatever their background (Ravoira & Cherry 1992). Use of contraception is more likely among adolescent females who are high academic achievers and have a future orientation (Humenick et al 1991).

SOURCE: Adapted from Steinberg L: *Adolescence*, 3rd ed. New York: McGraw Hill, 1993.

she has someone to love and to love her. As a result some young teenagers consciously plan to get pregnant (Holt & Johnson 1991). A few develop close relationships with their "mothers-in-law" and new extended family. For these few pregnancy provides the opportunity for a more stable family experience than is available with the girl's family of origin (Flanigan et al 1990).

Pregnancy may be a young woman's form of delinquency. Pregnant adolescents often have troubled family relationships, poor school achievement, and exposure to drug abuse (Humenick et al 1991; Ravoira & Cherry 1992).

Pregnancy risk taking has also been linked to lack of knowledge about contraception. Because of this, many health care providers advocate sex education in schools. Others feel that sex education is the responsibility of the parents and are concerned that sex education in the schools will promote sexual activity. Review of research on sex education, however, demonstrates that generally there is a lack of association with increased sexual activity (Humenick et al 1991).

Ethnographic research that examined African American teenage mothers' perspectives of teenage pregnancy suggests that teens in inner-city neighborhoods are socialized to a single parenthood (Williams 1991). Childbearing female role models include mothers, sisters, cousins, aunts, and peers who become single mothers as teenagers. The teenage mothers who were interviewed identified completion of high school and living independently as more important than marriage. They saw themselves as capable of raising children without a father in the household because their mother and their aunts had done it. The stigma of unwed motherhood has been removed not only from this subculture, but also from the broad cultural perspective throughout the United States (Williams 1991). The percent of African American female-headed families nearly doubled (from 22% to 42%) between 1960 and the late 1980s, with one factor contributing to this change identified as an increased community tolerance of the female single parent (Rosenheim & Testa 1992).

Cultural values may cause a young woman to desire pregnancy. Many cultures, such as the Latino culture (including individuals from all Spanish-speaking countries), equate evidence of fertility with adult status. Duany and Pittman (1990) suggest that the formation of families and the onset of employment occur at an earlier age for Latinos than for either White or Black youths and are marks of adult success.

Teenage pregnancy can result from an incestuous relationship. The psychologic turmoil experienced by the incest victim may obliterate thought of the risk of pregnancy, especially for the young adolescent. Older adolescents may fear the possibility of pregnancy, but for a variety of psychologic reasons may deny the reality. In the very young adolescent incest or sexual abuse should be suspected as a possible cause of pregnancy. Teenage pregnancy could also be caused by other nonvoluntary sexual experiences such as date rape.

The decision to terminate the pregnancy is not uncommon among the teenage population. Statistics indicate that 39% of pregnancies in mothers under age 15 resulted in live births, 51% ended in induced abortions, and 10% involved fetal losses. In mothers between the ages of 15 and 19, 48% resulted in live births, 40% ended in induced abortions, and 12% involved fetal losses. When abortion rates for Whites and other races were compared, the percentages were essentially the same during the teenage years (US Bureau of the Census 1993).

Much controversy surrounds abortion laws. Proponents of increased parental involvement (notification or consent of parents prior to an abortion) believe this would lead to a decrease in sexual activity among teens (Horner & Hilde 1991). Others predict that more restrictive abortion laws nationwide would increase the numbers of teens giving birth, increase perinatal morbidity and mortality, and lead to a significant increase in illegal abortion with its many tragedies (Horner & Hilde 1991). Relinquishment of babies for adoption could increase with enactment of restrictive abortion laws, but little research is available on relinquishment because of the small numbers currently involved (Bachrach et al 1992).

Overview of the Adolescent Period

Physical Changes

Puberty, that period during which an individual becomes capable of reproduction, is a maturational process that can last from 1½ to 6 years. The major physical changes of puberty include a growth spurt, weight change, and the appearance of secondary sexual characteristics. Menarche, or the time of the first menstrual period, usually occurs in the last half of this maturational process, with the average age between 12 and 13 (Steinberg 1993).

The initial menstrual cycles are usually irregular and often anovulatory for the first 12 to 18 months; however, this is not true for all females. Some adolescents do not use contraception during this time because they falsely assume that they cannot get pregnant. Even if their initial menstrual cycles are anovulatory, there is no certainty about when the first ovulatory cycle will occur; thus contraception is important during this time for all adolescents who are sexually active.

Psychosocial Development

Although it is well documented that the onset of puberty now occurs at a younger age, there are no data to indicate that psychosocial development, particularly cognitive development, occurs at an earlier age. In fact authorities believe that there is a widening gap between psychologic and biologic maturation in adolescents (Rosenheim & Testa 1992).

Developmental tasks of adolescence have been described by many writers and are based on a variety of classic theories. These tasks are issues that individuals may struggle with at other times in their lives, but they are especially significant during adolescence for a successful transition from childhood to adulthood. The following are major developmental tasks of this period (Steinberg 1993):

- Developing an identity
- Gaining autonomy and independence
- Developing intimacy in a relationship
- Developing comfort with one's own sexuality
- Developing a sense of achievement

Resolution of these tasks is a developmental process that occurs over time. This developmental process is reflected in the behaviors of youths during early, middle, and late adolescence. Although average ages for the completion of tasks have been identified, these ages are somewhat arbitrary and are affected by many factors such as culture, religion, and socioeconomic status.

In **early adolescence** (age 14 and under) the teen still sees authority in the parents. However, she begins the process of "leaving the family" by spending more time with friends, especially friends of the same sex. Conformity to peer group standards is reflected in her behavior and in the clothes she wears. During this phase the adolescent has a rich fantasy life. In addition she is struggling to become comfortable with her changing body and body image and to fit this image with her fantasy life. Much time is spent in front of the mirror. The adolescent in this phase is very egocentric and is a concrete thinker. She has only minimal ability to see herself in the future or foresee the consequences of her behavior. She perceives her locus of control as external; that is, her destiny is controlled by others such as parents and school authorities.

TABLE 16-2 Initial Reaction to Awareness of Pregnancy

Age	Adolescent Behavior	Nursing Implications
Early adolescent (14 and under)	Fears rejection by family and peers. Enters health care system with an adult, most likely mother (parents still seen as locus of control). Value system still closely reflects that of parents, so still turns to parents for decision or approval of decision. Pregnancy probably not result of intimate relationship. Self-conscious about normal adolescent changes in body. Self-consciousness and low self-esteem likely to increase with rapid breast enlargement and abdominal enlargement of pregnancy.	Nonjudgmental in approach to care. Focus on needs and concerns of adolescent teenager, but if parent accompanies daughter, parent needs to be included in plan of care. Encourage both to express concerns and feelings regarding pregnancy and options: abortion, maintaining pregnancy, adoption. Be realistic and concrete in discussing implications of each option. During physical exam of adolescent respect increased sense of modesty. Explain in simple and concrete terms physical changes that are produced by pregnancy versus puberty. Explain each step of physical exam in simple and concrete terms.
Middle adolescent (15–17 years)	Fears rejection by peers and parents. Unsure in whom to confide. May seek confirmation of pregnancy on own with increased awareness of options and services, such as over-the-counter pregnancy kits and Planned Parenthood. If in an ongoing, caring relationship with partner (peer), may choose him as confidant. Economic dependence on parents may determine if and when parents are told. Future educational plans, perception of parental support or lack of support are significant factors in decision regarding termination or maintenance of the pregnancy. Possible conflict in parental and own developing value system.	Nonjudgmental in approach to care. Reassure regarding confidentiality. Help adolescent identify significant individuals in whom she can confide to help make a decision about the pregnancy. Need to be aware of state laws regarding requirement of parental notification if abortion intended. Also need to be aware of state laws regarding requirements for marriage: usually minimum age 18 for both parties; 16- and 17-year-olds only with consent of parents. Encourage adolescent to be realistic about parental response to pregnancy.
Older adolescent (18–19 years)	Most likely to confirm pregnancy on own and at an earlier date due to increased acceptance and awareness of consequences of behavior. Likely to use pregnancy kit for confirmation. Relationship with father of baby, future educational plans, own value system are among significant determinants of decision about pregnancy.	Nonjudgmental in approach to care. Reassure regarding confidentiality. Encourage adolescent to identify significant individuals in whom she can confide. Refer to counseling as appropriate. Encourage adolescent to be realistic about parental response to pregnancy.

Middle adolescence (15 to 17 years) is the time for challenging: Experimenting with drugs, alcohol, and sex is a common avenue for rebellion. The middle adolescent seeks independence and turns increasingly to her peer group. Peer group identification is obvious in her choice of dress, makeup, hair style, and music. During this phase the adolescent may believe that she is invincible and will not suffer negative consequences from risk-taking behaviors. These years are often a time of great turmoil for the family as the adolescent struggles for independence and challenges the family's values and expectations.

The middle adolescent wants to be treated as an adult. However, fear of adult responsibility may cause fluctuation in behavior. At times she seems like a child; at other times she is surprisingly mature. She is beginning to move from concrete thinking to formal operational thought but is not yet able to anticipate the long-term implications of all her actions.

In **late adolescence** (18 to 19 years) the young woman is more at ease with her individuality and decision-making ability. She can think abstractly and anticipate consequences. During this time she becomes more confident of her personal identity. The late adolescent is capable of formal operational thought. She is learning to solve problems, to conceptualize, and to make decisions. These abilities help her see herself as having control, which leads to the ability to understand and accept the consequences of her behavior.

Table 16–2 suggests typical behaviors of the early, middle, and late adolescent when she becomes aware of her pregnancy. In reviewing these behaviors it is important to realize that other factors may influence the age at which these behaviors are seen.

The Adolescent Mother

Physiologic Risks

Several studies in the last decade indicate that young age by itself is not a risk factor for poor outcome of pregnancy. Those teens at highest risk tend to be from lower socioeconomic backgrounds and fail to receive early prenatal care (Humenick et al 1991; Santelli & Jacobson 1990). Unfortunately, many adolescents fail to seek early prenatal care. Those who do may fail to cooperate with recommendations, especially those focusing on dietary practices, either because of a lack of understanding of the importance of good nutrition or because of concerns related to body image. Thus risks for pregnant adolescents include preterm births, low-birth-weight (LBW) infants, pregnancy-induced hypertension (PIH) and its sequelae, and iron-deficiency anemia. Various studies indicate that early prenatal care, with emphasis on nutrition counseling and coordination of agencies providing comprehensive services, significantly improves birth weights of babies of pregnant adolescents (Humenick et al 1991).

Pregnancy-induced hypertension represents the most prevalent medical complication in adolescents. It is not clear whether this is related to such factors as poor nutrition, low weight gain, or parity, rather than age itself (Humenick et al 1991). Iron-deficiency anemia is a problem in all pregnant women. The adolescent who begins her pregnancy already anemic, however, is at increased risk and must be followed closely and counseled carefully regarding nutrition during pregnancy.

The increased risk of cephalopelvic disproportion (CPD) is a concern in adolescent pregnancy, especially with the younger adolescent because of a lack of pelvic maturity.

Teenagers 15 to 19 years old have a high incidence of sexually transmitted infections. The presence of herpes virus or gonorrhea during a pregnancy greatly increases the risk to the fetus. The incidence of chlamydial infection is also increased in this age group. Other problems seen in adolescents are cigarette smoking and drug use. The damage may be already done to the fetus by smoking or drug use by the time pregnancy is confirmed in young women.

Psychologic Risks

The most profound psychologic risk to the adolescent who maintains her pregnancy is the interruption of progress on her developmental tasks. Although adolescents have become sexually active at an earlier age and the incidence of adolescent pregnancy has increased, the developmental tasks of this age group remain the same. Add to this the tasks of pregnancy, and the young woman has an overwhelming amount of psychologic work to do, the success of which will affect her own and her newborn's future.

Sociologic Risks

A substantial body of research indicates that the adolescent mother is at higher risk for social and economic disadvantages than her teenage counterpart who is not pregnant and lives in the same social environment. Being forced into adult roles before completing adolescent developmental tasks causes a series of events that affects the adolescent's entire life. These events may result in a prolonged dependence on parents, lack of stable relationships with the opposite sex, and lack of economic and social stability. In addition the closer that pregnancy occurs to the changes of puberty and menarche, the more difficulty the teenager will have in becoming comfortable with her body image, given the continuing physical changes that do not fit her image of a "normal" teenager.

Many teenage mothers drop out of school during their pregnancy, as described in Table 16–1. This tendency may have as much to do with low academic achievement and low academic commitment as it does with the pregnancy. Many never complete their education. Lack of education reduces the quality of jobs available to these individuals. Childbearing at an early age is a strong predictor for need for public assistance, especially in lower socioeconomic groups and when the pregnant adolescent's family will not support her (Grogger & Bronars 1993; Humenick et al 1991).

There is evidence that in the United States the younger the adolescent at her first pregnancy, the more likely she is to become pregnant again while still an adolescent (Howard & Mitchell 1993). These young women frequently fail to establish a stable family. Their family structure tends to be a single-parent, matriarchal family structure, often the same type in which the adolescent herself was raised.

Some pregnant adolescents choose to marry the father of the baby, who is often also a teenager. Unfortunately, the majority of adolescent marriages end in divorce (Rosenheim & Testa 1992; Steinberg 1993). This fact should not be surprising because pregnancy and marriage interrupt their "childhood" and basic education. Failure to be self-supporting logically follows lack of education and lost career goals. Lack of maturity in dealing with an intimate relationship also contributes to marital breakdown in this age group.

In general children of teenage mothers are found to be at a developmental disadvantage compared to children whose mothers were older at the time of their birth. Many factors contribute to these differences, but the strongest evidence indicates that the adverse social and economic conditions facing teenage mothers are significant factors. These factors result in high rates of family instability, disadvantaged neighborhoods, and poor educational experiences for these children (Humenick et al 1991).

The increased incidence of maternal complications, premature birth, and low-birth-weight babies among adolescent mothers also has an impact on society because many of these mothers are on welfare. The need for increased financial support for good prenatal care and nutritional programs remains critical.

Table 16–3 identifies the early adolescent's response to the developmental tasks of pregnancy. The early adolescent's response reflects her level of development, with pregnancy as an interruption of the normal process of development. The middle and late adolescents respond differently, reflecting their maturational progress through the developmental tasks. In addition to her maturational level, the amount of nurturing the pregnant adolescent receives is also a critical factor in the way in which she handles pregnancy and motherhood.

The Adolescent Father

The adolescent father must complete the developmental tasks of his age group and is no better prepared psychologically to deal with the consequences of pregnancy than his female counterpart. Consequently, the adolescent who attempts to assume his responsibility as a father faces

Stage	Developmental Tasks of Pregnancy	Early Adolescent's Response to Pregnancy	Nursing Implications
First trimester	Pregnancy confirmation. Seeking early prenatal care as a confirmation tool. Begins to evaluate her diet and general health habits. Initial ambivalence common. Usually supportive partner.	May delay confirmation of pregnancy until late part of first trimester—unaware of pregnancy, fear of confiding in anyone, or denial. Rapid enlargement and sensitivity of breasts embarrassing and frightening to early adolescent—may be perceived as changes of puberty. If confiding in mother, may be experiencing family turmoil in response to pregnancy.	Explain physiologic changes of pregnancy versus those associated with puberty. Explain that ambivalence is normal with any pregnancy, but recognize it as a much greater concern with adolescent pregnancy. Emphasize need for good nutrition as important for her well-being as much as infant's (prevention of PIH and anemia). Use simple explanations and lots of audiovisuals. Have adolescent listen to FHR with Doppler.
Second trimester	Changes in physical appearance begin, and fetal movement is experienced, causing pregnancy to be experienced as a reality. Begins wearing maternity clothes to accommodate the physical changes. As a result of quickening she perceives her fetus as a real baby and begins preparing for the maternal role and new relationships with her partner and members of her family.	Some teenagers may delay validation of pregnancy until now, with family turmoil occurring at this time. Abdominal enlargement and quickening may be perceived as loss of control over body image. May try to maintain prepregnant weight and wear restrictive clothing to control and conceal changing body. Becomes dependent on her own mother for support. Egocentric; unable to develop a maternal role at this time.	Continue to discuss importance of good nutrition and adequate weight gain as noted above. Discuss ways of utilizing common teenage clothing (large sweatshirts, blouses) to promote comfort but preserve adolescent image to some degree. Discuss plans being made for baby, continued educational plans, and role of teen's parents.
Third trimester	At end of second trimester begins to view fetus as separate from self. Buys baby clothes and supplies. Prepares a place for the baby. Realistic about what baby is like. Prepares to give birth to infant. Anxiety increases as labor and birth approach and has concerns about well-being of fetus.	May focus on "wanting it to be over." May have trouble individuating fetus. May have fantasies, dreams, or nightmares about childbirth. Natural fears of labor and birth greater than with older primigravida. Probably has not been in a hospital, and may associate this with negative experiences.	Need to assess if preparing for baby by buying supplies and preparing a place in the home. Childbirth education important. Provide hospital tour. Need to assess for discomforts of pregnancy, such as heartburn and constipation. Adolescent may be uncomfortable mentioning these and other problems.

many of the same psychologic and sociologic risks as the adolescent mother.

Because he is not yet mature, his level of cognitive development and decision-making skills influence whether he remains supportive of the mother of the child or flees the situation. His educational and career goals may be threatened as he anticipates marrying or quitting school to support the young woman and his child. Data indicate that high school dropout rates are higher for adolescents who are aware of their role in fathering the forthcoming child than for other youths (Steinberg 1993). The job skills of the adolescent father, particularly when he quits school, are minimal and unlikely to contribute significantly to the economic support of the pregnant adolescent.

The unwed adolescent father often faces negative reactions from people in his environment, including his own family and the family of the young woman. Feelings of anger, shame, and disappointment may be aimed at him. He may feel isolated and alone, and if the young woman's parents refuse to allow him to see her, his sole source of emotional support may be gone.

The conscientious adolescent father faces a serious situation that may be overwhelming for him. The unresolved stress may lead to a crisis, manifested by abnormal adaptive behavior, marked depression, somatic symptoms, and/or deviant behavior. He has the same concerns about being rejected by family and peers as does the pregnant adolescent female.

Adolescent fathers are usually within 3 or 4 years of age of the adolescent mother. The mother and father are generally from similar socioeconomic backgrounds and have similar education. Many are involved in meaningful relationships. Frequently, the fathers are involved in the decision making regarding abortion or adoption. Many fathers are very involved in the pregnancy and in the child-rearing.

Adolescent fathers do become sexually active at an earlier age than adolescent mothers, but many know less about contraception and reproduction, feeling this is a woman's domain (Marsiglio 1993).

Psychologic and sociologic risks to the adolescent father are in many ways similar to the adolescent mother's risks. Adolescent fathers tend to achieve less formal education than older fathers, and they enter the labor force earlier with less education. They tend to pursue less prestigious careers and have less job satisfaction. Adolescent fathers often marry at a younger age and have larger families than older fathers. In addition the divorce rate of marriages with an adolescent spouse at the time of birth is greater than that of couples who postpone childbearing and marriage (Fielding & Williams 1991).

The lack of responsibility shown by some unwed fathers is a reflection of our cultural and community attitudes. Unfortunately, in some instances young men who seek to assume parental responsibility are discouraged by the agencies with which they deal. This attitude may be in the process of changing. Fathers are being included on birth certificates far more frequently today than in the past. This helps ensure the father's rights and encourages him to meet his responsibilities to his child. In addition, legal paternity gives children access to military and social security benefits and to medical information about their fathers (Humenick et al 1991).

In some situations the pregnant adolescent female may not want to identify or contact the father of the baby, and the male may not readily acknowledge paternity. Those situations include rape, exploitative sexual relations, incest, and casual sexual relations. If health care providers suspect any of the first three causes, further investigation into the situation is important for the well-being of the pregnant adolescent, and referral to other resources should be done as appropriate.

In situations in which the adolescent father wants to assume some responsibility, he should be supported in his behavior by health care providers as appropriate. It is important, however, that the pregnant adolescent have the opportunity to make the decision about whether she wants the father to participate in her health care.

If the adolescents perceive that they have a caring relationship, the adolescent father may want to be supportive and protective but probably does not understand the physical and psychologic changes his female partner is experiencing. The young man will need education regarding pregnancy, childbirth, child care, and parenting. Some clinics have couples attend classes together; others offer special classes just for fathers. In becoming a parent the adolescent male needs to learn rates of growth and development so he can understand the newborn's potential and does not become frustrated and dissatisfied with the child's behavior because of unrealistic expectations.

Although the adolescent father may have been included in the health care of the young woman throughout the pregnancy, it is not unusual for the female adolescent to want her mother as her primary support person during labor and birth. This is especially true with younger adolescents. It is important to support her wishes, but it is also important that the adolescent father not be ignored.

As a part of counseling, the nurse should assess the young man's stressors, his support systems, his plans for involvement in the pregnancy and childbearing, and his future plans. He should be referred to social services for an opportunity to be counseled regarding his educational and vocational future. When the father is involved in the pregnancy, the young mother feels less deserted, more confident in her decision making, and better able to discuss her future.

Reactions of Family and Social Supports to Adolescent Pregnancy

Perhaps the first, most intense crisis of the pregnant adolescent is telling her parents that she is pregnant. The young woman may not talk about her pregnancy until it is obvious. Her mother is usually the first to find out.

Parents' initial reactions to the news are usually shock, anger, shame, guilt, and sorrow. The angry mother

---

RESEARCH IN PRACTICE

Adolescent health status has declined in the past two decades, primarily related to increased risk-taking behavior. Pregnancy may be one result of risk-taking that has long-term consequences for mother and baby. Many adolescents also delay entry into the health care system for prenatal care, increasing their potential for complications. Even though they take risks, adolescents also express concern about self-care issues. Using this conceptual framework, Sally Hughes Lee and Laurie Grubbs explored how pregnant teenagers care for themselves during their pregnancy, and attempted to determine whether a relationship existed between early or late entry into prenatal care and stated self-care practices.

Forty-six pregnant teenagers (aged 14–18 years) made up the sample. Thirty-four entered prenatal care prior to the 14th week of gestation and 12 sought care after the 27th week. Data were collected by interview and analyzed by developing categories related to self-care. The authors compared the two groups by reporting frequency of similar responses within developed categories.

Categories of self-care activities that emerged for both groups included nutrition, rest, exercise, abstinence from addictive substances, and physical safety. Nutritional issues included eating healthy food and fear of gaining too much or too little weight. Safety concerns centered on avoiding strenuous sports. The groups provided similar responses, but showed some differences in frequency of responses. The primary differences involved the time and source of self-care information about diet, exercise, rest, and other pregnancy related concerns and whether the group identified prenatal care as a self-care activity. The early group reported receiving pregnancy related self-care information from formal prenatal classes and from educational materials, while the late-entering group obtained information through informal channels, such as from mothers or sisters. The late group did not perceive prenatal care as a self-care activity while the early group did.

Clinical Application of Study

Having bar graphs comparing the results of the two groups would have been helpful to readers. Because delay in obtaining care may increase risk during a teen pregnancy, nurses who have contact with pregnant adolescents might focus on early prenatal care as a self-care activity.

SOURCE: Lee S, Grubbs L: A comparison of self-reported self-care practices of pregnant adolescents. *Nurse Practitioner* 1993; 18(9):25.

---

may accompany her daughter to the clinic. The nurse needs to assess the disharmony that is occurring and explain the process of adaptation that follows.

Mothers frequently feel guilty about their daughters' pregnancies. They wonder what they have done wrong and feel they have been inadequate parents. They are also angry because they are concerned about themselves. Just as their children are growing up and they see a new sense of freedom coming, they now have the responsibility of helping their daughters deal with a crisis. They may also feel angry at "being made a grandmother," perhaps at a young age. Once these reactions are dealt with, a calmer atmosphere generally develops, which supports necessary decision making. The mother may become involved in decision making regarding abortion, adoption, marriage, and dealing with the father-to-be and his family. Family input in these matters is important in the adolescent's decision making.

As the pregnancy progresses, the mother begins to take on the grandmother role. She may begin to buy presents for the newborn and plan for the future. She may participate in prenatal care and classes and can be an excellent support system for her daughter. She should be encouraged to participate if the mother-daughter relationship is positive. If the baby's father is involved in the pregnancy, he and the pregnant teen's mother may be able to work together to support the teenage mother. The mother should be updated on obstetric practice to clarify any misconceptions she might have. During labor and birth, the mother will be a key figure for her daughter. Drawing on her own experience, she can offer reassurance and instill confidence in the adolescent.

The last stages of a mother's acceptance occur after her daughter's child is born. As the mother attempts to integrate her role of grandmother, an initial blurring of roles occurs. The grandmother now sees her daughter as a mother, and the daughter begins to identify herself as a mother. Role confusion may develop and sometimes continues for years—the new grandmother may essentially do all the mothering and caretaking activities for the newborn while her daughter remains only a daughter and becomes a sibling of her newborn. The degree of role confusion is influenced by the age and maturity of the adolescent mother. Until the daughter is able to internalize her role as mother, her own mother will be unable to identify completely as a grandmother.

This new role development is clouded by the young woman's struggle to complete her tasks of adolescence. The wise mother will gently encourage a balance between helping her daughter learn to be a parent and allowing her daughter to complete the tasks of adolescence. As her daughter becomes more confident in the role of parent, the mother can gradually encourage more independence for the daughter.

The pregnant adolescent must also deal with the reactions of siblings and other family members and friends who form her support network. Their concern and caring can be a significant factor in her ability to deal with the pregnancy and make needed decisions. If the father of the child is involved, he too can be a source of support for the young woman. Those teens who decide not to tell anyone of the pregnancy face a stressful period without normal support systems. This increases the crisis nature of the situation unless the young woman is able to develop a new support network during the pregnancy.

Nursing Assessment

The nurse needs to establish a data base to plan interventions for the adolescent mother-to-be. Areas of assessment include a history of family and personal physical health, developmental level and impact of pregnancy, and a thorough assessment of emotional and financial support. The nurse also assesses the family and social support network and the father's degree of involvement in the pregnancy.

Physical Health

As with all pregnant women, it is important prenatally to have information on general physical health. This may be the first time many adolescents have ever provided a health history. The nurse may find it helpful to ask very specific questions and give examples if the young woman appears confused about a question.

The following areas should be assessed:

- Family and personal health history
- Medical history
- Menstrual history
- Obstetric and gynecologic history
- Substance abuse history

Developmental Level and the Impact of Pregnancy

It is important to assess the maturational level of each individual. Assessment of the adolescent's development level and the impact of pregnancy is reflected in the degree of recognition of the realities and responsibilities involved in teenage pregnancy and parenting (Table 16–3). The mother's self-concept (including body image), her relationship with the significant adults in her life, her attitude toward her pregnancy, and her coping methods in the situation are just a few of the significant factors that need to be assessed.

Support Systems

The socioeconomic status of the pregnant adolescent often places the baby at risk throughout life, beginning with conception. It is essential also to assess family and social support systems as well as the extent of financial support available.

Adolescent life-styles and support systems vary tremendously. It is imperative that the interdisciplinary health team have information regarding the expectant adolescents' feelings and perceptions about themselves, their sexuality, and the coming baby; their knowledge of, attitude toward, and anticipated ability to care for and support the infant; and their maturational level and needs.

Nursing Diagnosis

The nursing diagnoses that are applicable to any pregnant woman apply to the pregnant adolescent. Other nursing diagnoses are influenced by the adolescent's age, support systems, socioeconomic situation, health, and maturity. Examples of nursing diagnoses more specific to the pregnant adolescent may include the following:

- Altered nutrition: Less than body requirements related to poor eating habits.

- Self-esteem disturbance related to unanticipated pregnancy.

Nursing Plan and Implementation

Early, thorough prenatal care is the strongest and most critical determinant for reducing risk for the adolescent mother and her newborn. The nurse needs to understand the special needs of the adolescent mother to meet this challenge successfully. See Nursing Care Plan: Unplanned Adolescent Pregnancy on page 404.

Issue of Confidentiality

Most states in the United States have passed legislation that confirms the right of some minors to assume the rights of adults. These adolescents are referred to as **emancipated minors.** An adolescent may be considered emancipated if he or she is self-supporting and living away from home, married, pregnant, a parent, or in the military service (Cohn 1991). The pregnant adolescent, even if very young, is considered emancipated and has the right and responsibility to consent to health care for herself and later for her child. She is entitled to respect and confidentiality in her dealings with health care providers (Reedy 1991). Only with her agreement can other adults, including her parents, be included in communication.

Development of a Trusting Relationship with the Pregnant Adolescent

The nurse needs to be attentive to the special problems of adolescents. The first visit to the clinic or office may be fraught with extreme anxiety on the part of the young woman. Not only will she be nervous because of her situation, but also this may well be her first exposure to the

health care system since early childhood. Making this first experience as positive as possible for the young woman will encourage her cooperation in returning for follow-up care and ensure a favorable attitude toward the importance of health care whether she chooses to terminate or maintain the pregnancy.

Depending on how young the adolescent is, this may be her first pelvic examination, an anxiety-provoking experience for any woman. The nurse can help provide a thorough explanation of the procedure. A gentle and thoughtful examination technique will help the young woman to relax. A mirror is helpful in allowing the client to see her cervix, educating her about her anatomy, and giving her a part in the exam.

Developing a trusting relationship with the pregnant adolescent is essential. Honesty and respect for the individual and a caring attitude promote self-esteem. As the nurse develops a trusting relationship with the young woman, his or her attitudes about self-care and responsibility affect the adolescent's maturation process.

Critical Thinking Question

Imagine that you are a nurse in a clinic caring for a young adolescent who recently learned that she is pregnant and is trying to decide what to do. What are your own beliefs about adolescent pregnancy, abortion, relinquishment, and single parenting? How would you approach your discussion of choices with the adolescent?

Promotion of Self-Esteem and Problem-Solving Skills

The nurse assists the adolescent in her decision-making and problem-solving skills so that she may proceed with her developmental tasks and begin to assume responsibility for her life as well as her newborn's life. An overview of what the young woman will experience over the prenatal course, along with thorough explanations and rationale for each procedure as it occurs, will foster the adolescent's understanding and give her some measure of control. Actively involving the young woman in her care will give her a sense of participation and responsibility (Figure 16–1).

Adolescents tend to be egocentric, and even the realization that their health and habits affect the fetus may not be regarded as important by them. It is often helpful to emphasize the effects of these practices on the client herself. Because of their immature cognitive development, adolescents need help in problem solving, in visualizing themselves in the future, and in imagining what the consequences of their actions might be. In addition the nurse needs to understand that the developmental tasks of pregnancy must be met by the adolescent in addition to the stage-related developmental tasks she is already coping with. Table 16–3 identifies the developmental tasks of pregnancy and the early adolescent's response to pregnancy, with implications for nursing care.

Promotion of Physical Well-Being

Baseline weight and blood pressure measurements will be valuable in assessing weight gain and predisposition to pregnancy-induced hypertension. The adolescent may be encouraged to take part in her care by measuring and recording her weight. The nurse may use this time as an opportunity for assisting the young woman in problem solving: "Have I gained too much or too little weight?" "What influence does my diet have on my weight?" "How can I change my eating habits?"

Another way to introduce the subject of nutrition is during measurement of baseline and subsequent hemoglobin and hematocrit values. Because the adolescent is at risk for anemia, she will need education regarding the importance of iron in her diet. A nutritional consultation is indicated for all adolescents. Group classes are helpful because peer pressure is strong among this age group. If the expense of proper food is an issue, the nurse or nutritionist should refer the teen to available community resources.

The nurse needs to keep in mind that adolescents may fear laboratory tests, which can evoke early child-

hood memories of being "stuck" with needles or hurt. Explanations help ease nerves, and coordination of services will avoid multiple venous punctures.

Pregnancy-induced hypertension represents the most prevalent medical complication of pregnant adolescents. Blood pressure readings of 140/90 mm Hg are not acceptable as the determinant of PIH in adolescents. Women aged 14 to 20 years without evidence of high blood pressure usually have diastolic readings between 50 and 66 mm Hg. Gradual increases from the prepregnant diastolic readings, along with excessive weight gain, must be evaluated as precursors to PIH. This is one reason why early prenatal care is vital to management of the adolescent.

Adolescents have an increased incidence of sexually transmitted diseases (STDs). The initial prenatal examination should include gonococcal and chlamydial cultures and wet prep for *Candida*, *Trichomonas*, and *Gardnerella*. Tests for syphilis should also be done. Education about STDs is important, as is careful observation of herpetic lesions or other symptoms throughout the young woman's pregnancy. Research indicates that although today's teens are knowledgeable about AIDS, they know much less about other STDs, especially with regard to symptoms and risk reduction (Witwer 1990). If the adolescent's history indicates that she is at increased risk for HIV, she should be given information about it and offered HIV screening.

Substance abuse should also be discussed with adolescents. It is important to review the risks associated with the use of tobacco, caffeine, drugs, and alcohol. The young woman should be aware of the effects of these substances on her development as well as on the development of the fetus.

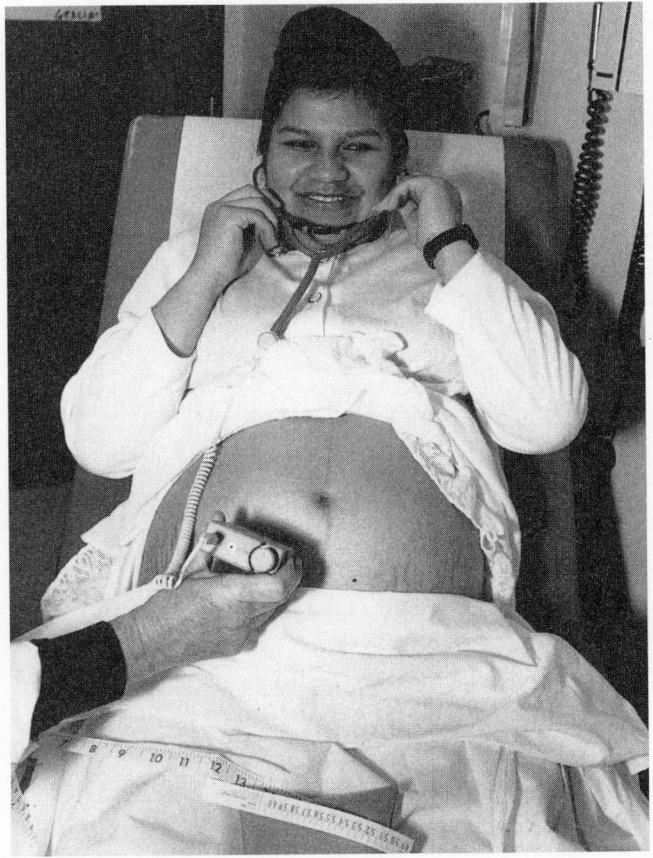

FIGURE 16-1 The nurse provides this young mother with an opportunity to listen to her baby's heartbeat.

Text continues on page 406

UNPLANNED ADOLESCENT PREGNANCY

Nursing Assessment

Nursing History

1. Age
2. Subjective symptoms of pregnancy, LMP, gravida, parity, and menstrual history
3. Her perception of her pregnancy and her anxiety level
4. Family structure/support system

Physical Examination

1. Review results of pelvic examination to assess uterine changes associated with pregnancy.

Diagnostic Studies

1. Urine hCG
2. Other prenatal lab work as appropriate

NURSING DIAGNOSIS: Anxiety related to fear of parental reaction secondary to unplanned adolescent pregnancy

EXPECTED OUTCOME: Adolescent will identify her support system and demonstrate reduction in anxiety.

Nursing Interventions	Rationale
Encourage the adolescent to express her own feelings and concerns, including her perception regarding parental response to the pregnancy as well as reaction of sexual partner.	Helps to identify specific areas where guidance in problem solving is needed. Her age as well as her relationship with her parents and her sexual partner are important factors in helping her identify a support system.
Assess relationship with sexual partner and explore possible consequences of contacting him.	The adolescent may want her sexual partner involved in decision making but may be concerned about parental reaction to his involvement.
If the adolescent is evasive and uncomfortable about discussing sexual partner, investigate the possibility of incest and/or other situations of forced sex.	Incest as a cause of pregnancy is possible, especially in very young adolescents. If client was forced to have intercourse, additional counseling will be critical.
In those states where appropriate, reassure client that decision to share news of pregnancy with parents is hers.	Most states do not require parental notification of pregnancy.
Encourage client to identify a support system to help her make decisions about how to deal with her unplanned pregnancy.	Important for adolescent to have support from significant individuals in her life in making decisions and in followthrough.

OUTCOME MET IF:

- Adolescent expresses her feelings and concerns regarding the pregnancy.
- Adolescent verbalizes her understanding of confidentiality regarding her pregnancy.
- Adolescent verbalizes a plan to tell or not to tell her parents of the pregnancy.
- Adolescent identifies a support system to help her in decision making.
- Adolescent verbalizes a decision regarding involvement of the baby's father.
- Adolescent demonstrates decreased anxiety.

NURSING DIAGNOSIS: Anxiety related to decisional conflict secondary to unplanned pregnancy

EXPECTED OUTCOME: Adolescent will understand the alternatives in dealing with her unplanned pregnancy.

Nursing Interventions	Rationale
If adolescent is accompanied by a parent or boyfriend, visit with her initially by herself to assess her concerns without the presence of another person.	This may be the only way to find out how the adolescent feels and to discuss any special concerns she has. Because incest is a concern in the early adolescent, it is important to explore family relationships.
Present the alternatives: terminating the pregnancy, maintaining the pregnancy, and choosing whether or not to parent.	Many adolescents are not aware of all the alternatives available in dealing with an unplanned pregnancy. Health care providers do not impose their own values on their clients. If necessary, refer client to a more objective counselor.
Encourage her to share her feelings about each alternative and projected consequences as it relates to her situation in life.	It is important to assess the client's perception of projected consequences in her own life in order to help her do more effective problem solving in arriving at a

UNPLANNED ADOLESCENT PREGNANCY *continued*

Identify agency resources with help for each of the alternatives.

decision most comfortable for her. In addition her beliefs about abortion may be in conflict with her parents and/or boyfriend.

Many adolescents are unaware of resources available to support them in the choices they may make, especially if they decide to maintain their pregnancy and give the baby up for adoption.

OUTCOME MET IF:

- Adolescent is able to discuss all options and the consequences of each in regard to the pregnancy.
- Adolescent is able to identify appropriate resources for each alternative.

NURSING DIAGNOSIS: Knowledge deficit related to lack of information about voluntary interruption of pregnancy (VIP)

EXPECTED OUTCOME: The adolescent is able to discuss termination of pregnancy in an informed manner.

Nursing Interventions	Rationale
Assess client's perceptions and knowledge about VIP.	Clients frequently have many misconceptions about induced abortions. It is important to clarify misconceptions before explaining procedure.
Explain what to expect with an abortion done in the first trimester, including procedure, where it is done, what most women experience.	The adolescent is usually unaware of what is actually involved with an abortion, including physical consequences and what to expect regarding the products of conception in the first trimester.
Discuss how second-trimester abortions differ.	Adolescent may not realize that all factors related to induced abortion change as pregnancy progresses.
Discuss cost considerations related to an abortion.	Adolescents often have unrealistic ideas about health costs. Cost considerations may be an important factor in the adolescent's decision to share news of pregnancy with parents if parental notification is not required by state law.
Explain state law requirements related to parental notification with induced abortion.	Many states require parental notification but not parental consent for a termination of a pregnancy.
Discuss with adolescent the importance of her feeling comfortable with her final decision, stressing that some ambivalence would be experienced with any of the decisions. In addition, if she is leaning toward termination of the pregnancy, inform the adolescent that it is safest when done as early in the pregnancy as possible.	Most adolescents are unaware of the limited time frame in which a first-trimester abortion can be done, especially if they have delayed confirmation of their pregnancy. If delayed too long, procedure for a first-trimester abortion may not be usable.
Encourage adolescent to examine closely her own values and beliefs about abortion.	Examination of her beliefs is important for the adolescent to be comfortable with her decision. The beliefs of her parents or peers may be in conflict with her own beliefs.

OUTCOME MET IF:

- Adolescent verbalizes understanding of the termination procedure in first and second trimester of a pregnancy.
- Adolescent discusses cost associated with termination of a pregnancy.
- Adolescent verbalizes understanding of state laws in regard to parental notification.
- Adolescent verbalizes positive feelings in regard to decision to terminate pregnancy.

Essential Nursing Activities to Achieve Outcomes

1. Begin establishing rapport with the adolescent.
2. Assess the adolescent's knowledge in regard to options, community resources available, understanding of state laws, and financial resources available.
3. Assess the adolescent's support system, including parental involvement, partner involvement, and other support.
4. Provide information regarding the pregnancy, options, and available resources with appropriate contacts.
5. Assess the adolescent's anxiety level.
6. Provide an opportunity for the adolescent to express concerns and apprehensions regarding the pregnancy.
7. Provide a nonthreatening atmosphere to allow for questions and expression of feelings.

Ongoing care should include the same assessments that the older woman receives. Special attention should be paid to evaluating fetal growth by determining when quickening occurs and by measuring fundal height, fetal heart tones, and fetal movement. The corresponding dates of auscultating fetal heart tones with the date of last menstrual period and quickening can be helpful in determining correct estimates of time of birth. If there is a question of size-date discrepancy by 2 cm either way, an ultrasound is warranted to establish fetal age so that instances of IUGR may be diagnosed and treated early.

Promotion of Family Adaptation

The nurse assesses the family situation during the first prenatal visit and finds out the level of involvement the adolescent desires from each of her family members and the father of the child as well as her perception of their present support. A sensitive approach to daughter-mother relationships helps motivate their communication. If the mother and daughter agree, the mother should be included in the client's care. Encouraging the mother to become part of the maternity team, to join grandmother crisis support groups, and to obtain counseling aids the mother in adapting to her role and in supporting her daughter.

The nurse should also help the mother assess her daughter's needs and assist her in meeting them. Some adolescents become more dependent during pregnancy, and some become more independent. The mother can ease and encourage her daughter's self-growth by understanding how best to respond and support the adolescent.

The adolescent's relationship with her father will also be affected by the pregnancy. The nurse can provide information to the father and encourage his involvement to the degree that is acceptable for both daughter and father.

Finally, the father of the adolescent's infant should not be forgotten in promoting the family's adaptation to the pregnancy (Humenick et al 1991). He should be included to the extent that he wishes and that is acceptable to the teenage mother.

Facilitation of Prenatal Education

Prenatal education programs should include the clinic and the school system (Figure 16–2). Many adolescents cite the school as the preferred agency for education during pregnancy and early parenting. School systems are currently attempting to meet this need in a variety of ways. The most effective method appears to be mainstreaming the pregnant adolescent in academic classes with her peers and adding classes appropriate to her needs during pregnancy and initial parenting experiences. Classes about growth and development beginning with the newborn and early infancy can help teenage parents have more realistic expectations of their infants and may help decrease child abuse. Mainstreaming pregnant

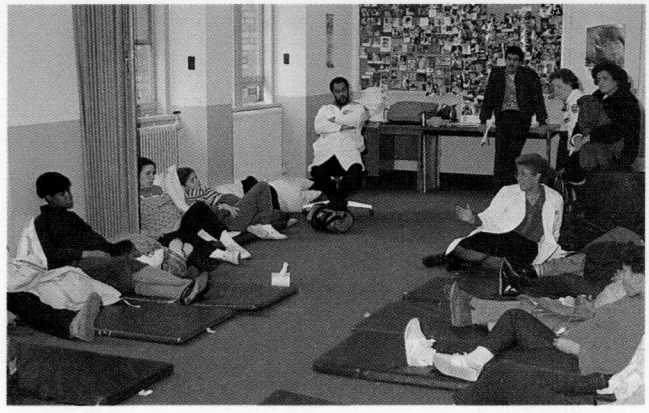

FIGURE 16-2 Young adolescents may benefit from prenatal classes designed for them.

adolescents in school is also an ideal way to help them complete their education while learning the skills they need to cope with childbearing and parenting. Vocational guidance in this setting is also most beneficial to their future.

Regardless of the sponsorship or setting of prenatal classes for pregnant teenagers and adolescent fathers, the developmental tasks of the adolescent need to be considered. For example, the methods of teaching this age group should be somewhat different from regular prenatal classes. The younger adolescent tends to be a more concrete thinker than the older and more mature pregnant adult. Increased use of audiovisuals that are appropriate to their social situation and age is helpful. More demonstrations may be required, and they need to be simple and direct.

Areas that might be included in prenatal classes are anatomy and physiology, sex education, exercises for pregnancy and postpartum, maternal and infant nutrition, growth and development of the fetus, labor and birth, family planning, and infant development. Adolescents may want to participate in the teaching of these classes and should be encouraged to do so. Peer support and friendships can blossom among these young women, helping them all to mature.

The clinic can offer rap sessions, pamphlets, or films in the waiting room. Giving the clients something to do while they wait for their appointments may encourage them to return and also may help them learn. Decorating the clinic with attractive educational posters and creating an informal atmosphere establishes an environment where adolescents feel free to interact with professionals.

Ideally, prenatal classes for the adolescent are oriented to more than just pregnancy, childbirth, and immediate newborn care. The goals of many of these classes are expanding to deal with more complex social issues that result from adolescent pregnancies. A multidisciplinary team approach is important in planning and implementing these classes. Goals for many of these classes now include promoting self-esteem; helping participants identify the problems and conflicts of teenage parenting and how to prepare for them; educating participants about sexuality, relationships, and contraception to deter unwanted pregnancies; teaching participants parenting skills; providing information about community resources and other resources available to teenage parents; and helping participants develop more adaptive coping skills.

Evaluation

Anticipated outcomes of nursing care include:

- A trusting relationship is established with the pregnant adolescent.

- The adolescent is able to use her problem-solving abilities to make appropriate choices.

- The adolescent complies with the recommendations of the health care team and receives effective health care throughout her pregnancy and birth and during the postpartum period.

- The adolescent, her partner (if he is involved), and their families are able to cope successfully with the effects of the pregnancy.

- The adolescent is knowledgeable about pregnancy and makes appropriate health care choices.

- The adolescent demonstrates developmental and pregnancy progression within established normal parameters.

- The adolescent develops skills in child care and parenting.

CARE OF THE EXPECTANT COUPLE OVER 35

Today an increasing number of women are choosing to have their first baby after age 35. In fact the rate of first births to women between the ages of 35 and 39 more than doubled between 1980 and 1992 in the United States. For women between the ages of 40 and 44, the birth rate increased by 40% during the same period (US Bureau of the Census 1993). Many factors contribute to this trend, including the following:

- Ability of women to choose to delay childbirth because of the availability of effective birth control methods

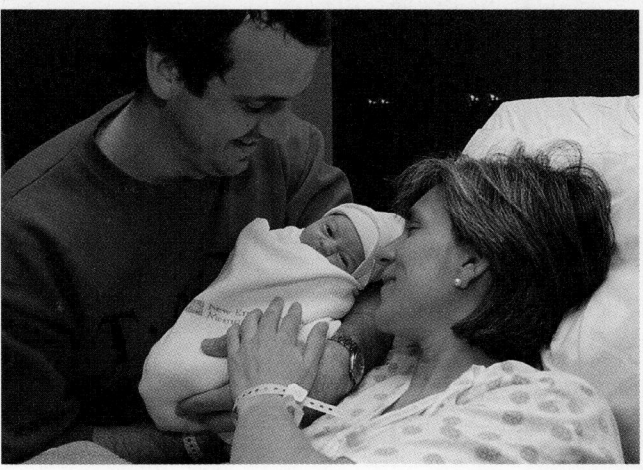

FIGURE 16-3 For many older couples the decision to have a child may be very rewarding.

- A changed emphasis on the maternal role because of the women's liberation movement and its stress on expanded roles for women

- The desire of women to delay pregnancy until they have obtained advanced education and established themselves professionally

- The reality that some women are older when they first consider childbirth because of the increased incidence of later marriage and second marriage

- The higher cost of living and need for two salaries, which cause some young couples to delay childbearing until they are more secure financially

- The increased number of women in this older age group coupled with the fact that the number of women expected to conceive at a younger age is decreasing, resulting in an increased number of women over age 35 who are conceiving (Maroulis 1993)

- The increased availability of specialized fertilization procedures, which offers opportunities for women who had previously been considered infertile

There are advantages to having a first baby after the age of 35. Single women or couples who delay childbearing until they are older tend to be well educated and financially secure. Usually their decision to have a baby was deliberately and thoughtfully made. Given their greater life experiences, they are much more aware of the realities of having a child and what it means to have a baby at their age (Figure 16-3). Many of the women have experienced fulfillment in their careers and feel secure enough to take on the added responsibility of a child. Some women are ready to make a change in their lives, desiring to stay home with a new baby. Those who plan to continue working are able to afford good child care.

Medical Risks

Historically, medical professionals considered women who were over 30 at the time of their first pregnancy, and especially those who were 35 or older, at higher risk for maternal or fetal complications than younger women. This age-related concern began to change during the 1980s when studies comparing healthy pregnant women over 35 years of age with healthy younger pregnant women did not confirm these beliefs. These studies suggest that preexisting medical problems such as hypertension or diabetes play a more significant role than age in maternal well-being and outcome of pregnancy (Mansfield 1986; Redwine 1988).

A study using a sample composed of private clients who were predominantly White, married, and college educated found an increased incidence of PIH, gestational diabetes, abruptio placentae, gestational bleeding, and placenta previa in women over age 35. Although the older mothers were more likely to have specific complications during the antepartal and intrapartal periods, the rate of poor neonatal outcome was not increased appreciably over that of mothers between ages 20 and 29 (Berkowitz et al 1990). Another study of White first-born infants suggests a modest increase of low birth weight and preterm birth with increase in maternal age when high-risk factors were not present (Aldous & Edmonson 1993).

Fibroid tumors (leiomyoma) occur with greater frequency in women over age 35. Fibroids located inside the uterus may interfere when they increase in size, which can occur as a result of estrogen stimulation during pregnancy. This increased size can lead to malpresentations, premature labor, dystocia, or problems in the third stage of labor. Fibroid tumors may also increase the incidence of early postpartum hemorrhage if they prevent the uterus from contracting completely after childbirth.

The risk of conceiving a child with Down syndrome does increase with age, especially over age 35 (see Table 7–10). The use of amniocentesis or chorionic villus sampling (CVS) is routinely offered to all women over age 35 to permit the early detection of several chromosomal abnormalities including Down syndrome.

The incidence of cesarean births also rises sharply after the age of 35. This practice may occur because of obstetricians' preset expectations of higher risk with women they may refer to as an "elderly primipara" and concern about the increased value of this long-awaited child. Many physicians do not want to take any chances with the outcome of pregnancy in this age group. The research of Berkowitz et al (1990) supports this possibility.

Special Concerns of the Expectant Couple Over 35

No matter what their age, most expectant couples have concerns regarding the well-being of the fetus and their ability to parent. The older couple has additional concerns related to their age, especially the closer they are to 40. Some couples are concerned about whether they will have enough energy to care for a new baby. Of greater concern is their ability to deal with the needs of the child in 10 years when they too are 10 years older.

The financial concerns of the older couple are usually different from those of the younger couple. The older couple is generally more financially secure than the younger couple. However, when their "baby" is ready for college, the older couple may be close to retirement, when they might not have the means to provide for their child.

While considering their financial future and future retirement, the older couple may be forced to face their own mortality. Certainly this is not uncommon in midlife, but instead of confronting this issue at 40 to 45 years of age or later, the older expectant couple may confront the issue several years earlier as they consider what will happen as their child grows.

Couples who choose to delay childbearing often have friends who have made similar choices, so they have a support network available. The older couple facing pregnancy following a late or second marriage or after therapy for infertility may find themselves somewhat isolated socially. They may feel "different" because they are often the only couple in their peer group expecting their first baby. In fact many of their peers are likely to be parents of adolescents or young adults and may be grandparents as well.

The response of older couples who already have children to learning that the woman is pregnant may vary greatly depending on whether the pregnancy was planned or unexpected. Other factors influencing their response include the attitudes of their children, family, and friends to the pregnancy; the impact on their life-style; and the financial implications of having another child. Sometimes couples who had previously been married to other mates will choose to have a child together. The concept of **blended family** applies to situations in which "her" children, "his" children, and "their" children come together as a new family group.

Health care professionals may treat the older expectant couple differently than they would a younger couple. Older women may be asked to submit to more medical procedures, such as amniocentesis and ultrasound, than younger women. An older woman may be prevented from using a birthing room or birthing center even if she is healthy because her age is considered to put her at risk.

The woman who has delayed pregnancy may be concerned about the limited amount of time that she has to bear children. When pregnancy does not occur as quickly as she hoped, the older woman may become increasingly anxious as time slips away on her "biological clock." When an older woman becomes pregnant but experiences a spontaneous abortion, her grief for the loss of her unborn child is exacerbated by her anxiety about her ability to conceive again in the time remaining to her.

Nursing Assessment

In working with a woman in her 30s or 40s who is pregnant the nurse makes the same assessments as are appropriate in caring for any woman who is pregnant. These include assessment of physical status, the woman's understanding of pregnancy and the changes that accompany it, any health teaching needs that exist, the degree of support the woman has available to her, and her knowledge of infant care. In addition the nurse explores the woman's and her partner's attitudes about the pregnancy and their expectations of the impact a baby will have on their lives.

Nursing Diagnosis

The nursing diagnoses that are applicable to any pregnant woman apply to the pregnant woman who is over the age of 35. Examples of other nursing diagnoses that may apply include the following:

- Decisional conflict related to unexpected pregnancy
- Impaired social interaction related to unplanned pregnancy

Nursing Plan and Implementation

Once an older couple has made the decision to have a child, it is the nurse's responsibility to respect and support the couple in this decision. As with any client, risks need to be discussed, concerns need to be identified, and strengths need to be promoted. The woman's age should not be made an issue. To promote a sense of well-being, the nurse should treat the pregnancy as "normal" unless specific health risks are identified. See Nursing Care Plan: Genetic Counseling for the Older Pregnant Woman on page 410.

As the pregnancy continues, the nurse should identify and discuss concerns the woman may have related to her age or to specific health problems. The older woman who has made a conscious decision to become pregnant often has carefully thought through potential problems and may actually have fewer concerns than a younger woman or one with an unplanned pregnancy.

Childbirth education classes are important in promoting adaptation to the event of childbirth for expectant couples of any age. However, older expectant couples, who are still in the minority, often feel uncomfortable in classes where the majority of participants are much younger. Because of the differences in age and life experiences, many of the needs of the older couple may not be met in the class. The nurse teaching a childbirth education class should try to anticipate the informational needs of the older couple. At the same time the nurse should not make the couple feel any more uncomfortable by drawing attention to their age. As the number of expectant older couples increases, the nurse may find it useful to offer an "over 30" childbirth education class to accommodate the specific needs of older couples. Such classes are being developed in some larger urban areas.

Women who are over 35 years of age and having their first baby tend to be better educated than other health care consumers. These clients frequently know the kind of care and services they want and are assertive in their interactions with the health care system. The nurse should neither be intimidated by these individuals nor assume that anticipatory guidance and support are not needed. Instead the nurse should support the couple's strengths and be sensitive to their individual needs.

Provision of Support if Amniocentesis Is Advised

In working with older expectant couples the nurse needs to be sensitive to their special needs. A particularly difficult issue these couples face is the possibility of bearing an unhealthy child. Because of the risk of Down syndrome in these families, amniocentesis is encouraged. Chorionic villus sampling may also be suggested if available in the area. The decision to have amniocentesis can be difficult to make merely on the basis of its possible risks to the fetus. But that becomes almost a minor concern when the couple thinks of the implications of the possible findings of Down syndrome or other chromosomal abnormalities. The finding of abnormalities means that the couple may be faced with an even more difficult decision about continuing the pregnancy.

A couple's decision to have amniocentesis is usually related to their beliefs and attitudes about abortion. Amniocentesis is usually not even considered by couples who are strongly opposed to abortion for any reason. Health professionals must respect their decision and take a nonjudgmental approach to their continued care.

The decision to have an abortion is a painful one even when couples are not opposed to abortion on political or philosophic grounds. Even though the couple may believe that terminating a high-risk pregnancy is right for their family, they may feel a great deal of ambivalence about amniocentesis. If the results are such that the couple elects to have an abortion, they will feel much grief for their loss.

Many health professionals assume that the couple who agrees to amniocentesis will also elect to have an abortion if Down syndrome or another condition is diagnosed. This is not necessarily the case. Some couples choose not to have an abortion after being informed that their unborn child has genetic abnormalities.

For the couple who agrees to amniocentesis the first few months of pregnancy are a difficult time. Amniocentesis cannot be done until 14 weeks of pregnancy, and the chromosomal studies take roughly 2 weeks to complete. Their fear that the fetus is at risk may delay the successful completion of the psychologic tasks of early pregnancy.

GENETIC COUNSELING FOR THE OLDER PREGNANT WOMAN

Nursing Assessment

Nursing History
1. Age
2. Gravida
3. Parity
4. LMP
5. Religious preference

Physical Examination
1. Pelvic examination to assess uterine changes associated with pregnancy

Diagnostic Studies
1. Urine hCG
2. Other prenatal laboratory work as appropriate

NURSING DIAGNOSIS: Knowledge deficit related to lack of information about increase in genetic risks in the older pregnant woman

EXPECTED OUTCOME: Woman/family will obtain all information regarding pregnancy in the woman over 35 years of age.

Nursing Interventions	Rationale
Explain increased risk of Down syndrome after age 35.	Cannot assume that all clients are aware of this risk.
Share statistics that demonstrate incidence of Down syndrome in different age groups and how incidence increases at 35 and dramatically increases over age 40.	Helps woman/family develop a more realistic perspective of the increased risk with age.
Discuss realities of having a Down syndrome baby and lifelong prognosis for adults with Down syndrome.	Important for woman/family to understand lifelong implications and variations in severity of problems.
Assess for concerns and questions. Clarify as appropriate.	May uncover additional questions or concerns of the woman/family.

OUTCOME MET IF:
- Woman/family can describe increased risk of Down syndrome with pregnancy over the ages of 35 and 40.
- Woman/family can discuss problems and strengths related to individuals with Down syndrome and possible consequences related to their decision.
- Woman/family verbalize that all questions have been answered to their satisfaction at this time.

NURSING DIAGNOSIS: Knowledge deficit related to lack of information about amniocentesis

EXPECTED OUTCOME: Woman/family will have accurate information related to amniocentesis.

Nursing Interventions	Rationale
Assess woman/family's knowledge or ideas related to amniocentesis.	Woman/family may have no knowledge of amniocentesis or may have misconceptions that increase their anxiety and fear about the procedure.
Clarify misconceptions about procedure with factual information.	Difficult for woman/family to listen if concerns and misconceptions are not addressed initially.
Explain each step of the procedure and its effect on the mother and the fetus.	Most couples do not know what to expect and have fears about risks to mother and fetus.
Assess for further questions or concerns.	New questions and concerns may arise as procedure is explained.

OUTCOME MET IF:
- Woman/family verbalizes understanding of what information the amniocentesis can provide, the risks and benefits of having an amniocentesis, and the amniocentesis procedure.

Essential Nursing Activities to Achieve Outcomes

Assess the woman/family's knowledge regarding
1. Risks of pregnancy in woman over the age of 35
2. Statistics on possible Down syndrome pregnancy
3. Implications of birth of a baby with Down syndrome
4. The risks, benefits, and procedure of an amniocentesis

The nurse can support couples who decide to have amniocentesis in several ways:

- The nurse should make sure that the couple is aware of the risks of amniocentesis and why it is being performed.

- The nurse who is present during the amniocentesis procedure can offer comfort and emotional support to the expectant woman. The nurse can also provide information about the procedure as it is being performed.

- The nurse can facilitate a support group for women during the difficult waiting period between the procedure and the results.

- If the results indicate that the fetus has Down syndrome or another genetic abnormality, the nurse can ensure that the couple has complete information about the condition, its range of possible manifestations, and its developmental implications.

- The nurse can support the couple in their decision about continuing or terminating the pregnancy. It is essential that the nurse and other health professionals involved with the couple not impose their philosophic or political beliefs about abortion on the couple. The decision is the couple's, and it should be based on their belief system and a nonbiased presentation of risks and choices from care givers.

Evaluation

Anticipated outcomes of nursing care include:

- The woman and her partner are knowledgeable about the pregnancy and make appropriate health care choices.

- The expectant couple (and their children) are able to cope successfully with the pregnancy and its implications for the future.

- The woman receives effective health care throughout her pregnancy and during birth and the postpartum period.

- The woman and her partner develop skills in child care and parenting as necessary.

KEY CONCEPTS

Many factors contribute to the increase in the teenage pregnancy rate, including earlier onset of menarche, earlier age of first sexual intercourse, lack of knowledge related to conception, lack of easy access to contraception, and lessened stigma associated with adolescent pregnancy in some populations.

Factors affecting an adolescent's response to pregnancy include her degree of achievement of the developmental tasks of adolescence (which can be closely associated with age), as well as cultural, religious, and socioeconomic factors.

The adolescent father who wants to be involved is often overlooked by health care providers. If he assumes accountability, however, he is also at increased risk for social and economic problems.

Often the adolescent has little understanding of pregnancy, childbirth, or parenting. Consequently, education is a primary responsibility of the nurse.

Childbirth among women over 35 is becoming increasingly common. It poses fewer health risks than previously believed and offers advantages for the woman or couple who make the choice.

A major risk for the older expectant couple relates to the increased incidence of Down syndrome in children born to women over age 35 or 40. Amniocentesis can provide information as to whether the fetus has Down syndrome. The couple can then decide whether they wish to continue the pregnancy.

REFERENCES

Abma JC, Mott FL: Substance use and prenatal care during pregnancy among young women. *Fam Plan Perspectives* May/June 1991; 23:117.

Adolescent unintended pregnancy: The scope of the problem. *Contracep Rep* May 1994; 5(2):4.

Aldous MB, Edmonson MB: Maternal age at first childbirth and risk of low birth weight and preterm delivery in Washington state. *JAMA* December 1993; 270:2574.

Bachrach CA, Stolley KS, London KA: Relinquishment of premarital births: Evidence from national survey data. *Fam Plan Perspectives* January/February 1992; 24:27.

Berkowitz GS et al: Delayed childbearing and the outcome of pregnancy. *N Engl J Med* March 1990; 322:659.

Blankson ML et al: Health behavior and outcomes in sequential pregnancies of black and white adolescents. *JAMA* March 1993; 269:1401.

Boyer D, Fine D: Sexual abuse as a factor in adolescent pregnancy and child maltreatment. *Fam Plan Perspectives* January/February 1992; 24:4.

Burnhill MS: Adolescent pregnancy rates in the US. *Contemp OB/GYN* February 1994; 39(2):27.

Cheng TL et al: Confidentiality in health care: A survey of knowledge, perceptions and attitudes among high school students. *JAMA* 1993; 269:1404.

Children's Defense Fund: Teenage pregnancy in the Latino community factsheet. Washington, DC: Children's Defense Fund, 1991.

Cohn SD: The evolving law of adolescent health care. *NAACOG's Clin Issues Perinatal Women's Health Nurs* 1991; 2(2):201.

Crooks R, Baur K: *Our Sexuality.* Redwood City, CA: Benjamin/Cummings, 1993.

Duany L, Pittman K: *Latino Youths at a Crossroads*. Washington, DC: Children's Defense Fund, 1990.

East PL, Felice ME: Pregnancy risk among the younger sisters of pregnant and childbearing adolescents. *J Develop Behav Pediatr* April 1992; 13:128.

Fielding JE, Williams CA: Adolescent pregnancy in the United States: A review and recommendations for clinicians and research needs. *Am J Prev Med* 1991; 7:47.

Flannigan B et al: Alcohol use as a situational influence on young women's pregnancy risk-taking behaviors. *Adolescence* Spring 1990; 25:205.

Grogger J, Bronars S: The socioeconomic consequences of teenage childbearing: Findings from a natural experiment. *Fam Plan Perspectives* 1993; 25:156.

Holt JL, Johnson SD: Developmental tasks: A key to reducing teenage pregnancy. *J Pediatr Nurs* 1991; 6:191.

Horner SD, Hilde ED: A tree of impact model evaluation of consequences of repeal of the abortion law on teenage pregnancy. *J Am Acad Nurse Pract* July/September 1991; 3:116.

Howard M, Mitchell ME: Preventing teenage pregnancy: Some questions to be answered and some answers to be questioned. *Pediatr Annals* February 1993; 22:109.

Humenick SS, Wilkerson NN, Paul NW: *Adolescent Pregnancy: Nursing Perspectives on Prevention* (Original article series 17:1). White Plains, NY: March of Dimes Birth Defects Foundation, 1991.

Kahn JR, Anderson KE: Intergenerational patterns of teenage fertility. *Demography* 1992; 29:39.

Mansfield PK: *Pregnancy for Older Women*. New York: Praeger, 1986.

Maroulis G: Fertility, pregnancy, and the older woman. *Contemp OB/GYN* May 1993; 38(5):101.

Marsiglio W: Adolescent males' orientation toward paternity and contraception. *Fam Plan Perspectives* January/February 1993; 25:22.

Mosher WD, McNally JW: Contraceptive use at first premarital intercourse: United States, 1965–1988. *Fam Plan Perspectives* May/June 1991; 23:108.

National Center for Health Statistics: Advance report of final natality statistics, 1989. *Monthly Vital Stat Rep* 40 1991; 8:1.

Peckham S: Preventing unintended teenage pregnancies. *Pub Health* 1993; 107:125.

Ravoira L, Cherry AL: *Social Bonds and Teen Pregnancy*. Westport, CT: Praeger, 1992.

Redwine FO: Pregnancy in women over 35. *Female Patient* May 1988; 135:30.

Reedy NJ: The very young pregnant adolescent. *NAACOG's Clin Issues Perinatal Women's Health Nurs* 1991; 2(2):209.

Rosenheim MK, Testa MF: *Early Parenthood and Coming of Age in the 1990s*. New Brunswick, NJ: Rutgers Univ Press, 1992.

Santelli JS, Jacobson MS: Birth weight outcomes for repeat teenage pregnancy. *J Adol Health Care* May 1990; 11:240.

Steinberg L: *Adolescence*, 3rd ed. New York: McGraw-Hill, 1993.

Teens and contraception: Encouraging compliance. *Contracep Rep* 1992; 2(6):4.

US Bureau of the Census: *Statistical Abstract of the United States 1993*, 113th ed. Washington, DC: 1993.

Williams CW: *Black Teenage Mothers*. Lexington, MA: Lexington Books, 1991.

Witwer M: Survey finds teenagers know more about AIDS than about other STDs. *Fam Plan Perspectives* May/June 1990; 22:138.

CHAPTER 17

MATERNAL NUTRITION

I'm trying to be very careful about what I eat. I've had more salads and fresh fruit than I can remember. Sometimes, though, I get a "cookie attack" and indulge myself. My husband said I should eat oatmeal cookies so I could feel that my cravings were nutritionally sound!

KEY TERMS

Calorie

Folic acid

Kilocalorie

Lactase deficiency

Lacto-ovovegetarians

Lactose intolerance

Lactovegetarians

Pica

Recommended dietary allowance (RDA)

Vegans

OBJECTIVES

Identify the role of specific nutrients in the diet of the pregnant woman.

Compare nutritional needs during pregnancy, postpartum, and lactation with nonpregnant requirements.

Discuss effects of maternal nutrition on fetal outcomes.

Evaluate adequacy and pattern of weight gain during different stages of pregnancy.

Plan adequate prenatal vegetarian diets based on nutritional requirements of pregnancy.

Describe ways in which various physical, psychosocial, and cultural factors can affect nutritional intake and status.

Compare recommendations for weight gain and nutrient intakes in the pregnant adolescent with those for the mature pregnant adult.

Describe basic factors a nurse should consider when offering nutritional counseling to a pregnant adolescent.

Compare nutritional counseling issues for nursing and nonnursing mothers.

Formulate a nutritional care plan for pregnant women based on a diagnosis of nutritional problems.

woman's nutritional status prior to and during pregnancy can significantly influence her health and that of her unborn child. In most prenatal clinics and offices nurses provide nutritional counseling directly or work closely with dietitians in providing any necessary nutritional assessment and teaching.

This chapter focuses on the nutritional needs of a normal pregnant woman. Special sections consider the nutritional needs of the pregnant adolescent and the woman after birth.

Good prenatal nutrition is the result of proper eating throughout life, not just during pregnancy, although pregnancy may motivate a woman to improve poor eating habits. Many factors influence the ability of a woman to achieve good prenatal nutrition.

- *General nutritional status prior to pregnancy.* Nutritional deficits at the time of conception and the early prenatal period may influence the outcome of the pregnancy.

- *Maternal age.* An expectant adolescent must meet the nutritional needs for her own growth in addition to the nutritional needs of pregnancy. This may be especially difficult because teenagers often have nutritional deficiencies. Such deficiencies may be due to a variety of causes such as chronic dieting, frequent intake of fast foods, attempts to conceal pregnancy, and other life-style habits.

- *Maternal parity.* The mother's nutritional needs and the outcome of the pregnancy are influenced by the number of pregnancies she has had and the intervals between them.

A mother's nutritional status does affect her fetus. Factors influencing fetal well-being are interrelated, but nutrient deficiency can produce measurable effects on cell and organ growth of the developing fetus.

Fetal growth occurs in three overlapping stages: (1) growth by increase in cell number, (2) growth by increase in cell number and cell size, and (3) growth by increase in cell size alone. The nutritional problems that interfere with cell division may have permanent consequences. If the nutritional insult occurs when cells are mainly enlarging, the changes are usually reversible when normal nutrition resumes.

Growth of fetal and maternal tissues requires increased quantities of essential dietary components. Typi-

---

TABLE 17-1 Recommended Dietary Allowances (RDAs) for Nonpregnant, Pregnant, and Lactating Females, revised 1989*

Age (years) and Sex Group	Weight† kg	lb	Height† cm	in	Protein g	Vitamin A μgR‡	Vitamin D μg§	Vitamin E mgα-TE‖	Vitamin K μg	Vitamin C mg	Thiamine mg	Riboflavin mg	Niacin mg NE¶	Vitamin B_6 mg	Folate μg	Vitamin B_{12} μg	Calcium mg	Phosphorous mg	Magnesium mg	Iron mg	Zinc mg	Iodine μg	Selenium μg
Females																							
11–14	46	101	157	62	46	800	10	8	45	50	1.1	1.3	15	1.4	150	2.0	1200	1200	280	15	12	150	45
15–18	55	120	163	64	44	800	10	8	55	60	1.1	1.3	15	1.5	180	2.0	1200	1200	300	15	12	150	50
19–24	58	128	164	65	46	800	10	8	60	60	1.1	1.3	15	1.6	180	2.0	1200	1200	280	15	12	150	55
25–50	63	138	163	64	50	800	5	8	65	60	1.1	1.3	15	1.6	180	2.0	800	800	280	15	12	150	55
51+	65	143	160	63	50	800	5	8	65	60	1.0	1.2	13	1.6	180	2.0	800	800	280	10	12	150	55
Pregnant					60	800	10	10	65	70	1.5	1.6	17	2.2	400	2.2	1200	1200	320	30	15	175	65
Lactating																							
1st 6 months					65	1300	10	12	65	95	1.6	1.8	20	2.1	280	2.6	1200	1200	355	15	19	200	75
2nd 6 months					62	1200	10	11	65	90	1.6	1.7	20	2.1	260	2.6	1200	1200	340	15	16	200	75

*The allowances, expressed as average daily intakes over time, are intended to provide for individual variations among most normal persons as they live in the United States under usual environmental stresses. Diets should be based on a variety of common foods in order to provide other nutrients for which human requirements have been less well defined.

†Weights and heights of reference adults are actual medians for the US population of the designated age, as reported by NHANES II. The median weights and heights of those under 19 years of age were taken from Hamill PVV et al: Physical growth. National Center for Health Statistics Percentiles.

Am J Clin Nutr 1979; 32:607. The use of these figures does not imply that the height-to-weight ratios are ideal.

‡Retinol equivalents. 1 retinol equivalent = 1 μg retinol or 6 μg β-carotene.

§As cholecalciferol. 10 μg cholecalciferol = 400 IU of vitamin D.

‖α-Tocopherol equivalents. 1 mg d-α tocopherol = 1 α-TE.

¶1 NE (niacin equivalent) is equal to 1 mg of niacin or 60 mg of dietary tryptophan.

SOURCE: *Recommended Dietary Allowances*, 10th ed. 1989 National Academy of Sciences, National Research Council, Washington, DC.

cally these have been listed as percentage increases in the **recommended dietary allowances (RDA)** over those for nonpregnant women. However, the tenth edition of the Recommended Dietary Allowances now provides absolute, specific figure allowances for pregnant and lactating women (Table 17–1). In addition the RDAs are now provided for the first and second 6-month periods of lac-

tation to reflect the differences in the amount of milk produced (750 mL and 600 mL, respectively) (National Research Council 1989).

Most of the recommended nutrients can be obtained by eating a well-balanced diet each day. The basic food groups and recommended amounts during pregnancy and lactation are presented in Table 17–2.

TABLE 17-2 Daily Food Plan for Pregnancy and Lactation

Food Group	Nutrients Provided	Food Source	Recommended Daily Amount During Pregnancy	Recommended Daily Amount During Lactation
Dairy products	Protein; riboflavin; vitamins A, D, and others; calcium; phosphorous; zinc; magnesium	Milk—whole, 2%, skim, dry, buttermilk Cheeses—hard, semisoft, cottage Yogurt—plain, low-fat Soybean milk—canned, dry	Four (8 oz) cups (5 for teenagers) used plain or with flavoring, in shakes, soups, puddings, custards, cocoa Calcium in 1 cup milk equivalent to 1 1/2 cups cottage cheese, 1 1/2 oz hard or semisoft cheese, 1 cup yogurt, 1 1/2 cups ice cream (high in fat and sugar)	Four 8 oz cups (five for teenagers); equivalent amount of cheese, yogurt and so forth
Meat and meat alternatives	Protein; iron; thiamine, niacin, and other vitamins; minerals	Beef, pork, veal, lamb, poultry, animal organ meats, fish, eggs; legumes; nuts, seeds, peanut butter, grains in proper vegetarian combination (vitamin B_{12} supplement needed)	Three servings (one serving = 2 oz), combination in amounts necessary for same nutrient equivalent (varies greatly)	Two servings
Grain products, whole grain or enriched	B vitamins; iron; whole grain also has zinc, magnesium, and other trace elements; provides fiber	Breads and bread products such as cornbread, muffins, waffles, hotcakes, biscuits, dumplings, cereals, pastas, rice	Six to 11 servings daily: one serving = one slice bread, 3/4 cup or 1 oz dry cereal, 1/2 cup rice or pasta	Same as for pregnancy
Fruits and fruit juices	Vitamins A and C; minerals; raw fruits for roughage	Citrus fruits and juices, melons, berries, all other fruits and juices	Two to four servings (one serving for vitamin C): one serving = one medium fruit, 1/2–1 cup fruit, 4 oz orange or grapefruit juice	Same as for pregnancy
Vegetables and vegetable juices	Vitamins A and C; minerals; provides roughage	Leafy green vegetables; deep yellow or orange vegetables such as carrots, sweet potatoes, squash, tomatoes; green vegetables such as peas, green beans, broccoli; other vegetables such as beets, cabbage, potatoes, corn, lima beans	Three to five servings (one serving of dark green or deep yellow vegetable for vitamin A): one serving = 1/2–1 cup vegetable, two tomatoes, one medium potato	Same as for pregnancy
Fats	Vitamins A and D; linoleic acid	Butter, cream cheese, fortified table spreads; cream, whipped cream, whipped toppings; avocado, mayonnaise, oil, nuts	As desired in moderation (high in calories): one serving = 1 tbsp butter or enriched margarine	Same as for pregnancy
Sugar and sweets		Sugar, brown sugar, honey, molasses	Occasionally, if desired	Same as for pregnancy
Desserts		Nutritious desserts such as puddings, custards, fruit whips, and crisps; other rich, sweet desserts and pastries	Occasionally, if desired	Same as for pregnancy
Beverages		Coffee, decaffeinated beverages, tea, bouillon, carbonated drinks	As desired, in moderation	Same as for pregnancy
Miscellaneous		Iodized salt, herbs, spices, condiments	As desired	Same as for pregnancy

NOTE: The pregnant woman should eat regularly, three meals a day, with nutritious snacks of fruit, cheese, milk, or other foods between meals if desired. (More frequent but smaller meals are also recommended.) Four to 6 (8 oz) glasses of water and a total of 8 to 10 (8 oz) cups total fluid intake should be consumed daily. Water is an essential nutrient.

MATERNAL WEIGHT GAIN

Maternal weight gain is an important factor in fetal growth and infant birth weight. An adequate weight gain over time indicates an adequate caloric intake. It does not, however, ensure that the woman has a sufficient nutrient intake. The diet may not be of high enough quality even though its caloric content supports the recommended weight gain. The pregnant woman must maintain the nutritional quality of her diet as her weight gain progresses.

Optimal weight gain depends on the woman's weight for height (body mass index, BMI) and her prepregnant nutritional state. The Institute of Medicine (1992) recommends weight gain in terms of optimum ranges based on prepregnant BMI (Table 17–3).

The pattern of weight gain during pregnancy is also important. The recommended pattern consists of a gain of 1.6 to 2.3 kg (3.5 to 5 lb) during the first trimester, followed by an average gain of 0.5 kg (1 lb) per week during the last two trimesters. The rate of weight gain needs to be slightly higher for underweight women and slightly lower for overweight women (Institute of Medicine 1990). During the second trimester most of the weight gain reflects an increase in blood volume; enlargement of breasts, uterus, and associated tissue and fluid; and deposit of maternal fat. In the last trimester the maternal weight gain is mainly that of the fetus, placenta, and amniotic fluid.

The average maternal weight gain is distributed as follows:

5 kg (11 lb)	Fetus, placenta, amniotic fluid
0.9 kg (2 lb)	Uterus
1.8 kg (4 lb)	Increased blood volume
1.4 kg (3 lb)	Breast tissue
2.3 to 4.5 kg (5 to 10 lb)	Maternal stores

Inadequate gains (less than 1 kg [2.2 lb] per month during the second and third trimesters of pregnancy) or excessive gains (more than 3 kg [6.6 lb] per month) should be evaluated and the need for nutritional counseling considered. Inadequate weight gain has been associated with low-birth-weight infants and a higher incidence of infant morbidity and mortality.

Because of the association between inadequate weight gain and low-birth-weight infants, most care givers pay particular attention to weight gain during pregnancy. A woman should generally gain 4.5 to 6 kg (10 to 13 lb) by 20 weeks' gestation. If she has not, further nutritional evaluation and counseling should be offered.

Monitoring the weight gain of the obese woman (one who weighs 20% or more above her recommended prepregnant weight) during pregnancy is very important. Obese women, even if not diabetic, have an increased risk of having a large baby. Women who weigh 50% above the recommended weight also have an increased risk of chronic hyptertension, increased blood lipids, and gestational diabetes (Jovanovic-Peterson 1990). One should not assume that because a woman is overweight and even gaining weight that her diet is nutritionally sound. Weight gain alone does not guarantee adequate nutrition. A diet may be high in energy (calories) but low in vitamins, minerals, or even complex carbohydrates and protein. Pregnancy is not a time for dieting, and severe weight restriction during pregnancy can result in maternal ketosis, a threat to fetal well-being. Counseling for the obese pregnant woman usually focuses on encouraging her to eat according to the Food Guide Pyramid (Figure 17–1). Less emphasis is placed on the amount of weight gain and more on the quality of her intake.

Women who are 10% or more below their recommended weight prior to conception have an increased risk of giving birth to a low-weight infant and may have an increased risk of developing PIH (Institute of Medicine 1990). Merely advocating the average weight gain is not adequate counseling for the underweight woman who is pregnant. The nurse first assesses why the woman is underweight. Once the cause is determined, intervention can be planned with the woman. The underweight woman is usually advised to increase her caloric intake by 500 kilocalories (kcal) above the nonpregnant RDA (as opposed to the usual 300 kcal increase). She should also consume 20 g additional protein. This is often difficult for the underweight woman, especially if she has a small appetite, and she will require support and encouragement from family and health care providers.

TABLE 17-3	Recommended Total Weight Gain Ranges for Pregnant Women

	Recommended Total Gain	
Prepregnancy Weight-for-Height Category	lb	kg
Low (BMI <19.8)	28–40	12.5–18
Normal (BMI 19.8–26)	25–35	11.5–16
High (BMI >26.0–29.0)	15–25	7.0–11.5
Obese (BMI >29.0)	≥15	≥7.0

NOTE: For singleton pregnancies. The range for women carrying twins is 16–20 kg (35–45 lb). Young adolescents (<2 years after menarche) and African American women should strive for gains at the upper end of the range. Short women (<157 cm or <62 in) should strive for gains at the lower end of the range.

SOURCE: Food and Nutrition Board, Institute of Medicine: *Nutrition During Pregnancy and Lactation.* Washington, DC: National Academy Press, 1992, p 44.

NUTRITIONAL REQUIREMENTS

Critical Thinking Question

In counseling a pregnant woman about nutrition, what role do the RDAs play?

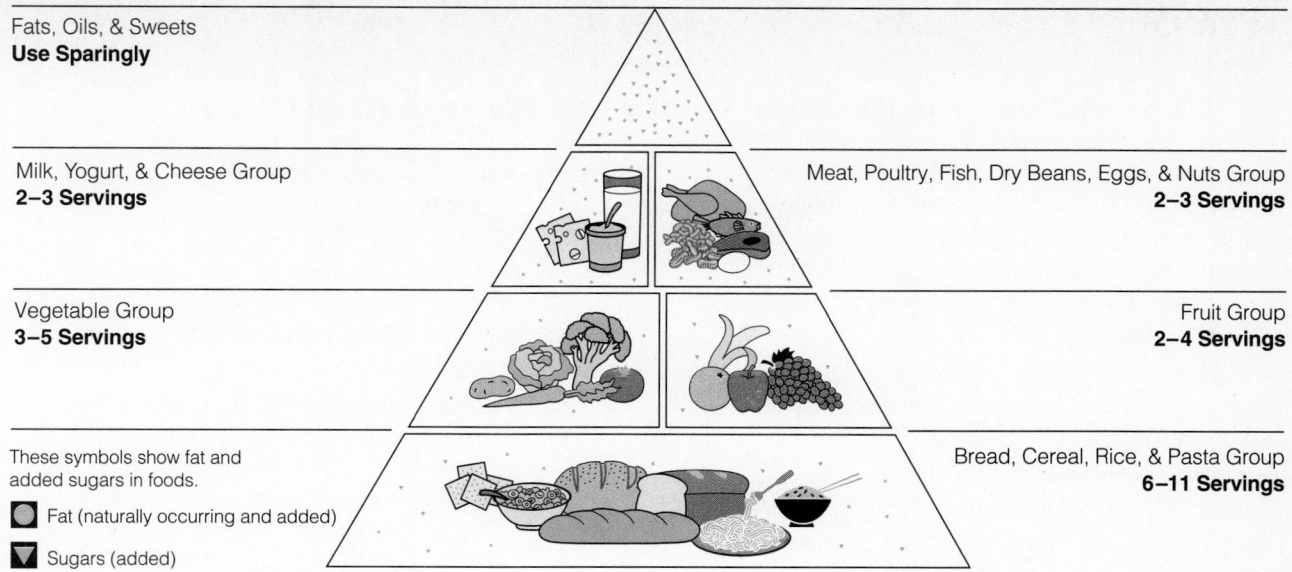

FIGURE 17-1 The Food Guide Pyramid provides a quick reference for people interested in healthy eating. The largest portion of the pyramid is devoted to grains, rice, bread, and pasta, while the smallest portion of the pyramid is devoted to fats, oils, and sweets, which should be used sparingly.

SOURCE: US Dept of Agriculture; US Dept of Health and Human Services.

The RDA for calories and almost all nutrients increases during pregnancy, although the amount of increase varies with each nutrient. These increases reflect the additional requirements of both the mother and the developing fetus (Table 17–1).

Calories

The term **calorie** (cal) stands for the amount of heat required to raise the temperature of 1 g of water 1 C. The **kilocalorie** (kcal) is equivalent to 1000 cal and is the unit used to express the energy value of food.

The RDA for energy is no caloric increase during the first trimester and a daily increase of 300 kcal during the second and third trimesters. Weight gains should be monitored regularly, and diets should be individualized for caloric needs. Prepregnant weight, height, maternal age, activity, and health status all affect caloric needs.

The Teaching Guide: Helping the Pregnant Woman Add 300 kcal to Her Diet on page 418 offers suggestions for providing basic nutritional information to pregnant women.

Carbohydrates

Carbohydrates provide protective functions, fiber, and energy. Carbohydrates contribute to the total caloric intake required. If the total caloric intake is not adequate, the body uses protein for energy. Protein then becomes unavailable for growth needs. In addition protein breakdown leads to ketosis. Ketosis can be a problem, especially in diabetic women, due to glycosuria, reduced alkaline reserves, and lipidemia.

The carbohydrate and caloric needs of the pregnant woman increase, especially during the last two trimesters. Carbohydrate intake promotes weight gain and growth of the fetus, placenta, and other maternal tissues. Dairy products, fruits, vegetables, and whole grain cereals and breads all contain carbohydrates and other important nutrients.

Protein

During pregnancy protein is needed in increased amounts to provide amino acids for fetal development, blood volume expansion, and growth of other maternal tissues such as breasts and uterus. Protein also contributes to the body's overall energy metabolism. The RDA for protein during pregnancy is 60 g, an increase of about 14 g (Table 17–1).

The quality of dietary protein is as important as the total amount consumed. The quality is determined by the complex of amino acids that makes up the protein. Proteins of animal origin generally have a greater combination of amino acids than those of plant origin. Proteins are said to be complete when they are made up of the amino acids necessary to sustain growth and are considered incomplete when they lack some of the necessary amino acids.

To obtain high-quality protein in the diet, it is best to eat a variety of foods. Animal products such as meat, fish, poultry, and eggs are sources of high-quality protein. Dairy products are also important protein sources. A quart of milk supplies 32 g of protein, more than half the average daily protein requirement (see Table 17–4). Milk

HELPING THE PREGNANT WOMAN ADD 300 KCAL TO HER DIET

Assessment: The nurse recognizes that the notion of "eating for two" may cause a woman to overestimate the amount of food she should consume during pregnancy. The nurse assesses the pregnant woman's knowledge of basic nutrition, including the use of the Food Guide Pyramid (Figure 17–1), and assesses her awareness of the best way to increase the nutrients in her diet.

Nursing Diagnosis: The key nursing diagnosis will probably be: Knowledge deficit related to lack of information about nutritional needs during pregnancy.

Nursing Plan and Implementation: The teaching plan focuses on providing information about the Food Guide Pyramid and about the most effective way to use the additional 300 kcal that a woman needs daily during pregnancy.

Client Goals: At the completion of the teaching the woman will:

1. Identify the Food Guide Pyramid categories and the foods included in each
2. Cite the increase in kcal indicated during pregnancy
3. Discuss the most nutritionally sound way to use the additional calories
4. Use the information she has gained to plan a nutritionally sound sample menu

---

Teaching Plan

Content: The food groups include the following:

Grains: Six to 11 servings (one serving = one slice bread, 1/2 hamburger roll, 1 oz dry cereal, 1 tortilla, 1/2 cup pasta, rice, grits)

Fruits: Two to four servings, one should be a good source of vitamin C (one serving = 1 medium-sized piece of fruit, 1/2 cup juice)

Vegetables: Three to five servings (one serving = 1 cup raw vegetable, 1 cup green leafy vegetable, 1/2 cup cooked vegetable)

Dairy: Two to three servings (one serving = 1 cup milk or yogurt, 1.5 oz hard cheese, 2 cups cottage cheese, 1 cup pudding made with milk)

Meats and alternatives: Two to three servings (one serving = 2 oz cooked lean meat, poultry, or fish; 2 eggs; 1/2 cup cottage cheese; 1 cup cooked legumes [kidney, lima, garbanzo, or soy beans, split peas]; 6 oz tofu; 2 oz nuts or seeds; 4 tbsp peanut butter)

Not all foods that are nutritionally equivalent have the same number of calories; it is important to consider that when making food choices.

The Food Guide Pyramid is designed to represent the food groups needed to make a balanced diet. The grain, fruit, and vegetable groups are at the base of the pyramid and should account for the majority of the food selections. Fewer servings of dairy and meat or meat alternative are required in the diet, and these groups fall in the middle portion of the pyramid. The very top of the pyramid represents fats, oils, and sweets. These items do not have a high nutritional value and should be used sparingly.

Emphasize that a woman only has to add 300 kcal/day during pregnancy. This can be achieved by adding two milk servings and one serving of meat or alternative. Because of the varying caloric value a woman needs

Teaching Method: *Ask woman if she has received nutritional information using this approach before. Discuss her understanding of it. Use that information to plan the amount of detail you will use.*

Use a chart or colorful handout to explain the basic food groups and to give examples of equivalent foods.

Use a calorie-counting guide to compare the calories in a variety of foods that are equivalent, such as 2 oz beef and 2 oz fish or 1 cup low-fat milk and 1 cup whole milk.

Use a similar approach to evaluate the calories in fats, oils, and sweets, but also evaluate their nutrient content, especially levels of nutrients such as vitamin C, iron, and calcium.

In planning the woman's diet to get optimum nutrition without too many additional calories, it is often helpful to ask her to plan and evaluate a sample menu.

to consider the advisability of using low-fat milk, lean cuts of meat, or fish broiled or baked instead of fried.

Foods can be combined. For example, 1 cup spaghetti with a 2 oz meatball would count as 1 serving meat, 3/4 cup spaghetti = 1 grain, and 1/4 cup tomato sauce = 1/2 serving vegetable.

Evaluation: Teaching has been effective if all the identified goals are achieved and if the woman seems comfortable planning her diet to provide for the best nutrition possible.

Provide handouts on which the woman can list the foods she has eaten and check off the corresponding nutrient categories. Have her bring her completed handouts to a subsequent visit.

can be incorporated into the diet in a variety of dishes, including soups, puddings, custards, sauces, yogurt and beverages such as hot chocolate and milk and fruit drinks. Various kinds of hard and soft cheeses and cottage cheese are excellent protein sources, although cream cheese is categorized as a fat source only. Table 17–4 provides information on the protein content of commonly used foods.

Women who have allergies to milk, who have lactose intolerance, or who practice vegetarianism may find dried or canned soy milk acceptable. It can be used in cooked dishes or as a beverage. Tofu, or soybean curd, can replace cottage cheese.

If little or no protein comes from animal sources, it will be necessary to combine foods of plant origin to obtain the amino acids necessary for a complete protein. Examples of combined proteins are beans and rice, peanut butter on whole grain bread, and whole grain cereal and milk. Adequate dietary protein can be obtained by consuming a varied diet, and protein and amino acid supplements are not recommended (Institute of Medicine 1990).

Fat

Fats are valuable sources of energy for the body. Fats are more completely absorbed during pregnancy, resulting in a marked increase in serum lipids, lipoproteins, and cholesterol and decreased elimination of fat through the bowel. Fat deposits in the fetus increase from about 2% at midpregnancy to almost 12% at term. The US Dietary Guidelines recommend that fat calories should not exceed 30% of the total daily caloric intake, and less than 10% should be saturated fat (USDA/USDHHS 1990).

When dairy products are used as a regular part of the diet, it may be helpful to select items that have a reduced fat content. Selecting lean cuts of meats, fish, and poultry will also help decrease dietary fat.

Minerals

Increased minerals needed for the growth of new tissue during pregnancy are obtained by improved mineral absorption and an increase in mineral allowances.

Calcium and Phosphorus

Calcium and phosphorus are involved in mineralization of fetal bones and teeth, energy and cell production, and acid-base buffering. Calcium is absorbed and used more efficiently during pregnancy. Some calcium and phosphorus are required early in pregnancy, but most of the fetus's bone calcification occurs during the last 2 or 3

TABLE 17–4	Amount of Protein in Commonly Used Foods

Food	Protein (g)
Dairy	
Milk, 8 oz	8
Cheese, cheddar, Swiss, and so forth, 1 oz	7
Cottage cheese, 1/4 cup	7
Meat and meat alternatives	
Meat, fish, poultry, 1 oz	7
Egg, 1	7
Cooked dry beans & peas, 1/2 cup	7
Cooked soybeans, 1/2 cup	11
Peanut butter, 2 tbsp	7
Peanuts (3 tbsp), cashews/almonds (5 tbsp)	7
Breads and cereals	
Bread, 1 slice	2
Buns, biscuits, muffins, 1	2
Cooked cereals & grain, 1/2 cup	2
Breakfast cereal, 1 oz	2
Vegetables and fruits	
Vegetables, 1/2 cup	0.5–1
Fruits & juices, 1/2 cup	0.5

months. Teeth begin to form at about 8 weeks' gestation and are formed by birth. The 6-year molars begin to calcify just before birth. This means that calcium is particularly important as a structural element. Additional calcium is stored in the maternal skeleton as a reserve for lactation.

The RDA for calcium for the pregnant or lactating woman, regardless of age, is 1200 mg/day. If calcium intakes are low, fetal needs will be met at the mother's expense by demineralization of maternal bone.

A diet that includes 4 cups of milk or an equivalent dairy alternate (Table 17–2) will provide sufficient calcium. Smaller amounts of calcium are supplied by legumes, nuts, dried fruits, and dark green leafy vegetables (such as kale, cabbage, collards, and turnip greens). It is important to remember that some of the calcium in beet greens, spinach, and chard is bound with oxalic acid, which makes it unavailable to the body. Larger amounts of these foods need to be consumed if they are used as a substitute for dairy sources of calcium (Table 17–5).

Because caffeine increases urinary excretion of calcium, women who consume large quantities of caffeine-containing beverages such as coffee, tea, or colas may be advised to increase dietary calcium to 1500 mg and reduce caffeine intake.

The RDA for phosphorus is the same as the RDA for calcium: 1200 mg/day for the pregnant or lactating woman. Phosphorus is readily supplied through calcium- and protein-rich foods, especially milk, eggs, and meat.

Because phosphorus is so widely available in foods, the dietary intake of phosphorus frequently exceeds the calcium intake. An excess of phosphorus can result in a disturbance of the calcium-phosphorus ratio in the body, decreased calcium absorption, and increased excretion of calcium. Excess phosphorus can be reduced by limiting the snack foods, processed meats, and cola drinks in which it abounds. However, if vitamin D and magnesium are adequate, most adults can tolerate relatively wide variations in dietary calcium-phosphorus ratios.

Iodine

Inorganic iodine is excreted in the urine during pregnancy. Enlargement of the thyroid gland may occur if iodine is not replaced by adequate dietary intake or additional supplement. Iodine deficiency is the most widespread nutritional cause of impaired brain development. This can result in cretinism and lesser degrees of retardation (DeLong 1993).

The iodine allowance of 175 μg/day can be met by using iodized salt. When sodium is restricted, the physician may prescribe an iodine supplement.

Sodium

The sodium ion is essential for proper metabolism and the regulation of fluid balance. Sodium intake in the form of salt is never entirely curtailed during pregnancy, even

TABLE 17-5	Foods that Provide Comparable Amounts of Calcium

Food	Amount
Dairy	
Milk	8 oz
Cheese, cheddar	1 1/2 oz
Pudding, vanilla	1 cup
Fruits	
Figs	10
Raisins	2 cups
Vegetables	
Broccoli	2 1/2 cups
Collards	1 cup
Kale	3 cups
Mustard greens	3 1/2 cups
Turnip greens	1 1/2 cups
Fish	
Salmon, canned, with bones	2/3 cup
Sardines	6
Nuts	
Almonds	4 oz
Brazil	1/2 cup
Miscellaneous	
Molasses, blackstrap	2 tbsp

SOURCE: Data from Pennington JAT: *Bowes and Church's Food Values of Portions Commonly Used*, 15th ed. Philadelphia: Lippincott, 1989.

when hypertension or PIH is present. A moderate sodium intake (2–3 g) can be obtained by using fresh food seasoned to taste during cooking. The use of extra salt at the table should be avoided. Salty foods such as potato chips, ham, sausages, and sodium-based seasonings can be eliminated to avoid excessive intake.

Zinc

Zinc is involved in protein metabolism and the synthesis of DNA and RNA. The RDA during pregnancy is 15 mg. Sources include milk, liver, shellfish, and wheat bran. Zinc deficiency during pregnancy may affect embryonic growth and result in malformation (Rosso 1990).

Magnesium

Magnesium is essential for cellular metabolism and structural growth. The RDA for pregnancy is 320 mg. Sources include milk, whole grains, beet greens, nuts, legumes, and tea.

Iron

Iron requirements increase during pregnancy due to the growth of the fetus and placenta and the expansion of maternal blood volume (Luke & Keith 1992). Anemia in pregnancy is mainly caused by low iron stores, although it may also be caused by inadequate intake of other nutrients, such as vitamins B_6 and B_{12}, folic acid, ascorbic acid, copper, and zinc. Women with poor diet histories, frequent conceptions, or records of prior iron depletion are particularly at risk.

Iron deficiency anemia is generally defined as a decrease in the oxygen-carrying capacity of the blood. This significantly reduces the hemoglobin per decaliter of blood, the volume of packed red cells per decaliter of blood (hematocrit), or the number of erythrocytes.

The normal hematocrit in the nonpregnant woman is 38% to 47%. In the pregnant woman the level may drop to as low as 34%, even when nutrition is adequate. This condition is called the *physiologic anemia of pregnancy* (see Chapter 13).

Fetal demands for iron further contribute to symptoms of anemia in the pregnant woman. The fetal liver stores iron, especially during the third trimester. The infant needs this stored iron during the first 4 months of life to compensate for the normally inadequate levels of iron in breast milk and non–iron-fortified formulas.

To prevent anemia, the woman must balance iron requirements and intake. Doing so is a problem for nonpregnant women and a greater one for pregnant women. By carefully selecting foods high in iron, the woman can increase her daily iron intake considerably. Lean meats, dark green leafy vegetables, eggs, and whole grain and enriched breads and cereals are the foods usually depended on for their iron content. Other iron sources include dried fruits, legumes, shellfish, and molasses.

Iron absorption is generally higher for animal products than for vegetable products. However, absorption of iron from nonmeat sources may be enhanced by combining them with meat or a food rich in vitamin C.

The most iron that can reasonably be obtained from the average diet is about 15 to 18 mg/day. However, the RDA for iron during pregnancy is 30 mg. Thus during pregnancy a supplement of simple iron salt, such as ferrous gluconate, ferrous fumarate, or ferrous sulfate is needed. The Institute of Medicine recommends a daily supplement of 30 mg elemental iron. Iron deficiency anemia is treated with a daily ferrous iron supplement of 60–120 mg (Institute of Medicine 1992). Unfortunately, iron supplements often cause gastrointestinal discomfort, especially if taken on an empty stomach. Supplements are not usually given during the first trimester because the increased demand is still minimal, and iron may increase the woman's nausea. Once an iron supplement is begun, taking it after a meal may help reduce gastrointestinal discomfort.

Vitamins

Vitamins are organic substances necessary for life and growth. They are found in small amounts in specific foods and generally cannot be synthesized by the body in adequate amounts.

Vitamins are grouped according to solubility. Those that dissolve in fat are A, D, E, and K; those soluble in water include C and the B complex. An adequate intake of all vitamins is essential during pregnancy; however, several are required in larger than normal amounts to fulfill specific needs.

A balanced diet generally provides necessary vitamins without the need for supplementation. Despite this, many people who are concerned about nutrition have become involved in the practice of taking exceptionally large doses—megadoses—of vitamins. However, in vitamin therapy more is not necessarily better. Megadoses of vitamins, especially vitamins A, D, C, and B_6, have had a negative effect on the fetus. Furthermore, excessive intake of one vitamin may interfere with the body's use of another vitamin. For example, excessive intake of vitamin C may block the body's use of vitamin B_{12}. Consequently, although it is important to meet the RDA of vitamins during pregnancy, megadoses are best avoided.

Fat-Soluble Vitamins

The fat-soluble vitamins A, D, E, and K are stored in the liver and thus are available should the dietary intake become inadequate. The major complication related to these vitamins is not deficiency but toxicity due to overdose because excess amounts of A, D, E, and K are not excreted in the urine. Symptoms of vitamin toxicity include nausea, gastrointestinal upset, dryness and cracking of the skin, and loss of hair.

Vitamin A is involved in the growth of epithelial cells, which line the entire gastrointestinal tract and compose the skin. Vitamin A plays a role in the metabolism of carbohydrates and fats. The body cannot synthesize glycogen in the absence of vitamin A, and the body's ability to handle cholesterol is also affected. The protective layer of tissue surrounding nerve fibers does not form properly if vitamin A is lacking.

Probably the best-known function of vitamin A is its effect on vision in dim light. A person's ability to see in the dark depends on the eye's supply of retinol, a form of vitamin A. In this manner vitamin A prevents night blindness. Vitamin A is associated with the formation and development of healthy eyes in the fetus.

If maternal stores of vitamin A are adequate, the overall effects of pregnancy on the woman's vitamin A requirements are not remarkable. The blood serum level of vitamin A decreases slightly in early pregnancy, rises in late pregnancy, and falls before the onset of labor. Thus the RDA for vitamin A (800 μg) does not increase during pregnancy.

Deficiencies of vitamin A are not common. However, an inadequate maternal intake has been associated with preterm birth, intrauterine growth retardation, and decreased birth weight (Institute of Medicine 1990). Excessive intake of preformed vitamin A is toxic to both children and adults. There are indications that excessive intake of vitamin A in the fetus can cause eye, ear, and bone malformations, cleft palate, possible renal anomalies, and central nervous system damage (Luke & Keith 1992).

Rich plant sources of vitamin A include deep green and yellow vegetables and some fruits; animal sources include liver, liver oil, kidney, egg yolk, cream, butter, and fortified margarine.

Vitamin D is best known for its role in the absorption and utilization of calcium and phosphorus in skeletal development. To supply the needs of the developing fetus, the pregnant woman should have a vitamin D intake of 10 μg/day.

Various degrees of vitamin D deficiency can affect the development of the fetus. Symptoms can range from a reduction of fetal bone calcification to hypoplasia of the dental enamel or, in cases of severe deficiency, intrauterine rickets (Rosso 1990).

Main food sources of vitamin D include fortified milk, margarine, butter, liver, and egg yolks. Drinking a quart of vitamin D–fortified milk daily provides the vitamin D needed during pregnancy.

Excessive intake of vitamin D is not usually a result of eating but of taking high-potency vitamin preparations. Overdoses during pregnancy can cause hypercalcemia or high blood calcium levels due to withdrawal of calcium from the skeletal tissue. In the fetus, cardiac defects, especially aortic stenosis, may occur (Luke & Keith 1992). Continued overdose in adults or children can also cause hypercalcemia and eventually death, especially in young children. Symptoms of toxicity are excessive thirst, loss of appetite, vomiting, weight loss, irritability, and high blood calcium levels.

The major function of *vitamin E*, or tocopherol, is as an antioxidant. Vitamin E takes on oxygen, thus preventing another substance from undergoing chemical change. For example, vitamin E helps spare vitamin A by preventing its oxidation in the intestinal tract and the tissues. It decreases the oxidation of polyunsaturated fats, thus helping to retain the flexibility and health of the cell membrane. In protecting the cell membrane vitamin E affects the health of all cells in the body.

Vitamin E is also involved in certain enzymatic and metabolic reactions. It is an essential nutrient for the synthesis of nucleic acids required in the formation of red blood cells in the bone marrow. Vitamin E is beneficial in treating certain types of muscular pain and intermittent claudication, in surface healing of wounds and burns, and in protecting lung tissue from the damaging effects of smog. These functions may help explain the abundant claims and cures attributed to vitamin E, many of which have not been scientifically proved.

The newborn's need for vitamin E has been widely recognized. Human milk provides adequate vitamin E, whereas cow's milk is lower in E content. Deficiency symptoms of vitamin E are related to long-term inability to absorb fats. In humans, malabsorption problems exist in cases of cystic fibrosis, liver cirrhosis, postgastrectomy, obstructive jaundice, pancreatic problems, and sprue.

The recommended intake of vitamin E increases from 8 IU for nonpregnant females to 10 IU for pregnant women. The vitamin E requirement varies with the polyunsaturated fat content of the diet. Vitamin E is widely distributed in foodstuffs, especially vegetable fats and oils, whole grains, greens, and eggs.

Some pregnant women massage vitamin E oil on the abdominal skin to make it supple and possibly prevent permanent stretch marks. It is questionable whether taking high doses orally will accomplish this goal or satisfy any other claims related to vitamin E's role in reproduction or virility. In addition, excessive intake of vitamin E has been associated with abnormal coagulation in the newborn.

Vitamin K, or menadione as used synthetically in medicine, is an essential factor for the synthesis of prothrombin; its function is thus related to normal blood clotting. Synthesis occurs in the intestinal tract by the *Escherichia coli* normally inhabiting the large intestine. However, the body's need for vitamin K is not totally met through synthesis. Green leafy vegetables and liver are excellent sources. The RDA for vitamin K does not increase during pregnancy. Newborn infants, having a sterile intestinal tract and receiving sterile feeding, lack vitamin K. Thus newborns often receive a dose of menadione as a protective measure to prevent hemorrhage.

Intake of vitamin K is usually adequate in a well-balanced prenatal diet. Secondary problems may arise if an illness results in malabsorption of fats or if antibiotics are used for an extended period. Antibiotics inhibit vitamin K synthesis by destroying intestinal *E coli*.

Water-Soluble Vitamins

Water-soluble vitamins are excreted in the urine. Only small amounts are stored, so there is little protection from dietary inadequacies. Thus adequate amounts must be ingested daily. During pregnancy the concentration of water-soluble vitamins in the maternal serum falls, whereas high concentrations are found in the fetus.

The requirement for *vitamin C* (ascorbic acid) is increased in pregnancy from 60 to 70 mg. The major function of vitamin C is to aid the formation and development of connective tissue and the vascular system. Ascorbic acid is essential to the formation of collagen. Collagen is like a cement that binds cells together, just as mortar holds bricks together. If the collagen begins to disintegrate due to lack of ascorbic acid, cell functioning is disturbed, and cell structure breaks down, causing muscular weakness, capillary hemorrhage, and eventual death. These are symptoms of scurvy, the disease caused by vitamin C deficiency. Infants fed mainly cow's milk become deficient in vitamin C. Newborns of women who have taken megadoses of vitamin C may experience a rebound form of scurvy.

Maternal plasma levels of vitamin C progressively decline throughout pregnancy, with values at term being about half those at midpregnancy. It appears that ascorbic acid concentrates in the placenta; levels in the fetus are 50% or more above maternal levels.

A nutritious diet should meet the pregnant woman's needs for vitamin C without additional supplementation. Common food sources of vitamin C include citrus fruit, tomatoes, cantaloupe, strawberries, potatoes, broccoli, and other leafy green vegetables. Ascorbic acid is readily destroyed by water and oxidation. Therefore foods containing vitamin C should have limited exposure to air, heat, and water during storage and cooking.

The *B vitamins* include thiamine (B_1), riboflavin (B_2), niacin, folic acid, pantothenic acid, vitamin B_6, and vitamin B_{12}. These vitamins serve as vital coenzyme factors in many reactions, such as cell respiration, glucose oxidation, and energy metabolism. The quantities needed therefore invariably increase as caloric intake increases to meet the metabolic and growth needs of the pregnant woman.

The *thiamine* requirement increases from the prepregnant level of 1.1 mg/day to 1.5 mg/day. Sources include pork, liver, milk, potatoes, enriched breads, and cereals.

Riboflavin deficiency is manifested by cheilosis (fissures and cracks of the lips and the corners of the mouth) and other skin lesions. During pregnancy women may excrete less riboflavin and still require more because of increased energy and protein needs. An additional 0.3 mg/day is recommended. Sources include milk, liver, eggs, enriched breads, and cereals.

An increase of 2 mg daily in *niacin* intake is recommended during pregnancy and 5 mg during lactation. Sources of niacin include meat, fish, poultry, liver, whole grains, enriched breads, cereals, and peanuts.

Folic acid promotes adequate fetal growth and prevents the macrocytic, megaloblastic anemia of pregnancy. Folic acid is directly related to the outcome of pregnancy and to maternal and fetal health. Inadequate intake of folic acid has been associated with neural tube defects (NTD) (spina bifida, meningomyelocele). The use of folic acid supplementation before conception and during pregnancy can reduce the risk of spina bifida and other neural tube defects in the fetus. All women of childbearing age should consume 0.4 mg of folic acid daily to reduce the risk of a pregnancy affected by neural tube defects (CDC 1992). Large dose supplementation (4 mg/day) is recommended only for women who have had a previous NTD-affected pregnancy and are planning another pregnancy. Supplementation should begin, if possible, 1 month before conception and should continue for the first 3 months of pregnancy (Contraception Report 1993). This level of folic acid should be taken only by prescription and under the supervision of a qualified health care provider.

Megaloblastic anemia due to folate deficiency is rarely found in the United States, but those caring for pregnant women must be aware that it does occur. Folate deficiency can also be present in the absence of overt anemia.

The best food sources of folates are fresh green leafy vegetables, kidney, liver, food yeasts, and peanuts. Many foods contain small amounts of folic acid. Cow's milk contains a small amount of folic acid, but goat's milk has none. Therefore, infants and children who are given goat's milk must receive a folate supplement to prevent a deficiency.

Folic acid content of foods can be altered by preparation methods. Because folic acid is a water-soluble nutrient, care must be taken in cooking. Loss of the vitamin from vegetables and meats can be considerable when they are cooked in large amounts of water or simply overcooked.

No allowance has been set for *pantothenic acid* in pregnancy, but 5 mg/day is considered a safe, adequate intake. Sources include meats, egg yolk, legumes, and whole grain cereals and breads.

Vitamin B_6 (pyridoxine) has long been associated biochemically with pregnancy. The RDA for vitamin B_6 during pregnancy is 2.2 mg, an increase of 0.6 mg over the allowance for nonpregnant women. Because pyridoxine is associated with amino acid metabolism, a higher than average protein intake requires increased pyridoxine intake. The slightly increased need can generally be supplied by dietary sources, which include wheat germ, yeast, fish, liver, pork, potatoes, and lentils.

Vitamin B_{12}, or cobalamin, is the cobalt-containing vitamin found only in animal sources. Rarely is B_{12} deficiency found in women of reproductive age. Vegans can develop a deficiency, however, so it is essential that their dietary intake be supplemented with this vitamin. Occasionally, vitamin B_{12} levels decrease during pregnancy but increase again after birth. The RDA during pregnancy is 2.2 μg/day, an increase of 0.2 μg.

A deficiency may also be due to a congenital inability to absorb vitamin B_{12} resulting in pernicious anemia; infertility is a complication of this type of anemia.

Folic acid and iron are the only nutritional supplements generally recommended during pregnancy. The increased need for other vitamins and minerals can usually be met with an adequate diet. To avoid possible deficiencies, however, many health care professionals still recommend a daily vitamin supplement. As the new recommendations become more well known this practice may change.

Fluid

The nutrient water is essential for life and is found in all body tissues. It is necessary for many biochemical reactions. It also serves as a lubricant, acts as a medium of transport for carrying substances in and out of the body, and aids in the regulation of body temperature. A pregnant woman should consume at least 8 to 10 (8 oz) glasses of fluid each day, of which 4 to 6 glasses should be water.

Other beverages such as juices and milk can contribute water as well as other nutrients to the diet. Sodas and diet sodas should be used in moderation because they do not contribute to the nutritional value of the diet.

A moderate use of caffeine during pregnancy has not been shown to increase the risk of spontaneous abortion, intrauterine growth retardation, or microcephaly (Mills et al 1993). However, caffeine does pass readily to the fetus, who is unable to metabolize it effectively (Institute of Medicine 1990). Caffeinated beverages have a diuretic effect, which may be counterproductive to increasing fluid intake. Two (8 oz) glasses of caffeinated beverages per day is considered a safe level of consumption (Narod et al 1991).

VEGETARIANISM

Vegetarianism is the dietary choice of many people, for religious (Seventh-Day Adventists), health, and ethical reasons. There are several types of vegetarians. **Lacto-ovovegetarians** include milk, dairy products, and eggs in their diet. **Lactovegetarians** include dairy products but no eggs in their diet. **Vegans** are "pure" vegetarians who will not eat any food from animal sources.

In their position statement on vegetarian diets the American Dietetic Association stated that "vegetarian diets are healthful and nutritionally adequate when appropriately planned" (ADA 1988a). People following vegetarian diets tend to have lower blood pressure; a lower incidence of coronary artery disease, osteoporosis, gallstones, kidney stones, and diverticulitis; and weights closer to desirable levels than do nonvegetarians (ADA 1988b).

The expectant woman who is vegetarian must eat the proper combination of foods to obtain adequate nutrients. If her diet allows, a woman can obtain ample and complete proteins from dairy products and eggs. Plant protein quality may be improved if consumed with these animal proteins. If the diet contains less than four servings of milk and dairy products, calcium supplementation may be necessary.

If a vegan diet is followed, careful planning is necessary to obtain sufficient calories and complete proteins. Obtaining sufficient calories to achieve adequate weight gains can be difficult because vegan diets tend to be higher in fiber and therefore filling. Low prepregnancy weight and optimum pregnancy weight gains are often a problem. Supplementation with energy-dense foods helps provide increased energy intake to prevent the body from using protein for caloric needs.

If energy needs are met adequately, protein needs can usually be met if recommendations for complementing proteins are followed. An adequate vegan diet contains protein from unrefined grains (brown rice and whole wheat), legumes (beans, split peas, lentils), nuts in large quantities, and a variety of cooked and fresh vegetables and fruits. Complete protein may be obtained by eating different types of complementary proteins, such as legumes and whole grain cereals, nuts and whole grain cereals, or nuts and legumes, over the course of a day (ADA 1988b). Seeds may be used in the vegetarian diet if the quantity is large enough.

Because vegans use no animal products, a daily supplement of 4 μg of vitamin B$_{12}$ is necessary. If soy milk is used, only partial supplementation may be needed. If no soy milk is taken, daily supplements of 1200 mg of calcium and 10 μg of vitamin D are needed.

Because the best sources of iron and zinc are found in animal products, vegan diets may also be low in these minerals. In addition a high fiber intake may reduce mineral (calcium, iron, and zinc) bioavailability (Rosso 1990). Emphasis should be placed on the use of foods containing these nutrients. A vegetarian food group guide is given in Table 17–6.

FACTORS INFLUENCING NUTRITION

Besides having knowledge of nutritional needs and food sources, the nurse needs to be aware of other factors that affect a client's nutrition. What are the age, life-style, dietary practices, and culture of the pregnant woman? What food beliefs and habits does she have? What a person eats is determined by availability, economics, and symbolism. These factors and others influence the expectant mother's acceptance of the nurse's intervention.

Lactase Deficiency (Lactose Intolerance)

Some individuals have difficulty digesting milk and dairy products. This condition, known as **lactase deficiency (lactose intolerance),** results from an inadequate amount of the enzyme lactase, which breaks down the milk sugar lactose into smaller digestible substances.

Lactase deficiency is found in many people of African, Mexican American, Native American, Ashkenazic Jewish, and Asian descent (Institute of Medicine 1990). People who are not affected are mainly of Northern European heritage. Symptoms may include abdominal distention, discomfort, nausea, vomiting, loose stools, and cramps. When counseling pregnant women who might be intolerant of milk and milk products, the nurse should be aware of the following:

- Tolerances vary with the individual.
- Even a partial glass of milk can produce symptoms.
- Milk is sometimes tolerated in cooked form, such as in custards.
- Cultured or fermented dairy products such as buttermilk, cheese, and yogurt are sometimes tolerated.

TABLE 17-6	Vegetarian Food Groups			
Food Group	**Mixed Diet**	**Lacto-ovovegetarian**	**Lacto-vegetarian**	**Vegan**
Grain	Bread, cereal, rice, pasta	Bread, cereal, rice, pasta	Bread, cereal, rice, pasta	Bread, cereal, rice, pasta
Fruit	Fruit, fruit juices	Fruit, fruit juices	Fruit, fruit juices	Fruit, fruit juices
Vegetable	Vegetables, vegetable juices	Vegetables, vegetable juices	Vegetables, vegetable juices	Vegetables, vegetable juices
Dairy	Milk, yogurt, cheese	Milk, yogurt, cheese	Milk, yogurt, cheese	Fortified soy milk
Meat and meat alternatives	Meat, fish, poultry, eggs, legumes, tofu, nuts, nut butters	Eggs, legumes, tofu, nuts, nut butters	Legumes, tofu, nuts, nut butters	Legumes, tofu, nuts, nut butters

- In some instances the enzyme lactase may be used to alleviate the problem. It is available in several forms: as a tablet to be chewed before ingesting milk or milk products and as a liquid to add to milk itself. Lactase-treated milk is also available commercially in some grocery stores, although it may be more expensive than regular milk.

- Alternative sources of calcium such as calcium fortified orange juice, green leafy vegetables, and Tums antacids may be recommended. Supplementation is also recommended.

Pica

Pica is the persistent eating of substances such as dirt, clay, starch, freezer frost, burnt matches, or ashes that are not ordinarily considered edible or to have nutritive value. Most women who practice pica in pregnancy eat such substances only during that time.

Iron deficiency anemia is the most common concern in pica. The ingestion of laundry starch or certain types of clay may contribute to iron deficiency by replacing iron-containing foods from the diet or by interfering with iron absorption. The ingestion of large quantities of clay could fill the intestine and cause fecal impaction. The ingestion of starch may be associated with excessive weight gain.

Nurses should be aware of pica and its implications for the woman and her fetus. Often pica is part of the tradition of certain communities or families. Assessment for pica is an important part of the nutritional history. However, women may be embarrassed about their cravings or reluctant to discuss them for fear of criticism. It is helpful if the nurse uses a nonjudgmental approach. Reeducation of the expectant woman is important in helping her to decrease or eliminate this practice.

Common Discomforts of Pregnancy

Gastrointestinal functioning can be altered at various times throughout pregnancy. Although these changes can be uncomfortable for the woman, they are seldom a major problem. Minor dietary modifications may provide relief for some individuals (see also Chapter 15).

Many women experience nausea and vomiting during the first few months of their pregnancy. For most the symptoms last only a few months. Dietary modifications for nausea and vomiting encourage the use of easy-to-digest foods and the avoidance of spicy and fatty food.

Heartburn is an uncomfortable, burning sensation that results when stomach contents back up into the esophagus. It is usually caused by the expanding uterus pushing against the digestive tract. Dietary modifications that control the amount and type of food in the stomach may help control the symptoms.

Constipation may occur in pregnancy as a result of hormonal influence on the muscles of the digestive tract and pressure exerted on the intestines by the expanding uterus. Iron supplements may also contribute to constipation. Adequate fluid and fiber intake are recommended dietary modifications. Laxatives are to be avoided unless they are recommended by a health care provider.

Cultural, Ethnic, and Religious Influences

Cultural, ethnic, and occasionally religious backgrounds determine one's experiences with food and influence food preferences and habits (Figure 17–2). People of different nationalities are accustomed to eating different foods because of the kinds of foodstuffs available in their countries of origin. The way food is prepared varies, depending on the customs and traditions of the ethnic and cultural group. In addition the laws of certain religions sanction particular foods, prohibit others, and direct the preparation and serving of meals.

In each culture certain foods have symbolic significance. Generally, these symbolic foods are related to major life experiences such as birth, death, or developmental milestones. Although generalizations have been made about the food practices of ethnic and religious groups, there are many variations. Food customs will differ among groups in various regions of the same country, families within local regions, and individuals within the

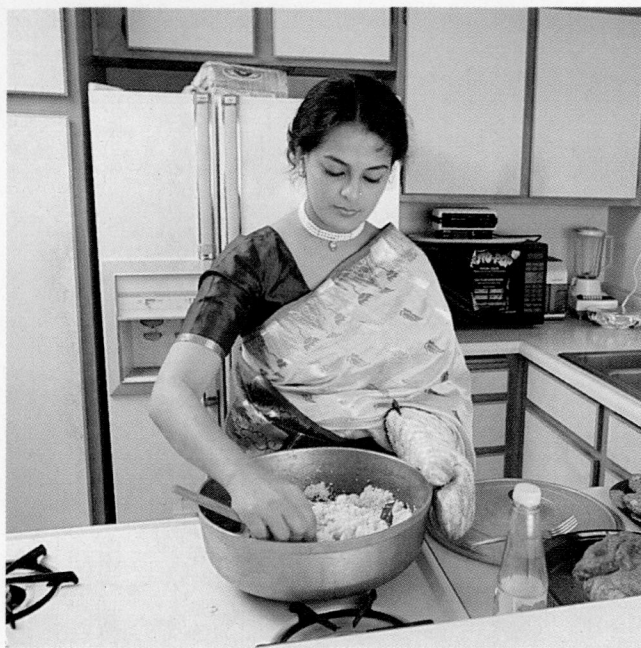

FIGURE 17-2 Food preferences and habits are affected by cultural factors.

same family. The extent to which traditional ethnic foods and customs are continued is affected by the recency of immigration, the extent of exposure to other cultures, and the availability, quality, and cost of the traditional foods.

The relationship of food to pregnancy is reflected in beliefs or sayings. Nurses frequently hear that the pregnant woman must eat for two or that the fetus takes from the mother all the nutrients it needs. Less frequently, nurses may learn that some women believe that craving one food excessively can cause the baby to be "marked," that the shape of the birthmark echoes the shape of the food the mother craved during pregnancy. In other cases milk is omitted from the diet because of the belief that drinking it makes babies too big, thereby causing difficult births.

It is common for health care providers to give dietary advice from the cultural context of their own views (Way 1991). When working with a pregnant woman from any ethnic background, it is important to understand the significance of cultural influences on her eating habits and to identify any beliefs she may have about foods and pregnancy.

The nurses can use generalizations about ethnic food preferences as an introduction to customs of an unfamiliar culture. The level of adherence to the traditional food customs must be determined by talking with the client. Dietary advice can then be given in a manner that is meaningful to the client.

Psychosocial Factors

The sharing of food has long been a symbol of friendliness, warmth, and social acceptance in many cultures. Food is also symbolic of motherliness; that is, taking care of the family and feeding them well is a part of the traditional mothering role. The mother influences her chil-

RESEARCH IN PRACTICE

Even though Saudi Arabia has promising economic resources and is a rapidly developing country, its population still experiences a high rate of maternal and infant mortality. Malnutrition contributes to this problem according to Ahlam Mansour and Shadia Hassan. These authors interviewed Saudi women to determine what factors influence the women's knowledge about nutrition as it relates to pregnancy and lactation.

The systematically chosen sample of 150 Saudi mothers were married, pregnant, and had experienced at least one previous pregnancy. Data collection consisted of a three-part structured interview. The first part of the interview obtained demographic information. The second part ascertained knowledge of nutrition related to needs during pregnancy and lactation. The third part identified the sources from which the mothers obtained nutritional information. The knowledge base of each woman, obtained from the second part of the interview, was quantified and used to cluster the mothers into three groups. The classifications of level of knowledge included poor, good, and very good. Because only three mothers had scores high enough to be classified as very good, the top two categories were collapsed into one group.

Results of the study showed that 48% of these women had experienced 7 or more pregnancies. The mothers scored an average of 3.95 out of a possible 10 on questions about nutrition and pregnancy, and 5.35 out of 10 on questions pertaining to nutrition during lactation. Only 25% had completed elementary school or higher education. More than half (56%) identified friends as their most important source of nutrition information, and only 5% mentioned nurses or physicians.

Chi-square analysis identified relationships between nutritional knowledge scores and the demographic variables of (1) age; (2) level of education; and (3) numbers of pregnancies, births, abortions, stillbirths, and living children. Results of the analysis showed a direct relationship between knowledge score and level of education, and a decreasing relationship between knowledge score and number of pregnancies, births, and living children.

Clinical Application of Study

The authors suggest an accurate and thorough assessment of current health education programs and sensitization of health care providers to the importance of nutritional education for pregnant women in all developing countries.

SOURCE: Mansour A, Hassan S: Factors that influence women's nutrition knowledge in Saudi Arabia. *Health Care for Women International* 1994; 15:213.

dren's likes and dislikes by what she prepares and by her attitude about foods. Certain foods are assigned positive or negative values, as reflected in the statements "Milk helps you grow" and "Coffee stunts your growth."

Some foods and food-related practices are associated with status. Some foods are prepared "just for company." Other foods are served only on special occasions—for example, holidays such as Thanksgiving.

Socioeconomic Factors

Socioeconomic level may be a determinant of nutritional status. Poverty-level families are unable to afford the same foods that higher-income families can. Thus pregnant women with low incomes are frequently at risk for poor nutrition.

Education

Knowledge about the basic components of a balanced diet is essential. Often educational level is related to economic status, but even people on very limited incomes can prepare well-balanced meals if their knowledge of nutrition is adequate.

Psychologic Factors

Emotions directly affect nutritional well-being. For example, anorexia nervosa, a psychologic disorder that occurs primarily in adolescent girls, is manifested as self-inflicted starvation, resulting in malnutrition and ultimately death if not treated. Loss of appetite is also a common symptom of serious depression.

The expectant woman's attitudes and feelings about her pregnancy may influence her nutritional status. The woman who is depressed or who does not wish to be pregnant may manifest these feelings by loss of appetite or by improper food practices, such as overindulgence in sweets or alcohol.

THE PREGNANT ADOLESCENT

Nutritional care of the pregnant adolescent is of particular concern to health care professionals. Many adolescents are nutritionally at risk due to a variety of complex and interrelated emotional, social, and economic factors that may adversely affect dietary intake.

Nutritional Concerns

General Concerns

In their position statement the ADA stated, "pregnant adolescents as a group are nutritionally at risk and require nutritional intervention early and throughout the duration of their pregnancies" (ADA 1989a, p 104). Nutritional status is an important, modifiable variable in any pregnancy, but especially adolescent pregnancy, because teens are more likely than older women to be under-

weight at the onset of pregnancy and to gain less weight during pregnancy. Good maternal weight gain during adolescent pregnancy significantly improves fetal growth and reduces mortality without increasing overall risk of cesarean birth or complications.

Important nutrition-related factors to assess in pregnant adolescents include low prepregnant weight, low weight gain during pregnancy, younger age with regard to menarche, smoking, excessive prepregnant weight, anemia, unhealthy life-style (drugs, alcohol use), chronic disease, and history of an eating disorder (ADA 1989b).

Each of these factors can independently affect the adolescent's nutrient intake and consequently the status of the pregnancy. The high incidence of low-birth-weight infants born to pregnant adolescents (age 14 to 17) is more likely a result of the number of risk factors present than their maternal age. These risk factors seem to have more impact on pregnant adolescents than on the pregnant nonadolescents (Johnston et al 1991).

The psychosocial development of adolescents often results in a compromised nutritional intake. As adolescents become more independent, they make more of their own food choices; these may be influenced, either positively or negatively, by peer acceptance.

Physiologic maturation plays a role in the development of a body image and self-concept. Weight gain and changes in body appearance occur as growth and development progress. This may be difficult for some adolescent girls to accept and can lead to a negative self-concept and possible restrictive food choices. In some cases it can be a contributing factor in the development of eating disorders.

The weight gain of pregnancy can be affected by the adolescent's attitudes. She may have trouble consuming a diet that will support the desired increase in pounds. Negative attitudes about gaining weight during pregnancy are most common among heavier or depressed adolescents and those who do not perceive their families as supportive (Stevens-Simon et al 1993).

In determining nutrient needs for pregnant adolescents it is important to consider the number of years that have passed since menstruation began. Adolescent females generally are considered physiologically mature about 4 years after menarche because linear growth is usually completed by this time. Their nutritional needs would be similar to other "adult" women.

Adolescents who become pregnant fewer than 4 years after menarche, however, are at a high biologic risk due to their physiologic and anatomic immaturity. They are most likely to be growing, which can impact the fetus's development. Growing adolescents have infants who weigh less than those of nongrowing adolescents and adults 19 to 29 years of age (Scholl & Hediger 1993). Nutritional needs for these young women will be higher than for those whose growth has been completed.

Very little information is currently available on the nutritional needs of adolescents. Estimates are usually obtained by using the RDA for nonpregnant teenagers (age 11 to 14 or 15 to 18) and adding nutrient amounts recommended for all pregnant women (Table 17–1). Although the RDA is based on chronologic age, it is probably the best available figures to use if the pregnant female is still growing. If mature, the pregnant adolescent has nutritional needs approaching those reported for pregnant adults. However, young adolescents (13 to 15 years) need to gain more weight than older adolescents (16 years or older) to produce babies of equal size. Thus in determining the optimum weight gain for a pregnant adolescent it is important to consider the following:

- Recommended weight gain for a normal pregnancy
- Amount of weight gain expected during the postmenarcheal year during which the pregnancy occurs

The issue of recommended weight gain during pregnancy was addressed earlier in this chapter (in "Maternal Weight Gain"). Weight gain needs to be higher for adolescents than for adults to reduce the risk of low birth weight.

The weight gain for a normal pregnancy and the expected weight gain due to growth would be added together to obtain a recommended weight gain for the pregnant adolescent. Young adolescents (2 years after menarche) should strive for a weight gain at the upper end of the range of weight gain for adults (Table 17–3).

Specific Nutrient Concerns

Caloric needs of pregnant adolescents vary widely. Major factors in determining caloric needs include whether growth has been completed and the physical activity level of the individual. Figures as high as 50 kcal/kg have been suggested for young, growing teens who are very active physically. A satisfactory weight gain will confirm adequacy of caloric intake in most cases.

Inadequate iron intake is a main concern with the adolescent diet. Iron needs are high for the pregnant teen due to the requirement for iron by the enlarging muscle mass and blood volume. Iron supplements—providing 30 to 60 mg of elemental iron—are definitely indicated.

Calcium is another nutrient that demands special attention from pregnant adolescents. Inadequate intake of calcium is frequently a problem in this age group. Adequate calcium intake is needed to support normal growth and development of the fetus as well as growth and maintenance of calcium stores in the adolescent. To provide for these needs an intake of 1200 to 1600 mg/day of calcium is recommended to promote bone mineralization in the adolescent as well as to support fetal skeletal growth (Matkovic 1991). Calcium supplementation is indicated for teens with an aversion to or intolerance of milk unless other dairy products or significant calcium sources are consumed in sufficient quantities.

Because folic acid plays a role in cell reproduction, it is also an important nutrient for pregnant teens. As previously indicated, a supplement is often suggested for pregnant females, whether adult or teenager.

Other nutrients and vitamins must be considered when evaluating the overall nutritional quality of the teenager's diet. Nutrients that have frequently been found to be deficient in this age group include zinc and vitamins A, D, and B_6. Inclusion of a wide variety of foods—especially fresh and lightly processed foods—is helpful in obtaining adequate amounts of trace minerals, fiber, and other vitamins. A low-dose vitamin and mineral supplement may be necessary when the diet is not adequate (Institute of Medicine 1990).

Eating Disorders

Eating disorders are most common in adolescent girls and young women. They are psychologic disorders that can have a major impact on physiologic well-being.

Anorexia nervosa is an eating disorder characterized by an extreme fear of weight gain and fat. People with this problem have distorted body images and perceive themselves as fat even though they are extremely underweight. Their dietary intake is very restricted in both variety and quantity. In addition to their restrictive eating they may engage in excessive exercise to prevent weight gain.

Individuals with anorexia nervosa do not often become pregnant because of the physiologic changes that affect their reproductive systems. If they do, they may suffer from hypokalemia, ketosis, and weight loss. In most cases the infant's birth weight is severely depressed (Rosso 1990).

The eating disorder bulimia is characterized by binging (secretly consuming large amounts of food in a short time) and purging. Self-induced vomiting is the most common method of purging; laxatives and/or diuretics may also be used. Individuals with bulimia often maintain a normal or close to normal weight for their height, so it is difficult to know if binging and purging occur. The self-induced vomiting of bulimia may even mimic hyperemesis gravidarum (Rosso 1990).

In both anorexia nervosa and bulimia the treatment needs to be a team approach involving medical, dietetic, and psychiatric practitioners. The pregnant adolescent or young woman with an eating disorder needs to be closely monitored and supported throughout her pregnancy.

Dietary Patterns

Healthy adolescents often have irregular eating patterns. Many skip breakfast, and most tend to be frequent snackers. Teens rarely follow the traditional three meals a day pattern, their day-to-day intake often varies drastically, and they eat food combinations that may seem bizarre to adults. Despite this, adolescents usually achieve a better nutritional balance than most adults would expect.

In assessing the diet of the pregnant adolescent the nurse should consider the eating pattern over time, not simply a single day's intake. This pattern is critical because of the irregularity of most adolescent eating patterns. Once the pattern is identified, counseling can be directed toward correcting deficiencies.

Counseling Issues

Critical Thinking Question

In counseling a pregnant adolescent, what approaches might be most effective in helping the teenager develop a more nutritionally sound eating pattern?

A positive approach to nutritional counseling for the pregnant adolescent is more effective than a negative one. The nurse must be ready to suggest valuable foods that pregnant teens can choose in many places and at any time. If the adolescent's mother does most of the meal preparation, it may be useful to include her in the discussion if the adolescent agrees. Involving the expectant father in counseling may be beneficial. If the teen is remaining in school, cooperation can also be sought from school lunch personnel (ADA 1989b).

The pregnant teenager will soon become a parent, and her understanding of nutrition will influence not only her well-being but also that of her child. However, teens tend to live in the present, and counseling that stresses long-term changes may be less effective than more concrete approaches. In many cases group classes are effective, especially those with other teens. In a group atmosphere adolescents often work together to plan adequate meals including foods that are special favorites.

POSTPARTUM NUTRITION

Nutritional needs will change following the birth. Nutrient requirements will vary depending on whether the mother decides to breastfeed. An assessment of postpartal nutritional status is necessary before nutritional guidance is given.

Postpartal Nutritional Status

Determination of postpartal nutritional status is based primarily on the new mother's weight, hemoglobin and hematocrit levels, clinical signs, and dietary history.

As previously discussed, an ideal weight gain for the normal-weight woman during pregnancy is between 11.5 and 16 kg (25 and 35 lb). After birth there is a weight loss of approximately 10 to 12 lb. Additional weight loss will be most rapid during the first few weeks after birth as the uterus returns to normal size, tissue fluids are released, and maternal blood volume returns to normal. The mother's weight will then begin to stabilize. Weight loss may also be affected by lactation. Weight loss of women who breastfeed tends to be greater than that of those who do not if breastfeeding continues for at least 6 months (Dewey et al 1993). However, this will vary among individuals; not all women who breastfeed will lose weight, or the weight loss may be negligible (Schauberger et al 1992).

The rate of postpartum weight loss is influenced by many factors. Some women approach their prepregnancy weight several weeks after birth; most approach this weight about 6 months later. The amount of weight gained during pregnancy is a major determinant of weight loss after childbirth. Generally, the more weight gained during pregnancy, the more is lost postpartum. Other factors that have been shown to increase weight loss are the return to work outside the home, parity (multiparous women lose less weight), and smoking (Schauberger et al 1992).

It is important to evaluate the mother's current weight, ideal weight for her height, weight before pregnancy, and weight before the birth. Women who are interested in weight reduction should be referred to a dietitian. Different guidelines for weight loss are used for nursing mothers and nonnursing mothers.

Hemoglobin and erythrocyte values vary after birth, but they should return to normal levels within 2 to 6 weeks. Hematocrit levels should rise gradually due to hemoconcentration as extracellular fluid is excreted. The hematocrit is usually checked at the postpartum visit to detect any anemia. Mothers can be encouraged to eat a diet high in iron. Iron supplements are generally prescribed for 2 to 3 months following birth to replenish supplies depleted by pregnancy.

Clinical symptoms the new mother may be experiencing are assessed. Food cravings and aversions typically drop significantly during the postpartal period and are not usually problematic. However, constipation is a common problem following birth. The nurse can encourage the woman to maintain a high fluid intake to keep the stool soft. Dietary sources of fiber and physical exercise are also helpful in preventing constipation.

Specific information on diet and eating habits is obtained directly from the woman. Visiting the mother during mealtimes provides an opportunity for unobtrusive nutritional assessment. Which foods has a woman selected? Has she avoided fruits and vegetables? Is her diet nutritionally sound? A comment focusing on a positive aspect of her meal selection may initiate a discussion of nutrition.

The dietitian should be informed about any woman whose cultural or religious beliefs require specific foods. Appropriate meals can then be prepared for her. The nurse may also refer women with unusual eating habits or numerous questions about food or nutrition to a dietitian. In all cases the nurse should provide literature on nutrition so that the woman will have a source of appropriate information at home.

Nutritional Care of Nonnursing Mothers

After birth the nonnursing mother's dietary requirements return to prepregnancy levels (Table 17–1). If the mother has a good understanding of nutritional principles, it is sufficient to advise her to reduce her daily caloric intake by about 300 kcal and to return to prepregnancy levels for other nutrients.

If the mother has a poor understanding of nutrition, this is an opportunity to teach her the basic principles and the importance of a well-balanced diet. Her eating habits and dietary practices will eventually be reflected in the diet of her child.

If the mother has gained excessive weight during pregnancy (or perhaps was overweight before pregnancy), referral to a dietitian is appropriate. The dietitian can design weight-reduction diets to meet nutritional needs and food preferences. Weight loss goals of 1 to 2 lb/week are usually suggested.

In addition to learning how to meet her own nutritional needs, the new mother will usually be interested in learning how to provide for her infant's nutritional needs. A discussion of infant feeding, which includes topics such as selecting infant formulas, formula preparation, and vitamin/mineral supplementation, is appropriate and generally well received.

Nutritional Care of Nursing Mothers

Nutrient Needs

Nutrient needs are increased during breastfeeding. Table 17–1 lists the RDA during breastfeeding for specific nutrients. Table 17–2 provides a sample daily food guide for lactating women. A few key nutrients need further discussion.

Calories One of the most important factors in the diet while breastfeeding is calories. An inadequate caloric intake can reduce milk volume. However, milk quality generally remains unaffected.

The nursing mother should increase her caloric intake by 200 kcal over the pregnancy requirements (that is, a 500 kcal increase from her prepregnancy requirement). This results in a total of about 2500 to 2700 kcal/day for most women.

The nursing mother can use the food guide pyramid to assess her dietary intake. She should strive to include a variety of foods from each food group. Her caloric intake needs to provide enough energy to sustain lactation. After her weight stabilizes several weeks following childbirth, weight loss should not exceed more than 1 lb/week for nursing mothers.

Protein Because protein is an important ingredient in breast milk, an adequate intake is essential while breast-feeding. An intake of 65 g/day during the first 6 months of breastfeeding and 62 g/day during the second 6 months is recommended. As in pregnancy, it is important to consume adequate nonprotein calories in order to prevent the use of protein as an energy source.

Calcium Calcium is also an important ingredient in milk production, and increases over nonpregnancy needs are expected. Requirements during breastfeeding remain the same as requirements during pregnancy: 1200 mg/day. An inadequate intake of calcium from food sources necessitates the use of calcium supplements.

Iron Because iron is not a principal mineral component of milk, needs during lactation are not substantially different from those of nonpregnant women. However, as previously mentioned, continued supplementation of the mother for 2 to 3 months after parturition is advisable in order to replenish maternal stores depleted by pregnancy.

Fluids Liquids are especially important during lactation because inadequate fluid intake may decrease milk volume. Fluid recommendations while breastfeeding are 8 to 10 (8 oz) glasses daily and can be fulfilled with water, juices, milk, and soups.

Counseling Issues

In addition to counseling nursing mothers on how to meet their increased nutrient needs during breastfeeding, nurses should discuss a few issues related to infant feeding.

For example, many mothers are concerned about how specific foods they eat will affect their babies during breastfeeding. Generally, there are no foods the nursing mother must avoid except those to which she might be allergic. Occasionally, however, some nursing mothers find that their babies are affected by certain foods. Onions, turnips, cabbage, chocolate, spices, and seasonings are commonly listed as offenders. The best advice to give the nursing mother is to avoid those foods she suspects cause distress in her infant. For the most part, however, she should be able to eat any nourishing food she wants without fear that her baby will be affected. For further discussion of successful infant feeding see Chapter 30.

APPLYING THE NURSING PROCESS

Nursing Assessment

Assessment of nutritional status is necessary in order to plan an optimal diet with each woman. Data may be gathered from the woman's chart and by interviewing her. Information is obtained about (1) the woman's height and weight and her weight gain during pregnancy; (2) pertinent laboratory values, especially hemoglobin and hematocrit; (3) clinical signs that have possible nutritional implications, such as constipation, anorexia, or heartburn; and (4) diet history to determine the woman's views on nutrition as well as her specific nutrient intake.

A diet history may be obtained by asking the woman to complete a 24-hour diet recall, in which she lists everything consumed in the previous 24 hours, including foods, fluids, and any supplements. Diet may also be evaluated using a food summary. The woman is given a list of common categories of foods and asked how frequently in a day (or week) she consumes foods from the list. Common categories include vegetables, fruits, milk or cheese, meat or poultry, fish, desserts or sweets, coffee or tea, and alcoholic beverages. This method may be less reliable because it requires the individual to be accurate in generalizing about her intake.

In some instances the nurse will ask the woman to keep a food record or diary of everything she eats for a specified period of time (such as a week). This provides a clearer picture of nutritional patterns and may prompt the woman to make changes if the diary reveals areas of deficiency or excess.

During the data-gathering process the nurse has an opportunity to determine what the woman is interested in learning. Health care providers often perceive that their clients are more interested in certain topics than they actually are (Freda et al 1993). Nursing plans developed on this basis would be less successful than ones that address the client's primary interests. Once this has been determined, the nurse can discuss important aspects of nutrition in the context of the family's needs and lifestyle. The nurse also seeks information about psychologic, cultural, and socioeconomic factors that may influence food intake.

The nurse can use a nutritional questionnaire such as the one shown in Figure 17–3 to gather and record important facts. This information provides a database the nurse can use to develop an intervention plan to fit the woman's individual needs. The sample questionnaire has been filled in to demonstrate this process.

Nursing Diagnosis

Once the data are obtained the nurse begins to analyze the information, formulate appropriate nursing diagnoses, and develop client goals. For a woman during the first trimester, for example, the diagnosis may be "Altered nutrition: Less than body requirements related to nausea and vomiting." In many cases the diagnosis may be related to excessive weight gain. In such cases the diagnosis might be "Altered nutrition: More than body requirements related to excessive intake of calories." Although these diagnoses are broad, the nurse must be specific in addressing issues such as inadequate intake of nutrients

CRITICAL THINKING IN PRACTICE

Jane is 14 weeks pregnant. The rate and total amount of her weight gain during the first trimester have been consistent with recommendations. She has gained an average of 0.5 kg (1 lb) per week during both of the past 2 weeks. Her appetite is good, and she consumes three meals per day and snacks between meals on occasion.

Jane has altered her diet because she is concerned about her weight gain becoming excessive. She told the nurse that she has decreased her intake from the bread and dairy groups in order to limit her calorie intake. Since she has omitted most dairy products, she has increased her consumption of salads and broccoli to provide sources of calcium.

A diet history revealed the following:

Grain	3–4 servings, mainly cereal and rice
Fruit	2–4 servings, fresh fruit
Vegetables	3–5 servings, salads, peas, corn, broccoli
Meat	4–5 servings, beef, pork, chicken
Dairy	occasionally cheese, ice cream, pudding
Fats, oils, sweets	occasionally salad dressings, margarine, desserts
Beverages	8–10 servings, soda, juices, water

After assessing her diet history, what is your evaluation of Jane's diet? How could you counsel her?

Answers can be found in Appendix I.

such as iron, calcium, or folic acid; problems with nutrition due to a limited food budget; problems related to physiologic alterations such as anorexia, heartburn, or nausea; and behavioral problems related to excessive dieting, anorexia nervosa, or bulimia. In some instances the category "Knowledge deficit" may seem most appropriate.

Nursing Plan and Implementation

After the nursing diagnosis is made, the nurse can plan an approach to correct any nutritional deficiencies or improve the overall quality of the diet. In counseling the pregnant woman it is important to avoid "talking down to" her or "preaching" to her. Information should be presented in a clear, logical way, using appropriate language, but avoiding jargon. Examples are often helpful in clarifying material. All questions should be answered appropriately and clearly.

When a person requires nutritional counseling, it usually indicates that a dietary change is necessary. Change is often difficult for people, however. Counseling

NUTRITIONAL QUESTIONNAIRE

Name ___Susan Longmont___   Date ___12-16-96___

Age ___20___

Ethnic group ___Caucasian___

Religion ___Protestant___

Gravida ___1̇___   Para ___0̇___

Age of youngest child? ___NA___   EDC ___7-7-88___

Birth weights of previous children? ___NA___

Usual nonpregnant weight ___115___   Present weight ___125___

Weight gain during last pregnancy? ___NA___

Vitamin supplements? ___none___

Current medications? ___aspirin for headache___

Do you smoke? ___yes___   How much per day? ___1-1½ packs___

Eating patterns:

1. How many meals per day? ___2___   when ___12:30 pm   6:30 pm___

2. How many snacks per day? ___3___   when ___10:30 am 4:00 pm 10:00 pm___

3. What other foods are important to your usual diet? ___chocolate and candy bars___

4. Amount per day ___4 bars/week___

5. Do you have any different food preferences now? ___no___

6. Do you eat nonfoods such as:

		Amount
laundry starch	no	NA
ice	yes	10 cubes/day
other (name)	no	NA

7. What foods do you dislike or do not eat? ___spinach and dried beans___

8. For added information complete a typical daily intake (24 hour recall is suggested).

Do you have special problems in food preparation such as:

1. Physical disability   yes ___   no ___✓___   Explain

2. Cooking appliances   yes ___   no ___✓___   Explain

3. Refrigeration of food   yes ___   no ___✓___   Explain

Who does the meal planning? ___I do.___   shopping? ___We both do.___

cooking? ___I do most of the time but my husband likes to help.___

Are there transportation problems? ___We have only one car but we go in the evening.___

Financial situation: ___My husband is working and going to school.___

___I am not working.___   Foodstamps ___Yes___   W/c ___no___

Do you have any previous nutritional problems? ___No. I have never paid much attention___

___to food before, but now I have lots of questions.___

Are there any problems with this pregnancy? Nausea ___Yes, in the morning.___

Constipation ___No___   Other ___NA___

Assessment by the nurse following the completion of the questionnaire.

Basic estimated nutrient and caloric value of typical daily intake.

Please circle one of the following:

Protein intake was   low   adequate   high

Caloric intake was   (low)   adequate   high

Calcium intake was   (low)   adequate   high

Iron intake was   low   adequate   (high)

Vitamin C intake was   low   (adequate)   high

FIGURE 17-3   Sample nutritional questionnaire used in nursing management of a pregnant woman.

will be more effective if the nurse understands the client's values and explains the needed change in a way that is meaningful to the client. Because the pregnant woman must follow the plan, it should be developed in cooperation with her, be suitable for her financial level and background, and be based on reasonable, achievable goals.

The following example demonstrates one way a nurse can implement a plan with a client based on the nursing diagnosis.

Diagnosis: Altered nutrition: Less than body requirements related to low intake of calcium
Client goal: The woman will increase her intake of calcium to RDA levels.
Implementation:

1. Plan with the woman additional milk or dairy products that can reasonably be added to the diet (specify amounts).

2. Encourage the use of other calcium sources such as leafy green vegetables and legumes.

3. Plan for the addition of powdered milk in cooking and baking.

4. If none of the above are realistic or acceptable, consider the use of calcium supplements.

Counseling Families About Good Nutrition

Food is a significant portion of a family's budget, and meeting nutritional needs may be a challenge for families on limited incomes. Some families qualify for special assistance to meet their nutritional needs. The *Food Stamp Program* provides stamps or coupons for participating households whose net monthly income is below a specified level. These stamps can be used to purchase food for the household each month.

The *Special Supplemental Food Program for Women, Infants, and Children (WIC)* is designed to assist pregnant or breastfeeding women with low incomes and their children under 5 years of age. The program provides food assistance, nutrition education, and referrals to health care providers. The food distributed, including dried beans and peas, peanut butter, eggs, cheese, milk, fortified adult and infant cereals, juice, and iron-fortified infant formula, is designed to provide good sources of iron, protein, and certain vitamins for individuals with an inadequate diet. The WIC program is credited with helping reduce the incidence of low birth weight in infants and in decreasing the incidence of anemia in the infants and young children of low-income families (General Accounting Office 1992).

Most families can benefit from guidance about food purchasing and preparation. Women should be advised to plan food purchases thoughtfully by preparing general menus and a list before shopping. It is also helpful to advise clients to monitor sales, compare brands, and be se-

lective when purchasing processed foods, which tend to be expensive. Other techniques for keeping food costs down without jeopardizing quality include buying food in season, using bulk foods when appropriate, using whole grain or enriched products, buying lower-grade eggs (grading has no relation to the egg's nutritional value but indicates color of the shell and delicacy of flavor), and avoiding fancy grades of food and foods in elaborate packaging.

Evaluation

Once a plan has been developed and implemented, the nurse and client may wish to identify ways of evaluating its effectiveness. Evaluation may involve keeping a food journal, writing out weekly menus, returning for weekly weighing, and the like. If anemia is a special problem, periodic hematocrit assessments are also indicated.

Women with serious nutritional deficiencies are referred to a dietitian. The nurse can then work closely with the dietitian and the client to improve the pregnant woman's health by modifying her diet.

KEY CONCEPTS

Maternal weight gains averaging 11.5 to 16 kg (25 to 35 lb) for a normal-weight woman are associated with the best reproductive outcomes.

If the diet is adequate, folic acid and iron are the only supplements generally recommended during pregnancy.

Caloric restriction to reduce weight should not be undertaken during pregnancy.

Pregnant women should be encouraged to eat regularly and to eat a wide variety of foods, especially fresh and lightly processed foods.

Taking megadoses of vitamins during pregnancy is unnecessary and potentially dangerous.

In vegetarian diets special emphasis should be placed on obtaining ample complete proteins, calories, calcium, iron, vitamin D, vitamin B_{12}, and zinc through food sources or supplementation if necessary.

Evaluation of physical, psychosocial, and cultural factors that affect food intake is essential before nutritional status can be determined and nutritional counseling planned.

Adolescents who become pregnant less than 4 years after menarche have higher nutritional needs and are considered to be at high biologic risk.

Weight gains during adolescent pregnancy must accommodate recommended gains for a normal pregnancy plus necessary gains due to growth.

After childbirth the nonnursing mother's dietary requirements return to prepregnancy levels.

Nursing mothers require an adequate caloric and fluid intake to maintain ample milk volume.

REFERENCES

American Dietetic Association: Nutrition management of adolescent pregnancy: Technical support paper. *J Am Diet Assoc* January 1989a; 89:105.

American Dietetic Association: Position of the American Dietetic Association: Nutrition management of adolescent pregnancy. *J Am Diet Assoc* January 1989b; 89:104.

American Dietetic Association: Position of the American Dietetic Association: Vegetarian diets. *J Am Diet Assoc* March 1988a; 88:351.

American Dietetic Association: Position of the American Dietetic Association: Vegetarian diets—technical support paper. *J Am Diet Assoc* March 1988b; 88:352.

Barclay BA: Experience with enteral nutrition in the treatment of hyperemesis gravidarum. *Nutr Clin Pract* 1990; 5:153.

Belizán JM et al: Calcium supplementation to prevent hypertensive disorders of pregnancy. *N Engl J Med* November 1991; 325:1399.

Centers for Disease Control and Prevention: Recommendations for use of folic acid to reduce number of spina bifida cases and other neural tube defects. *MMWR* 1992; 41:RR-14.

Cunningham FG, Lindheimer MD: Hypertension in pregnancy. *N Engl J Med* April 1992; 326:927.

DeLong GR: Effects of nutrition on brain development in humans. *Am J Clin Nutr* 1993; 57(suppl):286S.

Dewey KG et al: Maternal weight-loss patterns during prolonged lactation. *Am J Clin Nutr* August 1993; 58:162.

Folic acid for prevention of neural tube defects. *Contracep Rep* July 1993; 4(3):11.

Freda MC et al: What pregnant women want to know: A comparison of client and provider perceptions. *JOGNN* May/June 1993; 22:237.

General Accounting Office: Early intervention: Federal investments like WIC can produce savings. *Document HRD 92-18.* Washington, DC, May 1992.

Horner RD et al: Pica practices of pregnant women. *J Am Diet Assoc* January 1991; 91:34.

Institute of Medicine, Subcommittee for a Clinical Application Guide. *Nutrition During Pregnancy and Lactation: An Implementation Guide.* Washington, DC: National Academy Press, 1992.

Institute of Medicine, Subcommittee on Dietary Intake and Nutrient Supplements During Pregnancy, Committee on Nutrition Status During Pregnancy and Lactation, Food and Nutrition Board: *Nutrition During Pregnancy: Weight Gain and Nutrient Supplements.* Washington, DC: National Academy Press, 1990.

Johnston CS et al: Pregnancy weight gain in adolescents and young adults. *J Am Coll Nutr* 1991; 10:185.

Luke B, Keith L: *Principles and Practice of Maternal Nutrition.* Park Ridge, NJ: Parthenon, 1992.

Matkovic V: Calcium metabolism and calcium requirements during skeletal modeling and consolidation of bone mass. *Am J Clin Nutr* 1991; 54:245S.

Medical Research Council Vitamin Research Group: Prevention of neural tube defects: Results of the medical research council vitamin study. *Lancet* July 1991; 338:131.

Mills JL et al: Moderate caffeine use and the risk of spontaneous abortion and intrauterine growth retardation. *JAMA* February 1993; 269:593.

Narod SA et al: Coffee during pregnancy: A reproductive hazard? *Am J Obstet Gynecol* April 1991; 164:1109.

National Research Council, Food and Nutrition Board: *Recommended Dietary Allowances,* 10th ed. Washington, DC: National Academy Press, 1989.

Rosso P: *Nutrition and Metabolism in Pregnancy.* New York: Oxford Univ Press, 1990.

Schauberger CW et al: Factors that influence weight loss in the puerperium. *Obstet Gynecol* March 1992; 79:424.

Scholl TO, Hediger ML: A review of the epidemiology of nutrition and adolescent pregnancy: Maternal growth during pregnancy and its effect on the fetus. *J Am Coll Nutr* 1993; 12:101.

Stevens-Simon C et al: Weight gain attitudes among pregnant adolescents. *J Adoles Health* 1993; 14:369.

US Department of Agriculture, US Department of Health and Human Services: Nutrition and your health: Dietary guidelines for Americans, 3rd ed. *Home and Garden Bulletin no. 232,* Washington, DC, 1990.

Way S: Food for Asian mothers-to-be. *Nurs Times* December 1991; 87:50.

CHAPTER 18

PREGNANCY AT RISK: PREGESTATIONAL PROBLEMS

I've been a nurse for 25 years now, and I've never seen anything change nursing practice more than AIDS has. Nursing students today will take universal precautions for granted because they won't know any other way, but I can remember when we could touch more freely. I remember drying a newly born infant and stroking him—my hands warm against his skin. I remember a time when people didn't think twice before trying to stop bleeding or give other first aid at an accident scene. I know this way is safer, but a part of me mourns what we have lost.

KEY TERMS

Acquired immunodeficiency syndrome (AIDS)

Crack

Gestational diabetes mellitus

Macrosomia

OBJECTIVES

Describe the effects of various heart disorders on pregnancy, including their implications for nursing care.

Discuss the pathology, treatment, and nursing care of pregnant women with diabetes.

Discriminate among the four major types of anemia associated with pregnancy with regard to signs, treatment, and implications for pregnancy.

Discuss acquired immunodeficiency syndrome (AIDS), including care of the pregnant woman with AIDS, neonatal implications, and ramifications for the childbearing family.

Summarize the effects of alcohol and illicit drugs on the childbearing woman and her fetus/newborn.

Compare the effects of selected gestational medical conditions on pregnancy.

*E*ven though it is a normal process, pregnancy is biologically, physiologically, and psychologically stressful. For some women pregnancy may even be a life-threatening event. Prenatal care is aimed toward identification, assessment, and management of women whose pregnancies are at risk because of potential or existing complications.

Disruptive conditions that arise during the gestational period are the result of many high-risk factors, such as age, blood type, socioeconomic status, parity, psychologic well-being, and predisposing chronic illnesses. The major thrust of prenatal nursing care should be toward screening women for these complications and developing supportive therapies that will promote optimal health for mother and fetus.

This chapter focuses on women with pregestational medical disorders and the possible effects of these on the outcome of pregnancy.

CARE OF THE WOMAN WITH HEART DISEASE

A healthy woman with a normal heart has adequate cardiac reserve to adjust to the demands of pregnancy with little difficulty. The woman with heart disease has decreased cardiac reserve, making it more difficult for her heart to accommodate the higher work load of pregnancy.

Approximately 1% of pregnant women are at risk because of pregestational heart disease. Heart disease ranks fourth after hypertension, hemorrhage, and infection as a cause of maternal mortality. Although rheumatic heart disease used to predominate, congenital heart defects now constitute at least half of all cases of heart disease encountered during pregnancy (Cunningham et al 1993). Other less common causes of heart disease in pregnancy include Marfan syndrome, peripartum cardiomyopathy, and Eisenmenger syndrome. All cause significant maternal mortality. Mitral valve prolapse is usually asymptomatic but is addressed here because of its frequent occurrence during pregnancy.

Congenital heart defects have become a more common finding in pregnant women as improved surgical techniques enable females born with heart defects to live to childbearing age. The exact pathology depends on the specific defect. Congenital defects most often seen in pregnant women include tetralogy of Fallot, atrial septal defect, ventricular septal defect, patent ductus arteriosus, and coarctation of the aorta. When surgical repair can be accomplished with no remaining evidence of organic heart disease, pregnancy may be undertaken with confidence. In such cases antibiotic prophylaxis is recommended to prevent subacute bacterial endocarditis at the time of birth. When congenital heart disease is associated with cyanosis, whether the defect was originally uncorrected or the correction failed to relieve the cyanosis, the woman should be counseled to avoid pregnancy because the risk to both her and the fetus would be high. She also needs to know that there is a 2% to 5% chance of the baby inheriting the disorder because most congenital heart defects are believed to be polygenetic and multifactorial in origin.

Rheumatic heart has declined rapidly in the last four decades, primarily because of prompt identification of pharyngeal infections caused by group A beta-hemolytic streptococcus and the availability of penicillin for treatment. Rheumatic fever, which may develop in untreated streptococcal infections, is an inflammatory connective tissue disease that can involve the heart, joints, central nervous system, skin, and subcutaneous tissue. When the heart is affected, mitral valve stenosis is the most common and serious lesion. Aortic valve involvement, manifested by aortic insufficiency, is the second most common problem. The tricuspid and pulmonic valves are rarely affected.

Recurrent acute inflammation from bouts of rheumatic fever causes scar tissue formation on the valves. The scarring results in stenosis (narrowing) of the mitral valve, which may be accompanied by mitral regurgitation. Obstructed blood flow across the narrow valve from the left atrium to the left ventricle can lead to elevated left atrial pressure and elevated pulmonary venous and capillary pressures.

The increased blood volume of pregnancy, coupled with the pregnant woman's need for increased cardiac output, stresses the heart of a woman with mitral valve stenosis. She may develop dyspnea, orthopnea, and pulmonary edema and is at increased risk for congestive heart failure (CHF). Even the woman who has no symptoms at the onset of her pregnancy is at increased risk for CHF.

When the aortic valve is involved, the scarring usually leaves the valve unable to close completely (aortic incompetence or insufficiency) during diastole. Blood then regurgitates back into the left ventricle, leading to volume overload of the left ventricle and inadequate perfusion of the coronary arteries. Occasionally, there is both aortic stenosis and regurgitation.

With mild aortic insufficiency the woman may be asymptomatic. But if the valve dysfunction worsens, she may experience dyspnea and even chest pain (due to inadequate blood flow to the heart muscle) with exertion.

Marfan syndrome is an autosomal dominant disorder of connective tissue in which there may be serious cardiovascular involvement—usually dissection or rupture of the aorta. Because maternal mortality rate may be as high as 25% to 50%, a pregnant woman with Marfan syndrome needs very careful cardiovascular assessment and counseling regarding her prognosis for a successful pregnancy (Cruikshank 1994). Because of the inheritance pattern of the disease, there is a 50% chance of its being passed on to offspring.

Mitral valve prolapse (MVP) is usually an asymptomatic condition that is found in as many as 5% of women of childbearing age (Cunningham et al 1993). The condition is more common in women than in men and seems to run in families. In MVP the mitral valve leaflets tend to prolapse into the left atrium during ventricular systole because the chordae tendineae that support them are long and thin. As a result some mitral regurgitation may occur. On auscultation a midsystolic click and a late systolic murmur are heard.

Women with MVP usually tolerate pregnancy well, and the prognosis is excellent. Most women require assurance that they can continue with normal activities. A few women experience symptoms—primarily palpitations, chest pain, and dyspnea—which are usually due to arrhythmias. They are often treated with propranolol hydrochloride (Inderal). Limiting caffeine intake also helps decrease palpitations. Women should be given antibiotic prophylaxis if there is mitral valve regurgitation, valvular damage, or any other risk factors (Cunningham et al 1993).

Peripartum cardiomyopathy is a dysfunction of the left ventricle that occurs in the last month of pregnancy or the first 5 months postpartum in a woman with no previous history of heart disease. The symptoms are related to congestive heart failure: dyspnea, orthopnea, chest pain, palpitations, weakness, and edema. The cause is unknown. Treatment includes digitalis, diuretics, anticoagulants, and bed rest. The condition may resolve with bed rest as the heart gradually returns to normal size. Subsequent pregnancy is strongly discouraged because the disease tends to recur during pregnancy.

Eisenmenger syndrome is not a congenital defect, but a complication that can develop with any cardiac lesion when right to left shunting causes increased pulmonary vascular resistance. This condition cannot be corrected surgically and is associated with a high maternal mortality rate (Cunningham et al 1993).

Medical Therapy

The primary goal of medical management is early diagnosis and ongoing treatment of the woman with cardiac disease. Echocardiogram, chest x-ray, electrocardiogram, auscultation of heart sounds, and sometimes cardiac catheterization are essential for establishing the type and severity of the heart disease. The severity of heart disease can also be determined by the individual's ability to perform ordinary physical activity. The following classification of functional capacity has been standardized by the Criteria Committee of the New York Heart Association (1955):

- Class I. No limitation of physical activity. Ordinary physical activity causes no discomfort; anginal pain is not present.
- Class II. Slight limitation of physical activity. Ordinary physical activity causes fatigue, dyspnea, palpitation, or anginal pain.
- Class III. Moderate to marked limitation of physical activity. During less than ordinary physical activity the person experiences excessive fatigue, dyspnea, palpitation, or anginal pain.
- Class IV. Inability to carry on any physical activity without experiencing discomforts. Even at rest the person experiences symptoms of cardiac insufficiency or anginal pain.

Women in classes I and II usually experience a normal pregnancy and have few complications, whereas those in classes III and IV are at risk for more severe complications, which may affect both maternal and fetal outcomes.

Because anemia increases the work of the heart, it should be diagnosed early and treated if present. Infection also increases the cardiac work load, so even minor infections should be treated thoroughly. To reduce the risk of pyelonephritis, monthly screening for asymptomatic bacteriuria is indicated, with antibiotic therapy as needed (Cruikshank 1994).

Drug Therapy

Besides the iron and vitamin supplements prescribed during pregnancy, the pregnant woman with heart disease may need additional drug therapy to maintain health. Antibiotics, usually penicillin if not contraindicated by allergy, are used during pregnancy to prevent recurrent bouts of rheumatic fever and subsequent heart valve damage. Antibiotics are also recommended during labor and the early postpartum period for either acquired or congenital disease to prevent bacterial endocarditis. If the woman develops coagulation problems, the anticoagulant heparin may be used. Heparin offers the greatest safety to the fetus because it does not cross the placenta. The thiazide diuretics and furosemide (Lasix) may be used to treat congestive heart failure if it develops. Digitalis glycosides and common antiarrhythmic drugs may be used to treat cardiac failure and arrhythmias. These agents do cross the placenta but have no reported teratogenic effect; however, they have not been adequately studied to establish their safety in pregnancy (Cunningham et al 1993).

Labor

Spontaneous natural labor with adequate pain relief is usually recommended for clients in classes I and II. Those in classes III and IV may need to be hospitalized prior to onset of labor for cardiovascular stabilization. They may also require invasive cardiac monitoring during labor.

Childbirth

Use of low forceps provides the safest method of birth, with lumbar epidural anesthesia to reduce the stress of pushing. Cesarean is used only if fetal or maternal indications exist, not on the basis of heart disease alone.

Critical Thinking Question

What specific information does the nurse need to help the pregnant woman with heart disease plan her schedule to avoid stress and allow sufficient time for rest?

APPLYING THE NURSING PROCESS

Nursing Assessment

The stress of pregnancy on the functional capacity of the heart is assessed during every antepartal visit. The nurse notes the category of functional capacity assigned to the woman, takes the woman's pulse, respirations, and blood pressure, and compares them to the normal values expected during pregnancy and to the woman's previous values. The nurse then determines the woman's activity level, including rest, and any changes in the pulse and respirations that have occurred since previous visits. The nurse also identifies and evaluates other factors that would increase strain on the heart. These might include anemia, infection, anxiety, lack of support system, and household and career demands.

The following symptoms, if they are progressive, are indicative of congestive heart failure, the heart's signal of its decreased ability to meet the demands of pregnancy:

- Cough (frequent, with or without hemoptysis)
- Dyspnea (progressive, upon exertion)
- Edema (progressive, generalized, including extremities, face, eyelids)
- Heart murmurs (heard on auscultation)
- Palpitations
- Rales (auscultated in lung bases)

This cycle is *progressive* because some of these same behaviors are seen to a minor degree in a pregnancy without cardiac problems.

Nursing Diagnosis

Nursing diagnoses that might apply to the pregnant woman with heart disease include the following:

- Decreased cardiac output: easy fatigability

- Impaired gas exchange related to pulmonary edema secondary to cardiac decompensation
- Fear related to the effects of the maternal cardiac condition on fetal well-being

Nursing Plan and Implementation

Nursing care is directed toward maintaining a balance between cardiac reserve and cardiac work load.

Antepartal Nursing Care

Nursing actions are designed to meet the physiologic and psychosocial needs of the pregnant woman with heart disease. The priority of nursing actions varies based on the severity of the disease process and the individual needs of the woman as determined by nursing assessment.

The woman and her family should thoroughly understand her condition and its management and should recognize signs of potential complications. This will increase their understanding and decrease anxiety. When the nurse provides thorough explanations, uses printed material, and provides frequent opportunities to ask questions and discuss concerns, the woman is better able to meet her own health care needs and seek assistance appropriately.

As part of health teaching the nurse explains the purposes of the dietary and activity changes that are required. A diet is instituted that is high in iron, protein, and essential nutrients but low in sodium, with adequate calories to ensure normal weight gain. Such a diet best meets the nutrition needs of the client with cardiac disease. Excessive weight gain is avoided because it taxes the heart. To help preserve her cardiac reserves, the woman may need to restrict her activities. In addition, 8–10 hours of sleep, with frequent daily rest periods, is essential. The nurse can encourage the woman to rest in the side-lying position to promote optimal placental perfusion. Because upper respiratory infections may tax the heart and lead to decompensation, the woman must avoid contact with sources of infection.

During the first half of pregnancy the woman is seen approximately every 2 weeks to assess cardiac status. During the second half of pregnancy the woman is seen weekly. These assessments are especially important between weeks 28 and 30, when the blood volume reaches maximum amounts. If symptoms of cardiac decompensation occur, prompt medical intervention is indicated to correct the cardiac problem.

Intrapartal Nursing Care

Labor and birth exert tremendous stress on the woman and her fetus. This stress could be fatal to the fetus of a woman with cardiac disease because the fetus may be receiving a decreased oxygen and blood supply. Thus the intrapartal care of a woman with cardiac disease is aimed at reducing the amount of physical exertion and accompanying fatigue.

The nurse evaluates maternal vital signs frequently to determine the woman's response to labor. A pulse rate greater than 100 beats per minute or respirations greater than 25 per minute may indicate beginning cardiac decompensation and require further evaluation. The nurse also auscultates the woman's lungs frequently for evidence of rales and carefully observes for other signs of developing decompensation.

To ensure cardiac emptying and adequate oxygenation, the nurse encourages the laboring woman to assume either a semi-Fowler's or side-lying position with her head and shoulders elevated. Oxygen by mask, diuretics to reduce fluid retention, sedatives and analgesics, prophylactic antibiotics, and digitalis may also be used as indicated by the woman's status.

The nurse remains with the woman to support her. It is essential that the nurse keep the woman and her family informed of labor progress and management plans, collaborating with them to fulfill their wishes for the birth experience as much as possible. The nurse needs to maintain an atmosphere of calm to lessen the anxiety of the woman and her family.

Continuous electronic fetal monitoring is used to provide ongoing assessment of the fetus's response to labor. To prevent overexertion and the accompanying fatigue, the nurse encourages the woman to sleep and relax between contractions and provides her with emotional support and encouragement. During pushing, the nurse encourages the woman to use shorter, more moderate open glottis pushing (see Chapter 23), with complete relaxation between pushes. Vital signs are monitored closely during the second stage.

Postpartal Nursing Care

The postpartal period is a significant time for the woman with cardiac disease. After birth the intra-abdominal pressure and the venous pressure are reduced, the splanchnic vessels engorge, and blood flow to the heart increases. As extravascular fluid returns to the bloodstream for excretion, cardiac output and blood volume increase. This physiologic adaptation places great strain on the heart and may lead to decompensation, especially in the first 48 hours postpartum.

So that the health care team can detect any possible problems, the woman remains in the hospital for approximately 1 week to rest and recover. Her vital signs are monitored frequently, and she is assessed for signs of decompensation. She stays in the semi-Fowler's or side-lying position, with her head and shoulders elevated, and begins a gradual, progressive activity program. Appropriate diet and stool softeners facilitate bowel movement without undue strain.

The postpartum nurse gives the woman opportunities to discuss her birth experience and helps her deal with any feelings or concerns that cause her distress. The nurse also encourages maternal-infant attachment by providing frequent opportunities for the mother to interact with her child.

Because there is no evidence that cardiac output is compromised during lactation, the only concern about breastfeeding for women with cardiovascular disease is related to medications that the mother may be taking (Lawrence 1989). These must be evaluated for their ability to pass into the milk and for any effect of the drug on lactation. The nurse can assist the breastfeeding mother to a comfortable side-lying position with her head moderately elevated or to a semi-Fowler's position. To conserve the mother's energy, the nurse should position the newborn at the breast and be available to burp the baby and reposition him or her at the other breast.

In addition to providing the normal postpartum discharge teaching, the nurse should ensure that the woman and her family understand the signs of possible problems resulting from her heart disease or from other postpartal complications. The nurse plans with the woman an activity schedule that is gradual, progressive, and appropriate to her needs and home environment. The nurse provides appropriate health teaching, including information about resumption of sexual activity and contraception. Visiting nurse or homemaker assistance referrals may be necessary, depending on the woman's status.

Evaluation

Anticipated outcomes of nursing care include:

- The woman clearly understands her condition and its possible impact on pregnancy, labor and birth, and the postpartal period.

- The woman participates in developing an appropriate health care regimen and follows it throughout her pregnancy.

- The woman gives birth to a healthy infant.

- The woman avoids congestive heart failure.

- The woman identifies signs and symptoms of possible complications postpartally.

- The woman is comfortable caring for her newborn infant.

CARE OF THE WOMAN WITH DIABETES MELLITUS

Diabetes mellitus, an endocrine disorder of carbohydrate metabolism, results from inadequate production or utilization of insulin. Insulin, produced by the beta cells of the islets of Langerhans in the pancreas, lowers blood glucose levels by enabling the glucose to move from the blood into muscle and adipose tissue cells.

Pathophysiology of Diabetes Mellitus

In diabetes mellitus the pancreas does not produce sufficient amounts of insulin to allow necessary carbohydrate metabolism. With inadequate amounts of insulin glucose cannot enter the cells but remains outside in the blood. The body cells become energy depleted while the blood glucose level remains elevated. Fats and proteins in the body tissues are then oxidized by the cells as a source of energy. This results in wasting of fat and muscle tissue of the body, negative nitrogen balance due to protein breakdown, and ketosis due to fat metabolism. The strong osmotic force of the glucose concentration in the blood pulls water from the cells into the blood, which results in cellular dehydration. The high level of glucose in the blood eventually spills over into the urine, producing glycosuria. Osmotic pressure of the glucose in the urine prevents reabsorption of water into the kidney tubules, causing extracellular dehydration.

These pathologic developments cause the four cardinal signs and symptoms of diabetes mellitus: polyuria, polydipsia, weight loss, and polyphagia. *Polyuria* (frequent urination) results because water is not reabsorbed by the renal tubules due to the osmotic activity of glucose. *Polydipsia* (excessive thirst) is caused by dehydration from polyuria. *Weight loss* (seen in insulin-dependent diabetes, also called type I diabetes) is due to the use of fat and muscle tissue for energy. *Polyphagia* (excessive hunger) is caused by tissue loss and a state of starvation, which results from the inability of the cells to utilize the blood glucose. Diagnosis of diabetes is based on the presence of clinical symptoms and laboratory tests showing elevated glucose levels in the blood.

Classification of Diabetes Mellitus

States of altered carbohydrate metabolism have been classified several different ways. Table 18–1 shows the current accepted classification, a result of the 1979 report of a special committee of the National Institutes of Health (National Diabetes Data Group 1979). This classification contains three main categories: diabetes mellitus (DM), impaired glucose tolerance (IGT), and gestational diabetes mellitus (GDM).

Table 18–2 shows White's classification of diabetes in pregnancy. This classification is useful for describing the extent of the disease.

Gestational Diabetes Mellitus

Gestational diabetes mellitus is defined as carbohydrate intolerance of variable severity with onset or first recognition during pregnancy. It results from (1) an

TABLE 18-1	Classification of Diabetes Mellitus (DM) and Other Categories of Glucose Intolerance

Diabetes mellitus
    Type I, insulin-dependent (IDDM)
    Type II, noninsulin-dependent (NIDDM)
        Nonobese NIDDM
        Obese NIDDM
    Secondary diabetes
Impaired glucose tolerance (IGT)
Gestational diabetes mellitus (GDM)

SOURCE: National Diabetes Data Group of National Institutes of Health, *Diabetes* 1979; 28:1039. Adapted with permission from the American Diabetes Association Inc.

unidentified preexistent disease, (2) the unmasking of a compensated metabolic abnormality by the added stress of pregnancy, or (3) a direct consequence of the altered maternal metabolism stemming from changing hormonal levels. Diet therapy is the cornerstone of intervention for GDM, but insulin therapy is indicated when dietary management is inadequate (Ratner 1993).

In most instances the overt diabetic manifestation disappears postpartum, though subtle manifestations of impaired insulin secretory capacity may remain. Although gestational diabetes mellitus incidence rates vary, many of these individuals progress to overt type II diabetes mellitus with time (O'Sullivan 1991).

Carbohydrate Metabolism in Pregnancy

The changes in carbohydrate, protein, and fat metabolism in normal pregnancy are profound. Carbohydrate metabolism is affected early in pregnancy by a rise in serum levels of estrogen, progesterone, and other hormones. These hormones stimulate increased insulin production by the maternal pancreatic beta cells and increased tissue response to insulin early in pregnancy. Therefore an anabolic (building up) state exists during the first half of pregnancy with storage of glycogen in the liver and other tissues.

The second half of pregnancy is characterized by increased resistance to insulin, which appears to be due to secretion of human placental lactogen (hPL) and elevated levels of estrogen, progesterone, and other hormones (Spellacy 1994). This diminished effectiveness of insulin results in a catabolic state during fasting periods (eg, during the night and after meal absorption). Because increasing amounts of circulating maternal glucose and amino acids are being diverted to the fetus, maternal fat is metabolized during fasting periods much more readily than in a nonpregnant person. This process is called *accelerated starvation*. Ketones may be present in the urine as a result of lipolysis (maternal metabolism of fat).

A rise in the glomerular filtration rate in the kidneys in conjunction with decreased tubular glucose reabsorp-

TABLE 18-2 — White's Classification of Diabetes in Pregnancy

Class	Criterion
A	Chemical diabetes
B	Maturity onset (age over 20 years), duration under 10 years, no vascular lesions
C_1	Age 10 to 19 years at onset
C_2	10 to 19 years' duration
D_1	Under 10 years at onset
D_2	Over 20 years' duration
D_3	Benign retinopathy
D_4	Calcified vessels of legs
D_5	Hypertension
E	No longer sought
F	Nephropathy
G	Many failures
H	Cardiopathy
R	Proliferating retinopathy
T	Renal transplant (added by Tagatz and colleagues of the University of Minnesota)

SOURCE: White P: Classification of obstetric diabetes. *Am J Obstet Gynecol* 1978; 130:228. Used with permission.

tion results in glycosuria. A decrease in the normal fasting blood glucose occurs in pregnancy, but free fatty acids and ketones are increased. The fed state is also altered by a more pronounced and prolonged elevation in plasma glucose (Cunningham et al 1993).

In summary, the delicate system of checks and balances that exists between glucose production and glucose utilization is stressed by the growing fetus, who derives energy from glucose taken solely from maternal stores. This stress is referred to as the *diabetogenic effect* of pregnancy. Thus any preexisting disruption in carbohydrate metabolism is augmented by pregnancy, and any diabetic potential may precipitate gestational diabetes mellitus.

Influence of Pregnancy on Diabetes

Pregnancy can affect diabetes significantly. First, the physiologic changes of pregnancy can drastically alter insulin requirements. Second, pregnancy may accelerate the progress of vascular disease secondary to diabetes.

The disease may be more difficult to control during pregnancy because insulin requirements are changeable. Insulin need frequently decreases early in the first trimester. Levels of hPL, an insulin antagonist, are low, energy demands of the embryo are minimal, and the woman may be consuming less food due to nausea and vomiting. Nausea and vomiting may also cause dietary fluctuations, which can increase the risk of hypoglycemia or insulin shock. Insulin requirements usually begin to

rise late in the first trimester as glucose use and glycogen storage by the woman and fetus are increased. As a result of placental maturation and production of hPL and other hormones, insulin requirements may double or quadruple by the end of pregnancy.

Increased energy needs during labor may require more insulin to balance intravenous glucose. After delivery of the placenta, insulin requirements usually decrease abruptly with loss of hPL in the maternal circulation.

Other factors contribute to the difficulty in controlling the disease. As pregnancy progresses the renal threshold for glucose decreases. There is also an increased risk of ketoacidosis, which may occur at lower serum glucose levels in the pregnant woman with diabetes than in the nonpregnant diabetic. The vascular disease that accompanies diabetes may progress during pregnancy. Hypertension may occur. Nephropathy may result from renal impairment, and retinopathy may also occur.

The primary concern for the pregnant woman who has diabetes is control of circulating blood glucose levels. If control can be achieved and maintained, diabetes generally does not worsen during pregnancy. The woman's health status may even improve due to close medical supervision.

ESSENTIAL PRECAUTIONS IN PRACTICE

A PREGNANT WOMAN WITH DIABETES MELLITUS

In caring for a pregnant woman with diabetes mellitus all the precautions apply that are established for any hospitalized pregnant, laboring, or postpartal woman. In addition, remember the following specifics:

- Gloves should be worn when doing finger sticks for glucose levels, when starting IVs, when testing urine for ketones, or when drawing blood for other laboratory tests.

- When teaching a woman to do her own blood glucose testing, gloves should be available and put on if it becomes necessary for the nurse to help the woman obtain a blood sample. The woman does not need to wear gloves during the procedure.

- Needles, syringes, lancets, and other sharp objects should be disposed of in appropriately labeled containers.

REMEMBER to wash your hands prior to putting the disposable gloves on and AGAIN immediately after you remove the gloves.

For further information consult OSHA and CDC guidelines.

Influence of Diabetes on Pregnancy Outcome

The discovery of insulin in 1921 allowed women with diabetes to survive to adulthood and bear children. Since then, maternal mortality from diabetes has been minimal. However, the pregnancy of a woman who has diabetes carries a higher risk of complications, especially perinatal mortality and congenital anomalies. The risk of perinatal mortality has been reduced by the recent recognition of the importance of tight metabolic control (blood glucose between 70 mg/dL and 120 mg/dL). New techniques for monitoring blood glucose, delivering insulin, and monitoring the fetus have also reduced perinatal mortality.

Maternal Risks

Maternal health problems in diabetic pregnancy have been greatly reduced with the team approach to early prenatal care and emphasis on maintaining control of blood glucose levels. The prognosis for the pregnant woman with gestational, type I, or type II diabetes that has not resulted in significant vascular damage is positive. However, diabetic pregnancy still carries higher risks for complications than normal pregnancy.

Hydramnios, or an increase in the volume of amniotic fluid, occurs in 10% to 20% of pregnant diabetics. Hydramnios is thought to be a result of excessive fetal urination because of fetal hyperglycemia (Mandeville 1992). Premature rupture of membranes and onset of labor may result, but only occasionally does this pose a threat.

Pregnancy-induced hypertension (PIH) occurs more often in diabetic pregnancies, especially when diabetes-related vascular changes already exist.

Hyperglycemia due to insufficient amounts of insulin can lead to *ketoacidosis* as a result of the increase in ketone bodies (which are acidic) in the blood released when fatty acids are metabolized. Ketoacidosis usually develops slowly, but it may develop more rapidly in the pregnant woman because of the hyperketonemia associated with accelerated starvation in the nonfed state. The tendency for higher postprandial glucose levels because of decreased gastric motility and the contrainsulin effects of hPL also predispose the woman to ketoacidosis. If the ketoacidosis is not treated, it can lead to coma and death of both mother and fetus.

In pregnancy, particularly in the presence of prolonged vomiting, carbohydrate deficiency may lead to ketosis as fat cells are metabolized for energy needs. Measurement of blood glucose levels will easily differentiate starvation ketosis (a hypoglycemic state treated with glucose solution) from diabetic ketoacidosis (a hyperglycemic state treated with insulin).

Another risk to the pregnant woman with diabetes is *dystocia*, caused by fetopelvic disproportion if fetal macrosomia exists. *Anemia* may develop as a result of vascular involvement and poor nutritional intake. The pregnant woman with diabetes is at increased risk for monilial vaginitis and urinary tract infections because of increased glycosuria, which contributes to a favorable environment for bacterial growth. If untreated, asymptomatic bacteriuria can lead to pyelonephritis, a serious kidney infection.

During pregnancy about 15% of diabetic women will have some increase in retinopathy. Severe proliferative retinopathy can lead to blindness if not treated with laser coagulation (Spellacy 1994).

Fetal-Neonatal Risks

Maintaining maternal glucose in the normal range has resulted not only in decreased perinatal mortality but also in reduced perinatal morbidity. It is now clear that many of the problems of the neonate result directly from high maternal plasma glucose levels. In the presence of severe maternal ketoacidosis the risk of fetal death increases to 50% (Spellacy 1994). Fetal enzyme systems cease functioning in an acidic environment.

The incidence of congenital anomalies in diabetic pregnancies is three to four times higher than in the general population and is related to high glucose levels during the 3rd to 6th week of gestation. Studies have demonstrated the cost-effectiveness of preconception care to prevent congenital anomalies in this high-risk population (Elixhauser et al 1993). The anomalies often involve the heart, central nervous system, and skeletal system. Septal defects, coarctation of the aorta, and transposition of the great vessels are the most common heart lesions seen. Ventricular septal hypertrophy was reported in 75% of fetuses of diabetic mothers studied (Veille et al 1992). Central nervous system anomalies include hydrocephalus, meningomyelocele, and anencephaly. One anomaly, sacral agenesis, appears only in infants of diabetic mothers.

Characteristically, infants of type I diabetic mothers (or classes A, B, and C, see Table 18–2) are large for gestational age (LGA) as a result of high levels of fetal insulin production stimulated by the high levels of glucose crossing the placenta from the mother. Sustained fetal hyperinsulinism and hyperglycemia ultimately lead to excessive growth (**macrosomia**) and deposition of fat. If born vaginally, the macrosomic infant is at increased risk for birth trauma such as fractured clavicle or brachial plexus injuries due to shoulder dystocia. To prevent such injuries, cesarean birth may be necessary if macrosomia is confirmed (Spellacy 1994).

After birth the umbilical cord is severed, and thus the generous maternal blood glucose supply is eliminated. However, continued islet cell hyperactivity leads to excessive insulin levels and depleted blood glucose (hypoglycemia) in 2 to 4 hours. Macrosomia can be significantly reduced by tight maternal blood glucose control.

Infants of diabetic mothers with vascular involvement may demonstrate intrauterine growth retardation (IUGR). This occurs because vascular changes in the mother decrease the efficiency of placental perfusion, and the fetus is not as well sustained in utero.

Respiratory distress syndrome appears to result from inhibition, by high levels of fetal insulin, of some fetal enzymes necessary for surfactant production. *Polycythemia* in the neonate is due primarily to the diminished ability of glycosylated hemoglobin in the mother's blood to release oxygen. *Hyperbilirubinemia* is a direct result of the inability of immature liver enzymes to metabolize the increased bilirubin resulting from the polycythemia. *Hypocalcemia*, characterized by signs of irritability or even tetany, may occur. The cause of these low calcium levels in infants of diabetic mothers is not known (Spellacy 1994).

Medical Therapy

Detection and Diagnosis of Gestational Diabetes

Gestational diabetes is more common than pregestational diabetes. It is estimated to occur in 3% to 6% of pregnancies. Therefore screening for the detection of diabetes is a standard part of prenatal care. If the possibility of diabetes is suspected, further testing is undertaken for diagnosis.

Two screening tests are commonly administered to pregnant women:

1. *Urine testing.* The pregnant woman's urine is tested for glucose at her first prenatal visit and again on subsequent visits. Glycosuria is not diagnostic of diabetes mellitus, but the presence of glycosuria is an indication for glucose tolerance testing. In the nonpregnant adult, glucose is not generally spilled into the urine until the blood sugar level is 180 mg/dL or greater. During pregnancy the renal threshold is lower, and glucose may spill into the urine when blood glucose levels are 130 mg/dL.

    Tes-Tape and Diastix are methods of choice in urine testing. They are specific for glucose and do not show positive readings in the presence of lactose or fructose. Single-specimen urine tests are used in routine screening at each antenatal visit.

    Urine is also tested for ketones using Ketostix or Acetest. Both are simple tests for detecting ketones in the urine and are usually done routinely for type I (ketosis-prone) diabetes.

2. *50 g oral glucose tolerance test.* All pregnant women, regardless of risk factors, should be screened for diabetes toward the end of the second trimester (24–28 weeks) (American Diabetes Association 1991; Spellacy 1994). Women with risk factors (age over 30; family history of diabetes; a prior macrosomic, malformed, or stillborn infant; obesity; hypertension; or glycosuria) should be screened when first seen for prenatal care (Spellacy 1994).

The oral glucose load is administered without regard to time of day or time of last meal, and venous plasma glucose is measured 1 hour later. A plasma level that exceeds 140 mg/dL indicates a need for further diagnostic testing.

Diagnosis

Oral Glucose Tolerance Test (OGTT) A 100 g oral glucose load is administered in the morning after an overnight fast for at least 8 hours but not more than 14 hours and after at least 3 days of unrestricted diet ($\geq$ 150 g carbohydrate) and physical activity. Venous plasma glucose is measured fasting and at 1, 2, and 3 hours. The woman should remain seated and not smoke throughout the test. Two or more of the following venous plasma concentrations must be met or exceeded for a diagnosis of diabetes (American Diabetes Association 1991):

Fasting	105 mg/dL
1 hour	190 mg/dL
2 hour	165 mg/dL
3 hour	145 mg/dL

The result is considered borderline abnormal if only one value is elevated, and the OGTT is repeated in 1 month (Spellacy 1994).

Laboratory Assessment of Long-Term Glucose Control

Glycosylated hemoglobin (HbA_{1c}) is a laboratory test that loosely reflects glucose control over the previous 4 to 8 weeks. It measures the percentage of glycohemoglobin in the blood. Glycohemoglobin or HbA_{1c} is the hemoglobin to which a glucose molecule is attached. The test is not reliable for screening for gestational diabetes or for close daily control, but it is useful as an indicator of overall blood glucose control (Mandeville 1992). Among women with abnormal HbA_{1c} values no critical level was identified that provided predictive power for fetal congenital heart disease (Shields et al 1993).

Antepartal Management of Diabetes

The major goals of medical care for a pregnant woman with diabetes—whether gestational or pregestational—are: (1) to maintain a physiologic equilibrium of insulin availability and glucose utilization during pregnancy and (2) to deliver an optimally healthy mother and newborn. To achieve these goals, good prenatal care using a team approach is a top priority. The team consists of an obstetrician, an endocrinologist, a perinatologist, a diabetes nurse-educator, a perinatal nurse, a nutritionist, a social worker, and, most importantly, the diabetic woman and her partner. Education of the couple and their active involvement in managing her care are essential for a good outcome.

For the woman with gestational diabetes the diagnosis may be a shock, leaving her frightened and anxious (Mandeville 1992). She needs clear explanation and teaching to enlist her participation in ensuring a good outcome. The diabetes nurse-educator plays a major role in this counseling.

The woman with pregestational diabetes needs to understand changes she can expect during pregnancy; thus she should receive such teaching in preconception counseling. At the initial prenatal visit, height, weight, and vital signs are assessed along with a thorough assessment of thyroid and cardiac function. Special attention is given to dating the pregnancy. Laboratory data are obtained, and the diabetes is classified using White's criteria. Women should be screened for diabetic neuropathy, and a fundoscopic examination is done to detect any retinopathy. In some cases the woman may be referred to an opthalmologist for further evaluation.

Dietary Regulation The pregnant woman requires about 300 calories per day more than she does when she is not pregnant to meet increased metabolic demands (Mandeville 1992). In general, women need approximately 30 kcal/kg of ideal body weight (IBW) during the first trimester and 35 to 36 kcal/kg IBW during the second and third trimesters. If ketonuria develops or the woman complains of hunger, the number of calories may be increased. Dietary guidelines are similar for women with gestational and pregestational diabetes. Approximately 50% to 60% of the calories should come from complex carbohydrates with adequate fiber to slow down absorption, about 12% to 20% of calories (or 1.5 g/kg body weight) should be protein, and 20% to 30% should be fat (Cunningham et al 1993). This caloric intake is divided among three meals and three snacks. The prebedtime snack is the most important and must include both protein and complex carbohydrates to prevent hypoglycemia at night. Because it is so important that the pregnant woman follow these guidelines, a nutritionist works out meal plans based on the woman's life-style, culture, and food preferences and teaches her food exchanges so she can vary and plan her own meals. Cookbooks for diabetics are available and can be a great help.

Glucose Monitoring Glucose monitoring is an essential part of diabetes management for determining the need for insulin and assessing glucose control. Many physicians have the woman come in for weekly assessment of her fasting glucose levels and one or two postprandial levels. Other physicians recommend home monitoring for most of their clients. In some centers home monitoring of blood glucose levels has become a standard and routine part of pregnancy management for both gestational and pregestational diabetes.

Home Care Home blood glucose monitoring should be taught at the first visit after the diagnosis of gestational diabetes has been established. The woman with pregesta-

tional diabetes may already be monitoring her own blood sugar.

It is usually recommended that monitoring be done at least four times per day, a fasting blood sugar before breakfast, then a postprandial test 2 hours after each meal. Women are encouraged to maintain blood sugars in the normal ranges as follows: fasting (before eating or taking insulin), 60 to 100 mg/dL; 2 hours after each meal, 100 to 140 mg/dL. Some recommend more rigid control of blood glucose, with the goal of fasting blood sugar of 70 to 95 mg/dL and 2-hour postprandial blood sugar of less than 120 mg/dL, if this can be done without frequent hypoglycemic reactions (Ratner 1993).

Insulin Administration Whether or not the woman with gestational diabetes needs additional insulin (over her own body production) depends on how well her blood glucose levels can be maintained by diet alone. Individuals with pregestational diabetes usually have type I diabetes, requiring insulin administration. Whether the client has gestational or pregestational diabetes, the type of insulin used should be human. Human insulin is the least likely to cause an allergic response. If the woman has previously used bovine or porcine insulin, she may require smaller doses of human insulin to achieve the same pharmacologic effect. She is instructed to take an initial glucose reading at 2 AM to avoid nocturnal or early morning hypoglycemic episodes.

The insulin program should be kept as simple as possible while still achieving the goals of normal fasting and postprandial blood glucose levels. A single dose of intermediate (NPH or lente) insulin in the morning may be sufficient. Most women will need a mixture of intermediate and regular insulin twice daily (Mandeville 1992). Often two-thirds of the total insulin dose is taken with breakfast in a ratio of intermediate to regular of 2:1. The remaining third is taken with the evening meal in a 1:1 ratio. It is important to remember that the amount of insulin needed usually increases during each trimester of pregnancy.

Insulin pumps, providing continuous subcutaneous insulin infusion, are not as widely used during pregnancy as it was thought they might be when they were first introduced. These pumps are effective in improving glucose control, but the woman must be guarded against recurrent hypoglycemia and the possibility of the pump becoming dislodged. With experience these problems are lessened. However, conventional insulin administration seems to produce similar glucose outcomes (Cunningham et al 1993).

Oral hypoglycemics are never used during pregnancy because they cross the placenta, may be teratogenic, and stimulate fetal insulin production (Piacquadio 1991).

Evaluation of Fetal Status Information about the well-being, maturation, and size of the fetus is important for planning the course of the pregnancy and the timing of birth. Because pregnancies complicated by diabetes are at increased risk of neural tube defects, maternal *serum α-fetoprotein (AFP)* screening is done during weeks 16 to 18 of gestation (see Chapter 20).

Daily maternal evaluation of *fetal activity*, begun at about 28 weeks, is effective and simple to perform. The woman is taught a particular method for counting fetal movement (see Chapter 15), records the results on a special card, and brings the card to each subsequent office visit.

Nonstress testing (NST) is usually begun weekly at about 30 weeks. If evidence of IUGR, PIH, oligohydramnios, or poorly controlled blood glucose exists, testing may begin as early as 26 weeks and may be done more often (Mandeville 1992). Some researchers recommend twice-weekly NSTs beginning after 32 weeks' gestation (Landon & Gabbe 1991). If the woman requires hospitalization (for example, to control glycemia or for complications), NST may be done daily.

Contraction stress testing is used primarily after 32 weeks' gestation if there is a nonreactive NST or if some variable decelerations are seen on the tracing (see Chapter 20).

Ultrasound at 18 weeks establishes gestational age and diagnoses multiple pregnancy or congenital anomalies. It is repeated at 28 weeks to monitor fetal growth for IUGR or macrosomia. Some agencies do *biophysical profiles* (ultrasound evaluation of fetal well-being in which fetal breathing movements; fetal activity, reactivity, and muscle tone; and amniotic fluid volume are assessed) as part of an ongoing evaluation of fetal status.

Intrapartal Management of Diabetes Mellitus

During the intrapartal period medical therapy includes the following:

- *Timing of birth.* Most diabetic pregnancies are allowed to go to term, with spontaneous labor, thereby decreasing the risk of respiratory distress in the neonate. In pregnancies in which there is evidence of fetal macrosomia, fetal compromise, or elevated maternal HbA_{1c}, amniocentesis is done for lecithin/sphingomyelin (L/S) ratio and the concentration of saturated phosphatidylcholine (SPC). Whereas levels of 2:1 ratio for the L/S ratio and > 500 µg/dL of SPC indicate fetal lung maturity in the nondiabetic pregnancy, levels of up to 3.5:1 L/S ratio and >1000 µg/dL of SPC have been found necessary at some centers before low risk of respiratory distress syndrome (RDS) is achieved. The presence of phosphatidylglycerol (PG) seems to enhance lecithin activity, and its presence is considered favorable for lung maturity. Fetal lung maturity must be weighed against other considerations when deciding time of childbirth (Cunningham et al 1993).

- *Labor management.* The degree of prenatal maintenance of normal maternal glucose levels (euglycemia) and the maintenance of maternal euglycemia during labor are important in preventing neonatal hypoglycemia. Maternal insulin requirements often decrease dramatically during labor (Mandeville 1992). Consequently, maternal glucose levels are measured hourly to determine insulin need. Often two intravenous lines are used, one with a 5% dextrose solution and one with a saline solution. The saline solution is then available if a bolus is needed or for piggybacking insulin. Insulin clings to the plastic intravenous bag and tubing. To ensure that the woman receives the desired dose, the intravenous tubing must be flushed with insulin before the prescribed amount is added. During the second stage of labor and the immediate postpartum period the woman may not need additional insulin. The intravenous insulin is discontinued with the completion of the third stage of labor.

Postpartal Management of Diabetes Mellitus

Maternal insulin requirements fall significantly postpartally because the levels of hPL, progesterone, and estrogen fall after placental separation, and their anti-insulin effect ceases, resulting in decreased blood glucose levels. The diabetic mother may require no insulin for the first 24 hours or only one-fourth to one-half her previous dose. Then reestablishment of insulin needs based on blood glucose testing is necessary. Diet and exercise levels must also be redetermined.

Diabetic control and the establishment of parent-child relationships in light of neonatal needs are the priorities of this period. If her newborn must be cared for in a special care nursery, the mother needs support and information about the baby's condition. Every effort must be made to provide as much contact as possible between the parents and their newborn.

Other components of postpartal care include:

- *Breastfeeding.* Breastfeeding is encouraged as beneficial to both mother and baby. The composition of breast milk is not altered by diabetes, and infants of mothers with diabetes gain weight appropriately. The lactating mother with diabetes often has a sense of well-being and diminished insulin needs even while increasing caloric intake (Lawrence 1989). Blood glucose levels may be lower because glucose is transferred from serum to breast to be converted to lactose, and energy is expended in milk production. Calorie needs increase during lactation to 500 to 800 kcal above prepregnant requirements. Insulin must be adjusted according to individual needs. Home blood glucose monitoring should continue for the insulin-dependent diabetic.

Initial breastfeeding should take place soon after birth, as with all breastfeeding mothers. The mother and infant should not be separated if at all possible because this interferes with the establishment of normal lactation. If the baby cannot nurse right away, the mother can be taught to express her milk with a pump or manually to prevent engorgement. Research indicates that for insulin-dependent diabetic women, maintaining good diabetic control during breastfeeding requires great effort and flexibility (Gagne 1992).

- *Contraception.* Barrier methods of contraception (diaphragm and condom) used with spermicide are safe, effective, and inexpensive. They are recommended for the client with diabetes. The use of oral contraceptives by diabetic women is controversial. There is some evidence that women with diabetes who take oral contraceptives have a higher risk of cardiovascular disease (Cunningham et al 1993). Many physicians prescribe only lower-dose pills to women with diabetes, and they may restrict their use to women who have no vascular disease and who do not smoke. The progesterone-only pill has a higher failure rate but is otherwise safer. Elective sterilization is chosen by many couples who have completed their families.

APPLYING THE NURSING PROCESS

Nursing Assessment

Whether diabetes (usually type I) has been diagnosed before pregnancy occurs or the diagnosis is made during pregnancy (GDM), careful assessment of the disease process and the woman's understanding of diabetes is important. Thorough physical examination, including assessment for vascular complications of the disease, any

CRITICAL THINKING IN PRACTICE

Patti Chang is a 35-year-old, gravida 3, para 2, well-educated, active Chinese American woman with no history of glucose intolerance. Her two children were born healthy at 36 weeks' gestation. She receives the usual 50 g glucose tolerance test at 26 weeks gestation, and her plasma level is 160 mg/dL. She seems irritated and frustrated when her obstetrician tells her that it would be best to perform a 3-hour fasting glucose tolerance test. After the physician leaves the room, Patti asks the nurse the following questions: Will the glucose hurt my baby? What will the treatment be? How will the nurse answer the questions? Why does Patti seem so upset?

Answers can be found in Appendix I.

signs of infectious conditions, and urine and blood testing for glucose, is essential on the first prenatal visit. Follow-up visits are usually scheduled twice a month during the first two trimesters and once a week during the last trimester.

Assessment is also needed to yield information about the woman's ability to cope with the combined stress of pregnancy and diabetes and her ability to follow a recommended regimen of care. Determination of the woman's knowledge about diabetes and self-care is needed before formulating a teaching plan.

Nursing Diagnosis

Nursing diagnoses that may apply are identified in the Nursing Care Plan: Care of the Woman with Diabetes Mellitus on page 448.

Nursing Plan and Implementation

Provision of Prepregnancy Counseling

Prepregnancy counseling may be provided by a nurse and a physician, using a team approach. Ideally, the couple is seen prior to pregnancy so that the diabetes can be assessed by ophthalmologic evaluation, electrocardiographic study, and a 24-hour urine collection for creatinine clearance and protein excretion. Prepregnancy counseling about the importance of tight glucose control has been shown to be cost-effective in preventing congenital anomalies (Elixhauser et al 1993). If the diabetes is of recent onset without vascular complications, the outcome of pregnancy should be good provided that glucose levels are controlled.

Promotion of Effective Home Blood Glucose Monitoring

The diabetes nurse-educator teaches the client how and when to monitor her blood sugar, the desired range of blood sugar levels, and the importance of good control (Figure 18–1). The woman may opt for either a visual method of blood testing or the use of a glucose meter. With either method the client is taught to follow the manufacturer's directions exactly, to wash hands thoroughly before puncturing her finger, and to touch the blood droplet, not her finger, to the test pad on the strip. With the visual method she waits the prescribed time and then compares the color on the strip with a color chart provided on the strip bottle. The test strips must be stored as directed, and unused strips should be discarded after their expiration date.

If the client is using a blood glucose meter, an electronic eye measures the blood sugar, and a digital reading is given. The blood droplet should cover the test pad because uncovered portions are read as low sugar. The glucose meter is a portable pocket-sized device that is more accurate than the visual, color comparison method. Some meters are able to store and recall a specified number of readings.

The nurse may offer the client the following tips regarding finger puncture: (1) Various spring-loaded devices are available that make puncturing easier. (2) Hanging the arm down for 30 seconds increases blood flow to the fingers. (3) The sides of fingers should be punctured instead of the ends because ends contain more pain-sensitive nerves.

Diabetic clients need to keep a record of each blood sugar reading as a guide for management. Specific record sheets are available for this purpose. The woman is instructed to bring the record sheet with her for each visit.

Promotion of Effective Insulin Use

The nurse ensures that the couple understands the purpose of the insulin, the types of insulin the woman is to use, and the correct procedure for its administration. The woman's partner is also instructed about insulin administration in case it should be necessary for him to give it.

For some highly motivated women whose glucose levels are not well controlled with multiple injections, the continuous insulin infusion pump may improve glucose control. A needle is secured in the subcutaneous tissue of the anterior abdominal wall and connected by cannula to a syringe filled with regular insulin. A pump that automatically resets to the basal infusion rate after giving the preprandial bolus is important for preventing problems of hypoglycemia. The woman needs to learn to use the insulin pump and become confident in coordinating the dosages with her glucose readings to achieve euglycemia. The diabetes nurse-educator works with her to achieve these goals.

Promotion of a Planned Exercise Program

Exercise is encouraged for the woman's overall well-being. If she is used to a regular exercise program, she is encouraged to continue. She is advised to exercise after meals when blood sugar levels are high, to wear diabetic identification, to carry a simple sugar such as hard candy, to monitor her blood glucose levels regularly, and to avoid injecting insulin into an extremity that will soon be used during exercise.

If she has not been following a regular exercise plan, she is encouraged to begin gradually. Due to alterations in metabolism with exercise, the woman's blood glucose should be well controlled before she begins an exercise program.

Teaching for Self-Care

Using the information gained during the nursing assessment of the pregnant woman with diabetes, the nurse provides appropriate teaching to the woman and her family so that the woman can meet her own health care needs as much as possible.

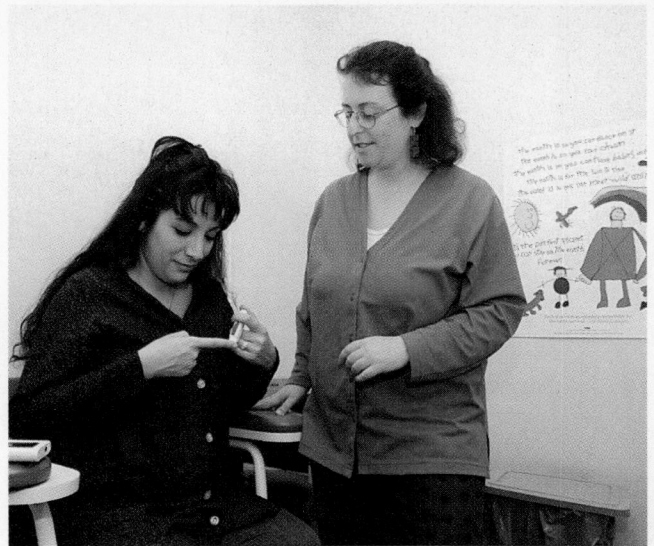

FIGURE 18-1   The nurse teaches the pregnant woman with gestational diabetes mellitus how to do home glucose monitoring.

- *Symptoms of hypoglycemia and ketoacidosis.* The pregnant diabetic woman must recognize symptoms of changing glucose levels and take appropriate action by immediately checking her capillary blood glucose level. If it is less than 60 mg/dL, she is advised to take 20 g of carbohydrate, wait 20 minutes, and then retest her glucose level. The necessary carbohydrate can be obtained by drinking 13.3 oz cola, 14.5 oz whole milk, or 12 oz orange or apple juice (Mandeville 1992). Many people overtreat their symptoms by continuing to eat. This can cause a rebound hyperglycemia. The woman should carry a snack at all times and should have other fast sources of glucose (simple carbohydrates) at hand so that she can treat an insulin reaction when milk is not available. Family members are also taught how to inject glucagon in the event that food does not work or is not feasible, for instance, in the presence of severe morning sickness.

- *Smoking.* Smoking has harmful effects on both the maternal vascular system and the developing fetus and is contraindicated for both pregnancy and diabetes.

- *Travel.* Insulin can be kept at room temperature while traveling. Insulin supplies should be kept with the traveler and not packed in the baggage. Special meals can be arranged by notifying most airlines a few days before departure. A diabetic identification bracelet or necklace should be worn. In addition the woman should check with her physician for any instructions or advice before leaving.

- *Hospitalization.* Hospitalization may become necessary during the pregnancy to evaluate blood glucose levels and adjust insulin dosages.

Text continues on page 451

CARE OF THE WOMAN WITH DIABETES MELLITUS

Nursing Assessment

Nursing History

1. Complete client and family history
2. Client's predisposition to diabetes, including
   a. Recurrent PIH
   b. Previous LGA infants (>4000 g)
   c. Hydramnios
   d. Unexplained fetal death
   e. Obesity
   f. Family history of diabetes

Physical Examination

1. Length of gestation
2. Complaints of thirst and hunger
3. Recurrent monilial vaginitis or urinary tract infection (UTI)
4. Frequent urination beyond first trimester and before the third trimester
5. Fundal height greater than expected for gestation
6. Obesity
7. Fundoscopic examination to detect any vascular changes

Diagnostic Studies

1. Fasting plasma glucose (FPG)
2. Three-hour GTT
3. Urine test for glucose, ketones
4. Ultrasound to evaluate fetal growth and detect hydramnios
5. If woman has IDDM, glycosylated hemoglobin level (HbA$_{1c}$)
6. Maternal serum α-fetoprotein (AFP) screen
7. Doppler blood flow studies to evaluate vascular changes and placental perfusion

Third-Trimester Fetal Assessments

1. Serial NSTs
2. CST as necessary
3. Serial ultrasound
4. Biophysical profile to determine fetal maturity
5. Amniocentesis for L/S ratio and phosphatidyglycerol (PG)

NURSING DIAGNOSIS: Risk for altered nutrition: More than body requirements related to imbalance between intake and available insulin

EXPECTED OUTCOME: Woman will discuss and follow her prescribed diet.

Nursing Interventions	Rationale
Discuss importance of strict dietary control. Work with nutritionist and client to plan an individualized diet.	Dietary management is designed to ensure optimum fetal growth and normalize blood glucose levels. The greatest success occurs when a dietary plan is individualized to meet client needs and preferences.

Inform the client of the recommended intakes:
    30–35% kcal/kg body weight
    12–20% protein
    50–60% carbohydrate
    25–30% fat
Sodium intake may be restricted somewhat.
	Recommended intake is designed to permit the following weight gain (Kitzmiller et al 1988):
	    Underweight, 13.6+ kg (30+ lb)
	    Desirable weight, 11–13 kg (24–30 lb)
	    Overweight, 9–11 kg (20–24 lb)
	    Very overweight, 6.8–9 kg (15–20 lb)

OUTCOME MET IF:
- Woman verbalizes understanding of prescribed diet by discussing food groups and appropriate portions of carbohydrates, proteins, and fats and keeps a good diary that reflects appropriate intake.
- Woman maintains weight gain within the desired range based on prepregnancy weight.
- Woman's glycosylated hemoglobin (HbA$_{1c}$) remains in normal range (<7%).

NURSING DIAGNOSIS: Risk for injury related to possible complications secondary to hypoglycemia or hyperglycemia

EXPECTED OUTCOME: Woman avoids injury associated with hypoglycemia or hyperglycemia.

Nursing Interventions	Rationale
Determine insulin needs: 1. Check lab results of FPG and 2-hour postprandial. 2. Test blood four times daily using Dextrostix.	Sufficient insulin must be present to enable proper carbohydrate metabolism to take place. Pregnancy requires a marked increase in circulating insulin to maintain normal blood glucose.

CARE OF THE WOMAN WITH DIABETES MELLITUS *continued*

Nursing Interventions	Rationale
Teach use of home blood glucose monitoring device. Determine amount of insulin based on sliding scale.	Fasting glucose level tends to be lower than nonpregnant value.
Administer regular or NPH insulin or combination as ordered.	Effectiveness of insulin may be reduced by presence of hPL.
Teach early signs of hypoglycemia including sweating, periodic tingling, disorientation, shakiness, pallor, clammy skin, irritability, hunger, headache, blurred vision, and, if untreated, coma or convulsions.	Insulin requirements fluctuate widely during pregnancy because of many factors, including lowered glucose tolerance, especially in second half of pregnancy, and fluctuate during intrapartal period due to depletion of glycogen stores during labor. In addition, during lactation, conversion of blood glucose into lactose may cause marked changes in glucose tolerance and/or hypoglycemia.
Teach woman/family that insulin requirements will increase during pregnancy.	Insulin requirements increase due to an increase in hPL, estrogen, and progesterone, which have an anti-insulin effect.
Teach appropriate interventions if hypoglycemia occurs.	Self-care at home in the event of hypoglycemia may save the client's life or prevent brain damage.
Treat hypoglycemia per standing orders or agency protocol within minutes of onset and notify physician:	
1. Obtain immediate blood glucose level.	Provides baseline information on glucose levels.
2. If <60 mg/dL, have client drink 15 oz milk or 12 oz orange juice.	Liquids are absorbed from the GI tract faster than solids.
3. If woman is not alert enough to swallow, give 1 mg glucagon subcutaneously or intramuscularly.	Glucagon triggers the conversion of glycogen stored in the liver to glucose.
4. If the woman is in labor with intravenous lines in place, give 10–20 mL of 50% dextrose IV. Standing order should be available.	
Teach early signs of hyperglycemia and treatment.	Woman can recognize signs and administer self-treatment.
	Woman can also report any symptoms that may occur.
Observe for signs of hyperglycemia such as polyuria, polydipsia, dry mouth, increased appetite, fatigue, nausea, hot flushed skin, rapid deep breathing, abdominal cramps, acetone breath, headache, drowsiness, depressed reflexes, oliguria or anuria, stupor, or coma.	
Administer treatment for hyperglycemia and notify physician:	
1. Obtain frequent measurement of blood glucose; measure urine acetone.	Need to establish a baseline and to determine additional dosage and prevent overtreatment; urine acetone indicates development of ketoacidosis.
2. Administer prescribed amount of regular insulin subcutaneously or intravenously or combination of routes.	Insulin restores the body's normal metabolism of carbohydrates, proteins, and fats. Regular insulin is used because it acts immediately and is of short duration.
3. Replace fluids IV, orally, or in combination.	Fluids are depleted in the process of ketoacidosis; hypotension can result from decreased blood volume due to dehydration.
4. Measure intake and output.	Polyuria is an early sign of hyperglycemia; oliguria develops with hypotension and decreased blood flow to the kidneys.
5. Observe for symptoms of circulatory collapse; monitor BP and pulse.	Circulatory collapse can result from hypotension.

OUTCOME MET IF:
- No episode of hypoglycemia as evidenced by no sweating, tingling, disorientation, shakiness, clammy skin, hunger, headache, or blurred vision
- No episode of hyperglycemia as evidenced by no polyuria, polydipsia, dry mouth, increased appetite, fatigue, nausea, hot flushed skin, rapid deep breathing, acetone breath, or drowsiness
- Blood glucose levels remain <100 mg/dL fasting; <140 mg/dL 2-hour postprandial.

NURSING DIAGNOSIS: Risk for infection related to UTI secondary to glycosuria

EXPECTED OUTCOME: Woman identifies signs of developing UTI and appropriate self-care measures to help prevent UTI.

Nursing Interventions	Rationale
Review preventive measures such as voiding frequently, voiding immediately following intercourse, wiping from front to back, wearing cotton underpants, drinking cranberry juice.	Preventive measures are designed to remove bacteria from the bladder, avoid contamination from the rectal area or outside sources, facilitate air flow in the perineal area, and acidify the urine.

CARE OF THE WOMAN WITH DIABETES MELLITUS *continued*

Nursing Interventions	Rationale
Teach signs of developing UTI, including urgency, frequency, dysuria, and hematuria; low back pain with kidney involvement. Obtain clean-catch urine for culture and sensitivity.	Incidence of UTI is increased in diabetes, possibly because the existence of glycosuria provides rich medium for bacterial growth.
Administer prescribed antibiotics.	Antibiotic prescribed is specific to causative organism.
Encourage fluids to 2000–3000 mL/day. Measure intake and output.	Increased fluid intake promotes urinary removal of organisms.

OUTCOME MET IF:
- Woman verbalizes preventive measures to avoid a UTI.
- Woman verbalizes signs and symptoms of a developing UTI.

NURSING DIAGNOSIS: Knowledge deficit related to lack of information about diabetes mellitus, its treatment, its implications for the woman, her baby, and the birth process.

EXPECTED OUTCOME: Woman/family discusses the diabetes and its possible implications for the pregnancy.

Nursing Interventions	Rationale
Provide teaching as indicated, based on an assessment of woman/family's knowledge level: 1. Explain procedures. 2. Allow for questions. 3. Develop a teaching plan to discuss and provide opportunities to practice administering insulin. Provide written information. Include family as appropriate so others can administer insulin if necessary. 4. Provide information about possible changes to expect during labor and birth due to DM. Explain about IV insulin and continuous monitoring of fetal status. Stress unchanged aspects of the experience.	Decreasing fear and increasing knowledge will make the client a more effective member of the health care team. Anticipatory guidance helps the woman/family prepare for the experience.

OUTCOME MET IF:
- Woman/family verbalizes/demonstrates understanding of disease process, insulin administration, childbirth process, and differences and similarities to expect in labor and birth.

NURSING DIAGNOSIS: Risk of injury to fetus related to the effects of diabetes on uteroplacental functioning and fetal growth

EXPECTED OUTCOME: Woman discusses rationale for antepartal testing and cooperates with scheduled appointments.

Nursing Interventions	Rationale
Explain purpose of all scheduled tests and procedures: 1. Ultrasound as ordered to provide periodic assessment of fetal size 2. Fetal activity diary 3. Serial NSTs 4. CST if indicated 5. Measurement of L/S ratio and PG levels to determine fetal lung maturity 6. Biophysical profile 7. Doppler blood flow studies to evaluate placental circulation	Cooperation is increased when the client understands the purpose of the tests. Information about fetal growth and activity helps care givers evaluate placental functioning, anticipate the need for cesarean birth, determine fetal maturity, and decide on best time for birth.

OUTCOME MET IF:
- Woman verbalizes understanding of the rationale for the various antepartal tests to be performed and what to expect during the procedures.
- Woman verbalizes understanding of importance of keeping accurate records, such as the fetal activity diary, and attending all scheduled appointments.

CARE OF THE WOMAN WITH DIABETES MELLITUS *continued*

NURSING DIAGNOSIS: Altered family processes related to client's DM and the need for hospitalization

EXPECTED OUTCOME: Family copes successfully with the woman's illness, plans for changes as necessary following discharge, and shares their thoughts, feelings, and concerns with each other.

Nursing Interventions	Rationale
Encourage visits from family members, including older siblings.	Illness in one family member impacts the entire family.
Discuss with woman/family changes that are necessary following discharge regarding insulin, diet, exercise, and so forth.	
Assist family to make specific plans.	
Arrange for social services to visit or for homemaker assistance if necessary following discharge.	Sometimes outside support is necessary to help the family deal with feelings and identify ways of dealing with the illness.
Give the family members information about the frustration that can occur when a family member is ill. Provide opportunities for them to discuss their feelings. Offer suggestions for coping.	

OUTCOME MET IF:
- Woman/family verbalizes feelings and concerns in regard to the diabetes and the pregnancy and specific plans for dealing with possible hospitalization.

Essential Nursing Activities To Achieve Outcomes

Antepartum

1. Provide nutritional counseling, including calorie requirements, recommended intakes, meal schedules, and meal plans.
2. Assess the woman/family's understanding of
   a. How to monitor glucose levels
   b. How to administer insulin
   c. Appropriate weight gain
   d. Signs and symptoms to report regarding hypoglycemia, hyperglycemia, and UTI
   e. Need for all antepartal maternal and fetal tests
   f. Importance of attending all scheduled visits
   g. Expectations for labor and birth

Intrapartum

1. Monitor glucose hourly.
2. Start IVs: one D5 solution and one LR.
3. Provide continuous fetal monitoring assessing for late decelerations and/or decreased variability.
4. Be alert for signs and symptoms of hypoglycemia or hyperglycemia.

Postpartum

1. Be aware of decreased insulin requirements postpartum.
2. Be alert for signs and symptoms of hypoglycemia.
3. If the client is breastfeeding, stress the importance of proper latch on to prevent cracked nipples and/or engorgement that may lead to mastitis.
4. Be aware that insulin requirements may remain decreased during lactation.
5. Inform the client of the importance of continued home glucose monitoring.
6. Teach the client about signs and symptoms to report for UTI, mastitis, and infection of incision.

- *Support groups.* Many communities have diabetes support groups or education classes, which can be most helpful to women with newly diagnosed diabetes.

- *Cesarean birth.* Chances for a cesarean birth are increased if the pregnant woman is diabetic. This possibility should be anticipated—enrollment in cesarean birth preparation classes may be suggested. Many hospitals offer classes, and information is available through organizations such as Cesarean/Support Education and Concern (C/Sec, Inc); Cesarean Birth Council; or the Cesarean Association for Research, Education, Support and Satisfac-

tion in Birthing (Caress). The couple may prefer simply to discuss cesarean birth with the nurse and their obstetrician and read some books on the topic.

Evaluation

Anticipated outcomes of nursing care include:

- The woman clearly understands her condition and its possible impact on her pregnancy, labor and birth, and postpartal period.

- The woman cooperates and participates in developing a health care regimen to meet her needs and follows it throughout her pregnancy.
- The woman gives birth to a healthy newborn.
- The woman avoids developing hypoglycemia or hyperglycemia.
- The woman is able to care for her newborn.

CARE OF THE WOMAN WITH ANEMIA

Anemia indicates inadequate levels of hemoglobin (Hb) in the blood. In 1990 the CDC defined anemia as hemoglobin less than 11 g/dL in the first and third trimesters and less than 10.5 g/dL in the second trimester. The common anemias of pregnancy are due either to insufficient hemoglobin production related to nutritional deficiency in iron or folic acid during pregnancy or to hemoglobin destruction in inherited disorders, specifically sickle cell anemia and thalassemia.

Iron Deficiency Anemia

Dietary iron is needed to synthesize hemoglobin. Because hemoglobin is necessary to transport oxygen, a deficiency of iron may affect the body's transport of oxygen.

Iron deficiency anemia is the most common medical complication of pregnancy, primarily as a consequence of expansion of plasma volume without normal expansion of maternal hemoglobin mass (Cunningham et al 1993). About 15% to 30% of Western women of childbearing age are iron deficient. Of pregnant women not taking iron supplements, 84% are iron deficient at term. Approximately 200 mg of iron will be conserved due to the functional amenorrhea of pregnancy, but a pregnant woman needs approximately 1000 mg more iron intake during the pregnancy. Between 300 and 400 mg of iron is transferred to the fetus; 500 mg is needed for the increased red blood cell mass in the woman's own increased circulating blood volume; another 100 mg is needed for the placenta; and about 280 mg is needed to replace the 1 mg of iron lost daily through feces, urine, and sweat.

The greatest need for increased iron intake is in the second half of pregnancy. When the iron needs of pregnancy are not met, maternal hemoglobin falls below 11 g/dL. Serum ferritin levels, indicating iron stores, are below 12 μg/L.

Many women begin pregnancy in a slightly anemic state. In pregnancy mild anemia can rapidly become more severe; therefore it needs immediate treatment.

Maternal Risks

The woman with iron deficiency anemia may be asymptomatic, but she is more susceptible to infection, may tire easily, has an increased chance of PIH and postpartal hemorrhage, and tolerates poorly even minimal blood loss during birth. Healing of an episiotomy or an incision may be delayed. If the anemia is severe (Hb less than 6 g/dL), cardiac failure may ensue.

Fetal-Neonatal Risks

There is evidence of increased risk of low birth weight, prematurity, stillbirth, and neonatal death in infants of women with severe iron deficiency (maternal Hb less than 6 g/dL) (Scholl et al 1992). The infant is not iron deficient at birth due to active transport of iron across the placenta, even when maternal iron stores are low. However, these babies do have lower iron stores and are at increased risk for developing iron deficiency during infancy.

Medical Therapy

The first goal of health care is to prevent iron deficiency anemia. If it occurs, the goal is to return low iron and hemoglobin levels to normal.

Home Care Iron supplements are essential during pregnancy because dietary sources cannot meet the extra requirements. Oral doses of ferrous salt such as ferrous sulfate 300 mg (60 mg of elemental iron) are taken daily to prevent anemia. The dose is increased to three times daily to treat deficiency and restore hemoglobin to 12 g/dL. With a twin pregnancy a larger dose is needed. If a large dose of oral iron causes vomiting, diarrhea, or constipation or if the anemia is discovered late in pregnancy, parenteral iron may be needed.

APPLYING THE NURSING PROCESS

Nursing Assessment

The main presenting symptom of iron deficiency anemia may be fatigue. Nutritional history usually gives evidence of poor dietary intake of iron. Physical examination reveals pallor of skin and conjunctiva. Laboratory studies show Hb values below 11 g/dL, serum ferritin levels below 12 μg/L, and possibly microcytic and hypochromic red blood cells (a late finding).

Nursing Diagnosis

Nursing diagnoses that might apply to a pregnant woman with iron deficiency anemia include the following:

- Altered nutrition: Less than body requirements related to inadequate intake of iron-containing foods
- Constipation related to daily intake of iron supplements

Nursing Plan and Implementation

Critical Thinking Question

In addition to iron supplements, what other sources of iron can the nurse recommend to a woman with iron deficiency anemia?

The woman is taught to take iron tablets with vitamin C (eg, orange juice) to increase absorption. Iron absorption is reduced 40% to 50% if the tablets are taken with meals. However, gastrointestinal upset is more likely if they are taken on an empty stomach. The client may tolerate the iron better if she starts with small doses and gradually increases the dosage over several days. She is informed that her stool will turn black and may be more formed. She is also advised to keep the tablets out of the reach of children because ingestion may be fatal to a young child.

Evaluation

Anticipated outcomes of nursing care include:

- The woman is able to identify the risks associated with iron deficiency anemia during pregnancy.
- The woman takes her iron supplements as recommended.
- The woman's hemoglobin levels remain normal or return to normal levels during her pregnancy.

Folic Acid Deficiency Anemia

Folate deficiency is the most common cause of megaloblastic anemia during pregnancy, affecting between 1% and 4% of pregnant women in the United States. It is more prevalent with twin pregnancies.

Folic acid is needed for DNA and RNA synthesis and cell duplication. In its absence immature red blood cells fail to divide, become enlarged (megaloblastic), and are fewer in number. With the tremendous cell multiplication that occurs in pregnancy an adequate amount of folic acid is crucial. However, increased urinary excretion of folic acid and fetal uptake can rapidly result in folic acid deficiency. It is usually diagnosed late in pregnancy or the early puerperium. Hemoglobin levels as low as 3 to 5 g/dL may be found.

RESEARCH IN PRACTICE

Inadequate prenatal care may predispose to low birth weight babies and preterm births, especially in women from a low income background. Although adequate prenatal care might improve pregnancy outcomes, some women wait to seek prenatal care until late in the pregnancy. Health status may be a predictor of health care utilization. Therefore Mary-Clayton Enderlein and her colleagues developed a study to determine whether prior medical or obstetrical problems and current symptoms could predict when a woman with low income would seek prenatal care.

The sample consisted of 473 pregnant women eligible for care at a community health center network. Eligibility requirements included having a family income under 185% of the federal poverty level and being without private insurance. Of the total sample, 237 women sought care on or before week 14 of their pregnancy, and the remaining 236 began prenatal care between weeks 15 and 32 weeks' gestation. All women beyond 32 weeks or at very high medical risk were referred elsewhere.

The researchers examined demographic variables and the health status of each woman. Health status encompassed evaluation of (1) medical history, such as allergies, diabetes mellitus, and seizure disorders; (2) obstetric history, typified by prior ectopic pregnancy, cesarean birth, or eclampsia; (3) gynecologic history, characterized by infertility, gynecologic surgery, or genital herpes; and (4) current obstetric problems, exemplified by nausea and vomiting, gonorrhea, and preeclampsia. By summing the number of conditions within each category, the authors obtained an indicator of the severity for each category.

Results of the study characterized late registrants for prenatal care as more likely to be slightly younger, employed, white, and primigravidas compared to the early registrants. Logistical regression provided an estimate of relative risk of late prenatal care based on health status. Women with no significant condition (none or one) in their medical history, obstetric history, or current obstetric status had a higher relative risk of late entry into prenatal care. Gynecologic conditions showed no significant impact on timing of entry into care.

Clinical Application of Study

Based on this study, health care providers need to be aware that a healthy low-income woman may put off early entry into prenatal care and should counsel any woman of childbearing age that current health status may not predict pregnancy outcome.

SOURCE: Enderlein M-C et al: Health status and timing of onset of prenatal care: Is there an association among low-income women? *Birth* 1994; 21(2):71.

Medical Therapy

Diagnosis of folic acid deficiency anemia may be difficult. Serum folate levels typically fall as pregnancy progresses. Even though folate levels are lower with deficiency, they will fluctuate with diet. Measurement of erythrocyte folate status is more reliable but indicates folate status of several weeks previously. Bone marrow biopsy is diagnostic but rarely used due to the discomfort it causes the woman.

Folic acid deficiency during pregnancy is prevented by a daily supplement of 0.4 mg of folate. Treatment of deficiency consists of 1 mg folic acid supplement. Because iron deficiency anemia almost always coexists with folic acid deficiency, the woman also needs iron supplements.

Nursing Care

The nurse can help the pregnant woman avoid folate deficiency by teaching her food sources of folic acid and cooking methods for preserving folic acid. The best sources are fresh leafy green vegetables, red meats, fish, poultry, and legumes. As much as 50% to 90% of folic acid can be lost by cooking in large volumes of water. Microwave cooking destroys more folic acid than conventional cooking.

Sickle Cell Anemia

Sickle cell anemia (HbSS) is a recessive autosomal disorder in which the normal adult hemoglobin, hemoglobin A (HbA), is abnormally formed. It occurs primarily in people of African descent and occasionally in people of Mediterranean origin (ie, Greeks, Italians, Arabs, and Turks) (Cruikshank 1994). The anemia is characterized by acute, recurring, painful episodes. Individuals with the disorder are homozygous for the sickle cell gene. They inherit from each parent an allele causing an amino acid substitution in the two beta protein chains in the hemoglobin molecule. This abnormal hemoglobin is called hemoglobin S (HbS). Heterozygous individuals are carriers for sickle cell anemia but are usually asymptomatic. This condition is called sickle cell trait (HbSA). One of the beta protein chains formed in their hemoglobin is normal; the other has the amino acid substitution. Sickle cell trait occurs in 1 out of 10 African Americans; sickle cell anemia is found in 1 out of 400 (Cruikshank 1994).

Hemoglobin S causes the red blood cells to be sickle or crescent shaped. Whereas normal hemoglobin is soluble, in conditions of low oxygenation, HbS becomes semisolid and distorts the red blood cell shape. These erythrocytes easily interlock and clog capillaries, particularly in organs characterized by slow flow and high oxygen extraction, such as the spleen, bone marrow, and placenta. This phenomenon, called *sickling*, varies in frequency depending upon the amount of the S hemoglobin in the red blood cells (there is seldom a crisis with levels below 40%) and other hemoglobin factors. Diagnosis is confirmed by hemoglobin electrophoresis or a test to induce sickling in a blood sample.

Maternal Risks

Women with sickle cell trait have a good prognosis for pregnancy if they have adequate nutrition and prenatal care. They are, however, at increased risk for nephritis, bacteriuria, and hematuria, and they tend to become anemic (Pollack 1993).

Women with sickle cell anemia have considerably more risk during pregnancy. Low oxygen pressure—caused by high temperature, dehydration, infection, or acidosis, for example—may precipitate a vaso-occlusive crisis. The crisis produces sudden attacks of pain that may be general or localized in bones or joints, lungs, abdominal organs, or the spinal cord. The pain is due to ischemia in the tissues from occluded capillaries. Vaso-occlusive crises occur more often in the second half of pregnancy.

The woman with sickle cell anemia has increased susceptibility to certain infections due to impaired immune functioning. Congestive heart failure or acute renal failure may also occur. The maternal mortality rate has been reduced to about 2% with improved antepartal care (Koshy & Burd 1991).

Fetal-Neonatal Risks

The incidence of fetal death during and immediately following an attack has decreased greatly in recent years but is still high. Prematurity and IUGR are also associated with sickle cell anemia. Fetal death is believed to be due to sickling attacks in the placenta.

Medical Therapy

Vaso-occlusive crisis is best treated by a perinatal team in a medical center. Partial exchange transfusion of HbA for HbS red cells is most important. With erythrocytophoresis the woman's blood is removed, the HbS is separated out, and the woman's plasma and other blood factors are returned to her through another vein. The crisis and pain subsides more quickly with this technique.

Rehydration with intravenous fluids, administration of antibiotics and analgesics, and fetal heart rate monitoring are also important aspects of therapy. Antiembolism stockings are used postpartally.

If vaso-occlusive crisis occurs during labor, the previous therapies are instituted. The woman is also given oxygen and kept in a left lateral position. Oxytocics may be used if needed. Episiotomy and outlet forceps are recommended to shorten the second stage.

Several antisickling agents are being researched, and in the future sickle cell crisis may be prevented.

APPLYING THE NURSING PROCESS

Nursing Assessment

The woman with sickle cell anemia usually relates a history of frequent illnesses and recurrent abdominal and joint pains and is found to be extremely anemic. The woman may appear undernourished and have long, thin extremities. Ulcers are often present on her ankles. Anemia may be severe.

A diagnosis of sickle cell anemia is confirmed by hemoglobin electrophoresis or a test to induce sickling in a blood sample. The woman should be assessed for infection, which is associated with one-third of sickle cell crises in adults. Those most commonly seen during pregnancy or postpartum are pneumonia, urinary tract infections, puerperal endomyometritis, and osteomyelitis.

Fetal status is assessed during a crisis by electronic fetal monitoring. During labor the woman's vital signs and the FHR are assessed frequently. Compatible blood should be available for transfusion. Oxygen is administered if necessary. The woman is assessed for joint pains and other signs of sickle cell crisis.

Nursing Diagnosis

Nursing diagnoses that might apply to the pregnant woman with sickle cell anemia include the following:

- Acute pain related to the effects of sickle cell crisis

- Knowledge deficit related to lack of knowledge of the need to avoid exposure to infection secondary to the risk of a sickle cell crisis

Nursing Plan and Implementation

Teaching for Self-Care

The nursing goal when working with a pregnant woman with sickle cell disease is to provide effective health teaching to help prevent a sickle cell attack (crisis), improve the anemia, and prevent infection. The woman is taught to increase hydration, use good hygiene practices, avoid people with infections, seek immediate treatment for infection, and take folic acid supplements. Folic acid is important because of its role in red blood cell production. The woman with sickle cell anemia maintains her hemoglobin levels by intense erythropoiesis and thus requires folic acid supplements. Bed rest is sometimes recommended to decrease the chance of preterm labor. Other nursing interventions are aimed at facilitating the medical therapy and alleviating anxiety through support and education.

Genetic counseling is recommended when both parents have the disease or are known carriers.

Evaluation

Anticipated outcomes of nursing care include:

- The woman is able to describe her condition and identify its possible impact on her pregnancy, labor and childbirth, and postpartal period.

- The woman takes appropriate health care measures to avoid a sickle cell crisis.

- The woman gives birth to a healthy infant.

- The woman and her care givers quickly identify and successfully manage any complications that arise.

Thalassemia

The thalassemias are a group of autosomal recessive disorders characterized by a defect in the synthesis of the α or β chains in the hemoglobin molecule. The one most frequently encountered in the United States is β-thalassemia. Symptoms are caused by the shortened life span of the red blood cells resulting in active erythropoiesis in the liver, spleen, and bones. This produces hepatosplenomegaly and sometimes bony malformations. The thalassemias are seen most often in persons from Greece, Italy, or southern China and are also known as Mediterranean anemia and Cooley's anemia. Early identification avoids unnecessary treatment of anemia (Esposito 1992).

If the woman is heterozygous for β-thalassemia, half of the β chains are formed normally. This is β-thalassemia minor or β-thalassemia trait. Mild anemia is usually the only symptom.

Persons born homozygous for the disease have β-thalassemia major, with severe anemia that appears several months after birth. Newborns have fetal hemoglobin (HbF), which does not have β chains; therefore there is a delay in onset of the anemia. Once they start producing adult type hemoglobin (HbA), such infants are dependent on transfusions, from which they eventually develop iron overload. Iron chelation therapy must be instituted soon after chronic transfusions are begun because excess iron damages the liver and heart. Without chelation therapy these infants do not live past the second or third decade, and those who reach puberty are often amenorrheic and infertile (Giardina & Hilgartner 1992).

Maternal-Fetal-Neonatal Risks

The woman with β-thalassemia minor has mild anemia with small (microcytic) red cells. This mild anemia must be distinguished from iron deficiency anemia because a woman with β-thalassemia minor should not receive iron therapy. The pregnancy is otherwise uncomplicated by the disease.

Beta-thalassemia major increases the woman's risk for PIH and other complications. The risk of fetal loss and the incidence of low birth weight are also increased.

Medical Therapy

Women with thalassemia may need folic acid supplements. Those with thalassemia major may need transfusion and chelation therapy. They should avoid exposure to infections and seek treatment promptly if an infection develops. Amniocentesis to determine the presence of the disease in the fetus is offered to the woman.

Nursing Care

The woman with thalassemia needs to understand her disease, the possibility of transmitting it to her offspring, and the amniocentesis procedure. These clients have lived with thalassemia since childhood but may have questions regarding its effect on pregnancy outcome and their own prognosis.

CARE OF THE WOMAN WITH ACQUIRED IMMUNODEFICIENCY SYNDROME (AIDS)

Acquired immunodeficiency syndrome (AIDS), caused by the human immunodeficiency virus (HIV), is one of today's major health concerns. HIV is a retrovirus that targets the CD4+ T-lymphocyte. The CD4+ T-lymphocyte coordinates a number of important immunologic functions, and a loss of these functions results in progressive impairment of the immune response. Studies of the natural history of HIV infection have documented a wide spectrum of disease manifestations, ranging from asymptomatic infection to life-threatening conditions characterized by severe immunodeficiency, serious opportunistic infections, and cancers (CDC 1992).

The diagnosis of AIDS is made when an individual is HIV positive and is identified as having one of several specific opportunistic infections. AIDS can also be diagnosed without laboratory evidence of HIV infection when one of the opportunistic infections is definitively diagnosed and there is no other known cause for the immune deficiency.

As of September 30, 1993, there was a total of 339,250 cases of AIDS reported in the United States (CDC 1993). Homosexual and bisexual males are still the largest group of infected individuals. Women accounted for 40,702 (11%) of the cases. In one US study, rates among Black women were 3 to 35 times higher than in White women in nine states, regardless of urbanicity (Wasser et al 1993). Pediatric cases total 4,906 (1.4%), which includes both males and females under the age of 13. Of these pediatric cases 4,325 (88%) were infants born to mothers with AIDS or at risk for AIDS during the prenatal or intrapartum period or during the time of breastfeeding.

Although once most infants and children who acquired HIV perinatally lived in urban areas with a high incidence of drug abuse, it is no longer confined to the nation's urban areas. The National Research Council (1990) has noted epidemiologic patterns that show increasing geographic diffusion of the virus.

HIV found in blood, semen, vaginal fluid, and breast milk has been implicated in disease transmission, although the virus has been isolated in urine, tears, cerebrospinal fluid, lymph nodes, brain tissue, and bone marrow. HIV shedding has also been detected in the genital tract of women (Clemetson et al 1993). Homosexual intercourse is the primary method of transmission in men (65%). Intravenous drug use is the means of transmission for 20% (Cohn 1993). More than 51% of women with AIDS acquired the infection through intravenous drug use; approximately 32% contracted HIV through heterosexual activity. The fastest growing category of HIV-infected women consists of those who acquired the disease through heterosexual sex (Stratton 1994). Transmission can also occur through exposure to contaminated blood or blood products or through organ transplants.

Perinatal transmission of HIV, which is the primary cause of pediatric AIDS in the United States, can occur transplacentally, during birth, or via breast milk. HIV infection has occurred in some infants despite cesarean birth, suggesting that use of this childbirth method does not prevent intrapartum transmission (Cohn 1993).

Once infected with the virus, the individual develops antibodies that can be detected with enzyme-linked immunosorbent assay (ELISA) and confirmed with the Western blot test. Antibodies can be detected in most individuals 6 to 12 weeks after exposure, but in rare circumstances the latent period is longer. An asymptomatic period of variable length generally follows seroconversion. The CDC (1992) estimates that in the United States 1 to 1.5 million people are HIV-positive but asymptomatic. In the adult population fewer than 5% of infected persons develop AIDS within 3 years; the mean time from infection to the development of AIDS is about 10 years.

As the incidence of AIDS increases, a growing number of health care providers have begun questioning their ethical responsibilities with regard to clients who test HIV-positive. Some physicians have refused to provide care to people with AIDS. The Committee on Ethics of the American College of Obstetricians and Gynecologists (1990, p 1043) has formulated a position statement on physicians' responsibilities. It states, ". . . it is unethical for an obstetrician-gynecologist to refuse to accept or continue to care for persons solely because they are or are thought to be seropositive for HIV. To avoid or delay treatment of a seropositive person is ethically equivalent to refusal of care."

Maternal Risks

Studies evaluating the impact of HIV infection on pregnancy results are mixed, and the American College of Obstetricians and Gynecologists (1992) reports that there is no definitive evidence that preterm birth, low birth weight, or pregnancy complications are increased in seropositive women. On the other hand, a study by Temmerman et al (1994) reported significantly lower birth weight and increased prematurity in women who were HIV-positive. The HIV-infected women in their study also experienced a higher incidence of postpartum endometritis. Similarly, there is no definitive evidence that pregnancy affects the clinical progression of HIV disease (Cohn 1993; Hankins et al 1992). More large, gender-specific studies are necessary to more accurately evaluate these and other health-related issues.

AIDS-defining diseases that are more common in women than in men include wasting syndrome, esophageal candidiasis, and herpes simplex virus disease. Kaposi's sarcoma is rare in women. Non–AIDS-defining gynecologic conditions such as vaginal candida infections and cervical pathology are prevalent among women at all stages of HIV infection. Associations have been documented between the presence of human papillomavirus, lower genital tract neoplasia, and HIV-related immunosuppression (Hankins et al 1992).

Fetal-Neonatal Risks

Although AIDS may develop in the infants of seropositive mothers, transmission does not always occur. Often infants will have a positive antibody titer, which reflects the passive transfer of maternal antibodies. Infected infants are usually asymptomatic at birth. More than half the children born antibody-positive lose maternal antibody by 15 months of age and remain asymptomatic (Jones et al 1993).

Infected newborns are likely to be small for gestational age (SGA) at birth. Facial characteristics that may indicate the newborn had been infected with HIV early in gestation include microcephaly; patulous lips; a prominent, boxlike forehead; increased distance between the inner canthus of the eyes; a flattened nasal bridge; and a mild obliquity of the eyes. The mortality rate for these infants is especially high.

The signs of AIDS in infants may include failure to thrive, hepatosplenomegaly, interstitial lymphocytic pneumonia, recurrent infections, cell-mediated immunodeficiency, evidence of Epstein-Barr virus, and neurologic abnormalities. Recurrent bacterial infections are common in children with AIDS; Kaposi's sarcoma is rare. Awareness of these signs in infants is extremely important. One recent study found that HIV testing that relied heavily on maternal risk assessment resulted in delayed diagnosis of AIDS in children (Hsu et al 1992). The prognosis for an infected child remains poor; those with clinical illness in the first 6 months often do not survive beyond 1 year of age.

Encephalopathy, characterized by delayed developmental milestones or the loss of acquired skills, including cognitive abilities, is found in 50–90% of children with AIDS. Treatments that prevent the central nervous system effects of HIV have yet to be identified. Well-controlled developmental studies are needed to clarify the relationship between HIV and child development to help professionals design appropriate, school-based educational plans (Armstrong et al 1993).

Medical Therapy

The goal for antenatal care is identification of the pregnant woman at risk for AIDS. Women at risk who are pregnant or planning a pregnancy should be offered HIV antibody testing. Testing is done using ELISA. The Western blot test is used to confirm the diagnosis with positive ELISA results. Women who test positive should be counseled about the implications of the diagnosis for themselves and their fetus in order to ensure an informed reproductive choice. A woman who chooses to continue her pregnancy needs excellent prenatal care with special attention to her psychosocial and teaching needs (Porcher 1992).

HIV-infected women should be evaluated and treated for other sexually transmitted infections and for conditions occurring more commonly in women with HIV such as tuberculosis, cytomegalovirus, toxoplasmosis, and cervical dysplasia. HIV-infected women with no history of hepatitis B should receive the hepatitis vaccine, which is not contraindicated prenatally, as well as the pneumococcal vaccine and an annual flu shot (Stratton 1994). In addition to routine prenatal laboratory tests, a platelet count and a complete blood count with differential should be obtained at the first prenatal visit and repeated each trimester to identify anemia, thrombocytopenia, and leukopenia, which are associated both with HIV infection and with antiviral therapy.

The woman with HIV also should be assessed regularly for serologic changes that indicate the disease is progressing. This is determined by the absolute CD4+ T-lymphocyte count, which provides the number of helper T4 cells. When the CD4+ count drops below 500/mm^3, many physicians institute antiviral therapy with zidovudine (Retrovir, formerly called azidothymidine [AZT]) (Wiesenfeld & Sweet 1994). Others prefer to wait until the postpartum period. Most clinicians prescribe zidovudine for pregnant women with CD4+ counts approaching or below 200/mm^3 (DeFerrari et al 1993). Its use during the first trimester is discouraged, however, because its possible effects on the fetus are not known.

In the woman, zidovudine suppresses bone marrow function and has major side effects such as thrombocytopenia, anemia, and granulocytopenia. These hematologic side effects may be increased if the woman takes acetaminophen, and she should be advised to avoid it (Cox et al 1990). When CD4+ counts fall to 200/mm^3 or lower, opportunistic infections such as *Pneumocystis carinii* pneumonia are more likely to develop, and prophylaxis should be instituted. The drug of choice for both prophylaxis and treatment of *Pneumocystis carinii* pneumonia is oral trimethoprim-sulfamethoxazole (TMP-SMX), also called co-trimoxazole.

At each prenatal visit asymptomatic HIV-infected women should be monitored for early signs of complications, such as weight loss in the second or third trimesters or fever. The mouth should be inspected for signs of infections such as thrush (candidiasis) or hairy leukoplakia; the lungs should be auscultated for signs of pneumonia; the lymph nodes, liver, and spleen should be palpated for signs of enlargement. Each trimester the woman should have a visual examination and a fundoscopic examination to detect such complications as toxoplasmosis retinitis. Further discussion of the most advanced therapy for the pregnant woman who is HIV-positive or who has symptomatic AIDS may be found in journal articles and specialty texts.

A pregnancy complicated by HIV infection, even if asymptomatic, is considered high risk, and the fetus is monitored closely. Weekly nonstress testing is begun at 32 weeks' gestation, and serial ultrasounds are done to detect intrauterine growth retardation. Biophysical profiles are also indicated (see Chapter 20). Invasive procedures such as amniocentesis are avoided when possible to prevent the contamination of a noninfected infant.

Intrapartal care is similar to that for all pregnant women, although strict adherence to universal precautions is crucial to avoid nosocomial infection. To prevent exposure of an uninfected infant to HIV during labor and birth, invasive procedures such as vaginal examinations following rupture of the membranes, fetal scalp electrode monitoring, fetal scalp sampling, and vacuum extraction should be done only after carefully evaluating the risks and benefits (DeFerrari et al 1993). Studies to date do not indicate that cesarean birth decreases the risk of fetal infection; as a result cesarean is used only for obstetric reasons (ACOG 1992).

Women who are HIV-positive are at increased risk for complications such as intrapartal or postpartal hemorrhage, postpartal infection, poor wound healing, and infections of the genitourinary tract. Thus they need careful monitoring and appropriate therapy as indicated.

Following childbirth, the HIV-positive woman should be referred to a physician knowledgeable about treating individuals with HIV infection (ACOG 1992).

Because of the profound implications of HIV infection for the woman, her family, the fetus/newborn, and her health care providers, screening is recommended for women at increased risk, including the following: prostitutes; women whose current or previous sex partners have been bisexual, abused IV drugs, had hemophilia, or tested positive for HIV; and women from countries where heterosexual transmission is common. In addition clinics located in areas with a large HIV-positive population may require routine HIV screening of all prenatal clients.

Nursing Assessment

A woman who tests positive for HIV may be asymptomatic or may present with any of the following signs of symptoms: fatigue, anemia, malaise, progressive weight loss, lymphadenopathy, diarrhea, fever, neurologic dysfunction, cell-mediated immunodeficiency, or evidence of Kaposi's sarcoma (purplish, reddish-brown lesions either externally or internally).

If a woman tests HIV-positive or is involved in a relationship that places her at high risk, the nurse should assess the woman's knowledge level about the disease, its implications for her and her fetus, and self-care measures the woman can take.

Nursing Diagnosis

Examples of nursing diagnoses that might apply for an HIV-positive pregnant woman are included in the Nursing Care Plan: Care of the Woman with AIDS on page 460. Other examples include the following:

- Knowledge deficit related to lack of information about AIDS and its long-term implications for the woman and her unborn child
- Risk for infection related to altered immunity secondary to AIDS
- Ineffective family coping related to the implications of a positive HIV test in one of the family members

Nursing Plan and Implementation

Provision of Anticipatory Guidance

Nurses need to help women understand that AIDS is a fatal disease. The incidence of AIDS is increasing so significantly that it is the fifth leading cause of death for women of childbearing age (Wiesenfeld & Sweet 1994). AIDS can be avoided if women avoid sharing IV drug needles and practice safe sex, including insisting that their sex partners wear a latex condom for each act of intercourse.

Women at risk for AIDS should be offered premarital and prepregnancy screening for HIV antibodies (ACOG 1992). They should be given clear information about the implications of a diagnosis of HIV, including societal attitudes. Access to information about the disease and about the test results empowers women by enabling them to make informed decisions about their sexual activities and about becoming pregnant.

A detailed drug and sexual history of each prenatal client is the first step in perinatal AIDS prevention. Women at risk for AIDS should be offered HIV counseling. The following are counseling and education guidelines for HIV testing:

- HIV testing discussion should be incorporated into the normal prenatal assessment.

- The woman should be assured of confidentiality (the difference between anonymity and confidentiality should be explained).

- An educational environment that is private, comfortable, and nonjudgmental should be provided.

- The woman should be given information about AIDS, including pathophysiology, mode of transmission of HIV, high-risk behaviors, and methods of decreasing transmission, such as practicing safe sex and not sharing needles.

- If the woman chooses to have an antibody test for HIV (ELISA, Western blot), written consent should be obtained.

- Posttest counseling should be provided. A negative test means that no HIV antibodies were found. It does not ensure that the woman has not been infected with the virus because antibodies may not be detected for 6 weeks to 6 months after exposure.

- If test results are positive, supportive follow-up is necessary. This includes an explanation of the implications for the woman and her unborn child, recommended medical therapy, follow-up of sex partners, transmission prevention, discussion of immediate posttest plans, and referral to appropriate psychologic and educational services. The woman should be told not to donate blood or blood products and not to share toothbrushes, razors, and other implements that could be contaminated with blood.

This information can be overwhelming to the woman who is HIV-positive and should be provided orally and in writing. She will need more than one counseling session to absorb the information. The initial reaction may be one of shock or denial, so it is important to allow her a little time to think and to give her empathy and support. The nurse needs to stress that being HIV-positive does not mean that the woman has AIDS but that she can transmit the virus to others by sexual contact, sharing IV drug needles, and donating blood and to her fetus during pregnancy. Most people do develop AIDS within 10 years. It is currently impossible to prevent AIDS from developing in people who are HIV-positive or to predict when they will develop the disease.

Monitoring the Asymptomatic Pregnant Woman

In monitoring the asymptomatic HIV-positive pregnant woman the nurse should be alert for nonspecific symptoms such as fever, weight loss, fatigue, persistent candidiasis, diarrhea, cough, skin lesions, and behavior changes. Laboratory findings such as decreased hemoglo-

bin, hematocrit, and T4 lymphocytes; elevated erythrocyte sedimentation rate (ESR); and abnormal complete blood count, differential, and platelets may indicate complications such as infection or progression of the disease.

Education about optimal nutrition and maintenance of wellness are important and should be reviewed frequently with the woman.

Reducing the Risk of Transmission

The nurse is faced with the important task of taking the precautions necessary to protect staff, other clients, and families from exposure to AIDS while meeting the needs of the childbearing woman with AIDS.

In 1987 the CDC stated that the increasing prevalence of AIDS and the risk of exposure faced by health care workers is significant enough that *precautions should be taken with all clients* (not only those with known HIV infection), especially in dealing with blood and body fluids. These are now called *universal precautions.*

Nurses who deal with childbearing families are exposed frequently to blood and body fluids and should pay careful attention to the CDC guidelines, including the following:

1. Care givers should wear disposable latex gloves when having contact with a client's mucus membranes, nonintact skin, body fluids, or blood. Contact includes, for example, changing chux pads, peripads, diapers, or dressings; starting or discontinuing intravenous fluids; and drawing blood.

2. After giving care to a client, gloves should be removed and hands should be washed before caring for another client.

3. In addition to gloves, protective coverings such as a plastic apron, gown, mask, and eye or face shield should be worn during any procedures that frequently result in contamination from splashing of body fluids. These include amniotomy, vaginal examination, vaginal or cesarean birth, suctioning, and care of the newborn until after the initial bath has been done. (Note: Full-sized glasses are considered sufficient eye protection. Although agencies are required to provide eye shields, nurses may choose to purchase their own eye goggles and clean them with soap and water.)

4. At birth the newborn should be suctioned with a disposable bulb syringe or mucus extractor attached to wall suction at a low setting. DeLee mucus traps with mouth suction are not used because of the risk of inadvertently ingesting secretions.

5. Similar care should be taken during any resuscitation procedures. To avoid the need for mouth-to-mouth resuscitation, sufficient mouthpieces and ventilation equipment should be available. Disposable resuscitation masks are recommended.

CARE OF THE WOMAN WITH AIDS

Nursing Assessment

Nursing History

1. Course of the present pregnancy
2. Estimated gestational age
3. Sensitivity to medications
4. History of infections

Physical Examination

1. Fetal size, fetal status (FHR), and fetal maturity
2. Signs of fatigue, weakness, recurrent diarrhea, pallor, night sweats
3. Lymphadenopathy
4. Present weight and amount of weight gain or weight loss
5. Presence of nonproductive cough, fever, sore throat, chills, shortness of breath (*Pneumocystis carinii* pneumonia)

6. Dark purplish marks or lesions, especially on the lower extremities (Kaposi's sarcoma)
7. Oral, gingival lesions

Diagnostic Studies

1. Ultrasound
2. Fetal maturity studies (L/S ratio, PG, creatinine)
3. Hemoglobin and hematocrit
4. WBC
5. HIV-1
6. CD4+ T lymphocyte count
7. ESR
8. Differential
9. Platelet count

NURSING DIAGNOSIS: Altered nutrition: Less than body requirements related to decreased appetite

EXPECTED OUTCOME: Woman maintains current body weight or gains weight.

Nursing Interventions	Rationale
Weigh woman.	Establishes baseline weight.
Obtain food history.	Helps identify food likes and dislikes and plan meals.
Plan high-protein, high-calorie diet.	Provides for nutrition of woman and fetus.
Provide teaching regarding nutritional needs.	Nutritional education and support may help the woman plan her daily diet.

OUTCOME MET IF: • Woman maintains weight or gains weight.

NURSING DIAGNOSIS: Fear related to outcome of pregnancy and disease

EXPECTED OUTCOME: Woman verbalizes her fears in regard to the pregnancy and disease process.

Nursing Interventions	Rationale
Establish rapport.	Establishment of rapport helps create a therapeutic relationship.
Provide opportunities to talk without interruption.	
Provide support and counseling.	
Discuss disease process, impact on pregnancy, and pregnancy options.	The nurse presents factual, appropriate data and then supports the woman/family in whatever decisions are made.
Assess support system.	
Refer to community resources.	

OUTCOME MET IF: • Woman verbalizes understanding of disease process, impact of the disease on the pregnancy, possible impact of the pregnancy on the disease, and available resources.

---

6. Syringes and needles are disposed of in a special puncture-resistant container. Needles are *never* recapped using two hands; a one-handed scoop technique is acceptable. Needles should never be twisted or broken by hand.

7. In the event that a glove is torn it should be removed, the hands should be cleansed, and new gloves should be applied.

8. Gloves and protective coverings should also be worn during any cleaning procedures.

CARE OF THE WOMAN WITH AIDS *continued*

NURSING DIAGNOSIS: Knowledge deficit related to lack of information about appropriate precautions to prevent transmission of HIV infection

EXPECTED OUTCOME: Woman identifies necessary precautions to prevent spread of HIV infection.

Nursing Interventions	Rationale
Provide information on transmission of HIV and measures to prevent infection. Discuss household safety issues (eg, it is acceptable to use same dishes, safe to sleep in same bed, safe to use same bathroom, can hold and hug children, should avoid using razors and toothbrushes and should wear gloves and use 10% bleach-solution to clean spills of body fluids or disinfect bathroom). Inform the woman that sexual abstinence is safest; otherwise latex condoms should be used. Discuss the implications of breastfeeding.	Information regarding how HIV is spread is an important basis for medical asepsis. As the woman understands more about the disease, she will be able to take precautions to protect against the spread of HIV. Current information suggests that the virus may be spread in breast milk.

OUTCOME MET IF: • Woman discusses methods of transmission, precautions to prevent spread of infection, and possible implication for newborn if breastfeeding is desired.

NURSING DIAGNOSIS: Risk for infection related to suppressed immune status

EXPECTED OUTCOME: Woman does not develop infections during the hospital stay.

Nursing Interventions	Rationale
Monitor for signs of infection (fever, cough, sore throat, night sweats).	Any pathogen may be able to establish itself in an immunosuppressed body. *Pneumocystis carinii* pneumonia is an infection frequently associated with AIDS.
Maintain appropriate isolation precautions (see Appendix H).	Isolation precautions are advised for all clients who are hospitalized based on method of transmission and presence of epidemiologically important microorganisms such as HIV.

OUTCOME MET IF: • On discharge the woman shows no signs of fever, cough, sore throat, night sweats, diarrhea, or oral sores.

Essential Nursing Activities To Achieve Outcomes

If the client is asymptomatic, the primary nursing activity is client teaching regarding

1. Disease process
2. Screening and health care for sex partners as appropriate
3. Impact of disease on pregnancy
4. Methods of HIV transmission
5. Precautions to take in preventing the spread of infection
6. Options in regard to pregnancy
7. Available community resources
8. Signs and symptoms to report to health care provider, including common discomforts of pregnancy such as nausea and fatigue and complications such as premature rupture of membranes, vaginal bleeding, and preterm labor.
9. Importance of regular prenatal visits

10. Importance of compliance with health care providers' recommendations
11. Possible need for antepartal testing in the third trimester, including NST and BPP

If the client is symptomatic, the nurse

1. Provides client teaching as for the asymptomatic client
2. Assesses for cardiac, renal, pulmonary, and hepatic involvement
3. Schedules prenatal visits according to the client's needs
4. Discusses with the woman/family the management of labor and birth, including possible need for a cesarean if the woman is unable to tolerate labor, and influence of the woman's medication on the type of anesthesia used
5. Assesses the woman's support system

Provision of Emotional Support

The psychologic implications of AIDS for the childbearing family are staggering. The woman is faced with the knowledge that she and her newborn have decreased chances for survival. She may have feelings of fear, help-lessness, anger, and isolation. If she shares her diagnosis with others, she may face rejection and condemnation. The couple must deal with the impact of the illness on the partner, who may or may not be infected, and on other children. Dealing with the tasks and responsibilities of a newborn may be especially difficult if the woman is physically depleted or if she is trying to come to grips with the long-term implications of her condition.

The nonjudgmental, supportive nurse plays an essential role in preserving confidentiality and the client's right to privacy. In addition the nurse can help ensure that the woman receives complete, accurate information about her condition and ways she might cope. This usually involves a referral to social services for follow-up care. The hospitalized woman will often welcome the opportunity to talk with someone about her fears and desires.

Evaluation

Anticipated outcomes of nursing care include:

- The woman discusses the implications of her positive HIV antibody screen (or diagnosis of AIDS), its implications for her unborn child and for herself, the method of transmission, and treatment options.

- The woman uses information regarding social services (or other agency) referral for follow-up assistance and counseling.

- The woman begins to verbalize her feelings about her condition and its implications in an atmosphere she finds supportive.

- The woman implements health-focused self-care practices.

CARE OF THE SUBSTANCE-ABUSING WOMAN

Substance abuse occurs when an individual experiences difficulties with work, family, social relations, and health as a result of alcohol or drug use. According to the National Institute on Drug Abuse (NIDA) National Household Survey on Drug Abuse, 48.6% of the female population surveyed aged 12 to 35+ admitted to using drugs (NIDA 1991). Studies have shown that illicit drug users seldom use only one drug.

Because women of childbearing age (15–44 years) make up a substantial proportion of the drug-using population, the problem has major significance for women and children. In testimony to these statistics is the increasing number of drug-exposed infants being born throughout the United States. Indiscriminate use of drugs during pregnancy, particularly in the first trimester,

| TABLE 18-3 | Possible Effects of Selected Drugs of Abuse/Addiction on Fetus and Neonate |

Maternal Drug	Effect on Fetus/Neonate
Depressants	
Alcohol	Cardiac anomalies, IUGR, potential teratogenic effects, FAS, FAE
Narcotics	
Heroin	Withdrawal symptoms, convulsions, death, IUGR, respiratory alkalosis, hyperbilirubinemia
Methadone	Fetal distress, meconium aspiration; with abrupt termination of the drug, severe withdrawal symptoms, neonatal death
Barbiturates	Neonatal depression, increased anomalies; teratogenic effect(?); withdrawal symptoms, convulsions, hyperactivity, hyperreflexia, vasomotor instability
Phenobarbital	Bleeding (with excessive doses)
"T's and Blues" (combination of the following)	
Talwin (narcotic)	Safe for use in pregnancy; depresses respiration if taken close to time of birth
Amytal (barbiturate)	See barbiturates
Tranquilizers	
Phenothiazine derivatives	Withdrawal, extrapyramidal dysfunction, delayed respiratory onset, hyperbilirubinemia, hypotonia or hyperactivity, decreased platelet count
Diazepam (Valium)	Hypotonia, hypothermia, low Apgar score, respiratory depression, poor sucking reflex, possible cleft lip
Antianxiety drugs	
Lithium	Congenital anomalies; lethargy and cyanosis in the newborn
Stimulants	
Amphetamines	
Amphetamine sulfate (Benzedrine)	Generalized arthritis, learning disabilities, poor motor coordination, transposition of the great vessels, cleft palate
Dextroamphetamine sulfate (dexedrine sulfate)	Congenital heart defects, hyperbilirubinemia
Cocaine	Learning disabilities, poor state organization, decreased interactive behavior, CNS anomalies, cardiac anomalies, genitourinary anomalies, SIDS
Caffeine (more than 600 mg/day)	Spontaneous abortion, IUGR, increased incidence of cleft palate; other anomalies suspected
Nicotine (half to one pack cigarettes/day)	Increased rate of spontaneous abortion, increased incidence of placental abruption, SGA, small head circumference, decreased length, SIDS
Psychotropics	
PCP ("angel dust")	Flaccid appearance, poor head control, impaired neurologic development
LSD	Chromosomal breakage?
Marijuana	IUGR, potential impaired immunologic mechanisms

may adversely affect the health of the woman and the growth and development of her fetus. Drugs that are commonly misused include alcohol, cocaine, marijuana, amphetamines, barbiturates, hallucinogens, heroin, and other narcotics. Table 18–3 identifies common addictive drugs and their effects on the fetus and newborn. Abuse of these drugs poses a major threat to the successful completion of pregnancy.

Drug use during pregnancy may be the most frequently missed diagnosis in all of maternity care. Substance-abusing women typically do not seek prenatal care until late in their pregnancy, may be noncompliant, or may present in labor with no prenatal care.

Providing prenatal care to chemically dependent women presents multiple dilemmas and challenges to clinicians. However, it must be viewed as an opportunity to bring these alienated women into the health care system. Pregnancy represents a period in most women's lives when they recognize the need for and are receptive to caring and responsive interventions. By optimizing the prenatal experience of chemically dependent women, maternal-fetal outcomes will be improved and the groundwork laid for the ongoing therapeutic services that are needed to maintain the health and well-being of the mother and child (Atlen 1993).

The substance-abusing woman who seeks prenatal care may not voluntarily reveal her addiction, so care givers should be alert for a history or physical signs that suggest substance abuse (Table 18–4). Because substance abuse has increased rapidly in the past decade, it is helpful to discuss the specific substances that are abused to increase understanding of this serious problem.

Substances Commonly Abused During Pregnancy

Alcohol

Alcohol abuse has increased dramatically among women in the United States. The incidence is highest among women 20–40 years old; alcoholism is also seen in teenagers. Chronic abuse of alcohol can undermine maternal health by causing malnutrition (especially folic acid and thiamine deficiencies), bone marrow suppression, increased incidence of infections, and liver disease. As a result of alcohol dependence the woman may have withdrawal seizures in the intrapartal period as early as 12–48 hours after she stops drinking. Delirium tremens may occur in the postpartal period, and the newborn may suffer a withdrawal syndrome.

The effects of alcohol on the fetus may result in a group of signs referred to as *fetal alcohol syndrome (FAS)*. The syndrome has characteristic physical and mental abnormalities that vary in severity and combination. (See discussion in Chapter 31.) There is no definitive answer to how much alcohol a woman can safely consume during pregnancy. The expectant woman should "play it safe" by avoiding alcohol completely during the early weeks of

TABLE 18-4	Factors Associated with the Substance Abuser

Appearance and Physical Signs	**Maternity History (Previous Pregnancies)**
Pupils dilated or constricted	
Marked fatigue or exhaustion	Abruptio placentae
Abscesses, track marks, or edema of arms and legs	Low-birth-weight infant
	Sudden infant death syndrome
Inflamed nasal mucosa	Fetal death
Inappropriate or disoriented behavior	Preterm birth
	Spontaneous abortion
Medical History	
	Current Pregnancy
HIV positive	
Cirrhosis	Abruptio placentae
Endocarditis	Sexually transmitted infection
Sexually transmitted infection	Vaginal spotting or bleeding
Hepatitis	IUGR
Pancreatitis	Low weight gain
Pneumonia	Fetal bradycardia
Cellulitis	Fetal hyperactivity

SOURCE: Adapted from MacGregor SN, Keith LG: Substance abuse in pregnancy: A practical management plan. *Female Patient* January 1989; 14:49; Chashoff IJ: Perinatal effects of cocaine. *Contemp OB/GYN* 1987; 29:163.

pregnancy when organogenesis is occurring. During the remainder of the pregnancy she may have an occasional drink, although none at all is safest.

The nursing staff in the maternity unit must be aware of the manifestations of alcohol abuse so that they can prepare for the client's special needs. The care regimen includes sedation to decrease irritability and tremors, seizure precautions, intravenous fluid therapy for hydration, and preparation for an addicted neonate. Although high doses of sedatives and analgesics may be necessary for the woman, caution is advised because these can cause fetal depression.

Breastfeeding generally is not contraindicated, although alcohol is excreted in breast milk. Excessive alcohol consumption may intoxicate the infant and inhibit maternal let-down reflex. Discharge planning for the alcohol-addicted mother and newborn should be correlated with the social service department of the hospital.

Cocaine/Crack

Cocaine use is one of the most serious epidemics affecting the childbearing family. Approximately 1 in 10 pregnant women is believed to use cocaine, with even higher rates reported in urban areas (Weathers et al 1993). Cocaine acts at the nerve terminals to prevent the reuptake of dopamine and norepinephrine, which in turn results in vasoconstriction, tachycardia, and hypertension. Placental vasoconstriction decreases blood flow to the fetus.

Cocaine is usually taken in three ways: snorting, smoking, and intravenous injection. **Crack** is a form of free base cocaine that is made up of baking soda, water, and cocaine mixed into a paste and microwaved to form a rock. The rock can then be smoked. Many women, especially those in low-income areas, favor this form of the drug over other forms because it is readily available and cheaper. In addition smoking crack leads to a quicker, more intense high because the drug is absorbed through the large surface area of the lungs.

The onset of effects of cocaine occurs rapidly, but the euphoria lasts only about 30 minutes. This profound euphoria and excitement is usually followed by irritability,

CONTEMPORARY ISSUE

FREEDOM OF CHOICE OR CHILD ABUSE?

Substance abuse during pregnancy is fast becoming a major health issue. It is related to a variety of preventable health risks, including preterm birth, intrauterine growth retardation, birth defects, neonatal addiction, and AIDS. Attitudes toward pregnant women who abuse drugs vary widely from understanding and sympathy to scorn and condemnation. Some suggest that a woman's rights to privacy and freedom of choice are so basic that nothing should override them. Others see the substance-abusing mother as a victim, just as her fetus is a victim. Still others suggest that the rights of the fetus are paramount. Those supporting fetal rights may go so far as to suggest that, by choosing to become pregnant, a woman has an enhanced duty to ensure the well-being of her fetus even at increased risk to herself. Some also stress the cost to society of substance abuse, both in caring for the woman and in meeting the needs of her children, especially if the children are born addicted.

States approach the issue in a variety of ways. Some view substance abuse during pregnancy as child abuse and, if the child is born addicted, may also accuse the mother of drug trafficking. Such an approach subjects the woman to arrest and penalty. Other states view the problem as a social issue rather than a criminal one and provide treatment programs and supportive care.

This issue raises several questions:

- If fetal rights take such precedence that a woman can be penalized for life-style choices, what pregnant woman can be totally free from worry about prosecution? What of the obese woman? The smoker? The woman who never exercises? The woman who refuses any prenatal testing?

- Does it serve society to penalize pregnant women who abuse substances, or are they being held to an unfairly high standard of behavior?

- Does the actual conflict become one of the fundamental right to privacy versus the authority of the state?

- Should the state ever be able to force an addicted woman to terminate a pregnancy?

- Is prosecution counterproductive? Will women who fear criminal prosecution for substance abuse avoid the health care system and increase their risk?

- Should mandatory drug screening of all pregnant women be instituted to detect the problem early, mandate treatment, and decrease the incidence of addicted neonates?

depression, pessimism, fatigue, and a strong desire for more cocaine. This pattern often leads the user to take repeated doses to sustain the effect. Cocaine metabolites may be present in the urine of a pregnant woman for up to 4 to 7 days following use.

The cocaine user is difficult to identify prenatally. Because cocaine is an illegal substance, many women are reluctant to volunteer information about their drug use. The nurse who is familiar with the woman may recognize subtle signs of cocaine use, including mood swings and appetite changes, and withdrawal symptoms such as depression, irritability, nausea, lack of motivation, and psychomotor changes.

Major adverse maternal effects of cocaine use include seizures and hallucinations, pulmonary edema, respiratory failure, and cardiac problems. Women who use cocaine have an increased incidence of spontaneous first-trimester abortion, abruptio placentae, IUGR, preterm birth, and stillbirth.

Exposure of the fetus to cocaine in utero increases the risk of IUGR, small head circumference, shorter body length, altered brain development, malformations of the genitourinary tract, and lower Apgar scores. Newborns who were exposed to cocaine in utero may have neurobehavioral disturbances, marked irritability, an exaggerated startle reflex, labile emotions, and an increased risk of sudden infant death syndrome (SIDS). These newborns have poor interactive behaviors, have difficulty responding appropriately to voices, and fail to respond well to consoling behaviors. These complications may interfere with maternal-infant attachment and increase the infant's risk of abuse and neglect (Zaichkin et al 1993).

Cocaine does cross into the breast milk and may cause such symptoms in the breastfeeding infant as extreme irritability, vomiting, diarrhea, dilated pupils, and apnea. Thus women who continue to use cocaine following childbirth should avoid nursing.

Marijuana

Approximately 15% of pregnant women use marijuana, often in conjunction with alcohol and tobacco. Men who smoke marijuana may have decreased sperm counts and may develop gynecomastia (enlarged breasts); women may experience menstrual cycle irregularities. To date, however, there is no evidence that marijuana has any teratogenic effects. One study has reported an increase in precipitous labors (less than 3 hours) in heavy marijuana users (Niebyl 1991), but these results have not been confirmed. The impact of heavy marijuana use on pregnancy is difficult to evaluate because of the variety of social factors that may influence the results.

Infants exposed to marijuana in utero have been reported to have increased fine tremors, prolonged startles, irritability, and poor habituation to visual stimuli, but these symptoms were not present in follow-up at 12 and 24 months of age (Cunningham et al 1993).

Phencyclidine (PCP)

Phencyclidine (PCP) is a popular hallucinogen that can be smoked, taken orally, or injected intravenously. The onset of effects occurs in 2 to 4 minutes and lasts about 4 to 6 hours, with no withdrawal state. The drug causes confusion, delirium, and hallucinations and may produce feelings of euphoria. Signs of PCP use include constricted pupils, ataxia, nystagmus, double vision (diplopia), dizziness, and diaphoresis. The greatest risk for the pregnant woman is overdose or a psychotic response. Signs of overdose include hypertension, hyperthermia, diaphoresis, and possible coma, which may jeopardize fetal well-being.

PCP has been associated with facial abnormalities in the newborn (Cunningham et al 1993) and neurobehavioral problems including wild behavior states, flaccid appearance, and poor head control.

Heroin

Heroin is an illicit CNS depressant narcotic that alters perception and produces euphoria. It is an addictive drug that is generally administered intravenously, although a snortable form of heroin called Karachi is available. Pregnancy in women who use heroin is considered high risk because of the increased incidence in these women of poor nutrition, iron deficiency anemia, and PIH. There is also an increased rate of breech position, abnormal placental implantation, abruptio placentae, preterm labor, premature rupture of the membranes (PROM), and meconium staining. These women also have a higher incidence of sexually transmitted infection because many rely on prostitution to support their drug habit.

The fetus of a heroin-addicted woman is at increased risk for IUGR, meconium aspiration, and hypoxia. The newborn frequently shows signs of heroin addiction such as restlessness; shrill, high-pitched cry; irritability; fist sucking; vomiting; and seizures. Signs of withdrawal usually appear within 72 hours and may last for several days. The newborn may exhibit poor consolability for 3 months or more. These behaviors may interfere with successful maternal-infant attachment and increase the potential for parenting problems in an already high-risk mother.

Methadone

Methadone is the most commonly used drug in the treatment of women who are dependent on opioids such as heroin. Methadone blocks withdrawal symptoms and the craving for street drugs. Dosage should be individualized at the lowest possible therapeutic level. Methadone does cross the placenta and has been associated with problems such as PIH, hepatitis, placental problems, and abnormal fetal presentation (Hans 1989).

Prenatal exposure to methadone may result in reduced head circumference, poor motor coordination, increased body tension, and delayed achievement of motor skills. The neonate may experience withdrawal symptoms that are more severe than those associated with heroin.

Medical Therapy

Antepartal care of the pregnant addict involves medical, socioeconomic, and legal considerations. The use of a team approach allows for the comprehensive management necessary to provide safe labor and childbirth for woman and fetus.

The management of drug addiction may include hospitalization as necessary to initiate detoxification. "Cold turkey" withdrawal is not advisable during pregnancy because of potential risk to the fetus. Maintenance and support therapy are given during weekly prenatal visits.

Urine screening is also done regularly throughout pregnancy if the woman is a known or suspected substance abuser. This testing is helpful in identifying the type and amount of drug being abused.

Critical Thinking Question

What psychosocial factors contribute to the onset of substance abuse?

APPLYING THE NURSING PROCESS

Nursing Assessment

The nurse should be alert for clues in the history or appearance of the woman that suggest substance abuse (Table 18–4). If abuse is suspected, the nurse needs to ask direct questions, beginning with less threatening questions about use of tobacco, caffeine, and over-the-counter medications. The nurse can then progress to questions about alcohol consumption and finally questions focusing on past and current use of illicit drugs. The nurse who is matter-of-fact and nonjudgmental in approach is more likely to elicit honest responses.

Nursing assessment of the woman who is a known substance abuser focuses on her general health status, with specific attention to nutritional status, susceptibility to infections, and evaluation of all body systems. The nurse also assesses the woman's understanding of the impact of substance abuse on herself and her pregnancy. Some women are reluctant to discuss their substance abuse; others are quite open about it. Once the nurse establishes a relationship of trust, he or she can gain information that can be used to plan the woman's ongoing care.

Nursing Diagnosis

Nursing diagnoses that may apply are listed in the Nursing Care Plan: Care of the Substance-Abusing Woman.

Text continues on page 468

NURSING CARE PLAN

CARE OF THE SUBSTANCE-ABUSING WOMAN

Nursing Assessment

Nursing History

1. Course of the present pregnancy
2. Estimated gestational age, late prenatal care, missed appointments
3. Prior abruptio placentae, stillbirths, miscarriages, neonatal deaths
4. Irregular menses, amenorrhea
5. Sensitivity to medications
6. Drug use: kind of drugs, duration, frequency and route of administration, symptoms during withdrawal
7. History of infections: STDs, hepatitis, HIV, AIDS
8. History of child abuse, neglect, sexual abuse

Physical Examination

1. Fetal size, fetal status (FHR), fetal maturity
2. Present weight, amount of weight gain or weight loss
3. Bloodshot eyes, dilated or constricted pupils
4. Rhinitis, nasal or sinus irritation, septal erosion, loss of sense of smell
5. Poor dental hygiene
6. Shortness of breath, slurred speech
7. Needle marks, ecchymotic spots or scars, subcutaneous abscesses
8. Jaundice, hepatomegaly
9. Unsteady walk, impaired coordination, slowed reflexes

Diagnostic Studies

1. Ultrasound
2. CBC, VDRL, HIV
3. Urinalysis, urine toxicologic screen
4. Cervical culture for gonorrhea, chlamydia, Pap smear
5. Tuberculin skin test

NURSING DIAGNOSIS: Altered nutrition: Less than body requirements related to pregnancy and drug abuse

EXPECTED OUTCOME: Woman maintains current weight or gains weight.

Nursing Interventions	Rationale
Weigh woman.	Establishes baseline weight.
Obtain food history.	Helps identify food likes and dislikes and assists in meal planning.
Plan high-protein, high-calorie diet.	Provides for nutrition of woman and fetus.
Provide supplemental vitamins.	
Provide teaching regarding nutritional needs.	Nutritional education and support may help the woman plan her daily diet.
Reinforce information with printed material to take home.	

OUTCOME MET IF:
- Woman maintains or gains weight.

NURSING DIAGNOSIS: Knowledge deficit related to lack of information about the effects of substance abuse on self and pregnancy

EXPECTED OUTCOME: Woman describes the effects of substance abuse during pregnancy.

Nursing Interventions	Rationale
Give accurate and specific information on complications associated with drug use in a nonjudgmental way.	Information regarding drug use is an important basis for changing behaviors.
Explain that quitting or decreasing drug use at any time in pregnancy improves outcome.	
Help family members or significant other develop skills necessary to support the woman.	The woman needs those around her to participate in the change.
Identify drug withdrawal programs and written material for pregnant woman.	Additional programs will reinforce the information.

OUTCOME MET IF:
- Woman discusses effects of substance abuse on self and developing fetus.

CARE OF THE SUBSTANCE-ABUSING WOMAN *continued*

NURSING DIAGNOSIS: Altered family process related to developmental transition of pregnancy

EXPECTED OUTCOME: Woman is prepared for the birth of the baby.

Nursing Interventions	Rationale
Assess the woman's perception of her pregnancy.	Substance-abusing women often deny the pregnancy or don't believe that they can get pregnant because of irregular menses.
Help the woman identify support systems.	These women often feel guilty and are sensitive to criticism.
Help the woman identify stresses in her life.	
Promote attachment by encouraging attendance at childbirth and parenting classes with significant other(s).	This will help make the pregnancy seem more real and will help the woman begin the parenting process.
Encourage listening to fetal heart rate by the woman and significant other(s) at each visit.	
Show sonogram to the woman to help her visualize the fetus.	
Help the woman identify major areas in her life that will be affected by the new infant.	

OUTCOME MET IF:
- Woman verbalizes acceptance of pregnancy and identifies support system.

NURSING DIAGNOSIS: Risk for noncompliance related to difficulty in following prenatal recommendations

EXPECTED OUTCOME: Woman participates actively in prenatal care.

Nursing Interventions	Rationale
Emphasize the positive information about the fetal growth and development that is determined from your physical assessment.	Make the prenatal visits a valued time for the woman.
Identify barriers to compliance and strategies to overcome them.	Timing and travel to the office are often among the reasons they miss appointments.
Refer the woman to social services and other supportive agencies.	
Ensure that the woman feels she gets something out of the visit.	These women typically have low self-esteem and do not recognize the importance of their own needs.

OUTCOME MET IF:
- The woman keeps her appointments and verbalizes the importance of prenatal care.

Essential Nursing Activities To Achieve Outcomes

1. Screen for signs/symptoms of withdrawal.
2. Provide teaching about the effects of substance abuse on the fetus/neonate.
3. Teach the woman about good nutrition. Work with her to plan a balanced diet using foods she enjoys and has access to following discharge.
4. Include the family and the father, if he is involved, in teaching and discussion.
5. Provide information on community resources.
6. Avoid a critical or judgmental attitude.

Nursing Plan and Implementation

Prevention of substance abuse during pregnancy is the ideal nursing goal and is best accomplished through client education. Unfortunately, many women who are substance abusers do not receive regular health care and may not seek care until they are far along in pregnancy.

The nurse's role in providing prenatal care for the woman who is a substance abuser focuses on ongoing assessment and client teaching. The nurse can provide information about the relationship between substance abuse and existing health problems and the implications for the woman's unborn child. By establishing a relationship of trust and support the nurse may ensure the woman's cooperation.

TABLE 18-5	Less Common Medical Conditions and Pregnancy		
Condition	**Brief Description**	**Maternal Implications**	**Fetal/Neonatal Implications**
Rheumatoid arthritis	Chronic inflammatory disease believed to be caused by a genetically influenced antigen-antibody reaction. Symptoms include fatigue, low-grade fever, pain and swelling of joints, morning stiffness, pain on movement. Treated with salicylates, physical therapy, and rest. Corticosteroids used cautiously if not responsive to above.	Usually there is remission of rheumatoid arthritis symptoms during pregnancy, often with a relapse postpartum. Anemia may be present due to blood loss from salicylate therapy. Mother needs extra rest, particularly to relieve weight-bearing joints, but needs to continue range-of-motion exercises. If in remission, may stop medication during pregnancy.	Possibility of prolonged gestation and longer labor with heavy salicylate use. Possible teratogenic effects of salicylates.
Epilepsy	Chronic disorder characterized by seizures; may be idiopathic or secondary to other conditions, such as head injury, metabolic and nutritional disorders such as PKU or vitamin B_6 deficiency, encephalitis, neoplasms, or circulatory interferences. Treated with anticonvulsants.	Seizure frequency often increases during pregnancy, with slightly higher incidence of hyperemesis gravidarum, preeclampsia, and vaginal hemorrhage. A woman who has been seizure free for a year should be withdrawn from medication prior to conception; a woman who requires medication has a 90% chance of having a normal child; women who seek advice after the first trimester should be maintained on their medication. Folic acid, iron, and vitamin D therapy needed during pregnancy (Meadow 1989).	Three times higher incidence of congenital anomalies (ten times higher for cleft lip and palate, four times higher for septal heart defects) if mother on anticonvulsive medications (Meadow 1989).
Hepatitis B	Hepatitis B, caused by the hepatitis B virus (HBV), is a major, growing health problem. There was a 37% increase of acute hepatitis B between 1979 and 1989, when the immunization plan targeted only those at risk for hepatitis. Groups at risk include those from areas with a high incidence (primarily developing countries), illegal IV drug users, prostitutes, homosexuals, those with multiple sex partners, or occupational exposure to blood, although many infected people have no identifiable source of infection. HBV transmission is blood borne, primarily sexually and perinatally transmitted. Because of the dramatic increase and the difficulty of vaccinating high-risk individuals before they become infected, the CDC now recommends (1) testing all pregnant women for the presence of hepatitis B surface antigen (HBsAG), (2) providing immunoprophylaxis to the newborns of HBsAg-positive women, (3) providing routine vaccinations to all neonates born to HBsAg-negative women (CDC 1991).	Hepatitis B does not usually affect the course of pregnancy. However, chronic HBV carriers have a great potential for infecting others when exposure to blood and bodily fluids occurs. In addition chronic carriers may develop long-term sequelae, such as chronic liver disease and liver cancer. Approximately 4000 to 5000 deaths are caused annually by liver disease associated with chronic HBV infection. It is now recommended that all pregnant women be tested for the presence of hepatitis B surface antigen (HBsAg). A woman who is negative may be given the hepatitis vaccine.	Perinatal transmission most often occurs at or near the time of childbirth. More important, the risk of becoming a chronic carrier of the HBV is inversely related to the age of the individual at the time of initial infection (Crawford & Pruss 1993). Therefore infants infected perinatally have the highest risk of becoming chronically infected if not treated. Recommendations now include routine vaccination of all neonates born to HBsAg-negative women and immunoprophylaxis to all newborns of HBsAg-positive women.

Preparation for labor and birth should be part of the prenatal planning. Fear, tension, or discomfort may be relieved through nonnarcotic psychologic support and careful explanation of the labor process. If pain medication is necessary, it should not be withheld, however, because the notion that it will contribute to further addiction is mistaken (Lynch & McKeon 1990). Preferred methods of pain relief include the use of psychoprophylaxis and regional or local anesthetics such as pudendal block and local infiltration. These techniques decrease risk of additional fetal respiratory depression. Immediate intensive care should be available for the newborn, who will probably be depressed, SGA, and premature. For care of the addicted newborn see Chapter 31.

TABLE 18-5 _continued_			
Condition	**Brief Description**	**Maternal Implications**	**Fetal/Neonatal Implications**
Hyperthyroidism (thyrotoxicosis)	Enlarged, overactive thyroid gland; increased T_4:TBG ratio and increased BMR. Symptoms include muscle wasting, tachycardia, excessive sweating, and exophthalmos. Treatment by antithyroid drug propylthiouracil (PTU) while monitoring free T_4 levels. Surgery used only if drug intolerance exists.	Mild hyperthyroidism is not dangerous. Increased incidence of PIH and postpartum hemorrhage if not well controlled. Serious risk related to thyroid storm characterized by high fever, tachycardia, sweating, and congestive heart failure. Now occurs rarely. When diagnosed during pregnancy, may be transient or permanent.	Neonatal thyrotoxicosis is rare. Even low doses of antithyroid drug in mother may produce a mild fetal/neonatal hypothyroidism; higher dose may produce a goiter or mental deficiencies. Fetal loss not increased in euthyroid women. If untreated, rates of abortion, intrauterine death, and stillbirth increase. Breastfeeding contraindicated for women on antithyroid medication because it is excreted in the milk (may be tried by woman on low dose if neonatal T_4 levels are monitored).
Hypothyroidism	Characterized by inadequate thyroid secretions (decreased T_4:TBG ratio), elevated TSH, lowered BMR, and enlarged thyroid gland (goiter). Symptoms include lack of energy, excessive weight gain, cold intolerance, dry skin, and constipation. Treated by thyroxine replacement therapy.	Long-term replacement therapy usually continues at same dosage during pregnancy as before. Weekly NST after 35 weeks' gestation.	If mother untreated, fetal loss 50%; high risk of congenital goiter or true cretinism. Therefore newborns are screened for T_4 level. Mild TSH elevations present little risk because TSH does not cross the placenta.
Maternal phenylketonuria (PKU) (hyperphenylalaninemia)	Inherited recessive single gene anomaly causing a deficiency of the liver enzyme needed to convert the amino acid phenylalanine to tyrosine resulting in high serum levels of phenylalanine. Brain damage and mental retardation occur if not treated early.	Low phenylalanine diet is mandatory prior to conception and during pregnancy. The woman should be counseled that her children will either inherit the disease or be carriers, depending on the zygosity of the father for the disease. Treatment at a PKU center is recommended.	Risk to fetus if maternal treatment not begun preconception. In untreated women increased incidence of fetal mental retardation, microcephaly, congenital heart defects, and growth retardation. Fetal phenylalanine levels are approximately 50% higher than maternal levels.
Multiple sclerosis	Neurologic disorder characterized by destruction of the myelin sheath of nerve fibers. The condition occurs primarily in young adults, is marked by periods of remission, progresses to marked physical disability in 10 to 20 years.	Associated with remission during pregnancy, but with 50% relapse rate postpartum (Birk & Rudick 1989). Rest is important; help with child care should be planned. Uterine contraction strength is not diminished, but because sensation is frequently lessened, labor may be almost painless.	Increased evidence of a genetic causal effect (Birk & Rudick 1989). Therefore reproductive counseling is recommended.
Systemic lupus erythematosus (SLE)	Chronic autoimmune collagen disease, characterized by exacerbations and remissions; symptoms range from characteristic rash to inflammation and pain in joints, fever, nephritis, depression, cranial nerve disorders, and peripheral neuropathies.	Mild cases—little risk to mother or fetus. Severe cases—because of extra burden on the kidneys, therapeutic abortion may be indicated. Woman must be careful to avoid fatigue, infection, and strong sunlight.	Increased incidence of spontaneous abortion, stillbirth, prematurity, and SGA neonates. Infants with neonatal lupus syndrome without cardiac involvement respond well to supportive therapy, and the condition resolves during the first year of life (Dombrowski 1989). The prognosis for those with heart lesions (about 25%) depends on their severity but may be guarded (Dombrowski 1989).
Tuberculosis (TB)	Infection caused by _Mycobacterium tuberculosis;_ inflammatory process causes destruction of lung tissue, increased sputum, and coughing. Associated primarily with poverty and malnutrition and may be found among refugees from countries where TB is prevalent. Treated with isoniazid and either ethambutol or rifampin or both.	The incidence of tuberculosis has begun to increase significantly since the late 1980s, and it is increasingly associated with HIV infection (Margono et al 1994). If TB inactive due to prior treatment, relapse rate no greater than for nonpregnant women. When isoniazid is used during pregnancy, the woman should take supplemental pyridoxine (vitamin B_6). Extra rest and limited contact with others is required until disease becomes inactive.	If maternal TB is inactive, mother may breastfeed and care for her infant. If TB is active, neonate should not have direct contact with mother until she is noninfectious. Isoniazid crosses the placenta, but most studies show no teratogenic effects. Rifampin crosses the placenta. Possibility of harmful effects still being studied.

Evaluation

Anticipated outcomes of nursing care include:

- The woman is able to describe the impact of her substance abuse on herself and her unborn child.

- The woman successfully participates in a drug therapy program.

- The woman successfully gives birth to a healthy infant.

- The woman agrees to cooperate with a referral to social services (or another appropriate community agency) for follow-up care after discharge.

OTHER MEDICAL CONDITIONS AND PREGNANCY

A woman with a preexisting medical condition should be aware of the possible impact of pregnancy on her condition, as well as the impact of her condition on the successful outcome of her pregnancy. Table 18–5 on page 468 discusses some of the less common medical conditions vis-à-vis pregnancy.

KEY CONCEPTS

The diagnosis of high-risk pregnancy can shock an expectant couple. Providing emotional support, teaching about the condition and prognosis, and educating for self-care are important nursing measures that help the client cope.

Cardiac disease during pregnancy requires careful assessment, limitation of activity, and knowing and reporting signs of impending cardiac decompensation by both client and nurse.

The key point in the care of the pregnant woman with diabetes is scrupulous maternal plasma glucose control. This is best achieved by home blood glucose monitoring, multiple daily insulin injections, and a careful diet. To reduce incidence of congenital anomalies and other problems in the neonate, the woman should be euglycemic prior to conception and throughout the pregnancy. Diabetic clients more than most other clients need to be educated about their conditions and involved with their own care.

Almost any health problem that a person can have when not pregnant can coexist with pregnancy. Some problems, such as anemias, may be exacerbated by pregnancy. Others, such as collagen disease, may go into temporary remission with pregnancy. Regardless of the health problem, careful health care is needed throughout pregnancy to improve the outcome for mother and fetus.

Substance abuse (either drugs or alcohol) not only is detrimental to the mother's health but also may have profound lasting effects on the fetus.

REFERENCES

Ades AE et al: Vertically transmitted HIV infection in the British Isles. *Brit Med J* 1993; 15:306.

American College of Obstetricians and Gynecologists: *Human Immunodeficiency Virus Infections.* ACOG technical bulletin no. 169. Washington, DC: American College of Obstetricians and Gynecologists, 1992.

American College of Obstetricians and Gynecologists: *Management of Diabetes Mellitus in Pregnancy.* ACOG technical bulletin no. 92. Washington, DC: American College of Obstetricians and Gynecologists, 1986.

American Diabetes Association: Summary and recommendations of the 3rd international workshop-conference on gestational diabetes mellitus. *Diabetes* 1991; 40 (suppl 2):197.

Armstrong FD et al: Pediatric HIV infection: A neuropsychological and educational challenge. *J Learn Disab* 1993; 26(2):92.

Atlen PM et al: Critical components of obstetric management of chemically dependent women. *Clin Obstet Gynecol* 1993; 36(2):347.

Barbour BG: Alcohol and pregnancy. *J Nurse-Midwifery* 1990; 35(2):78.

Bendell A, Efantis-Potter J: Acquired immune deficiency syndrome in pregnancy. In: *High-Risk Intrapartum Nursing.* Mandeville L, Troiano N (editors). Philadelphia: Lippincott, 1992.

Birk KA, Rudick RA: Caring for the ob patient who has multiple sclerosis. *Contemp OB/GYN* July 1989; 34:58.

Centers for Disease Control: Public health service guidelines for counseling and antibody testing to prevent HIV infection and AIDS. *MMWR* 1987; 36:509.

Centers for Disease Control: 1993 Revised classifications system for HIV infection and expanded surveillance case definition for AIDS among adolescents and adults. *MMWR* 1992; 41:RR17.

Chashoff IJ: Perinatal effects of cocaine. *Contemp OB/GYN* 1987; 29:163.

Clemetson DB et al: Detection of HIV DNA in cervical and vaginal secretions: Prevalence and correlates among women in Nairobie, Kenya. *JAMA* 1993; 9:269(22):2860.

Cohn JA: Human immunodeficiency virus and AIDS: 1993 Update. *J Nurse-Midwifery* March/April 1993; 38(2):65.

Committee on Ethics, American College of Obstetricians and Gynecologists: Human immunodeficiency virus infection: Physicians' responsibilities. *Obstet Gynecol* June 1990; 75(6):1043.

Cox PH et al: Outcome of treatment with AZT of patients with AIDS and symptomatic HIV infection. *Nurse Pract* 1990; 15:36.

Crawford N, Pruss A: Preventing neonatal hepatitis B infection during the perinatal period. *JOGNN* 1993; 22(6):491.

Criteria Committee of the New York Heart Association: *Nomenclature and Criteria for Diagnosis of Diseases of the Heart and Blood Vessels,* 5th ed. New York: New York Heart Association, 1955.

Cruikshank DP: Cardiovascular, pulmonary, renal, and hematologic diseases in pregnancy. In: *Danforth's Obstetrics and*

Gynecology, 7th ed. Scott JR et al (editors). Philadelphia: Lippincott, 1994.

Cunningham FG et al: *Williams Obstetrics*, 19th ed. Norwalk, CT: Appleton & Lange, 1993.

Damm P et al. Predictive factors for the development of diabetes in women with previous gestational diabetes mellitus. *Am J Obstet Gynecol* 1992; 167:607.

DeFerrari E et al: Nurse-midwifery management of women with human immunodeficiency virus disease. *J Nurse-Midwifery* March/April 1993; 38(2):86.

Dombrowski MP, Sokol RJ: Cocaine and abruption. *Contemp OB/GYN* April 1990; 35:13.

Dombrowski RA: Autoimmune disease in pregnancy. *Med Clin North Am* May 1989; 73:605.

Elixhauser A et al: Cost-benefit analysis of pre-conception care for women with established diabetes mellitus. *Diabetes Care* 1993; 16(8):1146.

Engel NS: Insulin therapy in pregnancy. *MCN* January/February 1989; 14:19.

Esposito NW: Thalassemias: Simple screening for hereditary anemias. *Nurse Pract* 1992; 17(2):50.

Fadden RR et al: Reproductive preferences of pregnant woman under shifting probabilities of vertical HIV transmission. *Women's Health Issues* Winter 1993; 3(4):216.

Ferris AM et al: Perinatal lactation protocol and outcome in mothers with and without insulin-dependent diabetes mellitus. *Am J Clin Nutr* 1993; 58(1):43.

Funkhouser AW et al: Prenatal care and drug use in pregnant women. *Drug Alcohol Dep* 1993; 33(1):1.

Gagne MP et al: The breast-feeding experience of women with type 1 diabetes. *Health Care Women Int* 1992; 13(3):249.

Gianopoulos JG: Cardiac disease in pregnancy. *Med Clin North Am* May 1989; 73:639.

Giardina PJ, Hilgartner MW: Update on thalassemia. *Pediatr in Rev* 1992; 13(2):55.

Hankins CA et al: HIV disease and AIDS in women: Current knowledge and a research agenda. *J Acq Immunodef Synd* 1992; 5(10):957.

Hans SL: Developmental consequences of prenatal exposure to methadone. *Ann NY Acad Sci* 1989; 562:195.

Hessol NA et al: Prevalence, incidence and progression of human immunodeficiency virus infection in homosexual and bisexual men in hepatitis B vaccine trials, 1978–1988. *Am J Epidemiol* 1989; 130:1167.

Hsu HW et al: Perinatally acquired human immunodeficiency virus infection: Extent of clinical recognition in a population-based cohort. *Ped Infect Dis J* 1992; 11(11):941.

Janke JR: Prenatal cocaine use: Effects on perinatal outcome. *J Nurse-Midwifery* 1990; 35(2):75.

Jones DS et al: Lack of detectable human immunodeficiency virus infection in antibody-negative children born to human immunodeficiency virus-infected mothers. *Ped Infect Dis J* 1993; 12(3):222.

Jovanic-Peterson L: Nutritional management of the obese gestational diabetic pregnant woman. *J Am Coll Nutr* 1992; 11:246.

Keohane N, Lacey L: Preparing the woman with gestational diabetes for self-care. *JOGNN* 1991; 20(3):189.

Kitzmiller JL et al: Managing diabetes and pregnancy. *Curr Probl Obstet Gynecol Fertil* July/August 1988; 11:125.

Koshy M, Burd L: Management of pregnancy in sickle cell syndromes. *Hematol Oncol Clin North Am* 1991; 5(3):585.

Landon MB, Gable SG: Fetal surveillance in the pregnancy complicated by diabetes mellitus. *Clin Obstet Gynecol* 1991; 34:535.

Lawrence RA: Breastfeeding and medical disease. *Med Clin North Am* May 1989; 73:583.

Lynch M, McKeon VA: Cocaine use during pregnancy. *JOGNN* July/August 1990; 19:285.

Mandeville L: Diabetes mellitus in pregnancy. In: *High-Risk Intrapartum Nursing*. Mandeville L, Troiano N (editors). Philadelphia: Lippincott, 1992.

Margono F et al: Resurgence of active tuberculosis among pregnant women. *Obstet Gynecol* June 1994; 83(6):911.

McCain GC, Deatrick JA: The experience of high-risk pregnancy. *JOGNN* June 1994; 23(5):421.

Meadow SR: Epilepsy in pregnancy: What are the hazards? *Contemp OB/GYN* November 1989; 34:51.

Mello NK et al: Neuroendocrine consequences of alcohol abuse in women. *Ann NY Acad Sci* 1989; 562:211.

Morbidity and Mortality Weekly Report, Supplement: Recommendations for prevention of HIV transmission in health care settings. August 21, 1987; 36(25):2.

National Diabetes Data Group: *Classification of Diabetes Mellitus and Other Categories of Glucose Intolerance*. Washington, DC: NIH, 1979.

National Institute on Drug Abuse: *National Household Survey on Drug Abuse: Population Estimates of 1990*. Rockville, MD: National Institute on Drug Abuse, 1991.

National Research Council: State of the epidemic. In: *AIDS: The Second Decade*. Washington, DC: National Academy Press, 1990, pp 38–80.

Niebyl JR: Drugs in pregnancy and lactation. In: *Obstetrics: Normal and Problem Pregnancies*, 2nd ed. Gabbe SG et al (editors). New York: Churchill Livingstone, 1991.

Norlander E et al: Factors influencing neonatal morbidity in gestational diabetic pregnancy. *Brit J Obstet Gyn* June 1989; 96:671.

O'Sullivan JB: Diabetes mellitus after GDM. *Diabetes* 1991; 40(suppl 2):131.

Petitti DBK, Coleman C: Cocaine and the risk of low birth weight. *Am J Pub Health* 1990; 80(1):25.

Piacquadio K et al: Effects of in-utero exposure to oral hypoglycemic drugs. *Lancet* 1991; 338:866.

Pollack CV: Emergencies in sickle cell disease. *Em Med Clin North Am* 1993; 11(2):365.

Porcher FK: HIV-infected pregnant women and their infants: Primary health care implications. *Nurse Pract* 1992; 17(11):46.

Racine A et al: The association between prenatal care and birth weight among women exposed to cocaine in NYC. *JAMA* 1993; 270(13):1581.

Ratner R: Gestational diabetes mellitus: After three international workshops, do we know how to diagnose and manage it yet? *J Clin Endocrin Metab* 1993; 77(1):1.

Roberts AB et al: Fructosamine compared with a glucose load as a screening test for gestational diabetes. *Obstet Gynecol* November 1990; 76:773.

Sacks DA et al: How reliable is the fifty-gram, one-hour glucose screening test? *Am J Obstet Gynecol* September 1989; 161:642.

Scholl TO et al: Anemia vs iron deficiency: Increased risk of preterm delivery in a prospective study. *Am J Clin Nutr* 1992; 55(5):985.

Shaw FE, Maynard JE: Hepatitis B: Still a concern for you and your patients. *Contemp OB/GYN* March 1986; 27:27.

Shields LE et al: The prognostic value of hemoglobin A_{1c} in predicting fetal heart disease in diabetic pregnancies. *Obstet Gynecol* 1993; 81(6):954.

Spellacy WN: Diabetes mellitus and pregnancy. In: *Danforth's Obstetrics and Gynecology*, 7th ed. Scott JR et al (editors). Philadelphia: Lippincott, 1994.

Stratton P: Treatment options for HIV pregnancies. *Contemp OB/GYN* May 1994; 39(5):99.

Temmerman M et al: Maternal human immunodeficiency virus-1 infection and pregnancy outcome. *Obstet Gynecol* April 1994; 83(4):495.

Veille JC et al: Interventricular septal thickness in fetuses of diabetic mothers. *Obstet Gynecol* 1992; 79:51.

Wasser SC et al: Urban-nonurban distribution of HIV infection in childbearing women in the United States. *J Acq Immunodef Synd* 1993; 6(9):1035.

Weathers WT et al: Cocaine use in women from a defined population: Prevalence at delivery and effects on growth in infants. *Pediatrics* 1993; 91(2):350.

White WBK: Management of hypertension during lactation. *Hypertension* 1984; 6:297.

Wiesenfeld HC, Sweet RL: Perinatal infections. In: *Danforth's Obstetrics and Gynecology*, 7th ed. Scott JR et al (editors). Philadelphia: Lippincott, 1994.

Wiley K, Grohar J: Human immunodeficiency virus and precautions for obstetric, gynecologic, and neonatal nurses. *JOGNN* May/June 1988; 17:165.

Winn HN, Reece EA: Integrating management of diabetic pregnancies. *Contemp OB/GYN* January 1989; 33:91.

Zaichkin J et al: The drug-exposed mother and infant: A regional center experience. *Neonatal Network* 1993; 12(3):41.

CHAPTER 19

PREGNANCY AT RISK: GESTATIONAL ONSET

A short while ago, my husband and I happily found out that we were expecting our second child, and although we had experienced it before, we anxiously looked forward to each exciting step along the way. On my second routine prenatal visit, however, we were informed that no heartbeat was evident and that I appeared to be nowhere near my then estimated 14 weeks. An ultrasound verified what my doctor had suspected: There was no viable pregnancy—I had miscarried. I was suddenly overwhelmed with a feeling of great loss. But after my D&C, that feeling of loss turned to one of fear and uncertainty as my doctor informed me that no fetal development had existed; I had had a molar pregnancy.

As my doctor told me about the disease and explained the potential risks, it occurred to me that the possibility existed that I might never have another child. Suddenly, my healthy, happy toddler became the most important element in my life—how blessed I was to have her!

Although some anxiety still exists, I now approach my weekly follow-up visits with a renewed sense of being. It will be at least another year before my husband and I might again rejoice in the anticipation of a second child; but for now we rejoice more fully in the precious one we have.

KEY TERMS

Abortion

Eclampsia

Ectopic pregnancy

Erythroblastosis fetalis

Gestational trophoblastic disease (GTD)

HELLP syndrome

Hydatidiform mole

Hydrops fetalis

Hyperemesis gravidarum

Incompetent cervix

Miscarriage

Preeclampsia

Pregnancy-induced hypertension (PIH)

Premature rupture of membranes (PROM)

Preterm labor

Rh immune globulin (RhoGAM)

Tocolysis

OBJECTIVES

Discuss the medical therapy and nursing care of a woman with hyperemesis gravidarum.

Contrast the etiology, medical therapy, and nursing interventions for the various bleeding problems associated with pregnancy.

Identify the medical therapy and nursing interventions indicated in caring for a woman with an incompetent cervix.

Delineate the nursing care needs of a woman experiencing premature rupture of the membranes or preterm labor.

Describe the development and course of hypertensive disorders associated with pregnancy.

Explain the cause and prevention of hemolytic disease of the newborn secondary to Rh incompatibility.

Compare Rh incompatibility to ABO incompatibility with regard to occurrence, treatment, and implications for the fetus/newborn.

Summarize the effects of surgical procedures on pregnancy and explain ways in which pregnancy may complicate diagnosis of conditions that require surgery.

Discuss the implications of trauma due to accidents or battering for the pregnant woman and her fetus.

Describe the effects of infections on the pregnant woman and her unborn child.

$\mathscr{P}$regnancy is usually a normal, uncomplicated experience. In some cases, however, problems arise during the pregnancy that place the woman and her unborn child at risk. Regular prenatal care serves to detect these potential complications quickly so that effective care can be provided. This chapter focuses on problems that primarily occur during pregnancy, those with a gestational onset.

CARE OF THE WOMAN WITH HYPEREMESIS GRAVIDARUM

Morning sickness, nausea, and vomiting of mild to moderate intensity are common during early pregnancy. **Hyperemesis gravidarum,** a relatively rare condition, is excessive vomiting during pregnancy. Hyperemesis can progress to a point at which the woman not only vomits everything she swallows but retches between meals. Dehydration, acidosis, starvation, and eventually death of the mother, the fetus, or both are the result of untreated hyperemesis (Newman et al 1993).

The cause of hyperemesis during pregnancy is still unclear but may be related to increased levels of human chorionic gonadotropin (hCG) and estradiol (Long & Russell 1993). Hyperemesis gravidarum occurs more often with molar pregnancies (discussed later in this chapter) and multiple gestations. Elevated thyroid function occurs in a significant number of cases and has recently received attention, but has not been found to be the cause or result of hyperemesis. Psychologic factors, such as ambivalence toward the pregnancy and stress, may also be causative (Newman et al 1993).

In severe cases the pathology of hyperemesis begins with dehydration. This leads to fluid-electrolyte imbalance and alkalosis from the loss of hydrochloric acid. More prolonged vomiting can result in loss of predominantly alkaline intestinal juices and the occurrence of acidosis. Hypovolemia from dehydration leads to hypotension and increased pulse rate, with increased hematocrit and blood urea nitrogen levels and decreased urine output. Severe potassium loss (hypokalemia) interferes with the ability of the kidneys to concentrate urine and disrupts cardiac functioning. Starvation causes muscle wasting and severe protein and vitamin deficiencies.

Characteristic symptoms include jaundice, hemorrhage, and peripheral neuropathy due to deficiencies of vitamin C and B-complex vitamins, and bleeding from mucosal areas due to hypothrombinemia. Fetal or embryonic death may result, and the woman may suffer irreversible metabolic changes or death.

The differential diagnosis may involve infectious diseases such as encephalitis or viral hepatitis, intestinal obstruction, hydatidiform mole, peptic ulcer, or drug reaction. The diagnostic criteria for hyperemesis include a history of intractable vomiting in the first half of pregnancy, dehydration, ketonuria, and a weight loss of 5% of prepregnancy weight (Long & Russell 1993).

Medical Therapy

The goals of treatment include control of vomiting, correction of dehydration, restoration of electrolyte balance, and maintenance of adequate nutrition. Initially, the woman is given nothing orally, with administration of intravenous fluids of 3000 mL in the first 24 hours. This therapy provides fluid, glucose, vitamin (B-complex, C, A, and D), and electrolyte replacement. Desired urine output is a minimum of 1000 mL/24 hours. Agents commonly used to control nausea and vomiting of hyperemesis gravidarum are phenothiazines (prochlorperazine, chlorpromazine, promethazine, perphenazine) and antihistamines (meclizine, dimenhydrinate, diphenhydramine) (Long & Russell 1993).

Usually nothing is given by mouth for 48 hours. IV therapy is continued until all vomiting ceases. If the woman's condition does not respond to this management, total parenteral nutrition may be needed.

When the woman's condition has improved, oral feedings can be given. Six small dry feedings followed by clear liquids is one suggested treatment. Another method is 1 oz of water offered each hour, followed as tolerated by clear, then nourishing liquids, progressing on succeeding days to low-fat soft and regular diets. Outpatient or home care is available to help the woman maintain enteral and parenteral nutritional therapies while staying at home. This option has the added benefit of giving the home care nurse the opportunity to observe family interactions and the home environment.

APPLYING THE NURSING PROCESS

Nursing Assessment

When a woman is hospitalized for control of vomiting, the nurse must regularly assess the amount and character of further emesis, intake and output, fetal heart rate, maternal vital signs, initial weight, evidence of jaundice or bleeding, and the woman's emotional state.

Nursing Diagnosis

Nursing diagnoses that may apply to the woman with hyperemesis gravidarum include the following:

- Altered nutrition: Less than body requirements related to persistent vomiting secondary to hyperemesis

- Fear related to the effects of hyperemesis on fetal well-being

Nursing Plan and Implementation

Treatment of nausea and vomiting begins early in pregnancy when the complaints first arise. The woman is counseled regarding remedies she can try at home, including such tactics as resting with her feet up and head elevated or slowly sipping carbonated beverages when nauseated. Herbal tea such as spearmint, peppermint, raspberry, chamomile, or ginger root may be helpful. Avoiding odors and exposure to fresh air is also helpful (Newman et al 1993). If the nausea and vomiting progress to a point where oral intake is not tolerated and dehydration is evident, medical intervention is required.

Nursing care should be supportive and directed at maintaining a relaxed, quiet environment away from food odors or offensive smells. Once oral feedings are started, food should be attractively served. Oral hygiene is important because the mouth is dry and may be irritated from vomitus. Weight gain or loss should be monitored regularly. Because emotional factors have been found to play a major role in this condition, psychotherapy may be recommended. With proper treatment, the prognosis is favorable.

Evaluation

Anticipated outcomes of nursing care include:

- The woman is able to explain hyperemesis gravidarum, its therapy, and its possible effects on her pregnancy.
- The woman's condition is corrected, and possible complications are avoided.

CARE OF THE WOMAN WITH A BLEEDING DISORDER

During the first and second trimesters of pregnancy the major cause of bleeding is **abortion.** This is the expulsion of the fetus prior to viability, which is considered 20 weeks' gestation. Abortions are either *spontaneous*, occurring naturally, or *induced*, occurring as a result of artificial or mechanical interruption. **Miscarriage** is a lay term applied to spontaneous abortion.

Other complications that can cause bleeding in the first half of pregnancy are ectopic pregnancy and gestational trophoblastic disease. In the second half of pregnancy, particularly in the third trimester, the two major causes of bleeding are placenta previa and abruptio placentae.

General Principles of Nursing Intervention

Spotting is relatively common during pregnancy and can occur following sexual intercourse or exercise due to trauma to the highly vascular cervix. However, the woman is advised to report any spotting or bleeding that occurs during pregnancy so that it can be evaluated.

It is often the nurse's responsibility to make the initial assessment of bleeding. In general the following nursing measures should be implemented for pregnant women being treated for bleeding disorders:

- Monitor blood pressure and pulse frequently.
- Observe woman for behaviors indicative of shock, such as pallor, clammy skin, perspiration, dyspnea, or restlessness.
- Count pads to assess amount of bleeding over a given time period; save any tissue or clots expelled.
- If pregnancy is of 12 weeks' gestation or beyond, assess fetal heart tones with a Doppler.
- Prepare for intravenous therapy. There may be standing orders to start IV therapy on bleeding clients.
- Prepare equipment for examination.
- Have oxygen therapy available.
- Collect and organize all data, including antepartal history, onset of bleeding episode, laboratory studies (hemoglobin, hematocrit, and hormonal assays).
- Obtain an order to type and cross-match for blood if there is evidence of significant blood loss.
- Assess coping mechanisms of woman in crisis. Give emotional support to enhance her coping abilities by continuous, sustained presence, by clear explanation of procedures, and by communicating her status to her family. Most importantly, prepare the woman for possible fetal loss. Assess her expressions of anger, denial, guilt, depression, or self-blame.

Spontaneous Abortion

Many pregnancies end in the first trimester as a result of spontaneous abortion. Statistics are inaccurate because some women may have aborted without being aware that they were pregnant during the early weeks of gestation, when the bleeding may be seen as a heavy menstrual period. If these very early abortions are included, the actual incidence of spontaneous abortion is approximately 50%. However, when only weeks 4 through 20 are considered, the rate is 10% to 17% (Blackburn & Loper 1992).

When a spontaneous abortion occurs, the woman and her family may search for a cause so that they may plan knowledgeably for future family expansion. However, even with current technology and medical advances a direct cause cannot always be determined.

About 50% of first trimester spontaneous abortions are related to chromosomal abnormalities (Simpson 1990). Other causes include teratogenic drugs, faulty implantation due to abnormalities of the female reproductive tract, a weakened cervix, placental abnormalities, chronic maternal diseases, endocrine imbalances, and maternal infections from the TORCH group. It is believed by some that psychic trauma and accidents are a primary cause of abortion, but statistics do not support this belief.

The pathophysiology of spontaneous abortion differs according to the cause. In most cases embryonic death occurs, which results in loss of hCG and decreased progesterone and estrogen levels. The uterine decidua is then sloughed off (vaginal bleeding), and the uterus becomes irritable, contracts, and usually expels the embryo/fetus. In late spontaneous abortion the cause is usually a maternal factor, for example, incompetent cervix or maternal disease, and fetal death may not precede the onset of abortion.

Spontaneous abortion can be extremely distressing to the couple desiring a child. Chances for carrying the next pregnancy to term after one spontaneous abortion are as good as they are for the general population. Thereafter, however, chances of successful pregnancy decrease with each succeeding spontaneous abortion.

Classification

Spontaneous abortions are subdivided into the following categories so that they can be differentiated clinically:

1. *Threatened abortion.* Unexplained bleeding, cramping, or backache indicate that the fetus may be in jeopardy. Bleeding may persist for days. The cervix is closed. It may be followed by partial or complete expulsion of pregnancy (Figure 19–1).

2. *Imminent abortion.* Bleeding and cramping increase. The internal cervical os dilates. Membranes may rupture. The term *inevitable abortion* also applies.

3. *Complete abortion.* All the products of conception are expelled.

4. *Incomplete abortion.* Part of the products of conception are retained, most often the placenta. The internal cervical os is dilated and will admit one finger.

5. *Missed abortion.* The fetus dies in utero but is not expelled. Uterine growth ceases, breast changes regress, and the woman may report a brownish vaginal discharge. The cervix is closed. Diagnosis is made based on history, pelvic examination, and a negative pregnancy test and may be confirmed by ultrasound if necessary. If the fetus is retained beyond 6 weeks, fetal autolysis results in the release of thromboplastin and disseminated intravascular coagulation (DIC) may develop.

6. *Habitual abortion.* Abortion occurs consecutively in three or more pregnancies.

Medical Therapy

One of the more reliable indicators of potential spontaneous abortion is the presence of pelvic cramping and backache. These symptoms are usually absent in bleeding caused by polyps, ruptured cervical blood vessels, or cervical erosion.

Laboratory evaluations to help determine the cause of vaginal bleeding include ultrasound scanning, for presence of gestational sac, and hCG level. The latter can confirm a pregnancy, but because the hCG level falls slowly after fetal death, it cannot confirm a live embryo/fetus. Hemoglobin and hematocrit levels are obtained to assess blood loss. Blood is typed and cross-matched for possible replacement needs.

The therapy prescribed for the pregnant woman with bleeding is bed rest, abstinence from coitus, and perhaps sedation. If bleeding persists and abortion is imminent or incomplete, the woman may be hospitalized, intravenous therapy or blood transfusions may be started to replace fluid, and dilation and curettage or suction evacuation is performed to remove the remainder of the products of conception. If the woman is Rh negative and not sensitized, Rh$_o$(D) immune globulin (RhoGAM) is given within 72 hours. (See discussion on Rh sensitization later in this chapter.)

In missed abortions the products of conception eventually are expelled spontaneously. If this does not occur within 1 month to 6 weeks after fetal death, hospitalization is necessary. Suction evacuation or dilation and curettage is done if the pregnancy is in the first trimester. Beyond 12 weeks' gestation, induction of labor by intravenous oxytocin and prostaglandins may be used to expel the dead fetus.

Critical Thinking Question

What questions would you ask a woman who is 8 weeks pregnant who calls to report that she is having a small amount of vaginal bleeding? What recommendations would you make to this woman?

APPLYING THE NURSING PROCESS

Nursing Assessment

The nurse assesses the amount and appearance of any vaginal bleeding and monitors the woman's vital signs and degree of discomfort. If the pregnancy is 10–12 weeks or more, fetal heart rate should be assessed by Doppler, fetoscope, or electronic fetal monitor. The nurse also assesses the responses of the woman and her family to this crisis and evaluates their coping mechanisms and ability to comfort each other.

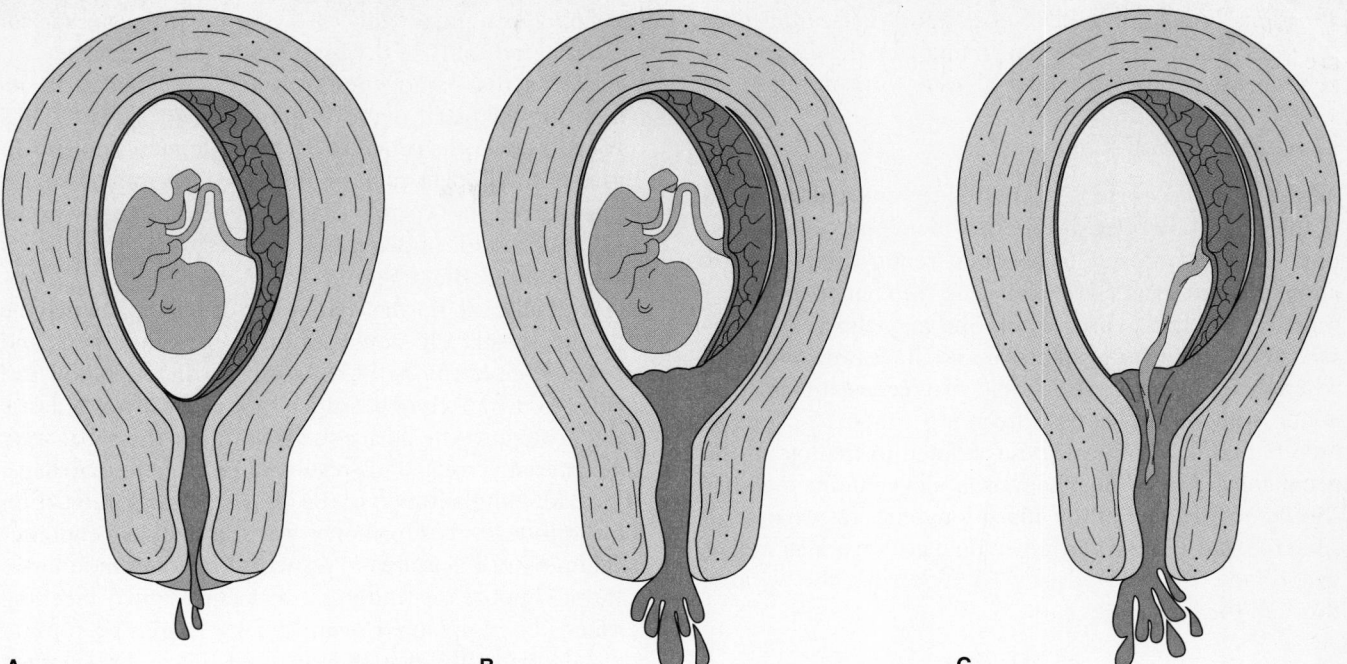

FIGURE 19-1 Types of spontaneous abortion. *A* Threatened. The cervix is not dilated, and the placenta is still attached to the uterine wall, but some bleeding occurs. *B* Imminent. The placenta has separated from the uterine wall, the cervix has dilated, and the amount of bleeding has increased. *C* Incomplete. The embryo/fetus has passed out of the uterus; however, the placenta remains.

Nursing Diagnosis

Nursing diagnoses that may apply include the following:

- Fear related to possible pregnancy loss
- Pain related to abdominal cramping secondary to threatened abortion
- Anticipatory grieving related to expected loss of unborn child

Nursing Plan and Implementation

Providing emotional support is an important task for nurses caring for women who have spontaneously aborted because the attachment process already begun is disrupted. Feelings of shock or disbelief are normal at first. Couples who approached the pregnancy with feelings of joy and a sense of expectancy now feel grief, sadness, and possibly anger.

Because many women, even with planned pregnancies, feel some ambivalence initially, guilt is a common emotion. These feelings may be even stronger for women who were negative about their pregnancies. The woman may harbor negative feelings about herself, ranging from lowered self-esteem, resulting from a belief that she is lacking or abnormal in some way, to a notion that the abortion may be a punishment for some wrongdoing.

The nurse can offer invaluable psychologic support to the woman and her family by encouraging them to verbalize their feelings, allowing them the privacy to grieve, and listening sympathetically to their concerns about this pregnancy and future ones. The nurse can aid in decreasing any feelings of guilt or blame by supplying the woman and her family with information regarding the causes of spontaneous abortion and possibly referring them to clergy or other health care professionals for additional help, such as a genetic counselor if there is a history of habitual abortions.

The grieving period following a spontaneous abortion usually lasts 6 to 24 months. Many couples can be helped during this period by an organization or support group established for parents who have lost a fetus or newborn.

We lost our baby together. I know, you could say I never really had a baby, except during those few hours when it was already over and done with, but I guess these things aren't entirely logical. I loved my baby. . . . Absorbed in pain and self-pity, still I was flooded with adoration for this tiny, not yet shaped baby who had lived in me.
~A MIDWIFE'S STORY~

The physical pain of the cramps and the amount of bleeding may be more severe than a couple anticipates, even when they are prepared for the possibility of an abortion. Nurses need to be aware that couples feel unprepared for their first experience of spontaneous abortion. Nurses should offer support in dealing with the physical experience by explaining why the discomfort is occurring and by offering analgesics for pain relief.

Teaching for Self-Care

The pregnant woman is instructed to report all episodes of bleeding to her health care provider. The woman hospitalized for spontaneous abortion requires information about possible causes of the loss and the chances of recurrence with a future pregnancy. She may also require information about the grief process so she is prepared for it when she goes home. She should also receive information about available resources, including support groups to help her cope with her feelings related to the loss of the pregnancy. The woman's partner or a family member should be included in the educational process when possible to assist him or her in personal grief work as well as to provide tools to assist in supporting the woman through the loss.

Evaluation

Anticipated outcomes of nursing care include:

- The woman is able to explain spontaneous abortion, the treatment measures employed in her care, and long-term implications for future pregnancies.

- The woman suffers no complications.

- The woman and her partner are able to begin verbalizing their grief and recognize that the grieving process usually lasts several months.

Ectopic Pregnancy

Ectopic pregnancy is an implantation of the blastocyst in a site other than the endometrial lining of the uterus. It may result from a number of different causes, including tubal damage caused by pelvic inflammatory disease; previous pelvic or tubal surgery; endometriosis; previous ectopic pregnancy; presence of an IUD; high levels of estrogen and progesterone, which can alter the motility of the egg in the fallopian tube; congenital anomalies of the tube; and blighted conceptus (Hammond & Bachus 1994).

The incidence of ectopic pregnancy has increased dramatically in the past several years. Currently there is 1 ectopic pregnancy for every 44 live births in the US (Hammond & Bachus 1994). This increased incidence may be related in part to improved diagnostic technology. Many of these early ectopic pregnancies probably went undiagnosed in the past and were reabsorbed (Pansky et al 1991). Because maternal mortality from other causes is declining, ectopic pregnancy is now the primary cause of maternal mortality in the first trimester of pregnancy.

The actual pathogenesis of ectopic pregnancy occurs when the fertilized ovum is prevented or slowed in its progress down the tube. The fertilized ovum implants in either the fallopian tube or the ovary, peritoneal cavity, cervix, or uterine cornua (Figure 19–2). The most common location for implantation of an ectopic pregnancy is the ampulla of the tube.

Initially, the normal symptoms of pregnancy may be present, specifically, amenorrhea, breast tenderness, and nausea. The hormone hCG is present in the blood and urine. With an ectopic implantation the trophoblastic cells grow into the adjacent tissue, often the tubal wall, and arterial vessels. This results in internal hemorrhage. The faulty implantation of the placenta causes fluctuation of hormone levels. Hormones first stimulate the endometrial lining of the uterus to grow, but fluctuation in levels cannot support the endometrium, and vaginal bleeding ensues. The implanted ovum quickly begins to rupture the fallopian tube if it is implanted there. The woman may experience one-sided lower abdominal pain or diffuse lower abdominal pain and vasomotor disturbances such as fainting or dizziness. About 50% of the time referred right shoulder pain occurs from blood irritating the subdiaphragmatic phrenic nerve (Hayashi & Castillo 1993).

In many instances the symptoms are not obvious. One-fourth of ectopic pregnancies may involve uterine enlargement. Physical examination usually reveals adnexal tenderness; an adnexal mass is palpable in approximately one-half of the cases.

If internal hemorrhage is profuse, the woman rapidly develops signs of hypovolemic shock. More commonly, the bleeding is slow (chronic), and the abdomen gradually becomes rigid and very tender. If bleeding into the pelvic cavity has been extensive, vaginal examination causes extreme pain, and a mass of blood may be palpated in the cul-de-sac of Douglas.

Laboratory tests may reveal low hemoglobin and hematocrit levels and rising leukocyte levels. The hCG titers are lower than in intrauterine pregnancy.

Medical Therapy

It is important to differentiate an ectopic pregnancy from other disorders with similar clinical presenting pictures. Consideration must be given to possible spontaneous abortion, ruptured corpus luteum cyst, appendicitis, salpingitis, torsion of the ovary, ovarian cysts, and urinary tract infection.

The following measures are used to establish the diagnosis of ectopic pregnancy and assess the woman's status:

- A careful assessment of menstrual history, particularly the LMP.

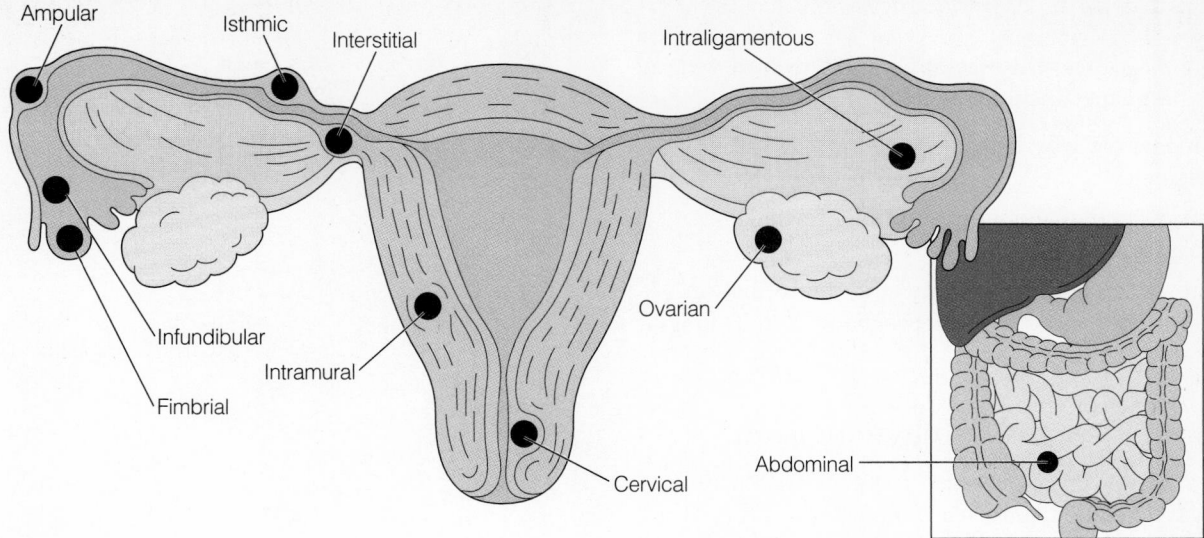

FIGURE 19-2 Various implantation sites in ectopic pregnancy. The most common site is within the fallopian tube, hence the name "tubal pregnancy."

- Careful pelvic exam to identify any abnormal pelvic masses and tenderness.

- Culdocentesis. (The woman is positioned with her legs in stirrups, and a needle is inserted through the posterior vaginal vault into the cul-de-sac of Douglas. If free-flowing blood without clots is aspirated, it is indicative of ectopic pregnancy, and prompt surgical intervention is mandatory.)

- Laparoscopy may reveal an extrauterine pregnancy and is especially helpful in diagnosing an unruptured tubal pregnancy. (If culdocentesis reveals free abdominal blood, laparoscopy is not necessary.)

- Ultrasound may be useful in identifying a gestational sac in an unruptured tubal pregnancy. (Its most common value is in confirming an intrauterine pregnancy, which usually rules out an ectopic one.)

- Laparotomy will give a confirmed diagnosis and allow opportunity for immediate treatment.

Once the diagnosis of ectopic pregnancy has been made, surgery is usually done. Excision of the affected tube is the treatment of choice to avoid recurrent ectopic pregnancy in that tube. If the woman has previously had damage to the other tube and desires future pregnancies, a linear salpingostomy will be performed to gently evacuate the ectopic pregnancy and preserve the tube. If the tube is badly damaged, a total salpingectomy is performed, leaving the ovary in place unless it is damaged. If massive infection is found, a complete removal of uterus, tubes, and ovaries may be necessary.

Intravenous therapy and blood transfusion are used to replace fluid loss. During surgery the most important risk to be considered is potential hemorrhage. Bleeding must be controlled, and replacement therapy should be on hand. The Rh-negative nonsensitized woman is given $Rh_o(D)$ immune globulin to prevent sensitization.

Recently, drug therapy to induce dissolution of the ectopic pregnancy has been attempted when the diagnosis of tubal pregnancy is made before rupture occurs (Stovall et al 1991). The drug used is usually methotrexate, a folinic acid antagonist, which acts by inhibiting cell division. The drug has the advantage over surgery of being less expensive when used on an outpatient basis. Tubal healing is improved, and there is a greater chance of maintaining fertility (Hammond & Bachus 1994). Research on this treatment option is ongoing.

APPLYING THE NURSING PROCESS

Nursing Assessment

When the woman with a suspected ectopic pregnancy is admitted to the hospital, the nurse assesses the appearance and amount of vaginal bleeding. The nurse monitors vital signs, particularly blood pressure and pulse, for evidence of developing shock.

It is also the nurse's responsibility to assess the woman's emotional status and coping abilities and to evaluate the couple's informational needs. If surgery is necessary, the nurse performs the ongoing assessments appropriate for any client postoperatively.

Nursing Diagnosis

Nursing diagnoses that may apply for a woman with an ectopic pregnancy include the following:

- Anticipatory grieving related to the loss of the pregnancy
- Pain related to abdominal bleeding secondary to tubal rupture
- Knowledge deficit related to lack of information about treatment of ectopic pregnancy and its long-term implications

Nursing Plan and Implementation

Once a diagnosis of ectopic pregnancy is made and surgery is scheduled, the nurse starts an IV as ordered and begins preoperative teaching. Signs of developing shock should be reported immediately. If the woman is experiencing severe abdominal pain, the nurse can administer appropriate analgesics and evaluate their effectiveness.

Teaching for Self-Care

Teaching is an important part of nursing care. The woman may want her condition and various procedures explained. She may need instruction regarding measures to prevent infection, symptoms to report (pain, bleeding, fever), and her follow-up visit.

The woman and her family will need emotional support during this difficult time. Their feelings and responses to this crisis will probably be similar to those that occur in cases of spontaneous abortion. As a result, similar nursing actions are required.

Evaluation

Anticipated outcomes of nursing care include:

- The woman is able to explain ectopic pregnancy, treatment alternatives, and implications for future childbearing.
- The woman and her care givers detect possible complications of therapy early and manage them successfully.
- The woman and her partner are able to begin verbalizing their loss and recognize that the grieving process usually lasts several months.

Gestational Trophoblastic Disease

Gestational trophoblastic disease (GTD) includes hydatidiform mole, invasive mole (chorioadenoma destruens), and choriocarcinoma.

Hydatidiform mole (molar pregnancy) is a disease in which (1) abnormal development of the placenta oc-

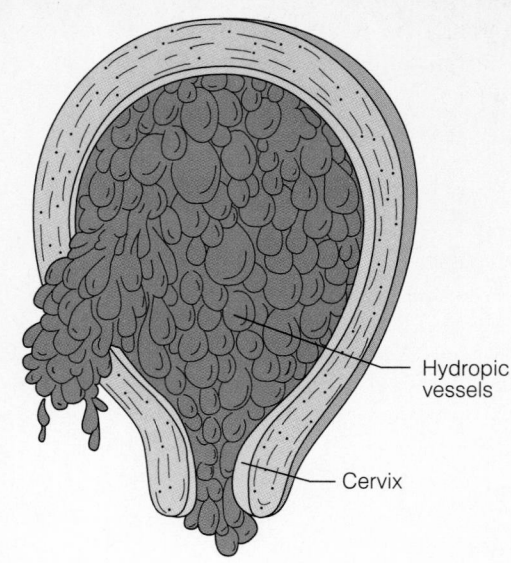

FIGURE 19-3 Hydatidiform mole. Vaginal bleeding, often brownish (the characteristic "prune juice" appearance) but sometimes bright red, is a common sign. In this figure some of the hydropic vessels are being passed. This occurrence is diagnostic for hydatidiform mole.

curs, resulting in fluid-filled, grapelike clusters (Figure 19-3), and (2) the trophoblastic tissue proliferates. The significance of this disease for the woman who has it is the loss of the pregnancy and the possibility, though remote, of developing choriocarcinoma, a form of cancer, from the trophoblastic tissue.

Molar pregnancies are classified into two types, complete and partial, both of which meet the above criteria. Little is known about the cause of either type, but some of the pathophysiology has been clarified. The *complete mole* develops from an ovum that contains no maternal genetic material, an "empty" egg. How the maternal chromosomes are lost is not known. In most cases a haploid sperm, 23X, fertilizes the egg and duplicates before the first cell division. The conceptus then contains in its cells a 46XX chromosomal set of totally paternal origin (Lawler et al 1991; Oi 1991). The embryo dies very early, when just a few millimeters long and before embryo-placental circulation has been established. Therefore the hydropic (fluid-filled) vesicles that form from the chorionic villi are avascular in the complete mole. No embryonic-fetal tissue or membranes are found. Choriocarcinoma seems to be associated primarily with the complete mole.

The *partial mole* has a triploid karyotype, ie, 69 chromosomes. Most often a normal ovum with 23 chromosomes is fertilized by two sperm (dispermy) or by a sperm that has failed to undergo the first meiosis and therefore contains 46 chromosomes. In about one-fifth of the cases the ovum did not undergo reduction division, so it contains 46 chromosomes and is fertilized by a normal sperm (Lawler et al 1991).

In partial molar pregnancy the villi are often vascularized and may be hydropic only in sections of the placenta rather than universally as with a complete mole. Often partial moles are recognized only after spontaneous abortion, or they may go unnoticed. Unlike the complete mole, the fetus usually survives to 8 or 9 weeks' gestation and occasionally longer. Twin pregnancies in which a normal fetus coexists with a molar pregnancy have been reported (Vejerslev 1991).

The incidence of GTD varies significantly worldwide. In the United States hydatidiform mole occurs in about 1 in 2000 pregnancies. In Southeast Asia and the Far East, however, the incidence may be as high as 1 in 200 pregnancies (Hayashi & Castillo 1993). The incidence of molar pregnancy increases with extremes in maternal age and has a familial tendency. The risk of repeat molar pregnancy has been reported as 0.6 to 2% of subsequent pregnancies (Vejerslev 1991).

Invasive mole (chorioadenoma destruens) is similar to a complete mole but involves the uterine myometrium. Treatment is the same as for a complete mole.

Medical Therapy

Diagnosis of hydatidiform mole is often suspected in the presence of the following signs:

- Vaginal bleeding is almost universal with molar pregnancies and may occur as early as the fourth week or as late as the second trimester. It is often brownish "like prune juice" due to liquefaction of the uterine clot, but it may be bright red.

- Anemia occurs frequently due to the loss of blood.

- Hydropic vesicles may be passed and if so are diagnostic (Figure 19–3). With a partial mole the vesicles are often smaller and may not be noticed by the woman.

- Uterine enlargement greater than expected for gestational age is a classic sign, present in about 50% of cases. In the remainder the uterus is appropriate or small for the gestational stage. Enlargement is due to the proliferating trophoblastic tissue and to a large amount of clotted blood.

- Absence of fetal heart sounds in the presence of other signs of pregnancy is a classic sign of molar pregnancy. (Only rarely has a viable fetus been born in a partial molar pregnancy.)

- Markedly elevated serum hCG may be present due to continued secretion by the proliferating trophoblastic tissue.

- Hyperemesis gravidarum may occur, probably as a result of the high levels of hCG.

- Pregnancy-induced hypertension (PIH) may be seen, especially if the molar pregnancy continues into the second trimester. Because PIH is a disease of late pregnancy, if symptoms occur in the first half of pregnancy, molar pregnancy must be considered as the first diagnosis (Vejerslev 1991).

Ultrasound is the primary means of diagnosing a molar pregnancy, usually after 6 to 8 weeks, when the vesicular enlargement of the villi can be identified.

Therapy begins with evacuation of the mole and curettage of the uterus to remove all fragments of the placenta. Early evacuation decreases the possibility of other complications. If the woman is older and has completed her childbearing, or if there is excessive bleeding, hysterectomy may be the treatment of choice to reduce the incidence of malignant sequelae.

Complications associated with hydatidiform mole that require medical recognition and therapy include the following:

- Anemia

- Hyperthyroidism

- Infection, usually seen with late diagnosis and spontaneous abortion of the mole

- Disseminated intravascular coagulation

- Trophoblastic embolization of the lung, usually seen after molar evacuation of a significantly enlarged uterus (this creates a cardiorespiratory emergency)

- Theca-lutein ovarian cysts, which may be small or large enough to displace the uterus.

Malignant GTD, usually choriocarcinoma, develops following evacuation of a mole in 20% of women. To detect this serious problem early and initiate treatment, follow-up care is essential. Follow-up consists of baseline chest x-ray exam to detect metastasis, physical examination including pelvic exam, and regular measurements of serum hCG levels. Initially, hCG levels are monitored weekly until a normal level is obtained; hCG levels are rechecked 2 to 4 weeks after the first normal level to confirm the finding; hCG levels are then monitored every 1 to 2 months for 6 to 12 more months (Hammond 1994).

Effective contraception is necessary during this time to prevent pregnancy and the resulting confusion about the cause of changes in hCG levels. In addition pregnancy could mask an hCG rise associated with malignant GTD.

Continued high or rising hCG levels in women who have had molar pregnancy but are not currently pregnant indicate malignant GTD (choriocarcinoma). Treatment at a center specializing in GTD is advised. Once pregnancy has been ruled out, full physical examination, chest x-ray exam, abdominopelvic CT scan, and brain CT scan are done to rule out metastatic spread. Chemotherapy is then begun using methotrexate alone or in combination with other chemotherapy agents.

After treatment careful follow-up monitoring of hCG levels is important. Malignant GTD is curable if diagnosed early and treated appropriately. Repeat moles range from 1 in 50 to 1 in 150. Malignant sequelae appear to be increased with repetitive moles (Oi 1991).

Nursing Assessment

It is important for nurses involved in antepartal care to be aware of symptoms of hydatidiform mole and observe for these at each antepartal visit. The classic symptoms used to diagnose molar pregnancy are found more frequently with the complete than with the partial mole. The partial mole may be difficult to distinguish from a missed abortion prior to evacuation.

When the woman is hospitalized for evacuation of the mole, the nurse should monitor vital signs and vaginal bleeding for evidence of hemorrhage. In addition the nurse determines whether abdominal pain is present and assesses the woman's emotional state and coping ability.

Nursing Diagnosis

Nursing diagnoses that may apply to a woman with a hydatidiform mole include the following:

- Fear related to the possible development of choriocarcinoma
- Knowledge deficit related to a lack of understanding of the need for regular monitoring of hCG levels
- Anticipatory grieving related to the loss of the pregnancy

Nursing Plan and Implementation

When molar pregnancy is suspected, the woman needs emotional support. The nurse can relieve some of the woman's anxiety by answering questions about the disease process and explaining what ultrasound and other diagnostic procedures will entail. If a molar pregnancy is diagnosed, the nurse supports the childbearing family as they deal with their grief about the lost pregnancy. Health care counselors, the hospital chaplain, or their own clergy may be of assistance in helping them deal with this loss.

When the woman is hospitalized for evacuation of the mole, explanation of the curettage procedure is necessary. Although the physician is responsible for providing this explanation, the woman and her partner may have many questions and concerns that the nurse can discuss with them. The nurse may also clarify areas of confusion or misunderstanding.

Typed and cross-matched blood must be available for surgery because of previous blood loss and the potential for hemorrhage. Oxytocin is administered to keep the uterus contracted and prevent hemorrhage. Prolonged therapy with oxytocin may result in water intoxication because of its slight antidiuretic effect (McKenry & Salerno 1992). In addition, acute renal failure, a syndrome of rapid onset, may occur when significant hemorrhage results in absolute loss of fluid volume (Kristensen 1991). Following surgery, the nurse carefully observes the woman's urinary output, watches for further signs of bleeding, and assesses for any signs of infection.

If the woman is Rh negative and not sensitized, she is given $Rh_o(D)$ immune globulin to prevent antibody formation. (See discussion on Rh sensitization later in this chapter.)

The woman needs to know the importance of the follow-up visits. She is advised to use contraception to delay becoming pregnant again until after the follow-up program is completed.

Evaluation

Anticipated outcomes of nursing care include:

- The woman has a smooth recovery following successful evacuation of the mole.
- The woman is able to explain GTD, its treatment, follow-up, and long-term implications for pregnancy.
- The woman and her partner are able to begin verbalizing their grief at the loss of their anticipated child.
- The woman understands the importance of follow-up assessment and indicates her willingness to cooperate with the regimen.

Placenta Previa

In placenta previa the placenta is improperly implanted in the lower uterine segment, sometimes over the internal os. As the lower uterine segment contracts and the cervix dilates in the later weeks of pregnancy, the placental villi are torn from the uterine wall, thus exposing the uterine sinuses at the placental site. Bleeding begins, but because its amount depends on the number of sinuses exposed, it may initially be either scanty or profuse. The classic symptom is painless vaginal bleeding usually occurring after 20 weeks' gestation. See Chapter 25 for an in-depth discussion of placenta previa.

Abruptio Placentae

Abruptio placentae is the premature separation of the placenta from the uterine wall. It occurs prior to birth, usually during the labor process. See Chapter 25 for an in-depth description of abruptio placentae.

CARE OF THE WOMAN WITH AN INCOMPETENT CERVIX

Incompetent cervix refers to the premature dilatation of the cervix, usually about the fourth or fifth month of pregnancy and is associated with repeated second trimester spontaneous abortion. It occurs in about 0.5% to 1.0% of pregnancies and is responsible for 15% to 20% of second trimester pregnancy losses (Heppard & Garite 1992). Congenital causes include cervical structural defects, uterine anomalies, and abnormal cervical development due to maternal exposure to diethylstilbestrol (DES). Acquired defects include previous traumatic birth or trauma to the cervix during D & C (dilatation and curettage), cervical conization, or cauterization.

A positive history of repeated, painless, and bloodless second trimester abortion is significant. Serial pelvic examinations early in the second trimester reveal progressive effacement and dilatation of the cervix and bulging of the membranes through the os with a characteristic hourglass appearance. Uterine contractions are usually absent until late in the process (Heppard & Garite 1992). If incompetent cervix is suspected, serial ultrasound provides information on dilatation of the internal cervical os before a dilated external os is detected (Niebyl 1990).

Incompetent cervix has been managed by a variety of surgical, mechanical, and medical methods. The treatment most commonly used is the Shirodkar-Barter operation (cerclage), or a modification of it by McDonald, which reinforces the weakened cervix by encircling it at the level of the internal os with suture material. If a woman has a history of cervical incompetence, a cerclage (purse-string suture) is placed in the cervix between 14 and 18 weeks' gestation. When cervical incompetence is diagnosed during the current pregnancy, the woman is placed in trendelenburg position to reduce pressure on the cervix and allow for the recession of the amniotic sac (bag of waters) back into the uterine cavity in situations where it has begun to prolapse. Cervical cultures for gonorrhea and vaginal cultures for group B strep should be obtained before the placement of a cerclage. The success of the procedure dramatically decreases if performed after 20 weeks' gestation.

The procedure should not be done if any of the following conditions exist: The diagnosis is in doubt, known fetal malformation exists, the fetus has died, amniotic membranes are ruptured, vaginal bleeding or hyperirritability of the uterus exists, or the cervix is dilated beyond 4 cm. Once the suture is in place, a cesarean birth may be planned (to prevent repeating the procedure in subsequent pregnancies), or the suture may be cut with sterile scissors at term (after 37 complete weeks' gestation) and vaginal birth permitted. The woman must understand the importance of contacting her physician immediately if her membranes rupture or labor begins. The physician can remove the suture to prevent possible complications. The success rate for carrying the pregnancy to term is 80% to 90% (Scott 1994a).

CARE OF THE WOMAN WITH PREMATURE RUPTURE OF MEMBRANES

Controversy surrounds the definition of **premature rupture of membranes (PROM).** Some authorities define PROM as the spontaneous rupture of the bag of waters any time before the onset of labor; others require that a specific period elapse without labor, generally between 1 and 12 hours. Preterm PROM has been described as rupture before 36 weeks' gestation. Prolonged rupture of the membranes is rupture more than 24 hours before birth (Heppard & Garite 1992; Kappy et al 1993).

Although the cause of PROM is unknown, a variety of factors are correlated with its occurrence. An incompetent cervix may be the cause of second trimester PROM. Cervicitis, UTI, amniocentesis, placenta previa, abruptio placentae, hydramnios, trauma, multiple pregnancy, and maternal genital tract anomalies may also result in PROM. Studies suggest that in a substantial number of cases, premature rupture of the membranes may be the result of subclinical intrauterine infection or inflammation of the chorioamnion (Romero & Ghidini 1993).

PROM occurs in 8.1% to 18.5% of all births, with a significantly higher incidence associated with preterm births. In 90% of women at term the onset of regular uterine contractions occurs within 24 hours after membranes rupture (Heppard & Garite 1992).

Maternal Risks

Maternal risk is related to infection, specifically chorioamnionitis (intra-amniotic infection resulting from bacterial invasion and inflammation of the membranes before birth) and endometritis (infection of the endometrium postpartally that may be related to chorioamnionitis or may occur independently) (Garite & Spellacy 1994).

Fetal-Neonatal Risks

The most common neonatal complication in pregnancies involving PROM before 37 weeks' gestation is respiratory distress syndrome (RDS) (see Chapter 32), which occurs in 10% to 40% of newborns. Infection is documented in less than 10% of newborns. The preterm fetus is further jeopardized by the associated risks of malpresentation (especially breech) and prolapse of the umbilical cord (see Chapter 25). Perinatal mortality largely depends on gestational age (Kappy et al 1993).

Some research has suggested that a latent period following preterm rupture of the membranes may stimulate pulmonary maturation in the preterm infant and thereby reduce the rate of RDS. The stress of PROM acts as a fetal stimulus for the release of naturally occurring steroid, which in turn accelerates lung maturation. In contrast other reports have noted no significant effect on the preterm newborn (Hallak & Bottoms 1993; Kappy et al 1993).

Umbilical cord compression may occur related to decreased amniotic fluid volume and may result in fetal asphyxia and, in severe cases, death. When membranes rupture very early in gestation, marked oligohydramnios may result in intrauterine growth retardation, hypoplastic lungs, and limb deformities due to compression (Heppard & Garite 1992).

Medical Therapy

A sterile speculum exam is done to identify ruptured membranes. After confirming with nitrazine paper and a microscopic examination (ferning test) that the membranes have ruptured (Chapter 22), the gestational age of the fetus is calculated. Single or combination methods of calculation may be used, including Nagele's rule, early physical exam with uterine size consistent with LMP, early positive pregnancy test, fundal height, ultrasound to measure the fetal biparietal diameter, and amniocentesis to identify lung maturity (Chapter 20). The gestational age of the fetus and the presence or absence of infection determine the medical treatment for PROM (Table 19–1). If the fetus is preterm or if infection is present, more drastic medical therapy is necessary to prevent complications.

If maternal signs and symptoms of infection are evident, antibiotic therapy (usually intravenous) is begun immediately, and the fetus is born vaginally or by cesarean, regardless of the gestational age. Upon admission to the nursery the newborn is assessed for sepsis and started on antibiotics. Chapter 32 provides further information about the newborn with sepsis.

TABLE 19-1	Currently Used Plans for Women with Premature Rupture of Membranes

Preterm

Expectant management (observation); birth when labor or clinical infection develops

Fetal pulmonary status determined by amniotic fluid testing; birth if fetus is mature

Risk of infection determined by amniotic fluid Gram stain, white cell count, glucose and culture; maternal white cell count and C-reactive protein, assessment for maternal fever or uterine tenderness; assessment for fetal well-being through electronic fetal monitoring or ultrasound for biophysical profile scoring; birth if infection develops

Administration of corticosteroids, with or without birth in 48 hours after first dose; tocolytics as needed

Birth after an arbitrary latent period (eg, 16–72 hours)

Assess for group B streptococci (or *Neisseria gonorrhoeae*); treatment indicated if positive

Combinations of the above

Term

Induction if spontaneous labor does not begin in approximately 12 hours, or if cervix is ripe, or if there are other complications (eg, PIH)

Expectant management for women with uncomplicated pregnancies and cervix unfavorable for induction

Management of PROM in the absence of infection and gestation of less than 37 weeks is usually conservative. The woman is hospitalized on bed rest. An admission CBC, C-reactive protein (CRP), and urinalysis are obtained. Continuous electronic fetal monitoring may be ordered at the beginning of treatment but usually is discontinued after a few hours unless the fetus is estimated to be very low birth weight (VLBW). Regular nonstress tests (NSTs) and biophysical profiles are used to monitor fetal well-being until labor begins or cesarean birth becomes necessary (Kappy et al 1993). Maternal blood pressure, pulse, and temperature and FHR are assessed every 4 hours. A WBC and a CRP are ordered daily. Vaginal exams are avoided to decrease the chance of infection. As the gestation approaches 34 weeks, an amniocentesis may be done weekly to evaluate lecithin/sphingomyelin (L/S ratio) and phosphotidylglycerol (PG) (see Chapter 20). After initial treatment and observation, if leaking of fluid ceases, some women may be followed at home. The woman is advised to continue bed rest (with bathroom privileges), monitor her temperature four times a day, and avoid intercourse, douches, and tampons. The woman is advised to contact her physician and return to the hospital if she has fever, uterine tenderness and/or contractions, increased leakage of fluid, decreased fetal movement, or a foul vaginal discharge. Weekly NSTs should be continued (Kappy et al 1993).

Opinions of the value of administering glucocorticoids (betamethasone or dexamethasone) prophylactically for PROM are sharply divided (Garite & Spellacy

BETAMETHASONE (CELESTONE SOLUPAN)

Overview of Maternal-Fetal Action

Studies have provided ample evidence that glucocorticoids such as betamethasone are capable of inducing pulmonary maturation and decreasing the incidence of respiratory distress syndrome in preterm infants. The mechanism by which corticosteroids accelerate fetal lung maturity is unclear, but it is related to the stimulation of enzyme activity by the drug. The enzyme is required for biosynthesis of surfactant by the type II pneumocytes. Surfactant is of major importance to the proper functioning of the lung in that it decreases the surface tension of the alveoli. Glucocorticoids also increase the rate of glycogen depletion, which leads to thinning of the interalveolar septa and increases the size of the alveoli. The thinning of the epithelium brings the capillaries into closer proximity with the air spaces and improves oxygen exchange (Blackburn & Loper 1992). Black female newborns have shown the largest decrease in respiratory distress syndrome after this therapy; White males have been much less responsive (Williams 1991a). Only firstborn twin appears to benefit from antenatal steroid therapy (Briggs et al 1994).

Route, Dosage, Frequency

Prenatal maternal intramuscular injections of 12 mg of betamethasone are given once a day for 2 days. Dexamethasone may also be given in doses of 6 mg every 12 hours for four doses (NIH Development Conference 1994). To obtain maximum results, birth should be delayed for at least 24 hours after completing the first round of treatment. The effect of corticosteroids may be transient. Currently, it is suggested that the treatment regimen be repeated every week up to 34 weeks' gestation for the undelivered fetus with an immature lung profile.

Contraindications

Inability to delay birth for 24 to 48 hours
Adequate L/S ratio
Presence of a condition that necessitates immediate birth (eg, maternal bleeding)
Presence of maternal infection, diabetes mellitus, hypertension
Gestational age greater than 34 completed weeks

Maternal Side Effects

Bishop (1981) reports that suspected maternal risks include (1) initiation of lactation; (2) increased risk of infection; (3) augmentation of placental insufficiency in hypertensive women; (4) gastrointestinal bleeding; (5) inability to use estriol levels to assess fetal status; (6) possible pulmonary edema when used concurrently with tocolytics (such as ritodrine)
May cause Na^+ retention, K^+ loss, weight gain, edema, indigestion
Increased risk of infection if PROM present (Briggs et al 1994)
May mask signs and symptoms of infection

Effects on Fetus/Neonate

Lowered cortisol levels at birth, but rebound occurs by 2 hours of age (Briggs et al 1994)
Hypoglycemia
Increased risk of neonatal sepsis (Briggs et al 1994)
Animal studies have shown serious fetal side effects such as reduced head circumference, reduced weight of the fetal adrenal and thymus glands, and decreased placental weight (Briggs et al 1994). Human studies have not shown these effects, however.

Nursing Considerations

Assess for presence of contraindications.
Provide education regarding possible side effects.
Administer betamethasone deep into gluteal muscle, avoiding injection into deltoid (high incidence of local atrophy). (Dexamethasone may be administered I/M or I/V.)
Periodically evaluate BP, pulse, weight, and edema.
Assess lab data for electrolytes and blood glucose.
Although concomitant use of betamethasone and tocolytic agents has been implicated in increased risk of pulmonary edema, the betamethasone has little mineral corticoid activity; therefore it probably doesn't add significantly to the salt and water retention effects of beta-adrenergic agonists. Other causes of noncardiogenic pulmonary edema should also be investigated if pulmonary edema develops during administration of betamethasone to a woman in preterm labor.

1994; Williams 1991a). When gestation is between 34 and 36 weeks, medical practice has been to delay birth for 24 hours after PROM to allow natural elevation of maternal-fetal blood glucocorticoids, thereby contributing to fetal lung maturity. If gestation is between 28 and 32 weeks and labor can be delayed for 24 to 48 hours, betamethasone (Celestone) is frequently given. Glucocorticoids are not administered in the presence of uterine infection. (See Drug Guide: Betamethasone.) Some studies of the use of glucocorticoids with preterm PROM have not shown a reduction in the rate or severity of neonatal RDS in treated women. Meta-analysis of all research suggests that there is a modest decrease in RDS when corticosteroids are given and a slightly increased risk of maternal infection (Garite & Spellacy 1994). Prophylactic antibiotic therapy may decrease the likelihood of chorioamnionitis in PROM, particularly with colonization of group B streptococci (Williams 1991a).

Nursing Assessment

Determining the duration of the rupture of membranes is a significant component of the antepartal assessment. The nurse asks the woman when her membranes ruptured and when contractions began because the risk of infection may be directly related to the time involved. Gestational age is determined to prepare for the possibility of a preterm birth. The nurse observes the mother for signs and symptoms of infection, especially by reviewing her WBC, CRP, temperature, and pulse rate and the character of her amniotic fluid. If the mother has a fever, hydration status should be checked. Fetal heart rate tracings should be watched for tachycardia, loss of variability, and/or decelerations. When a preterm or cesarean birth is anticipated, the nurse evaluates the childbirth preparation and coping abilities of the woman and her partner.

Nursing Diagnosis

Nursing diagnoses that may be used with PROM include the following:

- Risk for infection related to premature rupture of membranes
- Impaired gas exchange in the fetus related to compression of the umbilical cord secondary to prolapse of the cord
- Risk for ineffective individual coping related to unknown outcome of the pregnancy

Nursing Plan and Implementation

Nursing actions should focus on the woman, her partner, and the fetus. Uterine activity and fetal response to the labor are evaluated, but vaginal exams are not done unless absolutely necessary. The woman is encouraged to rest on her right or left side to promote optimal uteroplacental perfusion. Comfort measures may help promote rest and relaxation. The nurse must also ensure that hydration is maintained, particularly if the woman's temperature is elevated.

Teaching for Self-Care

Education is another important aspect of nursing care. The couple needs to understand the implications of PROM and all treatment methods. It is important to address side effects and alternative treatments. The couple needs to know that although the membranes are ruptured, amniotic fluid continues to be produced.

Providing psychologic support for the couple is critical. The nurse may reduce anxiety by listening empathetically, relaying accurate information, and providing explanations of procedures. It may be necessary to prepare the couple for a cesarean birth, a preterm newborn, and the possibility of fetal or neonatal demise.

Evaluation

Anticipated outcomes of nursing care include:

- The woman's risk of infection and cord prolapse are decreased.
- The couple is able to discuss the implications of PROM and all treatment options.
- The pregnancy is maintained without trauma to the mother or the fetus.

CARE OF THE WOMAN AT RISK DUE TO PRETERM LABOR

Labor that occurs between 20 and 37 completed weeks of pregnancy is referred to as **preterm labor.** Prematurity continues to be the number one perinatal and neonatal problem in the United States today—it is estimated that 7%–10% of all live births occur prematurely (Parsons & Spellacy 1994). The causes may be maternal, fetal, or placental factors. Maternal factors include cardiovascular or renal disease, diabetes, PIH, abdominal surgery during pregnancy, a blow to the abdomen, uterine anomalies, cervical incompetence, DES exposure, history of cone biopsy, and maternal infection. Fetal factors include multiple pregnancy, hydramnios, and fetal infection. Placental factors include placenta previa and abruptio placentae (Lipshitz et al 1993).

A correlation exists between preterm birth and low socioeconomic status, a history of preterm births, poor antenatal care, and maternal smoking (especially more than one pack per day) (Lipshitz et al 1993).

Risk-scoring tools help identify a large proportion of pregnant women who are at risk for preterm birth. Table 19–2 presents a list of risk factors for spontaneous preterm birth. It is important to reassess the risks and observe cervical changes as the pregnancy progresses.

Maternal Risks

The major risks for the woman involve psychologic stress factors related to her concern for her unborn child. Physiologic maternal risks are related to possible medical treatments for preterm labor such as tocolysis and prolonged bed rest or are related to the cause of preterm labor such as hemorrhage from placental abruption or placenta previa.

TABLE 19-2 Risk Factors for Spontaneous Preterm Labor

Multiple gestation	Previous preterm birth
DES exposure	Previous preterm labor with a term birth
Known cervical incompetence	Abdominal surgery during pregnancy
Hydramnios	History of cone biopsy
Uterine anomaly	Cervical shortening < 1 cm at 32 weeks
Cervix dilated > 1 cm at 32 weeks	Uterine irritability
Second trimester abortion ×2	Age (<19 or >40)
Fetal abnormality	Low socioeconomic status
Febrile illness	Cigarettes—more than 10/day
Bleeding after 12 weeks	Substance abuse
History of pyelonephritis or other maternal infection	Second trimester abortion ×1
	Poor weight gain
Maternal medical disease	More than 2 first trimester abortions

Tocolysis is the use of therapeutic interventions in an attempt to stop labor; tocolytic agents are drugs used to stop labor.

Fetal-Neonatal Risks

Mortality increases for neonates born before 37 weeks' gestation. Although the preterm infant is faced with many maturational deficiencies (fat storage, heat regulation, immaturity of organ systems), the most critical factor is the lack of development of the respiratory system—to the extent that life cannot be supported. In some instances, such as severe maternal diabetes or serious isoimmunization, continuation of the pregnancy may be more life-threatening to the fetus than the hazards of prematurity. See Chapter 32 for in-depth consideration of the preterm newborn.

Medical Therapy

The goal of medical therapy is to prevent preterm labor from advancing to a point that no longer responds to medical treatment. If the cervix is dilated more than 3 to 4 cm and more than 50% effaced, the effects of tocolytics on labor is reduced. If labor cannot be arrested, the priority becomes successful preterm birth and management of its psychologic effect on the woman and her partner.

Due to the often subtle symptoms of preterm labor, the mother who is at risk for preterm labor may benefit from participating in a preterm birth prevention program. These programs, which have become increasingly popular, generally focus on three areas: (1) early identification of women at high risk for preterm birth, (2) education of these women about the often subtle signs and symptoms of preterm labor, and (3) appropriate and effective management by health care providers during prenatal visits and in the event that preterm labor occurs.

RESEARCH IN PRACTICE

Preterm labor, which affects 8% to 10% of all pregnancies, often results in activity restriction for the woman. Although in some cases the woman is hospitalized, often the activity restriction occurs at home. Katharyn May explored the impact of maternal activity restriction on the expectant father.

The final study sample consisted of two groups of 15 men whose partners experienced activity restriction during pregnancy. In one group the fathers were interviewed, with their partners present, twice during the pregnancy and once after birth. The second group of men had partners who had experienced an activity-restricted pregnancy in the previous 2 years. These 15 couples participated in focus group interviews during which the men and the women were separated.

Preliminary analysis of the interviews revealed five major themes for these fathers. In the first theme, fathers identified that they and their partners complied with the prescribed medical regimen but received little help from their health care providers. Second, participants expressed a sense of isolation, and they did not discuss the problem with co-workers or any other fathers who had a similar experience. Third, the theme of shock and worry occurred for the men because the development of a high-risk pregnancy did not comply with their expectations of a normal pregnancy. Also, the fathers reported a sense of constant worry about their partners, financial matters, or adequate child care. In the fourth theme, fathers described the stress of "having to do it all" including household chores, child care, work, and finding time to spend with their partners. The fifth theme encompassed maintenance of the relationship, which many expectant fathers found challenging. The fathers voiced understanding about the emotional irritability and lability of their partners and tended to respond with a mixture of exasperation and sympathy. The researcher noted findings of significant family stress in at least four of the households. However, results of the focus group suggested that long-term consequences of activity restriction during pregnancy are limited.

Clinical Application of the Study

Nurses in contact with expectant families in which the mother must undergo activity restriction need to encourage the father to express his worries and help him anticipate solutions to potential problems. Also the nurse needs to help him find some social support to alleviate the sense of isolation.

SOURCE: May K: Impact of maternal activity restriction for preterm labor on the expectant father. *JOGNN* 1994; 23(3):246.

If preterm labor is suspected, the diagnosis should be confirmed before therapy is begun. Common criteria used for diagnosis are found in Table 19–3. Any medical condition that may contribute to preterm labor should also be treated, and maternal or fetal contraindications to inhibiting labor should be identified.

TABLE 19-3	Criteria for Diagnosis of Preterm Labor

Gestation 20–37 weeks

and

Documented uterine contractions
(4/20 minute, 8/60 minute)

and

Ruptured membranes	*or*	Intact membranes
		and
		Documented cervical change
		or
		Cervical effacement of 80%
		or
		Cervical dilatation 2 cm

SOURCE: Creasy RK, Resnik R: *Maternal-Fetal Medicine*, 2nd ed. Philadelphia: WB Saunders, 1989, table 33–9, p 448.

The ACOG technical bulletin (1989) specifies the following contraindications to interrupting labor: severe PIH, eclampsia (convulsions), maternal hemodynamic instability, fetal anomalies incompatible with life, chorioamnionitis, hemorrhage, fetal maturity, fetal death, severe abruptio placentae, severe fetal growth retardation, or acute fetal distress.

Drugs currently used for tocolysis include beta-adrenergic agonists (also called β-mimetics), magnesium sulfate ($MgSO_4$), prostaglandin synthetase inhibitors, and calcium channel blockers. The β-mimetics (ritodrine [Yutopar] and terbutaline sulfate [Brethine]) and magnesium sulfate are the most widely used tocolytics. Although ritodrine is FDA approved for use in preterm labor, it is much less frequently employed than terbutaline, which is not FDA approved for this use. Terbutaline is preferred for treating preterm labor because it is effective and significantly less expensive than ritodrine (Narrigan 1993).

Although tocolytic drugs do suppress contractions and allow prolongation of pregnancy, the β-mimetics, $MgSO_4$, and prostaglandin synthetase inhibitors may cause significant side effects, the most serious of which is maternal pulmonary edema. Reducing the dose and duration of therapy sometimes decreases side effects (Lipshitz et al 1993).

Currently, preterm labor is treated with IV tocolytics, typically terbutaline or magnesium sulfate. Beta-adrenergic agonists and magnesium sulfate are comparable in their efficacy in stopping preterm labor. Initial therapy with $MgSO_4$ is indicated in women with cardiopulmonary disease, diabetes, or infection; in all other cases the selection of $MgSO_4$ or β-mimetics depends on the experience of the health care providers (Parsons & Spellacy 1994). Once uterine activity is stopped, the woman is placed on oral tocolysis or subcutaneous terbu-

taline via infusion pump for long-term maintenance (Figure 19–4).

Although preventing preterm labor is the primary goal of tocolysis, delaying birth can significantly reduce neonatal morbidity and mortality by providing time for fetal therapy and transfer to a tertiary care center if necessary. The ACOG Committee on Obstetric Practice (1994) recommends that corticosteroids (typically betamethasone or dexamethasone) be administered antenatally to women at risk of preterm birth because of their beneficial effect on fetal lung maturation. Any women who are candidates for tocolysis are candidates for antenatal corticosteroids, regardless of fetal gender, race, or availability of surfactant therapy for the newborn, especially between 24 and 34 weeks' gestation (ACOG 1994). Thyroid stimulators such as thyrotropin-releasing hormone (TRH) increase fetal thyroid function and thereby accelerate fetal lung maturation. They are often used in conjunction with glucocorticoids to reduce the incidence or severity of respiratory distress syndrome in the newborn (Parsons & Spellacy 1994).

Magnesium sulfate, long used in the treatment of PIH, has been gaining favor in the treatment of preterm labor because it is effective and has fewer side effects than beta-adrenergic agonists. The usual recommended loading dose is 4 to 6 g IV over 20 minutes. The constant dose is then 2 to 3 g/hour titrated to deep tendon reflexes and serum magnesium levels. The therapy is maintained for 12 to 24 hours at the lowest rate to maintain cessation of contractions. The maternal serum level that is important for tocolysis seems to be 5 to 8 mg/dL (Heppard & Garite 1992).

Side effects with the loading dose may include flushing, a feeling of warmth, headache, nystagmus, nausea, and dizziness. Other side effects include lethargy and sluggishness and a 2% risk of pulmonary edema if the woman has predisposing conditions such as multiple gestation, infection, or hydramnios. See Drug Guide: Magnesium Sulfate on page 490 for other side effects. Fetal side effects may include hypotonia and lethargy that persist for 1 or 2 days following birth (Lipshitz et al 1993).

In comparison with IV ritodrine, magnesium sulfate has less effect on systolic or diastolic blood pressure (mean blood pressure and uteroplacental perfusion are maintained), no alteration of maternal heart rate (though it may cause a slight decrease in the fetal heart rate), no effect on cardiac output, and only a slight increase in placental blood flow.

Long-term oral therapy may be accomplished with magnesium gluconate. The therapeutic dose is usually 1 g every 2–4 hours. This dose may be as effective as oral beta-agonists in preventing uterine contractions (Heppard & Garite 1992). In a study by Martin and Morrison (1987) the mean serum level of magnesium gluconate when 1 g was administered orally every 4 hours was 2.16 mg/dL. This is well below the current therapeutic clinical levels of magnesium that have been used in treating women ported. Because of the possibility of serious fetal side effects, indomethacin is not used after 34 weeks' gestation and is limited to a 48-hour course of therapy (Heppard & Garite 1992; Lipshitz et al 1993).

Home Care

In recent years programs have evolved involving home monitoring of uterine activity combined with daily contact between the woman and a nurse. The monitor consists of a contraction sensor belt the woman wears around her abdomen. A small electronic recorder worn at the waist collects and transmits uterine activity data via the telephone to be interpreted by a nurse at a receiving center. The woman also receives in-depth education about the signs and symptoms of preterm labor and how to palpate for contractions. These programs are intended for use by women at high risk for preterm labor or by those treated for preterm labor and discharged from inpatient care.

Although the combination of the electronic monitor and nursing care seems to be effective, it is not clear at this point whether the value lies in the electronic monitor or in the education and follow-up by a nurse. Research has demonstrated that women who receive intensive education and daily nursing contact alone experience no difference in incidence of preterm birth compared with a group that had electronic home monitoring of contractions in addition to the same education and nursing contact. Based on this information, the American College of Obstetricians and Gynecologists does not currently recommend the routine clinical use of the electronic uterine activity monitor at home (Merkatz & Merkatz 1991). In spite of this controversy, home uterine activity monitoring continues to be widely used.

After stabilization following treatment for preterm labor, many women require long-term oral tocolysis. It has been reported that half of these women will "break through," that is, have a recurrence of uterine activity (Lam 1989). It is suspected that sensitivity to beta-adrenergic agonists is lost over time. In 1988 Lam and others presented the continuous terbutaline infusion pump as an alternative to women who broke through oral therapy or who were unable to tolerate its side effects. The infusion pump, which has been used for continuous insulin infusion in diabetics, delivers low doses of terbutaline (basal rate) as well as intermittent boluses to coincide with predetermined peak periods of uterine contractility. The advantages of this regime seem to be an overall lower daily dose of terbutaline, which reduces drug desensitization, and reduced maternal side effects. The combined use of the terbutaline pump and home uterine activity monitoring has allowed some women who might otherwise require prolonged hospitalization to be managed at home.

Pump therapy is initiated in the hospital following treatment of preterm labor with intravenous tocolytics. The woman remains in the hospital anywhere from 1 to 3

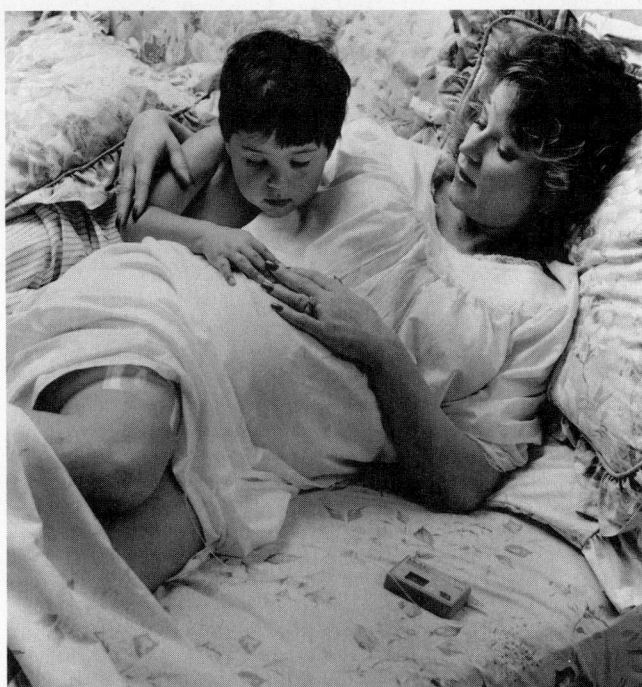

FIGURE 19-4 A pregnant woman who experienced an episode of preterm labor and remains at risk uses a subcutaneous terbutaline pump at home. (Note that the woman is lying on her left side to promote optimal placental perfusion.) (Courtesy Tokos Medical Corporation)

with preeclampsia and eclampsia. Therefore adequate serum levels for treating preterm labor may not necessarily be as high as those needed to treat preeclampsia.

Recently, calcium channel blockers have been used to inhibit preterm labor. Of the calcium channel blockers approved for use in the United States, nifedipine appears to have the most clinical promise as a tocolytic. The mechanism of action is to blockade the slow calcium channels at the cell surface and inhibit contractile activity. Nifedipine is well absorbed either orally or sublingually. The most common side effects are related to arterial vasodilation, that is, hypotension, tachycardia, facial flushing, and headache. Because the mechanism of action of nifedipine is different from the beta-adrenergic drugs, co-administration of nifedipine and terbutaline or ritodrine may prove beneficial in the treatment of preterm labor. Because both magnesium sulfate and nifedipine block calcium, however, co-administration of them has been implicated in serious maternal side effects related to low calcium levels.

In some centers prostaglandin synthetase inhibitors (PSI) such as indomethacin (Indocin) are being investigated and used in selected instances. However, potential fetal side effects, such as premature closure of the ductus arteriosus and decreased fetal urine output, have been re-

MAGNESIUM SULFATE (MgSO₄)

Pregnancy Risk Category: B

Overview of Obstetric Action

MgSO₄ acts as a CNS depressant by decreasing the quantity of acetylcholine released by motor nerve impulses and thereby blocking neuromuscular transmission. This action reduces the possibility of convulsion, which is why MgSO₄ is used in the treatment of preeclampsia. Because magnesium sulfate secondarily relaxes smooth muscle, it may decrease the blood pressure, although it is not considered an antihypertensive. MgSO₄ may also decrease the frequency and intensity of uterine contractions; as a result it is also used as a tocolytic in the treatment of preterm labor.

Route, Dosage, Frequency

MgSO₄ is generally given intravenously to control dosage more accurately and prevent overdosage. An occasional physician still prescribes intramuscular administration. However, it is painful and irritating to the tissues and does not permit the close control that IV administration does. The intravenous route allows for immediate onset of action. It must be given by infusion pump for accurate dosage.

For Treatment of Preterm Labor

Loading dose: 6 g MgSO₄ in 250 mL solution administered over a 30 minute period (Parsons & Spellacy 1994).
Maintenance dose: 2–4 g/hour via infusion pump (Parsons & Spellacy 1994).

For Treatment of Preeclampsia

Loading dose: 4–6 g MgSO₄ as a 20% solution is administered over a 15–20 minute period (Arias 1993).
Maintenance dose: 1–2 g/hour via infusion pump (Mandeville & Troiano 1992).
Note: MgSO₄ is excreted via the kidneys. Because women in preterm labor typically have normal renal function, they generally require higher levels of magnesium to achieve a therapeutic range that women who have preeclampsia and may have compromised renal function (Parsons & Spellacy 1994).

Maternal Contraindications

Diagnosed maternal myasthenia gravis is the only absolute contraindication to the administration of MgSO₄ (Mandeville & Troiano 1992). A history of myocardial damage or heart block is a relative contraindication to use of the drug because of the effects on nerve transmission and muscle contractility. Extreme care is necessary in administration to women with impaired renal function because the drug is eliminated by the kidneys, and toxic magnesium levels may develop quickly.

Maternal Side Effects

Most maternal side effects are dose related. Lethargy and weakness related to neuromuscular blockade are common. Sweating, a feeling of warmth, flushing, and nasal congestion may be related to peripheral vasodilation. Other common side effects include nausea and vomiting, constipation, visual blurring, headache, and slurred speech. Signs of developing toxicity include depression or absence of reflexes, oliguria, confusion, respiratory depression, circulatory collapse, and respiratory paralysis. Rapid administration of large doses may cause cardiac arrest.

Effects on Fetus/Neonate

The drug readily crosses the placenta. Some authorities suggest that transient decrease in FHR variability may occur; others report that no change occurred. In general MgSO₄ therapy does not pose a risk to the fetus. Occasionally, the newborn may demonstrate neurologic depression or respiratory depression, loss of reflexes, and muscle weakness (Briggs et al 1994). Ill effects in the newborn may actually be related to fetal growth retardation, prematurity, or perinatal asphyxia (Knuppel & Drukker 1993).

Nursing Considerations

1. Monitor the blood pressure closely during administration.

2. Monitor maternal serum magnesium levels as ordered (usually every 6–8 hours). Therapeutic levels are in the range of 4–8 mg/dL. Reflexes often disappear at serum magnesium levels of 8–10 mg/dL; respiratory depression occurs at levels of 10–15 mg/dL; cardiac conduction problems occur at levels above 15 mg/dL (Scott 1994b).

3. Monitor respirations closely. If the rate is less than 12/minute, magnesium toxicity may be developing, and further assessments are indicated. Many protocols require stopping the medication if the respiratory rate falls below 12/minute.

4. Assess knee jerk (patellar tendon reflex) for evidence of diminished or absent reflexes. Loss of reflexes is often the first sign of developing toxicity (Sibai 1990). Also note marked lethargy or decreased level of consciousness and hypotension.

5. Determine urinary output. Output less than 30 mL/hour may result in the accumulation of toxic levels of magnesium.

6. If the respirations or urinary output fall below specified levels or if the reflexes are diminished or absent, no further magnesium should be administered until these factors return to normal.

7. The antagonist of magnesium sulfate is calcium. Consequently, an ampule of calcium gluconate should be available at the bedside. The usual dose is 1 g given IV over a period of about 3 minutes.

8. Monitor fetal heart tones continuously with IV administration.

9. Continue MgSO₄ infusion for approximately 24 hours after birth as prophylaxis against postpartum seizures if given for PIH.

10. If the mother has received MgSO₄ close to birth, the newborn should be closely observed for signs of magnesium toxicity for 24–48 hours.

NOTE: Protocols for magnesium sulfate administration may vary somewhat according to agency policy. Consequently, individuals are referred to their own agency protocols for specific guidelines.

days to establish the most effective basal and bolus regime. The woman is educated regarding pump operation, changing the syringe, and rotating the site of subcutaneous infusion. She is also taught signs and symptoms of serious drug side effects and safety precautions such as checking the pulse before boluses are given.

Once at home the woman usually receives weekly or biweekly visits from the home care nurse, education regarding preterm labor, and home uterine activity monitoring. During visits from the home care nurse physical assessments similar to those done in the hospital take place. The pump regime is adjusted based on the daily uterine activity records. Weekly cervical exams may be performed to enhance detection of preterm labor. Incorporated into the woman's plan of care should be the psychologic impact of having a high-risk pregnancy. Consideration of her ability to care for herself, the impact of the changes in relationships that will occur, and care of any young children in the home are among the issues that affect the woman's ability to cope effectively with this situation. The home care nurse needs to be alert to any signs that the woman is failing to achieve the emotional and developmental tasks of pregnancy, such as lack of maternal attachment. An individualized nursing care plan helps focus on each woman's specific needs.

APPLYING THE NURSING PROCESS

Nursing Assessment

During the antepartal period the nurse identifies the woman at risk for preterm labor by noting the presence of predisposing factors. During the intrapartal period the nurse assesses the progress of labor and the physiologic impact of labor on the mother and fetus.

Nursing Diagnosis

Nursing diagnoses that may apply to the woman with preterm labor include the following:

- Knowledge deficit related to lack of information about causes, identification, and treatment of preterm labor

- Fear related to early labor and birth

- Ineffective individual coping related to need for constant attention to pregnancy

Nursing Plan and Implementation

Teaching for Self-Care

Once the woman at risk for preterm labor has been identified, she needs to be taught about the importance of recognizing the onset of labor. Increasing the woman's awareness of the subtle symptoms of preterm labor is one of the most important teaching objectives of the nurse (see Teaching Guide: Preterm Labor on page 492). The signs and symptoms of preterm labor include the following:

- Uterine contractions that occur every 10 minutes or less with or without pain

- Change in Braxton-Hicks contractions from irregular to a regular pattern

- Mild menstrual-like cramps felt low in the abdomen

- Constant or intermittent feelings of pelvic pressure that may feel like the baby pressing down

- Rupture of membranes

- Low, dull backache, which may be constant or intermittent

- Sudden increase in vaginal discharge (an increase in amount or a change to more clear and watery or a pinkish tinge)

- Abdominal cramping with or without diarrhea (Eganhouse & Burnside 1992)

The woman is also taught to evaluate contraction activity once or twice a day. She does so by lying down tilted to one side with a pillow behind her back for support. The woman places her fingertips on the fundus of the uterus (which is above the umbilicus after 20 weeks' gestation). She checks for contractions (hardening or tightening in the uterus) for about 1 hour. It is important for the pregnant woman to know that uterine contractions occur occasionally throughout the pregnancy. If they occur every 10 minutes for 1 hour, however, the cervix could begin to dilate, and labor could continue.

The nurse ensures that the woman knows when to report signs and symptoms. If contractions occur every 10 minutes (or less) for 1 hour, if any of the other signs and symptoms are present for 1 hour, or if clear fluid begins leaking from the vagina, she should telephone her physician/nurse-midwife, clinic, or hospital birthing unit and make arrangements to be checked for ongoing labor.

If the woman experiences any preterm labor symptoms for more than 15 minutes while physically active, she should be instructed to do the following:

- Empty her bladder

- Lie down tilted toward her side

- Drink 3 to 4 (8 oz) cups of fluid

- Palpate for uterine contractions, and if contractions occur 10 minutes apart or less for 1 hour, notify the health care provider (Lipshitz et al 1993)

- Rest for 30 minutes after the symptoms have subsided and gradually resume activity

- Call her health care provider if symptoms persist, even if uterine contractions are not palpable

Care givers need to be aware that the woman is knowledgeable and attuned to changes in her body, and her call must be taken seriously. When a woman is at risk

PRETERM LABOR

Assessment During the antepartal period the woman generally is screened for factors that place her at risk for preterm labor. The nurse then spends time with the woman and assesses her understanding of the danger of preterm labor, signs of preterm labor, and actions she can take to prevent it. If she is on a home monitoring program, the nurse assesses the woman's understanding of the purpose and rationale for the program.

Nursing Diagnosis The key nursing diagnosis will probably be: Knowledge deficit related to lack of information about the risks of preterm labor and self-care measures to prevent it.

Nursing Plan and Implementation Teaching will focus on the risks of preterm labor, the functions of and procedures for home monitoring, and self-care activities to decrease the risk of preterm labor.

Client Goals At the completion of the teaching the woman will be able to do the following:

1. Discuss the risks of preterm labor
2. Describe the purpose of home monitoring
3. Demonstrate the correct procedures for doing home monitoring
4. Explain self-care measures that help decrease the risk of preterm labor

Teaching Plan

Content Describe the dangers of preterm labor, especially the risk of prematurity in the infant, and all the potential problems.

Stress the value of home monitoring in evaluating uterine activity on a regular basis. Emphasize that many of the early symptoms of labor such as backache and increased bloody show may be subtle initially. Home monitoring can often detect increased uterine activity in the early stages before cervical changes progress to the point where it is impossible to stop labor.

Recent studies have demonstrated that home uterine monitoring programs offer little or no significant difference in preterm delivery compared with patients followed by daily patient-nurse contact and no home uterine monitoring (Grimes & Shultz 1992; Lipshitz et al 1993).

If the woman is to be part of a home monitoring program, the monitoring nurse will usually do the initial teaching. Be prepared to reinforce the information provided and answer questions that may arise.

Summarize self-care measures such as excellent fluid intake (2 to 3 quarts daily), voiding every 2 hours, avoiding lifting and overexertion, avoiding nipple stimulation or orgasm, limiting sexual activity, and cooperating with activity restrictions and bed rest requirements.

Evaluation At the end of the teaching session the woman will be able to discuss the risks of preterm labor, demonstrate home monitoring techniques and explain their rationale, and implement self-care activities to decrease the risks of preterm labor.

Teaching Method *Discuss the risks specifically. Many people understand in a general way that prematurity can be dangerous, but they fail to understand how the baby is affected.*

Use handouts during the discussion. Help the woman clearly understand the value of the program because, to be successful, it requires a real commitment on her part.

Teach the woman how to palpate for uterine contractions.

Do a demonstration, and ask for a return demonstration.

Use a handout during the discussion. Provide opportunities for discussion. If the woman has concerns about certain recommendations, try to modify the approach to best meet her needs.

for preterm labor, she may have many episodes of contractions and other signs or symptoms. If she is treated positively, she will feel freer to report problems as they arise.

Other preventive measures the woman could follow are presented in Table 19–4.

Promotion of Maternal-Fetal Well-Being During Labor

Provision of supportive nursing care to the woman in preterm labor is important during hospitalization. This care consists of promoting bed rest, monitoring vital

TABLE 19-4	Self-Care Measures to Prevent Preterm Labor

Rest two or three times a day lying on your left side.

Drink 2 to 3 quarts of water or fruit juice each day. Avoid caffeine drinks. Filling a quart container and drinking from it will eliminate the need to keep track of numerous glasses of fluid.

Empty your bladder at least every 2 hours during waking hours.

Avoid lifting heavy objects. If small children are in the home, work out alternatives for picking them up, such as sitting on a chair and having them climb on your lap.

Avoid prenatal breast preparation such as nipple rolling or rubbing nipples with a towel. This is not meant to discourage breastfeeding but to avoid the potential increase in uterine irritability.

Pace necessary activities to avoid overexertion.

Sexual activity may need to be curtailed or eliminated.

Find pleasurable ways to help compensate for limitations of activities and boost the spirits.

Try to focus on 1 day or 1 week at a time rather than on longer periods of time.

If on bed rest, get dressed each day and rest on a couch rather than becoming isolated in the bedroom.

SOURCE: Prepared in consultation with Susan Bennett, RN, ACCE, Coordinator of the Prematurity Prevention Program.

signs (especially blood pressure and respirations), measuring intake and output, and continuous monitoring of FHR and uterine contractions. Placing the woman on her left side facilitates maternal-fetal circulation. Vaginal examinations are kept to a minimum. If tocolytic agents are being administered, the mother and fetus are monitored closely for any adverse effects.

Provision of Emotional Support to the Family

Whether preterm labor is arrested or proceeds, the woman and her partner experience intense psychologic stress. Decreasing the anxiety associated with the unknown and the risk of a preterm newborn is a primary aim of the nurse. The nurse also recognizes the stress of prolonged bed rest and of lack of sexual contact and helps the couple find satisfactory ways of dealing with these stresses. With empathetic communication the nurse can facilitate the couple's expression of their feelings, which commonly include guilt and anxiety, thereby helping the couple identify and implement coping mechanisms. The nurse also keeps the couple informed about the labor progress, the treatment regimen, and the status of the fetus so that their full cooperation can be elicited. In the event of imminent vaginal or cesarean birth the couple should be offered brief but ongoing explanations to prepare them for the actual birth process and the events following the birth.

Evaluation

Anticipated outcomes of nursing care include:

- The woman understands the cause, identification, and treatment of preterm labor.

- The woman's fears about early labor and birth are lessened.

- The woman feels comfortable in her ability to cope with her situation and has resources to call on.

- The woman understands self-care measures and can identify characteristics that need to be reported to her care giver.

- The woman and her baby have a safe labor and birth.

CARE OF THE WOMAN WITH A HYPERTENSIVE DISORDER

A number of hypertensive disorders can occur during pregnancy. Various attempts have been made to classify these disorders. The following classification is recommended by the American College of Obstetricians and Gynecologists (Silver 1989):

- Pregnancy-induced hypertension (preeclampsia-eclampsia)

- Chronic hypertension

- Chronic hypertension with superimposed preeclampsia

- Late or transient hypertension

Pregnancy-Induced Hypertension

Pregnancy-induced hypertension (PIH) is the most common hypertensive disorder in pregnancy, comprising up to two-thirds of the cases. It is characterized by the development of hypertension, proteinuria, and edema. Because only hypertension may be present early in the disease process, that finding is therefore the basis for diagnosis.

The definition of PIH is an increase in systolic blood pressure of 30 mm Hg and/or of diastolic of 15 mm Hg over baseline. These blood pressure changes must be noted on at least two occasions 6 hours or more apart for the diagnosis to be made. Ideally, the blood pressures should be compared with a baseline established in the first trimester (Knuppel & Drukker 1993). In the absence of baseline values a blood pressure of 140/90 has been accepted as hypertension.

The cause of PIH remains unknown, despite much research over many decades. It has been called "the disease of theories" because so many theories have been proposed for its etiology. The condition's former name, "toxemia of pregnancy," was based on a theory that a toxin produced in a pregnant woman's body caused the disease.

The term is no longer applicable, however, because the theory has not been substantiated. Currently, the study of the pathogenesis of pregnancy-induced hypertension involves several areas such as immunologic phenomena, dietary factors, toxic relationships, a uterine stretch reflex, and a hemodynamic hypothesis.

Preeclampsia and eclampsia are the two categories of PIH. The term **preeclampsia** indicates that this is a progressive disease unless there is intervention to control it. **Eclampsia** means "convulsion." If a woman has a convulsion, she is considered "eclamptic." Most often PIH is seen in the last 10 weeks of gestation, during labor, or in the first 48 hours after childbirth. Although birth of the fetus is the only known cure for PIH, it can be controlled with early diagnosis and careful management.

PIH occurs in 6% to 8% of all pregnancies in the United States (Aumann & Baird 1993). Among Black primigravidas the incidence is 15% to 20%, and in young primigravidas with twin pregnancies it is 30% (Sibai 1989). It is seen more often in primigravidas; teenagers of lower socioeconomic class; and women over 35, especially if they are primigravidas. Women with a family history of PIH are at higher risk for it, as are women with a large placental mass associated with multiple gestation, hydatidiform mole, Rh incompatibility, and diabetes mellitus.

Today PIH seldom progresses to the eclamptic state due to early diagnosis and careful management. However, hypertension remains one of the most frequently occurring and potentially life-threatening complications of pregnancy in the United States (Blackburn & Loper 1992).

Normal Physiologic Changes in Pregnancy

Following is a brief review of the physiologic changes that occur normally, allowing for a healthy adaptation to pregnancy (see Chapter 13).

Blood volume increases 30% to 50%. Peripheral vascular resistance decreases, and pregnancy-induced arterial dilation occurs.

The increased blood volume is necessary to perfuse the placenta and the increased tissue mass of the uterus and breasts. The higher blood volume also helps protect the fetus from impaired circulation due to maternal supine position, and it compensates for blood loss during childbirth.

The lowered peripheral vascular resistance results in lower blood pressure from the middle of the first trimester through the second trimester. Gradually, blood pressure returns to normal or near normal values by term.

Pregnancy stimulates the increased production of various hormones and enzymes, which have varying and sometimes opposing effects. Plasma levels of the enzyme renin are elevated three to four times over nonpregnant levels. Renin is involved in the formation of angiotensin I, which is converted to angiotensin II. The plasma level of angiotensin II, an active vasoconstrictor that stimulates a rise in blood pressure, is therefore also elevated. But blood pressure does not rise in normal pregnancy because by 10 weeks' gestation the pregnant woman develops a resistance to the pressor effects of angiotensin II. This resistance is thought to be due in part to vasodilator prostaglandins, particularly prostacyclin, which increases during pregnancy.

Aldosterone, a potent mineralocorticoid hormone secreted by the adrenal cortex, stimulates the kidney tubules to reabsorb sodium and water. Progesterone blocks the effect of aldosterone. Progesterone levels are elevated early in pregnancy and remain so until term. The result is sodium loss by the renal tubules.

The glomerular filtration rate increases 50%. This results in faster clearance and decreased plasma levels of creatinine, urea, and uric acid, as well as increased urine levels of these chemicals. Thus plasma values that are considered normal for nonpregnant women may be pathologic in pregnancy.

Physiologic edema, located primarily in the ankles, is a normal occurrence during pregnancy. It is caused by the increased movement of fluid out of the intravascular hemodiluted blood, with its decreased colloid osmotic pressure, into extracellular spaces. This movement is aided by increased hydrostatic pressure in the venous capillaries of the dependent limbs, due to pressure of the gravid uterus on the inferior vena cava.

Pregnancy is described as a hypercoaguable state because of the increased levels of most clotting factors. Fibrinogen is elevated to levels of approximately 450,000 mg/dL. Platelets remain in the normal range of 150,000/μL to 400,000/μL. However, factor XIII (fibrin stabilizing factor) is decreased due to placental enzymes.

Pathophysiology of PIH

The pathophysiology of PIH is not well understood, but various models have been proposed. Two of these, vasospasm and early hemodynamic alterations (Figure 19–5), are based on research examining the response of pregnant women to the infusion of pressor agents. Women who develop PIH become more sensitive to pressor agents rather than less sensitive to them, as in normal pregnancy. This response has been linked to the ratio between the prostaglandins prostacyclin and thromboxane. Prostacyclin, a vasodilator, decreases blood pressure, prevents platelet aggregation, and promotes uterine blood flow. Prostacyclin is decreased in preeclampsia, allowing the potent vasoconstrictor and platelet-aggregating effects of thromboxane to dominate. These hormones are produced partially by the placenta, which would help explain the reversal of the condition when the placenta is removed and why the incidence is increased when there is a larger than normal placental mass, such as in hydrops, multiple pregnancy, or hydatidiform mole. There also seems to be an increased risk of pregnancy-induced hy-

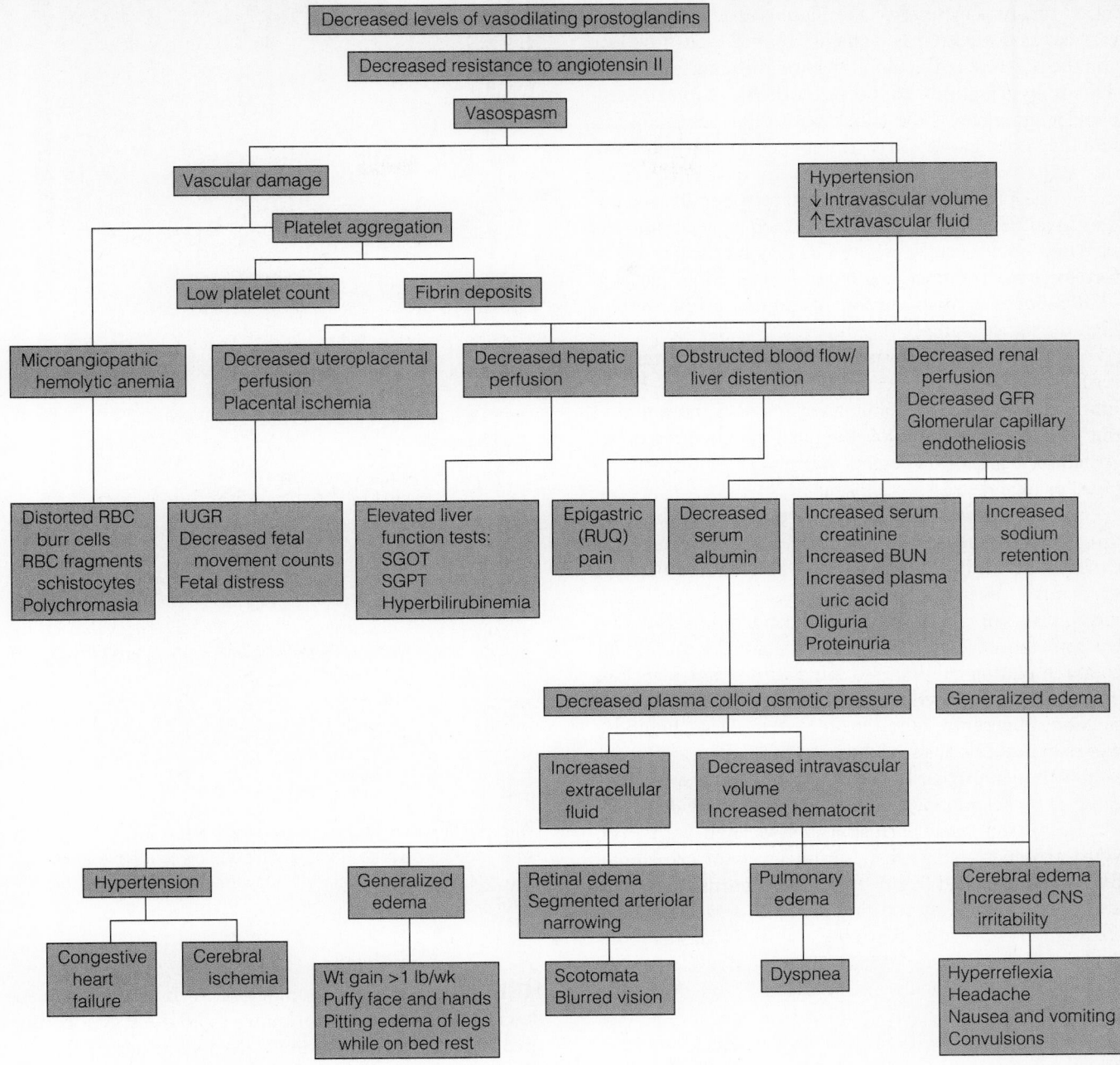

FIGURE 19-5 Clinical manifestations and possible pathophysiology of PIH.

pertension in women with preexisting vascular disease (Knuppel & Drukker 1993).

The underlying pathology in preeclampsia seems to be related to maternal vasospasm with alternating regions of constriction and dilation. The constricted and dilated areas occur throughout the arterial system as well as in major organs, the uterus, and placenta. Previously, it was thought that vascular endothelial injury was solely responsible for the vasoconstriction. Platelets adhere to the disrupted endothelial sites, decreasing the number of circulating platelets. The narrowed vessels reduce flow to any or all organ systems, thus destroying blood components attempting to push their way through the constricted areas.

New findings suggest another theory. Women who develop preeclampsia have been found to have an elevated cardiac output and an associated hyperdynamic vasodilation in the first trimester that causes endothelial damage (Krening 1992). The vasodilation acts as a compensatory mechanism, allowing maintenance of a normal blood pressure in spite of the high cardiac output. The vascular endothelium is damaged by the high flow rate and the pressure of the blood rushing through the vessels. The body responds to the endothelial damage with platelet aggregation and adherence to the damaged sites. Platelet aggregation may influence the prostacyclin: thromboxane ratio, affecting the course of the disease. As the disease progresses, the compensatory vasodilation begins to fail. The blood pressure starts to increase, and the systemic vascular resistance (SVR) may increase in an effort to protect end organs from damage. The elevated SVR reduces cardiac output, leading to a low output, high resistance state.

The loss of normal vasodilation of uterine arterioles results in decreased placental perfusion (Figure 19–6). Fibrin deposits and ischemic areas may also be found in the placenta. The effect on the fetus may be growth retardation, decrease in fetal movement, and chronic hypoxia or fetal distress.

Recently, attention has been directed to another theory, which postulates that uteroplacental ischemia acts as a trigger for PIH with other factors, such as immunologic mechanisms initiated by paternal genetic material, playing contributory roles. It has also been hypothesized that women who develop PIH do not sustain the normal increase in plasma volume associated with pregnancy. This may lead to decreased uteroplacental blood flow, which activates the renin-angiotensin system. This hemodynamic hypothesis suggests hypovolemia plays an important pathogenic role, but it is not seen as the primary cause of preeclampsia (Knuppel & Drukker 1993).

Decreased renal perfusion is associated with PIH. With a reduction in GFR, serum levels of creatinine, BUN, and uric acid begin to rise from normal pregnant levels, while urine output diminishes. For each 50% decrease in GFR, serum creatinine and BUN plasma levels double, while sodium is retained in increased amounts. Sodium retention results in increased extracellular volume and increased sensitivity to angiotensin II. The typical kidney lesion of PIH involves swollen glomerular capillary endothelial cells containing fibrin deposits. Stretching of the capillary walls allows the large protein molecules, primarily albumin, to escape into the urine, decreasing serum albumin.

Edema is usually more profound in PIH than in normal pregnancy. Its pathologic basis is twofold:

1. The higher salt retention draws out intravascular fluid.
2. Plasma colloid osmotic pressure decreases due to serum albumin loss through edematous renal glomeruli and damaged vascular endothelium. This causes fluid movement to extracellular spaces.

The decreased intravascular volume causes increased viscosity of the blood and a corresponding rise in hematocrit.

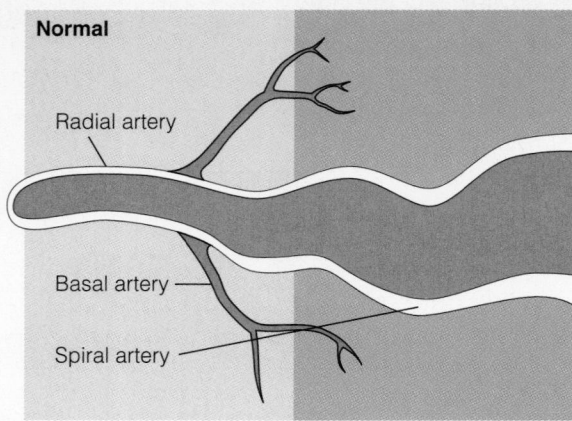

A

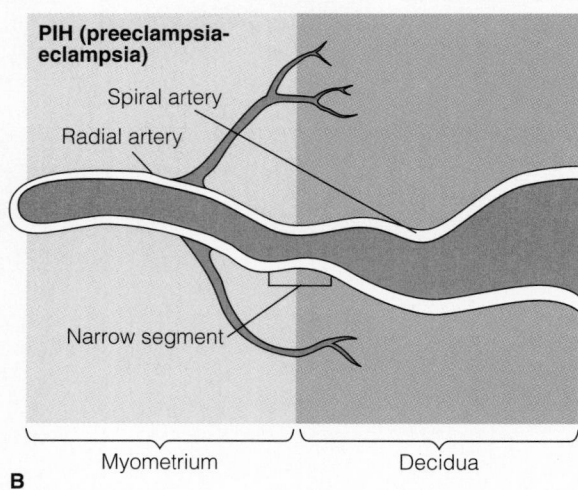

B

FIGURE 19-6   *A* In normal pregnancy the passive quality of the spiral arteries permits increased blood flow to the placenta. *B* In PIH vasoconstriction of the myometrial segment of the spiral arteries occurs.

HELLP Syndrome   A unique set of findings has been described. This syndrome, known as **HELLP syndrome**, involves <u>h</u>emolysis, <u>e</u>levated <u>l</u>iver enzymes, and <u>l</u>ow <u>p</u>latelet count. Although HELLP syndrome is usually associated with severe preeclampsia, it may occur before the signs and symptoms of preeclampsia develop. Ninety percent of women with HELLP syndrome present with symptoms before 36 weeks' gestation.

The hemolysis that occurs is termed *microangiopathic hemolytic anemia*. It is thought that red blood cells are distorted or fragmented during passage through small, damaged blood vessels. Elevated liver enzymes occur from blood flow that is obstructed due to fibrin deposits. Hyperbilirubinemia and jaundice may also be seen. Liver distention causes epigastric pain. Thrombocytopenia is a frequent finding in PIH. Vascular damage is associated with vasospasm, and platelets aggregate at sites of damage, resulting in low platelet count (less than 100,000).

Symptoms may include nausea, vomiting, malaise, flulike symptoms, or epigastric pain (Knuppel & Drukker

1993). This may lead to misdiagnoses of gastroenteritis, hepatitis, gall bladder disease, pyelonephritis, renal disease, or thrombocytopenia purpura. Regardless of their blood pressure or the presence of protein in their urine, women presenting with the above symptoms should have a CBC with platelet count and liver enzymes drawn. Perinatal morbidity and mortality with HELLP syndrome are high; therefore the possibility of HELLP should be considered carefully.

Women with HELLP syndrome are best cared for in a tertiary care center. Initially, the mother's condition should be assessed and stabilized, especially if her platelets are very low. Platelet transfusions are indicated for platelet counts below 20,000 mm^3. The fetus is also assessed using a nonstress test and biophysical profile. All women with true HELLP syndrome should give birth regardless of gestational age. Labor may be induced with oxytocin in women at 32 weeks' gestation or more. At less than 32 weeks' gestation cesarean birth is indicated (Sibai 1990).

Maternal Risks

Increased intraocular pressure due to PIH can cause retinal detachment, but spontaneous reattachment usually occurs with reduction in blood pressure and diuresis.

Central nervous system changes associated with PIH are hyperreflexia, headache, and convulsions. Hyperreflexia may be due to increased intracellular sodium and decreased intracellular potassium levels. Headaches are usually frontal and occipital, may be constant, and are caused by cerebral vasospasm. Cerebral edema and vasoconstriction are responsible for convulsions. Cerebral hemorrhage—either petechial or related to a large hematoma—is the most common cause of death following eclampsia.

Women who have preeclampsia complicated by HELLP syndrome do tend to have a somewhat longer clinical and hematologic recovery time than those who do not develop HELLP (Martin et al 1990).

Fetal-Neonatal Risks

Infants of women with hypertension during pregnancy tend to be small-for-gestational-age (SGA). The cause is related specifically to maternal vasospasm and hypovolemia, which result in fetal hypoxia and malnutrition. In addition the newborn may be premature because of the necessity for early birth.

Perinatal mortality associated with preeclampsia is approximately 10%, and that associated with eclampsia is 20%. When preeclampsia is superimposed on chronic hypertension, perinatal mortality may be higher.

At birth the newborn may be oversedated because of medications administered to the woman. The newborn may also have hypermagnesemia due to treatment of the woman with large doses of magnesium sulfate.

HOW SMALL IS TOO SMALL?

Advances in medical technology and obstetric/perinatal care have influenced our perception of when a fetus is considered viable. In the past many infants born prior to 28 weeks' gestation were considered nonviable. With aggressive perinatal management the limits of birth weight have been progressively lowered. Now fetuses born weighing 750 to 1000 g (approximately 24 to 26 weeks' gestation) are surviving in increasing numbers. The greatest strides have been made with infants weighing over 1000 g, whose survival has doubled in the last 15 years. Many states now consider a live-born fetus viable if it is at least 20 weeks' gestation or weighs 500 g or more. This change in the definition of viability raises many questions regarding obstetric management of premature labor and birth, decisions regarding initiation of resuscitation and provision of life support treatments, and long-term care needs. The long-term physiologic and psychologic implications for these tiny infants and their families are not known.

This dilemma has produced many philosophic, ethical, legal, and economic questions, such as the following:

- What is a reasonable definition of viability?

- Is there a need for a consensus on the lower limits of birth weight at which efforts at resuscitation will not be made?

- Should the parameters used as a guide for critical decisions involving preterm viability be gestational age or birth weight?

- Who is to be involved in the decision regarding the course of action for "nonviable" fetuses, and when is the decision to be made?

- What are the legal, ethical, social, and economic implications of the current concept of fetal viability?

Medical Therapy

The goals of medical management are prompt diagnosis of the disease; prevention of cerebral hemorrhage, convulsion, hematologic complications, and renal and hepatic diseases; and birth of an uncompromised newborn as close to term as possible. Reduction of elevated blood pressure is essential in accomplishing these goals.

Clinical Manifestations and Diagnosis

Mild Preeclampsia   The diagnosis of mild preeclampsia is made based on the following blood pressure findings: a rise in systolic blood pressure of 30 mm Hg or more, and/or a rise in diastolic blood pressure of 15 mm Hg or more above the baseline on two occasions at least 6 hours apart. If an early first trimester blood pressure reading is not available for a baseline parameter, 140/90 is used to designate mild preeclampsia. Generalized edema, seen as puffy face, hands, and dependent areas such as the ankles and lower legs, may be present. Edema is identified by a weight gain of more than 1.5 kg/month (3.3 lb) in the second trimester or more than 0.5 kg/week (1.1 lb) in the third trimester. Edema is assessed on a 1+ to 4+ scale. Proteinuria is often a late sign of preeclampsia. It may not be present until the disease has progressed to the severe or eclamptic stage. If proteinuria is present with mild preeclampsia, protein is generally between 300 mg/L (1+ dipstick) and 1 g/L (2+ dipstick). This is measured in a midstream clean-catch or catheter-derived urine specimen. Over a 24-hour period less than 5 g of protein would be lost in the urine.

Severe Preeclampsia   Severe preeclampsia may develop suddenly. The following clinical signs are often present:

- Blood pressure of 160/110 or higher on two occasions at least 6 hours apart while the woman is on bed rest

- Proteinuria ≥5 g/L in 24 hours

- Oliguria: urine output ≤400 mL/24 hours

- Other changes in laboratory values associated with severe preeclampsia (see Figure 19–5)

Other signs or symptoms that may be present include headache, blurred vision or scotomata (spots before the eyes), narrowed segments on the retinal arterioles when examined with an ophthalmoscope, retinal edema (retinas appear wet and glistening) on funduscopy, dyspnea due to pulmonary edema, moist breath sounds on auscultation, pitting edema of lower extremities while on bed rest, epigastric pain, hyperreflexia, nausea and vomiting, irritability, and emotional tension.

Eclampsia   Eclampsia, characterized by convulsion or coma, may occur before the onset of labor, during labor, or early in the postpartal period. Late postpartal eclampsia (convulsions occurring more than 48 hours following birth) occurs rarely but has been documented (Lubarsky et al 1994). Some women experience only 1 convulsion, especially if it occurs late in labor or during the postpartal period. Others may have from 2 to 20 or more. Unless they occur extremely frequently, the woman often regains consciousness between convulsions.

Antepartal Management   Currently, there is no known cure for PIH. Recent research has focused on preventing it in at-risk women through the use of low-dose (50–150 mg daily) aspirin. Aspirin is known to block the action of an enzyme, cyclooxygenase, essential to the production of prostaglandins. This results in lowered levels of thromboxane, the vasoconstrictor. At the same time levels of the vasodilator prostacyclin are not significantly affected (Hines & Jones 1994). Possible adverse effects of aspirin therapy for the newborn include intraventricular hemorrhage, cephalhematoma, and hematuria. To date

reports on the effectiveness of aspirin therapy are mixed, but two large studies are currently under way (Sibai 1994). The medical therapy for PIH depends on the severity of the disease.

Home Care of Mild Preeclampsia   In general, women with proteinuric preeclampsia should be admitted to the hospital. However, with changes in health care more attention has been given to decreasing inpatient hospital days for women whose symptoms allow. In response to that, several companies that provide home monitoring of uterine activity have developed similar programs for home blood pressure monitoring of mildly preeclamptic women. Day care for hypertension in pregnancy has also been examined as a means to reduce hospital admissions.

Selection of women eligible for home care is based on physician discretion. General recommendations are that only nonproteinuric, mildly hypertensive women be considered for home care. When being followed by a home care organization, women are given initial education about pregnancy-induced hypertension and its effects on both mother and fetus. Women must be able to recognize the signs and symptoms of worsening PIH (Table 19–5), be able to accurately count fetal movements, be cooperative, and know when to call the doctor. The importance of bed rest in a side-lying position is stressed, and the woman may be encouraged to keep a journal of occasions when she gets out of bed. The nurse then reviews this information with the woman to see if any modifications can be made in the household to reduce the temptation to be out of bed. For example, if a woman goes to the refrigerator several times a day, placing a cooler at her bedside may encourage better cooperation.

Physician orders will guide each woman's home care program. The physician determines how often the blood pressure is to be taken and what parameters are acceptable. Urine is dipped daily for protein, and the woman weighs herself daily. Weight gains of 1.4 kg (3 lb) in 24 hours or 1.8 kg (4 lb) in a 3-day period are generally cause for concern. Remote NSTs will be performed on a daily to biweekly basis. Some companies that provide this service have equipment that allows phone transmission of blood pressure readings as well as fetal monitor tracings. This eliminates concerns about inaccurate reporting on the part of the woman. Nursing contact varies from daily to weekly, depending on physician request. Laboratory testing regularly evaluates platelet counts, uric acid and BUN, liver enzymes, and 24-hour urine specimens for creatinine clearance and total protein.

If cooperation is lacking or a proper surveillance program does not exist, the woman should be hospitalized. Any woman with worsening symptoms or severe PIH should be managed in the hospital.

Physicians are often wary about managing even mild preeclampsia on an outpatient basis because it can rapidly progress to severe preeclampsia. Inpatient management

TABLE 19-5	Signs and Symptoms of Worsening PIH

Increasing edema, especially of hands and face
    (If on bedrest, observe for sacral edema.)
Worsening headache
Epigastric pain
Visual disturbances
Decreasing urinary output
Nausea/vomiting
Bleeding gums
Disorientation
Generalized complaints of not feeling well

goals are basically the same as home care. The possible disadvantage is separating the woman from her support system and placing her in an unfamiliar and possibly more stressful environment. The advantages are access to closer surveillance and faster intervention in the case of emergency.

Hospital Care of Mild Preeclampsia   Hospital care includes placing the woman on bed rest, primarily in the left lateral recumbent position, to decrease pressure on the vena cava, thereby increasing venous return, circulatory volume, and placental and renal perfusion. Improved renal blood flow helps decrease angiotensin II levels, promotes diuresis, and lowers blood pressure.

Diet should be well balanced and moderate to high in protein (80 to 100 g/day, or 1.5 g/kg/day) to replace protein lost in the urine. Sodium intake should be moderate, not to exceed 6 g/day. Excessively salty foods should be avoided, but strict sodium restriction and diuretics are no longer used in treating PIH.

Tests to evaluate fetal status are done more frequently as a pregnant woman's PIH progresses. Monitoring fetal well-being is essential to achieving a safe outcome for the fetus. The following tests are used:

- Fetal movement record
- Nonstress test
- Ultrasonography every 3–4 weeks for serial determination of growth
- Biophysical profile
- Serum creatinine determinations
- Amniocentesis to determine fetal lung maturity
- Doppler velocimetry beginning at 30–32 weeks to screen for fetal compromise

These tests are described in detail in Chapter 20.

Severe Preeclampsia   If the uterine environment is considered detrimental to fetal growth and maturation, birth may be the treatment of choice for both mother and fetus even if the fetus is immature. Other medical therapies for preeclampsia include the following:

- *Bed rest.* Bed rest must be complete. Stimuli that may bring on a convulsion should be reduced.

- *Diet.* A high-protein, moderate-sodium diet is given as long as the woman is alert and has no nausea or indication of impending convulsion.

- *Anticonvulsants.* Magnesium sulfate is the treatment of choice for convulsions. Its CNS-depressant action reduces the possibility of convulsion. Blood levels of $MgSO_4$ should be maintained at therapeutic levels (levels vary according to laboratory). Excessive blood levels may produce respiratory paralysis and/or cardiac arrest. (See Drug Guide: Magnesium Sulfate on page 490.)

TEACHING MOMENT

When caring for a woman with PIH who is receiving IV magnesium sulfate, it is imperative that you follow protocols for monitoring blood levels of magnesium. You are probably already aware of the common signs of increasing magnesium levels, such as diminished reflexes and decreased respiratory rate. However, there are some subtle clues you can also watch for that may suggest either the therapeutic or the toxic range. When a woman's magnesium level is in the therapeutic range, she usually has some slurring of speech, awkwardness of movement, and decreased appetite. If the woman begins to have difficulty swallowing and begins to drool, she may be approaching the toxic range.

- *Fluid and electrolyte replacement.* The goal of fluid intake is to achieve a balance between correcting hypovolemia and preventing circulatory overload. Fluid intake may be oral or supplemented with intravenous therapy. Intravenous fluids may be started "to keep lines open" in case they are needed for drug therapy even when oral intake is adequate. Criteria vary for determining appropriate fluid intake. Electrolytes are replaced as indicated by daily serum electrolyte levels.

- *Medication.* A sedative, such as diazepam (Valium) or phenobarbital, is sometimes given to encourage quiet bed rest.

- *Antihypertensives.* Aldomet (Methyldopa), normodyne (Labetelol), and nifedipine (Procardia) are antihypertensives that may be administered orally for the acute treatment of severe preeclampsia. In general, antihypertensive therapy is given for diastolic blood pressures of 110 or above. The therapeutic goal is to maintain the diastolic blood pressure between 90 and 100 mm Hg. Decreasing the diastolic below 90 may decrease uterine blood flow, causing fetal compromise. Intravenous antihypertensives are used for hypertension unresponsive to oral medication or for hypertensive crises.

Eclampsia   Approximately 5% of women with preeclampsia develop eclampsia. Convulsions may be focal, multifocal, or generalized. The etiology of the seizure is most likely related to cerebral vasospasm, edema, hemorrhage, ischemia, and hypertensive or metabolic encephalopathy. Many women experience an increase in deep tendon reflexes (DTRs) before seizure, but seizures may also occur without hyperreflexia. The woman with preeclampsia should be monitored for signs and symptoms of impending eclampsia: scotomata, which can appear as dark spots or flashing lights in the field of vision; blurred vision; epigastric pain; vomiting; persistent or severe headache, generally frontal in location; neurologic hyperactivity; pulmonary edema; or cyanosis.

If a seizure occurs, nursing assessment should consist of time of onset, progress of the seizure, body involvement, duration, incontinence, status of the fetus, and signs of placental abruption. The airway should be maintained and oxygen administered during the seizure. The woman is positioned on her side to avoid aspiration. Suctioning may be necessary to keep the airway clear; a tongue blade should not be inserted into the back of the throat because it may stimulate the gag reflex. To prevent injury, side rails should be up and padded, but the woman should not be restrained.

A bolus of 4 to 6 g magnesium sulfate is administered intravenously over 5 minutes in an attempt to break the seizure (Knuppel & Drukker 1993). Magnesium failures require the addition of a second agent such as 5–10 mg of diazepam or 125 mg of pentobarbital. Dilantin may be used for seizure prevention: A bolus of 10 mg/kg of body weight is piggybacked to a main line and infused at a rate no greater than 50 mg/minute. A second bolus of 5 mg/kg of dilantin is given 2 hours later with maintenance doses beginning 12 hours later and repeated every 8 to 12 hours based on serum levels of the drug. The therapeutic range of dilantin is 10–20 μg/mL (Heppard & Garite 1992).

During a seizure fetal bradycardia may occur. If possible, the fetus is allowed to recover before birth. The seizure increases uterine irritability and may cause a precipitous birth. Therefore a minimum ratio of one nurse to one client is imperative to assess fetal and maternal status. While she is still unconscious, the woman should be observed for onset of labor. The woman is observed for signs of placental separation (see Chapter 25). She should be checked every 15 minutes for vaginal bleeding, which may or may not be present with abruptio placentae. The abdomen is palpated for uterine rigidity.

Following a seizure, frequent auscultation of maternal lungs is required to assess for complications from aspiration and to rule out pulmonary edema, which is common in eclamptic clients. The woman is watched for circulatory and renal failure and for signs of cerebral hemorrhage. Furosemide (Lasix) may be given for pulmonary edema; digitalis may be given for circulatory failure. Intake and output are monitored hourly.

A woman may have a single convulsion or many convulsions, usually followed by a period of coma. She may be combative and confused as she arouses, but having a family member at her side helps to reduce her agitation. Also, avoid bright light, noises, and frequent disturbances.

The most serious complication, cerebral hemorrhage, arises from uncontrolled hypertension. Loss of vision, which is usually temporary, is a sign of impending hemorrhage. Blood pressure control with intravenous hydralazine has been the preferred treatment until after birth because of extensive experience with its use and rare reports of adverse fetal affects. Recently, hydralazine use in nonobstetric clients has given way to several new, very effective medications. The reduced call for the drug has led to hydralazine being less available for the obstetric population and a search for alternative therapies. Intravenous options are labetalol, diazoxide, or nitroprusside. Nitroprusside has been restricted to hypertensive crises when childbirth is imminent and other medications have not worked. Fetal cyanide poisoning may occur if the drug is continued and birth is delayed. Use of nitroprusside requires an arterial line because of its quick action and profound effects on blood pressure.

Intrapartal Management   Labor may be induced by intravenous oxytocin when there is evidence of fetal maturity and cervical readiness. In very severe cases cesarean birth may be necessary regardless of fetal maturity.

The woman may receive both intravenous oxytocin and $MgSO_4$ simultaneously. Because $MgSO_4$ has depressant action on smooth muscle, uterine contractions may diminish, and labor may be augmented with oxytocin. Equipment and intravenous lines for both fluids must be checked frequently to ensure that they are being administered at the proper rate. Infusion pumps should be used to guarantee accuracy. Bags and tubings must be labeled carefully.

Meperidine (Demerol) or fentanyl may be given intravenously for pain relief in labor. A pudendal block is often used for childbirth. An epidural block may be used if it is administered by a skilled anesthesiologist who is knowledgeable about PIH.

Childbirth in the Sims' or semisitting position should be considered. If the lithotomy position is used, a wedge should be placed under the right buttock to displace the uterus. The wedge should also be used if birth is by cesarean. Oxygen is administered to the woman during labor if need is indicated by fetal response to the contractions.

Eclampsia Often the woman with eclampsia is cared for in an intensive care unit until labor begins or is induced. Invasive hemodynamic monitoring of either central venous pressure (CVP) or pulmonary artery wedge pressure (PAWP) may be instituted using a Swan-Ganz catheter. Both these procedures carry risk to the woman, and the decision to use them should be made judiciously.

When the woman's vital signs have stabilized, urinary output is good, and the maternal and fetal hypoxic and acidotic states are alleviated, birth of the fetus should be considered. Birth is the only known cure for PIH. If the newborn will be preterm, it may be necessary to transfer the woman to a perinatal center for childbirth. The woman and her partner deserve careful explanation about the status of the fetus and woman and the treatment they are receiving. Plans for childbirth and further treatment must be discussed with them.

A pediatrician or neonatal nurse practitioner must be available to care for the newborn at birth. This care giver must be aware of all amounts and times of medication the woman has received during labor.

Postpartum Management The woman with PIH usually improves rapidly after childbirth, although seizures can still occur during the first 48 hours postpartum. A woman who has required $MgSO_4$ antepartally will continue to receive the infusion for about 24 hours postpartum. Antihypertensive medication may also be required for a time. Postpartum nurses should be acutely aware of the possibility of a worsening of the maternal condition in the immediate postpartum period. The potential for HELLP syndrome, liver rupture, or seizure continues, and one should not be lulled into a false sense of security once birth has occurred.

Women with PIH are not at greater risk for developing chronic hypertension later in life, but if blood pressure fails to return to normal parameters during the postpartum period, further evaluation is indicated to rule out underlying causes for hypertension. Young women are generally healthy and may not have sought regular health care before pregnancy, increasing the likelihood of a preexisting problem becoming evident during pregnancy or in the postpartum period.

Nursing Assessment

An essential part of nursing assessment is to obtain a baseline blood pressure early in pregnancy. Arterial blood pressure varies with position, being highest when the woman is sitting, intermediate when she is supine, and lowest when she is in the left lateral recumbent position.

ESSENTIAL PRECAUTIONS IN PRACTICE

A WOMAN WITH PIH

In caring for a woman with PIH, all the precautions established for any hospitalized pregnant, laboring, or postpartal woman apply. In addition remember the following specifics.

- Gloves should be worn when testing urine for proteinuria, when starting IV for $MgSO_4$ therapy, when doing finger sticks to test hematocrit, or when drawing blood for other laboratory tests.

- If eclampsia occurs and the woman convulses, gloves should be worn when removing the airway.

- If incontinence occurs during the convulsion, a splash apron and gloves should be worn when cleansing the woman and while changing the bedding.

- Needles, syringes, lancets, and other sharp objects should be disposed of in appropriately labeled containers.

REMEMBER to wash your hands prior to putting disposable gloves on and AGAIN immediately after you remove the gloves.

For further information, consult OSHA and CDC guidelines.

Therefore it is important that the woman be in the same position when the blood pressure is measured each visit.

Blood pressure is taken and recorded each antepartal visit. If the blood pressure rises or even if the normal slight decrease in blood pressure expected between 8 and 28 weeks of pregnancy does not occur, the woman should be followed closely.

When blood pressure and other signs indicate that the PIH has become severe, hospitalization is necessary to monitor the woman's condition closely. The nurse then assesses the following:

- *Blood pressure*. Blood pressure should be determined every 1 to 4 hours, more frequently if indicated by medication or other changes in the woman's status.

- *Temperature*. Temperature should be determined every 4 hours, every 2 hours if elevated.

- *Pulse and respirations*. Pulse rate and respiration should be determined along with blood pressure.

- *Fetal heart rate*. The fetal heart rate should be determined with the blood pressure or monitored continuously with the electronic fetal monitor if the situation indicates.

- *Urinary output*. Every voiding should be measured. Frequently, the woman will have an indwelling catheter. In this case hourly urine output can be assessed. Output should be 700 mL or greater in 24 hours or at least 30 mL per hour.

- *Urine protein.* Urinary protein is determined hourly if an indwelling catheter is in place or with each voiding. Readings of 3+ or 4+ indicate loss of 5 g or more of protein in 24 hours.

- *Urine specific gravity.* Specific gravity of the urine should be determined hourly or with each voiding. Readings over 1.040 correlate with oliguria and proteinuria.

- *Edema.* The face (especially eyelids and cheekbone area), fingers, hands, arms (ulnar surface and wrist), legs (tibial surface), ankles, feet, and sacral area are inspected and palpated for edema. The degree of pitting is determined by pressing over bony areas.

- *Weight.* The woman is weighed daily at the same time, wearing the same robe or gown and slippers. Weighing may be omitted if the woman is to maintain strict bed rest, or a bed scale may be used.

- *Pulmonary edema.* The woman is observed for coughing. The lungs are auscultated for moist respirations.

- *Deep tendon reflexes.* The woman is assessed for evidence of hyperreflexia in the brachial, wrist, patellar, or Achilles tendons (Table 19–6). The patellar reflex is the easiest to assess (Procedure 19–1: Assessing Deep Tendon Reflexes and Clonus). Clonus should also be assessed by vigorously dorsiflexing the foot

PROCEDURE 19-1
ASSESSING DEEP TENDON REFLEXES AND CLONUS

Nursing Action	Rationale
Objective: Assemble and prepare equipment.	
Obtain a percussion hammer. If one is not available, the side of the hand is also useful in assessing DTRs.	*A percussion hammer permits accurate delivery of a brisk tap.*
Objective: Prepare woman.	
Explain the procedure, indications for the procedure, and information that will be obtained. At a minimum the patellar reflex should be checked. Most nurses check a second reflex such as the biceps, triceps, or brachioradialis.	*Explanation decreases anxiety and increases cooperation. Deep tendon reflexes (DTRs) are assessed to gain information about CNS status and to assess the effects of MgSO$_4$ if the woman is receiving it.*
Objective: Elicit reflexes.	
Patellar reflex. The woman is positioned with her legs hanging over the edge of the bed (feet should not be touching the floor) (Figure 19–7). She may also lie supine with her knees slightly flexed and supported by the nurse. The nurse briskly strikes the patellar tendon, which is located just below the patella. Normal response is extension or a thrusting forward of the foot.	*Correct positioning and technique are essential to elicit the reflex. The correct position causes the muscle to be slightly stretched. Then when the tendon is stretched with the tap, the muscle should contract.*
Biceps reflex. The woman's arm is flexed at the elbow with the nurse's thumb placed on the biceps tendon. The nurse's thumb is struck in a slightly downward motion and response is assessed. Normal response is flexion of the arm.	
Objective: Grade reflexes.	
Reflexes are graded on a scale of 0 to 4+. See Table 19–6 on page 504.	*Normally reflexes are 1+ or 2+. With CNS irritation hyperreflexia may be present; with high magnesium levels reflexes may be diminished or absent.*

Nursing Action	Rationale

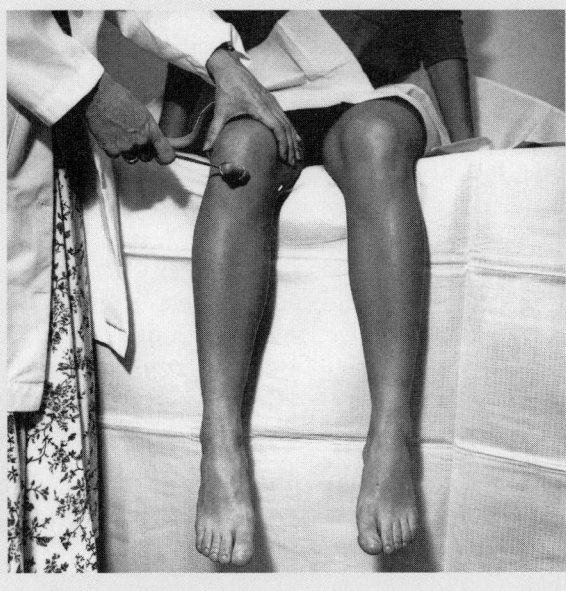

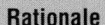

FIGURE 19-7   Correct position for eliciting patellar reflex: sitting.

Objective: Assess for clonus.

With the knee flexed and the leg supported, vigorously dorsiflex the foot, maintain the dorsiflexion momentarily, and then release (Figure 19–8).

Normal response: The foot returns to its normal position of plantar flexion. Clonus is present if the foot "jerks" or taps against the examiner's hand. If so, the number of taps or beats of clonus is recorded.

Clonus indicates more pronounced hyperreflexia and is indicative of CNS irritability.

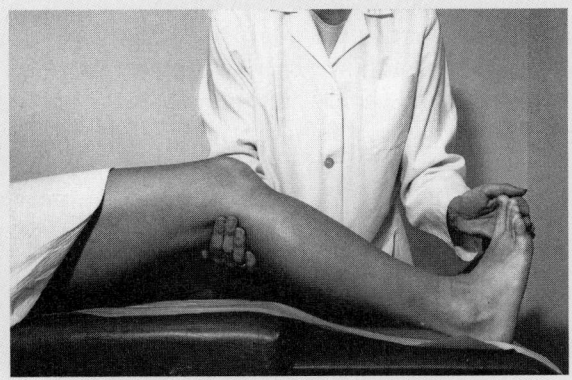

FIGURE 19-8   To elicit clonus, sharply dorsiflex the foot.

Objective: Report and record findings.

For example: DTRs 2+, no clonus or DTRs 4+, 2 beats clonus.

Provides a permanent record.

TABLE 19-6	Deep Tendon Reflex Rating Scale
Rating	**Assessment**
4+	Hyperactive; very brisk, jerky, or clonic response; abnormal
3+	Brisker than average; may not be abnormal
2+	Average response; normal
1+	Diminished response; low normal
0	No response; abnormal

while the knee is held in a fixed position. Normally no clonus is present. If it is present, it is measured as one to four beats and is recorded as such.

- *Placental separation.* The woman should be assessed hourly for vaginal bleeding and/or uterine rigidity.

- *Headache.* The woman should be questioned about the existence and location of any headache.

- *Visual disturbance.* The woman should be questioned about any visual blurring or changes, including scotomata. The results of the daily funduscopic exam should be recorded on the chart.

- *Epigastric pain.* The woman should be asked about any epigastric pain. It is important to differentiate it from simple heartburn, which tends to be familiar and less intense.

- *Laboratory blood tests.* Daily tests of hematocrit to measure hemoconcentration; blood urea nitrogen, creatinine, and uric acid levels to assess kidney function; clotting studies for any indication of thrombocytopenia or DIC; liver enzymes; and electrolyte levels for deficiencies are all indicated.

- *Level of consciousness.* The woman is observed for alertness, mood changes, and any signs of impending convulsion or coma.

- *Emotional response and level of understanding.* The woman's emotional response should be carefully assessed so that support and teaching can be planned accordingly.

In addition the nurse continues to assess the effects of any medications administered. Because the administration of prescribed medications is an important aspect of care, the nurse is, of course, familiar with the more commonly used medications, their purpose, implications, and associated untoward or toxic effects.

Nursing Diagnosis

Examples of nursing diagnoses that may apply are listed in the Nursing Care Plan: Care of the Woman with Pregnancy-Induced Hypertension (Preeclampsia-Eclampsia).

Nursing Plan and Implementation

Provision of Support and Teaching

A woman with PIH has several major concerns. She may fear losing the fetus. She may worry about her personal relationship with her other children and her personal and sexual relationship with her partner. She may be concerned about finances—health insurance does not always cover all the tests, prolonged hospitalization, and so on that may be associated with complications during pregnancy. Finally, the woman may be depressed or resentful about being left alone or may feel bored. If she has small children, she may have difficulty providing for their care. The woman who does not have children may worry that she never will.

The nurse should identify and discuss each of these areas with the couple. It is necessary to explain to them the reasons for bed rest. A woman with mild preeclampsia may feel very well and be unable to see the need for resting even a few hours a day. The nurse can refer the couple to many community resources such as homemaking services, a support group for the partner, or a hotline. Arrangements may be made for the partner to attend childbirth classes if both are not able to, or a nurse may be found to teach the classes privately.

The woman needs to know which symptoms are significant and should be reported at once. Usually, the woman with mild preeclampsia is seen once or twice a week, but she may need to come in earlier if symptoms indicate the condition is progressing. She must understand her diet plan, which must match her culture, finances, and life-style.

The development of severe preeclampsia is a cause for increased concern to the woman and her family. The most immediate concerns of the woman and her partner usually are about the prognosis for herself and the fetus. The nurse can offer honest and hopeful information. She can explain the plan of therapy and the reasons for procedures to the extent that the woman or her partner are interested. The nurse should keep the couple informed of the fetal status and should also take the time to discuss other concerns the couple may express. The nurse provides as much information as possible and seeks other sources of information or aid for the family as needed. Nurses can offer to contact a minister or hospital chaplain for additional support if the couple so chooses.

Prevention of Convulsion

The nurse should maintain a quiet, low-stimulus environment for the woman. The woman should be placed in a private room in a quiet location where she can be watched closely. Visitors are limited to close family or main support persons. The woman should maintain the left lateral recumbent position most of the time, with side rails up for her protection. Unlimited phone calls are

Text continues on page 508

CARE OF THE WOMAN WITH PREGNANCY-INDUCED HYPERTENSION (PREECLAMPSIA-ECLAMPSIA)

Nursing Assessment

Nursing History

1. Predisposing factors in the client history:
   a. Primigravida
   b. Presence of diabetes mellitus
   c. Multiple pregnancy
   d. Hydramnios
   e. Gestational trophoblastic disease
   f. Preexisting vascular or renal disease
   g. Adolescent or older maternal age
   h. Family history of PIH

Physical Examination

1. Blood pressure elevated (as compared to baseline, if available). Elevation of ≥ 30 mm Hg systolic and ≥ 15 mm Hg diastolic; ≥ 140/90 if baseline not available.
2. Presence of edema as indicated by weight gain or puffy hands and feet. Assessment of periorbital edema requires ongoing evaluation.
3. Presence of hyperreflexia and clonus.

4. Presence of headache, visual disturbances, drowsiness, epigastric pain, nausea and/or vomiting.
5. Vaginal bleeding, abdominal tenderness, or signs of labor.

Diagnostic Studies

1. Fluid intake and urinary output for quantity and specific gravity.
2. Urine for urinary protein: 1 g protein/24 hour = 1–2+; 5 g protein/24 hour = 3–4+.
3. Hematocrit: Elevation of hematocrit implies hemoconcentration, which occurs as fluid leaves the intravascular space and enters the extravascular space.
4. BUN: Not usually elevated except in women with cardiovascular or renal disease.
5. Blood uric acid appears to correlate well with the severity of the preeclampsia-eclampsia. (Note: Thiazide diuretics can cause significant increases in uric acid levels.)
6. Liver enzymes: elevated AST, ALT.
7. Antithrombin III: decreased.
8. Fetal assessment: fetal movement record, NSTs, ultrasound evaluation of fetal well-being.

NURSING DIAGNOSIS: Fluid volume deficit related to fluid shift from intravascular to extravascular space secondary to vasospasm

EXPECTED OUTCOME: Fluid volume deficit will be controlled, and intravascular volume will be maintained.

Nursing Interventions	Rationale
Assess BP every 1–4 hours using same arm with woman in same position.	Blood pressure can fluctuate hourly. Blood pressure increases as a result of increased peripheral resistance due to peripheral vasoconstriction and arteriolar spasm.
Weigh daily. A gain of 1 kg/week or more in the second trimester or a gain of 1/2 kg/week or more in the third trimester is suggestive of PIH.	Weight gain and edema are due to sodium and water retention.
Assess for edema: +(1+) Minimal: slight edema of pedal and pretibial areas ++(2+) Marked edema of lower extremities +++(3+) Edema of hands, face, lower abdominal wall, and sacrum ++++(4+) Anasarca with ascites	Decreased plasma colloid osmotic pressure causes movement of fluid from the intravascular to extravascular space.
Maintain on bedrest. Encourage the left lateral recumbent position.	Bedrest produces an increase in GFR.
Maintain moderate salt intake (2–3 g/24 hours).	Normal salt intake is now advised, but excessive salt intake may make the condition worse.
Report urine output <30 mL/hour or urine specific gravity >1.040.	Renal plasma flow and glomerular filtration are decreased in PIH. Increasing oliguria indicates a worsening condition.
Test urine for protein hourly or as ordered. Maintain indwelling catheter.	Proteinuria results from the escape of protein through edematous epithelium of the glomerular capillaries.
Evaluate hematocrit levels regularly.	Decreased intravascular fluid volume leads to increased hematocrit level because of change in proportion of RBCs to volume of fluid.
Provide adequate protein: 1.5 g/kg/24 hours for incipient and mild preeclampsia.	Plasma proteins affect movement of intravascular and extravascular fluids.

OUTCOME MET IF:

- Edema decreases and is no greater than 2+
- Urine output 30 mL/hour or 700 mL/24 hours
- Proteinuria decreasing (no greater than 2+ on dipstick or <1 g of protein in 24 hours)
- Normal specific gravity <1.040

- BP remains less than 30 mm Hg systolic and 15 mm Hg diastolic over baseline
- Hematocrit 32%–40%
- Lung sounds are clear

CARE OF THE WOMAN WITH PREGNANCY-INDUCED HYPERTENSION
(PREECLAMPSIA-ECLAMPSIA) *continued*

NURSING DIAGNOSIS: Knowledge deficit related to lack of information about PIH, its treatment, and the implications for the woman and her fetus

EXPECTED OUTCOME: Woman verbalizes her understanding of the condition and its implications.

Nursing Interventions	Rationale
Discuss PIH and its implications for the client and fetus/newborn.	Thorough information may help the woman/family better understand the condition and its implications.
Explain the purpose and importance of treatment measures.	
Work with the woman/family to plan ways for them to deal with the hospitalization.	Hospitalization during pregnancy is usually unanticipated and may cause a major disruption in the woman/family's life.

OUTCOME MET IF:
- Woman/family able to discuss PIH disease process, and verbalize implications for mother and fetus/newborn and importance of compliance with treatment measures

---

NURSING DIAGNOSIS: Risk for injury related to possibility of convulsion secondary to cerebral vasospasm or edema

EXPECTED OUTCOME: Woman will not develop seizures or signs that her condition is worsening.

Nursing Interventions	Rationale
Monitor knee, ankle, and biceps reflexes and clonus.	Hyperreflexia indicates CNS irritability.
Promote bed rest in the left lateral recumbent position in a darkened, quiet room.	
Limit visitors.	
Administer magnesium sulfate per physician order: IV dose: 4–6 g loading dose MgSO₄ followed by continuous infusion at a rate of 1–2 g/hour (Mandeville & Troiano 1992).	Magnesium sulfate is a cerebral depressant. It also reduces neuromuscular irritability and causes vasodilation and transient drop in BP.
Monitor magnesium levels frequently to prevent overdose (2 hours after beginning infusion and then every 2–4 hours).	The therapeutic blood level is 4–8 mg/dL (Mandeville & Troiano 1992).
Before administering subsequent doses of magnesium sulfate, check reflexes (knee, ankle, biceps), respirations, and urine output. Do not give magnesium sulfate if:	Knee jerk disappears when magnesium sulfate blood levels are 8–10 mg/dL. Toxic signs and symptoms develop with increased blood levels. Respiratory depression can occur at blood levels of 10–15 mg/dL. Cardiac conduction problems can occur at levels above 15 mg/dL (Scott 1994b).
1. Reflexes are absent.	
2. Respirations are <12/minute.	
3. Urine output in the past 4 hours is <100 mL.	Kidneys are the only route for excretion of magnesium sulfate.
Have calcium gluconate available.	Calcium gluconate is the antidote for magnesium sulfate.
Maintain seizure precautions:	
1. Keep room quiet, dark.	Quiet and dark reduce stimuli.
2. Instruct the woman to report any signs of headache or visual disturbances.	
3. Have emergency equipment available, including oxygen, suction, padded tongue blade if agency policy permits.	
4. Pad side rails.	Padding protects client.
5. Educate other care givers regarding the possibility of convulsions and appropriate actions.	
Provide supportive care during convulsion:	
1. Place tongue blade or airway in woman's mouth, if it can be done without force, according to agency policy.	Acts to maintain airway and to prevent the woman from biting her tongue.
2. Suction nasopharynx as necessary.	Removes mucus and secretions.
3. Administer oxygen.	Promotes oxygenation.
4. Note type of seizure and duration.	Precipitous labor may start during seizure.
After seizure, assess for uterine contractions and assess fetal status.	Continuous fetal monitoring until woman is stable is necessary to identify fetal stress.

OUTCOME MET IF:
- Woman develops no seizures
- Reflexes are 1+ or 2+ on a 4+ scale
- No clonus beats are noted
- Respirations are >12 breaths/minute
- Urine output is >30 mL/hour
- Woman reports no headaches or visual disturbances

CARE OF THE WOMAN WITH PREGNANCY-INDUCED HYPERTENSION (PREECLAMPSIA-ECLAMPSIA) *continued*

NURSING DIAGNOSIS: Risk for injury to fetus related to inadequate placental perfusion secondary to vasospasm or possible abruptio placentae

EXPECTED OUTCOME: Fetus will tolerate the stress of maternal condition without injury.

Nursing Interventions	Rationale
Encourage mother to assume left lateral recumbent position.	Avoids pressure on the vena cava and promotes optimal placental perfusion.
Evaluate results of serial fetal assessments such as NST, CST, ultrasound, and BPP.	Fetal assessment determines fetal status, placental sufficiency, and ability to withstand the stress of labor, as well as fetal maturity.
Report any signs of abruptio placentae such as uterine tenderness, vaginal bleeding, change in fetal activity, change in fetal heart rate, sustained abdominal pain.	Vasospasm and high blood pressure of PIH increase the risk of abruptio placentae.
Monitor the fetus closely with electronic fetal monitor. Report evidence of late decelerations, decreased variability, and normal FHR baseline.	Because of decreased placental perfusion due to vasospasm, the fetus may have difficulty tolerating the stress of labor, and cesarean birth may be necessary.

OUTCOME MET IF:
- Fetus has no late decelerations
- Average long- and short-term variabilities are present
- FHR 120–160 bpm

- Mother reports no abdominal tenderness or bleeding
- All tests performed are within normal limits: NST is reactive; CST is negative; BPP score is 8 or higher

NURSING DIAGNOSIS: Risk for injury to the mother related to hematologic and hepatic abnormalities secondary to the HELLP syndrome

EXPECTED OUTCOME: Woman will not develop injury from hematologic or hepatic complications.

Nursing Interventions	Rationale
Obtain blood samples as ordered to evaluate hemoglobin and hematocrit, SGOT, SGPT, and platelet count.	HELLP syndrome refers to hemolysis of RBCs causing signs of anemia, elevated liver enzymes because of liver damage (causing jaundice), and low platelet count related to severe vasospasm and developing DIC.
Monitor test results, and report abnormal findings.	
Report signs of hemolytic anemia, (eg, pallor, fatigue, anorexia, and dyspnea).	
Report signs of liver dysfunction, including nausea and vomiting, right upper quadrant pain, jaundice, and malaise.	
Report signs of developing DIC immediately (eg, epistaxis, hematuria, petechiae, bleeding gums, GI tract bleeding, and retinal or conjunctival hemorrhages).	

OUTCOME MET IF:
- Lab values stay within normal limits.
- No signs or symptoms of jaundice/bleeding are noted.

- Woman reports no nausea and vomiting, upper quadrant pain, fatigue, or anorexia.

Essential Nursing Activities To Achieve Outcomes

If the woman's condition is unstable:
BP: 160/110 or greater
Proteinuria: 5 g
Urine output: <30 g/hour
Edema: 3+ to 4+

1. Take BP, pulse, and respirations every 2 hours.
2. Record hourly I&O (indwelling catheter provides most accurate reading).
3. Monitor IV and possible Swan-Ganz.
4. Administer magnesium sulfate IV in 4–6 g loading dose followed by 1–2 g/hour (Arias 1993).
5. Assess reflexes and clonus every 2 hours.
6. Monitor fetus continually.
7. Auscultate lung sounds every 4 hours.

8. Assess for edema qid.
9. Follow seizure precautions.
10. Limit visitors.
11. Provide a quiet environment.

If the woman's condition is stable:
BP: 140/90 to 160/110.
Proteinuria: 3–4 gm
Urine output >30 g/hour
Edema: 1+ to 2+

1. Take BP, pulse, and respirations every 4 hours.
2. Record I&O every 4 hours.
3. Assess reflexes and clonus every 4 hours.
4. Perform fetal monitoring 30-minute reactive strip qid.
5. Weigh daily.

avoided because the phone ringing unexpectedly may be too jarring. To avoid a sense of isolation, however, some women find it preferable to limit calls to a certain time of the day.

Provision of Effective Care and Support if Eclampsia Develops

The occurrence of a convulsion is frightening to any family members who may be present, although the woman will not be able to recall it when she becomes conscious. Therefore offering explanations to family members, and to the woman herself later, is essential.

When the tonic phase of the convulsion begins, the woman should be turned to her side (if she is not already in that position) to aid circulation to the placenta. Her head should be turned face down to allow saliva to drain from her mouth. Attempting to insert a padded tongue blade has been questioned, and in many facilities it is no longer advocated. In others it is used if it can be done without force because it may prevent injury to the woman's mouth. The side rails should be padded or a pillow put between the woman and each side rail.

After 15 to 20 seconds the clonic phase starts. When the thrashing subsides, intensive monitoring and therapy begin. An oral airway is inserted, the woman's nasopharynx is suctioned, and oxygen administration is begun by nasal catheter. Fetal heart tones are monitored continuously. Maternal vital signs are monitored every 5 minutes until they are stable, then every 15 minutes.

Promotion of Maternal-Fetal Well-Being During Labor and Birth

The plan of care for the woman with PIH in labor depends on both maternal and fetal condition. The woman may have mild or severe preeclampsia, may become eclamptic during labor, or may have been eclamptic before the onset of labor. Therefore, careful monitoring of blood pressure and checking for edema and proteinuria are necessary for all women in labor. The prenatal record should be obtained so that current blood pressure readings may be compared with the baseline reading.

The woman with PIH in labor is kept positioned on her side as much as possible. Both woman and fetus are monitored carefully throughout labor. Signs of progressing labor are noted. In addition the nurse must be alert for indications of worsening PIH, placental separation, pulmonary edema, circulatory renal failure, and fetal distress.

During the second stage of labor the woman is encouraged to push while lying on her side. If she is unable to do so comfortably or effectively, she can be helped to a semisitting position for pushing and resume the lateral position between each contraction. Birth is in the side-lying position if possible. If the lithotomy position is used, a wedge is placed under the woman's hip.

A family member is encouraged to stay with the woman as long as possible throughout labor and childbirth. This is especially needed if the woman has been transferred to a high-risk center from another facility. The woman in labor and the family member or support person should be oriented to the new surroundings and kept informed of progress and plan of care. The woman should be cared for by the same nurses throughout her hospital stay.

Promotion of Maternal Well-Being During the Postpartal Period

The amount of postpartal vaginal bleeding should be noted carefully. Because the woman with PIH is hypovolemic, even normal blood loss can be serious. Rising pulse rate and falling urine output are indications of excessive blood loss. The uterus should be palpated frequently and massaged when needed to keep it contracted.

Blood pressure and pulse are checked every 4 hours for 48 hours. Hematocrit may be measured daily. The woman is instructed to report any headache or visual disturbance. No ergot preparations such as methergine are given because they have a hypertensive effect. Intake and output recordings are continued for 48 hours postpartum. Increased urinary output within 48 hours after birth is a highly favorable sign. With the diuresis edema recedes and blood pressure returns to normal.

Postpartal depression can develop after the long ordeal of the difficult pregnancy. Family members are urged to visit, and as much mother-infant contact as possible should be allowed. There may be fears about a future pregnancy. The couple needs information about the chance of PIH occurring again. They also should be given family planning information. Oral contraceptives may be used if the woman's blood pressure has returned to normal by the time they are prescribed (usually 4 to 6 weeks postpartum).

Evaluation

Anticipated outcomes of nursing care include:

- The woman is able to explain PIH, its implications for her pregnancy, the treatment regimen, and possible complications.

- The woman suffers no eclamptic convulsions.

- The woman and her care givers detect evidence of increasing severity of the PIH or possible complications early so that appropriate treatment measures can be instituted.

- The woman gives birth to a healthy newborn.

Chronic Hypertensive Disease

Chronic hypertension exists when the blood pressure is 140/90 or higher before pregnancy or before the 20th week of gestation or persists indefinitely following childbirth. If the diastolic blood pressure is greater than 80 mm Hg during the second trimester, chronic hypertension should be suspected. The cause of chronic hypertension has not been determined. For the majority of chronic hypertensive women the disease is mild. The goal of medical therapy is to prevent the development of preeclampsia and to ensure normal growth of the fetus. One of the challenges the health care team faces is differentiating chronic hypertension from preeclampsia. This is even more difficult if a woman arrives for her first prenatal visit during the second trimester when blood pressure is generally lower and preexisting hypertension is more difficult to recognize. When a woman with known hypertension becomes pregnant, she should start prenatal care as soon as possible. She will need to visit her health care provider at least every 2 weeks during pregnancy. During the woman's initial visit the usual prenatal assessment and laboratory tests are done. Additional laboratory tests include baseline serum creatinine, BUN, serum electrolytes, urine protein, and urine culture. Exams revealing optic fundi with hemorrhage or exudate, plasma creatinine > 20 mg/dL, or the presence of chronic conditions such as diabetes or collagen, vascular, or renal disease are suggestive of chronic hypertension. If the hypertension is significant, an EKG and chest x-ray are done to obtain baseline values.

Ultrasound is done at 8–12 weeks to date the pregnancy as accurately as possible. It is done again between 20 and 26 weeks and at 32 weeks to diagnose IUGR. Weekly nonstress tests or biophysical profiles should begin at 30–32 weeks' gestation (Knuppel & Drukker 1993). Creatinine clearance is determined early in pregnancy and repeated every 2 months if renal disease is suspected.

In addition to these ongoing assessments the following interventions are usually instituted:

- *Bed rest.* Frequent rest periods are advisable. At a minimum the woman should rest for two 1-hour periods, one at midday and one in the late afternoon.

- *Diet.* Protein intake of 1.5 g/kg body weight/day is recommended if proteinuria is significant. Moderate salt intake (2 g sodium or less/day) is advised (Scott 1994b).

- *Medication control.* Diuretic medication is gradually eliminated if the woman was on it prior to pregnancy. Antihypertensive medication may be continued, primarily to prevent maternal complications in women with severe chronic hypertension (blood pressure > 100 mm Hg diastolic). The drug of choice is methyldopa (Aldomet) (Scott 1994b).

- *Blood pressure.* The woman or her partner can monitor her blood pressure regularly and maintain a record. Home monitoring is often more accurate because the woman is more relaxed and in a familiar environment.

The primary nursing goal is to provide sufficient information so that the woman is able to meet her self-care needs. She is given information about her diet, the importance of regular rest, her medications, and the need for blood pressure control. She is taught to assess fetal movement daily during rest periods.

Chronic Hypertension with Superimposed PIH

Preeclampsia develops in approximately 25% of women previously found to have chronic hypertension. When elevations of systolic blood pressure 30 mm Hg above the baseline or of diastolic blood pressure 15 mm Hg above the baseline are discovered on two occasions at least 6 hours apart, proteinuria develops, or edema occurs in the upper half of the body, the woman needs close monitoring and careful management. Her condition may progress quickly to eclampsia, sometimes before 30 weeks of pregnancy.

Late or Transient Hypertension

Late hypertension exists when transient elevation of blood pressure occurs during labor or in the early postpartal period, returning to normal within 10 days postpartum.

CARE OF THE WOMAN AT RISK FOR RH SENSITIZATION

Rh sensitization results from an antigen-antibody immunologic reaction within the body. Sensitization most commonly occurs when an Rh negative woman carries an Rh positive fetus, either to term or terminated by spontaneous or induced abortion. It can also occur if an Rh negative nonpregnant woman receives an Rh positive blood transfusion or experiences an Rh positive tubal pregnancy.

A number of known red blood cell (RBC) antigens are involved in the Rh system, all of which are controlled by three pairs of genes: Cc, Dd, and Ee. Antigens in the D group are usually involved in incompatibility between the mother and fetus, although other RBC antigens can also cause isoimmunization. The factors implicated in pathogenesis, in order of antigenic potential, are D, C, E, c, e, and, hypothetically, d (d has never been demonstrated but is thought to exist). There are many genetic combinations (genotypes) possible, such as CDE, cDe, Cde, and so forth. Individuals who are homozygous for the D antigen (DD) or heterozygous (Dd) are Rh positive because the D antigen is dominant; those whose genotype is dd, homozygous for the recessive antigen, are Rh negative.

During a normal pregnancy, small amounts of fetal blood (<0.5 mL) may cross the placenta. If the fetus is Rh positive, some women develop anti-D antibodies in response to this exposure. During delivery of the placenta or due to trauma, even larger quantities of fetal blood can enter maternal circulation (Blackburn & Loper 1992). After exposure to the Rh positive antigen the primary response is development of gamma M immunoglobin (IgM). This primary response develops slowly over several weeks or months. IgM antibodies are large and do not cross the placenta. Once a woman is isoimmunized, she is immunized for life.

Following the primary response, the production of IgG anti-D antibody develops rapidly. IgG is capable of crossing the placenta and coating the fetal Rh (D) positive red cells, causing hemolysis. A second exposure to a very small amount of Rh (D) positive cells produces a rapid secondary immune response, developing in a few days and stronger than the primary response (Figure 19–9).

Thus although hemolysis is not generally a problem for the fetus during a first pregnancy, it may create problems during subsequent pregnancies.

The hemolysis caused by the IgG antibody in the fetus creates fetal anemia. The fetus responds by increasing red cell production. The presence of nucleated RBCs (erythroblasts) is why the term **erythroblastosis fetalis** was coined for this severe hemolytic disease of the fetus and newborn. Immune suppression with **Rh immune globulin (RhoGAM)** appears to be effective as long as it occurs before the development of IgG antibodies (Ingardia & Pitcher 1993).

Approximately 87% of White Americans, 92% to 93% of Black Americans, and 99% of Asian populations are Rh positive. An Rh-negative woman who gives birth to an Rh-positive, ABO compatible infant has a 16% risk of becoming sensitized as a result of her pregnancy (Ingardia & Pitcher 1993).

Fetal-Neonatal Risks

Critical Thinking Question

Would problems arise for a fetus if the mother is Rh positive and the father is Rh negative?

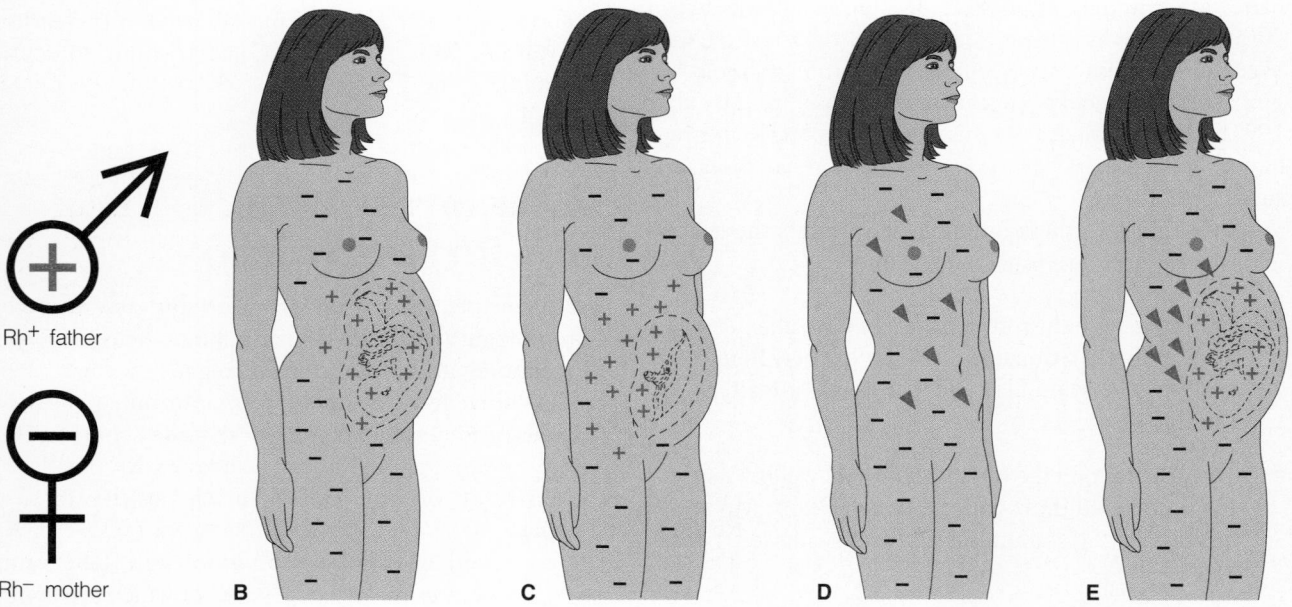

Rh⁺ father

A   Rh⁻ mother   B   C   D   E

FIGURE 19-9   Rh isoimmunization sequence. *A* Rh positive father and Rh negative mother. *B* Pregnancy with Rh positive fetus. Some Rh positive blood enters the mother's blood. *C* As the placenta separates, the mother is further exposed to the Rh positive blood. *D* The mother is sensitized to the Rh posi- tive blood; anti–Rh positive antibodies (triangles) are formed. *E* In subsequent pregnancies with an Rh positive fetus Rh positive red blood cells are attacked by the anti–Rh positive maternal antibodies, causing hemolysis of red blood cells in the fetus.

Although maternal sensitization can now be prevented by appropriate administration of Rh immune globulin (RhIgG), infants still die of hemolytic disease secondary to Rh incompatibility. In the fetus, red blood cell destruction leads to hyperbilirubinemia and anemia. If treatment is not initiated, this anemia can cause marked fetal edema, called **hydrops fetalis.** Congestive heart failure may result, as well as marked jaundice (called *icterus gravis*), which can lead to neurologic damage (*kernicterus*).

The possibility also exists that an Rh negative female fetus carried by an Rh positive mother may become sensitized in utero. This female would not demonstrate signs of hemolytic disease, but because she would be sensitized before even becoming pregnant, she would have a positive antibody screen when receiving prenatal care with her first Rh positive fetus.

Rh sensitization and the resultant hemolytic disease of the newborn are less common today because of the development of RhIgG. See Chapter 32 for treatment of the newborn affected by Rh sensitization.

Screening for Rh Incompatibility and Sensitization

At the first prenatal visit (1) a history is taken of previous sensitization, abortions, blood transfusions, or children who developed jaundice or anemia during the neonatal period; (2) maternal blood type (ABO) and Rh factor are determined, and a routine Rh antibody screen is done; and (3) other medical complications such as diabetes, infections, or hypertension are identified. An antibody screen (indirect Coombs' test) is done to determine if an Rh negative woman is sensitized (has developed isoimmunity) to the Rh antigen. The indirect Coombs' test measures the number of antibodies in the maternal blood. If the Rh negative woman is not D-isoimmunized, a repeat D antibody determination should be made at 28 weeks' gestation (ACOG 1990b).

If the woman is Rh negative (dd), the father of the unborn child is asked to come into the clinic or physician's office to be assessed for his Rh factor and blood type. If he is homozygous for Rh positive (DD), all his offspring will be Rh positive. If he is heterozygous (Dd), 50% of his offspring will be Rh negative and 50% heterozygous for Rh positive. If the father is Rh negative, all their children will be Rh negative, and no Rh incompatibility with the mother will occur. If the father is Rh positive or the mother is known to have previously carried an Rh positive fetus, further testing and careful management are needed.

Titers should be determined every 2–4 weeks beginning at 16–18 weeks, biweekly during the third trimester, and the week before the due date. If the test shows a maternal antibody titer of 1:16 or greater early in pregnancy, a delta optical density (ΔOD) analysis of the amniotic fluid is performed at 26 weeks. If the titer is 1:16 or less late in pregnancy, birth at 38 weeks or spontaneous labor at term can be anticipated.

Negative antibody titers can consistently identify the fetus *not* at risk. However, the titers cannot reliably point out the fetus in danger because the level of the titer does not correlate with the severity of the disease. For instance in a severely sensitized woman antibody titers may be moderately high and remain at the same level although the fetus is being more and more severely affected. Conversely, a woman sensitized by previous Rh positive fetuses may show a high fixed antibody titer during a pregnancy in which the fetus is Rh negative. Fetal assessment includes percutaneous umbilical cord blood sampling (PUBS), amniocentesis, amniotic fluid analysis, and ultrasound.

Ultrasound should be done at 14 to 16 weeks to determine gestational age. Then serial ultrasounds and amniotic fluid analysis should be done to follow fetal progress. The presence of ascites and subcutaneous edema are signs of severe fetal involvement (Scott & Branch 1994). Other indicators of the fetal condition include an increase in fetal heart size, hydramnios, and placental size and texture.

The concentration of bilirubin pigments in the amniotic fluid declines during normal pregnancy. Hemolysis would result in a higher ΔOD level, which is constant or rising. Amniotic fluid, obtained by transabdominal amniocentesis, is separated from its cellular components by centrifuge. The amount of pigment from the degradation of red blood cells can be measured in the amniotic fluid. The fluid is subjected to spectrophotometric studies to determine the severity of the fetal hemolytic process. The ΔOD value and gestational age determine the plan of obstetric-pediatric management.

If the spectrophotometric readings are in zone I (A) ΔOD at 450 nm, a normal or mildly anemic neonate may be anticipated, and birth at term may be permitted. Prognosis for this newborn is good, but phototherapy or exchange transfusion may be necessary. A reading in zone II (B) ΔOD at 450 nm indicates a moderately anemic fetus who may be hydropic or stillborn if born at term. Fetuses with a ΔOD in the upper zone II need to be followed with a PUBS or repeat amniocentesis within the week (ACOG 1990a). Once the fetus reaches viability, induced vaginal or cesarean birth is indicated. The exact timing of birth needs to be determined individually based on factors such as fetal well-being, lung maturity, and previous obstetric history. A fair prognosis and possible need for exchange transfusion are anticipated. Readings within zone III (C) ΔOD at 450 nm indicate a severely affected fetus who may require intrauterine transfusion every 1 to 2 weeks between weeks 26 and 32 until viability is reached, followed by birth, usually by cesarean. Neonatal exchange transfusion is anticipated. Prognosis is guarded.

Fetal monitoring may identify the very ill fetus by documenting less movement or lack of movement. The appearance of sinusoidal pattern suggests fetal anemia and a deteriorating fetal condition (see Chapter 22).

Medical Therapy

The goal of medical management is the birth of a mature fetus who has not developed severe hemolysis in utero. This requires early identification and treatment of maternal conditions that predispose to hemolytic disease, coordinated obstetric-pediatric treatment for the seriously affected newborn, and prevention of Rh sensitization if none is present.

Antepartal Management

Two primary interventions are used by the physician to aid the fetus whose blood cells are being destroyed by maternal antibodies: early birth of the fetus and intrauterine transfusion, both of which carry risks. Ideally, birth should be delayed until fetal pulmonary maturity is confirmed at about 36 to 37 weeks. This is possible for most pregnancies with spectrophotometric readings in zones I and II (A and B).

Intrauterine transfusion is done to correct the anemia produced by the red blood cell hemolysis. This may be done either intravascularly through PUBS or intraperitoneally as early as 18 weeks. Intravascular transfusion has greatly improved the outcome for severely affected fetuses. Under ultrasound visualization the umbilical vein is entered, and the fetus is temporarily paralyzed with 0.1 mg/kg estimated fetal weight of pancuronium bromide. A fetal hematocrit is obtained; then washed, irradiated Rh negative packed red blood cells (PRBCs) are transfused. The volume of PRBCs is determined by a formula based on estimated normal blood volume, the pretransfusion hematocrit, the hematocrit of the blood to be transfused, and the desired hematocrit (Ingardia & Pitcher 1993). Repeat transfusions can be scheduled as necessary until the fetus is sufficiently mature to tolerate birth. Prior to this technology transfusions were done by introducing the needle into the fetal abdomen and peritoneal cavity. Blood was transfused through a catheter into the peritoneal cavity, where diaphragmatic lymphatics absorbed the RBCs into fetal circulation.

About 80% to 90% of transfused fetuses survive. The procedure is hazardous to the fetus, however (Scott & Branch 1994). Complications include fetal distress, fetal hematoma, fetal-maternal hemorrhage, fetal death, and chorioamnionitis (Ingardia & Pitcher 1993). Birth is delayed until at least 32 weeks' gestation if possible. Premature newborns are generally more susceptible to damage from hemolytic disease. They often require exchange transfusion and usually require intensive nursery care.

TABLE 19-7   Rh Sensitization

When trying to work through Rh problems, the nurse should remember the following:

- A potential problem exists when an Rh negative mother and an Rh positive father conceive a child who is Rh positive.
- In this situation the mother may become sensitized or produce antibodies to her fetus' Rh positive blood.

The following tests are used to detect sensitization:

- Indirect Coombs' tests—done on the mother's blood to measure the number of Rh positive antibodies
- Direct Coombs' test—done on the infant's blood to detect antibody-coated Rh positive RBCs.

Based on the results of these tests, the following may be done:

- If the mother's indirect Coombs' test is negative and the infant's direct Coomb's test is negative (confirming that sensitization has not occurred), the mother is given RhIgG within 72 hours of birth.
- If the mother's indirect Coomb's test is positive and her Rh positive infant has a positive direct Coomb's test, RhIgG is *not* given; in this case the infant is carefully monitored for hemolytic disease.
- It is recommended that RhIgG be given at 28 weeks antenatally to decrease possible transplacental bleeding concerns.
- RhIgG is also administered after each abortion (spontaneous or therapeutic), ectopic pregnancy, amniocentesis, chorionic villi sampling (CVS), percutaneous umbilical blood sampling (PUBS), or maternal trauma.

Postpartal Management

The goals of postpartal care are to prevent sensitization in the as-yet-unsensitized pregnant woman and to treat the isoimmune hemolytic disease in the newborn.

The Rh negative mother who has no titer (indirect Coombs' negative, nonsensitized) and who has given birth to an Rh positive fetus (direct Coombs' negative) is given an intramuscular injection of 300 μg RhIgG globulin (RhoGAM, HypRho-D) within 72 hours so that she does not have time to produce antibodies to fetal cells that entered her bloodstream when the placenta separated. This protocol reduces the incidence of antenatal sensitization by 93%. RhIgG works to destroy the fetal cells in the maternal circulation before sensitization occurs, thereby blocking maternal antibody production. This provides temporary passive immunity for the mother, which prevents the development of permanent active immunity (antibody formation).

The normal dose of RhIgG should suppress the immune response to approximately 30 mL Rh positive whole blood. However, if a larger fetomaternal bleed may have occurred, a Kleihauer-Betke test can be performed. This test is used to obtain an estimate of the size of a fetomaternal bleed. Based on the findings an additional 300 μg of RhIgG is given for every 15 mL of fetal red blood cells in the woman's circulation at a rate of 300 μg every 12 hours until the total necessary dose is given (Scott & Branch 1994).

When the woman is Rh negative and not sensitized and the father is Rh positive or unknown, RhIgG is also given after each abortion, ectopic pregnancy, amniocentesis, PUBS, or external version. After any maternal trauma a Kleihauer-Betke test can be performed to identify the need for RhIgG administration. If abortion or ectopic pregnancy occurs in the first trimester, a smaller (50 μg) dose of RhIgG (MICRhoGAM or Mini-Gamulin Rh) is used. A full dose is used following second trimester amniocentesis. Occasionally, sensitization can occur antepartally due to small transplacental bleeds. To prevent this from occurring, an antibody screen is performed on an Rh negative woman at 28 weeks' gestation. If it is negative, 300 μg RhIgG is generally administered prophylactically (Queenan 1994). RhIgG is not given to the newborn or the father. It is not effective for and should not be given to a previously sensitized woman. However, sometimes after childbirth or an abortion the results of the blood test do not clearly show whether or not the mother is already sensitized to the Rh antigen. In such cases RhIgG should be given because it will cause no harm. Table 19–7 summarizes the major considerations in caring for an Rh negative woman. The treatment of the newborn with isoimmune hemolytic disease is discussed in Chapter 32.

APPLYING THE NURSING PROCESS

Nursing Assessment

As part of the initial prenatal history the nurse asks the mother if she knows her blood type and Rh factor. Many women are aware that they are Rh negative and that this status has implications for pregnancy. If the woman knows she is Rh negative, the nurse can assess the woman's knowledge of what that means. The nurse can also ask the woman if she ever received RhIgG, if she has had any previous pregnancies and their outcome, and if she knows her partner's Rh factor. Should the partner be Rh negative, there is no risk to the fetus, who will also be Rh negative.

If the woman does not know what Rh type she is, intervention cannot begin until the initial laboratory data are obtained. Once that is done, the nurse plans intervention based on the findings.

If the woman becomes sensitized during her pregnancy, nursing assessment focuses on the knowledge level and coping skills of the woman and her family. The nurse also provides ongoing assessment during procedures to evaluate fetal well-being, such as ultrasound and amniocentesis.

Postpartally, the nurse reviews data about the Rh type of the fetus. If the fetus is Rh positive, the mother is Rh negative, and no sensitization has occurred, nursing assessment reveals the need to administer RhIgG.

Nursing Diagnosis

Nursing diagnoses that might apply to the pregnant woman at risk for Rh sensitization include the following:

- Knowledge deficit related to a lack of understanding of the need to receive RhIgG and when it should be administered
- Ineffective individual coping related to depression secondary to the development of indications of the need for fetal exchange transfusion

Nursing Plan and Implementation

During the antepartal period the nurse explains the mechanisms involved in isoimmunization and answers any questions the woman and her partner may have. It is imperative that the woman understand the importance of receiving RhIgG after every spontaneous or therapeutic abortion or ectopic pregnancy if she is not already sensitized. The nurse also explains the purpose of the RhIgG administered at 28 weeks if the woman is not sensitized.

If the woman is sensitized to the Rh factor, it poses a threat to any Rh positive fetus she carries. The nurse provides emotional support to the family to help them deal with their grief and any feelings of guilt about the infant's condition. Should an intrauterine transfusion become necessary, the nurse continues to provide emotional support while also assuming his or her responsibilities as part of the health care team.

During labor the nurse caring for an Rh negative woman who has not been sensitized ensures that the woman's blood is assessed for any antibodies and also has been cross-matched for RhIgG. On the postpartum unit the nurse generally is responsible for administering the RhIgG (Procedure 19–2: Administration of Rh Immune Globulin [RhIgG] on page 514).

Evaluation

Anticipated outcomes of nursing care include:

- The woman is able to explain the process of Rh sensitization and its implications for her unborn child and for subsequent pregnancies.
- If the woman has not been sensitized, she is able to explain the importance of receiving RhIgG when necessary and cooperates with the recommended dosage schedule.
- The woman gives birth to a healthy newborn.
- If complications develop for the fetus (or newborn), they are detected quickly, and therapy is instituted.

Nursing Action	Rationale
Objective: Confirm that Rh immune globulin is indicated.	
Confirm that mother is Rh negative by checking her prenatal or intrapartal record. Then confirm that sensitization has not occurred—maternal indirect Coombs' negative.	*Sensitization occurs when an Rh negative woman is exposed to Rh positive blood. She develops antibodies to the Rh positive blood. These antibodies can attack the fetal red blood cells, causing profound anemia. If both the direct and indirect Coombs' tests are negative, sensitization has not occurred, and Rh immune globulin is indicated.*
Confirm that infant is Rh positive. (A sample of the infant's cord blood is generally sent to the lab immediately after birth for typing and cross-matching.) If infant is Rh positive, confirm that sensitization has not occurred—direct Coombs' negative.	
Objective: Confirm that the woman does not have a history of allergy to immune globulin preparations.	
Review entries on medication allergies in client chart, and ask woman specifically whether she has had any allergic reactions to medications, globulins, or blood products.	*Rh immune globulin is made from the plasma portion of blood. Allergic reactions are possible.*
Objective: Explain purpose and procedure. Have consent signed.	
Many agencies require informed consent before administering Rh immune globulin.	*The woman should clearly understand the purpose of the procedure, its rationale, and the procedure itself, including any risks. Generally, the primary side effects are erythema and tenderness at the injection site and allergic responses.*
Objective: Obtain correct medication.	
Rh immune globulin is available from the blood bank or pharmacy according to agency policy. Lot numbers for the drug and the cross-match should be the same.	*Because blood products are involved in the preparation, careful verification is essential.*
Objective: Confirm client identity, and administer medication in deltoid muscle.	
Medication is administered intramuscularly within 72 hours of childbirth. The normal dose of 300 μg provides passive immunity following exposure of up to 15 mL of transfused RBCs or 30 mL of fetal blood. If a larger bleed is suspected (as in cases of severe abruptio placentae), additional doses may be administered at one time using multiple sites or at regular intervals as long as all doses are given within 72 hours of childbirth.	*The medication causes passive immunity to occur and "tricks" the body into believing that it is not necessary to develop antibodies. Immunization is indicated any time there is a potential for maternal exposure to Rh positive blood. It is given prophylactically at 28 weeks' gestation, within 72 hours after the birth of an Rh positive Coombs' negative child, and following any spontaneous or therapeutic abortion, ectopic pregnancy, or amniocentesis.*
Objective: Complete education for self-care.	
Provide opportunities for the woman to ask questions and express concerns.	*Many women, especially primigravidas, are not aware of the risks for an Rh positive fetus of a sensitized Rh negative mother. They must understand the importance of receiving medication for each pregnancy to ensure continued protection.*
Objective: Complete client record.	
Chart according to agency procedure. Most agencies chart lot number, route, dose, client education.	*Provides a permanent record.*

CARE OF THE WOMAN AT RISK DUE TO ABO INCOMPATIBILITY

ABO incompatibility is rather common (occurring in 12% of pregnancies) but rarely causes significant hemolysis. In most cases ABO incompatibility is limited to type O mothers with a type A or B fetus. The group B fetus of an A mother and the group A fetus of a B mother are only occasionally affected. Group O infants, because they have no antigenic sites on the red blood cells, are never affected regardless of the mother's blood type. The incompatibility occurs as a result of the maternal antibodies present in her serum and interaction between the antigen sites on the fetal red blood cells.

Anti-A and anti-B antibodies are naturally occurring; that is, women are naturally exposed to the A and B antigens through the foods they eat and through exposure to infection by gram-negative bacteria. As a result some women have high serum anti-A and anti-B titers before they become pregnant. Once the woman becomes pregnant, the maternal serum anti-A and anti-B antibodies cross the placenta and produce hemolysis of the fetal red blood cells. With ABO incompatibility the first infant is frequently involved, and no relationship exists between the appearance of the disease and repeated sensitization from one pregnancy to the next.

Unlike the case of Rh incompatibility, treatment is never warranted antepartally. As part of the initial assessment, however, the nurse should note whether the potential for an ABO incompatibility exists. This alerts care givers so that following birth the newborn can be assessed carefully for the development of hyperbilirubinemia (Chapter 32).

CARE OF THE WOMAN REQUIRING SURGERY DURING PREGNANCY

Although elective surgery should be delayed until the postpartal period, essential surgery can generally be undertaken during pregnancy. Surgery does pose some risks. The incidence of spontaneous abortion is increased for women who have surgery in the first trimester. There is also an increased incidence of fetal mortality and of low-birth-weight (less than 2500 g) infants. When pelvic surgery is necessary, the incidence of premature labor and intrauterine growth retardation increases (Mazze & Källén 1989).

Medical Therapy

Although general preoperative and postoperative care is similar for gravid and nongravid women, special considerations must be kept in mind whenever the surgical client is pregnant. The early second trimester is the best time to operate because there is less risk of causing spontaneous abortion or early labor, and the uterus is not so large as to impinge on the abdominal field.

The preoperative chest radiograph and electrocardiogram, which are routine for persons over age 40, should be done on the same basis for the pregnant woman. If a chest radiograph is done, the fetus should be shielded from the radiation. Because of decreased intestinal motility and decreased free gastric acid secretion during pregnancy, stomach emptying time is delayed, which increases risk of vomiting during induction of anesthesia and during the postoperative period. Therefore a nasogastric tube is recommended prior to major surgery. An indwelling urinary catheter prevents bladder distention, decreases risk of injury to the bladder, and promotes ease of monitoring output. Support stockings during and after surgery help prevent venous stasis and the development of thrombophlebitis. Fetal heart tones must be monitored before, during, and after surgery.

Pregnancy causes increased secretions of the respiratory tract and engorgement of the nasal mucous membrane, often making breathing through the nose difficult. Because of this, pregnant women often need an endotracheal tube for respiratory support during surgery. Care givers must guard against maternal hypoxia during surgery because uterine circulation will be decreased and fetal oxygenation can decline very quickly. During surgery and the recovery period the woman is positioned to allow optimal uteroplacental-fetal circulation. A wedge is placed under her hip to tip the uterus and thereby avoid pressure by the fetus on the maternal vena cava.

Spinal or epidural anesthesia is preferred because local anesthetics are not associated with birth defects. Caution must be exercised because this type of anesthesia may produce hypotension and respiratory apnea in the pregnant woman. The frequency and degree of the hypotension increase with higher anesthetic levels. This can be prevented in many cases with a preanesthetic infusion of 900 to 1000 mL of fluid.

Blood loss during surgery is monitored carefully. Measurement of fetal heart tones gives the best indication of blood loss. Because of the normal increased blood volume of pregnancy, uterine blood flow may be reduced significantly before the maternal blood pressure begins to fall. Fluid replacement should be done with balanced electrolyte solution and, if needed, with whole blood.

APPLYING THE NURSING PROCESS

Nursing Assessment

During the preoperative period the nurse assesses the pregnant woman's health status in the same way that any preoperative client is assessed. Is there any sign of respiratory infection, fever, urinary tract infection, or anemia? Are laboratory values all within normal limits for surgery (except in the case of emergency surgery, which may, of necessity, be done even with abnormal laboratory values)? Do the woman and her family understand the surgical procedure? Do they know what to expect postoperatively? Do they have any questions or concerns?

The nurse also considers the impact of surgery on the woman's pregnancy. Is the fetal heart rate normal? Does the woman understand the implications of surgery with regard to her pregnancy? How is she coping?

Postoperatively, the nurse completes all necessary postoperative assessments and also continues to assess fetal status, primarily by monitoring the fetal heart rate.

Nursing Diagnosis

Nursing diagnoses that might apply to the pregnant woman who requires surgery include the following:

- Altered tissue perfusion (fetal) related to the effects of general anesthesia on fetal oxygenation
- Anxiety related to lack of knowledge of preoperative and postoperative procedures

Nursing Plan and Implementation

Much of the nurse's care during the preoperative period is directed toward the educational needs of the woman and her family. The nurse plans time to review the procedure and answer any questions the family may have. The nurse recognizes that the need for surgery during the woman's pregnancy is probably very distressing for the family. The nurse works to help decrease their anxiety by providing information and emotional support.

Postoperatively, the nurse is caring for two clients: the mother and her unborn child. In addition to monitoring the status of both, the nurse considers both in providing care. If surgery is done in the first trimester, the nurse should be aware of the potential teratogenic effect of any medications prescribed and should discuss the implications with the surgeon and obstetrician. During the third trimester the nurse, recognizing the potential for vena caval syndrome if the woman lies flat on her back, helps the woman maintain a side-lying position. To avoid inadequate oxygenation, the nurse also encourages the woman to turn, breathe deeply, and cough regularly and also to use any ventilation therapy, such as incentive spirometry, to avoid developing pneumonia. The pregnant woman is also at increased risk for thrombophlebitis, so the nurse applies antiembolism stockings, encourages leg exercises while the woman is confined to bed, and begins ambulation as soon as possible. The nurse also encourages the woman to maintain or resume an adequate diet as soon as possible. If cultural factors influence the woman's dietary practices, the nurse and dietitian should work together to meet the woman's needs.

Discharge teaching is especially important. The woman and her family should have a clear understanding of what to expect regarding activity level, discomfort, diet, medications, and any special considerations. In addition they should know any warning signs that they should report to their physician immediately.

Evaluation

Anticipated outcomes of nursing care include:

- The woman is able to explain the surgical procedure, its risks and benefits, and its implications for her pregnancy.
- Care givers maintain adequate oxygenation throughout surgery and postoperatively.
- Potential complications are avoided or detected early and treated successfully.
- The woman is able to describe any necessary post-discharge activities, limitations, and follow-up and agrees to cooperate with the recommended regimen.
- The woman maintains her pregnancy successfully.

CARE OF THE WOMAN SUFFERING TRAUMA FROM AN ACCIDENT

Accidents and injury are the leading cause of death in women of reproductive age. Accidental injury has been estimated to complicate approximately 7% of all pregnancies and account for 200,000 injuries to pregnant women each year (Leiserowitz & Smith 1991; Pimentel 1991). Domestic abuse may be the etiology of trauma and is discussed in the next section.

In early pregnancy body changes increase the potential for injury through fatigue, fainting spells, and hyperventilation. Late in pregnancy the woman has less balance and coordination and may fall. Her protruding abdomen is vulnerable to a variety of minor injuries. The fetus is usually well protected by the amniotic fluid, which distributes the force of a blow equally in all directions, and by the muscle layers of the uterus and abdominal wall. In early pregnancy, while the uterus is still in the pelvis, it is shielded from blows by the surrounding pelvic organs, muscles, and bony structures. Trauma that causes concern includes blunt trauma, from an automobile accident, for example; penetrating abdominal injuries, such as knife and gunshot wounds; and the complications of maternal shock, premature labor, and spontaneous abortion.

Maternal mortality most often occurs from head trauma or hemorrhage. Uterine rupture may result from strong deceleration forces in an automobile accident with or without seat belts. However, seat belts worn low under the abdomen are recommended. Traumatic separation of the placenta can occur; it results in a high rate of fetal mortality. Premature labor is another serious hazard to the fetus, often following rupture of membranes during an accident. Premature labor can ensue even if the woman is not injured.

Maternal fractures, even of the pelvis, are tolerated well. However, ruptured bladder, retroperitoneal hemorrhage, and shock are complications to watch for with a fractured pelvis.

Complications caused by trauma are more common after assault than after motor vehicle accidents. Fetal or placental injury occurs in 89% of gunshot wounds to the abdomen, with a 66% chance of perinatal mortality. Stab wounds tend to cause less damage than bullet wounds.

Medical Therapy

The goal of medical therapy is to stabilize the injury and promote well-being for both mother and fetus. Thus medical therapy initially focuses on ensuring airway adequacy, maintaining ventilation and adequate circulatory volume, controlling acute bleeding, and splinting fractures to prevent vascular or tissue injury. Once the mother is stabilized, fetal status is assessed.

Care must be taken at the scene of the injury to avoid the development of supine hypotensive syndrome. A wedge is generally placed under the woman's right hip. A neck brace is used if a neck injury is suspected, or the woman is placed on a backboard, and the entire board is tilted to displace the uterus. Prompt treatment of maternal hypotension or hypovolemia also averts poor fetal oxygenation. Obstetric consultation is necessary to ensure that the needs of both mother and fetus are met.

In cases of noncatastrophic trauma, that is, where the mother's life is not directly threatened, fetal monitoring for 4 hours should be sufficient if there is no vaginal bleeding, uterine tenderness, contractions, or leaking amniotic fluid. Abruptio placentae may occur following a blow to the abdomen as the flexible myometrium of the uterus sustains a contour-changing impact that the relatively inelastic placenta cannot match. The increased intrauterine pressure during the blow further shears the placenta from the underlying decidua basalis. Abruptio placentae may occur in up to 5% of women who sustain minor injuries (ACOG 1991) and in up to 66% of women who sustain major abdominal trauma (Rosenfeld 1990). Increased uterine irritability in the first few hours following trauma helps identify women who may be at high risk for this potentially catastrophic complication. If the woman is bleeding, contracting, or has uterine tenderness or a nonreassuring fetal heart rate tracing, a 24–48 hour observation is recommended.

Fetomaternal hemorrhage occurs four to five times more often in pregnant women who have experienced trauma. A Kleihauer-Betke test may be useful in helping identify unsensitized, Rh negative women who have experienced fetal-maternal bleeds due to trauma. RhIgG should be given to any unsensitized Rh negative woman to be certain she is covered for small fetal hemorrhages that may be below the sensitivity of the Kleihauer-Betke test.

There has been controversy regarding the use of beta-adrenergic tocolytics in pregnant women following trauma because of the concerns regarding hemodynamic instability and the potential for masking uterine irritability or contractions that forewarn of abruptio placentae. Radiographic studies should be performed as needed to evaluate injuries regardless of fetal exposure.

When CPR is performed on the pregnant woman late in gestation, perimortem cesarean birth is advocated if CPR is unsuccessful in the first 4 minutes. Chest compressions are less effective in the third trimester due to compression of the inferior vena cava by the gravid uterus. Cesarean birth alleviates this compression and improves resuscitation efforts in both the fetus and the mother.

APPLYING THE NURSING PROCESS

Nursing Assessment

Each individual must be assessed according to the type and extent of her injuries. As with all trauma victims initial assessments focus on adequacy of the airway, evidence of breathing, existence of cardiovascular stability, and extent of injury. When an injured woman is pregnant, it is necessary to assess fetal status as well in order to avoid fetal hypoxia. Frequent maternal blood gas determinations are indicated if respiratory function is compromised.

Assessment should include a review of the specific history of past and present pregnancies to avoid incorrect interpretation of vital signs. Care givers do diagnostic tests as necessary, avoiding radiology in favor of ultrasonography whenever possible.

Ongoing assessments include evaluation of intake and output and other indicators of shock, normal postoperative evaluation in those women requiring surgery, determination of neurologic status, and assessment of mental outlook and anxiety level.

Nursing Diagnosis

Nursing diagnoses that might apply to the pregnant woman suffering trauma include the following:

- Pain related to the effects of the trauma experienced

- Constipation related to immobility secondary to the effects of the accident
- Fear related to the effects of the trauma on fetal well-being

Nursing Plan and Implementation

As a member of the health care team the nurse is actively involved in the ongoing assessment of the status of the woman and fetus. The nurse also has a primary responsibility to assess the childbearing woman's emotional state. The trauma victim must be oriented to her situation and receive explanation and reinforcement as necessary to help her understand any interventions. Family members should be involved as appropriate. The nurse also gives the pregnant woman an opportunity to discuss her feelings and concerns.

Evaluation

Anticipated outcomes of nursing care include:

- The woman and her family are able to understand the effects of the trauma on her and on her unborn child.
- Adequate oxygenation is maintained to promote fetal well-being.
- The woman's pain is adequately relieved, and her trauma is treated.
- Potential complications are quickly identified, and appropriate interventions are instituted.
- The woman gives birth to a healthy newborn.
- If the trauma results in fetal demise, the woman is able to verbalize her feelings and begin working through the grief process.

CARE OF THE BATTERED PREGNANT WOMAN

Domestic violence is an "overwhelming moral, economic, and public health burden" according to former Surgeon General C. Everett Koop (ACOG 1989a). Such violence often begins or increases during pregnancy. Physical abuse may result in loss of pregnancy, preterm labor, low-birth-weight infants, injury to the fetus, and fetal death (Bohn 1990). The first step toward helping the battered woman is to identify her. She needs support, confidence in her decision making, and the recognition that she can help herself.

Chronic psychosomatic symptoms can be an indicator of abuse. The woman may have nonspecific or vague complaints. It is important to assess old scars around the head, chest, arms, abdomen, and genitalia. Any bruising or evidence of pain is also evaluated. The nurse should be especially alert for signs of bruising or injury to the woman's breasts, abdomen, or genitalia because these areas are common targets of violence during pregnancy. Other indicators include a decrease in eye contact, silence when the partner is in the room, and a history of nervousness, insomnia, drug overdose, or alcohol problems. Frequent visits to the emergency room and a history of accidents without understandable causes are possible indicators of abuse.

The goals of treatment are to identify the woman at risk, increase her decision-making abilities to decrease the potential for further abuse, and provide a safe environment for the pregnant woman and her unborn child.

It is important to provide an environment that is private, accepting, and nonjudgmental so the woman can express her concerns. She needs to be aware of community resources available to her, such as emergency shelters; police, legal, and social services; and counseling. Nurses need to recognize that, ultimately, it is the woman's decision to either seek assistance or return to old patterns.

Because abuse often begins during pregnancy, it may be a new and unexpected experience for the woman. She may believe that it is an isolated incident, which will occur only during the pregnancy. She needs to know that battering may well occur following childbirth and may extend to the child as well. This is an important time for the nurse to provide information and establish a trusted link for the woman with a health care professional. Although the nurse may feel unsuccessful if the woman chooses to return to her partner, in the long term the information the nurse provides may help the woman make choices that end the violence. For further discussion see Chapter 11.

CARE OF THE WOMAN WITH A TORCH INFECTION

Infectious diseases in the TORCH group are those identified as causing serious harm to the embryo-fetus. These are toxoplasmosis, rubella, cytomegalovirus, and herpes simplex virus. (Some sources identify the O as "other infections.") The TORCH identification assists health team members to assess quickly the potential risk to each woman in pregnancy.

The importance of understanding what these infections are and identifying risk factors cannot be overemphasized. Exposure of the woman during the first 12 weeks of gestation may cause developmental anomalies. The three major viral infections are rubella, cytomegalovirus, and herpes simplex virus. Toxoplasmosis is a protozoal infection.

Toxoplasmosis

Toxoplasmosis is caused by the protozoan *Toxoplasma gondii*. It is innocuous in adults, but when contracted in pregnancy, it can profoundly affect the fetus. The pregnant woman may contract the organism by eating raw or poorly cooked meat or by contact with the feces of infected cats, either through the cat litter box or by gardening in areas frequented by cats. The percentage of childbearing women in North America who are seropositive for toxoplasmosis varies. In the United States approximately 20–25% of women in the reproductive age group are seropositive (Faro & Pastorek 1993). In Canada serologic surveys have shown rates in pregnant women to be about 40% (McDonald et al 1990).

Fetal-Neonatal Risks

Maternal infection during the first trimester is associated with the lowest incidence of fetal infection but often results in a spontaneous abortion if the fetus contracts the infection. The highest rate of fetal infection (65%) occurs when the mother contracts the infection in the third trimester, but almost 90% of infants are born without clinical signs of infection. In very mild cases retinochoroiditis may be the only recognizable damage, and it and other manifestations may not appear until adolescence or young adulthood. Severe neonatal disorders associated with congenital infection include convulsions, coma, microcephaly, and hydrocephalus. The infant with a severe infection may die soon after birth. Survivors are often blind, deaf, and severely retarded. Treatment of the mother can reduce the incidence of fetal infection by 60% (Cohen & Goldstein 1991).

Medical Therapy

The goal of medical treatment is to identify the woman at risk for toxoplasmosis and to treat the disease promptly if diagnosed. Diagnosis can be made by serologic testing, including the IgM and IgG fluorescent antibody tests. Elevated titers are detectable 5 days after infection and are usually present for 3 to 4 months. The indirect florescent Ab test (IFAT), the indirect hemagglutination test (IHAT), or the Sabin-Feldman dye test are also used to establish the diagnosis.

If diagnosis can be established by physical findings, history, and positive serologic results, the woman may be treated with sulfadiazine, pyrimethamine, and spiramycin. If toxoplasmosis is diagnosed before 20 weeks' gestation, therapeutic abortion should be considered because although the incidence of fetal transmission is lower in early pregnancy, damage to the fetus is generally more severe than if the disease is acquired later in the pregnancy.

APPLYING THE NURSING PROCESS

Nursing Assessment

The incubation period for the disease is 10 days. The woman with acute toxoplasmosis may be asymptomatic, or she may develop myalgia, malaise, rash, splenomegaly, and enlarged posterior cervical lymph nodes. Symptoms usually disappear in a few days or weeks.

Nursing Diagnosis

Nursing diagnoses that might apply to the pregnant woman with toxoplasmosis include the following:

- Risk for altered health maintenance related to lack of knowledge about ways in which a pregnant woman can contract toxoplasmosis
- Anticipatory grieving related to potential effects on infant of maternal toxoplasmosis

Nursing Plan and Implementation

The nurse caring for women during the antepartal period has the primary opportunity to discuss methods of prevention of toxoplasmosis with the childbearing woman. The woman must understand the importance of avoiding poorly cooked or raw meat, especially pork, beef, lamb, and, in the arctic region, caribou. Fruits and vegetables should be washed. She should avoid contact with the cat litter box by having someone else clean it. In addition, because it takes approximately 48 hours for the cat's feces to become infectious, the litter should be cleaned frequently. The nurse should also discuss the importance of wearing gloves when gardening and of avoiding garden areas frequented by cats.

Evaluation

Anticipated outcomes of nursing care include:

- The woman is able to discuss toxoplasmosis, its methods of transmission, the implications for her fetus, and measures she can take to avoid contracting it.
- The woman implements health measures to avoid contracting toxoplasmosis.
- The woman gives birth to a healthy newborn.

Rubella

The effects of rubella (German measles) are no more severe for pregnant women, nor are there greater complications in pregnant women, than in nonpregnant women of comparable age. However, the effects of this infection on the fetus and newborn are great because rubella causes a chronic infection that begins in the first trimester of pregnancy and may persist for months after birth.

An assessment of risk factors (Kaplan et al 1990) showed that first-time mothers were at highest risk of infection, although 39% of women giving birth to infants with congenital rubella syndrome (CRS) had had at least one previous live birth. Young, Black, and Hispanic first-time mothers are at higher risk for bearing an infant with CRS. Therefore nurses need to be aware of the importance of postpartum immunization to decrease unnecessary perinatal transmission. These figures also emphasize the need for routine immunization programs in the total population, targeting the high-risk populations (young, Black, Hispanic, and immigrants from Southeast Asia).

Fetal-Neonatal Risks

The period of greatest risk for the teratogenic effects of rubella on the fetus is during the first trimester, when 50%–90% of the fetuses exposed will be affected, resulting in spontaneous abortion or serious abnormalities. If infection occurs early in the second trimester, the resultant fetal effect is most often permanent hearing impairment, microcephaly, or psychomotor retardation (Faro & Pastorek 1993).

Clinical signs of congenital infection are congenital heart disease, IUGR, and cataracts. Cardiac involvements most often seen are patent ductus arteriosus and narrowing of peripheral pulmonary arteries. Cataracts may be unilateral or bilateral and may be present at birth or develop in the neonatal period. A petechial rash is seen in some infants, and hepatosplenomegaly and hyperbilirubinemia are frequently seen. Other abnormalities, such as mental retardation or cerebral palsy, may become evident in infancy. Diagnosis in the newborn can be conclusively made in the presence of these conditions and with an elevated rubella IgM antibody titer at birth.

Infants born with congenital rubella syndrome are infectious and should be isolated. These infants may continue to shed the virus for months.

The expanded rubella syndrome relates to effects that may develop for years after the infection. These include an increased incidence of insulin-dependent diabetes mellitus; sudden hearing loss; glaucoma; and a slow, progressive form of encephalitis.

Medical Therapy

The best therapy for rubella is prevention. Live attenuated vaccine is available and should be given to all children. Women of childbearing age should be tested for immunity and vaccinated if susceptible and if it is established that they are not pregnant. Health counseling in high school and in premarital clinic visits can emphasize the importance of screening prior to planning a pregnancy.

As part of the prenatal laboratory screen the woman is evaluated for rubella using hemagglutination inhibition (HAI), a serology test. The presence of a 1:16 titer or greater is evidence of immunity. A titer less than 1:8 indicates susceptibility to rubella.

Because the vaccine is made with attenuated virus, pregnant women are not vaccinated. However, it is considered safe for newly vaccinated children to have contact with pregnant women.

If a woman who is pregnant becomes infected during the first trimester, therapeutic abortion is an alternative.

APPLYING THE NURSING PROCESS

Nursing Assessment

A woman who develops rubella during pregnancy may be asymptomatic or may show signs of a mild infection, including a maculopapular rash, lymphadenopathy, muscular achiness, and joint pain. The presence of IgM antirubella antibody is diagnostic of a recent infection. These titers remain elevated for approximately 1 month following infection.

Nursing Diagnosis

Nursing diagnoses that may apply to the woman who develops rubella early in her pregnancy include:

- Ineffective family coping due to an inability to accept the possibility of fetal anomalies secondary to maternal rubella exposure
- Risk for altered health maintenance related to lack of knowledge about the importance of rubella immunization prior to becoming pregnant

Nursing Plan and Implementation

Nursing support and understanding are vital for the couple contemplating abortion due to a diagnosis of rubella. Such a decision may initiate a crisis for the couple who have planned their pregnancy. They need objective data to understand the possible effects on their fetus and the prognosis for the offspring.

Evaluation

Anticipated outcomes of nursing care include:

- The woman is able to describe the implications of rubella exposure during the first trimester of pregnancy.

- If exposure occurs in a woman who is not immune, she is able to identify her options and make a decision about continuing her pregnancy that is acceptable to her and her partner.

- The nonimmune woman receives the rubella vaccine during the early postpartal period.

- The woman gives birth to a healthy infant.

Cytomegalovirus

Cytomegalovirus (CMV) belongs to the herpes simplex virus group and causes both congenital and acquired infections referred to as *cytomegalic inclusion disease* (CID). The significance of this virus in pregnancy is related to its ability to be transmitted by asymptomatic women across the placenta to the fetus or by the cervical route during birth.

CID is probably the most prevalent infection in the TORCH group. Nearly half of adults have antibodies for the virus. The virus can be found in urine, saliva, cervical mucus, semen, and breast milk. It can be passed between humans by any close contact such as kissing, breastfeeding, and sexual intercourse. Asymptomatic CMV infection is particularly common in children and gravid women. It is a chronic, persistent infection in that the individual may shed the virus continually over many years. The cervix can harbor the virus, and an ascending infection can develop after birth. Although the virus is usually innocuous in adults and children, it may be fatal to the fetus.

Accurate diagnosis in the pregnant woman depends on the presence of CMV in the urine, a rise in IgM levels, and identification of the CMV antibodies within the serum IgM fraction. At present no treatment exists for maternal CMV or for the congenital disease in the newborn.

Fetal-Neonatal Risks

The cytomegalovirus is the most frequent agent of viral infection in the human fetus. It infects 0.5% to 2.5% of newborns. Ninety-five percent of infected fetuses will be asymptomatic at birth, but 5–10% of these infants will go on to develop significant neurologic complications (Faro & Pastorek 1993). Subclinical infections in the newborn are capable of producing mental retardation and auditory deficits, sometimes not recognized for several months, or learning disabilities not seen until childhood. CMV may be the most common cause of mental retardation.

For the fetus this infection can result in extensive intrauterine tissue damage that leads to fetal death; in survival with microcephaly, hydrocephaly, cerebral palsy, or mental retardation; or in survival with no damage at all.

The infected neonate is often SGA. The principal tissues and organs affected are the blood, brain, and liver. However, virtually all organs are potentially at risk. Hemolysis leads to anemia and hyperbilirubinemia. Thrombocytopenia and hepatosplenomegaly may also develop.

Herpes Simplex Virus

Herpes simplex virus (HSV-I or HSV-II) infection can cause painful lesions in the genital area. Lesions may also develop on the cervix. This condition and its implications for nonpregnant women are discussed in Chapter 10. However, because the presence of herpes lesions in the genital tract may profoundly affect the fetus, herpes infection as it relates to a pregnant woman is discussed here as part of the TORCH complex of infections.

Fetal-Neonatal Risks

The risk of transmission to the newborn is highest among women who contract their first herpes infection near the time of birth. It is lower among women with recurrent herpes (CDC 1993). Transmission of the herpes simplex virus to the fetus almost always occurs after the membranes rupture, as the virus ascends from active lesions or during vaginal birth, when the fetus comes in contact with genital lesions. Transplacental infection is rare.

If active HSV infection occurs during the first trimester, there is a 20% to 50% rate of spontaneous abortion or stillbirth (Stagno & Whitley 1985). Infection after 20 weeks of gestation is associated with an increased risk of preterm labor.

Approximately 50% of all infants who are born vaginally when the mother is shedding HSV in her vagina or cervix develop some form of herpes infection. Of these infants approximately half will die if untreated, and half will have severe complications (Faro & Pastorek 1993). Asymptomatic women may also harbor the virus. In a recent long-term study, over one-half of infants who developed neonatal herpes infection were born to women with no known history of the infection (Harger 1990).

The infected infant is often asymptomatic at birth but after an incubation period of 2 to 12 days develops symptoms of fever (or hypothermia), jaundice, seizures, and poor feeding. Approximately one-half of infected infants develop the characteristic vesicular skin lesions. Vidarabine has been useful in decreasing serious effects from neonatal herpes, but no definitive treatment exists as yet. Some experts treat asymptomatic infants who were exposed to herpes simplex virus during birth with acyclovir. Positive herpes cultures taken 24 to 48 hours after birth should be obtained before treatment (CDC 1989).

Medical Therapy

Although the vesicular lesions of herpes have a characteristic appearance, they rupture easily. Thus definitive diagnosis is made by culturing active lesions. Because cultures are expensive and not always available, many care givers obtain a discharge from the lesion and prepare a slide as for a Pap test. The presence of multinucleated giant cells indicates herpes.

Treatment is directed first toward relieving the woman's vulvar pain. If the attack is severe, walking, sitting, and even wearing clothing may be painful. The woman may be most comfortable in bed during the peak of the infection. Sitz baths three to four times daily, followed by drying of the vulva with a hair dryer or a light bulb, may promote healing and help prevent secondary infection. Cotton underwear helps keep the genital area dry.

Although acyclovir (Zovirax) does not cure the infection or prevent recurrence, it does reduce healing time of the initial attack and shortens the time that the live virus is in the lesions, thereby reducing the infectious period. Currently, however, it is not recommended for use during pregnancy.

HSV has not been found in breast milk. Present experience shows that breastfeeding is acceptable if the mother washes her hands well to prevent any direct transfer of the virus.

Because most infants become infected when they pass through a birth canal containing HSV, it was previously the practice to do serial cervical cultures. Recently, the Infectious Disease Society for Obstetrics and Gynecology issued new guidelines for the management of HSV in pregnancy. It recommends that a history of HSV infection in the woman or her partner be obtained and recorded at the first prenatal visit. Weekly cultures are not recommended for women with a history of HSV but with no visible lesions. Routine cultures in the last month of pregnancy are of little value because they would have to be performed daily. However, weekly examinations looking for the presence of lesions are recommended. For women with no visible lesions at the time of labor (or rupture of the membranes) vaginal birth should be attempted. For women with visible lesions cesarean birth is indicated to reduce the risk of neonatal infection. Cesarean birth is best attempted within 4 to 6 hours of rupture of membranes to decrease the risk of ascending infection. If membranes have been ruptured more than 12 hours, a vaginal birth is planned. The infant is treated with acyclovir (Faro & Pastorek 1993).

Nursing Assessment

During the initial prenatal visit it is important to learn whether the woman or her partner have had previous herpes infections. If so, ongoing assessment is indicated as pregnancy progresses.

Nursing Diagnosis

Nursing diagnoses that may apply to the pregnant woman with HSV include the following:

- Pain related to the presence of lesions secondary to herpes infection
- Sexual dysfunction related to unwillingness to engage in sexual intercourse secondary to the presence of active herpes lesions
- Ineffective individual coping related to depression secondary to the risk to the fetus if herpes lesions are present at birth

Nursing Plan and Implementation

Nurses need to be particularly concerned with client education about this fast-spreading disease. Women should be informed about what herpes is, how it is spread, and preventive measures. Women should also receive information about the association of genital herpes with spontaneous abortion, neonatal mortality and morbidity, and the possibility of cesarean birth. A woman needs to inform her future health care providers of her infection. She also should know of the possible association of genital herpes with cervical cancer and the importance of a yearly Pap smear.

The woman who acquired HSV as an adolescent may be devastated as a mature young adult who wants to have a family. Clients may be helped by counseling that allows expression of the anger, shame, and depression so often experienced by women with herpes. Literature may be helpful and is available from Planned Parenthood and many public health agencies. The American Social Health Association has established the HELP program to provide information and the latest research results on genital herpes. The association has a quarterly journal, *The Helper*, for nurses and herpes clients.

Evaluation

Anticipated outcomes of nursing care include:

- The woman is able to describe her infection with regard to its method of spread, expected medical therapy, comfort measures, implications for her pregnancy, and long-term implications.

- The woman has appropriate cultures done as recommended throughout her pregnancy.
- The woman gives birth to a healthy infant.

OTHER INFECTIONS IN PREGNANCY

In addition to the TORCH infections, other infections contribute to risk during pregnancy (Table 19–8). Spontaneous abortion is frequently the result of a severe maternal infection. Evidence exists that links infection and prematurity. In addition, if the pregnancy is carried to term in the presence of infection, the risk of maternal and fetal morbidity and mortality increases. Thus it is essen-

---

TABLE 19-8 Infections That Put Pregnancy at Risk

Condition and Causative Organism	Signs and Symptoms	Treatment	Implications for Pregnancy
Urinary Tract Infections			
Asymptomatic bacteriuria (ASB): *E coli, Klebsiella, Proteus* most common	Bacteria present in urine on culture with no accompanying symptoms.	Oral sulfonamides early in pregnancy, ampicillin and nitrofurantoin (Furadantin) in late pregnancy.	Women with ASB in early pregnancy may go on to develop cystitis or acute pyelonephritis by third trimester if not treated. Oral sulfonamides taken in the last few weeks of pregnancy may lead to neonatal hyperbilirubinemia and kernicterus.
Cystitis (lower UTI): Causative organisms same as ASB	Dysuria, urgency, frequency; low-grade fever and hematuria may occur. Urine culture (clean catch) show ↑ leukocytes. Presence of 10^5 (100,000) or more colonies bacteria per mL urine.	Same.	If not treated, infection may ascend and lead to acute pyelonephritis.
Acute pyelonephritis: Causative organisms same as ASB	Sudden onset. Chills, high fever, flank pain. Nausea, vomiting, malaise. May have decreased urine output, severe colicky pain, dehydration. Increased diastolic BP, positive FA test, low creatinine clearance. Marked bacteremia in urine culture, pyuria, WBC casts.	Hospitalization; IV antibiotic therapy. Other antibiotics safe during pregnancy include carbenicillin, methenamine, cephalosporins. Catheterization if output is ↓. Supportive therapy for comfort. Follow-up urine cultures are necessary.	Increased risk of premature birth and IUGR. These antibiotics interfere with urinary estriol levels and can cause false interpretations of estriol levels during pregnancy.
Vaginal Infections			
Vulvovaginal candidiasis (yeast infection): *Candida albicans*	Often thick, white, curdy discharge, severe itching, dysuria, dyspareunia. Diagnosis based on presence of hyphae and spores in a wet mount preparation of vaginal secretions.	Intravaginal insertion of miconazole or clotrimazole suppositories at bedtime for 1 week. Cream may be prescribed for topical application to the vulva if necessary.	If the infection is present at birth and the fetus is born vaginally, the fetus may contract thrush.
Bacterial vaginosis: *Gardnerella vaginalis*	Thin, watery, yellow-gray discharge with foul odor often described as "fishy." Wet mount preparation reveals "clue cells." Application of KOH (potassium hydroxide) to a specimen of vaginal secretions produces a pronounced fishy odor.	Nonpregnant women treated with metronidazole (Flagyl). In first trimester, pregnant women treated with clindamycin. In second and third trimesters, metronidazole vaginal gel or clindamycin cream preferred (CDC 1993).	Metronidazole has potential teratogenic effects. Possible ↑ risk of PROM and preterm birth. Confirmatory studies needed (CDC 1993).
Trichomoniasis: *Trichomonas vaginalis*	Occasionally asymptomatic. May have frothy greenish-gray vaginal discharge, pruritus, urinary symptoms. Strawberry patches may be visible on vaginal walls or cervix. Wet mount preparation of vaginal secretions shows motile flagellated trichomonads.	During early pregnancy symptoms may be controlled with clotrimazole vaginal suppositories. Both partners are treated, but no adequate treatment exists. After first trimester, a single 2 g dose of metronidazole may be used (CDC 1993).	Metromidazole has potential teratogenic effects. Associated with ↑ risk of PROM and preterm birth (CDC 1993).

TABLE 19-8 *continued*

Condition and Causative Organism	Signs and Symptoms	Treatment	Implications for Pregnancy
Sexually Transmitted Infections			
Chlamydial infection: *Chlamydia trachomatis*	Women are often asymptomatic. Symptoms may include thin or purulent discharge, urinary burning and frequency, or lower abdominal pain. Lab test available to detect monoclonal antibodies specific for *Chlamydia*.	Although nonpregnant women are treated with tetracycline, it may permanently discolor fetal teeth. Thus pregnant women are treated with erythromycin ethyl succinate.	Infant of woman with untreated chlamydial infection may develop newborn conjunctivitis, which can be treated with erythromycin eye ointment (but not silver nitrate). Infant may also develop chlamydial pneumonia. May be responsible for premature labor and fetal death.
Syphilis: *Treponema pallidum*, a spirochete	Primary stage: chancre, slight fever, malaise. Chancre lasts about 4 weeks, then disappears. Secondary stage: occurs 6 weeks to 6 months after infection. Skin eruptions (condyloma lata); also symptoms of acute arthritis, liver enlargement, iritis, chronic sore throat with hoarseness. Diagnosed by blood tests such as VDRL, RPR, FTA-ABS. Dark-field examination for spirochetes may also be done.	For syphilis less than 1 year in duration: 2.4 million U benzathine penicillin G IM. For syphilis of more than 1 year's duration: 2.4 million U benzathine penicillin G once a week for 3 weeks. Sexual partners should also be screened and treated.	Syphilis can be passed transplacentally to the fetus. If untreated, one of the following can occur: second trimester abortion, stillborn infant at term, congenitally infected infant, uninfected live infant.
Gonorrhea: *Neisseria gonorrhoeae*	Majority of women asymptomatic; disease often diagnosed during routine prenatal cervical culture. If symptoms are present they may include purulent vaginal discharge, dysuria, urinary frequency, inflammation and swelling of the vulva. Cervix may appear eroded.	Nonpregnant women are treated with ceftriaxone plus doxycycline. Pregnant women are treated with ceftriaxone plus erythromycin (CDC 1993). If the women is allergic to ceftriaxone, spectinomycin is used. All sexual partners are also treated.	Infection at time of birth may cause ophthalmia neonatorum in the newborn.
Condyloma acuminata: caused by a papovavirus	Soft, grayish-pink lesions on the vulva, vagina, cervix, or anus.	Podophyllin not used during pregnancy. Trichloroacetic acid, liquid nitrogen, or cryotherapy CO_2 laser therapy done under colposcopy is also successful (CDC 1993).	Possible teratogenic effect of podophyllin. Large doses have been associated with fetal death.

tial to maternal and fetal health that infection be diagnosed and treated promptly.

Urinary tract, vaginal, and sexually transmitted infections are discussed in detail in Chapter 10. Table 19–8 provides a summary of these infections and their implications for pregnancy.

KEY CONCEPTS

Hyperemesis gravidarum, excessive vomiting during pregnancy, may cause fluid and electrolyte imbalance, dehydration, and signs of starvation in the mother and, if severe enough, death of the fetus. Treatment is aimed at controlling the vomiting, correcting fluid and electrolyte imbalance, correcting dehydration, and improving nutritional status.

Several health problems associated with bleeding arise from the pregnancy itself, such as spontaneous abortion, ectopic pregnancy, and gestational trophoblastic disease. The nurse needs to be alert to early signs of these situations, to guard the woman against heavy bleeding and shock, to facilitate the medical treatment, and to provide educational and emotional support.

Incompetent cervix, the premature dilatation of the cervix, is the most common cause of second trimester abortion. It is treated surgically with a Shirodkar-Barter operation (cerclage), which involves placing a purse-string suture in the cervix to keep it closed.

Premature rupture of the membranes and preterm labor both place the fetus at risk. Women with PROM and no signs of infection are managed conservatively with bed rest and careful monitoring of fetal well-being. Women with a history of preterm labor may be placed on home fetal monitoring programs. If preterm labor develops, tocolytics are often effective in stopping labor but do have associated side effects.

Hypertension may exist prior to pregnancy or, more often, may develop during pregnancy. Pregnancy-induced hypertension can lead to growth retardation for the fetus and, if untreated, may lead to convulsions (eclampsia) and even death for the mother and fetus. A woman's understanding of the disease process helps motivate her to maintain the required rest periods in the left lateral position. Antihypertensive or anticonvulsive drugs may be part of the therapy.

Rh incompatibility can exist when an Rh negative woman and an Rh positive partner conceive a child who is Rh positive. The use of RhIgG has greatly decreased the incidence of severe sequelae due to Rh incompatibility because the drug "tricks" the body into thinking antibodies have been produced in response to the Rh antigen.

The impact of surgery or trauma on the pregnant woman and her fetus is related to timing in the pregnancy, seriousness of the situation, and other factors influencing the situation.

Physical violence often begins or continues during pregnancy. The nurse needs to be alert for signs of abuse, including bruising or injury to the breasts, abdomen, and genitalia. The woman should be given information about violence and about community resources available to assist her.

Urinary tract infections are a common problem in pregnancy. If untreated, the infection may ascend, causing more serious illness for the mother. Urinary tract infections are also associated with an increased risk of premature labor.

TORCH is an acronym standing for toxoplasmosis, rubella, cytomegalovirus, and herpes, all of which pose a grave threat to the fetus.

Sexually transmitted infections pose less of a threat to the fetus if detected and treated as soon as possible.

REFERENCES

American College of Obstetricians and Gynecologists: *Doctors Announce Campaign to Combat Domestic Violence.* ACOG news release, January 3, 1989a.

American College of Obstetricians and Gynecologists: *Preterm Labor.* ACOG Technical Bulletin no. 133. Washington, DC: ACOG, 1989b.

American College of Obstetricians and Gynecologists: *Management of Isoimmunization in Pregnancy.* ACOG Technical Bulletin no. 148. Washington, DC: ACOG, 1990a.

American College of Obstetricians and Gynecologists: *Prevention of D Isoimmunization.* ACOG Technical Bulletin no. 147. Washington, DC: ACOG, 1990b.

American College of Obstetricians and Gynecologists: *Trauma During Pregnancy.* ACOG Technical Bulletin no. 161. Washington, DC: ACOG, 1991.

American College of Obstetricians and Gynecologists: *Antenatal Corticosteroid Therapy for Fetal Maturation.* ACOG Committee Opinion no. 147. Washington, DC: ACOG, 1994.

Andrusdo KT: The role of oral magnesium in treating PTL: "Normalizer." *OB Pharm* 1988; 1(4):13.

Arias F: *Practical Guide to High-Risk Pregnancy and Delivery*, 2nd ed. St Louis: Mosby-Year Book, 1993.

Aumann GM-E, Baird MM: Risk assessment for pregnant women. In: *High-Risk Pregnancy: A Team Approach*, 2nd ed. Knuppel RA, Drukker JE (editors). Philadelphia: WB Saunders, 1993.

Besinger RE, Niebyl JR: The safety and efficacy of tocolytic agents in the treatment of preterm labor. *Obstet Gynecol Survey* 1990; 45(7):415.

Bishop EH: Acceleration of fetal pulmonary maturity. *Obstet Gynecol* 1981; 58(suppl):48.

Blackburn ST, Loper DL: *Maternal, Fetal, and Neonatal Physiology: A Clinical Perspective.* Philadelphia: WB Saunders, 1992.

Bohn DK: Domestic violence and pregnancy: Implications for practice. *J Nurse-Midwifery* March/April 1990; 35:86.

Bowman JM: Antenatal suppression of Rh alloimmunization. *Clin Obstet Gynecol* 1991; 34(2):296.

Briggs GC et al: *Drugs in Pregnancy and Lactation*, 4th ed. Baltimore: Williams & Wilkins, 1994.

Caritis SN, Kuller JA, Watt-Morse ML: Pharmacologic options for treating preterm labor. In: *Drug Therapy in Obstetrics and Gynecology.* Rayburn WF, Zuspan FP (editors). St Louis: Mosby-Year Book, 1992.

Centers for Disease Control: 1993 Sexually transmitted disease treatment guidelines. *MMWR* 1993; 42(RR-14):4.

Cohen SH, Goldstein E: Infectious disease complications. In: *Manual of Obstetrics: Diagnosis and Therapy.* Niswander KR, Evans AT (editors). Boston: Little, Brown, 1991.

Eganhouse DJ, Burnside SM: Nursing assessment and responsibilities in monitoring the preterm pregnancy. *JOGNN* 1992; 21(5):355.

Faro S, Pastorek JG: Perinatal infections. In: *High-Risk Pregnancy: A Team Approach*, 2nd ed. Knuppel RA, Drukker JE (editors). Philadelphia: WB Saunders, 1993.

Garite TJ, Spellacy WN: Premature rupture of membranes. In: *Danforth's Obstetrics and Gynecology*, 7th ed. Scott JR et al (editors). Philadelphia: Lippincott, 1994.

Giacoia GP, Yaffe S: Perinatal pharmacology. In: *Gynecology and Obstetrics*, vol 3. Sciarri JJ (editor). Philadelphia: Harper & Row, 1992.

Grimes DA, Shultz KF: Randomized controlled trials of home uterine activity monitoring: A review and critique. *Obstet Gynecol* 1992; 79(1):137.

Hallak M, Bottoms S: Accelerated pulmonary maturation from preterm premature rupture of membranes: A myth. *Am J Obstet Gynecol* 1993; 169:1045.

Hammond CB: Gestational trophoblastic neoplasms. In: *Danforth's Obstetrics and Gynecology*, 7th ed. Scott JR et al (editors). Philadelphia: Lippincott, 1994.

Hammond CB, Bachus KE: Ectopic pregnancy. In: *Danforth's Obstetrics and Gynecology*, 7th ed. Scott JR et al (editors). Philadelphia: Lippincott, 1994.

Hankins GVD: Complications of beta-sympathomimetic tocolytic agents. In: *Critical Care Obstetrics.* Clark SL et al (editors). Boston: Blackwell, 1991.

Harger JH: Infection protocols: Genital herpes. *Contemp OB/GYN* May 1990; 35:83.

Hayashi RH, Castillo MS: Bleeding in pregnancy. In: *High-Risk Pregnancy: A Team Approach*, 2nd ed. Knuppel RA, Drukker JE (editors). Philadelphia: WB Saunders, 1993.

Hendricks SK et al: Electrocardiographic changes associated with ritodrine-induced maternal tachycardia and hypokalemia. *Am J Obstet Gynecol* 1986; 154:921.

Heppard MCS, Garite TJ: *Acute Obstetrics: A Practical Guide*. St Louis: Mosby-Year Book, 1992.

Hines T, Jones MB: Can aspirin prevent and treat preeclampsia? *MCN* September/October 1994; 19:258.

Ingardia CJ, Pitcher EF: Additional complications in pregnancy. In: *High-Risk Pregnancy: A Team Approach*, 2nd ed. Knuppel RA, Drukker JE (editors). Philadelphia: WB Saunders, 1993.

Kaplan KM et al: A profile of mothers giving birth to infants with congenital rubella syndrome: An assessment of risk factors. *Am J Dis Child* 1990; 144:118.

Kappy KA, McTigue M, Guzman ER: Premature rupture of the membranes. In: *High-Risk Pregnancy: A Team Approach*, 2nd ed. Knuppel RA, Drukker JE (editors). Philadelphia: WB Saunders, 1993.

Knuppel RA, Drukker JE: Hypertension in pregnancy. In: *High-Risk Pregnancy: A Team Approach*, 2nd ed. Knuppel RA, Drukker JE (editors). Philadelphia: WB Saunders, 1993.

Kochenour N: Normal pregnancy and prenatal care. In: *Danforth's Obstetrics and Gynecology*, 7th ed. Scott JR et al (editors). Philadelphia: Lippincott, 1994.

Krening C: Perinatal hype+rtensive crisis. *NAACOG's Clin Issues Perinatal Women Health Nurs* 1992; 3(3):413.

Kristensen CG: Renal complications. In: *Manual of Obstetrics: Diagnosis and Therapy*. Niswander KR, Evans AT (editors). Boston: Little, Brown, 1991.

Lam F: Miniature pump infusion of terbutaline: An option in preterm labor. *Contemp OB/GYN* January 1989; 34:133.

Lawler SD, Fisher RA, Dent J: A prospective genetic study of complete and partial hydatidiform moles. *Am J Obstet Gynecol* 1991; 164:1270.

Leiserowitz GS, Smith LH: Surgical and gynecologic complications. In: *Manual of Obstetrics: Diagnosis and Therapy*. Niswander KR, Evans AT (editors). Boston: Little, Brown, 1991.

Lipshitz J, Pierce PM, Arntz M: Preterm labor. In: *High-Risk Pregnancy: A Team Approach*, 2nd ed. Knuppel RA, Drukker JE (editors). Philadelphia: WB Saunders, 1993.

Long P, Russell L: Hyperemesis gravidarum. *Perinatal Neonatal Nurs* 1993; 6(4):21.

Lubarsky SL et al: Late postpartum eclampsia revisited. *Obstet Gynecol* April 1994; 83:502.

Mandeville L, Troiano N: *High-Risk Intrapartum Nursing*. Philadelphia: Lippincott, 1992.

Martin JN et al: Pregnancy complicated by preeclampsia-eclampsia with the syndrome of hemolysis, elevated liver enzymes, and low platelet count: How rapid is postpartum recovery? *Obstet Gynecol* November 1990; 76:737.

Martin RW, Morrison JC: Oral magnesium for tocolysis. *Contemp OB/GYN* October 1987; 111.

Mazze RI, Källén B: Reproductive outcome after anesthesia and operation of 5405 cases. *Am J Obstet Gynecol* 1989; 161:1178.

McDonald JC et al: An outbreak of toxoplasmosis in pregnant women in northern Quebec. *J Infect Dis* 1990; 161:769.

McKenry LM, Salerno E: *Pharmacology in Nursing*. St Louis: Mosby-Year Book, 1992.

Merkatz RB, Merkatz IR: The contributions of the nurse and the machine in home uterine activity monitoring systems. *Am J Obstet Gynecol* 1991; 164(4):1159.

Morbidity and Mortality Weekly Report: Congenital syphilis—New York City 1986–88. *MMWR* December 8, 1989; 38:835.

Morbidity and Mortality Weekly Report: Progress toward achieving the 1990 objectives for the nation for sexually transmitted diseases. *MMWR* February 2, 1990; 39:52.

Narrigan D: Preterm labor: Miracle drug revisited. *Network News* 1993; 18(2):6.

Newman V, Fullerton JT, Anderson PO: Clinical advances in the management of severe nausea and vomiting during pregnancy. *JOGNN* 1993; 22(6):483.

Niebyl JR: Detecting incompetent cervix. *Contemp OB/GYN* October 1990; 35:37.

NIH: Effect of corticosteroids for fetal maturation on perinatal outcomes. *National Institutes of Health Consensus Development Conference Statement*. February 28–March 2, 1994.

Oi RH: Diseases of the placenta. In: *Manual of Obstetrics: Diagnosis and Therapy*. Niswander KR, Evans AT (editors). Boston: Little, Brown, 1991.

Pansky M et al: Nonsurgical management of tubal pregnancy. *Am J Obstet Gynecol* 1991; 164:888.

Parsons MT, Spellacy WN: Causes and management of preterm labor. In: *Danforth's Obstetrics and Gynecology*, 7th ed. Scott JR et al (editors). Philadelphia: Lippincott, 1994.

Pimentel L: Mother and child: Trauma in pregnancy. *Emerg Med Clin North Am* 1991; 9(3):549.

Queenan JT: Diagnosis and treatment of Rh-erythroblastosis fetalis. *Contemp OB/GYN* July 1994; 39:48.

Romero R, Ghidini A: Premature rupture of membranes: Amniotic fluid infection. *Obstet Gynecol* 1993; 38(11):75.

Rosenfield JA: Abdominal trauma in pregnancy: When is fetal monitoring necessary? *Postgrad Med* 1990; 88(6):89.

Scott JR: Early pregnancy loss. In: *Danforth's Obstetrics and Gynecology*, 7th ed. Scott JR et al (editors). Philadelphia: Lippincott, 1994a.

Scott JR: Hypersensitive disorders of pregnancy. In: *Danforth's Obstetrics and Gynecology*, 7th ed. Scott JR et al (editors). Philadelphia: Lippincott, 1994b.

Scott JR, Branch DW: Immunologic disorders in pregnancy. In: *Danforth's Obstetrics and Gynecology*, 7th ed. Scott JR et al (editors). Philadelphia: Lippincott, 1994.

Sibai BM: Benefits of low-dose aspirin during pregnancy. *Contemp OB/GYN* March 1994; 39:25.

Sibai BM: Preeclampsia-eclampsia. In: *Gynecology and Obstetrics*, vol 2. Sciarri JJ (editor). Philadelphia: Lippincott, 1989.

Sibai BM: Preeclampsia-eclampsia: Valid treatment approaches. *Contemp OB/GYN* August 1990; 35:84.

Silver HM: Acute hypertensive crisis in pregnancy. *Med Clin North Am* May 1989; 73:623.

Simpson JL: In: *Obstetrics: Normal and Problem Pregnancies*, 2nd ed. Gabbe SG et al (editors). New York: Churchill Livingstone, 1991.

Stagno S, Whitley RJ: Herpesvirus infections of pregnancy. Part II: Herpes simplex virus and varicella zoster virus infections. *N Engl J Med* 1985; 313(21):1327.

Stovall TG et al: Methotrexate treatment of unruptured ectopic pregnancy: A report of 100 cases. *Obstet Gynecol* 1991; 77(5):749.

Vejerslev LO: Clinical management and diagnostic possibilities in hydatidiform mole with coexistent fetus. *Obstet Gynecol Survey* 1991; 46(9):577.

Williams MC: Premature rupture of membranes. In: *Manual of Obstetrics: Diagnosis and Therapy*. Niswander KR, Evans AT (editors). Boston: Little, Brown, 1991a.

Williams MC: Preterm labor. In: *Manual of Obstetrics: Diagnosis and Therapy*. Niswander KR, Evans AT (editors). Boston: Little, Brown, 1991b.

Zuspan FP: Chronic hypertension in pregnancy. *Clin Obstet Gynecol* December 1984; 27:854.

CHAPTER 20

ASSESSMENT OF FETAL WELL-BEING

*M*y first pregnancy was so tenuous that I didn't know from one moment to the next how it would end. I hoped for our baby's safety, but in the end the baby died. When I became pregnant the next time, I was very nervous. Being able to see the baby on ultrasound helped me so much. I knew then that our baby was alive and growing.

KEY TERMS

Amniocentesis

Biophysical profile (BPP)

Chorionic villus sampling (CVS)

Contraction stress test (CST)

Fetal acoustic stimulation test (FAST)

Fetoscopy

Lecithin/sphingomyelin (L/S) ratio

Nonstress test (NST)

Percutaneous umbilical blood sampling (PUBS)

Phosphatidylglycerol (PG)

Surfactant

Ultrasound

OBJECTIVES

Identify indications for antenatal fetal surveillance.

Relate indications for ultrasound examination to the information that can be obtained from this procedure.

Outline pertinent information regarding assessment of fetal activity to be discussed with the woman.

Compare the procedures for the nonstress test, contraction stress test, and biophysical profile, including the indications, contraindications, and predictive value of each.

Describe components of a biophysical profile used to evaluate fetal well-being.

Discuss the nipple stimulation contractions stress test, including important factors to assess evaluation of fetal heart rate response.

Contrast genetic amniocentesis and chorionic villus sampling in evaluation of chromosomes.

Summarize counseling regarding triple screen testing and the implications of abnormal values.

Discuss the nurse's role in antenatal surveillance with regard to high-risk pregnancy management.

*D*uring the past two decades increasing interest has been focused on the problems of the at-risk pregnant woman, both for her health management and for conditions that may affect her unborn child. High-risk women and infants have a significantly greater chance of morbidity and mortality both before and after childbirth. Perinatal morbidity and mortality can be considerably reduced by early, skillful diagnosis and highly intensive antepartum care of the pregnant woman.

Several tests of fetal status are valuable in monitoring the well-being of the fetus. These include ultrasound, computerized tomography, magnetic resonance imaging, fetoscopy, percutaneous umbilical blood sampling, chorionic villus sampling, amniocentesis, and fetal stress tests (Table 20–1). Although the tests have been made as safe as possible, they involve various levels of risk. Fetal and maternal morbidity, mortality, and health status must be considered before antenatal diagnostic and antenatal surveillance tests are discussed with the woman. The woman must be informed of the risks and limitations of each diagnostic procedure. She must be given the opportunity to ask questions concerning the information presented and give her consent to the procedure.

Each pregnancy must be considered individually in terms of what diagnostic and antenatal surveillance test would provide information for the best outcome of the woman and her fetus. One must be certain the advantages outweigh the potential risks and expense. Each of these tests has its limitations in terms of screening, diagnostic accuracy, and applicability. Combining information obtained from various diagnostic and antenatal surveillance tests can provide an overall assessment of fetal well-being during the management of the high-risk pregnancy.

NURSING PROCESS DURING DIAGNOSTIC TESTING

The nurse's role during antepartal testing has continued to expand. The nurse uses the nursing process to guide nursing care during these interactions.

APPLYING THE NURSING PROCESS

Nursing Assessment

The nursing assessment begins with a history, the present pregnancy, and identification of possible indications for the particular diagnostic test. The nurse assesses the

| TABLE 20-1 | Summary of Screening and Diagnostic Tests | |

Goal	Test	Timing
To validate the pregnancy	Ultrasound: gestational sac volume	5 and 6 weeks after LMP by endovaginal ultrasound
To determine how advanced the pregnancy is	Ultrasound: crown-rump length	6 to 10 weeks' gestation
	Ultrasound: biparietal diameter, femur length, abdomen circumference	13 to 40 weeks' gestation
To identify normal growth of the fetus	Ultrasound: biparietal diameter	Most useful from 20 to 30 weeks' gestation
	Ultrasound: head:abdomen ratio	13 to 40 weeks' gestation
	Ultrasound: estimated fetal weight	About 24 to 40 weeks' gestation
To detect congenital anomalies and problems	Ultrasound	18 to 40 weeks' gestation
	Chorionic villus sampling	8 to 12 weeks' gestation
	Fetoscopy	Second and third trimesters
	Percutaneous blood sampling	
To localize the placenta	Ultrasound	Usually in third trimester or before amniocentesis
To assess fetal status	Biophysical profile	Approximately 28 weeks to birth
	Maternal assessment of fetal activity	About 28 weeks to birth
	Nonstress test	Approximately 28 weeks to birth
	Contraction stress test	After 28 weeks
To diagnose cardiac problems	Fetal echocardiography	Second and third trimesters
To assess fetal lung maturity	Amniocentesis	33 to 40 weeks
	L/S ratio	33 weeks to birth
	Phosphatidylglycerol	33 weeks to birth
	Phosphatidylcholine	33 weeks to birth
To obtain more information about breech presentation	Computerized tomography	Just before labor is anticipated or during labor
	X-ray	
	Ultrasound	

information that the woman and her support person have regarding the test, their questions and concerns, and the presence of any psychosociocultural factors that may influence the teaching process. During the test the nurse completes needed assessments to monitor the status of the woman and her fetus.

Nursing Diagnosis

The primary nursing diagnoses are directed toward providing information regarding the diagnostic test and minimizing any risks to the woman and her unborn child. The woman may also be fearful of the outcome of the tests, and nurses can play an important role in providing education, support, and counseling. Examples of nursing diagnoses that may be applicable include the following:

- Knowledge deficit related to insufficient information about the fetal assessment test and its purpose, benefits, risks, and alternatives
- Fear related to the specific test and/or possible unfavorable test results

Nursing Plan and Implementation

The nursing plan of care will be directed toward each specific nursing diagnosis. The nurse generally plays a vital role in providing information about the diagnostic test. The nurse assesses the woman's knowledge of the test and then provides information as needed. Some of the tests require written informed consent, and in these cases the physician or certified nurse-midwife is responsible for informing the woman about all risks and limitations of the test. In this instance the nurse can reinforce and clarify information (Table 20–2).

Because most of the tests are done on an outpatient basis, the interaction time is limited. The nurse therefore uses all basic knowledge of communication, developmental psychology, cultural factors, and so forth to quickly establish a trusting relationship with the woman and her support person.

The nurse also functions as an advocate for the expectant woman by helping her clarify question areas and obtain needed information. The nurse frequently knows the areas about which most women have questions and can anticipate many of their fears. When the woman is not able to verbalize questions, the nurse can assist by bringing up questions that other women have had.

During the testing sessions the nurse addresses the woman's fear by providing support and comfort measures such as relaxation techniques. The presence of the nurse reassures the woman and helps her cope with the tests.

Evaluation

The expected outcomes for the woman who is having diagnostic testing are that she understands the reasons for the test, understands the test results, and has had support during the tests. In addition the tests have been done without complication and the safety of the mother and her unborn child has been maintained.

TABLE 20-2 Sample Nursing Approaches to Pretest Teaching

Assess whether the woman knows the reason the screening or diagnostic test is being recommended.
Examples:
"Has your doctor/nurse-midwife told you why this test is necessary?"
"Sometimes tests are done for many different reasons. Can you tell me why you are having this test?"
"What is your understanding about what the test will show?"

Provide an opportunity for questions.
Examples:
"Do you have any questions about the test?"
"Is there anything that is not clear to you?"

Explain the test procedure, paying particular attention to any preparation the woman needs to do prior to the test.
Example:
"The test that has been ordered for you is designed to . . ." (Add specific information about the particular test. Give the explanation in simple language.)

Validate the woman's understanding of the preparation.
Example:
"Tell me what you will have to do to get ready for this test."

Give permission for the woman to continue to ask questions if needed.
Example:
"I'll be with you during the test. If you have any questions at any time, please don't hesitate to ask."

INDICATIONS FOR ANTENATAL TESTING

Women who are considered to be at risk and for whom the physician/certified nurse-midwife may order assessment of fetal well-being include women with the following complications:

- Decreased fetal movement
- Elevated maternal serum α-fetoprotein (MSAFP)
- Fetal heart rate arrhythmias
- Hemoglobinopathies
- History of preterm labor or birth, risk of preterm labor with current pregnancy, chromosomal or inherited biochemical disorders, and unexplained stillborn or intrapartal fetal death
- Hydramnios or oligohydramnios
- Infections, immunodeficiencies
- Maternal systemic disease such as anemia, antiphospholipid syndrome, chronic hypertension, cyanotic heart disease, gestational or insulin-dependent diabetes, hyperthyroidism, or lupus

- Multiple gestation
- Pregnancy past 41 completed weeks of gestation (postdate)
- Pregnancy-induced hypertension
- Preterm premature rupture of membranes (prior to 37 completed weeks of gestation)
- Suspected intrauterine growth retardation
- Vaginal bleeding

Each of these complications may increase the risk to the expectant woman and her fetus. The list is not complete; other preexisting medical diseases may place the woman at risk and necessitate diagnostic assessment of the fetus.

ULTRASOUND

The introduction of **ultrasound** to the practice of obstetrics in the 1950s dramatically influenced the clinical management of the fetus and mother during pregnancy. Recent improvements in "real-time" ultrasound equipment have permitted continuous immediate visualization of fetal structure and function and made it an indispensable tool for assessment of fetal age, health, and growth (Figure 20–1). As many as 90% of women seeking obstetric care in the United States will probably have at least one ultrasound examination during their pregnancy (Hagen-Ansert 1989).

Ultrasound studies produce continuous images by transmitting sound waves via a transducer applied to the woman's abdomen or labia or an endovaginal transducer inserted into the woman's vagina (Figure 20–2). Echoes from the sound waves are reflected from tissues back to the crystals in the transducer and converted to electrical signals, which are then amplified and displayed on an oscilloscope or television monitor. The difference in the signals reflected from tissues of varying thickness and

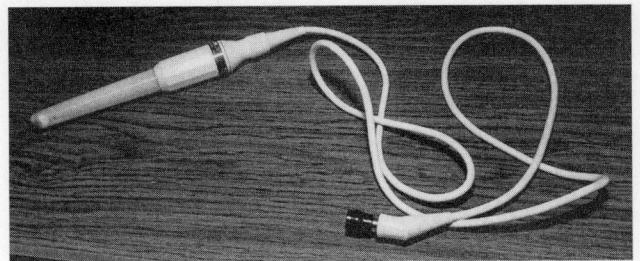

FIGURE 20-2 Endovaginal ultrasound transducer.

density creates the ultrasound image. Real-time imaging gives the impression of motion as the computer continually updates incoming fixed images in the ultrasound machine. The resulting visual images of the fetus may be used to evaluate both structural and functional characteristics, including fetal breathing movements, tone, limb movement, urination, eye movements, and cardiac activity (Figure 20–3).

In the past ultrasound scanning has been categorized as either level I (basic screening) or level II (comprehensive diagnostic). However, the American College of Obstetricians and Gynecologists (1993) has recently suggested that levels I and II be replaced. In order to standardize the content of an ultrasound exam, guidelines have been established for basic screening (level I), limited (no level designation), and comprehensive (level II) ultrasound exams.

A *basic screening ultrasound* examination (now called level I) is adequate for the majority of pregnant women. The ultrasound exam may be done by a nurse, certified nurse-midwife, obstetrician, or ultrasound technician who has had specialized training in performing the exam. The ultrasound exam is intended to yield the following information:

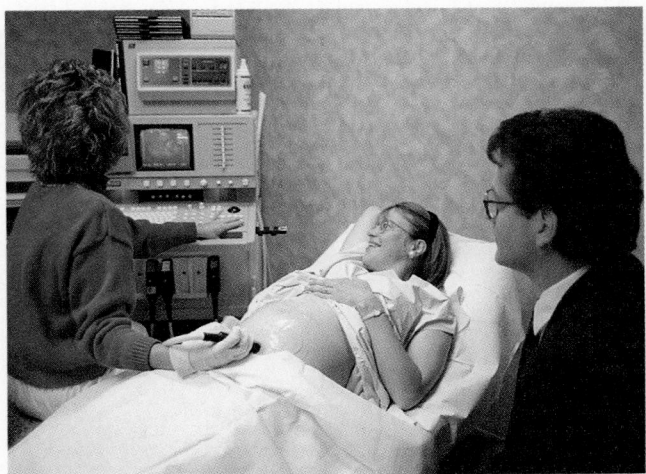

FIGURE 20-1 Ultrasound scanning permits visualization of the fetus in utero.

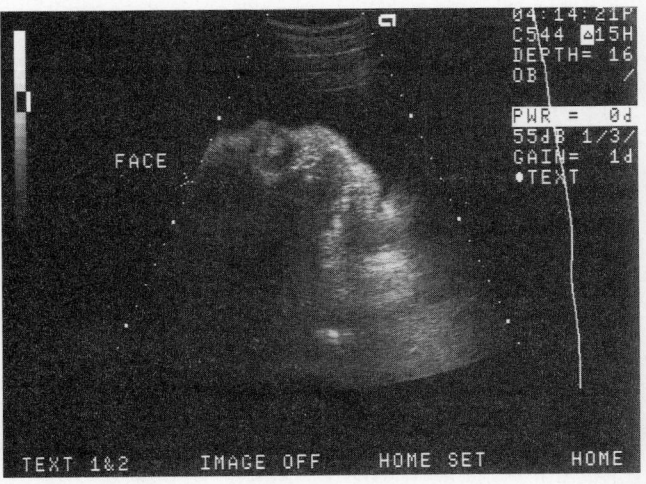

FIGURE 20-3 Ultrasound of fetal face.

- Documentation of fetal life early in the pregnancy
- Fetal number
- Assessment of gestational age
- Survey of fetal anatomy for gross malformations
- Fetal presentation
- Placental location
- Assessment of amniotic fluid volume
- Evaluation for maternal pelvic masses

A *limited ultrasound* examination is more involved than the basic screening examination and may be done in antepartum and/or intrapartum settings. It may include the following:

- More detailed assessment of amniotic fluid volume
- Fetal biophysical profile testing
- Ultrasonography-guided amniocentesis
- Ultrasound used with external cephalic version
- Examination to determine fetal life or death in the presence of complications or cessation of fetal movement
- Localization of placenta in the presence of antepartum hemorrhage
- Confirmation of fetal presentation near term or in the intrapartal area

AWHONN (Association of Women's Health, Obstetric, and Neonatal Nurses) (1993) has set educational guidelines and nursing practice competencies (expectations) for experienced obstetric nurses to perform limited ultrasound examinations. The guidelines indicate that the nurse must complete an educational program that includes didactic presentations and a clinical practicum. Limited ultrasound exams may also be performed by obstetricians and certified nurse-midwives.

A *comprehensive ultrasound* examination (now called level II) may be indicated for a woman who, from previous ultrasound examination or clinical evaluation, is suspected of carrying a fetus with a physiologic or anatomic defect. The comprehensive examination should be conducted by a professional (usually an obstetrician) with extensive training and experience in performing this examination and interpreting findings. Serial ultrasound (more than one ultrasound done over a period of time) may be used to assess and compare structural abnormalities or masses.

Ultrasound safety has been investigated over the course of 15 years in clinical, in vitro, and animal studies. A safe level of ultrasound has been defined arbitrarily as less than 100 mW/cm. Most instruments used in diagnostic ultrasonography produce energies no greater than 10–20 mW/cm. Ultrasound exposure at this intensity has not been found to cause any harmful biologic effects on ultrasound operators (the person who does the exam), pregnant women, fetuses, or other clients. Infants ex-

posed in utero have shown no significant differences in birth weight or length, childhood growth, cognitive function, acoustic or visual ability, or rates of neurologic deficits (Lyons et al 1988).

Procedures

There are three methods of ultrasound scanning: transabdominal, endovaginal, and translabial scanning.

Transabdominal Ultrasound

In the transabdominal approach mineral oil or a transmission gel is applied to the woman's abdomen, and a transducer is moved across the abdomen when the woman has a full or partially full bladder. The woman is advised to drink 1 quart of water within 1 hour before the examination, and she is asked to refrain from emptying her bladder. The bladder is used as an acoustic window for the sound waves to travel through when assessing cervical length, the vagina, placental location, and such. Visualization and location of the placenta are particularly important when vaginal bleeding is noted and placenta previa is the suspected cause.

The woman should always be positioned with a hip roll (right or left) so that her uterus is tilted off the main pelvic blood vessels. Because the uterus enlarges during the pregnancy, lying flat may decrease the blood supply to the uterus and fetus. If she is lying flat, she may experience shortness of breath, nausea, or diaphoresis along with fetal bradycardia. These symptoms may be relieved by having the woman roll over to her side.

Endovaginal Ultrasound

The endovaginal approach utilizes a small lightweight probe inserted into the vagina. Once inserted, the endovaginal probe is close to the structures being imaged and so produces clearer images than those obtained by transabdominal ultrasound. As a result endovaginal ultrasound is used to identify structures and fetal characteristics earlier in pregnancy (Hallak et al 1992).

After the procedure is fully explained to the woman, she is prepared in lithotomy position. The vaginal transducer is covered with a specially fitted sterile sheath, a condom, or one finger of a glove. Coupling gel is then applied to the covering, making insertion into the vagina easier and providing a medium for enhancing the ultrasound image (Goldstein 1992). In addition to providing a clearer image than the transabdominal method, the endovaginal procedure can be accomplished with an empty bladder.

Most women do not feel discomfort during the endovaginal ultrasound exam. The probe is smaller than a speculum, so insertion is usually completed with ease. The woman may feel some movement of the probe during the exam as various structures are imaged. Some women may want to insert the probe themselves to en-

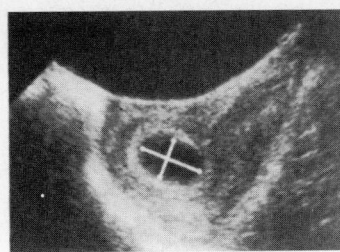

FIGURE 20-4   Measurement of the gestational sac. The ultrasound shows the uterus; the blackened oval area is the gestational sac. The fluid in the gestational sac does not generate echoes from the ultrasound and thus appears dark in contrast to the uterine tissue surrounding it. The lines through the gestational sac represent measurements that are taken. SOURCE: Callen PW: *Ultrasonography in Obstetrics and Gynecology*, 2nd ed. Philadelphia: WB Saunders, 1988, p 49.

hance their comfort; others may feel embarrassed even to be asked. The certified nurse-midwife/physician or ultrasonographer offer the choice based on their comfort level and the rapport they have with the woman.

Translabial Ultrasound

This method of ultrasound may be used in conjunction with transabdominal ultrasound. The transducer with a protective probe cover is placed on the woman's labia. It is not inserted into the vaginal vault. Translabial ultrasound is particularly useful for assessing cervical length, identifying the presenting part of the fetus, and confirming placenta previa (Ruffin et al 1992).

Clinical Application

ACOG (1993) has established guidelines regarding the information that should be obtained by ultrasound in each trimester, including biometry (fetal measurements) and a survey of fetal anatomy.

First Trimester Pregnancy

Transvaginal ultrasound often provides better and earlier first trimester assessment of pregnancy. With either abdominal or transvaginal methods the following information should be obtained:

- Presence of absence of the intrauterine gestational sac (Figure 20–4)
- Identification of the embryo or fetus

- Fetal number
- Presence or absence of fetal cardiac activity
- Crown-rump length (Figure 20–5)
- Evaluation of the uterus and adnexal structures

With abdominal ultrasound the gestational sac is visible at 6 weeks' gestation by menstrual dates. Transvaginal ultrasound allows the gestational sac to be identified by 5 menstrual weeks' gestation. Similarly, fetal heart activity can be detected with abdominal scanning at 7 weeks' gestation by menstrual dating and at 6 weeks' gestation with transvaginal scanning.

First trimester bleeding is the most common indication for early ultrasonography. Blighted ovum or an embryonic pregnancy can be diagnosed by the failure to detect a fetus within a normal gestational sac after 6 weeks' gestation by menstrual dating. Missed abortion is diagnosed by the absence of cardiac activity in an embryo after 7 weeks' gestation. In women with suspected ectopic pregnancy the main contribution of ultrasonography is demonstration of a gestational sac within the uterus, thereby confirming intrauterine pregnancy. Multiple pregnancy can be diagnosed only when multiple fetuses have documented cardiac activity. Variability in the fusion of the amnion and chorion in early pregnancy may give the appearance of more than one gestational sac.

During the first trimester measurement of the crown-rump length (CRL) of the fetus is most useful for accurate dating of a pregnancy. The correlation between fetal length and age is excellent because pathologic disorders will minimally affect fetal growth in the first

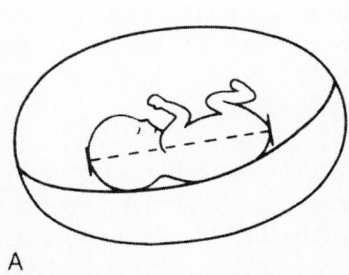

A

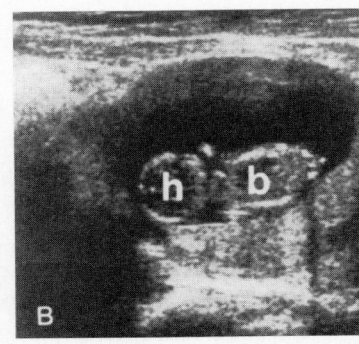

B

FIGURE 20-5   Measurement of the crown-rump length. *A* Schematic diagram. Dotted line shows the measurement from the top of the crown (head) to the bottom of the rump. *B* Ultrasound scan of the pregnant uterus, showing the longest length of a 9-week fetus. The head (h) can be differentiated from the body (b), but the internal anatomy cannot be clearly distinguished. SOURCE: Callen PW: *Ultrasonography in Obstetrics and Gynecology*, 2nd ed. Philadelphia: WB Saunders, 1988, p 50.

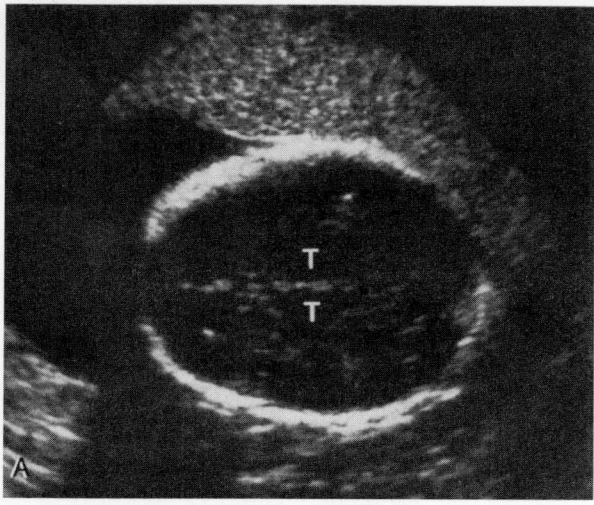
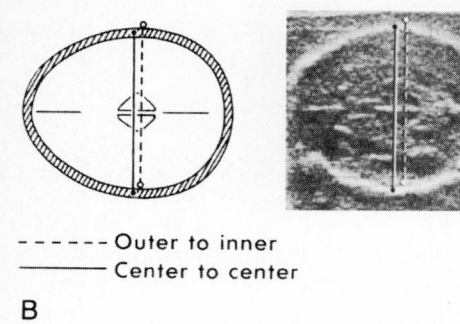

------ Outer to inner
——— Center to center

B

FIGURE 20-6 Measurement of the fetal biparietal diameter. *A* Ultrasound transaxial image of the fetal head, taken with the thalami (T) imaged in the midline, equidistant from the temporoparietal tables of the calvarium. *B* Diagram and image showing the leading edge (outer) to leading edge (inner) measurements of the fetal head, taken at the level of the thalami. SOURCE: Callen PW: *Ultrasonography in Obstetrics and Gynecology,* 2nd ed. Philadelphia: WB Saunders, 1988, p 51.

trimester. The measurement should be taken from the top of the fetal head to the outer rump, excluding limbs or yolk sac. A general formula is gestational age in weeks = CRL in cm + 6.5. CRL is no longer accurate after 12 weeks due to the extension and flexion of the active fetus (Callen 1994).

Second Trimester Pregnancy

In the second trimester the ultrasound measurements of the fetal biparietal diameter, femur length, and abdominal and head circumferences are used to estimate gestational age and fetal weight. The average of the gestational age predictions generated by each of these measurements provides the best estimate of fetal age. However, utilizing the averaging method may adversely affect the gestational age estimate if one of the measurements is grossly incompatible with the others. For example, measurements may show a small biparietal diameter secondary to compression of the fetal head in oligohydramnios or breech presentation. When this occurs, the abnormal value is deleted from the calculation of the mean gestational age.

Biparietal Diameter In the second trimester the biparietal diameter (BPD) is the most accepted means of measuring the fetal head and is the single most common measurement for estimating gestational age. Between 17 and 24 weeks' gestation is the optimal time for this measurement; at this point it has a predictive value of ± 5–7 days. The BPD should be measured at the level of the thalamus and the cavum septi pelludidi (Figure 20–6). Several tables that correlate the BPD with fetal gestational age are available. Serial ultrasounds enable the

practitioner to assess fetal growth according to the normal growth curve. If the curve begins to flatten, the physician must assess the fetus for fetal growth retardation. In this case additional antenatal surveillance, including Doppler flow studies and biophysical profile with nonstress tests, may be used to assess fetal well-being.

The BPD measurements can be obtained beginning at 11 weeks' gestation, but the BPD is too small for nomograms to be reliable until about 17 weeks. Detection of IUGR and an accurate prediction of fetal age can be most reliably achieved between 20 and 30 weeks' gestation, when the most rapid growth in the BPD occurs. After 40 weeks' gestation the BPD shows a growth of less than 1mm/week; thus sonograms obtained at this point are of no value. The BPD measurement generally correlates closely with gestational age, especially if serial determinations were obtained beginning early in the pregnancy. However, if only one determination is made late in pregnancy, the gestational age is less accurate and may vary by ± 4 weeks.

Head Circumference The BPD is accurate only if the head is the appropriate ovoid shape. Compression of the fetal skull occurs commonly in fetal malpresentation, such as breech, or in cases of oligohydramnios or multiple gestation. The head circumference is less affected by head compression and is therefore a valuable tool to assess gestational age (Figure 20–7).

Cephalic Index After 28 weeks the BPD alone should not be relied on to determine gestational age. After this time the *cephalic index* (the ratio of BPD to occipitofrontal [OF] diameter) should be evaluated to assess head shape.

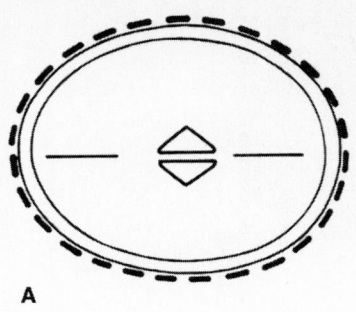

A

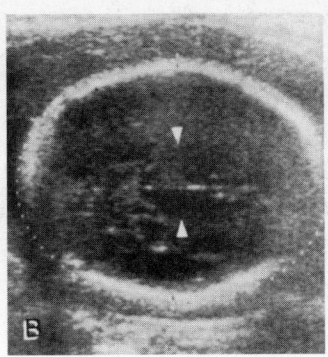

B

FIGURE 20-7 Measurement of head circumference. *A* Diagram showing a dotted line outlining the head, which indicates the correct place to make a circumference measurement. *B* Ultrasound transaxial scan showing the thalami (arrowheads), positioned in the midline. A dotted line created by a digitizer outlines the correct perimeter, just outside the hyperechoic calvarium, to obtain a circumference measurement. SOURCE: Callen PW: *Ultrasonography in Obstetrics and Gynecology,* 2nd ed. Philadelphia: WB Saunders, 1988, p 55.

The fetal head is normally oval, but there are variations. If the OF diameter is shortened and the BPD is elongated so that the head is unusually round, the alteration is known as brachycephaly. If the OF diameter is elongated and the BPD is shortened so that the head is unusually elongated, the condition is known as dolichocephaly. If the cephalic index is abnormal, gestational age should be determined by other parameters, and head abnormalities should be considered and further assessed (Figure 20–8).

Femur Length   Although any long bone may be used to determine gestational age, the femur is the easiest to image. Femur length is as accurate as BPD in determining gestational age (Callen 1994). Femur length measurement is made from the major trochanter to the external condyle. Femur length is shortened in the presence of osteogenesis imperfecta or dwarfism (Hadlock 1990b) (Figure 20–9).

Abdominal Measurements   Measurement of the fetal abdominal circumference is useful for monitoring fetal growth and detecting IUGR, macrosomia, and isoimmunization (due to ascites). Fetal abdominal girth ceases to increase in IUGR due to the depletion of glycogen in the fetal liver and diminished accumulation of subcutaneous tissue overlying the fetal abdomen. If the estimated date of birth has been established with early ultrasound measurements, the abdominal circumference measurement may be sufficient to monitor fetal growth. If abdominal circumference is the only measurement that has been taken during the pregnancy, it is meaningless (Figure 20–10).

Head/Abdomen Ratio   The head circumference (H) to abdomen circumference (A) ratio is used to assess disproportion between the fetal head and body. Disproportion may be observed in asymmetric IUGR (caused by

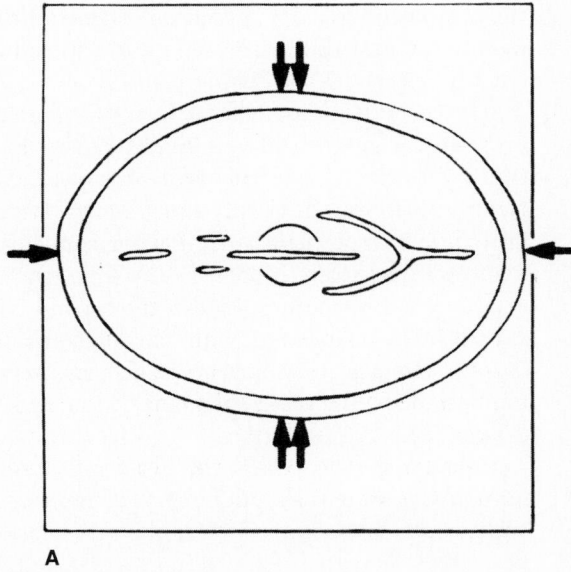

A

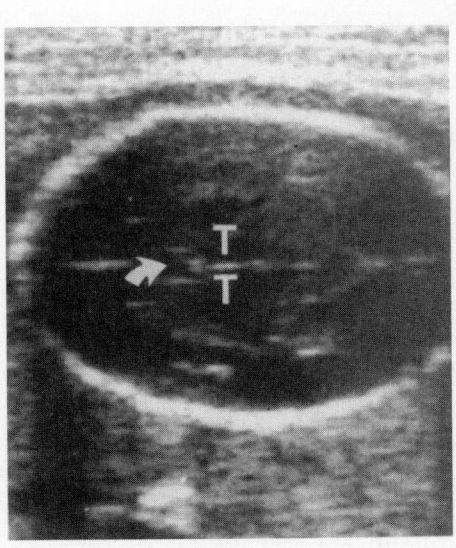

B

FIGURE 20-8   Measurement of the cephalic index. *A* The biparietal diameter denoted by the double arrows and the fronto-occipital diameter denoted by single arrows are both taken outer edge to outer edge. A ratio of the two gives the cephalic index. *B* Ultrasound transaxial scan of the fetal head at the level of the thalami (T) and cavum septi pellucidi (curved arrow). SOURCE: Callen PW: *Ultrasonography in Obstetrics and Gynecology,* 2nd ed. Philadelphia: WB Saunders, 1988, p 53.

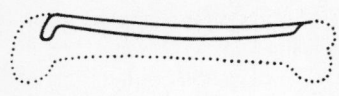

A

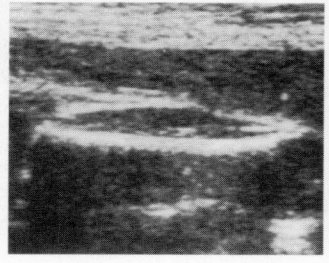

B

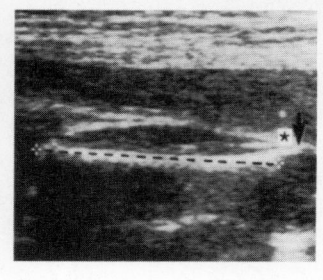

C

FIGURE 20-9 Measurement of the femur length. *A* Schematic diagram. *B* Ultrasound image. The hyperechoic line in the ossified lateral margin of the femoral diaphysis. The ends of the bone are the epiphyseal cartilages that have not yet calcified and are therefore hypoechoic. *C* The hyperechoic diaphysis is measured from one end to the other, denoted by the cursors and a dotted line. The "distal femoral point" (* and arrow) is a nonossified extension of the distal epiphyseal cartilage. It should not be included in the measurement. SOURCE: Callen PW: *Ultrasonography in Obstetrics and Gynecology,* 2nd ed. Philadelphia: WB Saunders, 1988, p 58.

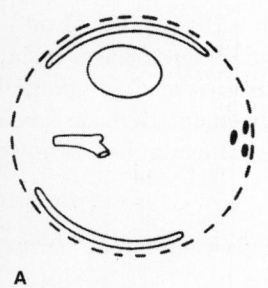

A

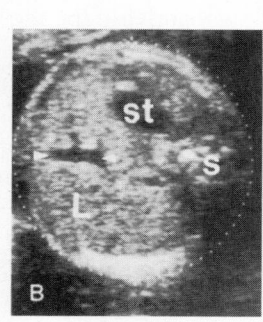

FIGURE 20-10 Measurement of the abdominal circumference. *A* Diagram showing the abdominal circumference as a dotted line traced at the outer margin of the abdomen. *B* Ultrasound transaxial image showing the umbilical portion of the left portal vein (arrowheads) correctly positioned within the liver and equidistant from the lateral walls. (s, spine; L, liver; st, stomach). A dotted line, created by a digitizer, outlines the outer margins of the abdomen, the correct place to obtain an abdominal circumference measurement. SOURCE: Callen PW: *Ultrasonography in Obstetrics and Gynecology,* 2nd ed. Philadelphia: WB Saunders, 1988, p 57.

uteroplacental insufficiency) and congenital anomalies such as microcephaly. The H/A ratio may also be used to estimate fetal weight (Hadlock 1990b).

Third Trimester Pregnancy

The ability to initially establish gestational age by ultrasound is lost in the third trimester because fetal growth rate is not uniform as it was in the first two trimesters. Without earlier ultrasound measurements ultrasound measurements obtained in the third trimester would vary by ± 3 weeks.

Uses of Fetal Ultrasound

Fetal Growth Determination

Serial ultrasound offers a valuable means of assessing intrauterine growth. IUGR is classified as symmetric (primary) or asymmetric (secondary). In symmetric IUGR all organs are reduced in size with equal reduction in body weight and head size; therefore the fetus has normal head circumference/abdominal circumference (HC/AC) and femur length/abdominal circumference (FL/AC) ratios. At birth all measurements fall below the tenth percentile. Such fetuses comprise approximately 20–25% of cases of IUGR. These cases usually are detected by ultrasonography when all growth parameters lag significantly behind those expected based on gestational age confirmed by accurate menstrual history or early ultrasound dating (ACOG 1993).

It has been estimated that 75% of symmetric IUGR or small for gestational age (SGA) fetuses are constitutionally small, 15%–20% have uteroplacental insufficiency due to various causes, and 5%–10% have impaired growth due to perinatal infections or congenital malformations (Manning & Hohler 1991). This growth retardation is noted in the first half of the second trimester. It may also be associated with chromosomal disorders, chronic hypoxia, teratogens, vascular and renal disease, multiple gestation, maternal malnutrition, and dwarf syndromes.

In asymmetric IUGR the head and brain sizes are normal, but there is a reduction in abdominal size, apparently caused by a compromise in the uteroplacental blood flow. The decreased blood flow is associated with PIH, chronic hypertension, diabetes mellitus, and chronic renal disease. This is the more common type of IUGR and is usually not evident prior to the third trimester. Fetuses with asymmetric IUGR are particularly at risk for perinatal asphyxia, hypocalcemia, polycythemia, and hypoglycemia in the neonatal period. Birth weight will be reduced to the tenth percentile, whereas cephalic size is spared and is in the normal range. Perinatal mortality is ten times that of average for gestational age babies (Faranoff & Martin 1992).

The earlier the gestational age is accurately assessed, the more accurate the prediction of IUGR. If a growth-retarded fetus is suspected, serial ultrasounds should be done every 2 to 3 weeks.

On first examination the estimated fetal weight (EFW) is figured as a percentile for that fetus. If the percentile is low, serial sonograms are warranted. If on repeat scan the fetus is at the same percentile, no abnormal growth has occurred. If the percentile increases, growth of the fetus has improved. If the fetus is at a lower percentile, fetal growth is slowing, and this fetus should be further assessed with intense antenatal surveillance, including biophysical profiles and Doppler flow studies. Cordocentesis may be done to obtain chromosomes and fetal blood gases (Pardi et al 1993).

Management of the growth-retarded fetus depends on fetal well-being and gestational age. After a comprehensive ultrasound survey for structural abnormalities and amniotic fluid index, amniocentesis may be used to evaluate chromosomes and lung maturity. Maternal oxygen therapy may be considered to increase fetal oxygenation; increased oral fluids may also be ordered (Battaglia et al 1992). The fetus will be assessed with at least weekly biophysical profiles with amniotic fluid index and some type of fetal activity assessment technique.

Serial ultrasounds for EFW growth curve, Doppler flow studies, and antenatal surveillance will help determine the optimal timing for birth (Chang et al 1993). The timing of birth may depend on gestational age and fetal well-being. If the gestational age of the fetus is greater than 37 weeks, the woman's cervical status will be assessed using Bishop's scoring system (Chapter 26). An amniocentesis to confirm fetal lung maturity may be done before labor is induced.

Detection of Congenital Anomalies

Ultrasound evaluation of fetal anatomy can detect many major and minor structural anomalies, though not with 100% accuracy. A basic ultrasound of fetal anatomy should include evaluation of the following:

- Head shape; size of ventricles to detect hydrocephalus, microcephalus, anencephalus, encephalocele; face for clefts; neck for presence of cystic hygroma
- Spine to detect meningomyelocele or spina bifida
- Chest and heart to detect diaphragmatic hernia, hypoplasia, pericardial teratoma, pleural effusion, congenital heart disease
- Abdomen to detect omphalocele, gastroschisis, tracheoesophageal fistula, hydronephrosis, dilated renal pelves, polycystic kidneys
- Extremities for skeletal dysplasia

Evaluation of the Placenta and Cervix

Placental Maturity The placenta should be evaluated to assess maturity. Grannum, Berkowitz, and Hobbins (1979) noted that throughout gestation the placenta undergoes maturational changes that may be visualized by ultrasound. These morphologic changes in the basal layer, chorionic plate, and intervening placental substance have been classified in terms of grades (0 to III), with increasing changes occurring from 12 weeks' gestation until term. The grade is described according to the presence of echogenic areas in the placental substance, basal layer, and chorionic plate: Grade 0 has a smooth chorionic plate. Grade I has some calcification, which is reflected as some irregularity of the chorionic plate. Grade II has larger indentations that extend down toward the uterine wall. Grade III has extensive calcifications and indentations of the chorionic wall that reach down to the uterine wall (Reed 1994) (Figure 20–11).

Placental Location The placental site should be evaluated in relationship to the cervix. The appearance of the placenta completely covering the internal os of the cervix is called *placenta previa*.

Cervical Length The cervical length can be measured by endovaginal or translabial ultrasound. This assessment has proved to be a more precise means of measuring the length of the cervical canal than a digital cervical exam. It has been used to follow women with cervical cerclage or preterm labor (Anderson et al 1990).

Deciding Whom To Screen

Controversy continues regarding whether ultrasound screening of all obstetric clients improves pregnancy outcome. A consensus development conference convened by the National Institute of Child Health and Human Development in 1984 concluded that no clinical benefit is derived from routine obstetric ultrasonography. However, this workshop did propose 27 indications for ultrasonography during pregnancy (Table 20–3).

Commonly advanced arguments in favor of routine scanning include early detection of unsuspected fetal anomalies and multiple gestation; accurate determination of gestational age, leading to improved diagnosis and management of postdatism and fetal growth retardation; and decreased perinatal mortality rate (Saari-Kemppainen et al 1990). Routine ultrasonography early in pregnancy can reduce the incidence of labor induction for suspected postdatism and decrease the frequency of undiagnosed major fetal anomalies and undiagnosed twins.

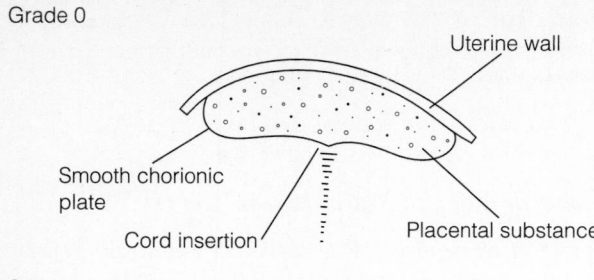

Grade 0

Uterine wall

Smooth chorionic plate

Cord insertion

Placental substance

A

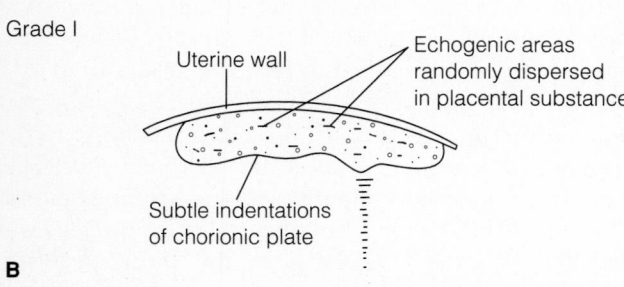

Grade I

Uterine wall

Echogenic areas randomly dispersed in placental substance

Subtle indentations of chorionic plate

B

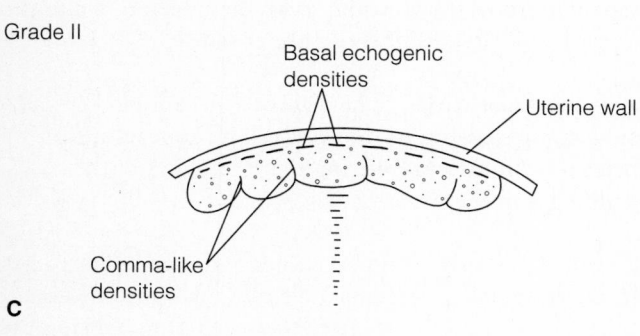

Grade II

Basal echogenic densities

Uterine wall

Comma-like densities

C

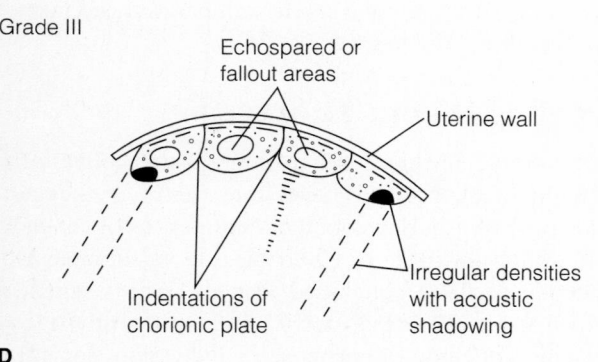

Grade III

Echospared or fallout areas

Uterine wall

Indentations of chorionic plate

Irregular densities with acoustic shadowing

D

FIGURE 20-11 Placental grading. *A* Diagram showing the ultrasonic appearance of a grade 0 placenta. *B* Diagram showing the ultrasonic appearance of a grade I placenta. *C* Diagram showing the ultrasonic appearance of a grade II placenta. *D* Diagram showing the ultrasonic appearance of a grade III placenta.

However, significant effects on infant outcome are not confirmed by randomized, controlled trials. Although obstetric ultrasound studies are performed routinely in many European countries, in the United States the routine use of ultrasonography cannot be supported from a cost-benefit standpoint.

ANTENATAL FETAL SURVEILLANCE

The major goal of antepartum fetal surveillance is the reduction of fetal demise in those populations at highest risk. Various techniques appear to be effective in reducing perinatal mortality in selected populations. Although antepartum fetal surveillance protocols may in the future also prove effective in reducing perinatal morbidity and improving long-term neurologic outcome, convincing data to support these effects presently do not exist (ACOG 1994).

Amniotic Fluid Assessment

The volume of amniotic fluid in the uterus serves as an important indicator of fetal well-being. Amniotic fluid volume abnormalities are associated with adverse perinatal outcomes. Polyhydramnios may indicate a fetal malformation. Oligohydramnios may be encountered with premature rupture of membranes, fetal urinary tract abnormalities, and placental insufficiency, often associated with IUGR or postdate pregnancy. Oligohydramnios has also often been associated with umbilical cord compression and thickened meconium-stained fluid (Fischer et al 1993; Moore 1995).

The amount of amniotic fluid can be evaluated by a technique called *amniotic fluid volume (AFV)* or *amniotic fluid index (AFI)*. AFV is determined by using ultrasound and looking throughout the uterus for pockets of amniotic fluid. (Because the fetus is completely surrounded by amniotic fluid, a pocket of fluid can be visualized in the bend of the fetal arm or between the fetal arm and the face, for example.) When a pocket is visualized, it is measured from top to bottom in centimeters. A pocket of amniotic fluid that measures at least 2 cm across is associated with a normal amount of fluid; a pocket of less than 2 cm is associated with oligohydramnios.

AFI is obtained by measuring pockets of amniotic fluid in four quadrants of the uterus. The landmarks for the quadrants are the maternal umbilicus and the linea nigra (a pigmented vertical line that extends upward from the center of the symphysis pubis to the umbilicus and sometimes beyond the uterus). Within each quadrant the largest pocket of amniotic fluid is identified and measured; then these measurements are added to obtain the AFI. An AFI greater than 20 cm indicates hydramnios; an AFI less than 5 cm indicates oligohydramnios. These cutoff values, which were derived from pregnancies ranging from 36–42 weeks, have also been applied, perhaps appropriately, throughout gestation. Because AFV fluctua-

TABLE 20-3 Circumstances Under Which Ultrasound Can Be of Benefit

Estimation of gestational age for clients (1) with uncertain clinical dates, (2) verification of dates of clients who are to undergo scheduled elective repeat cesarean birth, induction of labor, or for other elective termination of pregnancy. Ultrasound confirmation of dating permits proper timing of cesarean birth or labor induction to avoid premature birth.

Evaluation of fetal growth (eg, when the client has an identified etiology for uteroplacental insufficiency, such as severe preeclampsia, chronic hypertension, chronic renal disease, severe diabetes mellitus, or for other medical complications of pregnancy where fetal malnutrition, ie, IUGR or macrosomia, is suspected). Following fetal growth permits assessment of the impact of a complicating condition on the fetus and guides pregnancy management.

Vaginal bleeding of undetermined etiology in pregnancy. Ultrasound often allows determination of the source of bleeding and status of the fetus.

Determination of fetal presentation when the presenting part cannot be adequately determined in labor or the fetal presentation is variable in late pregnancy. Accurate knowledge of presentation guides management of childbirth.

Suspected multiple gestation based upon detection of more than one fetal heartbeat pattern, fundal height larger than expected for dates, and/or prior use of fertility drugs. Pregnancy management may be altered in multiple gestation.

Adjunct to amniocentesis. Ultrasound permits guidance of the needle to avoid the placenta and fetus, to increase the chance of obtaining amniotic fluid, and to decrease the chance of fetal loss.

Significant uterine size/clinical dates discrepancy. Ultrasound permits accurate dating and detection of such conditions as oligohydramnios and polyhydramnios, as well as multiple gestation, IUGR, and anomalies.

Pelvic mass detected clinically. Ultrasound can detect the location and nature of the mass and aid in diagnosis.

Suspected hydatidiform mole on the basis of clinical signs of hypertension, proteinuria, and/or the presence of ovarian cysts felt on pelvic examination or failure to detect fetal heart tones with a Doppler ultrasound device after 12 weeks. Ultrasound permits accurate diagnosis and differentiation of this malignancy from fetal death.

Adjunct to cervical cerclage placement. Ultrasound aids in timing and proper placement of the cerclage for patients with incompetent cervix.

Suspected ectopic pregnancy or when pregnancy occurs after tuboplasty or prior ectopic gestation. Ultrasound is a valuable diagnostic aid for this complication.

Adjunct to special procedures, such as fetoscopy, intrauterine transfusion, shunt placement, in vitro fertilization, embryo transfer, or chorionic villi sampling. Ultrasound aids instrument guidance that increases safety of these procedures.

Suspected fetal death. Rapid diagnosis enhances optimal management.

Suspected uterine abnormality (eg, clinically significant leiomyomata or congenital structural abnormalities such as bicornate uterus or uterus didelphys). Serial surveillance of fetal growth and state enhances fetal outcome.

Intrauterine contraceptive device localization. Ultrasound guidance facilitates removal, reducing chances of IUD-related complications.

Ovarian follicle development surveillance. This facilitates treatment of infertility.

Biophysical evaluation for fetal well-being after 28 weeks of gestation. Assessment of amniotic fluid, fetal tone, body movements, breathing movements, and heart rate patterns assists in assessment of high-risk pregnancies.

Observation of intrapartum events (eg, version/extraction of second twin, manual removal of placenta). These procedures may be done more safely with the visualization provided by ultrasound.

Suspected hydramnios or oligohydramnios. Confirmation of the diagnosis is permitted, as well as identification of the cause of the condition in certain pregnancies.

Suspected abruptio placentae. Confirmation of diagnosis and extent assists in clinical management.

Adjunct to external version from breech to vertex presentation. The visualization provided by ultrasound facilitates performance of this procedure.

Estimation of fetal weight and/or presentation in premature rupture of membranes and/or premature labor. Information provided by ultrasound guides management decisions on timing and method of birth.

Abnormal serum α-fetoprotein value for clinical gestational age when drawn. Ultrasound provides an accurate assessment of gestational age for the AFP comparison standard and indicates several conditions (eg, twins, anencephaly) that may cause elevated AFP values.

Follow-up observation of identified fetal anomaly. Ultrasound assessment of progression or lack of change assists in clinical decision making.

History of previous congenital anomaly. Detection of recurrence may be permitted, or psychologic benefit to patients may result from reassurance of no recurrence.

Serial evaluation of fetal growth in multiple gestation. Ultrasound permits recognition of discordant growth, guiding client management and timing of birth.

Evaluation of fetal condition in late registrants for prenatal care. Accurate knowledge of gestational age assists in pregnancy management decisions of this group.

SOURCE: Shearer MH: Revelations: A summary and analysis of the NIH consensus development conference on ultrasound imaging in pregnancy. *Birth* 1984; 11(1):27.

tions have been observed, gestational-age-dependent norms for the AFI were developed. The 5th and 95th percentiles are used to define abnormal AFVs (Moore & Cayle 1993; Moore 1995).

The AVI is a valid and reproducible measurement. It should be one component of a composite fetal assessment that also includes Doppler flow studies and a biophysical profile. The presence of oligohydramnios indicates possible fetal compromise and need for assessment and management, including maternal rest and hydration (Williams 1993).

Nursing Care

It is important for the nurse to ascertain whether the woman understands the reason the ultrasound has been ordered. The nurse can provide an opportunity for the woman to ask questions and can act as an advocate if there are questions or concerns that need to be addressed prior to the ultrasound examination. The nurse explains the preparation needed and ensures that adequate preparation is done. If certified to perform a basic or limited ultrasound exam, the nurse provides information regarding the purpose of this particular exam and performs it. After the exam, the nurse can assist with clarifying or interpreting test results for the woman and her partner or other support person.

Biophysical Profile (BPP)

The **biophysical profile (BPP)** represents an assessment of five fetal biophysical variables: breathing movement, body movement, tone, amniotic fluid volume, and FHR reactivity. The BPP is used to assess the fetus at risk for intrauterine compromise. The first four variables are

TABLE 20-4 Biophysical Profile Scoring: Technique and Interpretation

Biophysical Variable	Normal (Score = 2)	Abnormal (Score = 0)
Fetal breathing movements	≥1 episode of ≥30 seconds in 30 minutes	Absent or no episode of ≥30 seconds in 30 minutes
Gross body movements	≥3 discrete body/limb movements in 30 minutes (Episodes of active continuous movement considered as single movement.)	≤2 episodes of body/limb movements in 30 minutes
Fetal tone	≥1 episode of active extension with return to flexion of fetal limb(s) or trunk (Opening and closing of hand considered normal tone.)	Either slow extension with return to partial flexion or movement of limb in full extension or absent fetal movement
Reactive fetal heart rate	≥2 episodes of acceleration of ≥15 bpm and of ≥15 seconds associated with fetal movement in 20 minutes	<2 episodes of acceleration of fetal heart rate or acceleration of <15 bpm in 20 minutes
Qualitative amniotic fluid volume	≥1 pocket of fluid measuring ≥1 cm in two perpendicular planes	Either no pockets or a pocket <1 cm in two perpendicular planes

Management Based on Biophysical Profile Score

Attained Score	Intervention
10 of 10 or 8 of 10, with normal amniotic fluid volume	No intervention is needed, normal finding.
8 of 10 with abnormal amniotic fluid volume	If fetal renal function is normal and membranes are intact, delivery is indicated.
6 of 10 with normal amniotic fluid volume	Deliver fetus if it is mature. If immature, repeat test within 24 hours. If score is 6 of 10 or below, deliver fetus.
4 of 10, 2 of 10, or 0 of 10	Deliver fetus.

SOURCES: Manning FA et al: Fetal assessment based on fetal biophysical profile scoring: Experience in 12,620 referred high-risk pregnancies. *Am J Obstet Gynecol* 1985; 151(3):344; Manning FA: The biophysical profile: Contemporary use. *Tenth International Symposium on Perinatal Medicine and Obstetrical Ultrasound, April 9–12, 1990, Las Vegas, NV.*

assessed by ultrasound scanning; FHR reactivity is assessed with the nonstress test. By combining these five assessments, the BPP helps to identify the compromised fetus and confirm the healthy fetus.

Specific criteria for normal and abnormal assessments are delineated in Table 20–4 with a score of 2 being assigned to each normal finding and 0 to each abnormal one for a maximum score of 10. The absence of a specific activity is difficult to interpret because it may be indicative of CNS depression or simply the resting state of a healthy fetus. Scores of 8 to 10 are considered normal (Manning 1990). A score of 6 is considered equivocal (questionable). The fetus should be retested in 12–24 hours if it is immature; if the fetus is 38 weeks' or more gestation, birth should occur. A score of 4 or less is abnormal and indicates that the fetus should be born immediately (Table 20–4).

In the presence of oligohydramnios further evaluation may be warranted (Manning 1990). The correlation of BPP score and perinatal mortality has been studied extensively by Manning (1990), and the implications of each BPP score are illustrated in Table 20–5. If the BPP test score is 10/10 (a score of 2 on all five biophysical variables), the perinatal mortality rate in the next 7 days is less than 1/1000 for the fetus. If the BPP score is 2/10, the perinatal mortality rate is greatly increased. Table 20–5 indicates that the perinatal mortality rate in this case

is 125/1000, which means that if intervention does not occur, the fetus is 125 times as likely to die in the next 7 days than if the score were 10/10.

As noted by Vintzileos et al (1987), increasing use of the BPP has led to recognition of errors in interpretation and subsequent use of this assessment technique. These authors encourage management that is not based solely on BPP score but that includes evaluation of specific biophysical components of the test in order to decrease false-positive and false-negative tests. They note that the biophysical activities of the fetus that develop first are the last to disappear when all activities are arrested due to asphyxia; those that are the last to develop are the most sensitive to hypoxia, and their disappearance can be noted first. For example, fetal tone (exhibited by flexion of the extremities) is the first to develop and the last activity to cease during asphyxia. Other activities in the normal developmental sequence are fetal movement, followed by fetal breathing, and then reactivity of the FHR. Therefore FHR reactivity is the most sensitive to hypoxia. One of the first indications of fetal compromise is a nonreactive nonstress test.

Indications for BPP include those situations in which the NST and CST would be done. Assessment of these fetal biophysical activities is most useful in the evaluation of women who experience decreased fetal movement (who might subsequently have a nonreactive NST) and in

Test Score	Interpretation	Perinatal Mortality Within 1 Week Without Intervention	Management
10/10 8/10 (normal fluid) 8/8 (NST not done)	Risk of fetal asphyxia extremely rare	< 1/1000	Intervene only for obstetric and maternal factors. No indication for intervention for fetal disease.
8/10 (abnormal fluid)	Probable chronic fetal compromise	89/1000	Determine that there is functioning renal tissue and intact membranes. If so, birth is indicated for fetal indications.
6/10 (normal fluid)	Equivocal test, possible fetal asphyxia	Variable	If the fetus is mature, birth is indicated. In the immature fetus repeat test within 24 hours. If < 6/10, then birth is indicated.
6/10 (abnormal fluid)	Probable fetal asphyxia	89/1000	Birth is indicated for fetal indications.
4/10	High probability of fetal asphyxia	91/1000	Birth is indicated for fetal indications.
2/10	Fetal asphyxia almost certain	125/1000	Birth is indicated for fetal indications.
0/10	Fetal asphyxia certain	600/1000	Birth is indicated for fetal indications.

SOURCE: Manning FA: The biophysical profile: Contemporary use. *Tenth International Symposium on Perinatal Medicine and Obstetrical Ultrasound. April 9–12, 1990, Las Vegas, NV.*

the management of IUGR, preterm, diabetic, and postterm pregnancies, and premature rupture of the membranes (PROM) (Manning 1995).

Fetal Echocardiography

Among its many uses, ultrasound may be employed to examine fetal cardiac structures. Through echocardiography, treatment of fetal arrhythmias prior to birth is possible, and cases of congenital heart disease have been diagnosed prenatally and managed accordingly.

Fetal echocardiography is recommended for women who have a family history of congenital heart disease, maternal disease that may affect the fetus, history of maternal drug use, evidence of other fetal anomalies, or fetal hydrops. The best timing for fetal echocardiography is 18–22 weeks' gestation. There is a 15% occurrence of fetal cardiac arrythmias in this selected population. Premature atrial or ventricular contractions are commonly seen and usually require no treatment. Supraventricular tachycardia can result in hydrops and require in utero treatment to prevent fetal death. Complete heart block, particularly in association with structural heart disease, has poor prognosis for fetal survival (Brook et al 1993).

The advantage of being able to obtain information prenatally is that parents, as well as the medical and nursing staff, can be alerted for possible problems that may occur at birth or shortly thereafter and can thus plan appropriate interventions. Fetuses with diagnosed problems are serially evaluated to provide ongoing assessment. When cardiac malformations are diagnosed, comprehensive sound is performed to assess other fetal structures. Genetic amniocentesis may be recommended if cardiac malformations are noted because the risk of chromosomal abnormalities in these fetuses is about 5%.

Doppler Ultrasound Velocimetry

Recent advances in ultrasound technology have made it possible to noninvasively study blood flow changes that occur in maternal and fetal circulations to assess placental function. An ultrasound beam, like that provided by the pocket Doppler (a hand-held ultrasound device), is directed at the umbilical artery. The signal is reflected off the red blood cells (RBCs) moving within the vessels, and the subsequent "picture" (waveform) that is received looks like a series of waves. The highest velocity peak of the waves is the systolic measurement, and the lowest point is the diastolic velocity. The umbilical artery waveform can then be analyzed to provide information regarding velocity of blood flow in the vessel. The most common evaluation of blood flow velocity is the systolic to diastolic (S/D) ratio. The S/D ratio normally decreases as the fetus nears term. This phenomenon reflects the decreasing resistance of placental and umbilical vasculature to allow for greater umbilical blood flow to meet the needs of a growing fetus. The normal range for the S/D ratio is < 3 after 28 weeks' gestation. An elevated S/D ratio may be associated with fetal growth retardation (Shulman 1990), although Maulik (1995) notes that the S/D ratio may remain normal (Figures 20–12 and 20–13).

The absence of diastolic flow is abnormal, indicating impaired uteroplacental or umbilical circulation. The worst scenario is reverse end diastolic flow in which the blood flow regurgitates back toward the placenta at each heartbeat.

A decrease in fetal cardiac output or an increase in resistance of placental vessels will reduce umbilical artery blood flow. Clinical applications of Doppler flow analysis have included studies of fetal growth retardation associated with maternal hypertension. It has been noted that

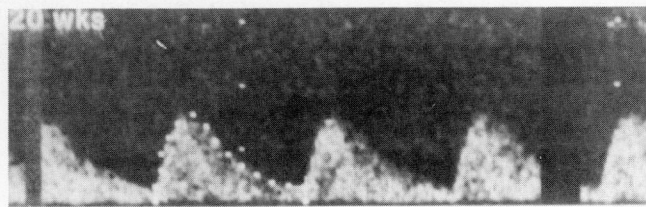

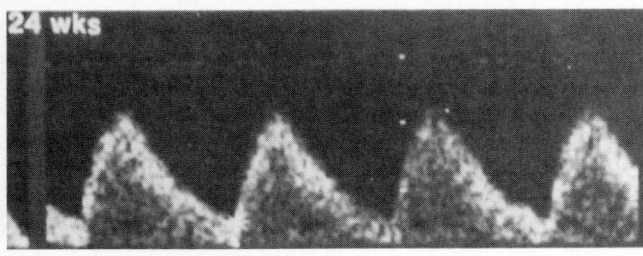

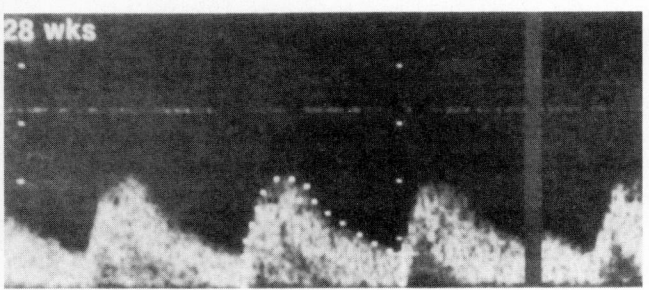

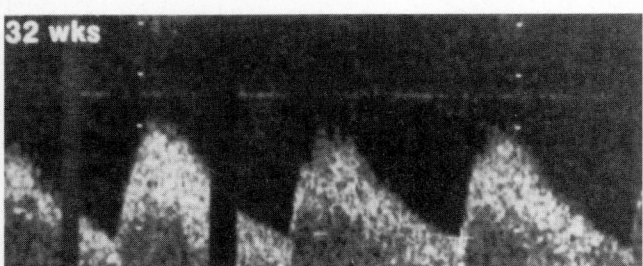

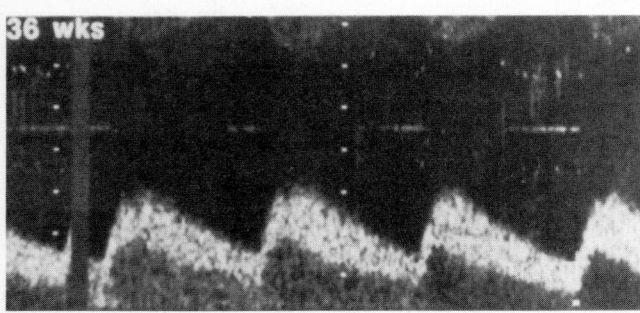

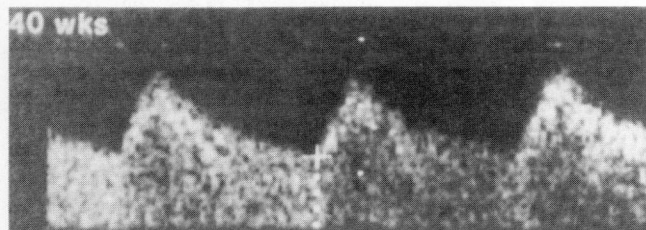

FIGURE 20-12   Serial studies of the umbilical artery velocity waveforms in a normal pregnancy from one client. SOURCE: Cundiff JL, Haybrich KL, Hinzman NG: Umbilical artery Doppler flow studies during pregnancy. *JOGNN* November/December 1990; 19(6):475, fig 3.

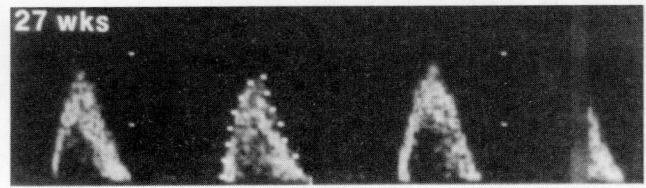

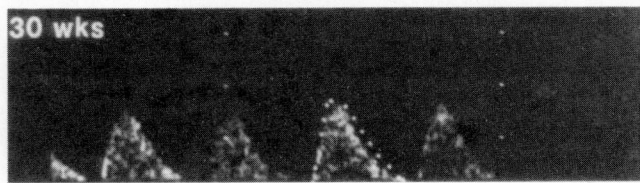

FIGURE 20-13   Two examples of abnormal umbilical artery velocity waveforms taken from a client with intrauterine growth retardation. SOURCE: Cundiff JL, Haybrich KL, Hinzman HG: Umbilical artery Doppler flow studies during pregnancy. *JOGNN* November/December 1990; 19(6):475, fig 4.

hypertensive or preeclamptic mothers giving birth to growth-retarded infants have abnormal Doppler flow velocity waveforms. In most cases decreased maternal blood flow has been shown to precede a decrease in fetal blood flow.

Doppler blood flow studies are also helpful in the assessment and management of multiple gestation, diabetes, prolonged pregnancy, sickle cell disease, and twin-to-twin transfusion. Umbilical velocimetry must be used along with the NST, AFI, CST, and BPP. Some investigators have suggested that there is a progressive and proportional increase in umbilical artery resistance with hypoxia, hypercapnia, and acidosis (Bonnin et al 1992). Arduini and colleagues (1992) have found changes of Doppler flow studies in the fetal vessels preceding the onset of late decelerations in the growth-retarded fetus.

Investigators are currently studying other fetal arteries, such as the internal carotid, descending aortic, intracerebral, renal, internal iliac, and femoral, and the umbilical vein in an attempt to improve the sensitivity of Doppler blood flow study (Reed 1990).

MATERNAL ASSESSMENT OF FETAL ACTIVITY

Assessment of fetal movement patterns has been used as a screening procedure in the evaluation of fetal status since 1971, when the clinical significance of various types of fetal activity was first described (Sadovsky 1985b). Clinicians now generally agree that vigorous fetal activity provides reassurance of fetal well-being and that marked decrease in activity or cessation of movement may indicate possible fetal compromise requiring immediate follow-up evaluation. Fetal movements are usually assessed by the woman but may also be assessed by BPP or NST.

Sadovsky (1985a) noted that although there is considerable variation among individuals, the average number of daily movements rises from about 200 at 20 weeks to a maximum of 575 at 32 weeks and gradually decreases to an average of 282 at term. In women with a multiple gestation daily fetal movements are significantly higher. Although women report periods of markedly decreased fetal movement, this has been found to be associated with periods of fetal sleep, medications, smoking, and other factors. It has also been noted that some women are not as aware of fetal activity and that more fetal movements are usually noted on ultrasound assessment than by the woman herself. Although there are various types of fetal movements, women at high risk for fetal hypoxia have noted a reduction in or disappearance of fetal movements or changes in the type of fetal activity with a predominance of only weak movements prior to fetal death.

Daily fetal movement assessment by the woman can be done in a variety of ways. One method is the Cardiff count-to-ten method. The woman begins counting fetal movements at the same time each day and continues counting until she has noted ten movements. She records the movements on a special graph. If it takes longer each day to note ten movements or if fetal movements are notably decreased, the woman is instructed to contact her certified nurse-midwife/physician. See Teaching Guide: What To Tell the Pregnant Woman About Assessing Fetal Activity in Chapter 15 for further information.

Sudden, strong, vigorous movements followed by cessation are characteristic signs of acute fetal distress and impending death. Women should immediately notify their certified nurse-midwife/physician if they note this type of fetal activity.

Although maternal assessment of fetal activity is a subjective means of evaluating fetal status, it has been found to be an excellent screening test for diagnosing chronic fetal distress. Furthermore, it is simple for the woman to perform, does not interfere with her normal routines, costs nothing, provides reassurance, and may enhance maternal attachment (Rayburn 1995). Pregnant women need to understand that fetal movements are significant, that fetal activity changes during pregnancy, and that when movements weaken or cease, they should contact their care giver for further evaluation. Women should be reassured that there are fetal rest-sleep states during which minimal or no movement may occur. Gross fetal movements may be absent for at least an hour as the fetus rests.

Nursing Care

The nurse assists in teaching the technique for monitoring daily fetal movement (such as the Cardiff count-to-ten method). The nurse can also help the woman devise a daily record or method by which she can report fetal movements. The nurse is available for questions and to clarify areas of concern. The main message should be

HOW TO HELP COUPLES MAKE INFORMED DECISIONS REGARDING FETAL ASSESSMENT TECHNIQUES

Diagnostic assessment and testing techniques increase in number and complexity with every passing year. The availability of these techniques has changed the outlook for pregnancies at risk or pregnancies with special problems. Using the new technology, the presence of the fetus can be confirmed and some congenital problems can be identified very early in the pregnancy. Indeed, fetal well-being can be assessed at various times throughout the pregnancy in order to identify problems and make treatment decisions. Because of these advantages, tests are used ever more frequently.

The childbearing couple needs to have as much information as possible in order to make well-founded decisions when faced with the array of new assessment technologies. Parents need to be clear about the purpose of the proposed test, the information that may be obtained, the risks and benefits for both the mother and the baby, and the alternatives that are available.

Although the majority of the diagnostic tests currently used are administered by physicians, nurses have an integral role in this arena as client educators and advocates. The nurse assesses the informational needs of the couple, provides the information, and ensures that the couple understands the diagnostic technique being used. The nurse does this in preparation for each test, even though the physician will still need to provide required information when obtaining a signed informed consent.

The provision of information and the securing of informed consent are essential, but occasionally problems can get in the way:

- To ensure that the couple has a real choice about having the diagnostic test, the pertinent information needs to be provided ahead of time. It is difficult for parents to make other decisions or to refuse the test once they are in the actual test setting.

- It is often a challenge for nurses to obtain complete information regarding each new technique, and this may stand in the way of comprehensive and accurate teaching.

- Some nurses are unaware of the value they can bring to couples faced with diagnostic testing, and thus they ignore potential educational and advocacy roles.

- Often tests are done without any explanation to the couple. In some instances only the sketchiest information is provided. This makes it difficult for the couple to understand the situation and does not enable them to participate in their own care.

- Some physicians prefer that the couple not have much information because this may cause them to worry unnecessarily. This approach can quickly lead to conflict when unanticipated problems arise and the couple feels they were not made aware of the potential risks.

clear: Fetal movement and the mother's reporting of it are very important. This empowers the pregnant woman to be responsible for her own fetal surveillance.

NONSTRESS TEST (NST)

The **nonstress test (NST)** has become a widely accepted method of evaluating fetal status. The test involves using an electronic fetal monitor to obtain a tracing of the fetal heart rate and observation of acceleration of the FHR with fetal movement. The test is based on the knowledge that the fetus is normally active throughout pregnancy and that good fetal activity will result in acceleration of the fetal heart rate when the normal fetus moves. Accelerations of the FHR imply an intact central and autonomic nervous system that is not being affected by intrauterine hypoxia.

The advantages of the NST are that it is relatively quick, inexpensive, and easy to interpret; it can be done in an outpatient setting; and there are no known side effects. The disadvantages are that it is sometimes difficult to obtain a suitable tracing, the woman has to sit or lie relatively still for 20 to 30 minutes, and the fetus may be in a sleep cycle at the time the test is performed.

Fetal age must be considered in the use and evaluation of NSTs. The central nervous system (parasympathetic and sympathetic nervous systems) of the fetus usually matures sufficiently by the 30th week of gestation to allow frequent accelerations of the heart rate when fetal movement occurs (Soffici & Eden 1994). The NST can be used as an assessment tool in any pregnancy but is especially useful in the presence of diabetes, pregnancy-induced hypertension, intrauterine growth retardation, spontaneous rupture of membranes, multiple gestation, and other high-risk pregnancy problems. Testing intervals may vary, depending on the condition of the mother and baby and recommendations of various experts. Puder and Sokol (1994) suggest twice weekly testing for high-risk clients and weekly testing for other conditions.

Currently, a *modified NST* may also be used. In this test a device that sends sound into the fetus (called fetal acoustical stimulation [FAST]) is used after 5 minutes of testing. If there is no acceleration of the fetal heart rate, the sound stimulus is used again (see Fetal Acoustic Stimulation Test [FAST] and Vibroacoustic Stimulation Test [VST] for further discussion).

The NST is a good indicator of fetal well-being but is not an accurate predictor of poor outcomes. The false-negative rate (a reactive NST followed by an unexpected fetal death within 1 week) is 2.5 deaths per 1000. A nonreactive NST is fairly consistent in identifying at-risk fetuses. However, it has a false-positive rate of 40–80% (DeVoe 1990). The false-positive rate may be related to inadequate testing time; hypotension in the mother during the testing session; or maternal medications such as narcotics, magnesium sulfate, barbiturates, methadone, or antihypertensives (Puder & Sokol 1994).

NST Procedure

The NST is usually scheduled during the daytime hours, and the woman is asked to eat approximately 2 hours prior to the test. The woman is positioned in a semi-Fowler's position with a small pillow or blanket under the right hip to displace the uterus to the left. Many facilities use a recliner chair, which permits a semi-Fowler's position while providing a leg and foot rest. An electronic fetal monitor is applied (see discussion in Chapter 22). The examiner applies two belts around the woman's abdomen. One belt holds a tocodynamometer that detects uterine or fetal movement. The other belt holds an external transducer that detects the FHR.

Recordings of the FHR are obtained for approximately 30 to 40 minutes (minimum of 20 minutes and maximum of 40 minutes [Puder & Sokol 1994]). The woman or nurse notes each fetal movement as it is recorded by pushing a button that will record on the monitor strip. If no fetal movements occur after 30 or 40 minutes of observation, the woman is given orange or other fruit juice or a light meal. Fetal movements often increase due to distension of the maternal stomach and elevation in blood glucose. Other stimulation of the fetus may involve the use of FAST, a loud noise near her abdomen, or asking the mother to place her hands on her abdomen and gently push on her fetus.

Interpretation of NST

The results of the NST are interpreted as follows:

- A *reactive NST* shows at least two 15 bpm accelerations of FHR lasting 15 seconds or more with fetal movements over 20 minutes (Figure 20–14). Note that NST criteria vary somewhat among experts. Some define a reactive test as two accelerations of FHR in 20 minutes; others require two in 10 minutes. The nurse must be aware of institutional guidelines for interpretation of the NST.

- In a *nonreactive test* the reactive criteria are not met. For example, the accelerations are not as much as 15 beats per minute or do not last 15 seconds (Figure 20–15).

- An *unsatisfactory NST* has an inadequate external monitor tracing of the fetal heart rate.

It is particularly important that anyone who performs the NST also understands the significance of any spontaneous decelerations of the FHR during testing. If spontaneous decelerations are noted, the physician/certified nurse-midwife should be notified for further evaluation of fetal status (Paul & Miller 1995).

The NST may also show more subtle signs of fetal deterioration before the interpretation is nonreactive. With increasing levels of anoxia sleep cycles lengthen, accelerations become more uniform, the interval between accelerations increases, variability decreases, and the

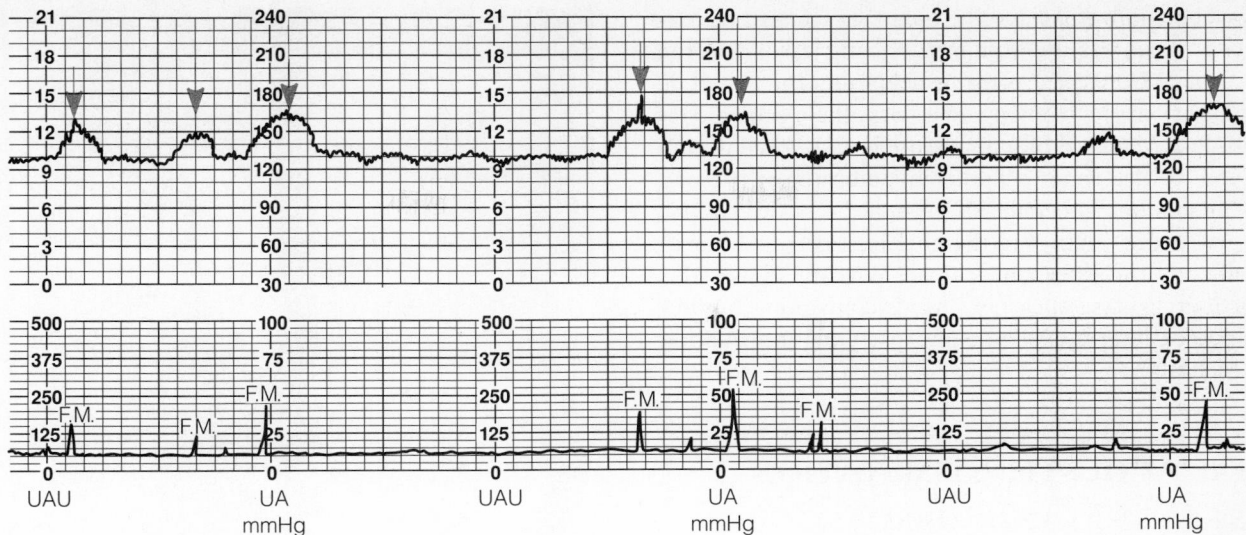

FIGURE 20-14 Example of a reactive nonstress test (NST). Accelerations of 15 bpm lasting 15 seconds with each fetal movement (FM). Top of strip shows fetal heart rate; bottom of strip shows uterine activity tracing. Note that FHR increases (above the baseline) at least 15 beats and remains at that rate for at least 15 seconds before returning to the former baseline.

FHR baseline may increase. This type of subtle change can be noted when serial NSTs are compared (Schifrin 1990). It is important that in this case the fetus be evaluated further with biophysical profile (BPP)/amniotic fluid index (AFI), biometry, and Doppler flow studies to assess fetal well-being.

Management

The clinical management may vary somewhat among different clinicians. Devoe (1989) recommends the following: If the NST is reactive in less than 30 minutes, the test is concluded and rescheduled as indicated by the condition that is present. If nonreactive, the test time is extended for 30 minutes at a time until the results are reactive; then the test is rescheduled as indicated. If the fetal heart rate is still nonreactive, additional testing such as diagnostic ultrasound and BPP/AFI or CST or immediate birth is considered. If the NST is nonreactive and spontaneous decelerations are present, diagnostic ultrasound and BPP/AFI are recommended.

Nursing Care

The nurse ascertains the woman's understanding of the NST, including fetal acoustic stimulation test (FAST) and

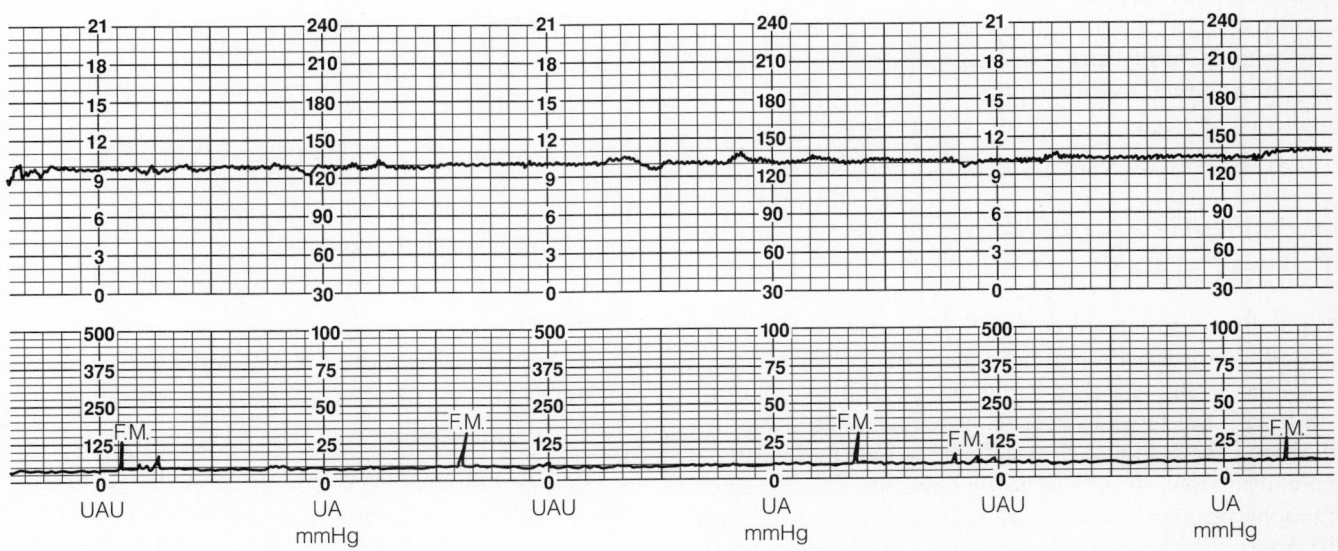

FIGURE 20-15 Example of a nonreactive NST. There are no accelerations of FHR with fetal movement (FM). Baseline FHR is 130 bpm. The tracing of uterine activity is on the bottom of the strip.

VST when appropriate and the possible results. The reasons for the NST, the equipment being used, and the procedure are reviewed prior to beginning the test. The nurse positions the woman and applies the electronic fetal monitor. Maternal blood pressure is monitored during the NST to determine whether hypotension is present. The nurse administers the NST, interprets the results, and reports the findings to the physician/certified nurse-midwife and the expectant woman. The nurse uses this opportunity to assess learning needs concerning the importance of fetal movement and provides information and teaching.

FETAL ACOUSTIC STIMULATION TEST (FAST) AND VIBROACOUSTIC STIMULATION TEST (VST)

Use of acoustic (sound) and vibroacoustic (vibration and sound) stimulation of the fetus is becoming more common as an adjunct to the NST. Several methods have been used (for example, loudspeakers, bells, artificial larynx). Figure 20–16 shows one example. A hand-held, self-contained, battery-operated device is applied to the maternal abdomen over the area of the fetal head. This device generates a low-frequency vibration and a buzzing sound, which are intended to induce accelerations of FHR in response to movement in those fetuses who demonstrate nonreactivity during the NST. Advantages of the **fetal acoustic stimulation test (FAST)** and vibroacoustic stimulation test (VST) are that they are noninvasive techniques, results are rapidly available, time for the NST is shortened, and the tests are easy to perform. A common FHR response to FAST or VST is tachycardia (FHR over 160 beats per minute). It is important to document the return of FHR to baseline. Caution must be exercised when using FAST or VST on a fetus that is already compromised. The response to the stimulation may include bradycardia and fetal distress. The FHR baseline and fetal well-being must be assessed before using FAST or VST.

CONTRACTION STRESS TEST (CST)

The **contraction stress test (CST)** is a means of evaluating the respiratory function (oxygen and carbon dioxide exchange) of the placenta. It enables the health care team to identify the fetus at risk for intrauterine asphyxia by observing the response of the FHR to the stress of uterine contractions (spontaneous or induced). During contractions intrauterine pressure increases. Blood flow to the intervillous space of the placenta is reduced momentarily, thereby decreasing oxygen transport to the fetus. A healthy fetus usually tolerates this reduction well. If the

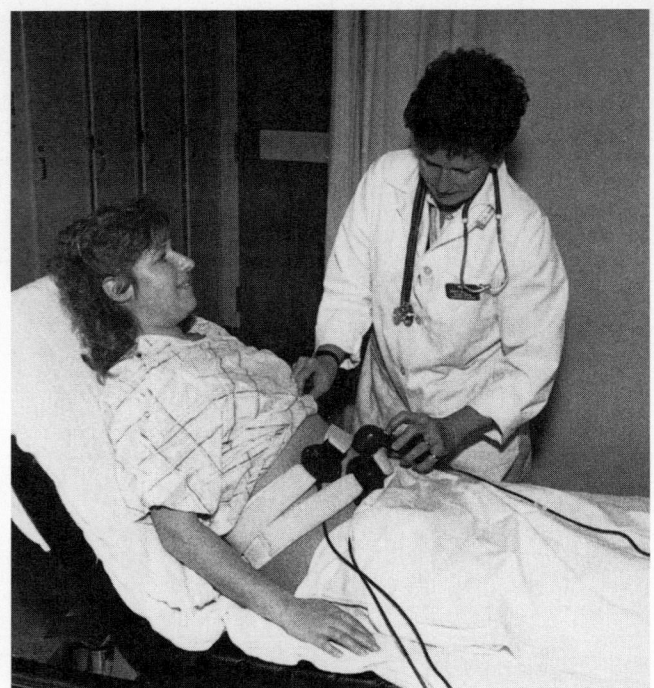

FIGURE 20-16   Fetal acoustic stimulation testing.

placental reserve is insufficient, fetal hypoxia, depression of the myocardium, and a decrease in FHR occur.

Indications and Contraindications

The CST is indicated for pregnancies at risk for placental insufficiency or fetal compromise because of any of the following:

- IUGR
- Diabetes mellitus
- Postdates (42 or more weeks' gestation)
- Nonreactive NST
- Abnormal or suspicious BPP

Contraindications for the CST are the following:

- Third trimester bleeding (placenta previa or marginal abruptio placentae)
- Previous cesarean birth with classical uterine incision
- Instances in which the risk of possible preterm labor outweighs the advantage of the CST, including:
  a. Premature rupture of the membranes
  b. Incompetent cervix or Shirodkar-Barter operation (cerclage—surgical procedure in which an incompetent cervix is encircled with suture to prevent it from dilating before term)
  c. Multiple gestation

CST Procedure

A necessary component of the CST is the presence of three uterine contractions of at least 40 seconds' duration in 10 minutes. The contractions may occur spontaneously, or they may be induced by oxytocin or nipple stimulation. The most common method of stimulating uterine contractions for a CST has been intravenous administration of oxytocin (Pitocin). This kind of CST is called the *oxytocin challenge test* (OCT). Many facilities now use *breast self-stimulation* to obtain a CST. This method is based on the fact that endogenous oxytocin is produced in response to stimulation of the breasts or nipples.

The CST is performed on an outpatient basis by qualified obstetric nurses well acquainted with fetal monitoring and the interpretation of various FHR patterns. Most facilities require the tests be administered in or near the labor and birth unit so that treatment is available in the event that adverse reactions to oxytocin stimulation occur. In many settings the physician/certified nurse-midwife must be present. The procedure, reasons for administering the test, equipment, and normal variations in monitoring that occur during the test should be clearly explained prior to the test to alleviate the woman's apprehension. A consent form may be signed. The woman should empty her bladder prior to beginning the CST because she may be confined to bed for 1½ to 2 hours.

During the test the woman assumes a semi-Fowler's or side-lying position to avoid supine hypotension. The ultrasonic transducer (from the electronic fetal monitor) is placed on the woman's abdomen over the area of the fetal back or chest so that the FHR may be accurately recorded on the monitoring strip. (See Chapter 22 for further discussion of fetal monitoring.) To record uterine contractions, the tocodynamometer (pressure transducer) is placed over the area of the uterine fundus. For the first 15 minutes the nurse records baseline measurements, including blood pressure, fetal activity, variations of the FHR during fetal movement, and spontaneous contractions. In addition pertinent medical and obstetric information may be obtained from the woman to aid in her further management.

After a 15-minute baseline recording an intravenous oxytocin contraction stress test is done. In the event that three spontaneous contractions of good quality lasting 40 to 60 seconds have occurred in a 10-minute period, the results are evaluated, and the test is concluded.

Intravenous Oxytocin Contraction Stress Test

A CST can also be done by using intravenous oxytocin. This test is also called an oxytocin challenge test (OCT). In this test an electrolyte solution such as lactated Ringer's solution is started as a primary infusion. A piggyback infusion of oxytocin in a similar solution is attached. An infusion pump is used so that the amount of oxytocin

RESEARCH IN PRACTICE

Clinical findings may be biased by observer expectancy. When examining a client, clinicians may find what they hope or expect to find based on review of the client's chart. Janet Engstrom, Claudia Sittler, and Karen Swift designed a study to determine whether such a bias exists for fundal measurements. They hypothesized that fundal height measurements would be biased by the clinician's ability to see the numeric markings on the tape measure being used and by the clinician knowing the fetus's gestational age.

This study was part of a larger research project examining four methods of determining fundal height. Ten certified nurse-midwives and four student nurse-midwives made fundal measurements. Each measured fundal height twice using each of four tools: marked tape measures, unmarked tape measures, pelvimetry calipers, and fundal height calipers. The measurements were obtained at prenatal visits, so each client also was examined by her regular care giver at this time. Each nurse obtained measurements from 10 pregnant women who had been selected for the study according to gestational age and body mass requirements. The researchers randomized the order of the measurements of each woman and established rigorous standards for collection and evaluation of the measurements.

To determine whether measurements were influenced by marked tape measures, the differences between the first and second unmarked measurements were calculated and compared with the differences between the first and second marked measurements. The researchers concluded that the ability to see the marks biased the clinicians, because the mean absolute difference (MAD) for the marked tape measure ($n = 335$, MAD = .61 cm) was smaller than that of the unmarked measurements ($n = 335$, MAD = .97 cm).

To determine whether a clinician's knowledge of the gestational age of a fetus biased fundal measurement, the researchers calculated the relationships between the number of of gestational weeks and three measurements of fundal height: marked tapes, unmarked tapes, and the measurement obtained by the care giver. The difference for each comparison was as follows: care giver, $n = 237$, MAD = 1.51 cm; marked tape, $n = 670$, MAD = 1.89 cm; unmarked tape, $n = 670$, MAD = 2.15 cm. The relatively low MAD for the care givers suggests that knowledge of gestational age prejudices fundal height measurements by clinicians.

Clinical Application of Study

As these authors suggest, clinicians should blind themselves to markings by using the blank side of measurement tapes to assess fundal height. Also, clinicians should consider making one measurement prior to reviewing the client's chart so that they are unaware of the pregnancy's stage in terms of gestational weeks.

SOURCE: Engstrom J, Sittler C, Swift K: Fundal height measurement: Part 5. The effect of clinician bias on fundal height measurements. *J Nurse-Midwifery* 1994; 39(3):130.

being infused can be measured accurately. The administration procedure is the same as for inducing labor through oxytocin administration (see Chapter 26). Oxytocin is administered until three uterine contractions lasting 40 to 60 seconds occur in a 10-minute period. If late decelerations are repetitive or occur more than three times, the oxytocin infusion should be discontinued and the physician notified immediately.

CST with Breast Self-Stimulation Test (BSST)

In BSST the woman stimulates one nipple through her clothing for 2 minutes. The procedure is stopped for 2 minutes and then repeated on the opposite breast. The complete cycle is repeated four times. If contractions do not occur, bilateral stimulation may be used for 10 minutes. When three contractions occur in 10 minutes, breast stimulation ceases (Lagrew 1995). The results are reviewed, recorded, and explained to the woman.

If a decrease in the fetal heart rate occurs with a uterine contraction, nipple stimulation is discontinued, the left lateral position is maintained, oxygen is begun via mask at 7–10 L per minute, and the certified certified nurse-midwife/physician is notified.

Interpretation and Management

A CST is usually not done prior to 28 weeks' gestation primarily for two reasons: First, in light of a positive test, birth and extrauterine survival would be questionable at such an early gestational age. Second, sufficient research has not been done to determine whether the same test results apply to a fetus of this gestation.

CSTs are usually begun at 32 to 34 weeks' gestation and are repeated once or twice a week until the woman gives birth. Should the woman's condition deteriorate, the CST should be repeated as soon as possible.

Interpretation of CST

A *negative CST* shows no late decelerations (Table 20–6 and Figure 20–17) is rarely associated with intrauterine fetal death (2.2 per 1000), so the test is usually repeated in 7 days (Sacks & Sokol 1989).

A *positive CST* displays late decelerations (Table 20–6 and Figure 20–18) may indicate the possibility of insufficient placental respiratory reserve (Devoe 1989). The fetus in this case is at higher risk for increased perinatal morbidity and mortality (75 to 100 per 1000) (Sacks & Sokol 1989). The fetus also has an increased risk of fetal distress, low 5-minute Apgar scores after birth, and IUGR (Devoe 1989). Less than 10% of CSTs in high-risk populations are positive (Devoe 1989).

The positive CST is associated with a 20% to 50% false-positive rate, which is attributed to aortocaval compression during uterine contractions, increased uterine tone during intravenous oxytocin-induced contractions, and the lack of any standardization of the "stress" that is

TABLE 20-6	Interpretation of the Contraction Stress Test

Result	Interpretation
Negative	No late decelerations occur with a minimum of three uterine contractions (lasting 40–60 seconds) in 10-minute period.
Positive	Late decelerations occur with 50% or more of the uterine contractions.
Equivocal	
Suspicious	Late decelerations occur with fewer than 50% of the uterine contractions once an adequate contraction pattern has been established.
Hyperstimulation	Late decelerations occur with excessive uterine activity (contractions closer than every 2 minutes, lasting for longer than 90 seconds, or a persistent increase in uterine tone).
Unsatisfactory	Uterine contraction pattern is inadequate, or FHR tracing is too poor to interpret.

SOURCE: Sacks AJ, Sokol RJ: Clinical use of antepartum fetal monitoring techniques. In: *Gynecology and Obstetrics,* vol. 2. Dilts PV, Sciarra JJ (editors). Philadelphia: Lippincott, 1989, Table 1, p 4.

produced by the uterine contractions (Sacks & Sokol 1989). Additional information may be obtained by performing an NST and assessing the variability of the FHR. When a reactive NST is present and the FHR has average variability, the outcome of the fetus during labor and birth is usually good. If a nonreactive NST and decreased variability are present, the obstetrician may consider a trial induction of labor or cesarean birth.

An *equivocal* (suspicious or difficult to interpret) test result may be managed by continuing the CST until the results are either negative or positive, or by rescheduling the test for after 1–2 hours of rest or for after performing BPP/AFI. Approximately 7% of CST results are equivocal.

A *hyperstimulation* pattern occurs in less than 3% of CSTs. This pattern is not reassuring in terms of providing information about the fetus, nor is the result useful (Devoe 1989).

An *unsatisfactory* result has fewer than three contractions per 10 minutes or a poor quality tracing. Repeat testing may be done after a period of rest, or another fetal assessment test may be done (Devoe 1989).

Regardless of the test result, if variable decelerations occur, ultrasound examination for amniotic fluid volume and localization of the umbilical cord is recommended (Devoe 1989).

Nursing Care

The nurse ascertains the woman's understanding of the CST and the possible results. The reasons for the CST and the procedure are reviewed before beginning the test.

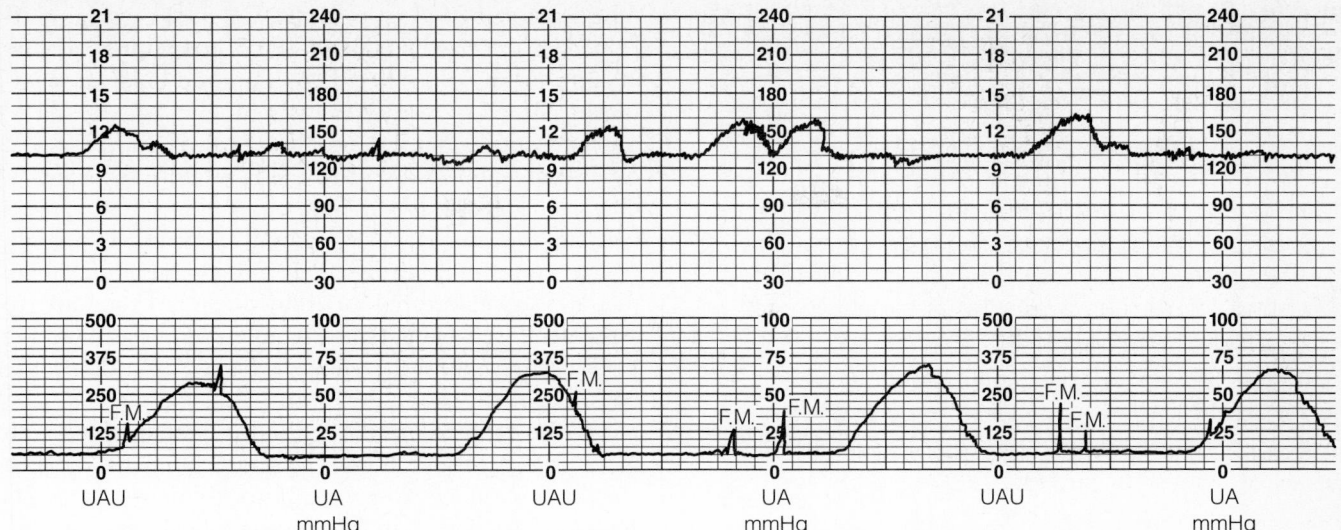

FIGURE 20-17 Example of a negative CST (and reactive NST). The baseline FHR is 130 bpm with acceleration of FHR of at least 15 bpm lasting 15 seconds with each fetal movement (FM). Uterine contractions recorded on bottom half of strip indicate three contractions in 8 minutes.

Written consent is required in some settings. In this case the physician/CNM is responsible for fully informing the woman about the test. The nurse administers the CST, interprets the results, and reports the findings to the physician/CNM and the expectant woman. The nurse is available to clarify any further treatment ordered by the physician/CNM.

AMNIOCENTESIS

Amniocentesis involves inserting a needle through the maternal abdomen into the uterine cavity to withdraw a sample of amniotic fluid. Amniocentesis is a fairly simple procedure, although complications do occur rarely (less than 1% of cases).

Early in the pregnancy (usually 16–18 weeks' gestation) amniocentesis can make chromosomal and biochemical determinations (enzyme analysis and α-fetoprotein measurement for neural tube defects) and can delineate abnormalities detected by ultrasound. Later in pregnancy (from about 30–35 weeks' gestation) amniocentesis may be done for lung maturity studies such as L/S ratio and the presence of phosphatidylglycerol and phosphatidylcholine. This procedure is also used to determine the presence or absence of intrauterine infection with premature rupture of the membranes in preterm labor before tocolytic therapy is considered.

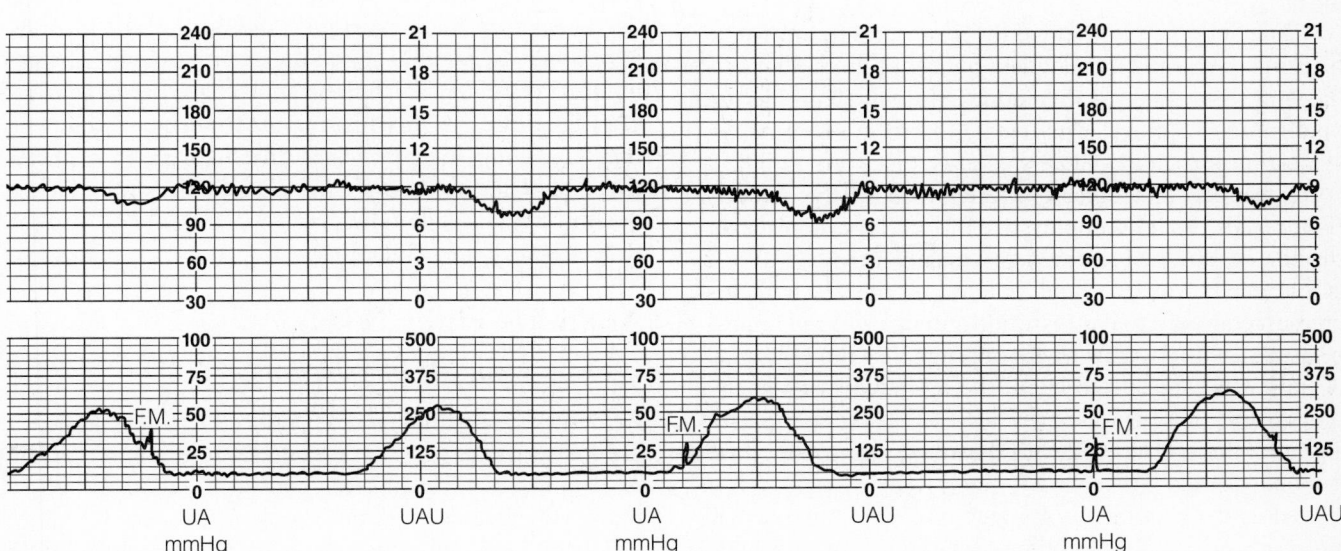

FIGURE 20-18 Example of a positive contraction stress test (CST). Repetitive late decelerations occur with each contraction. Note that there are no accelerations of FHR with three fetal movements (FM). The baseline FHR is 120 bpm. Uterine contractions (bottom half of strip) occurred four times in 12 minutes.

Amniotic fluid is obtained by transabdominal amniocentesis. The fetus, umbilical cord, or placenta may be punctured inadvertently, causing injuries ranging from minor scratches of fetal parts to intrauterine hemorrhage, leading to fetal distress and intrauterine fetal death. Placental perforation could result in hemorrhage from the fetal circulation, which could lead to fetal anemia or to increased sensitization of an Rh negative mother. Intra-amniotic infection and induction of preterm labor are also hazards. Complications are rare (0.5% to 1%), but the woman does need to be informed of them. A consent form is signed for this procedure.

Procedure

Amniocentesis is done on an outpatient basis but needs to be performed near a birthing area in case acute fetal distress is encountered. The pregnant woman should have a left lateral tilt to prevent hypotension during the procedure.

The abdomen is scanned by ultrasound to locate the placenta, fetus, and an adequate pocket of fluid. The amniocentesis, or "tap," is then done before the fetus has the opportunity to move. The needle insertion site is of the utmost importance because the fetus, placenta, umbilical cord, bladder, and uterine arteries must all be avoided (Figure 20–19). The importance of locating the placenta cannot be stressed enough, especially in cases of Rh isoimmunization, in which trauma to the placenta increases fetal-maternal transfusion and worsens the immunization. In the last few weeks of pregnancy the fetus may occupy what appears to be all the available space in the uterus, and there is a normal decrease in the amount of amniotic fluid. However, with the aid of ultrasound, fluid can be located.

After the abdomen is scanned, the abdominal skin is cleansed with povidone-iodine (Betadine). The woman is given the option of a local anesthetic for the insertion site. A 22-gauge spinal needle is inserted into the uterine cavity. Generally, fluid immediately flows into the needle.

The first few drops are discarded, and then a syringe is attached to the needle, and the fluid is aspirated (Figure 20–20). From 15 to 20 mL of amniotic fluid are withdrawn, placed in test tubes covered with tape (to shield the fluid from light to prevent breakdown of bilirubin and other pigments), and sent to the laboratory for analysis. The needle is withdrawn using ultrasound, and the insertion site is evaluated for streaming (movement of fluid), which would indicate bleeding into the amniotic fluid. The FHR is monitored for approximately 15 minutes to assess fetal well-being. If the woman's vital signs and the FHR are normal, she is allowed to leave (see Procedure 20–1).

If the collected amniotic fluid is contaminated with blood, the fluid should be centrifuged immediately. The woman is observed closely for 30 to 40 minutes for alterations in the FHR. The blood should be tested to determine whether it is maternal or fetal.

Rh negative women are given Rh immune globulin after amniocentesis, provided that they are not already sensitized. If the amniotic fluid from these women is contaminated with blood, the sample should be tested to identify fetal cells. In this situation a larger dose of immune globulin is required.

Nursing Care

The nurse assists the physician during the amniocentesis (Procedure 20–1: Nursing Responsibilities During Amniocentesis on page 552). In addition the nurse supports the woman undergoing amniocentesis. Women are usually apprehensive about what is about to happen as well as about the information that will be obtained by amniocentesis. The physician explains the procedure before the woman signs the consent form. As it is being performed, the woman may need additional emotional support. She may become anxious during the procedure. She may also become lightheaded, nauseated, and diaphoretic from lying on her back with a gravid uterus compressing the abdominal vessels, so it is important to have her in a lateral tilt. The nurse can provide support to the woman by further clarifying the physician's instructions or explanations, by relieving the woman's physical discomfort when possible, and by responding verbally and physically to the woman's need for reassurance.

Amniotic Fluid Tests

α-Fetoprotein (AFP) Screening

AFP is a fetal serum protein produced in the yolk sac for the first 6 weeks of gestation and then by the fetal liver. AFP concentration in fetal plasma peaks at about 15 weeks and then declines until term as it is excreted in fetal urine and subsequently into the amniotic fluid (Kochenour 1994). AFP is found in the amniotic fluid and maternal serum. The concentration of amniotic fluid AFP (AFAFP) parallels the rise and gradual decline of

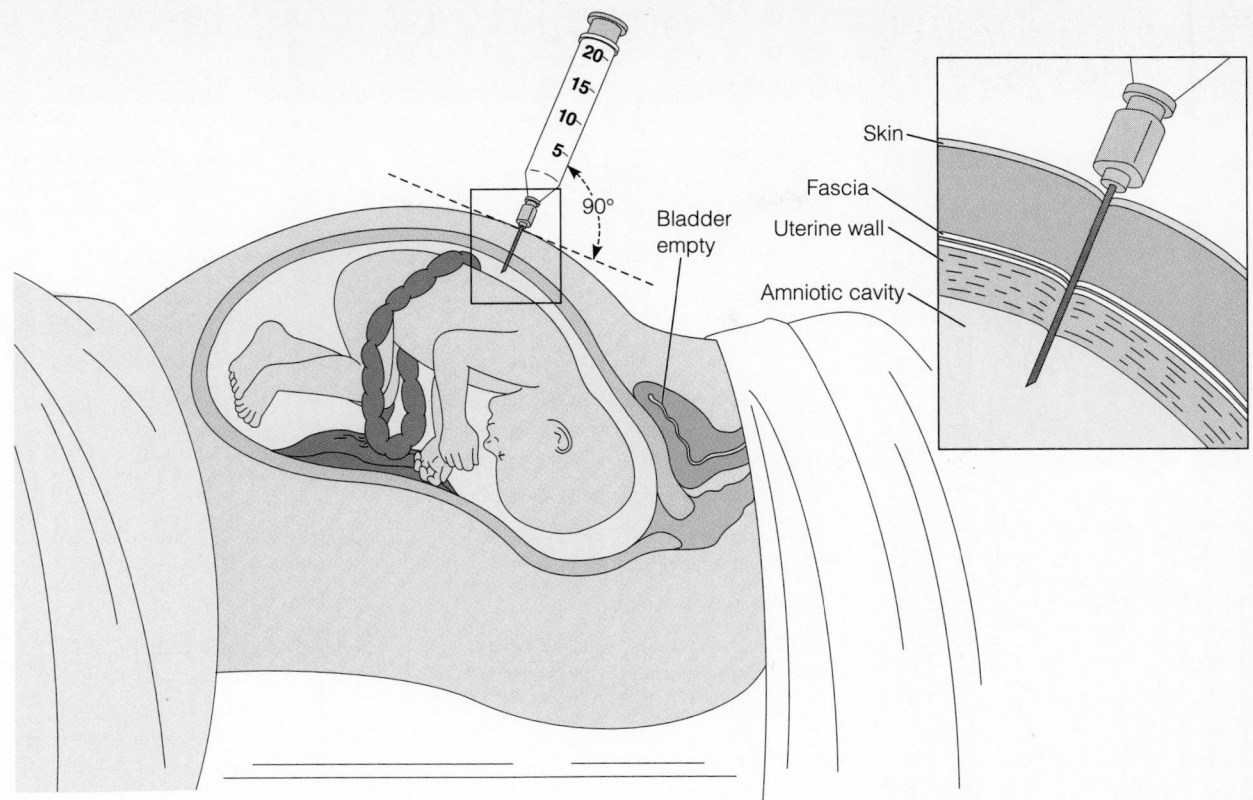

FIGURE 20-19 The woman is usually scanned by ultrasound to determine the placental site and to locate a pocket of fluid. As the needle is inserted, three levels of resistance are felt when the needle penetrates the skin, fascia, and uterine wall. When the needle is placed within the uterine cavity, amniotic fluid is withdrawn.

AFP in the fetal serum, but is at a lower level. Maternal serum AFP (MSAFP) rises slowly throughout pregnancy until it peaks at about the 30th week of gestation. Elevated MSAFP levels have been found in women whose fetus has an open neural tube defect (spina bifida or anencephaly), abdominal wall defect (gastroschisis or omphalocele), congenital nephrosis, cystic hygroma, incorrect gestational age (is more advanced in gestation than previously thought), fetal death, and multiple gestation (Kochenour 1994).

The incidence of neural tube defect (NTD) is approximately 1 in 1000 to 1 in 2000 in the United States. It occurs more frequently in the east than the west and is highest in the Appalachian area (Kochenour 1994). The incidence in other countries varies, reaching 10 in 1000 (1%) in Ireland, Wales, and the Punjab. In the United States the recurrence risk for a family with a child with NTD is 2% to 3%; if there have been two affected children, the risk is 6.4%; and if there are three or more affected children the risk is 25% (Kochenour 1994).

AFAFP peak concentration occurs at about 15 weeks' gestation, and the widest margin between normal and abnormal levels occurs between 16 and 18 weeks. Because concentrations vary at different weeks of gestation, a particular level (called a cutoff level) has been established at

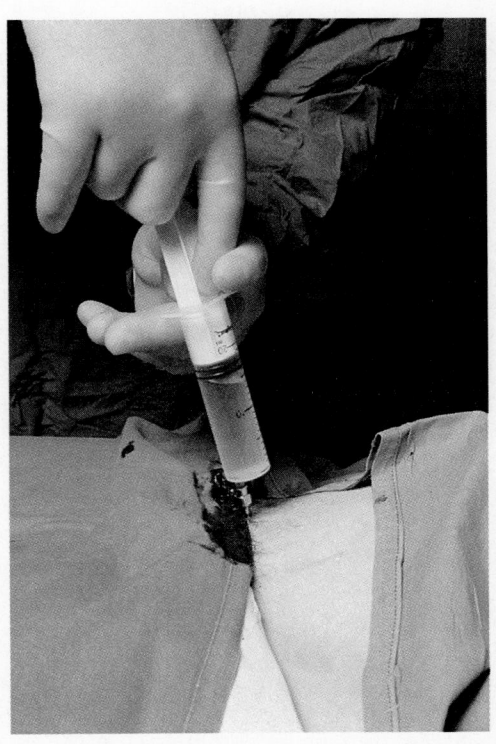

FIGURE 20-20 During amniocentesis amniotic fluid is aspirated into a syringe.

Objective	Nursing Action	Rationale
Prepare woman.	Explain procedure and reassure woman.	*Information will decrease anxiety.*
	Have woman sign consent form.	*It is the physician's responsibility to provide informed consent. Signing indicates woman's awareness of risks and consent to procedure.*
Prepare equipment.	Collect supplies: 22-gauge spinal needle with stylet; 10 mL and 20 mL syringes; 1% xylocaine; Betadine; three 10 mL test tubes with tops (amber colored or covered with tape)	*Amniotic fluid must be shielded from light to prevent breakdown of bilirubin.*
Monitor vital signs.	Obtain baseline data on maternal BP, pulse, respiration, and FHR.	*Status of woman and fetus is assessed.*
Locate fetus and placenta.	Monitor every 15 minutes.	
	Assist with real-time ultrasound to assess needle presentation during the procedure.	*Real-time ultrasound is used to identify fetal parts and placenta and locate pockets of amniotic fluid. Amniocentesis is usually performed laterally in the area of fetal small parts where pockets of amniotic fluid are usually seen.*
Cleanse abdomen.	Prep abdomen with cleansing agent.	*Incidence of infection is decreased.*
Collect specimen of amniotic fluid. (See Essential Precautions in Practice: During Amniocentesis.)	Obtain test tubes from physician; provide correct identification; send to lab with appropriate lab slips.	
Reassess vital signs.	Determine woman's BP, pulse, respirations, and FHR; palpate fundus to assess for uterine contractions; monitor woman with external fetal monitor for 20–30 minutes after amniocentesis.	*Fetus may have been inadvertently punctured. Uterine contractions may ensue following procedure; treatment course should be determined to counteract any supine hypotension and to increase venous return and cardiac output.*
	Assess blood type and need for RhoGAM.	
	Have woman rest on left side.	
Complete client record.	Record type of procedure done, date, time, name of physician performing test, maternal-fetal response, and disposition of specimen.	*Client records will be complete and current.*
Educate woman.	Reassure woman; instruct her to report any of the following side effects to her primary caretaker: unusual fetal hyperactivity or lack of movement; vaginal discharge—clear drainage or bleeding; uterine contractions or abdominal pain; fever or chills.	*Client will know how to recognize side effects or conditions that warrant further treatment.*
	Encourage light activity for 24 hours.	*Decrease in maternal activity will decrease uterine irritability and increase uteroplacental circulation.*
	Encourage increased oral fluids.	*Increased hydration will replace the amniotic fluid through uteroplacental circulation.*

each week of gestation. As long as the gestational age assessment is accurate, the identified cutoff level at each week in pregnancy results in an NTD detection rate of 98% and a 0.8% false-positive rate (an abnormality is thought to exist and it does not) (Kochenour 1994). The number of false-positive results depends on the cutoff level; the higher the cutoff level, the greater the proportion of women who will be suspected of having an abnormal fetus requiring additional testing. Therefore routine screening and cutoff levels depend on the particular population's risk for NTD. There is controversy regarding the necessity for mass screening due to expense of testing, problems related to assay and interpretation of results, the number of false-positive results, and the need for counseling. Women who may choose to be tested include those with a child with an NTD, with a strong family history of NTD, pregnant women with diabetes, and those residing in areas where NTD is prevalent.

MSAFP screening is most accurate when done between weeks 16 and 18. Using the appropriate cutoff number 95% of anencephalic fetuses, 80% of open spina bifida fetuses, and approximately 5% of closed spina bifida (hydrocephalus) fetuses are detected. The levels of MSAFP vary, depending on specific maternal characteristics. Therefore corrected levels must be established for maternal weight, race, multiple gestation, and diabetes.

Decreased levels of MSAFP have been associated with Down syndrome (Kochenour 1994). Women at increased risk for having a baby with Down syndrome may benefit from MSAFP screening to help detect a fetus with Down syndrome.

In the search for an improved screening test for Down syndrome (trisomy 21), trisomy 18, and NTD, the *triple test* was developed. The triple test assesses AFP, human chorionic gonadotrophin (hCG), and unconjugated estriol (UE3), in relation to maternal age. The hCG is a glycoprotein produced by the placenta, peaking at 10 weeks' gestation. Elevated levels of hCG have been associated with Down syndrome, hydrops fetalis, and Turner syndrome. Low levels of hCG have been associated with trisomy 18 and fetal demise. UE3 is a short-acting estrogen secreted by the placenta that increases linearly with gestation. Low levels of UE3 have been associated with anencephaly, Down syndrome, trisomy 18, hydrops fetalis, Turner syndrome, and fetal demise.

Evaluation of Rh-Sensitized Pregnancies

The first studies of amniotic fluid were done in the early 1950s for the evaluation of bilirubin pigment in the amniotic fluid of Rh-sensitized mothers. The analyst could determine the degree to which the fetus was affected by looking at the optical density of the fluid. Liley (1961) produced a graph that is now universally used in determining the severity of hemolytic disease in the fetus.

If a sensitized Rh negative woman produces an incompatible Rh positive fetus, antibodies cross the placenta and cause hemolytic anemia in the fetus. Concentrations of bilirubin and other breakdown products from destroyed red blood cells can be detected in amniotic fluid by spectrophotometry. By plotting their concentration or optical density at ΔOD 450 mu on a Liley curve, the physician can ascertain the degree to which the fetus is affected and the need for intervention or intrauterine transfusion (see Chapter 19).

Liley categorized the degree of hemolytic disease in three zones on the curve. If the optical density falls in zone I (low zone) at 28 to 31 weeks' gestation, the fetus will either be unaffected or have only mild hemolytic disease. Amniocentesis should be repeated in 2 or 3 weeks. When the optical density falls in zone II (midzone), amniocentesis is repeated frequently so that the trend can be determined. The age of the fetus and the trend in optical density indicate the necessity for fetal transfusion via percutaneous umbilical blood sampling (PUBS) or preterm birth. Optical densities falling in zone III (high zone) indicate that the fetus is severely affected and death is a possibility. Today fetal anemia may be directly assessed through PUBS, and red cells and platelets may be transfused directly into the fetal circulation rather than into the fetal peritoneal space as was done with intrauterine transfusion. Exact degrees of hemolysis can be determined by this method, earlier transfusion is possible, and complete reversal of hydrops fetalis has been reported after direct transfusion (Moise 1993).

The decision about whether to initiate birth or fetal transfusion depends on the gestational age of the fetus. If the fetal lungs are not mature, packed red blood cells compatible with the mother's serum are transfused into the fetus through the umbilical artery. Fetal transfusions are repeated whenever the fetal hematocrit falls below 30%. After about 32 or 33 weeks of gestation, early birth and extrauterine treatment are probably preferred to performing fetal transfusion.

Evaluation of Fetal Maturity

In managing the woman and fetus at risk the physician is constantly faced with the possibility of having to induce the birth of an infant prior to term and before the onset of labor. There are many indications for early termination of pregnancy, including repeat cesarean birth, premature rupture of the membranes, diabetes, hypertensive conditions in the pregnant woman, and placental insufficiency. Unfortunately, the most common cause of perinatal mortality is prematurity, especially in infants weighing 1500 g or less and with particular complications arising from pulmonary immaturity (Pernoll et al 1986). Birth of an infant with immature pulmonary function frequently results in respiratory distress syndrome (RDS), also known as hyaline membrane disease (Chapter 32).

Because gestational age, birth weight, and the rate of development of organ systems do not necessarily correspond, it may be necessary to determine the lung maturation of the fetus by amniotic fluid analysis before elective delivery. Concentrations of certain substances in the amniotic fluid reflect the pulmonary condition of the fetus (see below). In many cases birth of the infant can be delayed until the lungs show maturity.

L/S Ratio The alveoli of the lungs are lined by a substance called **surfactant,** which is composed of phospholipids. Surfactant lowers the surface tension of the alveoli during extrauterine respiratory exhalation. By lowering the alveolar surface tension, surfactant stabilizes the alveoli, and a certain amount of air always remain in the alveoli during expiration. When a newborn with mature pulmonary function takes its first breath, a tremendously high pressure is needed to open the lungs. Upon breathing out the lungs do not collapse, and about half the air in the alveoli is retained. An infant born too early in his or her development, when synthesis of surfactant is incomplete, is unable to maintain lung stability, resulting in underinflation of the lungs and development of RDS.

Fetal lung maturity can be assessed by determining the ratio of two components of surfactant—lecithin and sphingomyelin. Early in pregnancy the lecithin concentration in amniotic fluid is less than that of sphingomyelin (0.5:1 at 20 weeks), resulting in a low **lecithin/sphingomyelin (L/S) ratio.** At about 30 to 32 weeks' gestation, the amounts of the two substances become equal (1:1). The concentration of lecithin begins to exceed that of sphingomyelin, and at 35 weeks the L/S ratio is 2:1. When at least two times as much lecithin as sphingomyelin is found in the amniotic fluid, respiratory distress syndrome is very unlikely. Infants of diabetic mothers are an exception to this finding and have a high incidence of false-positive results; the L/S ratio of 2:1 may not indicate lung maturity in these infants. Delayed maturation is often seen in infants of diabetic mothers because the high blood sugars interfere with biochemical development.

Some types of chronic intrauterine fetal stress cause an acceleration of lung maturation in the fetus. Prolonged rupture of membranes (over 24 hours) results in acceleration of lung maturation by approximately 1 week and therefore has a protective effect. Amnionitis and vaginal bleeding more than 24 hours before birth also have a protective effect for the fetus (White et al 1986). Although the L/S ratio is the most universally used assay in evaluating pulmonary maturity, the results are not accurate when blood contaminates the amniotic fluid.

Phosphatidylglycerol Phosphatidylglycerol (PG) is the second most abundant phospholipid in surfactant. Phosphatidylglycerol appears at about 36 weeks' gestation and increases in amount until term. In instances of diabetes complicated by premature rupture of the membranes, vascular disease, or severe PIH, phosphatidylglycerol may be present before 35 weeks' gestation. PG is not measured in specific concentrations; rather, the mere presence of this substance is associated with very low risk of RDS, and the absence of PG is associated with the development of RDS.

Phosphatidylglycerol determination is also useful in blood-contaminated specimens. Because PG is not present in blood or vaginal fluids, its presence in a vaginal specimen is reliable for indicating lung maturity (Jobe 1989).

In recent years lung maturity has been most frequently assessed by a combination of L/S ratio and PG. Lung maturity apparently can be confirmed in most pregnancies if PG is present in conjunction with an L/S ratio of 2:1.

Identification of Meconium Staining

Any episode of hypoxia in utero may result in an increased fetal peristalsis, relaxation of the anal sphincter, and passage of meconium into the amniotic fluid. The amniotic fluid is normally clear, but the presence of meconium makes the fluid greenish.

Meconium staining may also be observed when amniocentesis is done. After the membranes have ruptured, meconium staining may be observed in the drainage from the vagina.

Once meconium staining is identified, more assessments must be made to determine if the fetus is suffering ongoing episodes of hypoxia.

OTHER DIAGNOSTIC TECHNIQUES

Chorionic Villus Sampling

Chorionic villus sampling (CVS) involves obtaining a sample of chorionic villi from the edge of the developing placenta. CVS is performed in some medical centers for first trimester diagnosis of genetic disorders. Villi in the chorion frondosum, present from 8–12 weeks' gestation, are believed to reflect fetal chromosome, enzyme, and DNA content, thereby permitting earlier diagnosis than can be obtained by amniocentesis.

There is an increased risk of pregnancy loss associated with CVS. The Medical Research Council (1991) reported a 4.6% higher loss rate for CVS than for amniocentesis. There is also an association between CVS and fetal limb reduction defects (a portion of a finger or toe missing), with the majority of defects occurring when procedures were performed before 9.5 weeks' gestation. The woman should be aware of the risks and benefits of CVS. Because CVS makes possible earlier diagnosis of congenital defects, first trimester (prior to 14 weeks' gestation) therapeutic abortion is possible if indicated and desired.

Before CVS an ultrasound is done to evaluate placental location, uterine position (retroverted or anteverted), and presence of intervening structures (ie, bowel, blood vessels). Various equipment has been used to aspirate chorionic villi from the placenta. The procedure can be done by transcervical placement of a catheter, transabdominal insertion of a needle into the placenta, or insertion of a needle through the posterior wall of the vagina and uterus into the placenta (Schulman et al 1992).

After counseling regarding diagnosis and procedure technique, preliminary blood work may be obtained. The morning of the procedure the woman is asked to fill her bladder because displacement of an anteverted uterus may aid in positioning the uterus for catheter insertion. A high-resolution linear-array or sector ultrasound is used to determine uterine position, cervical position, gestational sac size, and CRL measurement and to identify the area of placental formation and cord insertion. For the transcervical CVS the woman is then placed in lithotomy position; the vulva is cleansed with povidone-iodine solution (Betadine); and a sterile speculum is inserted into the vagina. The vaginal vault and cervix are cleansed with the same solution to decrease contamination from the vagina into the uterus. The anterior lip of the cervix is sometimes grasped with a tenaculum to aid in straightening anteflexion of the uterus. The catheter (or cannula) is slowly inserted under ultrasound guidance through the endocervix to the sampling site at the extra-amniotic placental edge (outside the gestational sac). The obturator is withdrawn from the catheter. A 30 mL syringe, containing 3 to 4 mL of tissue culture medium with heparin, is attached, and a sample of villi is aspirated by using a pressure of 20–30 mL (Elias & Simpson 1991). The contents of the syringe are flushed into a petri dish containing nutrient medium, and the villi are inspected microscopically and prepared for cell culture.

For the transabdominal sampling the woman is placed in the supine position. After the skin is cleansed with Betadine and local anesthesia given, an 18- or 20-gauge needle is inserted percutaneously through the maternal abdominal wall and uterine myometrium. The tip of the needle is advanced into the long axis of the chorion frondosum under ultrasound guidance. Chorionic villi are obtained by repeated, rapid aspirations of the syringe containing tissue culture medium and heparin. Transvaginal sampling is similar to the transcervical method except the needle is inserted into the vaginal mucosa overlying the cul-de-sac of Douglas.

Risks of CVS include failure to obtain tissue, rupture of membranes, leakage of amniotic fluid, bleeding, intrauterine infection, spontaneous abortion, maternal tissue contamination of the specimen, and Rh isoimmunization. Rh negative women are given $Rh_o(D)$ immune globulin to cover the risk of immunization from the procedure (Elias & Simpson 1991).

Fetal karyotype, diagnosis of hemoglobinopathies (eg, sickle cell anemia and α- and some β-thalassemias), phenylketonuria, α-antitrypsin deficiency, Down syndrome, Duchenne's muscular dystrophy, and factor IX deficiency can be detected by this technique. Rapid sex determination can be made so that pregnancies with a male fetus who would be affected in X-linked conditions can be identified early.

One of the greatest advantages to a mother undergoing this procedure is earlier diagnosis and decreased waiting time for results. Whereas amniocentesis is not done until at least 16 weeks' gestation, CVS is performed between 8 and 12 weeks. The CVS results are obtained in 24 hours if the direct preparation method is used and 7–10 days when tissue culture is used. Earlier diagnosis may relieve many of the personal, social, and psychologic concerns of families, particularly if therapeutic abortion is being considered. There may be less emotional stress involved with having an abortion at an earlier stage of gestation. First trimester abortions are also easier to perform, require less time, and are less costly.

Follow-up ultrasound and lab evaluation of each pregnancy must be done after performance of this procedure to evaluate fetal status. Further neonatal follow-up studies are necessary to evaluate the long-term effects of this technique.

Nursing Care

Before the test the nurse ascertains the woman's understanding of the CVS, its uses, the procedure, and the possible results. The nurse provides opportunities for questions and acts as an advocate when additional questions or concerns are raised. The nurse completes assessments following the procedure.

The nurse plays an important supportive role in helping the woman or couple express any feelings and fears regarding the procedure and also regarding the decision-making process if abortion is being considered. That supportive role continues if abortion is chosen, even though the nurse may not be present for the procedure. It is important that support be provided following the procedure by the nurse who established a relationship with the couple previously.

Fetoscopy

Fetoscopy is a procedure for directly observing the fetus and obtaining a sample of blood or skin. It enables the physician to diagnose such conditions as fetal hemoglobinopathies, immunodeficient diseases, coagulation and metabolic disorders, chromosome abnormalities, Rh isoimmunization, and serious skin defects (Quintero et al 1994b).

Prior to fetoscopy, women at risk for abnormalities are counseled by the genetic team. Indications, risks, and limitations of the procedure are thoroughly explained, and a consent form is signed for the procedure, which may be done from 11 to 36 weeks' gestation.

Ultrasound is performed prior to and during fetoscopy to determine the gestational age, fetal position, placental location and thickness, location of umbilical cord insertion into the placenta, location of pockets of amniotic fluid, position of the part of the fetus or tissue to be viewed or sampled, and placement of the cannula (Quintero et al 1994b). Following rapid intravenous sedation of the woman to decrease fetal activity, the abdomen is cleansed with povidone-iodine solution (Betadine), a local anesthetic solution may be injected into the maternal abdomen, and a 0.5 cm incision is made through the abdomen to the peritoneum.

A cannula containing a trochar is inserted through the incision into the uterus and the amniotic cavity to the site previously determined by ultrasound. The trochar is removed, and amniotic fluid is withdrawn for genetic cell analysis and AFP level. A light source is connected to a 15 cm fiber-optic endoscope, which is about the diameter of a 16-gauge needle, and introduced through the cannula to visualize the fetus on a video monitor. Custom-designed miniature (2 mm diameter) surgical instruments have been developed and are used in this procedure. A technique for rapid amniotic fluid exchange with lactated ringers keeps the amniotic fluid pressure change at a minimum through constant monitoring. Simultaneous display of ultrasound and fetoscopic images on a single monitor through a video mixer is helpful (Quintero et al 1994a).

If fetal blood sampling is to be performed, a 26- to 27-gauge needle is inserted through the side channel of the cannula and advanced until the vessel in the umbilical cord is pierced and a sample of blood is obtained.

The numerous indications for fetal blood sampling include suspicion of problems with hemoglobin or coagulation factors and need to assess for rubella, toxoplasmosis, and cytomegalovirus. In those facilities where percutaneous umbilical blood sampling is performed, fetoscopy is rarely performed for these purposes. During fetoscopy blood samples can be taken from vessels in that portion of the cord that is a few centimeters from the placental insertion site. This is usually difficult, however, so a sample (approximately 0.5 mL) is collected from blood that leaks into the amniotic cavity after the needle is withdrawn from the vessel. Because blood aspirated by this method is mixed with amniotic fluid and diagnosis of various inherited diseases requires a pure fetal blood sample, in questionable situations blood is aspirated from a cord vessel at the placental insersion site.

Mother and fetus are monitored for several hours following the procedure for alterations in blood pressure and pulse, FHR abnormalities, uterine activity, vaginal bleeding, and loss of amniotic fluid. The woman is hospitalized until care givers are sure that no immediate complications have arisen. Rh negative mothers are given Rh$_o$(D) immune globulin unless the fetal blood is found to be Rh negative; antibiotics and tocolytics may or may not be given prophylactically. The following day, prior to discharge, a repeat ultrasound is performed to confirm the adequacy of amniotic fluid and fetal viability. Women are advised to avoid strenuous activity for 1 to 2 weeks following fetoscopy and to report any pain, bleeding, leakage of amniotic fluid, or fever.

Although amniocentesis permits the prenatal diagnosis of many sex-linked diseases, chromosome defects, and metabolic disturbances, the majority of fetal cells obtained by this procedure are not found to be viable, and culture is difficult and lengthy. Furthermore, many severe congenital abnormalities may be diagnosed only by direct visualization of the fetus or by analyzing fetal blood or skin tissue. Fetoscopy has been used to view the extremities, spine, genitalia, and face in situations where the fetus is at risk for development of external abnormalities—such as limb and digital deformities, cleft lip and palate, and hereditary skin disorders—or genetic diseases affecting these structures.

As amniocentesis, ultrasound, and percutaneous umbilical blood sampling techniques become more sophisticated and conclusive for diagnosis of fetal conditions and more widely used, the need for fetoscopy will decrease except in unusual situations, such as tissue biopsy for diagnosis of genetic skin disorders not detectable by biochemical means, or as a backup measure when other procedures are inadequate.

Nursing Care

The nurse clarifies the woman's understanding of fetoscopy, providing time for questions and acting as an advocate when additional areas of concern arise. Following the test, the nurse completes assessments and continues to provide support.

Percutaneous Umbilical Blood Sampling

Percutaneous umbilical blood sampling (PUBS) (also called cordocentesis) is a technique used to obtain pure fetal blood from the umbilical cord while the fetus is in utero. This procedure is beginning to replace fetoscopy in major centers and has been used for diagnosis of hemophilias, hemoglobinopathies, fetal infections, chromosome abnormalities, fetal distress in labor, level of maternal drugs in the fetus, nonimmune hydrops, isoimmune hemolytic disorders, and immunodeficiencies and assessment of fetal hemoglobin and hematocrit for calculation of transfusion requirements in the second and third trimesters (Petrikovsky & Klein 1993).

The indications for fetal blood sampling include:

- Rapid fetal karyotyping
- Diagnosis of fetal infection (CMV, toxoplasmosis, parvovirus, rubella)
- Platelet disorders
- Fetal blood grouping
- Diagnosis and treatment of isoimmunization
- Assessment of fetal well-being (pH, PO$_2$)
- Fetal metabolic disorders

The woman is scanned with a linear-array ultrasound transducer with sterile probe cover, and a 25-gauge spinal needle is inserted into her abdomen through the skin alongside the transducer and into the fetal umbilical vein approximately 1 to 2 cm from the insertion of the cord into the placenta. The stylet is removed from the needle, and fetal blood is aspirated into a syringe containing an anticoagulant. Red blood cell size is determined to distinguish fetal from maternal cells. A paralytic agent, such as pancuronium bromide (Pavulon), may be given to prevent fetal movement during the procedure.

Within the last 10 years the improvements in ultrasonographic technique have made PUBS a relatively safe procedure with overall fetal loss rate less than 2%. The complication rate after PUBS is less than 0.5%. Complications include failure to obtain a sample, bleeding from the sampling site, premature rupture of membranes, chorioamnionitis, and fetal bradycardia (Feinn et al 1989). The risks are higher in obese mothers, in cases of a posterior placenta, and when gestational age is less than 19 weeks (Nicolaides et al 1992).

Nursing Care

The nurse plays an important role in helping women for which PUBS is recommended. Although a genetic counselor explains the risks for genetic defects and chromosome disorders, many women and their partners need to be helped to understand the procedure and its risks. They may need anticipatory guidance to help lessen their anxiety, as well as emotional support during the procedure and follow-up evaluation and testing. The nurse may need to assist with coordination of financial and social service resources. The nurse can help promote relaxation during the procedure by instructing the woman in breathing techniques. The nurse completes assessments during and immediately following the procedure and in some cases performs the NST following the procedure.

Magnetic Resonance Imaging (MRI)

A recent advance in maternal-fetal assessment has been magnetic resonance imaging (MRI). A major advantage of MRI is its ability to reveal previously inaccessible areas of the body without invasive techniques or risk of ionizing radiation. In addition MRI can accurately distinguish between normal and impaired or diseased tissues and between fetal and maternal anatomy. Although used in only a few selected regional perinatal centers and still undergoing considerable research for use during pregnancy, this imaging technology is a promising complementary procedure for specific maternal or fetal diseases.

MRI is similar to computerized tomography (CT) and ultrasound scanning. However, its advantages include the following:

- Images can be obtained in different planes.
- Fat and other soft tissues can be differentiated easily.
- Assessment does not require the woman to have a distended bladder.

- The entire fetus can be imaged in one scan.

Disadvantages of MRI are its extreme expense to the woman, equipment expense, incapacity for real-time imaging, necessity of having a radiologist interpret findings, unavailability of imaging in the labor and birth unit, longer performance time than ultrasound, difficulty in scanning when the fetus is moving a great deal, and occasional claustrophobia or intolerance by the woman of the confines of the magnetic unit for the extended periods of time required for scanning (45 to 60 minutes).

Currently, MRI can be used for confirmation of fetal abnormalities suggested by ultrasound examination, for pelvimetry, and for assessment of placental localization and size and maternal pelvic masses. No harmful effects have been reported in the literature, and clinical evidence to date indicates that MRI is safe. Even so, informed consent is required prior to this procedure.

Critical Thinking Question

Take a few moments and think about what your reaction would be to seeing your fetus by ultrasound. Would it make you feel anxious, or more comfortable? Relate your personal feelings to situations you have seen in your clinical facility.

PSYCHOLOGIC REACTIONS TO DIAGNOSTIC TESTING

Little is written regarding the impact of antepartum diagnostic testing on women's anxiety levels; however, the need for testing usually provokes fear.

Ultrasound use during pregnancy has become almost routine, and many women view this antepartum test as an expected part of the prenatal care. They approach the ultrasound with anticipation because it may provide confirmation of the pregnancy through visualization of the fetus with heartbeat or may even identify the sex of the fetus. However, when more invasive testing is recommended, it may evoke fear and anxiety in the woman and her partner as they consider the reason for the test, the risk to the fetus and woman during the test, and the implications of the test results.

One study (Campbell et al 1982) noted that being able to see the fetus early in the pregnancy through the use of ultrasound led to more positive attitudes toward the ultrasound procedure and decreased feelings of stress related to the ultrasound. The women who were able to view their fetus on the monitor screen displayed more positive health behavior changes after the ultrasound than those women who were not allowed to view the fetus when the ultrasound was performed. Reading and Platt (1985) studied the reactions of women who had ultrasound examinations for decreased fetal movement. All women approached the ultrasound with anxiety; however, the women who were allowed to view their fetus on the ultrasound screen had a reduction in their anxiety level over other women in the study who were given only verbal communication that their fetus was "okay." This study confirmed that prenatal testing does influence anxiety level (Reading and Platt 1985, p 910) and provides information for care givers regarding the importance of the test for the woman. The findings also emphasize the importance of providing visual feedback during ultrasound examinations.

Magnetic resonance imaging (MRI) can be used to assess previously inaccessible areas of the body via a noninvasive process without the risk of ionizing radiation. This procedure can accurately distinguish between normal and impaired or diseased tissues and between fetal and maternal anatomy and pathology.

KEY CONCEPTS

Ultrasound offers a valuable means of assessing intrauterine fetal growth because the growth can be followed over a period of time. It is noninvasive and painless, allows the physician to study the gestation serially, is nonradiating to both the woman and her fetus, and to date has no known harmful effects.

Using ultrasound, the gestational sac may be detected as early as 5 or 6 weeks after the LMP. Measurement of the CRL in early pregnancy is most useful for accurate dating of a pregnancy. The most important and frequently used ultrasound measurements are BPD, HC, AC, and femur length.

A fetal biophysical profile (BPP) includes five fetal variables (breathing movement, body movement, tone, amniotic fluid volume, and FHR reactivity). It assesses the fetus at risk for intrauterine compromise.

Maternal assessment of fetal activity is very useful as a screening procedure in evaluation of fetal status.

A nonstress test (NST) measures fetal heart rate during fetal activity; FHR normally increases in response to fetal activity. The desired result is a reactive test.

A contraction stress test (CST) provides a method for observing the response of the fetal heart rate to the stress of uterine contractions. The desired result is a negative test.

Amniocentesis can be used to obtain amniotic fluid for testing. A variety of tests is available to evaluate the presence of disease, genetic conditions, and fetal maturity.

The L/S ratio of the amniotic fluid can be used to assess fetal lung maturity. The presence of PG may also provide information about fetal lung maturity.

Chorionic villus sampling is a procedure that obtains fetal karyotyping in the first trimester.

Fetoscopy is a procedure for observing the fetus directly and obtaining a sample of blood or skin.

Percutaneous umbilical blood sampling (PUBS) is a technique used in the second and third trimesters for fetal diagnosis, assessment, and therapy.

Triple screening of AFP, hCG, and estriol in maternal serum provides information about the possibility of open neural tube defects and chromosome abnormalities (trisomy 13, 18, or 21) in the fetus.

REFERENCES

American College of Obstetricians and Gynecologists: *Ultrasonography in Pregnancy*. ACOG Technical Bulletin no. 187. Washington, DC: ACOG, 1994.

American Institute of Ultrasound in Medicine: *Bioeffects and Safety of Diagnostic Ultrasound*. Rockville, MD: AIUM, 1993.

Anderson FH et al: Prediction of risk for preterm delivery by ultrasonic measurement of cervical length. *Am J Obstet Gynecol* 1990; 163(3):859.

Antsaklis AJ et al: Fetoscopy: Fetal visualization and blood sampling in prenatal diagnosis. In: *Human Prenatal Diagnosis*. Filkins K, Russo JF (editors). New York: Marcel Dekker, 1985.

Arduini D et al: Changes of pulsatility index from fetal vessels preceding the onset of late decelerations in growth-retarded fetuses. *Obstet Gynecol* 1992; 79:605.

Association of Women's Health, Obstetrical and Neonatal Nurses: *Nursing Practice Competencies and Educational Guidelines for Limited Ultrasound Examinations in Obstetric and Gynecologic/Infertility Settings*. AWHONN, 1993.

Barford DA, Dickerman LH, Johnson WE: α-Fetoprotein: Relationship between maternal serum and alphafetoprotein levels. *Am J Obstet Gynecol* 1985; 151(8):1038.

Battaglia C et al: Maternal hyperoxygenation in the treatment of intrauterine growth retardation. *Am J Obstet Gynecol* 1992; 167:430.

Bonnin PH et al: Relationship between umbilical and fetal cerebral blood flow velocity waveforms and umbilical venous blood gases. *Ultrasound Obstet/Gynecol* 1992; 18(2):18.

Brook MM, Silverman NH, Villegas M: Cardiac ultrasonography in structural abnormalities and arrhythmias: Recognition and treatment. *West J Med* 1993; 159:286.

Broussard P: Antepartum surveillance: What tests to use, how to do the test. *Tenth International Symposium on Perinatal Medicine and Obstetrical Ultrasound. April 9–12, 1990. Las Vegas, NV.*

Callen PW: *Ultrasonography in Obstetrics and Gynecology*, 3rd ed. Philadelphia: WB Saunders, 1994.

Campbell S et al: Ultrasound scanning in pregnancy: The short term psychological effects of early realtime scans. *J Psychosom Obstet Gynecol* 1982; 1:57.

Chang TC et al: Identification of fetal growth retardation: Comparison of Doppler waveform indices and serial ultrasound measurements of abdominal circumference and fetal weight. *Obstet Gynecol* 1993; 82(2):230.

Clark SL: Antepartum fetal surveillance: Choice of tests. *Tenth International Symposium on Perinatal Medicine and Obstetrical Ultrasound. April 9–12, 1990. Las Vegas, NV.*

Crane JP: Routine obstetrical ultrasound: Should all pregnancies be screened? *Tenth International Symposium on Perinatal Medicine and Obstetrical Ultrasound. April 9–12, 1990. Las Vegas, NV.*

Cunningham FG et al: *Williams Obstetrics*, 19th ed. Norwalk, CT: Appleton & Lange, 1993.

Davis RO et al: Decreased levels of amniotic fluid α-fetoprotein associated with Down syndrome. *Am J Obstet Gynecol* 1985; 153(5):541.

Devoe LD: Nonstress and contraction stress testing. In: *Gynecology and Obstetrics*, vol. 3. Depp R, Eschenbach DA, Sciarra JJ (editors). Philadelphia: Harper & Row, 1989.

Devoe LD: The nonstress test. In: *Assessment and Care of the Fetus.* Eden HD, Boehm FH (editors). Norwalk, CT: Appleton & Lange, 1990.

Drugan A et al: Counseling for low maternal serum alpha-fetoprotein should emphasize all chromosome anomalies, not just Down syndrome! *Obstet Gynecol* 1989; 73:271.

Druzin ML et al: The relationship of the nonstress test to gestational age. *Am J Obstet Gynecol* 1985; 153:386.

Eik-Nes SH et al: Ultrasound screening in pregnancy: A randomized control trial. *Lancet* 1984; 1:1347.

Elias S, Simpson JL: Sampling the chorionic villi. *Contemp OB/GYN Technology Issue* 1991; 36:11.

Faranoff AA, Martin RJ: *Neonatal-Perinatal Medicine.* St Louis, MO: Mosby-Year Book, 1992.

Feinn D, Amon E, Petrie R: Funicentesis: A review of sonographically guided umbilical cord sampling. *Female Patient* 1989; 14:74.

Fischer RL et al: Amniotic fluid volume estimation in the postdate pregnancy: A comparison of techniques. *Obstet Gynecol* 1993; 81:698.

Freda MC et al: Fetal movement counting "which method." *MCN* November/December 1993; 18:314.

Freeman RK: The contraction stress test. In: *Assessment and Care of the Fetus.* Eden HD, Boehm FH (editors). Norwalk, CT: Appleton & Lange, 1990.

Gebauer C, Lowe N: The biophysical profile: Antepartal assessment of fetal well-being. *JOGNN* March/April 1993; 22(2):115.

Goldstein SR: Significance of cardiac activity in endovaginal ultrasound in very early embryos. *Obstet Gynecol* 1992; 80(4):670.

Grannum PAT, Berkowitz RI, Hobbins JC: The ultrasonic changes in the maturing placenta and their relation to fetal pulmonic maturity. *Am J Obstet Gynecol* 1979; 133:915.

Hadlock FP: Evaluation of fetal growth and size. *Tenth International Symposium on Perinatal Medicine and Obstetrical Ultrasound. April 9–12, 1990a. Las Vegas, NV.*

Hadlock FP: Ultrasound: Content of the basic U/S examination. *Tenth International Symposium on Perinatal Medicine and Obstetrical Ultrasound. April 9–12, 1990b. Las Vegas, NV.*

Hagen-Ansert S: *Textbook of Diagnostic Ultrasonography*, 3rd ed. St Louis, MO: Mosby, 1989.

Hallak M et al: Chorionic villus sampling: Transabdominal versus transcervical approaches in more than 4000 cases. *Obstet Gynecol* 1992; 80(3):349.

Hobbins JC et al: Percutaneous umbilical blood sampling. *Am J Obstet Gynecol* 1985; 152(1):1.

Jeanty P, Romero R: *Obstetrical Ultrasound.* New York: McGraw-Hill, 1984.

Jobe A: Amniotic fluid tests of fetal lung maturity. In: *Maternal-Fetal Medicine: Principles and Practice*, 2nd ed. Creasy RK, Resnik R (editors). Philadelphia: WB Saunders, 1989.

Johnson JM et al. Biophysical profile scoring in the management of the postterm pregnancy: An analysis of 307 patients. *Am J Obstet Gynecol* 1986; 154(2):269.

Kochenour NK: Normal pregnancy and prenatal care. In: *Danforth's Obstetrics and Gynecology*, 7th ed. Scott JR et al (editors). Philadelphia: Lippincott, 1994.

Lagrew DC: The contraction stress test. *Clin OB/GYN* 1995; 38(1):11.

Liley AW: Liquor amnii analysis in the management of the pregnancy complicated by rhesus sensitization. *Am J Obstet Gynecol* 1961; 32:1359.

Lyons EA et al: In utero exposure to diagnostic ultrasound: A 6-year follow-up. *Radiology* 1988; 166:687.

Manning FA: The biophysical profile: Contemporary use. *Tenth International Symposium on Perinatal Medicine and Obstetrical Ultrasound. April 9–12, 1990. Las Vegas, NV.*

Manning FA: Dynamic ultrasound-based fetal assessment: The fetal biophysical profile score. *Clin OB/GYN* 1995; 38(1):26.

Manning FA, Hohler C: Intrauterine growth retardation: Diagnosis, prognostication, and management based on ultrasound methods. In: *The Principles and Practices of Ultrasonography in Obstetrics and Gynecology*, 4th ed. Fleisher AC et al (editors). Norwalk, CT: Appleton & Lange, 1991.

Manning FA et al: Fetal assessment based on fetal biophysical profile scoring: IV. An analysis of perinatal morbidity and mortality. *J Obstet Gynecol* 1990; 162:703.

Marshall C: The nipple stimulation contraction stress test. *JOGNN* 1986; 15:459.

Maulik D: Doppler ultrasound velocimetry for fetal surveillance. *Clin OB/GYN* 1995; 38(1):91.

MCR: Medical Research Council European trial of chorion villus sampling. *Lancet* June 22, 1991; 337:1491.

Medearis AL et al: Coming of age: Twenty-one years of antepartum testing. *Am J Obstet Gynecol* 1993; 170(1):part 2. (SPO Abstract #26).

Moise K: Intrauterine transfusion with red cells and platelets. *Fetal Med* 1993; 159:318.

Moore TR: Assessment of amniotic fluid volume in at-risk pregnancies. *Clin OB/GYN* 1995; 38(1):78.

Moore TR, Cayle JE: The amniotic fluid index in normal human pregnancy. *Am J Obstet Gynecol* 1993; 81:698.

Nicolaides KH, Snijders R, Abbas A: Cordocentesis in operative obstetrics. In: *Operative Obstetrics.* Iffy L, Appussio J, Vinzileos A (editors). New York: McGraw-Hill, 1992.

Pardi G et al: Diagnostic value of blood sampling in fetuses with growth retardation. *N Engl J Med* 1993; 328(10):692.

Paul RH, Miller DA: Nonstress test. *Clin OB/GYN* 1995; 38(1):3.

Pernoll ML, Benda GI, Babson SG: *Diagnosis and Management of the Fetus and Newborn at Risk.* St Louis, MO: Mosby, 1986.

Petrikovsky B, Klein V: Fetal umbilical blood sampling. *Neo Int Care* March/April 1993; p 20.

Pinette MG et al: Maternal smoking and accelerated placental maturation. *Obstet Gynecol* 1989; 73:379.

Puder KS, Sokol RJ: Clinical use of antepartum fetal monitoring techniques. In: *Gynecology and Obstetrics.* Dilts PV, Sciarra JJ (editors). Philadelphia: Lippincott, 1994.

Queenan JT: Maternal serum α-fetoprotein screening. In: *Management of High-Risk Pregnancy*, 2nd ed. Queenan JT (editor). Oradell, NJ: Medical Economics Books, 1985.

Quintero RA et al: Transabdominal thin-gauge embryofetoscopy in continuing pregnancies. *Am J Obstet Gynecol* 1994a; 170(1): part 2. (SPO Abstract # 73).

Quintero RA et al: Operative fetoscopy: A new frontier in fetal medicine. *Am J Obstet Gynecol* 1994b; 170(1): part 2. (SPO Abstract # 76).

Rayburn WF: Fetal movement monitoring. *Clin OB/GYN* 1995; 38(1):59.

Reading AE, Platt LD: Impact of fetal testing on maternal anxiety. *J Reprod Med* December 1985; 30:907.

Reed KL: Ultrasound: Doppler flow—where does it fit in? *Tenth International Symposium on Perinatal Medicine and Obstetrical Ultrasound.* April 9–12, 1990. Las Vegas, NV.

Reed KL: Ultrasound during pregnancy. In: *Danforth's Obstetrics and Gynecology*, 7th ed. Scott JR et al (editors). Philadelphia: Lippincott, 1994.

Robinson L et al: Pregnancy outcomes after increasing maternal alpha-fetoprotein levels. *Obstet Gynecol* 1989; 74:17.

Ruffin JD, Pearson J, Woods KT: The fundamentals of transperineal ultrasound. *JDMS* July/August 1992; 8:188.

Saari-Kemppainen A et al: Ultrasound screening and perinatal mortality: Controlled trial of systematic one-stage screening in pregnancy. *Lancet* 1990; 336:387.

Sacks AJ, Sokol RJ: Clinical use of antepartum fetal monitoring techniques. In: *Gynecology and Obstetrics*, vol. 2. Dilts PV, Sciarra JJ (editors). Philadelphia: Harper & Row, 1989.

Sadovsky E: Fetal movement. In: *Management of High-Risk Pregnancy*, 2nd ed. Queenan JT (editor). Oradell, NJ: Medical Economics Books, 1985a.

Sadovsky E: Monitoring fetal movement: A useful screening test. *Contemp OB/GYN* April 1985b; 25:123.

Schifrin BS, Clement D: Why fetal monitoring remains a good idea. *Contemp OB/GYN* 1990; 35:70.

Shulman H: Doppler ultrasound. In: *Assessment and Care of the Fetus.* Eden RD, Boehm RH (editors). Norwalk CT: Appleton & Lange, 1990.

Shulman LP et al: Transvaginal chorionic villus sampling using transabdominal ultrasound guidance: A new technique for 1st trimester prenatal diagnosis. *ACOG* 1992.

Simpson JL, Elias S: Prenatal diagnosis of genetic disorders. In: *Maternal-Fetal Medicine: Principles and Practice*, 2nd ed. Creasy RK, Resnik R (editors). Philadelphia: WB Saunders, 1989.

Soffici AR, Eden RD: Assessment of fetal well-being. In: *Danforth's Obstetrics and Gynecology*, 7th ed. Scott JR et al (editors). Philadelphia: Lippincott, 1994.

Stark CR et al: Short and long term risks after exposure to diagnostic ultrasound in utero. *Obstet Gynecol* 1984; 63:194.

Vintzileos AM: The use and misuse of the fetal biophysical profile. *Am J Obstet Gynecol* 1987; 157:527.

Vintzileos AM et al: The use of fetal biophysical profile improves pregnancy outcome in premature rupture of the membranes. *Am J Obstet Gynecol* 1987; 157:236.

White E, Shy KK, Benedetti TJ: Chronic fetal stress and the risk of infant respiratory distress syndrome. *Obstet Gynecol* 1986; 67:57.

Williams K: Amniotic fluid assessment. *Obstet Gynecol Survey* 1993; 48(12):795.

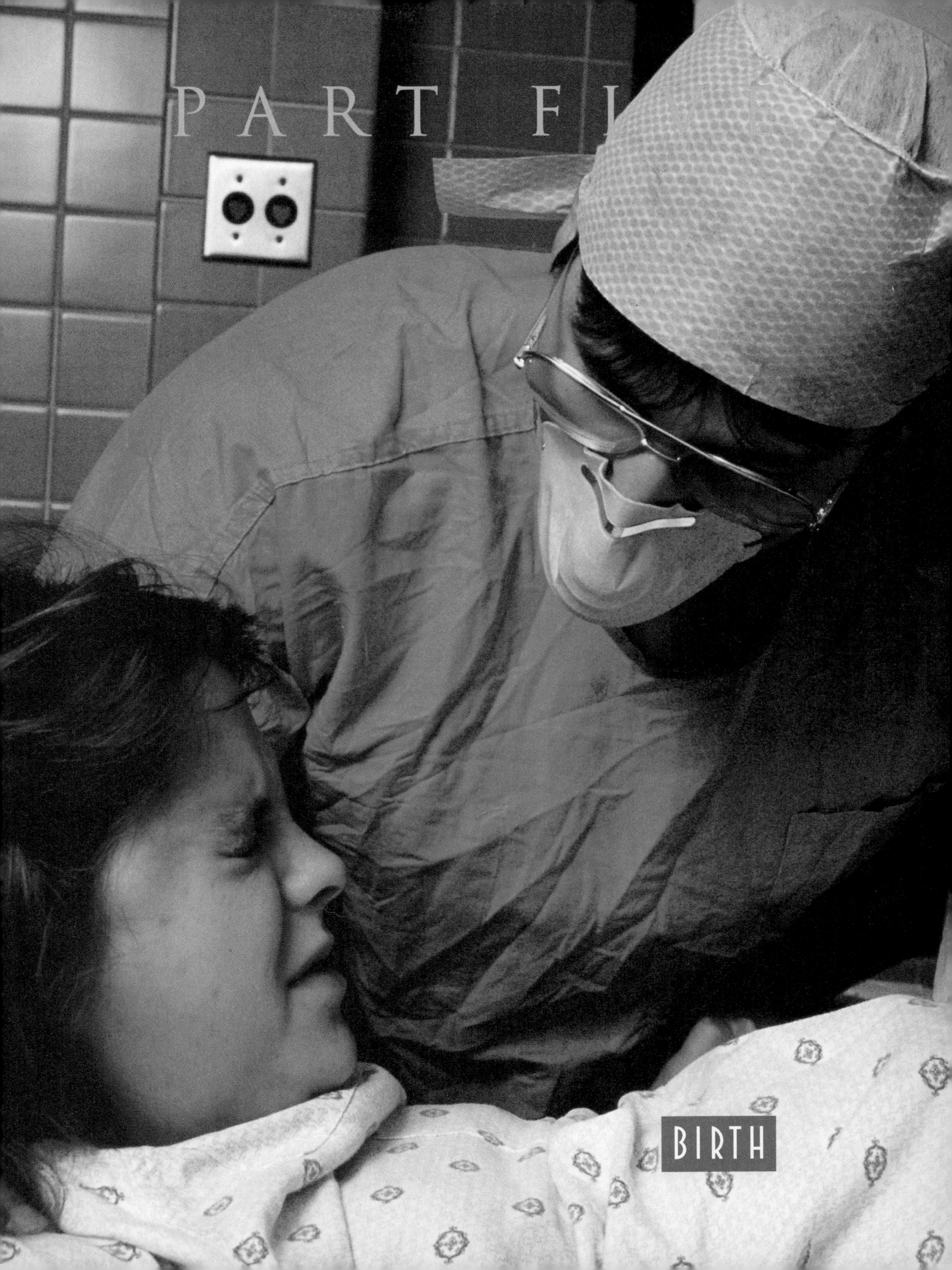

BIRTH

CHAPTER 21

PROCESSES AND STAGES OF LABOR AND BIRTH

*B*irth usually feels like a steamy kitchen—similar to holiday preparations, except that the smells are different. The smell of sweat is more acrid, there are some fetid odors, there is the smell and steam rising from blood. The air is thick, pungent, fertile. It is hard not to be reminded of fresh straw and night stars. There is near and heady promise.

~ A MIDWIFE'S STORY ~

KEY TERMS

Bloody show

Cardinal movements

Cervical dilatation

Crowning

Duration

Effacement

Engagement

Fetal attitude

Fetal lie

Fetal position

Fetal presentation

Fontanelles

Frequency

Intensity

Lightening

Malpositions

Malpresentations

Molding

Presenting part

Rupture of membranes (ROM)

Station

Sutures

OBJECTIVES

Examine the four critical factors that influence labor.

Describe the physiology of labor.

Discuss premonitory signs of labor.

Differentiate between false and true labor.

Describe the physiologic and psychologic changes occurring in each of the stages of labor.

Summarize maternal systemic responses to labor.

Discuss fetal responses to labor.

uring the weeks of gestation the fetus and the expectant woman prepare themselves for birth. The fetus progresses through various stages of growth and development in readiness for the independence of extrauterine life. The expectant woman undergoes various physiologic and psychologic adaptations during pregnancy that gradually prepare her for childbirth and the role of mother. The onset of labor marks a significant change in the relationship between the woman and the fetus.

CRITICAL FACTORS IN LABOR

Four factors are important in the process of labor and birth: the birth passage, the fetus, the primary forces of labor, and the woman's psychosocial considerations. Within these areas the following factors are significant:

1. Birth passage
   a. Size of the pelvis (diameters of the pelvic inlet, midpelvis, and outlet)
   b. Type of pelvis (gynecoid, android, anthropoid, platypelloid, or a combination)
   c. Ability of the cervix to dilate and efface and ability of the vaginal canal and the external opening of the vagina (the *introitus*) to distend

2. Fetus
   a. Fetal head (size and presence of molding)
   b. Fetal attitude (flexion or extension of the fetal body and extremities)
   c. Fetal lie
   d. Fetal presentation (the body part of the fetus entering the pelvis in a single or multiple pregnancy)
   e. Fetal position (relationship of the presenting part to one of the four quadrants of the maternal pelvis)
   f. Placenta (implantation site)

3. Primary forces of labor
   a. Frequency, duration, and intensity of uterine contractions as the fetus moves through the passage
   b. Effectiveness of the maternal pushing effort
   c. Duration of labor

4. Psychosocial considerations
   a. Physical preparation for childbirth
   b. Sociocultural heritage
   c. Previous childbirth experience
   d. Support from significant others
   e. Emotional integrity

The progress of labor is critically dependent on the complementary relationship of these four factors. Abnormalities in the birth passage, the fetus, the forces of labor, or the psychosocial status of the woman can alter the outcome of labor and jeopardize both the pregnant woman and her fetus. Complications during labor and birth are discussed in Chapter 25.

THE BIRTH PASSAGE

The true pelvis, which forms the bony canal through which the fetus must pass, is divided into three sections: the inlet, the pelvic cavity (midpelvis), and the outlet. (See Chapter 5 for a discussion of each part of the pelvis and Chapter 14 for techniques to assess the pelvis.)

The four classic types of pelvis are gynecoid, android, anthropoid, and platypelloid. The *gynecoid*, or female, pelvis is most common. All diameters of the gynecoid are adequate for childbirth. The *android*, or male, pelvis is usually not adequate for vaginal birth. The *anthropoid* pelvis is narrow from side to side, but is usually adequate for vaginal birth. The *platypelloid* pelvis, which is narrow from front to back, is usually not adequate (see Table 21–1).

THE FETUS

Fetal Head

The fetal head is composed of bony parts that can either hinder childbirth or make it easier. Once the head (the least compressible and largest part of the fetus) has been born, the birth of the rest of the body is rarely delayed.

The fetal skull has three major parts: the face, the base of the skull (cranium), and the vault of the cranium (roof). The bones of the face and cranial base are well fused and are essentially fixed. The base of the cranium is composed of the two temporal bones, each with a sphenoid and ethmoid bone. The bones composing the vault are the two frontal bones, the two parietal bones, and the occipital bone (Figure 21–1). These bones are not fused, allowing this portion of the head to adjust in shape as the presenting part of the fetus passes through the narrow portions of the pelvis. The cranial bones overlap under pressure of the powers of labor and the demands of the unyielding pelvis. This overlapping is called **molding.**

The **sutures** of the fetal skull are membranous spaces between the cranial bones. The intersections of the cranial sutures are called **fontanelles.** These sutures allow for molding of the fetal head and help the clinician

TABLE 21-1 Implications of Pelvic Type for Labor and Birth

Pelvic Type	Pertinent Characteristics	Implications for Birth
Gynecoid	Inlet rounded with all inlet diameters adequate Midpelvis adequate with parallel side walls Outlet adequate	Favorable for vaginal birth
Android	Inlet heart-shaped with short posterior sagittal diameter Midpelvis diameters reduced Outlet capacity reduced	Not favorable for vaginal birth Descent into pelvis is slow Fetal head enters pelvis in transverse or posterior with arrest of labor frequent
Anthropoid	Inlet oval with long anteroposterior diameter Midpelvis diameters adequate Outlet adequate	Favorable for vaginal birth
Platypelloid	Inlet oval with long transverse diameters Midpelvis diameters reduced Outlet capacity inadequate	Not favorable for vaginal birth Fetal head engages in transverse Difficult descent through midpelvis Frequent delay of progress at outlet of pelvis

Note: Description of pelvic shape is exaggerated for easier comprehension.

identify the position of the fetal head during vaginal examination. The important sutures of the cranial vault are as follows (Figure 21–1).

- *Frontal (mitotic) suture:* Located between the two frontal bones; becomes the anterior continuation of the sagittal suture
- *Sagittal suture:* Located between the parietal bones; divides the skull into left and right halves; runs anteroposteriorly, connecting the two fontanelles
- *Coronal sutures:* Located between the frontal and parietal bones; extend transversely left and right from the anterior fontanelle

- *Lambdoidal suture:* Located between the two parietal bones and the occipital bone; extends transversely left and right from the posterior fontanelle

The anterior and posterior fontanelles are clinically useful in identifying the position of the fetal head in the pelvis and in assessing the status of the newborn after birth. The anterior fontanelle is diamond-shaped and measures 2×3 cm. It permits growth of the brain by remaining unossified for as long as 18 months. The posterior fontanelle is much smaller and closes within 8 to 12 weeks after birth. It is shaped like a small triangle and marks the meeting point of the sagittal suture and the lambdoidal suture.

Following are several important landmarks of the fetal skull (Figure 21–2):

- *Mentum:* The fetal chin
- *Sinciput:* The anterior area known as the brow
- *Bregma:* The large diamond-shaped anterior fontanelle
- *Vertex:* The area between the anterior and posterior fontanelles
- *Posterior fontanelle:* The intersection between posterior cranial sutures
- *Occiput:* The area of the fetal skull occupied by the occipital bone, beneath the posterior fontanelle

The diameters of the fetal skull vary considerably within normal limits. Some diameters shorten and others lengthen as the head is molded during labor. Fetal head diameters are measured between the various landmarks on the skull (Figure 21–3). For example, the suboccipito-bregmatic diameter is the distance from the undersurface of the occiput to the center of the bregma, or anterior fontanelle. Fetal skull measurements are given in Figure 21–3.

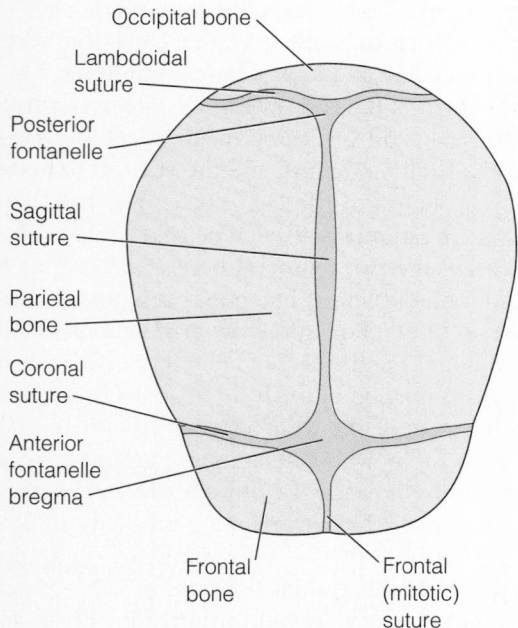

FIGURE 21-1 Superior view of the fetal skull.

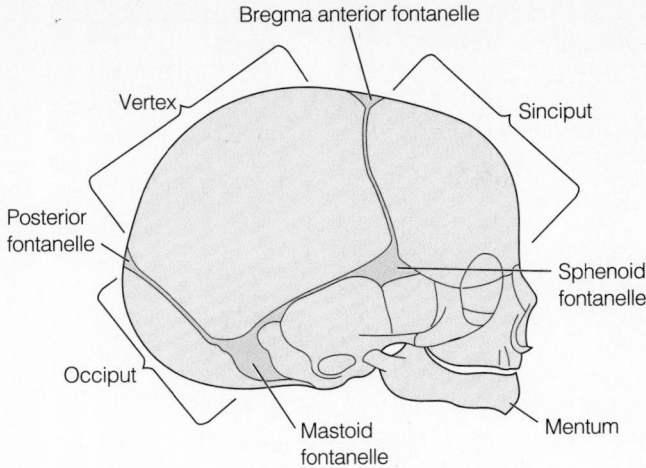

FIGURE 21-2   Lateral view of the fetal skull identifying the landmarks that have significance during birth.

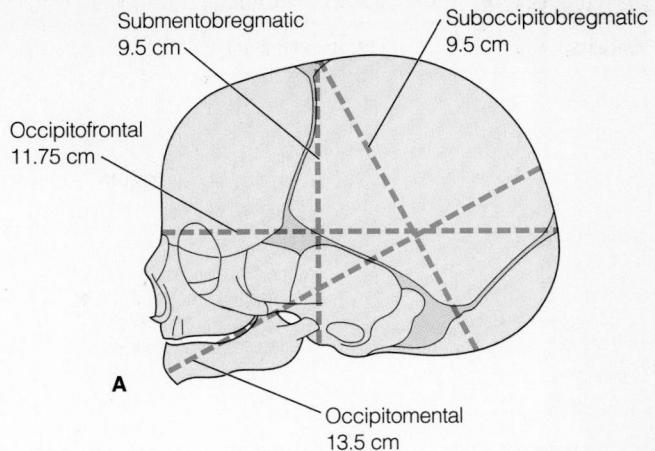

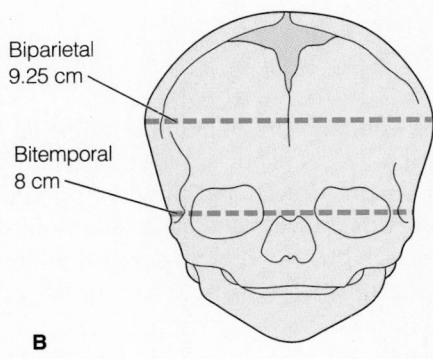

FIGURE 21-3   *A* Anteroposterior diameters of the fetal skull. When the vertex of the fetus presents and the fetal head is flexed with the chin on the chest, the smallest anteroposterior diameter (suboccipitobregmatic) enters the birth canal. *B* Transverse diameters of the fetal skull.

Fetal Attitude

Fetal attitude refers to the relation of the fetal parts to one another. The normal attitude of the fetus is one of moderate flexion of the head, flexion of the arms onto the chest, and flexion of the legs onto the abdomen.

Changes in fetal attitude, particularly in the position of the head, cause the fetus to present larger diameters of the fetal head to the maternal pelvis. These deviations from a normal fetal attitude often contribute to difficult labor (Figure 21–4).

Fetal Lie

Fetal lie refers to the relationship of the cephalocaudal axis (spinal column) of the fetus to the cephalocaudal axis of the woman. The fetus may assume either a longitudinal or a transverse lie. A *longitudinal lie* occurs when the cephalocaudal axis of the fetus is parallel to the woman's spine. A *transverse lie* occurs when the cephalocaudal axis of the fetal spine is at right angles to the woman's spine.

Fetal Presentation

Fetal presentation is determined by fetal lie and by the body part of the fetus that enters the maternal pelvis first. This portion of the fetus is referred to as the **presenting part**. Fetal presentation may be cephalic, breech, or shoulder (Table 21–2).

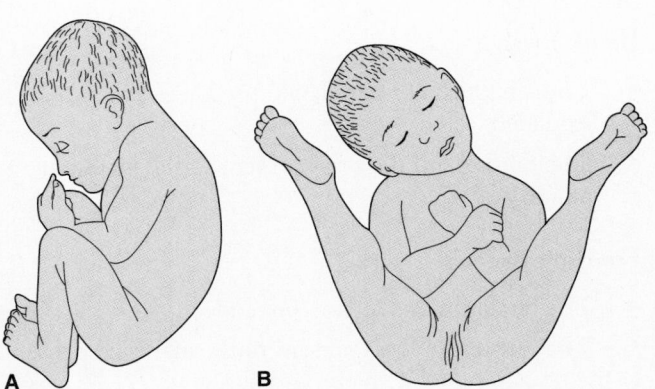

FIGURE 21-4   Fetal attitude. *A* The attitude (or relationship of body parts) of this fetus is normal. The head is flexed forward with the chin almost resting on the chest. The arms and legs are flexed. *B* In this view the head is tilted to the right. Although the arms are flexed, the legs are extended.

TABLE 21-2 Relationship of Fetus to Maternal Pelvis

Presentation	Attitude	Presenting Part	Landmark
Longitudinal lie (99.5%)			
Cephalic (96% to 97%)	Flexion of fetal head onto chest	Vertex (posterior part—occiput)	Occiput (O)
	Military (no flexion, no extension)	Vertex (median part)	Occiput (O)
	Partial extension	Brow	Forehead (frontum) (Fr)
	Complete extension of the head	Face	Chin (mentum) (M)
Breech (3% to 4%)			
Complete	Flexed hips and knees	Buttocks	Sacrum (S)
Frank	Flexed hips, extended knees	Buttocks	Sacrum (S)
Footling: single, double	Extended hips and knees	Feet	Sacrum (S)
Kneeling: single, double	Extended hips, flexed knees	Knees	Sacrum (S)
Transverse or oblique lie (0.5%)			
Shoulder	Variable	Shoulder, arm, trunk	Scapula (Sc or A)

SOURCE: Adapted from Oxorn H: *Human Labor and Birth*, 5th ed. Norwalk, CT: Appleton & Lange, 1986, p 54.

The most common presentation is cephalic. When this presentation occurs, labor and birth are more likely to proceed normally. Breech and shoulder presentations are associated with difficulties during labor and do not proceed as normal; therefore they are called **malpresentations.** (See Chapter 25 for discussion of malpresentations.)

Cephalic Presentation

The fetal head presents to the birth passage in approximately 97% of term births. The cephalic presentation can be further classified according to the degree of flexion or extension of the fetal head (attitude).

Vertex Presentation

- Vertex is the most common type of presentation.
- The fetal head is completely flexed onto the chest.
- The smallest diameter of the fetal head (suboccipitobregmatic) presents to the maternal pelvis (Figure 21–5A).
- The occiput is the presenting part.

Military Presentation

- The fetal head is neither flexed nor extended.
- The occipitofrontal diameter presents to the maternal pelvis (Figure 21–5B).
- The top of the head is the presenting part.

Brow Presentation

- The fetal head is partially extended.
- The occipitomental diameter, the largest anteroposterior diameter, is presented to the maternal pelvis (Figure 21–5C).

- The sinciput (see Figure 21–2) is the presenting part.

Face Presentation

- The fetal head is hyperextended (complete extension).
- The submentobregmatic diameter presents to the maternal pelvis (Figure 21–5D).
- The face is the presenting part.

Breech Presentation

Breech presentations occur in 3% of term births. These presentations are classified according to the attitude of the fetus's hips and knees. In all variations of the breech presentation the sacrum is the landmark to be noted (see Figure 21–8).

Complete Breech

- The fetal knees and hips are both flexed, the thighs are on the abdomen, and the calves are on the posterior aspect of the thighs.
- The buttocks and feet of the fetus present to the maternal pelvis.

Frank Breech

- The fetal hips are flexed, and the knees are extended.
- The buttocks of the fetus present to the maternal pelvis.

Footling Breech

- The fetal hips and legs are extended.
- The feet of the fetus present to the maternal pelvis.

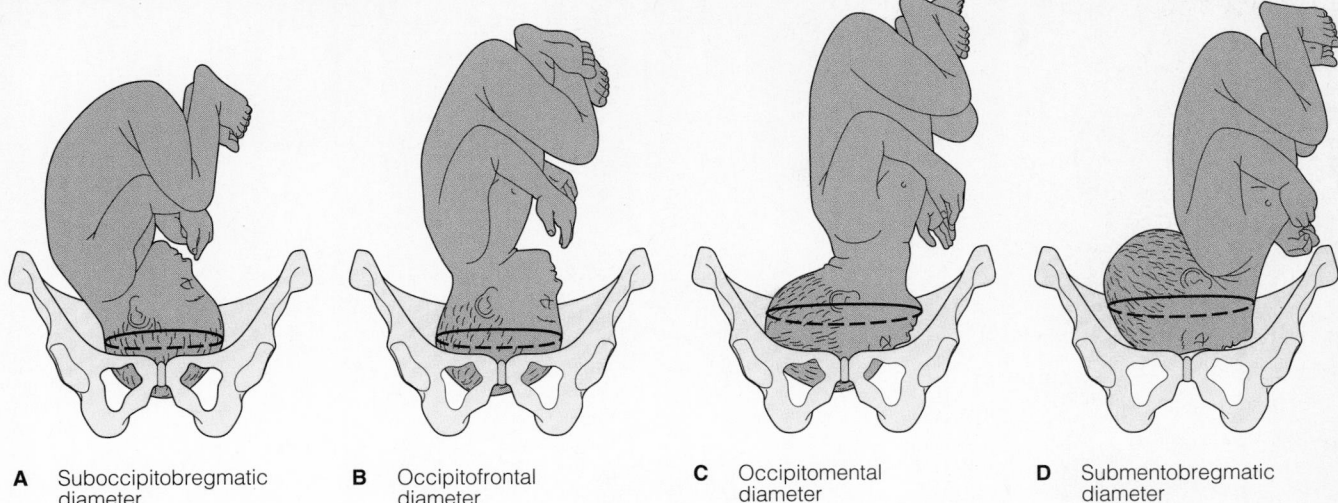

A Suboccipitobregmatic diameter

B Occipitofrontal diameter

C Occipitomental diameter

D Submentobregmatic diameter

FIGURE 21-5 Cephalic presentation. *A* Vertex presentation. Complete flexion of the head allows the suboccipitobregmatic diameter to present to the pelvis. *B* Military (median vertex) presentation with no flexion or extension. The occipitofrontal diameter presents to the pelvis. *C* Brow presentation. The fetal head is in partial (halfway) extension. The occipitomental diameter, which is the largest diameter of the fetal head, presents to the pelvis. *D* Face presentation. The fetal head is in complete extension, and the submentobregmatic diameter presents to the pelvis.

- In a single footling one foot presents; in a double footling both feet present.

Shoulder Presentation

A shoulder presentation is also called a *transverse lie*. Most frequently, the shoulder is the presenting part, and the acromion process of the scapula is the landmark to be noted. However, the fetal arm, back, abdomen, or side may present in a transverse lie. See Chapter 25 for further discussion of transverse lie.

FUNCTIONAL RELATIONSHIPS OF PRESENTING PART AND MATERNAL PELVIS

Engagement

Engagement of the presenting part occurs when the largest diameter of the presenting part reaches or passes through the pelvic inlet (Figure 21–6). When the fetal head is flexed, the biparietal diameter is the largest dimension of the fetal skull to pass through the pelvic inlet in a cephalic presentation. The intertrochanteric diameter (transverse diameter that is located between the right and left trocanter) is the largest to pass through the inlet in a breech presentation.

Engagement can be determined by vaginal examination. In primigravidas engagement usually occurs 2 weeks before term. Multiparas, however, may experience engagement several weeks before the onset of labor or during the process of labor. Engagement confirms the adequacy of the pelvic inlet. Engagement does not, however, indicate whether the midpelvis and outlet are also adequate.

The presenting part is said to be *floating* (or ballottable) when it is freely movable above the inlet. When the presenting part begins to descend into the inlet, before engagement has truly occurred, it is said to be *dipping* into the pelvis (Figure 21–6).

Station

Station refers to the relationship of the presenting part to an imaginary line drawn between the ischial spines of the maternal pelvis. In a normal pelvis the ischial spines mark the narrowest diameter through which the fetus must pass. These spines are not sharp protrusions that harm the fetus but rather blunted prominences at the midpelvis. The ischial spines as a landmark have been designated as zero station (Figure 21–7). If the presenting part is higher than the ischial spines, a negative number is assigned, noting centimeters above zero station. Station −5 is at the inlet, and station +4 is at the outlet. If the presenting part can be seen at the woman's perineum, birth will occur momentarily. During labor the presenting part should move progressively from the negative stations to the midpelvis at zero station and into the positive stations. Failure of the presenting part to descend in the presence of strong contractions may be due to disproportion between the maternal pelvis and fetal presenting part or to a short and/or entangled umbilical cord.

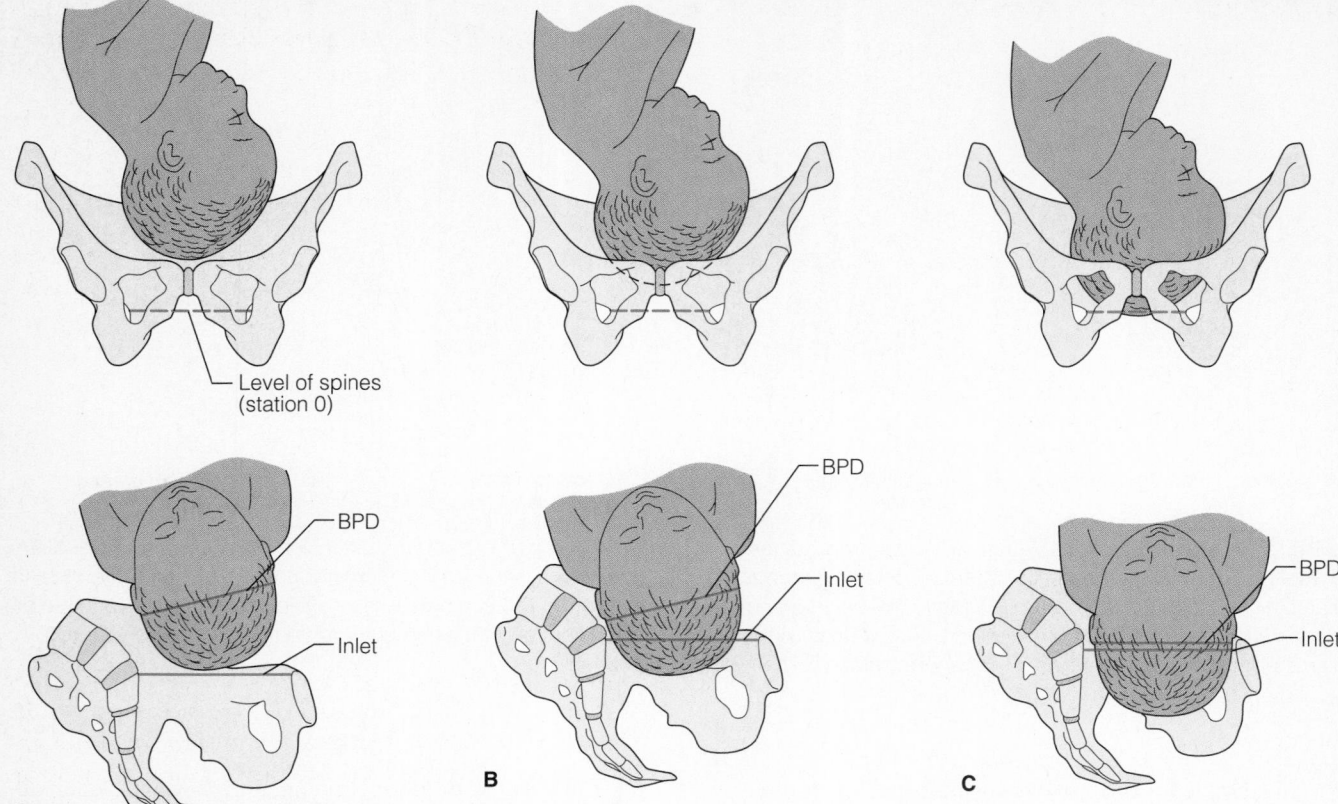

FIGURE 21-6 Process of engagement in cephalic presentation. *A* Floating. The fetal head is directed down toward the pelvis but can still easily move away from the inlet. *B* Dipping. The fetal head dips into the inlet but can be moved away by exerting pressure on the fetus. *C* Engaged. The biparietal diameter (BPD) of the fetal head is in the inlet of the pelvis. In most instances the presenting part (occiput) will be at the level of the ischial spines (0 station).

Fetal Position

Fetal position refers to the relationship of the landmark on the presenting fetal part to the front (anterior), back (posterior), or sides (right or left) of the maternal pelvis. The landmark on the fetal presenting part is related to four imaginary quadrants of the maternal pelvis: left anterior, right anterior, left posterior, and right posterior. These quadrants designate whether the presenting part is directed toward the front, back, left, or right of the maternal pelvis. The landmark chosen for vertex presentations is the occiput, and the landmark for face presentations is the mentum. In breech presentations the sacrum is the designated landmark, and the acromion process on the scapula is the landmark in shoulder presentations. If the landmark is directed toward the center of the side of the pelvis, fetal position is designated as *transverse*, rather than anterior or posterior. Three notations are used to describe the fetal position:

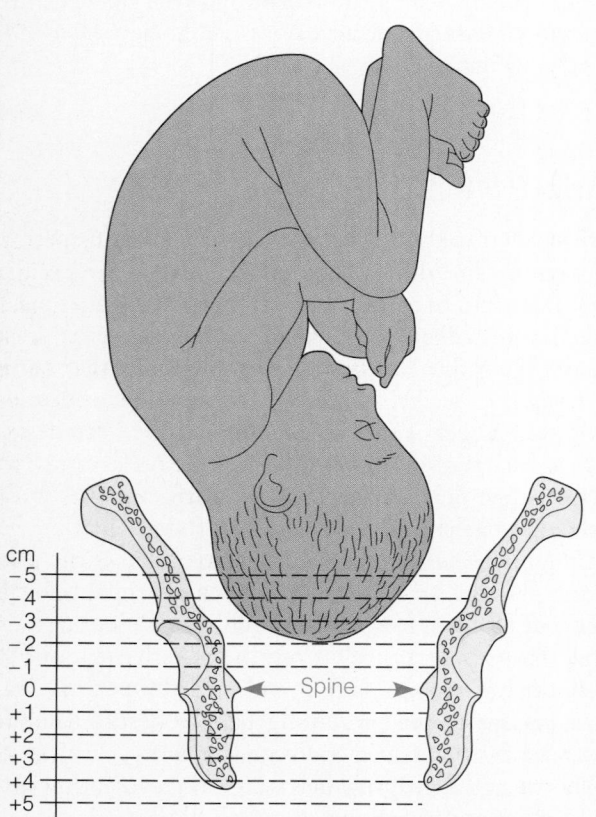

FIGURE 21-7 Measuring the station of the fetal head while it is descending. In this view the station is −2/−3.

1. Right (R) or left (L) side of the maternal pelvis
2. The landmark of the fetal presenting part: occiput (O), mentum (M), sacrum (S), or acromion process (A)
3. Anterior (A), posterior (P), or transverse (T), depending on whether the landmark is in the front, back, or side of the pelvis

The abbreviations of these notations help the health care team communicate the fetal position. Thus when the fetal occiput is directed toward the back and to the left of the passage, the abbreviation used is LOP (left-occiput-posterior). The term *dorsal* (D) is used when denoting the fetal position in a transverse lie; it refers to the fetal back. Thus the abbreviation RADA indicates that the acromion process of the scapula is directed toward the woman's right, and the fetus's back is anterior.

Following is a list of positions for various fetal presentations, some of which are illustrated in Figure 21–8.

Positions in vertex presentation:
ROA	Right-occiput-anterior
ROT	Right-occiput-transverse
ROP	Right-occiput-posterior
LOA	Left-occiput-anterior
LOT	Left-occiput-transverse
LOP	Left-occiput-posterior

Positions in face presentation:
RMA	Right-mentum-anterior
RMT	Right-mentum-transverse
RMP	Right-mentum-posterior
LMA	Left-mentum-anterior
LMT	Left-mentum-transverse
LMP	Left-mentum-posterior

Positions in breech presentation:
RSA	Right-sacrum-anterior
RST	Right-sacrum-transverse
RSP	Right-sacrum-posterior
LSA	Left-sacrum-anterior
LST	Left-sacrum-transverse
LSP	Left-sacrum-posterior

Positions in shoulder presentation:
RADA	Right-acromion-dorsal-anterior
RADP	Right-acromion-dorsal-posterior
LADA	Left-acromion-dorsal-anterior
LADP	Left-acromion-dorsal-posterior

The fetal position influences labor and birth. For example, in a posterior position the fetal head presents a larger diameter than in an anterior position. A posterior position increases the pressure on the maternal sacral nerves, causing the laboring woman to experience backache and pelvic pressure, which may lead her to bear down or feel the urge to push earlier than needed. The most common fetal position is occiput anterior. When this position occurs, the labor and birth are more likely to proceed normally. Positions other than occiput anterior are more frequently associated with problems during labor; therefore they are called **malpositions.** (See Chapter 25 for discussion of malpositions and their management.)

Assessment techniques to determine fetal position include inspection and palpation of the maternal abdomen and vaginal examination. (See Chapter 22 for further discussion of assessment of fetal position.)

Critical Thinking Question

As you look at the various positions, think about how each would feel if you could place your hands on the outside of the mother's abdomen.

THE FORCES OF LABOR

Primary and secondary powers work together to deliver the fetus, the fetal membranes, and the placenta from the uterus into the external environment. The *primary force* is uterine muscular contractions, which cause the changes of the first stage of labor—complete effacement and dilatation of the cervix. The *secondary force* is the use of abdominal muscles to push during the second stage of labor. The pushing adds to the primary power after full dilatation has occurred.

In labor, uterine contractions are rhythmic but intermittent. Between contractions is a period of relaxation. This period of relaxation allows uterine muscles to rest and provides respite for the laboring woman. It also restores uteroplacental circulation, which is important to fetal oxygenation and adequate circulation in the uterine blood vessels.

Each contraction has three phases: (1) *increment*, the "building up" of the contraction (the longest phase); (2) *acme*, or the peak of the contraction; and (3) *decrement*, or the "letting up" of the contraction. When describing uterine contractions during labor, care givers use the terms *frequency*, *duration*, and *intensity*. **Frequency** refers to the time between the beginning of one contraction and the beginning of the next contraction.

The **duration** of each contraction is measured from the beginning of the increment to the completion of decrement (Figure 21–9). In beginning labor the duration is about 30 seconds. As labor continues, duration increases to an average of 60 seconds with a range of 45 to 90 seconds (Varney 1987).

Intensity refers to the strength of the uterine contraction during acme. In most instances the intensity is estimated by palpating the contraction, but it may be measured directly with an intrauterine catheter attached to an electronic fetal monitor. Intensity of uterine contractions cannot be accurately measured by external monitoring with an electronic fetal monitor. When estimating intensity by palpation, the nurse determines whether it is mild, moderate, or strong by judging the amount of

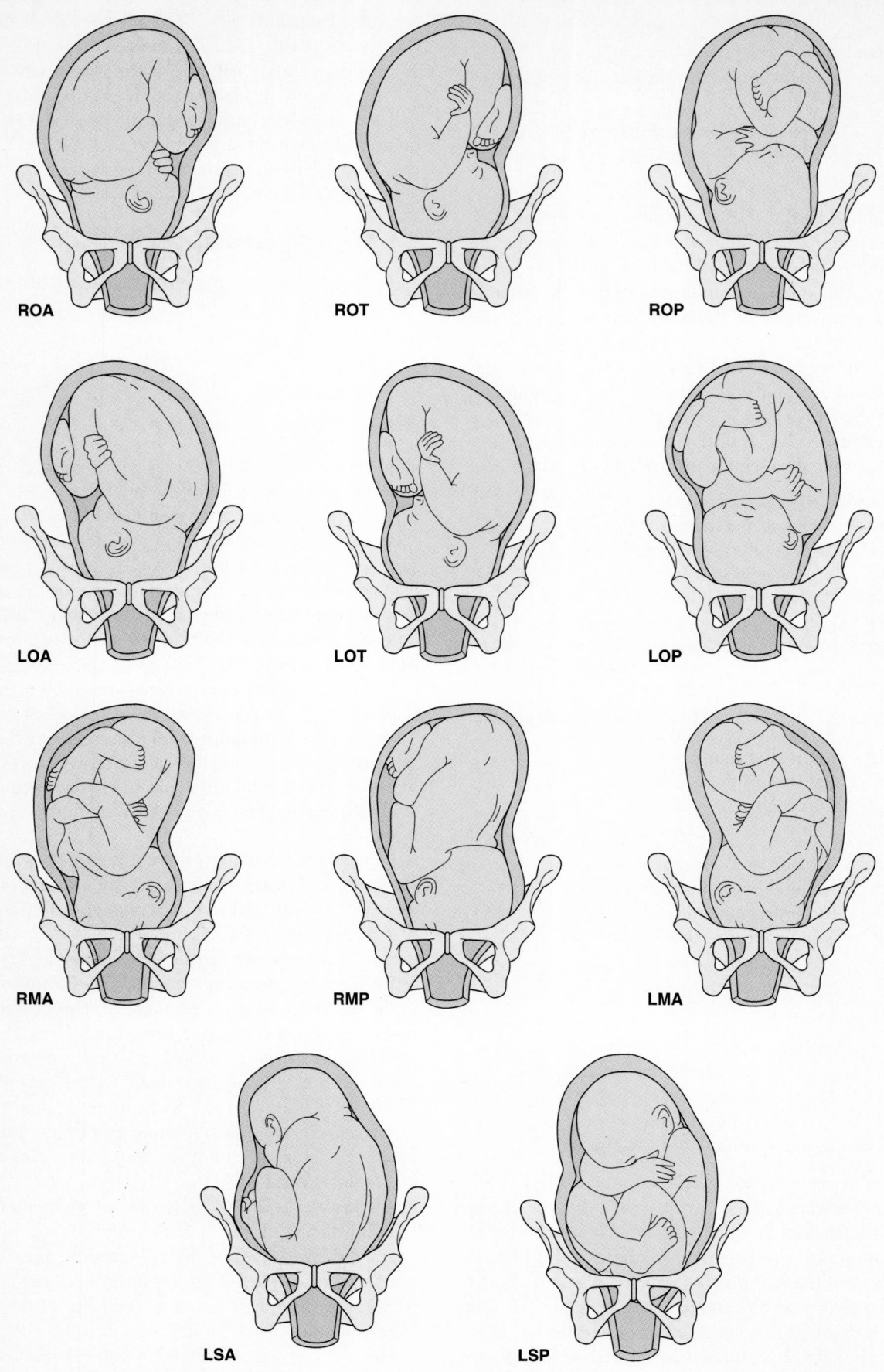

ROA **ROT** **ROP**

LOA **LOT** **LOP**

RMA **RMP** **LMA**

LSA **LSP**

FIGURE 21-8   Categories of presentation. SOURCE: Courtesy Ross Laboratories, Columbus, OH.

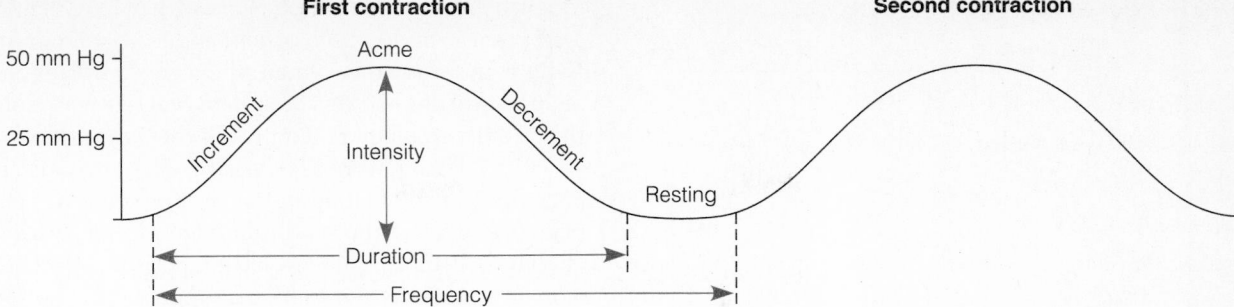

FIGURE 21-9   Characteristics of uterine contractions.

indentability of the uterine wall during the acme of a contraction. If the uterine wall can be indented easily, the contraction is considered mild. Strong intensity exists when the uterine wall cannot be indented. Moderate intensity falls between these two ranges. When intensity is measured with an intrauterine catheter, the normal resting tonus (between contractions) is about 10 to 12 mm Hg of pressure. During acme the intensity ranges from 25 to 30 mm Hg in early labor, 25 to 70 mm Hg in active labor, 40 to 80 mm Hg during transition, and 80 to 110 mm Hg while the woman is pushing in the second stage (Murray 1989; Zlatnik 1994). (See Chapter 22 for further discussion of assessment techniques.)

At the beginning of labor the contractions are usually mild, of short duration, and relatively infrequent. As labor progresses, duration of contractions lengthens, the intensity increases, and the frequency is every 2 to 3 minutes. Because the contractions are involuntary, the laboring woman cannot control their duration, frequency, or intensity.

PSYCHOSOCIAL CONSIDERATIONS

Similar psychosocial factors affect both the mother and the father. Both are transitioning into new roles and have expectations of themselves during the labor and birth experience, as care givers for their child, and for their new family. Although many prospective mothers and fathers attend childbirth preparation classes, both tend to be concerned about what labor will be like, whether they will each be able to perform the way they expect, whether the discomfort and pain will be more than the mother expects or can cope with, and whether the father can provide helpful support (McKay & Smith 1993; Nichols 1993).

Rubin (1984, p 52) notes that childbearing "requires an exchange of a known self in a known world for an unknown self in an unknown world. This is an act of courage." And no part of the childbearing period reflects this more than labor. Every woman is uncertain about what her labor will be like: A woman anticipating her first

labor faces a totally new experience, and even multiparas cannot be certain what each new labor will bring. The woman does not know whether she will live up to her expectations for herself in relation to her friends and relatives, whether she will be physically injured through laceration, episiotomy, or cesarean incision, or whether significant others will be as supportive as she hopes (Mercer 1985). The woman faces an irrevocable event—the birth of a new family member—and, consequently, disruption of life-style, relationships, and self-image. Finally, the woman must deal with concerns about her loss of control of bodily functions, emotional responses to an unfamiliar situation, and reactions to the pain associated with labor.

Information regarding the transition into the fathering role is rather limited at this time. Henderson and Brouse (1991) report that most of the information new fathers receive about their role comes from their friends, family, prenatal classes, and personal experience.

Various factors influence the couple's reaction to the physical and emotional crisis of labor (Table 21–3). Their usual coping mechanisms in response to stressful life events, support system, preparation for childbirth, and cultural influences are all significant factors.

Preparation for Labor

In her study of the psychosocial adaptations of pregnancy, Lederman (1984) found that certain psychosocial factors of pregnancy were predictive of progress in labor. One such factor was related to a woman's psychologic preparation for labor. Lederman found that expectant women prepared for labor through actions and through imaginary rehearsal. The actions frequently consisted of "nesting behavior" (housecleaning, decorating the nursery) and a "psyching up" (getting psychologically ready) for the labor, which seemed to vary depending on the woman's sense of self-confidence, self-esteem, and previous experiences with stress. Specific actions to prepare for labor are usually focused on becoming better informed and prepared. Nichols and Humenick (1988) suggest that

TABLE 21-3	Factors Associated with a Positive Birth Experience

Motivation for the pregnancy

Attendance at childbirth education classes

A sense of competence or mastery

Self-confidence and self-esteem

Positive relationship with mate

Maintaining control during labor

Support from mate or other person during labor

Not being left alone in labor

Trust in the medical/nursing staff

Having personal control of breathing patterns, comfort measures

Choosing a physician/certified nurse-midwife who has a similar philosophy of care

Receiving clear information regarding procedures

mastery, or control, of the childbearing experience is the key factor in perceived satisfaction. Childbirth education helps increase positive reactions to the birth experience by giving the laboring woman and her support persons greater opportunities to control the experience of labor.

An important developmental step for expectant women is to anticipate the labor in fantasy. Just as a woman "tries on" the maternal role during pregnancy, fantasizing about labor seems to help her understand and become better prepared for it. Fantasies about the excitement of the baby's birth and the sharing of the experience involve the woman in constructive preparation, even though she may still have some fears of labor. Women who have a great deal of apprehension about becoming a mother or a high fear of pain during labor are not able to fantasize the labor in positive ways and may have many disturbing thoughts (Lederman 1984).

Positive fantasies seem to involve many areas. The woman thinks about the contractions and the work and pain that will be involved, and this seems to provide a stimulus to becoming more prepared for labor. Lederman (1984) found that women who were able to visualize themselves as active participants in labor were usually well prepared and had positive self-images. Fantasy and thoughts about labor help the woman to have realistic ideas about the work, pain, and risks involved and to develop a sense of confidence in her ability to cope.

Many women fear the pain of contractions. They not only see the pain as threatening but also associate it with a loss of control over their bodies and emotions. Our society seems to value control and cooperation with established routines in health care settings. When a woman is facing labor, especially for the first time, she may worry about her ability to withstand the pain of labor and maintain control over herself. Women are afraid of becoming

fatigued and unable to relax because they may then act in a way that is undesirable or may induce bodily injury. In Lederman's study the women who were confident of their abilities usually had less fear than women who doubted their ability to maintain control of themselves.

The laboring woman's support system may also influence the course of labor and birth. For some women the presence of the father and other significant persons, including the nurse, tends to have a positive effect. Other women may prefer not to have a support person or family with them.

Preparation for childbirth is another factor that influences a woman's reaction to childbirth. Much attention has been focused on preparation during pregnancy as a way of increasing the woman's ability to cope during childbirth, decreasing her stress, anxiety, and pain, and imparting satisfaction with the childbearing experience. Although opinions vary concerning whether the amount of pain or discomfort is actually decreased, there is agreement that preparation tends to increase perceived satisfaction. Nichols and Humenick (1988) suggest that *mastery*, or control, of the childbearing experience is the key factor in perceived satisfaction. Childbirth education helps to increase positive reactions to the birth experience because education gives the laboring woman and her support persons greater opportunities to control the experience of labor.

DiMatteo et al (1993) report that mothers in the early postpartal period describe some common themes regarding the labor and birth experience: loss of autonomy and control, unexpected physical pain, unexpected emotional reactions, financial pressures, and support during labor and birth. Although the women attended childbirth preparation classes, they found that their wishes were not always possible in the birth setting and that many procedures were performed as if the decision-making authority rested with the medical/nursing personnel. For instance, because the nurse may tend to depend on the electronic fetal monitoring tracing for reassurance regarding the fetus's condition, the monitor may be left on for an extended period of time; the physician may order an IV; or bed rest may be imposed and movement restricted, without information to support the need for these interventions. Women in this situation report that their concern is for the baby, but it would be helpful to understand the need for the intervention and to be informed. DiMatteo et al (1993) suggest that women need to be prepared to face both areas that are under their *personal control*, such as patterned breathing and some comfort measures, and also *situational control* issues, which include some procedures requested by the certified nurse-midwife/physician or birth setting institutional protocols.

The women reported surprise at the amount of pain they experienced during labor and birth and that they felt poorly prepared. One study participant felt the pain was a "well-kept secret" (DiMatteo et al 1993, p 206). Others reported that women just don't talk about how painful it is until it is all over.

The third theme that emerged regarded unexpected emotional reactions. Many women felt emotionally drained at the end of the birth process, and some even described a feeling of detachment and disassociation. They felt that they did not "do enough" or "did not perform in the way that they should have" and had feelings of disappointment and sadness. Interestingly, Berry (1988) reported that fathers often felt they had not been able to provide the type of support they had wanted and voiced feelings of failure in their expected role during the labor and birth.

Financial concerns focused on which procedures or practices during labor and birth would be covered by insurance if unexpected problems occurred (DiMatteo et al 1993). Lack of coverage clearly may affect the type of care and pain relief measures available to a woman during labor and birth.

Concern for support during labor and birth was the last theme identified. Some women welcomed their partner's support and found these efforts very helpful; others felt that inexperience, anxiety, or other factors affected the partner's ability to be as supportive as needed. The women also spoke to the importance of support and information from the nurse. One reported, "[The nurse] was with me all the time, touching my hands. I think about her, and I wanted to go to find her to thank her because she was an incredible help" (DiMatteo et al 1993, p 207).

In a study by Khazoyan and Anderson (1994) Latina women were asked what they wanted from their partners during the birth experience. The women identified the need for the partner at the bedside, for communication, and for showing love. They desired the partner's presence throughout the entire labor and birth, and this presence was all that was necessary. The partner did not have to be actively involved in comforting and caretaking. Communication needs included talking and "affectionate and understanding words" from their partner. They looked to the partner for support and comfort. Showing love was described as holding their hand, hugging, or touching and did not always have to be demonstrative because the presence at the bedside was also interpreted as a "loving" gesture.

How the woman views the childbirth experience after the birth may have implications for mothering behaviors. Mercer (1985) and Walker and Montgomery (1994) found a significant relationship between the birth experience and mothering behaviors. It appears that any activities—by the expectant woman or by maternal-child health care providers—that enhance the birth experience will be beneficial as the woman prepares for labor, experiences labor, and begins her new role as a mother. The father's experience of childbirth and his opportunities for bonding may also have important implications for fathering (Henderson & Brouse 1991).

THE PHYSIOLOGY OF LABOR

Possible Causes of Labor Onset

The process of labor usually begins between the 38th and the 42nd week of gestation, when the fetus is mature and ready for birth. Although the exact cause of onset is not clearly understood, researchers do know that labor is precipitated by complex interactions of progesterone, estrogen, oxytocin, prostaglandins, fetal cortisol, and uterine distention. The relationship of some of these factors is presented in Figure 21–10.

Progesterone

Progesterone exerts a relaxant effect on the uterine smooth muscle by interfering with conduction of impulses from one cell to the next. During pregnancy, progesterone exerts a quieting effect, and the uterus generally is without contractions. The placenta produces progesterone, and toward the end of gestation biochemical changes occur that result in decreased availability of progesterone to myometrial cells (Blackburn & Loper 1992). With the decreased availability of progesterone, estrogen is better able to exert its effects.

Estrogen

Estrogen stimulates the smooth muscle of the uterus to contract. During pregnancy the stimulatory effects of estrogen are counterbalanced by the relaxant effects of progesterone. The balance between these two hormones keeps the uterine muscles from contracting in a regular pattern during pregnancy. At about 34–35 weeks' gestation estrogen levels rise. Estrogen exerts an effect on the

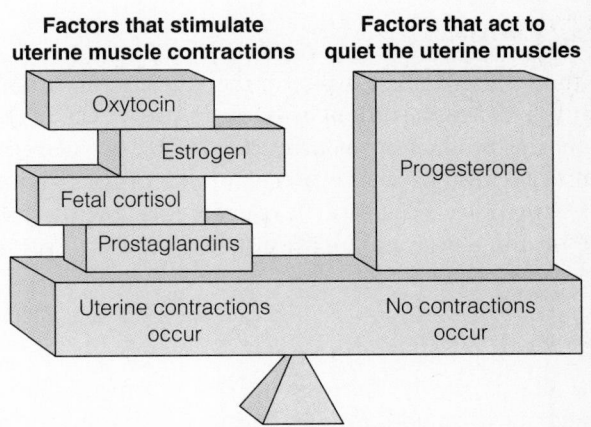

FIGURE 21-10   Factors affecting initiation of labor. The factors listed on the left have all been identified as providing stimulus to the beginning of labor. Progesterone exerts a relaxing effect, and a balance between all factors keeps the uterus quiet, without contraction. When the relationship of factors changes, the balance is tipped, and uterine labor begins.

formation of gap junctions (which help propagate the contraction from one cell to the next), stimulates an increase in the sensitivity of the myometrium to oxytocin, and stimulates prostaglandin formation (Blackburn & Loper 1992). This leads first to increased irritability (a readiness to contract) of the uterine smooth muscle and then to the promotion of actual uterine contractions.

The stimulatory effect is increased further because estrogen promotes the synthesis of prostaglandin in the decidua and the fetal membranes (amnion and chorion). Prostaglandins also stimulate the smooth muscle of the uterus.

Oxytocin

Oxytocin is produced by the maternal posterior pituitary. One of the effects of oxytocin is to stimulate contractions of the smooth muscle of the uterus. The uterus becomes increasingly sensitive (responsive) to the effects of oxytocin as the pregnancy nears term (40 weeks). This increased responsiveness is due to a marked change in the sensitivity of the myometrial cells to oxytocin (Blackburn & Loper 1992).

Prostaglandin

Although the exact relationship between prostaglandin and the onset of labor is not yet established, there is growing evidence that prostaglandin involvement is significant. Prostaglandin is known to stimulate smooth muscle contractions. It may also stimulate the production and release of oxytocin and lower the uterine threshold to oxytocin. The production of prostaglandins increases just before labor begins (Challis 1994), most likely as a result of the interaction of such factors as increased estrogen and decreased progesterone, increased fetal cortisol (Nathanielsz 1994), and increased distention of the uterus.

Fetal Cortisol

As the woman approaches term the fetus produces more cortisol. Cortisol is thought to exert two effects: (1) It slows the production of progesterone by the placenta, and (2) it stimulates the precursors to prostaglandins. These two effects decrease the relaxant effect of progesterone on the uterus and increase the stimulatory effect of prostaglandins.

Uterine Distention

The uterus slowly increases in size during gestation, stretching its smooth muscle. Most smooth muscle contracts when stretched, but the uterine smooth muscle does not because of the effect of progesterone. As the woman approaches term the decreased amount or effectiveness of progesterone increases uterine irritability and contractions. The irritability of the smooth muscle is enhanced by uterine distention, which stimulates the production of prostaglandins.

Myometrial Activity

In true labor the uterus divides into two portions. This division is known as the *physiologic retraction ring*. The upper portion, which is the contractile segment, becomes progressively thicker as labor advances. The lower portion, which includes the lower uterine segment and cervix, is passive. As labor continues the lower uterine segment expands and thins out.

With each contraction the muscles of the upper uterine segment shorten and exert a longitudinal traction on the cervix, causing effacement. **Effacement** is the taking up (or drawing up) of the internal os and the cervical canal into the uterine side walls. The cervix changes progressively from a long, thick structure to a structure that is tissue-paper thin (Figure 21–11). In primigravidas effacement usually precedes dilatation. The uterine muscle remains shorter and thicker and does not return to its original length. This phenomenon is known as brachystasis. The space in the uterine cavity decreases as a result of brachystasis, and this places downward pressure on the fetus (Cunningham et al 1993).

The uterus elongates with each contraction, decreasing the horizontal diameter. This elongation causes a straightening of the fetal body, pressing the part of the fetus in the upper portion of the uterus against the fundus and thrusting the presenting part down toward the lower uterine segment and the cervix. The pressure exerted by the fetus is called *fetal axis pressure*. As the uterus elongates the longitudinal muscle fibers are pulled upward over the presenting part. This action and the hydrostatic pressure of the fetal membranes cause **cervical dilatation.** The cervical os and cervical canal widen from less than a centimeter to approximately 10 cm, allowing birth of the fetus. When the cervix is completely dilated and retracted up into the lower uterine segment, it can no longer be palpated.

The round ligament pulls the fundus forward, aligning the fetus with the bony pelvis.

Intra-Abdominal Pressure

After the cervix is completely dilated, the maternal abdominal musculature contracts as the woman pushes. This pushing is called *bearing down*. The pushing aids in the expulsion of the fetus and the placenta. If the cervix is not completely dilated, bearing down can cause cervical edema (which retards dilatation), possible tearing and bruising of the cervix, and maternal exhaustion.

Musculature Changes in the Pelvic Floor

The levator ani muscle and fascia of the pelvic floor draw the rectum and vagina upward and forward with each contraction, along the curve of the pelvic floor. As the fetal head descends to the pelvic floor, the pressure of the

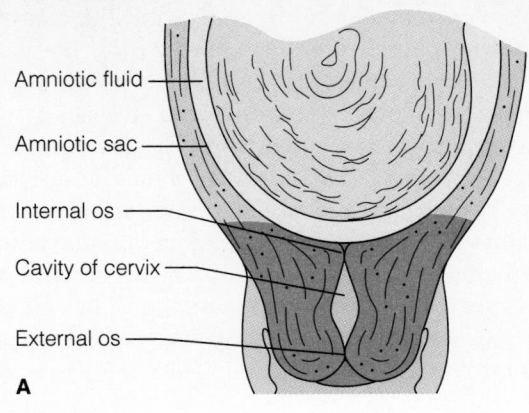

A

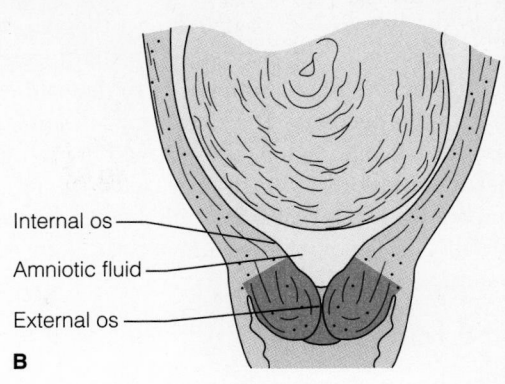

B

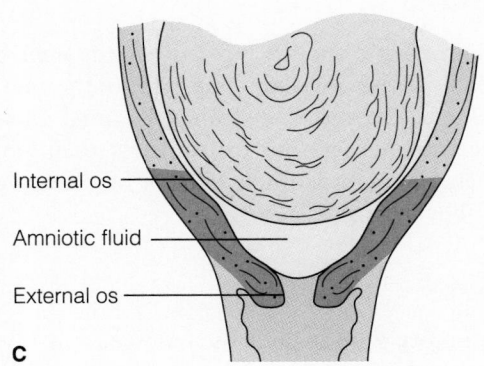

C

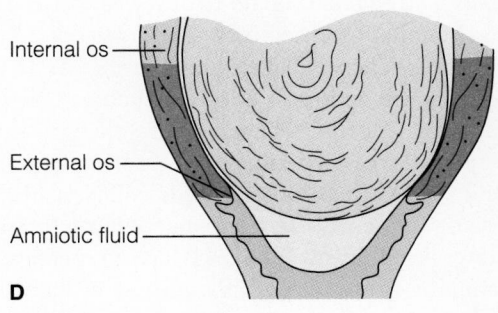

D

FIGURE 21-11   Effacement of the cervix in the primigravida. *A* At the beginning of labor there is no cervical effacement or dilatation. The fetal head is cushioned by amniotic fluid. *B* Beginning cervical effacement. As the cervix begins to efface, more amniotic fluid collects below the fetal head. *C* Cervix is about one-half effaced and slightly dilated. The increasing amount of amniotic fluid exerts hydrostatic pressure. *D* Complete effacement and dilatation.

presenting part causes the perineal structure, which was once 5 cm in thickness, to change to a structure less than a centimeter thick. A normal physiologic anesthesia is produced as a result of the decreased blood supply to the area. The anus everts, exposing the interior rectal wall as the fetal head descends forward (Cunningham et al 1993).

PREMONITORY SIGNS OF LABOR

Most primigravidas and many multiparas experience the following signs and symptoms of impending labor.

Lightening

Lightening describes what happens when the fetus begins to settle into the pelvic inlet (engagement). With its descent the uterus moves downward, and the fundus no longer presses on the diaphragm.

The woman can breathe more easily after lightening. With increased downward pressure of the presenting part, however, she may notice the following:

- Leg cramps or pains due to pressure on the nerves that course through the obturator foramen in the pelvis
- Increased pelvic pressure
- Increased venous stasis leading to edema in the lower extremities
- Increased urinary frequency
- Increased vaginal secretions resulting from congestion of the vaginal mucous membranes

Braxton Hicks Contractions

Prior to the onset of labor, Braxton Hicks contractions—the irregular, intermittent contractions that have been occurring throughout the pregnancy—may become uncomfortable. The pain seems to be in the abdomen and groin but may feel like the "drawing" sensations experienced by some women with dysmenorrhea. When these contractions are strong enough for the woman to believe she is in labor, she is said to be in false labor. *False labor* is uncomfortable and may be exhausting as the woman wonders if "this is it." Because the contractions can be fairly regular, she has no way of knowing if they are the beginning of true labor. She may come to the hospital/birthing center for a vaginal examination to determine if cervical dilatation is occurring. Frequent episodes of false labor and trips back and forth to the certified nurse-midwife/physician's office or hospital may frustrate or embarrass the woman, who feels that she should know when she is really in labor. Reassurance by nursing staff can ease embarrassment.

Cervical Changes

Considerable change occurs in the cervix during the prenatal and intrapartal period. At the beginning of pregnancy the cervix is rigid and firm, and it must soften so that it is able to stretch and dilate to allow the fetus passage. This softening of the cervix is called *ripening*.

As term approaches, collagen fibers in the cervix are broken down by the action of enzymes such as collagenase and elastase. As the collagen fibers change, their ability to bind is decreased because of increasing amounts of hyaluronic acid (which loosely binds collagen fibrils) and decreasing amounts of dermatan sulfate (which tightly binds collagen fibrils). There is also an increase in the water content of the cervix, and all these changes result in a weakening and softening of the cervix (Blackburn & Loper 1992, p 121).

Bloody Show

During the pregnancy cervical secretions have accumulated in the cervical canal to form a mucous plug. With softening and effacement of the cervix the mucous plug is often expelled, resulting in a small amount of blood loss from the exposed cervical capillaries. The resulting pink-tinged secretions are called **bloody show.**

Bloody show is considered a sign of impending labor, usually within 24–48 hours. Vaginal examination that includes manipulation of the cervix may also result in a blood-tinged discharge (may be more brownish in color), which is sometimes confused with bloody show.

Rupture of Membranes

In approximately 12% of women the amniotic membranes rupture before the onset of labor. This is called **rupture of membranes (ROM).** After membranes rupture, 80% of women will experience spontaneous labor within 24 hours. If membranes rupture and labor does not begin spontaneously within 12–24 hours, labor may be induced to avoid infection (once the membranes have ruptured there is an open pathway up into the uterine cavity). An induction of labor is done only if the pregnancy is near term.

When the membranes rupture, the amniotic fluid may be expelled in large amounts. If engagement has not occurred, the danger exists of the umbilical cord washing out with the fluid *(prolapsed cord)*. Because of these poten-

tial problems, the woman is advised to notify her certified nurse-midwife/physician and proceed to the hospital/birthing center. In some instances the fluid is expelled in small amounts and may be confused with episodes of urinary incontinence associated with urinary urgency, coughing, or sneezing. The discharge should be checked to ascertain its source and to determine further action. (See Chapter 22 for assessment techniques used to establish whether membranes are ruptured, for precautions the nurse uses to avoid exposure to amniotic fluid, and for guidelines regarding whether the woman should remain ambulatory.)

Sudden Burst of Energy

Some women report a sudden burst of energy approximately 24–48 hours before labor. The cause of the energy spurt is unknown. In prenatal teaching the nurse should warn prospective mothers not to overexert themselves during this energy burst so they will not be excessively tired when labor begins.

Other Signs

Other premonitory signs include the following:

- Weight loss of 2.2–6.6 kg (1–3 lb) resulting from fluid loss and electrolyte shifts produced by changes in estrogen and progesterone levels
- Increased backache and sacroiliac pressure from the influence of relaxin hormone on the pelvic joints
- Diarrhea, indigestion, or nausea and vomiting just prior to the onset of labor

The causes of these signs are unknown.

DIFFERENCES BETWEEN TRUE AND FALSE LABOR

The contractions of true labor produce progressive dilatation and effacement of the cervix. They occur regularly and increase in frequency, duration, and intensity. The discomfort of true labor contractions usually starts in the back and radiates around to the abdomen. The pain is not relieved by ambulation (in fact walking may intensify the pain).

The contractions of false labor do not produce progressive cervical effacement and dilatation. Classically, they are irregular and do not increase in frequency, duration, and intensity. The contractions may be perceived as a hardening or "balling up" without discomfort, or discomfort may occur mainly in the lower abdomen and groin. The discomfort may be relieved by ambulation.

The woman will find it helpful to know the characteristics of true labor contractions as well as the premonitory signs of ensuing labor. However, many times the only way to differentiate accurately between true and false labor is to assess dilatation. The woman must feel free to come in for accurate assessment of labor and should never be allowed to feel foolish if the labor is false. The nurse must reassure the woman that false labor is common and that it often cannot be distinguished from true labor except by vaginal examination (Table 21–4).

STAGES OF LABOR AND BIRTH

There are three stages of labor. The *first stage* begins with the beginning of true labor and ends when the cervix is completely dilated at 10 cm. The *second stage* begins with complete dilatation and ends with the birth of the infant. The *third stage* begins with the expulsion of the infant and ends with the expulsion of the placenta.

Some clinicians identify a *fourth stage* of labor. During this stage, which lasts 1 to 4 hours after expulsion of the placenta, the uterus effectively contracts to control bleeding at the placental site (Cunningham et al 1993).

The care of the laboring woman is discussed in Chapter 23.

First Stage

The first stage of labor is divided into the *latent*, *active*, and *transition* phases (Table 21–5). Each phase of labor is characterized by physical and psychologic changes.

Latent Phase

The *latent phase* begins with the onset of regular contractions. As the cervix begins to dilate it also effaces, although little or no fetal descent is evident. For a woman in her first labor (nullipara) the latent phase averages 8.6 hours but should not exceed 20 hours. The latent phase in multiparas averages 5.3 hours but should not exceed 14 hours.

Uterine contractions become established during the latent phase and increase in frequency, duration, and intensity. They may start as mild contractions lasting 15 to 20 seconds with a frequency of 10 to 20 minutes and progress to moderate ones lasting 30 to 40 seconds with a frequency of 5 to 7 minutes. They average 40 mm Hg during acme from a baseline tonus of 10 mm Hg (Varney 1987).

In the early or latent phase of the first stage of labor contractions are usually mild. The woman feels able to cope with the discomfort. She may be relieved that labor has finally started. Although she may be anxious, she is able to recognize and express those feelings of anxiety. The woman is often talkative and smiling and is eager to talk about herself and answer questions. Excitement is high, and her partner or other support person is often as elated as she is.

TABLE 21-4 Comparison of True and False Labor

True Labor	False Labor
Contractions are at regular intervals.	Contractions are irregular.
Intervals between contractions gradually shorten.	Usually no change.
Contractions increase in duration and intensity.	Usually no change.
Discomfort begins in back and radiates around to abdomen.	Discomfort is usually in abdomen.
Intensity usually increases with walking.	Walking has no effect on or lessens contractions.
Cervical dilatation and effacement are progressive.	No change.

TABLE 21-5 Characteristics of Labor

	First Stage			Second Stage
	Latent Phase	Active Phase	Transition Phase	
Nullipara	8 1/2 hours	6 hours		1 hour
Multipara	5 hours	4 1/2 hours		15 minutes
Cervical dilatation	0 to 3–4 cm	4–8 cm	8–10 cm	
Contractions				
Frequency	Every 10–20 minutes at the beginning and progressing to every 5–7 minutes	Every 2–3 minutes	Every 1 1/2–2 minutes	Every 1 1/2–2 minutes
Duration	15–20 seconds progressing to 30–40 seconds	60 seconds	60–90 seconds	60–90 seconds
Intensity	Begin as mild and progress to moderate	Begin as moderate and progress to strong	Strong	Strong

Nursing support during labor may influence the client's feelings about her birth experience and enhance her coping skills. Janet Bryanton, Heather Fraser-Davey, and Patricia Sullivan used a conceptual framework of social support to examine the helpfulness of selected nursing behaviors in assisting the pregnant woman to cope with labor. The primary categories of support that were considered included emotional, informational, and tangible support.

The sample consisted of 80 women: 34 primiparas and 46 multiparas. Criteria for inclusion in the study consisted of: ability to read and write English, having an uncomplicated birth and delivery in the previous 48–72 hours, delivery of a healthy baby at 37 or more weeks' gestation, attendance at prenatal classes, having a husband or other partner present during delivery, and being admitted at least 2 hours before delivery. The researchers collected data by having the women complete a revised, previously published questionnaire about what nursing behaviors had been most helpful to them during their labor and delivery. The authors established face and content validity for the instrument and reported reliability scores for both pilot and actual studies.

Results indicated that each of the 25 nursing support behaviors identified received mean ratings of 4.00 or greater on a scale of 1.00 to 5.00. The 5 top-rated behaviors included: making me feel cared about as an individual; praising me; appearing calm and confident with care; assisting in breathing and relaxing; and treating me with respect. Four of the top 5 behaviors incorporated an element of emotional support, suggesting that this is one of the most important components of support for a laboring woman. Three of the bottom 5 behaviors (although they also received relatively high ratings, ranging from 4.21 to 4.36), related to providing support for the partner rather than the mother. Helpful behaviors most frequently identified from open-ended questions entailed showing a sense of humor, using a low quiet voice, and acting professional. Findings from this study were consistent with prior studies about support for laboring women.

Clinical Application of Study

This study provides confirmation for caring as a critical component of nursing practice. Feeling cared for as an individual was ranked the highest by new mothers in this study about nursing support. Nurses may want to identify the caring behaviors that they exemplify during client care and determine how to more fully implement these behaviors in specific clinical situations.

SOURCE: Bryanton J, Fraser-Davey H, Sullivan P: Women's perceptions of nursing support during labor. *JOGNN* 1994; 23(8): 638.

At the beginning of labor the amniotic membranes bulge through the cervix in the shape of a cone. Spontaneous rupture of membranes (SROM) generally occurs at the height of an intense contraction with a gush of the fluid out of the vagina. In many instances the membranes are ruptured by the certified nurse-midwife/physician. This is called *amniotomy,* or artificial rupture of membranes (AROM).

Active Phase

During the *active phase* the cervix dilates from about 3 or 4 cm to 8 cm. Fetal descent is progressive. The cervical dilatation should be at least 1.2 cm/hour in nulliparas and 1.5 cm/hour in multiparas (Cunningham et al 1993).

Transition Phase

The *transition phase* is the last part of the first stage. Cervical dilation slows as it progresses from 8 to 10 cm and the rate of fetal descent increases. The average rate of descent is at least 1 cm/hour in nulliparas and 2 cm/hour in multiparas. The transition phase should not be longer than 3 hours for nulliparas and 1 hour for multiparas (Cunningham et al 1993). The total duration of the first stage may be increased by approximately 2 hours if epidural anesthesia is used (Kilpatrick & Laros 1989).

During the active and transition phases contractions become more frequent, are longer in duration, and increase in intensity. At the beginning of the active phase the contractions have a frequency of 2 to 3 minutes, a duration of 60 seconds, and are strong in intensity. During transition contractions have a frequency of 1½ to 2 minutes, a duration of 60 to 90 seconds, and are strong in intensity (Varney 1987).

When the woman enters the early active phase, her anxiety tends to increase as she senses the fairly constant intensification of contractions and pain. She begins to fear a loss of control and may use coping mechanisms to maintain control. Some women exhibit decreased ability to cope and a sense of helplessness. Women who have support persons available, particularly the baby's father, experience greater satisfaction and less anxiety throughout the birth process than those without these supports (Doering et al 1980).

When the woman enters the transition phase, she may demonstrate significant anxiety. She becomes acutely aware of the increasing force and intensity of the contractions. She may become restless, frequently changing position. She may fear being left alone, and it is crucial that the nurse be available as backup and relief for the support person. By the time the woman enters the transition phase she is inner directed and often tired. At the same time the support person may be feeling the need for a break. The woman should be reassured that she will not be left alone and should always be told where her support people are and how to reach the nurse.

The woman may also fear that she will be "torn open" or "split apart" by the force of the contractions.

Many clients experience a sensation of pressure so great with the peak of a contraction that it seems to them that their abdomens will burst open. The woman should be informed that this is a normal sensation and reassured that such bursting will not happen.

During transition the woman will most likely withdraw into herself. Increasingly she may doubt her ability to cope with labor. The woman may become apprehensive and irritable. She may be terrified of being left alone, though she does not want anyone to talk to her or touch her. However, with the next contraction she may ask for verbal and physical support. She may need help regaining focus and her breathing pattern. Other characteristics that may accompany this phase include the following:

- Hyperventilation, as the woman increases her breathing rate
- Restlessness
- Difficulty understanding directions
- A sense of bewilderment and anger at the contractions
- Statements that she "can't take it anymore"
- Requests for medication
- Hiccupping, belching, nausea, or vomiting
- Beads of perspiration on the upper lip
- Increasing rectal pressure

The woman in this phase is anxious to "get it over with." She may be amnesic and sleep between her now frequent contractions. Her support persons may start to feel helpless and may turn to the nurse for increased participation as their efforts to alleviate her discomfort seem less effective.

As dilatation approaches 10 cm there may be increased rectal pressure, an uncontrollable desire to bear down, increased amount of bloody show, and rupture of membranes.

Second Stage

The second stage of labor begins when the cervix is completely dilated (10 cm) and ends with birth of the infant. The second stage should be completed within 2 hours after the cervix becomes fully dilated for primigravidas (multiparas average 15 minutes). The use of conduction anesthesia may extend the duration of the second stage an additional 20 to 30 minutes (Kilpatrick & Laros 1989). Contractions continue with a frequency of 1½ to 2 minutes, a duration of 60 to 90 seconds, and strong intensity (Varney 1987). Descent of the fetal presenting part continues until it reaches the perineal floor.

As the fetal head descends the woman has the urge to push because of pressure of the fetal head on the sacral and obturator nerves. As she pushes intra-abdominal pressure is exerted from contraction of the maternal abdominal muscles. As the fetal head continues its descent the perineum begins to bulge, flatten, and move anteriorly. The amount of bloody show may increase. The labia begin to part with each contraction. Between contractions the fetal head appears to recede. With succeeding contractions and maternal pushing effort the fetal head descends farther. **Crowning** occurs when the fetal head is encircled by the external opening of the vagina (introitus) and means birth is imminent.

Usually, a childbirth-prepared woman feels relieved that the acute pain she felt during the transition phase is over (see Table 21–5). She also may be relieved that the birth is near and she can now push. Some women feel a sense of control now that they can be actively involved. Others, particularly those without childbirth preparation, may become frightened. They tend to fight each contraction and any attempt of others to persuade them to push with contractions. Such behavior may be frightening and disconcerting to her support persons. The woman may feel she has lost control and become embarrassed and apologetic, or she may demonstrate extreme irritability toward the staff or her supporters in an attempt to regain control over external forces against which she feels helpless. Some women feel acute, increasingly severe pain and a burning sensation as the perineum distends. The woman may continue to fear that she will tear apart.

Spontaneous Birth (Vertex Presentation)

As the head distends the vulva with each contraction the perineum becomes extremely thin, and the anus stretches and protrudes.

As extension occurs under the symphysis pubis the head is born. When the anterior shoulder meets the underside of the symphysis pubis, a gentle push by the mother aids in birth of the shoulders. The body then follows (Figure 21–12).

Birth of infants in breech presentation is discussed in Chapter 25.

Positional Changes

For the fetus to pass through the birth canal the fetal head and body must adjust to the maternal pelvis by certain positional changes. These changes, called **cardinal movements** or *mechanisms of labor*, are described in the order in which they occur (Figure 21–13).

Descent

Descent is thought to occur because of four forces: (1) pressure of the amniotic fluid, (2) direct pressure of the fundus of the uterus on the breech of the fetus, (3) contraction of the abdominal muscles, and (4) extension and straightening of the fetal body. The head enters the inlet in the occiput transverse or oblique position because the pelvic inlet is widest from side to side. The sagittal suture is an equal distance from the maternal symphysis pubis and sacral promontory.

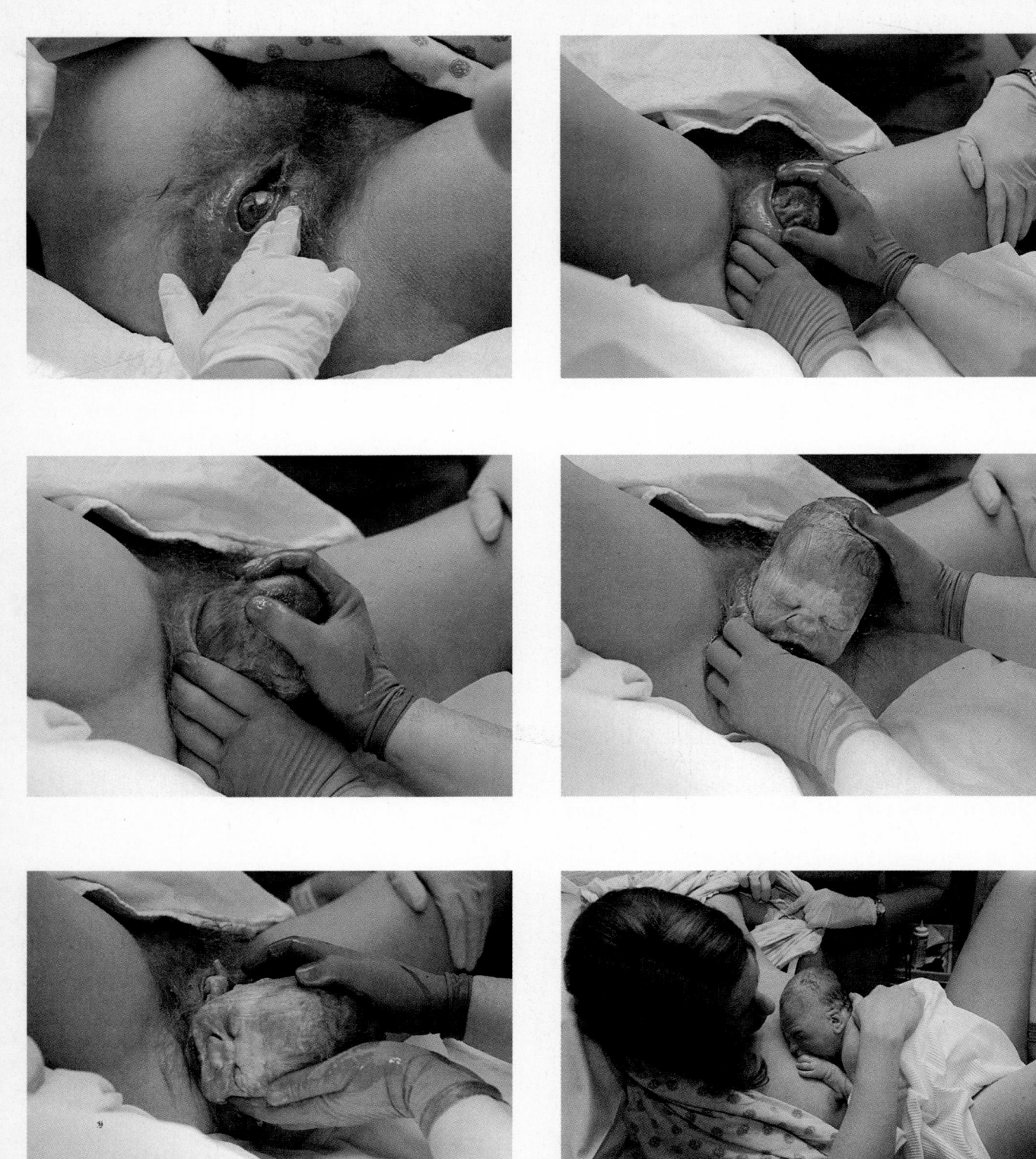

FIGURE 21-12   The birth sequence.

ONE FAMILY'S STORY

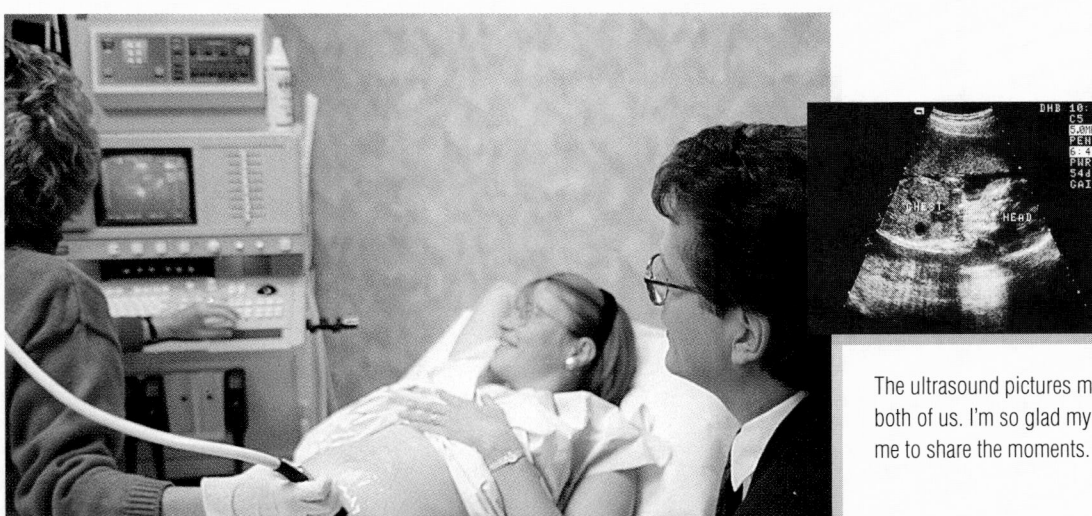

The ultrasound pictures made the baby seem real for both of us. I'm so glad my husband was able to be with me to share the moments.

$\mathcal{W}$e were so excited when we learned that I was pregnant. We had been waiting for this moment for some time, and we were ready to become parents. During the first trimester, I didn't look or feel pregnant, but when reading about the fetus' amazing development inside of me, I became very conscious of doing the best for our baby. I wonder if all parents feel the same?

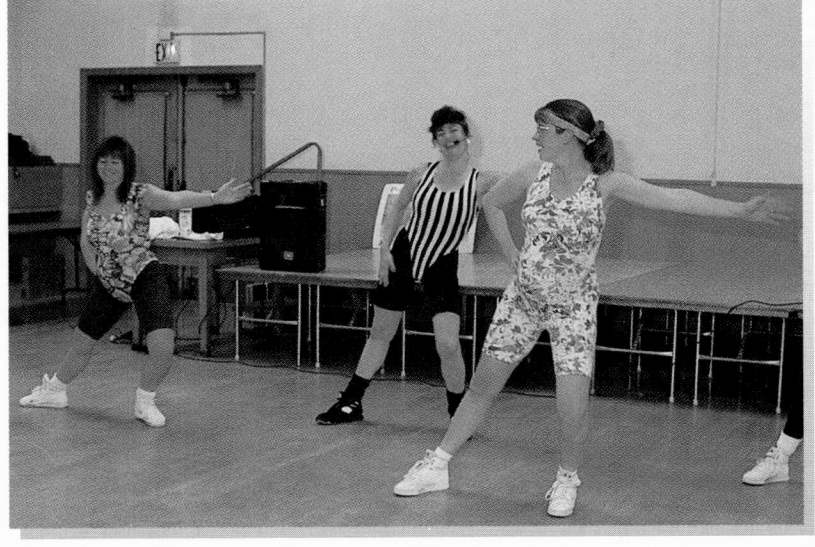

Exercise classes kept me fit and active. The instructor had me monitor my pulse to ensure that I didn't overdo.

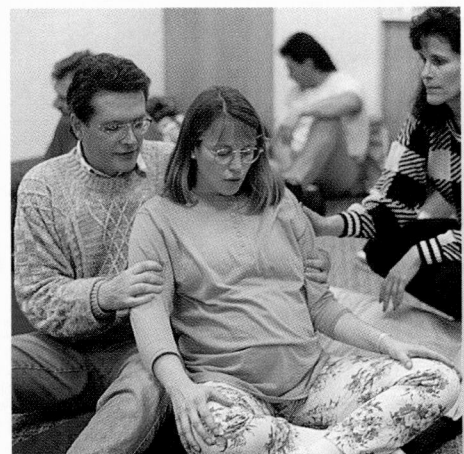

Childbirth preparation classes helped us learn to be a real team.

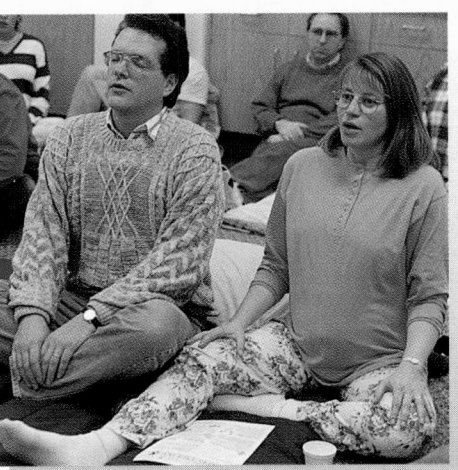

I was amazed at how fully involved my husband was. He did better at the breathing than I did!

Development is rapid; heart begins to pump blood; limb buds are well developed. Facial features and major divisions of the brain are discernible. Ears develop from skin folds; tiny bones and muscles are formed beneath the thin skin.

Embryo becomes a fetus, its beating heart discernible by ultrasound. Assumes a more human shape as lower body develops. At week 12, first movements begin. Sex is determinable. Kidneys produce urine.

Musculoskeletal system has matured; nervous system begins to exert control. Blood vessels rapidly develop. Fetal hands can grasp; legs kick actively. All organs begin to mature and grow. Fetus weighs about 7 oz (½ lb). FHT discernible with Doppler. Pancreas produces insulin.

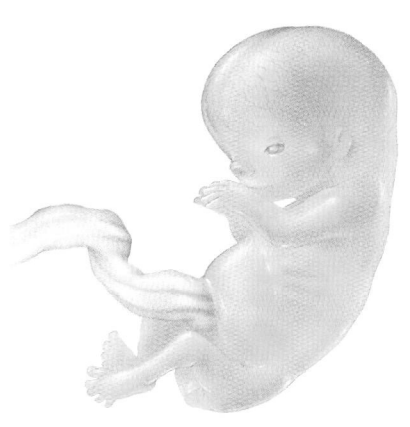
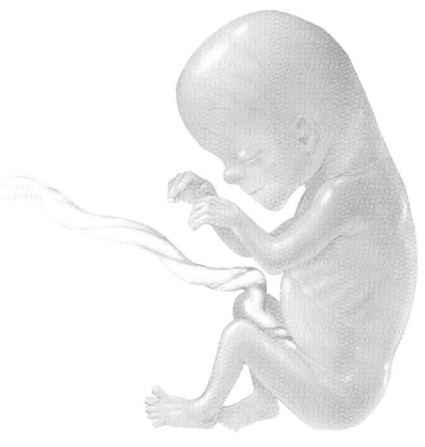
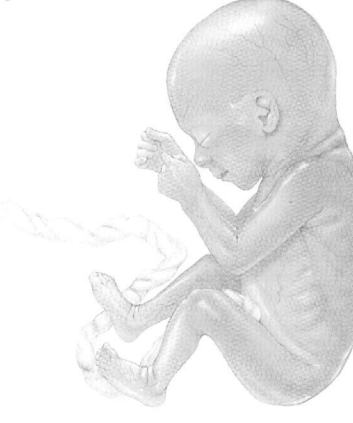

Morning sickness, may persist to 12 weeks. Uterus changes from pear to globular shape. Hegar's, Goodell's and Piskacek's signs appear. Cervix flexes; leukorrhea increases. Surprise and ambivalence about pregnancy may occur. No noticeable weight gain.

Chadwick's sign appears. Uterus rises above pelvic brim by 12 weeks. Braxton Hicks contractions may begin and continue throughout pregnancy. Potential for urinary tract infection (UTI) increases and exists throughout pregnancy. Weight gain of about 2½ to 4 lb during first trimester.

Placenta now fully functioning and producing hormones.

Fundus halfway between symphysis and umbilicus. Woman gains slightly less than 1 lb per wk for remainder of pregnancy. May feel more energetic. BPD measurement on ultrasound. Vaginal secretions increase. Itching, irritation, malodor suggest infection. Woman may begin wearing maternity clothes. Pressure on bladder lessens and urinary frequency decreases.

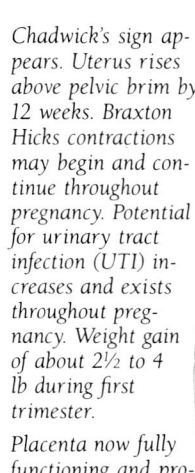

Eat dry crackers before arising; try frequent small, dry, low-fat meals with fluids taken between meals. Avoid use of hot tubs, saunas, and steam rooms throughout pregnancy.

Discuss attitudes toward pregnancy. Discuss value of early pregnancy classes that focus on what to expect during pregnancy. Provide information about childbirth preparation classes.

Adequate fluid intake and frequent voiding (every 2 hr while awake) help prevent UTI. Also helpful to void following intercourse. Wipe from front to rear.

Discuss nutrition and appropriate weight gain. Stress value of regular physical exercise, especially non-weightbearing activities or walking. Discuss possible effects of pregnancy on sexual relationship.

Daily shower or bath and thorough drying of vulva helpful; avoid douching during pregnancy. Consult caregiver if infection suspected; use only prescribed medications.

Review danger signs of pregnancy. Discuss infant feeding options; provide information on the value of breast-feeding. Provide information about clothing, shoes.

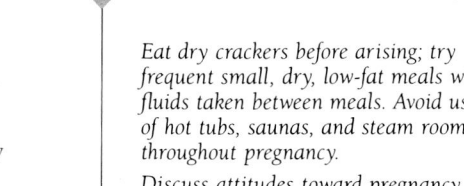

MATERNAL-FETAL DEVELOPMENT

FETAL DEVELOPMENT

The sperm fertilizes the ovum, which then divides and burrows into the uterus.

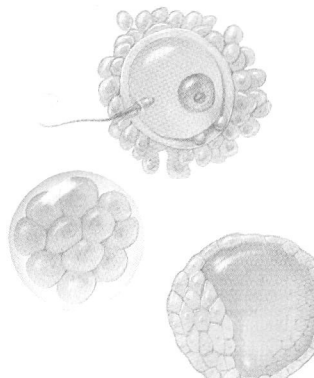

From the embryonic disk (ec[to]derm, entoderm, mesoderm) first body segments appear th[at] will eventually become the sp[ine,] brain, and spinal cord. Heart[,] blood circulation, and digesti[ve] tract take shape. Embryo is l[ess] than a quarter-inch long.

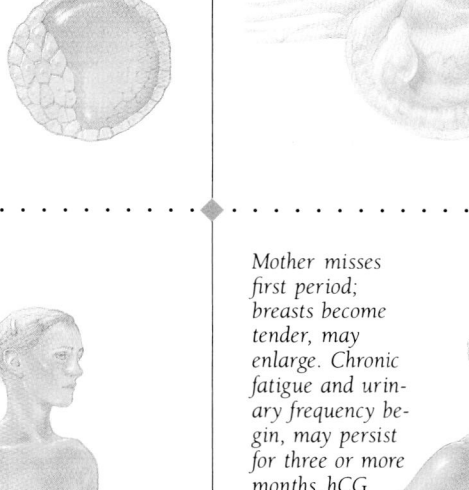

MATERNAL CHANGES

Mother misses first period; breasts become tender, may enlarge. Chronic fatigue and urinary frequency begin, may persist for three or more months. hCG in urine and serum 9 days after conception.

CLIENT TEACHING/ ANTICIPATORY GUIDANCE

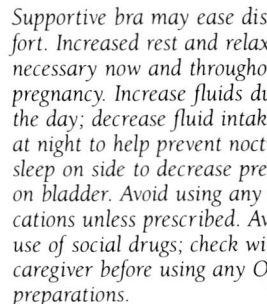

Supportive bra may ease disc[om]fort. Increased rest and relax[ation] necessary now and throughou[t] pregnancy. Increase fluids du[ring] the day; decrease fluid intake at night to help prevent noct[uria;] sleep on side to decrease pres[sure] on bladder. Avoid using any [medi]cations unless prescribed. Av[oid] use of social drugs; check wit[h] caregiver before using any O[TC] preparations.

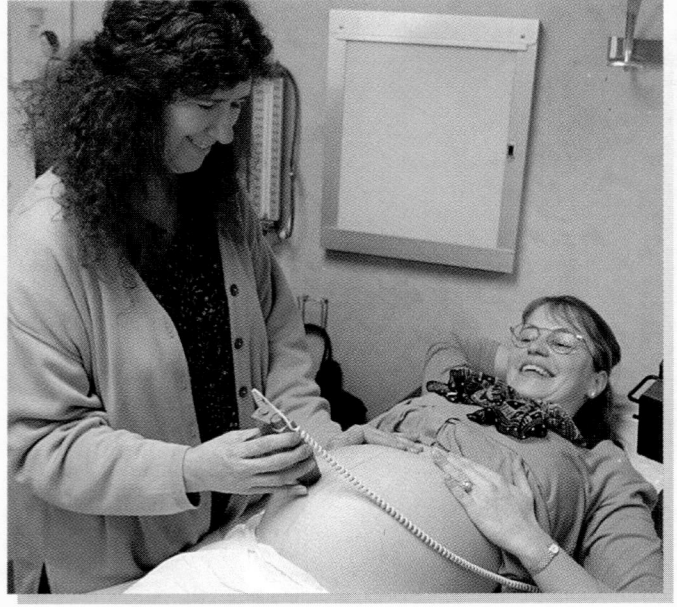

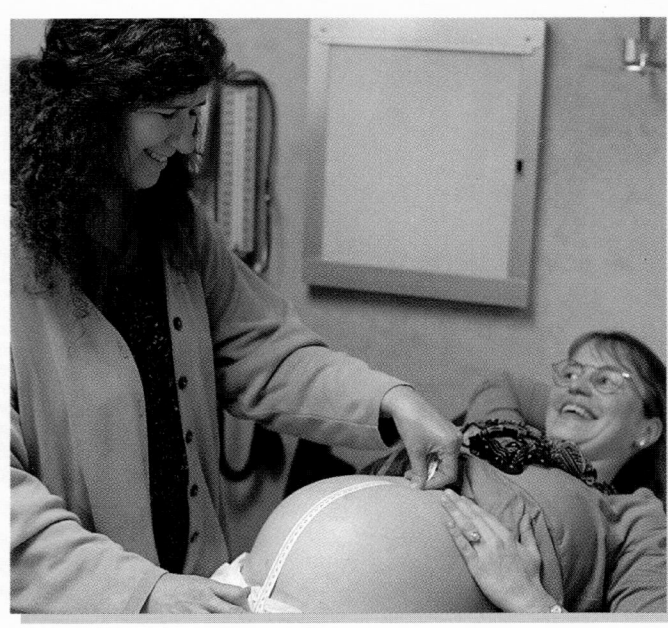

The regular exams by my midwife indicated that our baby was growing normally.

As the pregnancy progressed I learned about how the baby was growing and what to expect during labor and birth. The nurses were especially good about sharing information. They really seemed to want us to understand the process.

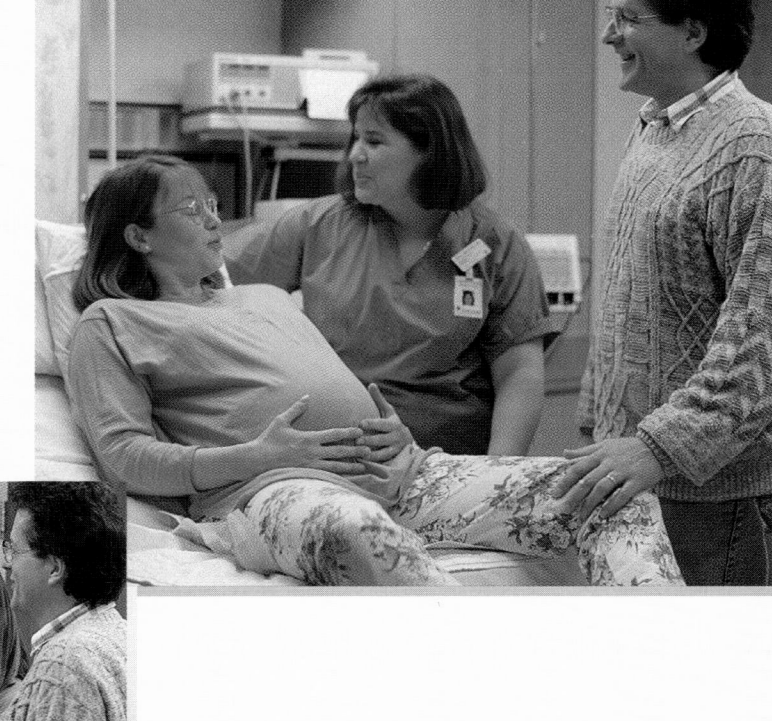

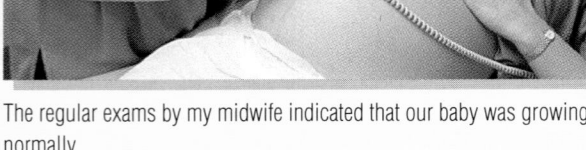

I loved listening to my baby's heartbeat.

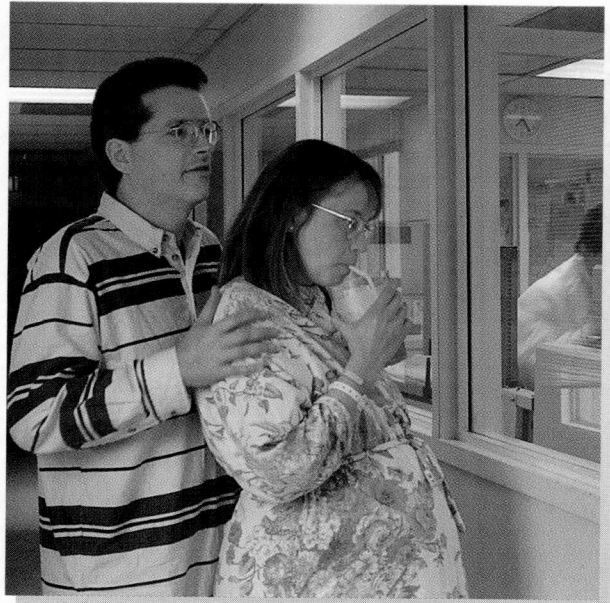

Early in my labor we walked the halls and visited the nursery to see the babies.

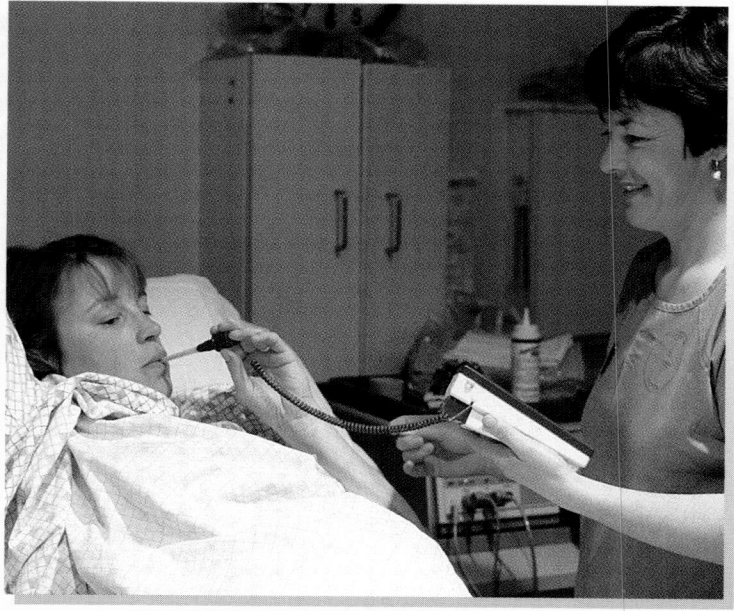

The nurses monitored my progress carefully.

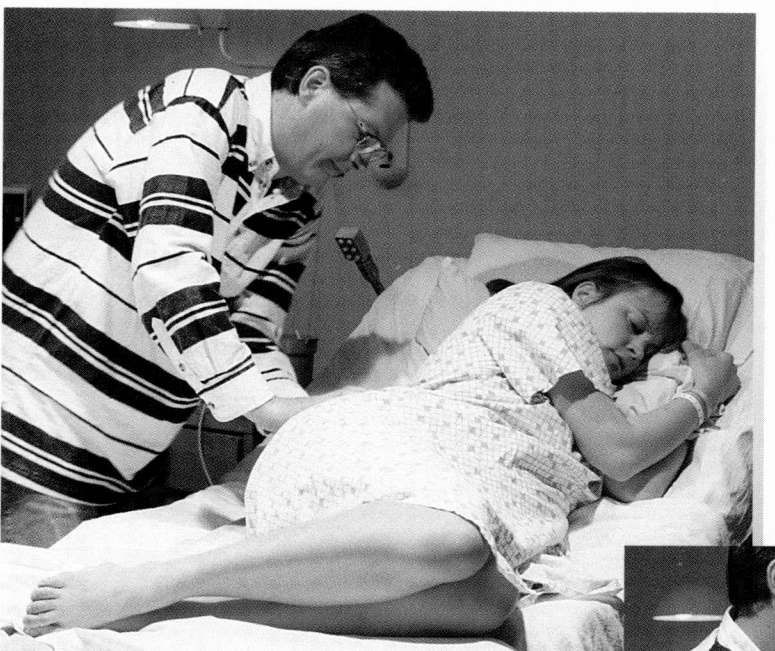

*L*abor was a challenge. While I felt mentally prepared, the intensity of some of my feelings came as a surprise. I'm so glad we were able to face the experience as a couple. It must have been harder in the past when loved ones weren't able to be present for the labor and birth.

The comfort techniques we had learned in the childbirth preparation classes really did help. At times I felt afraid and a little overwhelmed. Then it helped to talk.

Brown fat deposits are developing beneath the skin to insulate the baby following birth. Baby has grown to about 15–17 in. Begins storing iron, calcium, and phosphorus.

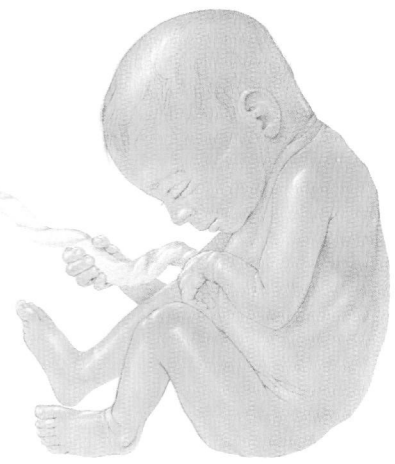

The entire uterus is occupied by the baby, thus restricting its activity. Maternal antibodies are transferred to the baby. This provides immunity for about 6 months until the infant's own immune system can take over.

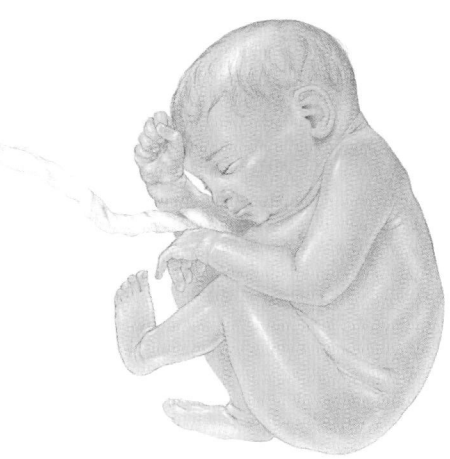

© 1996 Addison-Wesley Nursing, A Division of The Benjamin/Cummings Publishing Company, Inc.

From Olds et al, *Maternal-Newborn Nursing*, Fifth Edition

Illustrations by Charles W. Hoffman, MA, AMI

Fundus reaches xyphoid process; breasts full and tender. Urinary frequency may return. Swollen ankles and sleeping problems may develop. Dyspnea may develop.

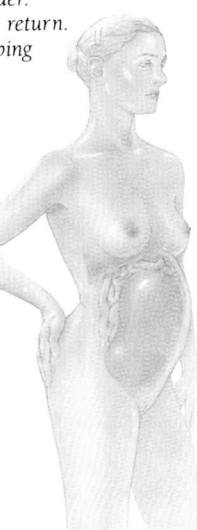

The fetus descends deeper into the mother's pelvis (lightening). The placenta is nearly 4 times as thick as it was 20 weeks ago, weighing nearly 20 oz. Mother is eager for birth, may have final burst of energy. Backaches, urinary frequency increase. Braxton Hicks contractions intensify as cervix and lower uterine segment prepare for labor. Couple may tour labor and delivery area.

Wear well-fitting supportive bra. Elevate legs once or twice daily for an hour or so. Sleep on left side if possible. Use naturally occurring diuretics such as 2 tbsp lemon juice in 1 cup water or a generous serving of watermelon if available. Avoid most diuretics unless specifically prescribed. Maintain proper posture; use extra pillows at night for severe dyspnea. Following culture and personal preference, may begin preparing nursery now.

Review signs of labor. Discuss plans for other children (if any), transportation to agency.

Continue pelvic tilt exercises. Wear low-heeled shoes or flats. Avoid heavy lifting. Sleep on side to relieve bladder pressure. Urinate frequently. Avoid all analgesics except acetominophen. Pack suitcase for delivery.

Discuss postpartum period including decisions such as circumcision, rooming-in. Discuss common postpartum discomforts; mention postpartum blues. Discuss family planning methods, infant care. Stress need for adequate rest postpartally. Provide support, especially if baby is overdue.

ADDISON-WESLEY NURSING
A Division of The Benjamin/Cummings Publishing Company, Inc.
Menlo Park, California • Reading, Massachusetts • New York
Don Mills, Ontario • Wokingham, UK • Amsterdam • Bonn
Paris • Milan • Madrid • Sydney • Singapore • Tokyo

20 WEEKS (column 1 — partially cut off at left edge)

...nix protects the body; fine hair
...nugo) covers the body and keeps the
...on the skin. Eyebrows, eyelashes,
...d head hair develop. Fetus develops
...egular schedule of sleeping, sucking
...d kicking.

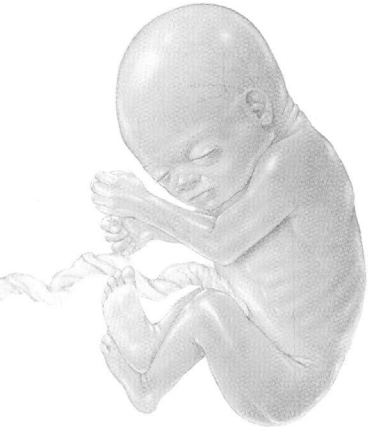

...ndus reaches level
...umbilicus. Breasts
...gin secreting co-
...trum. Amniotic
...c holds about
...0mL fluid.
...intness and diz-
...ess may occur,
...pecially with sud-
...n position changes.
...ricose veins may
...gin to develop.
...oman experiences
...al movement, and
...egnancy may sud-
...nly seem more
...eal." Areola
...rken. Nasal stuff-
...ess may develop.
...g cramps may
...gin to occur. Con-
...pation may
...velop.

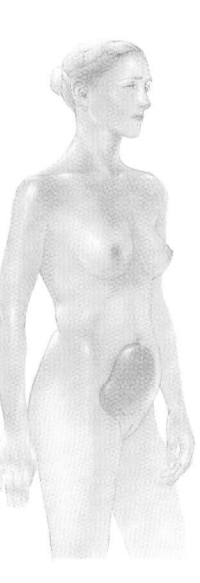

...t with feet elevated when possible;
...se slowly and carefully. Avoid pres-
...re on lower thighs. Support stockings
...ay be helpful. Cool-air vaporizer
...ay help. Eat foods containing fiber,
...ch as raw fruits, vegetables, cereals
...ith bran; drink liquids and exercise
...equently.

...iscuss breast care. Discuss dorsiflex-
...n of foot to relieve cramps; heat to
...fected muscle.

24 WEEKS (column 2)

Skeleton develops rapidly as bone-forming
cells increase activity. Respiratory movements
begin. Fetus weighs about 1 lb, 10 oz.

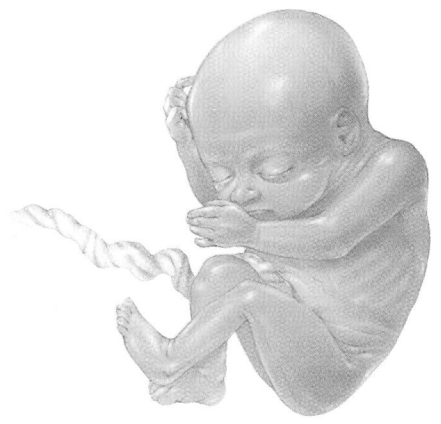

Fundus above umbilicus.
Backache and leg cramps
may begin. Skin changes
can include striae grav-
idarum, chloasma, linea
negra, acne, redness on
palms of hands and soles of
feet. Nosebleeds can occur.
May experience abdominal
itching as uterus enlarges;
will continue until end
of pregnancy.

Assure woman that skin changes generally
subside soon after birth. Discuss specific exercises such as pelvic tilt to help strengthen
back and abdominal muscles, and stress importance of good body mechanics. Reiterate
importance of avoiding medications, caffeine,
alcohol and smoking.

Woman may choose to apply petroleum jelly
in nostrils to relieve nosebleeds. Cool vaporizer may also help. Lanolin-based cream can
relieve itching. Mild soap can remove excess
oil associated with acne.

28 WEEKS (column 3)

Fetus can breathe, swallow, regulate temperature. Surfactant forms in lungs. Eyes begin to
open and close. Baby is ⅔ the size it will be
at birth.

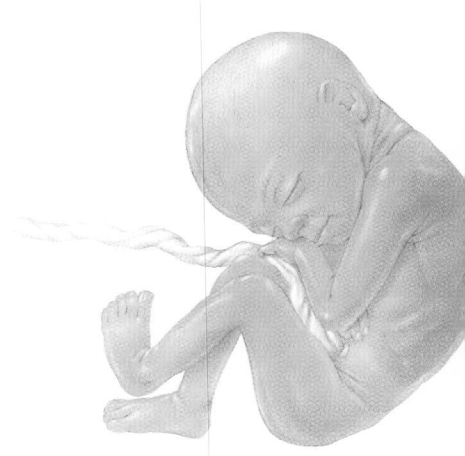

Fundus halfway between
umbilicus and xyphoid
process. May develop hem-
orrhoids. Thoracic breathing
replaces abdominal breathing. Fetal outline palpable.
May be tired of pregnancy
and eager for the mothering
role. Heartburn may begin
to occur. May begin taking
childbirth preparation
classes with partner or
support person.

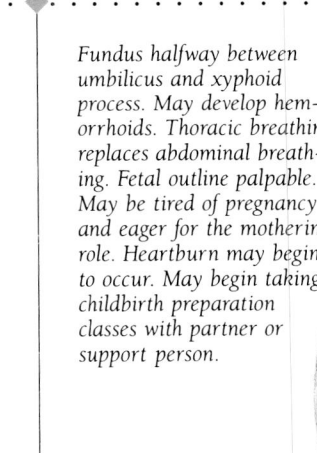

Avoid constipation; use sitz baths, gentle reinsertion of hemorrhoids with a fingertip as
necessary. Topical anesthetic agents may offer
relief of hemorrhoids. Stool softeners may be
prescribed by caregiver. Elevate legs and assume sidelying position when resting. Eat
small, more frequent meals; avoid fatty foods,
lying down after eating. Maalox or mylanta
may be helpful; Avoid sodium bicarbonate.
Discuss expectations about labor and delivery, caring for an infant.

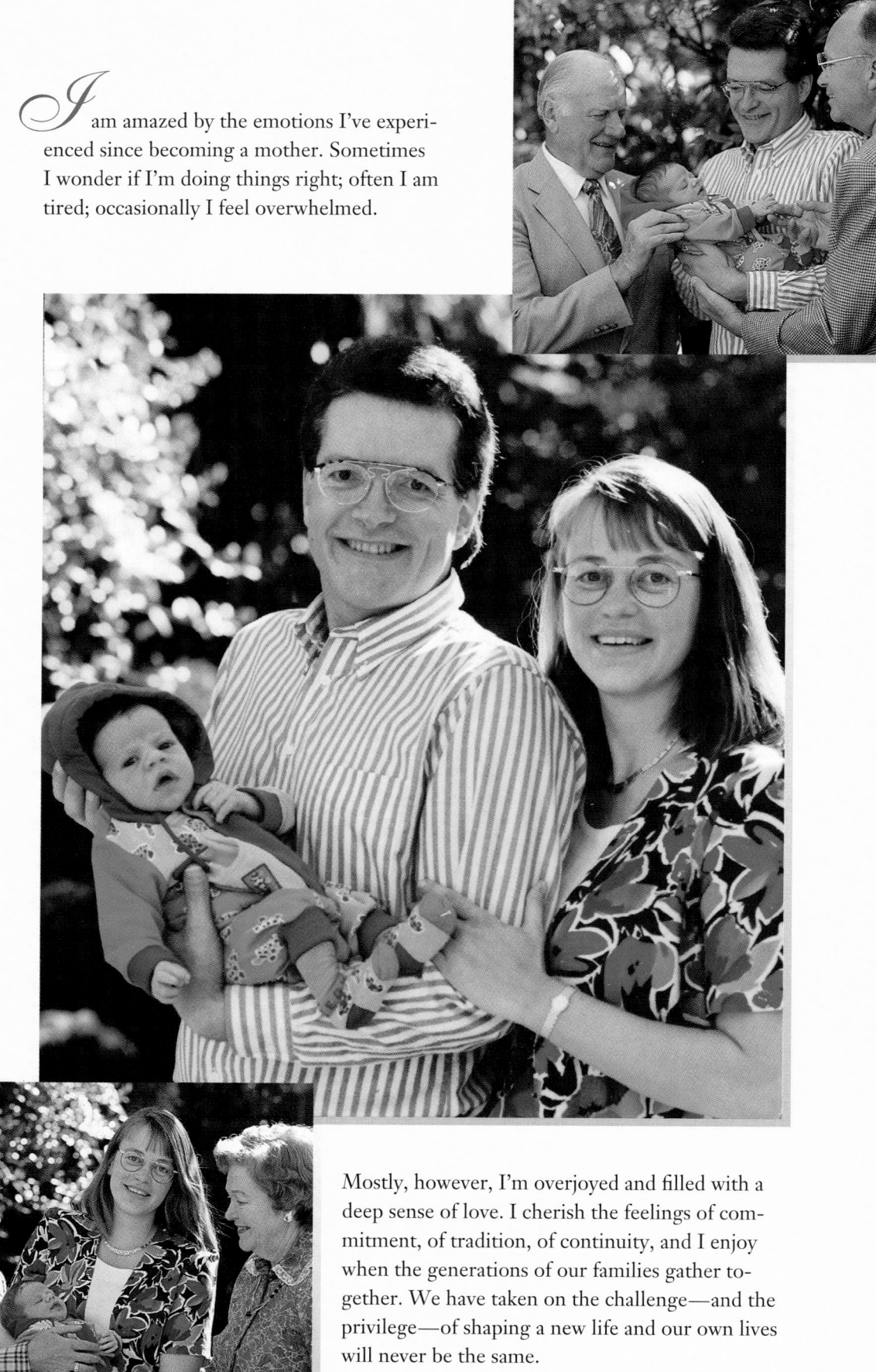

I am amazed by the emotions I've experienced since becoming a mother. Sometimes I wonder if I'm doing things right; often I am tired; occasionally I feel overwhelmed.

Mostly, however, I'm overjoyed and filled with a deep sense of love. I cherish the feelings of commitment, of tradition, of continuity, and I enjoy when the generations of our families gather together. We have taken on the challenge—and the privilege—of shaping a new life and our own lives will never be the same.

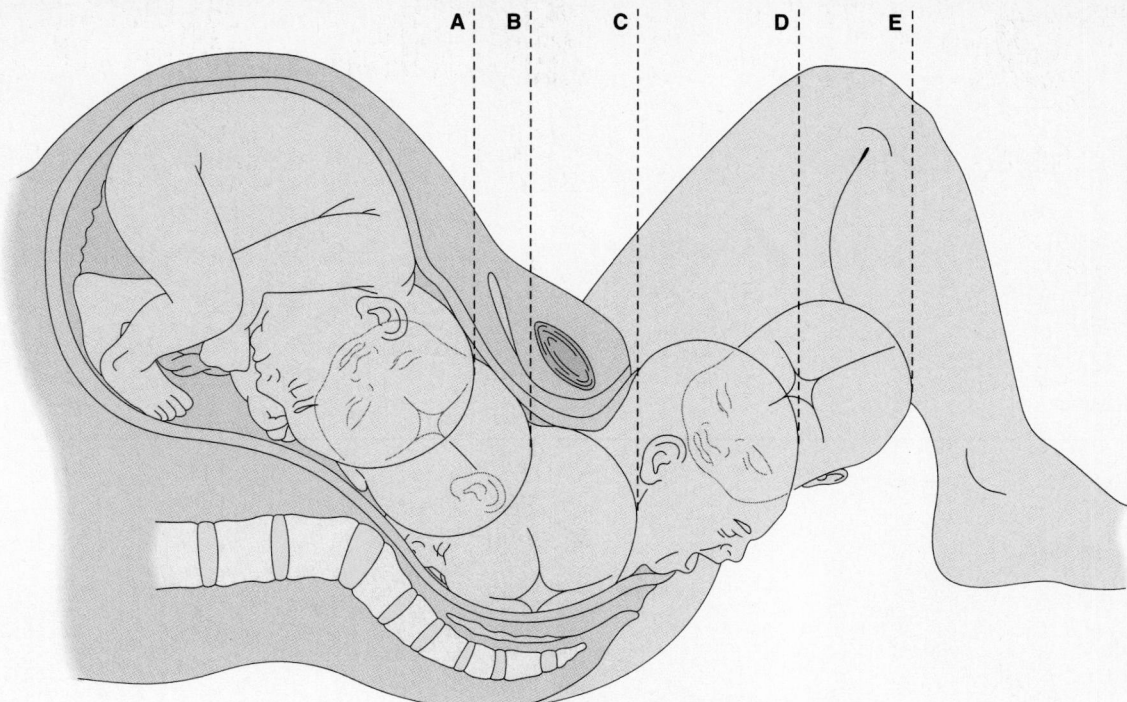

FIGURE 21-13 Mechanisms of labor. *A, B* Descent. *C* Internal rotation. *D* Extension. *E* External rotation.

Flexion

Flexion occurs as the fetal head descends and meets resistance from the soft tissues of the pelvis, the musculature of the pelvic floor, and the cervix.

Internal Rotation

The fetal head must rotate to fit the diameter of the pelvic cavity, which is widest in the anteroposterior diameter. As the occiput of the fetal head meets resistance from the levator ani muscles and their fascia, the occiput rotates from left to right, and the sagittal suture aligns in the anteroposterior pelvic diameter.

Extension

The resistance of the pelvic floor and the mechanical movement of the vulva opening anteriorly and forward assist with extension of the fetal head as it passes under the symphysis pubis. With this positional change the occiput, then brow and face, emerge from the vagina.

Restitution

The shoulders of the infant enter the pelvis obliquely and remain oblique when the head rotates to the anteroposterior diameter through internal rotation. Because of this rotation the neck becomes twisted. Once the head emerges and is free of pelvic resistance the neck untwists, turning the head to one side (restitution), and aligns with the position of the back in the birth canal.

External Rotation

As the shoulders rotate to the anteroposterior position in the pelvis, the head is turned farther to one side (external rotation).

Expulsion

After the external rotation and through expulsive efforts of the laboring woman the anterior shoulder meets the under surface of the symphysis pubis and slips under it. As lateral flexion of the shoulder and head occurs, the anterior shoulder is born before the posterior shoulder. The body follows quickly. The adaptations of the newborn to extrauterine life are discussed in Chapter 27.

Third Stage

Placental Separation

After the infant is born the uterus contracts firmly, diminishing its capacity and the surface area of placental attachment. The placenta begins to separate because of this

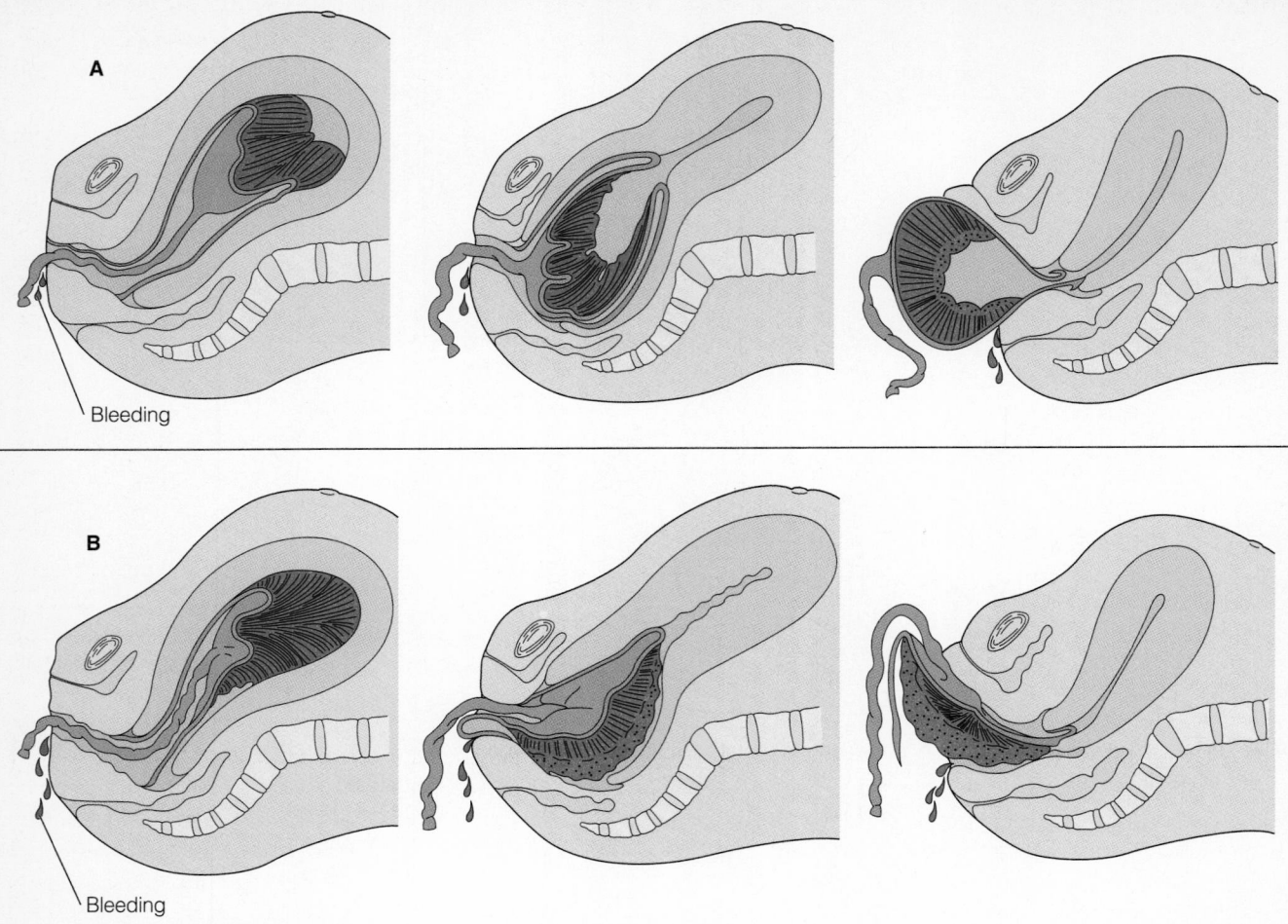

FIGURE 21-14 Placental separation and expulsion. *A* Schultze mechanism. *B* Duncan mechanism.

decrease in surface area. As this separation occurs, bleeding results in the formation of a hematoma between the placental tissue and the remaining decidua. This hematoma accelerates the separation process. The membranes are the last to separate. They are peeled off the uterine wall as the placenta descends into the vagina.

Signs of placental separation usually appear around 5 minutes after birth of the infant. These signs are (1) a globular-shaped uterus, (2) a rise of the fundus in the abdomen, (3) a sudden gush or trickle of blood, and (4) further protrusion of the umbilical cord out of the vagina.

Placental Delivery

When the signs of placental separation appear, the woman may bear down to aid in placental expulsion. If this fails and the certified nurse-midwife/physician has ascertained that the fundus is firm, gentle traction may be applied to the cord while pressure is exerted on the fundus. The weight of the placenta as it is guided into the placental pan (a basin that holds the placenta once it is expelled) aids in the removal of the membranes from the uterine wall. A placenta is considered to be *retained* if 30 minutes have elapsed from completion of the second stage of labor.

If the placenta separates from the inside to the outer margins, it is expelled with the fetal (shiny) side presenting (Figure 21–14). This is known as the *Schultze mechanism* of placental delivery or more commonly *shiny Schultze*. If the placenta separates from the outer margins inward, it will roll up and present sideways with the maternal surface delivering first. This is known as the *Duncan mechanism* of placental delivery and is commonly called *dirty Duncan* because the placental surface is rough.

Nursing and medical interventions during the third stage of labor are discussed in Chapter 23.

Fourth Stage

The fourth stage of labor is the time from 1 to 4 hours after birth in which physiologic readjustment of the mother's body begins. With the birth hemodynamic changes occur. Blood loss at birth ranges from 250 to 500 mL. With this blood loss and the weight of the pregnant uterus off of the surrounding vessels, blood is redistributed into venous beds. This results in a moderate drop in both systolic and diastolic blood pressure, increased pulse pressure, and moderate tachycardia (Albright et al 1986).

The cerebrospinal fluid pressure, which increased during labor, now drops and rapidly returns to normal values (Albright et al 1986).

The uterus remains contracted and is in the midline of the abdomen. The fundus is usually midway between the symphysis pubis and umbilicus. Its contracted state constricts the vessels at the site of placental implantation. Immediately after birth of the placenta the cervix is widely spread and thick.

Nausea and vomiting the woman may have experienced during transition usually cease. The woman may be thirsty and hungry. She may experience a shaking chill, which is thought to be associated with the ending of the physical exertion of labor. The bladder is often hypotonic due to trauma during the second stage and/or the administration of anesthetics that may decrease sensations. Hypotonic bladder leads to urinary retention. Nursing care of this stage is discussed in Chapter 23.

My whole life has been spent working with mothers and fathers during labor and birth. After all this time and so many wonderful moments I am still absolutely amazed at the wonder of this process. At the moment of birth the parents and I watch the baby's head appear, and we know that technically it is the result of a process of uterine contractions and movements of the fetus through the pelvis, but really, we know that it is truly a miraculous process.

MATERNAL SYSTEMIC RESPONSE TO LABOR

Cardiovascular System

The woman's cardiovascular system is stressed both by the uterine contractions and by the pain, anxiety, and apprehension the woman experiences. During labor there is a significant increase in cardiac output. Each strong contraction greatly decreases or completely stops the blood flow in the branches of the uterine artery that supply the intervillous space (in the placenta). This leads to a redistribution of about 300–500 mL of blood into the peripheral circulation and an increase in peripheral resistance, resulting in increased systolic and diastolic blood pressure, a slowing of the pulse rate, and an increase of about 31% in cardiac output (Blackburn & Loper 1992).

Maternal position also affects cardiac output, blood pressure, and pulse. When the laboring woman turns to a side-lying position, cardiac output increases by about 22%, the pulse rate decreases by about 6 beats per minute, and stroke volume increases by 27% (Blackburn & Loper 1992). When the woman is supine, cardiac output increases 25%, stroke volume increases 33%, pulse pressure increases more than 26%, blood pressure rises significantly, and pulse rate decreases by 15% (Ueland & Ferguson 1990).

There is an additional effect on hemodynamics during the bearing down efforts in the second stage. When the laboring woman holds her breath and pushes against a closed glottis (Valsalva maneuver), intrathoracic pressure rises. As intrathoracic pressure increases, the venous return is interrupted, which leads to a rise in the venous pressure. In addition the blood in the lungs is forced into the left atrium, which leads to a transient increase in cardiac output, blood pressure, and pulse pressure and causes bradycardia. As venous return to the lungs continues to be diminished while the breath is held, a decrease in blood pressure, pulse pressure, and cardiac output occurs.

When the next breath is taken (Valsalva maneuver is interrupted), the intrathoracic pressure is decreased. Venous return increases, which leads to refilling of the pulmonary bed and results in recovery of the cardiac output and stroke volume. This process is repeated with each pushing effort.

Immediately after birth cardiac output peaks with an 80% increase over prelabor values. Then in the first 10 minutes it decreases 20% to 25%. Cardiac output further decreases 20% to 25% in the first hour after the birth (Albright et al 1986). However, these decreases still leave the woman with an elevated cardiac output for at least 24 hours after the birth (Robson et al 1989).

Blood Pressure

As a result of increased cardiac output, systolic blood pressure rises during uterine contractions. In the first stage systolic pressure may increase by 35 mm Hg, and there may be further increases in the second stage during pushing efforts. Diastolic pressure also increases by about 25 mm Hg in the first stage and 65 mm Hg in the second stage. These increases begin just before the uterine contraction, with a return to baseline as soon as the contraction ends (Blackburn & Loper 1992).

Blood pressure may drop precipitously when the woman lies in a supine position and experiences supine hypotensive syndrome. In addition to hypotension there is an increase in the pulse rate, diaphoresis, nausea, weakness, and air hunger. These changes are attributed to the decreased cardiac output and a subsequent drop in stroke volume. Some researchers have suggested that in addition to venal caval compression from the weight of the pregnant uterus there is also aortocaval compression (Bottoms & Scott 1990).

Women with the highest risk of developing supine hypotensive syndrome are women in their first pregnancy with strong abdominal muscles and tightly drawn abdominal skin, women with hydramnios and/or multiple pregnancy, and obese women. Other predisposing factors include hypovolemia, dehydration, hemorrhage, metabolic acidosis, administration of narcotics (which results in vasodilation and inhibits compensatory mechanisms), and administration of regional anesthetics that results in *sympathetic blockade* (blocking of the sympathetic nervous system, which results in vasodilation and hypotension). A sympathetic blockade may occur with an epidural or a spinal block.

Fluid and Electrolyte Balance

Profuse perspiration (diaphoresis) occurs during labor. Hyperventilation also occurs, altering electrolyte and fluid balance from insensible water loss. The muscle activity elevates the body temperature, which increases sweating and evaporation from the skin. As the woman responds to the work of labor the rise in the respiratory rate increases the evaporative water volume because each breath of air must be warmed to the body temperature and humidified. With the increased evaporative water volume, maintaining adequate oral fluids/hydration is important. In some instances parenteral (IV) fluids are administered.

Respiratory System

Oxygen demand and consumption increase at the onset of labor because of the presence of uterine contractions. As anxiety and pain from uterine contractions increase hyperventilation frequently occurs. With hyperventilation there is a fall in $PaCO_2$, and respiratory alkalosis results (Blackburn & Loper 1992).

As labor progresses and contractions become more frequent, stronger, and prolonged, the work load, tension, and anxiety of the woman continue to change (Blackburn & Loper 1992).

By the end of the first stage most women have developed a mild metabolic acidosis compensated by respiratory alkalosis. As she pushes in the second stage of labor, the woman's $PaCO_2$ levels may rise along with blood lactate levels (due to muscular activity), and mild respiratory acidosis occurs. By the time the baby is born (end of second stage) there is metabolic acidosis uncompensated by respiratory alkalosis (Blackburn & Loper 1992).

The changes in acid-base status that occur in labor are quickly reversed in the fourth stage because of changes in the woman's respiratory rate. Acid-base levels return to pregnancy levels by 24 hours after birth, and nonpregnant values are attained a few weeks after birth (Blackburn & Loper 1992, p 269).

Renal System

During labor there is an increase in maternal renin, plasma renin activity, and angiotensinogen. This elevation is thought to be important in the control of utero-placental blood flow during birth and the early postpartal period (Blackburn & Loper 1992, p 345).

Structurally, the base of the bladder is pushed forward and upward when engagement occurs. The pressure from the presenting part may impair blood and lymph drainage from the base of the bladder, leading to edema of the tissues (Cunningham et al 1993).

Gastrointestinal System

During labor gastric motility and absorption of solid food are reduced. Gastric emptying time is prolonged, and gastric volume (amount of contents that remain in the stomach) remains over 25 mL, regardless of the time the last meal was taken. The acidity of the gastric contents increases, and more than half of laboring women have a gastric pH less than 2.5 (Blackburn & Loper 1992). Some narcotics also delay gastric emptying time and add to the risk of aspiration should general anesthesia need to be used (Blackburn & Loper 1992).

The fluid requirements of women in labor have not been clearly established. In some instances oral hydration is the primary goal. In other situations a heparin lock may be inserted so intravenous access is available if needed. If intravenous fluids are used, it is important to remember that when hypertonic glucose infusions are used, there is an increase in maternal blood glucose; this can lead to fetal hyperglycemia and hyperinsulinemia and to hypoglycemia in the newborn (Blackburn & Loper 1992).

Immune System and Other Blood Values

The WBC count increases to $25,000/mm^3$–$30,000/mm^3$ during labor and early postpartum (Kuhlmann & Cruikshank 1994). The change in WBC count is due mostly to increased neutrophils resulting from a physiologic response to stress. The increased WBC count makes it difficult to identify the presence of an infectious process.

Maternal blood glucose levels decrease because glucose is used as an energy source during uterine contractions. The decreased blood glucose levels lead to a decrease in insulin requirements (Blackburn & Loper 1992).

Pain

Theories of Pain

According to the *gate-control theory*, pain results from activity in several interacting specialized neural systems. The gate-control theory proposes that a mechanism in the dorsal horn of the spinal column serves as a valve or gate that increases or decreases the flow of nerve impulses from the periphery to the central nervous system. The gate mechanism is influenced by the size of the transmitting fibers and by the nerve impulses that descend from the brain. Psychologic processes such as past experiences, attention, and emotion may influence pain perception and response by activating the gate mechanism. The gates may be opened or closed by central nervous system activities, such as anxiety or excitement, or through selective localized activity.

The gate-control theory has two important implications for childbirth: Pain may be controlled by tactile stimulation and can be modified by activities controlled by the central nervous system. These include back rub, sacral pressure, effleurage, suggestion, distraction, and conditioning.

Pain During Labor

The pain associated with the first stage of labor is unique in that it accompanies a normal physiologic process. Even though perception of the pain of childbirth is greatly determined by cultural patterning, there is a physiologic basis for discomfort during labor. Pain during the first stage of labor arises from (1) dilatation of the cervix, (2) hypoxia of the uterine muscle cells during contraction, (3) stretching of the lower uterine segment, and (4) pressure on adjacent structures. The primary source of pain is dilatation or stretching of the cervix. Nerve impulses travel through the uterine plexus, inferior hypogastric (pelvic) plexus, middle hypogastric plexus, superior hypogastric plexus, and lumbar sympathetic and lower thoracic chain and enter the spinal cord through the posterior roots of the 12th, 11th, and 10th thoracic and 1st lumbar nerves (Figure 21–15). As with other visceral pain, pain from the uterus is referred to the dermatomes supplied by the 12th, 11th, and 10th thoracic nerves. The areas of referred pain include the lower abdominal wall and the areas over the lower lumbar region and the upper sacrum (Figure 21–16).

During the second stage of labor discomfort is due to (1) hypoxia of the contracting uterine muscle cells, (2) distention of the vagina and perineum, and (3) pressure on adjacent structures. The nerve impulses from the vagina and perineum are transmitted by way of the pudendal nerve plexus and enter the spinal cord through the posterior roots of the second, third, and fourth sacral nerves. The area of pain increases as shown in Figure 21–17.

Pain during the third stage results from uterine contractions and cervical dilatation as the placenta is expelled (Figure 21–18). The mechanism for the transmission of nerve impulses is the same as for the first stage of labor. The third stage of labor is short, and after this phase anesthesia is needed primarily for episiotomy repair.

Factors Affecting Response to Pain

Many factors affect the individual's perception of pain impulses. Some psychologic and environmental influences particularly appropriate to labor are discussed here.

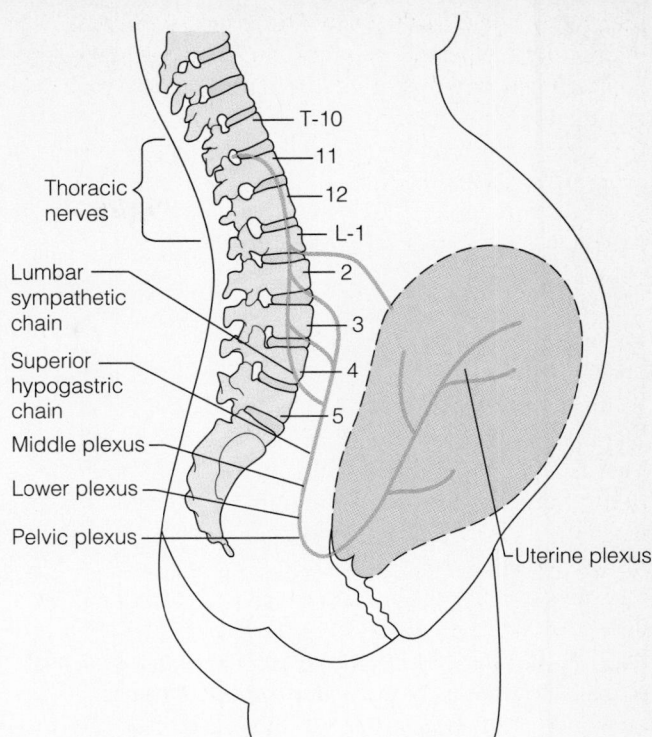

FIGURE 21-15 Pain pathway from uterus to spinal cord. Nerve impulses travel through the uterine plexus, pelvic plexus, inferior hypogastric plexus, middle and superior hypogastric plexus, and lumbar sympathetic chain and enter the spinal cord through the 12th, 11th, and 10th thoracic nerves. SOURCE: Modified from Bonica JJ: *Principles and Practice of Obstetric Analgesia and Anesthesia.* Philadelphia: Davis, 1972, p 492.

Effect of Childbirth Education Preparation for childbirth has been shown to reduce the need for analgesia and the subjective experience of tension and stress that occurs during labor. Crowe and Baeyer (1989) reported that women who demonstrated greater knowledge of childbirth and indicated they felt higher confidence after completing the classes reported a less painful childbirth.

Cultural Background Medical and nursing professionals have their own health care culture expectations of the woman in labor. She is expected to use a breathing technique and relaxation methods. Value is placed on maintaining self-control and knowing what to expect during labor and birth. It is important to know that the health care professional will interpret pain according to the health care culture norms although various other cultures have other ways of responding to pain (Bates 1987). The absence of crying and moaning does not necessarily mean that pain is absent, nor does the presence of crying and moaning necessarily mean that pain relief is desired at that moment. Some cultures believe it is natural to

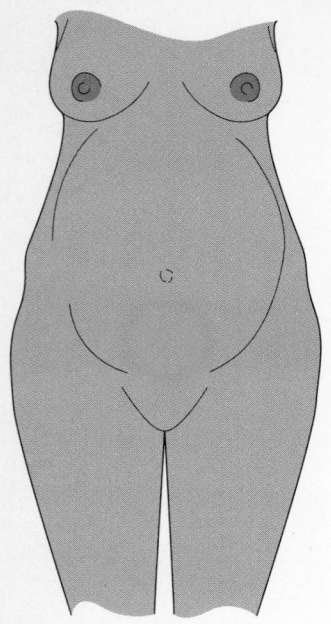
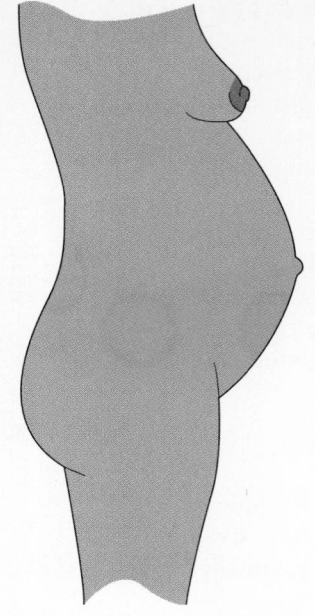
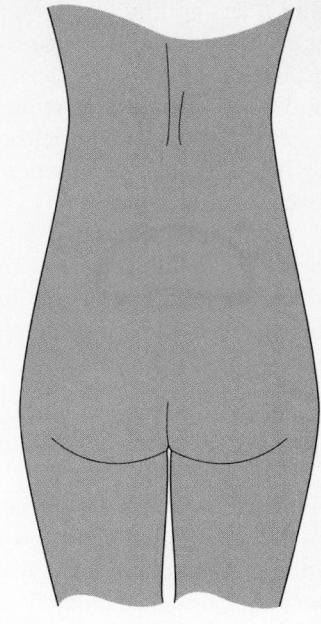

FIGURE 21-16 Area of reference of labor pain during the first stage. Pain is most intense in the darker colored areas.

SOURCE: Bonica JJ: *Principles and Practice of Obstetric Analgesia and Anesthesia.* Philadelphia: Davis, 1972, p 108.

communicate the pain experience, no matter how mild. Members of some cultures stoically accept pain out of fear or because it is expected of them.

An Asian woman may not outwardly express pain for fear of shaming herself and her family. Asian women may be anxious about losing face by their behavior (Engel

1989). Black women may also appear stoic in an effort to avoid showing weakness or calling undue attention to themselves (Kay 1982). Mexican women are taught to keep their mouths closed during labor and to avoid breathing in air that may cause the uterus to rise up. They cry out only during exhalation (Kay 1982). Navajo

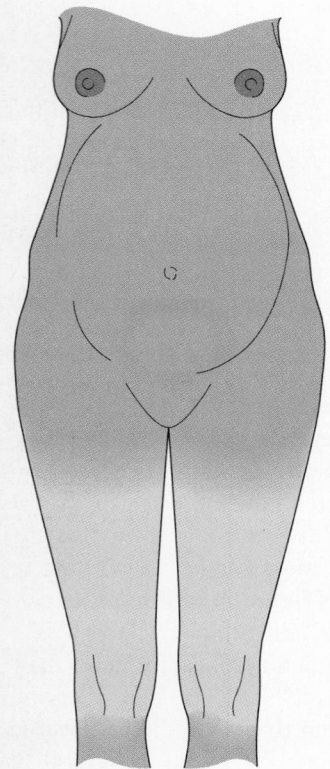
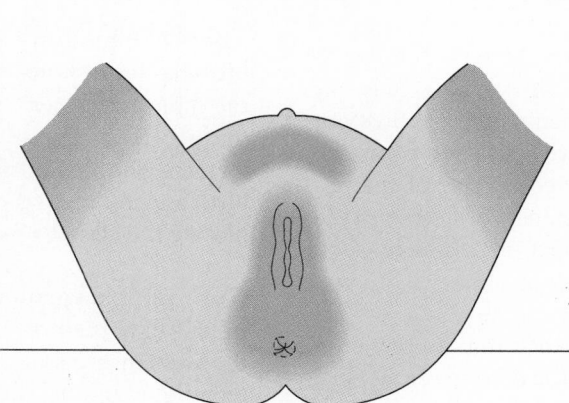
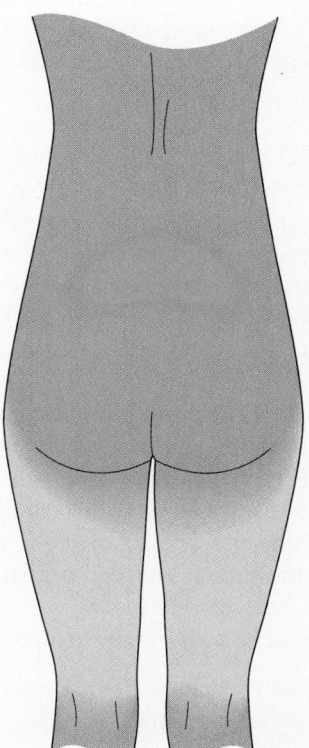

FIGURE 21-17 Distribution of labor pain during the later phase of the first stage and early phase of the second stage. The darkest colored areas indicate the location of the most intense pain; moderate color, moderate pain; and light color, mild pain. The uterine contractions, which at this stage are very strong, produce intense pain. SOURCE: Bonica JJ: *Principles and Practice of Obstetric Analgesia and Anesthesia.* Philadelphia: Davis, 1972, p 109.

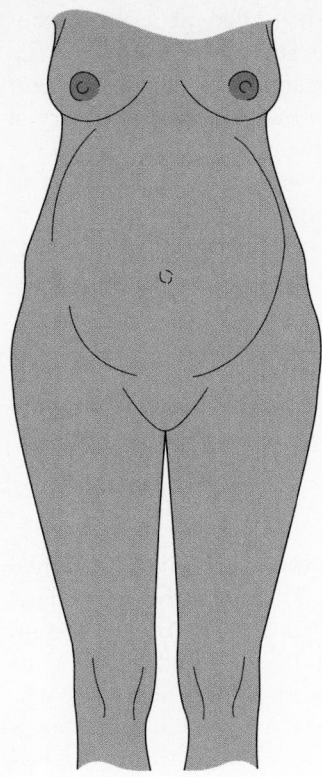
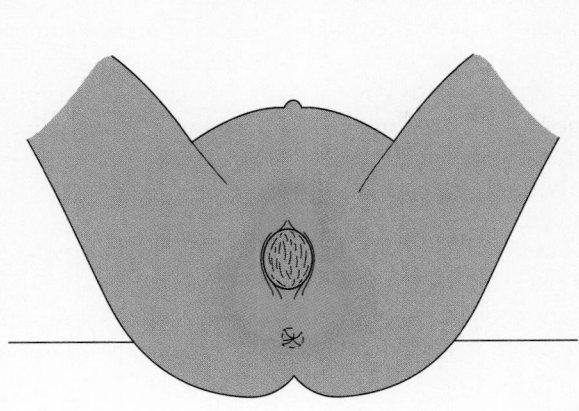
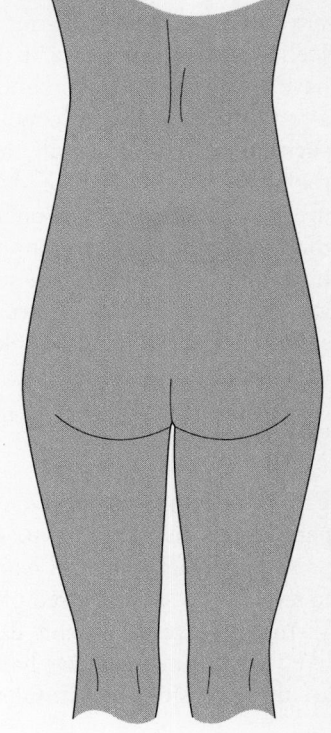

FIGURE 21-18 Distribution of labor pain during the later phase of the second stage and actual birth. The perineal component is the primary cause of discomfort. Uterine contractions contribute much less. SOURCE: Bonica JJ; *Principles and Practice of Obstetric Analgesia and Anesthesia*. Philadelphia: Davis, 1972, p 109.

women traditionally keep quiet to preserve the secrecy of the process (Kay 1982). The outward expression of the perceived pain may be difficult to interpret. Navajo women may be willing to receive pain medication but be hesitant to request it (Kay 1982). In a study by Senden et al (1988) it was noted that Dutch women both expected and received less pain medication than their American counterparts. In a different comparison Middle Eastern women with little education exhibited more pain behavior than those with higher education (Weisenberg & Caspi 1989). Interestingly, Senden et al (1988) and Weisenberg and Caspi (1989) found that all of the women expressed high satisfaction with their birth experience, which suggests that receiving the type of assistance (physical, medical) that the woman desired was more of an influence on her satisfaction than the pain actually experienced or expressed.

The health care culture may use touching and the support of others to decrease pain during labor. Various other cultural groups may or may not value the same comfort measures. The traditional Native American may want a female with her rather than her husband, and the Japanese woman may feel ashamed to be seen by her husband (Kay 1982). Hmong women usually prefer that their husbands remain with them in labor and be involved in comfort measures (Morrow 1986).

It is important, however, to avoid stereotyping women based on their ethnic backgrounds because exposure to North American culture and expectations may modify the behavioral response to pain. Nurses who are

providing support during labor must recognize that there are ways of reacting to pain that are different from the nurse's own personal views of appropriate behavior. Nurses need to be familiar with the cultural beliefs of those they are likely to assist during labor and use this knowledge along with assessment skills to verify the type of support that is needed.

Fatigue and Sleep Deprivation Exhaustion may be so great that a laboring woman's attention wanders from the physical stimuli of childbirth, or it may have the opposite effect, lowering the powers of resistance and self-control to produce an exaggerated response. Fatigue from sleep deprivation affects an individual's response to pain in several ways. The fatigued person has less energy and a decreased ability to use such strategies as distraction or imagination as coping mechanisms in dealing with pain. The fatigued woman in labor may choose a less demanding alternative, such as analgesia (McCaffery 1972). This is particularly important for a laboring woman who has a prolonged prodromal period, which may interfere with sleep. A woman may begin the active phase of labor in an exhausted state and have difficulty coping with the discomfort of frequent contractions.

Personal Significance of Pain The significance of pain is closely related to the woman's self-concept as well as to cultural expectations. She may view labor as a fearful event, one she has dreaded throughout pregnancy, or she may view it as the happiest event of her life. Pain may be interpreted by some women as punishment for perceived sins, such as engaging in premarital intercourse or feeling ambivalent toward the pregnancy. Others who have had preparation for childbirth may consider the pain a test of their ability to cope with a challenging event. If such women do not handle the pain of labor according to their expectations, they tend to experience a sense of failure, which threatens not only their self-concept but also their ability to mother. Consequently, it is vital that childbirth instructors and nurses stress to each woman that the reaction to childbirth is varied and individual. A woman should not feel a sense of failure if she requires analgesia to assist her in coping. The primary goal of childbirth preparation is a childbirth experience that is satisfying to both father and mother.

Previous Experience   One's previous experience with pain affects one's ability to manage current and future pain. Particularly painful experiences can condition one to expect the same degree of pain in a similar situation. Virtually all persons have experienced pain. It appears likely that those who have had more experience with pain are more sensitive to painful stimuli.

Anxiety   Anxiety related to pain must be approached on two levels, that associated with anticipation of pain and that associated with the presence of pain. Although a moderate degree of anxiety about impending pain is necessary for the person to handle the pain experience, anxiety during the pain experience should be reduced as much as possible by nursing intervention. Anxiety during labor produces tension, which increases the intensity of the pain.

Anxieties unrelated to the pain can also intensify the pain experience. For many young women admission for labor and birth is their first hospitalization. Routine procedures, rules and regulations, equipment, and the general environment are unfamiliar and anxiety provoking. For many women the spontaneous onset of labor has an element of surprise. Although the event is expected and even anticipated, few women are totally prepared for the actual onset of labor and hospitalization. Last-minute details must be completed. Arrangements for the care of other children have usually been made but now must actually be carried out. Having to leave young children for a few days is accompanied by varying degrees of anxiety for any mother.

Attention and Distraction   Both attention and distraction have an influence on the perception of pain. When pain sensation is the focus of attention, the perceived intensity is greater. The classic example is the football player who is unaware of an injury until the game is over and only then experiences painful sensations.

A sensory stimulus such as a back rub can serve as a distraction because the person's attention is focused on the stimulus rather than the pain. Cutaneous sensations are carried by large-diameter afferent fibers, which can inhibit the pain sensation carried by small-diameter fibers. This is a component of the gate-control theory of pain discussed earlier. Cutaneous stimulation to relieve pain may also be explained by the theory of extinction or perceptual dominance. This theory suggests that sensory input may extinguish pain or raise its threshold.

FETAL RESPONSE TO LABOR

When the fetus is normal, the mechanical and hemodynamic changes of normal labor have no adverse effects.

Heart Rate Changes

Fetal heart rate decelerations can occur with intracranial pressures of 40 to 55 mm Hg. The currently accepted explanation of this early deceleration is hypoxic depression of the central nervous system, which is under vagal control. The absence of these head compression decelerations (early decelerations) in some fetuses during labor is explained by the existence of a threshold that is reached more gradually in the presence of intact membranes and lack of maternal resistance. Early decelerations are harmless in the normal fetus.

Acid-Base Status in Labor

The blood flow to the fetus is slowed during the acme of the contraction, which leads to a slow decrease in the fetal pH. During the second stage, as uterine contractions become stronger and last longer and the woman pushes with each contraction, there is a more rapid decrease in fetal pH. There is also an increase in fetal base deficit and in PCO_2, and a drop in fetal oxygen saturation of about 10% (Creasy & Resnik 1994).

Fetal Movements

When the fetus is between 35 and 40 weeks, episodes of fetal breathing movements increase in the second and third hour following the mother's meals. There is also a marked increase during the night while the mother is asleep, which is thought to be part of a circadian rhythm in fetal breathing activity. In the healthy term fetus there are periods of no breathing movements that last up to 2 hours. It has been noted that the incidence of fetal breathing movements slows markedly and may cease about 3 days before the onset of spontaneous labor (Creasy & Resnik 1994).

Gross fetal body movements occur at a rate of about 20 to 50 per hour in the term fetus. The number of movements does not normally increase prior to or during labor (Creasy & Resnik 1994).

Behavior States

The human fetus develops behavioral states between 36 and 38 weeks of gestation. The behavioral states seem to continue during labor even in the presence of uterine contractions. Two sleep states (quiet and active) were most prevalent, although quiet and active awake states were occasionally observed. A decrease in fetal heart rate variability accompanies the quiet sleep state, and there is also a decrease in fetal breathing movements and other general body activity. The quiet sleep state lasted less than 40 minutes. Broussard (1990) suggests that as long as other fetal heart rate parameters are within normal limits, a decrease in variability will usually indicate a normal behavioral sleep state.

Hemodynamic Changes

The adequate exchange of nutrients and gases in the fetal capillaries and intervillous spaces depends in part on the fetal blood pressure. Fetal blood pressure is a protective mechanism for the normal fetus during the anoxic periods caused by the contracting uterus during labor. The fetal and placental reserve is enough to see the fetus through these anoxic periods unharmed (Creasy & Resnik 1994).

KEY CONCEPTS

Four factors that continually interact during labor and birth are the birth passage, the fetus, the forces of labor (contractions and pushing effort), and factors associated with the woman's psychosocial status.

Four types of pelves have been identified, and each has a different effect on labor. The diameters of gynecoid and anthropoid pelves are usually large enough for labor and birth to progress normally. In the android and platypelloid types the pelvic diameters are diminished (smaller than in gynecoid and anthropoid), and labor is more likely to be difficult (longer) and may result in a cesarean birth.

Important dimensions of the maternal pelvis include the diameters of the pelvic inlet, pelvic cavity, and pelvic outlet.

The fetal head contains bones in the top portion (cranial vault) that are not fused. This allows them to overlap somewhat in response to the pressures on the fetal head during labor. The pressure and overlapping of the sutures, which are membranous spaces between the cranial bones, result in a change in the shape of the head called molding.

Fetal attitude refers to the relation of the fetal parts to one another. The head is usually held in midline and not to one side or the other, and the extremities are usually flexed and held close to the body because there is little extra room within the uterine cavity.

Fetal lie refers to the relationship of the cephalocaudal (head to sacral area) axis of the fetus to the maternal spine. The fetal lie is either longitudinal (both the maternal and fetal spines are vertical) or transverse (the fetal spine is at a right angle to the maternal spine).

Fetal presentation is determined by the body part lying closest to the inlet of the maternal pelvis. In a longitudinal lie the fetal presentation is usually cephalic (head first) but may also be breech (buttocks or one or both feet first). In a transverse lie the presentation is called transverse, and the fetal shoulder is usually closest to the pelvic inlet.

Fetal position is the relationship of a specified landmark on the presenting fetal part to the sides, front, or back of the maternal pelvis. Once the position is known, the positions of the fetal head and back can be determined.

Engagement of the presenting part has occurred when the largest diameter of the fetal presenting part reaches or passes through the pelvic inlet.

Station refers to the relationship of the presenting part to an imaginary line drawn between the maternal ischial spines, which are in the midpoint of the pelvic cavity. The fetal presenting part enters the pelvic inlet at what is termed about a -5 and descends toward the ischial spines, where it is called a 0 station. Further descent from 0 to +4 occurs as the presenting part descends below the ischial spines toward the vaginal opening.

Each uterine contraction has an increment, acme, and decrement. Contraction frequency is the time from the beginning of one contraction to the beginning of the next contraction.

Duration of contractions refers to the period of time from the beginning to the end of one contraction.

Intensity of contractions refers to the strength of the contraction during acme. Intensity of contractions is termed mild, moderate, or strong.

Labor stresses the coping skills of women. Women with prenatal education about childbirth usually report more positive responses to labor.

Possible causes of labor include oxytocin stimulation, progesterone withdrawal, estrogen stimulation, fetal cortisol, and prostaglandin theory.

Factors that affect the response to labor pain include education, cultural beliefs, fatigue and sleep deprivation, personal significance of pain, previous experience, anxiety, and the availability of coping techniques.

Premonitory signs of labor include lightening, Braxton Hicks contractions, cervical softening and effacement, bloody show, sudden burst of energy, weight loss, and sometimes rupture of membranes.

True labor contractions occur regularly with an increase in frequency, duration, and intensity. The contractions usually start in the back and radiate around the abdomen. The discomfort is not relieved by ambulation. False labor contractions do not produce progressive cervical effacement and dilatation. They are irregular and do not increase in intensity. The discomfort may be relieved by ambulation.

There are four stages of labor and birth. The first stage is from beginning of true labor to complete dilatation of the cervix. The second stage is from complete dilatation of the cervix to birth. The third stage is from birth to expulsion of the placenta. The fourth stage is from expulsion of the placenta to a period of 1 to 4 hours after.

Placental separation is indicated by lengthening of the umbilical cord, a small spurt of blood, change in uterine shape, and a rise of the fundus in the abdomen.

The placenta is expelled by Schultze or Duncan mechanism. This is determined by the way it separates from the uterine wall.

The fetus accommodates to the maternal pelvis in a series of movements called the cardinal movements of labor, which include descent, flexion, internal rotation, extension, external rotation, expulsion, and restitution.

Maternal systemic responses to labor involve the cardiovascular, respiratory, renal, gastrointestinal, and immune systems.

The fetus is usually able to tolerate the labor process with no untoward changes.

REFERENCES

Albright GA et al: *Anesthesia in Obstetrics: Maternal, Fetal and Neonatal Aspects*, 2nd ed. Boston: Butterworths, 1986.

Bates MS: Ethnicity and pain: A biocultural model. *Soc Sci Med* 1987; 24(1):47.

Berry LM: Realistic expectations of the labor coach. *JOGNN* 1988; 18:354.

Blackburn ST, Loper DL: *Maternal, Fetal and Neonatal Physiology*. Philadelphia: WB Saunders, 1992.

Bottoms SF, Scott JR: Transfusion and shock. In: *Danforth's Obstetrics and Gynecology*, 6th ed. Scott JR et al (editors). Philadelphia: Lippincott, 1990.

Broussard P: Antepartum surveillance: What tests to use, how to do the test. *Tenth International Symposium in Perinatal Medicine and Obstetrical Ultrasound. April 9–12, 1990. Las Vegas, NV.*

Challis JRG: Characteristics of parturition. In: *Maternal-Fetal Medicine*, 3rd ed. Creasy RK, Resnik RR (editors). Philadelphia: WB Saunders, 1994.

Creasy RK, Resnik R: *Maternal-Fetal Medicine*, 3rd ed. Philadelphia: WB Saunders, 1994.

Crowe K, Baeyer C. Predictors of a positive childbirth experience. *Birth* June 1989; 16:2.

Cunningham FG, MacDonald PC, Gant NF: *Williams Obstetrics*, 19th ed. Norwalk, CT: Appleton & Lange, 1993.

DiMatteo, Kahn K, Berry SH: Narratives of birth and the postpartum: Analysis of the focus group responses of new mothers. *Birth* December 1993; 20(4):204.

Doering SG et al: Modeling the quality of women's birth experience. *J Health Social Behavior* March 1980; 21:12.

Engel NS: An American experience of pregnancy and childbirth in Japan. *Birth* June 1989; 16:81.

Henderson AD, Brouse AJ: The experience of new fathers during the first three weeks of life. *J Adv Nurs* 1991; 16:293.

Kay MA: *Anthropology of Human Birth*. Philadelphia: Davis, 1982.

Khazoyan CM, Anderson NLR: Latinas' expectations for their partners during childbirth. *MCN* July/Aug 1994; 19(4):226.

Kilpatrick SJ, Laros RK: Characteristics of normal labor. *Obstet Gynecol* 1989; 74:85.

Kuhlmann RS, Cruikshank DP: Maternal trauma during pregnancy. *Clin Obstet Gynecol* June 1994; 37(2):274.

Lederman RP: *Psychosocial Adaptation in Pregnancy: Assessment of Seven Dimensions of Maternal Development*. Englewood Cliffs, NJ: Prentice Hall, 1984.

McCaffery M: *Nursing Management of the Patient with Pain*. Philadelphia: Lippincott, 1972.

McKay S, Smith SY: "What are they talking about? Is something wrong?" Information sharing during the second stage of labor. *Birth* September 1993; 20(3):142.

Mercer RT: Relationship of the birth experience to later mothering behaviors. *J Nurse-Midwifery* 1985; 30:204.

Morrow K: Transcultural midwifery: Adapting to Hmong birthing customs in California. *J Nurse-Midwifery* 1986; 31:285.

Murray M: *Antepartal and Intrapartal Fetal Monitoring*. Washington, DC: NAACOG, 1989.

Nathanielsz PW: A time to be born: Implications of animal studies in maternal-fetal medicine. *Birth* September 1994; 21(3):163.

Nichols FH, Humenick SS: *Childbirth Education: Practice, Research, and Theory*. Philadelphia: WB Saunders, 1988.

Nichols MR: Paternal perspectives of the childbirth experience. *MCN* 1993; 21(3):99.

Robson SC et al: Maternal hemodynamics after normal delivery and delivery complicated by postpartum hemorrhage. *Obstet Gynecol* 1989; 74:234.

Rubin R: *Maternal Identity and the Maternal Experience*. New York: Springer, 1984.

Senden IPM et al: Labor pain: A comparison of parturients in a Dutch and an American teaching hospital. *Obstet Gynecol* April 1988; 71:541.

Ueland K, Ferguson JE: Cardiorespiratory physiology of pregnancy. In: *Gynecology and Obstetrics*, vol. 3. Depp R, Eschenbach DA, Sciarra JJ (editors). Philadelphia: Lippincott, 1990.

Varney H: *Nurse Midwifery*. Boston: Blackwell Scientific Publications, 1987.

Walker LO, Montgomery E: Maternal identity and role attainment: Long-term relations to children's development. *Nurs Res* March/April 1994; 43(2):105.

Weisenberg M, Caspi Z: Cultural and educational influences on pain of childbirth. *J Pain Symptom Mgmt* March 1989; 4:13.

Zlatnik FJ: Normal labor and delivery and its conduct. In: *Danforth's Obstetrics and Gynecology*, 7th ed. Scott JR et al (editors). Philadelphia: Lippincott, 1994.

CHAPTER 22

INTRAPARTAL NURSING ASSESSMENT

*W*e knew that everything was going OK and that I was making progress, but it was so good to have our nurse come check me to see if I was dilating. It was not very comfortable, but he was as gentle as he could be, and when he told me that I had dilated another two centimeters, I felt that I could keep going on. It was nice for us to know that the birth was getting closer with every contraction.

KEY TERMS

Accelerations

Baseline rate

Baseline variability

Decelerations

Fetal scalp blood sample

Intrauterine catheter

Leopold's maneuvers

Long-term variability (LTV)

Percutaneous umbilical blood sampling

Saltatory pattern

Scalp stimulation test

Short-term variability (STV)

Sinusoidal pattern

OBJECTIVES

Summarize intrapartal physical, psychosocial, and cultural assessments necessary for optimum maternal-fetal outcome.

Define and identify the outer limits of normal progress of each of the phases and stages of labor.

Compare the various methods of monitoring fetal heart rate and contractions, giving advantages and disadvantages of each.

Differentiate between baseline and periodic changes in the FHR, and describe the criteria and significance of each.

Outline the steps to be performed in the systematic evaluation of fetal heart rate tracings, and list factors to consider in evaluation of abnormal findings.

Identify nonreassuring fetal heart rate patterns and the interventions that should be carried out in the management of each.

Delineate the indications for fetal blood sampling and guidelines for management of labor for related pH values.

Discuss information to be taught when electronic fetal monitoring is used, and provide rationale for teaching.

Discuss psychologic reactions to electronic fetal monitoring and the role of the nurse.

he physiologic events that occur during labor call for many adaptations by the mother and fetus. Accurate and frequent assessment is crucial because the changes are rapid and involve two individuals, mother and child.

The nurse in the birth setting uses a wide variety of assessment skills to provide care to the mother and her child. The skills of observation, palpation, and auscultation are important as the nurse watches for subtle clues that may indicate a problem is developing. The nurse's presence with the laboring woman provides an opportunity for ongoing assessment, even as the nurse quietly provides comfort measures and assists the woman's coach in offering support.

In current practice the "hands-on" techniques are enhanced by the use of ultrasound and electronic monitoring. These techniques can be used to gather additional data and to validate the hands-on assessments. As with any advanced technological developments, it is tempting to let the machine become an important focus of care. In the birth setting where the contact between the couple and the nurse is so intense, "high-tech" assessments are easily meshed with "high-touch" assessments.

This chapter presents the assessments that are important in the birth setting.

MATERNAL ASSESSMENT

History

The woman's physiologic history may be obtained in an abbreviated format when the woman is admitted to the labor and birth area. Each agency has its own admission form, but similar information is usually obtained. Relevant data include the following:

- Name and age
- Attending physician or certified nurse-midwife (CNM)
- Personal data: blood type; Rh factor; results of serology testing, HIV testing, Rubella titer; prepregnant and present weight; allergies to medications, foods, or substances; and drug and alcohol consumption during pregnancy
- History of previous illness, such as TB, heart disease, diabetes, convulsive disorders, thyroid disorders
- Problems in the prenatal course, for example, elevated blood pressure, bleeding problems, recurrent urinary tract infection

- Pregnancy data: gravida, para, abortions, term and preterm infants, number of living children, neonatal deaths
- The method chosen for infant feeding
- Type of prenatal education (childbirth preparation classes)
- Requests regarding labor and birth (no enema, no analgesic or anesthetic, father and/or other support persons in attendance, and so on)
- History of special tests such as NST or ultrasound and reasons for test administration
- History of any preterm labor requiring tocolytic therapy
- Pediatrician/family practice physician
- Onset of labor
- Amniotic fluid membrane status (intact or spontaneously ruptured)
- Brief description of previous labor and birth

Assessment of psychosocial history is a critical component of intrapartal nursing assessment. The nurse begins the assessment when the woman is admitted into the birthing area by obtaining information such as the following:

- What is her marital status? Who are her support people?
- Is she safe in her relationship with the baby's father? Has there been any physical or emotional abuse prior to or during the pregnancy? If so, what interventions were made? In questioning the woman about safety and abuse issues it is important for the nurse to be aware that abuse affects one in six adult women and one in five teenagers during pregnancy (McFarland & Parker 1994). It is important to ensure that the woman is alone when the questions are asked so that she can answer freely. If she indicates there has been a problem, the questions from the Abuse Assessment Screen by McFarland and Parker (1994, p 322) could be used. The questions include:

1. Have you ever been emotionally or physically abused by your partner or someone important to you?
2. Within the last year, have you been hit, slapped, kicked, or otherwise physically hurt by someone? If yes, by whom? Total number of times?
3. Since you've been pregnant, were you hit, slapped, kicked, or otherwise physicaly hurt by someone? If yes, by whom? Total number of times?

4. Within the last year has anyone forced you to have sexual activities? If yes, who? Total number of times?
5. Are you afraid of your partner or anyone you listed above?

- Has she had difficulty or problems with previous pregnancies, labors, or births that would increase her anxiety now?
- Have emotional problems been present during the past few months? What interventions have occurred?

With the prevalence of sexual violence against women in our society (reported incidence is one in three women, regardless of age) the nurse needs to consider that the woman may have experienced sexual violence at some point in her life. In this case she may be anxious about the labor process, or anxiety may arise during labor. Because psychosocial factors may be complex, the woman's history may not be apparent until later in the labor and birth. The nurse must be aware of the following aspects of psychosocial history:

- Has the woman experienced rape or sexual abuse?
- Is there evidence of support between the woman and her partner?
- Is the partner controlling? Does the partner make decisions unilaterally?

It is important for the nurse to obtain the history in a setting that promotes trust and the establishment of a relationship. Some of the questions are straightforward, but others require care and privacy to assure that the woman has a safe environment in which to address them.

I will never forget the 16-year-old single mom who came into the birthing unit. She came in because it was her due date and she thought her labor had started. As I began to work with her, it was difficult to establish rapport. With each question and each action on my part, she seemed to become more uncomfortable. Even my suggestion of placing my hand on her abdomen to palpate contractions became frightening to her. We seemed to be dealing with something far beyond the anxiety that some young women have. She recoiled from me at the mention of any physical assessments.

It took every skill that I had to quietly stay with her, to establish a relationship, and to begin to gain her trust. She was finally able to tell me that the pregnancy was the result of a rape and that there had been continued sexual violence against her throughout the pregnancy. The labor and birth were so very difficult for both of us, each in our own way. She held onto my hand and pleaded with me not to leave her, and together we got through it.

As nurses, if we think of sexual abuse at all, it seems that it is about someone else—a person we read about in the newspaper or in another neighborhood. But we also need to realize that it

RESEARCH IN PRACTICE

The aftermath of childhood sexual abuse can manifest as problems with sexual identity, symptoms of posttraumatic stress disorder, and many other concerns. The experience of labor may force the woman to relive the abusive episode(s). Naomi Rhodes and Sally Hutchinson explored and described the labor experiences of childhood sexual abuse survivors using an ethnographic method. Care givers may recognize cues during labor that indicate prior abuse even if the client has repressed or not chosen to share the abusive incident. The study incorporated data from interviews of 7 mothers who were incest survivors, as well as 5 nurse midwives and 3 labor and delivery nurses who had observed the effects of sexual abuse on labor. Field notes collected over 6 years by Naomi Rhodes also served as participant observation data.

Findings resulting from ethnographic data analysis included four themes: forgetting and remembering, forced remembering, labor styles of sexually abused women, and connecting labor and sexual abuse. *Forgetting and remembering* encompasses repressing the memory of the abuse. This may be a psychologically protective mechanism, but it may also create difficulties during labor. For example, some women exhibit terror or panic during labor but cannot remember the abuse. *Forced remembering* occurs when labor triggers a reexperience of the abuse through body memory. *Labor styles of sexually abused women* include fighting, taking control, surrendering, and retreating. Fighting may manifest as a panic response, misdirection of pushing energy, or outbursts of irritability and anger. Taking control can be demonstrated by well prepared and organized behavior, or may appear desperate. Hypervigilance may occur as a form of taking control for the laboring woman. Surrendering may involve a sense of anything being allowed. In these cases women do not express vulnerability and, in fact, have probably dissociated themselves from the abuse and the labor. Retreating occurs when the woman removes herself emotionally from the labor situation. She may not react to contractions or interact with care givers, or she may have a flat affect. *Connecting labor and sexual abuse* can occur in an extreme form in which the laboring woman relives the abusive episode.

Clinical Application of Study

As the authors note, all nurses in labor and delivery need to be alert for the cues of past abuse in the laboring woman. If signs are observed, the nurse must avoid triggering traumatic memories and keep the woman focused on the birth. Any nurse who has contact with a pregnant abuse victim should help the woman and her partner prepare for the experience of labor by explaining common concerns such as potential control issues and how to cope with them.

SOURCE: Rhodes N, Hutchinson S: Labor experiences of childhood sexual abuse survivors. *Birth* 1994; 21(4): 213.

is us. I teach maternal-child nursing, and each fall as I pre-pare myself to go back into the birthing area with students, I seem to have to deal again with memories of my own past. There are so many aspects of labor and birthing that are triggers for memories, and I continue to work on dealing with the impact of the memories. In many ways I am lucky because my experience helps keep me in touch with the difficulty that some of the students may have in this area of nursing. It is something that we all work on, one day at a time.

Intrapartal High-Risk Screening

Screening for intrapartal high-risk factors is an integral part of assessing the normal laboring woman. As the history is obtained, the nurse notes the presence of any factors that may be associated with a high-risk condition. For example, the woman who reports a physical symptom such as intermittent bleeding needs further assessment to rule out abruptio placentae or placenta previa before the admission process continues. In addition to identifying the presence of a high-risk condition the nurse must recognize the implications of the condition for the laboring woman and her fetus. For example, in the case of an abnormal fetal presentation, the nurse understands that the labor may be prolonged, prolapse of the umbilical cord may be more likely, and the possibility of a cesarean birth is increased.

Although physical conditions are frequently listed as the major factors that increase risk in the intrapartal period, sociocultural variables such as poverty, nutrition, the amount of prenatal care, cultural beliefs regarding pregnancy, and communication patterns may also precipitate a high-risk situation in the intrapartal period. The nurse can begin gathering data regarding sociocultural factors as the woman enters the birthing area. The nurse observes the communication pattern between the woman and her support person(s) and their responses to admission questions and initial teaching. If the woman and her support person(s) do not speak English and translators are not available within the birthing room staff, the course of labor and the nurse's ability to interact and provide support and education are affected. The ability of the couple to make informed decisions is severely affected; therefore information in their primary language needs to be provided. Communication may also be affected by cultural practices such as beliefs regarding when to speak, who should ask questions, or whether it is acceptable to let others know if discomfort is occurring. The prenatal record may be quickly reviewed for number of prenatal visits, weight gain during pregnancy, progression of fundal height, assistance such as Medicaid and Women, Infants, and Children (WIC), and exposure to environmental agents.

A partial list of intrapartal risk factors is presented in Table 22–1. The factors precede the Intrapartal Assessment Guide because they must be kept in mind during the assessment.

Intrapartal Physical and Psychosociocultural Assessment

A physical examination is part of the admission procedure and part of the ongoing care of the client. Although the intrapartal physical assessment is not as complete and thorough as the initial prenatal physical examination (Chapter 14), it does involve assessment of some body systems and the actual labor process. The Intrapartal Assessment Guide, on pages 596–601, provides a framework the maternity nurse can use when examining the laboring woman.

The physical assessment portion includes assessments performed immediately on admission as well as ongoing assessments. When labor is progressing very quickly, the nurse may not have time for a complete assessment. In this case the critical physical assessments include maternal vital signs, labor status, fetal status, sterile vaginal examination, and laboratory findings (Procedure 22–1: Intrapartal Vaginal Examination on page 602).

The second section of the Intrapartal Assessment Guide addresses psychosocial aspects. The laboring woman's psychosocial status is an important part of the total assessment. The woman has previous ideas, knowledge, and fears about childbearing. By assessing her psychosocial status the nurse can meet the woman's needs for information and support. The nurse can then support the woman and her partner; in the absence of a partner the nurse may become the support person.

Individualized nursing care can best be planned and implemented when the values and beliefs of the laboring woman are known and honored. Frequently, however, the nurse feels uncertain about knowing what to ask or what to consider, perhaps because there has not been a personal opportunity to become aware of varying cultural values and beliefs. The cultural assessment portion of the Intrapartal Assessment Guide provides a place to start.

While performing the intrapartal assessment, the nurse must follow CDC guidelines to prevent exposure to body substances. The nurse can provide information in a factual manner regarding the precautions. A statement such as the following is helpful: "I will be wearing gloves when I change the Chux on which you are lying. This is to protect my hands from the discharge you are having and to protect you from any organisms that I may have on my hands." Sharing information with the laboring woman and her support person(s) will promote a supportive, caring environment. See Essential Precautions in Practice: During Intrapartal Assessment, on page 604, for further information.

Text continues on page 605

TABLE 22-1   Intrapartal High-Risk Factors

Factor	Maternal Implication	Fetal-Neonatal Implication
Abnormal presentation	↑ Incidence of cesarean birth ↑ Incidence of prolonged labor ↑ Hypertension risk ↑ Nausea and vomiting	↑ Incidence of placenta previa Prematurity ↑ Risk of congenital abnormality Neonatal physical trauma ↑ Risk of intrauterine growth retardation
Multiple gestation	↑ Uterine distension → ↑ risk of postpartum hemorrhage ↑ Risk of cesarean birth ↑ Risk of preterm labor	Low birth weight Prematurity ↑ Risk of congenital anomalies Feto-fetal transfusion
Hydramnios	↑ Discomfort ↑ Dyspnea ↑ Risk of preterm labor Edema of lower extremities	↑ Risk of esophageal or other high alimentary tract atresias ↑ Risk of CNS anomalies (myelocele)
Oligohydramnios	Maternal fear of "dry birth"	↑ Incidence of congenital anomalies ↑ Incidence of renal lesions ↑ Risk of IUGR ↑ Risk of fetal acidosis ↑ Risk of cord compression Postmaturity
Meconium staining of amniotic fluid	↑ Psychologic stress due to fear for baby	↑ Risk of fetal asphyxia ↑ Risk of meconium aspiration ↑ Risk of pneumonia due to aspiration of meconium
Premature rupture of membranes	↑ Risk of infection (chorioamnionitis) ↑ Risk of preterm labor ↑ Anxiety Fear for the baby Prolonged hospitalization ↑ Incidence of tocolytic therapy	↑ Perinatal morbidity Prematurity ↓ Birth weight ↑ Risk of respiratory distress syndrome Prolonged hospitalization
Induction of labor	↑ Risk of hypercontractility of uterus ↑ Risk of uterine rupture ↑ Length of labor if cervix not ready ↑ Anxiety	Prematurity if gestational age not assessed correctly Hypoxia if hyperstimulation occurs
Abruptio placentae-placenta previa	Hemorrhage Uterine atony	Fetal hypoxia/acidosis Fetal exsanguination ↑ Perinatal mortality
Failure to progress in labor	Maternal exhaustion ↑ Incidence of augmentation of labor ↑ Incidence of cesarean birth	Fetal hypoxia/acidosis Intracranial birth injury
Precipitous labor (< 3 hours)	Perineal, vaginal, cervical lacerations ↑ Risk of PP hemorrhage	Tentorial tears
Prolapse of umbilical cord	↑ Fear for baby Cesarean birth	Acute fetal hypoxia/acidosis
Fetal heart aberrations	↑ Fear for baby ↑ Risk of cesarean birth, forceps, vacuum Continuous electronic monitoring and intervention in labor	Tachycardia, chronic asphyxic insult, bradycardia, acute asphyxic insult Chronic hypoxia Congenital heart block
Uterine rupture	Hemorrhage Cesarean birth for hysterectomy ↑ Risk of death	Fetal anoxia Fetal hemorrhage ↑ Neonatal morbidity and mortality
Postdates (> 42 weeks)	↑ Anxiety ↑ Incidence of induction of labor ↑ Incidence of cesarean birth ↑ Use of technology to monitor fetus ↑ Risk of shoulder dystocia	Postmaturity syndrome ↑ Risk of fetal-neonatal mortality and morbidity ↑ Risk of antepartum fetal death ↑ Incidence/risk of large baby
Diabetes	↑ Risk of hydramnios ↑ Risk of hypoglycemia or hyperglycemia ↑ Risk of pregnancy-induced hypertension	↑ Risk of malpresentation ↑ Risk of macrosomia ↑ Risk of intrauterine growth retardation ↑ Risk of respiratory distress syndrome ↑ Risk of congenital anomalies
Pregnancy-induced hypertension	↑ Risk of seizures ↑ Risk of stroke ↑ Risk of HELLP	↑ Risk of small for gestational age baby ↑ Risk of preterm birth ↑ Risk of mortality
AIDS/STD	↑ Risk of additional infections	↑ Risk of transplacental transmission

FIRST STAGE OF LABOR

Physical Assessment/ Normal Findings	Alterations and Possible Causes*	Nursing Responses to Data†
Vital Signs		
Blood pressure (BP): < 130 systolic and < 85 diastolic in adult 18 years of age or older or no more than 15–20 mm Hg rise in systolic pressure over baseline BP during early pregnancy (Johannsen 1993)	High blood pressure (essential hypertension, preeclampsia, renal disease, apprehension or anxiety) Low blood pressure (supine hypotension)	Evaluate history of preexisting disorders and check for presence of other signs of preeclampsia. Do not assess during contractions; implement measures to decrease anxiety and then reassess. Turn woman on her side and recheck blood pressure. Provide quiet environment. Have O_2 available.
Pulse: 60–90 bpm	Increased pulse rate (excitement or anxiety, cardiac disorders, early shock)	Evaluate cause, reassess to see if rate continues; report to physician.
Respirations: 14–22/minute (or pulse rate divided by 4)	Marked tachypnea (respiratory disease), hyperventilation in transition phase	Assess between contractions; if marked tachypnea continues, assess for signs of respiratory disease.
	Hyperventilation (anxiety)	Encourage slow breaths if woman is hyperventilating.
Temperature: 36.2–37.6 C (98–99.6 F)	Elevated temperature (infection, dehydration)	Assess for other signs of infection or dehydration.
Weight		
15–30 lb greater than prepregnant weight	Weight gain > 30 lb (fluid retention, obesity, large infant, diabetes mellitus, PIH), weight gain < 15 lb (SGA)	Assess for signs of edema. Evaluate pattern from prenatal record.
Lungs		
Normal breath sounds, clear and equal	Rales, rhonchi, friction rub (infection), pulmonary edema, asthma	Reassess; refer to physician.
Fundus		
At 40 weeks' gestation located just below xyphoid process	Uterine size not compatible with estimated date of birth (SGA, large for gestational age [LGA], hydramnios, multiple pregnancy)	Reevaluate history regarding pregnancy dating. Refer to physician for additional assessment.
Edema		
Slight amount of dependent edema	Pitting edema of face, hands, legs, abdomen, sacral area (preeclampsia)	Check deep tendon reflexes for hyperactivity; check for clonus; refer to physician.
Hydration		
Normal skin turgor, elastic	Poor skin turgor (dehydration)	Assess skin turgor; refer to physician for deviations.

*Possible causes of alterations are placed in parentheses.

†This column provides guidelines for further assessment and initial nursing interventions.

FIRST STAGE OF LABOR *continued*

Physical Assessment/ Normal Findings	Alterations and Possible Causes*	Nursing Responses to Data†
Perineum		
Tissues smooth, pink color (see Prenatal Initial Physical Assessment Guide, Chapter 14)	Varicose veins of vulva, Herpes lesions	Exercise care while doing a perineal prep; note on client record need for follow-up in postpartal period; reassess after birth; refer to physician.
Clear mucus, may be blood tinged, earthy or human odor	Profuse, purulent, foul-smelling drainage	Suspected gonorrhea; report to physician; initiate care to newborn's eyes; notify neonatal nursing staff and pediatrician.
Presence of small amount of bloody show that gradually increases with further cervical dilatation	Hemorrhage	Assess BP and pulse, pallor, diaphoresis; report any marked changes. (Note: Gaping of vagina or anus and bulging of perineum are suggestive signs of second stage of labor.) Universal precautions.
Labor Status		
Uterine contractions: regular pattern	Failure to establish a regular pattern, prolonged latent phase Hypertonicity Hypotonicity	Evaluate whether woman is in true labor; ambulate if in early labor. Evaluate client status and contractile pattern. Obtain a 20-minute EFM monitor strip. Notify physician/CNM.
Cervical dilatation: progressive cervical dilatation from size of fingertip to 10 cm (Procedure 22–1)	Rigidity of cervix (frequent cervical infections, scar tissue, failure of presenting part to descend)	Evaluate contractions, fetal engagement, position, and cervical dilatation. Inform client of progress.
Cervical effacement: progressive thinning of cervix (Procedure 22–1)	Failure to efface (rigidity of cervix, failure of presenting part to engage); cervical edema (pushing effort by woman before cervix is fully dilated and effaced, trapped cervix)	Evaluate contractions, fetal engagement, and position. Notify physician/certified nurse-midwife if cervix is becoming edematous; work with woman to prevent pushing until cervix is completely dilated. Keep vaginal exams to a minimum.
Fetal descent: progressive descent of fetal presenting part from station −5 to +4 (Figure 22–3 in Procedure 22–1)	Failure of descent (abnormal fetal position or presentation, macrosomic fetus, inadequate pelvic measurement)	Evaluate fetal position, presentation, and size. Evaluate maternal pelvic measurements.
Membranes: may rupture before or during labor	Rupture of membranes more than 12–24 hours before initiation of labor	Assess for ruptured membranes using Nitrazine test tape before doing vaginal exam. Follow BSI precautions. Instruct woman with ruptured membranes to remain on bed rest if presenting part is not engaged and firmly down against the cervix. Keep vaginal exams to a minimum to prevent infection. When membranes rupture in the birth setting, **the nurse immediately assesses FHR** to detect changes associated with prolapse of umbilical cord (FHR slows).

*Possible causes of alterations are placed in parentheses.

†This column provides guidelines for further assessment and initial nursing interventions.

FIRST STAGE OF LABOR continued

Physical Assessment/ Normal Findings	Alterations and Possible Causes*	Nursing Responses to Data†
Labor Status continued		

Findings on Nitrazine test tape: Membranes probably intact
  yellow   pH 5.0
  olive   pH 5.5
  olive green   pH 6.0
 	
Membranes probably ruptured
  blue-green   pH 6.5
  blue-gray   pH 7.0
  deep blue   pH 7.5
	False-positive results may be obtained if large amount of bloody show is present, previous vaginal examination has been done using lubricant, or tape is touched by nurse's fingers.	Assess fluid for consistency, amount, odor; assess FHR frequently. Assess fluid at regular intervals for presence of meconium staining. Follow BSI precautions while assessing amniotic fluid.
		
		Teach woman that amniotic fluid is continually produced (to allay fear of "dry birth"). Teach woman that she may feel amniotic fluid trickle or gush with contractions. Change Chux pads often.

Amniotic fluid clear, with earthy/human odor, no foul-smelling odor	Greenish amniotic fluid (fetal stress)	Assess FHR; do vaginal exam to evaluate for prolapsed cord; apply fetal monitor for continuous data; report to physician.
	Strong odor (amnionitis)	Take woman's temperature and report to physician.
Fetal Status		
FHR: 120–160 bpm	<120 or >160 bpm (fetal stress); abnormal patterns on fetal monitor: decreased variability, late decelerations, variable decelerations	Initiate interventions based on particular FHR pattern.
Presentation: Cephalic, 97% Breech, 3%	Face, brow, or shoulder presentation	Report to physician; after presentation is confirmed as face, brow, or shoulder, woman may be prepared for cesarean birth.
Position: LOA most common	Persistent occipital-posterior (OP) position; transverse arrest	Carefully monitor maternal and fetal status.
Activity: fetal movement	Hyperactivity (may precede fetal hypoxia)	Carefully evaluate FHR; may apply fetal monitor.
	Complete lack of movement (fetal distress or fetal demise)	Carefully evaluate FHR; may apply fetal monitor. Report to physician/CNM.
Laboratory Evaluation		
Hematologic tests Hemoglobin: 12–16 g/dL	<12 g/dL (anemia, hemorrhage)	Evaluate woman for problems due to decreased oxygen-carrying capacity caused by lowered hemoglobin.

CBC
  Hematocrit: 38%–47%
  RBC: 4.2–5.4 million/μL
  WBC: 4500–11,000/μL, although leukocytosis to 20,000/μL is not unusual
  Platelets 150,000–400,000/mm³
	Presence of infection or blood dyscrasias, loss of blood (hemorrhage, DIC)	Evaluate for other signs of infection or for petechia, bruising, or unusual bleeding.

*Possible causes of alterations are placed in parentheses.

†This column provides guidelines for further assessment and initial nursing interventions.

FIRST STAGE OF LABOR *continued*

Physical Assessment/ Normal Findings	Alterations and Possible Causes*	Nursing Responses to Data†
Laboratory Evaluation *continued*		
Serologic testing STS or VDRL test: nonreactive.	Positive reaction (Chapter 14, Initial Prenatal Physical Assessment Guide)	For reactive test notify newborn nursery and pediatrician.
Rh	Rh positive fetus in Rh negative woman	Assess prenatal record for titer levels during pregnancy. Obtain cord blood for direct Coombs' at birth.
Urinalysis		Assess blood glucose; test urine for ketones; ketonuria and glycosuria require further assessment of blood sugars.‡
Glucose: negative	Glycosuria (low renal threshold for glucose, diabetes mellitus)	
Ketones: negative	Ketonuria (starvation ketosis)	
Proteins: negative	Proteinuria (urine specimen contaminated with vaginal secretions, fever, kidney disease); proteinuria of 2+ or greater found in uncontaminated urine may be a sign of ensuing preeclampsia	Instruct woman in collection technique; incidence of contamination from vaginal discharge is common.
Red blood cells: negative	Blood in urine (calculi, cystitis, glomerulonephritis, neoplasm)	Assess collection technique (may be bloody show).
White blood cells: negative	Presence of white blood cells (infection in genitourinary tract)	Assess for signs of urinary tract infection.
Casts: none	Presence of casts (nephrotic syndrome)	

Cultural Assessment§	Variations to Consider	Nursing Responses to Data†
Cultural influences determine customs and practices regarding intrapartal care.	Individual preferences may vary.	
Ask the following questions: Who would you like to remain with you during your labor and birth?	She may prefer only her coach to remain or may also want family and/or friends.	Provide support for her wishes by encouraging desired people to stay. Provide information to others (with the woman's permission) who are not in the room.
What would you like to wear during labor?	She may be more comfortable in her own clothes.	Offer supportive materials such as Chux if needed to protect her own clothing. Avoid subtle signals to the woman that she should not have chosen to remain in her own clothes. Have other clothing available if the woman desires. If her clothing becomes contaminated, it will be simple to place it in a plastic bag. The nurse can soak soiled clothing in cool water. The nurse needs to remember to wear disposable gloves and a plastic apron if splashing is anticipated.

*Possible causes of alterations are placed in parentheses.

†This column provides guidelines for further assessment and initial nursing interventions.

‡Glycosuria should not be discounted. The presence of glycosuria necessitates follow-up.

§These are only a few suggestions. We do not mean to imply that this is a comprehensive cultural assessment; rather, it is a tool to encourage cultural sensitivity.

FIRST STAGE OF LABOR continued

Cultural Assessment[§]	Variations to Consider	Nursing Responses to Data[†]
What activity would you like during labor?	She may want to ambulate most of the time, stand in the shower, sit in the jacuzzi, sit in a chair or on a stool, remain on the bed, and so forth.	Support the woman's wishes by providing encouragement and completing assessments in a manner so that the woman's activity and positional wishes are disturbed as little as possible.
What position would you like for the birth?	She may feel more comfortable in lithotomy with stirrups and her upper body elevated, or side-lying, or sitting in birthing bed.	Collect any supplies and equipment needed to support her in her chosen birthing position. Provide information to the coach regarding any changes that may be needed based on the chosen position.
Is there anything special you would like?	She may want the room darkened or to have curtains and windows open, music playing, a Leboyer birth, her coach to cut the umbilical cord, to save a portion of the umbilical cord, to save the placenta, to videotape the birth, and so forth.	Support requests, and communicate requests to any other nursing or medical personnel (so requests can continue to be supported and not questioned). If another nurse or physician does not honor the request, act as advocate for the woman by continuing to support her unless her desire is truly unsafe.
Ask the woman if she would like fluids, and ask what temperature she prefers.	She may prefer clear fluids other than water (tea, clear juice). She may prefer iced, room-temperature, or warmed fluids.	Provide fluids as desired.
Observe the woman's response when privacy is difficult to maintain and her body is exposed.	Some women do not seem to mind being exposed during an exam or procedure; others feel acute discomfort.	Maintain privacy and respect the woman's sense of privacy. If the woman is unable to provide specific information, the nurse may draw from general information regarding cultural variation: Southeast Asian women may not want any family member in the room during exam or procedures. Her partner may not be involved with coaching activities during labor or birth. Saudi woman may need to remain covered during the labor and birth and avoid exposure of any body part. The husband may need to be in the room but remain behind a curtain or screen so he does not view his wife at this time.
If the woman is to breastfeed, ask if she would like to feed her baby immediately after birth.	She may want to feed her baby right away or may want to wait a little while.	

Psychosocial Assessment	Variations to Consider	Nursing Responses to Data[†]
Preparation for Childbirth		
Woman has some information regarding process of normal labor and birth.	Some women do not have any information regarding childbirth.	Add to present information base.

[†]This column provides guidelines for further assessment and initial nursing interventions.

[§]These are only a few suggestions. We do not mean to imply that this is a comprehensive cultural assessment; rather, it is a tool to encourage cultural sensitivity.

FIRST STAGE OF LABOR continued

Psychosocial Assessment	Variations to Consider	Nursing Responses to Data[†]
Preparation for Childbirth *continued*		
Woman has breathing and/or relaxation techniques to use during labor.	Some women do not have any method of relaxation or breathing to use, and some do not desire them.	Support breathing and relaxation techniques that client is using; provide information if needed.
Response to Labor		
Latent phase: relaxed, excited, anxious for labor to be well established	May feel unable to cope with contractions because of fear, anxiety, or lack of information	Provide support and encouragement; establish trusting relationship.
Active phase: becomes more intense, begins to tire	May remain quiet and without any sign of discomfort or anxiety, may insist that she is unable to continue with the birthing process	Provide support and coaching if needed.
Transitional phase: feels tired, may feel unable to cope, needs frequent coaching to maintain breathing patterns		
Coping mechanisms: Ability to cope with labor through utilization of support system, breathing, relaxation techniques	May feel marked anxiety and apprehension, may not have coping mechanisms that can be brought into this experience, or may be unable to use them at this time	Support coping mechanisms if they are working for the woman; provide information and support if woman is exhibiting anxiety or needs additional alternative to present coping methods. Encourage participation of coach/significant other.
Anxiety		
Some anxiety and apprehension is within normal limits	May show anxiety through rapid breathing, nervous tremors, frowning, grimacing, clenching of teeth, thrashing movements, crying, increased pulse and blood pressure	Provide support, encouragement, and information. Teach relaxation techniques; support controlled breathing efforts. May need to provide a paper bag to breathe into if woman says her lips are tingling. Note FHR.
Sounds During Labor		
	Some women are very quiet and others moan or make a variety of noises.	Provide a supportive environment. Encourage woman to do what is right for her.
Support System		
Physical intimacy of mother-father (or mother-support relationship): caretaking activities such as soothing conversation, touching	Some women would prefer no contact, others may show clinging behaviors.	Encourage caretaking activities that appear to comfort the woman; encourage support to the woman; if support is limited, the nurse may take a more active role.
Support person stays in close proximity	Limited interaction may come from a desire for quiet.	Encourage support person to stay close (if this seems appropriate).
Relationship of mother-father (or support person): involved interaction	The support person may seem to be detached and maintain little support, attention, or conversation.	Support interactions; if interaction is limited, the nurse may provide more information and support. Assure that coach/significant other has short breaks, especially prior to transition.

[†]This column provides guidelines for further assessments and initial nursing interventions.

Nursing Action	Rationale
Objective: Set the stage for the exam.	
Explain the procedure, indications for the exam, what the exam may feel like, that it may cause discomfort or pain, and information that may be obtained.	*Explanation of exam can decrease the implied authority of the caregiver, decrease anxiety, and increase relaxation.*
Objective: Assemble and prepare supplies.	
Have the following equipment easily accessible:	*Examination is facilitated and can be done quickly.*
• Sterile disposable gloves	
• Lubricant	
• Nitrazine test tape	
Objective: Position the woman.	
Position the woman with thighs flexed and abducted; instruct her to put the heels of her feet together.	*Prevent contamination of area during examination and allow for visualization of external signs of labor progress.*
Drape her so that only the perineum is exposed.	*Provide as much privacy as possible.*
Encourage her to relax her muscles and legs during the procedure.	
Objective: Use aseptic technique during the exam.	
Inform the woman prior to touching her. Use gentleness.	*Communicate regard for the woman.*
If leakage of fluid has been noted or if woman reports leakage of fluid, use Nitrazine test tape before doing vaginal exam.	*Nitrazine test tape registers a change in pH if amniotic fluid is present (unless a lubricant has already been used).*
Put on both gloves; using thumb and forefinger of the nondominant hand, spread labia widely, insert well-lubricated second and index fingers of the dominant hand into vagina until they touch the cervix.	*Avoid contaminating hand by contact with the anus; positioning of hand with wrist straight and elbow tilted downward allows fingertips to point toward umbilicus and find cervix.*
If woman verbalizes discomfort, acknowledge it and apologize.	*Maintain "realness" of the situation and decrease passive role of the woman.*
Objective: Determine status of fetal membranes.	
Palpate for movable bulging sac through the cervix; observe for expression of amniotic fluid during exam.	*If intact, bag of waters feels like a bulge.*
Objective: Determine status of labor progress during and after contractions.	
Carry out the vaginal examination during and between contractions.	*Examination varies.*
Objective: Identify degree of cervical dilatation.	
Palpate for opening or what appears as a depression in the cervix (Figure 22–1).	*Estimation of the diameter of the depression identifies degree of dilatation.*

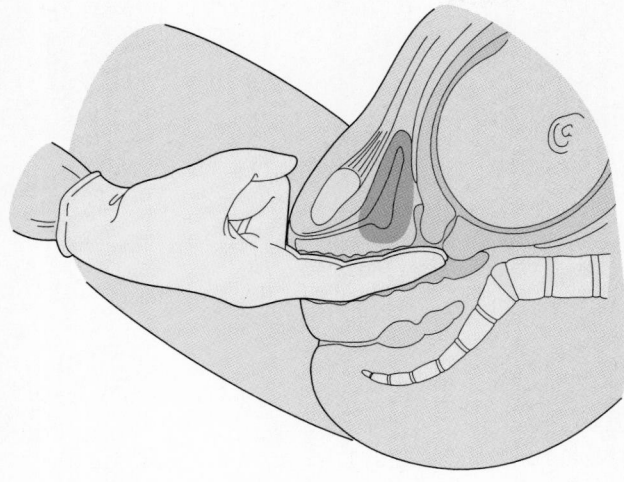

FIGURE 22-1   To gauge cervical dilatation, the nurse places the index and middle fingers against the cervix and determines the size of the opening. Before labor begins the cervix is long (approximately 2.5 cm), the sides feel thick, and the cervical canal is closed, so an examining finger cannot be inserted. During labor the cervix begins to dilate, and the size of the opening progresses from 1 cm to 10 cm in diameter.

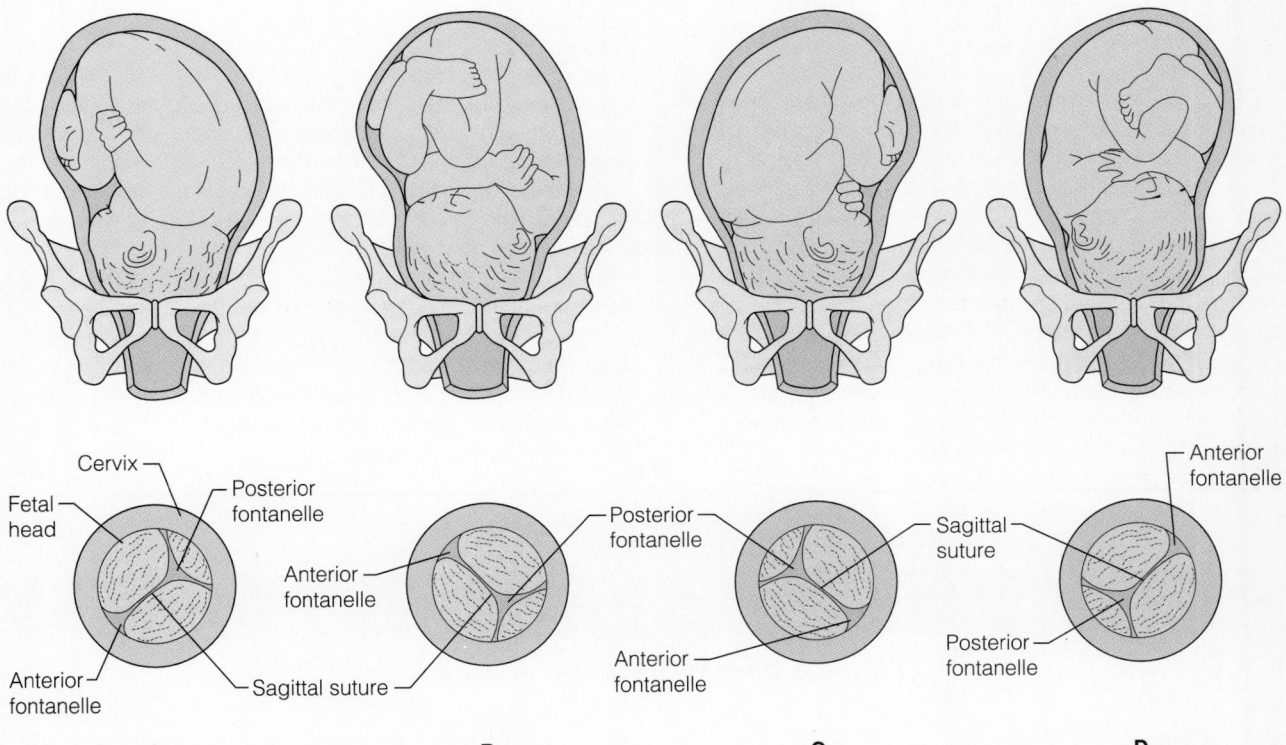

A   B   C   D

FIGURE 22-2   Palpation of the presenting part (portion of the fetus that enters the pelvis first). *A* Left occiput anterior (LOA). The occiput (area over the occipital bone on the posterior part of the fetal head) is in the left anterior quadrant of the woman's pelvis. When the fetus is in LOA, the posterior fontanelle (located just above the occipital bone and triangular in shape) is in the upper left quadrant of the maternal pelvis. *B* Left occiput posterior (LOP). The posterior fontanelle is in the lower left quadrant of the maternal pelvis. *C* Right occiput anterior (ROA). The posterior fontanelle is in the upper right quadrant of the maternal pelvis. *D* Right occiput posterior (ROP). The posterior fontanelle is in the lower right quadrant of the maternal pelvis. Note: The anterior fontanelle is diamond shaped. Because of the roundness of the fetal head, only a portion of the anterior fontanelle can be seen in each of the views, so it appears to be triangular in shape.

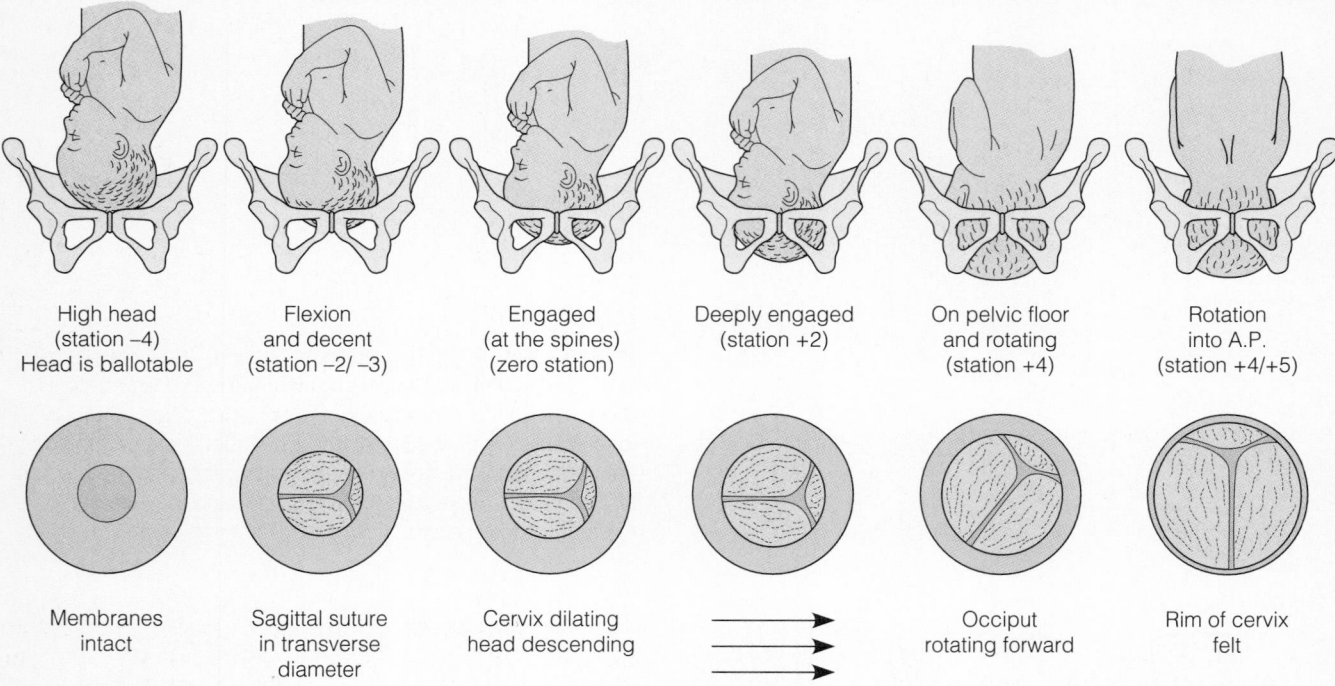

High head (station −4) Head is ballotable	Flexion and decent (station −2/ −3)	Engaged (at the spines) (zero station)	Deeply engaged (station +2)	On pelvic floor and rotating (station +4)	Rotation into A.P. (station +4/+5)
Membranes intact	Sagittal suture in transverse diameter	Cervix dilating head descending		Occiput rotating forward	Rim of cervix felt

FIGURE 22-3   Descent of the fetus through the maternal pelvis can be assessed by determining station (the relationship of the presenting part to an imaginary line between the maternal ischial spines). As the fetus moves downward, cardinal movements occur (See Chapter 21). The nurse assesses the station and can identify the cardinal movements by determining the position of the posterior fontanelle. The upper panels depict the fetal head progressing downward through the pelvis. From left to right the first four views depict descent and flexion of the fetal chin onto the fetal chest. In the last two views internal rotation is occurring. Each view also depicts downward movement of the fetal head through the maternal pelvis as measured by the change in station.

The lower panels of the illustration depict the cervix, which is still rather thick (little effacement has occurred). The amniotic membranes are still intact over the fetal head. When the fetus is at −4 station, the fetal head is ballotable (when it is touched by the examining nurse's finger, the head floats upward and then resettles downward). In the second view note the thinner cervix (which indicates more effacement has occurred). The sagittal suture and posterior fontanelle can be palpated. The next two views depict further effacement and descent of the fetal head from 0 station to +2. The last two views depict continuing effacement and the position that would be felt on vaginal exam of the presenting part while the fetal head is completing internal rotation.

ESSENTIAL PRECAUTIONS IN PRACTICE

DURING INTRAPARTAL ASSESSMENT

Examples of times when disposable gloves should be worn include:

- Assisting the woman as she removes any garments moist with bloody show and/or amniotic fluid

- Handling Chux and bedding that are moist with bloody show and/or amniotic fluid

- Checking amniotic fluid–soaked materials with Nitrazine test tape

- Placing the elastic straps for the electronic monitor around a woman who has been lying in bedding moist with bloody show and/or amniotic fluid

- Assisting with fetal blood sampling and handling the lab tubes

Sterile gloves are worn when the nurse does a sterile vaginal exam and when fetal scalp electrodes are placed. The sterile gloves are used to maintain sterile asepsis. They protect the nurse from exposure to vaginal secretions, bloody show, and amniotic fluid.

REMEMBER to wash your hands prior to pulling the disposable gloves on and AGAIN immediately after you remove the gloves.

For further information consult OSHA and CDC guidelines.

Methods of Evaluating Labor Progress

Contraction Assessment

Uterine contractions may be assessed by palpation and continuous electronic monitoring.

Palpation Contractions are assessed for frequency, regularity, duration, and intensity by placing one hand on the uterine fundus. To determine duration of the contraction (the length of a particular contraction), the time is noted when hardening of the fundus is first felt (beginning of the contraction) and relaxation occurs (end of the contraction). During the acme (peak) of the contraction, intensity can be evaluated by estimating the indentability of the fundus. At least three successive contractions should be assessed to provide enough data to determine the contraction pattern. Because frequency is determined by noting the time from the beginning of one contraction to the beginning of the next, if contractions began at 0700, 0704, and 0708, the frequency would be every 4 minutes.

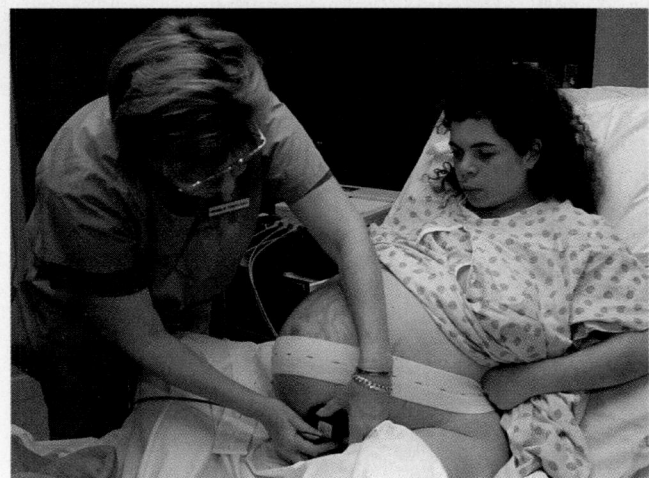

FIGURE 22-4 Woman in labor with external monitor applied. The toco placed on the uterine fundus is recording uterine contractions. The lower belt holds the ultrasonic device that monitors the fetal heart rate. The belts can be adjusted for comfort.

Electronic Monitoring with External Tocodynamometer Electronic monitoring of the uterine contractions provides continuous data. In many facilities it may be routinely done for all high-risk women and all women who are having oxytocin-induced labor. An indirect method of monitoring uterine activity is by use of the tocodynamometer (or "toco"), which contains a flexible disk that responds to pressure. This disk is placed against the fundus of the uterus (the area of greatest contractility) and is held in place by an elastic belt. As the uterus contracts pressure is exerted against the toco, transmitted to the monitor, and recorded on graph paper (Figure 22–4 and also Figure 22–11 on page 616). Uterine contractions can be assessed for frequency and duration but not for intensity. The intensity (as displayed on the graph

paper) is a reflection of how tightly the belt is applied around the maternal abdomen. When the belt is tight enough, the nurse should be able to note the beginning of contractions on the monitor just before or at the same time the woman begins to feel them.

The advantages to this method are that it may be used prior to rupture of membranes antepartally and intrapartally and it provides a continuous recording of the duration and frequency of contractions. The major disadvantage of this method is that it cannot assess the intensity of contractions (because the obtained tracing is influenced by how snugly the elastic belt is applied). Another disadvantage is that sometimes the belt bothers the woman because it must be snug to monitor uterine contractions accurately—the belt may require frequent readjustment as she changes position, or the woman may feel she needs to remain in one position as not to disturb the belt.

A beltless tocodynamometer has been developed. This system consists of an adhesive transducer that is applied to the most prominent part of the woman's abdomen with a double-sided adhesive film (Figure 22–5). The advantages of the nonbelted tocodynamometer include acceptance by the laboring woman due to increased freedom of movement and not having to wear a belt around the abdomen, easy application, infrequent readjustment, and convenience.

Electronic Monitoring by Internal Means In addition to providing information regarding uterine contraction frequency and duration, the **intrauterine catheter** method also assesses intensity. One type of intrauterine catheter consists of small polyethylene tubing that is inserted directly into the uterine cavity. The guide tube encasing the catheter is advanced as far as the internal

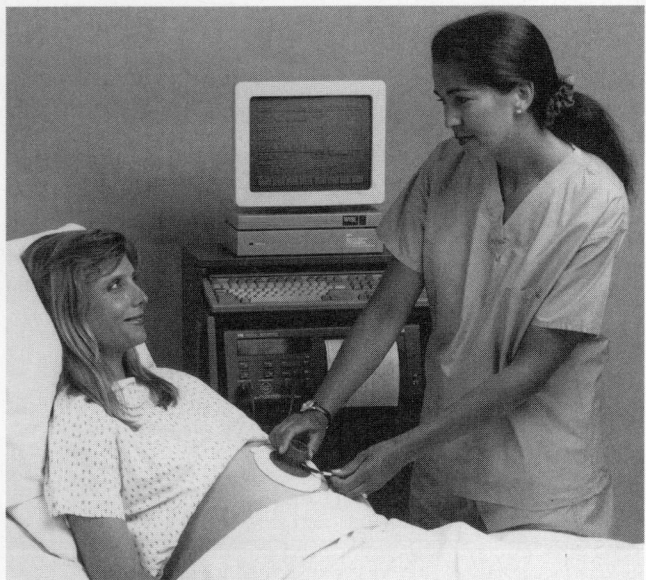

FIGURE 22-5 Beltless tocodynamometer system with adhesive transducer support plate and pressure transducer unit.
SOURCE: Courtesy of Corometrics Medical Systems, Inc, Wallingford, CT.

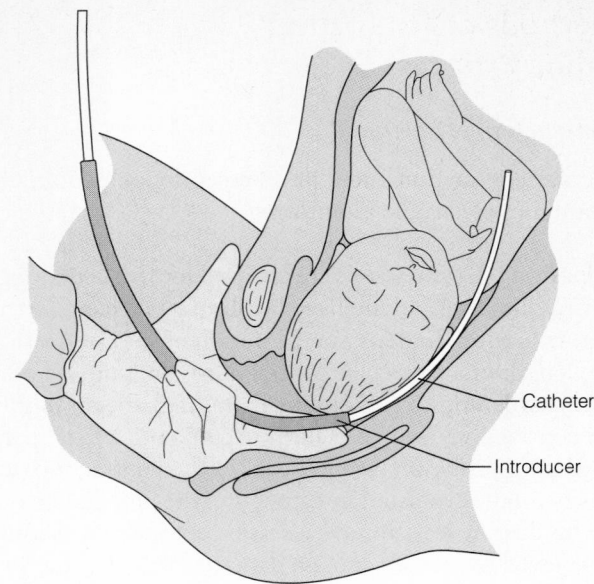

FIGURE 22-6 Technique of uterine catheter insertion. Note that the introducer (catheter guide) is inserted no farther than beyond the fingertips.

cervical os, and then the tubing is slowly threaded into the uterine cavity, usually in the area where fetal small parts are located. It is advanced only as far as the black marking indicated on the catheter, which should be visualized at the opening to the vagina (Figure 22–6). The catheter and strain gauge are filled with sterile water (not saline, which will corrode the transducer). The gauge is then connected to the monitor. For measurement of accurate baseline resting tone of the uterus the strain gauge should be adjusted to the height of the maternal xiphoid process. With the woman in the supine position this will approximate the level of the tip of the intrauterine catheter. By this means, a closed pressure system is maintained so that increases in intrauterine pressure with uterine contractions or hypertonus may be visualized.

The catheter is periodically flushed with sterile water to ensure patency and accurate resting tone. If the catheter becomes clogged with vernix or meconium, it will show an increase in baseline resting tone. If the woman changes position, the catheter should be flushed, the strain gauge readjusted, and the system recalibrated.

An intrauterine pressure catheter that functions without being filled with fluid is also available. The IN-TRAN Plus has a micropressure transducer (electronic sensor) at the tip of the catheter. The catheter is inserted into the uterine cavity and then connected by a cable to the electronic fetal monitor. This catheter incorporates a second lumen and a port for amnioinfusion (an infusion of fluid into the amniotic cavity to provide additional fluid or to dilute amniotic fluid that has thick meconium in it). The second port permits amnioinfusion while

simultaneously providing accurate monitoring of intrauterine pressure. This catheter has several advantages over fluid-filled systems: It does not require flushing to prevent obstruction by blood or meconium in the amniotic fluid; it is simple to equilibrate and easy to insert without assistance; it provides good quality recordings; and it can be zeroed at any time (Figure 22–7).

In many institutions the intrauterine catheter is used only during oxytocin augmentation, induction, or vaginal birth after cesarean. It is particularly important to quantitate the intensity and frequency of contractions to avoid hyperstimulation and possible uterine rupture due to overadministration of oxytocin. If the woman's labor is prolonged, internal monitoring should be used to accurately assess the frequency and strength of contractions and resultant FHR pattern response. When an intrauterine catheter is used, there is a 1% risk of infection, but this seems to depend on the duration of ruptured membranes and length of labor.

It is of particular importance that the nurse evaluate the woman's labor status by means other than the fetal monitor. As with any type of technology, no machine is flawless, and the monitor cannot fill the role of the nurse. One should never rely solely on data recorded by a machine. Technology is useful only as an adjunct to good nursing assessment. All too often women are in active labor with adequate contractions that are regarded as being of "poor quality" because the monitor is not functioning properly. The nurse should routinely palpate the intensity of the contractions and compare the assessment with data recorded by the monitor.

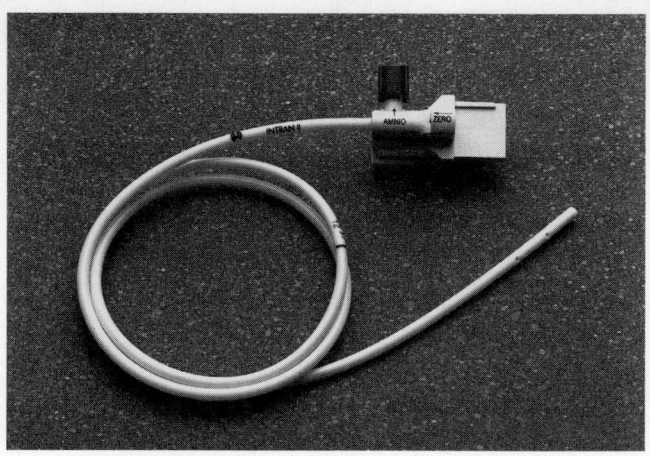

FIGURE 22-7 INTRAN intrauterine pressure catheter. There is a micropressure transducer (electronic sensor) located at the tip of the catheter and a port for amnioinfusion at the distal end of the catheter.

Trying to figure out if I was in labor was quite a task. Here I was, a labor and delivery nurse, and I couldn't decide if my contractions were the real thing. I timed them, and about the time I decided this was It, they would slow down. How exasperating not to be able to really know! It was hard on me because I felt surely a labor and delivery nurse should know for herself. But now I see that all women are in this spot. They want so much to be right, and we often treat them as if they should be able to know absolutely when it's the real thing. I'd like labor and delivery nurses to remember this.

Cervical Assessment

Cervical dilatation and effacement are evaluated directly by sterile vaginal examination (see Procedure 22–1: Intrapartal Vaginal Examination). The vaginal examination can also provide information regarding membrane status, fetal position, and station of the presenting part (Procedure 22–2: Assessing for Amniotic Fluid).

PROCEDURE 22-2
ASSESSING FOR AMNIOTIC FLUID

Nursing Action	Rationale
Objective: Assemble equipment. Gather Nitrazine test tape and a pair of disposable gloves.	*Nitrazine test tape reacts to alkaline fluids and confirms presence of amniotic fluid.*
May need microscope and glass slide if determining ferning of obtained fluid.	*Microscope is used to detect ferning pattern.*
Objective: Set the stage for the assessment. Explain the procedure, indications for the procedure, what she will feel, and information that may be obtained. Determine whether she has noted the escape of any clear fluid from the vagina.	*Explanation of the procedure decreases anxiety and increases relaxation.*
Objective: Test fluid. Prior to doing a vaginal exam that uses lubricant, put on gloves. With one gloved hand, spread the labia, and with the other hand place a small section of Nitrazine tape (approx. 2 in long) against the vaginal opening. You may also place the test tape against any clothing or pads that have been soaked with possible amniotic fluid. Take care not to touch tape with bare fingers prior to the test.	*Contamination of the Nitrazine test tape with lubricant can make the test unreliable.*
Compare the color on the test tape to the guide on the back of the Nitrazine test tape container to determine the test results.	*Enough fluid needs to be placed on the test tape to make it wet. Amniotic fluid is alkaline, and an alkaline fluid turns the Nitrazine test tape a dark blue. If the test tape remains a beige color, the test is negative for amniotic fluid.*
Amniotic fluid may also be obtained by speculum exam. Some labor and birth nurses are using this technique. If fluid is present in sufficient amount to draw some into a syringe, a small amount of fluid can be placed on a glass slide, allowed to dry, and then looked at under a microscope. A ferning pattern confirms the presence of amniotic fluid. See Figure 7–4 for an example of ferning.	*Obtaining a specimen by speculum exam reduces the contamination of the fluid with other substances such as blood.*
Objective: Record information on client's record. Record on labor record (eg, SROM, Nitrazine positive).	*Nurse documents status of membranes, intact or ruptured.*

Sterile vaginal examinations are thought to be an important yet rather routine assessment during the first and second stages of labor. Some clinicians have questioned whether sterile vaginal exams need to be done as frequently as current practice indicates and whether they are done in as comfortable and woman-centered manner as possible. Bergstrom and colleagues (1992) conducted a study in which labors were videotaped, then evaluated. They found that the method of communicating with the woman and enlisting her consent, the information shared about the procedure and the sensations it may cause, and the sharing of the exam's findings vary greatly among different nurses, certified nurse-midwives, and physicians. McKay and Smith (1993) conclude that the exam is sometimes done in a manner that suggests control by the care giver and emphasizes passivity in the woman and her inability to give consent in the situation.

Suggestions for improvement include asking the care giver to reconsider the need for each sterile vaginal exam by asking what information is needed at this time and keeping the number of exams to a minimum; talking with the woman prior to the exam and explaining how it will be done and that it may cause no discomfort, mild discomfort, or much pain; avoiding the practice of gloving and waiting with fist clenched (an action many clinicians take to keep from inadvertently contaminating the glove) because of the inherent nonverbal message of power that a gloved fist implies; telling the woman during the exam that her cervix will be palpated and she'll feel the pressure of the examining fingers; acknowledging and validating any pain the woman feels and suggesting comfort measures; reevaluating the need to keep the examining fingers in the vagina during a series of contractions because they may cause discomfort and emphasize a more authoritative care giver role; telling the woman before removing the examining fingers; and explaining the findings of the exam (Bergstrom et al 1992). Most of all, the care giver can acknowledge that it is the woman's body and that the exam can be consistently performed in a caring, respectful manner.

Evaluation of Labor Progress

Consistent progress in labor depends on a number of factors. The uterine contractions must be of sufficient frequency, duration, and intensity and the fetus must descend into and through the maternal pelvis. The maternal tissues need to provide enough resistance that the fetus can move through the pelvis, yet distend as the birth approaches. Once the first stage is completed, maternal pushing effort becomes a factor that affects the progress of labor.

The nurse can look to general guidelines to evaluate each woman's progress through labor and birth (Table 22-2). When dilatation and descent are not occurring as expected, the nurse needs to explore factors that may be affecting progress. For instance, if uterine contractions

---

TABLE 22-2 Contraction and Labor Progress Characteristics

Contraction Characteristics

Latent phase:	Every 10–20 minutes × 15–20 seconds; mild, progressing to Every 5–7 minutes × 30–40 seconds; moderate
Active phase:	Every 2–3 minutes × 60 seconds; moderate to strong
Transition phase:	Every 2 minutes × 60–90 seconds; strong

Labor Progress Characteristics

Primipara:	1.2 cm/hour dilatation 1 cm/hour descent <2 hours in second stage
Multipara:	1.5 cm/hour dilatation 2 cm/hour descent <1 hour in second stage

---

are not of the expected frequency, duration, and intensity for the point in labor, the nurse will consider factors such as the following:

1. Uterine exhaustion (Long labor process, large fetus, fetal malposition or malpresentation affect the contractibility of the uterine muscles.)

2. Overstretching of the uterus (Causes include large fetus, multiple gestation, hydramnios [excessive amniotic fluid].)

3. Anxiety and pain (Anxiety due to the labor or because the labor is not as expected. The woman experiences decreased ability to cope with increasing pain and discomfort, pain that is not relieved by interventions, fear of the actual birth, flashbacks to previous traumatic situations in other birth experiences or sexual violence or other situations in which she was very vulnerable and unable to control the circumstances.)

If fetal descent is not occurring within expected guidelines, the nurse considers the following:

1. Fetal malposition or malpresentation (The fetal presenting part does not exert the expected pressure on the cervix and does not proceed through the maternal pelvis as expected. An example is occiput posterior presentation, in which the occiput is directed toward the maternal back instead of downward and forward. This slows fetal descent as measured by assessing station.)

2. Fetal size and possible cephalopelvic disproportion (Fetal descent is slowed or stopped.)

3. Anxiety and pain (These cause tension in the maternal muscles, which may affect fetal position.)

If the second stage is not completed within the expected guidelines, the nurse considers the following:

1. Maternal exhaustion (The woman may be able to push, but exhaustion affects the amount of effort she has left to exert.)

2. Maternal anxiety (The woman may be unable to respond to the natural pushing urges of her body or may resist others' efforts to coach and/or assist her.)

3. Maternal position (Her position may not be conducive to combining pushing effort and gravity forces.)

4. Analgesia and/or anesthesia (Analgesia makes maternal effort difficult because of relaxation. Regional anesthesia blocks the urge or muscular ability to push.)

The nurse completes all assessments and evaluates the labor to determine whether it is progressing within normal parameters. Identification of abnormal labor progress is important in determining the need for additional assessments and treatments.

FETAL ASSESSMENT

Determination of Fetal Position and Presentation

Fetal position is determined in several ways. The woman's abdomen is inspected and palpated to determine fetal position; auscultation of fetal heart tones also helps determine fetal position. A vaginal examination may be done to determine the presenting part, and ultrasound examination may be used.

Inspection

The nurse should observe the woman's abdomen for size and shape. The lie of the fetus should be assessed by noting whether the uterus projects up and down (longitudinal lie) or left to right (transverse lie).

Palpation: Leopold's Maneuvers

Leopold's maneuvers are a systematic way to evaluate the maternal abdomen (Figure 22–8). Frequent practice increases the examiner's skill in determining fetal position by palpation. Leopold's maneuvers may be difficult to perform on an obese woman or on a woman who has excessive amniotic fluid (hydramnios).

Care should be taken to ensure the woman's comfort during Leopold's maneuvers. The woman should have recently emptied her bladder and should lie on her back with her abdomen uncovered. To aid in relaxation of the abdominal wall, the shoulders should be raised slightly on a pillow and the knees drawn up a little. The procedure should be completed between contractions. The examiner's hands should be warm.

Consideration should be given to several questions while inspecting and palpating the maternal abdomen:

- Is the fetal lie longitudinal or transverse?
- What is in the fundus? Am I feeling buttocks or head?

- Where is the fetal back?
- Where are the small parts or extremities?
- What is in the inlet? Does it confirm what I found in the fundus?
- Is the presenting part engaged, floating, or dipping into the inlet?
- Is there fetal movement?
- How large is the fetus (appropriate, large, or small for gestational age)?
- Is there one fetus or more than one?
- Is fundal height proportionate to the estimated gestational age?

First Maneuver While facing the woman, the nurse palpates the upper abdomen with both hands (Figure 22–8). The nurse determines the shape, size, consistency, and mobility of the form that is found. The fetal head is firm, hard, and round and moves independently of the trunk. The breech feels softer and symmetrical and has small bony prominences; it moves with the trunk.

Second Maneuver After ascertaining whether the head or the buttocks occupies the fundus, the nurse tries to determine the location of the fetal back and notes whether it is on the right or left side of the maternal abdomen. Still facing the woman, the nurse palpates the abdomen with deep but gentle pressure, using her palms (Figure 22–8). The right hand should be steady while the left hand explores the right side of the uterus. The maneuver is then repeated, probing with the right hand and steadying the uterus with the left hand. The fetal back should feel firm and smooth and should connect what was found in the fundus with a mass in the inlet. Once the back is located, the nurse validates the finding by palpating the fetal extremities (small irregularities and protrusions) on the opposite side of the abdomen.

Third Maneuver Next the nurse should determine what fetal part is lying above the inlet by gently grasping the lower portion of the abdomen just above the symphysis pubis with the thumb and fingers of the right hand (Figure 22–8). This maneuver yields the opposite information from what was found in the fundus and validates the presenting part. If the head is presenting and is not engaged, it may be gently pushed back and forth.

Fourth Maneuver For this portion of the examination the nurse faces the woman's feet and attempts to locate the cephalic prominence or brow. Location of this landmark assists in assessing the descent of the presenting part into the pelvis. The fingers of both hands are moved gently down the sides of the uterus toward the pubis (Figure 22–8). The cephalic prominence (brow) is located on the side where there is greatest resistance to the descent of the fingers toward the pubis. It is located on

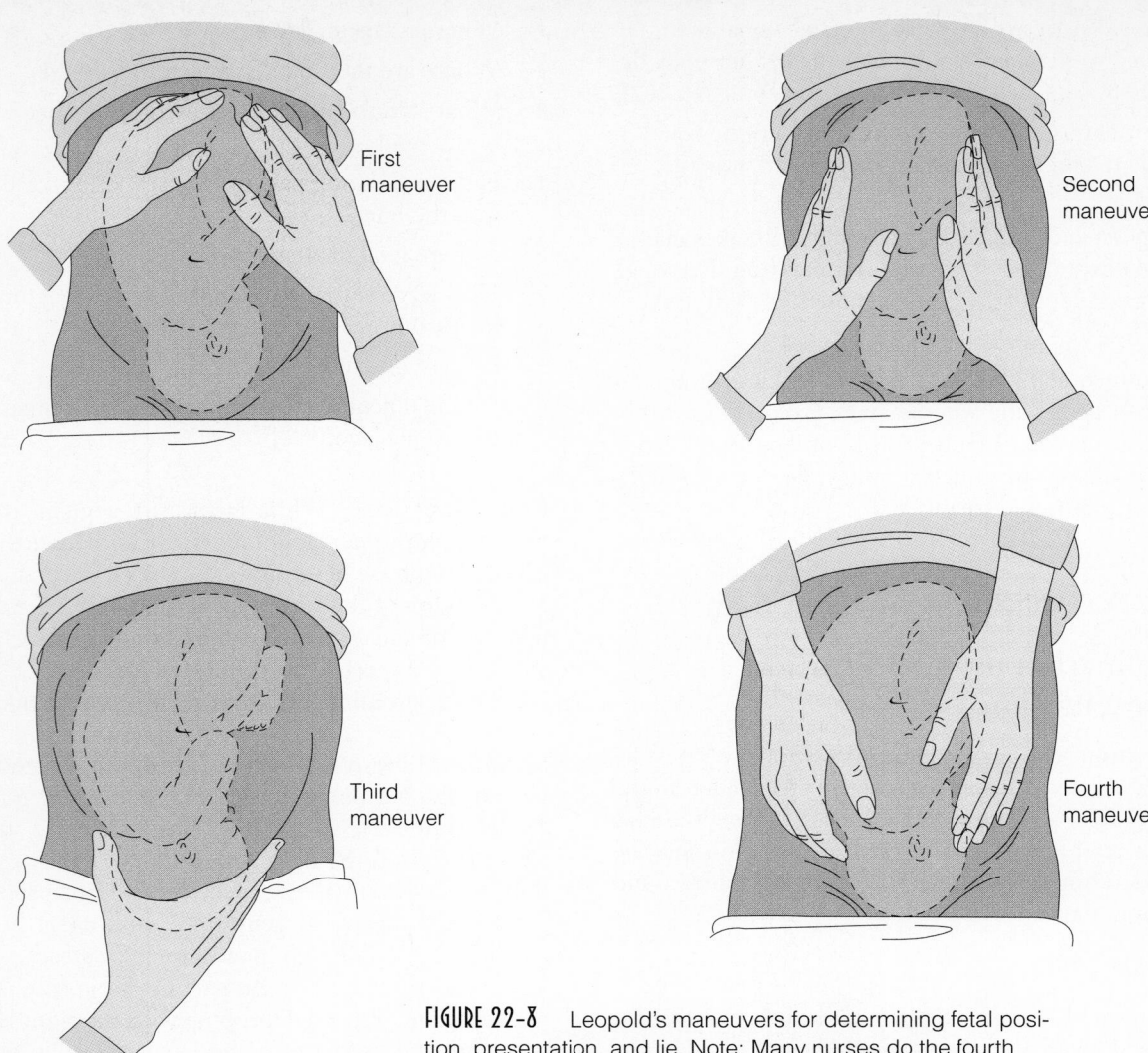

FIGURE 22-8   Leopold's maneuvers for determining fetal position, presentation, and lie. Note: Many nurses do the fourth maneuver first in order to identify the part of the fetus in the pelvic inlet.

the opposite side from the fetal back if the head is well flexed. However, when the fetal head is extended, the occiput is the first cephalic prominence felt, and it is located on the same side as the back. Therefore when completing the fourth maneuver, if the first cephalic prominence palpated is on the same side as the back, the head is not flexed. If the first prominence found is opposite the back, the head is well flexed.

Critical Thinking Question

The fetus in Figure 22–8 is in ROA position. Describe what you would feel during Leopold's maneuvers if the fetus were LOA.

Vaginal Examination

The vaginal examination reveals information regarding the fetus such as presentation, position, station, degree of flexion of the fetal head, and any swelling that might be present on the fetal scalp (caput succedaneum).

Ultrasound

Real-time ultrasound is frequently available in the birth setting and may be used to obtain specific information regarding the fetus. A real-time ultrasound may be done at this time to assess fetal lie, presentation, and position; obtain measurements of biparietal diameter to estimate gestational age; assess for anomalies when a vaginal examination reveals suspicious findings; assess placement of the placenta; and sometimes confirm the presence of more than one fetus. (See Chapter 20 for further discussion of the use of ultrasound for fetal assessment.)

Evaluation of Fetal Status During Labor

Auscultation of Fetal Heart Rate

The fetoscope or a hand-held ultrasound device is used to auscultate the fetal heart rate (FHR) between, during, and immediately after uterine contractions (Figure 22–9).

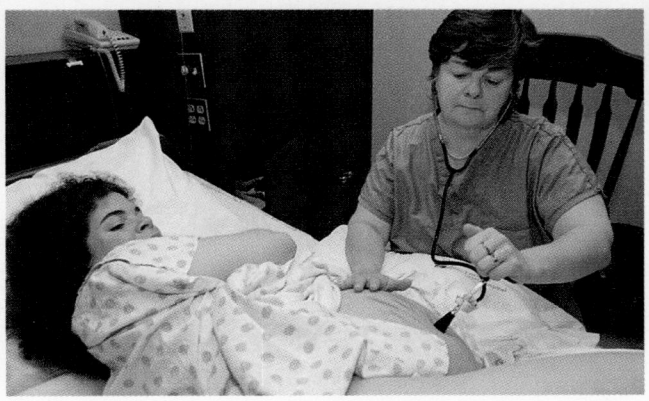

A

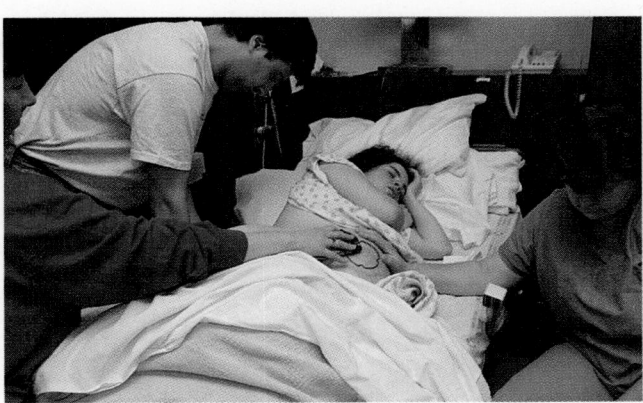

B

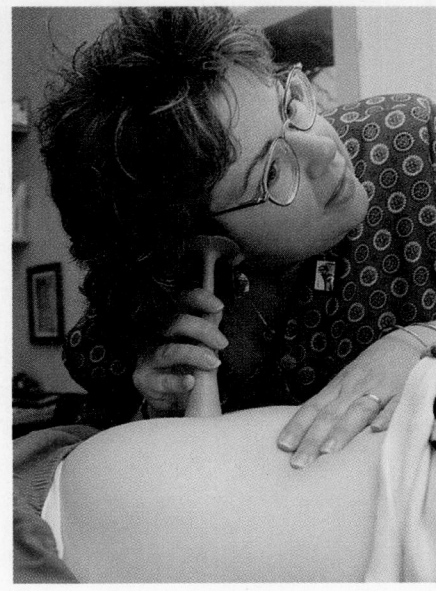

C

FIGURE 22-9 *A* The nurse holds the fetoscope as she places it against the maternal abdomen and then removes her fingers from the fetoscope while counting the fetal heartbeats. *B* When the fetal heart rate is picked up by the electronic monitor, the sound of the heartbeat can be heard by all persons in the room. *C* The Penar fetoscope can be easily used in outpatient or community setting.

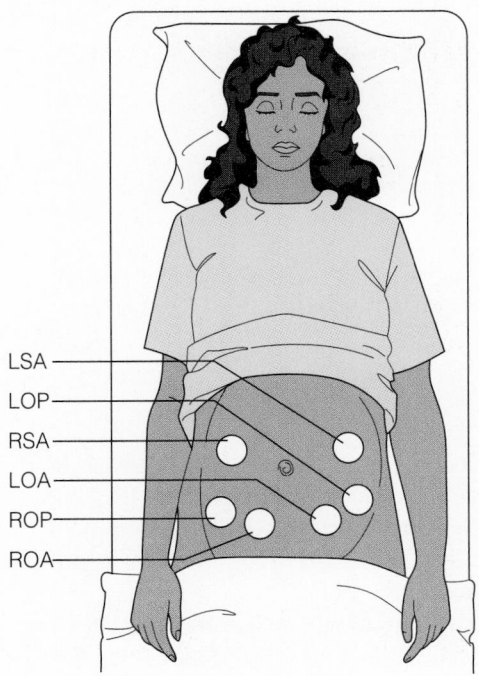

LSA
LOP
RSA
LOA
ROP
ROA

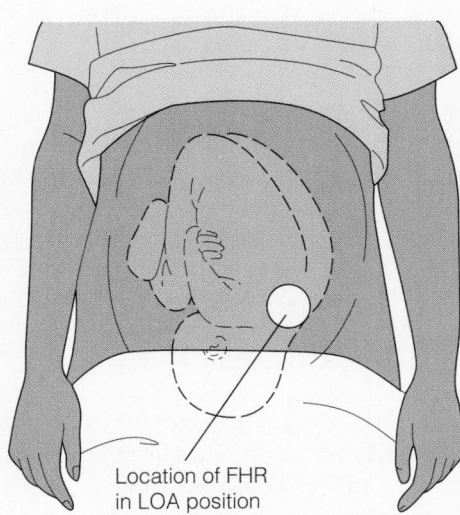

Location of FHR
in LOA position

FIGURE 22-10 Location of FHR in relation to the more commonly seen fetal positions. The fetal heart rate is heard more clearly over the fetal back.

Before listening to the FHR the first time, the nurse may choose to perform Leopold's maneuvers and check the maternal heart rate. Leopold's maneuvers not only indicate the probable location of the FHR, but also help determine the presence of multiple fetuses, fetal lie, and fetal presentation. FHR is heard most clearly at the fetal back (Figure 22–10). Thus, in a cephalic presentation

FHR is best heard in the lower quadrant of the maternal abdomen. In a breech presentation it is heard at or above the level of the maternal umbilicus. In a transverse lie FHR may be heard best just above or just below the umbilicus. As the presenting part descends and rotates through the maternal pelvis during labor, FHR tends to descend and move toward the midline.

Nursing Action	Rationale
Objective: Assemble equipment. Obtain a fetoscope or Doppler.	*The fetoscope is a special type of stethoscope that amplifies sound. The Doppler uses ultrasound.*
Objective: Prepare woman. Explain the procedure, indications for the procedure, and the information that will be obtained. Uncover the woman's abdomen.	*Explanation of the procedure decreases anxiety and increases relaxation.*
To use the fetoscope: Locate area of FHR using Leopold's maneuvers. Place the metal band of the fetoscope on your head; the diaphragm should extend out from your forehead. Place the diaphragm on the woman's abdomen halfway between the umbilicus and symphysis and in the midline. Without touching the fetoscope listen carefully for the sounds of the fetal heart, which are called fetal heart tones (FHTs). If the FHTs are not heard, move the fetoscope laterally about an inch, and then in a circle. Repeat in ever-widening circles until the FHTs are heard.	*The fetoscope is an older assessment tool; however, some clinicians prefer it because it is "natural" and does not rely on ultrasound. The metal band conducts sound.* *The FHR is most likely to be heard in this area.*
To use the Doppler: Place "ultrasonic gel" on the diaphragm of the Doppler. Note: Some Dopplers have a plastic cap over the diaphragm that will need to be removed to expose the diaphragm. Place diaphragm on the woman's abdomen halfway between the umbilicus and symphysis and in the midline. Listen carefully for the FHR (Figure 22–9C).	*Gel is used to maintain contact with the maternal abdomen and to enhance conduction of ultrasound.* *The FHR is most likely to be heard in this area.* *Sound level may be controlled with a volume knob.*
For both methods: Check the woman's pulse against the sounds heard. If the rates are the same, you have probably located maternal pulses (in abdominal vessels or in the placenta) and need to readjust the fetoscope or ultrasound device. If the rates are not similar, count the FHR for 1 full minute. Note	*Ensures the FHR, not the woman's pulse, is being heard.*

After FHR is located, it is counted for 30 seconds and multiplied by two to obtain the number of beats per minute. The nurse should occasionally listen for 1 full minute, through and just after a contraction, to detect any abnormal heart rate, especially if the FHR is over 160 (tachycardia) or under 120 (bradycardia) or irregular beats are heard. Listening through a contraction may be difficult because of maternal movement or a muffling of the FHR sounds. If the FHR is irregular or has changed markedly from the last assessment, the nurse should listen for 1 full minute through and immediately after a contraction. It is especially important to listen during and after the contraction to detect any deceleration that might occur. It is also important to listen immediately after each contraction when the woman is pushing during

second stage because fetal bradycardia frequently occurs as pressure is exerted on the fetal head during descent. See Procedure 22–3: Auscultation of Fetal Heart Rate and Table 22–3 for guidelines regarding how often to auscultate FHR.

The American Academy of Pediatrics and the American College of Obstetricians and Gynecologists Guidelines for Perinatal Care (1992) has indicated that auscultation as outlined is equivalent to electronic fetal monitoring. Albers (1994, p 109) notes that "electronic fetal monitoring is not more effective than intermittent auscultation in reducing perinatal mortality or morbidity." Some nurses may feel that the one-on-one nursing required to follow the guidelines and the use of nonelectronic equipment is not desirable; however, auscultation

Nursing Action	Rationale
that the fetal heart has a double rhythm (like an adult's heart), and just one sound is counted. If the FHR is not found, move the fetoscope or ultrasound device laterally.	
Tell parents what the FHR is; offer to help them listen if they would like.	
Objective: Provide systematic evaluation.	
Auscultate between, during, and for 30 seconds following a uterine contraction. For low-risk women NAACOG (1990) recommends an auscultation frequency of every 1 hour in the latent phase, every 30 minutes in the active phase, and every 15 minutes in the second stage. For high-risk women the recommended frequency is every 30 minutes in the latent phase, every 15 minutes in the active phase, and every 5 minutes in the second stage.	*Evaluation provides the opportunity to assess the fetal status and response to the labor process.*
Objective: Record information on client's record.	
Document FHR data (rate and rhythm), characteristics of uterine activity, and any actions taken as a result of the FHR.	*Complete documentation is mandatory.*
Sample nurse's entry:	
1/1/96 FHR 140 by auscultation, regular rhythm. Maternal pulse 78. 0730 UC q3min × 60 sec, strong. No increase or decrease in FHR noted during or following UC. J. Smith RN	*Nurse's entry documents FHR rate, rhythm, and response to the labor process.*
Sample nurse's entry for baseline and slowing of FHR after uterine contraction.	
1/1/96 FHR 136 by auscultation with slowing noted during the acme 0730 of UC and for 10 sec following the UC. Client turned to left side. Maternal pulse 80. FHR 140, regular rhythm with no decrease during or following the next two UC. UC q3min × 60 sec, strong. J. Smith RN	*Nurse's entry documents FHR rate, response to UC, nursing intervention, and fetal response.*

TABLE 22-3   Frequency of Auscultation: Assessment and Documentation

Low-Risk Patients

First stage of labor:
q 1 hour in latent phase
q 30 minutes in active phase

Second stage of labor:
q 15 minutes

Labor Events

Assess FHR prior to:
Initiation of labor-enhancing procedures (eg, artificial rupture of membranes)
Periods of ambulation
Administration of medications
Administration or initiation of analgesia/anesthesia

High-Risk Patients

First stage of labor:
q 30 minutes in latent phase
q 15 minutes in active phase

Second stage of labor:
q 5 minutes

Labor Events *continued*

Assess FHR following:
Rupture of membranes
Recognition of abnormal uterine activity patterns, such as increased basal tone or tachysystole
Evaluation of oxytocin (maintenance, increase, or decrease of dosage)
Administration of medications (at time of peak action)
Expulsion of enema
Urinary catheterization
Vaginal examination
Periods of ambulation
Evaluation of analgesia and/or anesthesia (maintenance, increase, or decrease of dosage)

SOURCE: NAACOG: *OGN Nursing Practice Resource, Fetal Heart Rate Auscultation.* Washington, DC: NAACOG, 1990, p 5.

Nursing Action	Rationale
Objective: Prepare woman.	
Explain the procedure, the indications for the EFM, and the information that will be obtained. Explain the monitor so that the woman and support person will know what they are seeing and hearing.	*Explanation of the procedure decreases anxiety and increases relaxation.*
Place the external fetal monitor. Turn on the monitor.	
Place two elastic belts around the woman's abdomen. Place the "toco" over the uterine fundus in the midline and secure it with a belt so that it fits snugly. Note the UC tracing. The resting tone tracing (without uterine contraction) should be recording on the 10 or 15 mm Hg pressure line.	*The uterine fundus is the area of greatest contractility.*
	If the tracing is on the zero line, there may be a constant grinding noise.
Apply ultrasonic gel to the diaphragm of the ultrasound transducer. Place the diaphragm on the maternal abdomen between the umbilicus and symphysis pubis, in the midline. Listen for the FHR (which will have a "whiplike" sound). When the FHR is located, attach the elastic belt snugly.	*Ultrasonic gel is used to maintain contact with the maternal abdomen. The ultrasonic beam is directed toward the fetal heart.*
	Firm contact is necessary to maintain a continuous tracing.
Objective: Identify the tracing.	
Place the following information on the beginning of the fetal monitor paper: date, time, client name, gravida, para, membrane status, physician/CNM name. (Note: Each birthing area may have specific guidelines regarding additional information that is to be included.)	*Assures accurate identification.*
Objective: Evaluate EFM tracing.	
For high-risk women NAACOG (1988) recommends evaluating the EFM tracing every 15 minutes in the first stage and every 5 minutes in the second stage. For low-risk women specific time intervals have not been recommended by NAACOG (now known as AWHONN). However, evaluation every 15–30 minutes in the first stage and every 5–15 minutes in the second stage (as long as the FHR has reassuring characteristics) is frequently done. The time interval for evaluation needs to be shortened if any nonreassuring characteristics occur.	*Evaluation provides the opportunity to assess the fetal status and response to the labor process. The presence of reassuring characteristics is associated with good fetal outcome. Rapid identification of nonreassuring characteristics allows interventions to be initiated and then to determine the fetal response to the interventions.*
Objective: Record information on client record.	
Sample nurse's entry:	
1/1/96 FHR BL 135–140. STV and LTV present. Two accelerations of 0700 20 bpm × 20 sec with fetal movement in 10 minutes. UC q3min × 50–60 sec of moderate intensity by palpation. No decelerations noted.	*Nurse's entry documents reassuring FHR characteristics and response to UCs. (Note: STV is the abbreviation for short-term variability, and LTV is long-term variability. See discussion later in this chapter).*
Sample nurse's entry if slowing is noted.	
1/1/96 FHR BL 135–144. STV and LTV present. Late deceleration 0730 noted with decrease of FHR to 130 bpm for 20 sec. UC q3min × 50–60 sec of moderate intensity by palpation. Client turned to left side. No further deceleration with three subsequent UC. Two accelerations of 20 bpm × 20 sec noted with fetal movement. Client instructed to remain on left side.	*Nurse's entry documents FHR rate, presence of variability, response of FHR to UC, intervention used, and subsequent positive fetal response to the intervention.*

by fetoscope is still a viable assessment that provides usable information.

If decelerations (discussed later in this chapter) are noted, the woman should be electronically monitored to rule out abnormalities in the FHR.

Electronic Fetal Monitoring

Electronic fetal monitoring (EFM) provides a visual assessment of fetal heart rate. A continuous tracing of the FHR can be obtained, allowing many characteristics of the fetal heart rate to be observed and evaluated. (See Procedure 22–4: Electronic Fetal Monitoring.)

When the FHR is monitored electronically, the interval between two successive fetal heartbeats is measured, and the rate is displayed as if the beats occurred at the same interval for 60 seconds. For example, if the interval between two beats is 0.5 second, the rate for 1 full minute would be 120 beats per minute.

EFM has major advantages over auscultation with the fetoscope. Electronic monitoring is an objective means of evaluating fetal well-being. Fetal distress can be detected by observing the continuous FHR and the periodic changes that occur during and after uterine contractions. Therefore, interventions can be timely and thus more effective.

Indications for Electronic Fetal Monitoring Any woman with previous history of medical or obstetric problems that might affect labor or the health of the fetus should be monitored by continuous electronic fetal monitoring. Some physicians advocate monitoring only those women considered to be at risk or at high risk, but many feel the procedure is mandatory for all women in labor. Table 22–4 lists specific indications for monitoring.

External Monitoring *External monitoring* of the fetus is usually accomplished by the use of ultrasound. A transducer, which emits continuous sound waves, is placed on the maternal abdomen. A water-soluble gel is applied to the underside of the transducer to aid in conduction of fetal heart sounds. When the transducer is placed correctly, the sound waves bounce off the fetal heart and are picked up by the electronic monitor. The actual moment-by-moment FHR is displayed simultaneously on a screen and on graph paper (Figure 22–11).

The transducer may inadvertently be directed toward a pulsating maternal vessel. In this case there will be a soft swooshing sound (uterine souffle), and the rate will be the same as the maternal pulse.

Disadvantages of monitoring fetal heart rate by external means are similar to those of external uterine contraction monitoring. In addition, a poor quality tracing may be obtained if the fetus is quite active, if more than a normal amount of amniotic fluid is present, if the woman is obese, or if the woman is moving about frequently.

TABLE 22-4	Indications for Electronic Monitoring

Fetal Factors

Decreased fetal movement
Abnormal auscultory FHR
Meconium passage
Abnormal presentations/positions
IUGR or SGA fetus
Postdates (>41 weeks)
Multiple gestation

Maternal Factors

Fever
Infections
PIH
Disease conditions (eg, hypertension, diabetes)
Anemia
Rh isoimmunization
Previous perinatal death
Grand multiparity
Previous cesarean birth
Borderline/contracted pelvis

Uterine Factors

Dysfunctional labor
Failure to progress in labor
Oxytocin induction/augmentation
Uterine anomalies

Complications of Pregnancy

Prolonged rupture of membranes
Premature rupture of membranes
Preterm labor
Marginal abruptio placentae
Partial placenta previa
Occult/frank prolapse of cord
Amnionitis

Regional Anesthesia

Elective Monitoring

Internal Monitoring Internal monitoring is accomplished through use of an internal spinal electrode, which is attached to the skin of the fetal head or buttocks (Figure 22–12). To insert the spinal electrode, the cervix must be dilated at least 2 cm, the presenting fetal part must be accessible by vaginal examination, and the membranes must be ruptured. Even though it is not possible to apply the electrode and catheter under strict sterile conditions, the procedure should be performed as aseptically as possible. The perineum should be cleaned with povidone-iodine solution (Betadine) or another cleansing agent. After determining fetal position by vaginal examination, the examiner (physician or nurse) inserts the electrode, which is encased in a plastic guide, to the level of the internal cervical os and attaches it to the presenting part, being careful not to apply it to the face, suture lines, fontanelles, or perineum if the fetus is in a breech presentation. The electrode is rotated clockwise until it is attached to the presenting part and is then disengaged from the guide tube. The guide tube is removed, and the end wires are connected to a leg plate that is attached to the woman's

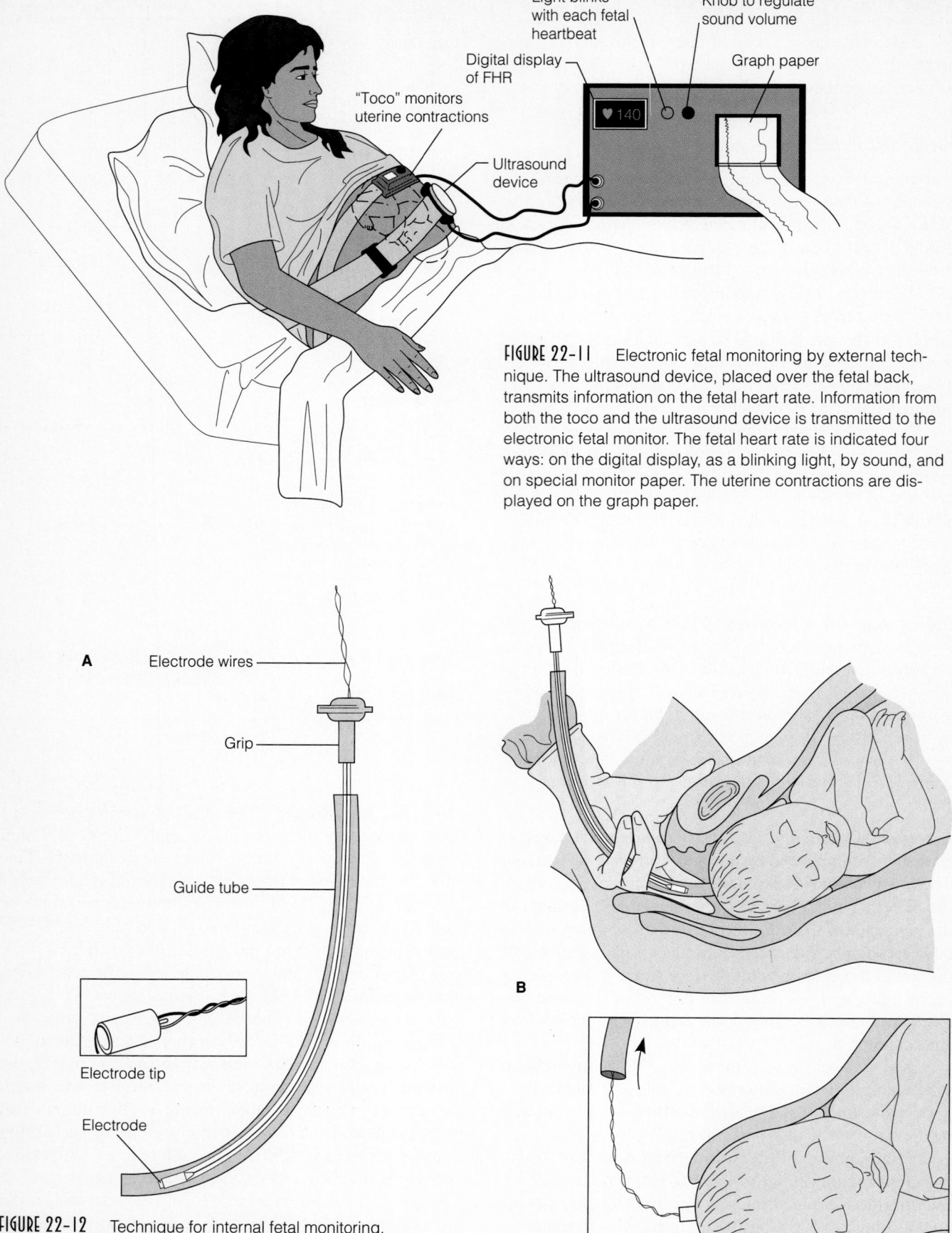

Light blinks
with each fetal
heartbeat

Knob to regulate
sound volume

Digital display
of FHR

Graph paper

"Toco" monitors
uterine contractions

Ultrasound
device

♥ 140

FIGURE 22-11 Electronic fetal monitoring by external technique. The ultrasound device, placed over the fetal back, transmits information on the fetal heart rate. Information from both the toco and the ultrasound device is transmitted to the electronic fetal monitor. The fetal heart rate is indicated four ways: on the digital display, as a blinking light, by sound, and on special monitor paper. The uterine contractions are displayed on the graph paper.

A

Electrode wires

Grip

Guide tube

Electrode tip

Electrode

B

C

FIGURE 22-12 Technique for internal fetal monitoring. *A* Spiral electrode. *B* Attaching the spiral electrode to the scalp. *C* Attached spiral electrode with guide tube removed.

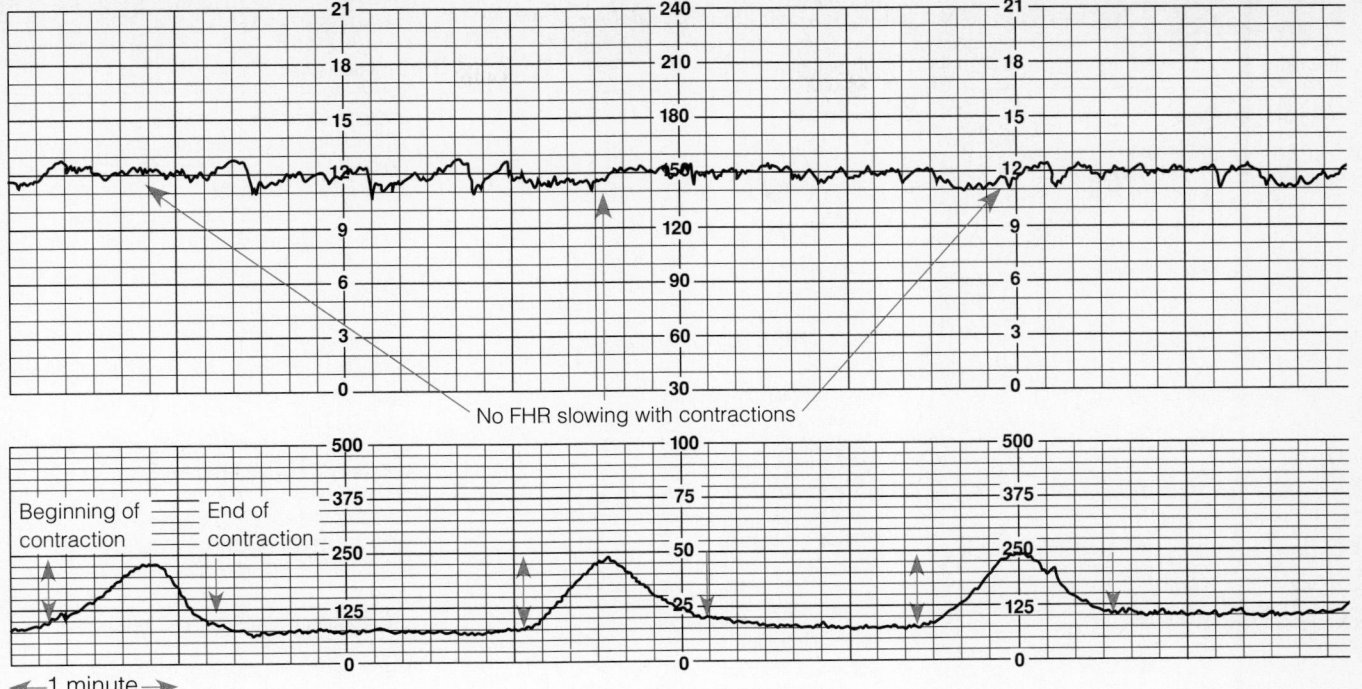

No FHR slowing with contractions

Beginning of contraction   End of contraction

←—1 minute—→

FIGURE 22-13   Normal FHR range is from 120 to 160 beats per minute. The FHR tracing in the upper portion of the graph indicates an FHR range of 140–155 bpm. The bottom portion depicts uterine contractions. Each dark vertical line marks 1 minute, and each small rectangle is 10 seconds. The contraction frequency is about every 3 minutes, and the duration of the contractions is 50–60 seconds.

thigh. The cable from the leg plate is connected to the monitor.

The FHR tracing at the top of Figure 22–13 was obtained by internal monitoring, and the uterine contraction tracing at the bottom by external monitoring. The spiral electrode provides an instantaneous and continuous recording of FHR that is clearer than data provided by external monitoring. Note that the FHR is variable (the tracing moves up and down instead of in a straight line), and the tracing stays close to the line numbered 150. If the graph paper moves through the monitor at 3 cm per minute, each vertical dark line represents 1 minute. On Figure 22–13 note that the frequency of the uterine contractions is every 2½ to 3 minutes. The duration of the contractions is 50 to 60 seconds.

Telemetry   Fetal heart rate and uterine activity may also be monitored by a telemetry system. Ultrasound, or fetal EKG, and external uterine pressure transducers are connected to a small battery-operated transducer. Signals are transmitted to a receiver connected to the monitor. The monitor displays FHR and uterine activity data on the oscilloscope and prints it out on graph paper to provide documentation. This system, which can be worn by means of a shoulder strap, allows the woman to ambulate, helping her to feel more comfortable and less confined during labor, yet provides for continuous monitoring. Telemetry provides for direct as well as indirect monitor-

ing of FHR, indirect monitoring of uterine pressure, and dual FHR monitoring of twins. (See a comparison of different methods in Table 22–5).

Fetal Heart Rate Patterns

Fetal heart rate is evaluated by assessing both baseline and periodic changes. Normal FHR ranges from 120 to 160 beats per minute. More important than FHR are the periodic changes that occur in response to the intermittent stress of uterine contractions and the baseline beat-to-beat variability of the fetal heart rate. A compromised fetus may have a normal heart rate but demonstrate slight periodic changes and decreased variability (the change in FHR over a few seconds to a few minutes) indicative of intrauterine hypoxia.

Baseline Rate   The **baseline rate** refers to the range of FHR observed between contractions during a continuous 10-minute period of monitoring. The range does not include the rate during decelerations. There are two abnormal variations of the baseline rate—those above 160 bpm (tachycardia) and those below 120 bpm (bradycardia). Variability also affects the baseline.

Tachycardia   Tachycardia is defined as a rate of 160 beats per minute or more for 10 minutes. Moderate tachycardia has rates of 160 to 179 bpm. Marked or severe tachycardia

TABLE 22-5 Advantages and Disadvantages of Various Monitoring Methods

Method	Advantages	Disadvantages
Fetoscope	Inexpensive Noninvasive Easy to use Easily transported	Intermittent information Gives no information regarding contractions Cannot assess variability or periodic changes in FHR unless moderate to severe Cannot hear FHT until 17–20 weeks' gestation More difficult to hear during a contraction
Doppler (pocket-sized ultrasound)	Inexpensive Noninvasive Easily transported Can hear FHT as early as 10–12 weeks	Gives no information regarding contractions Cannot assess variability Cannot assess periodic changes in FHR unless moderate to severe Intermittent information
External monitoring (by EFM)	Continuous information Noninvasive Uses: antepartal testing and during labor Gives permanent record Can assess relative frequency of contractions Can assess decreased variability and periodic changes Useful for client teaching	Equipment is expensive Subject to artifact Cannot assess variability unless decreased and then must confirm with internal monitoring Cannot quantitate contractions Belts uncomfortable to some women Subject to double- and half-counting Needs qualified and knowledgeable personnel to interpret
Internal monitoring (by EFM)	Accurate, continuous information Monitors fetal EKG Not subject to artifact Client more mobile in bed, chair Can quantitate contractions Can assess short-term and long-term variability Accurate assessment of periodic changes Useful for client teaching	Will measure maternal heart rate if fetus is dead Equipment is expensive Needs qualified and knowledgeable personnel to interpret Presenting part must be accessible, membranes must be ruptured, and cervix must be dilated enough for application of scalp electrode Requires knowledgeable personnel to apply equipment Client confined to bed or chair Slight increased risk of maternal or fetal infection Subject to double- and half-counting Invasive
Telemetry	Accurate, continuous information Client can be mobile (out of bed or in hall) Same advantages as internal monitoring	Equipment is expensive Invasive Not widely used at the present time Same disadvantages as internal monitoring

is defined as 180 bpm or more. Although tachycardia may occur without apparent reason, possible causes include the following (Tucker 1992, p 67):

- Early fetal hypoxia (This leads to stimulation of the sympathetic system as the fetus compensates for reduced blood flow.)

- Maternal fever (Metabolism of the fetus is accelerated because of increased maternal temperature.)

- Parasympatholytic drugs such as atropine or Vistaril (These drugs block the parasympathetic nervous system, so the heart rate rises.)

- Betasympathomimetic drugs such as ritodrine, terbutaline, atropine, and isoxsuprine (These drugs have a cardiac stimulant effect.)

- Amnionitis (Fetal myocardium metabolism is accelerated because of increased maternal temperature. Intrauterine temperature is higher than maternal body temperature, so fetal tachycardia may be the first sign of developing intrauterine infection [Murray 1989].)

- Maternal hyperthyroidism (Thyroid-stimulating hormones may cross the placenta and stimulate the fetal heart rate.)

- Fetal anemia (The heart rate is increased as a compensatory mechanism to improve tissue perfusion.)

Tachycardia is considered an ominous sign if it is accompanied by other FHR patterns such as late deceleration, severe variable decelerations, or decreased variability (Tucker 1992). If tachycardia is associated with maternal fever, treatment may consist of antipyretics, cooling measures, and antibiotics. Fetal arrhythmia needs to be ruled out. The pediatrician should be notified because tachycardia may cause heart failure in the newborn (Shifrin 1990).

Bradycardia   Fetal bradycardia is defined as a rate of less than 120 beats per minute for a 10-minute segment of time. Mild bradycardia ranges from 100 to 119 beats per minute and is considered benign. Moderate bradycardia is a fetal heart rate less than 100 beats per minute. Marked or severe bradycardia is an FHR less than 70 beats per minute and is associated with a rapidly occurring fetal acidosis. According to Tucker (1992, p 70), causes of fetal bradycardia include the following:

- Late (profound) fetal asphyxia (There is depression of myocardial activity.)

- Maternal hypotension (Maternal hypotension results in decreased blood flow to fetus.)

- Prolonged umbilical cord compression (Fetal baroceptors are activated by cord compression, and this produces vagal stimulation, which results in decrease in FHR.)

- Fetal arrhythmia (This is associated with complete heart block in fetus.)

Bradycardia may be a benign or ominous (preterminal) sign. If there is average variability present, the bradycardia is considered benign. When bradycardia is accompanied by decreased variability and late decelerations, it is considered ominous and a sign of advanced fetal distress (Tucker 1992).

Baseline Variability　One of the most important parameters of fetal well-being is noted in FHR variability. **Baseline variability** is a measure of the interplay (the "push-pull") effect between the sympathetic nervous system (which acts to increase heart rate) and the parasympathetic nervous system (which acts to decrease heart rate). There are two major types of fetal heart rate variability—short term and long term (Figure 22–14).

Long-term variability (LTV) refers to the larger rhythmic fluctuations of the FHR that occur from two to six times per minute with a normal range of six to ten beats per minute. The range refers to the difference between the lowest FHR and the highest FHR within 1 minute. Long-term variability is increased by fetal movement and decreased or absent when the fetus is in a sleep cycle. Long-term variability has been classified as follows (Hon 1976):

No variability	0–2 bpm
Minimal variability	3–5 bpm
Average variability	6–10 bpm
Moderate variability	11–25 bpm
Marked variability (*saltatory*)	>25 bpm

The **saltatory pattern** of marked or excessive variability is characterized by rapid variations in FHR that have a bizarre appearance. LTV occurs with a cycle frequency of three to six per minute, and the amplitude is greater than 25 beats per minute (Figure 22–15). The etiology of this pattern is uncertain. However, it frequently follows moderate to severe variable decelerations (Shifrin 1990).

An unusual pattern referred to as **sinusoidal** is occasionally seen. It is characterized by an undulant sine wave that is equally distributed above and below the baseline.

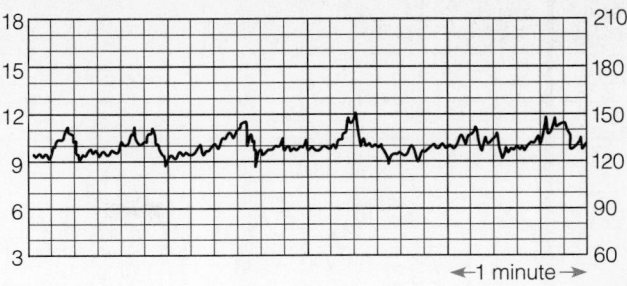

A

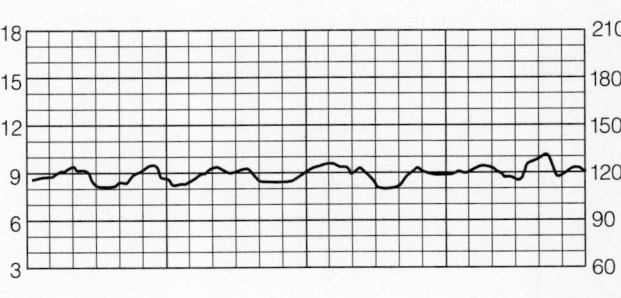

B

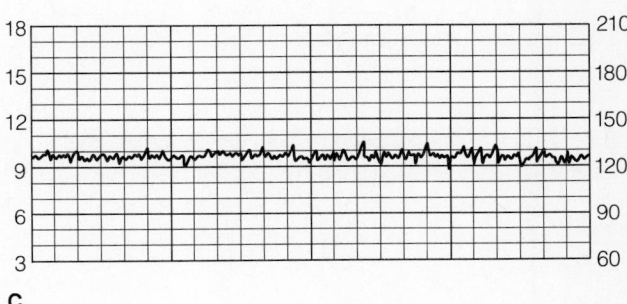

C

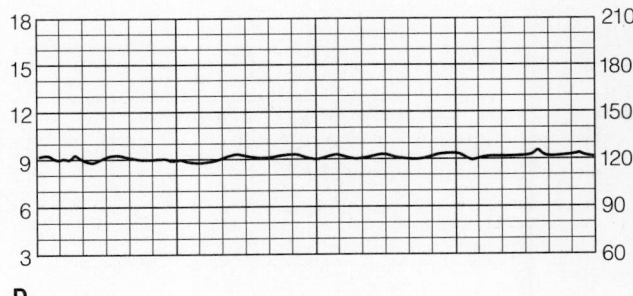

D

FIGURE 22-14　Short- and long-term variability. *A* Increased LTV; STV present. *B* Average LTV; STV absent. *C* Absent LTV; STV present. *D* Absent LTV; STV absent.

The FHR usually ranges between 120 and 160 beats per minute. This wavelike baseline FHR usually has an amplitude of 5 to 15 beats per minute and appears to oscillate in a regular, uniform pattern of two to six cycles per minute; there are differences of opinion about whether this is LTV. Fetal activity may be minimal or absent, and FHR accelerations are lacking. There is no beat-to-beat short-term variability (Figure 22–16).

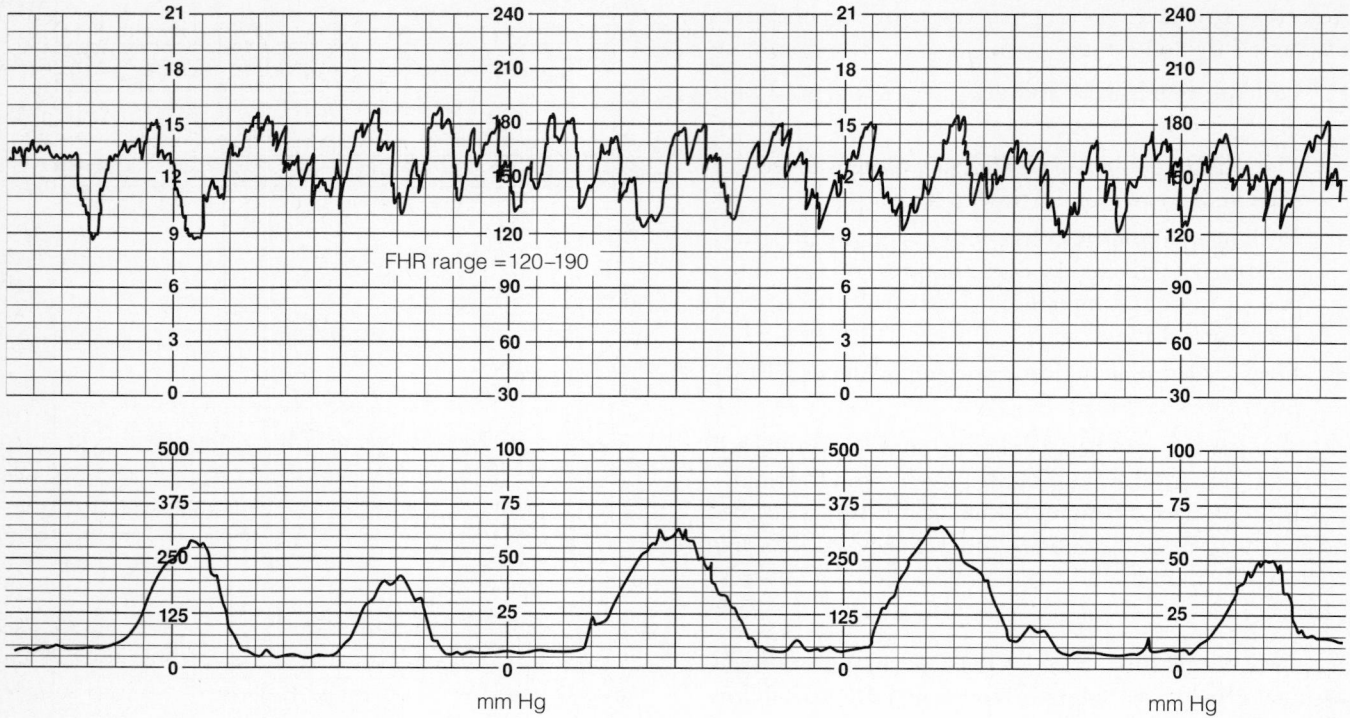

FIGURE 22-15 Saltatory pattern. Note the pattern of marked LTV. FHR varies markedly between 120 and 190 beats per minute. With this type of pattern it is not possible to determine an average baseline FHR because of the wide, marked variations. STV is present.

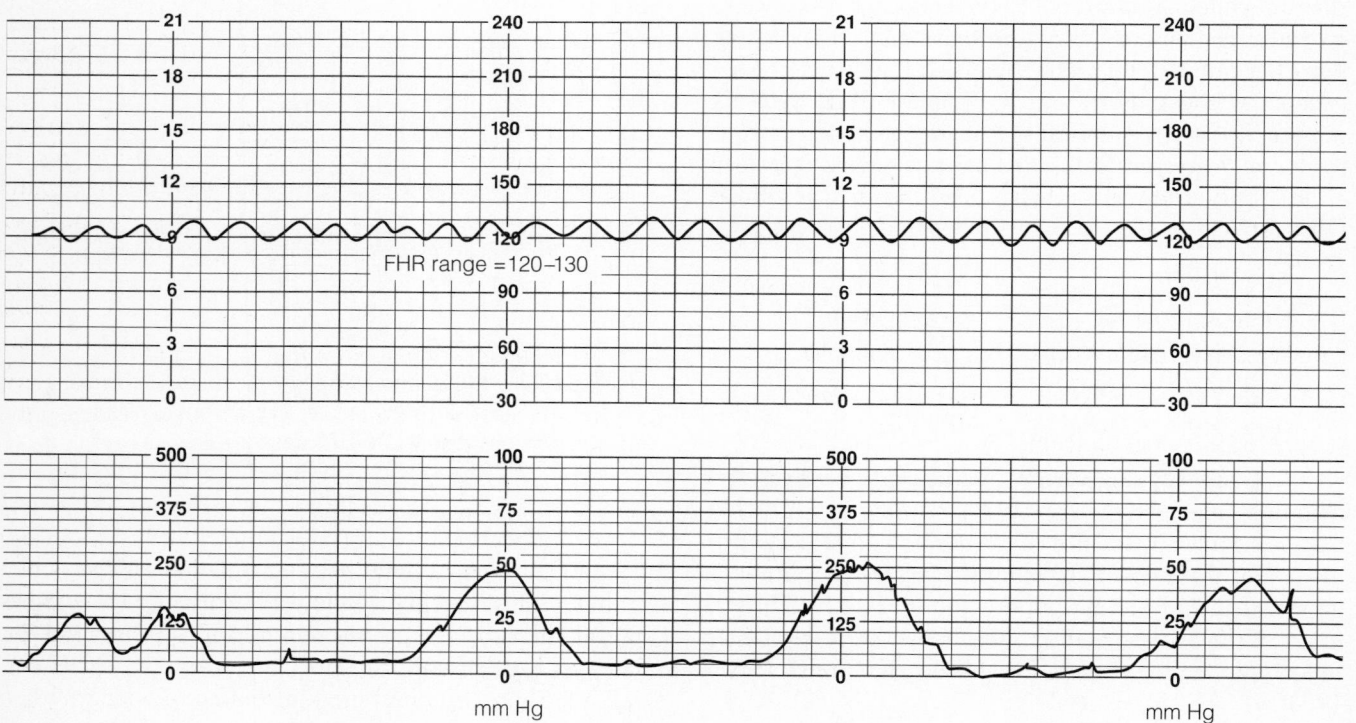

FIGURE 22-16 Sinusoidal pattern. Note the undulating waveform evenly distributed between the 120 and 130 bpm baseline. There is no STV; accelerations or decelerations are not present.

The sinusoidal pattern is associated with Rh iso-immunization, severe anemia, and occasionally asphyxiation (Parer 1994).

In the absence of analgesia-related occurrences, true sinusoidal FHR patterns noted intrapartally suggest fetal anemia or severe asphyxia. If noted by external monitoring, internal fetal monitoring should be instituted, and cesarean birth should be considered if the pattern is confirmed. Fetal blood sampling for determination of pH and hematocrit, ultrasound scan for signs of congestive heart failure and hydrops, and biophysical profile may aid in assessment, evaluation, and management of the fetus with this FHR pattern (Schneider & Tropper 1986).

Short-term variability (STV) refers to the differences between successive heartbeats as measured by the R–R wave interval of the QRS cardiac cycle and therefore represents actual beat-to-beat fluctuations in FHR. STV refers to the tiny fluctuations in FHR noted within the 10-second intervals of the electronic fetal monitoring tracing. These fluctuations average two to three beats per minute. Short-term variability is classified as either present or absent.

Rather than counting specific beats, with practice one can usually become skillful in "eyeballing" the FHR variability. When decreased LTV is noted, one must suspect some compromise of these mechanisms. Increased variability has not been as well defined, and the causes are unknown. The most important aspect of variability is that even in the presence of abnormal or questionable FHR patterns, if the ST variability is normal, the fetus is not suffering from cerebral asphyxia (Parer 1994a). During prolonged bradycardia or severe periodic changes (eg, late or severe variable decelerations, discussed later in this chapter), the fetus may decompensate and suffer cerebral and myocardial asphyxia and consequently demonstrate a decrease or loss of variability. If loss of ST variability accompanies tachycardia, fetal prognosis is usually poor (Parer 1994a), and immediate birth of the fetus should be considered if fetal blood acid-base determination is not feasible.

The nurse needs to keep in mind that STV can be evaluated only by internal monitoring. The external monitoring may demonstrate "normal" variability due to the presence of artifact when in fact it is decreased. An appearance of decreased variability warrants application of an internal electrode. Decreased variability may be seen with the following conditions (Shifrin, 1990; Tucker 1992, p 75):

- Asphyxia and acidosis (decreased blood flow to the fetus)
- Administration of drugs such as Demerol, Valium, Vistaril, Atropine, diazepam and local anesthetics (depress the fetal central nervous system)
- Fetal sleep cycle (usually lasts for 20–30 minutes, during which long-term variability is decreased)
- Fetus of less than 32 weeks' gestation (immature fetal neurologic control of heart rate)

Increased variability may be seen with the following conditions (Tucker 1992, p 74):

- Early mild hypoxia (Variability increases as a result of compensatory mechanism.)
- Fetal stimulation (The autonomic nervous system is stimulated because of abdominal palpitation, maternal vaginal examination, application of spiral electrode on the fetal head, or acoustic stimulation.)

Decreasing variability that does not appear to be associated with a fetal sleep cycle or the administration of drugs is a warning sign of fetal distress. It is especially ominous if decreased variability is accompanied by late decelerations.

External electronic fetal monitoring is not an adequate method to assess and evaluate short-term variability. If decreased variability is noted on external monitoring, application of a spiral electrode should be considered to obtain more accurate information.

Periodic Changes   Periodic changes are transient decelerations or accelerations of the FHR from the baseline that occur in response to contractions and fetal movement.

Acceleration   **Accelerations** are transient increases in the FHR normally caused by fetal movement. As the fetus moves in utero the heart rate increases as it does in adults when they exercise. When the fetus quiets down, the heart rate returns to normal. Acceleration often accompanies contractions, usually as a result of fetal movement in response to pressure of the contracting uterine musculature. Accelerations of this type are thought to be a sign of fetal well-being and adequate oxygen reserve.

Spontaneous accelerations are symmetric, uniform increases in FHR. They are benign, represent an intact CNS response to fetal movements or stimulation, and are not associated with contractions or decelerations. This type of acceleration serves as the criterion for a reactive nonstress test (NST) (Figure 22–17A). *Uniform accelerations* are symmetric, occur with contractions, and reflect the shape of the contraction. They are frequently seen in early labor before the membranes have ruptured, are commonly seen with nonvertex presentations, and are apparently benign (Figure 22–17B).

Variable accelerations are of variable shape and do not reflect the shape of contractions. They may be noted as short periods of increased variability that appear at the beginning and the end of a uterine contraction. The shape of the increased variability appears like "shoulders" around the contraction. These accelerations may also occur before and after variable decelerations and are associated with normal baseline variability. They are apparently benign (Figure 22–17C).

Rebound accelerations ("overshoot") are uniform in shape, immediately follow variable decelerations, and are accompanied by absent baseline variability. Tachycardia is

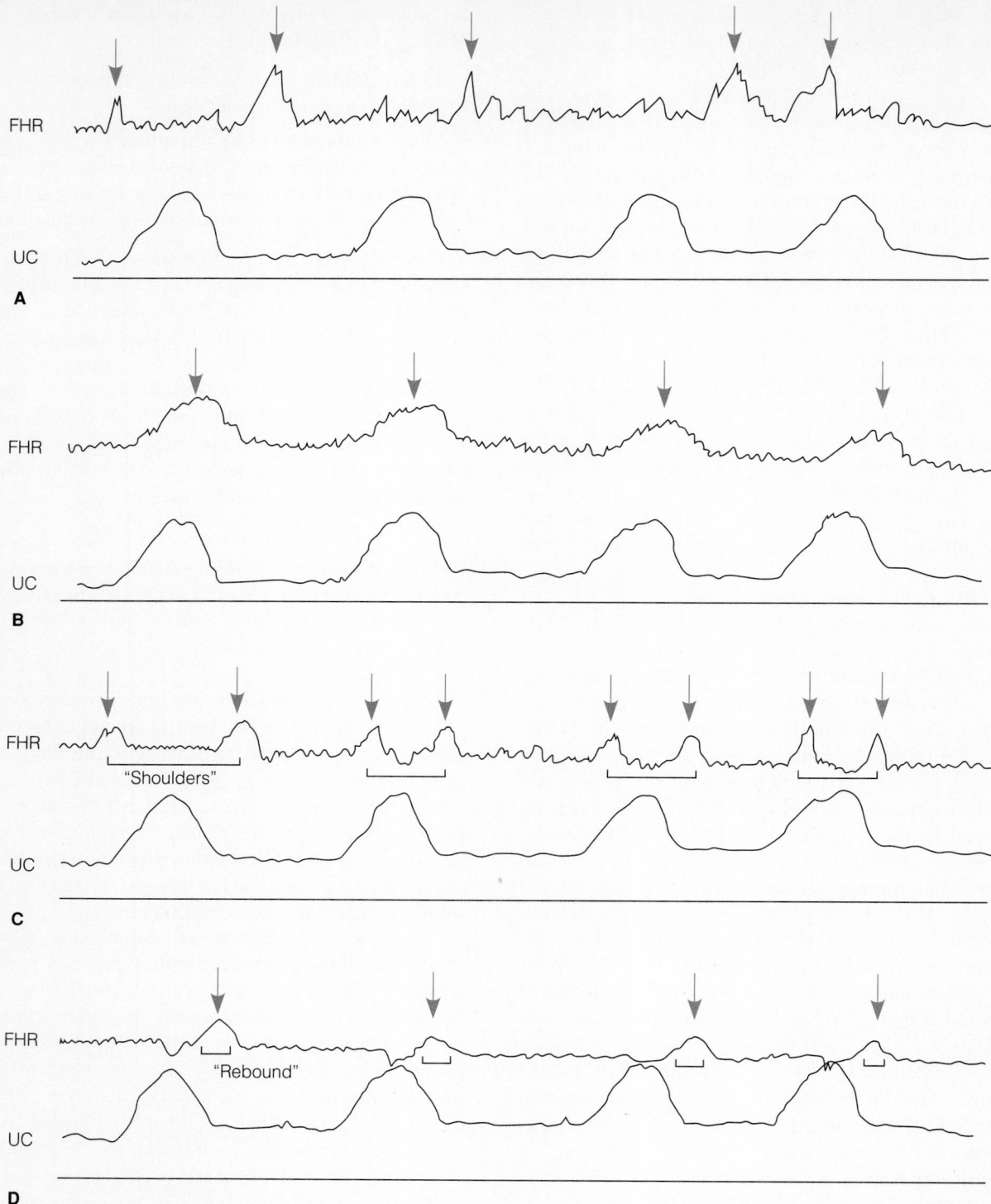

FIGURE 22-17 Types of accelerations. *A* Spontaneous accelerations. *B* Uniform accelerations. *C* Variable accelerations ("shoulders"). *D* Rebound accelerations ("overshoot").

frequently noted with "overshoot." This type of acceleration suggests autonomic nervous system imbalance or exhaustion of fetal compensatory mechanisms. It may be seen in asphyxiated or premature fetuses. Except in the case of prematurity, rebound accelerations should be considered an ominous sign with a deteriorating fetus (Figure 22–17D) (Shifrin 1990).

Deceleration **Decelerations** are periodic decreases in FHR from the normal baseline. Hon and Quilligan (1967) categorized them as early, late, and variable, according to when they occur in the contraction cycle and to their waveform (Figure 22–18).

Early decelerations are due to pressure on the fetal head as it progresses down the birth canal. They have a

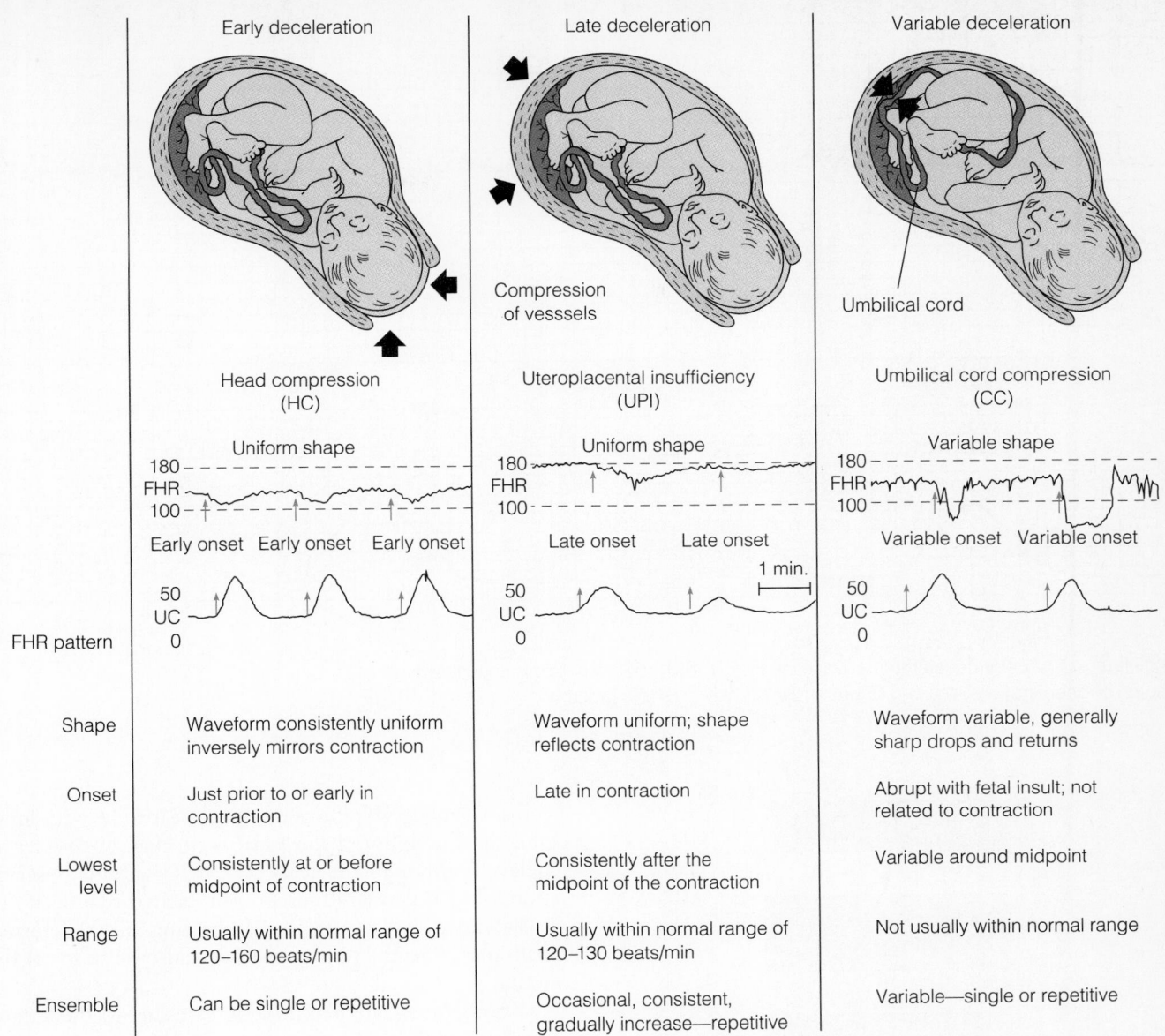

FHR pattern	Early deceleration	Late deceleration	Variable deceleration
	Head compression (HC)	Uteroplacental insufficiency (UPI)	Umbilical cord compression (CC)
Shape	Waveform consistently uniform inversely mirrors contraction	Waveform uniform; shape reflects contraction	Waveform variable, generally sharp drops and returns
Onset	Just prior to or early in contraction	Late in contraction	Abrupt with fetal insult; not related to contraction
Lowest level	Consistently at or before midpoint of contraction	Consistently after the midpoint of the contraction	Variable around midpoint
Range	Usually within normal range of 120–160 beats/min	Usually within normal range of 120–130 beats/min	Not usually within normal range
Ensemble	Can be single or repetitive	Occasional, consistent, gradually increase—repetitive	Variable—single or repetitive

FIGURE 22-18 Types and characteristics of early, late, and variable decelerations.
SOURCE: Hon *E: An Introduction to Fetal Heart Rate Monitoring,* 2nd ed. Los Angeles: University of Southern California School of Medicine, 1972, p 65.

uniform, smooth waveform that inversely mirrors that of the corresponding contraction. Beginning at the onset of the contraction and ending as the contraction ends, the nadir (lowest point) occurs at the peak of the contraction. The nadir is usually within the normal fetal heart rate range (Figure 22–19).

Early decelerations are generally benign and seen late in labor when the fetal head is on the perineum. Increased intracranial pressure results in local changes in cerebral blood flow, which in turn results in stimulation of vagal centers and produces a slowing of heart rate through the vagus nerve (Figure 22–20). If this pattern occurs early in labor, it may be due to head compression from cephalopelvic disproportion. A nurse must take great care in differentiating this type of deceleration from

late decelerations: They look identical yet differ in time of onset.

Early decelerations are not associated with loss of variability, tachycardia, or other FHR changes or with fetal hypoxia, acidosis, or low Apgar scores. Early decelerations are viewed as a reassuring FHR pattern unless seen in early labor or with lack of descent of the fetal head.

Late decelerations are due to uteroplacental insufficiency as the result of decreased blood flow and oxygen transfer to the fetus through the intervillous space during uterine contractions causing hypoxemia (Figure 22–21). They have a smooth, uniform shape that inversely mirrors the contractions (as do early decelerations) but are late in their onset and recovery. They begin at or within a few seconds after the peak of the contraction; the nadir is

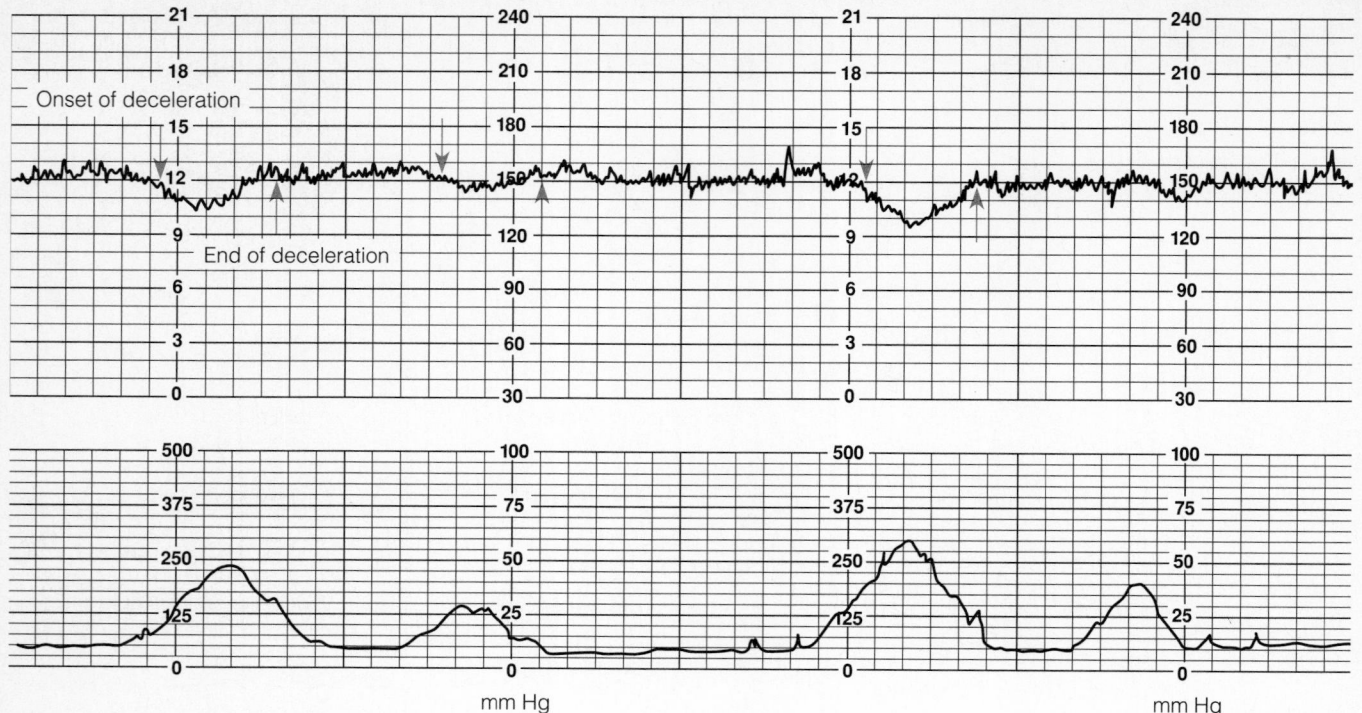

FIGURE 22-19 Early decelerations. Baseline FHR is 150–155 bpm. Nadir (the lowest point) of decelerations is 130–145 bpm. LTV is absent; STV is present.

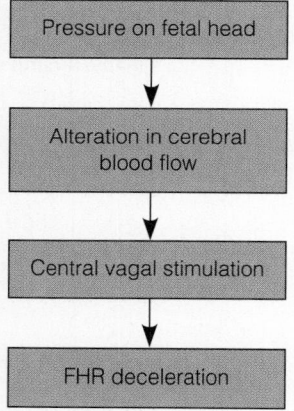

FIGURE 22-20 Mechanism of early deceleration (head compression). SOURCE: Adapted from Freeman RK, Garite TJ: The physiologic basis of fetal monitoring. In: *Fetal Heart Rate Monitoring*. Baltimore: Williams & Wilkins, 1981, p 13.

noted near the end of the contraction. They tend to occur with every contraction. When uteroplacental reserve is adequate, the fetus normally tolerates the transient stress of repetitive contractions. If fetal hypoxia occurs because of a decrease in uteroplacental blood flow (for example, from maternal hypotension or excessive uterine activity), late decelerations generally occur (Figure 22–22).

This pattern is always considered an ominous sign but does not necessarily require immediate birth of the fetus. If late decelerations do not appear to be worsening and the variability of the FHR is normal, birth may be delayed, although the fetus warrants constant observation. Should decelerations worsen, tachycardia occur, or variability decrease, fetal blood sampling for pH determination is indicated to evaluate the acid-base status of the fetus.

Sometimes late decelerations are due to the supine position of the laboring woman. In this case decreased uterine blood flow to the fetus may be alleviated by raising the woman's upper trunk or turning her to the side to displace pressure of the gravid uterus on the inferior vena cava. If the woman remains flat on her back, the fetus will continue to have decelerations due to oxygen compromise.

Late decelerations normally occur within the normal heart rate range (120–160 bpm) and may be quite obvious or very subtle and almost indistinguishable. Some fetuses at highest risk demonstrate a flat FHR baseline with late decelerations that are barely noticeable. It must be kept in mind that the depth of the deceleration does not indicate the severity of the insult.

Chronic uteroplacental insufficiency during pregnancy results in intrauterine growth retardation and, if severe enough, antenatal death. When uteroplacental insufficiency is acute due to factors occurring during labor, fetal distress may ensue. If not properly treated, intrapartal fetal death may occur.

Variable decelerations are appropriately named in that they vary in their onset, occurrence, and waveform. They

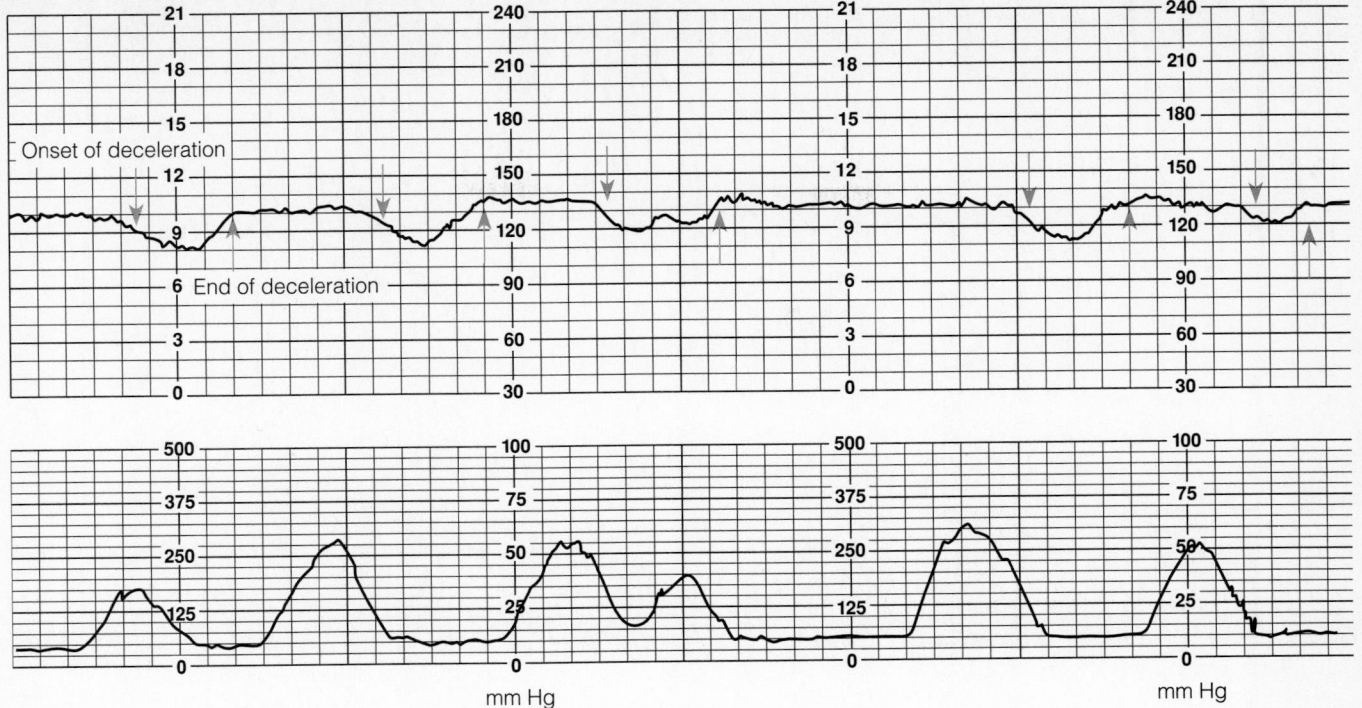

FIGURE 22-21 Late decelerations. Baseline FHR is 130–148 bpm. Nadir (lowest point) of decelerations is 110–120 bpm. LTV and STV are absent.

are thought to be due to umbilical cord occlusion, which decreases the amount of blood flow (therefore oxygen supply) to the fetus (Figure 22–23). Either the fetus squeezes the cord or rolls over onto it, transient pressure is exerted on the cord from compression, or the cord is around the neck of the fetus. An occasional or isolated variable deceleration is usually benign. Variable decelerations that are repetitive and begin to worsen during the course of labor are a cause for concern. Variable decelerations usually fall outside the normal FHR range and are classified as mild, moderate, and severe. They are acute in onset, vary in duration and intensity, and abruptly disappear when the insult of cord compression is relieved (Figure 22–24).

With repetitive decelerations one should suspect nuchal cord (umbilical cord around the neck), short cord, or occult prolapse of the cord. If this pattern becomes evident early in labor, variable decelerations may subsequently demonstrate a slow return to baseline due to repetitive stress. Acid-base status of the fetus should be assessed because cesarean birth, forceps birth, or vacuum extraction might be indicated.

Decelerations that seem to deviate more from the baseline and widen are ominous and warrant further investigation. When they are prolonged and severe, a significant oxygen deficit develops from myocardial depression (Shifrin 1990).

With progressively worsening variable decelerations an overshoot may occur. This is a blunt, smooth acceleration following the contraction and suggests autonomic

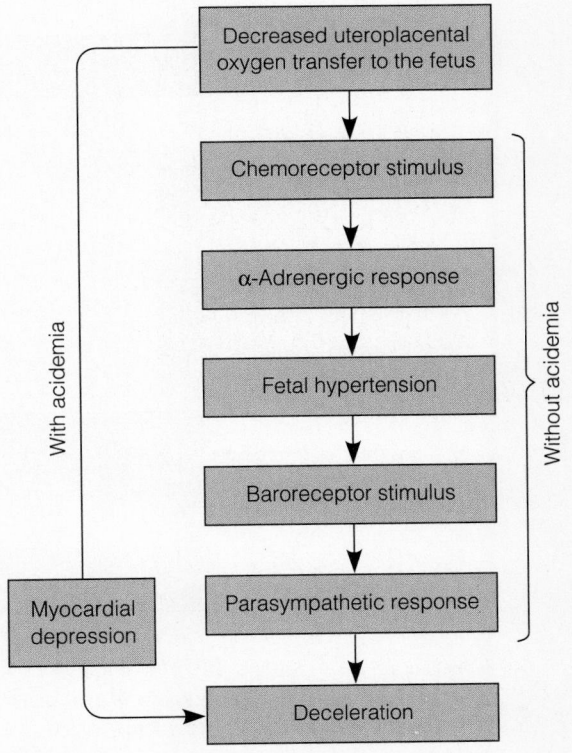

FIGURE 22-22 Mechanism of late deceleration. SOURCE: Freeman RK, Garite TJ: The physiologic basis of fetal monitoring. In: *Fetal Heart Rate Monitoring.* Baltimore: Williams & Wilkins, 1981, p 15.

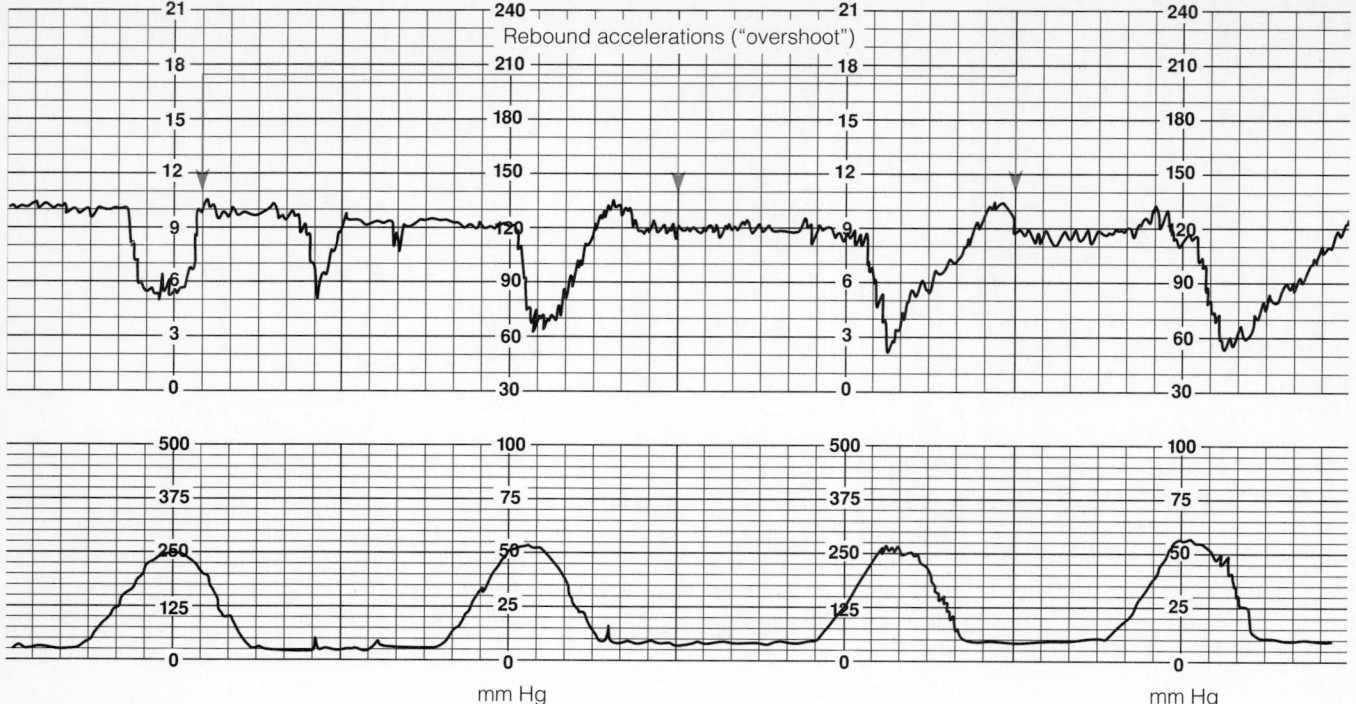

FIGURE 22-23 Variable decelerations with overshoot. The timing of the decelerations is variable, and most have a sharp decline. A rebound acceleration (overshoot) occurs after most of the decelerations. Baseline FHR is 115–130 bpm. Nadir of decelerations is 55–80 bpm. LTV is absent; STV is present.

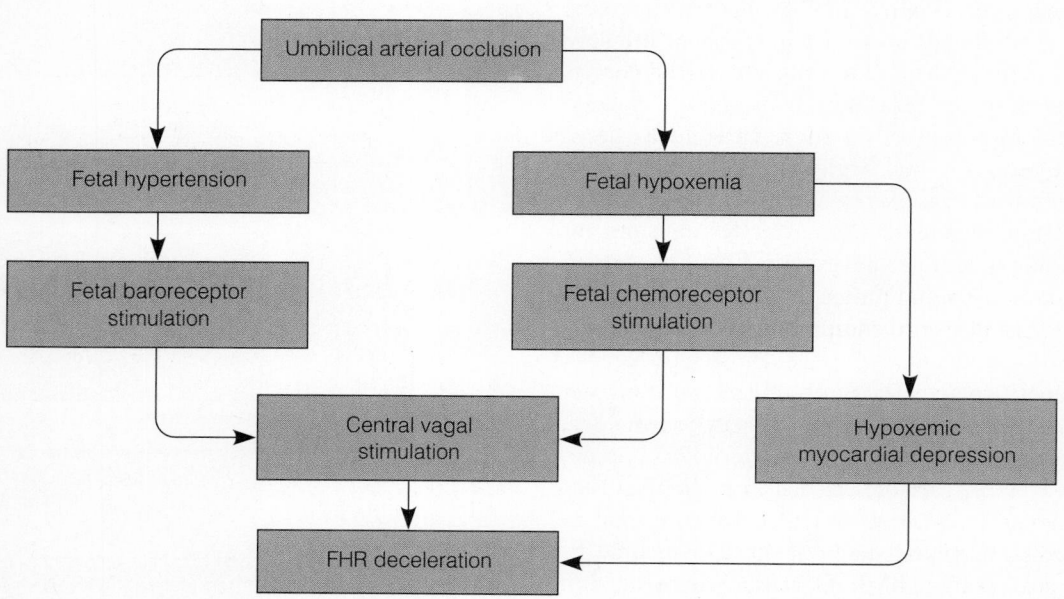

FIGURE 22-24 Mechanism of variable deceleration. SOURCE: Adapted from Freeman RK, Garite TJ: The physiologic basis of fetal monitoring. In: *Fetal Heart Rate Monitoring.* Baltimore: Williams & Wilkins, 1981, p 15.

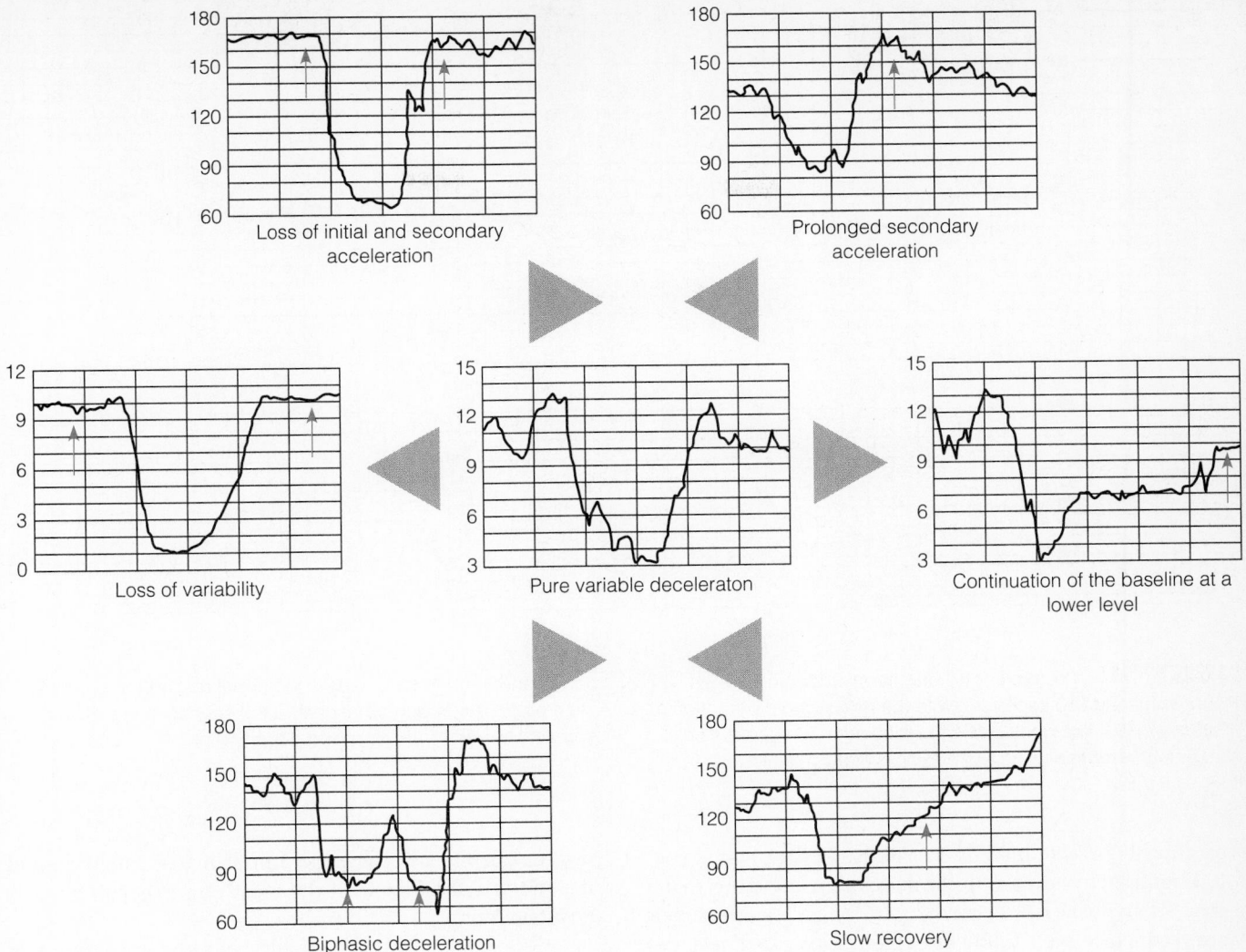

FIGURE 22-25 Atypical variable decelerations. The presence of any of these types of variable decelerations strongly suggests fetal hypoxia, especially when variability is decreased.

SOURCE: Krebs HB, Petrie RE, Dunn LJ: Atypical variable decelerations. *Am J Obstet Gynecol* 1983; 145(3):298.

imbalance of the fetus. It may be seen in neurologically impaired or severely asphyxiated fetuses (Shifrin 1990).

Criteria for evaluation of variable decelerations vary from one author to another, and the very nature of these periodic changes can pose considerable anxiety regarding management. Dr Robert Goodlin's "rule of the 60s" (Parer 1994b, p 285) describes severe variable decelerations as having the following characteristics: variable decelerations below 60 beats per minute, 60 beats per minute below baseline FHR, or variable decelerations lasting more than 60 seconds in duration. These criteria seem to be the easiest to remember and perhaps the most practical.

Variable decelerations are frequently seen in labor when the membranes are ruptured. This decreases protection to the cord especially as the fetus descends down the birth canal. Variable decelerations usually do not warrant immediate birth unless a rising baseline, loss of variability, and other ominous signs accompany them. Repo-

sitioning the woman often corrects this type of pattern. If it does not, the clinician may attempt to alleviate this pattern by insertion of sterile saline via intrauterine catheter (amnioinfusion) to help take pressure off the umbilical cord.

Krebs et al (1983) describe various "atypical variable decelerations," noting that variable decelerations are probably innocuous unless these features are present (Figure 25–25). They note that the presence of these atypical decelerations should be regarded as signs of fetal hypoxia. The nurse should be cognizant of pattern interpretation and be able to recognize severe and "atypical" variables. A point to remember, however, is that in the presence of normal variability of the FHR these variables have not been found to be associated with fetal acidosis and poor outcome.

Prolonged decelerations are those in which the FHR decreases from the baseline for 2 or more minutes (Figure 22–26). They may occur suddenly, and if the pattern is

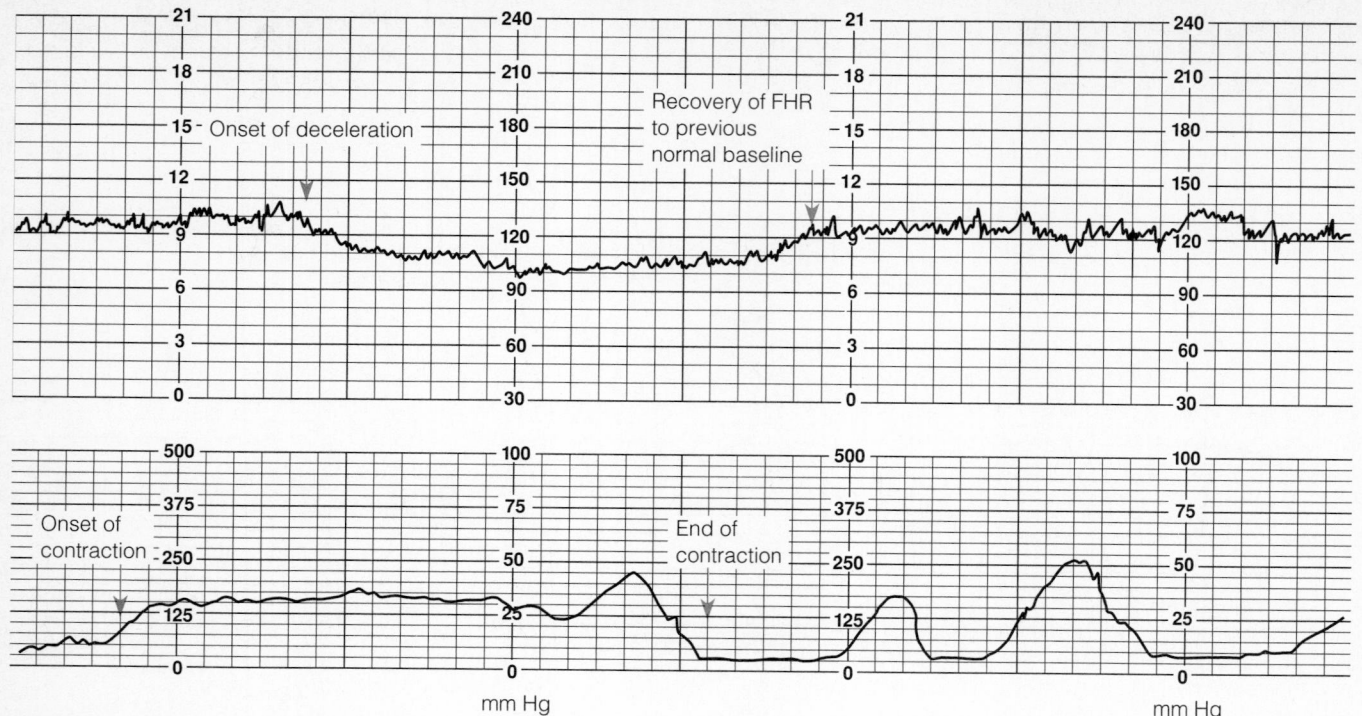

FIGURE 22-26 The prolonged deceleration depicted lasts approximately 160 seconds. Note the prolonged contraction of 120 seconds. The deceleration begins after 80 seconds of uterine contraction. Note the beginning return of FHR 30 sec- onds after uterine tone returns to normal resting tone (contraction ends). An important aspect of this tracing is that STV is present despite the prolonged deceleration.

promptly corrected, FHR variability will remain good. Rebound tachycardia is an ominous sign implying that a state of hypoxia has occurred. Prolonged decelerations are frequently seen following epidural block. These decelerations are thought to be due to fetal toxicity from fetal absorption of the drug through the uterine arteries or spasm of the uterine arteries resulting in decreased blood flow and hypoxia and reflex slowing of the FHR. Prolonged decelerations may often be seen with sudden occult or frank prolapse of the umbilical cord. When decelerations occur following administration of regional anesthesia, the woman should be turned on her side, evaluated for hypotension, and given a bolus of intravenous fluid (500 to 600 mL) to fill the dilated vascular space. This situation can usually be avoided by administering an IV bolus (800 to 900 mL) of lactated Ringer's or normal saline solution to the woman prior to administering regional anesthesia. Solutions containing dextrose should not be given because they may cause fetal hyperglycemia.

Combined decelerations may be seen occasionally when two different deceleration patterns occur together (for example, early/late, early/variable, or variable/late). The specific types of patterns must then be ascertained. For instance, variable decelerations with a slow return to baseline should be differentiated from a combined pattern of variable and late decelerations. The former is a sign that the compression of the umbilical cord is worsening; the latter is in indication of cord compression *plus*

uteroplacental insufficiency. Initial management should be aimed at treatment of the most ominous pattern first (Shifrin 1990).

Sporadic decelerations usually have the appearance of variable decelerations, are unrelated to contractions, and are generally short-lived. They usually appear with reassuring FHR patterns and are apparently of little clinical significance (Shifrin 1990).

Unclassified decelerations are uniform, often resemble late or early decelerations, may be preceded by accelerations, and are not usually repetitive or in proportion to the amplitude or duration of contractions. Treatment is unnecessary if the variability is normal. Scalp sampling should be considered if variability is poor, and the possibility of a fetus with a congenital anomaly should be considered (Shifrin 1990).

Psychologic Reactions to Electronic Monitoring

Many women have no knowledge of monitoring unless they have attended a prenatal class that dealt with this subject, and even then the type of prenatal class may affect the perception of fetal heart rate monitoring. Hansen et al (1985) found that women who attended classes provided by medical or nursing staff preferred electronic fetal monitoring (EFM), but women who attended non-nursing classes preferred auscultation (Syndal 1988).

Studies regarding reactions of women to electronic FHR monitoring reveal a variety of perceived advantages and disadvantages. Hansen et al (1985) found that women who had had a previous stillbirth or were currently in a high-risk pregnancy preferred EFM. While being monitored, women noted they felt constant reassurance that their baby was healthy and that problems would be identified quickly. Some women felt that use of the monitor helped them cope with contractions and even provided a diversion during labor. The monitor also provided a feeling of closeness to their baby and a sense of security. When questioned in the postpartum period, women noted that EFM promoted more involvement of the father during labor and birth (Syndal 1988).

Disadvantages of EFM were also experienced. Some women felt that the EFM increased their anxiety because of the monitor's frequent beeping and buzzing and a lack of understanding of how the monitor worked. The monitor became the focus of attention for many staff members, and some women felt that they had less attention from the nursing staff because a monitor was in place. In addition, some women did not like the hindrance of movement caused by the monitor (Syndal 1988).

Issues Surrounding EFM Use

Electronic fetal monitoring has been associated with some controversy. Experts have studied and debated its uses, advantages, and disadvantages; whether EFM increases cesarean birth rates and, if so, whether this increase is appropriate; and whether EFM improves perinatal morbidity and mortality. Overall in the United States approximately 60–70% of women have EFM during labor (Flamm 1994). In some birth settings all women are monitored continuously throughout their labor; in other settings EFM is used as a screening assessment or on an episodic basis, depending on the presence of risk factors.

In the past, EFM has been considered more effective than intermittent auscultation in reducing perinatal morbidity and mortality, but recent studies do not support this opinion (Albers 1994; Flamm 1994; Spencer 1994). However, looked at more specifically, it has been shown that EFM is more effective than auscultation in identifying abnormalities of the fetal heart (Neilson 1994). Despite its benefits, EFM has certain disadvantages: It is restrictive, requiring the woman to remain in bed, which can precipitate a cascade of problems (Albers 1994; Neilson 1994); and EFM has great potential to decrease the amount of personal care and personal time that the nurse expends on the laboring woman (Albers 1994; Spencer 1994). Albers (1994) identified additional clinical issues: if EFM is critical to intrapartal care, why is it not used for at least one-fourth of women?; preoccupation with EFM has the potential to focus on the needs of the fetus, overshadowing the known needs of the laboring woman; in spite of clinical research that shows no clear advantage of EFM over auscultation, many clinicians insist that EFM is the better method; the use of EFM has altered the staffing and the clinical practice of nurses within the birth area and has focused care on the gathering and interpretation of data, rather than on supportive care.

In light of the continued discussion regarding the relative merits of EFM and auscultation, it behooves professional maternal-child nurses to remain current regarding clinical research findings on these techniques and to examine their own feelings regarding related clinical practice issues. Laboring women need to be given accurate information and need an opportunity to talk about their feelings. The nurse's attitude may influence the woman's interpretation of information and thereby alter choice. When EFM is used, personal supportive care of the laboring woman must remain a priority.

Role of the Nurse

Prior to application of the monitor, the nurse should fully explain to the woman the reason for the monitor and the information that can be derived from its use. The nurse explains how the monitor can help identify the beginning of contractions and thus aid in breathing during the various phases of labor. Explanation of the information regarding the fetal heart rate is also important. An explanation alleviates apprehensions about equipment that may be totally unfamiliar to the woman. During labor it is advantageous to provide education regarding the use of the internal equipment because the care giver may quickly decide to convert to this method as a result of examination findings. Women who are informed about the possibility of internal monitoring are better prepared if a quick decision must be made to apply an electrode or catheter.

After the monitor is applied, basic information should be recorded on the monitor strip. The data included are the date, time, woman's name, physician, hospital or agency number, age, gravida, para, estimated date of birth, membrane status, maternal vital signs, and current medical problems. As the monitor strip continues to run and care is provided, it is important that documentation of occurrences during labor be recorded not only in the nurse's notes on the woman's hospital record, but also on the fetal monitor tracing. The following information should be included on the tracing (AAP-ACOG 1992):

1. Vaginal examinations (dilatation, effacement, station, and position)
2. Amniotomy or spontaneous rupture of membranes, color of amniotic fluid, presence and consistency of meconium
3. Maternal vital signs
4. Maternal position in bed and changes of position
5. Application of spiral electrode or intrauterine pressure catheter
6. Medications
7. Oxygen administration

8. Maternal behaviors (emesis, coughing, hiccups)

9. Fetal scalp stimulation or fetal scalp blood sampling

10. Vomiting

11. Pushing

12. Administration of anesthesia blocks

In addition, if the monitor does not automatically add the time on the strip at specific intervals, it is important to note the time when recording any information on the strip. If more than one nurse is adding information to the monitor strip, it is wise to initial each note. The tracing is considered a legal part of the woman's medical record and is submissible as evidence in court.

It is important for the laboring woman to feel that what is happening to her is the central focus. The nurse can acknowledge this by always speaking to and looking at the woman when entering the room, before looking at the monitor.

Evaluation of FHR Tracings

The nurse tends to use a systematic approach in evaluating FHR tracings to avoid interpreting findings on the basis of inadequate or erroneous data. With a systematic approach the nurse can make a more accurate and rapid assessment, easily communicate data to the woman, physician/certified nurse-midwife, and staff, and have a systematic, universal language for documenting the woman's record.

Evaluation of the electronic monitor tracing begins by looking at the uterine contraction pattern. To evaluate the contraction pattern, the nurse should:

1. Determine the uterine resting tone.

2. Assess the contractions:
    What is the frequency?
    What is the duration?
    What is the intensity (if internal monitoring)?

The next step is to evaluate the fetal heart rate tracing.

1. Determine the baseline:
    Is the baseline within normal range?
    Is there evidence of tachycardia?
    Is there evidence of bradycardia?

2. Determine FHR variability:
    Is short-term variability present or absent?
    Is long-term variability average, minimal, absent, moderate, or marked?

3. Determine if a sinusoidal pattern is present.

4. Determine if there are periodic changes.
    Are accelerations present?
    Do they meet the criteria for a reactive NST?
    Are decelerations present?
    Are they uniform in shape? If so, determine if they are early or late decelerations.

Are they nonuniform in shape? If so, determine if they are variable decelerations.

After evaluating the FHR tracing for the factors just listed, the nurse may further classify the tracing as reassuring (normal) or nonreassuring (worrisome). Reassuring patterns contain normal parameters and do not require additional treatment or intervention.

Characteristics of reassuring FHR patterns include the following:

• Baseline rate is 120–160 bpm.

• Short-term variability is present.

• Long-term variability ranges from three to five cycles per minute.

• Periodic patterns consist of accelerations with fetal movement, and early decelerations may be present.

Nonreassuring patterns indicate that the fetus is becoming stressed and intervention is needed. Characteristics of nonreassuring patterns include the following:

• Severe variable deceleration (FHR drops below 70 bpm for longer than 30–45 seconds and is accompanied by rising baseline or decreasing variability or slow return to baseline.)

• Late decelerations of any magnitude

• Absence of variability (No short-term or long-term variability is present.)

• Prolonged deceleration (Deceleration lasts 60–90 seconds or more.)

• Severe (marked) bradycardia (FHR baseline is 70 bpm or less.)

Nonreassuring patterns may require continuous monitoring and more involved treatment and intervention (Table 22–6).

It is important to provide information to the laboring woman regarding the FHR pattern and the interventions that will help her fetus. Most women are aware that something is happening, and sharing information with them provides reassurance that a potential or actual problem is identified and she is an active participant in the interventions. Occasionally, a problem arises that requires immediate intervention. In that case the nurse can say something like "It is important for you to turn on your left side right now because the baby is having a little difficulty. I'll explain what is happening in just a few moments." This type of response lets the woman know that although an action needs to be accomplished rapidly, information will soon be provided. In our haste to act quickly, we must not forget that it is the woman's body and her baby.

Labor and birth nurses must be skilled and competent in evaluating electronic fetal heart rate patterns. Competence can be maintained through frequent inservice and continuing education programs (Guild 1993; McRae 1993).

Pattern	Nursing Interventions
Variable decelerations Isolated or occasional Moderate	Report findings to physician/CNM and document in chart. Provide explanation to woman and partner. Change maternal position to one in which FHR pattern is most improved. Discontinue oxytocin if it is being administered and other interventions are unsuccessful. Perform vaginal examination to assess for prolapsed cord or change in labor progress. Monitor FHR continuously to assess current status and for further changes in FHR pattern.
Variable decelerations Severe and uncorrectable	Give oxygen if indicated. Report findings to physician/CNM and document in chart. Provide explanation to woman and partner. Prepare for probable cesarean birth. Follow interventions listed above. Prepare for vaginal birth unless baseline variability is decreasing and/or FHR is progressively rising—then cesarean, forceps, or vacuum birth is indicated. Assist physician with fetal scalp sampling if ordered. Prepare for cesarean birth if scalp pH shows acidosis or downward trend.
Late decelerations	Give oxygen if indicated. Report findings to physician/CNM and document in chart. Provide explanation to woman and partner. Monitor for further FHR changes. Maintain maternal position on left side. Maintain good hydration with IV fluids (normal saline or lactated Ringer's). Discontinue oxytocin if it is being administered and late decelerations persist despite other interventions. Administer oxygen by face mask at 7–10 L/minute. Monitor maternal blood pressure and pulse for signs of hypotension; possibly increase flow rate of IV fluids to treat hypotension. Follow physician's orders for treatment for hypotension if present. Increase IV fluids to maintain volume and hydration (normal saline or lactated Ringer's). Assess labor progress (dilatation and station). Assist physician with fetal blood sampling: If pH stays above 7.25, physician will continue monitoring and resample; if pH shows downward trend (between 7.25 and 7.20) or is below 7.20, prepare for birth by most expeditious means.
Late decelerations with tachycardia and/or decreasing variability	Report findings to physician/CNM and document in chart. Maintain maternal position on left side. Administer oxygen by face mask at 7–10 L/minute. Discontinue oxytocin if it is being administered. Assess maternal blood pressure and pulse. Increase IV fluids (normal saline or lactated Ringer's). Assess labor progress (dilatation and station). Prepare for immediate cesarean birth. Explain plan of treatment to woman and partner. Assist physician with fetal blood sampling (if ordered).
Prolonged decelerations	Perform vaginal examination to rule out prolapsed cord or to determine progress in labor status. Change maternal position as needed to try to alleviate decelerations. Discontinue oxytocin if it is being administered. Notify physician/CNM of findings/initial interventions and document in chart. Provide explanation to woman and partner. Increase IV fluids (normal saline or lactated Ringer's). Administer tocolytic if hypertonus noted and ordered by physician/CNM. Anticipate normal FHR recovery following deceleration if FHR previously normal. Anticipate intervention if FHR previously abnormal or deceleration lasts > 3 minutes.

ADDITIONAL ASSESSMENT TECHNIQUES

Scalp Stimulation Test

When there is a question regarding fetal status, the **scalp stimulation test** can be used before the more invasive fetal blood sampling. To use this technique, the examiner applies pressure to the fetal scalp while doing a vaginal examination. The fetus who is not in any stress or distress responds with an acceleration of the FHR (Miller 1990).

Fetal Scalp Blood Sampling

When nonreassuring or confusing FHR patterns are noted, additional information regarding the acid-base status of the fetus must be sought. This may be accomplished by the physician obtaining a **fetal scalp blood**

sample. The blood sample is usually drawn from the fetal scalp, but may be obtained from the fetus in the breech position (Boylan & Parisi 1994).

Boylan and Parisi (1994) suggest that fetal blood sampling may be of benefit in the following situations:

- Presence of thick meconium in the amniotic fluid (Thick meconium may be associated with fetal hypoxia, and the development of meconium aspiration syndrome is associated with the presence of acidosis at birth.)

- Absent short-term variability

- Decreased short-term variability that is present when the fetus is first monitored or that develops in the absence of administration of CNS depressants to the mother

- Later decelerations that persist for more than 10 minutes and do not respond to treatment measures

- Variable decelerations with decreased or absent short-term variability

- FHR patterns that are difficult to interpret

Fetal Blood Sampling Procedure

Equipment needed for fetal blood sampling is available in sterile disposable trays. Items included are heparinized capillary tubes, a short capillary tube holder, a 2 mm blade on long handle, a conical beveled endoscope, clay sealant, silicone gel, and long sponge swabs. An extra light source is needed. The woman's vulva and perineum should be thoroughly cleansed with povidone-iodine solution (Betadine) and sterile drapes arranged. A conical vaginal endoscope is inserted into the vagina and through the cervix to visualize the fetal site to be sampled (Figure 22–27). Working through the endoscope, the physician cleanses the site to remove vernix, blood, and amniotic fluid. Silicone gel is then applied to the site to provide a surface for the formation of a globule of blood. The site is punctured with a 2×2 mm microscalpel. A small amount (0.25 mL) of blood is then collected in a long heparinized capillary tube and immediately assessed for pH and base deficit values. Two or three samples should be collected during each procedure to confirm reliability of values. pH and base deficit determinations should be readily available in 10 to 15 minutes for this procedure to be of value.

The clotting mechanism is compromised when pH is lowered; therefore oozing at the site may occur for a period of time. Because loss of even minimal amounts of blood may be disastrous to the fetus, pressure is applied to the puncture site throughout two maternal contractions; then the site is observed through a third contraction. After the procedure the woman is observed for vaginal bleeding to assure that what may appear to be heavy bloody show is not a fetal hemorrhage from the puncture site.

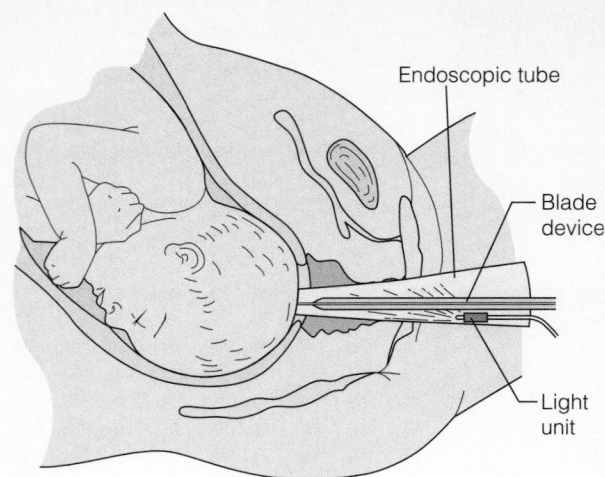

FIGURE 22-27 Technique of obtaining fetal blood from the scalp during labor. SOURCE: Creasy RK, Parer JT: Prenatal care and diagnosis. In: *Pediatrics,* 16th ed. Rudolph AM [editor]. Englewood Cliffs, NJ: Appleton-Century-Crofts, 1977.

The major fetal problem that may occur with fetal blood sampling is hemorrhage, especially if the fetus has blood dyscrasia such as hemophilia or von Willebrand's disease. In addition the use of a vacuum extractor to assist in vaginal birth following numerous punctures may be associated with bleeding problems. Infection of the scalp may occur about 1% of the time (Boylan & Parisi 1994).

Fetal Blood Sample Results

Normal pH values during labor are at or above 7.25, with 7.20 to 7.24 considered preacidotic. Values below 7.20 indicate serious acidosis. Most clinicians consider a pH value of 7.25 or more as normal and reassuring and resample only as indicated by FHR variability or periodic pattern. Values between 7.20 and 7.25 are evaluated on the basis of several factors, and sampling is usually repeated within 15 to 20 minutes (Depp 1990) to observe the trend in pH and base deficit. When a low pH is present, it is important to distinguish between respiratory and metabolic acidosis because management of each situation is different. Respiratory acidosis is indicated by a pH below 7.25 and a base deficit less than −6. Respiratory acidosis is associated with cord compression or uterine hyperstimulation, and the fetus may benefit from intrauterine resuscitation. Metabolic acidosis is indicated by a pH less than 7.25 and a base deficit of greater than −6. Metabolic acidosis is more frequently associated with a chronic condition of the fetus and indicates the need for immediate birth (Boylan & Parisi 1994). Values below 7.20 are considered acidotic and warrant immediate birth (Depp 1990) (Table 22–7).

TABLE 22–7	Review of Terms and Values Used in Acid-Base Measurements
pH	Is a measure of oxygen availability to the fetus.
P_{CO_2}	Is the respiratory component. Increased P_{CO_2} is associated with acidosis. Normal P_{CO_2} is associated with metabolic acidosis.
Base deficit	Is a metabolic component and provides a measure of bicarbonate deficit.
P_{O_2}	Refers to partial pressure of oxygen in blood.
Normal values:	pH: 7.25–7.40
	P_{CO_2}: 35–45 mm Hg
	Base deficit: 4–7 mEq/L
	P_{O_2}: 20–30 mm Hg

SOURCE: Shifrin BS: *Exercises in Fetal Monitoring.* St Louis: Mosby-Year Book, 1990.

Associated Factors

Some FHR patterns seem to be associated with abnormal fetal acid-base status. Short-term and long-term variability correlate better with fetal pH than deceleration patterns do. If STV and LTV are present, the pH will be in the normal range. If STV is present, the fetal pH is usually normal even in the presence of late decelerations. If STV is absent, however, the risk of acidosis increases. When STV is absent and variable decelerations are occurring, the pH will be in the preacidotic range. If late decelerations occur with no STV present, the pH will probably be in the acidotic range (Campbell et al 1986).

These findings are of particular significance when nonreassuring FHR patterns are observed and fetal acid-base determination is not feasible. One can be reassured that the fetus is not acidotic in almost 100% of cases if the variability remains normal (Parer 1994a). A pH above 7.25 predicts that the fetus will be vigorous in about 90% of cases; a pH below 7.15 predicts a depressed fetus with only 80% reliability (Parer 1994a). Fetal blood sampling seems unnecessary when variability is normal because the fetus will be vigorous despite the pH value.

Although not universally used at present, a pH electrode attached to the fetal scalp tissue can be used to monitor fetal pH continuously. This electrode does not measure fetal blood pH level per se, but rather the subcutaneous tissue pH level. In hypoxia an increase in alpha-adrenergic activity occurs initially with accompanying fetal hypertension, causing acidosis to occur in peripheral tissue more rapidly than in the central circulation. Conversely, as hypoxia is corrected, there may be a recovery lag of about 5 minutes in the pH value in the peripheral tissue (Boylan & Parisi 1994).

Considerable skill is required for both continuous and intermittent fetal blood sampling. As yet, even intermittent sampling is not widely done due to the difficulty of the procedure and the scarcity of blood gas microanalyzers on or near the birth unit to obtain immediate results.

Percutaneous Umbilical Blood Sampling

Percutaneous umbilical blood sampling (PUBS) or cordocentesis is a fetal assessment technique that involves obtaining a fetal blood sample from the umbilical cord. This entails inserting a needle through the maternal abdomen to access the umbilical vessels. Done under ultrasound guidance, the procedure can be performed at the bedside to assess fetal acid-base status during labor when fetal blood sampling may not be feasible and FHR patterns are confusing or worrisome (Hobbins et al 1985). See Chapter 20 for a description of the procedure. The procedure is also most helpful in the management of women with idiopathic thrombocytopenic purpura. Early assessment of fetal platelet count using this procedure may allow these women to give birth vaginally rather than by cesarean when the fetus cannot be assessed by fetal blood sampling because of inadequate dilatation of the cervix.

Cord Blood Analysis at Birth

In cases where there have been significant abnormal FHR patterns noted prior to birth, meconium-stained amniotic fluid, or a depressed infant at birth, analysis of umbilical cord blood may be done immediately after birth to assess the infants' respiratory status. The cord is usually clamped before the infant takes its first breath to provide evaluation of blood gas status before the infant interacts with the extrauterine environment because values can change after only a few seconds of neonatal breathing.

An 8- to 10-inch segment of the umbilical cord is double-clamped and cut, and a small amount of blood is aspirated from one of the umbilical arteries (arterial blood seems to provide the most reliable indication of blood gas status and fetal tissue pH). Blood is collected in a heparinized syringe unless it is to be analyzed immediately; it should not be allowed to remain in the segment of cord longer than 30 minutes. As noted by Depp (Chez & Depp 1987), the only reason for not doing routine cord blood analysis is the added expense. Other clinicians may collect a segment of cord and send samples only if the Apgar score is below 7 at 5 minutes, as recommended by the American College of Obstetricians and Gynecologists (1991). In this instance values might be used to clarify the cause of a low Apgar score while minimizing any medicolegal exposure and expense. Determination of pH and base deficit values can differentiate whether fetal acidemia is due to hypoperfusion of the placenta or cord compression.

Intrapartal assessment includes attention to both physical and psychosociocultural parameters of the laboring woman, assessment of the fetus, and ongoing assessment for conditions that place the woman and her fetus at increased risk.

A sterile vaginal examination determines the status of fetal membranes, cervical dilatation and effacement, and fetal presentation, position, and station.

Uterine contractions may be assessed by palpation or by an electronic monitor. The electronic monitor may be used for external or internal monitoring.

Leopold's maneuvers provide a systematic evaluation of fetal presentation and position.

Fetal presentation and position may also be assessed by vaginal examination or ultrasound.

The fetal heart rate may be assessed by auscultation (with a fetoscope) or electronic monitoring.

Electronic fetal monitoring is accomplished by indirect ultrasound or by direct methods that require the placement of a spiral electrode on the fetal presenting part.

Indications for electronic monitoring include fetal, maternal, and uterine factors; presence of pregnancy complications; regional anesthesia; and elective monitoring.

True variability of the FHR can be assessed only by direct electronic monitoring.

Baseline FHR refers to the range of FHR observed between contractions during a 10-minute period of monitoring.

The normal range of FHR is 120–160 beats per minute.

Baseline changes of the FHR include tachycardia, bradycardia, and variability.

Tachycardia is defined as a rate of 160 beats per minute or more for a 10-minute segment of time.

Bradycardia is defined as a rate of less than 120 beats per minute for a 10-minute segment of time.

Baseline variability is an important parameter of fetal well-being. It includes both long- and short-term variability.

Periodic changes are transient decelerations or accelerations of the FHR from the baseline. Accelerations are normally caused by fetal movement. Decelerations may be termed early, late, variable, or sinusoidal.

Early decelerations are due to compression of the fetal head during contractions and are considered reassuring.

Late decelerations are associated with uteroplacental insufficiency and are considered ominous.

Variable decelerations are associated with compression of the umbilical cord.

Sinusoidal patterns are characterized by an undulant sine wave.

Psychologic reactions to monitoring vary between feelings of relief and feelings of being tied down.

Birthing room nurses have responsibilities in recognizing and interpreting fetal monitoring patterns, notifying the physician/CNM of problems, and initiating corrective and supportive measures when needed.

Fetal scalp stimulation can be used when there is a question regarding fetal status.

Fetal acid-base status may be assessed by fetal blood sampling.

A sample of fetal blood may be obtained by a process called percutaneous umbilical blood sampling.

REFERENCES

ACOG: Committee opinion: Utility of umbilical cord blood acid-base assessment, 1991.

Albers LL: Clinical issues in electronic fetal monitoring. *Birth* 1994; 21(2):108.

American Academy of Pediatrics and American College of Obstetricians and Gynecologists: *Guidelines for Perinatal Care*, 2nd ed. Washington, DC: 1992.

Bergstrom L et al: "You'll feel me touching you, Sweetie": Vaginal examinations during the second stage of labor. *Birth* March 1993; 19:10.

Boesel RR et al: Umbilical cord blood studies help assess fetal respiratory status. *Contemp OB/GYN* November 1986; 28:(Medical Economics Co reprint, p 1).

Boylan PC, Parisi VM: Acid-base physiology in the fetus. In: *Maternal-Fetal Medicine: Principles and Practice*, 3rd ed. Creasy RK, Resnik R (editors). Philadelphia: WB Saunders, 1994.

Brady K et al: Reliability of fetal buttock blood sampling in assessing the acid-base balance of the breech fetus. *Obstet Gynecol* 1989; 74:886.

Cabaniss ML: *Fetal Monitoring Interpretation*. Philadelphia: Lippincott, 1993.

Campbell WA, Vintzileos AM, Nochimson DJ: Intrauterine versus extrauterine management/resuscitation of the fetus/neonate. *Clin Obstet Gynecol* 1986; 29(1):33.

Chez RA, Depp R: What cord blood analysis tells you (clinical dialogue). *Contemp OB/GYN* November 1987; 30:43.

Depp R: Clinical evaluation of fetal status. In: *Danforth's Obstetrics and Gynecology*, 6th ed. Scott JR et al (editors). Philadelphia: Lippincott, 1990.

Devoe LD et al: Monitoring intrauterine pressure during active labor. *J Reprod Med* October 1989; 34:811.

Flamm BL: Electronic fetal monitoring in the United States. *Birth* 1994; 21(2):105.

Freeman RK, Garite TJ: *Fetal Heart Rate Monitoring*. Baltimore: Williams & Wilkins, 1981.

Friedman EA: An objective method of evaluating labor. *Hosp Prac* 1970; 5:82.

Fukushima R et al: A beltless tocodynamometer: A preliminary report. *Obstet Gynecol* May 1989; 73:823.

Goyert GL, Sokol RJ, D'Angelo LJ: Practical fetal monitoring during labor. In: *Gynecology and Obstetrics*, vol 2. Dilts PV, Sciarri JJ (editors). Philadelphia: Lippincott, 1989.

Guild SD: A comprehensive fetal monitoring program for nursing practice and education. *JOGNN* 1993; 23(1):34.

Hansen PK et al: Maternal attitudes to fetal monitoring. *Eur J Obstet Gynecol Reprod Biol* 1985; 20:43.

Hobbins JC et al: Percutaneous umbilical blood sampling. *Am J Obstet Gynecol* 1985; 152(1):1.

Hon EH: *An Introduction to Fetal Heart Rate Monitoring*, 2nd ed. Los Angeles: University of Southern California School of Medicine.

Hon EH, Quilligan EJ: The classification of fetal heart rate: II. A revised working classification. *Conn Med* 1967; 31:779.

Johannsen JM: Update: Guidelines for treating hypertension. *AJN* March 1993; 93(3):42.

Krebs HB, Petrie RE, Dunn LJ: Atypical variable deceleration. *Am J Obstet Gynecol* 1983; 142:297.

Larson EB et al: Fetal monitoring and predictions by clinicians: Observations during a randomized clinical trial in very low birth weight infants. *Obstet Gynecol* October 1989; 74:584.

Martin CB, Gingerich B: Factors affecting the fetal heart rate: Genesis of FHR patterns. *JOGNN* 1976; 5(suppl):305s.

McKay S, Smith SY: "What are they talking about? Is something wrong?" Information sharing during the second stage of labor. *Birth* 1993; 20(3):142.

McFarland J, Parker B: Preventing abuse during pregnancy: An assessment and intervention protocol. *MCN* November/December 1994; 19:321.

McRae MJ: Litigation, electronic fetal monitoring, and the obstetric nurse. *JOGNN* 1993; 22(5):410.

Miller F: Fetal scalp stimulation. In: *Current Therapy in Obstetrics and Gynecology*. Quilligan EJ, Zuspan FP (editors). Philadelphia: WB Saunders, 1990.

Murray M: *Antepartal and Intrapartal Fetal Monitoring*. Washington, DC: NAACOG, 1989.

NAACOG: *Fetal Heart Rate Auscultation*. OGN Nursing Practice Resource. March 1990.

NAACOG: Statement: Nursing responsibilities in implementing intrapartum fetal heart rate monitoring. October 1988.

Neilson JP: Roundtable discussion: Controversies in electronic fetal heart rate monitoring during labor: Information from randomized trials. *Birth* 1994; 21(2):101.

Parer JT: Fetal acid-base balance. In: *Maternal-Fetal Medicine*. Creasy RK, Resnik R (editors). Philadelphia: WB Saunders, 1994a.

Parer JT: Fetal heart rate. In: *Maternal-Fetal Medicine*. Creasy RK, Resnik R (editors). Philadelphia: WB Saunders, 1994b.

Schneider EP, Tropper PJ: The variable deceleration, prolonged deceleration, and sinusoidal fetal heart rate. *Clin Obstet Gynecol* 1986; 29(1):64.

Shifrin BS: *Exercises in Fetal Monitoring*. St Louis: Mosby-Year Book, 1990.

Spencer J: Electronic fetal monitoring in the United Kingdom. *Birth* 1994; 21(2):106.

Strong TH, Paul RH: Intrapartum evaluation of an intrauterine pressure transducer. *Obstet Gynecol* March 1989; 73:432.

Syndal SH: Responses of laboring women to fetal heart rate monitoring. *J Nurse-Midwifery* September/October 1988; 33:208.

Thacker SB: The efficacy of intrapartum electronic fetal monitoring. *Am J Obstet Gynecol* November 1987; 156:4.

Tucker SM: *Pocket Guide Fetal Monitoring*. St Louis: Mosby, 1992.

Wilson RW, Shifrin BS: Is any pregnancy low risk? *Obstet Gynecol* 1980; 55:653.

CHAPTER 23

THE FAMILY IN CHILDBIRTH: NEEDS AND CARE

E ach birth is so special. When the new parents see their baby, it seems that time is suspended. I watch as they gaze at their baby and reach out with their fingers to touch the baby's hands and fingers. I have been so fortunate to be a birthing room nurse and to share this experience with so many new families, but each time is like no other.

KEY TERMS

Apgar score

Hyperventilation

Precipitous birth

OBJECTIVES

Compare the advantages and disadvantages of alternative settings for labor and birth.

Identify options that the childbearing family has during the intrapartal period.

Identify the data base to be created from information obtained upon admission to the birthing area.

Review the nursing care that is given during admission.

Plan strategies to meet the needs of the childbearing family.

Discuss nursing interventions to meet the needs of the laboring woman and the father during each stage of labor.

Integrate knowledge of nursing care of the family in the intrapartal period through the use of the nursing process.

Summarize immediate nursing care of the newborn following birth.

Discuss initial measures to assist the integration of the newborn into family life.

Delineate management of a nurse-managed precipitous birth.

*I*t is time for a child to be born. The waiting is over; labor has begun. The dreams and wishes of the past months fade as the expectant family faces the reality of the tasks of childbearing and childrearing that are ahead.

The family is about to undergo one of the most meaningful and stressful events in their life together. The adequacy of their preparation for childbirth will now be tested. The coping mechanisms, communication, and support systems that they have established will be put to the test. The childbearing family may feel that their psychologic and physical limits are about to be challenged. The laboring woman may question her ability to cope with the challenges of labor and to meet her expectations for herself. The father may wonder if he is really ready and able to provide the kind of support and assistance that will be needed. They may worry about the baby's health. Although they look forward to the birth of their baby, the realities of parenthood and incorporating a new family member also present challenges. They both enter a relatively unknown environment where, even with prenatal preparation, many challenges and unknown possibilities await them.

Maternal-newborn nursing has kept pace with the changing philosophy of childbirth. Nurses who choose positions in a birthing area are presented with many opportunities to interact with a wide variety of childbearing families, from one that wants maximal decision making and participation in their care to one that wants more interaction with the nurse, to a single woman who enters the birthing experience alone, without support. It is frequently a challenge to provide high-level care in a relaxed atmosphere as well as supportive, culturally sensitive care to such a wide variety of clients.

The previous two chapters present information that is basic to this chapter. Chapter 21 presents a database of information regarding physiologic and psychologic changes during labor and birth, and Chapter 22 discusses intrapartal assessment. This chapter discusses nursing care during labor and birth.

NURSING DIAGNOSIS DURING LABOR AND BIRTH

When a plan of care is devised for the intrapartal period, the nurse can develop a general plan that encompasses all of the process, from the beginning of labor through the fourth stage, or the plan can be developed for each stage of labor and birth. An overall plan presents an overview of the whole process, but it is usually general in nature. A plan of care that identifies nursing diagnoses for (at least) each stage provides an opportunity to identify more specific nursing care. In the first stage nursing diagnoses that

may be selected include (1) Fear related to discomfort of labor and unknown labor outcome, (2) Compromised, ineffective family coping related to labor process, (3) Pain related to uterine contractions, cervical dilatation, and fetal descent, (4) Knowledge deficit related to lack of information about normal labor process and comfort measures, and (5) Anxiety related to unknown birth outcome and anticipated discomfort. Nursing diagnoses for the second and third stages may include (1) Pain related to uterine contractions, birth process, and/or perineal trauma from birth, (2) Knowledge deficit related to lack of information about pushing methods prior to birth, (3) Ineffective individual coping related to birth process, and (4) Fear related to outcome of birth process. In the fourth stage, possible nursing diagnoses include (1) Pain related to perineal trauma, (2) Knowledge deficit related to lack of information about involutional process and self-care needs, and (3) Altered family processes related to incorporation of newborn into the family.

NURSING PLAN AND IMPLEMENTATION DURING ADMISSION

Families, especially fathers, are concerned about getting to the hospital on time. Sometimes labor occurs so rapidly that birth is imminent upon admission. Usually, family members plan to arrive at the birth setting at the beginning of the active phase of labor or when the following occur:

- Rupture of membranes (ROM)

- Regular, frequent uterine contractions (nulliparas, 5–10 minutes apart for 1 hour; multiparas, 10–15 minutes apart for 1 hour)

- Any vaginal bleeding

If time permits and the family is not familiar with what will occur during labor, the nurse can provide information. (See Teaching Guide: What To Expect During Labor on page 638.)

The families may be facing a number of unfamiliar procedures that are routine for health care providers. It is important to remember that all women have the right to determine what happens to their bodies. *Informed consent should be obtained prior to any procedure that involves touching the body.*

How the maternity nurse greets the woman and her partner influences the course of her hospital stay. The sudden environmental change and the sometimes impersonal and technical aspects of admission can produce emotional stress. If the family is greeted in a brusque, harried manner, they are less likely to look to the nurse

WHAT TO EXPECT DURING LABOR

Assessment   As each woman is admitted into the birthing area the nurse assesses the woman's knowledge regarding the childbirth experience. The woman's knowledge base will be affected by previous births, attendance at childbirth education classes, and the amount of information she has been able to gather during her pregnancy by asking questions or reading. The nurse also assesses the factors that affect communication and anxiety level. Labor progress is assessed so that decisions regarding what to teach and the time available for teaching can be ascertained. If the woman is in early labor and she needs additional information, the nurse proceeds with teaching.

Nursing Diagnosis   The key nursing diagnosis probably will be: Knowledge deficit related to lack of information about nursing care during labor.

Nursing Plan and Implementation   The teaching focuses on information regarding the assessments and support the woman will receive during labor.

Client Goals   At the completion of the teaching the woman will be able to do the following:

1. Verbalize the assessments the nurse will complete during labor

2. Discuss the support/comfort measures that are available

Teaching Plan

Content   Aspects of the admission process include the following:

*   Abbreviated history

*   Physical assessment (maternal vital signs [VS], fetal heart rate [FHR], contraction status, status of membranes)

*   Assessment of uterine contractions (frequency, duration, intensity)

*   Orientation to surroundings

*   Introductions to other staff who will be assisting her

*   Determination of woman's and family support person's expectations of the nurse

Present aspects of ongoing physical care, such as when to expect assessment of maternal VS, FHR, and contractions.

If electronic fetal monitor is used, orient the woman to how it works and the information it provides. Orient woman to sights and sounds of monitor. Explain what "normal" data will look like and what characteristics are being watched for.

Be sure to note that assessments will increase as the labor progresses; about the time the woman would like to be left alone (transition phase), the assessments increase in order to help keep the mother and baby safe by noting any changes from the normal course.

Explain the vaginal examination and what information can be obtained.

Review comfort techniques that may be used in labor, and ascertain what the woman thinks will be effective in promoting comfort.

Review breathing techniques the woman has learned so the nurse will be able to support her technique.

Review comfort/support measures such as: positioning, back rub, effleurage, touch, distraction techniques, ambulation.

If woman is in early labor, offer to give her a tour of the birthing area.

Teaching Method   *Provide information on the basic assessment and care activities. Allow time for questions and discussion as labor progress permits.*

Bring fetal monitor into the birthing room and demonstrate how it works.

Use cervical dilatation chart to illustrate the amount of dilatation.

Discussion.

Ask woman to demonstrate technique.

Discussion.

Provide a tour of birthing area, explaining equipment and routines. Include partner.

Evaluation   At the end of this teaching session, the woman will be able to verbalize assessments that will occur during her labor and to discuss comfort/support measures that may be used.

for support. A calm, pleasant manner indicates to the family that they are important. It helps instill in the couple a sense of confidence in the staff's ability to provide quality, caring, and safety during this critical time.

Following the initial greeting, the woman may be taken into a labor lounge for evaluation or admitted directly into a birthing room. Some couples prefer to remain together during the admission process, and others prefer to have the partner wait outside. As the nurse helps the woman undress and get into a hospital gown, the nurse can begin to develop rapport and establish the nursing data base. The experienced labor and birth nurse can obtain essential information regarding the woman and her pregnancy. By doing an admission assessment, the nurse can initiate any immediate interventions needed and establish individualized priorities. The nurse is then able to make effective nursing decisions regarding intrapartal care:

- Are there factors that put the laboring women or the fetus at risk?
- Should ambulation or bed rest be encouraged?
- Is more frequent monitoring needed?
- What does the woman want during her labor and birth?
- Who will be with her for social support?

The woman is made comfortable. If she wants to rest in bed, a side-lying or semi-Fowler's position rather than a supine position is most comfortable and avoids supine hypotensive syndrome (vena caval syndrome).

After obtaining the essential information from the woman and her records, the nurse begins the intrapartal assessment. (Chapter 22 considers intrapartal assessment in depth.) (See Essential Precautions in Practice: During Admission and Labor.)

Before assessments begin, it is important to establish rapport and to create an environment in which the family feels free to ask questions. The support and encouragement of the nurse in maintaining a caring environment has begun with the initial admission but needs to be attended to with all subsequent actions. Before completing assessments the nurse may provide the opportunity for questions and may explain the environment and the procedures that will be a part of the labor and birthing care. As the assessments begin, the nurse auscultates the fetal heart rate (FHR). (Detailed information on monitoring FHR is presented in Chapter 22.) The woman's blood pressure, pulse, respirations, and oral temperature are assessed. Contraction status (frequency, duration, and intensity), cervical dilatation and effacement, and fetal presentation and station are determined. (See Chapter 22 for discussion of sterile vaginal examinations [SVE].) After the SVE, the nurse shares the findings with the couple. If there are signs of advanced labor (frequent contractions, an urge to bear down, and so on), a vaginal examination must be done quickly after admission. If there are signs of excessive bleeding or if the woman reports episodes of

bleeding in the last trimester, a vaginal examination should *not* be done.

Results of FHR assessment, uterine contraction evaluation, and the vaginal examination help determine whether the rest of the admission process can proceed at a more leisurely pace or whether additional interventions have higher priority. For example, an FHR of 110 beats per minute (bpm) on auscultation indicates that an electronic fetal monitor should be applied immediately to obtain additional data. The woman's vital signs can be assessed after this is done (Table 23–1).

TEACHING MOMENT

If the monitor is no longer recording the fetal heart rate tracing, before you assume there is a problem with the baby, check that there is adequate gel under the transducer and reposition it.

After admission data are obtained, a clean-voided midstream urine specimen is collected. The woman with intact membranes may collect her specimen in the bathroom. If the membranes are ruptured and the presenting

TABLE 23-1	Indicators of Normal Labor Process on Admission

Indicator	Normal Characteristics
Uterine contractions	Frequency of not less than 2 minutes Duration of less than 75 seconds Uterine relaxation between contractions Most intense discomfort only with contractions (Some women, especially those with occiput posterior position, complain of less intense lower abdominal and/or back pain between contractions.)
Fetal heart rate	Rate 120 to 160 with average variability Absence of variability or late decelerations
Maternal vital signs	B/P below 140/90 or less than +30/+15 above prepregnancy readings Pulse 60 to 100 Temperature between 97.8 and 99.6 F
If membranes ruptured	Fluid clear without odor

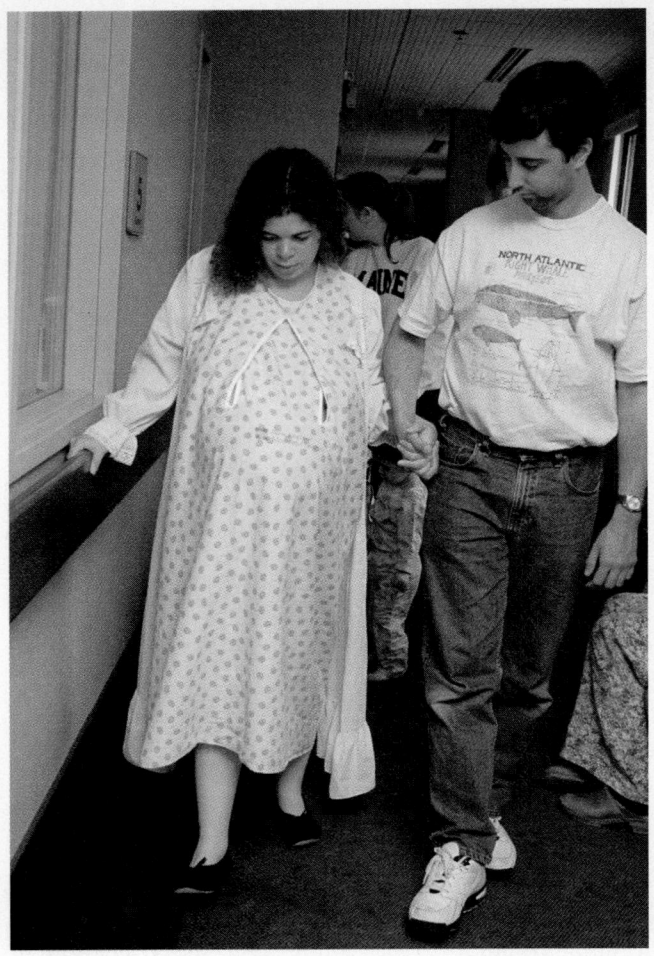

FIGURE 23-1 Woman and her partner walking in the hospital during labor.

part is *not* engaged, the woman is generally asked to remain in bed to avoid prolapse of the umbilical cord. If ambulation is desired to increase the labor contractions, it is generally safe for the woman to walk if the fetal head is well engaged and the monitor strip shows reassuring signs of fetal well-being (Figure 23–1).

The nurse can test the woman's urine for the presence of protein, ketones, and glucose by using a dipstick before sending the sample to the laboratory. This procedure is especially important if nondependent edema or elevated blood pressure is noted on admission. Proteinuria of 1+ or more may be a sign of impending preeclampsia. Glycosuria is found frequently in pregnant women because of the increased glomerular filtration rate in the proximal tubules and the inability of these tubules to increase glucose reabsorption. However, it may also be associated with gestational diabetes and should not be discounted.

After the woman has collected the urine specimen, the nurse can shave the pubic area (called a prep) and administer an enema if these procedures are indicated. A prep and enema are now done less frequently than in the past, but some physicians still order them. A prep usually means removing perineal hair below the vaginal orifice, where an episiotomy or repair of a laceration would be done. The area can be shaved or the perineal hair clipped with a pair of sterile scissors. A miniprep is usually considered removing perineal hair from the labia parallel to the upper aspect of the vaginal orifice and downward to the rectum.

The use of preps is controversial. Some certified nurse-midwives/physicians believe that this form of skin preparation facilitates their work during the birth, makes perineal repair easier, and prevents infection (Garforth & Garcia 1989). Others believe that a prep is unnecessary because hair is minimal between the vagina and rectum and shaving may actually increase the risk of infection. Many women question the need for a prep and request that it be omitted. The nurse needs to ascertain the woman's wishes in this matter. Hopefully, the woman has discussed her wishes with her physician/certified nurse-midwife during the prenatal period. If not, the nurse should act as her advocate in communicating the client's wishes to her provider.

When a prep is to be done, the nurse explains the procedure to the woman. Most women feel embarrassed and vulnerable during this procedure, so the nurse needs to exercise great care to provide privacy and support. The nurse performing the prep will need to observe body substance isolation (BSI) and universal precautions by washing hands and using disposable gloves. While performing a prep, the nurse places one hand just under the symphysis pubis to hold the skin taut, applies warmed soapy water with a sponge, and holding a disposable razor in the other hand, shaves off the perineal hair with short downward strokes.

Administration of an enema is also controversial. Currently, many certified nurse-midwives/physicians leave the decision up to the woman, as long as there is no vaginal bleeding present, the labor is not preterm, and labor is not far advanced. If the woman has been constipated and desires an enema, usually a small-volume enema (such as Fleets) is given. The woman may expel the enema in the bathroom unless membranes are ruptured; then she is usually asked to use a bedpan. Before leaving the woman, the nurse must be sure that the woman knows how to operate the call system so that she can obtain help if she needs it. After the enema is expelled, the nurse monitors the FHR again to assess any changes. If the woman's partner and other support people have been out of the labor/birthing room, they are reunited as soon as possible.

Laboratory tests are often performed in the outpatient setting prior to admission. Hemoglobin and hematocrit values help determine the oxygen-carrying capacity of the circulatory system and the ability of the woman to withstand blood loss at birth. Elevation of the hematocrit indicates hemoconcentration of blood, which occurs with edema or dehydration. A low hemoglobin, in the absence of other evidence of bleeding, suggests anemia. Blood may be typed and cross-matched if the woman is in a high-risk category. A serology test for syphilis is obtained if one has not been done in the last 3 months or if an antepartal serology result was positive.

In many hospitals the admission process also includes signing an informed consent for treatment, and the client is given information on arranging advanced directives or instructions about her wishes if she were to become critically ill. An identification bracelet is attached to her wrist.

Depending on how rapidly labor is progressing, the nurse notifies the certified nurse-midwife/physician before or after completing the admission procedures. The report should include the following information: cervical dilatation and effacement, station, presenting part, status of the membranes, contraction pattern, FHR, vital signs that are not in the normal range, the woman's wishes, and her reaction to labor.

A nursing admission note is entered into the computer or the charting system. The admission note should include the reason for admission, the date and time of the woman's arrival and notification of the certified nurse-midwife/physician, the condition of the woman and her baby, and labor and membrane status (AAP-ACOG 1992).

Screening for psychosocial risk factors is also an integral part of the admission process. Risk factors include family violence, sexual abuse, drugs, alcohol, and sexually transmitted diseases. Chapter 22 suggests ways to obtain a psychosocial history regarding family and sexual violence. Always ask questions regarding family and sexual violence when the woman is alone. The nurse should ask about alcohol and drug use in a straightforward, matter-of-fact manner. Questions such as "How many times per week do you drink alcohol?" is straightforward and sets the stage for the woman to be specific in her answer. If

the woman reports that she does have alcohol on a daily basis, then the amount can be determined. Drug use can be assessed in a similar manner. The nurse must maintain a nonjudgmental approach and collect only information relating to the labor and birthing process. This dialogue provides an opportunity for the nurse to continue to build support, to provide information when requested, and to be direct yet supportive.

NURSING PLAN AND IMPLEMENTATION DURING THE FIRST STAGE OF LABOR

Women who have had a chance to look back at their labor have important information to share with birthing nurses regarding the activities and qualities of nursing care that helped them cope with labor and increased their satisfaction with the process.

Recent research provides information regarding nursing interventions and qualities of the nurse that laboring women have found helpful. A study by Bryanton, Fraser-Davey, and Sullivan (1994) indicated that birthing nurses rated making the woman physically comfortable and providing pain medication as important nursing interventions, but laboring women rated these activities much lower in importance. The laboring women identified the most helpful nursing behaviors as "making the woman feel cared about as an individual, giving praise, appearing calm and confident, assisting with breathing and relaxing, treating the woman with respect, explaining hospital routines, answering questions truthfully in an understandable language, providing a sense of security and accepting what the woman said and did without judging her" (p 641).

Other researchers have validated many similar nursing behaviors that have been identified as helpful. Mackey and Stepans (1993) noted that laboring women wanted the nurse to participate in labor and be there for them, to accept them as individuals, to give information and encouragement, and to be present when the woman desired. Brown and Lumley (1994) in a study of 790 Australian women found that the most important factors regarding satisfaction with nursing care were the importance of information, participation in decision making, and relationships formed with the nurses.

Nurses should incorporate information from recent studies into the plan of care they develop for each family.

Integration of Family Expectations

Most would agree that a family comes into the birth setting with great anxiety about their capabilities to endure labor and about the safety of their baby. What do they expect of the nurse who will be with them during this important event in their life? Mackey and Lock (1989)

Text continues on page 644

INTRAPARTAL CRITICAL PATHWAY

Category	First Stage	Second and Third Stage	Fourth Stage Birth to 1 Hour Past Birth
Referral	**Review prenatal record** **Advise CNM/physician of admission**	**Labor record for first stage**	**Report to Recovery room nurse**
Assessments	Admission assessments: ask about problems since last prenatal visit; labor status (contraction frequency and duration), membrane status (intact or ruptured); coping level; support; woman's desires during labor and birth; ability to verbalize needs; laboratory testing (blood and UA) Intrapartal assessments: Cervical assessment: from 1 to 10 cm dilatation; nullipara (1.2 cm/h), multipara (1.5 cm/h) Cervical effacement: from 0% to 100% Fetal descent: progressive descent from -4 to +4 Membrane assessment: intact or ruptured; when ruptured, Nitrazine positive, fluid clear, no foul odor Comfort level: woman states is able to cope with contractions Behavioral characteristics: facial expressions, tone of voice and verbal expressions are consistent with comfort level and ability to cope Latent Phase: • B/P, P, R q1h if in normal range (B/P 90-140/60-90 or not >30 mm Hg systolic or 15 mm Hg diastolic over baseline; pulse 60–90; respirations 12-20/min, quiet, easy) • Temp q4h unless >37.6 C (99.6 F) or membranes ruptured then q1h • Uterine contractions q30min (contractions q5-10min, 15-40sec, mild intensity) • FHR q60min (for low-risk women) and q30 min (for high-risk women) if reassuring (reassuring FHR has: baseline 120-160, STV present, LTV average, accelerations with fetal movement, no late nor variable decelerations); if nonreassuring, position on side, start O₂, assess for hypotension, monitor continuously, notify CNM/physician Active Phase: • B/P, P, R, q1h if WNL • Temp as above • Uterine contractions q30min: contractions q2–3min, 60 sec, moderate to strong • FHR q30min (for low-risk women) and q15min (for high-risk women) if reassuring; if nonreassuring institute interventions Transition: • B/P, P, R, q30min • Uterine contractions q15-30min: contractions q2min, 60-75 sec, strong • FHR q30min (for low-risk women) and q15min (for high-risk women) if reassuring; if nonreassuring, see above	Second stage assessment: • B/P, P, R q5–15min • Uterine contractions palpated continuously • FHR q15min (for low-risk women) and q5min (for high-risk women) if reassuring; if nonreassuring, monitor continuously Fetal descent: descent continues to birth Comfort level: woman states is able to cope with contractions and pushing Behavioral characteristics: response to pushing, facial expressions, verbalization Third stage assessments: • B/P, P, R q5min • Uterine contractions, palpate occasionally until placenta is delivered, fundus maintains tone and contraction pattern continues to birth of placenta Newborn assessments: • Assess Apgar score of newborn • Respirations 30-60, irregular • Apical pulse: 120-160 and somewhat irregular • Temperature: Skin temp above 36.5 C (97.8 F) • Umbilical cord: two arteries, one vein (if one artery, assess for anomalies and urine output) • Gestational age: 38-42 weeks	Immediate post birth assessments of mother q15min for one hour: • B/P; 90-140/60-90; should return to pre-labor level • Pulse: slightly lower than in labor; range is 60-90 • Respirations: 12-20/min; easy; quiet • Temperature: 36.2-37.6 C (98-99.6 F) • Fundus firm, in midline, at the umbilicus • Lochia rubra; moderate amount; <1 pad/h; no free flow or passage of clots with massage • Perineum: sutures intact; no bulging or marked swelling; minimal bruising may be present; no c/o severe pain nor rectal pain • Bladder nondistended; spontaneous void of >100mL clear, straw colored urine; bladder nondistended following voiding • If hemorrhoids present; no tenseness or marked engorgement; <2 cm diameter Comfort level: <3 on scale of 1 to 10 Energy level: awake and able to hold newborn Newborn assessments if newborn remains with parents: • Respirations: 30–60; irregular • Apical pulse: 120-160 and somewhat irregular • Temperature: skin temp above 36.5 C (97.8 F); skin feels warm to touch • Skin color noncyanotic • Mucus: small amount, clear, easily suctioned with bulb syringe without skin color change • Behavioral: newborn opens eyes widely if room is slightly darkened • Movements rhythmic; no hand tremors present
Comfort	Institute comfort measures: ambulation, frequent position change, effleurage, focal point, patterned paced breathing, visualization, therapeutic touch, back rub, moist cloths to face, holding hand, words of	Institute comfort measures: • Second stage: cool cloth to forehead, encouragement, coaching, help support legs while pushing, position of comfort for pushing and birth	Institute comfort measures: • Perineal discomfort: gently cleanse and apply ice pack; position to decrease pressure on perineum • Uterine discomfort: palpate fundus gently

Category	First Stage *continued*	Second and Third Stage *continued*	Fourth Stage **Birth to 1 Hour Past Birth** *continued*
Comfort *continued*	encouragement, changing underpad, shower, whirlpool, staying with the woman/family, warmed blanket at back, sacral pressure Offer pain medication or administer if requested Assist with administration of regional block	• Third stage: cool cloth to forehead, assist parents to see newborn, position mother to hold newborn, provide encouragement	• Hemorrhoids: ice pack • General fatigue: position of comfort, encourage rest • Administer pain medication _____
Teaching/ psychosocial	Establish rapport Orient to environment, expected assessments & procedures Answer questions and provide information Orient to EFM if used Teach relaxation, visualization & breathing pattern if needed Explain comfort measures available Assume advocacy role for woman/family during labor & birth	Orient to expected assessments and procedures Answer questions and provide information Explain comfort measures available Continue advocacy role	Explain immediate assessments and care after this first hour Teach self-massage of fundus and expected findings Instruct to call for assistance if mother desires to get OOB Begin newborn teaching; bulb syringe, positioning; maintaining warmth Assist parents in exploring their newborn Assist with first breastfeeding experience
Therapeutic nursing interventions and reports	Straight cath prn if bladder distended If regional block administered monitor B/P, FGR, sensation per protocol Provide continuing status reports to CNM/physician Perineal clip per woman's request Small enema per woman's request Perform sterile vaginal examination as indicated	Straight cath prn if bladder distended Continue monitoring VS, FHR and sensation if regional block has been given	Straight cath if bladder distended Monitor return of motor ability and sensation if regional block has been given Weigh perineal pads if lochia flow >1 saturated pad in 1 hour; presence of boggy uterus and clots; ↓ B/P, ↑P
Activity	Encourage ambulation unless contraindicated Maintain bedrest immediately after administration of IV pain medication, or following regional block Woman rests comfortably between contractions	Position comfortably for birth Woman rests comfortably between pushing efforts & while awaiting birth of placenta	Position of comfort
Nutrition	Ice chips and clear fluids Evaluate for signs of dehydration	Ice chips and clear fluids	Regular diet if assessments are WNL Encourage fluids
Elimination	Voids at least q2h; urine clear, straw colored, negative for protein Bladder nondistended May have bowel movement Monitor I & O with IVs	May void spontaneously with pushing May pass stool with pushing	Voids spontaneously
Medications		Local infiltration of anesthetic agent for birth by CNM/physician Pitocin 10 units IM, IVP per IV tubing, or added to IV fluids	Continue Pitocin infusion Administer pain medication _____
Discharge planning	Evaluate knowledge of labor and birth process Evaluate support system and need for referral after birth		Provide information if mother to be moved from LDR room Provide opportunity for parents to ask questions regarding newborn Evaluate knowledge of normal postpartum, newborn care
Family involvement	Identify available support person(s) Recognize possible impact of culture on responses Observe interaction between woman and partner Create moment alone with woman to identify possible abuse Assess current parenting skills	Provide opportunities for woman and support person(s) to watch newborn assessments Perform newborn assessment on mother's abdomen/chest if possible	Provide opportunity for parents to be with baby Encourage skin to skin contact Darken room to encourage eye to eye contact Provide quiet time for new family Parenting: demonstrates early culturally expected parenting behaviors

conducted a study to identify couples' expectations of the labor and birth nurse. They wanted the nurse to be calm, considerate, compassionate, concerned, and friendly—a person who accepts feelings and is interested in the woman as a person. The study revealed seven aspects of a nurse's role to be important: (1) presence of the nurse in the room during labor, (2) decision making, whether they wanted to make all decisions regarding their care, wanted a collaborative role with the nurse, or expected the nurse to make most of the decisions, (3) assistance with aspects of care, (4) physical assessment by the nurse, (5) information regarding progress and procedures, (6) comfort measures, and (7) support. The study participants also revealed that they had different expectations regarding the amount or level of nursing involvement, and they were divided into three groups: limited, moderate, or extensive nurse involvement.

The limited-nurse-involvement group expected that nurses would complete the necessary assessments and needed procedures, but other than that they wanted to let nurses know when their presence was desired in the room. They wanted to have their decisions respected.

The couples in the moderate-nurse-involvement group wanted the nurses' presence intermittently and wanted to collaborate with nurses regarding decisions. They wanted direction, assistance, encouragement, and frequent support.

The couples in the extensive-nurse-involvement group wanted nurses to be present almost all the time. They wanted the nurses to take responsibility and do what was best. The women wanted a lot of physical contact and wanted the nurses to somehow instill confidence in them that they could handle the labor.

With information regarding a variety of expectations it becomes a challenge for nurses to provide individualized care. The expert nurse needs to assess the couple's needs and desires and respond in just that manner.

In this case the nurse can look for cues: When the woman and her coach are admitted, do they seem to take control and know what is going to happen? Do they have a birth plan that they have already worked out, or do they seem hesitant and unsure of the process?

Although these two ends of the spectrum are obvious, they are a starting point. It would be fairly safe to assume that the "situation-is-in-control" couple would want a little less involvement, and the couple that is hesitant and asking questions will want more extensive involvement. The nurse can also gain more information by asking questions such as: "Other than the assessments that I will be making, what kind of involvement would you like from me? Would you like to call me when you need something or have me pop in now and then, or would you be more comfortable if I stay in the room most of the time?" This gives the couple an opportunity to make their wishes known. It is also important for the nurse to let the couple know that she or he understands their wishes may change during labor and that the nurse will be available for them throughout the process.

Integration of Cultural Beliefs

Knowledge of values, customs, and practices of different cultures is as important during labor as it is in the prenatal period. Without this knowledge a nurse is less likely to understand a family's behavior and may impose personal values and beliefs upon them. As cultural sensitivity increases, so does the likelihood of providing high-quality care.

The following sections briefly present a few possible cultural responses to labor. It is difficult to present even such a limited discussion in a clear, nonjudgmental way because once a statement is made, it may appear stereotypical, and of course no statement of a specific behavior can accurately reflect the preference of all people in a group. The nurse must always remain aware that an individual example of birthing practice will never be pertinent to all women in that individual's group. Within every culture each person develops his or her own beliefs and value system. General information about any culture or belief system needs to be regarded as background knowledge in light of which we meet each individual and determine that person's own needs and desires.

Modesty

Modesty is an important consideration for women regardless of the cultural grouping; however, some women may be more uncomfortable than others with the degree of exposure needed for some procedures during labor and the birth process. Some women may be particularly uncomfortable when men are present and feel more comfortable with women; others may be uncomfortable with exposure of personal body parts regardless of the gender of the examiner or person who assists them. The nurse needs to be observant of the woman's responses to examinations and procedures and to provide the draping and privacy that the woman needs. It is more prudent to assume that embarrassment will occur with exposure and take measures to provide privacy than to assume that it will not matter to the woman to be exposed during procedures. For example, some Asian women are not accustomed to male physicians and attendants. Modesty is of great concern, and exposure of as little of the woman's body as possible is strongly recommended.

Pain Expression

How women deal with the discomfort of labor varies widely. Some turn inward and remain very quiet during the whole process. They speak only to ask others to leave the room or cease conversation. Others may be very vocal, with behaviors such as counting out loud, moaning quietly, crying, or cursing loudly. They may also turn from side to side or change positions frequently. In Asian cultures it is important for individuals to act in a way that will not bring shame on the family. Therefore the Asian woman may not express pain outwardly for fear of shaming herself and her family (Hollingsworth et al 1980).

Women of Mexican cultural heritage, by contrast, may be vocally expressive during labor. The nurse supports a woman's individual expression, whatever it may be, in order to enhance the birthing experience for mother, baby, and family.

Cultural Beliefs: Some Examples

In looking at specific practices related to position, food, and drink during labor, some differences between cultures are apparent. In most non-European societies uninfluenced by Westernization, women assume an upright position in childbirth. For example, Hmong women from Laos report that squatting during childbirth is common in their culture (LaDu 1985). Some traditional Native American women give birth in upright positions. For example, the Pueblo woman may give birth on her knees, and the Zuni woman may kneel or squat while a midwife kneads her abdomen. In some tribes teas made of juniper twigs may be given to relax the woman (Higgins & Wayland 1981).

Hmong women have special customs regarding childbirth. The beginning of labor signifies the beginning of a transition and entails certain dietary restrictions. The woman may want to be active and should be able to move about during labor. The husband is frequently present and actively involved in providing comfort. During labor the woman usually prefers only "hot" foods and warm water to drink. Traditionally, the woman prefers that the amniotic membranes not be ruptured until just before birth. It is thought that the escape of fluid at this time makes the birth easier. She may choose to kneel or squat for the birth of her baby. As soon as the baby is born, a soft-boiled egg must be given to the mother to restore her energy. During the postpartum period the mother prefers "warm" foods, such as chicken prepared with warm water and warm rice (Morrow 1986).

Vietnamese women also follow prescribed customs during pregnancy and birth (Calhoun 1986). While in labor, the woman usually maintains self-control and may smile throughout the labor. She may prefer to walk about during labor and to give birth in a squatting position. She may avoid drinking cold water and prefer fluids at room temperature. The newborn is protected from praise to prevent jealousy.

Latina women have identified expectations of their partner during labor and birth such as wanting their partner to stay with them and to reassure them that everything will be alright. The women wanted the partner to show caring and that they loved them as they went through labor and to speak to them using affectionate words (Khazoyan & Anderson 1994).

Muslim women may have their husband, a female friend or relative, or a male relative with them during childbirth. Family support may be particularly important but does not preclude the importance of the nurse also being present. The woman may want to retain her head covering (khimar), and two long-sleeved gowns can be of-

RESEARCH IN PRACTICE

Health professionals may expect more from the Latino (Spanish speaking Mexican male) than the Latina expects from her partner during labor. Expectations and beliefs about pregnancy and childbearing are culturally based, and many health professionals come from a culture other than Latino. Some Latinas hold and follow traditional Mexican beliefs and practices intended to protect the fetus and promote an easy delivery. These practices may include performing abdominal massage to correct the position of the baby for delivery and avoiding drafts of cold air or eclipses of the moon to prevent harm to the mother and child. Expectations of the male partner during labor and delivery are also impacted by the culture of the couple.

Cara Khazoyan and Nancy Anderson determined the expectations of 10 Latina women during labor using an ethnographic approach. The qualitative study was based on data collected during two indepth interviews with each participant, one in the third trimester and one after delivery. The interviews were conducted in Spanish. In the antenatal interview, the women discussed their expectations of their partners during labor. During the postpartum interview, the participants described their childbirth experiences. Data transcription and analysis resulted in the identification of categories leading to the development of themes.

Three themes emerged from the analysis: estar conmigo, hablar conmigo, and showing love. Estar conmigo (presence at the bedside) entailed the women's desire for their partners to be with them throughout labor and birth. The presence of the partner or just being there was important. The theme of hablar conmigo (communication with the partner) involved talking with the partner during labor and birth, as well as reassurance, encouragement, and patience. The third theme, showing love, developed from the women's expressed desire to have their partners demonstrate love by holding them, displaying other signs of affection, or just by staying at the bedside.

Clinical Application of Study

Nurses need to be cognizant of their own culturally based norms and expectations and avoid imposing them on persons from different cultures. Asking expectant couples about their expectations for the male partner during labor and delivery may help alleviate misunderstandings. However, as the authors note, more studies are needed to determine what nurses expect from fathers, and more cross cultural studies are needed to identify different expectations.

SOURCE: Khazoyan C, Anderson N: Latinas' expectations for their partners during childbirth. *MCN* 1994; July/August 19:226.

fered. It is important to have examinations done by a female nurse, physician, or CNM whenever possible. Some Muslim women are not comfortable in the presence of a male physician or nurse. If a male physician is involved with their care, they may wish for their husband to remain in the room during all care by the physician. It is important to recognize that modesty needs vary and each individual will need to be assessed. After the birth Muslim fathers traditionally call praise to Allah (adhan) in the newborn's right ear and clean the newborn. It is helpful if the birthing room personnel are aware of these practices so that this family's expectations and wishes may be incorporated into care (Hutchinson & Baqi-Aziz 1994).

In working with women from another culture an awareness of historical beliefs and practices helps the nurse understand and support their behavior. The maternity nurse would do well to make it a priority to become acquainted with the beliefs and practices of the various subcultures in the community. In the birthing situation the nurse supports the family's cultural practices as long as it is safe to do so.

Critical Thinking Question

What cultural beliefs do you bring to the birthing area? How have your beliefs been influenced by your family and friends? How might you establish the cultural expectations of the birth couple? To what extent should the birth couple control birth options?

Support of the Adolescent During Birth

Each adolescent in labor is different. The nurse must assess what each client brings to the experience by asking the following questions:

- Has the young woman received prenatal care?
- What are her attitudes and feelings about the pregnancy?
- How does her developmental stage influence her behavior, and how are her specific needs different?
- Who will attend the birth, and what is the person's relationship to her?
- What preparation has she had for the experience?
- What are her expectations and fears regarding labor and birth?
- How has her culture influenced her?
- What are her usual coping mechanisms?
- Does she have adequate social support?
- Does she plan to keep the newborn? If so, does she need to learn parenting skills?

Any adolescent who has not had prenatal care requires close observation during labor. Adolescents are at highest risk for pregnancy and labor complications and must be assessed carefully. The status of the fetus is monitored to assure its well-being. The young woman's prenatal record is carefully reviewed for risks. The adolescent is more likely to have pregnancy-induced hypertension (PIH), cephalopelvic disproportion (CPD), anemia, drugs ingested during pregnancy, sexually transmitted infections, and size-date discrepancies.

The nurse's support role depends on the young woman's support system during labor. When the client is not accompanied by someone who will stay with her during childbirth, it is even more important for the nurse to establish a trusting relationship with her. In this way the nurse can help her cope with labor and understand what is happening to her. Establishing rapport without recrimination will provide emotional support and encouragement. The adolescent who is given positive reinforcement for "work well done" will leave the experience with increased self-esteem, despite the emotional stress and difficulty of giving birth at so young an age.

The nurse must explain changes in the young woman's behavior and substantiate her wishes. The nursing staff should reinforce the adolescent's feelings that she is important by gentle caring.

The adolescent who has taken childbirth education classes is generally better prepared than the adolescent who has had no preparation. The nurse must keep in mind, however, that the younger the adolescent, the less she may be able to participate actively in the process.

The very young adolescent (under age 14) has fewer coping mechanisms and less experience to draw on than her older counterparts have. Because her cognitive development is incomplete, the younger adolescent may have fewer problem-solving capabilities. Her ego integrity may be more threatened by the experience, and she may be more vulnerable to stress and discomfort.

The very young woman needs someone to rely on at all times during labor. She may be more childlike and dependent than older teens. The nurse must be sure that instructions and explanations are simple and concrete. During the transition phase the young teenager may become withdrawn and unable to express her need to be nurtured. Touch, soothing encouragement, and measures to maintain her comfort help her maintain control and meet her needs for dependence. During the second stage of labor the young adolescent may feel as if she is losing control and may reach out to those around her. By remaining calm and giving directions the nurse helps her control feelings of helplessness.

The middle adolescent (age 14–16 years) often attempts to remain calm and unflinching during labor. If unable to break through the teenager's stoic barrier, the nurse needs to rise above frustration and realize that a caring attitude will still affect the young woman.

Many older adolescents feel that they "know it all," but they may be no more prepared for childbirth than younger counterparts. The nurse's reinforcement and nonjudgmental manner will help them save face. If the adolescent has not taken classes, she may require preparation and explanations. The older teenager's response to the stresses of labor, however, is similar to that of the adult woman.

Even if the adolescent is planning to relinquish her newborn, she should be given the option of seeing and holding the infant. She may be reluctant to do this at first, but the grieving process is facilitated if the mother sees the infant. However, seeing or holding the newborn should be the young woman's choice. (See Chapter 34 for further discussion of the relinquishing mother and the adolescent parent.)

Promotion of Comfort in the First Stage

During the first stage of labor the nurse plans ways to help the woman cope with the intensity of labor contractions. Women suffer much discomfort from uncomfortable position, diaphoresis, continual leaking of amniotic fluid, a full bladder, a dry mouth, anxiety, and fear. Nursing interventions can minimize the effects of these factors. These interventions are described later in this section.

There are many types of responses to pain, including tension and mental anguish. The most frequent physiologic manifestations are increased pulse and respiratory rates, dilated pupils, increased blood pressure, and muscle tension. In labor these reactions are transitory because the pain is intermittent. Increased muscle tension is most significant because it may impede the progress of labor. Women in labor frequently tighten skeletal muscles voluntarily during a contraction and remain motionless. As the intensity of the contraction increases with the progress of labor, the woman is less aware of the environment and may have difficulty hearing verbal instructions. The pattern of coping with labor contractions varies from the use of highly structured breathing techniques to grimacing, moaning, and loud vocalizations. Some women feel that making sounds helps them cope and do the work of labor; others begin to make loud sounds only as they lose their ability to cope.

Some women may want physical contact during contractions (Figure 23–2). They may provide verbal and nonverbal signs such as crying, moaning, and beseeching the coach and/or nurse to hold their hand or rub their back. They may reach out and grasp the support person or indicate their anxiety or fear through eye contact (Weaver 1990). A woman generally wants touching and physical contact at times during the first part of labor, but when she moves into the transition phase, she rebuffs all efforts and pulls away. However, some women do not want to be touched at all, regardless of the phase of labor.

Many nurses like to incorporate touch into their nursing care, and they readily respond to the women's cues. Others may be more hesitant, perhaps because of previous experience with being rebuffed or their own personal values regarding touch. Weaver (1990) notes that some labor and birthing nurses avoid the use of touch when caring for another nurse's client or when the woman has a communicable disease or poor hygiene.

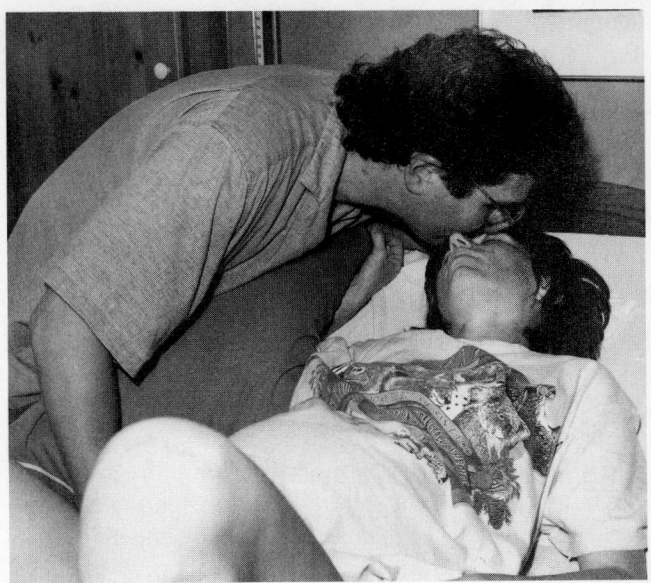

FIGURE 23-2   The woman's partner provides support and encouragement during labor.

A decrease in the intensity of discomfort is one of the goals of nursing support during labor. Nursing measures used to decrease pain include:

- Ensuring general comfort
- Decreasing anxiety
- Providing information
- Using specific supportive relaxation techniques
- Encouraging paced breathing
- Administering pharmacologic agents as needed

General Comfort

General comfort measures are of utmost importance throughout labor. By relieving minor discomforts the nurse helps the woman use her coping mechanisms to deal with pain.

The woman is encouraged to ambulate if it is not contraindicated. If she stays in bed, she may assume any position that she finds comfortable. A side-lying position is generally the most advantageous for the laboring woman, although frequent position changes seem to achieve more efficient contractions (Roberts et al 1983). Care should be taken that all body parts are supported, with the joints slightly flexed. For instance, when the woman is in a side-lying position, pillows may be placed against her chest and under the uppermost arm. A pillow or folded bath blanket is placed between her knees to support the uppermost leg and relieve tension or muscle strain. A pillow placed at the woman's midback also helps provide support. If the woman is more comfortable on her back, the head of the bed should be elevated to relieve the pressure of the uterus on the vena cava. Pillows may be placed under each arm and under the knees to provide support. Because a pregnant woman is at increased risk for thrombophlebitis, excessive pressure behind the knee and calf should be avoided, and frequent assessment of pressure points needs to be made. Back rubs and frequent changes of position contribute to comfort and relaxation.

Diaphoresis and the constant leaking of amniotic fluid can dampen the woman's gown and bed linen. Fresh, smooth, dry bed linen promotes comfort. To avoid having to change the bottom sheet following rupture of the membranes, the nurse may replace the underpads at frequent intervals (BSI precautions need to be followed). The perineal area should be kept as clean and dry as possible to promote comfort as well as to prevent infection. A full bladder adds to the discomfort during a contraction and may prolong labor by interfering with the descent of the fetus. The bladder should be kept as empty as possible. Even though the woman is voiding, urine may be retained because of the pressure of the fetal presenting part. A full bladder can be detected by palpation directly over the symphysis pubis. Some of the regional procedures for analgesia during labor contribute to the inability to void, and catheterization may be necessary. The woman should be encouraged to empty her bladder every 2–3 hours.

TEACHING MOMENT

Catheterizing a woman during a contraction is more uncomfortable for her and difficult to do because of the increased downward pressure. To avoid these problems, pass the catheter between contractions. If the baby's head is low in the pelvis, you have to change the direction of the catheter. Visualize passing it up and over the baby's head rather than straight into the urethra.

The woman may experience dryness of the oral mucous membranes. A lemon glycerine swab, popsicles, ice chips, or a wet 4 × 4 sponge may relieve the discomfort. Some prepared childbirth programs advise the woman to bring lollipops to help combat the dryness that occurs with some of the breathing patterns.

Some women feel discomfort from cold feet. Wearing socks or slippers may increase their comfort.

Some family members or support persons are able to assist the woman with comfort measures. They may help with position changes, provide ice chips, walk with the laboring woman, and give effleurage and/or back rubs. If the family is not already involved in providing comfort measures and seems to want to be, the nurse can act as a role model while providing comfort measures and then invite the support person(s) to join in if they would like.

Family members also need to be encouraged to maintain their own comfort. As their attention is directed toward the laboring woman, they may forget their own needs. The nurse may have to encourage them to take breaks, to maintain food and fluid intake, and to rest.

Handling Anxiety

The anxiety experienced by women entering labor is related to a combination of factors inherent to the process. A moderate amount of anxiety about the pain enhances the ability to deal with the pain. But an excessive degree of anxiety decreases her ability to cope with the pain. Wuitchik et al (1989) found that women in the latent phase of labor who were experiencing increased levels of anxiety regarding safety and their ability to cope were also much more likely to describe their pain as "horrible" or "excruciating." They were more likely to have FHR decelerations in labor, a slow second stage, and/or a cesarean birth and more likely to need pediatric assistance for neonatal resuscitation at birth.

Ways to decrease anxiety that is not related to pain are to give information (which eases fear of the unknown), establish rapport with the couple (which helps them preserve their personal integrity), express confidence in the couple's ability to work with the labor process, and assist with breathing and relaxation techniques. In addition to being a good listener the nurse must demonstrate genuine concern for the laboring woman. Remaining with the woman as much as possible conveys a caring attitude and dispels fear of abandonment. Praise for correct breathing, relaxation efforts, and pushing efforts not only encourages repetition of the behavior but also decreases anxiety about the ability to cope with labor (Mackey & Lock 1989).

Teaching for Self-Care

Providing information about the nature of the discomfort that will occur during labor is important and is best achieved in the early portion of labor. Stressing the intermittent nature and maximum duration of the contractions can be most helpful. The woman can cope with pain better when she knows how far she has progressed and that a period of relief will follow. Describing the type of discomfort and specific sensations that will occur as labor progresses helps the woman recognize these sensations as normal and expected when she does experience them.

During the second stage the woman may interpret rectal pressure as a need to move her bowels. The instinctive response is to tighten muscles rather than bear down (push). The woman may be frightened by a "splitting apart" sensation or an intense "ring of fire" feeling that prevents bearing down with contractions. The woman who expects these sensations and understands that bearing down contributes to progress at this stage is more likely to do so.

Descriptions of sensations should be accompanied with information on specific comfort measures. Some women experience the urge to push during transition when the cervix is not fully dilated and effaced. Usually, this sensation can be managed with patterned-paced breathing. The woman will need ongoing support and encouragement from her partner and nurse.

A thorough explanation of surroundings, procedures, and equipment being used also decreases anxiety, thereby reducing pain. Attachment to an electronic monitor can produce fear because equipment of this type is associated with critically ill people. For others hearing their infant's heartbeat is reassuring. The monitor should be explained, and a simplified explanation of the monitor strip should be given. The nurse can emphasize that the use of the monitor provides information to assess the well-being of the fetus during the course of labor. In addition the nurse can show the woman and her coach how the monitor can help them use controlled breathing techniques to relieve pain. The monitor may indicate the beginning of a contraction just seconds before the woman feels it. The woman and coach can learn how to read the tracing to identify the beginning of the contraction.

Supportive Relaxation Techniques

Tense muscles increase resistance to the descent of the fetus and contribute to maternal fatigue. This fatigue increases pain perception and decreases the woman's ability to cope with the pain. Comfort measures, massage, techniques for decreasing anxiety, and client teaching can conserve energy. The laboring woman needs to be encouraged to use the periods between contractions for rest and relaxation. A prolonged prodromal phase of labor may have prohibited sleeping.

Distraction is another method of increasing relaxation and coping with discomfort. During early labor, conversation or activities such as light reading, cards, or other games serve as distractions. One technique that is effective for relieving moderate pain is to have the woman concentrate on a pleasant experience she has had in the past.

Touch is another type of distraction. Although some women regard touching as an invasion of privacy or threat to their independence, others want to touch and be touched during a painful experience. Nurses can make themselves available to the woman who desires touch. The nurse can place a hand on the side of the bed within the woman's reach. The person who needs touch will reach out for contact, and the nurse can pick up and follow through with this behavioral cue.

Visualization techniques enhance relaxation; with this method the woman visualizes her body relaxing or the perineum relaxing (Nichols & Humenick 1988) (Table 23-2).

Mild to moderate abdominal discomfort during contractions may be relieved or lessened by effleurage. Back pain associated with labor may be relieved more effectively by firm pressure on the lower back or sacral area. To apply firm pressure, the nurse places her hand or a rolled, warmed towel or blanket in the small of the woman's back.

In addition to these measures, the nurse can enhance the woman's relaxation by providing encouragement and support for her controlled breathing techniques.

Patterned-Paced Breathing

Patterned-paced breathing may help the laboring woman. Used correctly, patterned-paced breathing increases the woman's pain threshold, encourages relaxation, enhances the ability to cope with uterine contractions, and allows the uterus to function more efficiently.

Many women learn Lamaze breathing during prenatal education classes. This type of patterned-paced breathing has three levels. The woman tends to begin with the first level and then proceed to the next when she feels the need. Regardless of the level of breathing used, a cleansing breath begins and ends each pattern. A cleansing breath involves only the chest. It consists of inhaling through the nose and exhaling through pursed lips (as if blowing on a spoonful of hot food). (See Table 23-3 for information regarding patterned-paced breathing.)

Women usually practice the breathing for a number of weeks before birth. If the woman has not learned a patterned-paced breathing method, teaching her may be difficult when she is admitted in active labor. In this instance the nurse can teach abdominal and pant-pant-blow breathing. In abdominal breathing the woman moves the abdominal wall upward as she inhales and downward as she exhales (Table 23-3). This method tends to lift the abdominal wall off the contracting uterus and thus may provide some pain relief. The breathing is deep and rhythmical. As transition approaches the woman may feel

TABLE 23-2	Simple Visualization Method

Direct a visualization by saying something like the following: "Think about a place you have been that has pleasant memories and feelings around it. A place that was relaxing, where all your stress disappeared. As you think about this place, take in a breath and remember the smells around it. If it was outside, feel the warmth of the sun or the way the breeze felt on your face. Sit in the place again in your mind. Let all your tension and tiredness leave your body as you feel the warmth and breezes."

Give the woman a few moments to think about her special place. Ask if she would like to share information about the setting. If the woman chooses to do this, add the information to help her with the visualization (for example, "Think about the mountain cabin and the warmth of the sun on your face as you sit in the rocking chair on the front porch.").

After the woman has a visualization set up, suggest thinking about it during contractions as a means of increasing relaxation and focusing concentration. You could say, "As each contraction begins, think about this special place for a moment, and let your body relax. Keep a picture of your place in your mind as you breathe with the contraction. When the contraction is over, let your body stay relaxed. Feel the comfort of this room and support of those around you."

TABLE 23-3 Nursing Support of Patterned-Paced Breathing

Determine which breathing method the woman (couple) has learned. Provide encouragement as needed in maintaining breathing pattern. Provide support to the labor coach and assist as needed.

Lamaze Breathing Pattern Levels

First level (slow paced)
Pattern begins and ends with a cleansing breath (in through the nose and out through pursed lips as if cooling a spoonful of hot food). While inhaling through the nose and exhaling through pursed lips, slow breaths are taken, moving only the chest. The rate should be approximately 6–9/minute or 2 breaths/15 seconds. The coach or nurse may assist by reminding the woman to take a cleansing breath, and then the breaths could be counted out if needed to maintain pacing. The woman inhales as someone counts "one one thousand, two one thousand, three one thousand, four one thousand." Exhalation begins and continues through the same count.

First level for use during uterine contractions (The level begins and ends with a cleansing breath [CB].)

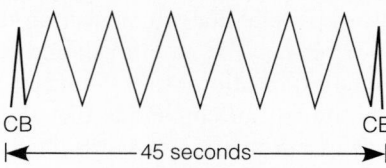

Second level (modified paced)
Pattern begins and ends with a cleansing breath. Breaths are then taken in and out silently through the mouth at approximately 4 breaths/5 seconds. The jaw and entire body need to be relaxed. The rate can be accelerated to 2–2 1/2 breaths/second. The rhythm for the breaths can be counted out as "one and two and one and two and…" with the woman exhaling on the numbers and inhaling on *and*.

Second level

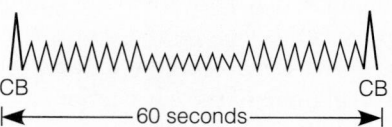

Third level (pattern paced)
Pattern begins and ends with a cleansing breath. All breaths are rhythmical, in and out through the mouth. Exhalations are accompanied by a "hee" or "hoo" sound in a varying pattern, 2:1, which begins as 3:1 (hee hee hee hoo) and can change to 2:1 (hee hee hoo) or 1:1 (hee hoo) as the intensity of the contraction changes. The rate should not be more rapid than 2–2 1/2/seconds. The rhythm of the breaths would match a "one and two and…" count.

Third level (Darkened spike represents "hoo.")

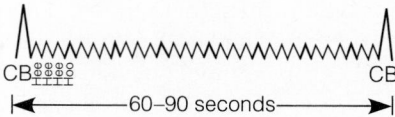

Abdominal Breathing Pattern Cues

The abdomen moves outward during inhalation and downward during exhalation. The rate remains slow with approximately 6–9 breaths/minute.

Breathing sequence for abdominal breathing

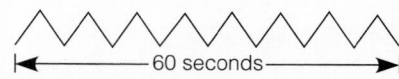

Quick Method

When the woman has not learned a particular method and is in active phase of labor, the nurse may teach her a combination of two patterns. Abdominal breathing may be used until labor is more advanced. Then a more rapid pattern consisting of two short blows from the mouth followed by a longer blow can be used. (This pattern is called "pant pant blow" even though all exhalations are a blowing motion.)

Pant-pant-blow breathing pattern

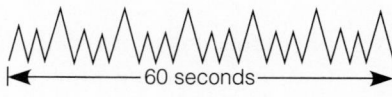

the need to breathe more rapidly. To avoid breathing too rapidly, which may occur with deep abdominal breathing, the woman can use the pant-pant-blow breathing pattern.

As the woman uses her breathing technique, the nurse can assess and support the interaction between the woman and her coach or support person. In the absence of a coach the nurse supports the laboring woman by helping to identify the beginning of each contraction and encouraging her as she breathes through it. Continued

encouragement and support with each contraction through labor have immeasurable benefits.

Hyperventilation may occur when a woman breathes very rapidly over a prolonged period of time. Hyperventilation is the result of an imbalance of oxygen and carbon dioxide (that is, too much carbon dioxide is exhaled, and too much oxygen remains in the body). The signs and symptoms of hyperventilation are tingling or numbness in the tip of nose, lips, fingers, or toes; dizzi-

TABLE 23-4 Normal Progress, Psychologic Characteristics, and Nursing Support During First and Second Stages of Labor

Phase	Cervical Dilatation	Uterine Contractions	Woman's Response	Support Measures
Stage 1 Latent phase	1–4 cm	Every 15–30 minutes, 15–30 seconds duration Mild intensity	Usually happy, talkative, and eager to be in labor Exhibits need for independence by taking care of own bodily needs and seeking information	Establish rapport on admission and continue to build during care. Assess information base and learning needs. Be available to consult regarding breathing technique if needed; teach breathing technique if needed and in early labor. Orient family to room, equipment, monitors, and procedures. Encourage woman and partner to participate in care as desired. Provide needed information. Assist woman into position of comfort; encourage frequent change of position; encourage ambulation during early labor. Offer fluids/ice chips. Keep couple informed of progress. Encourage woman to void every 1 to 2 hours. Assess need for an interest in using visualization to enhance relaxation and teach if appropriate.
Active phase	4–7 cm	Every 3–5 minutes, 30–60 seconds duration Moderate intensity	May experience feelings of helplessness Exhibits increased fatigue and may begin to feel restless and anxious as contractions become stronger Expresses fear of abandonment Becomes more dependent as she is less able to meet her needs	Encourage woman to maintain breathing patterns. Provide quiet environment to reduce external stimuli. Provide reassurance, encouragement, support; keep couple informed of progress. Promote comfort by giving back rubs, sacral pressure, cool cloth on forehead, assistance with position changes, support with pillows, effleurage. Provide ice chips, ointment for dry mouth and lips. Encourage to void every 1 to 2 hours. Offer shower/whirlpool/warm bath if available.
Transition	8–10 cm	Every 2–3 minutes, 45–90 seconds duration Strong intensity	Tires and may exhibit increased restlessness and irritability May feel she cannot keep up with labor process and is out of control Physical discomforts Fear of being left alone May fear tearing open or splitting apart with contractions	Encourage woman to rest between contractions. If she sleeps between contractions, wake her at beginning of contraction so she can begin breathing pattern (increases feeling of control). Provide support, encouragement, and praise for efforts. Keep couple informed of progress; encourage continued participation of support persons. Promote comfort as listed above but recognize many women do not want to be touched when in transition. Provide privacy. Provide ice chips, ointment for lips. Encourage to void every 1–2 hours.
Stage 2	Complete	Every $1\frac{1}{2}$–2 minutes	May feel out of control, helpless, panicky	Assist woman in pushing efforts. Encourage woman to assume position of comfort. Provide encouragement and praise for efforts. Keep couple informed of progress. Provide ice chips. Maintain privacy as woman desires.

ness; spots before the eyes; or spasms of the hands or feet (carpal-pedal spasms). If hyperventilation occurs, the woman should be encouraged to slow her breathing rate and to take shallow breaths. With instruction and encouragement many women are able to change their breathing to correct the problem. Encouraging the woman to relax and counting out loud for her so she can pace her breathing during contractions are also helpful. If the signs and symptoms continue or become more severe (that is, if they progress from numbness to spasms), the woman can breathe into a paper surgical mask or into her hands until symptoms abate. Breathing into a mask or her hands causes rebreathing of carbon dioxide. The nurse should remain with the woman to reassure her.

In some instances analgesics and/or regional anesthetic blocks may be used to enhance comfort and relaxation during labor. See Chapter 24 for a discussion of analgesia and anesthesia. Table 23–4 summarizes labor progress, possible responses of the laboring woman, and support measures.

Provision of Care in the First Stage of Labor

After the admission process is completed the nurse helps the laboring woman and her partner become comfortable with the surroundings. The nurse assesses the couple's

TABLE 23-5 Nursing Assessments in the First Stage

Phase	Mother	Fetus
Latent	Blood pressure, respirations each hour if in normal range Temperature every 4 hours unless over 37.5 C (99.6 F) or membranes ruptured, then every hour Uterine contractions every 30 minutes	FHR every 60 minutes for low-risk women and every 30 minutes for high-risk women if normal characteristics present (average variability, baseline in the 120–160 bpm range, without late or variable decelerations) (NAACOG 1990). Note fetal activity. If electronic fetal monitor in place, assess for reactive NST.
Active	Blood pressure, pulse, respirations every hour if in normal range Uterine contractions every 30 minutes	FHR every 30 minutes for low-risk women and every 15 minutes for high-risk women if normal characteristics are present (NAACOG 1990).
Transition	Blood pressure, pulse, respiration every 30 minutes	FHR every 30 minutes for low-risk women and every 15 minutes for high-risk women if normal characteristics are present (NAACOG 1990).

individual needs and plans for this experience. As long as there are no contraindications (such as vaginal bleeding or ROM with the fetus unengaged), the woman may be encouraged to ambulate because labor is shortened by upright positions. Many women feel much more at ease and comfortable if they can move around and do not have to remain in bed.

The nurse needs to evaluate physical parameters of the woman and her fetus. Maternal temperature is monitored every 4 hours unless the temperature is over 37.5 C (99.6 F); if it is, it must be taken every hour. Blood pressure, pulse, and respirations are monitored every hour. If the woman's blood pressure is over 140/90 mm Hg or her pulse is more than 100, the certified nurse-midwife/physician must be notified. The blood pressure and pulse are then reevaluated more frequently. Uterine contractions are palpated for frequency, intensity, and duration. The FHR is auscultated every 60 minutes for low-risk women and every 30 minutes for high-risk women as long as it remains between 120 and 160/bpm and is reassuring. The FHR should be auscultated throughout one contraction and for about 15 seconds after the contraction to assure that there are no decelerations. If the FHR is not in the 120–160 range and/or decelerations are heard, continuous electronic monitoring is recommended (Table 23–5).

The laboring woman may be feeling some discomfort during contractions. The nurse can assist with diversions or by repositioning her. The woman may begin to use her breathing method during contractions (see the preceding discussion of pain management).

If the laboring woman has not had childbirth education classes, the latent phase is a time when the nurse can give anticipatory guidance. Most women are not too uncomfortable with contractions at this time and are responsive to teaching about breathing and other techniques for coping with labor contractions. In fact many women in the latent phase seek information about what to expect. The unprepared woman may hesitate to ask questions and thus can benefit even more from anticipatory guidance by the nurse. If the woman's membranes are intact, a tour of the birthing facility can help decrease anxiety and distract her from her discomfort.

The nurse should offer fluids in the form of clear liquids and/or ice chips at frequent intervals. Because gastric emptying time is prolonged during labor, solid foods are usually avoided. However, fasting during labor is becoming a controversial practice. Some providers believe that eating and drinking in labor should be an option to women. Many nurse-midwifery practices are now encouraging mothers to eat and drink to toleration, based on the current literature (Ludka & Roberts 1993).

Active Phase

During this phase the contractions have a frequency of 2–3 minutes, a duration of 50–60 seconds, and moderate intensity. Contractions need to be palpated every 15–30 minutes. As the contractions become more frequent and intense, vaginal exams are done to assess cervical dilatation and effacement and fetal station and position. During the active phase the cervix dilates from 4 to 7 cm, and vaginal discharge and bloody show increase. Maternal blood pressure, pulse, and respirations should be monitored every hour for low-risk women (unless elevated, as previously noted) and every 30 minutes for high-risk women. The FHR is auscultated and evaluated every 30 minutes for low-risk women and every 15 minutes for high-risk women (NAACOG 1990).

A woman who has been ambulatory up to this point may now wish to sit in a chair or on a bed (Figure 23–3). If the woman wants to lie on the bed, she is encouraged to assume a side-lying position. The nurse can assist her to a position of comfort and may place pillows to support her body. To increase comfort, the nurse can give back rubs or effleurage or place a cool cloth on the woman's fore-

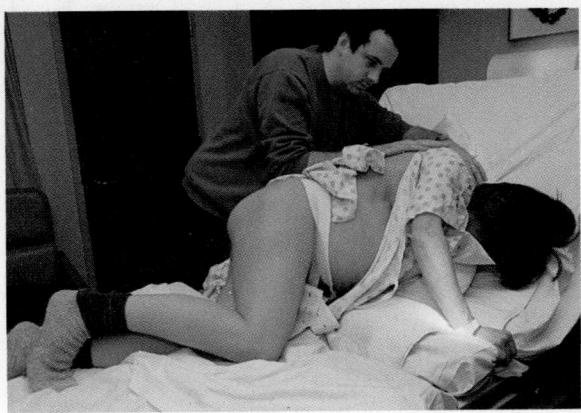
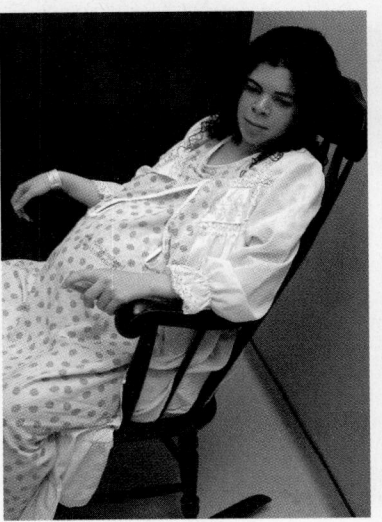
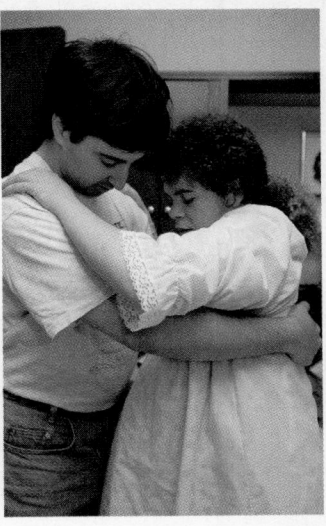

FIGURE 23-3   The laboring woman is encouraged to choose a position of comfort, and assessments and interventions are modified as necessary.

head or across her neck. The use of hydrotherapy during labor promotes maternal relaxation and pain management and decreases the length of labor (Brown 1982; Daniels 1989). Thus women can be encouraged to use a warm bath or whirlpool (Jacuzzi) to increase comfort during labor.

Because vaginal discharge increases, the nurse needs to change the Chux frequently. Washing the perineum with warm soap and water removes secretions and increases comfort. The nurse needs to use body substance isolation to avoid exposure to vaginal secretions.

Pharmacologic support may be administered at this time if the woman has a well-established contraction pattern and she is not expected to give birth within the next 1 or 2 hours. If an analgesic is given, the woman must remain in bed to promote her safety. If no one can be at the bedside with her, the side rails should be up.

For the woman experiencing slow progress of labor or the inability to tolerate fluids, an intravenous electrolyte solution may be started to provide energy and prevent dehydration (Keppler 1988; Newton et al 1988). If an IV is started, it becomes even more important to encourage voiding every 1 to 2 hours to prevent bladder distention.

If the amniotic membranes have not ruptured previously, they may during this phase. When the membranes rupture, the nurse notes the color and odor of the amniotic fluid and the time of rupture and immediately auscultates the FHR. The fluid should be clear with no odor. When the amniotic fluid contains meconium, it is called meconium-stained fluid. Meconium may be present when the fetus is in a breech presentation. In this case it may not indicate any fetal stress. In a cephalic presentation meconium staining may indicate fetal stress. Fetal stress leads to intestinal and anal sphincter relaxation, and meconium may be released into the amniotic fluid. Meconium turns the fluid greenish-brown. Whenever the nurse notes meconium-stained fluid, an electronic

monitor is applied to continuously assess the FHR. The time of rupture is noted because the incidence of amnionitis is increased with rupture over 24 hours. An additional concern is prolapse of the umbilical cord, which occurs when membranes rupture and the fetus is not engaged. The concern is that the amniotic fluid coming through the cervix will propel the umbilical cord through the cervix (prolapsed cord). This is assessed by monitoring for signs of fetal distress and/or performing a vaginal examination with a sterile glove. The FHR is auscultated because a drop in the rate might indicate an undetected prolapsed cord. Immediate intervention is necessary to remove pressure on a prolapsed umbilical cord until a cesarean birth can be performed (Chapter 25). See Table 23–6 for additional deviations from normal.

Transition

During transition the contraction frequency is every 2–3 minutes, duration is 60–90 seconds, and intensity is strong. Cervical dilatation increases from 8 to 10 cm, effacement is complete (100%), and there is usually a heavy amount of bloody show. Contractions are palpated at least every 15 minutes. Sterile vaginal examinations are done more frequently because this stage of labor usually is accompanied by rapid change. Maternal blood pressure, pulse, and respirations are taken at least every 30 minutes, and FHR is auscultated every 15 minutes.

Comfort measures become very important in this phase of labor, but continual assessment is required to intervene appropriately. The woman may rapidly change from wanting a back rub and other "hands-on" care to wanting to be left completely alone. The support person and the nurse need to follow her cues and change interventions as needed. Because the woman is breathing more rapidly, the nurse can offer small spoons of ice chips to moisten her mouth or apply petroleum jelly to dry lips. The nurse can encourage the woman to rest between

TABLE 23-6 Deviations from Normal Labor Process Requiring Immediate Intervention

Problem	Immediate Action
Woman admitted with vaginal bleeding or history of painless vaginal bleeding	Do not perform vaginal examination. Assess FHR. Evaluate amount of blood loss. Evaluate labor pattern. Notify physician/CNM immediately.
Presence of greenish or brownish amniotic fluid	Continuously monitor FHR. Evaluate dilatation of cervix and determine if umbilical cord is prolapsed. Evaluate presentation (vertex or breech). Maintain woman on complete bed rest on left side. Notify physician/CNM immediately.
Absence of FHR and fetal movement	Notify physician/CNM. Provide truthful information and emotional support to laboring couple. Remain with the couple.
Prolapse of umbilical cord	Relieve pressure on cord manually. Continuously monitor FHR; watch for changes in FHR pattern. Notify physician/CNM. Assist woman into knee-chest position. Administer oxygen.
Woman admitted in advanced labor; birth imminent	Prepare for immediate birth. Obtain critical information: EDB History of bleeding problems History of medical or obstetric problems Past and/or present use/abuse of prescription/OTC/illicit drugs Problems with this pregnancy FHR and maternal vital signs Whether membranes are ruptured and how long since rupture Blood type and Rh Direct another person to contact physician/CNM. Do not leave woman alone. Provide support to couple. Put on gloves.

contractions. If analgesics have been administered, a quiet environment enhances the quality of rest between contractions. The nurse can awaken the woman just before another contraction starts so that she can begin patterned-paced breathing.

Some women have difficulty coping with the intensity of labor during this time and need help with their breathing. Either the support person or the nurse can breathe along with the woman during each contraction to help her maintain her pattern. It is helpful to encourage her and assure her that she is doing a good job. The woman will begin to feel increased rectal pressure as the fetal presenting part moves down the birth canal and sometimes a burning sensation as the tissues become stretched. The nurse encourages the woman to refrain from pushing until the cervix is completely dilated. This measure helps prevent cervical edema.

The end of transition and beginning of the second stage may be indicated by involuntary passage of flatus

and the movement of the fetus from the side of the maternal abdomen to the midline. Other indications include a change in the woman's voice or the sounds she is making. As the fetus moves down and she feels increased pressure and a bearing-down sensation, her voice tends to deepen. A moan during a contraction takes on a more gutteral quality. Expert nurses recognize this sound as a sign of changes in the woman.

NURSING PLAN AND IMPLEMENTATION DURING THE SECOND STAGE OF LABOR

Provision of Care in the Second Stage

The second stage begins when the cervix is completely dilated (10 cm). The uterine contractions continue as in the transition phase. Frequent sterile vaginal examinations are done to assess progress. Maternal pulse, blood pressure, and FHR are assessed every 5–15 minutes; some protocols recommend assessment after each contraction (Table 23–7). As the woman pushes during the second stage she may make a variety of sounds. A low-pitched, grunting sound ("uhhh") usually indicates the woman is working with the pushing (McKay & Roberts 1990). If she begins to feel she is going to lose control, her sound may change to a high-pitched cry or whimper, or she may even cry out in pain.

Nursing responses to the woman may vary. At times the sounds are disturbing for nurses and physicians, and they feel the need to help or encourage her to be more quiet. Other nurses feel more comfortable with maternal sounds and use them as cues. The nurse provides support during the woman's pushing effort and stays sensitive to changes in the sounds for clues that the woman needs help coping with her pain. The nurse may encourage her to push harder and not let any breath out or to put all her effort into the push and not into making noise. Nurses and physicians seem to value staying in control, and for some, a childbearing women's loss of control is a source of embarrassment (McKay & Roberts 1990).

When the woman feels an uncontrollable urge to push (bear down), the nurse can help by encouraging her and by assisting with positioning (Figure 23–4). The woman can be propped up with pillows to a semireclining position. Other positions might include side-lying, squatting, or hands and knees.

When the contraction begins, the nurse tells the woman to take two short breaths, then to take a third breath and hold it while pulling back on her knees and pushing down with her abdominal muscles. Some women prefer to exhale slightly (*exhale breathing*) while pushing to avoid the physiologic effects of the Valsalva maneuver. With this method the woman takes several deep breaths and then holds her breath for 5–6 seconds. Then, through slightly pursed lips, she exhales slowly every 5–6

TABLE 23-7	Nursing Assessments in the Second Stage
Mother	**Fetus**
Blood pressure, pulse, respirations every 5–15 minutes.	FHR every 15 minutes for low-risk women and every 5 minutes for high-risk women (NAACOG 1990).
Uterine contraction palpated continuously.	

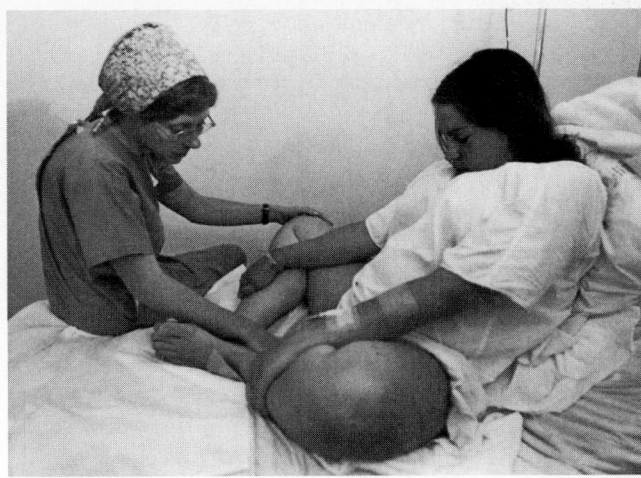

FIGURE 23-4   The nurse provides encouragement and support during pushing efforts.

seconds while continuing to hold her breath. The woman takes another breath and continues exhale breathing and pushing during the contraction.

> *I knew when I was completely dilated. I knew when to push and I did it without tearing. My body told me to listen. I knew what to do.*
> ~ HARRIETTE HARTIGAN, *WOMEN IN BIRTH* ~

The woman is encouraged to rest between contractions. Although the laboring woman may appear exhausted at this time, most experience relief at being able to push with contractions. Perspiration increases with the pushing efforts, and a cold washcloth for forehead and face is most soothing. The birthing woman may also appreciate sips of fluid or ice chips at this time.

> *When I began pushing, I felt in control because I could do something. . . . I could push the baby out. I knew he was ready to be born.*
> ~ HARRIETTE HARTIGAN, *WOMEN IN BIRTH* ~

Maternal positions such as standing, squatting while leaning back on a partner or on a birthing bar (Figure 23–5), lying in a lateral or Sims' position, and crouching on hands and knees may increase comfort and effectiveness of pushing. Some women feel that sitting on a toilet seat is a comfortable position that assists their pushing efforts. This position may cause anxiety in the care givers, however, for fear that the birth may occur quickly in this most inopportune place.

Additional comfort measures may be used during this stage. Hot perineal, abdominal, and back compresses may be used to increase muscle relaxation. Perineal massage and stretching with a lubricant (Lubafax) may relieve the tearing and burning sensation as the perineal tissue distends. (At this time perineal stretching is done by the CNM and not other nursing staff.)

Visualization techniques may be helpful (Simkin 1989). The woman can be encouraged to envision the infant descending the birth canal. Phrases such as "Open to your baby" and "Let the baby come; don't try to hold back" can be useful and calming.

Nurses frequently have learned one way for assisting the woman during pushing efforts and may hesitate to en-

courage unique positions. It is important to support the woman's needs and to encourage a change in position if anticipated progress is not made.

Throughout the second stage it remains important to continue to provide information regarding progress and what is happening in the labor. It is also imperative to

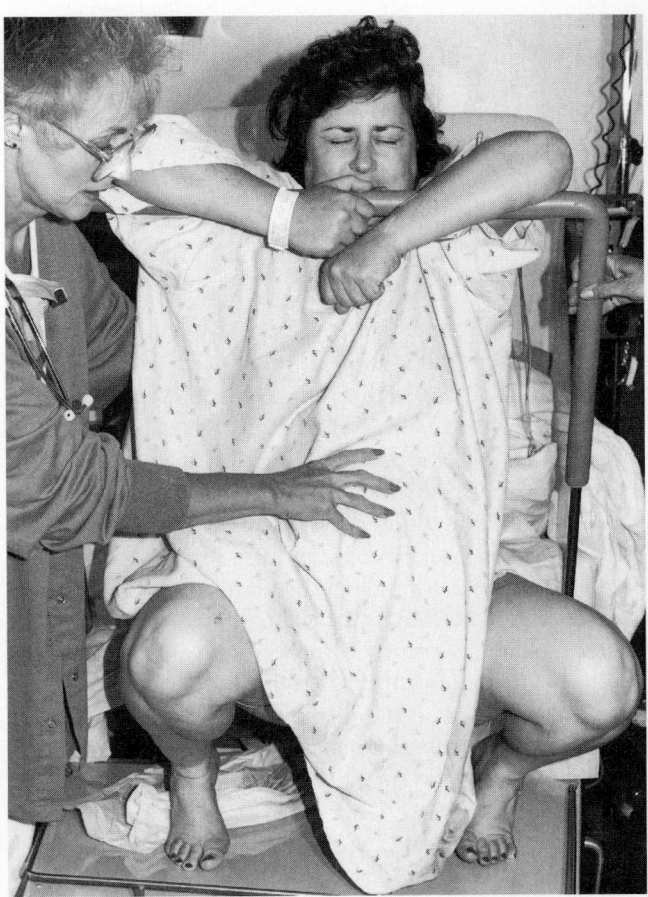

FIGURE 23-5   Using a birthing bar.

address the woman's questions honestly and to acknowledge her concerns. (McKay & Smith 1993).

A nullipara is usually prepared for birth when the perineum begins to bulge. A multipara usually progresses much more quickly, so she may be prepared for the birth when the cervix is dilated 7–8 cm.

The woman's blood pressure and the FHR are monitored between contractions, and the contraction are palpated until the birth. The nurse continues to assist the woman in her pushing efforts. Both the woman and the coach are kept informed of procedures and of progress, and both are supported throughout the birth.

In addition to assisting the woman and her partner, the nurse assists the physician or certified nurse-midwife in preparing for the birth. The physician/CNM dons a sterile gown and gloves and places sterile drapes over the woman's abdomen and legs. An episiotomy may be done just before birth if there is a need for one. See the discussion of episiotomy in Chapter 26.

Promotion of Comfort in the Second Stage

Most of the comfort measures that have been used during the first stage remain appropriate at this time. Cool cloths to the face and forehead may help provide cooling as the woman is involved in the intense physical exertion of pushing. If she has been diaphoretic, a dry gown may be comforting. The woman may feel hot and want to remove some of the covering. Care still needs to be taken to provide privacy even though covers are removed. The woman can be encouraged to rest and "let all muscles go" during the period between contractions. The nurse and support person(s) can assist the woman into a pushing position with each contraction to further conserve energy. Sips of fluid or ice chips may be used to provide moisture and relieve dryness of the mouth.

Assisting the Couple and Physician/CNM During Birth

Shortly before the birth the birthing room or delivery room is prepared with equipment and materials that may be needed. Family members do not need to change into other clothing if the birth occurs in a birthing room; they don a disposable scrub suit if the birth is to occur in a delivery room or surgery suite. Good handwashing is required of the nurses and certified nurse-midwife/physician. Nurses who will be in direct contact with the mother at the time of birth need to wear protective clothing such as an apron or gown with a splash apron, disposable gloves, and eye covering (see Essential Precautions in Practice: During Birth). The certified nurse-midwife/physician will also need to wear a gown with a splash apron, or plastic apron, eye covering, and sterile gloves.

If the laboring woman is to give birth in a delivery room, she will be moved shortly before birth on her bed or a cart. It is important to preserve her privacy during the transfer, and safety must be provided by raising the side rails into a locked position. In the delivery room the labor bed or transfer cart must be carefully supported against the delivery table; this ensures the woman's safety during the transfer.

It is important that the woman move from one bed to another between contractions. During the contraction the woman feels increased discomfort and may be involved in pushing efforts. Perineal bulging may be occurring, which adds to the discomfort and difficulty in moving. All of these factors make moving very uncomfortable. If birth seems imminent (within the next minute), it is safer for the woman to give birth in her labor bed or on the cart. Transfer to the delivery table is then delayed until after the baby is born and the cord has been clamped and cut.

Even though there are differences in the delivery room setting, the family can still be together during the

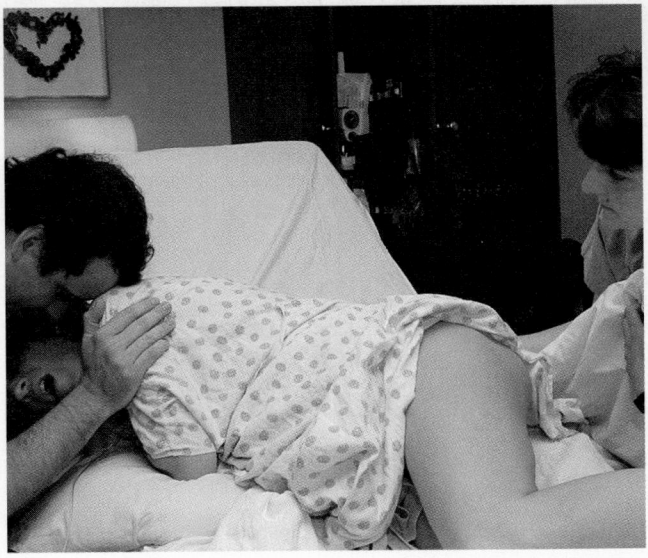 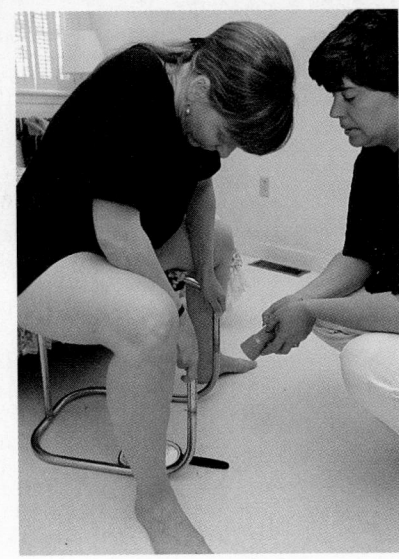

A

B

FIGURE 23-6 Birthing positions. *A* Side-lying position. *B* Using a birthing stool.

Maternal Birthing Positions

The woman is usually positioned for birth on a bed, birthing chair, or delivery table. In some instances she may give birth standing at the side of the bed or on her hands and knees on the floor. The position the woman assumes is determined not only by her individual wishes but also by the certified nurse-midwife/physician.

Stirrups are not often used, but if they are, they are padded to alleviate pressure, and both legs should be lifted simultaneously to avoid strain on abdominal, back, and perineal muscles. The stirrups should be adjusted to fit the woman's legs. The feet are supported in the stirrup holders. The height and angle of the stirrups are adjusted so there is no pressure on the back of the knees or the calf, which might cause discomfort and postpartal vascular problems. This is particularly true of women with epidural anesthesia. The birthing bed is elevated 30–60 degrees to help the woman bear down, and handles are provided so she may pull back on them.

The upright posture for birth was considered normal in most societies until modern times. Squatting, kneeling, standing, and sitting were variously selected by women for birth. Only within the last 200 years has the recumbent position become more usual in the Western world. Its use in this century has been reinforced because of the convenience it offers in applying new technology. The lithotomy position has thus become the conventional manner in which North American women give birth in hospitals. In searching for alternative positions consumers and professionals alike are refocusing on the comfort of the lobbying woman rather than on the convenience of the certified nurse-midwife/physician (Figure 23–6 and Table 23–8).

Recumbent Position The lithotomy position for birth is used sometimes to enhance the maintenance of asepsis, assessment of FHR, and performance of episiotomy and repair. In contrast, when the comfort and well-being of the woman and fetus are considered, the following disadvantages have been noted:

- There is a decrease of as much as 30% in the blood pressure of 10% of women.
- Many women experience difficulty breathing because of pressure of the uterus on the diaphragm.
- The uterine axis is directed toward the symphysis pubis instead of the pelvic inlet.
- Aspiration of vomitus is more likely.
- The woman may feel resentment at being forced to assume an "embarrassing" position.
- Tightening of the vagina and perineum as the thighs are flexed may increase the need for an episiotomy.
- The position may interfere with the frequency and intensity of contractions.
- Stirrups cause excessive pressure on the legs.
- The woman works against gravity.

birth. It is important to provide encouragement for family members to participate because the delivery room environment may be unfamiliar and seem less relaxed. The family member may be hesitant to continue to provide support for fear of interfering or being in the way.

TABLE 23-8   Comparison of Birthing Positions

Position	Advantages	Disadvantages	Nursing Actions
Sitting in birthing chair	Gravity aids descent and expulsion of infant. Does not compromise venous return from lower extremities. Chair can be tilted to various degrees. Woman can view birth process.	If woman is short, sitting with legs spread may increase tension on perineum, which may lead to lacerations. Position of body, legs, and feet cannot be altered. Potential for increased blood loss (Sleep et al 1989).	Encourage woman to tilt the chair to increase her comfort. Assess for pressure points on legs.
Semi-Fowler's	Does not compromise venous return from lower extremities. Woman can view birth process.	If legs are positioned wide apart, relaxation of perineal tissues is decreased.	Assess that upper torso is evenly supported. Increase support of body by changing position of bed or using pillows as props.
Left lateral Sims'	Does not compromise venous return from lower extremities. Increases perineal relaxation and decreases need for episiotomy. Appears to prevent rapid descent.	It is difficult for the woman to see the birth.	Adjust position so that the upper leg lies on the bed (scissor fashion) or is supported by the partner or on pillows.
Squatting	Size of pelvic outlet is increased. Gravity aids descent and expulsion of newborn. Second stage may be shortened (Sleep et al 1989).	It may be difficult to maintain balance while squatting.	Help woman maintain balance. Use a squatting bar if available.
Sitting in birthing bed	Gravity aids descent and expulsion of the fetus. Does not compromise venous return from lower extremities. Woman can view the birth process. Leg position may be changed at will.		Ensure that legs and feet have adequate support.
Hands and knees	Increases perineal relaxation and decreases episiotomies. Increases placental and umbilical blood flow and decreases fetal distress. Improves fetal rotation. Nurse is better able to assess perineum. Nurse has better access to fetal nose and mouth for suctioning at birth. Facilitates birth of infant with shoulder dystocia.	Woman cannot view birth. There is decreased contact with birth attendant. Care givers cannot use instruments. There is increased maternal fatigue.	Adjust birthing bed by dropping the foot down. Supply extra pillows for increased support.

These disadvantages may be lessened slightly if the woman is in a lithotomy position with her back elevated 30–40 degrees (Sleep et al 1989).

Left Lateral Sims' Position   A common position favored by some women and birth attendants is the left lateral Sims' position (Figure 23–6A on page 657). In assuming this position for birth the woman lies on her left side with her left leg extended and her right knee drawn against her abdomen or flexed by her side or with both legs bent at the knees. Those who favor this position find it increases overall comfort, does not compromise venous return from the lower extremities, and diminishes the chances of aspiration should vomiting occur. Women also perceive the lateral Sims' as a more natural and comfortable position and less intrusive with no stirrups or overhead lights required. Birth attendants have found the position has a positive effect on the management of fetal shoulder dystocias. Fewer episiotomies are required in this position because the perineum tends to be more relaxed. The disadvantages cited relate to the difficulty of cutting and repairing large episiotomies and problems with difficult forceps births (Gardosi et al 1989).

Squatting Position   Squatting is favored by some women primarily for the positive use it makes of gravity. Squatting is thought to facilitate the entrance of the presenting part into the pelvic inlet, thus hastening engagement. A squatting bar (birthing bar) may be used across a bed or on the floor to increase the woman's balance and provide some support (Figure 23–6B on page 657). During the second stage of labor, squatting increases the size of the pelvic outlet and helps in the woman's pushing efforts. Some birth attendants object to this position because the perineum is relatively inaccessible, and it is difficult for them to control the birth process. Squatting also increases the difficulty of administering analgesia, using instruments, and monitoring fetal status.

Semi-Fowler's Position A semi-Fowler's position is advocated by some as an appropriate middle ground between the recumbent and upright positions. This position enhances the effectiveness of the abdominal muscle efforts while the woman is pushing and thereby shortens the second stage of labor. Raising and supporting the torso helps the woman view the birth process. At the same time the birth attendant has access to the perineum. Supporting a woman in this position is not difficult with most birthing beds (Figure 23–7).

Sitting Position The sitting position is becoming an option for more women with the increased availability of birthing chairs. The use of birthing chairs or stools can be traced back to ancient Egypt and was broadly used in ancient Greek, Roman, and Incan civilizations. In the wake of the nineteenth-century battle against puerperal fever birthing chairs began to vanish on hygienic grounds. Birthing chairs are being used again during the second stage of labor and are perceived by some women who use them as a positive way to participate in the birth process. A supported sitting position may also be achieved in a birthing bed.

The upright sitting position offers advantages similar to squatting. It has been postulated that the weight of a term fetus is sufficient force in itself to supply much of what is needed to bring the newborn into the world. Proponents of the birthing chair state that it makes possible spontaneous births that would have required operative assistance in the recumbent position. Women experiencing severe back pain have found use of the chair can diminish or eliminate the pain. The woman can curl forward and grasp her knees and ankles during pushing efforts. She can usually see the birth without aid of mirrors, and following birth she can lift the baby up toward her face.

Duration of second stage and fetal outcome is not significantly affected by use of the birthing chair. However, a potential for increased blood loss may exist.

Hands and Knees Position The hands and knees position is more comfortable for a woman experiencing back labor because there is less pressure on the maternal back from the fetus, and the fetus may be able to rotate more easily from the posterior position. The mother can be well supported by dropping the foot of the birthing bed and supplying extra pillows upon which she can rest her forearms. Because there is less pressure on the perineum, there is less need for an episiotomy. The birth attendant is better able to assess the perineum for stretching and good access to the fetal nose and mouth for suctioning at the time of birth. This position may also increase placental and umbilical blood flow during episodes of fetal distress. Lastly, the hands and knees position may

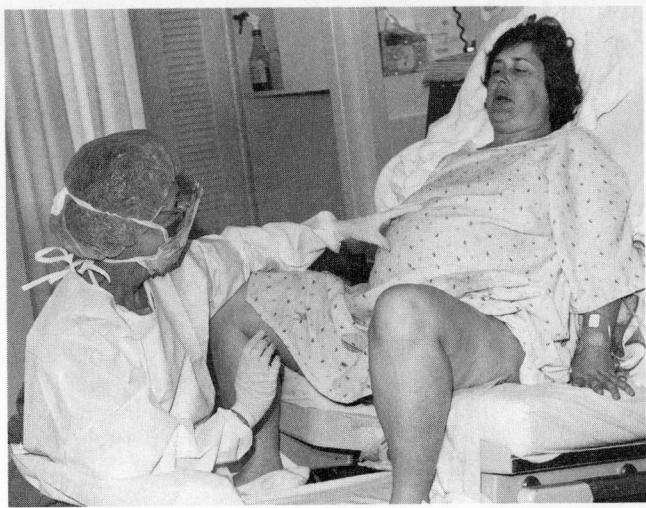

FIGURE 23-7 Observing standard precautions (universal precautions and body substance isolation) at the time of birth involves using a number of articles. In this high-risk situation the nurse wears disposable gloves, a disposable paper gown that ties in the back and is either impervious to fluids or has a plastic splash apron on it, and a disposable mask and eyeglasses or goggles to avoid splashes in the face and eyes at the time of birth to meet recommendations of both universal precautions and body substance isolation. This nurse has also donned a disposable hat, which is not required for universal or BSI precautions. The nurse must work hard to avoid the distancing that the mask and other garb may create. This nurse continues to maintain eye contact, to use touch, and to provide encouragement and support to the laboring woman.

increase the pelvic diameter and facilitate birth of the infant with shoulder dystocia. Disadvantages of this position include decreased eye-to-eye contact between the mother and birth attendant, the inability to use instruments, and the potential necessity of repositioning the mother for perineal repair. Women may also become easily fatigued in this position (Gannon 1992).

Critical Thinking Question

What factors might influence the birthing position that a woman chooses?

Cleansing the Perineum

After being positioned for the birth the woman's vulvar and perineal area is cleansed to increase her comfort and to remove the bloody discharge that is present prior to the actual birth. An aseptic technique such as the one that follows is recommended.

After a thorough hand washing, the nurse opens the sterile prep tray, dons sterile gloves, and cleans the vulva

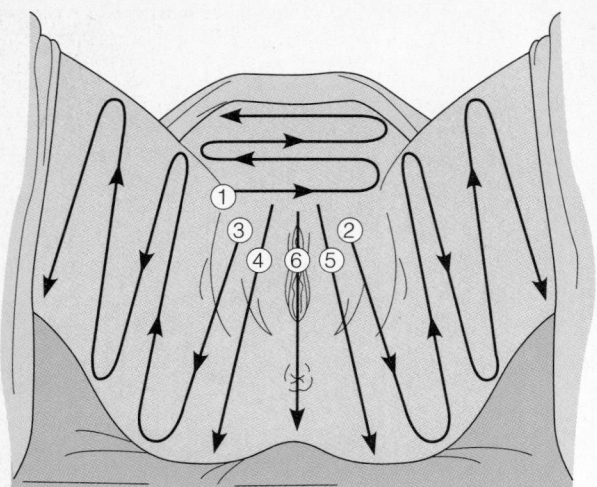

FIGURE 23-8   Cleansing the perineum prior to birth. The nurse follows the numbered diagram, using a new sponge for each area.

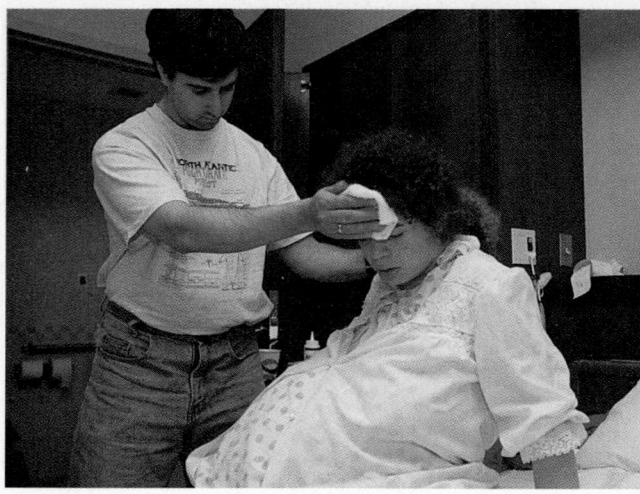

FIGURE 23-9   The partner can provide comfort and assistance during contractions.

and perineum with the cleansing solution (Figure 23–8). Some agency policy dictates the area be rinsed with sterile water. Beginning with the mons pubis, the area is cleansed up to the lower abdomen. A second sponge is used to clean the inner groin and thigh of one leg, and a third is used to clean the other leg, moving upward to avoid carrying material from surrounding areas to the vaginal outlet. The last three sponges are used to clean the labia and vestibule with one downward sweep each. The used sponges are discarded. Once the cleansing is completed, the woman returns to the desired birthing position.

Supporting the Couple

The labor coach and/or support person is made comfortable. Both the woman and the coach are kept informed of procedures and progress and are supported throughout the birth. In some birth settings there is a mirror that can be adjusted so that the couple may watch the birth.

The woman's blood pressure is monitored between contractions, and the contractions are palpated until the birth. FHR is auscultated every 15 minutes for low-risk women and every 5 minutes for high-risk women (NAACOG 1990). The nurse and support person continue to assist the woman (Figure 23–9).

In addition to assisting the woman and her partner, the nurse assists the physician or certified nurse-midwife in preparing for the birth.

Physician/CNM Interventions

When the fetal head has distended the perineum, the clinician may perform certain hand maneuvers that are believed to prevent undue trauma to the fetal head and maternal soft tissues. The woman may be asked to breathe rapidly to avoid too rapid a birth of the fetal head.

After the infant's head is born, the clinician palpates the neck for the presence of a cord, which can be slipped over the fetal head if it is loose. If the cord is tight, it is double-clamped and cut.

Restitution and external rotation occur after the head is born. The only assistance needed during this time is support of the maternal perineum. While awaiting completion of external rotation, the clinical suctions the newborn's nose and mouth to remove mucus. When the newborn's shoulder appears at the symphysis pubis, the clinician may use both hands to grasp the newborn's head gently and pull downward for release of the anterior shoulder. Gentle upward traction facilitates release of the posterior shoulder.

Birth of the newborn's body may be controlled by grasping the posterior shoulder with one hand, palm turned toward the perineum. The left hand may be used for this if the newborn is LOA. The right hand then follows along the infant's back, and the feet are grasped as they are expelled. The newborn's head is kept down and to the side as the newborn's feet, legs, and body are tucked under the clinician's left arm in a football hold. The clinician's right hand is then free for further care of the newborn and the newborn is securely held. Certified nurse-midwives often deliver the newborn directly to the mother's abdomen. The nose and mouth are suctioned with a bulb syringe, and respiratory passages are cleared. Figure 23–10 depicts an entire birthing experience.

There is considerable controversy about when to clamp and cut the cord. If the newborn is held at or below the vagina as cord clamping is delayed, as much as 50 to 100 mL of blood may be shifted from the placenta to the newborn. If the newborn is held 50 to 60 cm above the vagina, blood may be transferred from the neonate to the placenta. The extra amount of blood added to the new-

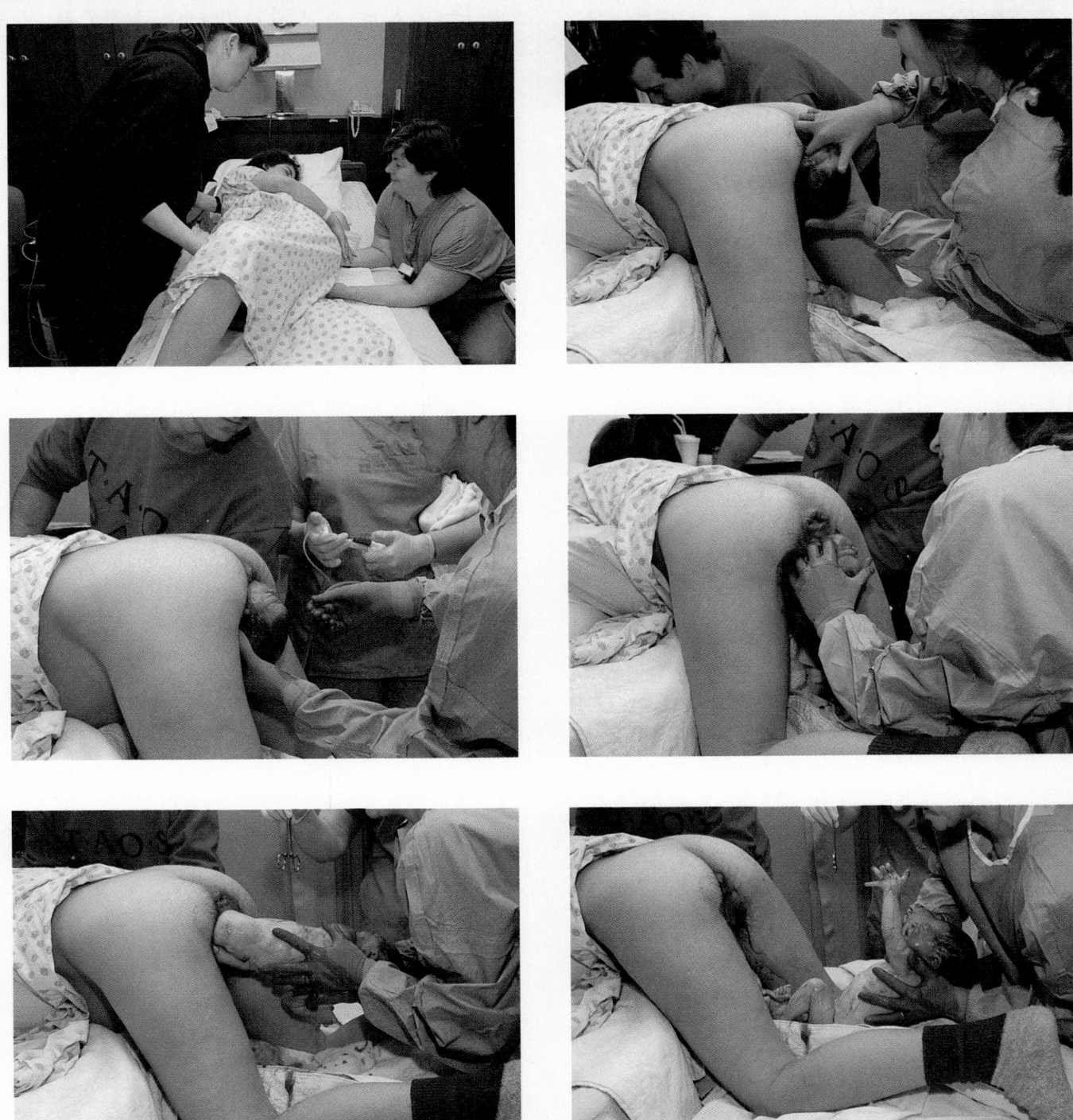

FIGURE 23-10   A birthing sequence.

born's circulation by holding the child below the vagina may reduce the frequency of iron-deficiency anemia, which can occur later in infancy—or the circulatory overload may produce polycythemia and favor hyperbilirubinemia. Cunningham et al (1993) advocate clamping the cord after clearing the newborn's airway, which takes about 30 seconds. The newborn is not elevated above the vagina.

The cord is usually clamped with two Kelly clamps and cut between them, although some birth attendants may ask that the cord be double-clamped so that a section is available for the collection of cord blood gases. The clamp on the placental side is placed on the mother's abdomen. A plastic cord clamp or umbilical tape may be applied on the newborn's cord about 2 cm from the newborn's abdomen, and then the Kelly clamp on the newborn's side may be removed. The father or other support person may wish to cut the cord after it has been clamped by the birth attendant.

> *The sheer pleasure of the feeling of a born baby on one's thighs is like nothing on earth.*
> ~ MARGARET DRABBLE, *EVER SINCE EVE* ~

NURSING PLAN AND IMPLEMENTATION DURING THE THIRD STAGE

Provision of Initial Care of the Newborn

The physician/certified nurse-midwife places the newborn on the mother's abdomen or in the radiant-heated unit to begin the initial care. If the newborn is not placed on the mother's abdomen, the radiant-heated unit is positioned so the parents can see the baby.

Because the first priority is to maintain respirations, the newborn is placed in a modified Trendelenburg position to aid drainage of mucus from the nasopharynx and trachea. The newborn is also suctioned with a bulb syringe or DeLee mucus trap as needed (Procedure 23–1: Nasal Pharyngeal Suctioning).

The second priority is to provide and maintain warmth, so the newborn is dried immediately with warmed soft infant blankets. It is important to begin drying the newborn's head first to minimize heat loss. Warmth can be maintained by putting the newborn in skin-to-skin contact with the mother and placing warmed blankets over both of them. If the newborn is placed in a radiant-heated unit, he or she is dried, laid on a dry blanket, and left uncovered under the radiant heat. Because radiant heat warms the outer surface of objects, a newborn wrapped in blankets will receive no benefit. In many settings a stocking cap is placed on the newborn's head to conserve heat.

Apgar Scoring System

The Apgar scoring system (Table 23–9) was designed in 1952 by Dr Virginia Apgar, an anesthesiologist. The purpose of the **Apgar score** is to evaluate the physical condition of the newborn at birth and the immediate need for resuscitation. The newborn is rated 1 minute after birth and again at 5 minutes and receives a total score ranging from 0 to 10 based on the following criteria:

1. The *heart rate* is auscultated or palpated at the junction of the umbilical cord and skin. This is the most important assessment. A newborn heart rate of less than 100 beats per minute indicates the need for immediate resuscitation.

2. The *respiratory effort* is the second most important Apgar assessment. Complete absence of respirations is termed *apnea*. A vigorous cry indicates good respirations.

3. The *muscle tone* is determined by evaluating the degree of flexion and resistance to straightening of the extremities. A normal newborn's elbows and hips are flexed, with the knees positioned up toward the abdomen.

4. The *reflex irritability* is evaluated by flicking the soles of the feet or by inserting a nasal catheter in the nose. A cry merits a full score of 2. A grimace is 1 point, and no response is 0.

5. The *skin color* is inspected for cyanosis and pallor. Newborns generally have blue extremities, and the rest of the body is pink, which merits a score of 1. This condition is termed *acrocyanosis* and is present in 85% of normal newborns at 1 minute after birth. A completely pink newborn scores a 2, and a totally cyanotic, pale infant is scored 0. Newborns with darker skin pigmentation will not be pink. Their skin color is assessed for pallor and acrocyanosis, and a score is selected based on the assessment.

A score of 8 to 10 indicates a newborn in good condition who requires only nasopharyngeal suctioning and perhaps some oxygen near the face. An Apgar score between 4 and 7 indicates the need for stimulation; a score under 4 indicates the need for resuscitation. See the discussion in Chapter 32.

Care of the Umbilical Cord

If the physician/certified nurse-midwife has not placed a cord clamp on the newborn's umbilical cord, it is the responsibility of the nurse to do so. Before applying the cord clamp, the nurse examines the cut end for the pres-

| TABLE 23-9 | The Apgar Scoring System |

Sign	Score		
	0	**1**	**2**
Heart rate	Absent	Slow—below 100	Above 100
Respiratory effort	Absent	Slow—irregular	Good crying
Muscle tone	Flaccid	Some flexion of extremities	Active motion
Reflex irritability	None	Grimace	Vigorous cry
Color	Pale blue	Body pink, blue extremities	Completely pink

SOURCE: Apgar V: The newborn (Apgar) scoring system, reflections and advice. *Pediatr Clin North Am* August 1966;13:645.

Nursing Action	Rationale
Objective: Clear secretions from newborn's nose and/or oropharynx if respirations are depressed and/or if amniotic fluid was meconium stained.	
Tighten the lid on the DeLee mucus trap or other suction device collection bottle.	*Avoids spillage of secretions and prevents air from leaking out of lid*
Connect one end of the DeLee tubing to low suction.	*Provides suction*
Insert other end of tubing in newborn's nose or mouth 3 to 5 inches (Figure 23-11).	*Clears nasopharynx*

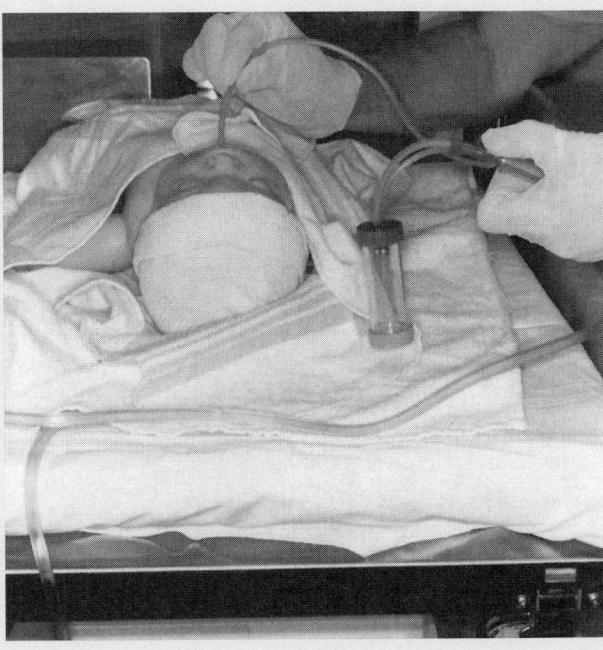

FIGURE 23-11   DeLee mucus trap.

Continue suction as tube is removed.	*Avoids redepositing secretions in newborn's nasopharynx*
Continue reinserting tube and providing suction for as long as fluid is aspirated.	*Facilitates removal of secretions*
Note: Excessive suctioning can cause vagal stimulation, which causes decreased heart rate.	
Occasionally, the tube may be passed into the newborn's stomach to remove secretions or meconium that was swallowed before birth. If this is necessary, insert tube into newborn's mouth and then into stomach. Provide suction and continue suction as tube is removed. Be careful not to aspirate the fluid yourself.	*If meconium was present in amniotic fluid, the baby may have swallowed some.* *Secretions and/or meconium aspirate may be removed from newborn's stomach to decrease incidence of aspiration of stomach contents.*
Objective: Record information on client's record. Document completion of procedure and amount and type of secretions obtained.	*Provides documentation of intervention and status at birth*

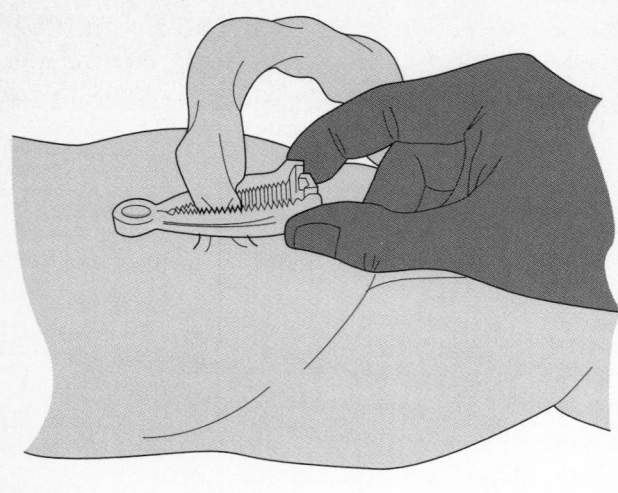

A

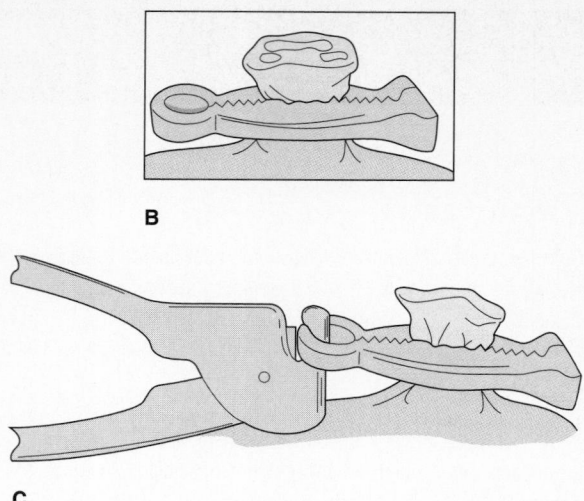

B

C

FIGURE 23-12 Hollister cord clamp. *A* Clamp is positioned ½ to 1 inch from the abdomen and then secured. *B* Cut cord. The one vein and two arteries can be seen. *C* Plastic device for removing clamp after cord has dried. After the cord is cut, the nurse grasps the Hollister clamp on either side of the cut area and gently separates it.

ence of two arteries and one vein. The umbilical vein is the largest vessel, and the arteries are smaller vessels. The presence of only one artery in the umbilical cord is associated with genitourinary abnormalities. The number of vessels is recorded on the birth and newborn records. The cord is clamped approximately ½ to 1 inch from the abdomen to allow room between the abdomen and clamp as the cord dries (Figure 23–12). Abdominal skin must not be clamped because this will cause necrosis of the tissue. The clamp is removed in the newborn nursery approximately 24 hours after birth if the cord has dried.

Newborn Physical Assessment by the Nurse

An abbreviated systematic physical assessment is performed by the nurse in the birthing area to detect any abnormalities (Table 23–10). First, the size of the newborn and the contour and size of the head in relationship to the rest of the body are noted. The newborn's posture and movements indicate tone and neurologic functioning.

The skin is inspected for discoloration, presence of vernix caseosa and lanugo, and evidence of trauma and desquamation (peeling of skin). Vernix caseosa is a white, cheesy substance found normally on newborns. It is absorbed within 24 hours after birth. Vernix is abundant on preterm infants and absent on postterm newborns. A large quantity of fine hair (lanugo) is often seen on preterm newborns, especially on their shoulders, foreheads, backs, and cheeks. Desquamation of the skin is seen in postterm newborns.

The nares are observed for flaring. As the newborn cries, the palate can be inspected for cleft palate. Mucus in the nose and mouth can be assessed and removed with the bulb syringe as needed. The chest is inspected for respiratory rate and the presence of retractions. If retractions are present, the newborn is assessed for grunting or stridor. A normal respiratory rate is 30–40 per minute. The lungs may be auscultated bilaterally for breath sounds. Absence of breath sounds on one side could mean pneumothorax. Rales may be heard immediately after birth because a small amount of fluid may remain in the lungs; this fluid will be absorbed. Rhonchi indicate aspiration of oral secretions.

The elimination of urine or meconium is noted and recorded on the newborn record.

Newborn Identification

To ensure correct identification, the nurse gives the mother and the newborn matching identification bands in the birthing or delivery room. One bracelet is placed on the mother's wrist and sometimes on the wrist of her partner or a support person who the mother designates. Two bracelets are placed on the newborn—one on the wrist and one on the ankle. The newborn bands must be applied snugly to prevent their loss.

Most hospitals footprint the newborn and fingerprint the mother for further identification purposes. To prepare the newborn for footprinting, the nurse wipes the soles of both the newborn's feet to remove any vernix caseosa.

Initiation of Attachment

The birth of the baby is usually an emotionally charged time for all members of the family. The sight of the new baby and the sounds of the first cry create an exhilarating

TABLE 23-10 Initial Newborn Evaluation

Assess	Normal Findings
Respirations	Rate 36–60, irregular
	No retractions, no grunting
Apical pulse	Rate 120–160 and somewhat irregular
Temperature	Skin temp above 36.5 C (97.8 F)
Skin color	Body pink with bluish extremities
Umbilical cord	Two arteries and one vein
Gestational age	Should be 38–42 weeks to remain with parents for extended
	time
Sole creases	Sole creases that involve the heel

In general expect scant amount of vernix on upper back, axilla, groin; lanugo only on upper back; ears with incurving of upper 2/3 of pinnae and thin cartilage that springs back from folding; male genitalia—testes palpated in upper or lower scrotum; female genitalia—labia majora larger; clitoris nearly covered

In the following situations newborns should generally be stabilized rather than remaining with parents in the birth area for an extended period of time:

Apgar less than 8 at 1 minute and less than 9 at 5 minutes or baby requires resuscitation measures (other than whiffs of oxygen)

Respirations below 30 or above 60, with retractions and/or grunting

Apical pulse below 120 or above 160 with marked irregularities

Skin temperature below 36.5 C (97.8 F)

Skin color pale blue or circumoral pallor

Baby less than 38 or more than 42 weeks' gestation

Baby very small or very large for gestational age

Congenital anomalies involving open areas in the skin (meningomyelocele)

and emotional moment for the new parents. They may be filled with utter amazement, and as the baby is placed on the mother's abdomen or chest, she frequently reaches out to touch and stroke her baby. When the newborn is placed in this position, the father also has a very clear, close view and can also reach out to touch his baby. When the parents feel comfortable in the environment, they may talk to the newborn, and some mothers talk to their babies in a high-pitched voice, which seems to soothe newborns. Some couples verbally express amazement and pride when they see they have produced a beautiful, healthy baby. Their verbalization enhances feelings of accomplishment and ecstasy. If lights in the birthing area can be dimmed, the newborn will probably open his or her eyes wide and gaze at the surroundings. In this first hour after birth the newborn is usually quiet and continues to gaze. This is a wonderful opportunity for eye-to-eye contact with the parents, and many parents are content to gaze quietly at their newborn.

Even though the baby is on the mother's abdomen or chest, the nurse can complete any needed assessments or interventions such as footprinting and applying an identification bracelet to the child. As soon as possible the nurse can assist the mother to a more comfortable position for holding the newborn. Newborns have highly developed sensory skills that allow them to be active partic-

ipants in interactions from birth (Righard & Alade 1990). Breastfeeding can be encouraged if the mother and baby desire. Various researchers emphasize that the baby will seek out the mother's breast and that early contact between the two can greatly impact breastfeeding success (Kennell 1994; Righard & Alade 1990). Even if the newborn does not actively nurse, she or he can lick, taste, and smell the mother's skin. This activity stimulates the maternal release of prolactin, which promotes the onset of lactation.

The initial parental-newborn attachment period can be enhanced if the care providers keep routine investigations to a minimum, delay instillation of ophalmic antibiotic for 1 hour, keep the room slightly darkened, avoid loud noises, talk in quiet tones, and provide privacy. Both parents need to be encouraged to do whatever they feel most comfortable doing. Parents may have differing wishes concerning contact with their newborn: Some want immediate and unlimited time; some prefer to wait until all birth-related activities are completed (the placenta is expelled and episiotomy repair is completed); others prefer limited contact immediately after birth and quiet time later. Although immediate contact may be important for attachment and initiation of breastfeeding, the parents' wishes need to be supported.

I was hungry for the baby as he was born. I wanted to see, hold him. It was hours before I realized or even thought love in relation to him.

~ HARRIETTE HARTIGAN, *WOMEN IN BIRTH* ~

CNM/Physician Interventions

After the cord has been clamped and cut, the physician/certified nurse-midwife observes for the following signs of placental separation:

1. The uterus rises upward in the abdomen because the placenta settles downward into the lower uterine segment.

2. As the placenta proceeds downward, the umbilical cord lengthens.

3. A sudden trickle or spurt of blood appears.

4. The uterus changes from a discoid to a globular shape.

While waiting for these signs, the nurse gently palpates the uterus to check for ballooning caused by uterine relaxation and subsequent bleeding into the uterine cavity.

After the placenta has separated it may be expelled by various techniques such as maternal bearing down effort, controlled cord traction, and fundal pressure. Maternal effort allows the placenta to be expelled spontaneously and is best accomplished in an upright position. When the mother is in a dorsal recumbent or lithotomy position, she or the nurse can help the process by splinting or supporting her abdominal muscles. The mother or nurse can place her palms over the lower abdomen, or the mother can flex her thighs over her abdomen. The mother then bears down to expel the placenta.

To help the woman expel her placenta, the physician/CNM first ensures that separation has occurred and then places one hand above the symphysis pubis with the palm against the anterior surface of the uterus. The uterus is displaced upward and backward as the mother is asked to relax her abdominal muscles and breathe through an open mouth. The elevation of the uterus straightens out the birth canal and facilitates expulsion of the placenta, as well as protecting the uterus from invasion. Gentle traction is exerted on the umbilical cord. Excessive pulling may result in increased risk of uterine involution. During this procedure the nurse encourages the mother to continue breathing through an open mouth and to relax her abdominal muscles.

Fundal pressure is not a method of choice because it is very uncomfortable for the mother, may damage uterine supports, and may invert the uterus. If this method is needed, the mother is asked to relax her abdominal muscles, and then the physician's/certified nurse-midwife's hand is placed behind the uterus with the fingers directed downward toward the maternal spine. With a quick "scooping" motion the contracted uterus is pressed downward in an arc. This motion is different from direct downward pressure, which folds the uterus over the lower segment and does not enhance movement of the placenta. During the procedure the nurse provides continued encouragement to maintain abdominal relaxation. This is very difficult due to the discomfort of the procedure.

After expulsion of the placenta the physician/certified nurse-midwife inspects the placental membranes to make sure they are intact and that all cotyledons are present. This inspection is especially important with placentas expelled via the Duncan mechanism (the chance of tearing off a portion of a cotyledon is greatest with this mechanism of placental separation). If there is a defect or a part missing from the placenta, a digital uterine examination is done. The vagina and cervix are inspected for lacerations, and any necessary repairs are made. An episiotomy may be repaired now if it has not been done previously. (See further discussion of episiotomy in Chapter 26.) The fundus of the uterus is palpated; normal position is at the midline and below the umbilicus. If the fundus is displaced, it may be because of a full bladder or a collection of blood in the uterus.

The time and mechanism (Schultze or Duncan) of expulsion of the placenta are noted on the birth record.

Use of Oxytocics

Some certified nurse-midwives/physicians advocate the use of an oxytocic drug (Pitocin) to stimulate uterine contractions after birth and to reduce the incidence of third-stage hemorrhage (Long 1986).

The physician/certified nurse-midwife may request that 10 units of oxytocin be given intramuscularly to the

woman when the anterior shoulder of the infant appears at the vaginal opening. Others question whether this method increases the incidence of neonatal hyperviscosity because an additional bolus of blood may be infused into the fetus when the uterus contracts in response to the oxytocin. At other times 10 units of oxytocin may be administered IM at the time of placental expulsion. Some physicians are injecting oxytocin into the umbilical vein immediately after the cord is clamped and cut (Reddy & Carey 1989). Both techniques are thought to facilitate expulsion of the placenta. An IV bolus of oxytocin may cause profound hypotension and tachycardia (Prendiville & Elbourne 1989). Some prefer to add 10 units of oxytocin to IV fluids administered over a period of hours. Additional information and associated nursing implications are presented in the Drug Guide: Oxytocin (Pitocin) in Chapter 26.

Methylergonovine maleate (Methergine) or prostaglandin F$_2$ alpha (Prendiville & Elbourne 1989) may be given IM after expulsion of the placenta to cause contraction of the uterus. Information regarding Methergine and associated nursing implications are presented in the Drug Guide: Methergine in Chapter 34.

NURSING PLAN AND IMPLEMENTATION DURING THE FOURTH STAGE

The period immediately following expulsion of the placenta is referred to as the fourth stage of labor and birth. Actually, the label is misleading because labor and birth are completed with delivery of the placenta, and the next few hours are actually the immediate recovery phase. The fourth stage is usually defined as lasting 1 to 4 hours after the birth or until vital signs are stable. Nursing care in this phase involves the basics of postpartum nursing care. (See Essential Precautions in Practice: During the Fourth Stage.)

Immediately after the placenta is expelled, repair of an episiotomy or vaginal lacerations is done. The uterus is palpated at frequent intervals to ensure that it remains firmly contracted. If the mother has not held her baby yet, immediate newborn care should be completed at her side and within her reach so that she can touch her baby during this time. As soon as immediate care is completed, the new mother is usually eager to cuddle and explore her baby. If she plans to breastfeed and the baby is interested, she should be encouraged and helped to do so right after birth while the baby is awake and alert. Care should be taken not to try to force an uninterested baby to breastfeed because it will just lead to frustration for both mother and baby.

Behavioral characteristics of the mother vary, depending on such factors as the length of labor and the extent of interruption in normal sleep patterns. After the initial excitement of becoming acquainted with their new

TABLE 23-11	Maternal Adaptations Following Birth
Characteristic	**Normal Finding**
Blood pressure	Returns to prelabor level
Pulse	Slightly lower than in labor
Uterine fundus	In the midline at the umbilicus or 1–2 fingerbreadths below the umbilicus
Lochia	Red (rubra), small to moderate amount (from spotting on pads to $\frac{1}{4}-\frac{1}{2}$ of pad covered in 15 minutes) Doesn't exceed saturation of one pad in first hour
Bladder	Nonpalpable
Perineum	Smooth, pink, without bruising or edema
Emotional state	Wide variation, including excited, exhilarated, smiling, crying, fatigued, verbal, quiet, pensive, and sleepy

baby and notifying others of the birth, many new mothers are very tired and want to rest. Others are wide awake, eager to talk about their labor and satisfy basic body needs, such as hunger and thirst. Although labor is completed, the uterus is sensitive to touch. Palpation of the uterine fundus will be uncomfortable for the woman.

Provisions of Care

As soon as the certified nurse-midwife/physician completes the repair of any perineal lacerations or an episiotomy, drapes (if used) are removed. If the mother is to remain in the birthing bed, the nurse places clean absorbent pads beneath her and applies maternity pads. A cold pack may be placed directly on the perineum if perineal edema is present or an episiotomy has been done. If a mother prefers to shower immediately after birth, the nurse can assist her as needed and change the bed linens while the mother is up.

If stirrups were used, her perineum is cleansed and maternity pads applied before her legs are removed from the stirrups. In order to avoid muscle strain both legs are removed from the stirrups at the same time. The legs may be "bicycled" to promote circulation return. The woman is transferred to a recovery room bed. If the mother has not had a chance to hold her infant, she may do so before she is transferred from the birthing room. The nurse ensures that the mother and father and newborn are given time to begin the attachment process.

In addition to encouraging family celebration of the birth, the immediate recovery period involves assessing both maternal bleeding and newborn stabilization. The most significant source of bleeding is from the site where the placenta was implanted and where uterine vessels previously provided pooling of maternal blood to nourish the fetus. It is therefore critical that the fundus stay well contracted in order to clamp off these uterine vessels and prevent hemorrhage. It is the nurse's responsibility to assess the mother's blood pressure, pulse, firmness, and position of fundus, and amount and character of vaginal blood flow every 15 minutes for the first 1 or 2 hours. Deviations from the normal ranges require more frequent checking (Table 23–11). Blood pressure should return to the prelabor level, and pulse rate should be slightly lower than it was in labor. The return of the blood pressure is due to an increased volume of blood returning to the maternal circulation from the uteroplacental shunt. Baroreceptors cause a vagal response, which slows the pulse. The physiologic slowing may be offset by excitement, increased temperature, and/or dehydration. A rise in the blood pressure may be a response to oxytocic drugs or may be caused by PIH. Blood loss may be reflected by a lowered blood pressure and a rising pulse rate.

The fundus should be firm at the umbilicus or lower and in the midline. The uterus should be palpated (Figure 23–13) but not massaged unless boggy (atonic). When a uterus becomes boggy, pooling of blood occurs within it, resulting in the formation of clots. Anything left in the uterus prevents it from contracting effectively. Thus if it becomes boggy or appears to rise in the abdomen, the fundus should be massaged until firm; then with one hand supporting the uterus at the symphysis pubis, the nurse should attempt to express retained clots. The uterus at this time is very tender, and palpation and massage cause discomfort. All palpation and massage should be done as gently as possible.

A boggy uterus feels very soft instead of firm and hard. In some cases the uterus has relaxed so much that it cannot be found when the nurse attempts to palpate it. In this case the nurse places her hand in the midline of the

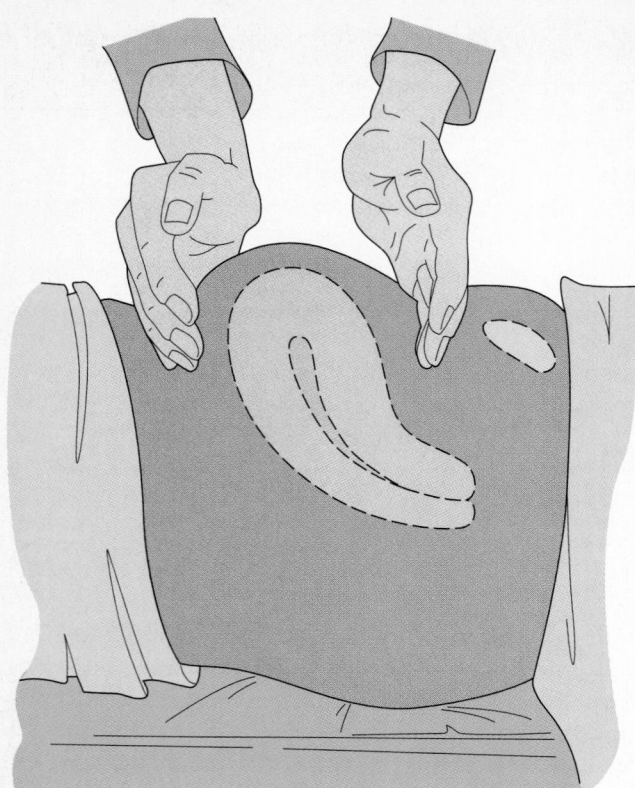

FIGURE 23-13 Suggested method of palpating the fundus of the uterus during the fourth stage. The left hand is placed just above the symphysis pubis, and gentle downward pressure is exerted. The right hand is cupped around the uterine fundus.

abdomen about at the level of the umbilicus and begins to make kneading motions. This motion stimulates the uterine fundus to contract, and the nurse will feel the fundus tighten to a firm, hard object.

The nurse inspects the bloody vaginal discharge for amount and charts it as minimal, moderate, or heavy. It should be bright red. Because different brands of maternity pads absorb varying amounts of blood, it may be necessary to weigh the maternity pad to determine actual blood loss. A gram scale is used, and 1 g is equivalent to approximately 1 mL of blood. If the perineal pad becomes soaked in a 15-minute period or if blood pools under the buttocks, continuous observation is necessary. As long as the woman remains in bed during the first hour, bleeding should not exceed saturation of one pad (Long 1986). Laceration of the vagina, cervix, or an unligated vessel in the episiotomy may be indicated by a continuous trickle of blood even though the fundus remains firm. (See Procedure 23–2: Evaluating Lochia After Birth.)

If the fundus rises and displaces to the right, the nurse palpates the bladder to determine whether it is distended. All measures should be taken to enable the mother to void. If she is unable to void, catheterization is necessary. Postpartal women have decreased sensations to

void as a result of the decreased tone of the bladder due to the trauma imposed on the bladder and urethra during childbirth. The bladder fills rapidly as the body attempts to rid itself of the extra fluid volume returned from the uteroplacental circulation and of intravenous fluid that may have been received during labor and birth. If the mother is unable to void, a warm towel placed across the lower abdomen or warm water poured over the perineum or spirits of peppermint poured into a bedpan may help the urinary sphincter relax and thus facilitate voiding. A distended bladder can cause uterine atony, thus increasing postpartal bleeding.

The perineum is inspected for edema and hematoma formation. With an episiotomy or laceration an ice pack often reduces swelling and alleviates discomfort (Hill 1989; LaFoy & Geden 1989).

The following conditions should be reported to the CNM/physician: hypotension, tachycardia, uterine atony, excessive bleeding, or a temperature over 38 C (100 F). The nurse should be aware that the blood pressure may not fall rapidly in the presence of dangerous bleeding in postpartal mothers because of the extra systemic volume. However, an increasing pulse rate may be noted before a decrease in blood pressure is detected. A normal blood pressure with the mother in the Fowler's position is a good confirmation of a normotensive woman.

Women frequently have tremors in the immediate postpartal period. It has been proposed that this shivering response is caused by a difference in internal and external body temperatures (higher temperature inside the body than on the outside). Another theory is that the woman is reacting to the fetal cells that have entered the maternal circulation at the placental site. A heated bath blanket placed next to the woman and perhaps a warm drink tend to alleviate the problem.

The couple may be tired, hungry, and thirsty. Some hospitals serve the couple a meal. The tired mother will probably drift off into a welcome sleep. The father should also be encouraged to rest because his supporting role is physically and mentally tiring. The mother is usually transferred from the birthing unit to the postpartal unit after 2 hours or more, depending on agency policy and if the following criteria are met: stable vital signs, no bleeding, nondistended bladder, firm fundus, sensations fully recovered from any anesthetic agent received during childbirth.

NURSING PLAN AND IMPLEMENTATION DURING NURSE-ATTENDED BIRTH

Occasionally, labor progresses so rapidly that the maternity nurse is faced with the task of managing the birth of the baby. This is called a **precipitous birth.** The attend-

Nursing Action	Rationale
Objective: Prepare woman.	
Explain the procedure, the reason for carrying out the procedure, and information that will be obtained.	*Decreases anxiety and increases relaxation*
Objective: Obtain and evaluate maternal vital signs.	
Assess maternal temperature, blood pressure, and pulse.	*Provides information regarding physiologic status*
Objective: Accurately evaluate the amount of lochia after birth.	
Put on disposable gloves prior to the assessment.	*Universal precautions and body substance isolation require use of gloves when exposed to body secretions such as lochia.*
Lower perineal pad so amount of lochia can be visualized.	*Allows nurse to view amount of lochia collected during the assessment*
Palpate uterine fundus by placing one hand on the fundus and the other hand just over the symphysis pubis and press downward. With the other hand palpate the uterine fundus.	*The fundus is located in the midlines at the umbilicus or one to two fingerbreadths below the umbilicus.* *Downward pressure exerted just above the symphysis pubis will prevent excessive downward movement of the uterus during assessment.*
Determine firmness of fundus.	*The uterus needs to remain firmly contracted to prevent excessive blood loss.*
If fundus is boggy, massage by rubbing in circular motion.	*Manual pressure stimulates uterine contractions.*
Evaluate the color and amount of lochia, and observe for the presence of clots. The following guidelines may be used to evaluate and describe the amount of lochia:	*Provides information regarding expected status. After birth a moderate amount of lochia rubra, without clots, is expected.*
Small: smaller than a 4 in stain on the pad; 10 to 25 mL	
Moderate: smaller than a 6 in stain; 25 to 50 mL	
Large: Larger than 6 in stain; 50 to 80 mL (Leugenbiehl et al 1990)	
If blood loss exceeds above guidelines, the perineal pads and the Chux may be weighed to more accurately estimate blood loss.	*An estimate may be obtained by using the equivalent of 1 g of weight equals 1 mL.* *Weighing the pads and Chux can provide important information because amounts of blood loss may be underestimated due to the expectation that some blood will be lost normally.*

ing maternity nurse has the primary responsibility for providing a physically and psychologically safe experience for the woman and her baby.

A woman whose physician or certified nurse-midwife is not present may feel disappointed, frightened, and abandoned, especially if she is not prepared through childbirth education. The nurse can support the woman by keeping her informed about the labor progress and assuring her that the nurse will stay with her. If birth is imminent, the nurse must not leave the mother alone. Auxiliary personnel can be directed to contact the attending physician or certified nurse-midwife, or other physicians/CNMs who are in the facility. The auxiliary personnel should also retrieve the emergency pack ("precip pack"), which should be readily accessible to the labor rooms. A typical pack contains the following items: a small drape that can be placed under the woman's buttocks to provide a sterile field; a bulb syringe to clear mucus from the newborn's mouth; two sterile clamps (Kelly or Rochester) to clamp the umbilical cord before applying a cord clamp; sterile scissors to cut the umbilical cord; a sterile umbilical cord clamp, either Hesseltine or

Hollister; a baby blanket to wrap the newborn in after birth; a package of sterile gloves.

As the materials are being gathered, the nurse must remain calm. The woman is reassured by the nurse's composure and feels that the nurse is competent. The primary goal of nursing care is the safe birth of the fetus.

Birth of Infant in Vertex Presentation

The nurse manages precipitous birth in the hospital by encouraging the woman to assume a comfortable position. If time permits, the nurse scrubs her hands with soap and water and puts on sterile gloves. Sterile drapes are placed under the woman's buttocks.

At all times during the birth the nurse gives clear instructions to the woman, supports her efforts, and provides reassurance. The nurse needs to remain calm and proceed in a slow, confident manner.

When the infant's head crowns, the nurse instructs the woman to breathe rapidly, which decreases her urge to push. The nurse checks whether the amniotic sac is intact. If it is, the nurse tears the sac with a clamp so the newborn will not breathe in amniotic fluid with the first breath.

The nurse may place an index finger inside the lower portion of the vagina and the thumb on the outer portion of the perineum and *gently* massage the area to aid in stretching of perineal tissues and to help prevent perineal lacerations. This is called "ironing the perineum."

With one hand the nurse applies gentle pressure against the fetal head to maintain flexion and prevent it from popping out rapidly. *The nurse does not hold the head back forcibly.* Rapid birth of the head may tear the woman's perineal tissues. The rapid change in pressure within the fetal head may cause subdural or dural tears. The nurse supports the perineum with the other hand and allows the head to be delivered between contractions.

As the woman continues to breathe rapidly, the nurse inserts one or two fingers along the back of the fetal head to check for the umbilical cord. If the cord is around the neck, the nurse bends her fingers like a fish hook, grasps the cord, and pulls it over the baby's head, loosens it, or slips it down over the shoulders. It is important to check that the cord is not wrapped around more than one time. If the cord is tightly looped and cannot be slipped over the baby's head, the nurse places two clamps on the cord, cuts it between the clamps, and unwinds the cord.

Immediately after birth of the head, first the mouth, throat, and then the nasal passages are suctioned. The nurse places the hand on each side of the head and instructs the woman to push gently so that the rest of the body can be expelled quickly. The newborn must be supported as it emerges.

The newborn is held at the level of the uterus to facilitate blood flow through the umbilical cord. The combination of amniotic fluid and vernix makes the newborn very slippery, so the nurse must be careful to avoid dropping the newborn. The nose and mouth of the newborn are suctioned again, using a bulb syringe. The nurse then dries the newborn quickly to prevent heat loss.

As soon as the nurse determines that the newborn's respirations are adequate, the infant can be placed on the mother's abdomen. The newborn's head should be slightly lower than the body to aid drainage of fluid and mucus. The weight of the newborn on the mother's abdomen stimulates uterine contractions, which aid in placental separation. The umbilical cord should not be pulled. The Apgar is assessed at 1 and 5 minutes.

The nurse is alert for signs of placental separation. When these signs are present, the nurse places one hand just above the symphysis pubis to guard the uterus and uses the other hand to maintain *gentle* downward traction on the cord while instructing the mother to push so that the placenta can be expelled. In some instances the mother can squat, and this usually helps expel the placenta. The nurse inspects the placenta to determine whether it is intact.

The nurse checks the firmness of the uterus. The fundus may be gently massaged to stimulate contractions and decrease bleeding. Putting the newborn to breast also stimulates uterine contractions through release of oxytocin from the pituitary gland.

The umbilical cord may now be cut. Two sterile clamps are placed approximately 2 to 4 inches from the newborn's abdomen. The cord is cut between them with sterile scissors. A sterile cord clamp (Hollister or Hesseltine) can be placed adjacent to the clamp on the newborn's cord, between the clamp and the newborn's abdomen. The clamp *must not* be placed snugly against the abdomen because the cord will dry and shrink.

The area under the mother's buttocks is cleaned, and her perineum is inspected for lacerations. Bleeding from lacerations may be controlled by pressing a clean perineal pad against the perineum and instructing the woman to keep her thighs together.

If the physician's/certified nurse-midwife's arrival is delayed or if the newborn is having respiratory distress, the newborn should be transported immediately to the nursery. *The newborn must be properly identified before he or she leaves the birthing area.*

Record Keeping

The following information is noted and placed on a birth record:

1. Position of fetus at birth
2. Presence of cord around neck or shoulder (nuchal cord)
3. Time of birth
4. Apgar scores at 1 and 5 minutes after birth
5. Gender of newborn
6. Time of expulsion of placenta

7. Method of placental expulsion
8. Appearance and intactness of placenta
9. Mother's condition
10. Any medications that were given to mother or newborn (per agency protocol)

Postbirth Interventions

Postbirth interventions are the same as those listed under Nursing Plan and Implementation During the Third Stage.

Birth of Infant in Breech Presentation

A significant factor in a breech birth is that the smallest part of the fetus presents first; succeeding parts are progressively larger. The cervix is not as effectively dilated when the fetus is in breech presentation as it is when the fetus is in the vertex position. Therefore descent is usually slow and may not occur until the cervix is fully dilated and the membranes rupture.

The primary concern in a breech birth is to prevent the entrapment of the head in the cervix. The nurse is advised to avoid intervening until the buttocks are born. Then the nurse pulls down a loop of cord (to avoid stress on its point of insertion) and supports the breech in both hands. The infant's body is lifted slightly upward for birth of the posterior shoulder and arm. The newborn may then be lowered, and the anterior shoulder and arm will pass under the symphysis pubis.

Suprapubic pressure should be applied to maintain the normal flexion of the baby's head and should be continued until the baby is born. The nape of the neck pivots under the symphysis, and the rest of the head is born over the perineum by a movement of flexion (Varney 1987).

The remaining birth and postbirth interventions for breech birth are described in the preceding section on precipitous birth of an infant in vertex presentation.

EVALUATION

Evaluation provides an opportunity to determine the effectiveness of nursing care. As a result of comprehensive nursing care during the intrapartal period the following outcomes may be anticipated:

- The mother's physical needs and the psychologic well-being of the family have been maintained and supported.
- The baby's physical and psychologic well-being has been protected and supported.
- The family has had input into the birth process, and members have participated as much as they desired.
- The birth was safe and promoted family cohesiveness.

KEY CONCEPTS

Admission to the birth setting involves assessment of many physiologic and psychologic factors. The information gained helps the nurse establish priorities of care.

Before care is begun, it is important to explain what will be done, the reasons, potential benefits and risks, and possible alternatives if appropriate. This helps the woman determine what happens to her body and is a critical element in the process of obtaining informed consent.

Behavioral responses to labor vary with the phase of labor, the preparation the woman has had, and her previous experience, cultural beliefs, and developmental level.

Each woman's cultural beliefs affect her needs for privacy, expression of discomfort, and expectations for the birth and the role she wishes the father to play in the birth event.

The laboring woman's comfort may be increased by general comfort measures, supportive relaxation techniques, methods of handling anxiety, controlled breathing, and support by a caring person.

The laboring woman fears being alone during labor. Even though there is a support person available, the woman's anxiety may be decreased when the nurse remains with her.

Maternal birthing positions include a wide variety of possibilities from side-lying to sitting, squatting, and lying flat.

Immediate assessments of the newborn include evaluation of the Apgar score and an abbreviated physical assessment. These early assessments help determine the need for resuscitation and whether the newborn's adaptation to extrauterine life is progressing normally. The newborn who is not experiencing problems may remain with the parents for an extended period of time following birth.

Immediate care of the newborn following birth also includes maintenance of respirations, promotion of warmth, prevention of infection, and accurate identification.

The new parents and their baby are given time together as soon as possible after birth.

Nursing assessments continue after the birth and are important to ensure that normal physiologic adaptations are taking place.

The adolescent has special needs in the birth setting. Her developmental needs require specialized nursing care.

REFERENCES

American Academy of Pediatrics and The American College of Obstetricians and Gynecologists: *Guidelines for Perinatal Care*, 2nd ed. Washington, DC, 1992.

Brown C: Therapeutic effects of bathing during labor. *J Nurse-Midwifery* 1982; 27:13.

Brown S, Lumley J: Satisfaction with care in labor and birth: A survey of 790 Australian women. *Birth* March 1994; 21(1):4.

Bryanton J, Fraser-Davey H, Sullivan P: Women's perceptions of nursing support during labor. *JOGNN* 1994; 23(8):638.

Calhoun MA: The Vietnamese woman: Health/illness attitudes and behaviors. In: *Women, Health and Culture*. Stern PN (editor). Washington, DC: Hemisphere, 1986.

Cunningham FG et al (editors). *Williams Obstetrics*, 19th ed. Norwalk, CT: Appleton & Lange, 1993.

Daniels K: Water birth: The newest form of safe, gentle, joyous birth. *J Nurse-Midwifery* 1989; 34:198.

Gannon JM: Delivery on the hands and knees. *J Nurse-Midwifery* 1992; 37:48.

Gardosi J, Sylvester S, Lynch: Alternative positions in the second stage of labour: A randomized controlled trial. *Brit J Obstet Gynecol* November 1989; 96:1290.

Garforth S, Garcia J: Hospital admission practices. In: *Effective Care in Pregnancy and Childbirth*, vol 2: *Childbirth*. Chalmers I, Enkin M, Keirse MJNC (editors). New York: Oxford Univ Press, 1989.

Higgins PG, Wayland JR: Labour and delivery in North America. *Nurs Times* September 1981 (midwifery suppl) p 77.

Hill PD: Effects of heat and cold on the perineum after episiotomy/lacerations. *JOGNN* March/April 1989; 18:124.

Hollingsworth AO et al: The refugees and childbearing: What to expect. *RN* November 1980; 43:45.

Hutchinson MK, Baqi-Aziz M: Nursing care of the childbearing Muslim family. *JOGNN* 1994; 23(9):767.

Kennell JH: The time has come to reassess delivery room routines. *Birth* March 1994; 21(1):49.

Keppler AB: The use of intravenous fluids during labor. *Birth* June 1988; 15:75.

Khazoyan CM, Anderson NLR: Latinas' expectations for their partners during childbirth. *MCN* 1994; 19:226.

LaDu EB: Childbirth care for Hmong families. *MCN* November/December 1985; 10:382.

LaFoy J, Geden EA: Postepisiotomy pain: Warm versus cold sitz bath. *JOGNN* September/October 1989; 18:399.

Leboyer F: *Birth Without Violence*. New York: Knopf, 1976.

Long PJ: Management of the third stage of labor: A review. *J Nurse-Midwifery* May/June 1986; 31:135.

Ludka LM, Roberts CC: Eating and drinking in labor: A literature review. *J Nurse-Midwifery* 1993; 38:199.

Lugenbiehl DL et al: Standardized assessment of blood loss. *MCN* July/August 1990; 15:241.

Mackey MC, Lock SE: Women's expectations of the labor and delivery nurse. *JOGNN* November/December 1989; 18(6):505.

Mackey MC, Stepans ME: Women's evaluation of their labor and delivery nurses. *JOGNN* 1993; 23(5):413.

McKay S, Roberts J: Obstetrics by ear: Maternal and caregiver perceptions of the meaning of maternal sounds during second stage of labor. *J Nurse-Midwifery* September/October 1990; 35(5):266.

McKay S, Smith S: "What are they talking about? Is something wrong?" Information sharing during the second stage of labor. *Birth* 1993; 20(3):142.

Morrow K: Transcultural midwifery: Adapting to Hmong birthing customs in California. *J Nurse-Midwifery* November/December 1986; 31:285.

NAACOG OGN Nursing Practice Resource: *Fetal Heart Rate Auscultation*. March 1990.

Newton N, Newton M, Broach J: Psychologic, physical, nutritional, and technologic aspects of intravenous infusion during labor. *Birth* June 1988; 15:67.

Nichols FH, Humenick SS: *Childbirth Education: Practice, Research and Theory*. Philadelphia: WB Saunders, 1988.

Prendiville W, Ellbourne D: Care during the third stage of labour. In: *Effective Care in Pregnancy and Childbirth*, vol 2: *Childbirth*. Chalmers I, Enkin M, Keirse MJNC (editors). New York: Oxford Univ Press, 1989.

Reddy VV, Carey JC: Effect of umbilical vein oxytocin on puerperal blood loss and length of the third stage of labor. *Am J Obstet Gynecol* January 1989; 160:206.

Righard L, Alade MO: Effect of delivery room routines on success of first breastfeed. *Lancet* 1990; 336:1105.

Roberts JE et al: The effects of maternal position on uterine contractility and efficiency. *Birth* Winter 1983; 10(4):243.

Simkin P: Non-pharmacological methods of pain relief during labour. In: *Effective Care in Pregnancy and Childbirth*, vol 2: *Childbirth*. Chalmers I, Enkin M, Keirse MJNC (editors). New York: Oxford Univ Press, 1989.

Sleep J, Roberts J, Chalmers I: Care during the second stage of labor. In: *Effective Care in Pregnancy and Childbirth*, vol 2: *Childbirth*. Chalmers I, Enkin M, Keirse MJNC (editors). New York: Oxford Univ Press, 1989.

Varney H: *Nurse-Midwifery*, 2nd ed. Boston: Blackwell Scientific Publications, 1987.

Weaver DF: Nurses' views on the meaning of touch in obstetrical nursing practice. *JOGNN* March/April 1990; 19(2):157.

Wuitchik M, Bakal D, Lipshitz J: The clinical significance of pain and cognitive activity in latent labor. *Obstet Gynecol* January 1989; 73(1):35.

CHAPTER 24

MATERNAL ANALGESIA AND ANESTHESIA

*W*e had attended all of our classes and practiced through the last few weeks, but I was not ready for the amount of discomfort that I felt during my labor. I had hoped to go through the whole labor and birth without any medications, but we had talked about it and knew that if I felt I needed something, that it would be alright. My nurse was also helpful and supportive of my decision. She helped me feel that I was making a good decision and that I wasn't failing somehow.

KEY TERMS

Epidural block

Local anesthesia

Pudendal block

Spinal block

OBJECTIVES

Describe the use of systemic drugs to promote pain relief during labor.

Compare the major types of regional analgesia and anesthesia, including area affected, advantages, disadvantages, techniques, and nursing implications.

Discuss the complications of regional anesthesia that may occur.

Describe the major inhalation and intravenous anesthetics used to provide general anesthesia.

Delineate the major complications of general anesthesia.

The childbearing woman experiences many demanding sensations and discomforts during labor and birth. The nurse can assist her to have a positive childbirth experience by providing effective comfort measures. Nursing interventions directed toward pain relief begin with nonpharmacologic measures such as providing information, support, and physical comfort. Back rubs, the application of cool cloths to her forehead, showers, whirlpool (Jacuzzi), and encouragement as the woman practices breathing techniques are examples of comfort measures. Some laboring women need no further interventions. For other women the progression of labor brings increasing discomfort that interferes with their ability to perform breathing techniques and maintain a sense of control. Pharmacologic analgesics may be used to decrease this discomfort, increase relaxation, and reestablish the woman's sense of control. The nurse may need to remind her there is medication to take the edge off her pain and needs to reassure her it is alright to take pain medication.

METHODS OF PAIN RELIEF

Pain and discomfort during labor may be relieved by several different methods. In addition to the nursing measures and patterned-paced breathing discussed in Chapter 23, systemic drugs and regional nerve blocks are available.

The methods are not mutually exclusive, and any one may be used in combination with other comfort measures. Systemic drugs such as meperidine (Demerol) may help the laboring woman rest and cope with her labor contractions. Regional nerve blocks such as an epidural may be used to relieve the discomfort of labor contractions and still make it possible for the expectant couple to be involved in the labor and birth process.

Although systemic analgesics and local anesthetic agents affect the fetus, so do the pain and stress experienced by the laboring woman. During the pain and stress of labor there is an increase in maternal ventilation and oxygen consumption, which decreases the amount of oxygen available to the fetus. An increase in alveolar ventilation at term will cause the $PaCO_2$ to decrease to about 32 mm Hg and causes respiratory alkalosis to develop. Arterial pH remains normal because of a compensatory decrease in serum bicarbonate (Miller 1992). During labor and birth, the main causes of stress for the fetus are hypoxia and asphyxia. Fetal hypoxia is caused by the mother breathing a hypoxic mixture of gases; as a result, decreased oxygen tension presents to the uteroplacental unit. Fetal asphyxia is secondary to a reduction of at least 50% in uterine blood flow (Ostheimer 1992). Maternal respiratory alkalosis and acidosis tend to be easier to treat than fetal problems because treatment may require simply increasing or decreasing the maternal respiratory rate.

Plasma epinephrine and norepinephrine levels are higher during than in the last trimester of pregnancy. The body's response to the pain and stress of labor causes a release of high levels of catecholamines. When discussing medication alternatives with any couple, a positive approach should be taken to help them understand that maternal discomfort and anxiety may have as much adverse effect on the fetus as the administration of a small amount of an analgesic agent.

Many couples who have had childbirth education approach childbirth confident that the psychoprophylactic techniques they have learned will enable them to cope with the discomforts of labor. There is a good deal of peer pressure on expectant parents to have the "ideal" birth experience. They may plan a natural childbirth with perhaps local infiltration anesthesia for episiotomy repair. The necessity for analgesia may elicit a sense of inadequacy and a feeling of guilt. The nurse has a very special role in assisting a woman and her partner to accept alterations in their original plan. Reassurance that accepting analgesia for discomfort is not a failure is important in maintaining the woman's self-esteem. The emphasis should be placed on the goal of a healthy, satisfying outcome for the family.

SYSTEMIC DRUGS

The goal of pharmacologic pain relief during labor is to provide maximal analgesia with minimal risk for the woman and fetus. Three factors must be considered in the use of analgesic agents: (1) the effects on the woman, (2) the effects on the fetus, and (3) the effects on the labor contractions.

Maternal drug action is of primary importance because the well-being of the fetus depends on adequate functioning of the maternal cardiopulmonary system. Any alteration of function that disturbs the woman's homeostatic mechanism affects the fetal environment. Maintaining the maternal respiratory rate and blood pressure within normal range is thus of prime importance. The use of electronic fetal monitoring has provided a means of accurately assessing the effects of pharmacologic agents on uterine contractions.

All systemic drugs used for pain relief during labor cross the placental barrier by simple diffusion, with some agents crossing more readily than others. Drug action in the body depends on the rate at which the substance is metabolized by liver enzymes and excreted by the kidneys. The fetal liver enzymes and renal systems are inadequate to metabolize analgesic agents, so high doses remain active in fetal circulation for a prolonged period of time. The fetal brain receives a greater amount of the cardiac output than the neonatal brain. The percentage of blood volume flowing to the brain is increased even further during intrauterine stress, so the hypoxic fetus receives an even larger amount of a depressant drug. The blood-brain barrier is more permeable at the time of birth, a factor that also increases the amount of drug carried to the central nervous system.

Administration of Analgesic Agents

The optimal time for administering analgesia is determined after making a complete assessment of many factors. In general an analgesic agent is administered to nulliparas when the cervix has dilated to 5 or 6 cm and to multiparas when the cervix has reached 3 or 4 cm dilatation. This is only a generalization, however; the character of each labor must be taken into account. Analgesia given too early may prolong labor and depress the fetus. Analgesia given too late is of no value to the woman and may cause neonatal respiratory depression. In many institutions the nurse decides when to give the analgesic ordered by the physician/certified nurse-midwife (CNM) or certified registered nurse-anesthetist. This decision is based on a complete assessment of the woman and the progress of labor.

Maternal Assessment

- The woman is willing to receive medication after being advised about it.
- Vital signs are stable.

Fetal Assessment

- The fetal heart rate (FHR) is between 120 and 160 beats/minute, and no late or variable decelerations are present.
- Short-term variability is present, and long-term variability is average.
- The fetus exhibits normal movement, and accelerations are present with fetal movement.
- The fetus is at term.
- Meconium staining is not present.

Assessment of Labor

- The contraction pattern is well established.
- The cervix is dilated at least 4–5 cm in nulliparas and 3–4 cm in multiparas.
- The fetal presenting part is engaged.
- There is progressive descent of the fetal presenting part. No complications are present.

TABLE 24–1	What Women Need To Know About Pain Relief Medications

Type of medication administered
Route of administration
Expected effects of medication
Implications for fetus/newborn
Safety measures needed (for example, remain in bed with side rails up)

If normal parameters are not present, the nurse may need to complete further assessments with the physician/CNM.

Prior to administering the medication, the nurse once again validates whether the woman has a history of any drug reactions or allergies and provides information regarding the medication (Table 24–1). After giving the medication, the nurse records the drug name, dose, route, and site and the woman's BP and pulse on the electronic monitor strip and on the woman's record. If the woman is alone, side rails should be raised to provide safety. The FHR is assessed for possible effects of the medication. See Essential Precautions in Practice: During Administration of Analgesia and Anesthesia on page 676.

Currently, a minimal amount of an analgesic agent is given during labor. Oral analgesics are not used because of poor absorption and prolonged gastric emptying time. The intramuscular and intravenous routes are used instead. When the prescribed route is intramuscular, the needle must be of sufficient length to penetrate the muscle rather than only the subcutaneous fat. The intravenous route is preferred because it results in prompt, smooth, and more predictable action with a smaller total dose than the intramuscular route. When an agent is given intravenously, it should be administered by titrating the drug until the desired effect is achieved. It has been suggested that the intravenous injection be given with the onset of a contraction, when the blood flow to the uterus and the fetus is decreased.

When an analgesic medication is administered by intramuscular or subcutaneous route, it will take a few minutes for the effect to be felt. The nurse can continue with other supportive measures to enhance comfort, such as ensuring a quiet environment in the room, providing a back rub or cool cloth, assisting with relaxation exercises and visualizations, or providing therapeutic touch until the effect of the medication is felt. When the medication is felt, the woman may sleep between contractions. This short period of rest helps her relax and can restore her energy. When an intravenous route is ordered by the certified nurse-midwife/physician, the effect of the drug will be felt within a couple of minutes, so if any change of position is necessary or if the woman needs to void, the nurse may suggest that these activities be completed

TABLE 24-2 Opioids Used for Labor Analgesia and Common Doses

Narcotic	Intravenous Dose	Intramuscular Dose
Morphine	2.5–5.0 mg	5–10 mg
Meperidine (Demerol)	25–50 mg	50–100 mg
Pentazocin (Talwin)	10–20 mg	20–30 mg
Butorphanol (Stadol)	1–2 mg	1–2 mg
Nalbuphine (Nubain)	5–10 mg	10–20 mg

before the drug administration. Some women may be so uncomfortable that they do not want anything except the medication. In this case administering the medication first would be more helpful for the woman.

Narcotic Analgesics

Narcotics that are injected into the circulation have their primary action at sites in the brain. Specifically, a narcotic that diffuses out of cerebral capillaries and reaches the periventricular/periaquaductal gray area of the brain will activate the neurons that descend to the spinal cord and inhibit the transmission of pain impulses in the substantia gelatinosa (Paradise 1994). Nausea and vomiting are produced by stimulation of the medullary chemoreceptor trigger zone.

A brief discussion of some selected narcotic analgesics appears in the next section. Table 24–2 presents information regarding the common doses of various opioids that may be administered during labor.

Meperidine Hydrochloride (Demerol)

Meperidine hydrochloride (Demerol) is a pure agonist and narcotic analgesic that is effective for alleviating pain during the first stage of labor. It may be given by the intravenous or intramuscular route. The IV route provides effective analgesia within 5 to 10 minutes and has a duration of about 3 hours; the usual IV dose is 25 mg. When Demerol is given intramuscularly, the dose is usually between 50 and 75 mg; the duration of the effect is 2–4 hours. Neonatal depression *can* occur, particularly when Demerol has been administered 2–3 hours before birth. If the interval between injection and birth is less than

1 hour, there is no appreciable neonatal effect (McDonald 1992). If maternal or fetal depression occurs, naloxone may be ordered to reverse the effects. See Drug Guide: Meperidine Hydrochloride for further discussion and nursing implications.

Butorphanol Tartrate (Stadol)

Butorphanol tartrate (Stadol) is a mixed agonist-antagonist agent. This type of agent can exert an analgesic effect when other more powerful agonists (such as morphine or meperidine) are not present in the body. In the presence of a more powerful agonist the mixed agonist-antagonist reverses the analgesic effects. This action may precipitate withdrawal in drug-dependent adults.

Butorphanol tartrate (Stadol) can be given by the intramuscular or intravenous route. Its onset of action occurs 10 minutes after IV injection, and the duration is from 3 to 4 hours (McDonald 1992). The recommended initial dose is 2 mg IM every 3–4 hours. If it is given IV, the dosage is reduced. Respiratory depression of both the mother and fetus/newborn can occur. The effects of Stadol can also be reversed with naloxone. Stadol should not be used for women with a known opiate dependency and should be used with caution if drug dependence is suspected.

Urinary retention following administration of this drug is rare. The nurse should, however, be alert for bladder distention when a woman has received butorphanol for analgesia during labor, has intravenous fluids infusing, and receives regional anesthesia.

Nursing Implications The respiratory depression and other effects are additive when butorphanol is administered with other central nervous system depressants such as sedatives, phenothiazides, and other tranquilizers, hypnotics, and general anesthetics. The respiratory and cardiac status of the woman should be evaluated by careful observation of vital signs and pulse oximetry. The maternal level of consciousness should also be checked frequently. Continuous electronic monitoring of the fetal heart rate, pattern, and variability is recommended. Respiratory depression in the mother or fetus/newborn can be reversed by naloxone (Narcan), which is a specific an-

MEPERIDINE HYDROCHLORIDE (DEMEROL)

Overview of Action

Meperidine hydrochloride is a narcotic analgesic that interferes with pain impulses at the subcortical level of the brain. In addition it enhances analgesia by altering the physiologic response to pain, suppressing anxiety and apprehension, and creating a euphoric feeling. Meperidine hydrochloride is used during labor to provide analgesia. Peak analgesia occurs in 40–60 minutes with intramuscular and in 5 minutes with intravenous administration. Duration is 2–4 hours (Skidmore-Roth 1994). Administration after labor has reached the active phase does not appear to delay labor or decrease uterine contraction frequency or duration. Meperidine HCl crosses the placental barrier and appears in cord blood within 2 minutes and after maternal intravenous injection can be detected in amniotic fluid 30 minutes after IM injection (Briggs et al 1994).

Route, Dosage, Frequency

IM: 50–100 mg every 3–4 hours
IV: 25 mg by slow intravenous push every 3–4 hours

Maternal Contraindications

Hypersensitivity to meperidine, asthma
CNS depression
Respiratory depression
Fetal distress
Preterm labor if birth is imminent
Hypotension
Respirations <12 per minute
Concurrent use with anticonvulsants may increase depressant effects

Maternal Side Effects

Respiratory depression
Nausea and vomiting, dry mouth
Drowsiness, dizziness, flushing
Transient hypotension
Increased intracranial pressure (Skidmore-Roth 1994)

Effect on Fetus/Neonate

Possible neonatal respiratory depression if birth occurs 60 minutes or longer after administration of the drug to the mother; incidence of respiratory depression peaks at 2–3 hours after IM administration (Briggs et al 1994)
Neonatal hypotonia, lethargy, interference of thermoregulatory response
Neurologic and behavioral alterations for several days after birth; presence of meperidine in neonatal saliva up to 48 hours following birth (Briggs et al 1994)
May have depressed attention and social responsiveness for first 6 weeks of life (Briggs et al 1994)

Nursing Considerations

Assess the woman's history, labor and fetal status, maternal blood pressure, and respirations to identify contraindications to administration.
Intramuscular doses should be injected deeply to avoid irritation to subcutaneous tissue.
Intravenous doses should be diluted and administered slowly.
Provide for the woman's safety by instructing her to remain on bed rest, by keeping side rails up, and placing call bell within reach.
Evaluate effect of drug.
Observe for maternal side effects.
Assess for respiratory depression, notify physician/CNM if respirations are <12/minute (Skidmore-Roth 1994).
Observe newborn for respiratory depression; be prepared to initiate resuscitative measures and administer antagonist naloxone if needed.

tagonist for this agent. A slightly depressed newborn is not likely to have prolonged drowsiness or sluggishness because the metabolites of butorphanol are inactive.

Butorphanol should not be used for women with a known opiate dependency and should be used with caution if drug dependence is suspected.

Urinary retention following administration of butorphanol is rare. The nurse should, however, be alert for bladder distention when a woman has received this drug for analgesia during labor, has intravenous fluids infusing, and receives regional anesthesia (epidural or subarachnoid block) for the birth. Butorphanol should be pro-

tected from light and stored at room temperature. This agent is not federally controlled and has been placed in the nonscheduled category. Hospitals vary in their own control of the drug.

Nalbuphine (Nubain)

Nalbuphine (Nubain) is similar to butorphanol in that it is a synthetic agonist-antagonist narcotic analgesic. Nalbuphine crosses the placenta to the fetus and can cause fetal distress and neonatal respiratory depression (Briggs et al 1994; Levinson & Shnider 1993). The duration of action is 3–6 hours, and the half-life is 5 hours (Skidmore-Roth 1994). Nalbuphine may be given by subcutaneous, intravenous (by intravenous push or by patient-controlled analgesia method), or intramuscular routes. The usual single dose is 10–20 mg (Skidmore-Roth 1994). Side effects include maternal respiratory depression, drowsiness, dizziness, nausea, diaphoresis (Skidmore-Roth 1994), and, although rare, a sinusoidal pattern may develop (Briggs et al 1994).

Nursing Implications Intravenous doses should be given over 3–5 minutes (Skidmore-Roth 1994). Maternal respiratory rate, quality of respirations, and characteristics of the FHR must be carefully assessed. Respirations of less than 12 or any evidence of a sinusoidal pattern should be reported immediately to the physician.

Opiate Antagonists: Naloxone (Narcan)

Because naloxone is an antagonist with little or no agonistic effect, it exhibits little pharmacologic activity in the absence of narcotics. Naloxone can be used to reverse the mild respiratory depression following small doses of opiates. The drug is useful for respiratory depression caused by fentanyl, alpha-prodine, morphine, and meperidine as well as pentazocine and butorphanol. *Naloxone is the drug of choice when the depressant is unknown because it will cause no further depression.* An initial dose of 0.4 mg to 2.0 mg may be administered intravenously. The dose of naloxone for the neonate is 0.1 mg/kg given intravenously, intramuscularly, subcutaneously, or via the endotracheal tube. The use of the dilute neonatal naloxone concentration (0.02 mg/mL) is no longer recommended because unacceptable fluid volumes may be given. The adult concentrations of 0.4 mg/mL or 1 mg/mL are recommended (Ostheimer 1992). After naloxone administration, the neonate should be observed for at least 4 hours before transfer to the regular nursery.

Nursing Implications When naloxone is given, other resuscitative measures and trained personnel should be readily available. The duration of the drug is shorter (minutes to hours) than the analgesic drug it is acting as an antagonist for, so the nurse must be alert to the return of respiratory depression and the need for repeated doses. Naloxone should be given with caution in women with known or suspected opiate dependency because it may precipitate severe withdrawal symptoms in the newborn. For further discussion see Drug Guide: Naloxone Hydrochloride (Narcan) in Chapter 32.

Sedatives

The principal use of barbiturates in current obstetric practice is in false labor or in the early stages of beginning labor. An oral dose of secobarbital (Seconal) or pentobarbital (Nembutal) promotes relaxation and allows the woman to sleep for a few hours. The woman can then enter the active phase of labor in a more relaxed and rested state.

REGIONAL ANALGESIA AND ANESTHESIA

Regional analgesia and anesthesia are achieved by injecting anesthetic agents (called *local anesthetics*) into an area that will bring the agent into direct contact with nervous tissue. Local agents stabilize the cell membrane, which prevents initiation and transmission of nerve impulses and produces a temporary and reversible loss of sensation called a regional block. The regional blocks most commonly used in childbearing include peridural block (lumbar epidural), subarachnoid block (spinal for cesarean birth or low spinal for vaginal birth), pudendal block, and local infiltration. The regional blocks may be accomplished by a single injection or continuously by means of an indwelling plastic catheter. Before initiating any regional block, intravenous fluids should be infusing to provide hydration and direct access to the intravascular system in case of adverse effects. Also, oxygen—along with necessary equipment for rapid conversion to a general anesthetic—should be available prior to regional block administration. Regional blocks have gained widespread popularity in recent years and are particularly compatible with the goals of psychoprophylactic preparation for childbirth.

Essential prerequisites for the administration of regional analgesia and anesthesia are knowledge of the anatomy and physiology of pertinent structures, techniques for administration, the pharmacology of local anesthetics, and potential complications. With the exception of nurse-anesthetists and nurse-midwives, who may perform procedures for which they have been trained, nurses in the United States may *not* legally administer anesthetic agents. However, the nurse must have an adequate knowledge of all aspects of regional anesthesia to provide support and give appropriate reinforcement of the administrator's explanation to the woman. The nurse who has a thorough understanding of the techniques and agents can also provide more efficient assistance to the administrator. The woman's safety is increased when the nurse recognizes complications and immediately initiates appropriate intervention.

The relief of pain associated with the first stage of labor can be accomplished by blocking the sensory nerves supplying the uterus with the techniques of lumbar sympathetic and peridural (epidural and caudal) blocks. Pain associated with the second stage and with birth can be alleviated with pudendal, peridural, and subarachnoid (spinal and low spinal) blocks (Figure 24–1, Table 24–3).

It is important for the laboring woman to have information regarding the regional block that is to be admin-

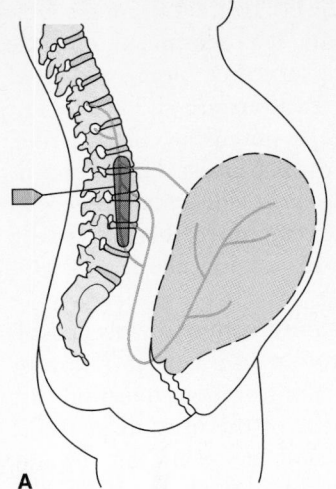 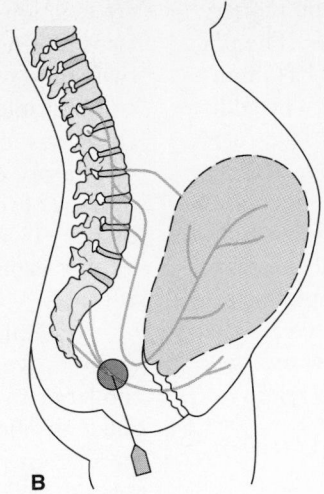 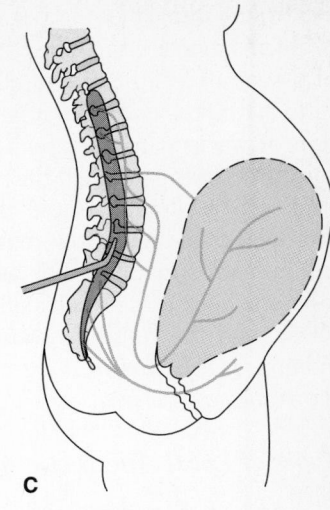

A   B   C

FIGURE 24-1   Schematic diagram showing pain pathways and
sites of interruption. *A* Lumbar sympathetic (spinal) block:
relief of uterine pain only. *B* Pudendal block: relief of perineal
pain. *C* Lumbar epidural block: Dark area demonstrates
peridural (epidural) space and nerves affected, and the gray

tube represents a continuous plastic catheter.
SOURCE: Bonica JJ: *Principles and Practice of Obstetric
Analgesia and Anesthesia.* Philadelphia: Davis, 1972, pp 492,
512, 521, 614.

istered. As with other procedures, the woman needs to
know how the block is given, the expected effect on her
and the fetus, advantages and disadvantages, and possible
complications. Many women discuss possible anesthetic
blocks with their care provider at some point in the pregnancy. If they have not, it will be important for them to
have an opportunity to ask questions and obtain information prior to receiving the block while in labor.

Anesthetic Agents for Regional Blocks

Local anesthetics block nerve conduction by impairing
propagation of the action potential in axons. They interact directly with specific receptors on the sodium chan-

nel, inhibiting sodium ion influx (Firestone et al 1993).
The types of nerve fibers are differentially sensitive to the
various anesthetic agents. In general the smaller the fiber,
the more sensitive it is to local agents. For example, it is
possible to block the small C and A delta fibers, which
transmit pain and temperature, without blocking the
larger A alpha, A beta, and A gamma fibers, which continue to maintain a sense of pressure, muscle tone, position sense, and motor function.

Absorption of local anesthetics depends primarily on
the vascularity of the area of injection. The agents also
contribute to increased blood flow by causing vasodilation. High concentrations of drugs cause greater vasodilation. Good maternal physical condition or a high metabolic rate aids absorption. Malnutrition, dehydration,

TABLE 24-3	Summary of Commonly Used Regional Blocks		
Type of Block	**Areas Affected**	**Use During Labor and Birth**	**Nursing Actions**
Lumbar epidural	Vagina and perineum	Given in first stage and second stage of labor	Assess woman's knowledge regarding the block. Act as advocate to help her obtain further information if needed. Monitor maternal blood pressure to detect the major side effect, which is hypotension. Provide support and comfort. See Nursing Care Plan: Regional Anesthesia—Lumbar Epidural for further nursing actions.
Pudendal	Perineum and lower vagina	Given in the second stage just prior to birth to provide anesthesia for episiotomy or for low forceps birth	Assess woman's knowledge regarding the block. Act as advocate to help her obtain further information if needed.
Local infiltration	Perineum	Administered just before birth to provide anesthesia for episiotomy	Assess woman's knowledge regarding the block. Provide information as needed. Provide comfort and support. Observe perineum for bruising or other discoloration in the recovery period.

electrolyte imbalance, and cardiovascular and pulmonary problems increase the potential for toxic effects. The pH of tissues affects the rate of absorption, which has implications for fetal complications such as acidosis. The addition of vasoconstrictors such as epinephrine delays absorption and prolongs the anesthetic effect. Recent studies have demonstrated that epinephrine decreases uteroplacental blood flow, making it an undesirable additive in many situations. The breakdown of local anesthetics in the body is accomplished by the liver and plasma esterase, and the resulting substance is eliminated by the kidneys. *It is important to use the weakest concentration and the smallest amount necessary to produce the desired results.*

Types of Local Anesthetic Agents

Three types of local anesthetic agents are currently available—esters, amides, and opiates. The ester type includes procaine hydrochloride (Novocain), chloroprocaine hydrochloride (Nesacaine), and tetracaine hydrochloride (Pontocaine). Esters are rapidly metabolized; therefore toxic maternal levels are not as likely to be reached, and placental transfer to the fetus is prevented. Amide types include lidocaine hydrochloride (Xylocaine), mepivacaine hydrochloride (Carbocaine), and bupivacaine hydrochloride (Marcaine). Amide types are more powerful and longer-acting agents. They readily cross the placenta, can be measured in the fetal circulation, and affect the fetus for a prolonged period.

The use of intrathecal and epidural routes for opiate-type agents is relatively new in obstetric analgesia and anesthesia. Some of the agents being used include morphine and fentanyl. The mechanism of action seems to involve specific opiate receptors in the spinal cord (Paradise 1994).

A variety of agents and a wide range of doses have been used for epidural anesthesia with varying results. The most commonly used agents are lidocaine 2% with epinephrine 1:200,000, bupivacaine 0.5%, and 2-chloroprocaine 3%. Each agent provides adequate anesthesia with 15 to 20 mL of the solution, but each has been identified with side effects. The pharmacology of each drug must be understood before it is used.

Epidural anesthesia can provide prolonged pain relief by intraspinal injection of an opioid. Some of the opioids used are morphine, butorphanol, hydromorphone, fentanyl, and sufentanil. The woman must be carefully monitored when these drugs are administered. Some of the side effects include pruritus, nausea and vomiting, vertigo, drowsiness, respiratory depression, and urinary retention.

Adverse Maternal Reactions to Anesthetic Agents

Reactions to local anesthetic agents range from mild symptoms to cardiovascular collapse. Mild reactions include palpitations, vertigo, tinnitus, apprehension, confusion, headache, and a metallic taste in the mouth. Moderate reactions include more severe degrees of mild symptoms plus nausea and vomiting, hypotension, and muscle twitching, which may progress to convulsions and loss of consciousness. The severe reactions are sudden loss of consciousness, coma, severe hypotension, bradycardia, respiratory depression, and cardiac arrest. High concentrations of the agents may also cause local toxic effects on tissues. It is important to remember that when the mother experiences an adverse reaction, the fetus is also affected.

Systemic toxic reactions most commonly occur with an excessive dose through too great a concentration or too large a volume. Accidental intravenous injection that suddenly increases the amount of the drug in maternal circulation results in depression of vasomotor, respiratory, and other medullary centers of the brain. It also depresses the heart and peripheral vascular bed. A massive intravascular dose can result in sudden circulatory collapse within 1 minute. Reactions to subcutaneous and extradural injection occur in 5 to 40 minutes. The short-acting agents (procaine) can produce toxic reactions in 10 to 15 minutes and the long-acting agents (mepivacaine), in 20 to 40 minutes. *It is imperative that the woman be under close supervision by knowledgeable personnel throughout the time that the agent is being used and that an intravenous line is in place.*

If epinephrine has been added to the anesthetic agent to prolong the anesthesia, it is necessary to differentiate between reaction to the anesthetic agent and to the epinephrine. Reaction to epinephrine is characterized by pallor, perspiration, a greater increase in blood pressure and pulse than occurs with reactions to anesthetic agents, and dyspnea.

Psycogenic reactions can occur, with symptoms similar to systemic toxic reactions. This phenomenon may occur as the procedure is begun and prior to the injection of the anesthetic agent. Regardless of the cause, the symptoms must be treated.

Allergic reactions to anesthetic agents may also occur. The manifestations of the antigen-antibody reaction include urticaria, laryngeal edema, joint pain, swelling of the tongue, and bronchospasm.

Interventions

Treatment of Systemic Toxicity In the treatment of mild toxicity the administration of oxygen by mask and intravenous injection of a short-acting barbiturate to decrease anxiety is advocated. Preparation must be made to treat convulsion or cardiovascular collapse. Specific nursing interventions in the treatment of systemic toxicity are included in the Nursing Care Plan: Regional Anesthesia—Lumbar Epidural on pages 681–684.

Treatment of Convulsions The best treatment for convulsions is establishing the airway and administering 100% oxygen (Barash et al 1993). Thiopental or diazepam may be administered to stop convulsions. Small

Text continues on page 684

REGIONAL ANESTHESIA—LUMBAR EPIDURAL

Nursing Assessment

Nursing History

1. Allergies to drugs (especially anesthetic agents)
2. Psychologic status:
   a. What kind of anesthesia does the woman want? What kind will she accept?
   b. Does she understand the procedure?
   c. What does she expect it to accomplish?
   d. Is she able to cope with the labor process? Can she follow directions?
3. Prenatal preparation and education, including the type of childbirth classes and her degree of involvement
4. Presence of disease states or physical problems including:
   a. Cardiovascular disorders
   b. Pulmonary disorders
   c. CNS disorders
   d. Metabolic problems
   e. Scoliosis
   f. Kyphosis
   g. Spinal fusion
5. Course of current pregnancy
6. Availability of support person
7. When woman last ate or took fluids
8. What other drugs woman has taken recently
9. Estimated gestational age of the fetus, based on calendar dates and ultrasound data

Physical Examination

1. Maternal vital signs and FHR to establish baselines
2. Evaluation of pregnant uterus (Leopold's maneuvers to determine fetal size, presentation, and position)
3. Quality of contractions, including frequency, duration, and intensity
4. Vaginal examination to determine:
   a. Status of cervix
      i. Dilatation   ii. Effacement
   b. Maternal-fetal pelvic relationship
      i. Presentation and position   ii. Station of presenting part
   c. Rate of progress in labor
5. Determination whether site to be used for injection is free from infection
6. Determination of the status of the fetus, using the stability of FHR and the result of assessments of fetal well-being

Diagnostic Studies

1. Screening lab tests for coagulation disorders

Test	Normal Value
Bleeding time	1–5 minutes
Platelet count	150,000–400,000/μL
Thrombin time	16–20 seconds
Partial thromboplastin time	24–36 seconds
Prothrombin time	11–12 seconds

2. Fetal scalp blood samples if fetal distress occurs

NURSING DIAGNOSIS: Knowledge deficit related to lack of information about regional anesthetic and analgesia

EXPECTED OUTCOME: Woman will be able to discuss the regional block.

Nursing Interventions	Rationale
Determine current knowledge level.	Allows nurse to provide individual teaching.
Evaluate factors related to learning, such as primary language spoken, ability to hear and interpret information, and/or presence of anxiety.	These factors may affect the woman's ability to process information.
Provide information regarding the reason for the block, effect of the block, possible side effects, possible alternative pain relief measures, and associated nursing care that may be expected.	Understanding the anticipated effects, side effects, and nursing care will help the woman be informed, participate in decision making, and give informed consent.

OUTCOME MET IF:

- Woman verbalizes her understanding of type of regional block to be given, expected effects, possible side effects, alternative comfort measures, and expected nursing care.

NURSING DIAGNOSIS: Risk for injury related to hypotension secondary to vasodilation and pooling of blood in the extremities

EXPECTED OUTCOME: Woman remains normotensive.

Nursing Interventions	Rationale
Have legal consents signed.	Regional block is an invasive procedure and method of providing anesthetic. Written consent is strongly recommended.
Have woman empty bladder.	Regional anesthesia interferes with the woman's urge to void, so it is best to begin with an empty bladder.

REGIONAL ANESTHESIA—LUMBAR EPIDURAL *continued*

Nursing Interventions	Rationale
Initiate intravenous infusion.	Intravenous fluids maintain adequate hydration and provide systemic access in the event of maternal hypotension or other untoward events.
Hydrate the woman receiving an epidural block with 500–1000 mL fluid prior to procedure. Dextrose-free solution is recommended.	Increased intravenous fluid intake increases blood volume and cardiac output to help minimize hypotension. Rapid infusion of fluids containing dextrose causes fetal hyperglycemia with rebound hypoglycemia in the first 2 hours after birth.
Position woman correctly for procedure (see text for proper positioning for individual procedures).	Proper positioning opens the lumbar space and avoids compression of epidural space.
Assess maternal status:	
1. Obtain baseline vital signs before any anesthetic agent is given.	Baseline reading allows more complete evaluation of maternal status.
2. Monitor blood pressure every 1–2 minutes for 10 minutes and then every 5–15 minutes following administration of anesthetic agent.	Hypotension is a frequent complication of regional anesthesia.
3. Monitor pulse and respiration.	Pulse may slow following spinal anesthesia due to decreases in venous return, venous pressure, and right heart pressure. Respiratory paralysis is a potential complication of regional anesthesia.
Observe, record, and report complications of anesthesia, including hypotension, fetal stress, respiratory paralysis, changes in uterine contractility, decrease in voluntary muscle effort, trauma to extremities, nausea and vomiting, and loss of bladder tone.	The most common complications of the epidural are related to hypotension of the mother.
Observe, record, and report symptoms of hypotension, including systolic pressure <100 mm Hg or a 20–30% fall in systolic pressure, apprehension, restlessness, dizziness, tinnitus, headache.	
Initiate treatment measures:	
1. Place woman in left lateral position with the foot of the bed elevated.	Gravity increases venous filling of the heart and the pulmonary blood volume, resulting in an increase in stroke volume and cardiac output with a rise in blood pressure. Side-lying position maximizes blood flow to the placenta.
2. Increase IV fluid rate.	Blood volume increases and circulation improves.
3. Administer oxygen by face mask at 7–10 L/minute.	Oxygen content of circulating blood increases.
4. Administer vasopressors as ordered (usually ephedrine 5–15 mg IV).	Vasoconstriction occurs. Vasopressors are not used in pregnant women unless absolutely necessary because they may further compromise the fetus. Ephedrine's primary action is by stimulation of cardiac muscle, which leads to increased uterine blood flow. Vasopressors that act primarily by vasoconstriction will decrease uterine blood flow and should be avoided (Taylor 1993).
5. Manually displace uterus laterally to left.	Increases venous return (vena cava is usually to the right).
6. Keep woman supine (semireclining) for 5–10 minutes following administration of block to allow drug to diffuse bilaterally. After 5–10 minutes position woman on side.	Allows anesthetic drug to diffuse bilaterally. Increases venous return.
Observe, record, and report fetal bradycardia (FHR <120 bpm) and loss of beat-to-beat variability	Maternal hypotension causes decreased blood circulation to fetus and results in fetal hypoxia. Amide group of anesthetic agents (bupivacaine, mepivacaine, and lidocaine) have potential to produce direct fetal myocardial depression; bradycardia may be caused by reduced placental blood flow.

OUTCOME MET IF:
- BP remains above 110/70 and pulse within 60–80 bpm.
- FHR is between 120 and 160 bpm with average LTV and STV present.
- Accelerations of FHR are present with fetal movement.
- No late decelerations or prolonged variable decelerations.

NURSING DIAGNOSIS: Impaired gas exchange in fetus related to effects of anesthetic agent

EXPECTED OUTCOME: Fetus will show no signs of fetal stress.

Nursing Interventions	Rationale
Observe, record, and report symptoms of hypotension: BP <100 mm Hg or 20 to 30% fall in systolic pressure; nausea, apprehension. If hypotension occurs, institute treatment measures as previously discussed.	Maternal hypotension will decrease oxygenation of fetus. Early detection and immediate treatment decrease hypoxia in fetus.
Monitor BP and pulse following birth.	Hypotension due to anesthetic agent may be delayed in onset.

REGIONAL ANESTHESIA—LUMBAR EPIDURAL continued

Nursing Interventions	Rationale
Explain possible delayed effects of anesthetic agents on fetus.	Anesthetic agents may produce neonatal neurobehavioral effects that could interfere with bonding.
Assist woman to assume left lateral position.	Left lateral position prevents compression of the vena cava, assisting venous return from extremities.
Monitor fetal status: 1. Use fetal monitoring to establish a baseline reading of FHR.	Maternal hypotension may interfere with fetal oxygenation and is evidenced by fetal bradycardia or prolonged deceleration.
2. Monitor FHR continuously.	Local anesthetic agents may cause loss of variability and late decelerations.

OUTCOME MET IF:
- FHR remains at 120–160 bpm.
- Fetal heart rate tracing shows average long-term variability with short-term variability present and no late or prolonged variable decelerations.

- There are accelerations of the fetal heart rate with fetal movement or scalp stimulation.

NURSING DIAGNOSIS: Altered urinary elimination related to effects of epidural

EXPECTED OUTCOME: Woman will have normal urinary elimination.

Nursing Interventions	Rationale
Assess bladder for distention and encourage the woman to void hourly.	Urinary retention frequently accompanies epidural block; client may be unaware of need to void.
Catheterize if necessary.	Client has been overhydrated, and distention may impede the progress of labor, increase the chance of bladder trauma, and cause lack of postpartum bladder tone. Because anesthetic agents may decrease frequency of contractions, return of uncomfortable contractions is an indication of need for reinjection of epidural catheter. Optimal time is prior to the return of painful contractions.

OUTCOME MET IF:
- Bladder is not distended per palpation.
- Urination occurs without difficulty.

- No urinary retention is present.
- Voiding in amounts >125 cc per voiding.

NURSING DIAGNOSIS: Risk for injury related to decreased motor control

EXPECTED OUTCOME: Woman will experience no neurologic injury from lack of extremity support.

Nursing Interventions	Rationale
Assess and inform woman of progress of labor. Provide reassurance throughout labor.	Woman who chooses epidural wants to experience and participate in labor and birth.
During second stage coordinate woman's pushing efforts with increased uterine pressure of contractions.	Loss of sensation may decrease awareness of the urge to push and the ability to push. Pushing without contraction will be ineffective and cause maternal exhaustion.
Assist with "sitting close" reinjection for birth.	Additional anesthesia is necessary for perineal relaxation, birth, and episiotomy repair.
Support extremities during movement.	Epidural block should not produce motor paralysis, but the client may not have full control of the extremities.
Ensure woman understands need for assistance with ambulation.	Motor control of the legs may be weak following epidural. Ambulation is delayed until complete sensation and ability to control legs has returned.

OUTCOME MET IF:
- Woman verbalizes understanding of need for assistance with ambulation in recovery period and early postpartum until full return of sensation.

- Woman experiences return of movement and sensation.

REGIONAL ANESTHESIA—LUMBAR EPIDURAL *continued*

NURSING DIAGNOSIS: Risk for injury related to toxic systemic reaction

EXPECTED OUTCOME: Woman will remain free of signs and symptoms of toxic systemic reaction.

Nursing Interventions	Rationale
Observe for and report symptoms of toxic reaction: excitement, disorientation, incoherent speech, muscle twitching, nausea and vomiting, and convulsions or severe reactions of sudden loss of consciousness, severe hypotension, bradycardia, respiratory depression, and cardiac arrest.	Larger volume of anesthetic agent used with epidural increases likelihood of toxic reaction. Continuous flow epidural or small, more frequent doses of analgesic agent are recommended to avoid severe reactions.
Institute treatment immediately: 1. Support ventilation. 2. Increase IV fluids. 3. Administer muscle relaxant for convulsions as ordered. 4. Be prepared for respiratory and cardiac resuscitation.	Immediate treatment will lessen the effects of toxic systemic reactions on fetus.

OUTCOME MET IF: • Woman does not display signs and symptoms of excitement, disorientation, incoherent speech, nausea, vomiting, loss of consciousness, severe hypotension, bradycardia, respiratory arrest, or cardiac arrest.

Essential Nursing Activities to Achieve Outcomes

Before Epidural

1. Provide individualized teaching regarding epidural.
2. Obtain baseline information:
   a. Reactive fetal monitoring strip, 20–30 minutes
   b. Maternal vital signs, including BP, R, P, T
   c. Vaginal exam, including dilatation, effacement, station, and position
3. Document all findings.
4. Have woman empty bladder.
5. Start IV.
6. Hydrate woman with at least 500 cc IV fluid.

During Epidural Injection

1. Help position woman for epidural insertion: either left side, legs slightly flexed, or sitting upright, leaning forward at the waist.
2. Continue to answer questions.
3. Give emotional support.

4. If woman is placed in sitting position, stand in front of her to assist with physical support.

After Epidural Injection

1. Assist woman to reposition in semi-Fowler's position or supine with wedge under hip.
2. Assess BP every 1–2 minutes for 10 minutes, then every 5–15 minutes until stable.
3. Assess fetal monitor for reassuring strip: baseline 120–160 bpm, average long-term variability, short term present, no late or prolonged decelerations.
4. Assess bladder at frequent intervals. Have woman void every hour.
5. Instruct woman to maintain bed rest until full function of lower extremities returns.
6. Assess for potential problems of epidural infusion: sedation, nausea, vomiting, pruritis, hypotension, and "breakthrough pain."

---

doses are adequate and help avoid cardiorespiratory depression. Typical intravenous doses are 75–100 mg for thiopental and 5–10 mg for diazepam (Ostheimer 1992).

Treatment of Sudden Cardiovascular Collapse   In sudden collapse an airway must be established as cardiopulmonary resuscitation begins. The airway of choice is an endotracheal tube with 100% oxygen for ventilations. Intravenous fluids are increased, and emergency cesarean birth may be started immediately (Barash et al 1993).

Peridural Block—Lumbar Epidural

Peridural anesthesia, or **epidural block,** can provide pain relief throughout the course of labor. The peridural or *epidural space* is a potential space between the dura mater and the ligamentum flavum extending from the base of the skull to the end of the sacral canal (Figure 24–2). It contains areolar tissue, fat lymphatics, and the internal vertebral venous plexus. Access to the space is through the lumbar area. The technique is most often used as a con-

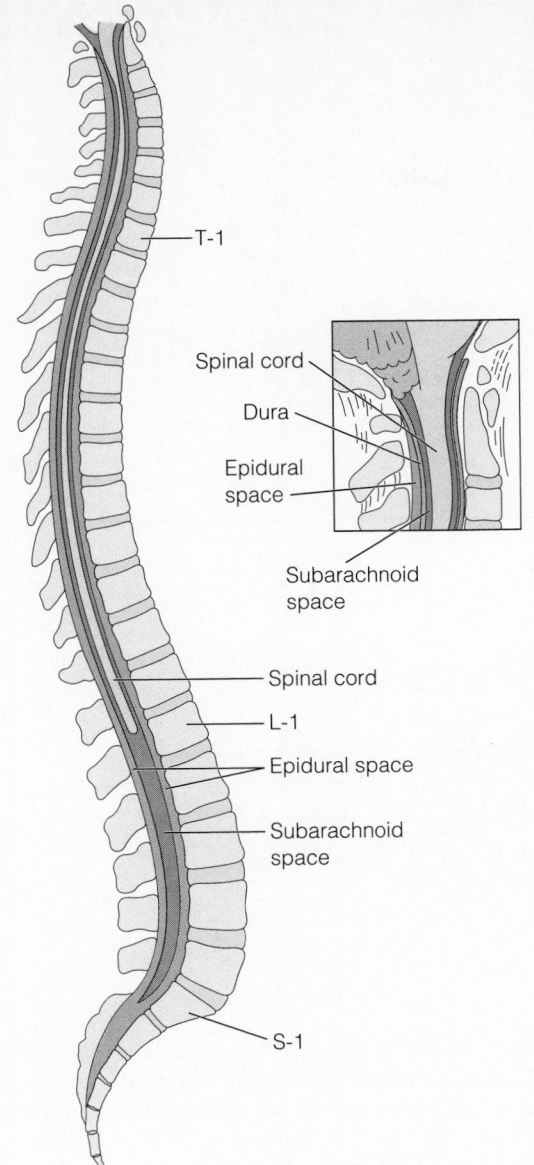

FIGURE 24-2   The epidural space is between the dura mater and the ligamentum flavum, extending from the base of the skull to the end of the sacral canal.

Labels on figure: T-1, Spinal cord, Dura, Epidural space, Subarachnoid space, Spinal cord, L-1, Epidural space, Subarachnoid space, S-1

Advantages

The lumbar epidural block produces good analgesia that alters maternal physiologic responses to pain. The woman is fully awake during labor and birth. The continuous technique allows different blocking for each stage of labor so that internal rotation of the fetus can be accomplished, and many times the dose of anesthetic agent can be adjusted so that the woman's reflex urge to bear down is preserved.

Disadvantages

The most common complication of an epidural block is maternal hypotension. This is generally prevented by preloading with a rapid infusion of intravenous fluids, then providing intravenous fluids continuously. Other disadvantages are that the onset of analgesia may be delayed 10 to 20 minutes. Epidural block requires skilled personnel for administration and close observation of the woman and her fetus. The anesthesiologist must be careful while administering the block to avoid perforating the dura mater, which would place the needle in the subarachnoid space and, if not recognized, would result in the anesthestic agent being injected into the spinal canal. Skilled nurses are also required to maintain close observation of the laboring woman and her fetus. Variability of the FHR may decrease, and late decelerations may occur if maternal hypotension develops. Epidural analgesia does not prolong the first stage of labor and may even shorten the active and transition phases because of the pain relief.

The influence of the epidural block on the second stage of labor remains controversial. Some believe that with adequate management the woman's ability to push can be maintained, so the second stage will be essentially the same length as it would be without a block. Others believe that the pushing urge is disturbed, affecting the woman's actual ability to push and prolonging the second stage (Ostheimer 1992).

Contraindications

The absolute contraindications for epidural block are lack of client consent, localized infections on the skin, coagulopathy, allergy to a specific class of local anesthetic agents, and raised intracranial pressure (Firestone et al 1993).

Technique for Lumbar Epidural Block

The following steps must be taken by the anesthesiologist in administering a lumbar epidural block:

1. Maternal and fetal status and labor progress are evaluated. Because maternal blood pressure and pulse will be taken frequently, an automatic blood pressure device may be useful. FHR is continuously monitored by an electronic fetal monitor.

tinuous block to provide analgesia and anesthesia from active labor through the birth and episiotomy repair.

Lumbar epidural block, particularly continuous lumbar epidural block, has become fairly common during childbirth in the United States. The block can be administered as a single dose to be used as anesthesia for a cesarean birth, or it can be administered for analgesia and anesthetic effect during labor and vaginal birth. When used during labor, the block may be administered as soon as active labor is established and is usually given when a nullipara has dilated 5 to 6 cm or a multipara has dilated 3 to 4 cm.

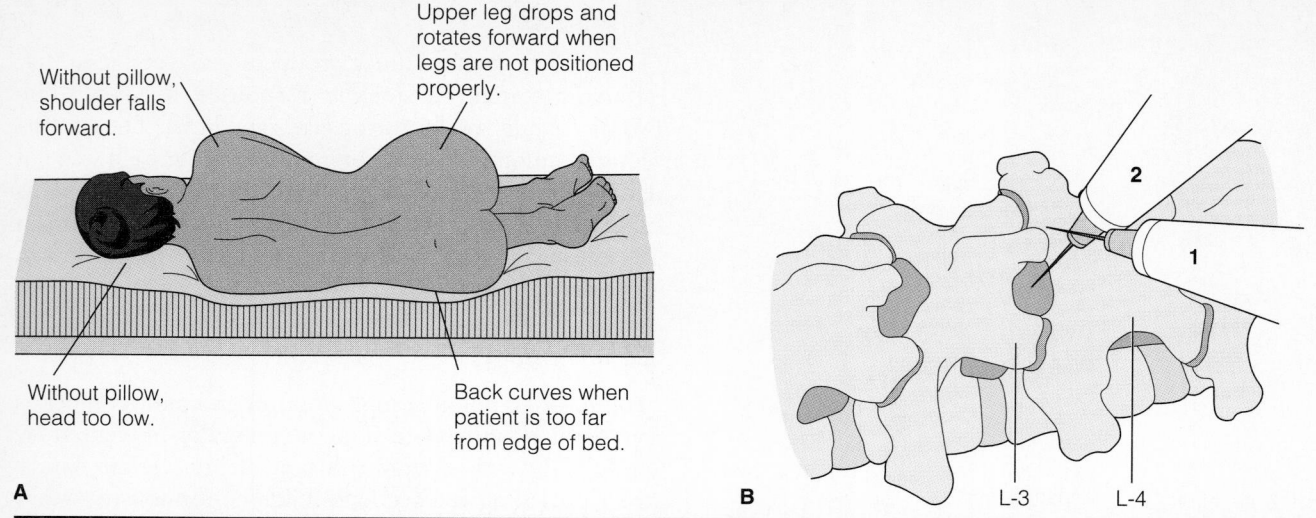

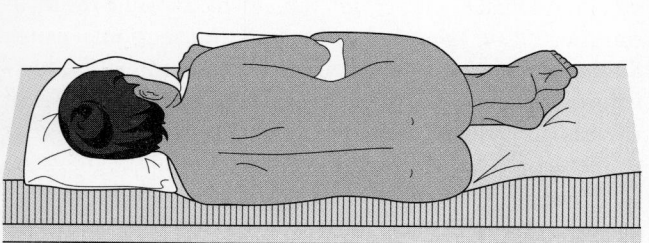

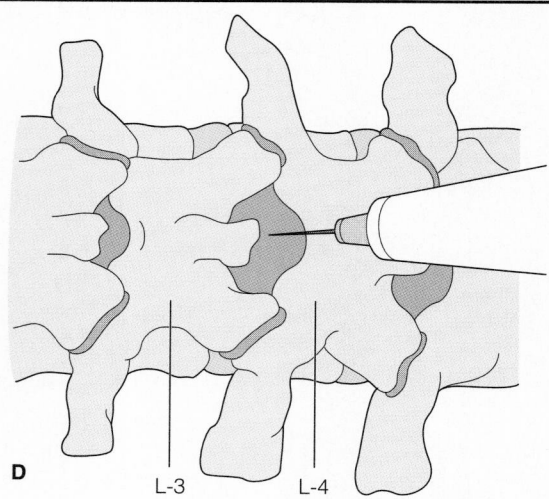

FIGURE 24-3 Positioning woman for epidural anesthesia block. *A* Incorrect maternal positioning for placing subarachnoid or epidural block. The upper shoulder has fallen forward, upper leg has rotated forward, and the client is positioned on the center of the bed so that there is no support from the edge and the back can curve. *B* Vertebral position with client in incorrect position. The vertebrae rotate forward, and if the needle is inserted in the usual way (1), the apophyseal joints are encountered. The direction the needle must follow is shown in *D. C* Correct maternal positioning. The back is straight and vertical, the shoulders are square, and the upper leg is prevented from rolling forward. *D* Vertebral position with the woman correctly positioned. SOURCE: Shnider SM, Levinson G: *Anesthesia for Obstetrics,* 3rd ed. Baltimore: Williams & Wilkins, 1993, figs 9.0, 9.10, 9.11, 9.12.

Labels in figure A:
- Without pillow, shoulder falls forward.
- Upper leg drops and rotates forward when legs are not positioned properly.
- Without pillow, head too low.
- Back curves when patient is too far from edge of bed.

Labels in figures B and D: L-3, L-4

2. Oxygen and resuscitative equipment is readied.

3. An intravenous infusion is begun, and a preload of 500 to 1000 mL of balanced salt solution is given over approximately 15 to 30 minutes.

4. The woman is placed on her left side, at the edge of the bed (the mattress is firmer and provides more support), with her legs slightly flexed. *The spinal column is not kept convex, as it is for a spinal block, because the convex position reduces the peridural space to a greater degree and stretches the dura mater, making it more susceptible to puncture.* (The epidural space is decreased during pregnancy because of venous engorgement. It is also smaller in obese and short individuals.) A small pillow may be placed under her head and in front of her chest to provide support for her arms. A sitting position may be used for obese women (Shnider & Levinson 1993) (Figure 24–3).

5. The skin is prepared with an antiseptic agent.

6. A skin wheal is made to anesthetize the supraspinous and interspinous ligaments.

7. A short, beveled 16- to 18-gauge needle with stylet is passed to the ligamentum flavum in the widest interspace below the second lumbar vertebrae (usually in the third or fourth lumbar interspace) (Figure 24–4). The ligamentum flavum is identified by its resistance to injection of saline or air (called loss of resistance technique). Resistance disappears as the peridural space is entered.

8. Aspiration for blood (indicating that a vessel has been inadvertently entered) and cerebrospinal fluid

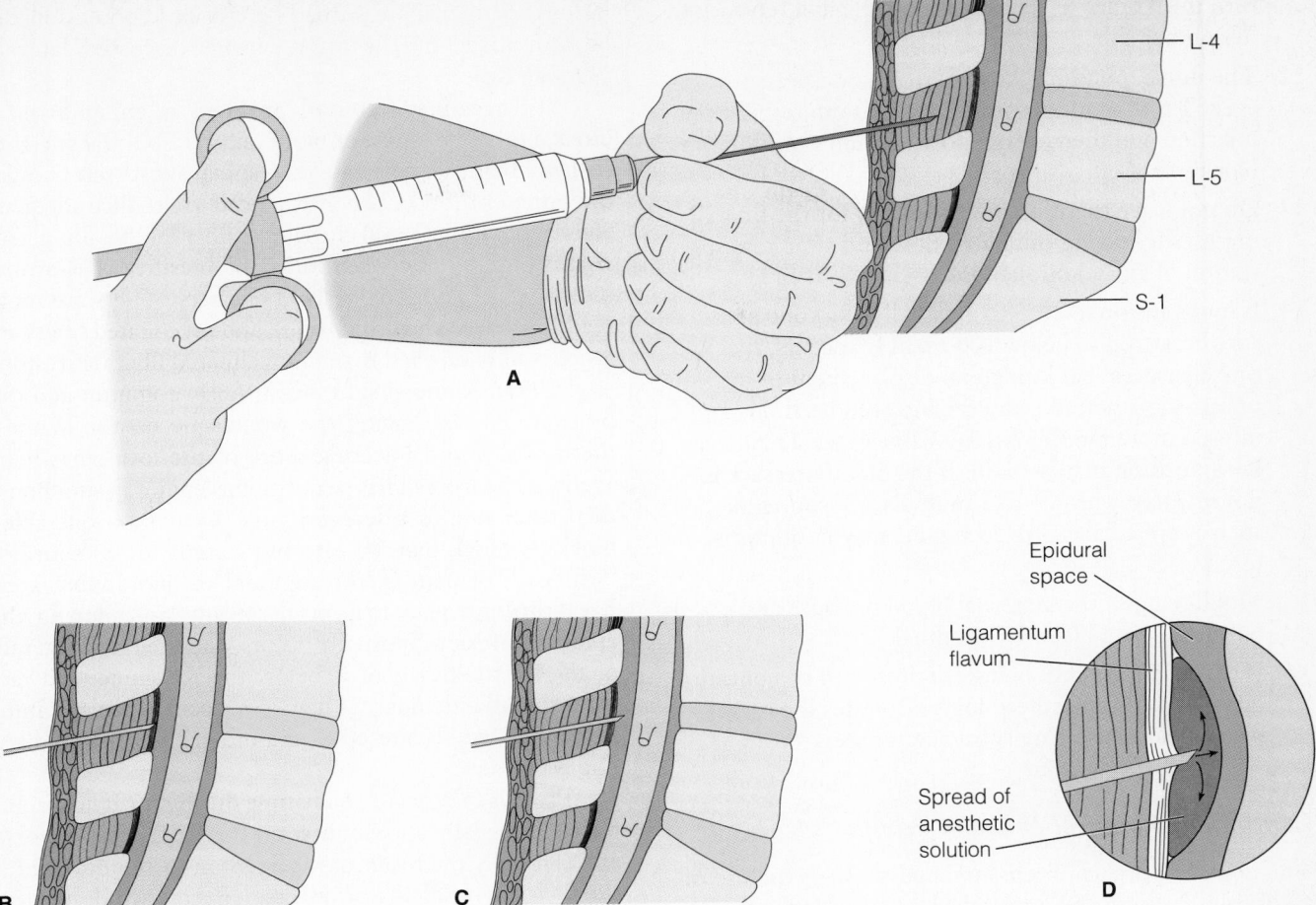

FIGURE 24-4 Technique for lumbar epidural block. *A* Proper position of insertion. *B* Needle in the ligamentum flavum. *C* Tip of needle in epidural space. *D* Force of injection push-ing dura away from tip of needle. SOURCE: Bonica JJ: *Principles and Practice of Obstetric Analgesia and Anesthesia.* Philadelphia: Davis, 1972, p 631.

(indicating the dura mater has been punctured) is done.

9. A test dose of 2 to 3 mL of anesthetic agent is injected to make sure the dura mater has not been penetrated.

10. After checking again to confirm the dura mater has not been perforated, a single dose of 10 to 12 mL is injected to provide anesthesia for the birth. (Note: The subsequent care is described in Technique for Continuous Lumbar Epidural Block.)

Technique for Continuous Lumbar Epidural Block

The procedure of a continuous lumbar epidural block is the same as for the lumbar block just described through step 8, after which the following steps are taken (Shnider & Levinson 1993):

9. Inject 5 mL of preservative-free saline in order to pass the catheter into the epidural space more easily.

10. Insert the catheter approximately 1 to 2 cm into the epidural space. Remove the needle. Aspirate for blood or cerebrospinal fluid, and, if negative, inject a test dose of local anesthetic agent containing epinephrine 1:200,000 concentration. If the catheter is intravascular, there will be a 20–30% increase in maternal pulse rate (Taylor 1993). If the subarachnoid space has been entered, sensory and motor changes in the woman's extremities will occur within 3–5 minutes (Taylor 1993). If there are not untoward effects, additional anesthetic agent is injected. The catheter is securely taped so that its placement will not be disturbed.

11. The woman is placed in a semireclining position with left lateral tilt of uterus for 10 minutes to allow for distribution of the block and then maintained in a side-lying position to maximize uteroplacental perfusion. If she needs to be turned to a supine position for fetal blood sampling or other procedures,

turn the woman as quickly as possible and reposition her on her side.

12. The nurse monitors the maternal blood pressure every 1 to 2 minutes for the first 10 minutes past the injection and then every 5 to 15 minutes until the block wears off.

13. Do not leave the woman unattended for the first 20 minutes following the initial dose and after administration of any additional dose.

14. If hypotension (a 20% to 30% fall in systolic pressure or a drop to below 100 mm Hg) occurs, the nurse ensures that left lateral displacement of the uterus is maintained, and the intravenous fluids are infused more rapidly. A 10- to 20-degree Trendelenburg position may be used. If the blood pressure is not restored within 1 to 2 minutes, a vasopressor such as ephedrine, 5 to 15 mg IV, may be administered.

15. Monitoring of the maternal blood pressure and pulse and the FHR are continued.

16. If the epidural is not being administered by continuous pump, the anesthesiologist aspirates the catheter prior to administering subsequent doses.

Continuous Epidural Infusion Pumps

The newest approach in epidural anesthesia is the use of a continuous infusion pump developed specifically for epidurals. Some of its potential benefits include lower total dose to achieve anesthesia, gradual onsets of effect with less hemodynamic alteration (sympathetic blockade), and prolonged anesthesia made possible by the continuous injection of the local anesthetic agent and prevention of loss of block or decreased effect of the block during prolonged labors and births or procedures (such as cesarean birth) and recovery (Morgan et al 1992). With lower total doses the woman may have more control over her leg movements and still have adequate pain control. Administer continuous epidural infusions with the same precautions used for intermittent injections.

Many local anesthetic agents have been used for the continuous infusion epidural block. Drugs such as bupivacaine (Marcaine) and chloroprocaine (Nesacaine) have been used with success. However, narcotics are now being used more frequently. The narcotics do have maternal and therefore fetal side effects and need to be administered with caution. The use of narcotics during labor in continuous epidural infusions is still controversial.

Problems and Adverse Effects

The major side effect of epidural anesthesia is maternal hypotension caused by a spinal blockade, which lowers peripheral resistance, decreases venous return to the heart, and subsequently lessens cardiac output, resulting in lowered blood pressure. The risk of hypotension can be minimized by the interventions discussed later in Nursing Role.

A distressing maternal problem is an inadequate block, unilateral block, or block failure. Epidural anesthesia has a higher failure rate than spinal anesthesia because the catheter must be properly placed to produce adequate anesthesia. Fink (1989) cites nerve fiber length along with volume and weak concentration of anesthetics as probable causes of poor analgesia. Thin nerve fibers are more readily blocked than thick ones, and myelinated fibers are more readily blocked than unmyelinated fibers (Firestone et al 1993). A one-sided block is fairly common and can be overcome by having the woman lie on the unanesthetized side and injecting more of the local anesthetic agent. If the woman has a continuous epidural, she should turn from side to side every hour to avoid a one-sided block. A block may be effective except for a "spot" or "window" of pain in the inguinal or suprapubic area. Breakthrough pain may occur at any time during the epidural infusion. It usually occurs when the infusion rate of the anesthetic agent is below the recommended rate for a therapeutic dose. It may also occur when the infusion pump rate is altered or the integrity of the epidural line is broken.

Pruritis may occur at any time during the epidural infusion. It usually appears first on the face, neck, or torso and is usually the result of the agent in the epidural infusion. Other problems or adverse effects include urinary retention, shivering, nausea, vomiting, and pyrexia.

Complications

One of the most serious complications of regional anesthesia, systemic toxic reaction, has been discussed in Adverse Maternal Reactions to Anesthetic Agents. Toxic reactions following a lumbar epidural may be caused by unintentional placement of the drug in the arachnoid or subarachnoid space, excessive amount of the drug in the epidural space (massive epidural), or accidental intravascular injection. Because large quantities of anesthetic agent are used for epidural block, the likelihood of toxic reactions is higher than with some of the other regional procedures. The incidence of drug reactions is relatively low, but the possibility is always present.

Studies have identified other complications such as increased instrumental delivery rate, increased incidence of cesarean birth for dystocia, and persistent backache following birth (Howell & Chalmers 1992; MacArthur et al 1992; MacArthur et al 1993; Russell et al 1993; Thorpe et al 1993).

Nursing Role

The nurse assesses the maternal vital signs and FHR for baseline information and to ensure that both maternal and fetal vital signs are within normal limits. (Note: All information regarding assessments, procedures, and such are to be recorded on the electronic monitor strip as well as in the nursing notes.) Labor progress is also assessed. The procedure and expected results are explained, and the woman's questions are answered. If questions arise that indicate the need for the woman and/or the father or other support person to talk with the anesthesiologist, then the nurse will act as an advocate and arrange that conversation. The laboring woman will need to give informed consent for the epidural, so she must clearly understand all aspects of the procedure.

The nurse starts an IV if one is not already in place and preloads at a rapid infusion rate to increase both blood volume and cardiac output. The greater circulating blood volume will counteract the loss of peripheral resistance that occurs with sympathetic blockade (Marx & Rabin 1993). It is recommended that dextrose-free solutions be used because dextrose can cause fetal hyperglycemia with rebound hypoglycemia the first few hours after birth. It is helpful to provide an opportunity for the woman to void just before administering the block because her urge to urinate will be decreased. The nurse assists the woman with positioning on her left side as described under "Techniques for Lumbar Epidural Block" (see Figure 24–4). After the epidural block is given, the woman may be positioned in a semireclining position with left lateral tilt to assure equal distribution of the block; then she is turned to a side-lying position. If she is supine for procedures such as sterile vaginal examinations or fetal scalp blood sampling, place a wedge under her right hip to help eliminate aortocaval compression. The nurse takes maternal blood pressure and pulse on a frequent basis, so an automatic blood pressure measurement device may be used. The FHR is monitored and assessed by continuous electronic fetal monitor.

If hypotension (systolic blood pressure below 100 mm Hg) occurs, the nurse assists with corrective measures such as positioning the woman in a left-side-lying position, increasing the flow rate of the intravenous infusion, and placing the bed in a 10- to 20-degree Trendelenburg position. If maternal blood pressure does not increase within 1 to 2 minutes, 5 to 15 mg of ephedrine may be administered IV per physician or protocol order. These measures are usually sufficient; however, if hypotension persists, oxygen by mask at 7–10 L/minute and additional vasopressors may be needed (Shnider et al 1993). Administration of oxygen helps decrease the nausea associated with a drop in blood pressure, increases fetal oxygenation, and reassures the mother. With severe or prolonged hypotension added treatment includes elevating the woman's legs for 2 or 3 minutes to increase blood return from the extremities.

If additional local anesthetic agents are injected, the regimen of assessing maternal blood pressure and initial surveillance should be repeated each time the epidural catheter is reinjected. If the woman's legs have been in stirrups during a vaginal birth, her blood pressure should be assessed as soon as her legs are taken out of the stirrups. While the legs were elevated, circulating blood volume in the trunk increased. Restoring circulation to the legs decreases the overall blood volume and may precipitate hypotension.

Throughout the administration of the block the nurse provides continued support by offering information and reassurance and remaining with the woman. Additional nursing care following the block includes frequent assessment of the bladder to avoid bladder distention. Catheterization may be necessary because most women are unable to void. Shivering may be caused by heat loss from increased peripheral blood flow or alteration of thermal input to the central nervous system when warm but not cold sensations have been suppressed. Applying warmed blankets and reassuring her may make the woman feel more comfortable.

The nurse assesses the woman's comfort and whether she has adequate pain relief. If a "spot" or "window" of pain exists or a unilateral block, the woman may be turned to the unanesthetized side. It is important for the woman to turn from side to side every hour to promote equal distribution of the anesthetic agent. If positioning changes do not help and the woman has inadequate pain relief, the anesthetist needs to be notified.

Nausea and vomiting may be associated with hypotension, so the nurse needs to ensure that maternal blood pressure is within normal limits. In addition, an antiemetic may be ordered to increase the woman's comfort.

Respiratory rate and quality of the respirations should be assessed no less than every 15–30 minutes. The nurse should notify the anesthetist of any significant decreases in respiratory rate or respiratory pattern changes. If the respiratory rate falls below 14 respirations per minute, naloxone (Narcan) may be given to remove the effect of the anesthetic agent; respirations will then return to a normal rate.

The woman's face, neck, and torso are inspected on a frequent basis for pruritis. If present, it is usually treated with Benadryl, 25 mg IV, or 50 mg given intramuscularly. Should no standing order exist, the nurse should notify the anesthetist. The epidural infusion may need to be discontinued.

During the second stage of labor the woman may require assistance with pushing because she may not feel her contractions or experience the urge to push. She may also need assistance holding or controlling her legs in order to push. (Women with epidurals may have decreased sensation and decreased ability to move their legs or may have essentially no control over movement.)

Ambulation should be delayed until the anesthesia has worn off. This may take several hours, depending on the agent and the total dose. Motor control of the legs is weak but not totally absent after birth. Return of complete sensation and the ability to control the legs are essential before ambulation is attempted. The woman must also be able to maintain blood pressure in a sitting and then standing position. For further discussion of nursing care see Nursing Care Plan: Regional Anesthesia—Lumbar Epidural on page 681.

Epidural Narcotic Analgesia After Birth

To provide analgesia for approximately 24 hours after the birth, the anesthesiologist may inject morphine, 5.0 mg or 7.5 mg, into the epidural space immediately following the birth. The analgesic effect begins approximately 30 to 60 minutes after the injection. The side effects include pruritus, which occurs in 11% to 90% of clients. Nausea and vomiting affect between 12% and 50% of clients and most commonly occur between 4 and 7 hours after the morphine injection. Urinary retention occurs in 15% to 90% of clients. The onset seems to occur early and resolves within 14 to 16 hours following the birth.

Subarachnoid Block (Spinal)

In subarachnoid block, or **spinal block,** a local anesthetic agent is injected directly into the spinal fluid in the spinal canal to provide anesthesia for vaginal or cesarean birth. For vaginal birth blockade to the T_{10} dermatome is usually effective, whereas cesarean birth requires anesthesia to the T_8 dermatome (Figure 24–5).

The subarachnoid space is the fluid-filled area between the dura and the spinal cord. During pregnancy the space decreases because of the distention of the epidural veins. Thus a specific dose of anesthetic produces a much higher level of anesthesia in the pregnant woman than in the nonpregnant woman. When a low spinal block is properly administered, failure rate is low.

Advantages

The advantages are immediate onset of anesthesia, relative ease of administration, a smaller drug volume, and maternal compartmentalization of the drug.

Disadvantages

The primary disadvantage is intense blockade of sympathetic fibers, resulting in a high incidence of hypotension. This leads to a greater potential for fetal hypoxia. In addition, uterine tone is maintained, which makes intrauterine manipulation difficult, and the level of spinal blockage is less predictable in laboring women.

Contraindications

Spinal anesthesia is contraindicated for women with severe hypovolemia, regardless of cause; central nervous system disease; infection over the site of puncture; maternal coagulation problems; and allergy to local anesthetic agents. Sepsis and active genital herpes may be considered relative rather than absolute contraindications. It is also contraindicated for women who do not wish to have spinal procedures (Cunningham et al 1993).

Technique

The following steps are followed in administering a subarachnoid block:

1. The woman is placed in a sitting or left lateral position. This may be uncomfortable because the block is not done until the fetal head begins to distend the perineum.
2. Intravenous infusion should be checked for patency.
3. The woman places her arms between her knees, bows her head, and arches her back to widen the intervertebral space.
4. Careful skin preparation is done, maintaining sterility.
5. A skin wheal is made over L3 or L4.
6. A 25-gauge needle with stylet is passed through the wheal into the interspinous ligament, ligamentum

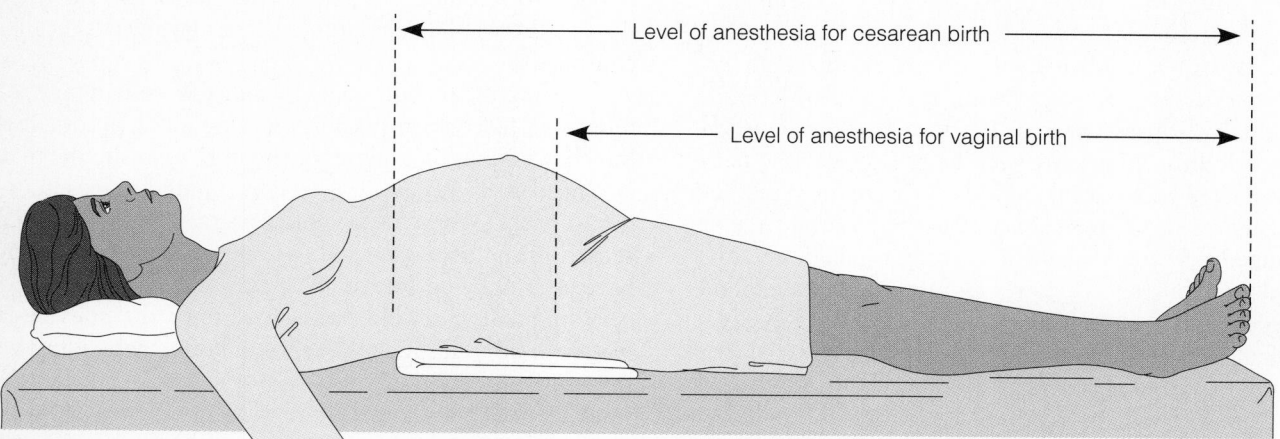

FIGURE 24-5 Levels of anesthesia for vaginal and cesarean births. SOURCE: Reprinted with permission of Ross Laboratories, Columbus, OH. From Clinical Education Aid no. 17.

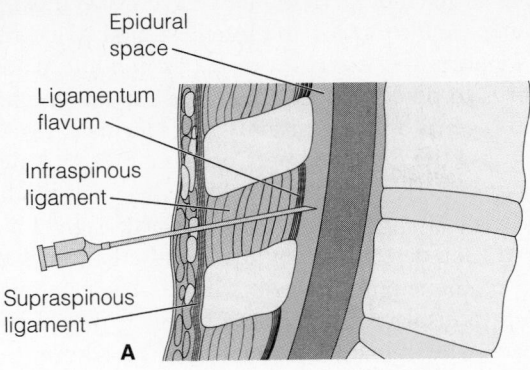

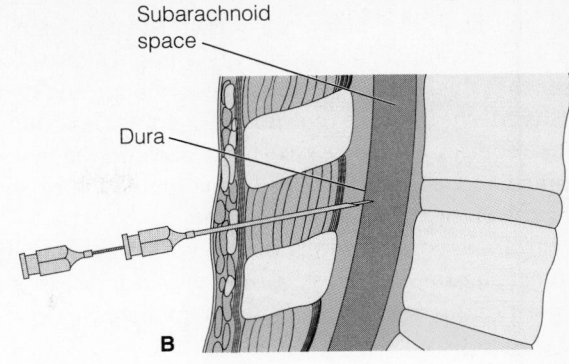

FIGURE 24-6 Double needle technique for spinal injection. *A* Large needle in epidural space. *B* 25-gauge needle in larger needle entering the spinal canal. SOURCE: Bonica JJ: *Principles and Practice of Obstetric Analgesia and Anesthesia.* Philadelphia: Davis, 1972, p 563.

flavum, and epidural space into the subarachnoid space (Figure 24–6).

7. Upon removal of the stylet, a drop of fluid can be seen in the hub of the needle if the spinal canal has been entered.

8. The appropriate amount of anesthetic agent is injected slowly, and both needles are removed.

9. With hyperbaric solutions the woman remains sitting up for 45 seconds.

10. The woman is placed on her back with a pillow under her head. Position changes can alter the dermatome level if done within 3 to 5 minutes. After 10 minutes a position change will not affect the level of anesthesia.

11. Blood pressure, pulse, and respiration must be monitored every 1 to 2 minutes for the first 10 minutes, then every 5 to 10 minutes.

A sitting or left lateral position may be used for the administration of spinal (subarachnoid block) anesthesia. Because the procedure is not done until the presenting part is on the perineum, sitting on the edge of the operating room bed may be very difficult for the laboring woman. The nurse helps the woman into position and provides encouragement and support during the procedure. The nurse informs the physician when a contraction is beginning so the anesthetic agent will not be injected at that time.

In the absence of maternal hypotension or toxic reaction there is no direct effect on the fetus with subarachnoid block. The amount of anesthetic used is too small to reach fetal circulation in a quantity that might cause fetal depression. Spinal anesthesia has been shown to be well tolerated by a healthy fetus when a maternal IV fluid load in excess of 1000 mL precedes the administration of the spinal.

Complications

The complications of spinal anesthesia include hypotension, drug reaction, total spinal, neurologic sequelae, and spinal headache. The side effects include nausea, shivering, and urinary retention as described in Peridural Block—Lumbar Epidural on page 684. The hypotension that occurs with spinal anesthesia seems more profound than with epidural anesthesia (Stoelting et al 1990).

Hypotension can be minimized by prehydrating with 500 to 1000 mL of non-dextrose-containing fluids and displacing the uterus to the left. The practice of placing an already hypotensive woman in a sitting position following injection to prevent upward spread of hyperbaric solution is dangerous because it will cause venous pooling in the lower extremities, further decreasing the maternal blood pressure. The normal curve of the thoracic spine prevents cranial spread of an intrathecal agent. A pillow is placed under the woman's head to exaggerate the curve.

Treatment of hypotension is the same as with an epidural: positioning the women in a left lateral, head-down position and rapidly infusing intravenous fluids. The prevention of cardiovascular collapse requires early detection, supplemental oxygen, assisted ventilation, and measures to maintain the blood pressure. The extent to which the fetus is affected relates to the degree of maternal hypotension. When maternal hypotension has been reversed, it is best to delay the birth for 4 to 5 minutes to allow the fetus to recover. Resuscitative equipment and trained personnel must be available to treat the mother and baby.

A total spinal occurs when there is paralysis of the respiratory muscles. It is a relatively rare but critical event. The symptoms are apnea, dilation of pupils, loss of consciousness, and absence of blood pressure. The onset of symptoms usually occurs within minutes of the injection but can occur in a span of time ranging from 30 seconds to 45 minutes. Resuscitative treatment, airway control, and support of blood pressure must begin immediately. If this complication occurs, it is important to remember that this woman is not asleep; although she may be paralyzed, she is aware of everything going on around her. She requires assurance that her respiration is being maintained and will continue to be maintained until she can breathe on her own.

Neurologic complications may occur coincidentally with spinal anesthesia such as with preexisting disease or faulty positioning of the woman. Genuine neurologic sequelae such as paralysis is extremely rare.

Although much less serious than other complications, headache may be an unpleasant aftermath of spinal anesthesia. It is the most frequent complication. Leakage of spinal fluid at the site of dural puncture is thought to be the cause. Several techniques have been suggested to decrease the possibility of headache. The use of a 25- or 26-gauge needle and entering the dura at a shallow angle rather than a right angle help reduce the incidence of leaking spinal fluid (Nicholson et al 1989). The incidence of spinal headache is only about 2% after puncture with a 25-gauge spinal needle, as opposed to 70% incidence if a larger gauge needle such as a 16-gauge needle is used. Hyperhydration and keeping the woman flat in bed for 6 to 12 hours after birth have been recommended as preventive measures, but there is no evidence that these procedures are effective.

The postspinal block headache usually begins on the second postpartal day and lasts several days to a week. It may be of varying degrees of severity. The pain occurs or becomes worse when the woman sits or stands and decreases or ceases when she lies down or flexes and extends her head.

Treatment consists primarily of bed rest, increased fluids, and analgesics for the mild or moderate forms. Severe and incapacitating headache has been treated successfully by saline injection. In another technique a "blood patch" is placed over the site of dural puncture. About 10 to 20 mL of blood is drawn from the woman and immediately injected, via sterile technique, into the epidural space over the site of the perforation; the clot applies pressure and seals off the leak. In many cases this procedure has dramatically relieved symptoms. The success rate ranges from 89% to 100%.

Nursing Role

The nurse should assist in positioning the patient, provide oxygen via nasal cannula or mask, record baseline vital signs of the mother and fetus and start an intravenous infusion prior to administration of block. After the block is instilled, the nurse should monitor vital signs every 5 minutes × 6, and assess level of block and respiratory status.

The nurse positions the woman correctly on the operating room table, usually upright with her legs on a stool. The woman places her arms between her knees, bows her head (shoulders should be even with hips), and arches her back to widen the intervertebral spaces. The nurse supports the woman in this position and palpates the uterus to detect the beginning of a contraction. Intrathecal agents are not administered during a contraction because the increased pressure could cause a higher level of anesthesia than desired. After the agent has been administered, the woman is asked to sit upright for the length of time determined by the anesthetist and is then assisted to the supine position with a wedge under her right hip to displace the uterus; a pillow is placed under her head. The spinal block may also be administered when the woman is in a side-lying position. The nurse monitors blood pressure, pulse, and respirations every 5 minutes until the birth. Some physicians administer oxygen as a prophylactic measure. The woman should be kept informed of everything that is going on in the birthing area, particularly if she is receiving mask oxygen. Placing her legs in stirrups will facilitate venous return from the extremities. Both legs should be raised at the same time to avoid undue tension and possible injury to back muscles.

If hypotension should occur, the intravenous fluids should be increased and the uterus displaced manually to the left. If the woman reports that she is having difficulty breathing, she needs to be assessed very carefully. Total spinal rarely occurs, but the possibility must always be kept in mind. The woman should be observed for apnea, unconsciousness, pupil dilation, and unobtainable blood pressure. Prompt treatment, which may include the use of a vasopressor (such as ephedrine), may avert a catastrophe for the woman and/or baby. It is essential to establish an airway and give oxygen with positive pressure until the woman can be intubated and other emergency measures instituted.

Following birth, the legs should be lowered slowly and simultaneously. A sudden movement of the extremities when vasomotor paralysis is present can precipitate a hypotensive episode. Although the effectiveness of the supine position to avoid headache following a spinal is controversial, the physician's orders may include lying flat for 6 to 12 hours.

The nursing interventions during administration of a spinal for cesarean birth will be the same except for placing the legs in lithotomy position. It is even more important that the woman be kept informed about activities around her and reminded of the fact that she may have sensations but will not have pain. Reassurance and support of the woman are essential in helping her participate in the birth experience.

Pudendal Block

The **pudendal block** technique provides perineal anesthesia for the second stage of labor, birth, and episiotomy repair. An anesthetic agent is injected below the pudendal plexus, which arises from the anterior division of the second and third sacral nerves and the entire fourth sacral nerve. The pudendal nerve crosses the sacrosciatic notch and passes the tip of the ischial spine, where it divides into the perineal, dorsal, and inferior hemorrhoidal nerves. The perineal nerve, which is the largest branch of the pudendal plexus, supplies the skin of the vulvar area, the perineal muscles, and the urethral sphincter. The dorsal nerve supplies the clitoris, and the inferior hemorrhoidal nerve supplies the skin and muscles of the perineal region as well as the internal anal sphincter. Pudendal block provides relief of pain from perineal distention but does not relieve pain of uterine contractions.

Pudendal block is a relatively simple procedure but requires a thorough knowledge of pelvic anatomy to block the pudendal nerve adequately.

Advantages and Disadvantages

The advantages of pudendal block are ease of administration and absence of maternal hypotension. It also allows the use of low forceps or vacuum extraction for birth.

A moderate dose of anesthetic agent (10 mL per side) has minimal ill effects on the woman and the course of labor. The urge to bear down during the second stage of labor may be decreased, but the woman is able to do so with appropriate coaching. There is usually little effect on the uncompromised fetus unless overly rapid or intravascular injection occurs. The block may be done by a transvaginal or transperineal approach. Transvaginal injection is simpler, safer, and more direct, making it the procedure of choice.

Technique

A pudendal block is administered as follows:

1. The woman is placed in a lithotomy or dorsal recumbent position with her knees flexed.

2. A 12.7 to 15.24 cm, 22-gauge needle with guide is used to protect the vaginal wall and control needle depth.

3. The instrument is guided into the vagina until the ischial spine is reached (Figure 24–7).

4. The needle is advanced through the vaginal wall into the space where the pudendal nerve passes.

5. Following aspiration to make sure that the needle is not in a blood vessel, 3 to 5 mL of solution is injected.

6. The needle is advanced 1 cm more, aspiration is repeated, and another 3 to 5 mL of the agent is injected.

7. Injection of the agent into the pudendal nerve on the opposite side follows the same procedure.

Chloroprocaine (Nesacaine), which has a low toxicity, may be used if prompt but brief anesthesia is needed. Lidocaine (Xylocaine) has prompt effect and intermediate action. Other agents used are mepivacaine (Carbocaine) and bupivacaine (Marcaine).

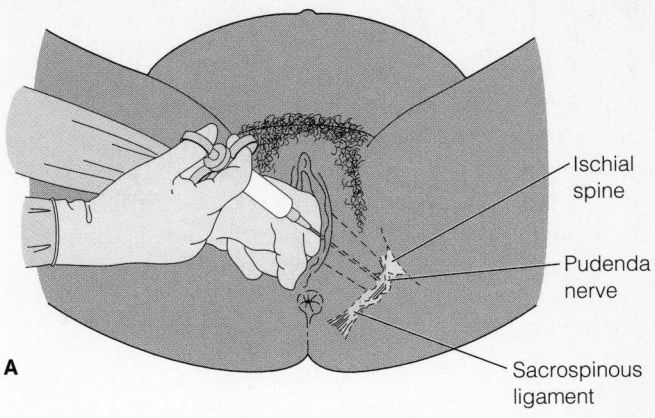

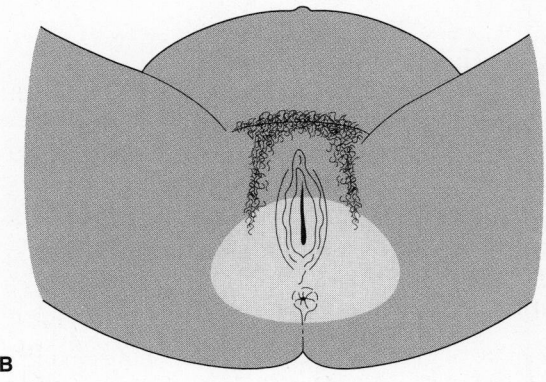

FIGURE 24-7 *A* Pudendal block by the transvaginal approach. *B* Area of perineum affected by pudendal block.

For most women the pudendal block is compatible with the goals of psychoprophylactic preparation for childbirth. The transvaginal technique must be done before the fetal head has advanced too far in the birth canal. Demonstrable blood levels of anesthetic agents have been documented in the fetus, but serious fetal complications are rare.

Complications

Systemic toxic reaction can occur from accidental vascular injection. Other possible maternal complications specific to pudendal block include broad ligament hematoma, perforation of the rectum, and trauma to the sciatic nerve. Following the birth, neonatal bradycardia, hypoventilation or apnea, hypotonia, tonic seizures, and reduced responsiveness have been reported. These difficulties can usually be attributed to accidental injection of the fetal scalp.

Nursing Role

The nurse explains the procedure and the expected effect and answers any questions. Pudendal block does not alter maternal vital signs or FHR, so assessments in addition to the expected ones are not necessary.

Local Infiltration Anesthesia

Local anesthesia is accomplished by injection of an anesthetic agent into the intracutaneous, subcutaneous, and intramuscular areas of the perineum. It is generally used at the time of birth for episiotomy repair and is especially useful for women giving birth by psychoprophylactic methods of childbirth. The procedure is technically simple and is practically free from complications.

Advantages

The major advantage of the local block is that it involves the use of the least amount of anesthetic agent. It can be done only if an episiotomy is needed just prior to the birth.

Disadvantages

A disadvantage is that large amounts of solution must be used. Although any local anesthetic may be used, chloroprocaine (Nesacaine), lidocaine (Xylocaine), and mepivacaine (Carbocaine) are the agents of choice in local infiltration because of their capacity for diffusion.

Technique

The technique of local anesthesia consists of injecting the agent with a long, beveled 22-gauge needle into the various fascial planes of the perineum (Figure 24–8). The procedure is deceptively simple; however, overdose may occur if the anesthetist does not wait for the anesthetic to take effect before injecting more solution. An excessive volume or concentration contributes to systemic toxic reactions and local toxic effects.

Nursing Role

The nurse explains the procedure and the expected effect and answers any questions. Local anesthetic agents have no effect on maternal vital signs or FHR, so additional assessments are unnecessary.

GENERAL ANESTHESIA

A general anesthesia may be needed for cesarean birth and surgical intervention with some obstetric complications. The method used to achieve general anesthesia may be intravenous injection, inhalation of anesthetic agents, or a combination of both methods.

Prior to induction of anesthesia the woman should have a wedge placed under her right hip to displace the uterus and avoid vena caval compression in the supine position. She should also be preoxygenated with 3 to 5 minutes of 100% oxygen. Intravenous fluids should be initiated so that access to the intravascular system is immediately available. The woman who has been in prolonged labor may also need to be hydrated if an infusion was not previously in place.

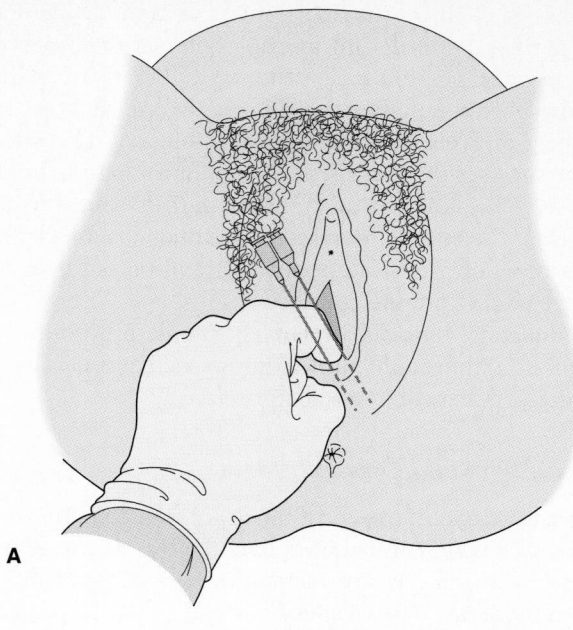

A

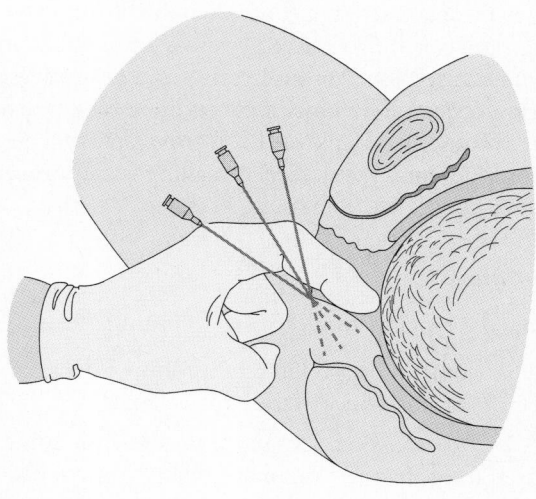

B

FIGURE 24-8   Local infiltration anesthesia. *A* Technique of local infiltration for episiotomy and repair. *B* Technique of local infiltration showing fan pattern for the fascial planes. SOURCE: Bonica JJ: *Principles and Practice of Obstetric Analgesia and Anesthesia.* Philadelphia: Davis, 1972, p 505.

Inhalation Anesthetics

A number of inhalation agents may be used for general anesthesia. Nitrous oxide is usually employed in combination with other agents for anesthesia. Nitrous oxide provides good analgesia but is a poor muscle relaxant. Isoflurane (Forane) is a good choice when uterine relax-

Luisa Silva, a 33-year-old G1 P0, is 32 weeks pregnant. She is trying to decide if she should accept any analgesia during her labor. She has finished childbirth education classes and wants an unmedicated labor and birth. She says, "I want to do this on my own, but I'm afraid it may be too much. Will it be OK if I need to take something?" What will you tell her?

Answers can be found in Appendix I.

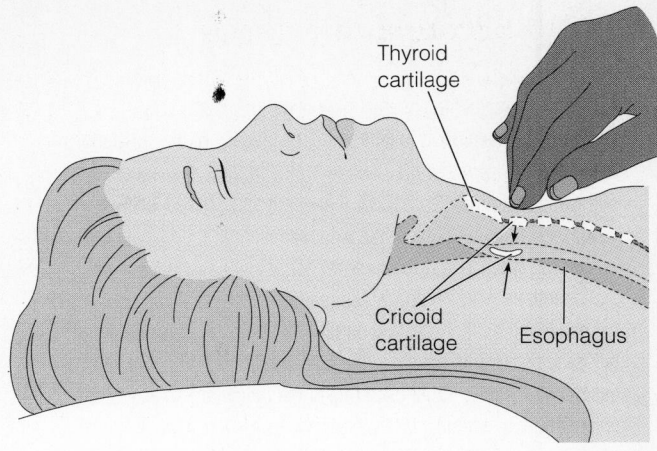

FIGURE 24-9 Proper position for fingers in applying cricoid pressure until a cuffed endotracheal tube is placed by the anesthesiologist/certified nurse-anesthetist. The cricoid cartilage is depressed 2–3 cm posteriorly so that the esophagus is occluded.

ation is essential (when the uterus is very irritable and tense or when there is anticipated difficulty in extracting a very large fetus from the uterus). Isoflurane provides relaxation while maintaining uterine blood flow and maternal blood pressure.

Intravenous Anesthetics

Sodium thiopental (Pentothal) is an ultra–short-acting barbiturate that produces narcosis within 30 seconds after intravenous administration. Sodium thiopental is most frequently used for induction of anesthesia. It differs from inhalation anesthetics in that little or no analgesia occurs and the method of administration is less controllable. Significant maternal complications include hypotension, vasodilation, laryngospasm, and inadequate muscle relaxation. Minimal use of sodium thiopental usually does not affect neonatal status at birth (in terms of Apgar scores and cord blood pH). However, the newborn may have slightly lessened muscle tone and decreased excitability in the first day of life (Capogna & Celleno 1993).

Complications

General anesthesia is not without risk. The leading cause of obstetric anesthetic death is regurgitation and aspiration of gastric contents. Other complications include fetal depression and uterine relaxation.

Vomiting and aspiration are problems because of decreased gastric motility and delayed gastric emptying associated with pregnancy. The gastric contents are highly acidic and produce chemical pneumonitis if aspirated. Prophylactic antacid therapy to reduce the acidic content of the stomach prior to general anesthesia has become common practice in the past decade. A nonparticulate oral antacid (such as polycitra or bicitra) may be administered (Cheek & Gutsche 1993).

Endotracheal intubation secures the maternal airway and prevents aspiration during general anesthesia. In or-

der to prevent possible regurgitation during intubation, cricoid pressure is applied as the woman loses consciousness and is maintained until the cuffed endotracheal tube is in place and the anesthesiologist/certified nurse-anesthetist has indicated the pressure can be released (Figure 24–9).

Fetal depression is directly proportional to the depth and duration of the anesthesia. Most general anesthetic agents reach the fetus in about 2 minutes. The poor fetal metabolism of anesthetic agents is similar to that of analgesic agents administered during labor. General anesthesia is not advocated when the fetus is at risk, particularly in preterm births.

Uterine relaxation is associated with most general anesthetic agents. The uterus must be carefully monitored for firmness, and the amount of lochial flow must be observed frequently.

NEONATAL NEUROBEHAVIORAL EFFECTS OF ANESTHESIA AND ANALGESIA

Studies have focused on the neurobehavioral effects on the newborn of pharmacologic agents used during labor and birth. Although analgesic and anesthetic agents may alter the behavioral and adaptive function of the newborn, physiologic factors such as hunger, degree of hydration, and time within the sleep-wake cycle may also exert an influence (Capogna & Celleno 1993). The long-range importance of these findings has not been well established.

Although aromatherapy as treatment is gaining popularity, little research has been done to determine the efficacy of the substances that are used. Lavender oil, used in aromatherapy, may act as an antiseptic and promote healing. Ailsa Dale and Sheila Cornwell developed a study to determine whether lavender oil relieved perineal discomfort when used following childbirth.

Mothers were randomly assigned to one of three groups of 119 women. Each mother added 6 drops of a particular odorous liquid to her daily bath for 10 days postpartum. Depending on her group assignment, each mother used one of the following: an extract of lavender oil; a synthetic lavender oil; or, as a control, an aromatic, inert placebo. Each mother recorded her mood and completed a visual analog scale rating her degree of perineal discomfort daily. Either a hospital- or community-based midwife assessed each woman's perineum daily as part of normal care. Both the investigators and the mothers were unaware of the type of additive being used by each woman until completion of the study. The authors also collected data on the women such as parity, delivery type, presence of perineal infection, and use of other pain medications.

The authors hypothesized that there would be no difference in the mean discomfort score among the three groups. They processed the data using analysis of variance for the discomfort and mood scores and chi-square for nominal variables. No difference in mood scores was found among the groups. Although the women using pure lavender oil had a lower mean discomfort score for the first 5 days postpartum, the difference was not large enough to be statistically significant, even when the authors attempted several additional statistical techniques. Neither the women in the study nor the attending midwives noted any side effects during the aromatherapy trial. The authors propose future study in which the amount of lavender oil used is varied.

Clinical Application of Study

Although the authors tried using several statistical tests to analyze the data, results of this study did not support the use of lavender oil to promote healing and reduce perineal discomfort postpartum. The use of several statistical tests may increase the risk of a type I error or the possibility of concluding that significant differences exist due to the research treatment when in fact the differences occurred by chance. Despite the mothers' slightly lower mean scores for discomfort with the use of lavender oil, and its lack of side effects, the difference was found to be insignificant, so the use of lavender oil should *not* be recommended as a healing agent based on this study.

SOURCE: Dale A, Cornwell S: The role of lavender oil in relieving perineal discomfort following childbirth: A blind randomized clinical trial. *J Adv Nurs 1994;* 19:89.

ANALGESIC AND ANESTHETIC CONSIDERATIONS FOR THE HIGH-RISK MOTHER AND FETUS

Up to this point the discussion of obstetric analgesia and anesthesia has dealt with the healthy woman and healthy fetus. Pain relief for high-risk women during labor and birth requires skill in decision making, close observation, and awareness of potential threats to the woman and fetus. Safety for all involved necessitates the close cooperation of obstetrician, anesthesiologist, pediatrician, and labor nurse. The pathophysiologic changes that accompany maternal disorders have a direct influence on the choice of agent or technique. It is difficult to separate maternal and fetal complications because whatever alters the woman's response will also affect the fetus. The effects on the woman cannot be considered without the potential effects on the fetus.

Preterm Labor

The preterm fetus has special risks and requirements. An immature fetus is more susceptible to depressant drugs because it has less protein available for binding; has a poorly developed blood-brain barrier, which increases the likelihood that pharmacologic agents will attain a higher concentration in the central nervous system; and has a decreased ability to metabolize and excrete drugs after birth. Analgesia during labor should be avoided whenever possible. If it becomes necessary, the smallest dose that will provide relief should be administered. Emotional support will be very valuable to the woman in this situation.

Pregnancy-Induced Hypertension

Pregnancies complicated by PIH are high-risk situations, as indicated in Chapter 19. The potential for chronic placental insufficiency and/or preterm birth are also present. The woman with mild PIH usually may have the analgesia or anesthesia of choice, although the incidence of hypotension with epidural anesthesia is increased. If hypotension occurs with the epidural, it provides further stress on an already compromised cardiovascular system. Hypotension can usually be managed with judicial fluid increase and positioning (Gutsche & Cheek 1993).

The woman with severe PIH is a real challenge. Regional anesthesia seems to be the preferred method as long as hypotension can be avoided. Raising the central venous pressure by 3 to 4 cm H_2O with intravenous fluids helps avoid hypotension, but it must be remembered that this woman is already threatened with heart failure. The effect of fluid intake can be monitored with a CVP line or pulmonary catheter. It is important to monitor and record the fluid intake and output. Some physicians use vasopressors; others avoid them because of the possible decrease in uterine blood flow to an already compromised fetus and the threat of a maternal cerebral vascular accident. Spinal anesthesia is rarely used because of the greater potential for hypotension.

With the use of general anesthesia there is a risk of aggravating maternal hypertension. The safest method for general anesthesia includes intubation, which may cause a hypertensive episode.

Diabetes Mellitus

The fetus of a mother with diabetes mellitus may have compromised placental reserve, and hypotension during regional anesthesia can deplete this reserve even further. If labor can be managed without fetal distress, small doses of intravenous narcotics with pudendal block at birth or the continuous epidural technique may be undertaken. If fetal distress occurs, cesarean birth may be necessary.

Anesthesia for cesarean birth requires special consideration in this case. The diabetic woman is more likely to experience cardiovascular depression during a regional block because of higher sympathetic blockade (Datta 1993). If a regional block is selected, it is recommended that acute hydration (preload) be provided by administering dextrose-free solution. In addition left uterine displacement is initiated prior to the administration of the block and maintained throughout the surgery. Hypotension is treated promptly with 10–30 mg ephedrine (Datta 1993).

Cardiac Disease

Pregnancy imposes significant risk for the woman with cardiac disease. With mild mitral stenosis the preferred anesthetic is continual epidural anesthesia with low forceps birth. This method avoids the cardiovascular changes associated with contractions and the Valsalva maneuver during bearing down in the second stage of labor. Hypotension can be avoided with carefully controlled intravenous fluids and measuring CVP to avoid overload. A cesarean birth may be done with epidural or general anesthesia. Ketamine should be avoided because it produces tachycardia.

Bleeding Complications

The current trend in treating bleeding complications during labor is toward scheduled cesarean birth when possible. When the maternal cardiovascular system is stable and there is no evidence of fetal distress, an epidural may be given for birth. However, when either of these conditions results in active bleeding, the threat of hypovolemia must be treated immediately. Maternal hypovolemia and shock produce fetal hypoxia, acidosis, and possible fetal death.

Regional blocks are contraindicated during active bleeding because the sympathetic block causes vasodilatation and further reduction of the vascular volume. General anesthesia is recommended for these cases. Sodium thiopental may be used, but it is a cardiac depressant and vasodilator, and ketamine may be a more appropriate choice for induction. Following birth of the infant and placenta, oxytocin should not be given as an intravenous bolus to contract the uterus because the vasodilatation produced causes a decrease in blood pressure and in total peripheral resistance. Oxytocin should be given as a dilute infusion to gain an oxytocic effect to treat uterine atony (relaxation) and to control postpartum bleeding (Biehl 1993).

KEY CONCEPTS

Pain relief during labor may be enhanced by psychoprophylactic methods and administration of analgesics and regional anesthesia blocks.

The goal of pharmacologic pain relief during labor is to provide maximal analgesia with minimal risk for the woman and fetus.

The optimal time for administering analgesia is determined after making a complete assessment of many factors. An analgesic agent is generally administered to nulliparas when the cervix has dilated 5 to 6 cm and to multiparas when the cervix has reached 3 to 4 cm dilatation.

The most common analgesic agents include meperidine (Demerol), butorphanol (Stadol), and nalbuphine (Nubain).

Opiate antagonists, such as naloxone, counteract the respiratory depressant effect of the opiate narcotics by acting at specific receptor sites in the CNS.

Regional anesthesia is achieved by injecting local anesthetic agents into an area that will bring the agent into direct contact with nerve tissue. Methods most commonly used in childbearing include peridural block (lumbar epidural), subarachnoid block (spinal or low spinal), pudendal block, and local infiltration.

Two types of local anesthetic agents used in regional blocks are amide and ester groups. The amides are absorbed quickly and can be found in maternal blood within minutes after administration. The esters are metabolized more rapidly and have only limited placental transfer.

New agents in use for intrathecal and epidural routes include morphine and fentanyl.

Untoward reactions of the woman to local anesthetic agents range from mild symptoms, such as palpitations, to cardiovascular collapse.

The goal of general anesthesia is to provide maximal pain relief with minimal side effects to the woman and her fetus.

Complications of general anesthesia include fetal depression, uterine relaxation, vomiting, and aspiration.

The choice of analgesia and anesthesia for the high-risk woman and fetus requires careful evaluation.

REFERENCES

Barash P et al: Epidural and spinal anesthesia. In: *Clinical Anesthesia* Covino BG, Lambert DH (editors). Philadelphia: Lippincott, 1993.

Biehl DR: Antepartum and postpartum hemorrhage. In: *Anesthesia for Obstetrics*, 3rd ed. Shnider SM, Levinson G (editors). Baltimore: Williams & Wilkins, 1993.

Briggs GG, Freeman RK, Yaffe SJ: *Drugs in Pregnancy and Lactation*, 4th ed. Baltimore: Williams & Wilkins, 1994.

Capogna G, Celleno D: The effects of anesthetic agents on the newborn. In: *The Effects on the Baby of Maternal Analgesia and Anesthesia*. Reynolds F (editor). London: WB Saunders, 1993.

Cheek TG, Gutsche BR: Pulmonary aspiration of gastric contents. In: *Anesthesia for Obstetrics*. Shnider SM, Levinson G (editors). Baltimore: Williams & Wilkins, 1993.

Cohen M: Continuous epidural infusions for acute postoperative pain, part 2. *Curr Rev Nurs Anes* 1990; 22:181.

Cunningham FG, MacDonald PC, Gant NF: *Williams Obstetrics*, 19th ed. Norwalk, CT: Appleton & Lange, 1993.

Datta S: Anesthesia for the pregnant diabetic patient. In: *Anesthesia for Obstetrics*, 3rd ed. Shnider SM, Levinson G (editors). Baltimore: Williams & Wilkins, 1993.

Davison J et al. Obstetric anesthesia. In: *Clinical Anesthesia Procedures of the Massachusetts General Hospital*, 4th ed. Boston: Little, Brown, 1993.

Fink BR: Mechanisms of differential axial blockade in epidural and subarachnoid anesthesia. *Anesthesiology* 1989; 70(5):855.

Firestone L et al: *Clinical Anesthesia Procedures by the Massachusetts General Hospital*, 3rd ed. Boston: Little, Brown, 1993.

Giacoia GP, Yaffee S: Perinatal pharmacology. In: *Gynecology and Obstetrics*, vol 3. Sciarri JJ (editor). Philadelphia: Harper & Row, 1982.

Gutsche BR, Cheek TG: Anesthetic considerations in preeclampsia-eclampsia. In: *Anesthesia for Obstetrics*, 3rd ed. Shnider SM, Levinson G (editors). Baltimore: Williams & Wilkins, 1993.

Howell CJ, Chalmers I: A review of prospectively controlled comparisons of epidural with non-epidural forms of pain relief during labour. *Int J Obstet Anaesth* 1992; 1:93.

Levinson G, Shnider SM: Systemic medication for labor and delivery. In: *Anesthesia for Obstetrics*, 3rd ed. Shnider SM, Levinson G (editors). Baltimore: Williams & Wilkins, 1993.

MacArthur C, Lewis M, Knox EG: An investigation of long-term problems after obstetric epidural anesthesia. *Brit Med J* 1992; 304:1279.

MacArthur C, Lewis M, Knox EG: Accidental dural puncture in obstetric patients and long term symptoms. *Brit Med J* 1993; 306:883.

MacDonald A: Epidural analgesia for labour (intermittent top up or continuous infusion). *Midwives Chronicle* 1992; 105:79.

Marx GF, Rabin JM: Anesthesia for cesarean section and neonatal welfare. In: *The Effects on the Baby of Maternal Analgesia and Anaesthesia*. Reynolds F (editor). London: WB Saunders, 1993.

Miller R: Obstetric anesthesia. In: *Anesthesia*, 3rd ed. New York: Churchill-Livingstone, 1992.

Morgan G et al. Obstetric anesthesia. In: *Clinical Anesthesiology*. Norwalk, CT: Appleton & Lange, 1992.

Nicholson C et al: Avoiding the pitfalls of epidural anesthesia in obstetrics. *J Am Assoc Nurse Anesth* 1989; 57(3):220.

Ostheimer G: *Manual of Obstetric Anesthesia*, 2nd ed. New York: Churchill-Livingstone, 1992.

Paradise NF: Personal communication. 1994.

Physicians' Desk Reference, 43rd ed. Oradell, NJ: Medical Economics, 1994.

Russel R et al: Assessing long-term backache after childbirth. *Brit Med J* 1993; 306:1299.

Shnider SM, Levinson G: *Anesthesia for Obstetrics*, 3rd ed. Baltimore: Williams & Wilkins, 1993.

Shnider SM, Levinson G, Ralston DH: Regional anesthesia for labor and delivery. In: *Anesthesia for Obstetrics*, 3rd ed. Shnider SM, Levinson G (editors). Baltimore: Williams & Wilkins, 1993.

Skidmore-Roth L: *Mosby's 1991 Nursing Drug Reference*. St Louis: Mosby-Year Book, 1991.

Skidmore-Roth L: *Mosby's 1994 Nursing Drug Reference*. St Louis: Mosby-Year Book, 1994.

Stoelting R et al: Spinal, epidural and caudal blocks. In: *Basics of Anesthesia*, 2nd ed. New York: Churchill-Livingstone, 1990.

Taylor T: Epidural anesthesia in the maternity patient. *MCN* March/April 1993; 18:86.

Thorpe JA et al: The effect of intrapartum epidural analgesia on nulliparous labor: A randomized, controlled, prospective trial. *Am J Obstet Gynecol* 1993; 169:851.

Vender JS, Spiess BD: *Post Anesthesia Care*. Philadelphia: WB Saunders, 1992.

CHAPTER 25

CHILDBIRTH AT RISK

*S*ince the day I began my nursing program, I had been
waiting for this rotation in the birthing center. At last I would
be able to be with a couple during their labor and birth. My first family
had such wonderful plans for the labor and birth. I was able to be with
them and could even assist with helping her breathe when she got to transition. Then suddenly the fetal heart rate dropped, and I recognized a variable
deceleration. It lasted 20 seconds, but it felt like it was forever. The nurse and
I helped the mother onto her other side, and we waited expectantly. I felt like
time had stopped, but I realized at that moment that if I was feeling like this,
so were the parents. I looked at them, and their faces were so tense. I reached
out and took her hand. I didn't know what to say, but I knew that at least I
could stay with her. There were no further problems, but I will never
forget that moment.

KEY TERMS

Abruptio placentae

Amniotic fluid embolism

Cephalopelvic disproportion
(CPD)

Dystocia

Hydramnios

Macrosomia

Oligohydramnios

Persistent occiput-posterior (OP)
position

Placenta previa

Postterm pregnancy

Precipitous labor

Prolapsed cord

Uterine inversion

OBJECTIVES

Describe the psychologic factors that
may contribute to complications during
labor and birth.

Discuss dysfunctional labor patterns.

Describe the impact of postterm pregnancy on the childbearing family.

Explore the causes and management of
uterine rupture.

Summarize various types of fetal metabolism and malpresentation and possible
associated problems.

Discuss the identification, management,
and care of fetal developmental abnormalities such as macrosomia and hydrocephalus.

Discuss the nursing care that is indicated
in the event of fetal distress.

Discuss intrauterine fetal death, including etiology, diagnosis, management,
and the nurse's role in assisting the
family.

Compare abruptio placentae and placenta previa.

Identify variations that may occur in the
umbilical cord and insertion into the
placenta.

Discuss the identification, management,
and nursing care of women with amniotic fluid embolus, hydramnios, and
oligohydramnios.

Delineate the effects of pelvic contractures on labor and birth.

Discuss complications of the third and
fourth stages.

The successful completion of the 40-week gestational period requires the harmonious functioning of four components: the psychosocial factors, the primary forces of labor, the fetus, and the birth passage. (These components are described in depth in Chapter 21.) The psychosocial factors are the intellectual and emotional processes of the pregnant woman as influenced by heredity and environment and include her feelings about pregnancy and motherhood. The primary forces of labor are the myometrial forces of the contracting uterus. The fetus in this case includes all the products of conception: the fetus, placenta, cord, membranes, and amniotic fluid. The birth passage comprises the vagina, introitus, and bony pelvis. Disruptions in any of the four components may affect the others and cause **dystocia** (abnormal or difficult labor). Some of the most common disruptions are discussed in this chapter.

COMPLICATED CHILDBIRTH: EFFECTS ON THE FAMILY AND THE ROLE OF THE NURSE

A complicated pregnancy and difficult labor and birth are crisis situations that can test the coping mechanisms of every individual involved. The family may respond to the crisis in relatively typical ways or may respond dysfunctionally.

During the antepartal period of a normal, low-risk pregnancy, resolution of any ambivalence about the pregnancy usually occurs when fetal movement is felt. With a complicated pregnancy, feelings of ambivalence may continue as the family experiences fear and anxiety about the woman's health and the health and welfare of the fetus. Hostile behaviors and feelings of guilt may be displayed as a woman questions her ability to bear healthy children, a father blames himself for the pregnancy, or the family accuses the health care team of poor management.

If a pregnancy is going well, the parents begin to develop a desire to nurture and love their child as they prepare for their parenting role. With a complicated pregnancy, the uncertainty about the outcome for the fetus inhibits their ability to adapt to the pregnancy and hinders the evolvement of feelings of adequacy as parents.

When an infant is stillborn or dies following birth, the couple must mourn and deal with the pain of detaching themselves. As the parents respond to their loss, they experience the anger, guilt, pain, and sadness associated with the grieving process.

Parents of an ill or deformed infant must not only resolve their feelings of guilt and grief, but they must also prepare themselves to care for that child. This couple may be unable to face the possibility that their infant may not survive. They may doubt their ability to care properly for the child. The great costs of caring for the high-risk child may create financial difficulties for the family. The emotional toll of caring for such a child may also be extreme.

The birth of an ill, abnormal, or stillborn infant presents the couple with the reality that they may have been fearing throughout the pregnancy. It is imperative that the medical and nursing staff responds in supportive ways. Maintaining communication and providing support for the woman and her family are important. At times nurses are reluctant to say anything to the parents because they are searching for the "right words." In reality it is reassuring to know that any words offered in genuine support and with a sense of caring are "right."

Providing emotional support to the family is a vital nursing role. When a labor is complicated or when the fetus dies, the woman should have consistent support and not be left alone. The partner should be encouraged to remain, and the nurse should be present to observe the woman or couple and to provide support. By attending and responding with empathy, the nurse helps the couple acknowledge their loss and begin their grieving process. Using comfort measures to meet basic needs also demonstrates a caring attitude.

CARE OF THE WOMAN AT RISK DUE TO EXCESSIVE ANXIETY AND FEAR

Stress, anxiety, and fear have a profound effect on labor, particularly when complications that imply maternal or fetal jeopardy occur. A labor process that was initially viewed with confidence and happiness may provoke anxiety and a variety of physiologic and psychologic responses once labor has begun.

Neural and endocrine changes are produced by stress and anxiety. The liver releases glucose to satisfy the body's increased energy needs. The bronchial tree dilates for increased oxygen intake. The anterior pituitary is stimulated, which results in an increase in production of glucocorticoids and mineralocorticoids by the adrenal cortex. These hormones promote the retention of sodium and the excretion of potassium and also stimulate the posterior pituitary to release antidiuretic hormone for the conservation of water. The loss of potassium is believed to assist in the reduction of myometrial activity. The reduction of glucose stores from stress and anxiety decreases the availability of glucose used by a contracting uterus.

The sympathetic nervous system stimulates the adrenal medulla to secrete epinephrine, which increases heart rate, cardiac output, and blood pressure. The sympathetic nervous system also stimulates the adrenals to release norepinephrine, which increases peripheral vasoconstriction and blood flow to the vital organs. This physiologic reaction can adversely affect the contracting uterus. The uterus responds to alpha-excitatory and beta-inhibitory effects of epinephrine. Through baroreceptor stimulation epinephrine inhibits myometrial activity (beta-receptors), uterine contractility decreases, and labor is prolonged (Lederman 1984).

The anxiety, fear, and pain experienced by the laboring woman may produce a vicious cycle, resulting in increased fear and anxiety because of continued central pain perception. This leads to enhanced catecholamine release, which in turn increases physical distress and may result in myometrial dysfunction and ineffectual labor (Lederman et al 1985) (Figure 25–1).

APPLYING THE NURSING PROCESS

Nursing Assessment

Unless birth is imminent or severe complications exist, the nurse begins the assessment by reviewing the woman's background. Factors such as age, parity, marital and socioeconomic status, culture, and knowledge and understanding of the labor process contribute to the woman's psychologic response to labor.

As labor progresses, the nurse is alert for the woman's verbal and nonverbal behavioral responses to the pain and anxiety coexisting with labor. The woman who is agitated and seems uncooperative or too quiet and compliant may require further appraisal for anxiety. Verbal statements such as "Is everything okay?" "I'm really nervous," or "What's going on?" usually indicate some degree of anxiety and concern. Other women may be irritable, require frequent explanations, or repeat the same questions. The nurse further observes for nonverbal cues, including a tense posture, clenched hands, or pain out of context to the stage of labor. Recognizing the impact of fatigue on pain and anxiety is another important nursing observation.

Nursing Diagnosis

Nursing diagnoses that may apply to the woman with excessive fear or anxiety include the following:

- Anxiety related to stress of the labor process
- Fear related to unknown outcome of labor
- Ineffective individual coping related to difficulty using relaxation techniques during labor

RESEARCH IN PRACTICE

The psychological benefits of vaginal delivery after a previous cesarean section (VBAC), were researched by Jacqueline Fawcett, Lorraine Tulman, and Jane Spedden. The purposes of the study included comparing the women's reactions to each of the two birth experiences, identifying influential factors in the women's decisions to try VBAC, and describing the factors involved in a successful outcome of VBAC as determined by the woman.

The theoretical framework of this study was derived from Sister Callista Roy's (1991) Adaptation Model. The researchers investigated the focal stimuli of the VBAC experience and the contextual stimuli of the demographic characteristics and prior experiences during delivery. They also examined the woman's adaptation using Roy's concepts of cognator coping mechanism and adaptive response modes of physiologic, self-concept, role function, and interdependence. The woman's decisions to try VBAC and determination of causes of success represented the cognator coping mechanism.

Thirty-two women who had experienced VBAC constituted the study sample. Sample characteristics were described in the study. Data were collected using an instrument to measure preceptions of birth and a 3 part birth experience questionnaire. Content analysis resulted in identification of adaptive and ineffective responses to both the current vaginal and previous cesarean birth experiences. Investigators found a statistically significant difference between the type of birth experience and the type of response using chi-square ($p < .0005$). The participants reported more ineffective responses to cesarean birth than to vaginal delivery in terms of self-concept, role function, and interdependence modes. Women provided many reasons for choosing VBAC including wanting to avoid the risk of surgery to themselves and to their babies, and wanting to have a vaginal birth experience. The women identified support from labor and delivery nurses as the number one factor in a successful outcome of VBAC. Support from the physician ranked number two.

Clinical Application of Study

This study provides an example of using a nursing theory to organize and guide a research study. The theory was an integral part of the conceptual framework and the analysis of results.

SOURCES: Fawcett J, Tulman L, Spedden J: Responses to vaginal birth after cesarean section. *JOGNN* 1994; 23(3):253.

Roy Sr C, Andrews H: *The Roy adaptation model: The definitive statement.* Norwalk, CT: Appleton & Lange, 1991.

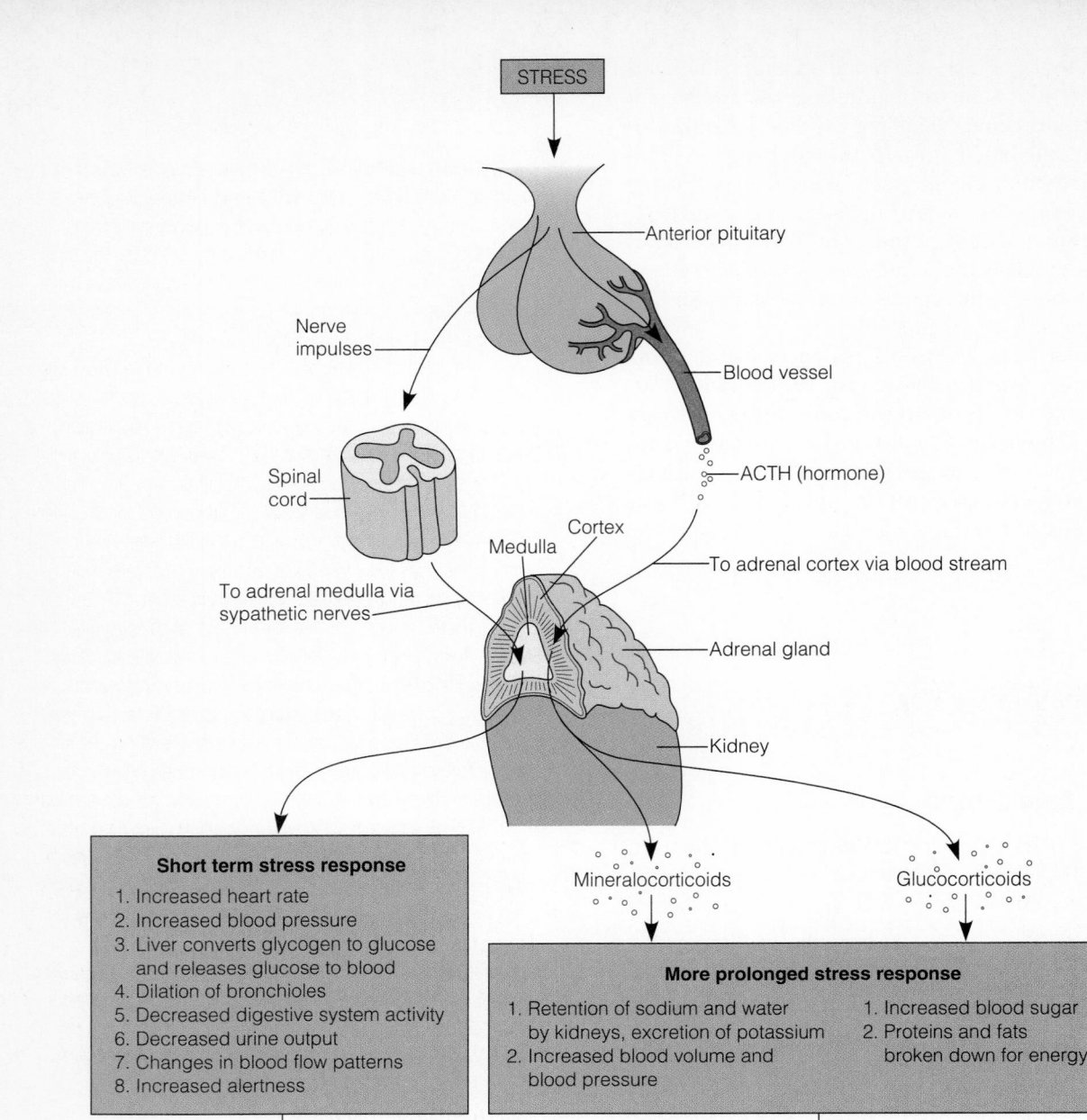

STRESS

Anterior pituitary

Nerve impulses

Blood vessel

Spinal cord

ACTH (hormone)

Cortex

Medulla

To adrenal medulla via sypathetic nerves

To adrenal cortex via blood stream

Adrenal gland

Kidney

Mineralocorticoids

Glucocorticoids

Short term stress response

1. Increased heart rate
2. Increased blood pressure
3. Liver converts glycogen to glucose and releases glucose to blood
4. Dilation of bronchioles
5. Decreased digestive system activity
6. Decreased urine output
7. Changes in blood flow patterns
8. Increased alertness

More prolonged stress response

1. Retention of sodium and water by kidneys, excretion of potassium
2. Increased blood volume and blood pressure

1. Increased blood sugar
2. Proteins and fats broken down for energy

Effects of stress on labor

1. Reduction of myometrial activity
2. Changes in glucose affect glucose stores needed by a contracting uterus
3. Increased blood pressure and vaso-constriction results in decreased blood flow to uterus, placenta and fetus
4. Decreases in uterine contractility due to increased circulation, decreased glucose availability, and inhibition of myometrial activity caused by increased amounts of epinephrine

STRESS

FIGURE 25-1   Effects of stress on labor. SOURCE: Adapted from Campbell N: *Biology,* 2nd ed. Redwood City, CA: Benjamin/Cummings, 1990.

Nursing Plan and Implementation

Anticipatory Education During the Prenatal Period

Prenatal classes provide relevant information about the developmental and psychologic changes that can be expected during childbirth and teach relaxation strategies to reduce the anxiety and pain of labor. Couples learn coping mechanisms in the form of physical and emotional comfort measures, controlled breathing exercises, and relaxation techniques.

Nursing research demonstrates that education is effective in minimizing the stress accompanying labor. Research findings indicate that women who participate in prenatal classes benefit by learning methods to decrease pain and promote psychologic well-being and satisfaction with health care (Koehn 1993, p 66).

Provision of Support During Labor and Birth

Prepared couples should be offered support and encouragement by the nurse as they employ the techniques they have learned. If the woman begins to lose control, the nurse can often assist the partner in helping the woman regain control. If anxiety is evident, the nurse should acknowledge and alleviate it, if possible, through comfort measures (see Chapter 23).

Unprepared couples can be taught many of these activities at the time of admission, especially if active labor has not begun. Clear but succinct information about the labor process, medical procedures, the environment, simple breathing exercises, and relaxation techniques can be given, thereby preventing or relieving some apprehension and fear. Even a woman in active labor who has had no prior preparation can achieve a great deal of relaxation from physical comfort measures, touch, frequent attention, therapeutic interaction, and possibly analgesics.

The nurse's ability to help the woman and her partner cope with the stress of labor is directly related to the rapport established among them. By employing a calm, caring, confident, nonjudgmental approach, the nurse not only is able to acknowledge the anxiety, but also is often able to identify the source of the distress. Once the causative factors are known, the appropriate interventions, such as information, comfort measures, touch, or therapeutic communication, can be implemented.

Provision of Support During the Postpartal Period

If possible, the nurse should follow up with the mother after the labor and birth to review the intrapartal process. Further explanations and reassurance may be offered as the woman's needs dictate. This is also an important time for the woman to share feelings about the labor.

Evaluation

Anticipated outcomes of nursing care include:

- The woman experiences a decrease in physiologic and psychologic signs of stress and an increase in physiologic and psychologic comfort.
- The woman uses effective coping mechanisms to manage her stress and anxiety in labor.
- The woman's and the family's fear is decreased.
- The woman verbalizes feelings regarding her labor.

CARE OF THE WOMAN EXPERIENCING DYSFUNCTIONAL LABOR

Hypertonic Labor Patterns

In **hypertonic** patterns the resting tone of the myometrium rises more than 15 mm Hg and may rise as much as 50 to 85 mm Hg. The frequency of contractions is usually increased, whereas the intensity may be decreased (Figure 25–2B). The hypertonic pattern usually occurs prior to the cervix reaching a dilatation of 4 cm or more.

Contractions are painful but ineffective in dilating and effacing the cervix, which may lead to a prolonged latent phase. Very anxious nulliparas at term or postterm are most commonly afflicted with hypertonic labor.

Maternal Risks

Hypertonic labor patterns are extremely painful because of uterine muscle cell anoxia. There is an increase in uterine muscle tone but little cervical dilatation and effacement. Because hypertonic labor often occurs in the latent phase of the first stage of labor, when dilatation may be no more than 2 or 3 cm, the woman may be suspected of overreacting to her labor. She may be aware of the lack of progress and become anxious and discouraged. A woman who has prepared for her labor and birth may feel frustrated as her coping mechanisms are severely tested.

Fetal-Neonatal Risks

Fetal distress occurs early because contractions interfere with the uteroplacental exchange. If this distress goes unidentified, the fetus may not survive. In addition, prolonged pressure on the fetal head may result in cephalhematoma, caput succedaneum, or excessive molding (Figure 25–3).

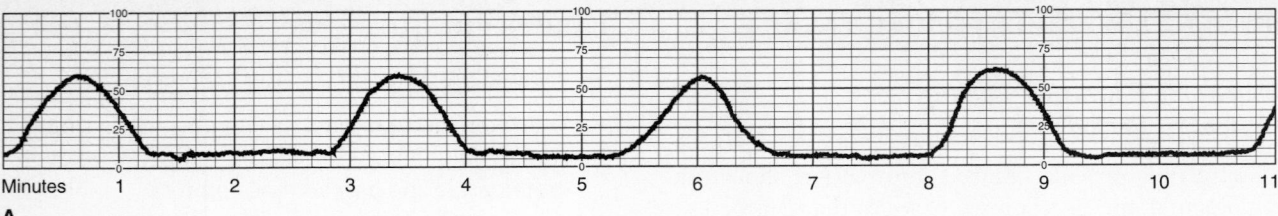

A

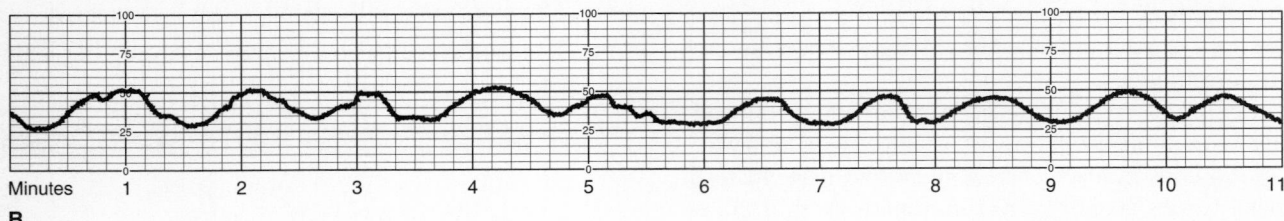

B

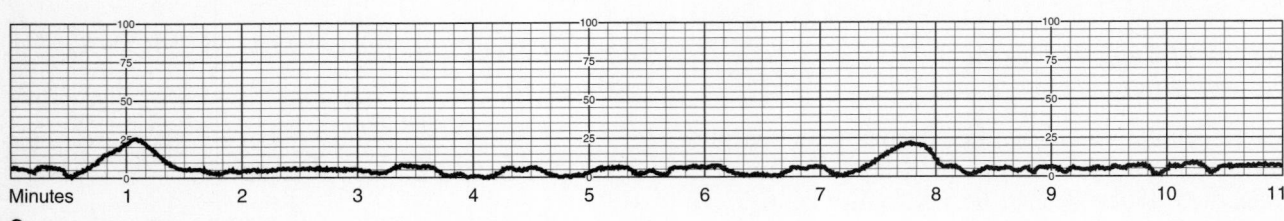

C

FIGURE 25-2   Comparison of labor patterns. *A* Normal uterine contraction pattern. Note contraction frequency is every 3 minutes; duration is 60 seconds. The baseline resting tone is below 10 mm Hg. *B* Hypertonic uterine pattern. Note in this example the contraction frequency is every minute, duration is 50 seconds (which allows only a 10-second rest between contractions), intensity increases approximately 25 mm Hg during the contraction, and the resting tone of the uterus is increased. *C* Hypotonic uterine contraction pattern. Note in this example the contraction frequency is every 7 minutes with some uterine activity between contractions, duration is 50 seconds, and intensity increases approximately 25 mm Hg during contractions.

Medical Therapy

As long as the membranes are intact and there are no indications of fetal stress, the goal of treatment is to arrest uterine activity and establish a more effective labor pattern. This is accomplished by promoting relaxation and reducing pain. Bed rest and sedation are common medical treatments. Oxytocin is not administered to a woman suffering from hypertonic uterine activity because it is likely to accentuate the abnormal labor pattern (Cunningham et al 1993). If the hypertonic pattern continues and develops into prolonged latent phase, an oxytocin infusion and/or amniotomy may be used as treatment methods (see Chapter 26). These methods are instituted only after cephalopelvic disproportion (CPD) and fetal malpresentation have been ruled out. When an oxytocin infusion is used to stimulate uterine contractions, the physician/certified nurse-midwife needs to assure that vaginal birth is possible; in other words, the maternal pelvis must be large enough for the fetus to pass through. If the maternal pelvic diameters are less than average or if the fetus is particularly large or is in a malpresentation or malposition, then **cephalopelvic disproportion (CPD)** is said to be present. In the presence of CPD labor will not be stimulated because vaginal birth is not possible.

APPLYING THE NURSING PROCESS

Nursing Assessment

The relationship between the intensity of pain being experienced and the degree to which the cervix is dilating and effacing should be evaluated as a part of the labor assessment. Whether anxiety is having a deleterious effect on labor progress should also be noted, especially if the mother is a primigravida or is postterm. Evidence of increasing frustration and discouragement on the part of the mother and her partner may become apparent as labor ensues and their birth plan cannot be followed.

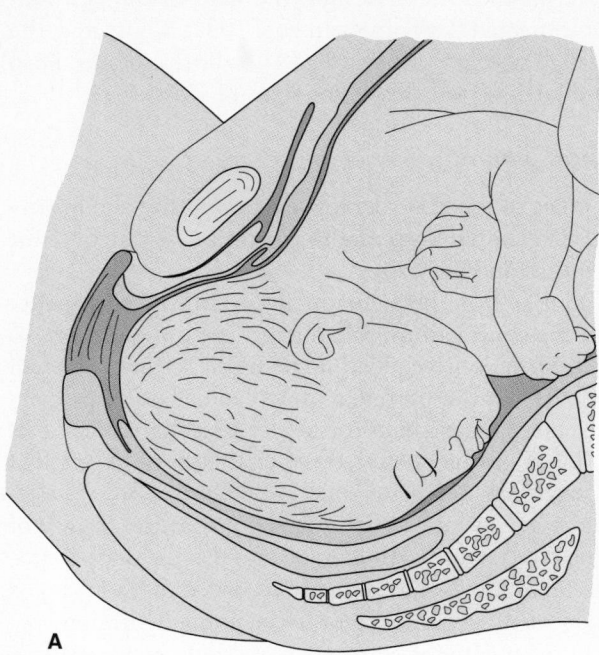

A

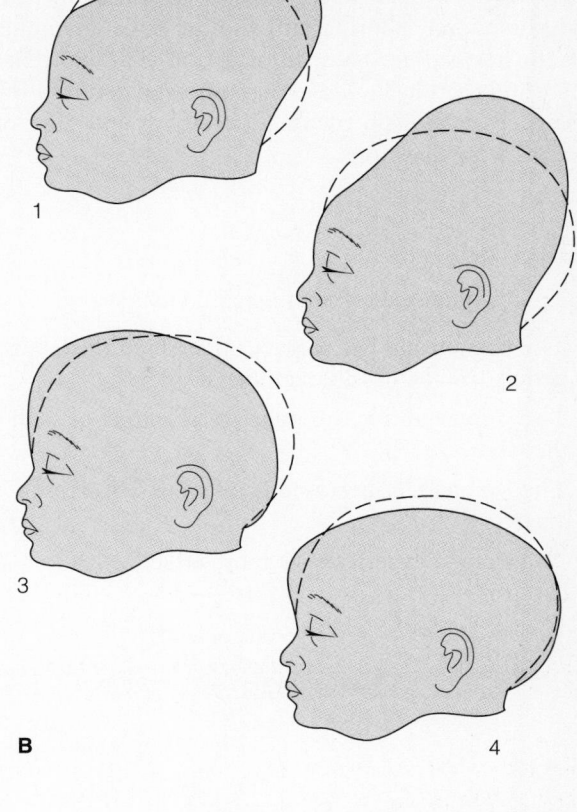

B

FIGURE 25-3   Effects of labor on the fetal head. *A* Caput succedaneum formation. The presenting portion of the scalp area is encircled by the cervix during labor, causing swelling of the soft tissue. *B* Molding of the fetal head in cephalic presentations: (1) occiput anterior, (2) occiput posterior, (3) brow, (4) face.

Nursing Diagnosis

Nursing diagnoses that may apply to the woman in hypertonic labor include the following:

- Pain related to woman's difficulty in relaxing secondary to hypertonic uterine contractions
- Risk for ineffective individual coping related to ineffectiveness of breathing techniques to relieve discomfort
- Anxiety related to slow labor progress
- Knowledge deficit related to lack of information about dysfunctional labor patterns

Nursing Plan and Implementation

Provisions of Comfort and Support to the Laboring Woman and Her Partner

The woman experiencing a hypertonic labor pattern will probably be very uncomfortable because of the increased force of contractions. Her anxiety level and that of her partner may be high. The nurse attempts to reduce the woman's discomfort and promote a more effective labor pattern.

The nurse may suggest supportive measures such as a change of position: left lateral side-lying, high Fowler's, on her knees in the bed with her arms up around the top of the bed while it is in high Fowler's, rocking in a rocking chair, sitting up, and walking. Soothing measures such as a warm shower, whirlpool, quiet environment, music the woman finds soothing, back rub, therapeutic touch, and visualization may also be helpful. Comfort measures may also be utilized: Mouth care, change of linens, effleurage, and relaxation exercises may provide more comfort. If sedation is ordered, the nurse ensures that the environment is conducive to relaxation. The labor coach may also need assistance in helping the woman cope. A calm, understanding approach by the nurse offers the woman and her partner further support. Provision of information about the cause of the hypertonic labor pattern and assurances that the woman is not overreacting to the situation are also important nursing actions.

Promotion of Maternal-Fetal Physical Well-Being

Fluid balance must be maintained through adequate hydration. Urine ketones should be monitored hourly. If possible, the couple should be informed of labor progress.

Providing Education

The laboring woman needs to have information about the dysfunctional labor pattern and the possible implications for her and her baby. Information will help relieve anxiety and thereby increase relaxation and comfort. The nurse needs to explain treatment methods and offer opportunities for questions.

Evaluation

Anticipated outcomes of nursing care include:

- The woman and her partner understand the labor pattern and its possible implications.
- The woman and her partner are able to cope with the labor.
- The woman has increased comfort and decreased anxiety.
- The woman experiences a more effective labor pattern.

Hypotonic Labor Patterns

In **hypotonic** *dysfunctional labor*, uterine activity in early labor has been within normal limits, but then a hypotonic pattern consisting of infrequent uterine contractions of mild to moderate intensity and a marked slowing or arrest of cervical dilatation and fetal descent occurs. In this pattern the myometrial resting tone is below 8 mm Hg. Fewer than two to three contractions occur in a 10-minute period (Figure 25–2*C*). The hypotonic pattern usually occurs after at least 4 cm of cervical dilatation. Hypotonic labor may occur when uterine fibers are overstretched from twins, large singletons, hydramnios, and grandmultiparity. Hypotonic uterine motility also occurs when sedation such as meperidine (Demerol) is given in the latent phase of labor or in the presence of various degrees of CPD. It may also occur with pelvic contraction and fetal malposition. Clinically, hypotonic uterine motility may occur in the latent or active phase, but it is most often seen in the active phase.

Maternal Risks

When labor is prolonged, the number of sterile vaginal examinations and other invasive interventions increases, and intrauterine infection may result. In addition, maternal exhaustion and physical and psychologic stress may occur. The risk of postpartal hemorrhage is increased because a pattern of inadequate uterine contractions has already been present and may persist after birth.

Fetal-Neonatal Risks

If maternal infection develops, the fetus or the newborn may be affected (Cunningham et al 1993). If affected, the fetus may develop tachycardia. After birth, the newborn should be observed closely for signs of sepsis.

Medical Therapy

The goals of medical therapy are to improve the quality of uterine contractions and to ensure a safe outcome for the woman and her baby.

Prior to beginning treatment to improve the quality of uterine contractions, rule out any contraindications to vaginal birth. The certified nurse-midwife/physician will reevaluate for the presence of cephalopelvic disproportion, fetal malpresentation (such as breech), or malposition (brow or face). After these factors have been ruled out, oxytocin (Pitocin) may be administered intravenously via an infusion pump to improve the quality of uterine contractions. An amniotomy may be done if amniotic membranes have not yet ruptured. The IV fluids are also useful in restoring or maintaining hydration.

As the quality of uterine contractions improves (frequency is at least 3 minutes, duration about 60 seconds, and strong intensity), there should be progressive cervical dilatation and fetal descent (measured by station). If the contraction pattern does not improve or fetal descent does not occur, cesarean birth may be necessary.

APPLYING THE NURSING PROCESS

Nursing Assessment

Assessing maternal vital signs, contractions, and cervical dilatation provides the nurse with data to evaluate maternal-fetal status, as do FHR and fetal descent. The nurse is also alert for signs and symptoms of infection and dehydration. The couple's stress and coping are assessed because the presence of a hypotonic labor pattern adds additional stress to the labor.

Nursing Diagnosis

Possible nursing diagnoses include the following:

- Pain related to difficulty in coping with uterine contractions secondary to dysfunctional labor
- Knowledge deficit related to lack of information about dysfunctional labor
- Ineffective individual coping related to difficult labor

Nursing Plan and Implementation

Promotion of Maternal-Fetal Physical Well-Being

Nursing measures include frequent monitoring of contractions, maternal vital signs, and FHR. If meconium is present in the amniotic fluid, observing fetal status closely becomes more critical, and in most instances an internal scalp electrode is placed in order to obtain more accurate data. Maintaining an intake and output record provides a way of determining maternal hydration or dehydration. The woman should be encouraged to void every 2 hours, and her bladder should be checked for distention. If the bladder is distended and the woman cannot void, catheterization will be necessary. Because her labor may be prolonged, the woman must continue to be monitored for signs of infection (elevated temperature, chills, changes in characteristics of amniotic fluid). Vaginal examinations should be kept to a minimum, but in this case they are done more often to be sure of dilatory progress, especially when it is suspected that cesarean birth will be necessary. The nursing implications of oxytocin infusion are presented in the Drug Guide: Oxytocin (Pitocin) in Chapter 26. See Essential Precautions in Practice: During Care of the Woman at Risk for Intrapartal Complications.

Provision of Emotional Support

The nurse helps the woman and her partner cope with this difficult labor. Important nursing measures include a warm, caring approach coupled with techniques to reduce anxiety, such as using comfort measures (position changes, encouragement to move about, shower, whirlpool, back rub, use of touch), encouraging stress-reducing activities (breathing patterns, relaxation techniques, visualizations), and not leaving the couple alone.

Providing Education

The nurse can provide additional information regarding coping techniques. It is particularly important to address the couple's concerns and questions with clear, accurate information. They need to be informed of progress and possible treatment measures. Disadvantages and treatment alternatives also need to be discussed and understood by the woman and her partner.

Evaluation

Anticipated outcomes of nursing care include:

- The woman/couple can verbally identify the type of labor pattern that is occurring and the treatment plan.
- The risk of infection to the woman and fetus has been reduced.

- The woman maintains comfort during labor.
- The father's supportive role is respected and maintained, and he is included in all planning if he chooses to be involved.

TEACHING MOMENT

As you know, normal cervical dilatation in a first-time mother—commonly known as a "primip"—is just over 1.0 cm/hour, and dilation in a "multip" is about 1.5 cm/hour. If your assessments reveal that this expected pattern is not occurring, consider that a problem may be developing. The most likely causes of the problem are related to either the contractions or the fetal position or size.

Precipitous Labor

Precipitous labor is extremely rapid labor that lasts for less than 3 hours. The most common causes are abnormally low resistance in maternal tissues, which allows for rapid cervical dilatation and fetal descent, and exceptionally strong uterine contractions (Cunningham et al 1993). Other contributing factors in precipitous labor are multiparity, large pelvis, previous precipitous labor, and a small fetus in a favorable position. Precipitous labor may also be caused by oxytocin overdose, which can occur during

ESSENTIAL PRECAUTIONS IN PRACTICE

DURING CARE OF THE WOMAN AT RISK FOR INTRAPARTAL COMPLICATIONS

Examples of times when disposable gloves should be worn include the following:

- Handling Chux and bedding that are moist with bloody show or amniotic fluid
- Cleansing the perineum
- Assessing the perineum

REMEMBER to wash your hands prior to putting the disposable gloves on and AGAIN immediately after you remove the gloves.

For further information consult OSHA and CDC guidelines.

induction of labor. In this case precipitous labor results from treatment error.

Precipitous labor and precipitous birth are not the same. A precipitous birth is an unexpected, sudden, and often unattended birth. See page 668 for discussion of precipitous birth.

Maternal Risks

The woman may have difficulty coping with this intense, rapid labor. If the cervix is effaced and the maternal soft tissues are not resistant to stretching, maternal complications may be few. However, if the cervix is firm and the maternal soft tissues are resistant, lacerations of the cervix, vagina, perineum, and periuretheral area may occur because the tissues do not stretch adequately. There is also a possibility of uterine rupture. When resistance is present, amniotic fluid embolism may occur (see page 748). The woman is also at risk for postpartal hemorrhage due to the altered labor pattern.

Fetal-Neonatal Risks

Rapid labor and birth cause increased pressures on and in the fetal head and may cause cerebral trauma to the newborn. If the birth is unattended and unassisted, the newborn may suffer from lack of care in the first few minutes of life.

Medical Therapy

Any woman with a history of precipitous labor requires close medical monitoring and preparation for precipitous birth to facilitate a safe outcome for the mother and fetus. Drugs such as magnesium sulfate or a tocolytic agent such as terbutaline may be used to slow the uterine contractions (Cunningham et al 1993). (See Drug Guide: Magnesium Sulfate in Chapter 19.)

APPLYING THE NURSING PROCESS

Nursing Assessment

During the intrapartal nursing assessment the nurse can identify a woman at increased risk of precipitous labor (for example, a previous history of precipitous or short labor places a woman at risk). During the labor the presence of one or both of the following factors may indicate potential problems:

- Accelerated cervical dilatation and fetal descent
- Intense uterine contractions with little uterine relaxation between contractions

Nursing Diagnosis

Nursing diagnoses that may apply to the woman with precipitous labor include the following:

- Risk for injury related to rapid labor and birth
- Pain related to rapid labor process

Nursing Plan and Implementation

Monitoring Labor Progress

If the woman has a history of precipitous labor, her contractions and cervical dilatation are closely monitored. The nurse stays in constant attendance if at all possible.

To avoid hyperstimulation of the uterus and possible precipitous labor during oxytocin administration, the nurse should be alert to the dangers of oxytocin overdosage (see Drug Guide: Oxytocin [Pitocin] in Chapter 26). If the woman who is receiving oxytocin develops an accelerated labor pattern, the oxytocin dosage is decreased or discontinued. (See Chapter 26 for further discussion.)

Promotion of Emotional Well-Being Comfort and rest may be promoted by assisting the woman to a comfortable position and providing a quiet environment. Information and support are given before and after the birth.

Assistance During Labor An imminent birth may be slowed by having the woman pant or blow with each contraction. It is also helpful for the nurse to breathe with the woman during this time to help her pace her breathing. If birth occurs, the nurse assists with it. (See page 668 in Chapter 23.)

Evaluation

Anticipated outcomes of nursing care include:

- The woman and her baby are closely monitored during labor, and a safe birth occurs.
- The couple feels support and enhanced comfort during labor and birth.

CARE OF THE WOMAN WITH POSTTERM PREGNANCY

Postterm pregnancy is one that extends more than 294 days or 42 weeks past the first day of the last menstrual period. The incidence is approximately 7–12% of all pregnancies, and about 5% continue beyond 43 weeks (Lake 1992; Resnik 1994). Some of the 7–12% are not truly postterm, but rather occur in a woman who has menstrual cycles that are variable (Kochenour 1992). Although many pregnancies extend beyond the anticipated due date, the true postterm pregnancy is associated with increased risk for asphyxia and trauma in the fetus.

The cause of postterm pregnancy is unknown. It does seem to occur more frequently in nulliparas between ages 15 and 20, in multigravidas over age 35, and when an anencephalic fetus is present (Lake 1992).

Maternal Risks

Although postterm pregnancy does not pose any significant risk to the woman during the pregnancy, the labor and birth process may be affected. In many instances labor is induced, and frequently the woman's cervix is unripe (cervix is firm, posterior, with minimal effacement and dilatation) which leads to a longer labor. There is an increased incidence of operative birth (use of forceps and need for episiotomy due to macrosomia) and cesarean birth.

Fetal-Neonatal Risks

True postterm pregnancies are frequently associated with placental changes that cause a decrease in the uterine-placental-fetal circulation. This decrease reduces the blood supply, oxygen, and nutrition for the fetus. Oligohydramnios (decreased amount of amniotic fluid) is frequently present and may increase the risk of umbilical cord compression (because the cord does not have as much fluid to float in). Macrosomia (fetal weight in excess of 4000 g) occurs three to seven times more frequently than in term infants and is more likely to be associated with birth trauma or shoulder dystocia (difficulty or inability to deliver the baby's shoulders) (Cunningham et al 1993). During labor the postterm fetus has a very high incidence of FHR baseline changes such as tachycardia, saltatory changes (marked variability) and variable decelerations (due to cord compression), meconium staining of the amniotic fluid, and neonatal depression at birth (Cucco et al 1989). Perinatal mortality doubles by 43 weeks' gestation and triples by 44 weeks (Kochenour 1992).

Medical Therapy

When the 40th week of gestation is completed and birth has not occurred, most obstetricians begin using the non-stress test (NST), biophysical profile (BPP) (especially the amniotic fluid volume portion of the BPP), and Doppler flow studies as assessment tools. The tests may be done two to three times a week, and some physicians advise a contraction stress test (CST) once a week (Resnik 1994). If the gestation extends into the 42nd week and the cervix is favorable (soft, with some effacement present),

then induction of labor is usually recommended and is 95% successful (Kochenour 1992). If the cervix is unfavorable, the tests are continued for 1 more week. Birth is accomplished at 43 weeks by induction if the cervix is favorable or by cesarean birth if it is not. If at any time the fetal assessment tests indicate a problem, interventions are taken to accomplish the birth. If oligohydramnios is present, an amnioinfusion may be done. (See Chapter 26 for further discussion.)

Nursing Assessment

When the woman is admitted into the birthing area, it is important to establish the EDB and ascertain the type of antenatal testing that has been completed. During labor ongoing assessments of the FHR by continuous electronic fetal monitoring are important to identify reassuring characteristics (presence of short-term and long-term variability, accelerations with fetal movement) and to determine the presence of variable decelerations so that corrective actions may be taken. When amniotic membranes rupture, the nurse assesses the fluid for the presence of meconium. Ongoing assessments of labor progress (contractions, progressive cervical dilatation and effacement, and fetal descent) may provide clues to the presence of a macrosomic fetus because labor may be lengthened.

Nursing Diagnosis

Possible nursing diagnoses for the woman with postterm pregnancy include the following:

- Knowledge deficit related to lack of information about postterm pregnancy
- Fear related to the unknown outcome for the baby
- Risk for anxiety related to unknown outcome for baby
- Risk for ineffective individual (or family) coping related to concern regarding the status of the baby

Nursing Plan and Implementation

Promotion of Fetal Well-Being

The woman may be taught to assess fetal activity each day to become more familiar with fetal movement and to detect any decrease in movement. (See Chapter 20 for further discussion of fetal movement records.)

In the birth setting careful attention is directed toward assessing the response of the fetus during labor.

Continuous electronic fetal monitoring of FHR is important to determine whether reassuring characteristics are present and to detect variable decelerations, especially if oligohydramnios is present. If variable decelerations are present, the laboring woman's position is changed to attempt to take pressure off the umbilical cord, and FHR is reevaluated. When an amnioinfusion is done, the nurse assists with the procedure and monitors the infusion and the response of the FHR. (See Chapter 26 for further discussion.)

Promotion of Emotional Support to the Mother

Women with pregnancies that extend past the due date frequently report that they would like more support from nursing personnel. In one study (Campbell 1986), women reported that they felt increased stress and anxiety and had more difficulty coping. Encouragement, support, and recognition of the woman's anxiety were all identified as helpful strategies by health personnel.

Providing Client Education

The woman needs to have information regarding the postdate pregnancy and the antenatal testing that will be indicated. The implications and associated risks for the baby need to be addressed as well as possible treatment plans. The woman and her partner need opportunities to ask questions and clarify information.

Evaluation

Anticipated outcomes of nursing care include:

- The woman has knowledge regarding the postdate pregnancy.
- The woman and her partner/family feel supported and able to cope with the labor and birth.
- Fetal problems are identified quickly.

CARE OF THE WOMAN WITH A RUPTURED UTERUS

A **ruptured uterus** involves the tearing of previously intact uterine muscle or of a uterine scar from a previous surgery. Rupture during pregnancy is usually in the upper segment of the uterus. If it occurs during labor, the rupture usually occurs in the lower segment. The incidence of uterine rupture is about 1 in 1230 to 6673 births (Phelan 1990).

Uterine rupture is classified as complete or incomplete. The complete rupture extends through the three muscle layers of the uterus, and there is direct communication between the uterine and abdominal cavities (Oxorn 1986). Incomplete rupture involves the whole myometrium, while the peritoneum that overlies the uterus remains intact (Oxorn 1986). A uterine rupture is also classified as spontaneous, which occurs during labor, or traumatic, which is associated with a manipulation or procedure—such as an external version—that puts stress on the uterus. The rupture can be caused by one or more of the following:

- A weakened cesarean scar, usually from a classic incision into the uterus (see Chapter 26)
- Obstetric trauma that may occur with a version or a difficult forceps-assisted birth
- Mismanagement of oxytocin induction or augmentation
- Obstructed labor (as with CPD)
- Trauma or a blow to the uterus
- Vaginal birth after previous cesarean birth

The signs and symptoms of a complete rupture include excruciating pain and cessation of contractions. Vaginal hemorrhage may occur, but vaginal bleeding is usually not profuse. Massive intraperitoneal hemorrhage and hematomas of the broad ligament are hidden sources of bleeding and may account for the scant vaginal bleeding. The woman exhibits signs of hypovolemic shock, and the fetal heart stops beating.

Maternal Risks

Uterine rupture is responsible for at least 5% of all maternal deaths (Hayashi & Castillo 1993). The main causes of death are shock and blood loss. If the rupture is recognized and treatment can be instituted, a hysterectomy is usually done.

Fetal-Neonatal Risks

When the blood supply to the uterus is interrupted, about 80% of fetuses demonstrate fetal distress such as FHR decelerations, developing bradycardia, and loss of variability (Rodriguez et al 1989). In a spontaneous rupture the fetus may be forced through the rupture into the abdominal cavity, where it quickly dies (Oxorn 1986). Overall, the fetal mortality rate ranges from 3% in labors that include the use of external EFM or an intrauterine pressure catheter, to 38% in labors with no uterine monitor (Rodriguez et al 1989).

Medical Therapy

In the presence of a threatened or actual rupture, emergency surgical intervention is done to save the mother and her baby. Delivery is by cesarean birth. If the rupture

(uterine tear) is small, the physician may be able to repair
it. If the rupture is large, the physician may do a hysterectomy.

Nursing Care

The nurse should be alert for warning signs of an impending rupture such as fetal distress, abdominal pain,
and hemorrhage.

The nurse may be the one to identify the warning
signs of impending rupture or maternal hemorrhage if
rupture has occurred. In acute rupture the nurse quickly
mobilizes the staff for emergency surgery. The nurse
continues to assess the maternal-fetal status and initiates
treatments to stabilize the woman during the hemorrhage.

When the physiologic needs of the woman and the
fetus are met, the nurse can focus on the emotional needs
of the family. The family must have a clear understanding
of the procedure and its implications for future childbearing. If fetal death has occurred, the mother and father
should also be given an opportunity to grieve and to see
their infant if they desire.

CARE OF THE WOMAN AND
FETUS AT RISK DUE TO
FETAL MALPOSITION

Occiput-Posterior Position

Persistent occiput-posterior (OP) position of the fetus is probably one of the most common complications
encountered in obstetrics. Although this position may be
normal in some races because of a genetically small transverse diameter of the midpelvis, it is considered a malposition because of the maternal and fetal difficulties that
may result. It should be remembered that the fetus generally rotates to conform with the orientation of the maternal pelvis. For a fetus in an occiput-posterior position

to rotate to an occiput-anterior position, it must rotate
135 degrees (ROP to ROT to ROA to OA), and in most
cases this rotation is accomplished. In others, however, it
is not. Labor progress may cease or the fetus may be born
in a posterior position.

Maternal-Fetal-Neonatal Risks

The woman may suffer a third- or fourth-degree perineal
laceration or extension of a midline episiotomy during
the second stage of labor. There is no increased risk of fetal mortality due to the occiput-posterior position unless
labor is protracted or an operative birth is performed.

Medical Therapy

Medical treatment focuses on close monitoring of maternal and fetal statuses and labor progress to determine
whether vaginal or cesarean birth is the safer method. According to Cunningham et al (1993), vaginal birth is possible as follows:

1. Await spontaneous birth
2. Forceps-assisted birth with the occiput directly
   posterior
3. Forceps rotation of the occiput to the anterior position and birth (Scanzoni maneuver; Figure 25–4)
4. Manual rotation to the anterior position followed by
   forceps-assisted birth (Figure 25–5)

If the pelvis is roomy and the perineum is relaxed, as
found in grandmultiparity, the fetus may have no particular problem emerging spontaneously in the occiput-posterior position. If, however, the perineum is rigid, the second stage of labor may be prolonged. A prolonged second
stage is one that lasts over an hour in multiparas and 2
hours or more in nulliparas. One complication of the fetus emerging in the occiput-posterior position is the possibility of a third- or fourth-degree perineal laceration or
extension of a midline episiotomy.

In the event of a prolonged second stage with arrest
of descent due to occiput-posterior position, a midforceps or manual rotation may be done if no CPD is
present. In cases of CPD cesarean birth is the preferred
treatment.

Nursing Assessment

The first sign of occiput-posterior position is intense
back pain in the first stage of labor. The back pain is
caused by the fetal occiput compressing the sacral nerves.

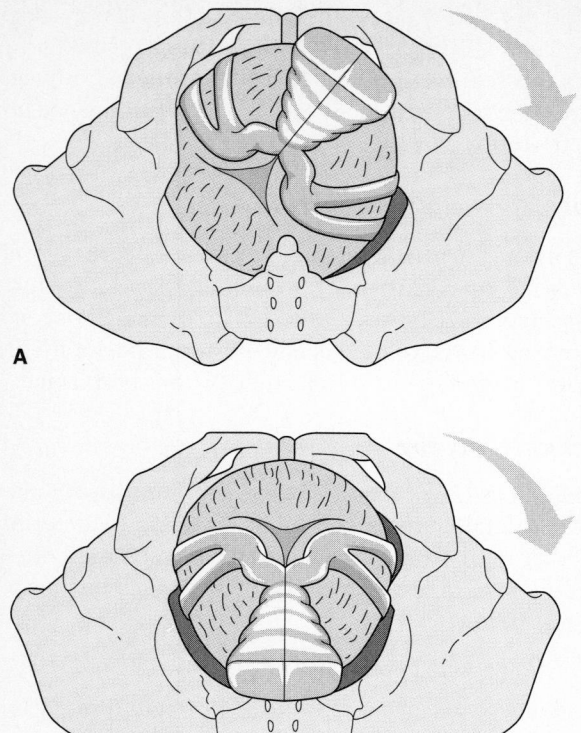

A

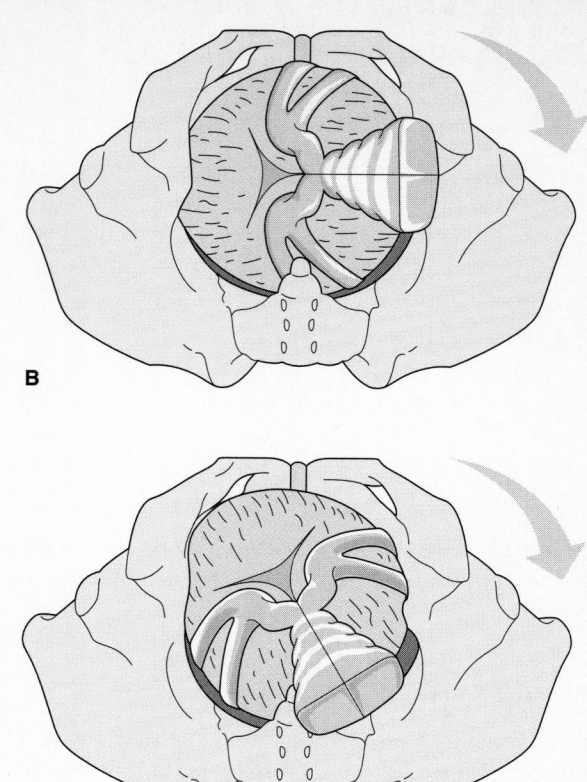

B

D

C

FIGURE 25-4 Scanzoni maneuver, anterior rotation. In clockwise order: *A* Forceps are applied to the fetal head, which is in ROP position. *B* Fetal head is rotated 45 degrees to ROT. *C* Fetal head is rotated another 45 degrees to ROA. *D* Fetal head is rotated another 45 degrees to OA. The fetal position

has changed from ROP to ROT to ROA to OA for a rotation of 135 degrees. The forceps are now upside down, so they are removed and reapplied to provide the traction necessary for a forceps-assisted birth. SOURCE: Oxorn J: Human Labor and Birth, 5th ed. Norwalk, CT: Appleton & Lange, 1986, p 401.

Other signs and symptoms may include a dysfunctional labor pattern, a prolonged active phase, secondary arrest of dilatation, or arrest of descent. Further assessment may reveal a depression in the maternal abdomen above the symphysis pubis (because the fetal face, rather than the back of its head, is turned up against the symphysis). Fetal heart tones may be heard far laterally on the maternal abdomen, and on vaginal examination the nurse will find the wide diamond-shaped anterior fontanelle in the anterior portion of the pelvis. This fontanelle may be difficult to feel because of molding of the fetal head.

Nursing Diagnosis

Nursing diagnoses that may apply to women with persistent OP position include the following:

- Pain related to back discomfort secondary to occiput-posterior position
- Ineffective individual coping related to persistent back pain

Nursing Plan and Implementation
Facilitation of Fetal Position Change

Changing maternal posture has been used for many years to enhance rotation of OP or OT to OA. The woman may be placed on one side and then asked to move to the other side as the fetus begins to rotate. This side-lying position may promote rotation; it also enables the support persons to apply counterpressure on the sacral area to decrease discomfort. A knee-chest position provides a downward slant to the vaginal canal, directing the fetal head downward on descent. Andrews and Andrews (1983) suggest that a hands-and-knees position is often effective in rotating the fetus. In addition to maintaining a hands-and-knees position on the bed, the woman may do pelvic rocking, and the support person may perform firm stroking motions on the abdomen. The stroking begins over the fetal back and swings around to the other side of the abdomen. After the fetus has rotated, the woman lies in a Sims' position on the side opposite the fetal back. In addition to these positions the woman may want to sit on

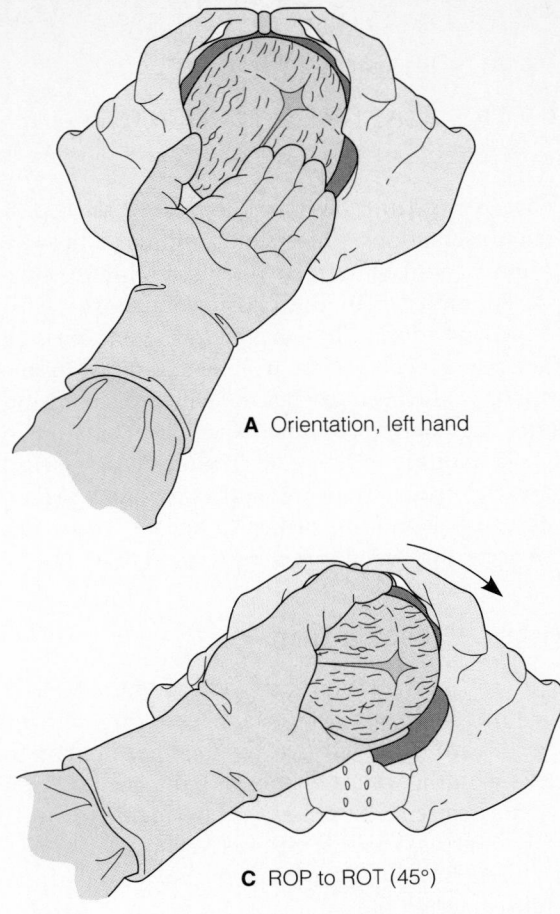

A Orientation, left hand

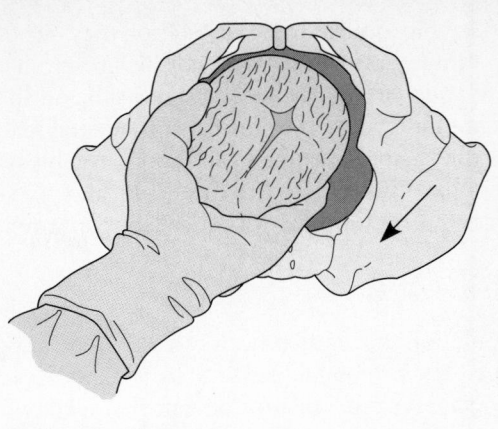

B Grasping the head

C ROP to ROT (45°)

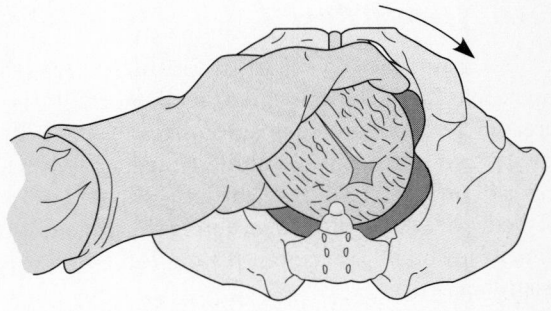

D Manual rotation using left hand: ROT to ROA (45°)

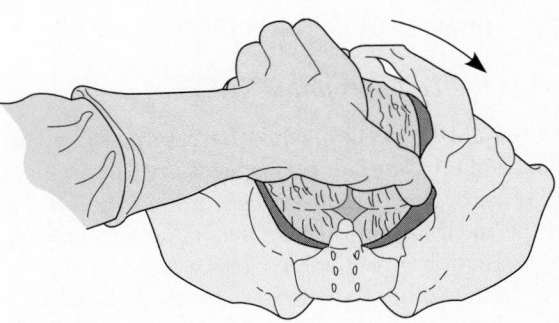

E The manual rotation is completed as the head is rotated another 45° from ROA to OA

FIGURE 25-5 Manual rotation of ROP to OA. *A* The physician's left hand is inserted into the vagina. *B* The back of the fetal head is grasped. *C* The head is flexed and then rotated 45 degrees to ROT. *D* The head is rotated another 45 degrees to ROA. *E* The manual rotation is completed as the head is rotated another 45 degrees from ROA to OA. During the manual rotation the physician's other hand is placed on the maternal abdomen, and the body is turned in the same direction by applying pressure to the fetal breech or shoulders.

the toilet, walk around the room, stand beside the bed and lean forward with her hands on the bed and do the pelvic rock, rest in a whirlpool, or lie on her side in the bed.

Evaluation

Anticipated outcomes of nursing care include:

- The woman's discomfort is decreased.
- The woman and her partner understand comfort measures and position changes that may assist her.

- The woman's coping abilities are strengthened.
- The woman and her partner feel supported and encouraged.

Transverse Arrest

In women with hypotonic labor or a diminished antero-posterior pelvic diameter (as seen with the platypelloid pelvis) or diminished transverse diameter (in the android pelvis), an incomplete internal rotation may occur, resulting in a transverse arrest. This may also result in arrest of descent and a prolonged second stage of labor. In cases of severe molding and caput formation the fetal scalp is visible at the vaginal opening even though the biparietal diameters have not entered the inlet. If labor is effective, spontaneous rotation may occur as labor continues.

Maternal Risks

Manipulation during birth can cause maternal soft tissue damage. Any prolonged pressure by the fetal head in one position may cause the woman later gynecologic problems, such as fistulas resulting from tissue anoxia. Postpartal hemorrhage may result from undetected lacerations or atony if the labor was hypotonic.

Fetal-Neonatal Risks

Unless a protraction or arrest disorder is present or an operative birth is performed, fetal mortality is not increased with transverse position because most fetuses do rotate spontaneously. Cerebral damage may be caused in cases of undetected CPD. The fetus should be closely observed in utero by the nurse, and at the time of birth a pediatrician should be present if a midforceps-assisted birth is anticipated.

Medical Therapy

The choice of medical treatment depends on the degree of fetal rotation. In the presence of a hypotonic labor pattern and no CPD, dilute oxytocin may be administered while closely monitoring the maternal-fetal response (Cunningham et al 1993). When rotation, uterine activity, and CPD are absent, birth is often accomplished by midforceps, manual rotation, or vacuum extraction. If deep transverse arrest exists, forceps may be applied as long as excessive force is avoided. Cesarean birth is preferred, however.

Nursing Care

After identifying women in whom transverse arrest may occur, the nurse continues careful assessment of labor progress. If the labor becomes prolonged or a cesarean birth is necessary, the nurse assesses the coping abilities and knowledge level of the woman and her partner.

The nurse continues efforts to support and comfort the laboring woman. Continuous monitoring of contractions (frequency, duration, and intensity), amount of maternal discomfort, maternal vital signs, and fetal response to labor are important nursing interventions. The nurse notifies the physician/certified nurse-midwife in case of distress or a change in the labor pattern.

The couple is prepared by the nurse for the extreme molding of the infant's head. The nurse remains alert for signs of postpartal hemorrhage.

CARE OF THE WOMAN AND FETUS AT RISK DUE TO FETAL MALPRESENTATION

Three vertex attitudes of the fetus are classified as abnormal presentations: the sinciput (military), brow, and face (Figure 25–6). The fetal body straightens out in these presentations from the classic fetal position to an S-shaped position. The sinciput presentation is probably the least difficult for the woman and fetus. In most cases as soon as the head reaches the pelvic floor, flexion occurs and a vaginal birth results.

In addition to the vertex malpresentation the breech, shoulder (transverse lie), and compound presentations can cause significant difficulty during labor. These and the vertex presentations are discussed here.

Brow Presentation

In a brow presentation the forehead of the fetus becomes the presenting part. The fetal neck is extended instead of flexed, with the result that the fetal head enters the birth canal with the widest diameter of the head (occipitomental) foremost (Figure 19–3). The incidence is 1:500 to 1:1000 births (Sokol & Brindley 1990).

The brow presentation occurs more often in the multipara than the nullipara and is thought to be due to lax abdominal and pelvic musculature. Two-thirds of brow presentations will spontaneously convert to face or occipital presentation (Sokol & Brindley 1990).

Maternal-Fetal-Neonatal Risks

Birth should be accomplished by cesarean birth in the presence of CPD or failure of a brow presentation to convert to an occiput or face presentation. With a vaginal birth perineal lacerations are inevitable and may extend into the rectum or vaginal fornices.

Fetal mortality is increased due to injuries received during the birth and/or infection because of prolonged labor. Trauma during the birth process can include tentorial tears, cerebral and neck compression, and damage to the trachea and larynx.

Medical Therapy

Active medical intervention is not necessary as long as cervical dilatation and fetal descent are occurring. In the presence of labor problems but no CPD a manual conversion may be attempted. Some medical experts advocate midforceps-assisted birth in the presence of complete dilatation and fetal station at +2. In the presence of failed conversions, CPD, or secondary arrest of labor cesarean birth is the preferred method of management. Adequate resuscitation equipment and pediatric assistance should be available at the time of birth.

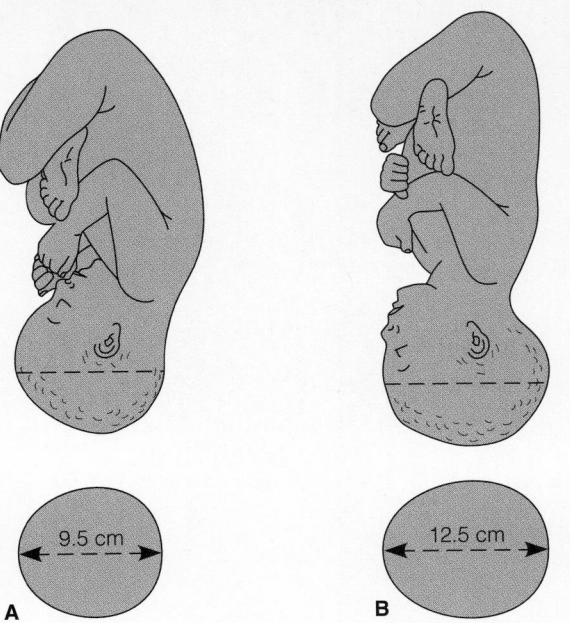

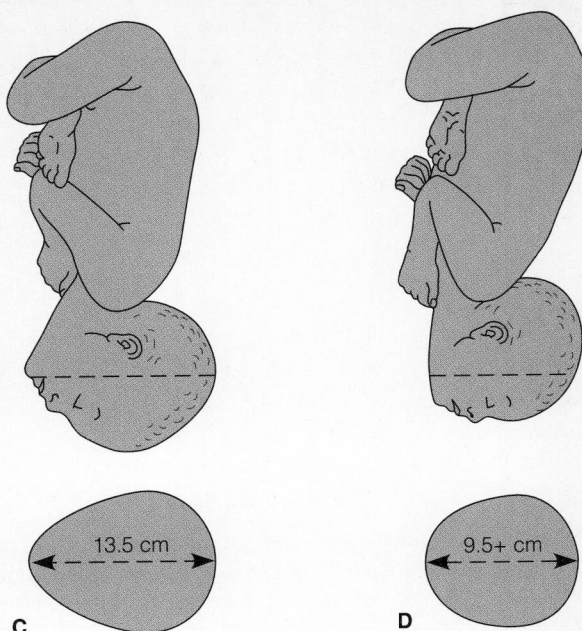

A 9.5 cm **B** 12.5 cm **C** 13.5 cm **D** 9.5+ cm

FIGURE 25-6   Types of cephalic presentations *A* The occiput is the presenting part because the head is flexed and the fetal chin is against the chest. The largest anteroposterior (AP) diameter that presents and passes through the pelvis is approximately 9.5 cm. *B* Military presentation. The head is neither flexed nor extended. The presenting AP diameter is approximately 12.5 cm. *C* Brow presentation. The largest diameter of the fetal head (approximately 13.5 cm) presents in this situation. *D* Face presentation. The AP diameter is 9.5 cm. SOURCE: Danforth DN, Scott JR (editors): *Obstetrics and Gynecology,* 5th ed. New York: Lippincott: 1990, Fig 8-9, p 170.

APPLYING THE NURSING PROCESS

Nursing Assessment

Leopold's maneuvers reveal a cephalic prominence on the same side as the fetal back. A brow presentation can be detected on vaginal examination by palpation of the diamond-shaped anterior fontanelle on one side and orbital ridges and root of the nose on the other side (Figure 25–7).

Nursing Diagnosis

Nursing diagnoses that may apply to brow presentation include the following:

- Anxiety/Fear related to outcome for fetus
- Knowledge deficit related to lack of information about possible maternal-fetal effects of brow presentation
- Risk for injury to the fetus related to pressure on fetal structures secondary to brow presentation

Nursing Plan and Implementation

Nursing management of abnormal cephalic presentations includes close observation of the woman for labor aberrations and of the fetus for signs of stress. The fetus should

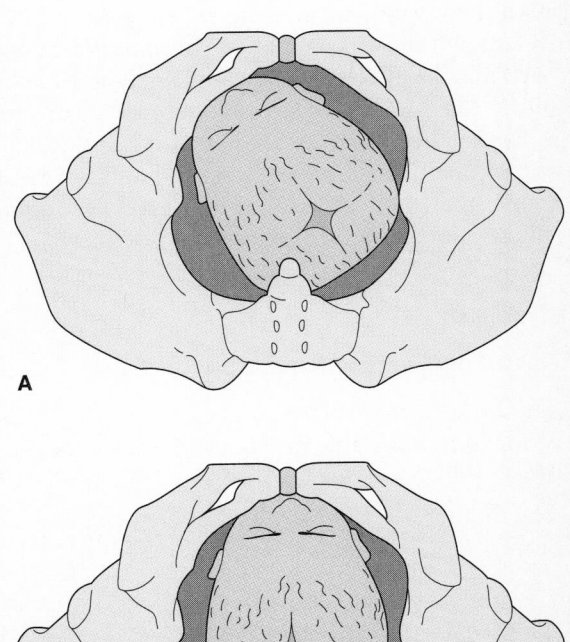

FIGURE 25-7   Brow presentation. *A* Descent. *B* Internal rotation in the pelvic cavity. SOURCE: Oxorn H: *Human Labor and Birth,* 5th ed. Norwalk, CT: Appleton & Lange 1986, p 211.

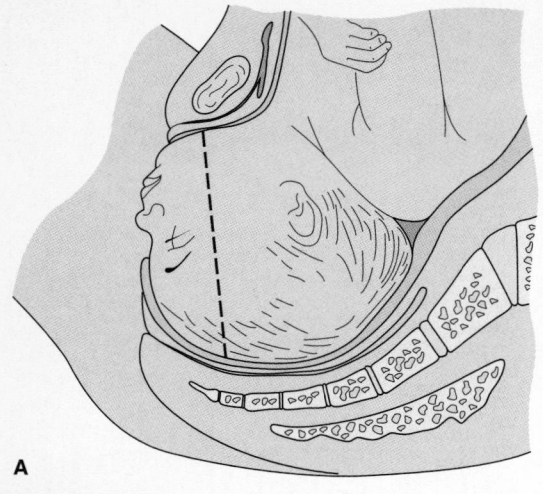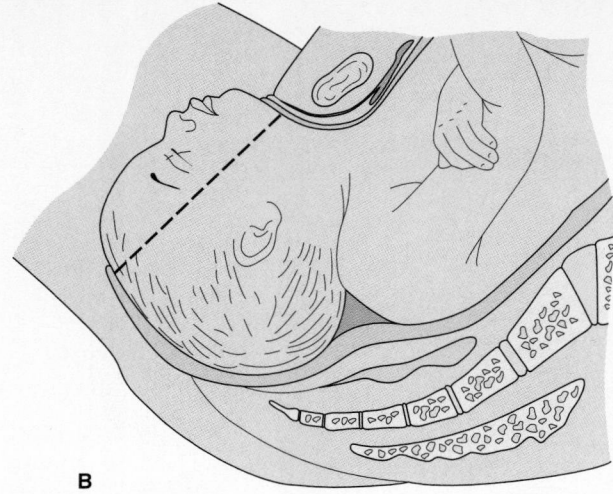

FIGURE 25-8 Mechanism of birth in face (mentoanterior) position. *A* The submetobregmatic diameter at the outlet. *B* The fetal head is born by movement of flexion.

be observed closely during labor for signs of hypoxia as evidenced by late decelerations and bradycardia.

The nurse may need to explain the position of the fetus to the laboring couple or to interpret what the physician/CNM has told them. The nurse should stay close at hand to reassure the couple, inform them of any changes, and assist them with labor-coping techniques.

In face and brow presentation the appearance of the newborn may be affected. The couple may need help in beginning the attachment process because of the newborn's facial appearance. After the infant is inspected for gross abnormalities, the pediatrician and nurse can assure the couple that the facial edema and excessive molding are only temporary and will subside in 3 or 4 days.

Evaluation

Anticipated outcomes of nursing care include:

- The woman and her partner understand the implications and associated problems of brow presentation.

- The mother and her baby have a safe labor and birth.

Face Presentation

In a face presentation the face of the fetus is the presenting part. The fetal head is hyperextended even more than in the brow presentation. Face presentation occurs most frequently in multiparas, in preterm birth, and in the presence of anencephaly. The incidence of face presentation is about 1 in 600 deliveries. (Sokol & Brindley 1990).

Maternal-Fetal-Neonatal Risks

The risks of CPD and prolonged labor are increased with face presentation. As with any prolonged labor, the chance of infection is increased.

The fetus may develop caput succedaneum of the face during labor, and after birth the edema gives the newborn an unusual appearance. As with the brow presentation, the neck and internal structures may swell due to the trauma received during descent. Petechiae and ecchymoses are often seen in the superficial layers of the facial skin because of the birth trauma.

Medical Therapy

If no CPD is present, the chin (mentum) is anterior, and the labor pattern is effective, the objective of medical treatment is a vaginal birth (Figure 25–8). Mentum posteriors can become wedged on the anterior surface of the sacrum (Figure 25–9). In this case as well as in the presence of CPD, cesarean birth is the preferred method of management.

Nursing Assessment

When performing Leopold's maneuvers, the nurse finds that the back of the fetus is difficult to outline, and a deep furrow can be palpated between the hard occiput and the

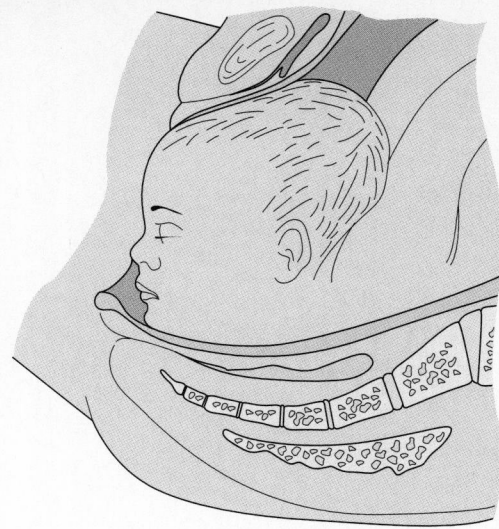

FIGURE 25-9   Face presentation. Mechanism of birth in mento-posterior position. Fetal head is unable to extend farther. The face becomes impacted.

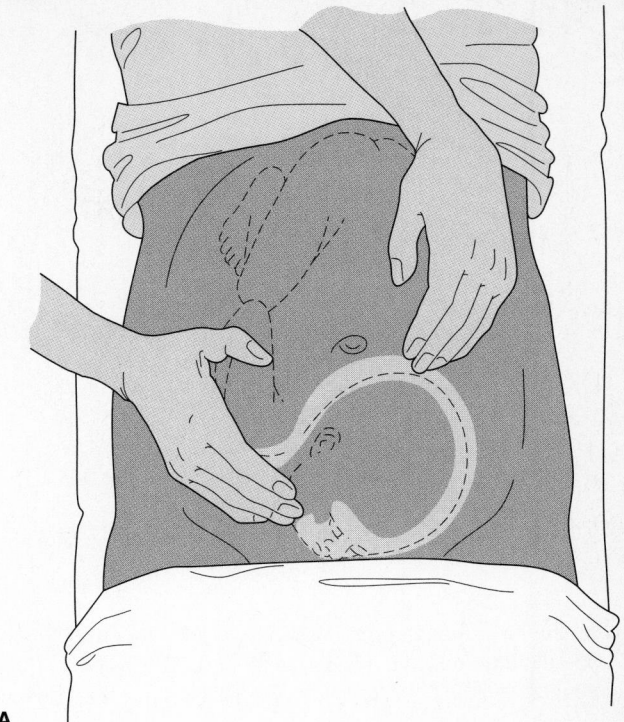

A

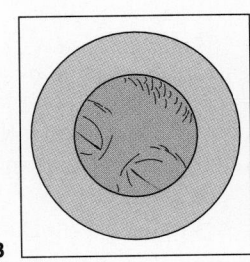

B

FIGURE 25-10   Face presentation. *A* Palpation of the maternal abdomen with the fetus in right mentum posterior (RMP). *B* Vaginal examination may permit palpation of facial features of the fetus.

fetal back (Figure 25–10). Fetal heart tones can be heard on the side where the fetal feet are palpated. It may be difficult to determine by vaginal examination whether a breech or face is presenting, especially if facial edema is already present. During the vaginal examination palpation of the saddle of the nose and the gums should be attempted. When assessing engagement, the nurse needs to remember that the face has to be deep within the pelvis before the biparietal diameters have entered the inlet.

Nursing Diagnosis

Nursing diagnoses that may apply to the woman with a fetus in face presentation include the following:

- Fear related to unknown outcome of the labor and appearance of the baby
- Risk for injury to the newborn's face related to edema secondary to the birth process

Nursing Plan and Implementation

Nursing interventions are the same as for the brow presentation.

Evaluation

Anticipated outcomes of nursing care include:

- The woman and her partner understand the implications and problems of face presentation.
- The mother and her baby have a safe labor and birth.

Breech Presentation

Breech presentation is the most common malpresentation, occurring in approximately 4% of births. The incidence of breech presentation is as high as 15% in infants weighing less than 2500 g, 30% in babies weighing 1000–1499 g, and 40% in babies under 1000 g (Cruikshank 1994). Almost 40% of term breech births are not identified until labor occurs (Gimovsky & Shifrin 1992).

Frank breech is the most common type of breech (especially at term) and occurs in about 60% of breech births. Single or double footling (incomplete breech) accounts for about 35% of breech births and occurs more frequently in preterm fetuses. The remaining 5% of breech presentations are complete breech presentations (Figure 25–11).

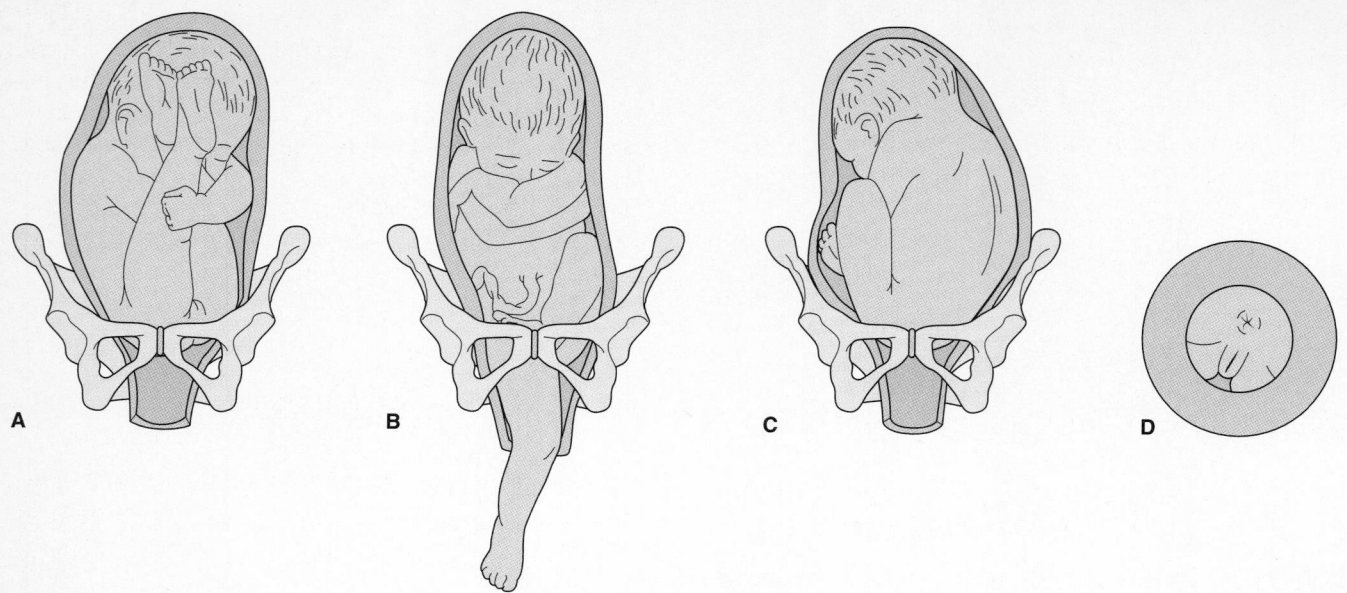

FIGURE 25-11 Breech presentation. *A* Frank breech. *B* Incomplete (footling) breech. *C* Complete breech in left sacral anterior (LSA) position. *D* On vaginal examination the nurse may feel the anal sphincter. The tissue of the fetal buttocks feels soft.

Maternal Risks

Breech presentation is most frequently associated with placenta previa, hydramnios, multiple gestation, and grandmultiparity (Cruikshank 1994).

There is a higher maternal morbidity and mortality rate because of the increased incidence of cesarean birth when the fetus is in breech presentation. The incidence of morbidity and mortality is even higher if the cesarean birth is an emergency (Cunningham et al 1993).

There is a difference of opinion regarding the implication of breech presentation on length of labor. Some believe that labor progresses at the same rate as cephalic presentation; others believe labor may be slowed because the buttocks do not exert as much pressure on the cervix as the fetal head.

Fetal-Neonatal Risks

Breech presentation has a fourfold increase in perinatal mortality than term cephalic presentation and a two- to threefold increase in preterm births. In addition to increased mortality, other major areas of risk are: (1) approximately 25% of breech presentations are premature at birth; (2) severe and lethal anomalies are present in 20% of preterm breech births and 6% to 7% of term breech births; and (3) birth trauma (especially of the head) may occur during either vaginal or cesarean breech birth (Gimovsky & Shifrin 1992). Head trauma is more likely in breech presentation because, unlike the slow molding that occurs as the fetal head moves through the birth canal in a cephalic presentation, the fetal head of a

breech is the last to come through the maternal pelvis, and molding does not occur. In the case of a preterm breech, although the body may deliver through a cervix that is not completely dilated, the larger head can be trapped by the cervix (called entrapment). This entrapment may also occur with cesarean birth if the incision is inadequate and/or there is less than optimum uterine relaxation (Cruikshank 1994).

Medical Therapy

Prior to the mid-1970s more than 90% of breeches were born vaginally. Through the 1980s, in an attempt to reduce fetal-neonatal morbidity and mortality associated with breech vaginal birth, the method of birth changed, and approximately 80% to 90% of breeches were born by cesarean. At this time efforts are being made to maintain safety for the mother and baby and yet decrease national cesarean birth rates. To accomplish this goal, an external version (changing a breech presentation to a cephalic presentation) is done when possible. Even if the breech presentation persists, a vaginal birth may still occur.

A woman who arrives in labor with a breech presentation needs to be carefully evaluated to determine if labor should continue and vaginal birth should occur. As long as the woman has not had a previous cesarean birth, the physician will first estimate fetal weight. If fetal weight is between 1500 g and 3800 g, the physician will use computed tomography (CT), ultrasound, and/or x-ray pelvimetry to evaluate extension of the fetal neck, extension of the fetal arms over the head, fetal measurements, presence of fetal anomalies, and maternal pelvic measurements. Contraindications for labor and vaginal birth include the following:

- Fetal weight less than 1500 g or more than 3800 g
- Hyperextension of the fetal neck of more than 90 degrees
- Extension of the fetal arms over the head
- Anomalies such as hydrocephalus
- Diminished maternal pelvic measurements (Average measurements are 11 cm for anteroposterior diameter of the pelvic inlet, 12 cm for the transverse diameter of the inlet and the anteroposterior diameter of the midpelvis, and 9.5 cm for the interspinous diameter.)

Once active labor is reached, the nullipara should have 1.2 cm cervical dilatation per hour, and the multipara, 1.5 cm per hour with progressive fetal descent. Unless an epidural regional block is used, the length of the second stage should not exceed 1 hour for a nullipara and 30 minutes for a multigravida (Cruikshank 1994).

Epidural anesthesia may be advantageous during the later portion of labor because it will help prevent the pushing sensation the woman may feel prior to complete dilatation. If the woman pushes before cervical dilatation is complete, the fetal body may be expelled and the head entrapped. At the time of birth the physician may have an assistant available in case forceps are needed. Once the fetal body is born, an assistant supports the fetal body as the physician applies Piper forceps to assist in birth of the fetal head (called aftercoming head) (Cruikshank 1994).

APPLYING THE NURSING PROCESS

Nursing Assessment

Frequently, the nurse is the first person to recognize a breech presentation. On palpation the hard vertex is felt in the fundus, and ballottement of the head can be done independently of the fetal body. The wider sacrum is palpated in the lower part of the abdomen. If the sacrum has not descended, on ballottement the entire fetal body will move. Furthermore, FHTs are usually auscultated above the umbilicus. Passage of meconium from compression of the infant's intestinal tract on descent is common.

Critical Thinking Question

Try to visualize what your hands would feel if you did Leopold's maneuvers when the fetus is in a breech presentation. Compare this to a transverse lie.

The nurse is particularly alert for a prolapsed umbilical cord, especially in incomplete breeches, because space through which the cord can slip is available between the cervix and presenting part. If the infant is small and the membranes rupture, the danger is even greater. This is one reason why any woman admitted to the birthing area with a history of ruptured membranes should not be ambulated until a full assessment, including vaginal examination, is performed.

Nursing Diagnosis

Nursing diagnoses that may apply to breech presentation include the following:

- Risk for impaired gas exchange in the fetus related to interruption in umbilical blood flow secondary to compression of the cord
- Knowledge deficit related to lack of information about implications and associated complications of breech presentation on the mother and fetus

Nursing Plan and Implementation

Promotion of Maternal-Fetal Well-Being

During labor the fetus is at increased risk for prolapse of the cord, so the nurse monitors the FHR by continuous EFM (see Prolapsed Umbilical Cord later in this chapter). Ongoing assessments of contractions, cervical dilatation, and effacement and fetal descent are also important to monitor labor progress. Emotional support and sharing of information are critical to the childbearing couple. They need to be kept apprised of the labor's current status as well as the possible treatment plans so they can continue to make informed choices.

Assistance During Vaginal Birth   During the birth the nurse continues to assess the FHR and to encourage the couple. Piper forceps need to be readily available to the physician, and the nurse may assist the physician if the forceps are needed for the birth.

Evaluation

Anticipated outcomes of nursing care include:

- The woman and her partner understand the implications and associated problems with breech presentation.
- The mother and baby have a safe labor and birth.
- Major complications are recognized early, and corrective measures are instituted.

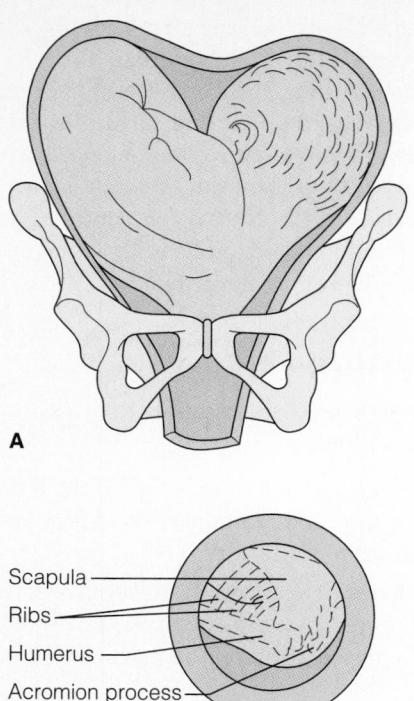

A

Scapula
Ribs
Humerus
Acromion process

B

FIGURE 25-12   Transverse lie. *A* Shoulder presentation. *B* On vaginal examination the nurse may feel the acromion process as the fetal presenting part.

Shoulder Presentation (Transverse Lie)

A transverse lie occurs in approximately 3 to 4 per 1000 term births (King 1994). The infant's long axis lies across the woman's abdomen, and on inspection the contour of the maternal abdomen appears widest from side to side (Figure 25–12).

Maternal conditions associated with a transverse lie are grandmultiparity with lax uterine musculature (the most common cause); obstructions such as bony dystocia, placenta previa, neoplasms, and fetal anomalies; hydramnios; and preterm labor. It is not uncommon in multiple gestations for one or more of the fetuses to be in a transverse lie.

Maternal Risks

Labor can be dysfunctional in the presence of a transverse lie. Uterine rupture, although rare, can occur (King 1994).

Fetal-Neonatal Risks

The stillbirth rate is two to three times higher for transverse lie than for cephalic presentation (King 1994). One danger of transverse lie is a prolapsed umbilical cord be-cause there is nothing in the pelvic inlet to serve as a blocking agent. Prolapse of a fetal arm may also occur. If the woman is allowed to labor in the presence of a transverse lie, the fetus may die from asphyxia and trauma.

Medical Therapy

Transverse lie may be diagnosed using Leopold's maneuvers and can then be confirmed by real-time ultrasound. At the time of the ultrasound exam it is important to confirm fetal position, fetal biparietal diameters (to confirm gestational age), and location of the placenta, and to carry out an examination for the presence of fetal anomalies and structural abnormalities of the uterus such as leimyomata (fibroid tumor) or adnexal tumors (King 1994).

Management varies, depending on the length of gestation, because many transverse lies convert to either cephalic or breech presentation by term (38 weeks). If the fetus is still in transverse lie at term, an external version may be done if: (1) there is no contraindication to vaginal birth (for example, a fetal anomaly, complete placenta previa, or a structural problem in the uterus); and (2) fetal pulmonary lung maturity is confirmed either by ultrasound measurements or by amniocentesis for assessment of phospholipids (2:1 L/S ratio and the presence of phosphotidylglycerol). An external version is accomplished with β-mimetic or magnesium sulfate tocolysis. After the fetus is turned to a cephalic presentation, labor is induced to keep the fetus from reverting to a transverse lie. A cesarean birth is planned at term and before rupture of membranes (to prevent prolapse of the umbilical cord) if the version is contraindicated or unsuccessful or if the woman refuses the version (King 1994). If membranes rupture and the cord prolapses prior to the planned cesarean birth, an emergency cesarean is done. Antibiotic therapy should be instituted and care taken to quickly identify any maternal hemorrhage (King 1994).

APPLYING THE NURSING PROCESS

Nursing Assessment

The nurse can identify a transverse lie by inspection and palpation of the abdomen, by auscultation of FHTs in the midline of the abdomen (not conclusive), and by vaginal examination.

On palpation no fetal part is felt in the fundal portion of the uterus or above the symphysis pubis. The head may be palpated on one side and the breech on the other. Fetal heart tones are usually auscultated just below the midline of the umbilicus. On vaginal examination, if a presenting part is palpated, it is the ridged thorax or possibly an arm that is compressed against the chest.

Nursing Diagnosis

Nursing diagnoses that may apply when transverse lie is present include the following:

- Knowledge deficit related to the lack of information about implications and problems associated with transverse lie
- Risk for impaired gas exchange in the fetus related to decrease in blood flow secondary to cord compression associated with prolapsed cord
- Risk for compromised, ineffective individual/family coping related to unknown outcome
- Fear related to unknown outcome of birth

Nursing Plan and Implementation

The primary nursing actions are to help evaluate the fetal presentation and to provide information and support to the couple. If an external version has been accomplished and an induction is done, the nurse completes all interventions related to the induction. (See discussion in Chapter 26.) If transverse lie is discovered when the woman is admitted to the birthing unit, the nurse provides information regarding the need for a cesarean birth and assists with preparation for the birth. Prior to the cesarean the nurse watches for rupture of membranes and the possibility of prolapse of the umbilical cord. (See Chapter 26 for further information regarding teaching with cesarean birth.)

Evaluation

Anticipated outcomes of nursing care include:

- The transverse lie is recognized promptly, and crucial assessments are completed.
- The mother and baby have a safe birth.
- The couple understands the implications and associated problems of transverse lie.

Compound Presentation

A **compound presentation** is one in which there are two presenting parts. It can occur when the pelvic inlet is not totally occluded by the primary presenting part. If the prolapsed part is a hand, the birth is generally not difficult. Sometimes the hand slips back, and occasionally it is born alongside the head. This may increase the chance of laceration. If the prolapsed part is left alone, the birth is generally not difficult. Cesarean birth is indicated in the presence of uterine dysfunction or fetal distress (Cunningham et al 1993).

CARE OF THE WOMAN AND FETUS AT RISK DUE TO DEVELOPMENTAL ABNORMALITIES

Macrosomia

Fetal **macrosomia** occurs when a newborn weighs more than 4000 g (8 lb, 14 oz) at birth. The incidence of macrosomia is 7.6% in the general population (Cunningham et al 1993). Overall the incidence of babies weighing over 4500 g (9 lb, 15 oz) is 1% in all births (Tamura & Sabbagha 1990).

Maternal Risks

The woman's pelvis that is adequate for an average-sized fetus may be disproportionately small for an oversized fetus. Distention of the uterus causes overstretching of the myometrial fibers, which may lead to dysfunctional labor and an increased incidence of postpartal hemorrhage. If the oversized fetus acts as an obstruction, the chance of uterine rupture during labor increases. During vaginal birth there is an increased risk of perineal lacerations.

Fetal-Neonatal Risks

Fetal prognosis is guarded. If a macrosomic fetus is unsuspected and labor is allowed to continue in the presence of disproportion, the fetus can receive cerebral trauma from intermittent forceful contact with the maternal bony pelvis. During difficult operative procedures performed at the time of vaginal birth, the fetus may become asphyxiated or experience neurologic damage from pressure exerted on its head.

Shoulder dystocia is a problem encountered when, following the delivery of the head, the anterior shoulder does not deliver either spontaneously or with gentle traction (Bowes 1994). If the fetus weighs more than 4000 g, the incidence of shoulder dystocia ranges from 13% to 31% (Keller et al 1990). Asphyxia is the most immediate danger to the baby, and if birth is not accomplished within a few minutes after the birth of the head, the baby will die (Sokol & Brindley 1990). If management of the shoulder dystocia is not accomplished correctly, there may be permanent injury to the baby. Brachial plexus injury (due to improper or excessive traction applied to the fetal head) and fractured clavicles occur in about 20% of shoulder dystocias (Mashburn 1988).

Medical Therapy

The occurrence of the maternal and fetal problems associated with macrosomic infants may be somewhat lessened by identifying macrosomia prior to the onset of labor. If a large fetus is suspected, the maternal pelvis should be evaluated carefully. An estimation of fetal size can be made by palpating the crown-rump length of the fetus in utero, but the greatest errors in estimation occur on both ends of the spectrum—the macrosomic fetus and the very small fetus. Fundal height can give some clue. Ultrasound or x-ray pelvimetry may give further information about fetal size. Whenever the uterus appears excessively large, hydramnios, an oversized fetus, or a multiple pregnancy must be considered.

Labor may proceed within normal limits, or there may be a slowing of fetal descent (change of station) and a prolonged second stage (Gross et al 1987). Even though these problems are present, it is still not possible to anticipate shoulder dystocia that results in trauma to the newborn. If difficulty extracting the shoulders occurs during the birth, the obstetrician/CNM may direct the woman to sharply flex her thighs up against her abdomen (McRoberts maneuver). This position is thought to change the maternal pelvic angle and therefore reduce the force needed to extract the shoulders and decrease the incidence of brachial plexus stretching and clavicular fracture (Figure 25-13) (Gonik et al 1989). In addition the obstetrician/CNM may incorporate other interventions such as checking the placement of the shoulder, enlarging the episiotomy, asking the labor and birth nurse to apply suprapubic pressure, and using the Woods Screw maneuver (consists of rotating the anterior shoulder 180 degrees to the posterior position).

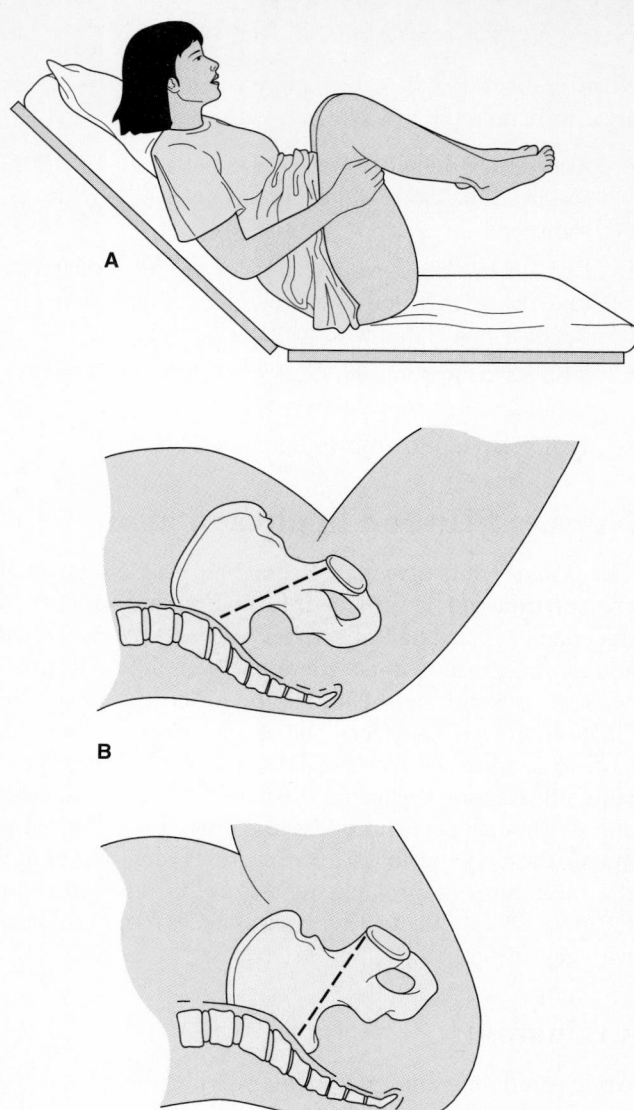

FIGURE 25-13   McRoberts maneuver. *A* The woman flexes her thighs up onto her abdomen. *B* The angle of the maternal pelvis prior to McRoberts maneuver. *C* The angle of the pelvis with McRoberts maneuver.

APPLYING THE NURSING PROCESS

Nursing Assessment

The nurse assists in identifying factors associated with macrosomic infants, which include multiparity, maternal obesity, excessive weight gain during this pregnancy, maternal diabetes, history of a large infant or previous shoulder dystocia, and pregnancy that extends to 42 weeks or beyond (Mashburn 1988). During the intrapartum period the risk factors include slow descent of the fetus and prolonged second stage. Because women with these risk factors are prime candidates for dystocia and its complications, the nurse frequently assesses the FHR for indications of fetal stress and evaluates the rate of cervical dilatation and fetal descent.

Nursing Diagnosis

Nursing diagnoses that may apply to the woman with a macrosomic fetus include the following:

- Risk for injury to the fetus related to trauma during the birth process

- Risk for infection related to traumatized tissue secondary to maternal tissue damage during birth
- Knowledge deficit related to lack of information about the implications and possible problems associated with birth of a macrosomic baby

Nursing Plan and Implementation

Promotion of Maternal-Fetal Physical Well-Being

The nurse monitors labor closely for a dysfunctional pattern. The fetal monitor is applied for continuous fetal evaluation. Early decelerations could mean disproportion at the bony inlet. Any sign of labor dysfunction or fetal stress should be reported to the physician.

If difficulty is encountered during the birth, as an emergency measure the physician/certified nurse-midwife may ask the nurse to apply suprapubic or fundal pressure in an attempt to aid the delivery of the fetal shoulders (Kline-Kaye & Miller-Slade 1990).

After the birth the nurse inspects the newborn for cephalhematoma, Erb palsy (caused by overstretching of the brachial plexus and damage to C5, C6, C7), and fractured clavicles (exhibited by nonmovement of one arm) and informs the admission nursery of any problems. The newborn will need to be observed closely for cerebral and neurologic damage.

Postpartally, the nurse checks the uterus for potential atony and the maternal vital signs for deviations suggesting shock.

Providing Emotional Support

The nurse provides support for the laboring woman and her partner and information regarding the implications and possible associated problems. During the birth the nurse continues to provide support and encouragement to the couple.

Evaluation

Anticipated outcomes of nursing care include:

- The woman and her partner understand the implications and possible associated problems.
- The mother and baby have a safe labor and birth.

CARE OF THE WOMAN WITH A MULTIPLE PREGNANCY

Twin Pregnancy

The incidence of naturally occurring twins in the United States is 1 per 80 pregnancies (Knuppel & Drukker 1993). Twins can develop from either the fertilization of two separate ova or from the division of one fertilized ovum. Twins that occur from two separate ova are called *dizygotic*, and they may be the same sex or different sexes. In this type of twinning there are two amnions (diamniotic) and two chorions (dichorionic).

Twins from one fertilized ovum are called *monozygotic* and are always of the same sex (Table 25–1). Monozygotic twins occur in 3 to 5 of each 1000 pregnancies (Wenstrom et al 1992). If the fertilized ovum (zygote) divides within the first 72 hours past fertilization, the twins will be diamniotic and dichorionic. If the division occurs from the fourth to the eighth day past fertilization, the embryos will develop with two separate amnions and one chorion (monochorionic). If the division happens after the eighth day, the two fetuses will share both a common amniotic sac and chorion (monoamniotic, monochorionic). The terminology is important because the perinatal morbidity and mortality rates differ greatly between different types of twins (Keith et al 1991).

The incidence of dizygotic twins is highest in women of African descent, women of higher age and parity, women with a family history of twins, and women experiencing a high frequency of coitus, as in the first 3 months of marriage (Hollenbach & Hickok 1990). The incidence of monozygotic twins is largely independent of age, parity, heredity, and race.

The perinatal morbidity and mortality rates for twins are almost twice that of singleton pregnancies, and the mortality rate for monozygotic twins is 3 times the rate for fraternal twins. The incidence of preterm birth is 12 times that of single births, and only 5% of twins reach 40 weeks of gestation (Hunter 1989).

During the prenatal period a fundal height greater than expected for the weeks of gestation and auscultation of two heartbeats that differ by at least 10 bpm are the most likely clues. Some women experience severe nausea and vomiting and develop severe anemia despite the intake of multiple-vitamin therapy. The α-fetoprotein level may be elevated (Kochenour 1992).

Maternal Risks

In addition to the normal physiologic changes in pregnancy the woman with twins has further changes in the cardiovascular system. The blood volume is increased an additional 500 mL. The heart does not enlarge, but cardiac output is increased in the second and third trimesters. The change in cardiac output is accomplished by an increase in heart rate and contractility. These changes probably reduce cardiac reserve, so maternal activity and exercise should be tailored to take these physiologic changes into consideration (Veille et al 1986).

Women with twin gestations have an 83% incidence of antenatal complications as compared to an incidence of 32% in singleton gestations (Makowski 1990). Some of the complications include the following:

- Spontaneous abortions are more common, possibly because of genetic defects or poor placental implantation or development.
- Maternal anemia occurs because the maternal system is nurturing more than one fetus.
- The increased incidence of pregnancy-induced hypertension (PIH) is thought to result from an oversized uterus and increased amounts of placental hormones.

TABLE 25-1   Characteristics of Twin Pregnancy

Type	Time of Division	Characteristics	Frequency	Mortality rate
Dizygous				
(Double ovum) Fraternal twins	Develop from two ova released at the same time.	Each twin has own placenta, chorion, amnion. Dizygous twins are called fraternal twins. They may be the same or different sex.	75% of all twins	
Monozygous				
(Single ovum) Identical twins				
Dichorionic-diamniotic twins	Division occurs at blastomere stage, 2 to 3 days past fertilization. Inner cell mass not yet developed.	Each twin has own chorion, amnion, placenta.	30% of monozygous twins	9%
Monochorionic-diamniotic twins	Division occurs at blastocyst stage, 4 to 6 days after fertilization. Inner cell mass divides in two.	Placenta has one chorion and two amnions. Each twin lies in own sac.	68% of monozygous twins	25%
Monochorionic-monoamniotic twins	Division occurs in primitive germ disk, 7 to 13 days past fertilization.	Twins lie in the same amniotic sac. Increased risk of umbilical cords becoming tangled or knotted.	2% of monozygous twins	>50%

- Third trimester bleeding from placenta previa and abruptio placentae occurs more frequently.

- Hydramnios may be due to increased renal perfusion from cross-vessel anastomosis of monozygotic twins.

Complications during labor include: (1) uterine dysfunction due to an overstretched myometrium; (2) abnormal fetal presentations; and (3) preterm labor. With rupture of membranes and hydramnios, abruptio placentae can occur. Danger of placental abruption after the birth of the first twin also exists because of a decrease in the surface area of the uterus to which the placenta is still attached.

The woman pregnant with twins may experience more physical discomfort during her pregnancy, such as shortness of breath, dyspnea on exertion, backaches, and pedal edema, because of the oversized uterus.

Occasionally, multiple pregnancies are not diagnosed until the time of birth; this occurs most often in cases of preterm labor. If the family has physically, psychologically, and financially prepared for one baby, problems can arise when they are suddenly confronted with more than one child. Infants of multiple pregnancies frequently require intensive care, and this may cause financial and emotional stress.

Fetal-Neonatal Risks

The perinatal mortality rate is approximately four times greater for twins than for a single fetus. The perinatal mortality rate for monoamniotic, monochorionic twins has been estimated as high as 50% (Kochenour 1992). Congenital anomalies are approximately twice as common in twin infants as in singleton infants (McLennan 1994). The fetus is preterm at a rate of five to ten times that of singletons, and 50% of twins weigh less than 2500 g (5 lb 8 oz) at birth (Theroux 1989).

Twins with monochorionic placentas may develop artery-to-artery anastomosis, which compromises fetoplacental circulation. One twin is overperfused and is born with polycythemia and hypervolemia and may have hypertension with an enlarged heart. This twin's amniotic sac exhibits hydramnios because of the increased renal perfusion and excessive voiding. The other twin has hypovolemia and exhibits intrauterine growth restriction (IUGR). In the newborn period the neonate with increased perfusion has an increased chance of hyperbilirubinemia as the system tries to rid itself of the extra red blood cells. The other twin is anemic, with all the problems that small-for-gestational-age (SGA) infants exhibit (Danskin & Neilson 1989).

Twins that share the same amniotic sac have some special problems. They have an increased chance of becoming entangled in each other's umbilical cords, and this problem is responsible for a stillborn rate of over 50%. They are also more likely to have developmental problems after birth. Their intelligence quotients are slightly lower than normal until the age of 11, and their physical growth continues to lag behind that of singletons (Theroux 1989).

Conjoined or Siamese twins occur when the division of the embryonic disk is incomplete. The incidence is 1 in

50,000 births and 1 in 400 pairs of monozygotic twins. The stillborn rate is 40% (Sakala 1986).

Medical Therapy

The goals of medical care are the promotion of normal fetal development for both fetuses, preventing the birth of preterm fetuses, and diminishing fetal trauma during labor.

Once the presence of twins has been detected, preventing and treating problems that infringe on the development and birth of normal fetuses is a significant medical activity. Prenatal care is comprehensive. The woman's visits are more frequent than those of the woman with one fetus. The childbearing woman needs to understand nutritional implications, assessment of fetal activity, signs of preterm labor, and danger signs.

Serial ultrasounds are done to assess the growth of each fetus and to provide early recognition of IUGR. Some physicians believe that bed rest in the lateral position enhances uterine-placental-fetal blood flow and decreases the risk of preterm labor. Others question the value of bed rest/hospitalization, especially for the prevention of uterine contractions, which seem to precede preterm labor (Crowther et al 1990).

Testing usually begins at 30 to 34 weeks' gestation and may include nonstress test (NST), biophysical profile, and Doppler ultrasound to assess umbilical blood waveforms. A reactive NST is associated with good fetal outcome if birth occurs within 1 week of the testing. The NST is done every 3 to 7 days until birth or until results become nonreactive (Hunter 1989). The biophysical profile is also accurate in assessing fetal status with twin pregnancies. A biophysical profile of 8 (as long as the amount of amniotic fluid measured is accurate) or better for each fetus is considered reassuring, and weekly or biweekly biophysical profiles and NSTs are continued (Hunter 1989).

Intrapartal management and assessment require careful attention to maternal and fetal status. The mother should have an IV in place with a large-bore needle. Anesthesia and cross-matched blood should be readily available. The twins are monitored by dual electronic fetal monitoring. The labor may progress very slowly or very quickly.

The decision regarding method of birth may not be made until labor occurs, and the method depends on a variety of factors. The presence of maternal complications such as placenta previa, abruptio placentae, or severe PIH usually indicates the need for cesarean birth. Fetal factors such as severe IUGR, preterm birth, fetal anomalies, fetal stress, or unfavorable fetal position or presentation also require cesarean birth.

Any combination of presentations and positions can occur with twins (Figure 25–14). Approximately 50% of twins are delivered by cesarean, which is chosen in the hope of reducing complications for the twins, especially birth asphyxia (Cunningham et al 1993).

Vaginal birth is planned when the following factors are present (Polin & Frangipane 1986):

- Gestation is greater than 32 weeks, and estimated fetal size is greater than 2000 g each
- Twin A (the fetus closest to the cervix) is the larger twin
- Twin A is vertex
- Twin B is vertex, breech, or transverse and smaller than twin A
- There is no evidence of fetal distress
- There is no CPD

Because most breech presentations are born by cesarean, many physicians choose cesarean birth if either of the twins is breech.

An anesthesiologist should be present during the vaginal birth in case a cesarean needs to be done. One additional obstetrician is usually available to assist in the event that complications occur. The presence of two pediatricians, two nurses to care for the babies, and two labor and delivery nurses is usually recommended.

Because labor is frequently preterm and the labor progress difficult to predict, the mother is usually not given analgesics. An epidural may be used for the last part of labor and birth, or local anesthesia may be given at the time of birth.

The twins are continually monitored by electronic fetal monitoring. After the birth of twin A, twin B is observed by ultrasound to assess position and descent into the pelvis. If twin B is in a transverse lie, the obstetrician converts it to a double footling breech by internal (podalic) version. The anesthesiologist administers general anesthesia such as halothane to effect good uterine relaxation during this procedure. Some physicians use external version to change the presentation of the second twin (Tchabo & Tomai 1992). If the baby weighs more than 1500 g (approximately 3 lb, 5 oz), there does not seem to be increased morbidity (Gocke et al 1989).

In some instances the second twin may need to be born by cesarean. Complications that would require this include profound fetal distress when vaginal birth is not imminent, prolapse of the cord, and contractions of the uterus that trap the second twin (Knuppel & Drukker 1993).

Birth in the presence of dysfunctional labor due to overstretched uterine fibers can be managed with cesarean birth or infusion of diluted oxytocin. There is little agreement on the benefits and dangers of the two methods or on the most beneficial type of analgesia and anesthesia to employ for labor and birth. In the presence of an unstable maternal circulatory system, as found with PIH, regional anesthetic agents such as epidurals or caudals can cause hypovolemic shock due to the blocking of the sympathetic nervous system. Large and continuous doses of narcotics can cause neonatal respiratory depression, especially if these infants are premature, as twins

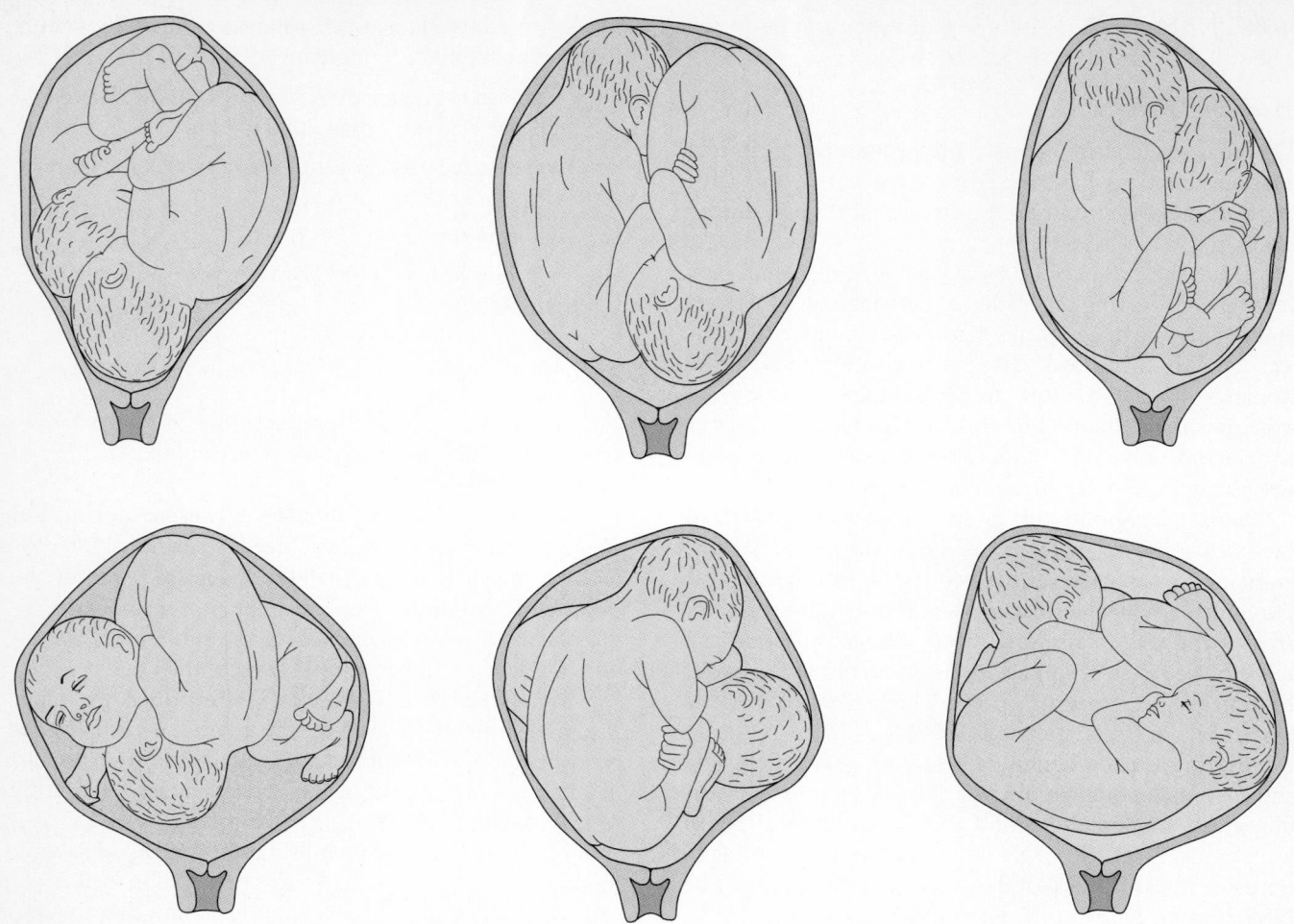

FIGURE 25-14   Twins may be in any of the above presentations while in utero.

frequently are. Cunningham et al (1993) advocate the use of pudendal block paired with the administration of nitrous oxide and oxygen at the time of vaginal birth. Others prefer epidural anesthesia, especially if external version of the second twin is contemplated (Jackson 1989).

The placentas are examined after the birth. If the twins are of the same sex, the placentas are sent to the pathology laboratory for examination to determine whether they are monozygotic or dizygotic twins.

Nursing Assessment

When obtaining a maternal history, it is important to identify a family history of twinning. Equally important is a history of medication taken to enhance fertility. These facts should be noted on the antepartal record.

At each antepartal clinic visit the nurse should measure the fundal height. Any growth, fetal movement, or heart tone auscultation out of proportion to gestational age by dates is indicative of twins. During palpation many small parts on all sides of the abdomen may be felt (Figure 25–15). If twins are suspected, the nurse should attempt to auscultate two separate heartbeats in different quadrants of the maternal abdomen. Use of the Doppler device may be helpful. Conclusive evidence of twins is found on sonography.

During the prenatal visits the nurse should determine the family's level of preparation for integrating more than one new member. Although the thought of having twins can be very exciting, the reality of the stress of attaching to two infants and the parental role may be a difficult adjustment (Niefert & Thorpe 1990).

During labor it is important to monitor both twins. An external electronic monitor can be applied to both twins, or if conditions permit, the internal monitor can be applied to twin A and the external monitor to twin B. The heart rates may be auscultated on different quadrants of the maternal abdomen, but continuous monitoring is

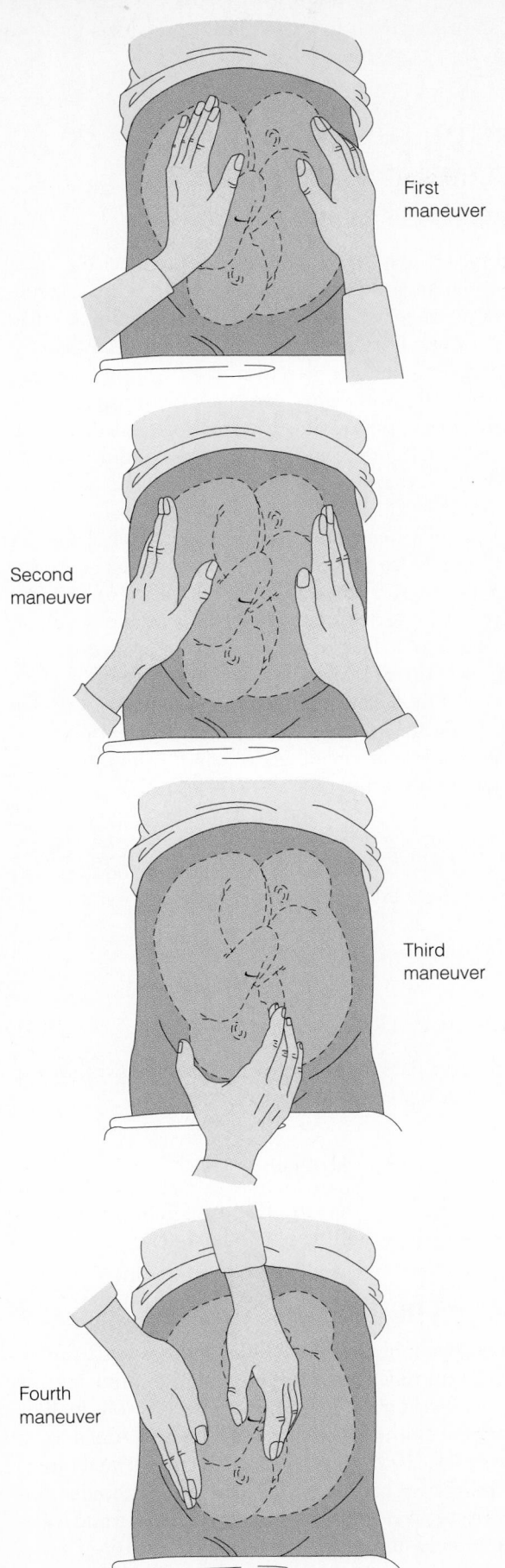

First maneuver

Second maneuver

Third maneuver

Fourth maneuver

more beneficial. Signs of distress should be reported to the obstetrician.

After a multiple birth the mother is closely monitored for postpartal hemorrhage.

Nursing Diagnosis

Nursing diagnoses that may apply to a woman with a twin pregnancy include the following:

- Fear related to unknown outcome of the birth process
- Ineffective individual coping related to uncertainty about the labor and birth plan
- Knowledge deficit related to implications and problems associated with twin pregnancy
- Risk for impaired gas exchange in the twins related to decreased oxygenation secondary to cord compression

Nursing Plan and Implementation

Teaching for Self-Care

Antepartally, the woman may need counseling about diet and daily activities. The nurse can help her plan meals to meet her increased needs. A daily intake of 4000 calories (minimum) and 135 g of protein is recommended for optimal weight gain and fetal growth. A prenatal vitamin and 1 mg of folic acid should also be taken daily. A weight gain of 40 to 60 lbs has been recommended with a 15 to 20 lb weight gain by 20 weeks (Hunter 1989).

Occasionally in multiple pregnancies women exhibit nausea and vomiting past the first trimester. A diet consisting of dry, nongreasy foods may be helpful. Antiemetics may be necessary to provide relief. The woman is more prone to have a feeling of fullness after eating, but this may be alleviated by eating small but frequent meals.

Maternal hypertension is treated with bed rest in the lateral position to increase uterine and kidney perfusion. The nurse can help the woman schedule frequent periods of rest during the day. Family members or friends may be willing to care for the woman's other children periodically to allow her time to get rest. Back discomfort can be alleviated by pelvic rocking, good posture, and good body mechanics.

Teaching regarding prevention and recognition of preterm labor is very important. For further discussion see Chapter 19.

FIGURE 25-15 Leopold's maneuvers in twin pregnancy. The fetus on the mother's right side is in cephalic presentation, and the fetus on the left is in breech presentation.

Preparation for Birth

The nurse needs to prepare to receive two neonates. This means a duplication of resuscitation equipment and newborn identification papers and bracelets. The newborns may be placed in individual radiant warmers or in the same one once they have an identification band applied. Two staff members should be available for newborn resuscitation.

If twins are discovered at the time of birth, the nurse must move quickly to prepare for the second newborn. The pediatric team may need to be notified at this time. While one nurse is monitoring the second twin in utero, the other nurse is caring for the first newborn and preparing to ensure correct identification of the neonates. Special precautions should be observed to ensure correct identification of the neonates. The first born is usually tagged Baby A and the second, Baby B.

Provision of Support to the Family

The nurse determines the woman's or family's need for referral to social welfare agencies, public health clinics, or other community agencies for follow-up care. The family may be unprepared financially and psychologically for the arrival of twins and thus at risk for further difficulties.

Evaluation

Anticipated outcomes of nursing care include:

- The woman is knowledgeable regarding the implications and problems associated with twin pregnancy.
- The woman feels she is able to cope with the pregnancy and birth.
- The woman understands the treatment plan and how to gain further information.
- The mother, father, and babies have a safe prenatal course, labor, and birth and a safe postpartal and newborn course.

Three or More Fetuses

When three or more fetuses are present, maternal and fetal problems are increased. The more fetuses conceived, the smaller they tend to be at the time of birth. Birth of three or more fetuses is best accomplished by cesarean because of the risk of fetal insult due to decreased placental perfusion and hemorrhage from the separating placenta during the intrapartal period (Cunningham et al 1993). Complicated obstetric maneuvers such as breech extraction and podalic version, the risk of prolapse of the cord, and an increase in fetal collision provide additional reasons for cesarean birth.

CARE OF THE WOMAN AND FETUS IN THE PRESENCE OF FETAL DISTRESS

When the oxygen supply is insufficient to meet the physiologic demands of the fetus, fetal distress may result. The condition may be acute, chronic, or a combination of both. A variety of factors may contribute to fetal distress. The most common are related to cord compression and uteroplacental insufficiency associated with placental abnormalities and preexisting maternal or fetal disease. If the resultant hypoxia persists and metabolic acidosis follows, the situation is potentially life threatening to the fetus.

The most common initial signs of fetal stress are meconium-stained amniotic fluid (in a vertex presentation) and changes in the FHR. The presence of ominous FHR patterns, such as late or severe variable decelerations, decrease or lack of variability, and progressive acceleration in the FHR baseline, are indicative of hypoxia. Fetal scalp blood samples demonstrating a pH value of 7.20 or less provide a more sophisticated indication of fetal problems and are generally obtained when questions about fetal status arise. (See also Chapter 22.)

Critical Thinking Question

Draw an FHR pattern that depicts late decelerations with minimal variability.

Maternal Risks

Indications of fetal stress greatly increase the psychologic stress a laboring woman must face.

Fetal-Neonatal Risks

Prolonged fetal hypoxia may lead to mental retardation or cerebral palsy and ultimately to fetal demise.

Medical Therapy

When there is evidence of possible fetal stress, treatment is centered on relieving the hypoxia and minimizing the effects of anoxia on the fetus. Initial interventions include changing the mother's position and administering oxygen by mask at 6 to 10 L per minute. If electronic fetal monitoring has not yet been used, it is usually instituted at this time. If oxytocin is in use, it should be discontinued. Fetal scalp blood samples are taken (Figure 25–16).

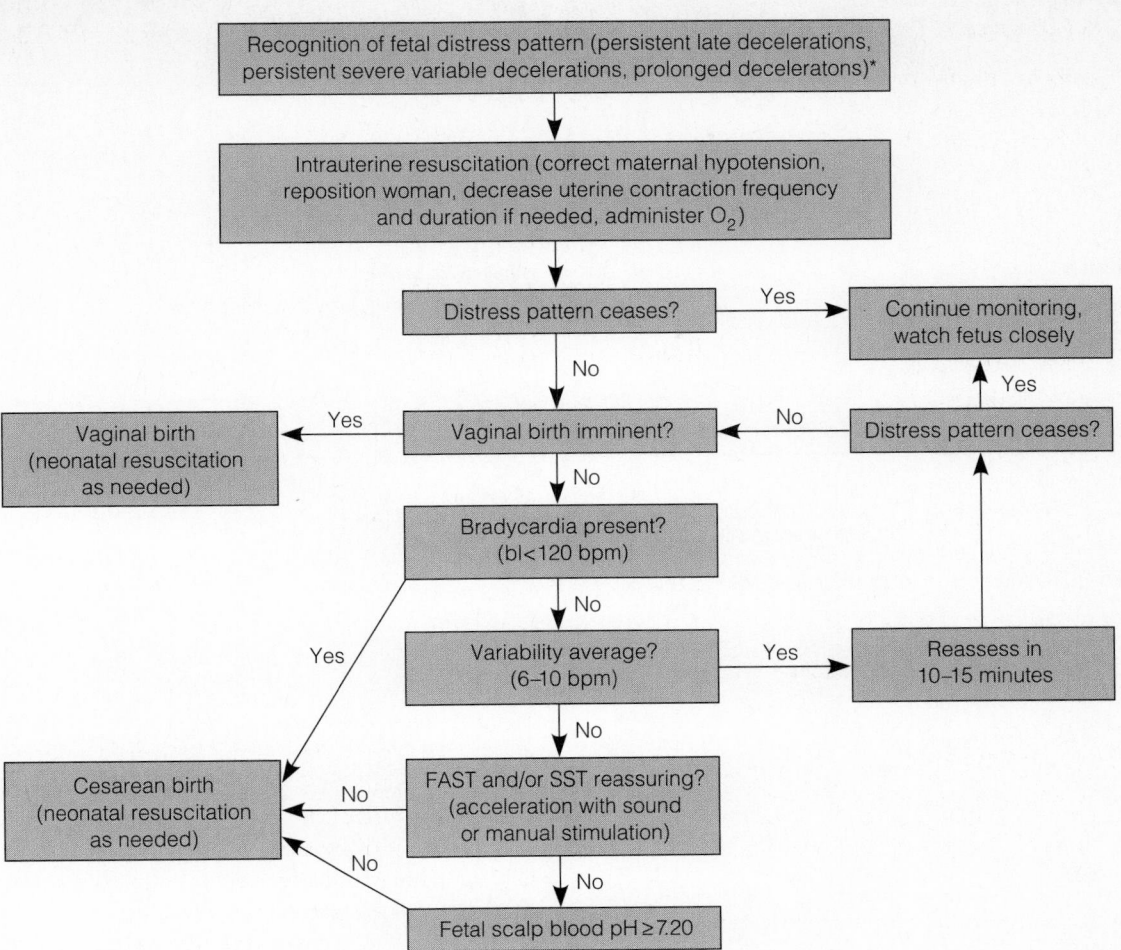

FIGURE 25-16 Intrapartum fetal distress management. Note: Bl = baseline; FAST = fetal acoustic stimulation test; SST = scalp stimulation test. SOURCES: Based on information from Strong TH: Fetal distress in the intrapartum period. In: *Current Therapy in Obstetrics and Gynecology,* 3rd ed. Quilligan EJ, Zuspan FP (editors). Philadelphia: WB Saunders, 1990; *Huddleston JF, Freeman RK: Estimation of fetal well-being. In: *Neonatal–Perinatal Medicine: Diseases of the Fetus and Newborn,* 5th ed. Fanroff AA, Martin RS (editors). St Louis: Mosby-Year Book, 1992.

Nursing Assessment

The nurse reviews the woman's prenatal history to anticipate the possibility of fetal distress. When the membranes rupture, it is important to assess FHR and to observe for meconium staining. As labor progresses, the nurse is particularly alert for even subtle changes in the FHR pattern and the fetal scalp pH, if available. Reports by the mother of increased or greatly decreased fetal activity may also be associated with fetal distress. For further discussion of FHR patterns and characteristics, see Evaluation of Fetal Status During Labor in Chapter 22.

Nursing Diagnosis

Nursing diagnoses that may apply are presented in the Nursing Care Plan: Fetal Stress on page 730.

Nursing Plan and Implementation

The professional staff may become so involved in assessing fetal status and initiating corrective measures that they fail to give explanations and emotional support to the woman, her partner, and other family members. It is imperative to provide both full explanations of the problem and comfort to the couple. In many instances, if birth is not imminent, the woman must undergo cesarean birth. This operation may cause fear and frustration for

FETAL STRESS

Nursing Assessment

Nursing History

1. Predisposing factors, including
   a. Preexisting maternal diseases
   b. Maternal hypotension, bleeding
   c. Placental abnormalities

Diagnostic Studies

1. Maternal hemoglobin and hematocrit
2. Urinalysis

NURSING DIAGNOSIS: Decreased cardiac output in fetus related to decreased uteroplacental perfusion secondary to maternal hypotension, decreased circulating blood volume, vasoconstriction associated with PIH

EXPECTED OUTCOME: Adequate placental and fetal perfusion is maintained.

Nursing Interventions	Rationale
Assess for early signs of fetal hypoxia:	Hypoxia is the reduction of oxygen to tissues. Fetal asphyxia implies profound hypoxia with resulting anaerobic glycolysis. This causes lactic acid buildup, resulting in metabolic acidosis. Gilstrap et al (1989) identified the following signs of asphyxia: 1. pH <7.00 and base deficit >20 2. Apgar score 0–3 at 5 minutes 3. Multiorgan system dysfunction 4. Neonatal neurologic sequelae, such as coma, seizures, or hypotonia
1. Decreased variability of fetal heart rate	Variability of FHR depends on intact sympathetic and parasympathetic nervous systems. When variability decreases, it indicates the fetus is no longer able to react or compensate for changes in the uterine environment.
2. Late decelerations in FHR	Vagal stimulation elicited through hypoxic brain tissues causes bradycardia.
3. Fetal hyperactivity	Fetus may initially become hyperactive in an attempt to increase circulation.
4. Presence of meconium in the amniotic fluid	Fetal hypoxia leads to increased intestinal peristalsis and anal sphincter relaxation, resulting in meconium release. Thick meconium may be an indicator of decreased amniotic fluid, which may be the result of a placental insufficiency.
If any of the above are found, initiate the following interventions:	
1. Administer oxygen to the woman with tight face mask at 7–10 L/minute, per physician order.	Administration of oxygen may increase amount of oxygen available for transport to the fetus. Tight face mask is used because the laboring woman tends to breathe through her mouth.
2. Change maternal position (lateral, left side preferred).	Changed maternal position may relieve compression of the maternal vena cava and the cord, thereby facilitating oxygen exchange.
3. Increase IV fluid (as per agency protocol).	Increases maternal circulating volume and cardiac output.
4. Discontinue oxytocin if infusing.	Decreases uterine activity.
5. Institute emergency measures for prolapse of cord: • Manually exert pressure on the presenting part. This must be done continuously. Woman may be maintained in supine position, Trendelenburg position, knee-chest position, or on her side with a pillow to elevate her hips. • If occult prolapse is suspected, change maternal position to side-lying. • Notify physician/certified nurse-midwife immediately.	Relieving the compression on the cord may alleviate fetal hypoxia. Prolonged compression can lead to CNS damage and even death.

OUTCOME MET IF:

- FHR 120–160 bpm
- Short-term variability present, average long-term variability
- Accelerations with fetal movement or on stimulation
- No late decelerations or prolonged variable decelerations

FETAL STRESS continued

NURSING DIAGNOSIS Anxiety related to knowledge of fetal stress

EXPECTED OUTCOME: Woman demonstrates decrease in anxiety.

Nursing Interventions	Rationale
Inform woman of fetal status.	*Anxiety is decreased when factual information is provided.*
Explain treatment plan. Provide accurate information.	

OUTCOME MET IF:

- Woman verbalizes understanding of current problem and interventions.

- Woman has no further questions.
- Woman appears less anxious.

Essential Nursing Activities to Achieve Outcomes

Nursing Assessment	Potential Fetal Stress If:	Nursing Interventions
1. Determine FHR baseline.	Tachycardia >160 bpm; bradycardia <110 bpm	1. Position changes: lateral; knee-chest.
2. Assess variability.	Decreased long-term variability; short-term variability absent	2. Increase infusion rate of IV fluids.
3. Monitor decelerations.		3. Oxygen at 6–10 L/minute with a tight face mask (as per agency protocol).
4. Monitor accelerations.	Persistent late decelerations; prolonged variable decelerations	4. Assess maternal vital signs.
5. Evaluate contraction pattern.	Absence of accelerations with fetal movement or scalp stimulation	5. Discontinue intravenous Pitocin.
6. Monitor uterine resting tone.	Contractions closer than every 2 minutes lasting >90 seconds	6. Notify physician of maternal and fetal assessment findings.
7. Take maternal vital signs.	Inadequate resting tone between contractions	7. Document assessments and specific information relayed to physician.
8. Evaluate amniotic fluid.	Temperature 100.4 F or >; hypotension	8. Reassure woman and family.
9. Assess the emotional status of the patient and family.	Meconium stained	9. Keep woman and family well informed through factual information.

the couple, especially if they were committed to a shared, prepared birth experience.

The nurse stays alert for clues of fetal stress, initiates corrective measures, and answers any questions the couple has. Additional information regarding nursing interventions are presented in the Nursing Care Plan: Fetal Stress. Also refer to Chapter 22 for discussion of fetal heart rate patterns.

Evaluation

Anticipated outcomes of nursing care include:

- The woman and her family feel supported and able to cope with their situation.

- The fetal heart rate remains in normal range, or supportive measures maintain the FHR as normal as possible.

CARE OF THE FAMILY AT RISK DUE TO INTRAUTERINE FETAL DEATH

Fetal death, often referred to as fetal demise, accounts for one-half of the perinatal mortality after 20 weeks' gestation. Intrauterine fetal death (IUFD) results from unknown causes or a number of physiologic maladaptations, including PIH, abruptio placentae, placenta previa, diabetes, infection, congenital anomalies, and isoimmune disease.

Maternal Risks

Prolonged retention of the fetus may lead to the development of disseminated intravascular coagulation (DIC) (also referred to a consumption coagulopathy). After the release of thromboplastin from the degenerating fetal tissues into the maternal bloodstream, the extrinsic clotting system is activated, triggering the formation of multiple tiny blood clots. Fibrinogen and factors V and VII are subsequently depleted, and the woman begins to display symptoms of DIC. Fibrinogen levels begin a linear descent 3 to 4 weeks after the death of the fetus and continue to decrease without appropriate medical intervention. An in-depth discussion of DIC is found later in this chapter.

Medical Therapy

Abdominal x-ray examination may reveal Spalding's sign (an overriding of the fetal cranial bones). In addition maternal estriol levels fall. Diagnosis of IUFD is confirmed by absence of heart action on real-time ultrasonography.

Most women have spontaneous labor within 2 weeks of fetal death. If other complications are not present, some physicians wait for labor to begin spontaneously (Cunningham et al 1993).

> APPLYING THE NURSING PROCESS

Nursing Assessment

Cessation of fetal movement reported by the mother to the nurse is frequently the first indication of fetal death. It is followed by a gradual decrease in the signs and symptoms of pregnancy. Fetal heart tones are absent, and fetal movement is no longer palpable. Once fetal demise is established by the physician, ongoing support and communication will become even more important. Open communication among the mother, her partner, and the health care team members contributes to a more realistic understanding of the medical condition and its associated treatments. The nurse may discuss prior experiences the family has had with stress and what they feel were their coping abilities at that time. Determining what social supports and resources the family has is also important.

Birth and death together. It's confusing and frightening enough for adults, but how are young children to understand it? For them the baby never really existed, or lived only briefly. What does this mean for them? Why are the parents so distraught? Too often, children's feelings about these issues are ignored or misunderstood. When parents are struggling to deal with their own feelings, they find it even harder to respond to the emotional needs of their other children.
~ WHEN PREGNANCY FAILS ~

Nursing Diagnosis

Nursing diagnoses that may apply to the woman experiencing intrauterine fetal death include the following:

- Grieving related to an actual loss

- Altered family processes related to loss of a family member
- Ineffective individual coping related to depression in response to loss of child
- Ineffective family coping related to death of a child

A friend asked if we had named our stillborn baby. After telling her the name, we both began referring to the baby by her name, Sarah. It felt good to call her a name.
~ WHEN PREGNANCY FAILS ~

Nursing Plan and Implementation

Provision of Emotional Support to the Family

The parents of a stillborn infant suffer a devastating experience, precipitating an intense emotional trauma. During the pregnancy the couple has already begun the attachment process, which now must be terminated through the grieving process. The behaviors that couples exhibit while mourning may be associated with the five stages of grieving described by Elizabeth Kübler-Ross (1969). Often the first stage is *denial* of the death of the fetus. Even when the initial health care provider suspects fetal demise, the couple is hoping that a second opinion will be different. Some couples may not be convinced of the death until they view and hold the stillborn infant. The second stage is *anger*, resulting from the feelings of loss, loneliness, and perhaps guilt. The anger may be projected at significant others and health care team members, or it may be omitted when the death of the fetus is sudden and unexpected. *Bargaining*, the third stage, may or may not be present, depending on the couple's preparation for the death of the fetus. If the death is unanticipated, the couple may have no time for bargaining. In the fourth stage *depression* is evidenced by preoccupation, weeping, and withdrawal. Physiologic postpartal depression appearing 24 to 48 hours after the stillbirth may compound the depression associated with grief. The final stage is *acceptance*, which involves the process of resolution. This is a highly individualized process that may take months to complete.

In some facilities a checklist is used to make sure important aspects of working with the parents are addressed. The checklist becomes a communication tool between staff members to share information particular to this couple (Brown 1992). Such a checklist might include the following items:

- When the fetal death is known before admission, inform the admission department and nursing staff so that inappropriate remarks are not made.
- Allow the woman and her partner to remain together as much as they wish. Provide privacy by assigning them to a private room.

- Stay with the couple, and do not leave them alone and isolated.

- As much as possible have the same nurse provide care to increase the support for the couple. Develop a care plan to provide for continuity of care. Encourage family members to visit support persons.

- Have the most experienced labor and birth nurse auscultate for fetal heart tones. This avoids the searching that a more inexperienced nurse might feel compelled to do. Avoid the temptation to listen again "to make sure."

- Listen to the couple; do not offer explanations. They require solace without minimizing the situation.

- Facilitate the woman and her partner's participation in the labor and birth process. When possible, allow them to make decisions about who will be present and what ritual will occur during the birth process. Allow the woman to make the decision regarding whether to have sedation during labor and birth. Provide a quiet supportive environment; ideally, the labor and birth should occur in a labor room or possibly a birthing room rather than the delivery room.

- Give parents accurate information regarding plans for labor and birth.

- Provide ongoing opportunities for the couple to ask questions.

- Arrange for the woman to be assigned to a room that is away from new mothers and babies if she requests it. It is important to let the woman decide if she wants to be on another unit. If early discharge is an option, allow the family to make that selection.

- Encourage the couple to experience the grief that they feel. Accept the weeping and depression. A couple may have intense feelings that they are unable to share with each other. Encourage them to talk together, and allow emotions to show freely. Help them understand that they may each experience different feelings (Cordell & Thomas 1989).

- Give the couple and family an opportunity to see and hold the stillborn infant in a private quiet location. (Advocates of seeing the stillborn believe that viewing assists in dispelling denial and enables the couple to progress to the next step in the grieving process.) If they choose to see their stillborn infant, prepare the couple for what they will see by saying "the baby is cold," "the baby is blue," "the baby is bruised," or other appropriate statements (Furrh & Copley 1989).

- Some families may elect to bathe or dress their stillborn; support them in their choice.

- Take a photograph of the infant, and let the family know it is available if they want it now or some time in the future.

- Offer a card with footprints, crib card, ID band, and possibly a lock of hair to the parents. These items may be kept with the photo if the parents do not want them at this time (Beckey et al 1985).

- Prepare the couple for returning home. If there are siblings, each will usually progress through age-appropriate grieving. Provide the parents with information about normal mourning reactions, both psychologic and physiologic.

- Furnish the mother with educational materials that discuss the changes she will experience in returning to the nonpregnant state.

- Provide information about community support groups, including group name, contact person if possible, and phone number. Use materials such as the book *When Hello Means Goodbye* by Schwiebert and Kirk (1985).

- Remember it is not so important to "say the right words." The caring support and human contact that a couple receives is important and can be conveyed through silence and your presence.

- Contact religious support systems if parents desire.

- Discuss further care of the stillborn baby (dress, rituals).

The nurse experiences many of the same grief reactions as the parents of a stillborn infant. It is important to have support persons and colleagues available for counseling and support.

Evaluation

Anticipated outcomes of nursing care include:

- The family members express their feelings about the death of their baby.

- The family participates in decisions regarding whether to see their baby and in other decisions regarding the baby.

- The family knows the community resources available and has names and phone numbers to use if they choose.

- The family is moving into and through the grieving process.

I knew something was wrong just by the way everyone was scurrying around in the delivery room and by that terrible silence. Then we knew the baby was dead. The doctor's only comment was, "It must be congenital," as if to say it certainly must be my fault, not his. Then a nurse said: "It would be worse if you had a five-year-old that died." I suppose she was right, but it certainly didn't make me feel any better. Later, the doctor said, "You're young, you'll have lots more kids." I was appalled—I was thirty-three already. Where do they learn all these stupid comments?
~ WHEN PREGNANCY FAILS ~

Care of the Woman and Fetus at Risk Due to Placental Problems

Maintenance of placental function is paramount to ensure fetal well-being and continuance of the pregnancy. Because the placenta is so vascular, problems that develop are usually associated with maternal and possible fetal hemorrhage. Causes and sources of hemorrhage are reviewed in Table 25–2.

Abruptio Placentae

Abruptio placentae is the premature separation of a normally implanted placenta from the uterine wall. Premature separation is considered a catastrophic event because of the severity of the hemorrhage that occurs. The incidence of abruptio placentae is 1 in 75 to 90 births (Lowe & Cunningham 1990) and is more frequent in pregnancies complicated by cocaine abuse (Dombrowski et al 1991). The risk of recurrence is much higher than for the general population. Karegaard and Gennser (1986) report a recurrence risk of tenfold—a 1 in 25 incidence in subsequent pregnancies.

The cause of abruptio placentae is largely unknown. Theories have been proposed relating its occurrence to decreased blood flow to the placenta through the sinuses during the last trimester. Excessive intrauterine pressure caused by hydramnios or multiple pregnancy, maternal hypertension, cigarette smoking, alcohol ingestion, increased maternal age and parity, trauma, and sudden changes in intrauterine pressure (as with amniotomy) have been suggested as contributing factors.

Pathophysiology

Premature separation of the placenta may be divided into three types (Figure 25–17):

1. *Marginal.* The blood passes between the fetal membranes and the uterine wall and escapes vaginally. Separation begins at the periphery of the placenta; this marginal sinus rupture may or may not become more severe.

2. *Central.* The placenta separates centrally, and the blood is trapped between the placenta and the uterine wall. Entrapment of the blood results in concealed bleeding.

3. *Complete.* Massive vaginal bleeding is seen in the presence of almost total separation.

The signs and symptoms of these three types of placental abruption are given in Table 25–3. In severe cases of central abruptio placentae a blood clot forms behind the placenta. With no place to escape the blood invades the myometrial tissues between the muscle fibers. This occurrence accounts for the uterine irritability that is a

| TABLE 25-2 | Causes and Sources of Hemorrhage |

Causes and Sources	Signs and Symptoms
Antepartal period	
Abortion	Vaginal bleeding
	Intermittent uterine contractions
	Rupture of membranes
Placenta previa	Painless vaginal bleeding after seventh month
Abruptio placentae	
Partial	Vaginal bleeding: no increase in uterine pain
Severe	May or may not be vaginal bleeding
	Extreme tenderness of abdominal area
	Rigid, boardlike abdomen
	Increase in size of abdomen
Intrapartal period	
Placenta previa	Bright red vaginal bleeding
Abruptio placentae	Same signs and symptoms as listed above
Uterine atony in stage III	Bright red vaginal bleeding
	Ineffectual contractility
Postpartal Period	
Uterine atony	Boggy uterus
	Dark vaginal bleeding
	Presence of clots
Retained placental fragments	Boggy uterus
	Dark vaginal bleeding
	Presence of clots
Lacerations of cervix or vagina	Firm uterus
	Bright red blood

significant sign of premature separation of the placenta. If hemorrhage continues, eventually the uterus turns entirely blue in color. After birth of the neonate the uterus contracts only with difficulty. This syndrome is known as a *Couvelaire uterus* and frequently necessitates hysterectomy.

As a result of the damage to the uterine wall and the retroplacental clotting with covert abruption, large amounts of thromboplastin are released into the maternal blood supply, which in turn triggers the development of disseminated intravascular coagulation (DIC) and the resultant hypofibrinogenemia. Fibrinogen levels, which are ordinarily elevated in pregnancy, may drop to incoagulable amounts within a matter of minutes as a result of rapidly developing premature separation of the placenta. Additional information on DIC is found later in this chapter.

Maternal Risks

Maternal mortality is now uncommon, although maternal morbidity is common (Cunningham et al 1993). Problems following the birth depend in large part on the

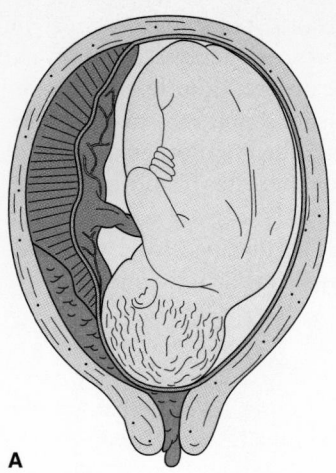 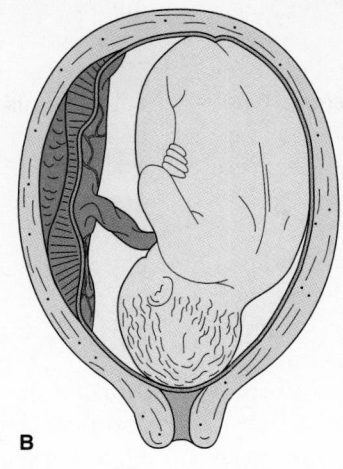 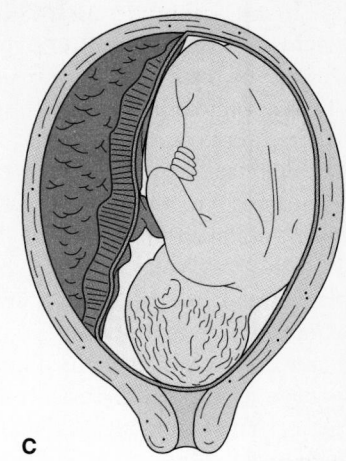

FIGURE 25-17 Abruptio placentae. *A* Marginal abruption with external hemorrhage. *B* Central abruption with concealed hemorrhage. *C* Complete separation.

severity of the intrapartal bleeding, coagulation defects (DIC), hypofibrinogenemia, and length of time between separation and the birth. Moderate to severe hemorrhage results in hemorrhagic shock, which ultimately may prove fatal to the mother if not reversed. In the postpartal period women who have suffered this disorder are at risk for hemorrhage and renal failure due to shock, vascular spasm, intravascular clotting, or a combination of the three. Another cause of renal failure is incompatible emergency blood transfusion. Failure is directly proportional to the number of units transfused.

Fetal-Neonatal Risks

Perinatal mortality associated with abruptio placentae ranges from 20% to 35% (Lowe & Cunningham 1990). In severe cases in which separation is almost complete, infant mortality is 100%. In less severe separation fetal outcome depends on the level of maturity. The most serious complications in the neonate arise from preterm labor, anemia, and hypoxia. If fetal hypoxia progresses unchecked, irreversible brain damage or fetal demise may result. With thorough assessment and prompt action on the part of the health care team, fetal and maternal outcome can be optimized.

Medical Therapy

Because of the risk of DIC, evaluating the results of coagulation tests is imperative. In DIC fibrinogen levels and platelet counts are usually decreased; prothrombin times and partial thromboplastin times are normal to prolonged. If the values are not markedly abnormal, serial testing may be helpful in establishing an abnormal trend that is indicative of coagulopathy. Another very sensitive test determines fibrin degradation products levels; these values rise with DIC.

After establishing the diagnosis, emphasis is placed on maintaining the cardiovascular status of the mother and developing a plan for effecting the birth of the fetus. Which birth method is selected depends on the condition of the woman and fetus; in many circumstances cesarean birth may be the safest option.

If the separation is mild and gestation is near term, labor may be induced, and the fetus may be born vaginally with as little trauma as possible. If the induction of labor by rupture of membranes and oxytocin infusion by pump do not initiate labor within 8 hours, a cesarean birth is usually done. A longer delay would increase the risk of increased hemorrhage, with resulting hypofibrinogenemia. Supportive treatment to decrease risk of DIC includes typing and cross-matching for blood transfusions (at least three units), clotting mechanism evaluation, and intravenous fluids.

TABLE 25-3	Differential Diagnosis	
	Placenta Previa	**Abruptio Placentae**
Onset	Quiet and sneaky	Sudden and stormy
Bleeding	External	External or concealed
Color of blood	Bright red	Dark venous
Anemia	= Blood loss	> Apparent blood loss
Shock	= Blood loss	> Apparent blood loss
Toxemia	Absent	May be present
Pain	Only labor	Severe and steady
Uterine tenderness	Absent	Present
Uterine tone	Soft and relaxed	Firm to stony hard
Uterine contour	Normal	May enlarge and change shape
Fetal heart tones	Usually present	Present or absent
Engagement	Absent	May be present
Presentation	May be abnormal	No relationship

SOURCE: Oxorn H: *Human Labor and Birth*, 5th ed. Norwalk, CT: Appleton & Lange, 1986, p 507.

In cases of moderate to severe placental separation, a cesarean birth is done after hypofibrinogenemia has been treated by intravenous infusion of cryoprecipitate or plasma. Vaginal birth is impossible in the event of a Couvelaire uterus because it could not contact properly in labor. Cesarean birth is necessary in the face of severe hemorrhage to allow an immediate hysterectomy to save both woman and fetus.

The hypovolemia that accompanies severe abruptio placentae is life threatening and must be combated with whole blood. If the fetus is alive but in distress, emergency cesarean birth is the method of choice. With a stillborn fetus vaginal birth is preferable unless shock from hemorrhage is uncontrollable. Intravenous fluids of a balanced salt solution such as lactated Ringer's are given through a 16- or 18-gauge cannula (Cunningham et al 1993). Central venous pressure (CVP) monitoring may be needed to evaluate intravenous fluid replacement. A normal CVP of 10 cm H_2O is the goal. The CVP is evaluated hourly, and results are communicated to the physician. Elevations of CVP may indicate fluid overload and pulmonary edema. The hematocrit is maintained at 30% through the administration of packed red cells and/or whole blood (Cunningham et al 1993).

Laboratory testing is ordered to provide ongoing data regarding hemoglobin, hematocrit, and coagulation status. A clot observation test may be done at the bedside to evaluate coagulation status. A glass tube containing 5 mL of maternal blood is inverted four to five times. If a clot fails to form in 6 minutes, a fibrinogen level of less than 150 mg/dL is suspected. If a clot is not formed in 30 minutes, the fibrinogen level may well be less than 100 mg/dL. A clot observation test may be completed by a physician or a nurse.

Measures are taken to stimulate labor to effect vaginal birth as indicated by the condition of the mother and fetus. The birth may be hastened by performing an amniotomy and by oxytocin stimulation. Previously, birth within 6 hours of the diagnosis of severe placental abruption was recommended to reduce maternal mortality and morbidity. Currently, changing medical practice directed to ensuring adequate fluid replacement, especially blood, appears to accomplish the same outcome (Cunningham et al 1993).

APPLYING THE NURSING PROCESS

Nursing Assessment

Electronic monitoring of the uterine contractions and resting tone between contractions provides information regarding the labor pattern and effectiveness of the oxytocin induction. Because uterine resting tone is fre-

quently increased with abruptio placentae, it must be evaluated frequently for further increase. Abdominal girth measurements may be ordered hourly and are obtained by placing a tape measure around the maternal abdomen at the level of the umbilicus. Another method of evaluating uterine size, which increases as more bleeding occurs at the site of abruption, is to place a mark at the top of the uterine fundus. The distance from the symphysis pubis to the mark may be evaluated hourly.

Nursing Diagnosis

Nursing diagnoses that may apply to the woman with abruptio placentae are presented in the Nursing Care Plan: Hemorrhage in Third Trimester and at Birth on page 738.

Nursing Plan and Implementation

The psychologic aspects of nursing care are very important. Maternal apprehension increases as the clinical picture changes. Factual reassurance and an explanation of the procedures and what is happening are essential for the emotional well-being of the expectant couple. The nurse can reinforce positive aspects of the woman's condition, such as normal FHR, normal vital signs, and decreased evidence of bleeding.

Other nursing care measures are addressed in the Nursing Care Plan: Hemorrhage in Third Trimester and at Birth on page 738.

Evaluation

Anticipated outcomes of nursing care include:

- The woman and her baby have a safe labor and birth without further complications for the mother or child.
- The woman and family verbalize understanding of reasons for medical therapy and risks.

Disseminated Intravascular Coagulation

Disseminated intravascular coagulation (DIC) is an abnormal overstimulation of the coagulation process, secondary to an underlying disease. The coagulation process remains essentially the same, but certain medical conditions hasten and intensify the response to the point that hemorrhage may be life threatening as coagulation factors are overconsumed (Figure 25–18).

Sepsis in the childbearing woman may activate the intrinsic coagulation pathway because of damage to the endothelial cells. The extrinsic pathway is activated by

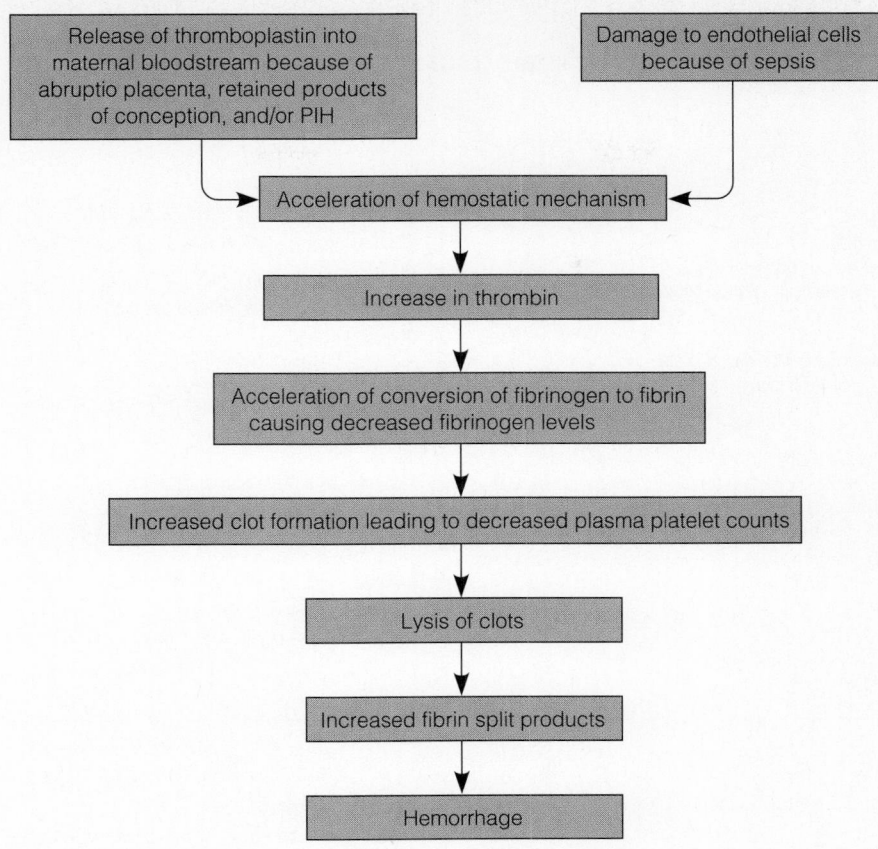

Activation of Extrinsic Coagulation Pathway

> Release of thromboplastin into maternal bloodstream because of abruptio placenta, retained products of conception, and/or PIH

Activation of Intrinsic Coagulation Pathway

> Damage to endothelial cells because of sepsis

> Acceleration of hemostatic mechanism

> Increase in thrombin

> Acceleration of conversion of fibrinogen to fibrin causing decreased fibrinogen levels

> Increased clot formation leading to decreased plasma platelet counts

> Lysis of clots

> Increased fibrin split products

> Hemorrhage

FIGURE 25-18 DIC coagulation process.

the release of thromboplastin from damaged tissues in such conditions as abruptio placentae, PIH, chorioamnionitis, and retained products of conception. The normally high levels of tissue thromboplastin in the placenta and decidua of the uterus may contribute to the occurrence of DIC. Amniotic fluid released into the bloodstream from amniotic fluid emboli and intra-amniotic saline infusions activates both pathways. With the initiation of the coagulation process massive numbers of clots form rapidly. Fibrinogen becomes depleted as it is converted to fibrin. Platelets are entrapped in the clots, leading to a decrease in the number of platelets. The coagulation process also activates plasminogen conversion to plasmin, which can lyse fibrinogen (dissolve clots). As the fibrin clots are destroyed, fibrin split products having an anticoagulant effect are released. Because of the elevated fibrin split products level, the decrease in the number of platelets, and the reduced fibrinogen level, the outcome is generalized bleeding. Ischemia of the organs follows from the vascular occlusion of the numerous fibrin thrombi. The multisite hemorrhages result in shock and can result in death.

The clinical manifestations of DIC begin subtly and become more overt with severity of the disease. The signs and symptoms are indicators of the degree of bleeding, which ranges from generalized hemorrhage to minor generalized bleeding to localized bleeding in the form of purpura and petechiae.

Medical Therapy

The goals of therapy are early diagnosis and supportive treatment of the woman with DIC. Confirmation of DIC is made with several blood tests. The prothrombin time (PT) test evaluates the extrinsic pathway in clotting. The PT is prolonged in DIC. The intrinsic pathway is evaluated by testing the partial thromboplastin time, which is also prolonged in DIC. Both platelets and fibrinogen levels decrease. Platelet counts below 50,000/µL result in spontaneous bleeding. Fibrinogen levels may be within normal ranges but will be lower than the initial level. The number of fibrin split products is elevated. The frequency of testing depends on the severity of the disease (Kelton & Cruikshank 1988).

Text continues on page 741

HEMORRHAGE IN THIRD TRIMESTER AND AT BIRTH

Nursing Assessment

Nursing History

1. Factors predisposing to hemorrhage:
   a. Presence of preeclampsia-eclampsia (PIH)
   b. Overdistension of the uterus; multiple pregnancy; hydramnios
   c. Grandmultiparity
   d. Advanced age
   e. Uterine contractile problems: hypotonicity; hypertonicity
   f. Painless vaginal bleeding after seventh month
   g. Presence of hypertension
   h. Presence of diabetes
   i. History of previous hemorrhage or bleeding problems, blood coagulation defects, abortion
   j. Retention of placental fragments
   k. Cervical and/or vaginal lacerations
2. Determine religious preference to establish whether client will permit a blood transfusion.

Physical Examination

1. Severe abdominal pain (central abruptio placentae)
2. External or concealed bleeding

3. Painless vaginal hemorrhage (placenta previa)
4. Shock symptoms (decreased blood pressure, increased pulse, pallor)
5. Uterine tetany or uterine atony
6. Portwine amniotic fluid with abruptio placentae
7. Degree of hemorrhage
8. Changes in FHR
9. Increased resting tone of uterus between contractions

Diagnostic Studies

1. Maternal hemoglobin and hematocrit
2. Type and cross-match
3. Fibrinogen levels
4. Platelets
5. Prothrombin time
6. Activated partial thromboplastin time
7. Fibrin split products

NURSING DIAGNOSIS: Fluid volume deficit related to hypovolemia secondary to excessive blood loss

EXPECTED OUTCOME: Woman maintains vital signs within normal limits and urine output >30 mL/hour.

Nursing Interventions	Rationale
Observe, record, and report blood loss.	Monitoring the amount of blood loss aids in determining appropriate interventions.
Evaluate using the following parameters:	
1. Monitor rate and quality of respirations frequently.	Initially, respiratory rate increases as a result of sympathoadrenal stimulation, resulting in increased metabolic rate; pain and anxiety may cause hyperventilation.
2. Measure pulse rate.	Increased pulse rate is an effect of increased epinephrine.
3. Assess pulse quality by direct palpation.	Reflects circulatory status.
4. Determine pulse deficit by comparing apical-radial rates.	Thready pulse indicates vasoconstriction and reflects decreased cardiac output; peripheral pulses may be absent if vasoconstriction is intense.
5. Compare present BP with woman's baseline BP; note pulse pressure.	Hypotension indicates loss of large amount of circulatory fluid or lack of compensation in circulatory system. As cardiac output decreases, there is usually a fall in pulse pressure. Peripheral vasoconstriction may make accurate readings difficult.
6. Monitor urine output (decrease to less than 30 mL/hour is sign of shock): a. Insert Foley catheter. b. Measure output hourly. c. Measure specific gravity to determine concentration of urine.	Vasoconstrictor effect of norepinephrine decreases blood flow to kidneys, which decreases GFR and the output of urine. Inability to concentrate urine may indicate renal damage from vasoconstriction and decreased blood perfusion.
7. Inspect skin for presence of pallor and cyanosis, coldness, and clamminess.	Skin reflects amount of vasoconstriction. Pallor is determined by intensity of vasoconstriction. Cyanosis occurs when the amount of unoxygenated hemoglobin in the blood is ≥ 5 g/dL blood. Coldness is caused by slow blood flow, and clamminess by sympathetic stimulation of sweat glands.
8. Evaluate state of consciousness frequently.	Diminished cerebral blood flow causes restlessness and anxiety. As shock progresses, state of consciousness decreases.
9. Measure CVP: normal CVP is 5–10 cm H_2O.	Provides estimation of volume of blood returning to heart to propel blood. Low CVP indicates a decrease in the circulating volume of blood (hypovolemia).
10. Assess amount of blood loss: a. Count pads. b. Weigh pads and Chux (1 g = approximately 1 mL blood). c. Record amount in a specific amount of time (eg, 50 mL bright red blood on pad in 20 minutes).	In pregnant and laboring clients blood is replaced according to estimates of actual blood loss, rather than using parameters of increased and decreased BP.

HEMORRHAGE IN THIRD TRIMESTER AND AT BIRTH *continued*

Nursing Interventions	Rationale
If hypovolemia is present:	
1. Relieve decreased blood pressure by administering whole blood per physician order.	*Hypotension results from decreased blood volume.*
2. While waiting for whole blood to be available, infuse isotonic fluids, plasma, plasma expanders, or serum albumin, per physician order.	*Degree of hypovolemia may be assessed by CVP, hemoglobin, and hematocrit.*
If marginal abruptio placentae is present:	
1. Evaluate blood loss.	*Provides information on type of abruption and maternal and fetal status. Bleeding often stops as shock develops but resumes as circulation is restored.*
2. Assess uterine contractile pattern, tenderness, and height.	*Provides information regarding uterine irritability.*
3. Start continuous monitoring of uterine contractions by EFM.	*Provides continuous data.*
4. Monitor maternal vital signs.	
5. Assess fetal status per continuous EFM.	*Assists in evaluating fetal status.*
6. Assess cervical dilatation and effacement to determine labor progress if uterine contractions are present.	
7. Rule out placenta previa.	*Ultrasound exam can confirm location of placenta.*
8. Assist with amniotomy, and begin oxytocin infusion per physician order if labor does not start immediately or is ineffective.	*Labor may be stimulated with oxytocin induction. If unsuccessful or condition worsens, cesarean birth will be done.*
9. Review and evaluate diagnostic lab tests (hemoglobin, hematocrit, PT, APPT, fibrin split products, fibrinogen, platelets).	*Provides information regarding hemodynamic status.*
If central abruptio placentae with severe blood loss is present:	*As above.*
1. Perform same assessments as for marginal abruptio placentae.	
2. Monitor CVP.	
3. Replace blood loss.	
4. Effect immediate birth.	
5. Observe for signs and symptoms of disseminated intravascular coagulation (DIC).	

OUTCOME MET IF:

- BP remains between 110/70 and 138/88.
- Pulse rate is within 60–90 bpm.
- Urine output is >30 cc/hour.
- Skin is warm and not clammy.
- Urine specific gravity is 1.010–1.025.

NURSING DIAGNOSIS: Risk for altered tissue perfusion related to blood loss secondary to uterine atony following birth

EXPECTED OUTCOME: Woman's uterus remains well contracted.

Nursing Interventions	Rationale
Assess contractility of uterus and amount of vaginal bleeding.	*Muscle fibers that have been overstretched or overused do not contract well; contraction of muscle fibers over open placental site is essential; slight relaxation of uterine muscle fibers leads to continuous oozing of blood.*
Postpartally, assess uterus every 15 minutes × 4, every 30 minutes × 2, every 60 minutes × 2–4. Evaluate more frequently if uterus is boggy or not in the midline. Administer oxytocin per protocol or physician order.	

OUTCOME MET IF:

- Fundus is firm, in the midline, at level of umbilicus or below.

HEMORRHAGE IN THIRD TRIMESTER AND AT BIRTH *continued*

NURSING DIAGNOSIS: Anxiety related to concern for own personal status and the baby's safety

EXPECTED OUTCOME: Woman verbalizes a decrease in anxiety.

Nursing Interventions	Rationale
Keep woman informed of present status. Provide accurate information. Provide opportunities for questions. Establish a trusting relationship. Encourage the woman to participate in decision making if at all possible.	*As hemorrhage occurs, the safety of the mother and baby are threatened. Anxiety and fear may be lessened somewhat when the woman is informed, understands what is happening, and has some part in the decision-making process.*

OUTCOME MET IF:

- Questions of woman/family are answered regarding fetal and maternal status.
- Woman/family verbalizes ability to make informed decisions based on information given.

NURSING DIAGNOSIS: Risk for impaired fetal gas exchange related to decreased blood volume and hypotension

EXPECTED OUTCOME: FHR will remain within normal limits without signs of stress or distress.

Nursing Interventions	Rationale
Assess and monitor fetal heart rate for baseline variability, decelerations, and accelerations. Observe for meconium in amniotic fluid. Assist in obtaining fetal blood sample (pH <7.20 indicates severe jeopardy), or perform scalp stimulation assessing for accelerations of the FHR.	*Hemorrhage from woman disrupts blood flow pattern to fetus, possibly compromising fetal status.* *Hypoxia causes increased motility of fetal intestines and relaxation of abdominal muscles, with release of meconium into amniotic fluid.* *An acceleration of the FHR of 15 beats above baseline with acceleration duration of 15 seconds is an indication of a fetal pH >7.24.*

OUTCOME MET IF:

- FHR 120–160 bpm.
- Short-term variability present, long-term variability average.
- No late or prolonged decelerations.
- Fetal scalp pH is >7.24.
- Accelerations with fetal scalp stimulation or acoustic stimulations.

Essential Nursing Activities to Achieve Outcomes

1. Assess BP, P, R every 2 hours and more frequently during active bleeding.

2. Assess urine output hourly during active bleeding.

3. Insert indwelling bladder catheter during active bleeding.

4. Measure specific gravity.

5. Assess skin color and temperature.

6. Assess contractions for frequency, duration, intensity.

7. Assess for uterine tenderness.

8. Assess level of consciousness.

9. Assess amount of blood loss.

10. Insert IV. May need a CVP line for accurate fluid replacement measurements.

11. Provide needed fluid volume replacement.

12. Obtain ordered lab work.

13. Assess for DIC.

14. Document all findings.

15. Provide emotional support to woman/family.

16. Answer all questions regarding treatment and therapy.

17. Monitor fetus continuously.

18. Assess FHR for baseline, variability, decelerations, and accelerations.

19. Do not perform vaginal exam with active bleeding.

20. Prepare for a possible cesarean.

Cases of DIC can frequently be resolved by correcting the underlying cause. In the childbearing woman terminating the pregnancy removes the causative factor. Until birth can be accomplished, supportive therapy is critical to maintain maternal-fetal status.

Initial treatment includes evaluation of vital signs; assessment of vaginal bleeding, uterine contractility, and resting tone; continuous FHR monitoring; and fetal blood studies. Intravenous infusions of lactated Ringer's are given through a 16- or 18-gauge cannula. An indwelling bladder catheter is used to allow better evaluation of urinary output, which should be maintained at 30 mL/hour to assure adequate renal perfusion. Anemia (hematocrit less than 30%) is treated by giving packed red cells. Each unit generally increases the hematocrit by 3 points and the hemoglobin by 1 to 1.5 g. Fresh frozen plasma may also be used to replace fibrinogen, factors V and VII, and antithrombin III. If fibrinogen levels are very low, cryoprecipitate is used. Each unit of cryoprecipitate provides approximately 250 mg of fibrinogen and raises the fibrinogen level by approximately 5 mg/dL (Cunningham et al 1993).

The administration of heparin is a controversial issue. Heparin is used to decrease thrombin generation and activity. When the causative factor cannot be removed, as with infection or in self-limiting cases in childbearing women, heparin is not used routinely. In some instances the use of heparin may even increase the hemorrhage (Cunningham et al 1993).

Vaginal birth without an episiotomy is the preferred birthing method because it avoids the surgical incision of numerous tissues and further stress on the hemostatic system. Conduction anesthesia should be avoided because of the chance of bleeding from injection puncture sites and the formation of hematomas.

APPLYING THE NURSING PROCESS

Nursing Assessment

The nurse should carefully observe for signs and symptoms of DIC in women who are candidates for this complication. Bleeding from injection sites, epistaxis, bleeding gums, and the presence of purpura and petechiae on the skin may be signs of developing DIC.

Clinical evidence may also be apparent in the results of laboratory blood tests specific to DIC. As appropriate, the nurse continues to assess maternal-fetal status by checking vital signs, uterine activity, FHR, and urinary output.

The nurse documents and reports signs and symptoms of DIC to the physician as well as any changes in the FHR, maternal vital signs, and uterine activity.

Nursing Diagnosis

Nursing diagnoses that may apply to the woman with DIC include the following:

- Fear related to unknown outcome of the labor and birth
- Risk for impaired gas exchange related to impaired oxygen-carrying ability of blood secondary to hemorrhage
- Risk for infection related to decreased hemoglobin

Nursing Plan and Implementation

In the event of major blood loss, nursing measures are directed toward assessment of maternal-fetal status and corrective or supportive treatment measures. The nurse is also responsible for monitoring administration of blood products.

Protecting the woman from further bleeding involves interventions such as padding the side rails, avoiding IM injections, assessing IV insertion sites, and placing the blood pressure cuff carefully to prevent bruising.

Meeting the woman's psychologic needs is another nursing priority. Accurate, informative explanations should be offered frequently. The nurse who listens and projects warmth and understanding is most likely to help the woman cope with her anxiety and frustration.

Evaluation

Anticipated outcomes of nursing care include:

- The woman's circulatory status is restored to normal, and blood loss is replaced.
- The mother and baby have a safe labor and birth, and further complications are quickly identified and treated.
- The parents understand the complication that occurred and are able to participate in decision making as much as possible.

Placenta Previa

In **placenta previa** the placenta is improperly implanted in the lower uterine segment. This implantation may be on a portion of the lower segment or over the internal os (Figure 25–19). As the lower uterine segment contracts and dilates in the later weeks of pregnancy, the placental villi are torn from the uterine wall, thus exposing the uterine sinuses at the placental site. Bleeding begins, but because its amount depends on the number of sinuses exposed, it may initially be either scanty or profuse.

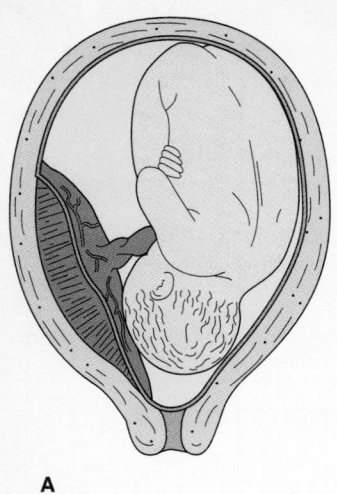 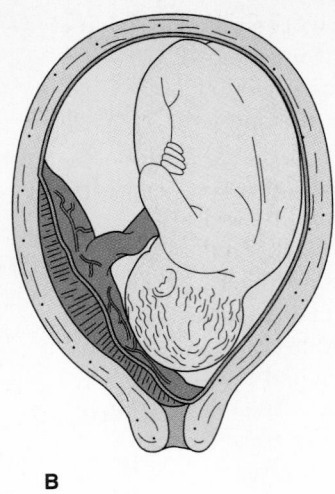 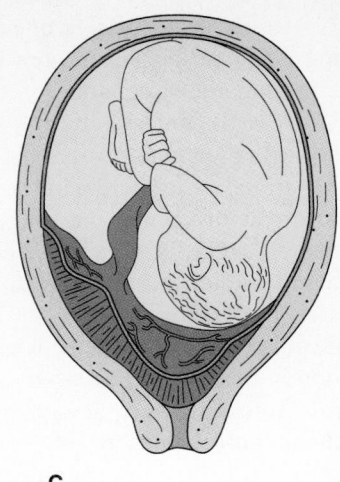

A   B   C

FIGURE 25-19   Placenta previa. *A* Low placental implantation. *B* Partial placenta previa. *C* Total placenta previa.

The cause of placenta previa is unknown. Statistically, it occurs in about 1 of every 250 births. Women with a previous history of placenta previa have a recurrence rate of 4% to 8% (Lavery 1990). Other factors associated with placenta previa are multiparity, increasing age, placenta accreta, defective development of blood vessels in the decidua, and a large placenta (Cunningham et al 1993).

Medical Therapy

The goal of medical care is to identify the cause of bleeding and to provide treatment that will ensure birth of a mature newborn. Indirect diagnosis is made by localizing the placenta through tests that require no vaginal examination. The most commonly employed diagnostic test is the transabdominal ultrasound scan (Figure 25–20). Transvaginal sonography is now being used to identify the presence of a placenta previa (Anderson 1992). If placenta previa is ruled out, a vaginal examination can be performed with a speculum to determine the cause of bleeding (such as cervical lesions).

Direct diagnosis of placenta previa can be made only by feeling the placenta inside the cervical os. However, such an examination may cause profuse bleeding due to tearing of tissue in the cotyledons of the placenta. Because of the danger of bleeding, a vaginal examination should be performed only if ultrasound is not available, the pregnancy is near term, and there is profuse vaginal bleeding. The examination may be done using a double setup procedure. In this situation it must be determined whether the cause of the bleeding is placenta previa or advanced labor with copious bloody show (which is normal). *Double setup* means that the delivery room is set up for the vaginal examination and normal vaginal birth and

for a cesarean birth should placenta previa be present and the examination precipitates brisk bleeding. Adequate personnel must be present to respond to treatment decisions.

The differential diagnosis of placental or cervical bleeding takes careful consideration. Partial separation of the placenta may also present with painless bleeding, and a true placenta previa may not demonstrate overt bleeding until labor begins, thus confusing the diagnosis. Another important fact to note is that the causes of slight to moderate antepartal bleeding episodes in 20% to 25% of women are never accurately diagnosed.

Care of the women with painless late gestational bleeding depends on (1) the week of gestation during

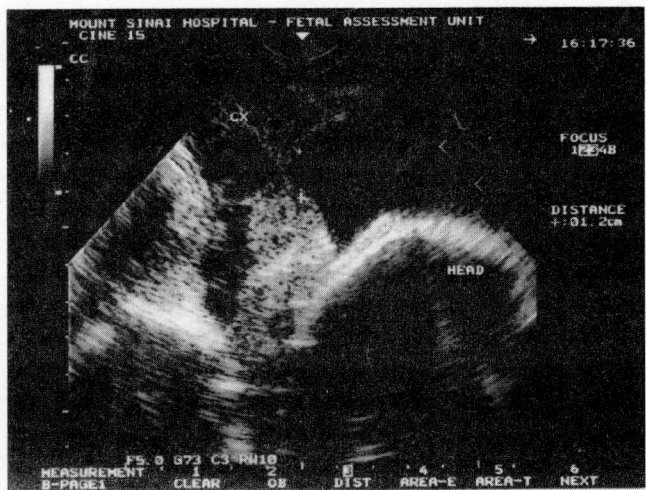

FIGURE 25-20   Ultrasound of placenta previa.

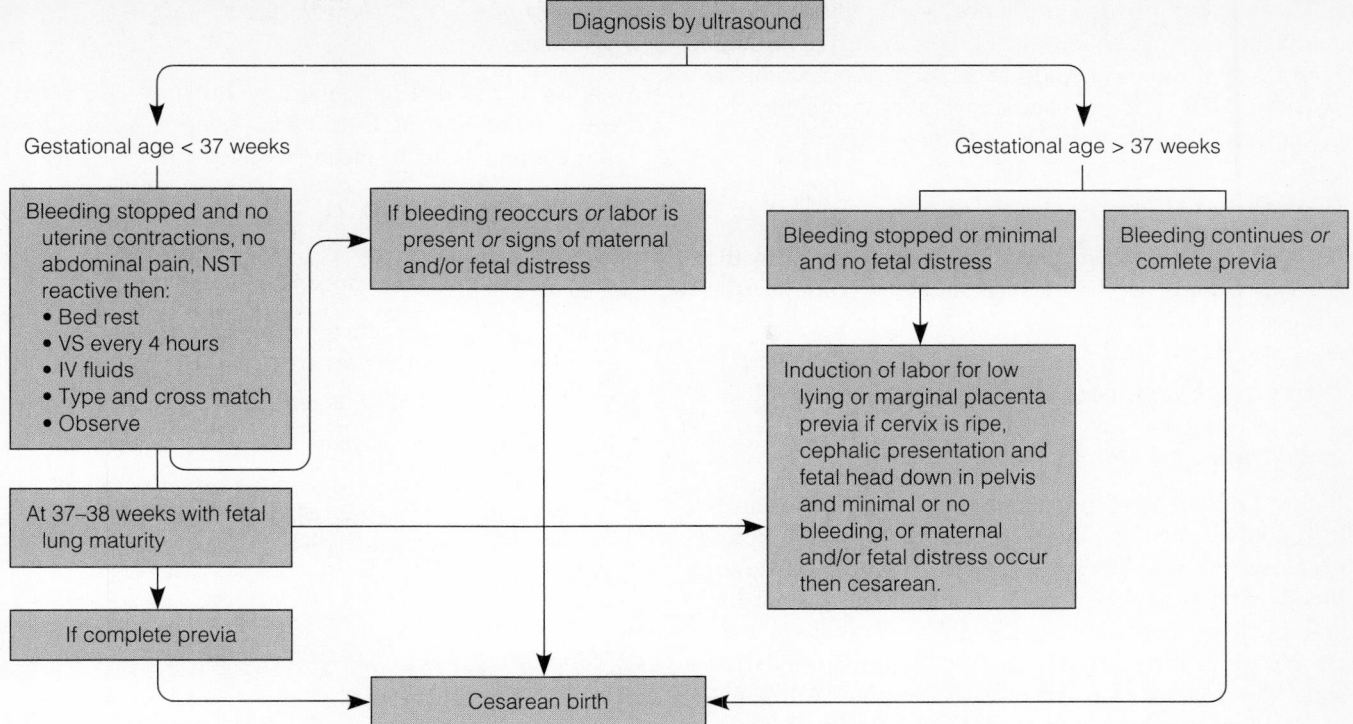

FIGURE 25-21 Management of placenta previa. SOURCE: Based on information from Barker RK, Fields DH, Kaufman SA: *Quick Reference to OB–GYN Procedures,* 3rd ed. New York: Lippincott/Harper & Row, 1990.

which the first bleeding episode occurs and (2) the amount of bleeding (Figure 25–21). If the pregnancy is less than 37 weeks' gestation, expectant management is employed to delay birth until about 37 weeks' gestation to allow the fetus to mature. Expectant management involves stringent regulations of the following:

1. Bed rest with bathroom privileges only as long as the woman is not bleeding

2. Absolutely no rectal or vaginal exams

3. Monitoring of blood loss, pain, and uterine contractility

4. Evaluating FHTs with external monitor

5. Monitoring vital signs

6. Complete laboratory evaluation: hemoglobin, hematocrit, Rh factor, and urinalysis

7. Intravenous fluid (lactated Ringer's) with drip rate monitored

8. Two units of cross-matched blood available for transfusion

If frequent, recurrent, or profuse bleeding persists or if fetal well-being appears threatened, a cesarean birth will need to be performed before 37 weeks.

Nursing Assessment

Assessment of the woman with placenta previa must be ongoing to prevent or treat complications that are potentially lethal to the mother and fetus. Painless, bright red vaginal bleeding is the best diagnostic sign of placenta previa. If this sign should develop during the last 3 months of a pregnancy, placenta previa should always be considered until ruled out by examination. The first bleeding episode is generally scanty. If no rectal or vaginal examinations are performed, it often subsides spontaneously. However, each subsequent hemorrhage is more profuse.

The uterus remains soft, and if labor begins, it relaxes fully between contractions. The FHR usually remains stable unless profuse hemorrhage and maternal shock occur. As a result of the placement of the placenta the fetal presenting part is often unengaged, and transverse lie is common.

Blood loss, pain, and uterine contractility are appraised by the nurse from both subjective and objective perspectives. Maternal vital signs and the results of blood and urine tests provide the nurse with additional data about the woman's condition. FHR is evaluated with an external fetal monitor. Another nursing responsibility is observing and verifying the family's ability to cope with the anxiety associated with an unknown outcome.

Nursing Diagnosis

Nursing diagnoses that may apply are presented in the Nursing Care Plan: Hemorrhage in Third Trimester and at Birth starting on page 738.

Nursing Plan and Implementation

Preparation for Double Setup Procedure

Before a double setup procedure is performed, the laboring couple should be physiologically and psychologically prepared for possible surgery (Chapter 26). A whole-blood setup should be readied for intravenous infusion and a patent intravenous line established before any intrusive procedures are undertaken. The maternal vital signs should be monitored every 15 minutes in the absence of hemorrhage and every 5 minutes with active hemorrhage. The external tocodynamometer should be connected to the maternal abdomen to monitor uterine activity continuously.

Promotion of Physical Well-Being

The nurse continues to monitor the woman and her fetus to determine the status of the bleeding and to determine the mother's and baby's responses. Vital signs, intake and output, and other pertinent assessments must be made frequently. The nurse evaluates the electronic monitor tracing to evaluate the fetal status.

Provision of Emotional Support to the Family During Expectant Management

Emotional support for the family is an important nursing care goal. When active bleeding is occurring, the assessments and management must be directed toward physical support. However, emotional aspects need to be addressed simultaneously. The nurse can explain the assessments being completed and the treatment measures that need to be done. Time can be provided for questions, and the nurse can act as an advocate in obtaining information for the family. Emotional support can also be offered by staying with the family and by the use of touch.

Promotion of Neonatal Physiologic Adaptation

The newborn's hemoglobin, cell volume, and erythrocyte count should be checked immediately and then monitored closely. The newborn may require oxygen and administration of blood and admission into a neonatal intensive care unit.

Provision of Care to the Woman with Bleeding

Additional information regarding nursing care is addressed in the Nursing Care Plan: Hemorrhage in Third Trimester and at Birth starting on page 738.

Evaluation

Anticipated outcomes of nursing care include:

- The cause of hemorrhage is recognized promptly, and corrective measures are taken.
- The woman's vital signs remain in the normal range.
- The woman and her baby have a safe labor and birth.
- The family understands what has happened and the implications and associated problems of placenta previa.

Other Placental Problems

Other problems of the placenta can be divided into those that are developmental and those that are degenerative. Developmental problems of the placenta include placental lesions, placenta succenturiata, circumvallate placenta, and battledore placenta (Figure 25–22). Degenerative changes include infarcts and placental calcification.

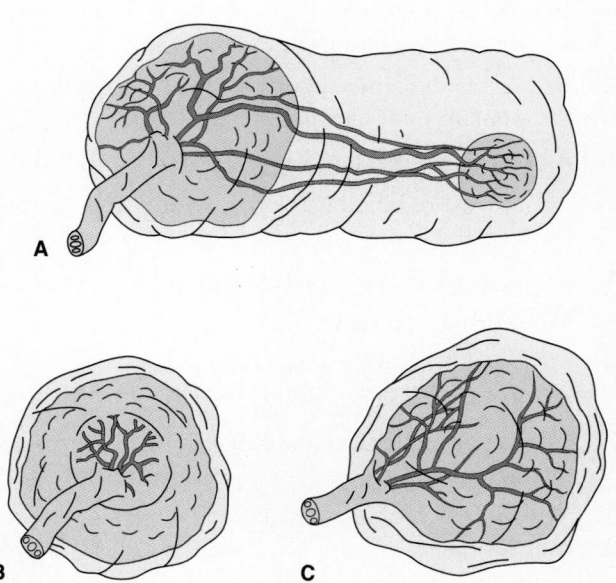

FIGURE 25-22   Placental variation. *A* Succenturiate placenta. *B* Circumvallate placenta. *C* Battledore placenta.

Succenturiate Placenta

In succenturiate placenta, one or more accessory lobes of fetal villi have developed on the placenta, with vascular connections of fetal origin (Figure 25–22A). Vessels from the major to the minor lobe(s) are supported only by the membranes, thus increasing the risk of the minor lobe being retained during the third stage of labor.

The gravest maternal danger is postpartal hemorrhage if this minor lobe is severed from the placenta and remains in the uterus. All placentas should be examined closely for intactness. If vessels appear to be severed at the margin of the placenta, the uterus should be explored for retained placental tissue. This condition is not usually diagnosed until after the birth of the placenta (Cunningham et al 1993). If the vascular connections rupture between the lobes, life-threatening fetal hemorrhage can result. At birth the infant should be inspected for pallor, cyanosis, retractions, tachypnea, tachycardia, and feeble pulse. The infant's cry will be weak and the muscle tone flaccid.

Circumvallate Placenta

In circumvallate placenta the fetal surface of the placenta is exposed through a ring opening around the umbilical cord (Figure 25–22B). The vessels descend from the cord and end at the margin of the ring instead of coursing through the entire surface area of the placenta. The ring is composed of a double fold of amnion and chorion with some degenerative decidua and fibrin between. The cause of this condition is unknown. Maternal-fetal problems include an increased incidence of late abortion or fetal death, antepartal hemorrhage, prematurity, and abnormal maternal bleeding during or following the third stage of labor, resulting from improper placental separation or shearing of membranes from the placenta.

Battledore Placenta

In the case of battledore placenta the umbilical cord is inserted at or near the placental margin (Figure 25–22C). As a result all fetal vessels transverse the placental surface in the same direction. The chances of preterm labor are high because of interference with fetal circulation and nutrition. Fetal distress or bleeding during labor is also likely because of cord compression or vessel rupture.

Placental Infarcts and Calcifications

In the aging process the placenta may develop infarcts and calcifications. They become significant if they cover a large enough area to interfere with the uterine-placental-fetal exchange. Altered exchange can also occur with certain maternal disease processes, such as hypertension. Infarcts are most often seen in cases of severe pregnancy-induced hypertension and in women who smoke.

CARE OF THE WOMAN AND FETUS AT RISK DUE TO PROBLEMS ASSOCIATED WITH THE UMBILICAL CORD

Prolapsed Umbilical Cord

When the umbilical cord precedes the fetal presenting part, it is known as a prolapsed cord. In this situation, pressure is placed on the umbilical cord as it is trapped between the presenting part and the maternal pelvis. Consequently, the vessels carrying blood to and from the fetus are compressed. The cord falls or is washed down through the cervix into the vagina and in rare circumstances may be visible at the lower edge of the vagina. In other cases the umbilical cord lies beside or just ahead of the fetal head; this is called *occult cord prolapse*.

Any time that the pelvic inlet is not completely filled by the fetus or when the presenting part is not firmly against the cervix, and the membranes rupture, the umbilical cord can be washed down into the birth canal in front of the presenting part (Figure 25–23). Prolapse of the cord is most likely to occur with a malpresentation (especially footling breech and shoulder presentations), low birth weight, a multipara with more than five previous births, multiple gestation, obstetric manipulation

> **Critical Thinking Question**
>
> Why do you think low birth weight, multiple gestation, presence of a long umbilical cord, and a multipara with more than five previous births create situations in which cord prolapse is more likely to occur?

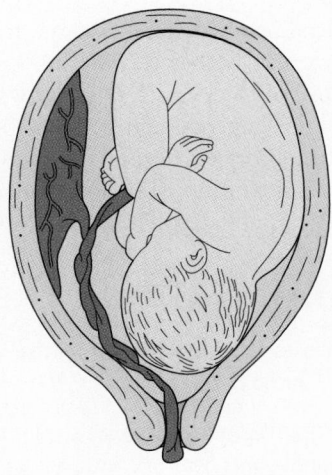

FIGURE 25-23   Prolapse of the umbilical cord.

(amniotomy), and the presence of a long cord (longer than 80 cm) (Cruikshank 1994). Approximately 50% of cord prolapses occur in the second stage (Cruikshank 1994). The incidence of cord prolapse is 0.2% to 0.6% of births (Cruikshank 1994).

Maternal-Fetal-Neonatal Risks

Although a prolapsed cord does not directly precipitate physical alterations in the woman, her immediate concern for the baby creates enormous stress. The woman may need to deal with some unusual interventions, a cesarean birth, and in some circumstances death of the baby.

The fetus is affected because compression of the umbilical cord occludes blood flow through the umbilical vessels. Bradycardia (FHR baseline below 120 beats per minute) and persistent variable decelerations may develop. If labor is occurring, the cord is compressed further with each contraction. If the pressure on the cord is not relieved, the fetus will die.

Medical Therapy

Preventing the occurrence of cord prolapse is the preferred medical approach. For all laboring women with a history of ruptured membranes, bed rest is usually indicated until engagement with no cord prolapse has been documented. If the prolapse does occur, it is most usually discovered by the nurse, and relieving the compression of the cord is critical for the fetus. The method of birth will most likely be cesarean.

APPLYING THE NURSING PROCESS

Nursing Assessment

In the intrapartal area the nurse reviews the nursing history and ascertains whether the woman is likely to be at risk for prolapse of the cord. Particularly when the presenting part is not engaged and spontaneous or artificial rupture of the membranes occurs, the nurse observes the perineum and assesses the FHR for bradycardia and severe, recurrent, variable decelerations.

Nursing Diagnosis

Nursing diagnoses that may apply to the woman with a prolapsed cord include the following:

- Risk for impaired gas exchange in the fetus related to decreased blood flow secondary to compression of the umbilical cord
- Fear related to unknown outcome

Nursing Plan and Implementation

Because there are few outward signs of cord prolapse, each pregnant woman is advised to call her physician or certified nurse-midwife when the membranes rupture and to go to the office, clinic, or birthing facility. A sterile vaginal examination determines if there is danger of cord prolapse. If the presenting part is well engaged, the risk is minimal, and ambulation may be encouraged. If it is not well engaged, bed rest is recommended to prevent cord prolapse. Maintenance of bed rest after rupture of membranes can lead to conflict if the laboring woman and her partner do not hold the same opinions. The nurse can ease this situation by helping communication between the physician/CNM and the couple.

If membranes have not yet ruptured when the woman arrives at the facility, at the time of spontaneous rupture or amniotomy (artificial rupture of the membranes) the FHR should be monitored by electronic fetal monitoring or auscultated for at least a full minute and again at the end of a contraction and after a few contractions. In the presence of cord prolapse EFM tracings show baseline bradycardia and/or severe, moderate, or prolonged variable decelerations. If these patterns are found, the nurse completes a sterile vaginal examination.

If a loop of cord is discovered, the nurse's gloved fingers are left in the vagina, and the presenting part is gently pushed upward to lift the fetal part off the cord and relieve cord compression until the physician/CNM arrives. This is a life-saving measure. Oxygen is administered, and FHR is monitored by EFM to see if the cord compression is adequately relieved (baseline will rise above 120 beats per minute and variable decelerations are lessened or relieved). The nurse may also feel pulsation in the cord; however, in some instances a pulsation cannot be felt, and FHR can be detected only by EFM.

In some cases another nurse may insert an indwelling bladder catheter and, using a sterile asepto syringe or infusion device, fill the bladder with approximately 350–500 mL of warmed, sterile, normal saline. The filled bladder lifts the fetal head upward and relieves pressure on the umbilical cord (Griese & Prickett 1993). Filling her bladder and maintaining the woman in a side-lying position may be all that is needed to relieve the pressure on the cord. If the bladder is not filled, the force of gravity can be incorporated. In this instance the nurse maintains pressure on the presenting part while doing a vaginal examination and instructs the woman to move into a knee-chest position or adjusts the bed to the Trendelenburg position. The nurse maintains pressure on the presenting part, and the woman is transported to the birthing or operating room in this position.

Evaluation

Anticipated outcomes of nursing care include:

- The FHR remains in normal range with supportive measures.

- The fetus is born safely.
- The woman and her partner feel supported.
- The woman and her partner understand the problem and the corrective measures that are undertaken.

Umbilical Cord Abnormalities

Umbilical cord abnormalities include congenital absence of an umbilical artery, insertion variations, cord length variations, and knots and loops of the cord. Insertion variations include velamentous insertion and vasa previa, and cord length problems include long and short cords.

Congenital Absence of Umbilical Artery

Absence of an umbilical artery may have serious fetal implications. The incidence of all types of fetal anomalies is 25% in infants born with two-vessel cords.

Immediately after the umbilical cord is cut it should be inspected to determine whether the correct number of vessels is present. If an artery is absent, the nurse should examine the newborn more closely for anomalies and gestational age problems.

Insertion Variations

In a *velamentous insertion* condition the vessels of the umbilical cord divide some distance from the placenta in the placental membranes (Figure 25–24). Velamentous insertions occur more frequently in multiple gestations than in singletons. Other placental anomalies, such as succenturiate placenta, often accompany this condition. The velamentous insertion is more easily compressed or kinked during pregnancy or labor because of the lack of Wharton's jelly to protect it. If the vessels become torn during labor, fetal hemorrhage can occur, and the blood can escape from the vagina. When fetal hemorrhage occurs, it results in FHR abnormalities.

When the vessels of a velamentous insertion transverse the internal os and appear in front of the fetus, a *vasa previa* has occurred. Fetal hemorrhage with asphyxia is likely to result because as the fetal blood escapes out of the vagina the hemorrhage will probably be diagnosed as maternal.

Cord Length Variations

The average length of the umbilical cord is 55 cm. Although short cords rarely cause complications directly, they have been associated with umbilical hernias in the fetus, abruptio placentae, and cord rupture. Long cords tend to twist and tangle around the fetus, causing transient variable decelerations. A long cord rarely causes fe-

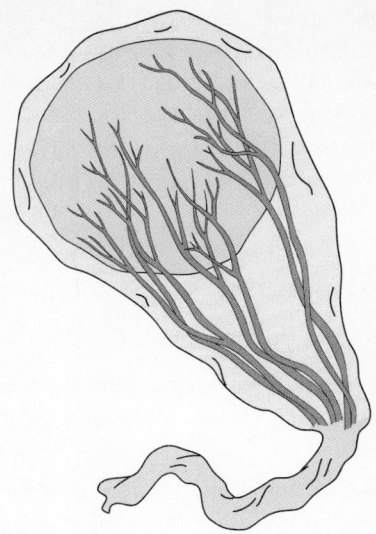

FIGURE 25-24 Placenta with a velamentous umbilical cord insertion.

tal death, however, because it is generally not pulled tight until descent at the time of birth. With a long cord and an active fetus one or more true knots can result. Again, these knots usually are not pulled tight enough to cause fetal stress until the infant has been born, and the cord can then be clamped and cut.

Medical Therapy

Preventing serious fetal complications and examining the newborn for anomalies that coexist with umbilical cord abnormalities are the goals of medical treatment.

In the presence of any vaginal bleeding during labor continuous monitoring of the fetus is imperative. Monitoring is best done with the aid of the external electronic monitor. Any signs of fetal stress should be reported immediately. In the presence of bleeding, laboratory tests may be used to differentiate fetal from maternal red blood cells. Fetal hemorrhage is resolved by termination of the pregnancy vaginally or through cesarean birth and by correction of neonatal anemia. Expediting the birth, whether vaginally or surgically, is paramount when severe fetal stress is apparent. Following the birth the pediatric team identifies and/or treats any neonatal complications or anomalies.

APPLYING THE NURSING PROCESS

Nursing Assessment

The presence of umbilical abnormalities may not become evident until the birth of the fetus. During labor the nurse should observe for signs of fetal distress and excessive bleeding (with velamentous and vasa previa).

Nursing Diagnosis

Nursing diagnoses that may apply include the following:

- Risk for impaired gas exchange in the fetus related to decreased blood flow secondary to placental abnormalities

- Knowledge deficit related to lack of information about implications and associated problems of placental abnormalities

Nursing Plan and Implementation

The nurse is alert for an unusual amount of bleeding during the labor and birth. Following the birth, the placenta is inspected for abnormalities.

Often any mild or moderate variable deceleration can be successfully managed by the nurse. Repositioning of the woman often alleviates pressure on the cord if this is the reason for the deceleration.

Evaluation

Anticipated outcomes of nursing care include:

- The mother and baby have a safe labor and birth.

- The woman's bleeding is assessed quickly, and corrective measures are taken.

- The family is able to cope successfully with fetal-neonatal anomalies if they exist.

CARE OF THE WOMAN AND FETUS AT RISK DUE TO AMNIOTIC FLUID–RELATED COMPLICATIONS

Amniotic Fluid Embolism

Amniotic fluid embolism can occur naturally after a tumultuous labor or from oxytocin induction with hypertonic uterine contractions. In the presence of a small tear in the amnion or chorion high in the uterus the fluid may leak into the chorionic plate and enter the maternal circulation through the gaping venous system. The fluid can also enter at areas of placental separation or cervical tears. Under pressure from the contracting uterus the fluid is driven into the maternal system. Amniotic fluid embolus occurs more often in multiparas. The incidence is 1 in 15,000 to 20,000 pregnancies, with a mortality rate of 80% (Chatelain & Quirk 1990; Clark 1994).

Maternal Risks

This condition frequently occurs during or after the birth when the woman has had a difficult, rapid labor. Suddenly, she experiences respiratory distress, circulatory collapse, acute hemorrhage, and cor pulmonale as the embolism blocks the vessels of the lungs. The more debris (such as meconium) in the amniotic fluid, the greater the maternal problems. The acute hemorrhage is a result of DIC, which is caused by the thromboplastinlike material found in amniotic fluid, in which factor VII is not essential. It has been demonstrated in vitro and in vivo that mucus, which is also found in amniotic fluid, induces coagulation by activation of factor X.

Maternal mortality is extremely high. In suspected cases in which the women survive it is difficult to determine whether an amniotic fluid embolism has actually occurred.

Fetal-Neonatal Risks

Birth must be facilitated immediately to ensure a live fetus. In many cases the birth has already occurred or the birth can be assisted vaginally with forceps. If labor has been tumultuous, the fetus may suffer problems associated with dysfunctional labor.

Medical Therapy

The goals of medical therapy are to maintain oxygenation, support the cardiovascular system and blood pressure, and assess coagulopathy (Clark 1990).

Any woman exhibiting chest pain, dyspnea, cyanosis, frothy sputum, tachycardia, hypotension, and massive hemorrhage needs the cooperation of every member of the health team if her life is to be saved. Medical and nursing interventions are supportive. Recovery is contingent upon the return of the mother's cardiovascular and respiratory stability. If necessary, the birth is assisted to enhance the health of the newborn.

APPLYING THE NURSING PROCESS

Nursing Assessment

The nurse must be especially observant for manifestations of amniotic fluid embolism when the labor has been short and difficult. Signs and symptoms of respiratory and circulatory collapse are sudden, acute, and severe and require immediate medical intervention.

Nursing Diagnosis

Nursing diagnoses that may apply in cases of amniotic fluid embolism include the following:

- Risk for impaired gas exchange related to anxiety, restlessness, and dyspnea secondary to amniotic fluid embolism
- Fear related to unknown outcome of the complication

Nursing Plan and Implementation

Maintenance of Oxygenation

In the absence of the physician, the nurse administers oxygen under positive pressure until medical help arrives. An intravenous line is quickly established. If respiratory and cardiac arrest occurs, cardiopulmonary resuscitation (CPR) is initiated immediately.

Provision of Cardiovascular Support

The nurse readies the equipment necessary for blood transfusion and for the insertion of the central venous pressure (CVP) line. As the blood volume is replaced, using fresh blood to provide clotting factors, the CVP is monitored frequently. In the presence of cor pulmonale fluid overload could easily occur.

When DIC is controlled with fibrinogen replacement, the nurse is responsible for obtaining fibrinogen and other medications needed. Intravenous heparin may be life saving.

Promotion of Fetal-Neonatal Well-Being

As one nurse helps the physician maintain maternal homeostasis, another nurse intervenes as necessary to maintain the well-being of the fetus in utero and the newborn after birth.

Evaluation

Anticipated outcomes of nursing care include:

- The woman's signs and symptoms are recognized and corrective measures taken quickly.
- Fetal distress is recognized and corrective measures taken early.
- The mother and her baby are stabilized, and no further complications develop.

Hydramnios

Hydramnios (also called polyhydramnios) occurs when there is over 2000 mL of amniotic fluid. The exact cause of hydramnios is unknown; however, it often occurs in cases of major congenital anomalies. It is postulated that a major source of amniotic fluid is found in special amnion cells that lie over the placenta (Cunningham et al 1993). During the second half of the pregnancy the fetus begins to swallow and inspire amniotic fluid and to urinate, which contributes to the amount present. In cases of hydramnios, no pathology has been found in the amniotic epithelium. However, hydramnios is associated with fetal malformations that affect the fetal swallowing mechanism and neurologic disorders in which the fetal meninges are exposed in the amniotic cavity.

This condition is also found in cases of anencephaly in which the fetus is thought to urinate excessively due to overstimulation of the cerebrospinal centers. When a monozygotic twin manifests hydramnios, it is possible that the twin with the increased blood volume urinates excessively. The weight of the placenta has been found to be increased in some cases of hydramnios, indicating that increased functioning of the placental tissue may be contributory.

There are two types of hydramnios: chronic and acute. In the chronic type the fluid volume gradually increases and is a problem of the third trimester. Most cases are of this variety. In acute cases the volume increases rapidly over a period of a few days. The acute type is usually diagnosed between 20 and 24 weeks' gestation (Queenan 1992).

Maternal Risks

When the amount of amniotic fluid is over 3000 mL, the woman experiences shortness of breath and edema in the lower extremities from compression of the vena cava. If hydramnios is severe enough, she can experience intense pain. The acute form of hydramnios tends to be more severe. Milder forms of hydramnios occur more frequently and are associated with minimal symptoms. Hydramnios is associated with such maternal disorders as diabetes and Rh sensitization.

Antepartally, if the amniotic fluid is removed too rapidly, abruptio placentae can result from a decreased attachment area. Because of these overstretched fibers, uterine dysfunction can occur intrapartally, and there is increased incidence of postpartal hemorrhage.

Fetal-Neonatal Risks

Fetal malformations and preterm birth are common with hydramnios; thus there is a fairly high rate of perinatal mortality. Prolapsed umbilical cord can occur when the membranes rupture, which adds a further complication for the fetus. The incidence of malpresentations is also increased.

Medical Therapy

Hydramnios is managed with supportive treatment unless the intensity of the woman's distress and symptoms dictate otherwise.

If the accumulation of amniotic fluid is severe enough to cause maternal dyspnea and pain, hospitalization and removal of the excessive fluid are required. This can be done vaginally or by amniocentesis. The dangers of performing the technique vaginally are prolapsed cord and the inability to remove the fluid slowly. If amniocentesis is performed, it should be done with the aid of sonography to prevent inadvertent damage to the fetus and placenta. The fluid should be removed slowly to prevent abruption (Cunningham et al 1993).

When performing amniocentesis, it is vital to maintain sterile technique. The nurse can offer support to the couple by explaining the procedure to them. The nurse assesses the clinician in interpreting sonographic findings. Prostaglandin synthesis inhibitor (indomethacin) is often utilized to treat hydramnios. Indomethacin has been shown to decrease amniotic fluid volume by decreasing fetal urine output (Moise 1991).

APPLYING THE NURSING PROCESS

Nursing Assessment

Hydramnios should be suspected when the fundal height increases out of proportion to the gestational age.

Critical Thinking Question

At 24 weeks' gestation what fundal height might indicate hydramnios? How will the pressure of hydramnios affect FHR assessment? How will it affect scoring of a biophysical profile?

As the amount of fluid increases, the nurse may have difficulty palpating the fetus and auscultating the FHR. In more severe cases the maternal abdomen appears extremely tense and tight on inspection. On sonography large spaces can be identified between the fetus and the uterine wall. An anencephalic infant or a dilated fetal stomach resulting from esophageal stress may also be identified, and multiple gestations may be confirmed. An x-ray fetogram will also show a radiolucent area of space and any fetal skeletal defects.

Nursing Diagnosis

Nursing diagnoses that may apply include the following:

- Risk for impaired gas exchange related to pressure on the diaphragm secondary to hydramnios

- Fear related to unknown outcome of the pregnancy

Nursing Plan and Implementation

When amniocentesis is performed, it is vital to maintain sterile technique to prevent infection. The nurse can offer support to the couple by explaining the procedure to them.

If the fetus has been diagnosed with a congenital defect in utero or is born with the defect, psychologic support is needed to assist the family. Often the nurse collaborates with social services to offer the family this additional help.

Evaluation

Anticipated outcomes of nursing care include:

- The woman and her partner understand the procedure, implications, risks, and characteristics that need to be reported to the care giver.

Oligohydramnios

Oligohydramnios is defined as a less-than-normal amount (approximately 500 mL is considered normal) of amniotic fluid. Although no exact amount of fluid has been identified, oligohydramnios is diagnosed when, on ultrasound examination, the largest vertical pocket of amniotic fluid is 5 cm or less (Marks & Divon 1992). The exact cause of this condition is unknown. It is found in cases of postmaturity, with IUGR secondary to placental insufficiency, and in fetal conditions associated with major renal malformations, including renal aplasia with dysplastic kidneys and obstructive lesions of the lower urinary tract (Queenan 1992). If oligohydramnios occurs in the first part of pregnancy, there is a danger of fetal adhesions (one part of the fetus may adhere to another part).

Maternal Risks

Labor may be dysfunctional; some women report that labor is more painful.

Fetal-Neonatal Risks

During the gestational period fetal skin and skeletal abnormalities may occur because fetal movement is impaired as a result of reduced amniotic fluid volume. Because there is less fluid available for the fetus to use during fetal breathing movements, pulmonary hypoplasia may develop. During the labor and birth the lessened amounts of fluid reduce the cushioning effect for the umbilical cord, and cord compression is more likely to occur.

Describe the FHR pattern associated with cord compression. What emergency nursing interventions are required?

Medical Therapy

During the antepartum period oligohydramnios may be suspected when the uterus does not increase in size according to the dates, the fetus is easily palpated and outlined by the examiner, and the fetus is not ballotable. The fetus can be assessed by biophysical profiles, nonstress tests, and serial ultrasound. During labor the fetus will be monitored by continuous electronic fetal monitoring to detect cord compression, which will be indicated by baseline bradycardia and/or moderate or severe variable decelerations. Some clinicians advocate the use of an amnioinfusion (a transcervical instillation of 200 to 300 mL or warmed sterile saline after membranes have ruptured) to decrease the frequency and severity of variable decelerations in the FHR during labor (Barber et al 1990). The infusion of saline provides more fluid for the umbilical cord to float in and thereby lessens or prevents cord compression.

Nursing Care

Continuous electronic fetal monitoring will be an important part of the assessment during the labor and birth. The nurse will evaluate the EFM tracing for presence of bradycardia and variable decelerations or other nonreassuring signs (such as increasing or decreasing baseline, decreased variability, or presence of late decelerations). If variable decelerations are noted, the woman's position can be changed (to relieve pressure on the umbilical cord), and the physician/CNM needs to be notified. If position changes are insufficient to relieve the pattern, an amnioinfusion may be done. After the birth the newborn is evaluated for signs of congenital anomalies, pulmonary hypoplasia, and/or postmaturity.

CARE OF THE WOMAN WITH CEPHALOPELVIC DISPROPORTION

The birth passage includes the maternal bony pelvis, beginning at the pelvic inlet and ending at the pelvic outlet, and the maternal soft tissues within these anatomic areas. A contracture in any of the described areas can result in cephalopelvic disproportion (CPD). Abnormal fetal presentations and positions occur in CPD as the fetus moves to accommodate to passage through the maternal pelvis.

The gynecoid and anthropoid pelvic types are usually adequate for vertex birth, but the android and platypelloid types predispose to CPD. Certain combinations of types also can result in pelvic diameters inadequate for vertex birth. (See Chapter 14 for a description of the types of pelves and their implications for childbirth.)

TABLE 25-4	Clues to Contractures of Maternal Pelvis

Diagonal conjugate <11.5 cm (contracture of inlet), outlet <8 cm (contracture of outlet)

Unengaged fetal head in early labor in primigravidas (consider contracture of inlet, malpresentation, or malposition)

Hypotonic uterine contraction pattern (consider contracted pelvis)

Deflexion of fetal head (fetal head not flexed on fetal chest; may be associated with occiput posterior)

Uncontrollable pushing prior to complete dilatation of cervix (may be associated with occiput posterior)

Failure of fetal descent (consider contracture of inlet, midpelvis, or outlet)

Edema of anterior portion (lip) of cervix (consider obstructed labor at the inlet)

Clues that may lead to suspicion of contractures of the maternal pelvis are presented in Table 25-4.

Types of Contractures

Contractures of the Inlet

The pelvic inlet is contracted if the shortest anterior-posterior diameter is less than 10 cm or the greatest transverse diameter is less than 12 cm. The anterior-posterior diameter may be approximately by measuring the diagonal conjugate, which in the contracted inlet is less than 11.5 cm. Clinical and x-ray pelvimetry are used to determine the smallest anterior-posterior diameter through which the fetal head must pass.

The treatment goal is to allow the natural forces of labor to push the biparietal diameter of the fetal head beyond the potential interspinous obstruction. Although forceps may be used, they cause difficulty because pulling on the head destroys flexion, and the space is further diminished. A bulging perineum and crowning indicate that the obstruction has been passed.

Contractures of the Outlet

An interischial tuberous diameter of less than 8 cm constitutes an outlet contracture. Outlet and midpelvic contractures frequently occur simultaneously. Whether vaginal birth can occur depends on the woman's interischial tuberous diameters and the fetal posterosagittal diameter.

Implications of Pelvic Contractures

Maternal Risks

Labor is prolonged and protracted in the presence of CPD, and premature rupture of the membranes (PROM) can result from the force of the unequally distributed contractions being exerted on the fetal membranes. In obstructed labor (the fetus is not able to pass through the birth canal) uterine rupture can also occur. With delayed descent necrosis of maternal soft tissues can result from pressure exerted by the fetal head. Eventually, necrosis can cause fistulas from the vagina to other nearby structures. Difficult forceps-assisted births can also result in damage to maternal soft tissue.

Fetal-Neonatal Risks

If the membranes rupture and the fetal head has not entered the inlet, there is a danger of cord prolapse. Extreme molding of the fetal head can result. Traumatic forceps-assisted births can damage the fetal skull and central nervous system.

Medical Therapy

Fetopelvic relationships can be assessed by comparing pelvic measurements obtained by a manual exam prior to labor and by computed tomography (CT), and estimated weight of the fetus as obtained by ultrasound measurements. Although it is no longer frequently used, an x-ray pelvimetry may be obtained. The x-ray pelvimetry provides measurements for the maternal pelvic inlet, mid-pelvis, outlet, degree of fetal descent, and selected diameters of the fetal head. Occasionally, in high-risk centers magnetic resonance imaging (MRI) is used to identify adequacy of pelvic diameters.

When the pelvic diameters are borderline or questionable, a trial of labor (TOL) may be advised. In this process the woman continues to labor, and careful assessments of uterine contractions, cervical dilatation, and fetal descent are made by the physician and nurse. As long as there is continued progress, the TOL continues. If progress ceases, the decision for a cesarean birth is made.

APPLYING THE NURSING PROCESS

Nursing Assessment

The adequacy of the maternal pelvis for a vaginal birth should be assessed intrapartally as well as antepartally. During the intrapartal assessment the size of the fetus and its presentation, position, and lie must also be considered. (See Chapter 22 for intrapartal assessment techniques.)

The nurse should suspect CPD when labor is prolonged, cervical dilatation and effacement are slow, and engagement of the presenting part is delayed.

Nursing Diagnosis

Nursing diagnoses that may apply include the following:

- Knowledge deficit related to lack of information about implications and associated complications of CPD
- Fear related to unknown outcome of labor

Nursing Plan and Implementation

Promotion of Maternal and Fetal Well-Being

Nursing actions during the TOL are similar to care during any labor with the exception that the assessments of cervical dilatations and fetal descent are more frequent. Contractions should be monitored continuously, and the labor progress may be charted on the Friedman graph. The fetus should also be monitored continuously. Any signs of fetal distress are reported to the physician/certified nurse-midwife immediately.

Position Changes to Increase Pelvic Diameters

The woman may be positioned in a variety of ways to increase the pelvic diameters. Sitting or squatting increases the outer diameters and may be effective in instances where there is failure of or slow fetal descent. Changing from one side to the other and/or maintaining a hands-and-knees position may assist the fetus in occiput-posterior position to change to an occiput-anterior position. The woman may instinctively want to assume one of these positions. If not, the nurse may encourage a change of position.

Provision of Emotional Support

A couple may need support in coping with the stresses of complicated labor. The nurse should keep the couple informed of what is happening and explain the procedures that are being used. This should reassure the couple that measures are being taken to resolve the problem.

Evaluation

Anticipated outcomes of nursing care include:

- The woman's fear is lessened.
- The woman has additional knowledge regarding the problems, implications, and treatment plans.

CARE OF THE WOMAN AT RISK DUE TO COMPLICATIONS OF THIRD AND FOURTH STAGES

Lacerations

Lacerations of the cervix or vagina may be indicated when bright red vaginal bleeding persists in the presence of a well-contracted uterus. The incidence of lacerations is higher when the childbearing woman is young or a nullipara, has an epidural, has forceps-assisted birth and an episiotomy (Bromberg 1986), and has not done perineal massage or preparation during pregnancy (Avery & Burket 1986). Vaginal and perineal lacerations are often categorized in terms of degree as follows:

- First-degree laceration is limited to the fourchet, perineal skin, and vaginal mucous membrane.

- Second-degree laceration involves the perineal skin, vaginal mucous membrane, underlying fascia, and muscles of the perineal body; it may extend upward on one or both sides of the vagina.

- Third-degree laceration extends through the perineal skin, vaginal mucous membranes, and perineal body and involves the anal sphincter; it may extend up the anterior wall of the rectum.

- Fourth-degree laceration is the same as the third degree but extends through the rectal mucosa to the lumen of the rectum; it may be called a third-degree laceration with a rectal wall extension.

Placenta Accreta

The chronic villi attach directly to the myometrium of the uterus in *placenta accreta*. Two other types of placental adherence are *placenta increta*, in which the myometrium is invaded, and *placenta percreta*, in which the myometrium is penetrated. The adherence itself may be total, partial, or focal, depending on the amount of placental involvement. The incidence of placenta accreta is 1 in 2000 to 3570 births (Zahn & Yeomans 1990). Placenta accreta is the most common type of adherent placenta and accounts for 80%, while 15% of adherent placentas are placenta increta, and 5% are placenta percreta (Zahn & Yeomans 1990).

The primary complication with placenta accreta is maternal hemorrhage and failure of the placenta to separate following birth of the infant. An abdominal hysterectomy may be the necessary treatment, depending on the amount and depth of involvement.

For further discussion of hemorrhage following birth see Chapter 36.

Inversion of Uterus

Uterine inversion occurs when the fundus of the uterus is prolapsed, inside out, through the cervix (Barber et al 1990). The incidence of uterine rupture is approximately 1 in 2500 births (Zahn & Yeomans 1990). It can be caused by a lax uterine wall coupled with undue tension on an umbilical cord when the placenta has not separated. Forceful pressure on the fundus with a dilated cervix and sudden emptying of the uterine contents may be contributing factors. Maternal bleeding occurs in 94% of women, and blood loss ranges from 800 to 1800 mL (Zahn & Yeomans 1990).

Restoration of the uterus to its normal position manually or by surgical intervention is the goal of medical treatment. The uterus is replaced manually by grasping the vaginal mass, spreading the cervical ring with the fingers and thumb, and steadily forcing the fundus upward. The woman is often placed under deep anesthesia for this procedure.

KEY CONCEPTS

Hypotonic labor patterns begin normally and then progress to infrequent, less intense contractions. If there are no contraindications, IV oxytocin is used as treatment.

Precipitous labor is extremely rapid labor that lasts less than 3 hours. It is associated with an increased risk to the mother and newborn infant.

Postterm pregnancy is one that extends more than 294 days, or 42 weeks past the first day of the last menstrual period.

Ruptured uterus is the tearing of previously intact uterine muscles or of an old uterine scar. The rupture can be caused by a weakened cesarean scar, obstetric trauma, CPD, and congenital defects of the birth canal.

The occiput posterior position of the fetus during labor prolongs the labor process, causes severe back discomfort in the laboring woman, and predisposes her to vaginal and perineal trauma and lacerations during birth.

The types of fetal malpresentations include face, brow, breech, and shoulder.

A fetus-newborn weighing more than 4000 g (8 lb, 13 oz) is termed macrosomic. Problems may occur during labor, birth, and in the early neonatal period.

Preventing and treating problems with infringe on the development and birth of normal fetuses are significant medical-nursing activities once the presence of twins has been detected.

Fetal distress is indicated by persistent late deceleration, persistent severe variable decelerations, and prolonged decelerations. If fetal distress is recognized and treated appropriately, the fetus may be spared any permanent damage.

Intrauterine fetal death poses a major nursing challenge to provide support and caring for the parents.

Major bleeding problems in the intrapartal period are abruptio placentae and placenta previa.

Abruptio placentae is the separation of the placenta from the side of the uterus prior to birth of the infant. Abruptio placentae may be central, marginal, or complete.

Placenta previa occurs when the placenta implants low in the uterus near or over the cervix. A low-lying or marginal placenta is one that lies near the cervix. In partial placenta previa part of the placenta lies over the cervix. In complete placenta previa the cervix is completely covered.

Prolapsed umbilical cord results when the umbilical cord precedes the fetal presenting part. When this occurs, pressure is placed on the umbilical cord, and blood flow to the fetus is diminished.

Amniotic fluid embolism occurs when a bolus of amniotic fluid enters the maternal circulation and then enters the maternal lungs. Maternal mortality is very high with this complication.

Hydramnios (also called polyhydramnios) occurs when there is over 2000 mL of amniotic fluid contained within the amniotic membranes. Hydramnios is associated with fetal malformations that affect fetal swallowing and with maternal diabetes mellitus, Rh sensitization, and multiple gestations.

Oligohydramnios is present when there is a severely reduced volume of amniotic fluid. Oligohydramnios is associated with IUGR, postterm, and fetal renal or urinary malfunctions. The fetus is more likely to experience variable decelerations because the amniotic fluid is insufficient to keep pressure off the umbilical cord.

Cephalopelvic disproportion (CPD) occurs when there is a narrowed diameter in the maternal pelvis. The narrowed diameter is called a contracture, and it may occur in the pelvic inlet, midpelvis, or outlet. If pelvic measurements are borderline, a trial of labor (TOL) may be attempted. Failure of cervical dilatation and/or fetal descent would then necessitate a cesarean birth.

Third- and fourth-stage complications usually involve a hemorrhage. Causes of hemorrhage include lacerations of the birth canal and/or cervix, placenta accreta, and uterine inversion.

REFERENCES

Anderson HF: Ultrasonography in labor. *Clin Obstet Gynecol* 1992; 35:527.

Andrews CM, Andrews EC: Nursing, maternal postures, and fetal positions. *Nurs Res* 1983; 32:6.

Avery MD, Burket MA: Effect of perineal massage on the incidence of episiotomy and perineal laceration in a nurse-midwifery service. *J Nurse-Midwifery* May/June 1986; 31:128.

Barber KRK, Fields DH, Kaufman SA: *Quick Reference to OB-GYN Procedures*, 3rd ed. Philadelphia: Lippincott, 1990.

Becky RD et al: Development of a perinatal grief checklist. *JOGNN* May/June 1985; 14:194.

Blackburn C, Copley R: One precious moment: What you can offer when a newborn infant dies. *Nursing* 1989; 19:52.

Bowes WA: Clinical aspects of normal and abnormal labor. In: *Maternal-Fetal Medicine*. Creasy RK, Resnik R (editors). Philadelphia: WB Saunders, 1994.

Bromberg MHP: Presumptive maternal benefits of routine episiotomy: A literature review. *J Nurse-Midwifery* May/June 1986; 11:70.

Brown Y: The crisis of pregnancy loss: A team approach to support. *Birth* June 1992; p 82.

Campbell G: Overdue delivery: Its impact on mother-to-be. *MCN* May/June 1986; 11:170.

Chatelain SM, Quirk JG: Amniotic and thromboembolism. *Clin Obstet Gynecol* 1990; 33:473.

Clark SL: Care of the critically ill obstetric patient. In: *Danforth's Obstetrics and Gynecology*, 7th ed. Scott JR et al (editors). Philadelphia: Lippincott, 1994.

Clark SL: New concepts of amniotic fluid embolism: A review. *Obstet Gynecol Survey* 1990; p 45.

Combs CA, Murphy EL, Laros RK: Factors associated with postpartum hemorrhage with vaginal birth. *Obstet Gynecol* January 1991; 77:69.

Cordell AS, Thomas N: Fathers and grieving: Coping with infant death. *J Perinatol* 1989; 10:75.

Crowther CA et al: The effects of hospitalization for rest on fetal growth, neonatal morbidity and length of gestation on twin pregnancy. *Brit J Obstet Gynecol* 1990; 97:872.

Cruikshank DP: Malpresentations and umbilical cord complications. In: *Danforth's Obstetrics and Gynecology*, 7th ed. Scott JR et al (editors). Philadelphia: Lippincott, 1994.

Cucco C, Osborne MA, Cibils LA: Maternal-fetal outcome in prolonged pregnancy. *Am J Obstet Gynecol* 1989; 161:916.

Cunningham FG et al: *Williams Obstetrics*, 19th ed. Norwalk, CT: Appleton-Century-Crofts, 1993.

Danskin FH, Neilson JP: Twin-to-twin treatment syndrome: What are appropriate diagnostic criteria? *Am J Obstet Gynecol* 1989; 161:365.

Dombrowski MP et al: Cocaine abuse is associated with abruptio placentae and decreased birth weight, but not shorter labor. *Obstet Gynecol* January 1991; 77(1):139.

Eden RD: Postdate pregnancy: Antenatal assessment of fetal wellbeing. *Clin Obstet Gynecol* June 1989; 32:235.

Eganhouse DJ: Fetal monitoring of twins. *JOGNN* January/February 1992; 21(1):17.

Gillogley K: Abnormal labor and delivery. In: *Manual of Obstetrics*. Niswander KR (editor). Boston: Little, Brown, 1991.

Gilson GJ et al: Prolonged pregnancy and the biophysical profile: A birthing center perspective. *J Nurse-Midwifery* July/August 1988; 33:171.

Gimovsky ML, Shifrin BS: Breech management. *J Perinatol* 1992; X11:143.

Gocke SE et al: Management of the nonvertex second twin: Primary cesarean section, external version or primary breech extraction. *Am J Obstet Gynecol* 1989; 161:111.

Gonik B, Allen R, Sorab J: Objective evaluation of the shoulder dystocia phenomenon: Effect of maternal pelvic orientation on force reduction. *Obstet Gynecol* 1989; 74:44.

Griese ME, Prickett SA: Nursing management of umbilical cord prolapse. *JOGNN* 1993; 22:311.

Gross TL et al: Shoulder dystocia: A fetal physician risk. *Am J Obstet Gynecol* June 1987; 156:408.

Hayashi RH, Castillo MS: Bleeding in pregnancy. In: *High Risk Pregnancy: A Team Approach*, 2nd ed. Knuppel RA, Drukker JE (editors). Philadelphia: WB Saunders, 1993.

Hollenbach KA, Hickok DE: Epidemiology and diagnosis of twin gestation. *Clin Obstet Gynecol* March 1990; 33:3.

Huddleston JF, Freeman RK: Estimations of fetal well-being. In: *Neonatal-Perinatal Medicine: Diseases of the Fetus and Newborn*, 5th ed. Fanaroff AA, Martin RJ (editors). St Louis: Mosby-Year Book, 1992.

Hunter LP: Twin gestation: Antepartum management. *J Perinatal Neonatal Nurs* 1989; 3:1.

Jackson VM: Delivery of the second twin. *J Perinatal Neonatal Nurs* 1989; 3(1):22.

Karegaard M, Gennser G: Incidence and recurrence rate of abruptio placentae in Sweden. *Obstet Gynecol* 1986; 67:523.

Keith LG, Lopez-Zeno JA, Luke B: Twin gestation. In: *Gynecology and Obstetrics*. Dilts PV, Sciarra JJ (editors). Philadelphia: Lippincott, 1991.

Keller JD et al: Infants of diabetic mothers with accelerated fetal growth by ultrasonography: Are they all alike? *Am J Obstet Gynecol* September 1990; 163(3):893.

Kelton JG, Cruikshank DP: Hematologic disorders of pregnancy. In: *Medical Complications During Pregnancy*. Burrow GN, Ferris TF (editors). Philadelphia: WB Saunders, 1988.

King JC: Transverse and oblique lie. In: *Gynecology and Obstetrics*, vol 2. Dilts PV, Sciarri JJ (editors). Philadelphia: Lippincott, 1994.

Kline-Kaye V, Miller-Slade D: The use of fundal pressure during the second stage of labor. *JOGNN* November/December 1990; 19(6):511.

Knuppel RA, Drukker JE: Twins and other multiple gestations. In: *High Risk Pregnancy: A Team Approach*, 2nd ed. Knuppel RA, Drukker JE (editors). Philadelphia: WB Saunders, 1993.

Kochenour NK: Postterm pregnancy. In: *Neonatal-Perinatal Medicine*. Fanaroff AA, Martin RJ (editors). St Louis: Mosby, 1992.

Koehn ML: The psychoeducational model of prepared childbirth education. *AWHONN Clin Issues Perinatal Women Health Nurs* 1993; 4:66.

Kovacs BW, Kirschbaum TH, Paul RH: Twin gestations. I: Antenatal care and complications. *Obstet Gynecol* 1989; 74:313.

Kübler-Ross E: *On Death and Dying*. New York: Macmillan, 1969.

Lake M: Prolonged Pregnancy. In: *High-Risk Intrapartum Nursing*. Mandeville LK, Troiano NH (editors). Philadelphia: Lippincott, 1992.

Langer O et al: Shoulder dystocia: Should the fetus weighing >4000 grams be delivered by cesarean section? *Am J Obstet Gynecol* 1991; 165(4):831.

Lavery JP: Placenta previa. *Clin Obstet Gynecol* September 1990; 33:414.

Lederer RP et al: Anxiety and epinephrine in multiparous women in labor: Relationship to duration in labor and fetal heart pattern. *Obstet Gynecol* 1985; 153:870.

Lederman RP, Lederman E, Work B: Anxiety and epinephrine in multiparous women in labor: Relationship to duration of labor and fetal heart rate pattern. *Obstet Gynecol* 1985; 153:870.

Lindell SG: Education for discharge: A time for change. *JOGNN* March/April 1988: 17(2):108.

Lowe TW, Cunningham FG: Placental abruption. *Clin Obstet Gynecol* September 1990; 33:406.

Makowski EL: Twin pregnancy. In: *Current Therapy in Obstetrics and Gynecology*, 3rd ed. Quilligan EJ, Zuspan FP (editors). Philadelphia: WB Saunders, 1990.

Marks AD, Divon MY: Longitudinal study of amniotic fluid index in postdated pregnancy. *Obstet Gynecol* 1992; 79:229.

Mashburn J: Identification and management of shoulder dystocia. *J Nurse-Midwifery* September/October 1988; 33(5): 225.

McLennan AH: Multiple gestation: Clinical characteristics and management. In: *Maternal-Fetal Medicine: Principles and Practice*, 3rd ed. Creasy RK, Resnik R (editors). Philadelphia: WB Saunders, 1994.

Moise KJ: Indomethacin therapy in the treatment of symptomatic polyhydramnios. *Clin Obstet Gynecol* 1991; 34:310.

Neifert M, Thorpe J: Twins: Family adjustment, parenting, and infant feeding in the fourth trimester. *Clin Obstet Gynecol* March 1990; 33:102.

Oxorn H: *Oxorn-Foote Human Labor and Birth*, 5th ed. Norwalk, CT: Appleton-Century-Crofts, 1986.

Phelan JP: Postdatism. *Clin Obstet Gynecol* June 1989; 32:219.

Phelan JP: Uterine rupture. *Clin Obstet Gynecol* September 1990; 33:432.

Pitkin RM: Fetal death: Diagnosis and management. *Am J Obstet Gynecol* September 1987; 157:583.

Polin JI, Frangipane WL: Current concepts in management of obstetric problems for pediatricians II: Modern concepts in the management of multiple gestation. *Pediatr Clin North Am* 1986; 33:649.

Queenan JT: Polyhydramnios, oligohydramnios and hydrops fetalis. In: *Neonatal-Perinatal Medicine*, 5th ed. Fanaroff AA, Martin RJ (editors). St Louis: Mosby-Year Book, 1992.

Quilligan EJ: Breech delivery. In: *Current Therapy in Obstetrics and Gynecology*. Quilligan EJ, Zuspan FP (editors). Philadelphia: WB Saunders, 1990.

Resnik R: Post-term pregnancy. In: *Current Therapy in Obstetrics and Gynecology*. Quilligan EJ, Zuspan FP (editors). Philadelphia: WB Saunders, 1990.

Resnik R: Post-term pregnancy. In: *Maternal-Fetal Medicine: Principles and Practice*, 3rd ed. Creasy RK, Resnik R (editors). Philadelphia: WB Saunders, 1994.

Rodriguez MH et al: Uterine rupture: Are intrauterine pressure catheters useful in the diagnosis? *Obstet Gynecol* 1989; 161:666.

Sakala EP: Obstetric management of conjoined twins. *Obstet Gynecol* 1986; 67:21S.

Schweibert P, Kirk P: *When Hello Means Goodbye*. Eugene, OR: Oregon Health Sciences University, 1985.

Sokol RJ, Brindley BA: Practical diagnosis and management of abnormal labor. In: *Danforth's Obstetrics and Gynecology*, 6th ed. Scott JR et al (editors). Philadelphia: Lippincott, 1990.

Spellacy WN: The postdate pregnancy. In: *Danforth's Obstetrics and Gynecology*, 6th ed. Scott JR et al (editors). Philadelphia: Lippincott, 1990.

Tamura RK, Sabbagha RE: Altered fetal growth. In: *Gynecology and Obstetrics*, vol 3. Depp R, Eshenbach DA, Sciara JJ (editors). Philadelphia: WB Saunders, 1990.

Tchabo JG, Tomai T: Selected intrapartum external cephalic version of the second twin. *Obstet Gynecol* March 1992; p 79.

Theroux R: Multiple birth: A unique parenting experience. *J Perinatal Neonatal Nurs* 1989; 3:35.

Veille JC et al: The effect of a calcium channel blocker (nifedipine) in uterine blood flow in the pregnant goat. *Am J Obstet Gynecol* 1986; 154:1160.

Watson WJ, Seeds JW: Diagnostic obstetric imaging. In: *Gynecology and Obstetrics.* Dilts PV, Sciarra JJ (editors). Philadelphia: Lippincott, 1990.

Weiner CP: Vaginal breech delivery in the 1990's. *Clin Obstet Gynecol* 1992; 35:559.

Wenstrom KD et al: Frequency, distribution and theoretical mechanisms of hematologic and weight discordance in monochorionic twins. *Obstet Gynecol* 1992; 80:257.

Wuitchik M, Bakal D, Lipshitz J: The clinical significance of pain and cognitive activity in latent labor. *Obstet Gynecol* January 1989; 73(1):35.

Zahn CN, Yeomans ER: Postpartum hemorrhage: Placenta accreta, uterine inversion, and puerperal hematomas. *Clin Obstet Gynecol* September 1990; 33:422.

CHAPTER 26

OBSTETRIC PROCEDURES: THE ROLE OF THE NURSE

*W*ith our first baby all of a sudden I had to have a cesarean. Everything happened so fast, but our son was OK and that's all that mattered. With our second baby I wanted to try a vaginal birth. Even though I wanted to, I was afraid. I don't know what I would have done without my nurse. She stayed with me the whole time and kept giving me support. She explained what was happening and gave me encouragement. I felt safe. I had a beautiful baby girl after 8 hours of labor. Everything went fine, and I am so glad that I was able to avoid another cesarean. We don't plan to have another baby, but if we did, I wouldn't be so afraid.

KEY TERMS

Amniotomy

Episiotomy

External version

Forceps

Induction of labor

Internal version

Vaginal birth after cesarean (VBAC)

OBJECTIVES

Examine the methods of external and internal version and the related nursing interventions.

Discuss the use of amniotomy in current maternal-newborn care.

Compare methods for inducing labor, explaining their advantages and disadvantages.

Discuss the use of transcervical intrapartum amnioinfusion.

Describe the types of episiotomies performed, the rationale for each, and the associated nursing interventions.

Summarize the indications for forceps-assisted birth, types of forceps that may be used, complications, and related interventions.

Discuss the use of vacuum extraction, including indications, procedure, complications, and related nursing interventions.

Explain the indications for cesarean birth, impact on the family unit, preparation and teaching needs, and associated nursing interventions.

Discuss vaginal birth following cesarean birth.

Most births occur without the need for operative obstetric intervention. In some instances, however, obstetric procedures are necessary to maintain safety for the woman and the fetus. The most common obstetric procedures are amniotomy, induction of labor, episiotomy, cesarean birth, and vaginal birth following a previous cesarean birth.

Generally, women are aware of the possible need for an obstetric procedure during their birth; however, some women expect to have a "natural" labor and birth and do not anticipate the need for any medical intervention. This conflict between expectation and the need for intervention presents a challenge to maternity nurses. The nurse can provide information regarding any procedure to make sure the woman and her partner understand what is proposed, the anticipated benefits and possible risks, and any possible alternative treatments.

CARE OF THE WOMAN DURING VERSION

Version, or turning the fetus, is a procedure used to change the fetal presentation by abdominal or intrauterine manipulation. The most common type of version is **external** (or cephalic) **version.** In an external version the presentation of the fetus is changed from a breech to a cephalic presentation by external manipulation of the maternal abdomen (Figure 26–1). The other type of version, called **internal** (or podalic) **version** is used only with the second twin during a vaginal birth. In an internal version the obstetrician places a hand inside the uterus and grabs the fetus' feet. The fetus is then turned from a transverse or cephalic to a breech presentation (Figure 26–2).

External Version

If breech or shoulder presentation (transverse lie) is detected in the later weeks of pregnancy, an external version may be attempted. The version is usually done after 37 weeks' gestation because most fetuses still in breech presentation at this time will not spontaneously change back to a vertex presentation. Successful external version rates over the past decade range from 60% to 75% (Kochenour 1994; Newman et al 1993).

The following criteria should be met prior to performing external version (Kochenour 1994):

- A single fetus (also called a singleton). If a multiple gestation exists, a variety of concerns preclude an external version. For example, a cesarean rather than vaginal birth may need to be considered, and

the fetuses might become entangled during a version.

- The fetal breech is not engaged. Once the presenting part is engaged, it is difficult to do a version.

- There must be an adequate amount of amniotic fluid. The amniotic fluid helps ease movement of the fetus and provides adequate room for the umbilical cord to float without being compressed.

- A reactive nonstress test (NST) should be obtained immediately prior to performing the version. A reactive NST indicates fetal well-being.

- The fetus must be 38 or more weeks gestation. A version may be accompanied by complications that require immediate birth by cesarean. If gestation is less than 38 weeks, a preterm birth would result. (Note: Occasionally, a physician may do an external version while the woman is in labor.)

Absolute contraindications include the following (Kochenour 1994):

- Marked or severe oligohydramnios. The decreased amount of amniotic fluid would increase the risk of

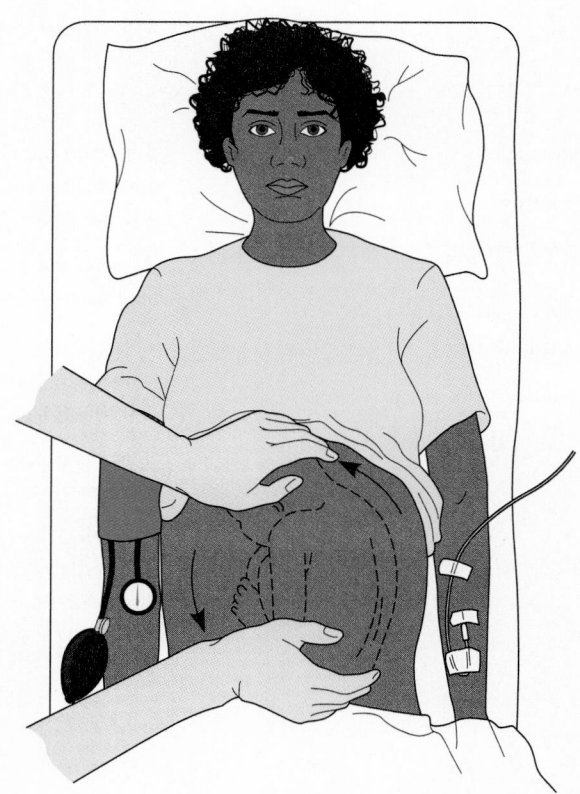

FIGURE 26-1 External (or cephalic) version of the fetus. A new technique involves pressure on the fetal head and buttocks so that the fetus completes a "backward flip" or "forward roll."

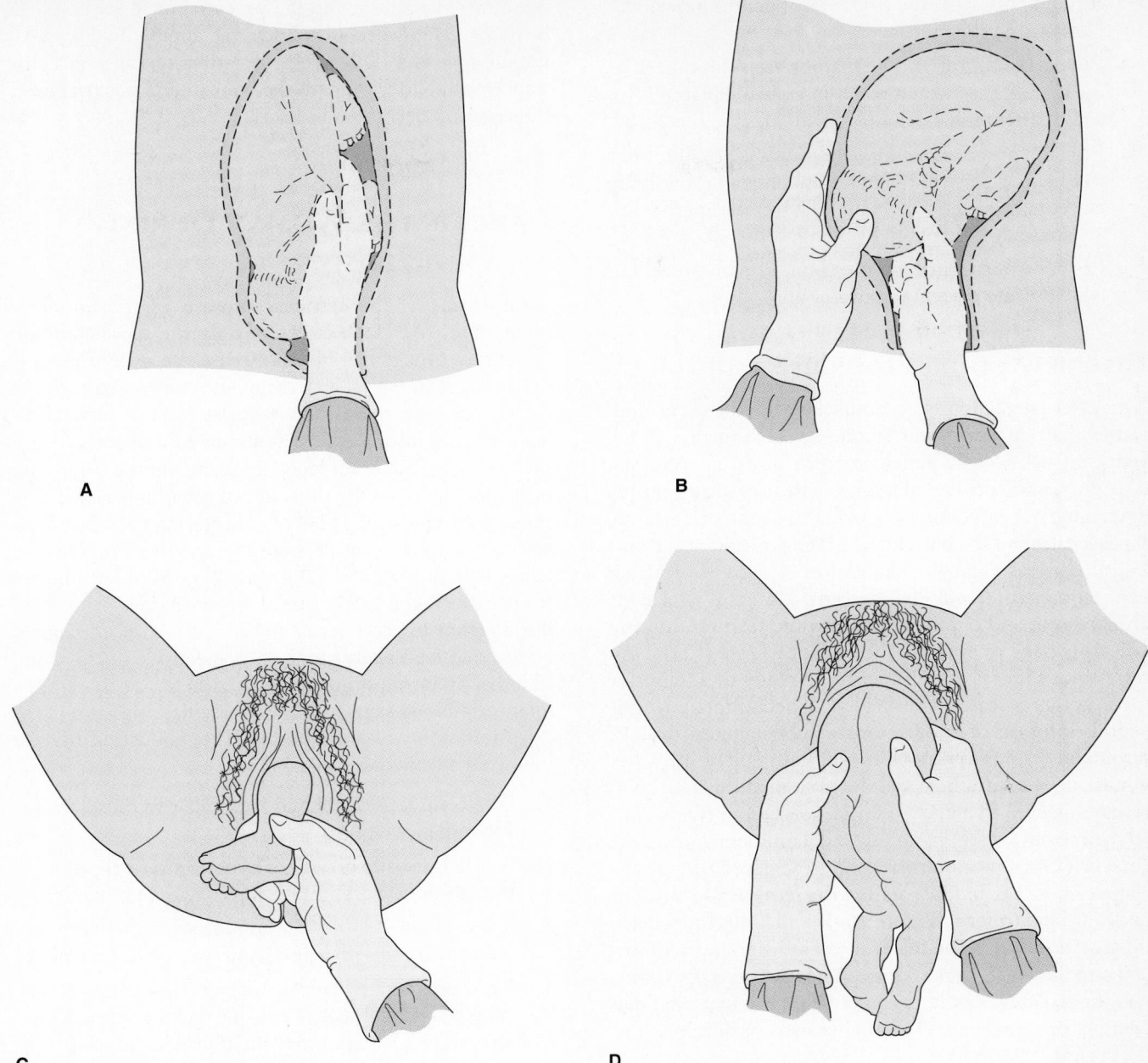

A

B

C

D

FIGURE 26-2 Podalic version and extraction of the fetus is used to assist in the vaginal birth of the second twin. *A* The physician reaches into the uterus and grasps a foot. Although a vertex birth is always preferred, in this instance of assisting in the birth of a second twin it is not possible to grasp any other fetal part. The fetal head would be too large to grasp and pull downward, and grasping the fetal arm would result in a trans-verse lie and make vaginal birth impossible. *B* While applying pressure on the outside of the abdomen to push the baby's head up toward the top of the uterus with one hand, the physi-cian pulls the baby's foot down toward the cervix. *C* Both feet have been pulled through the cervix and vagina. *D* The physi-cian now grasps the baby's trunk and continues to pull down-ward on the baby to assist the birth.

cord compression and make it difficult to move the fetus within the uterus.

- Premature rupture of the membranes. Rupture of the membranes would result in an inadequate amount of amniotic fluid.
- Placenta previa. If a complete previa is present, birth will be by cesarean. If a marginal previa or low-lying placenta is present, the manipulation during the version may precipitate bleeding.
- Previous third trimester bleeding. Previous bleeding may indicate placenta previa or abruption.

External Version Procedure

The external version is accomplished in a birthing unit, rather than an outpatient setting, in case further intervention (such as emergency cesarean birth) is necessary. The physician/certified nurse-midwife uses ultrasound to determine the number of fetuses, amount of amniotic fluid, location of the placenta, and the position of the umbilical cord. A vaginal examination is done to evaluate cervical dilatation and fetal descent. Maternal vital signs are assessed, and continuous electronic fetal monitoring (EFM) is done to evaluate the fetal heart rate (FHR). An intravenous line is established to be ready to administer medications in case of difficulty. A betamimetic (intravenous infusion of ritodrine or a subcutaneous dose of terbutaline) or intravenous magnesium sulfate (if a betamimetic is contraindicated due to a medical condition) is administered to achieve uterine relaxation. (Occasionally, some physicians do not use a betamimetic during the version.) Once uterine relaxation is achieved, the physician does the version by rotating the fetus in a forward or backward flip (refer to Figure 26–1) and holds the fetus in the new position as the intravenous infusion is discontinued and the uterus retains tone. The version is discontinued immediately in the presence of severe maternal discomfort or significant FHR bradycardia or decelerations (Clay et al 1993).

Nursing Care

The nurse completes the initial maternal and fetal assessments, provides ongoing evaluation of FHR, and performs the NST. The nurse continues to monitor maternal blood pressure and pulse about every 5 minutes throughout the version and for about 30 minutes after. Assessment of the maternal-fetal response to the ritodrine, terbutaline, or magnesium sulfate is also performed (see Magnesium Sulfate Drug Guide in Chapter 19). The nurse also provides information for the woman and her partner. The admission period and the time of the initial NST are excellent opportunities for client teaching. The woman should be encouraged to express her understanding and expectation of the procedure, verbalize her fears, and ask questions. The possibility of fail-

ure of the procedure and the potential need for cesarean birth if the fetus becomes distressed should be discussed. Explaining what will occur in either of these circumstances will better prepare the woman and her partner if intervention becomes necessary.

CARE OF THE WOMAN DURING AN AMNIOTOMY

Amniotomy is the artificial rupture of the amniotic membranes (AROM). It is probably the most common operative procedure in obstetrics. Because the amniotomy requires that an instrument be inserted through the cervix, there needs to be at least 2 cm of cervical dilatation present. The amniotomy may be performed as a method of induction of labor (to stimulate the beginning of labor), or it may be done at any time during the first stage of labor with the goal of accelerating the labor. If an amniotomy is done after 3 cm of cervical dilatation, the labor will probably be shortened by 90–120 minutes (Fraser & Sokol 1992). Amniotomy may also be done during labor to allow access to the fetus in order to apply an internal fetal heart monitoring electrode to the scalp, to insert an intrauterine pressure catheter, or to obtain a fetal scalp blood sample for acid-base determination.

Amniotomy as a method of labor induction has the following advantages:

1. The contractions elicited are similar to those of spontaneous labor.
2. There is usually no risk of hypertonus or rupture of the uterus, as with intravenous oxytocin induction.
3. The woman does not require the same intensive monitoring as with intravenous oxytocin induction.
4. EFM is facilitated because once the membranes are ruptured, a fetal scalp electrode may be applied, an intrauterine catheter may be inserted, and scalp blood sampling for pH determinations may be done to assist in evaluating a fetal heart rate pattern.
5. The color and composition of amniotic fluid can be evaluated.

The disadvantages of amniotomy are as follows:

1. Once an amniotomy is done, birth must occur because microorganisms can now invade the intrauterine cavity and cause amnionitis.
2. The danger of a prolapsed cord is increased once the membranes have ruptured, especially if the fetal presenting part is not firmly pressed down against the cervix.
3. Compression and molding of the fetal head are increased due to loss of the cushioning effect of the amniotic fluid for the fetal head during uterine contractions.

AROM Procedure

Before an amniotomy is performed, the fetus is assessed for presentation, position, and station. Unless the fetal head is well engaged in the pelvis, some obstetricians do not advocate an amniotomy because of the danger of prolapsed cord. Other risks are abruptio placentae (due to rapid decompression of the uterus with the rapid loss of amniotic fluid), infection (due to the introduction of organisms into the cervix and intrauterine cavity), and amniotic fluid embolus (due to rapid decompression of the uterus and small amounts of fluid entering the maternal vascular system from under the edge of the placenta). These complications may also be associated with spontaneous rupture of membranes.

While performing a sterile vaginal examination, the physician/CNM introduces an amnihook (or other rupturing device) into the vagina. A small tear is made in the amniotic membrane. Following rupture of the membranes, amniotic fluid is allowed to escape.

Nursing Care

The nurse explains the AROM procedure to the woman. The fetal presentation, position, and station are assessed because amniotomy is usually delayed until engagement has occurred. The woman is positioned in a semireclining position and draped to provide privacy. The FHR is assessed just prior to and immediately after the amniotomy, and the two FHR assessments are compared. If there are marked changes, the nurse should check for prolapse of

the cord. The amniotic fluid is inspected for amount, color, odor, and the presence of meconium or blood. While wearing disposable gloves, the nurse cleanses and dries the perineal area and changes the Chux pads. (See Essential Precautions in Practice: During Procedures.) Because there is now an open pathway for organisms to ascend into the uterus, strict sterile technique must be observed during vaginal examinations. In addition the number of vaginal examinations must be kept to a minimum in order to reduce the chance of introducing an infection, and the woman's temperature should be monitored every 2 hours. Bed rest is maintained unless the presenting part is engaged and is firmly against the cervix. The nurse needs to provide information regarding the amniotomy and the expected effects. Some couples may worry that all the amniotic fluid will be gone and that they will experience a "dry birth." It is important for them to know that amniotic fluid is constantly produced.

CARE OF THE WOMAN DURING PROSTAGLANDIN ADMINISTRATION AT TERM

The FDA has recently approved prostaglandin (PGE) gel for cervical ripening (softening the cervix) in pregnant woman at or near term when there is a medical or obstetric indication for induction of labor. The gel contains 0.5 mg of dinoprostone (a form of prostaglandin E_2) per 3 g of gel. Although the gel has been demonstrated to cause cervical ripening, shorter labor, and lower requirements for oxytocin during labor induction, most research has not found an improvement in the failed induction rate or a decrease in the overall cesarean birth rate when the gel is used (ACOG 1993).

Contraindications to the use of PGE gel include evidence of cephalopelvic disproportion (CPD), placenta previa, vasa previa, unexplained vaginal bleeding, and obstetric emergencies that may require surgical intervention (ACOG 1993). Prostaglandin should be used with caution in women with compromised cardiovascular, hepatic, or renal function and in women with asthma or glaucoma (Day & Snell 1993). Although some success has been reported, research must be done to investigate safe use of prostaglandin gel in women with a history of cesarean birth or major uterine surgery, grand multiparity, or premature rupture of membranes (ACOG 1993). Hypertension does not appear to be a contraindication to low-dose gel usage with close maternal and fetal monitoring (Rayburn et al 1991).

Possible maternal side effects of prostaglandin administration for cervical ripening prior to induction of labor include hyperstimulation of uterine contractions (more than five contractions in 10 minutes or two or more contractions lasting more than 2 minutes [Arias 1993]), nausea, and vomiting (Day & Snell 1993; Trofatter 1992).

Prostaglandin Gel Insertion Procedure

At this time it is recommended that prostaglandin gel be used only in a hospital birthing unit and that an obstetrician be readily available in case an emergency cesarean birth is needed. The use of PGE in outpatient settings and birth centers is currently under study (Day & Snell 1993). Prostaglandin is available in a prefilled syringe with a catheter attached to the hub. The catheter is inserted through the vagina and into the endocervix, where the gel is injected. The catheter has a small shield at the top so that the gel cannot be deposited above the internal os. Dinoprostone is also available as a gel that may be placed in a diaphragm and applied to the cervix and as a suppository that is placed in the posterior fornix (Day & Snell 1993).

Nursing Care

Physicians, certified nurse-midwives, and birthing room nurses who have had special education and training may administer PGE gels. Maternal vital signs are assessed for a baseline, and an electronic fetal monitor is applied to obtain an external tracing of uterine activity and FHR. After insertion the woman is instructed to remain supine (with a rolled blanket under her right hip to tip the uterus slightly to the left) for 15–30 minutes to minimize leakage of the gel from the endocervix (AWHONN 1993). The nurse monitors the woman for uterine hyperstimulation and FHR abnormalities (changes in baseline rate, variability, and presence of decelerations) for 30 minutes to 2 hours (AWHONN 1993). If uterine hyperstimulation occurs, the woman is positioned on her left side and oxygen is administered. The administration of a tocolytic agent (such as a subcutaneous injection of terbutaline) should be considered if the uterine hyperstimulation pattern continues (ACOG 1993). The gel may be removed if severe nausea, vomiting, or hyperstimulation of the uterus develops (Arias 1993).

CARE OF THE WOMAN DURING INDUCTION OF LABOR

The American College of Obstetricians and Gynecologists defines **induction of labor** as the stimulation of uterine contractions before the spontaneous onset of labor, with or without ruptured fetal membranes, for the purpose of accomplishing birth (ACOG 1991). Elective induction is defined as the initiation of labor for convenience. ACOG guidelines do not recommend elective induction (ACOG 1991). Conversely, indicated induction may be considered in the presence of the following:

- Diabetes mellitus
- Renal disease
- Pregnancy-induced hypertension (PIH)

- Premature rupture of membranes (PROM)
- Chorioamnionitis
- Fetal demise
- Postterm gestation
- Intrauterine fetal growth retardation (IUGR)
- Isoimmunization
- History of rapid labor (precipitous labor and birth)
- Mild abruptio placentae with no fetal stress or distress

The most frequently used methods of induction are amniotomy, intravenous oxytocin (Pitocin) infusion, or both. Oxytocin infusion is discussed later in this section. Amniotomy was discussed earlier in this chapter.

Contraindications

All contraindications to spontaneous labor and vaginal birth are contraindications to the induction of labor (Dunn 1990). Relative maternal contraindications include the following (ACOG 1991):

- Client refusal
- Placenta previa or vasa previa
- Abnormal fetal presentation
- Cord presentation
- Presenting part above the pelvic inlet
- Prior classic uterine incision
- Active genital herpes infection
- Pelvic structural deformities or cephalopelvic disproportion
- Invasive cervical carcinoma

Before induction is attempted, appropriate assessment must indicate that both the woman and fetus are ready for the onset of labor. This includes evaluation of fetal maturity and cervical readiness.

Labor Readiness

Fetal Maturity

Early diagnosis of pregnancy with adequate recorded data during the early months of pregnancy, including serial sonograms, is helpful in determining the expected date of birth. External abdominal examination of the growing uterus and amniotic fluid studies are also beneficial in assessing fetal maturity.

Cervical Readiness

The findings on vaginal examination will help determine whether cervical changes favorable for induction have occurred. Bishop (1964) developed a prelabor scoring system that is still helpful in predicting the inductibility of women (Table 26–1). Components evaluated are cervical

TABLE 26-1   Prelabor Status Evaluation Scoring System

Factor	Assigned Value			
	0	**1**	**2**	**3**
Cervical dilatation	Closed	1–2 cm	3–4 cm	5 cm or more
Cervical effacement	0%–30%	40%–50%	60%–70%	80% or more
Fetal station	−3	−2	−1, 0	+1, or lower
Cervical consistency	Firm	Moderate	Soft	
Cervical position	Posterior	Midposition	Anterior	

SOURCE: Modified from Bishop EH: Pelvic scoring for elective induction. *Obstet Gynecol* 1964; 24:266.

dilatation, effacement, consistency, and position, as well as the station of the fetal presenting part. A score of 0, 1, 2, or 3 is given to each assessed characteristic. The higher the total score for all the criteria, the more likely it is that labor will occur. The lower the total score, the higher the failure rate. A favorable cervix is the most important criterion for a successful induction.

The presence of a cervix that is anterior, soft, 50% effaced, and dilated at least 2 cm, with the fetal head at + 1 station or lower (Bishop score of 9) is favorable for successful induction (Dunn 1990).

Oxytocin Infusion

Intravenous administration of oxytocin is an effective method of initiating uterine contractions to induce labor. During administration the goal is to achieve two to three uterine contractions with a duration of 40 to 60 seconds in 10 minutes with good uterine relaxation and return to the baseline tone between contractions (Dunn 1990).

Medical Therapy

Ten units of oxytocin (Pitocin) are added to 1 L of intravenous fluid (usually 5% dextrose in balanced salt solution—for example, 5% dextrose in lactated Ringer's). The resulting mixture will contain 10 mU of oxytocin per milliliter (1 mU/minute = 6 mL/hour), and the prescribed dose can be calculated easily. Other dosage concentrations are presented in the Drug Guide: Oxytocin (Pitocin) on page 764.

A second bottle of intravenous fluid is prepared and used to start and maintain the infusion. This avoids infusing a large dose of oxytocin as the line is begun and provides additional fluids while the oxytocin solution is being kept at a low infusion rate. After the infusion is started, the oxytocin solution is piggybacked into the primary tubing port closest to the catheter insertion. This allows only a small amount of oxytocin to backflow into the tubing and ensures greater dosage accuracy. The oxytocin should be administered with a device that permits precise control of the flow rate. Over the past few years there have been differences in opinion regarding oxytocin

dosage. ACOG (1991) recommends two protocols for oxytocin infusion. The first utilizes an initial dose of 1–2 mU/minute with increases of 1 mU/minute every 15 minutes until the desired contraction pattern is obtained. The second protocol starts the initial dose at 0.5–1 mU/minute with increases every 40–60 minutes in increments of 1–2 mU/minute. The physician can choose either protocol.

A maximum oxytocin infusion rate of 2–8 mU/minute has been reported to be sufficient to achieve cervical dilatation of at least 1 cm/hour (ACOG 1991). Recent studies suggest that smaller dose regimens are as effective as previous larger dose regimens and that adverse effects of oxytocin are dose related (Brodsky & Pelzar, 1991). Once labor is established and cervical dilatation reaches 5 to 6 cm, oxytocin may be reduced by similar increments (ACOG 1988).

Oxytocin induction is not without some associated risks: hyperstimulation of the uterus, resulting in uterine contractions that are too frequent (more often than every 2 minutes), uterine contractions that are too intense, and/or an increased uterine resting tone. Other risks include uterine rupture and water intoxication (PDR 1994). See further discussion in the Drug Guide: Oxytocin (Pitocin) on page 764.

Researchers are studying a new method of labor induction with pulsatile oxytocin administration by a computer-controlled pump. In early studies (Willcourt et al 1994) pulsatile oxytocin was associated with decreased dosages and less risk of uterine hyperstimulation and fetal distress.

APPLYING THE NURSING PROCESS

Nursing Assessment

Close observation and accurate assessments are mandatory to provide safe, optimal care for both woman and fetus. Baseline data (maternal temperature, pulse, respiration, blood pressure, FHR, and NST) should be obtained

OXYTOCIN (PITOCIN)

Overview of Obstetric Action

Oxytocin (Pitocin) exerts a selective stimulatory effect on the smooth muscle of the uterus and blood vessels. Oxytocin affects the myometrial cells of the uterus by increasing the excitability of the muscle cell, increasing the strength of the muscle contraction, and supporting propagation of the contraction (movement of the contraction from one myometrial cell to the next). Its effect on the uterine contraction depends on the dosage used and on the excitability of the myometrial cells. During the first half of gestation little excitability of the myometrium occurs, and the uterus is fairly resistant to the effects of oxytocin. However, from midgestation on, the uterus responds increasingly to exogenous intravenous oxytocin. Cautious use of diluted oxytocin administered intravenously at term results in a slow rise of uterine activity.

The circulatory half-life of oxytocin is 3–5 minutes. It takes approximately 40 minutes for a particular dose of oxytocin to reach a steady-state plasma concentration (Arias 1993).

The effects of oxytocin on the cardiovascular system can be pronounced. There may be an initial decrease in the blood pressure, but with prolonged administration a 30% increase in the baseline blood pressure may be noted. Cardiac output and stroke volume are increased. With doses of 20 mU/minute or above the antidiuretic effect of oxytocin results in a decrease of free water exchange in the kidney and a marked decrease in urine output (Marshall 1985).

Oxytocin is used to **induce** labor at term and to **augment** uterine contractions in the first and second stages of labor. Oxytocin may also be used **immediately after birth to stimulate uterine contraction** and thereby control uterine atony.

Route, Dosage, Frequency

For induction of labor: Add 10 units Pitocin (1 mL) to 1000 mL of intravenous solution. (The resulting concentration is 10 mU oxytocin per 1 mL of intravenous fluid.) Using an infusion pump, administer IV, starting at 0.5–1 mU/minute and increase by 1–2 mU/minute every 40–60 minutes. Or start at 1–2 mU/minute and increase by 1 mU/minute every 15 minutes until a good contraction pattern (every 2–3 minutes and lasting 40–60 seconds) is achieved.

Maternal Contraindications

- Severe preeclampsia-eclampsia (PIH)
- Predisposition to uterine rupture (in nullipara over 35 years of age, multigravida 4 or more, overdistention of the uterus, previous major surgery of the cervix or uterus)
- Cephalopelvic disproportion
- Malpresentation or malposition of the fetus, cord prolapse
- Preterm infant
- Rigid, unripe cervix; total placenta previa
- Presence of fetal distress

Maternal Side Effects

Hyperstimulation of the uterus results in hypercontractility, which in turn may cause the following:

- Abruptio placentae
- Impaired uterine blood flow → fetal hypoxia
- Rapid labor → cervical lacerations
- Rapid labor and birth → lacerations of cervix, vagina, perineum, uterine atony, fetal trauma
- Uterine rupture
- Water intoxication (nausea, vomiting, hypotension, tachycardia, cardiac arrhythmia) if oxytocin is given in electrolyte-free solution or at a rate exceeding 20 mU/minute; hypotension with rapid IV bolus administration postpartum

Effect on Fetus-Neonate

- Fetal effects are primarily associated with the presence of hypercontractility of the maternal uterus. Hypercontractility causes a decrease in the oxygen supply to the fetus, which is reflected by irregularities and/or decrease in FHR.
- Hyperbilirubinemia (Arias 1993).
- Trauma from rapid birth.

Nursing Considerations

- Explain induction or augmentation procedure to client.
- Apply fetal monitor and obtain 15- to 20-minute tracing and NST to assess FHR before starting IV oxytocin.
- For induction or augmentation of labor, start with primary IV and piggyback secondary IV with oxytocin and infusion pump.
- Ensure continuous fetal and uterine contraction monitoring.
- The maximum rate is 40 mU/minute (ACOG 1988). Not all protocols recommend a maximum dose. When indicated, it is generally between 16 and 40 mU/minute (Owen & Hauth 1992). Decrease oxytocin by similar increments once labor has progressed to 5–6 cm dilatation (ACOG 1988; Arias 1993).

0.5 mU/minute	= 3 mL/hour	8 mU/minute	= 48 mL/hour
1.0 mU/minute	= 6 mL/hour	10 mU/minute	= 60 mL/hour
1.5 mU/minute	= 9 mL/hour	12 mU/minute	= 72 mL/hour
2 mU/minute	= 12 mL/hour	15 mU/minute	= 90 mL/hour
4 mU/minute	= 24 mL/hour	18 mU/minute	= 108 mL/hour
6 mU/minute	= 36 mL/hour	20 mU/minute	= 120 mL/hour

  Protocols may vary from one agency to another.

- Assess FHR, maternal blood pressure, pulse, and uterine contraction frequency, duration, and resting tone before each increase in oxytocin infusion rate.

OXYTOCIN (PITOCIN) continued

- Record all assessments and IV rate on monitor strip and on client's chart.

- Record oxytocin infusion rate in mU/minute and mL/hour (eg, 0.5 mU/minute [3 mL/hour]).

- Record all client activities (such as change of position, vomiting), procedures done (amniotomy, sterile vaginal examination), and administration of analgesics on monitor strip to allow for interpretation and evaluation of tracing.

- Assess cervical dilatation as needed.

- Apply nursing comfort measures.

- Discontinue IV oxytocin infusion and infuse primary solution when (1) fetal distress is noted (bradycardia, late or variable decelerations; (2) uterine contractions are more frequent than every 2 minutes; (3) duration of contractions exceeds more than 60 seconds; or (4) insufficient relaxation of the uterus between contractions or a steady increase in resting tone are noted (ACOG 1988); in addition to discontinuing IV oxytocin infusion, turn client to side, and if fetal distress is present, administer oxygen by tight face mask at 7–10 L/minute; notify physician.

- Maintain intake and output record.

For augmentation of labor:

Prepare and administer IV Pitocin as for labor induction. Increase rate until labor contractions are of good quality. The flow rate is gradually increased at no less than every 30 minutes to a maximum of 10 mU/minute (Cunningham et al 1993). In some settings or in a situation when limited fluids may be administered, a more concentrated solution may be used. When 10 U Pitocin is added to 500 mL IV solution, the resulting concentration is 1 mU/minute = 3 mL/hour. If 10 U Pitocin is added to 250 mL IV solution, the concentration is 1 mU/minute = 1.5 mL/hour.

For administration after delivery of placenta:

- One dose of 10 units Pitocin (1 mL) is given intramuscularly or by slow intravenous push or added to IV fluids for continuous infusion.

- Assess FHR, maternal blood pressure, pulse, and uterine contraction frequency, duration, and resting tone before each increase in oxytocin infusion rate.

- Record all assessments and IV rate on monitor strip and on client's chart. Record oxytocin infusion rate in mU/minute and mL/hour (eg, 0.5 mU/minute [3 mL/hour]).

- Record all client activities (such as change of position, vomiting), procedures done (amniotomy, sterile vaginal examination), and administration of analgesics on monitor strip to allow for interpretation and evaluation of tracing.

- Assess cervical dilatation as needed.

- Apply nursing comfort measures.

- Discontinue IV oxytocin infusion and infuse primary solution when (1) fetal stress or distress is noted (tachycardia or bradycardia, late or variable decelerations), (2) uterine contractions are more frequent than every 2 minutes, (3) duration of contractions exceeds 60 seconds, or (4) insufficient relaxation of the uterus between contractions or a steady increase in resting tone are noted (ACOG 1988). In addition to discontinuing IV oxytocin infusion, turn client to side, and if fetal distress is present, administer oxygen by tight face mask at 7–10 L/minute; notify physician.

- Maintain intake and output record. Assess intake and output every hour.

---

before beginning the infusion. A fetal monitor is used to provide continuous data. Many institutional protocols recommend obtaining a 20 minute EFM recording and NST before the infusion is started to obtain baseline data on uterine contractions and FHR.

Before each advancement of the infusion rate, assessments of the following should be made:

- Maternal blood pressure and pulse

- Uterine contraction status, including frequency, duration, intensity, resting tone between contractions, and maternal response to the contractions

- FHR baseline, variability (short term and long term), presence of accelerations and decelerations

As contractions are established, vaginal examinations are done to evaluate cervical dilatation, effacement, and station. The frequency of vaginal examinations primarily depends on the woman's parity and on characteristics of contractions. For example, a nullipara with contractions every 5 to 7 minutes, each lasting 30 seconds, who does not perceive her contractions does not usually require a vaginal examination. But when her contractions are every 2 to 3 minutes, lasting 50 to 60 seconds with good intensity, a vaginal examination will be needed to evaluate her progress.

When evaluating the need for analgesia, a vaginal examination should be performed to avoid giving the medication too early and increasing the risk of prolonging labor and to identify advanced dilatation and imminent birth.

Nursing Diagnosis

The nursing diagnoses that may be appropriate for labor induction are presented in the Nursing Care Plan: Induction of Labor starting on page 766.

Text continues on page 768

INDUCTION OF LABOR

Nursing Assessment

Nursing History

1. Previous pregnancies, present pregnancy, and childbirth preparation
2. Estimated gestational age of the fetus

Physical Examination

1. Examination of pregnant uterus (Leopold's maneuvers to determine fetal size and position)
2. Vaginal examination to evaluate cervical readiness:
   a. Ripe cervix feels soft to the examining finger, is located in a medial to anterior position, is more than 50% effaced, and is 2–3 cm dilated.
   b. Unripe cervix feels firm to the examining finger, is long and thick, is perhaps in a posterior position, and is dilated little or not at all.
3. Presence of contractions

4. Membranes intact or ruptured
5. Fetal size (Leopold's maneuvers, ultrasound)
6. Fetal readiness
7. CPD evaluation
8. Maternal vital signs and a 20 minute baseline fetal monitoring strip prior to induction

Diagnostic Studies

1. Fetal maturity tests (L/S ratio, creatinine concentrations, ultrasonography), NST, CST, BPP
2. Maternal blood studies (CBC, hemoglobin, hematocrit, blood type, Rh factor)
3. Urinalysis

NURSING DIAGNOSIS: Knowledge deficit related to lack of information about induction procedure

EXPECTED OUTCOME: Woman will verbalize understanding of the induction process.

Nursing Interventions	Rationale
Assess the woman's feelings regarding induction and answer her questions.	*Woman may be apprehensive about what will happen or feel a sense of failure that she cannot "go into labor by herself."*
Assess knowledge base regarding the induction process.	*After assessing knowledge base, appropriate information can be given to allay apprehension.*
Provide needed information (for example, when the cervix is ripe, contractions should begin in 30–60 minutes). Inform the woman that the length of labor depends on a number of factors.	
Assess knowledge of breathing techniques. If the woman does not have a method to use, teach breathing techniques before starting oxytocin infusion.	*Use of breathing techniques during contractions will help relaxation. Although a woman may be apprehensive about induction, teaching a new breathing method will be easier before contractions are present.*

OUTCOME MET IF:

- Woman verbalizes understanding of the medication utilized, the need for frequent vital signs, and the need for continuing fetal monitoring to evaluate contractions and fetal response.

NURSING DIAGNOSIS: Decreased cardiac output related to positional changes and the weight of the uterus on the vena cava

EXPECTED OUTCOME: Woman's vital signs will remain within normal limits.

Nursing Interventions	Rationale
Position woman on her left side and encourage her to avoid supine position. At a minimum assess maternal BP and FHR before every dosage increase or as indicated by patient status, risk factors, and institutional policy.	*Side-lying position maintains optimal blood flow to uterus and placenta.*
If the woman becomes hypotensive: 1. Keep her on her side. May change to other side. 2. Discontinue oxytocin infusion. 3. Increase rate of primary IV. 4. Monitor FHR. 5. Notify physician. 6. Assess for cause of hypotension.	*Hypotension is secondary to peripheral vasodilation induced by oxytocin, which causes diminished blood supply to placenta and resultant decrease in oxygen supply to fetus. Actions are directed toward improving blood flow and oxygenation of tissues.*

OUTCOME MET IF:

- BP and pulse stay within baseline limits with no significant increase or decrease.
- FHR shows no signs of tachycardia (>160 bpm) or late decelerations.

INDUCTION OF LABOR *continued*

NURSING DIAGNOSIS: Altered tissue perfusion (placenta) related to potential hypertonic contraction pattern

EXPECTED OUTCOME: Woman will maintain normal contraction pattern.

Nursing Interventions	Rationale
Apply monitor to obtain 20 to 30 minute tracing prior to starting induction to evaluate fetal status.	*Establishes baseline data.*
Start primary IV of lactated Ringer's.	
Administer oxytocin in electrolyte solution.	*Oxytocin has slight antidiuretic effect, especially when administered in electrolyte-free solutions.*
Piggyback oxytocin into primary IV at closest site to IV needle insertion.	*This prevents a bolus of fluid with Pitocin if the IV rate needs to be increased.*
Encourage voiding every 2 hours. Monitor and record I/O.	*Provides information on hydration status.*
Monitor for nausea, vomiting, hypotension, tachycardia, cardiac arrhythmias, headache, mental confusion, ↓ urinary output.	*These are signs and symptoms of water intoxication and must be differentiated from other problems.*
Monitor FHR by continuous electronic fetal monitoring. *Do not* start infusion or advance rate (if induction has already begun) if FHR is not in range of 120–160 bpm, if decelerations are present, or if variability decreases.	*Will provide continuous data regarding fetal response to induction.*
Evaluate and document maternal BP and pulse before beginning induction and then before each increase in infusion rate. *Do not* advance infusion rate in presence of maternal hypertension or hypotension or radical changes in pulse rate.	*Establishes baseline data and helps assess client response in induction. Client status may change rapidly.*
Evaluate and document contraction frequency, duration, and intensity prior to each increase in infusion rate.	*Evaluates uterine response to induction.*
The dosage of oxytocin should be documented with each increase or decrease and should be charted in milliunits.	
Oxytocin infusion rate does not need to be increased if contractions are every 2–3 minutes lasting 40–90 seconds with moderate intensity.	*The desired effect has been obtained. Further increase in rate may produce hypertonic labor pattern (eg, contractions with frequency of less than 2 minutes or more than five contractions in 10 minutes or a duration of >90 seconds).*
Discontinue oxytocin infusion if: 1. Contractions are more frequent than every 2 minutes 2. Contraction duration exceeds 90 seconds 3. Uterus does not relax between contractions	*Uterus is being overstimulated, and serious complications may develop for woman and fetus. Ruptured uterus or abruptio placentae can result from drug-induced hyperstimulation (more than five contractions in 10 minutes or two or more contractions lasting more than 2 minutes) (Arias 1993). Contractions lasting over 90 seconds with decreased resting tone may result in fetal hypoxia.*
Increase oxytocin IV infusion rate every 20 minutes until adequate contractions are achieved. *Do not exceed* an infusion rate of 20–40 mU/minute (Note: Protocols directing how often oxytocin is increased may vary from 15–60 minutes. See ACOG 1991 guidelines and institutional protocol.)	*Uterine response to oxytocin may be individualized.*
Check infusion pump to assure oxytocin is infusing. Check whether pump is on, chamber refills and empties, level of fluid in IV bottle becomes lower. If problem is found, correct it, and restart infusion at beginning dose. Check main IV site frequently. Check piggyback connection to primary tubing to assure solution is not leaking.	*Oxytocin may not be infusing due to pump, mechanical, or human error.*
Evaluate cervical dilatation by vaginal examination with each oxytocin dosage increase after labor is established.	*If vaginal exam reveals that the cervix seems to stretch easily, do not increase oxytocin dosage. Overdosage may occur, causing rapid labor with possible cervical lacerations and fetal damage. When there is no change in the cervix, additional oxytocin is needed.*
Monitor FHR continuously (normal range is 120–160 bpm). In episodes of bradycardia (<120 bpm) lasting for more than 30 seconds administer oxygen by face mask at 7–10 L/minute. Stop oxytocin infusion. Position woman on left side if quick recovery of FHR does not occur.	*Oxygen deficiency may occur over a long period of time. In cases of placental insufficiency or cord compression, compensated tachycardia may be evoked.*
Carefully evaluate fetal tachycardia (>160 bpm). Sustained tachycardia may necessitate discontinuation of oxytocin infusion. Assess for presence of meconium staining. Notify physician.	*Persistent fetal tachycardia causes more prominent oxygen deficiency (hypoxia) and carbon dioxide increase in fetal blood. Vasoconstriction occurs, with increased fetal blood flow through coronary arteries, brain, and placenta. This increased demand on myocardial performance leads to cardiac decompensation if oxygen exchange is impaired and hypoxia continues. Fetal hypoxia may also cause central vasomotor center to release adrenal catecholamines; at term this enhances depolarization of cardiac tachycardia oxygen deficiency.*

OUTCOME MET IF: • Woman's contraction pattern is established: contraction frequency 2–3 minutes, duration 40–90 seconds, relaxation of uterus between contractions is adequate per palpation and no greater than 20 mm Hg per monitor.

INDUCTION OF LABOR *continued*

NURSING DIAGNOSIS: Pain related to uterine contractions

EXPECTED OUTCOME: Woman will report reasonable comfort.

Nursing Interventions	Rationale
Provide support to woman as she uses breathing techniques.	*Contractions may build up more quickly with oxytocin infusion and may be more painful.*
Encourage use of effluerage, back rub, and other supportive measures.	*Techniques help maintain relaxation and thereby decrease pain sensation.*
Assess need for analgesia or anesthesia.	*After labor is well established analgesia or epidural anesthesia may be given without delaying progress.*

OUTCOME MET IF:

- Woman maintains breathing pattern and sense of control during labor.
- Woman reports a pain level of 5 or less (on a scale of 1–10) at all times during labor.

Essential Nursing Activities to Achieve Outcomes

Before Infusion

1. Perform 20 to 30 minute fetal reactive strip to validate fetal well-being and obtain baseline information.
2. Perform vaginal exam to obtain baseline data on dilatation, effacement, and station.
3. Assess for presence of contractions.
4. Obtain maternal vital signs: BP, P, R.
5. Provide emotional support through teaching and answering all questions.
6. Discuss comfort measures.

During Infusion

1. Start primary IV—piggyback oxytocin in electrolyte solution at closest IV insertion site.
2. Position woman in left lateral or semi-Fowler's position.

3. Adjust oxytocin rate no more often than 20 to 60 minute intervals at 1–2 mU/minute (See Drug Guide: Oxytocin [Pitocin].)
4. With each medication increase, assess maternal vital signs, contraction pattern, and fetal heart rate.
5. Discontinue oxytocin infusion if any of the following develop:
   a. Tachycardia or bradycardia
   b. Persistent late decelerations
   c. Prolonged variable decelerations
   d. Decreased long-term variability, absent short-term variability
   e. Contractions closer than every 2 minutes with a duration greater than 90 seconds
6. To restart oxytocin, all the above indications should have subsided for 30 minutes.
7. Oxytocin can be restarted at beginning rate or at half the dose when discontinued.

Nursing Plan and Implementation

During the oxytocin infusion the woman needs to be attented by nurses who are able to identify both maternal and fetal complications. A qualified obstetrician should be readily accessible to manage any complication that may occur (ACOG 1991).

Aspects to address during client teaching include the purpose and procedure for the induction, nursing care that will be provided, assessments during the induction procedure, comfort measures, and a review of breathing techniques that may be used during labor.

For additional information on nursing interventions see Drug Guide: Oxytocin (Pitocin) on page 764 and Nursing Care Plan: Induction of Labor on page 766.

Intravenous oxytocin may also be given for augmentation of labor; see Drug Guide: Oxytocin (Pitocin) on page 764 for further discussion.

Evaluation

Anticipated outcomes of nursing care include:

- The woman's labor is successfully induced.
- The labor and birth process are within normal limits, and the woman and her baby do not experience any complications.

CARE OF THE WOMAN DURING AMNIOINFUSION

Amnioinfusion is a technique by which approximately 250 mL to 300 mL of warmed, sterile, normal saline is introduced into the uterus. The normal saline is infused through an intrauterine catheter under the control of an infusion pump. Amnioinfusion is used in cases of oligohydramnios or thick, meconium-stained amniotic fluid and for intrauterine administration of antibiotics (Posner 1990). When oligohydramnios is present, there is not enough fluid to allow the umbilical cord to float freely, so it can become compressed against various parts of the fetus. When cord compression occurs, the blood supply to the fetus is diminished, and FHR bradycardia, variable decelerations, or both develop. Increasing the fluid volume of the uterus allows the cord to float and decreases the incidence and severity of variable decelerations.

If the fetus is stressed, meconium may be released into the amniotic fluid. If a small amount of meconium is released, light meconium staining of the amniotic fluid (light blackish-green discoloration) may occur. However, release of a large amount of meconium results in amniotic fluid that is more discolored and contains a high concentration of meconium. This concentrated fluid, if not expelled from the fetal mouth and throat during chest compression at birth, may be inspired by the fetus. Meconium aspiration and/or pneumonitis may occur. When thick, meconium-stained amniotic fluid is present during labor, amnioinfusion may be used to dilute the amniotic fluid and decrease the newborn's chances of inspiring meconium.

If chorioamnionitis (infection within the uterus) is present, an amnioinfusion may be used to instill antibiotics directly into the uterus.

CRITICAL THINKING IN PRACTICE

You are a birthing center nurse caring for Mary Johnson, gravida 2, para 1, during an oxytocin infusion to induce her labor. Mary has been receiving the medication via infusion pump for 4 hours and currently is receiving 6 mU/minute (36 mL/hour). You have just completed your assessments and found the following: BP 120/80, pulse 80, respirations 16; contractions every 3 minutes lasting 60 seconds and of strong intensity; the FHR baseline is 144–150 with average long-term variability; and cervical dilatation is 6 cm. Will you continue the same infusion rate, increase the rate, or decrease the rate?

Answers can be found in Appendix I.

Nursing Care

The nurse is frequently the first person to detect changes in FHR associated with cord compression or to observe thick, meconium-stained amniotic fluid. When cord compression is suspected, the immediate intervention is to assist the laboring woman to another position in an effort to relieve the compression (see Chapter 25 for further discussion). If this intervention is not successful, an amnioinfusion will be considered. The nurse helps with the amnioinfusion and monitors the woman's vital signs (blood pressure, pulse, and respiration) and contraction status (frequency, duration, intensity, resting tone, and associated maternal discomfort). FHR is monitored by continuous EFM. It is very important to provide ongoing information to the laboring woman and her partner and to answer questions as they arise. Comfort measures and positioning will be very important because the woman will now be on bed rest.

The amnioinfusion should not cause pain or discomfort for the laboring woman other than the need for bed rest. Depending upon the reason the amnioinfusion is done, it should result in decreased incidence and severity of variable decelerations, or the meconium-stained fluid should appear less thick and lighter in color.

CARE OF THE WOMAN DURING AN EPISIOTOMY

An **episiotomy** is a surgical incision of the perineal body that is done to protect the perineum, sphincter, and rectum from lacerations during the birth and to decrease the length of the second stage of labor (Bartscht & DeLancey 1992).

An episiotomy is one of the most common procedures in maternal-child care. Researchers estimate the rate of episiotomies as 60–90% of primigravidas (Crawford et al 1993). Even though the procedure is very common, its routine use has been questioned (Thorp & Bowes 1989). Current research suggests that rather than protecting the perineum from lacerations, the presence of an episiotomy makes it more likely that the woman will have deep perineal tears (Henriksen et al 1992). Borgatta et al (1989) reported that third- and fourth-degree perineal tears occurred in 27.9% of women who had an episiotomy and used stirrups during birth, as compared to 0.9% of women who gave birth without episiotomy or the use of stirrups. Additional complications associated with an episiotomy may be infection, blood loss, and pain and perineal discomfort that may continue for days or weeks past birth, including dyspareunia (painful intercourse) (Bartscht & DeLancey 1992).

Episiotomy Procedure

The episiotomy is performed with sharp scissors that have rounded points, just before birth, when approximately 3 to 4 cm of the fetal head is visible during a contraction (Cunningham et al 1993). There are two types in current practice: midline and mediolateral (Figure 26–3). A midline episiotomy is performed along the median raphe of the perineum. It extends down from the vaginal orifice to the fibers of the rectal sphincter. This type of episiotomy avoids muscle fibers and major blood vessels because it divides the insertions of the superficial perineal muscles. A midline episiotomy is preferred if the perineum is of adequate length and no difficulty is anticipated during the birth because the blood loss is less and the incision is easy to repair and heals with less discomfort for the mother. The major disadvantage is that a tear of the midline incision may extend through the anal sphincter and rectum.

In the presence of a short perineum, macrosomia, and instrumental delivery, a mediolateral episiotomy provides more room and decreases the possibility of a traumatic extension into the rectum (Crawford et al 1993). The mediolateral episiotomy begins in the midline of the posterior fourchette (in order to avoid incision into the Bartholin's gland) and extends at a 45-degree angle downward to the right or left (the direction depending on the handedness of the clinician). The mediolateral episiotomy may be complicated by greater blood loss, a longer healing period, and more postpartal discomfort.

The episiotomy is usually performed with regional or local anesthesia but may be performed without anesthesia in emergency situations. It is generally proposed that as crowning occurs, the distention of the tissues causes numbing. Adequate anesthesia must be given for the repair.

Repair of the episiotomy (episiorrhaphy) and any lacerations is accomplished either during the period between birth of the neonate and before expulsion of the placenta or after expulsion of the placenta.

Nursing Care

The woman needs to be supported during the repair because she may feel some pressure sensations. In the absence of adequate anesthesia she may feel pain. Placing a hand on her shoulder and talking with her can provide comfort and distraction from the repair process. If the

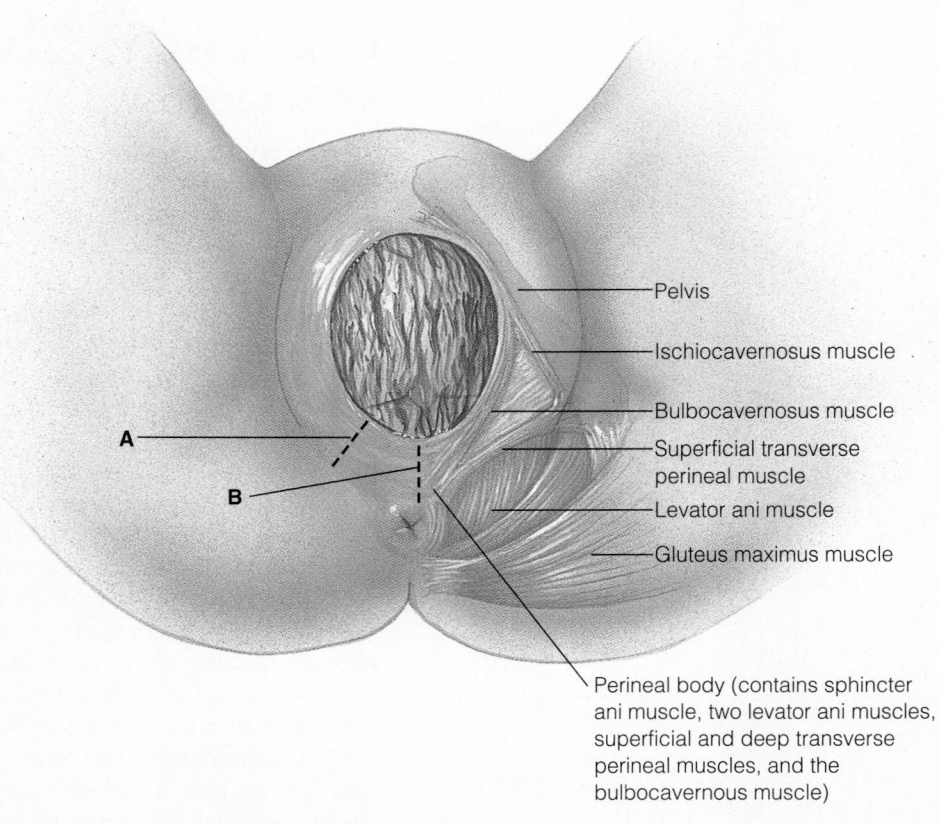

Pelvis

Ischiocavernosus muscle

Bulbocavernosus muscle

Superficial transverse perineal muscle

Levator ani muscle

Gluteus maximus muscle

Perineal body (contains sphincter ani muscle, two levator ani muscles, superficial and deep transverse perineal muscles, and the bulbocavernous muscle)

FIGURE 26-3   The two most common types of episiotomies are midline and mediolateral. *A* Right mediolateral. *B* Midline.

woman is having more discomfort than she can comfortably handle, the nurse needs to act as an advocate in communicating the woman's needs to the physician/CNM. At all times the woman needs to be the one who decides whether the amount of discomfort is tolerable, and she should never be told "This doesn't hurt." She is the person experiencing the discomfort, and her evaluation needs to be respected. If there are just a few (three to five) stitches left, she may choose to forego more local anesthesia, but she should be given the choice.

The type of episiotomy is recorded on the birth record. This information should also be included in a report to the recovery room so that adequate assessments can be made and relief measures can be instituted if necessary.

Pain relief measures may begin immediately after birth with application of an ice pack to the perineum. For optimal effect the ice pack should be applied for 20 to 30 minutes and removed for at least 20 minutes before being reapplied because the ice causes vasoconstriction, and if left in place more than 30 minutes, vasodilatation and subsequent edema may occur. The perineal tissues should be assessed frequently to prevent injury from the ice pack. The episiotomy site should be inspected every 15 minutes during the first hour after the birth for redness, swelling, tenderness, and hematomas. As a part of postpartal care the mother will need instruction in perineal hygiene care and comfort measures. (See Chapter 34 for additional discussion of relief measures.)

Critical Thinking Question

As a new mother's episiotomy is repaired, she says that she can feel the procedure and that it hurts. What will you do?

CARE OF THE WOMAN DURING FORCEPS-ASSISTED BIRTH

Forceps are designed to assist the birth of a fetus by providing traction or by providing the means to rotate the fetal head to an occiput-anterior position. A special type of forceps is designed to be used with a breech presentation, in which the forceps are applied to the aftercoming fetal head (called aftercoming because the head is born after the body). In 1988, after years of defining forceps applications as either low/outlet forceps or midforceps, the American College of Obstetricians and Gynecologists reclassified forceps applications into three categories: outlet, low, and midforceps. Criteria for outlet forceps application are as follows:

1. Forceps are applied when the fetal skull has reached the perineum. (There is bulging of the perineum.)

2. The scalp is visible between contractions. (Earlier in labor, as the woman pushes during the contraction,

the fetal scalp may be visible, but when the pushing effort ceases, the scalp recedes and is no longer visible. This criterion indicates that the scalp remains visible even when the woman is not pushing.)

3. The sagittal suture is not more than 45 degrees from the midline. The sagittal suture is the anterior-posterior suture on the top of the fetal head. At this point in a spontaneous birth, extension has almost been completed, external rotation is beginning, and the sagittal suture is between the midline and 45 degrees from the midline. (For example, think of a clock face. If 12 o'clock is the maternal symphysis pubis and the fetus is in LOA, the sagittal suture and the occiput are between 12 and 1:30.) The important aspect of this criterion is that with outlet forceps the fetal head is moving naturally from extension to external rotation, and the forceps are being used to guide or lift the head out.

The criterion for low forceps application is the leading edge (presenting part) of the fetal skull is at a station of +2 or more. The criterion for midforceps application is the fetal head is engaged (largest diameter of the head reaches or passes through the pelvic inlet), but the leading edge (presenting part) of the fetal skull is above +2 station. When midforceps are used, the goal is usually to rotate the head as well as to apply traction and facilitate the birth. Types of forceps used are depicted in Figure 26–4.

Indications

Indications for the use of forceps include the presence of any condition that threatens the mother or fetus and that can be relieved by birth. Conditions that put the woman at risk include heart disease, acute pulmonary edema, intrapartal infection, or exhaustion. Fetal conditions include premature placental separation and fetal distress. Forceps may be used electively to shorten the second stage of labor and spare the woman's pushing effort (when exhaustion and/or heart disease is present) or when regional anesthesia has affected the woman's motor innervation and she cannot push effectively. In the past, outlet forceps have been used to protect the head of a preterm infant during birth; however, the advantages of this practice are now being questioned (ACOG 1991; Cunningham et al 1993).

Neonatal Risks

Some neonates may develop a small area of ecchymosis and/or edema along the sides of the face as a result of forceps application. Caput succedaneum or cephalhematoma (and subsequent hyperbilirubinemia) may occur as well as transient facial paralysis. Previous studies suggested decreased IQ scores in children delivered by forceps. However, recent studies do not support these findings (Wesley et al 1993).

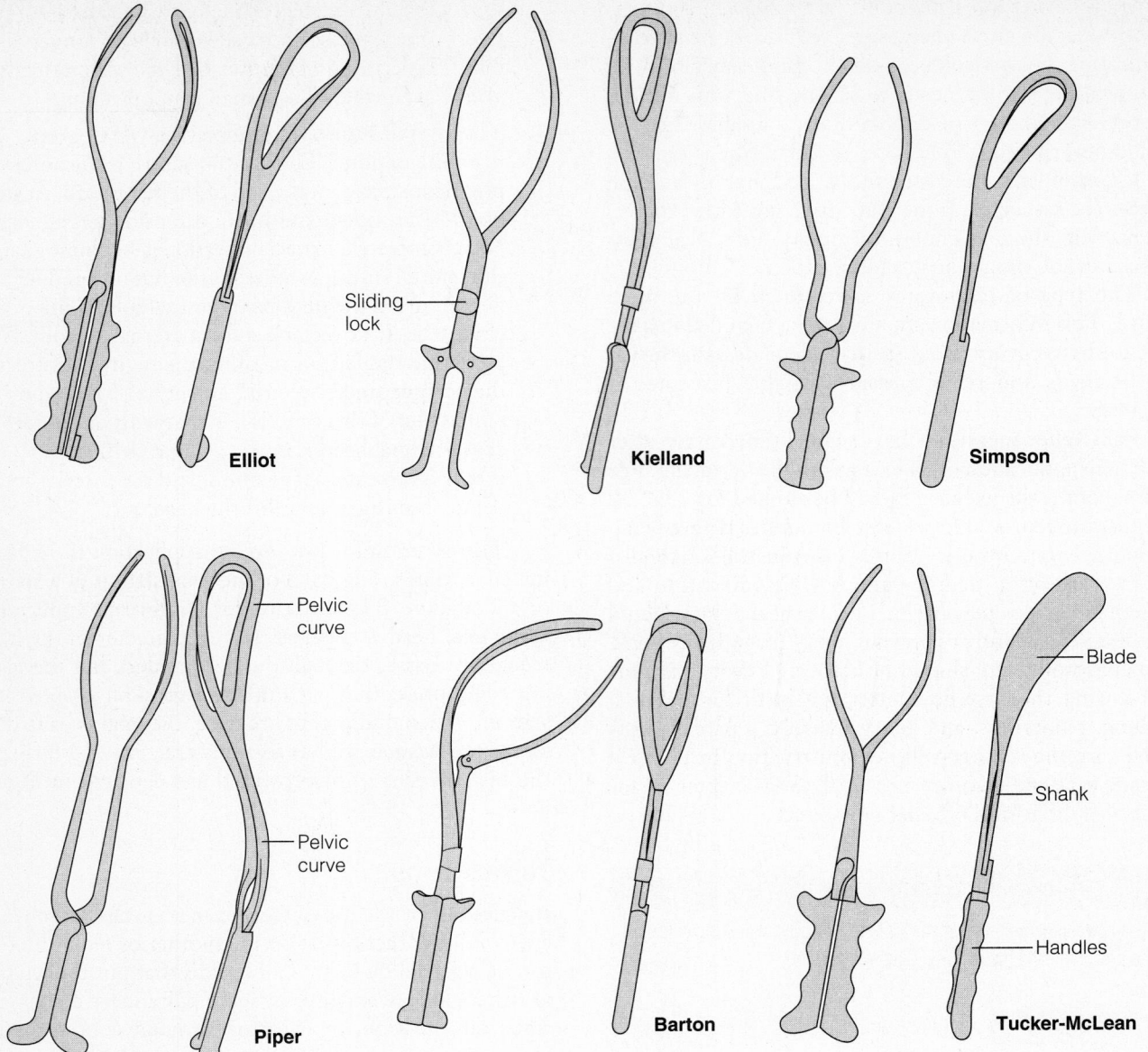

FIGURE 26-4 Forceps are composed of a blade, shank, and handle and may have a cephalic and pelvic curve. (Note labels on Piper and Tucker-McLean forceps.) The blades may be fenestrated (open) or solid. The front and lateral views of these forceps illustrate differences in blades, open and closed shank, and cephalic and pelvic curves. Elliot, Simpson, and Tucker-McLean forceps are used as outlet forceps. Kielland and Barton forceps are used for midforceps rotations. Piper forceps are used to provide traction and flexion of the after-coming head (the head comes after the body) of a fetus in breech presentation.

Prerequisites for Forceps Application

Use of forceps requires complete dilatation of the cervix and knowledge of the exact position and station of the fetal head. The membranes must be ruptured to allow a firm grasp on the fetal head. The presentation must be vertex or face with the chin anterior. In addition *there must be no disproportion between the fetal head and the maternal pelvis* (Cunningham et al 1993).

Trial or Failed Forceps Procedure

In a trial forceps procedure the physician attempts to use forceps with the knowledge that there is a degree of CPD. A complete setup for immediate cesarean birth needs to be available before the forceps are applied. If a good application cannot be obtained or if no descent occurs with the application, cesarean birth is the method of choice.

Nursing Care

The nurse can explain the procedure briefly to the woman. With adequate regional anesthesia the woman should feel some pressure but no pain. The nurse encourages her to maintain breathing techniques to prevent her from pushing during application of the forceps (Figure 26–5). The nurse monitors contractions. With each contraction the physician/CNM provides traction on the forceps as the woman pushes. The nurse monitors the FHR during each contraction until the birth. It is not uncommon to observe bradycardia as traction is being applied to the forceps. This bradycardia results from head compression and is transient.

The newborn is assessed for facial edema, bruising, caput succedaneum, cephalhematoma, and any sign of cerebral edema. In the fourth stage the nurse assesses the woman for perineal swelling, bruising, hematoma, and hemorrhage. In the postpartum period it is important to assess for signs of infection.

The nurse answers questions and reiterates explanations provided. Nursing assessments of the woman and her newborn are reviewed. Opportunities for questions are provided.

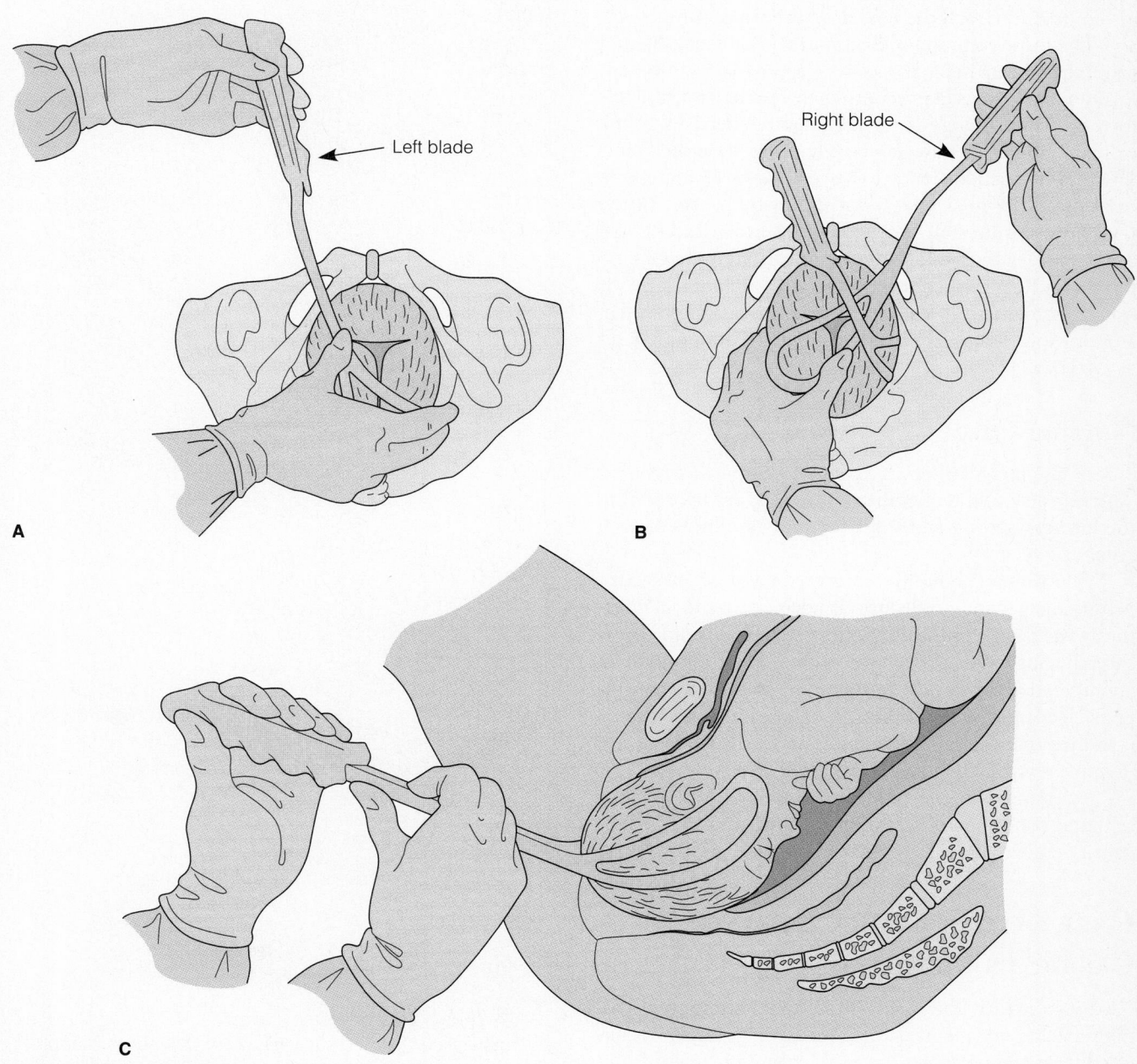

A

Left blade

Right blade

B

C

FIGURE 26-5 Application of forceps in occiput anterior (OA) position. *A* The left blade is inserted along the left side wall of the pelvis over the parietal bone. *B* The right blade is inserted along the right side wall of the pelvis over the parietal bone.

C With correct placement of the blades, the handles lock easily. During uterine contractions traction is applied to the forceps in a downward and outward direction to follow the birth canal.

CARE OF THE WOMAN DURING VACUUM EXTRACTION

Vacuum extraction is an obstetric procedure used to assist the birth of a fetus by applying suction to the fetal head. The vacuum extractor is composed of a soft suction cup attached to a suction bottle (pump) by tubing. The suction cup, which comes in various sizes, is placed against the occiput of the fetal head. Care must be taken to ensure that no cervical or vaginal tissue is trapped under the cup. The pump is used to create negative pressure (suction), and an artificial caput ("chignon") is formed. The physician then applies traction in coordination with uterine contractions, and the fetal head is born (Figure 26–6).

The most common indication for use of the vacuum extractor is a prolonged second stage of labor. Vacuum extraction is also used to relieve the woman of pushing effort or when analgesia or fatigue interfere with the woman's ability to push effectively (Niswander & Evans 1991). The vacuum extractor is preferred to forceps in cases of borderline CPD, when successful passage of the fetal head requires all potential space inside the vaginal canal. CPD is an absolute contraindication to vacuum extraction. Relative contraindications include face or breech presentation, extreme prematurity, macrosomia, and previous fetal scalp blood sampling (Cunningham et al 1993).

Nursing Care

There are many different types of vacuum extractors. The nurse should be familiar with the types used within the birthing setting and learn the pressure limits of each type.

The woman should be informed about what is happening during the procedure. If adequate regional anesthesia has been administered, the woman feels only pressure during the procedure. The FHR should be auscultated at least every 5 minutes or assessed by continuous electronic fetal monitoring. The parents need to be informed that the caput (chignon) on the baby's head will disappear within 2–3 days (Laufe et al 1990).

Assessment of the newborn should include inspection and continued observation for intracranial and subgaleal hemorrhage (Hall 1992).

CARE OF THE FAMILY DURING CESAREAN BIRTH

Cesarean birth is the birth of the infant through an abdominal and uterine incision. The word "cesarean" is derived from the Latin word *caedere*, meaning "to cut." Cesarean birth is one of the oldest surgical procedures known. Until the 20th century cesareans were primarily equated with an attempt to save the fetus of a dying

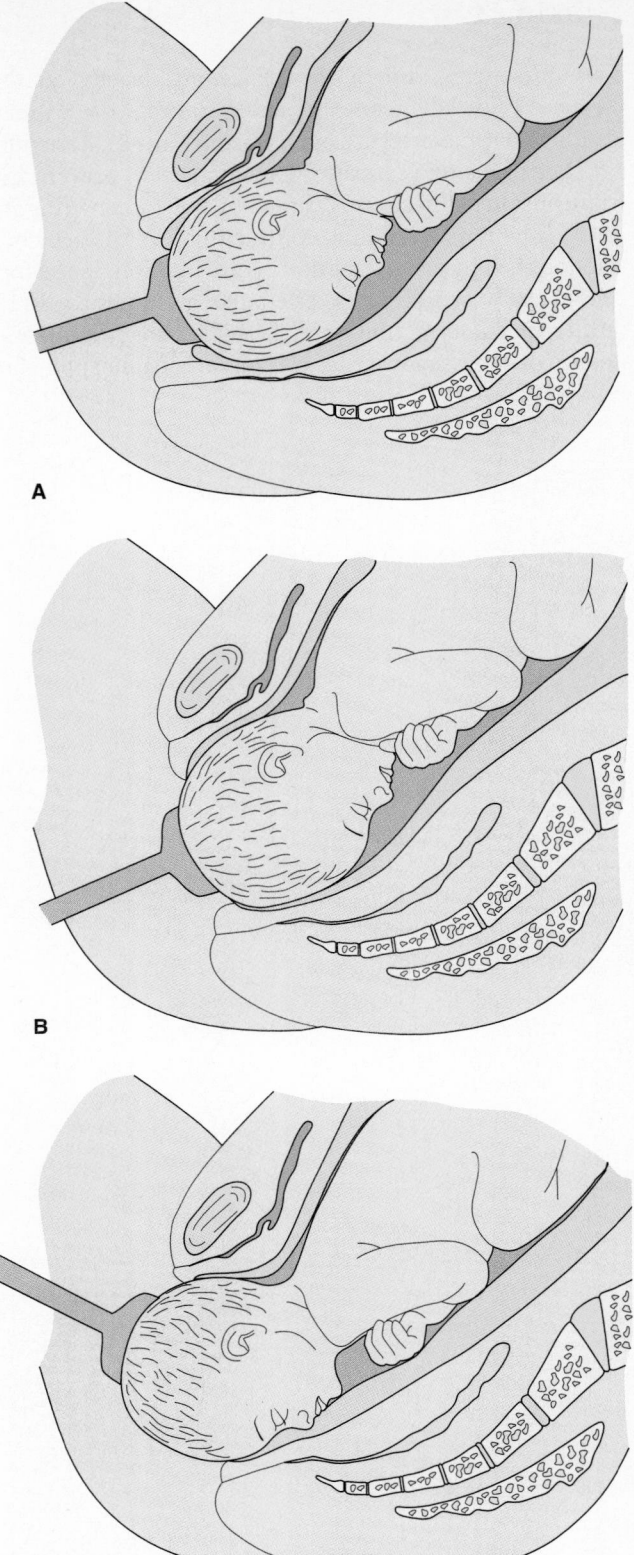

A

B

C

FIGURE 26-6 Vacuum extractor traction. *A* The cup is placed on the fetal occiput and suction is created. Traction is applied in a downward and outward direction. *B* Traction continues in a downward direction as the fetal head begins to emerge from the vagina. *C* Traction is maintained to lift the fetal head out of the vagina.

woman. As the maternal and perinatal morbidity and mortality rates associated with cesarean birth have steadily decreased throughout this century, the proportion of cesarean births has increased. In 1970 cesarean births comprised 5.5% of all births. Currently, approximately 23.5% of all births in the United States are by cesarean (Scott 1994). England has a cesarean birth rate of 12%; Wales, 13.5%; Scotland, 14.2% (Francome & Savage 1993); and Sweden, 10.8% (Nielsen et al 1994). International leaders in obstetric care suggest that a cesarean rate of no more than 12% is a realistic goal (some identify 7% as a target goal) and note that some countries have rates of just 2% with very low perinatal and maternal morbidity (Sakala 1993).

Many factors affect the cesarean birth rate, and they need to be considered in discussions about decreasing the current rate in the United States. Factors include changing philosophies regarding the best method of delivering breech presentation, interpretations of EFM tracings, and changing practice related to vaginal birth after cesarean birth (Nielsen et al 1994; Scott 1994). Many social, political, and gender issues also affect the cesarean birth rate. Women of higher socioeconomic class, who are better insured and cared for in private services with a physician, are more likely to have a cesarean birth than women who are of lower economic status, less healthy, and receiving public services (Sakala 1993). Other influencing factors include ethnicity, maternal age, maternal employment status, and the woman's ability to negotiate care (Sakala 1993).

Indications

Cesarean births are performed in the presence of a variety of maternal and fetal conditions. Commonly accepted indications include complete placenta previa, cephalic pelvic disproportion, placental abruption, active genital herpes, umbilical cord prolapse, failure to progress in labor, proven fetal distress, benign and malignant tumors that obstruct the birth canal, and cervical cerclage (Scott 1994). Indications that are more controversial include breech presentation, previous cesarean birth, major congenital anomalies, and severe Rh isoimmunization (Scott 1994). Of the current cesareans performed in the United States, 33% are for repeat cesarean birth, 30% are for dystocia, and the remaining 34% consist of all other indications (Scott 1994).

Maternal Mortality and Morbidity

Cesarean births have two to four times the maternal mortality of vaginal births. Although mortality is still low (approximately 1 to 2 deaths per 1000 cesareans as opposed to 0.06 deaths per 1000 live vaginal births), 25% of deaths are due to anesthesia complications (Dunn 1990). Morbidity occurs in 25% to 50% of women and is associated with a fairly wide variety of complications such as unexplained fever, endometritis, wound infection, urinary tract infection, atelectasis, thrombophlebitis, and pulmonary embolism (Scott 1994).

Surgical Techniques

Skin Incisions

The skin incision for a cesarean birth is either transverse (Pfannenstiel) or vertical and is not indicative of the type of incision made into the uterus. The transverse incision is made across the lowest and narrowest part of the abdomen. Because the incision is made just below the pubic hair line, it is almost invisible after healing. The limitations of this type of skin incision are that it does not allow for extension of the incision if needed. Because it usually requires more time, this incision is used when time is not of the essence (eg, with failure to progress and no fetal or maternal distress).

The vertical (infraumbilical midline) incision is made between the navel and the symphysis pubis. This type of incision is quicker and is therefore preferred in cases of fetal distress when rapid birth is indicated, preterm or macrosomic infants, or when the woman is obese (Cunningham et al 1993). The type of skin incision is determined by time factor, client preference, or physician preference.

Uterine Incisions

The type of uterine incision depends on the need for the cesarean. The choice of incision affects the woman's opportunity for a subsequent vaginal birth and her risks of a ruptured uterine scar with a subsequent pregnancy.

The two major types of uterine incisions are in the lower uterine segment or in the upper segment of the uterine corpus.

The lower uterine segment incision that is most commonly used is a transverse incision, although a vertical incision may also be used (Figure 26–7). The *transverse incision* is preferred for the following reasons (Cunningham et al 1993; Scott et al 1990):

1. The lower segment is the thinnest portion of the uterus and involves less blood loss.

2. It requires only moderate dissection of bladder from underlying myometrium.

3. It is easier to repair, although repair takes longer.

4. The site is less likely to rupture during subsequent pregnancies.

5. There is a decreased chance of adherence of bowel or omentum to the incision line.

The disadvantages include the following:

1. It takes longer to make a transverse incision.

2. It is limited in size because of the presence of major blood vessels on either side of the uterus.

3. It has a greater tendency to extend laterally into the uterine vessels.

4. The incision may stretch and become a thin win-

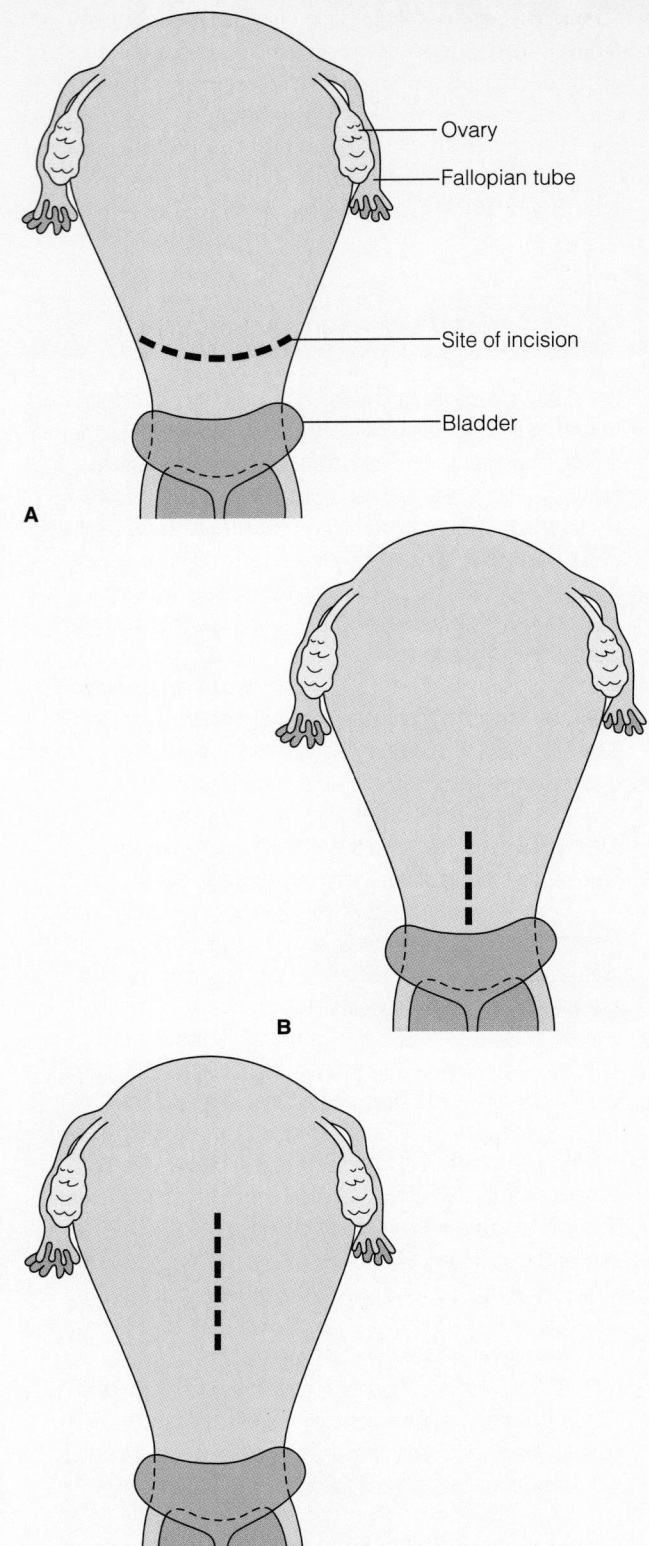

FIGURE 26-7 Uterine incisions for a cesarean birth. *A* This transverse incision in the lower uterine segment is called a Kerr incision. *B* The Sellheim incision is a vertical incision in the lower uterine segment. *C* This view illustrates the classic uterine incision that is done in the body (corpus) of the uterus. The classic incision was commonly done in the past and is associated with increased risk of uterine rupture in subsequent pregnancies and labor.

dow, but it usually does not create problems clinically until subsequent labor ensues.

The *lower uterine segment vertical incision* is preferred for multiple gestation, abnormal presentation, placenta previa, fetal distress, and preterm and macrosomic fetuses. Disadvantages of this incision are as follows:

1. The incision may extend downward into the cervix.
2. More extensive dissection of the bladder is needed to keep the incision in the lower uterine segment.
3. If it extends upward into the upper segment, hemostasis and closure are more difficult.
4. The chance of rupture with subsequent labor is increased (Martin et al 1993).

One other incision, the *classic incision*, was the method of choice for many years but is used infrequently now. This vertical incision was made into the upper uterine segment. More blood loss resulted, and it was more difficult to repair. Most important, there was an increased risk of uterine rupture with subsequent pregnancy, labor, and birth because the upper uterine segment is the most contractile portion of the uterus.

Nursing Care

Preparation for Cesarean Birth

Because one out of every three to four births is a cesarean, preparation for this possibility should be an integral part of prenatal education. *All* pregnant women and their partners should be encouraged to discuss with their obstetrician what the approach would be in the event of a cesarean. They can also discuss their needs and desires as a couple under those circumstances. Their preferences may include the following:

- Participating in the choice of anesthetic
- Father (or significant other) being present during the procedures and/or birth
- Father (or significant other) being present in the recovery or postpartum room
- Audio recording and/or taking pictures of the birth
- Delayed instillation of eye drops to promote eye contact between parent and infant in the first hours after birth
- Physical contact or holding the newborn while on the operating room table and/or in the recovery room (If the mother cannot hold the newborn, the father can hold the baby for her.)
- Breastfeeding immediately after birth

Information that couples need about cesarean birth includes the following:

- Preparation that may be done, such as abdominal prep, insertion of an indwelling bladder catheter, and starting an intravenous infusion

- Description or viewing of the delivery room
- Types of anesthesia for birth and analgesia available postpartum
- Sensations that may be experienced
- Roles of significant others
- Interaction with newborn
- Immediate recovery phase
- Postpartal phase

The context in which this information is given should be "birth oriented" rather than surgery oriented.

Preparation for Repeat Cesarean Birth

When a couple is anticipating a cesarean birth, they have time to analyze and synthesize the information they are given and to prepare for the experience. Many hospitals or local groups (such as C-Sec Inc) provide preparation classes for cesarean birth. The instructor should impart factual information and a feeling of normality, which will allow a couple to make choices and participate in their birth experience. Couples who have had previous negative experiences need an opportunity to describe what they felt contributed to these events. They should be encouraged to identify what they would like to have altered and to list interventions that would make the experience more positive. Those who have had positive experiences need reassurance that their needs and desires will be met in the same manner. In addition an opportunity should be given to discuss any fears or anxieties.

In a study by Reichert, Baron, and Fawcett (1993) women who had recently had a cesarean birth identified aspects of care that would have improved their experience. More support and information from nurses and physicians were major concerns. Nurses are in a position to provide additional information and to interpret explanations given by others if the couple does not understand. Women also wanted their partner with them more, especially during the administration of regional blocks, and more contact with the baby following the birth.

Preparation for Emergency Cesarean Birth

The period preceding surgery must be used to its greatest advantage. The couple needs some time for privacy to assimilate the information given to them and to ask for additional information. It is imperative that care givers use their most effective communication skills. The nurse must address what the couple may anticipate during the next few hours. Asking the couple "What questions do you have about the decision?" gives the couple an opportunity for further clarification. The nurse can prepare the woman in stages, giving her information and the rationale for each procedure before commencing. Before carrying out a procedure, it is essential to tell the woman (1) what is going to happen, (2) why it is being done, and (3) what sensations she may experience. This allows the woman to be informed and to consent to the procedure. The woman experiences a sense of control and therefore less helplessness and powerlessness.

Preparing the woman for surgery involves more than the procedures of establishing intravenous lines and urinary catheter or doing an abdominal prep. As discussed previously, good communication skills are very influential in helping the couple. Therapeutic touch and eye contact do much to maintain reality orientation and control. These measures reduce anxiety for the woman during the stressful preparatory period.

If the cesarean birth is scheduled and not an emergency, the nurse has ample time for preoperative teaching. The woman needs to practice her turning, coughing, and deep breathing. It is helpful if she is taught to splint her abdominal muscles when she coughs. An informed consent for surgery will need to be signed.

To prepare the woman for the surgery, she is given nothing by mouth. To reduce the likelihood of serious pulmonary damage should aspiration of gastric contents occur, antacids may be administered within 30 minutes of surgery. If epidural anesthesia is used, the nurse may assist with the procedure, monitor the woman's blood pressure and response, and continue EFM. An abdominal and perineal prep is done, and an indwelling catheter is inserted to prevent bladder distention. An intravenous line is started with a needle of adequate size to permit blood administration, and preoperative medication may be ordered. The pediatrician should be notified and adequate preparation made to receive the infant. The nurse should make sure that the infant warmer is functional and that appropriate resuscitation equipment is available.

The nurse assists in positioning the woman on the operating table. Fetal heart rate should be ascertained before surgery and during preparation because fetal hypoxia can result from aortocaval compression. The operating table may be adjusted so it slants slightly to one side, or a wedge (folded blanket or towels) may be placed under the right hip. The uterus should be displaced about 15 degrees from the midline. This helps relieve the pressure of the heavy uterus on the vena cava and lessens the incidence of vena caval compression and supine maternal hypotension. The suction should be in working order, and the urine collection bag should be positioned under the operating table to ensure proper urinary drainage. Auscultation or electronic monitoring of the fetal heart rate needs to continue until immediately prior to the surgery. A last-minute check is done to ensure that the fetal scalp electrode has been removed if the fetus was internally monitored.

Birth

Every effort should be made to include the father/partner in the birth experience. When the father attends the cesarean birth, he must scrub and wear a surgical gown and mask as do others in the operating suite. A stool can be placed beside the woman's head. The father can sit nearby to provide physical touch, visual contact, and verbal reassurance to his partner.

Other measures, such as the following, can be taken to promote the participation of the father who chooses not to be in the delivery room:

1. Allowing the father to be near the delivery/operating room, where he can hear the newborn's first cry

2. Encouraging the father to carry or accompany the infant to the nursery for the initial assessment

3. Involving the father in postpartal care in the recovery room

After birth the nurse assesses the Apgar score and completes the initial assessment and identification procedures as after a vaginal birth. Every effort must be made to assist the parents in bonding with the infant. If the mother is awake, one of her arms should be freed to enable her to touch and stroke the infant. The baby can be given to the father to hold until she or he must be taken to the nursery.

Analgesia and Anesthesia

There is no perfect anesthesia for cesarean birth. Each has its advantages, disadvantages, possible risks, and side effects. Goals for analgesia and anesthesia administration include safety, comfort, and emotional satisfaction for the client. See Chapter 24.

Immediate Postpartal Recovery Period

The nurse caring for the postpartal woman should check the mother's vital signs every 5 minutes until they are stable, then every 15 minutes for an hour, then every 30 minutes until she is discharged to the postpartal unit. The nurse should remain with the woman until she is stable.

The dressing and perineal pad must be checked every 15 minutes for at least an hour, and the fundus should be gently palpated to determine whether it is remaining firm. The fundus may be palpated by placing a hand to support the incision. Intravenous oxytocin is usually administered to promote the contractility of the uterine musculature. If the woman has been under general anesthesia, she should be positioned on her side to facilitate drainage of secretions, turned, and assisted with coughing and deep breathing every 2 hours for at least 24 hours. If she has received a spinal or epidural anesthetic, the level of anesthesia should be checked every 15 minutes. It is important to monitor intake and output and to observe the urine for bloody tinge, which could mean surgical trauma to the bladder. The physician prescribes medication to relieve the mother's pain and nausea, and this should be administered as needed. Some physicians use a single dose of epidural morphine (5 to 7.5 mg) for post-surgical pain relief. Facilitation of parent-infant interaction following birth and postpartal care is discussed in Chapter 35. Pertinent areas of nursing care are addressed in the Cesarean Birth Critical Pathway in Chapter 34.

CARE OF THE WOMAN UNDERGOING VAGINAL BIRTH AFTER CESAREAN (VBAC)

There is an increasing trend to have a trial of labor and **vaginal birth after cesarean (VBAC)** birth in cases of nonrecurring indications (for example, umbilical cord accident, placenta previa, fetal distress). This trend has been influenced by consumer demand and studies that support VBAC as a viable alternative (Leung et al 1993).

The 1988 ACOG guidelines state that the following aspects need to be considered for VBAC:

- A woman with one previous cesarean birth and a low transverse uterine incision should be counseled and encouraged to attempt VBAC.

- A woman with two or more previous cesareans may attempt VBAC.

- A classic uterine incision is a contraindication.

- It must be possible to do a cesarean in 30 minutes.

- A physician who is able to do a cesarean needs to be available.

The most common risks associated with VBAC are hemorrhage and uterine scar separation (uterine rupture). Leung et al (1993) reported that the risk of uterine rupture is increased in women who had excessive amounts of oxytocin, who had experienced dysfunctional labor, and who had a history of two or more previous cesarean births. Women who had macrosomia, a previous successful VBAC, unknown types of previous uterine incision, or a previous cesarean for CPD were not at increased risk.

Success rates for VBAC have been encouraging. Women whose previous cesarean was for fetal distress, twins, or breech presentation have been reported to have a 70% to 88% chance of success with VBAC (Scott 1993). Women who had recurrent problems, such as dystocia or failure to progress, had success rates that ranged from 60% to 70% (Scott 1994).

Nursing Care

The nursing care of a woman undergoing VBAC varies according to institutional protocols. Generally, if the woman is at very low risk (has had one previous cesarean with a lower uterine segment incision), her blood count, type, and screen are obtained on admission; a heplock is inserted for IV access if needed; continuous EFM is used; and clear fluids may be taken. If the woman is at higher risk, NPO status should be maintained and, in addition to the care listed above, an intrauterine catheter may be inserted to monitor intrauterine pressures during labor (Pridjian 1992).

Supportive and comfort measures are very important. The woman may be excited about this opportunity to experience labor and vaginal birth, or she may be hesitant and frightened about the possibility of complications. The presence of the nurse is important in providing information and encouragement for the laboring woman and her partner.

KEY CONCEPTS

An external (or cephalic) version may be done after 37 weeks' gestation to change a breech presentation to a cephalic presentation. The benefits of the version are that a lower-risk vaginal birth may be anticipated. The version is accomplished with the use of tocolytics to relax the uterus. An internal (podalic) version is used only when needed during the vaginal birth of a second twin.

Amniotomy (AROM) is performed to hasten labor. The risks are prolapse of the umbilical cord and infection.

Prostaglandin E_2 may be used before an induction of labor to soften the cervix (called cervical ripening). The gel is inserted into the vagina and held in place with a diaphragm.

Indicated induction of labor is done for many reasons. The methods include amniotomy and intravenous oxytocin infusion. Nursing responsibilities are heightened during an induced labor.

An episiotomy may be done just before birth of the fetus. Although in this country it is very prevalent, it is becoming somewhat controversial.

Forceps-assisted birth can be accomplished using outlet, low, or midforceps. Outlet forceps are the most common and are associated with few maternal-fetal complications. Midforceps are associated with more complications but, when needed, are an important aid to birth.

A vacuum extractor is a soft, pliable cup attached to suction that can be applied to the fetal head and used in much the same way as forceps.

At least one in four to five births is now accomplished by cesarean. The nurse has a vital role in providing information, support, and encouragement to the couple participating in a cesarean birth.

Vaginal birth after cesarean (VBAC) is becoming more popular. Overcoming the old fears of uterine rupture is a high priority for both the parents and the medical and nursing community.

REFERENCES

Affonso DD: *Impact of Cesarean Childbirth.* Philadelphia: Davis, 1981.

American College of Obstetricians and Gynecologists (ACOG): Guidelines for vaginal birth after previous cesarean birth. ACOG committee opinion no 64. Washington, DC, October 1988.

American College of Obstetricians and Gynecologists (ACOG): *Induction and Augmentation of Labor.* Technical bulletin no 157. Washington, DC: ACOG, 1991.

American College of Obstetricians and Gynecologists (ACOG): *Prostaglandin E Gel for Cervical Ripening*. ACOG committee opinion no 123. Washington, DC, October 1993.

Arias F: *Practical Guide to High-Risk Pregnancy and Delivery*. St Louis: Mosby-Year Book, 1993.

Association of Women's Health, Obstetric, and Neonatal Nurses (AWHONN): *Cervical Ripening and Induction and Augmentation of Labor*. Washington, DC: AWHONN, 1993.

Bartscht KD, DeLancey JOL: Episiotomy. In: *Gynecology and Obstetrics*, vol 2. Dilts PV, Sciarra JJ (editors). Philadelphia: Lippincott, 1992.

Bassel GM: Anesthesia for cesarean section. *Clin Obstet Gynecol* December 1985; 28:722.

Bishop EH: Pelvic scoring for elective induction. *Obstet Gynecol* 1964; 24:266.

Borgatta L, Piening SL, Cohen WR: Association of episiotomy and delivery position with deep perineal laceration during spontaneous delivery in nulliparous women. *Am J Obstet Gynecol* 1989; 160:294.

Brodsky PL, Pelzar EM: Rationale for the revision of oxytocin administration protocols. *JOGNN* November/December 1991; 20:440.

Clay LS, Criss K, Jackson UC: External cephalic version. *J Nurse-Midwifery* 1993; 38:72S.

Cox BE, Smith EC: The mother's self-esteem after a cesarean delivery. *MCN* September/October 1982; 7:309.

Crawford LA et al: Incontinence following rupture of the anal sphincter during delivery. *Obstet Gynecol* 1993; 82:527.

Cunningham FG, MacDonald PC, Gant NF: *Williams Obstetrics*, 19th ed. Norwalk, CT: Appleton & Lange, 1993.

Day ML, Snell BJ: Use of prostaglandins for induction of labor. *J Nurse-Midwifery* March/April 1993; 38:72S.

Dunn LJ: Cesarean section and other obstetric operations. In: *Danforth's Obstetrics and Gynecology*, 6th ed. Scott JR et al (editors). Philadelphia: Lippincott, 1990.

Francome C, Savage W: Cesarean section in Britain and the United States 12% or 24%: Is either the right rate? *Soc Sci Med* 1993; 37:1199.

Fraser WD, Sokol R: Amniotomy and maternal position in labor. *Clin Obstet Gynecol* 1992; 35:535.

Freeman RK: Can we lower the cesarean birth rate? *Tenth International Symposium on Perinatal Medicine and Obstetrical Ultrasound. April 9–12, 1990. Las Vegas, NV.*

Garite TJ et al: The influence of elective amniotomy on fetal heart rate patterns and the course of labor in term patients: A randomized study. *Am J Obstet Gynecol* June 1993; 168:1827.

Gould J, Davey B, Stafford F: Socioeconomic differences in rates of cesarean section. *N Engl J Med* 1989; 321:233.

Hall SL: Simultaneous occurrence of intracranial and subgaleal hemorrhages complicating vacuum extraction delivery. *J Perinatol* July/August 1992; 12:185.

Hangsleben KL, Taylor MA, Lynn NM: VBAC program in a nurse-midwifery service: Five years of experience. *J Nurse-Midwifery* July/August 1989; 34:179.

Henriksen TB et al: Episiotomy and perineal lesions in spontaneous vaginal deliveries. *Brit J Obstet Gynecol* December 1992; 99:950.

Jacobs MM: Prostaglandins for cervical ripening. In: *Antepartum and Intrapartum Management*. Parer JT (editor). Philadelphia: Lea & Febiger, 1989.

Kochenour NK: Normal pregnancy and prenatal care. In: *Danforth's Obstetrics and Gynecology*, 7th ed. Scott JR et al (editors). Philadelphia: Lippincott, 1994.

Laufe LE, Compton AA, Dilts PV: Forceps and vacuum delivery. In: *Gynecology and Obstetrics*, vol 2. Dilts PV, Sciarri JJ (editors). Philadelphia: Lippincott, 1990.

Leung AS et al: Risk factors associated with uterine rupture during trial of labor after cesarean delivery: A case-control study. *Am J Obstet Gynecol* 1993; 168:1358.

Marshall C: The art of induction/augmentation of labor. *JOGNN* January/February 1985; 14:22.

Martin RW, Wiser WL, Morrison JC: Cesarean birth—surgical techniques. In: *Gynecology and Obstetrics*, vol 2. Dilts PV, Sciarra JJ (editors). Philadelphia: Lippincott, 1990.

Miyazaki FS, Nevarez F: Saline amnioinfusion for relief of repetitive variable decelerations: A prospective randomized study. *Am J Obstet Gynecol* 1985; 153:301.

Miyazaki FS, Taylor NA: Saline amnioinfusion for relief of variable or prolonged decelerations. *Am J Obstet Gynecol* 1983; 146:670.

Newman RB et al: Predicting success of external cephalic version. *Am J Obstet Gynecol* August 1993; 169:245.

Nielsen TF, Olausson PO, Ingemarsson I: The cesarean section rate in Sweden: The end of the rise. *Birth* 1994; 21:34.

Niswander KR, Evans AT: *Manual of Obstetrics*. Boston: Little, Brown, 1991.

Nugent CE: Induction of labor. In: *Gynecology and Obstetrics*, vol 2. Dilts PV, Sciarri JJ (editors). Philadelphia: Lippincott, 1989.

O'Grady JP: *Modern Instrumental Delivery*. Baltimore: Williams & Wilkins, 1988.

Owen J, Hauth JC: Oxytocin for the induction or augmentation of labor. *Clin Obstet Gynecol* 1992; 35:464.

Petti DB: The ideal cesarean section rate. In: *Antepartum and Intrapartum Management*. Parer JT (editor). Philadelphia: Lea & Febiger, 1989.

Posner MD, Ballagh SA, Paul RH: The effect of amnioinfusion on uterine pressure and activity: A preliminary report. *Am J Obstet Gynecol* 1990; 163:813.

Pridjian G: Labor after prior cesarean section. *Clin Obstet Gynecol* 1992; 35:445.

Ramler D, Roberts J: A comparison of cold and warm sitz baths for relief of postpartum perineal pain. *JOGNN* November/December 1986; 15:471.

Rayburn W, Woods R, Ramadei C: Intravaginal prostaglandin E gel and cardiovascular changes in hypertensive pregnancies. *Am J Perinatol* July 1991; 8:233.

Reichert JA, Baron M, Fawcett J: Changes in attitudes toward cesarean birth. *JOGNN* 1993; 22:160.

Rockner G, Wahlberg V, Olund A: Episiotomy and perineal trauma during childbirth. *J Adv Nurs* 1989; 14:264.

Rosen DJD, Illeck JS, Greenspoon JS: Repeated external cephalic version at term. *Am J Obstet Gynecol* 1992; 167:508.

Sakala C: Medically unnecessary cesarean section births: Introduction to a symposium. *Soc Sci Med* 1993; 37:1177.

Scott JR et al: *Danforth's Obstetrics and Gynecology*, 7th ed. Philadelphia: Lippincott, 1994.

Scott JR et al: *Danforth's Obstetrics and Gynecology*, 6th ed. Philadelphia: Lippincott, 1990.

Sokol RK, Brindley BA: Practical diagnosis and management of abnormal labor. In: *Danforth's Obstetrics and Gynecology*, 6th ed. Scott JR et al (editors). Philadelphia: Lippincott, 1990.

Thorp JM, Bowes WA: Episiotomy: Can its routine use be defended? *Am J Obstet Gynecol* 1989; 160:1027.

Trofatter KF: Cervical ripening. *Clin Obstet Gynecol* 1992; 35:476.

Varner MW: Episiotomy: Techniques and indications. *Clin Obstet Gynecol* June 1986; 29:309.

Wenstrom KD, Parsons MT: The prevention of meconium aspiration in labor using amnioinfusion. *Obstet Gynecol* 1989; 73:647.

Wesley BD, van den Berg EJ, Reece EA: The effect of forceps delivery on cognitive development. *Am J Obstet Gynecol* 1993; 169:1091.

Willcourt RJ et al: Induction of labor with pulsatile oxytocin by a computer-controlled pump. *Obstet Gynecol* 1994; 170:603.

PART SIX

THE NEWBORN

CHAPTER 27

PHYSIOLOGIC RESPONSES OF THE NEWBORN TO BIRTH

*T*he incredible attributes of the newborn have a major purpose. They prepare the baby for interaction with the family and for life in the world.

~ THE AMAZING NEWBORN ~

KEY TERMS

Active acquired immunity

Brown adipose tissue (BAT)

Cardiopulmonary adaptation

Conduction

Convection

Evaporation

Habituation

Meconium

Neonatal transition

Orientation

Passive acquired immunity

Periodic breathing

Periods of reactivity

Physiologic anemia of infancy

Physiologic jaundice

Radiation

Self-quieting ability

Surfactant

Thermal neutral zone (TNZ)

Total serum bilirubin

OBJECTIVES

Summarize the respiratory and cardio-vascular changes that occur during the transition to extrauterine life.

Describe how various factors affect the newborn's blood values.

Summarize the major mechanisms of heat loss in the newborn and how the newborn produces heat.

Relate the processes by which a newborn produces heat to the major mechanisms of heat loss in the newborn.

Explain the steps involved in conjugation and excretion of bilirubin in the newborn.

Discuss the reasons why the newborn may develop jaundice.

Delineate the functional abilities of the newborn's gastrointestinal tract.

Identify the reasons the newborn's kidneys have difficulty maintaining fluid and electrolyte balance.

List the immunologic responses available to the newborn.

Explain the physiologic and behavioral responses of newborns during the periods of reactivity and identify possible interventions.

Describe the normal sensory-perceptual abilities and behavioral states present in the newborn period.

The newborn period is the time from birth through the first 28 days of life. During this period the newborn adjusts from intrauterine to extrauterine life. The nurse needs to be knowledgeable about a newborn's normal physiologic and behavioral adaptations and be able to recognize alterations from normal.

To begin life as a separate being, the baby must immediately establish respiratory gas exchange, which occurs in conjunction with marked circulatory changes. These radical and rapid changes are crucial to the maintenance of extrauterine life. The first few hours of life, in which the newborn stabilizes respiratory and circulatory functions, are called **neonatal transition.** All other newborn body systems change their level of functioning or become established over a longer period of time during the neonatal period.

RESPIRATORY ADAPTATIONS

Although the significant respiratory events occur at birth, certain intrauterine factors also enhance the newborn's ability to breathe.

Intrauterine Factors Supporting Respiratory Function

Fetal Lung Development

The respiratory system is in a continuous state of development during fetal life, and lung development continues into early childhood. During the first 20 weeks of gestation, lung development is limited to the differentiation of pulmonary, vascular, and lymphatic structures. At 20 to 24 weeks alveolar ducts begin to appear, followed by primitive alveoli at 24 to 28 weeks. During this time the alveolar epithelial cells begin to differentiate into type I cells (structures necessary for respiratory gas exchange) and type II cells (structures that provide for the synthesis and storage of surfactant). **Surfactant** is composed of a group of surface-active phospholipids (lecithin and sphingomyelin), which are critical for alveolar stability.

At 28 to 32 weeks the number of type II cells increases further. Lecithin production peaks at about 35 weeks' gestation and remains high until term, paralleling late fetal lung development. At this time the lungs are structurally developed enough to permit maintenance of good lung expansion and adequate exchange of gases.

Clinically, the peak production of lecithin corresponds closely to the marked decrease in incidence of idiopathic respiratory distress syndrome after 35 weeks' gestation. Production of sphingomyelin remains constant throughout gestation. The newborn born before the lecithin/sphingomyelin (L/S) ratio is 2:1 will have varying degrees of respiratory distress. (See discussion of L/S ratio in Chapters 20 and 32.)

Fetal Breathing Movements

The newborn's ability to breathe immediately upon exposure to air in the extrauterine environment appears to be the consequence of weeks of intrauterine practice. In this respect breathing can be perceived as a continuation of an intrauterine process as the lungs convert from being fluid-filled to gas-filled organs. Fetal breathing movements (FBM) occur as early as 11 weeks' gestation (see Chapter 20 for discussion). These breathing movements are essential for development of chest wall muscles, the diaphragm, and, to a lesser extent, for regulating lung fluid volume and therefore lung growth.

Initiation of Breathing

To maintain life, the lungs must function immediately after birth. Two radical changes must take place for the lungs to function:

1. Pulmonary ventilation must be established through lung expansion following birth.

2. A marked increase in the pulmonary circulation must occur.

The first breath of life—the gasp in response to mechanical, chemical, thermal, and sensory changes associated with birth—initiates the serial opening of the alveoli. Thus begins the transition from a fluid-filled environment to an air-breathing, independent, extrauterine life. Figure 27–1 summarizes the initiation of respiration.

Mechanical Events

During the latter half of gestation, the fetal lungs continuously produce fluid. This fluid production expands the lungs almost completely, filling the air spaces. Some of the lung fluid moves up into the trachea and into the amniotic fluid. The amniotic fluid is then swallowed by the fetus.

Production of lung fluid diminishes 2 to 4 days before onset of labor (Eden & Boehm 1990). However, approximately 80 to 110 mL of fluid remains in the respiratory passages of a normal term fetus at the time of birth. This fluid must be removed from the lungs to permit adequate movement of air.

The primary mechanical events that initiate respiration involve removal of fluid from the lungs as the fetus passes through the birth canal. The fetal chest is compressed during passage through the birth canal, thus increasing intrathoracic pressure. As a result approximately one-third of the fluid is squeezed out of the lungs. After

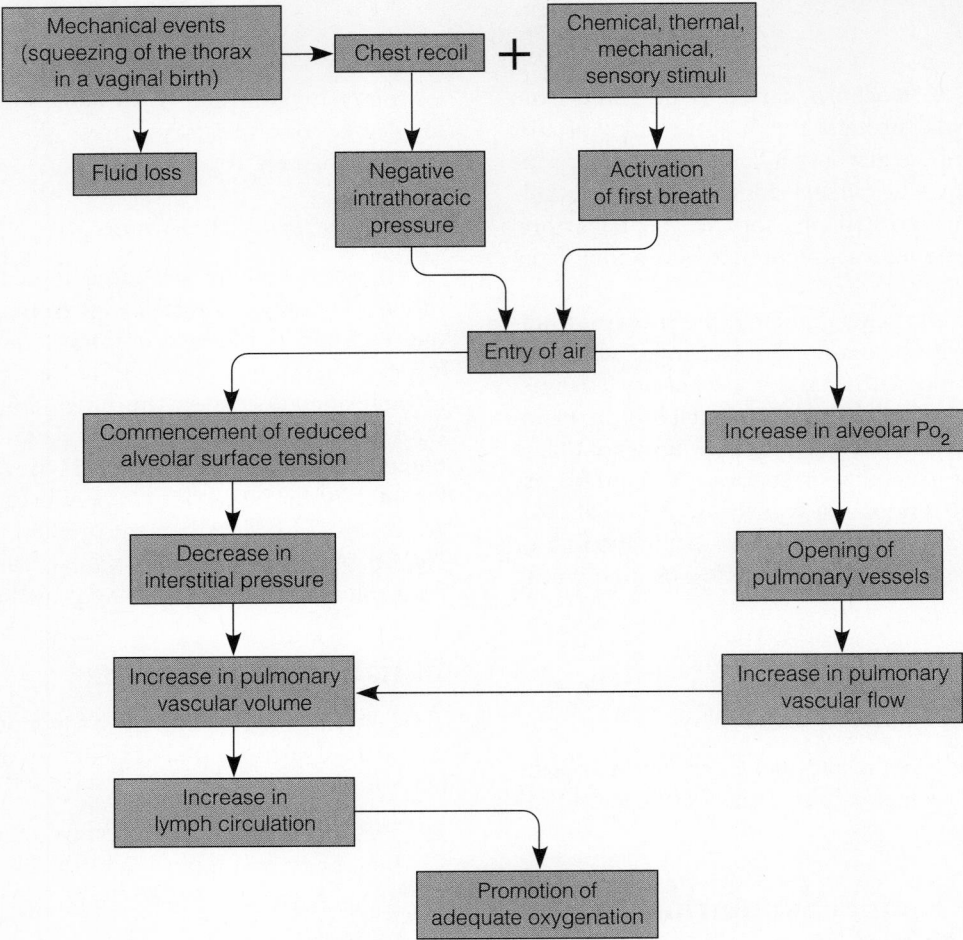

FIGURE 27-1 Initiation of respiration in the neonate.

the birth of the newborn's trunk, the chest wall recoils. This chest recoil creates negative intrathoracic pressure, which is thought to produce a small, passive inspiration of air that replaces the fluid that was squeezed out.

After this first inspiration, the newborn exhales, with crying, against a partially closed glottis, creating a positive intrathoracic pressure. The high positive intrathoracic pressure distributes the inspired air throughout the alveoli and begins the establishment of *functional residual capacity (FRC)* (the air left in the lungs at the end of a normal expiration). The higher intrathoracic pressure also increases absorption of lung fluid via the capillaries and lymphatic system. The negative intrathoracic pressure resulting from downward movement of the diaphragm with inspiration causes lung fluid to flow from the alveoli across the alveolar membranes into the pulmonary interstitial tissue.

With each succeeding breath the lungs expand, stretching the alveolar walls and increasing the alveolar volume. The expansion of the lung facilitates movement of the remaining lung fluid into the interstitial tissue. Because the protein concentration is higher in the pul-

monary capillaries, oncotic pressure draws the interstitial fluid into the capillaries and lymphatics. As pulmonary vascular resistance decreases, pulmonary blood flow increases, and more interstitial fluid is absorbed into the bloodstream. In the normal term newborn, movement of lung fluid to the interstitial tissue is rapid, but movement into lymph and blood vessels may take several hours. Figure 27–2 depicts the changes in fetal lung fluid with the first and subsequent breaths. About 80% of the fluid is reabsorbed within 2 hours after birth, and it is completely absorbed within 12 to 24 hours after birth.

Although the initial chest compression and recoil should clear the airways of accumulated fluid and permit further inspiration, most clinicians feel it is wise to suction mucus and fluid from the newborn's mouth and oropharynx. They use a mucus trap attached to suction as soon as the newborn's head and shoulders are born and again as the newborn adapts to extrauterine life and stabilizes (see Procedure 23–1, and Chapter 23).

Problems associated with lung fluid clearance and/or initiation of respiratory activity may be caused by a variety of factors. The lymphatics may be underdeveloped,

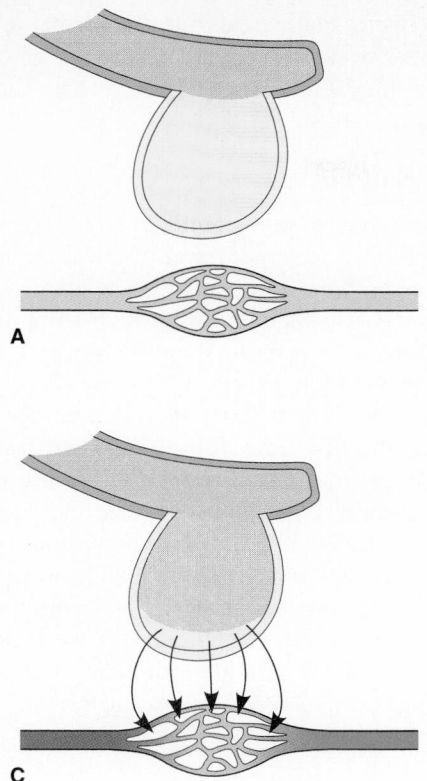

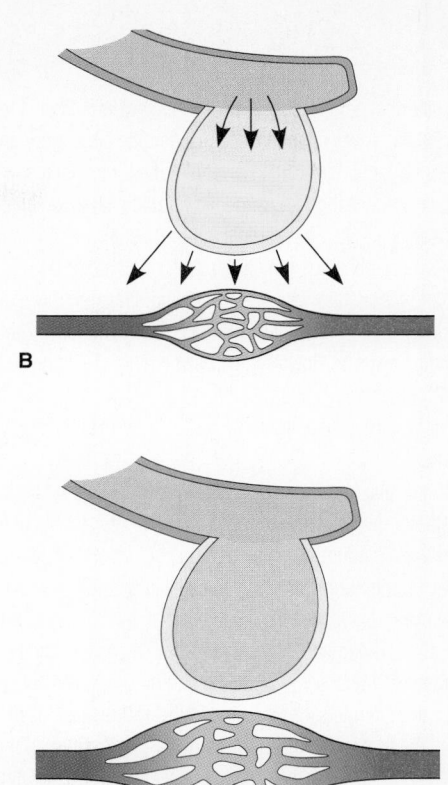

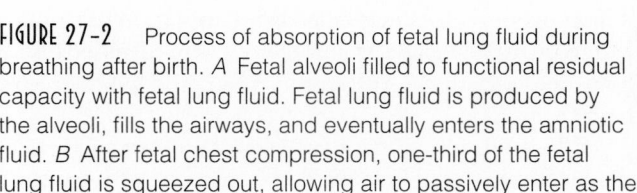

FIGURE 27-2 Process of absorption of fetal lung fluid during breathing after birth. *A* Fetal alveoli filled to functional residual capacity with fetal lung fluid. Fetal lung fluid is produced by the alveoli, fills the airways, and eventually enters the amniotic fluid. *B* After fetal chest compression, one-third of the fetal lung fluid is squeezed out, allowing air to passively enter as the chest recoils. *C* With each subsequent breath the lungs expand, facilitating the movement of the remaining fetal lung fluid into the capillaries and lymphatics. Pulmonary blood flow is increasing. *D* Normal alveoli after removal of fetal lung fluid and dilatation of pulmonary arteries. Surfactant has lined the inside of the alveoli to prevent collapse.

thus decreasing the rate at which the fluid is absorbed from the lungs. Complications that occur antenatally or during labor and birth can interfere with adequate lung expansion, causing failure to decrease pulmonary vascular resistance, resulting in decreased pulmonary blood flow. These complications include inadequate compression of the chest wall in a very small newborn, the absence of the chest wall compression in the newborn delivered by cesarean birth, respiratory depression secondary to maternal anesthesia, severe asphyxia at birth, or aspiration of amniotic fluid or meconium.

Chemical Stimuli

An important chemical stimulator that contributes to the onset of breathing is transitory asphyxia of the fetus and newborn. The first breath is really an inspiratory gasp triggered by the elevation in PCO_2 and decrease in pH and PO_2, which are the natural result of normal vaginal birth with cessation of placental gas exchange when the cord is clamped. These changes, which are present in all newborns to some degree, stimulate the aortic and carotid chemoreceptors, initiating impulses that trigger the medulla's respiratory center. Although brief periods of asphyxia are a significant stimulator, prolonged asphyxia is abnormal and acts as a central nervous system respiratory depressant.

Thermal Stimuli

A significant decrease in ambient temperature after birth (from 98.6 F to 70–75 F or 37 C to 21–23.9 C) is sufficient thermal stimulus for initiation of breathing. Skin nerve endings stimulated by the cold transmit impulses to the medullary respiratory control center, and the newborn responds with rhythmic respirations. Excessive

In the transitional period, during which the newborn adjusts to extrauterine life, many changes take place in the circulatory and respiratory systems. Fluid-filled alveoli in the lungs open and cardiac blood flow patterns change. Physiologic stressors can impact these changes. For example, crying, usually regarded as normal newborn behavior, may induce intrathoracic pressure changes and precipitate right-to-left intracardiac shunting. This shunting may result in hypoxemia, which further increases stress on the adapting newborn. However, the baby cannot cry while sucking on something. Donna Treloar used this framework to explore the effect of nonnutritive sucking on oxygenation in healthy, crying, full-term infants.

Nonnutritive sucking is defined as repetitive mouthing on a blind nipple or pacifier with no intake of food. The sample of 59 newborns were randomly assigned to one of two groups, controlled for gender assignment. The convenience sample met inclusion criteria relevant to age, weight, Apgar scores, health status, and ability to suck. The treatment group received a pacifier immediately after a prescribed heel stick, while the control group did not receive a pacifier until 7 minutes after the procedure. The researcher measured transcutaneous oxygen concentration ($tcPo_2$) and assessed the baby's behavioral state at the time of the heel stick. Observations made during the 5 minutes prior to the stick were considered baseline data. The "cry" period was defined as the 5 minutes immediately following the stick, and "postcry" referred to the period 5 to 7 minutes after the stick.

Using t-tests for data analysis, the author found statistically significant differences between the two groups in transcutaneous oxygen status. Differences were seen from the precry to cry periods ($t(57)=2.54$, $p=0.0136$) and from precry to postcry ($t(57)=3.63$, $p=0.0006$). The $tcPo_2$ for the control group decreased from precry to postcry by 2.2 mg Hg while the $tcPo_2$ for the treatment group increased by 5.6 mm Hg. Only 2 of the infants who received a pacifier were crying 3 minutes after the heel stick, but 16 infants from the control group were crying then.

Clinical Application of Study

This study demonstrated that using a pacifier to stop babies' crying was associated with increased $tcPo_2$. However, the study examined only healthy, full term infants. As the author notes, many compromised newborns may have pre-existing difficulties with oxygenation status. Therefore, the author suggests that allowing these compromised newborns to cry may reduce their already compromised oxygenation status.

SOURCE: Treloar D: The effect of nonnutritive sucking on oxygenation in healthy, crying, full-term infants. *Appl Nurs Res* 1994; 7(2):52.

cooling may result in profound respiratory depression and evidence of cold stress, but the normal temperature changes that occur at birth are apparently within acceptable physiologic limits. (See Chapter 32 for discussion of cold stress.)

Sensory Stimuli

As the fetus moves from a familiar, comfortable environment, a number of sensory and physical influences help initiate respiration. They include the numerous tactile, auditory, and visual stimuli of birth. During intrauterine life the fetus is in a dark, sound-dampened, fluid-filled environment and is nearly weightless. After birth the newborn experiences light, sounds, and the effects of gravity for the first time. Joint movement results in enhanced proprioceptive stimulation to the respiratory center to sustain respirations. Historically, vigorous stimulation was provided by slapping the buttocks or heels of the newborn, but today greater emphasis is placed on gentle physical contact. Thoroughly drying the newborn and placing it in skin-to-skin contact with the mother's chest and abdomen provides stimulation in a far more comforting way and also decreases heat loss.

Factors Opposing the First Breath

Three major factors may oppose the initiation of respiratory activity: (1) alveolar surface tension, (2) viscosity of lung fluid within the respiratory tract, and (3) degree of lung compliance.

The contracting force between the moist surfaces of the alveoli is called *alveolar surface tension*. This tension, which is necessary for healthy respiratory function, would nevertheless cause the small airways and alveoli to collapse after each inspiration were it not for the presence of surfactant. By reducing the attracting force between alveoli, surfactant prevents the alveoli from completely collapsing with each expiration and thus promotes lung expansion. Similarly, surfactant promotes lung *compliance*, the ability of the lung to fill with air easily. When surfactant is decreased, compliance is also decreased, and the pressure needed to expand the alveoli with air increases. Resistive forces of the fluid-filled lung combined with the small radii of the airways necessitates pressures of 20–25 cm of water to open the lung initially (James & Adamsons 1994).

The first breath usually establishes FRC that is 30% to 40% of the fully expanded lung volume. This FRC allows alveolar sacs to remain partially expanded on expiration. Thus the air that remains in the lung after expiration (FRC) decreases the need for continuous high pressures for each of the following breaths. Subsequent breaths require only 6–8 cm H_2O pressure to open alveoli during inspiration. Therefore, the first breath of life is usually the most difficult.

Cardiopulmonary Physiology

The onset of respiration stimulates in the cardiovascular system changes that are necessary for the successful transition to extrauterine life, hence the term **cardiopulmonary adaptation.** As air enters the lungs, PO_2 rises in the alveoli, which stimulates the relaxation of the pulmonary arteries and triggers a decrease in the pulmonary vascular resistance. As pulmonary vascular resistance decreases, the vascular flow in the lung increases very rapidly and achieves 100% normal flow volume at 24 hours of life. This delivery of greater blood volume to the lungs contributes to the conversion from fetal circulation to newborn circulation.

After pulmonary circulation is established, blood is distributed throughout the lung, although the alveoli may or may not be fully open. For adequate oxygenation to occur, sufficient blood must be delivered by the heart to the functioning open alveoli. Shunting of blood is common in the early newborn period. This occurs when blood perfuses unopen alveoli, there is decreased perfusion of open alveoli, or the ductus arteriosus or foramen ovale remains open. Shunting may divert a significant amount of blood away from the lungs, depending on the pressure changes of respiration, crying, and the cardiac cycle. This shunting in the newborn period is also responsible for the unstable transitional period in cardiopulmonary adaptation.

Oxygen Transport

The transportation of oxygen to the peripheral tissues depends on the type of hemoglobin in the red blood cell, the oxygen-carrying capacity of the blood and the cardiac output. In the fetus and newborn a variety of hemoglobins exists, the most significant being fetal hemoglobin (HbF) and adult hemoglobin (HbA). Approximately 70% to 90% of hemoglobin in the fetus and newborn is fetal hemoglobin. The greatest difference between HbF and HbA is related to the transport of oxygen.

The oxygen-carrying capacity of fetal hemoglobin is lower than that of adult hemoglobin. Though each gram of fetal hemoglobin carries less oxygen, it has a greater affinity for the oxygen molecules it carries. At any given arterial oxygen level, fetal hemoglobin has a greater saturation than adult hemoglobin. Thus the oxygen-hemoglobin dissociation curve for fetal hemoglobin lies to the left of that for adult hemoglobin (Figure 27–3). Fetal hemoglobin's greater affinity for oxygen benefits the fetus and newborn because it facilitates oxygen transfer across the placenta and into the newborn's tissues. In utero the fetus has an arterial oxygen tension (PaO_2) between 30 and 40 mm Hg. Due to the nature of the fetal hemoglobin as depicted in the curve, small changes in fetal PaO_2 result in a great amount of oxygen loading in the placenta or unloading to the tissues as compared to the adult. Fe-

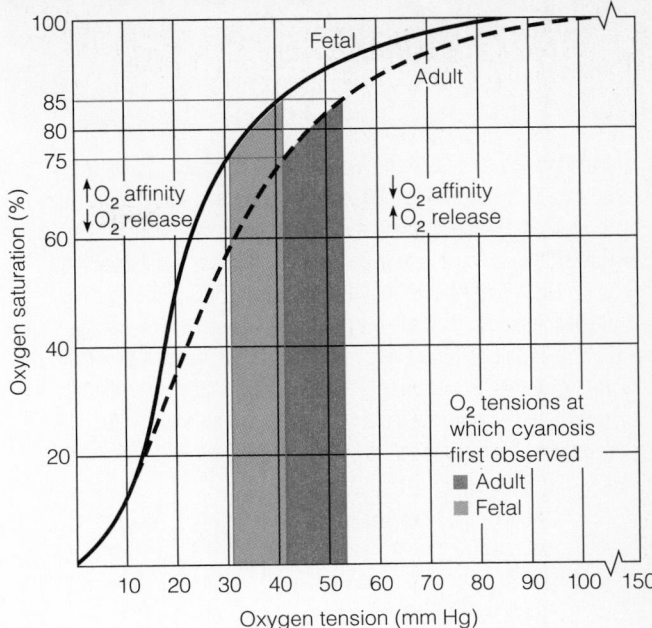

FIGURE 27-3 Fetal oxygen-hemoglobin dissociation curve. SOURCE: Modified from Klaus M, Fanaroff AA: *Care of the High Risk Infant,* 3rd ed. Philadelphia: WB Saunders, 1986, p 234.

tal hemoglobin's greater affinity for oxygen also requires that a lower tissue oxygen level exist prior to oxygen unloading than required by adult hemoglobin. Because of this phenomenon, the newborn will have both a lower arterial oxygen level and lower oxygen saturation than the adult before cyanosis becomes clinically apparent.

In addition to the specific characteristics of fetal hemoglobin, other conditions affect the transport of oxygen. Alkalosis and hypothermia result in increased oxygen affinity and thus less oxygen availability to the tissues; acidosis, hypercarbia, and hyperthermia result in decreased oxygen affinity, resulting in greater oxygen release to the tissues. Therefore, as blood is perfusing active tissues that are producing acids and carbon dioxide, hemoglobin's affinity for oxygen decreases, allowing oxygen unloading and carbon dioxide and acid uptake. This blood is then transferred to the placenta or the lungs, where its lower carbon dioxide and acid content results in uploading of these waste products from hemoglobin and the uptake of oxygen to be transferred to the tissues.

Other factors that regulate oxygen delivery to the tissues are oxygen-carrying capacity and cardiac output. The oxygen-carrying capacity of blood is defined as the product of the hemoglobin concentration and the maximum amount of oxygen that 1 g of hemoglobin can hold when it is fully saturated. The amount of oxygen bound to hemoglobin divided by the oxygen-carrying capacity gives a percent that signifies oxygen saturation. Oxygen saturation usually reaches a value between 96% and 98% after several hours of life. Although fetal hemoglobin can hold only 1.26 mL O_2 per gram of hemoglobin, compared to 1.34 mL O_2 per gram of adult hemoglobin, the newborn's hemoglobin level at birth (17 g/dL) is substantially greater than in adults (13 g/dL). Therefore the absolute oxygen-carrying capacity of fetal blood (21.42 vol%) is greater than in adult blood (17.42 vol%) and allows the fetus to tolerate the relatively hypoxic intrauterine environment.

A significant reduction in the oxygen-carrying capacity results in an increased cardiac output to compensate for hemoglobin's decreased oxygen concentration. Lastly, cardiac output of the fetus and newborn is relatively greater per body weight than in the adult, which contributes to the rapid delivery of oxygenated blood to tissues with high metabolic demands.

Maintaining Respiratory Function

The lungs' ability to maintain oxygen and carbon dioxide exchange (ventilation) is influenced by such factors as lung compliance and airway resistance. Lung compliance is influenced by the elastic recoil of the lung tissue and by anatomic variation. Anatomic differences in the newborn influence lung compliance. The infant has a relatively large heart and mediastinal structures that reduce available lung space. The large abdomen further encroaches on the high diaphragm to decrease lung space. Anatomically, the newborn chest is equipped with weak intercostal muscles, a rib cage with horizontal ribs, and a high diaphragm that restricts the space available for lung expansion. Another factor that limits ventilation is airway resistance, which depends on the radii, length, and number of airways.

Characteristics of Newborn Respiration

The normal newborn respiratory rate is 30–60 breaths per minute. Initial respirations may be largely diaphragmatic, shallow, and irregular in depth and rhythm. The abdomen's movements are synchronous with chest movements. When the breathing pattern is characterized by pauses lasting 5 to 15 seconds, **periodic breathing** is said to be occurring. Periodic breathing is rarely associated with differences in skin color or heart rate changes, and it has no prognostic significance. Tactile or other sensory stimulation stimulates the respiratory center and converts periodic breathing patterns to normal breathing patterns during neonatal transition. Newborn sleep states in particular influence respiratory patterns. During deep sleep the pattern is reasonably regular. Periodic breathing occurs with rapid eye movement (REM) sleep, and grossly irregular breathing is evident with motor activity, sucking, and crying. Cessation of breathing lasting more than 20 seconds is defined as *apnea* and is abnormal in term newborns. Apnea may or may not be associated with changes in skin color or heart rate (drop below 100 beats per minute). Apnea always needs to be further evaluated.

The newborn is an obligatory nose breather, and any obstruction will cause respiratory distress, so it is important to keep the throat and nose clear (Figure 32–6). If respirations drop below 30 or exceed 60 per minute when the infant is at rest, or if dyspnea, cyanosis, or nasal flaring and expiratory grunting occurs, the clinician should be notified. For about 2 hours after birth respiratory rates of 60 to 70 breaths per minute are normal. Some cyanosis and acrocyanosis is normal for several hours; thereafter, a steady improvement in color occurs. Any increased use of the intercostal muscle (retracting) may indicate respiratory distress. (See Chapter 32 and Table 32–2 for signs of respiratory distress.)

CARDIOVASCULAR ADAPTATIONS

As described earlier in this chapter, the onset of respiration triggers increased pulmonary blood flow after birth, which contributes to the transition from fetal to newborn circulation.

Fetal-Newborn Transitional Anatomy and Physiology

Due to the unique pattern of fetal circulation, blood with the highest oxygen content is directed to the heart and brain. Blood in the descending aorta is less oxygenated and supplies the kidneys and intestinal tract before it is returned to the placenta. Limited amounts of blood, pumped from the right ventricle toward the lungs, enters the pulmonary vessels. In the fetus increased pulmonary resistance forces most of the blood through the ductus arteriosus into the descending aorta (Table 27–1).

Marked changes occur in the cardiovascular system at birth. Expansion of the lungs with the first breath decreases the pulmonary vascular resistance and increases pulmonary blood flow. Left atrial pressure increases as blood returns from the pulmonary veins. Right atrial pressure drops, and systemic vascular resistance increases as umbilical venous flow is halted when the cord is clamped. As right atrial pressure falls below left atrial pressure, the foramen ovale closes.

These physiologic mechanisms mark the beginning of transition from fetal to neonatal circulation and show the interplay of the cardiovascular and respiratory systems (Figure 27–4). As the neonate adapts to extrauterine life, there are five major areas of change in circulatory function (Figure 27–5).

1. *Increased aortic pressure and decreased venous pressure.* With clamping of the umbilical cord the placental vascular bed is eliminated, and the intravascular space is reduced. Consequently, aortic (systemic) blood pressure is increased. At the same time, blood return via the inferior vena cava is decreased, resulting in decreased right atrial pressure and a small decrease in pressure within the venous circulation.

2. *Increased systemic pressure and decreased pulmonary artery pressure.* With the loss of the low-resistance

TABLE 27-1	Fetal and Neonatal Circulation	
System	**Fetal**	**Neonatal**
Pulmonary blood vessels	Constricted with very little blood flow; lungs not expanded	Vasodilation and increased blood flow; lungs expanded; increased oxygen stimulates vasodilation.
Systemic blood vessels	Dilated with low resistance; blood mostly in placenta	Arterial pressure rises due to loss of placenta; increased systemic blood volume and resistance.
Ductus arteriosus	Large with no tone; blood flow from pulmonary artery to aorta	Reversal of blood flow. Now from aorta to pulmonary artery due to increased left atrial pressure. Ductus is sensitive to increased oxygen and body chemicals and begins to constrict.
Foramen ovale	Patent with large blood flow from right atrium to left atrium	Increased pressure in left atrium attempts to reverse blood flow and shuts one-way valve.

placenta, systemic resistance increases, resulting in greater systemic pressure. At the same time lung expansion promotes increased pulmonary blood flow, and the increased blood PO_2 associated with initiation of respirations produces vasodilatation of pulmonary blood vessels. The combination of vasodilatation and increased pulmonary blood flow results in decreased pulmonary artery

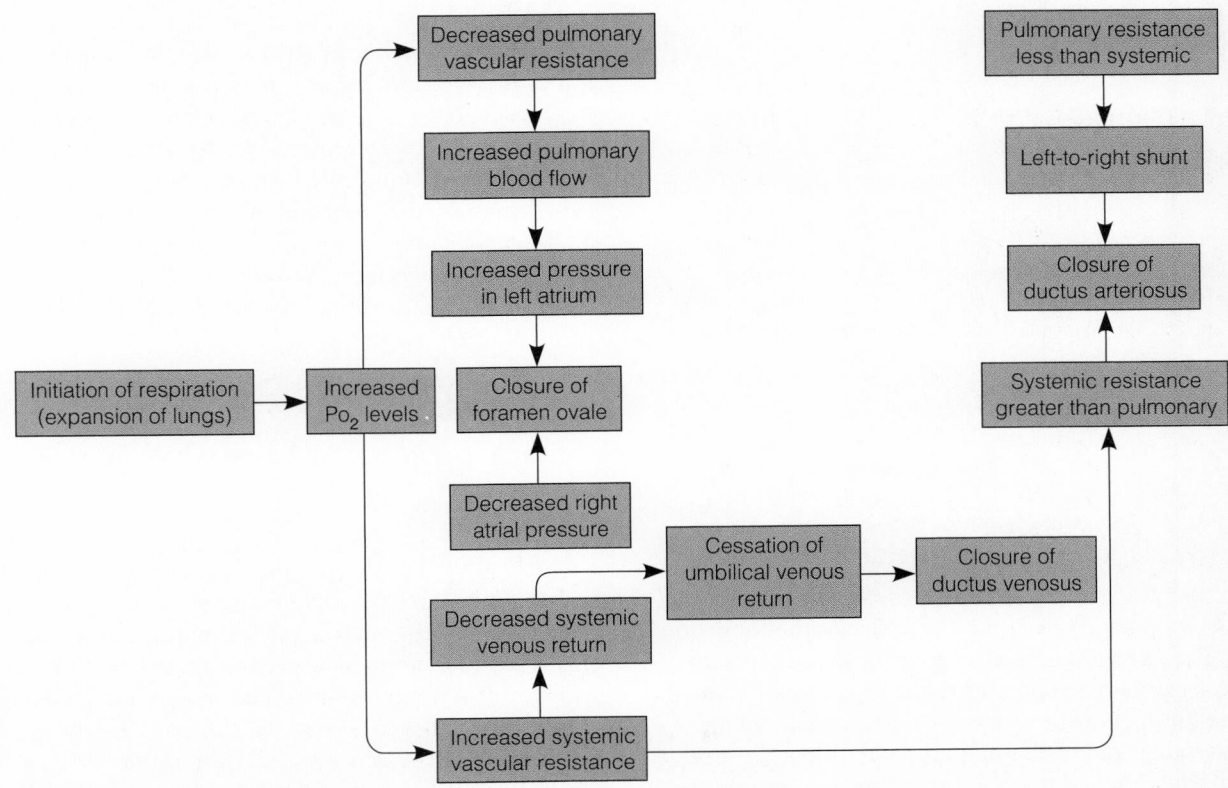

FIGURE 27-4   Transitional circulation: conversion from fetal to neonatal circulation.

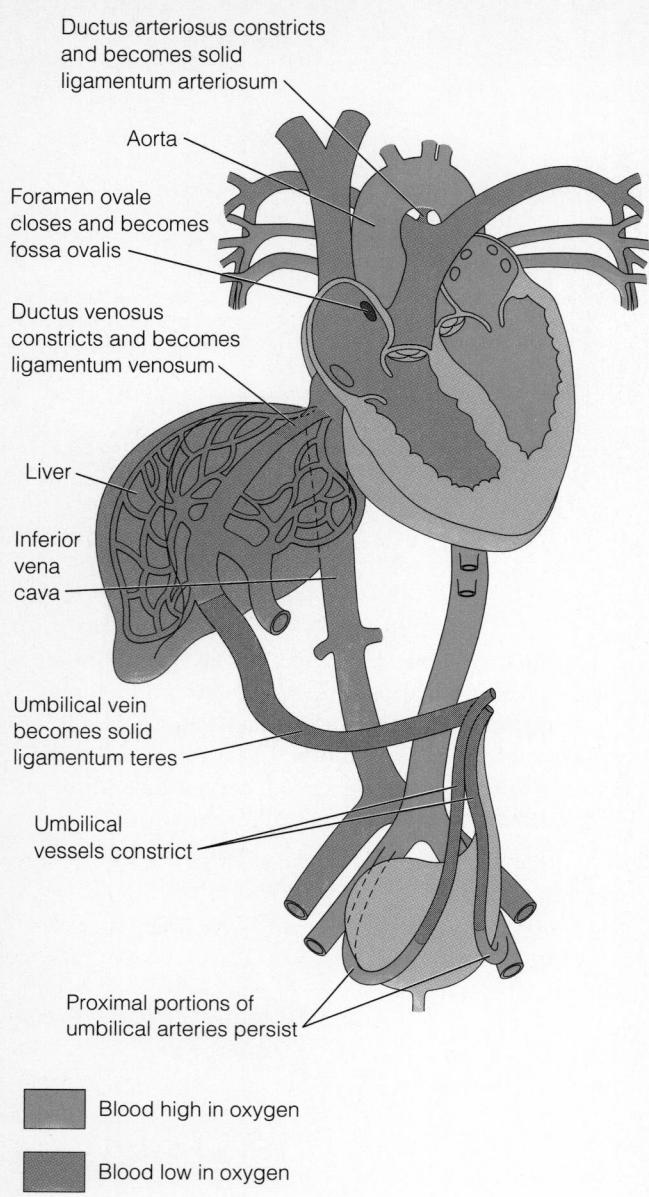

Ductus arteriosus constricts
and becomes solid
ligamentum arteriosum

Aorta

Foramen ovale
closes and becomes
fossa ovalis

Ductus venosus
constricts and becomes
ligamentum venosum

Liver

Inferior
vena
cava

Umbilical vein
becomes solid
ligamentum teres

Umbilical
vessels constrict

Proximal portions of
umbilical arteries persist

Blood high in oxygen

Blood low in oxygen

FIGURE 27-5   Major changes that occur in the newborn's circulatory system. SOURCE: Hole JW: *Human Anatomy and Physiology,* 5th ed. Dubuque, IA: William C Brown, 1990. All Rights Reserved.

resistance. As a result of opening the pulmonary vascular beds, the systemic vascular pressure increases, causing enhanced perfusion of the other body systems.

3. *Closure of the foramen ovale.* Closure of the foramen ovale is a function of changing atrial pressures. In utero, pressure is greater in the right atrium, and the foramen ovale is open. Decreased pulmonary resistance and increased pulmonary blood flow result in increased pulmonary venous return into the left atrium, thereby increasing left atrial pressure.

The decreased pulmonary vascular resistance and the decreased umbilical venous return to the right atrium also cause a decrease in right atrial pressure. The pressure gradients across the atria are now reversed, with left atrial pressure greater, and the foramen ovale is functionally closed 1–2 hours after birth. However, a slight right-to-left shunting may occur in the early neonatal period. Any increase in pulmonary resistance or right atrial pressure, such as occurs in crying, acidosis, cold stress, or induced hypoxia, may result in reopening of the foramen ovale, causing a right-to-left shunt. Permanent closure of the foramen ovale occurs within 6 months.

4. *Closure of the ductus arteriosus.* As the systemic vascular pressure exceeds the pulmonary vascular pressure, blood flow through the ductus arteriosus is reversed. Blood now flows from the aorta into the pulmonary artery. Furthermore, although the presence of oxygen causes the pulmonary arterioles to dilate, an increase in blood PO_2 triggers the opposite response: active construction in the ductus arteriosus.

In utero the placenta produces prostaglandin E_2 (PGE_2), which causes ductus vasodilatation. With the loss of the placenta and increased pulmonary blood flow, PGE_2 levels drop, leaving the active constriction by PO_2 unopposed. If the lungs fail to expand or if PO_2 levels drop, the ductus remains patent. Functional closure is accomplished within 15 hours of birth, and fibrosis of the ductus occurs within 3 weeks after birth (Nelson 1994; Long 1990).

5. *Closure of the ductus venosus.* Although the mechanism of initiating closure of the ductus venosus is not known, it appears to be related to mechanical pressure changes after severing of the cord, redistribution of blood, and cardiac output. Closure of the bypass forces perfusion of the liver. Fibrotic closure occurs within 2 months (Long 1990). Figure 27–6 depicts the changes in blood flow and oxygenation as the fetal cardiopulmonary circulation adapts to extrauterine life.

Characteristics of Cardiac Function

Heart Rate

Shortly after the first cry and the start of changes in the cardiopulmonary circulation the newborn heart rate accelerates to 175–180 beats per minute. The average resting heart rate in the first week of life is 125–130 bpm in a quiet, full-term newborn (Fanaroff & Martin 1992). The range of the heart rate in the full-term newborn is 100 bpm while asleep and 120–160 bpm while awake. Resting heart rates as low as 85–90 bpm and rates above 180 while crying may be seen (Taeusch et al 1991). Apical pulse

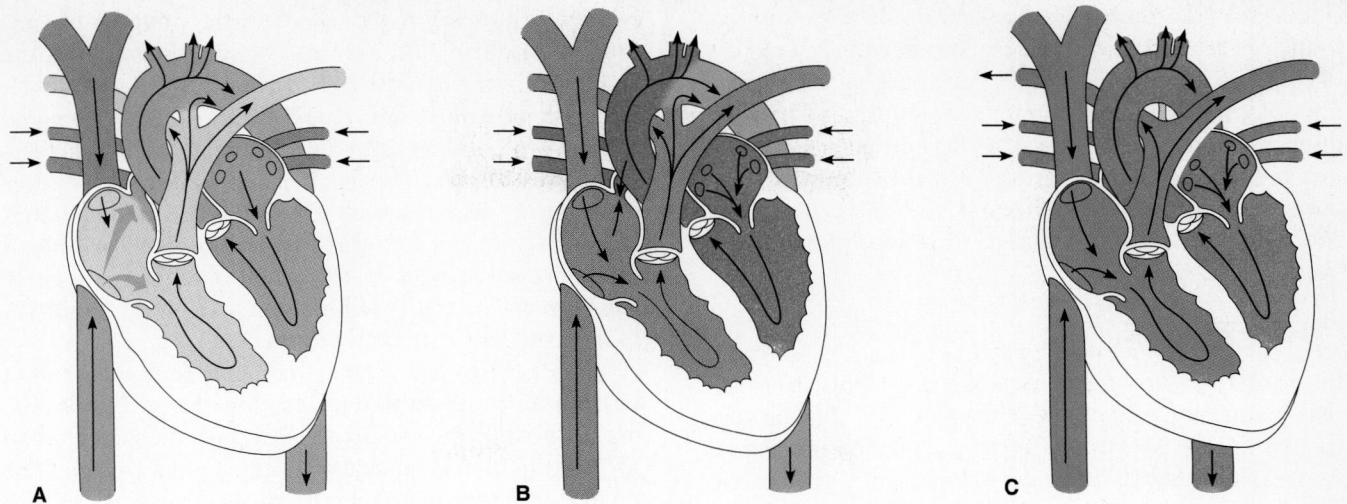

FIGURE 27-6 Fetal-neonatal circulation. *A* Pattern of blood flow and oxygenation in fetal circulation. *B* Pattern of blood flow and oxygenation in transitional circulation of the newborn. *C* Pattern of blood flow and oxygenation in neonatal circulation.

rates should be obtained by auscultation for a full minute, preferably when the newborn is asleep. The heart rate should be evaluated for abnormal rhythms or beats. Peripheral pulses of all extremities should also be evaluated to detect any lags or unusual characteristics. Peripheral radial pulses are difficult to palpate in the newborn. They can be assessed when blood pressure is measured if blood pressure readings are taken on all four extremities.

Blood Pressure

During the newborn period the blood pressure tends to be highest immediately after birth, and then it descends to its lowest level at about 3 hours of age. By 4 to 6 days of life the blood pressure rises and plateaus at a level approximately the same as the initial level. Blood pressure is sensitive to the changes in blood volume that occur in the transition to newborn circulation. Figure 27–7 diagrams this response. Peripheral perfusion pressure is a particularly sensitive indicator of the newborn's ability to compensate for alterations in blood volume prior to changes in blood pressure. Capillary refill should be less than 2–3 seconds when the skin is blanched.

Blood pressure values during the first 12 hours of life vary with the birth weight. In the full-term resting newborn the average blood pressure is 72/47 mm Hg and 64/39 mm Hg for the preterm newborn (Fanaroff & Martin 1992). Crying may cause an elevation of 20 mm Hg in both the systolic and diastolic blood pressure; thus accuracy is more likely in the quiet newborn. The measurement of blood pressure is best accomplished by using the Doppler technique or a 1–2 inch cuff and a stethoscope over the brachial artery.

Heart Murmurs

Murmurs are usually produced by turbulent blood flow. Murmurs may be heard when blood flows across an abnormal valve or across a stenosed valve, when there is an atrial septal or ventricular septal defect, or when there is increased flow across a normal valve.

In newborns 90% of all murmurs are transient and not associated with anomalies. They usually involve incomplete closure of the ductus arteriosus or foramen

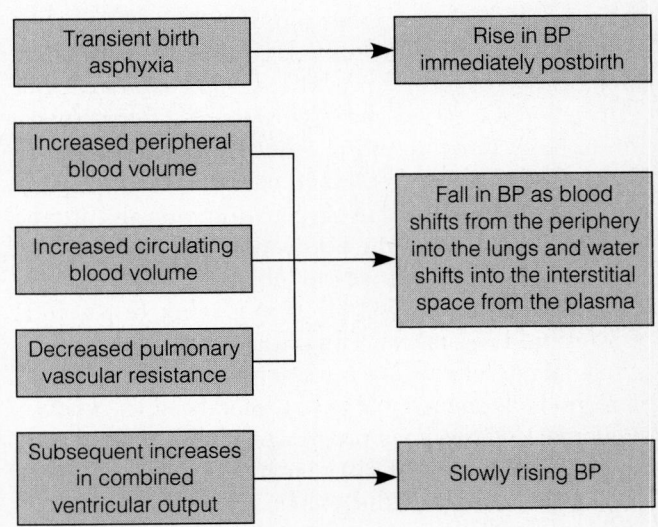

FIGURE 27-7 Response of blood pressure (BP) to changes in neonatal blood volume.

ovale. Soft murmurs may be heard as the pulmonary branch arteries increase their blood flow from 7% to 50% of combined ventricular output during transition, causing physiologic peripheral pulmonary stenosis. With early discharge, murmurs associated with ventricular septal defect and patent ductus arteriosus are not being picked up until the first well-baby checkup at 4–6 weeks of age. Murmurs are sometimes absent in seriously malformed hearts (Fletcher 1994).

Cardiac Work Load

In the first 2 hours after birth when the ductus arteriosus remains mostly patent, about one-third of the left ventricular output is returned to the pulmonary circulation. As a result the left ventricle has a significantly greater volume load than the right ventricle after birth. In the adult, right and left ventricular outputs are equal; in the newborn right ventricular output reflects systemic venous return, and left ventricular output reflects pulmonary venous return. Systemic blood volume and pulmonary blood volume are *not* equal in the neonate. The newborn's combined cardiac output (left and right ventricular) is greater per unit of body weight than it will be in later childhood.

Prior to birth, the right ventricle does approximately two-thirds of the cardiac work. This work load is seen in the increased size and thickness of the right ventricle at birth and may explain why right-sided heart defects are better tolerated than left-sided lesions after birth. After birth the left ventricle must assume a larger share of the cardiac work load, and it increases in size and thickness (Blackburn & Loper 1992). Thus left-sided heart defects rapidly become symptomatic after birth.

HEMATOLOGIC ADAPTATIONS

In the fetus, the hemoglobin and erythrocyte counts are high because of the nature of fetal circulation. Fetal blood (umbilical vein) in utero is 50% oxygen saturated; this relative hypoxia causes increased amounts of erythropoietin to be secreted, resulting in active erythropoiesis (an increase in nucleated red blood cells and reticulocytes). After birth the increases in oxygen saturation and arterial oxygen levels shut off the production of erythropoietin. In the first days of life, hemoglobin concentration may rise 1–2 g/dL above fetal levels as a result of placental transfusion, low oral fluid intake, and diminished extracellular fluid volume. By 1 week postnatally, peripheral hemoglobin is comparable to fetal blood counts. The hemoglobin level declines progressively thereafter during the first 2 to 3 months after birth (Polin & Fox 1992). During this period erythropoietin is again produced by the kidneys. The initial decline in hemoglobin creates a phenomenon known as **physiologic anemia of infancy.** A factor that influences the degree of physiologic anemia

is the nutritional status of the neonate. Supplies of vitamin E, folic acid, and iron may be inadequate given the amount of growth in the later part of the first year of life. Hemoglobin values fall, mainly from a decrease in red cell mass rather than from the dilutional effect of increasing plasma volume. The fact that red cell survival is lower in newborns than in adults, and that red cell production is less, also contributes to this anemia. Neonatal red blood cells have a life span of 80 to 100 days, approximately two-thirds of an adult's red blood cell life span. About 5% of neonatal RBCs retain their nucleus.

Leukocytosis is a normal finding because the stress of birth stimulates increased production of neutrophils during the first few days of life. Neutrophils then decrease to 35% of the total leukocyte count by 2 weeks of age. The thymus provides lymphoblasts to the lymph nodes and other lymphoid tissue. They then play a role in antibody formation. Lymphocytes eventually become the predominant type of leukocyte, and the total white blood count falls. Megakaryocytes appear in the liver and spleen as platelets at about 11 weeks' gestation and approach adult values by 30 weeks.

Blood volume of the term infant is estimated to be 80 to 85 mL/kg of body weight. For example, a 3.6 kg (8 lb) newborn has a blood volume of 290–309 mL. Blood volume varies based on the amount of placental transfusion received during the delivery of the placenta as well as other factors, including the following:

1. *Delayed cord clamping and the normal shift of plasma to the extravascular spaces.* Newborn hemoglobin and hematocrit values are higher when a placental transfusion occurs at birth. Placental vessels contain about 100 mL of blood at term, most of which can be transfused into the newborn by holding the newborn below the level of the placenta and by delaying clamping of the cord (Figure 27–8). Blood volume increases by 50% with delayed cord clamping (Polin & Fox 1992). The increase is reflected by a rise in hemoglobin level and an increase in the hematocrit to about 65% after birth (compared with 48% when the cord is clamped immediately). For greatest accuracy the initial hemoglobin and hematocrit levels should be measured in the cord blood, although this is not a routine practice.

2. *Gestational age.* There appears to be a positive association between gestational age, red blood cell numbers, and hemoglobin concentration.

3. *Prenatal and/or perinatal hemorrhage.* Occurrence of significant prenatal or perinatal bleeding decreases the hematocrit level and causes hypovolemia.

4. *The site of the blood sample.* Hemoglobin and hematocrit levels taken simultaneously are significantly higher in capillary blood than in venous blood during the neonatal period of life. Sluggish peripheral blood flow creates red blood cells stasis, thereby

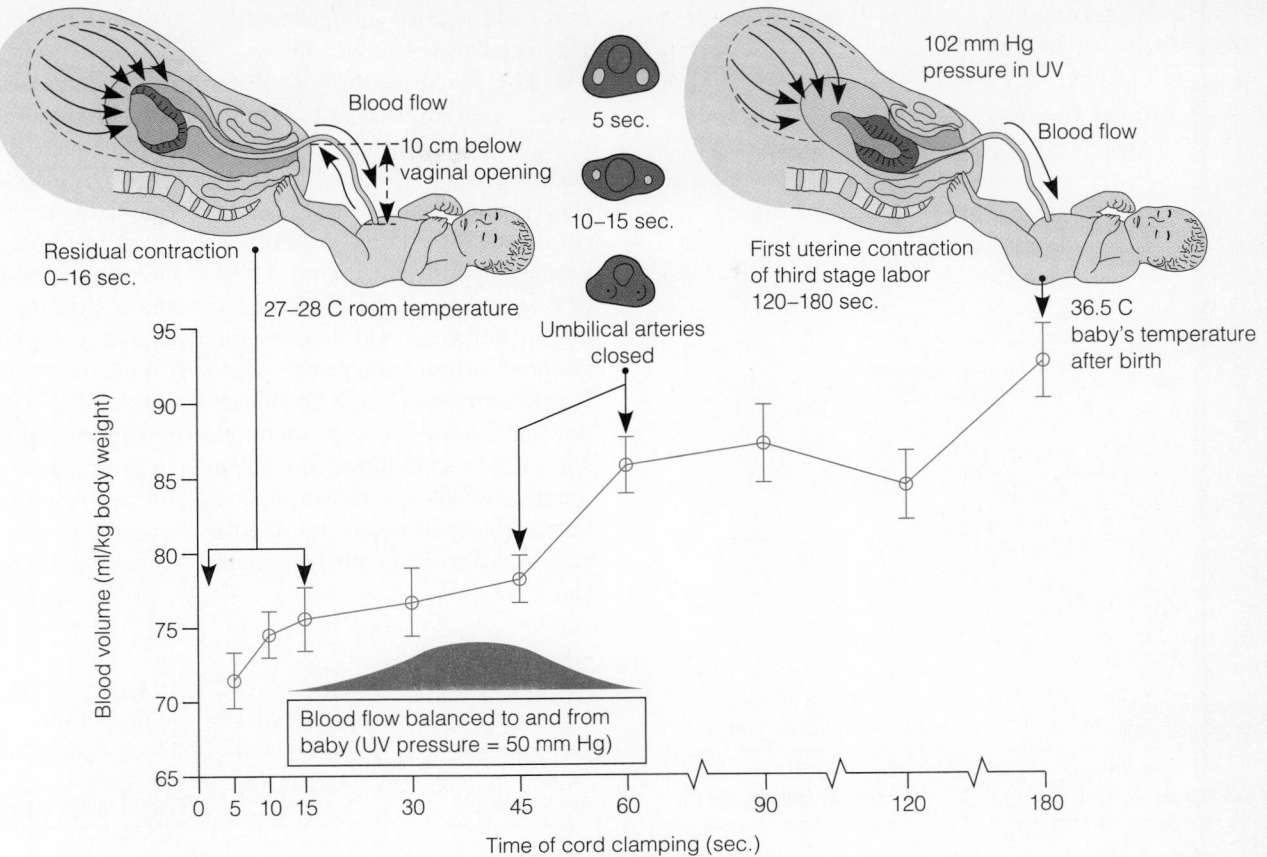

102 mm Hg pressure in UV

Blood flow

5 sec.

10–15 sec.

First uterine contraction of third stage labor 120–180 sec.

36.5 C baby's temperature after birth

Blood flow

–10 cm below vaginal opening

Residual contraction 0–16 sec.

27–28 C room temperature

Umbilical arteries closed

Blood flow balanced to and from baby (UV pressure = 50 mm Hg)

Blood volume (ml/kg body weight)

Time of cord clamping (sec.)

FIGURE 27-8 Schematic illustration of the mechanisms in placental transfusion (normal term births). The mean neonatal blood volume at 30 minutes is plotted against the time of cord clamping after birth (mean + SE, data from 114 full-term infants). Note episodic, stepwise increments in blood volume at 10, 60, and 180 seconds. SOURCE: Yao AC, Lind J: *Placental Transfusion: A Clinical and Physiological Study.* Springfield, IL: Charles C Thomas, 1982.

increasing their concentration in the capillaries. Because of this, blood samples taken from venous blood sites are more accurate.

The concentration of serum electrolytes in the blood indicates the fluid and electrolyte status of the newborn. See Table 27–2 for normal full-term newborn electrolyte and blood values.

TEMPERATURE REGULATION

Temperature regulation is the maintenance of balance between the loss of heat to the environment and the production of heat. Newborns are *homeothermic;* they attempt to stabilize their internal (core) body temperatures within a narrow range in spite of significant temperature variations in their environment. With birth the fetus moves from a warm intrauterine environment to the relatively colder extrauterine environment. The newborn's temperature may fall 2 C to 3 C after birth due mainly to

evaporative losses; this triggers cold-induced metabolic responses and heat production. Full-term newborns can increase their metabolic rate by 100% by 15–30 minutes after birth (Blackburn & Loper 1992).

Thermoregulation in the newborn is closely related to the rate of metabolism and oxygen consumption. Within a specific environmental range called the **thermal neutral zone (TNZ)** the rates of oxygen consumption and metabolism are minimal, and internal body temperature is maintained because of thermal balance (Table 27–3). For an unclothed full-term newborn the TNZ range is an ambient environmental temperature of 32–34 C (89.6–93.2 F). The limits for an adult are 26–28 C (78.8–82.4 F) (Polin & Fox 1992). Thus the normal newborn requires higher environmental temperatures to maintain a thermoneutral environment.

Several newborn characteristics affect the establishment of a TNZ. The newborn has decreased subcutaneous fat and a thin epidermis. Blood vessels are closer to the skin than those of an adult. Therefore, the circulating

TABLE 27-2 Normal Term Newborn Blood Values

Laboratory Data	Normal Range
Hemoglobin	15–20 g/dL
Hematocrit	43%–61%
WBC	10,000–30,000/mm³
Neutrophils	40%–80%
Immature WBC	3%–10%
Platelets	100,000–280,000/mm³
Reticulocytes	3%–6%
Blood volume	82.3 mL/kg (third day after early cord clamping)
	92.6 mL/kg (third day after delayed cord clamping)
Sodium	124–156 mmol/L
Potassium	5.3–7.3 mmol/L
Chloride	90–111 mmol/L
Calcium	7.3–9.2 mg/dL
Glucose	40–97 mg/dL

blood is influenced by changes in environmental temperature and in turn influences the hypothalamic temperature-regulating center.

The flexed posture of the term infant decreases the surface area exposed to the environment, thereby reducing heat loss. Other newborn characteristics such as size, surface area to body weight ratio, and age may also affect the establishment of a TNZ. Preterm small-for-gestational-age (SGA) newborns (due to decreased adipose tissue and hypoflexion) require higher environmental temperatures to achieve a thermal neutral environment. A larger, well-insulated newborn may be able to cope with lower environmental temperatures. If the environmental temperature falls below the lower limits of the TNZ, the newborn responds with increased oxygen consumption and raised metabolism, which results in greater heat production. Prolonged exposure to the cold may result in depleted glycogen stores and acidosis. Oxygen consumption also increases if the environmental temperature is above the TNZ.

TABLE 27-3 Neutral Thermal Environmental Temperatures

Age and Weight	Range of Temperature (C)	Age and Weight	Range of Temperature (C)
0–6 Hours		**72–96 Hours**	
Under 1200 g	34.0–35.4	Under 1200 g	34.0–35.0
1200–1500 g	33.9–34.4	1200–1500 g	33.0–34.0
1501–2500 g	32.8–33.8	1501–2500 g	31.1–33.2
Over 2500 (and >36 weeks)	32.0–33.8	Over 2500 (and >36 weeks)	29.8–32.8
6–12 Hours		**4–12 Days**	
Under 1200 g	34.0–35.4	Under 1500 g	33.0–34.0
1200–1500 g	33.5–34.4	1501–2500 g	31.0–33.2
1501–2500 g	32.2–33.8	Over 2500 (and >36 weeks)	
Over 2500 (and >36 weeks)	31.4–33.8	4–5 days	29.5–32.6
12–24 Hours		5–6 days	29.4–32.3
Under 1200 g	34.0–35.4	6–8 days	29.0–32.2
1200–1500 g	33.3–34.3	8–10 days	29.0–31.8
1501–2500 g	31.8–33.8	10–12 days	29.0–31.4
Over 2500 (and >36 weeks)	31.0–33.7	**12–14 Days**	
24–36 Hours		Under 1500 g	32.6–34.0
Under 1200 g	34.0–35.0	1500–2500 g	31.0–33.2
1200–1500 g	33.1–34.2	Over 2500 (and >36 weeks)	29.0–30.8
1501–2500 g	31.6–33.6	**2–3 Weeks**	
Over 2500 (and >36 weeks)	30.7–33.5	Under 1500 g	32.2–34.0
36–48 Hours		1500–2500 g	30.5–33.0
Under 1200 g	34.0–35.0	**3–4 Weeks**	
1200–1500 g	33.0–34.1	Under 1500 g	31.6–33.6
1501–2500 g	31.4–33.5	1500–2500 g	30.0–32.7
Over 2500 (and >36 weeks)	30.5–33.3	**4–5 Weeks**	
48–72 Hours		Under 1500 g	31.2–33.0
Under 1200 g	34.0–35.0	1500–2500 g	29.5–32.2
1200–1500 g	33.0–34.0	**5–6 Weeks**	
1501–2500 g	31.2–33.4	Under 1500 g	30.6–32.3
Over 2500 (and >36 weeks)	30.1–33.2	1500–2500 g	29.0–31.8

*Generally speaking, the smaller infants in each weight group will require a temperature in the higher portion of the temperature range.
Within each time range, the younger the infant, the higher the temperature required.

SOURCE: Adapted from Scopes and Ahmed (1966) (For his table Scopes had the walls of the incubator 1–2 degrees warmer than the ambient air temperatures.) Reproduced, with permission, from Klaus MH, Fanaroff, AA: *Care of the High-Risk Neonate,* 3rd ed. Philadelphia: WB Saunders, 1986, p 103.

Heat Loss

A newborn is at a distinct disadvantage in maintaining a normal temperature. With a large body surface in relation to mass and a limited amount of insulating subcutaneous fat, the full-term newborn loses about four times as much heat as an adult (Cunningham et al 1993). The newborn's poor thermal stability is primarily due to excessive heat loss rather than to impaired heat production. Because of the risk of hypothermia and possible cold stress, minimizing heat loss in the newborn after birth is essential. (See Chapters 23 and 29 for nursing measures.)

Two major routes of heat loss are from the internal core of the body to the body surface and from the external body surface to the environment. Usually the core temperature is higher than the skin temperature, resulting in continuous transfer or conduction of heat to the surface (Fanaroff & Martin 1992). The greater the difference in temperatures between core and skin, the more rapid the transfer. Infants losing heat from their skin surface must increase their core temperature to avoid hypothermia. This is accomplished by increasing oxygen consumption, depleting glycogen stores, and metabolizing brown fat.

Preventing heat loss from skin to the environment is essential to protecting the infant's core temperature and minimizing thermal stress. Heat loss from the body surface to the environment takes place by four avenues—convection, radiation, evaporation, and conduction (Figure 27–9).

- **Convection** is the loss of heat from the warm body surface to the cooler air currents. Air-conditioned rooms, air currents with a temperature below the infant's skin temperature, oxygen by mask, and removal of the infant from an incubator for procedures increases convective heat loss of the newborn.

- **Radiation** losses occur when heat transfers from the heated body surface to cooler surfaces and objects not in direct contact with the body. The walls of a room or of an incubator are potential causes of heat loss by radiation, even if the ambient temperature of the incubator is within the thermal neutral range for the infant. Placing cold objects (such as ice for blood gases) onto the incubator or near the infant in the radiant warmer will increase radiant heat losses.

- **Evaporation** is the loss of heat incurred when water is converted to a vapor. The newborn is particularly prone to heat loss by evaporation immediately after birth, when the infant is wet with amniotic fluid, as well as during baths and application of lotions or solutions to the skin.

- **Conduction** is the loss of heat to a cooler surface by direct skin contact. Chilled hands, cool scales, cold examination tables, and cold stethoscopes can cause heat loss by conduction. Even if objects are warmed to the incubator temperature, there still may be a

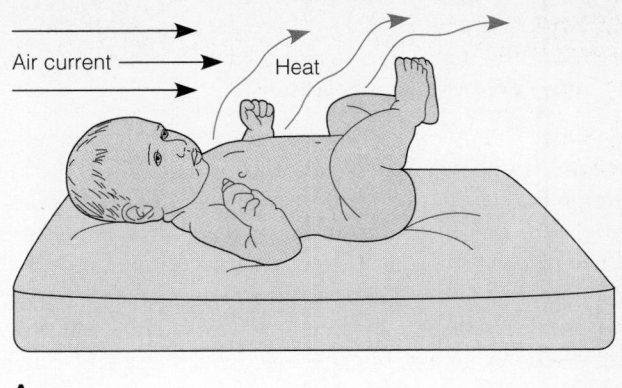

A

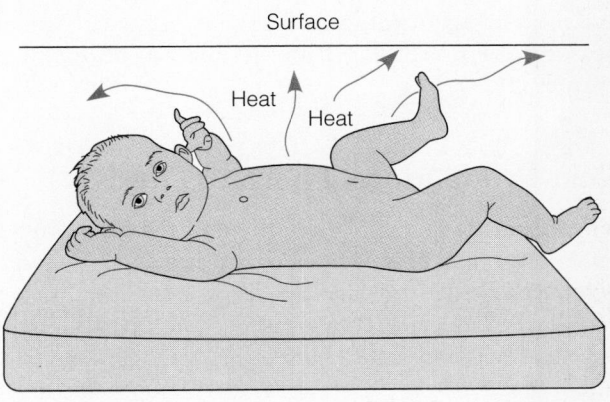

B

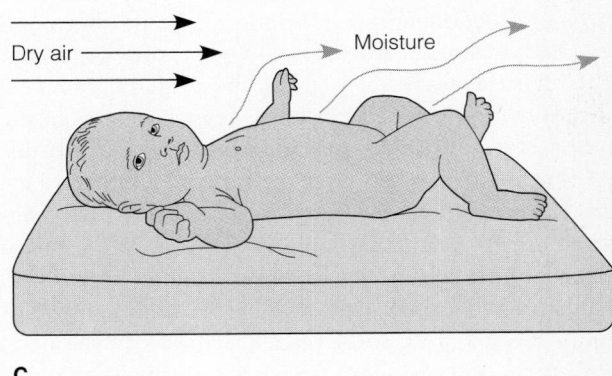

C

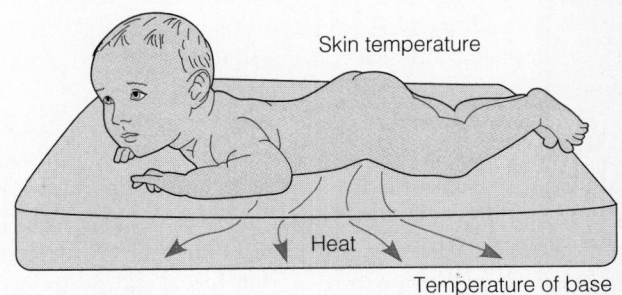

D

FIGURE 27-9 Methods of heat loss. *A* Convection. *B* Radiation. *C* Evaporation. *D* Conduction.

significant temperature difference between the infant's core temperature and the ambient temperature. This results in heat transfer.

Once the infant has been dried after birth, the highest losses of heat generally result from radiation and convection because of the newborn's large body surface compared with weight, and from thermal conduction because of the marked difference between core temperature and skin temperature. The newborn can respond to the cooler environmental temperature with adequate peripheral vasoconstriction, but this mechanism is less effective because of the minimal amount of fat insulation present, the large body surface, and ongoing thermal conduction. Because of these factors, minimizing the baby's heat loss and preventing hypothermia are imperative. Nursing measures for preventing hypothermia can be found in Chapter 29.

Heat Production (Thermogenesis)

When exposed to a cool environment, the newborn requires additional heat. The newborn has several physiologic mechanisms that increase heat production, or *thermogenesis*. These include increased basal metabolic rate, muscular activity, and chemical thermogenesis (also called *nonshivering thermogenesis [NST]*) mediated through the release of catecholamines such as norepinephrine (Hey 1994).

Nonshivering thermogenesis, an important mechanism of heat production, is unique to the newborn and uses the newborn's stores of **brown adipose tissue (BAT)** (also called brown fat) as the primary source of heat in the cold-stressed newborn. It first appears in the fetus at 26 to 30 weeks' gestation and continues to increase until 2 to 5 weeks after the birth of a full-term infant, unless it is depleted by cold stress. Brown fat is deposited in the midscapular area, around the neck, and in the axillas, with deeper placement around the trachea, esophagus, abdominal aorta, kidneys, and adrenal glands (Figure 27–10). BAT constitutes 2% to 6% of the newborn's total body weight. Brown fat receives its name from its dark color, which is due to its enriched blood supply, dense cellular content, and abundant nerve endings. These characteristics promote rapid metabolism, heat generation, and heat transfer to the peripheral circulation.

The large numbers of fat cells facilitate the speed with which triglycerides can be metabolized to produce heat. Energy is provided by glycogen and large numbers of mitochondria releasing adenosine triphosphate (ATP) for rapid metabolic turnover and production of heat. In addition, brown fat possesses a rich blood supply to enhance distribution of heat throughout the body and a nerve supply for initiation of metabolic activity.

NST occurs when skin receptors perceive a drop in environmental temperature and transmit sensations to

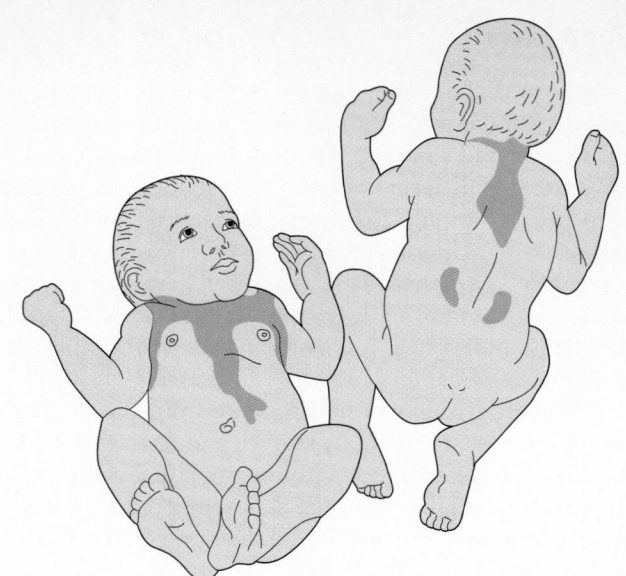

FIGURE 27-10   The distribution of brown adipose tissue (brown fat) in the neonate. SOURCE: Adapted from Davis V: Structure and function of brown adipose tissue in the neonate. *JOGNN* November/December 1980; 9:364.

the CNS, which in turn stimulates the sympathetic nervous system. Release of norepinephrine by the adrenal gland and at local nerve endings in the brown fat causes triglycerides to be metabolized into glycerol and fatty acids. The oxidation of fatty acids is highly exothermic (heat producing); thus heat is distributed to the body. Brown fat is a major producer of heat for the cold-stressed newborn.

Shivering, a form of muscular activity common in the cold adult, is rarely seen in the newborn, although it has been observed at ambient temperatures of 15 C (59 F) or less (Polin & Fox 1992). If shivering does appear, it means the newborn's metabolic rate has already doubled. The extra muscular activity does little to produce needed heat.

Thermographic studies of newborns exposed to cold show an increase in the skin heat over the brown fat deposits in the neonate between 1 and 14 days of age. If the brown fat supply has been depleted, the metabolic response to cold will be limited or lacking. An increase in basal metabolism as a result of hypothermia results in an increase in oxygen consumption. A decrease in the environmental temperature of 2 C, from 33 C to 31 C, is a drop sufficient to double the oxygen consumption of a term newborn.

The normal term neonate is usually able to cope with the increase, but the preterm neonate may be unable to increase ventilation to the necessary level of oxygen consumption. As a consequence, providing the newborn with an optimal thermal environment is absolutely necessary to prevent neonatal cold stress and the resulting metabolic physiologic responses. (See Chapter 32 for discussion of cold stress.)

Because oxidation of fatty acids depends on the availability of oxygen, glucose, and ATP, the newborn's ability to generate heat can be altered by pathologic events such as hypoxia, acidosis, and hypoglycemia or by medications that block the release of norepinephrine. The effect of certain drugs such as meperidine (Demerol) may also prevent metabolism of brown fat. Meperidine given to the laboring woman leads to a greater fall in the newborn's body temperature during the neonatal period. Neonatal hypothermia prolongs as well as potentiates the effects of many analgesic and anesthetic drugs in the newborn.

Response to Heat

Sweating is the usual initial response of the term newborn to hyperthermia. The newborn has six times as many sweat glands as the adult, but the capacity of the sweat gland is one-third that of the adult. The glands have limited function until after the fourth week of extrauterine life. Dissipation of heat is accomplished by peripheral vasodilatation and evaporation of insensible water loss. Sweat usually appears on the infant's forehead 35–40 minutes after exposure to an ambient temperature above 37 C (98.6 F). In term small-for-gestational-age infants the onset of sweating is delayed; it is virtually nonexistent in preterm infants less than 30 weeks' gestation due to the underdevelopment of the sweat glands (Hey 1994). Oxygen consumption and metabolic rate also increase in response to hyperthermia. Severe hyperthermia can lead to death or to gross brain damage if the baby survives.

HEPATIC ADAPTATIONS

In the newborn the liver is frequently palpable 2 to 3 cm below the right costal margin. It is relatively large and occupies about 40% of the abdominal cavity. The neonatal liver plays a significant role in iron storage, carbohydrate metabolism, conjugation of bilirubin, and coagulation.

Iron Storage and Red Blood Cell Production

As red blood cells are destroyed after birth, the iron is stored in the liver until needed for new red blood cell production. Newborn iron stores are determined by total body hemoglobin content and length of gestation. The term newborn has about 270 mg of iron at birth, and about 140 to 170 mg of this amount is in the hemoglobin. If the mother's iron intake has been adequate, enough iron will be stored to last until 5 months of age. After about 6 months of age, foods containing iron or iron supplements must be given to prevent anemia.

Carbohydrate Metabolism

At term the newborn's cord blood glucose is 70% to 80% of the maternal blood glucose level. Neonatal carbohydrate reserves are relatively low. One-third of this reserve is in the form of liver glycogen. Neonatal glycogen stores are twice that of the adult.

The newborn enters an energy crunch at the time of birth with the removal of the maternal glucose supply and the increased energy expenditure associated with the birth process and extrauterine life. Fuel sources are consumed at a faster rate because of the work of breathing, loss of heat when exposed to cold, activity, and activation of muscle tone. Glucose is the main source of energy in the first 4–6 hours after birth. The blood glucose level falls rapidly and then stabilizes at values of 50 to 60 mg/dL; by the third day postnatally the mean values increase to 60 to 70 mg/dL.

Assessment of glucose level using a Chemstrip method is done upon admission and at 4 hours of age. If the fetus or newborn experiences hypoxia, the glycogen stores are more rapidly used and may be depleted in order to meet metabolic requirements. As stores of liver and muscle glycogen and blood glucose decrease, the newborn compensates by changing from a predominantly carbohydrate metabolism to fat metabolism. Energy is derived from fat and protein as well as from carbohydrates. The amount and availability of each of these "fuel substrates" depends on the ability of immature metabolic pathways to function in the first few days of life.

Conjugation of Bilirubin

Conjugation of bilirubin is the conversion of yellow lipid-soluble pigment into water-soluble pigment. Unconjugated (indirect) bilirubin is a breakdown product derived from hemoglobin that is released primarily from destroyed red blood cells. Unconjugated bilirubin is not in an excretable form and is a potential toxin. **Total serum bilirubin** is the sum of conjugated (direct) and unconjugated (indirect) bilirubin.

The relatively immature fetal liver cannot conjugate bilirubin. However, unconjugated bilirubin can cross the placenta to be excreted by maternal processes, so conjugation is not required in the fetus. Total bilirubin at birth is less than 3 mg/mL unless an abnormal hemolytic process has been present. Postnatally, the newborn's liver must begin to conjugate bilirubin. The newborn's functionally immature hepatic enzyme systems and a relatively large bilirubin load produce an increase in serum bilirubin in the first few days of life.

The bilirubin formed after red blood cells are destroyed is transported in the blood bound to albumin. The bilirubin is transferred into the hepatocytes and bound to two intracellular proteins. These two proteins determine the amount of bilirubin that is held in the liver cells for processing. The clearance and conjugation of

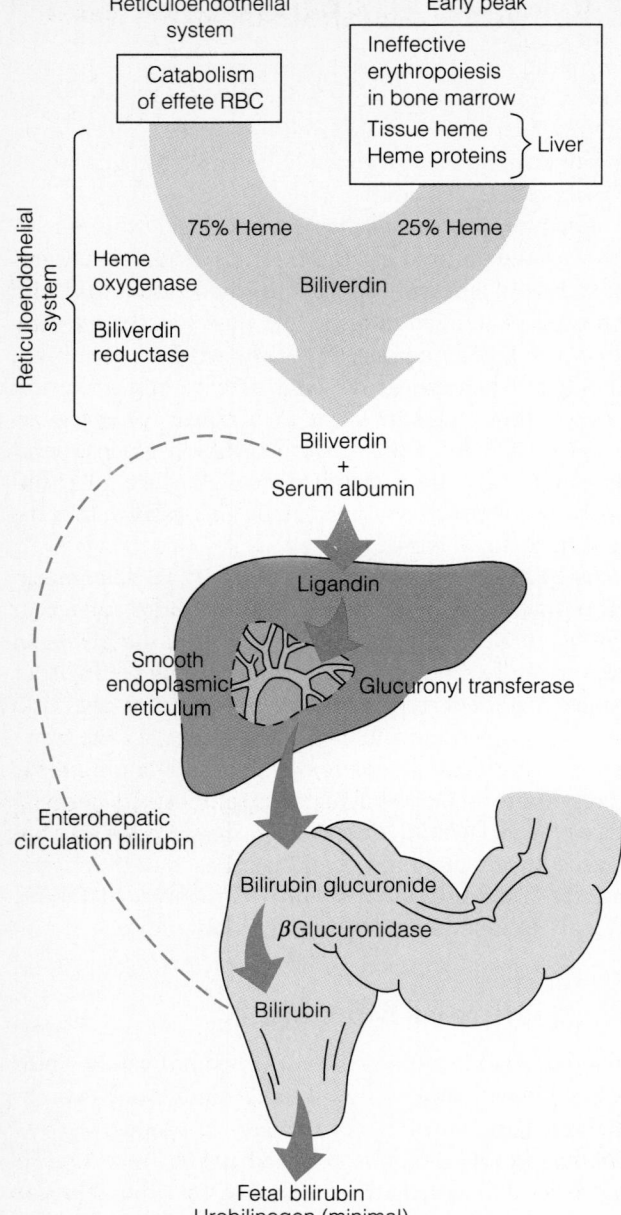

FIGURE 27-11 Conjugation of bilirubin in newborns. SOURCE: Avery GB, Fletcher MA, MacDonald MG: *Neonatology: Pathophysiology and Management of the Newborn,* 4th ed. Philadelphia: Lippincott, 1994, p 635.

bilirubin depend on the glucuronyl transferase enzyme that produces conjugated bilirubin. Conjugated bilirubin is excreted into the tiny bile ducts, then into the common duct and duodenum. The conjugated bilirubin then progresses down the intestines, where bacteria transform it into urobilinogen. This product is not reabsorbed but is excreted as a yellow-brown pigment in the stools.

The newborn liver has relatively less glucuronyl transferase activity at birth and in the first few weeks of life than an adult liver. This reduction in activity predisposes the newborn to decreased conjugation of bilirubin and increased susceptibility to jaundice.

Even after the bilirubin has been conjugated it can be converted back to unconjugated bilirubin by enterohepatic circulation. In the intestines, β-glucuronidase enzyme deconjugates the conjugated bilirubin if it has not yet been converted to urobiligen. The unconjugated bilirubin is then reabsorbed through the intestinal wall and brought back to the liver via portal vein circulation. This recycling of the bilirubin and decreased ability to clear bilirubin from the system are prevalent in babies who have very high β-glucuronidase activity levels as well as delayed bacterial colonization of the gut (Figure 27–11) and further increases the newborn's susceptibility to jaundice.

Physiologic Jaundice

Physiologic jaundice is caused by accelerated destruction of fetal RBCs, impaired conjugation of bilirubin, and increased bilirubin reabsorption from the intestinal tract. This condition does not have a pathologic basis, but rather is a normal biologic response of the newborn.

Maisels 1994 describes six factors whose interactions may give rise to physiologic jaundice:

1. *Increased amounts of bilirubin delivered to the liver.* The increased blood volume due to delayed cord clamping combined with faster RBC destruction in the newborn leads to an increased bilirubin level in the blood. A proportionately larger amount of nonerythrocyte bilirubin is formed in the newborn. Therefore newborns have two to three times greater production or breakdown of bilirubin. The use of forceps, which sometimes causes facial bruising and/or cephalhematoma (entrapped hemorrhage), can increase the amount of bilirubin to be handled by the liver.

2. *Defective uptake of bilirubin from the plasma.* If the newborn does not ingest adequate calories, the formation of hepatic intracellular binding proteins diminishes; this decreases bilirubin uptake from the blood and results in higher bilirubin levels.

3. *Defective conjugation of the bilirubin.* The hepatic enzyme glucuronyl transferase catalyzes the rate-limiting step in the conjugation and excretion of bilirubin. When this enzyme activity is decreased, the intracellular binding proteins remain saturated, and unconjugated bilirubin builds up in the blood. The fatty acids in maternal breast milk compete with bilirubin for albumin binding sites; this process is thought to impede bilirubin processing.

4. *Defect in bilirubin excretion.* A congenital infection may cause impaired excretion of conjugated bilirubin. Delay in introduction of bacterial flora and decreased intestinal motility can also delay excretion and increase enterohepatic circulation of bilirubin.

5. *Inadequate hepatic circulation.* Decreased oxygen supplies to the liver associated with neonatal hypoxia or

congenital heart disease lead to a rise in the bilirubin level.

6. *Increased reabsorption of bilirubin from the intestine.* Reduced bowel motility, intestinal obstruction, or delayed passage of meconium increases the circulation of bilirubin in the enterohepatic pathway, thereby resulting in higher bilirubin values.

About 50% of full-term and 80% of preterm newborns exhibit physiologic jaundice on about the second or third day after birth. The characteristic yellow color results from increased levels of unconjugated bilirubin, which are a normal product of RBC breakdown and reflect a temporary inability of the body to eliminate bilirubin. Serum levels of bilirubin are about 4–6 mg/dL before yellow coloration of the skin and sclera appears. The signs of physiologic jaundice appear *after* the first 24 hours postnatally. This differentiates physiologic jaundice from pathologic jaundice (Chapter 32), which is clinically seen at birth or within the first 24 hours of postnatal life.

In the past, the recommendation was that during the first week unconjugated bilirubin levels in physiologic jaundice should not exceed 13 mg/dL in the full-term or preterm newborn. Peak bilirubin levels are reached between days 3 and 5 in the full-term infant and between days 5 and 7 in the preterm infant. These values are established for European and American Caucasian newborns. Chinese, Japanese, Korean, and Native American newborns have considerably higher bilirubin levels that are not as apparent and that persist for longer periods with no apparent ill effects (Maisels 1994). Some recent studies propose levels up to 22 mg/dL (300–375 μmol/L) in well babies (Newman & Maisels 1992).

The nursery or postpartum room environment, including lighting, can hinder the early detection of the degree and type of jaundice. Pink walls and artificial lights mask the beginning of jaundice in newborns. Daylight assists the observer in early recognition by eliminating distortions caused by artificial light.

If jaundice is suspected, the nurse can quickly assess the newborn's coloring by pressing the skin, generally on the forehead or nose, with a finger. As blanching occurs, the nurse can observe the icterus (yellow coloring).

The following nursery or newborn care procedures are designed to decrease the probability of high bilirubin levels:

- The newborn's skin temperature is maintained at 36.5 C (97.8 F) or above because cold stress results in acidosis. Acidosis in turn decreases available serum albumin–binding sites, weakens albumin-binding powers, and causes elevated unconjugated bilirubin levels.

- Stool is monitored for amount and characteristics. Bilirubin is eliminated in the feces; inadequate stooling may result in reabsorption and recycling of bilirubin. Early breastfeeding is encouraged because the laxative effect of colostrum increases excretion of stool.

- Early feedings are also encouraged to promote intestinal elimination and bacterial colonization and to provide caloric and protein intake necessary for the formation of hepatic binding proteins (Wilkerson 1988).

If jaundice becomes apparent, nursing care is directed toward keeping the newborn well hydrated and promoting intestinal elimination. For specific nursing management and therapies see the Nursing Care Plan: Newborn with Jaundice in Chapter 32.

Physiologic jaundice may be very upsetting to parents; they require emotional support and thorough explanation of the condition. If the baby is placed under phototherapy, a few additional days of hospitalization may be required. This may also be disturbing to parents. They should be encouraged to provide for the emotional needs of their newborn by continuing to feed, hold, and caress the infant. If the mother is discharged, the parents should be encouraged to return for feedings and feel free to telephone or visit whenever possible. In many instances the mother, especially if she is breastfeeding, may elect to remain hospitalized with her newborn; this decision should be supported. As an alternative to continued hospitalization, some newborns are treated in home phototherapy programs.

Breastfeeding Jaundice

Breastfeeding is implicated in prolonged jaundice in some newborns. From 1% to 5% of newborns being breastfed will develop breastfeeding jaundice. The breastfed jaundiced newborn's bilirubin level begins to rise after the first week of life when physiologic jaundice is waning and the mother's mature milk has come in (Wilkerson 1988). The level peaks at 2–3 weeks of age and may reach 20–25 mg/dL without intervention (Maisels 1994).

It is theorized that some women's breast milk may contain several times the normal concentration of certain free fatty acids. These free fatty acids may compete with bilirubin for binding sites on albumin and inhibit the conjugation of bilirubin or increase lipase activity, which disrupts the red blood cell membrane. Increased lipase activity enhances absorption of bile across the gastrointestinal tract membrane, thereby increasing the enterohepatic circulation of bilirubin. In the past it was thought that the breast milk of women whose newborns have breastfeeding jaundice contained an enzyme that inhibited glucuronyl transferase.

Newborns with breastfeeding jaundice appear well, and at present there is an absence of documented kernicterus with this type of jaundice. Temporary cessation of breastfeeding may be advised if bilirubin reaches presumed toxic levels of approximately 20 mg/dL or if the interruption is necessary to establish the cause of the hyperbilirubinemia (Maisels 1994). Within 24 to 36 hours after discontinuing breastfeeding the newborn's serum bilirubin levels begin to fall dramatically, and breastfeeding should be resumed.

Many physicians believe that breastfeeding may be resumed once other causes of jaundice have been ruled out and breastfeeding is determined to be the cause. The bilirubin concentration may rise 2 to 3 mg/dL with a subsequent decline (Maisels 1994). Nursing mothers need encouragement and support in their desire to nurse their infants, assistance and instruction regarding pumping and expressing milk during the interrupted nursing period, and reassurance that nothing is wrong with their milk or their mothering abilities (Table 27–4).

Coagulation

The liver plays an important part in blood coagulation during fetal life and continues this function following birth. Coagulation factors II, VII, IX, and X (synthesized in the liver) are activated under the influence of vitamin K and therefore are considered vitamin K dependent. The absence of normal intestinal flora needed to synthesize vitamin K in the newborn gut results in low levels of vitamin K and creates a transient blood coagulation alteration between the second and fifth day of life. From a low point at about 2 to 3 days after birth these coagulation factors rise slowly but do not approach adult levels until 9 months of age or later. Other coagulation factors with low cord blood levels are XI, XII, and XIII. Fibrinogen and factors V and VII are near adult ranges (Eden & Boehm 1990).

Although newborn bleeding problems are rare, an injection of vitamin K (AquaMEPHYTON) is given prophylactically on the day of birth to combat potential clinical bleeding problems. (Hemorrhagic disease of the newborn is discussed in more depth in Chapter 32.)

Platelet counts at birth are in the same range as for older children, but newborns may manifest mild transient difficulty in platelet aggregation functioning. This platelet problem is accentuated by phototherapy (Eden & Boehm 1990).

Prenatal maternal therapy with phenytoin sodium (Dilantin) or phenobarbital also causes abnormal clotting studies and newborn bleeding in the first 24 hours after birth. Infants born to mothers receiving coumarin (warfarin) compounds may bleed because these agents cross the placenta and accentuate existing vitamin K–dependent factor deficiencies. Transient neonatal thrombocytopenia may occur in infants born to mothers with severe hypertension or HELLP syndrome (*h*emolysis, *e*levated *l*iver enzymes, and *l*ow *p*latelet count) and in mothers who have idiopathic isoimmune thrombocytopenic purpura.

GASTROINTESTINAL ADAPTATIONS

Fetal-Neonatal Transitional Physiology

Adequate maturity of the gastrointestinal tract is achieved by 36 to 38 weeks' gestation with the presence of enzymatic activity and the ability to transport most carbohydrate, fat, and protein nutrients across the intestinal membranes. Development of the secretory and absorptive surfaces is greater than that of the supporting musculature. All glandular elements found in the adult mucosa are present at birth, but the fetal structures are more shallow and less functional until 2–3 years of age.

By birth the newborn has experienced swallowing, gastric emptying, and intestinal propulsion. In utero, swallowing is accompanied by gastric emptying and peristalsis of the fetal intestinal tract. By the end of gestation peristalsis becomes much more active in preparation for extrauterine life. Fetal peristalsis is also stimulated by anoxia, causing the expulsion of meconium into the amniotic fluid in more mature fetuses.

Air enters the stomach immediately after birth. The small intestine is air-filled within 2 to 12 hours and the large bowel within 24 hours. The salivary glands are immature at birth, and little saliva is manufactured until the infant is about 3 months old. The newborn's stomach has a capacity of 50 to 60 mL. It empties intermittently, starting within a few minutes of the beginning of a feeding and ending between 2 and 4 hours after feeding.

The cardiac sphincter is immature, as is neural control of the stomach, so some regurgitation may be noted in the neonatal period. Regurgitation of the first few feedings during the first day or two of life can usually be lessened by avoiding overfeeding and by burping the newborn well during and after the feeding.

When no other signs and symptoms are evident, vomiting is limited and ceases within the first few days of life. Continuous vomiting or regurgitation should be ob-

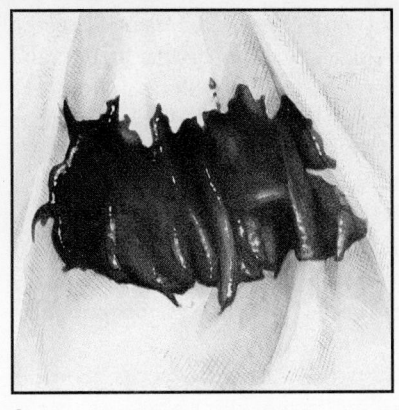
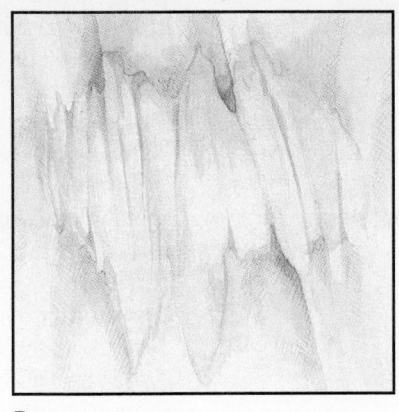
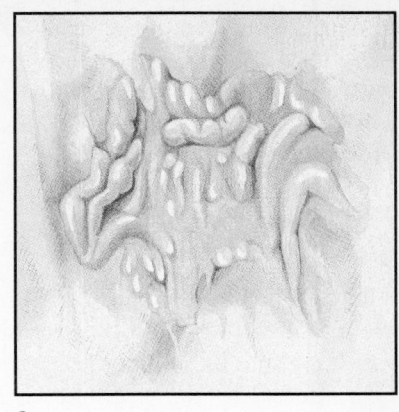

A   **B**   **C**

FIGURE 27-12   Newborn stool samples. *A* Meconium stool. *B* Breast milk stool. *C* Cow's milk stool.

served closely. If the newborn has swallowed bloody or purulent amniotic fluid, lavage of the stomach may be indicated in the term newborn to relieve the problem. Bilious vomiting is abnormal and must be evaluated thoroughly because it might represent a condition that warrants prompt surgical intervention.

Adequate digestion and absorption are essential for newborn growth and development. If optimal nutritional support is available, postnatal growth ideally should parallel intrauterine growth; that is, after 30 weeks of gestation the fetus gains 30 g per day and adds 1.2 cm to body length daily. To gain weight at the intrauterine rate, the term newborn requires 120 cal/kg/day. Following birth, caloric intake is often insufficient for weight gain until the newborn is 5 to 10 days old. During this time there may be a weight loss of 5% to 10% in term newborns. Shift of intracellular water to extracellular space and insensible water loss account for the 5% to 10% weight loss. Thus failure to lose weight when caloric intake is limited may indicate fluid retention.

Normal term newborns pass meconium within 8–24 hours of life—and almost always within 48 hours. **Meconium** is formed in utero from the amniotic fluid and its constituents, with intestinal secretions and shed mucosal cells. It is recognized by its thick, tarry, black (or dark green) appearance. Transitional (thinner brown to green) stools consisting of part meconium and part fecal material are passed for the next day or two, after which the stools become entirely fecal. Generally, the stools of a breastfed newborn are pale yellow (but may be pasty green); they are more liquid and more frequent than those of formula-fed newborns, whose stools are paler (Figure 27–12) (Salariya & Robertson 1993). Frequency of bowel movement varies but initially ranges from one every 2 to 3 days to as many as ten daily. Totally breastfed infants often progress to stools that occur every 5 to 7

TABLE 27-5	Physiologic Adaptations to Extrauterine Life

Periodic breathing may be present.
Desired skin temperature 36–36.5 C (96.8–97.7 F), stabilizes 4 to 6 hours after birth.
Desired blood glucose level reaches 60–70 mg/dL by third postnatal day.
Stools (progress from):
　　Meconium (thick, tarry, black)
　　Transitional stools (thin, brown to green)
　　Breastfed infants (yellow gold, soft, or mushy)
　　Bottle-fed infants (pale yellow, formed, and pasty)

days. Mothers should be counseled that this is not constipation as long as the bowel movement remains soft (Table 27–5).

When the nurse took my first child and put him to my breast his tiny mouth opened and reached for me as if he had known forever what to do.
　　　　　~LESLIE KENTON,
　　　　　ALL I EVER WANTED WAS A BABY~

Digestive Function

The term neonate has adequate intestinal and pancreatic enzymes to digest most simple carbohydrates, proteins, and fats. The newborn's gastric pH is neutral to slightly alkaline and becomes less acidic in about a week and remains less acidic than that of adults for 2 to 3 months. The stomach secretes pepsinogen, which is necessary for protein digestion and production of hydrochloric acid. Both pepsinogen and hydrochloric acid are necessary for the digestion of milk prior to its entrance into the small bowel. The digestion and absorption of nutrients are primarily functions of the small bowel, where pancreatic secretions digest starches and proteins. Bile secretions from the gallbladder through the bile duct aid in fat absorption, and duodenal secretions complete this complex process.

Digestion of Carbohydrates, Proteins, and Fats

The carbohydrates requiring digestion in the newborn are usually disaccharides (lactose, maltose, sucrose), which are split into monosaccharides (galactose, fructose, and glucose) by the enzymes of the intestinal mucosa. Lactose is the primary carbohydrate in the breastfeeding newborn and is generally easily digested and well absorbed. The only enzyme lacking at birth is pancreatic amylase, which remains relatively deficient during the first few months of life. Newborns have trouble digesting starches (changing more complex carbohydrates into maltose). Therefore, starches should not be introduced into the diet until after the first few months of life.

Although proteins require more digestion than carbohydrates, they are well digested and absorbed from the newborn intestine.

The newborn digests and absorbs fats less efficiently because of the minimal activity of pancreatic lipase. The neonate excretes 10% to 20% of the dietary fat intake, compared with 10% for the adult. The fat in breast milk is absorbed more completely by the newborn than is the fat in cow's milk because it consists of more medium-chain triglycerides and contains lipase. (See Chapter 30 for a more detailed discussion of infant nutrition.)

URINARY ADAPTATIONS

Kidney Development and Function

Certain physiologic features of the newborn's kidneys are important to consider when looking at the newborn's ability to handle body fluids and excrete urine.

1. The term newborn's kidneys have a full complement of functioning nephrons by 35 weeks of gestation.

2. The glomerular filtration rate of the newborn's kidneys is low in comparison with the adult rate. Because of this physiologic inefficiency, the newborn's kidneys are unable to dispose of water rapidly when necessary.

3. The juxtamedullary portion of the nephron has limited capacity to reabsorb Na^+ and H^+ and concentrate urine. The limitation of tubular reabsorption can lead to inappropriate loss of substances present in the glomerular filtrate, such as amino acids, bicarbonate, glucose, and sodium.

Full-term newborns are less able than adults to concentrate urine (reabsorb water back into the blood) because the tubules are short and narrow. There is a greater capacity for glomerular filtration than for tubular reabsorption-secretion. Although feeding practices may affect the osmolarity of the urine, the maximum concentrating ability of the newborn is a specific gravity of 1.025. The inability to concentrate urine is caused by the limited tubular reabsorption of water and limited excretion of solutes (principally sodium, potassium, chloride, bicarbonate, urea, and phosphate) in the growing newborn. The ability to concentrate urine fully is attained by 3 months of age.

Because the newborn has difficulty concentrating urine, the effect of excessive insensible water loss or restricted fluid intake is unpredictable. The newborn kidney is also limited in its dilutional capabilities. Maximal dilution ability is specific gravity of 1.001. Concentrating and dilutional limitations of renal function are important considerations in monitoring fluid therapy to avoid dehydration and overhydration (Blackburn 1994).

Characteristics of Newborn Urinary Function

Many newborns void immediately after birth and it frequently goes unnoticed. Among normal newborns 93% void by 24 hours after birth, and 98% void by 48 hours (Blackburn 1994). A newborn who has not voided by 48 hours should be assessed for adequacy of fluid intake, bladder distention, restlessness, and symptoms of pain. The appropriate clinical personnel should be notified if indicated.

The initial bladder volume is 6 to 44 mL of urine. Unless edema is present, normal urinary output is often limited, and the voidings are scanty until fluid intake increases. (The fluid of edema is eliminated by the kidneys, so infants with edema have a much higher urinary output.) The first 2 days postnatally the newborn voids two to six times daily, with a urine output of 15 mL per day. The newborn subsequently voids 5 to 25 times every 24 hours, with a volume of 25 mL/kg per day.

Following the first voiding, the newborn's urine frequently appears cloudy (due to mucous content) and has a high specific gravity, which decreases as fluid intake increases. Occasionally, pink stains ("brick dust spots") appear on the diaper. These are caused by urates and are innocuous. Blood may occasionally be observed on the diapers of female infants. This *pseudomenstruation* is related to the withdrawal of maternal hormones. Males may have bloody spotting from a circumcision. In the absence of apparent causes for bleeding, the physician/certified nurse-midwife/neonatal nurse practitioner should be notified. During early infancy normal urine is straw colored and almost odorless, although odor occurs when there is a metabolic disorder, when certain drugs are given, or when infection is present. Table 27–6 contains urinalysis values of the normal newborn.

TABLE 27-6 Newborn Urinalysis Values

Protein < 5–10 mg/dL
WBC < 2–3
RBC 0
Casts 0
Bacteria 0
Specific gravity 1.001–1.025
Color pale yellow

IMMUNOLOGIC ADAPTATIONS

With the transition to extrauterine life, newborns move from the sterile, protected environment of the uterus into a world filled with potential pathogens and antigens that challenge their still immature host defense mechanisms. The newborn possesses varying degrees of impairment of the nonspecific and specific immune responses. The inflammatory response and phagocytosis are altered in newborns primarily because functional limitations of their polymorphonuclear neutrophils (PMNs) affect leukocyte metabolic activities, mobilization, chemotaxis, opsonization, phagocytic activity, and intracellular killing. Newborns, particularly preterm infants, have decreased serum opsonization activity (the process of coating invasive bacteria to prepare them for phagocytic ingestion), resulting from low levels of immunoglobins and complement components. These limitations in the newborn's inflammatory response result in failure to recognize, localize, and destroy invasive bacteria. Thus the signs and symptoms of infection are often subtle and nonspecific in the newborn. The newborn also has a poor hypothalamic response to pyrogens; therefore fever is not a reliable indicator of infection. In the neonatal period, hypothermia is a more reliable sign of infection.

Preterm and term newborns experience significant alterations in humoral (antibody) and cell-mediated immunity and in the complement system. These combined developmental limitations increase the frequency and severity of neonatal infections.

Of the three major types of immunoglobulins primarily involved in immunity—IgG, IgA, and IgM—only IgG crosses the placenta. The pregnant woman forms antibodies in response to illness or immunization. This process is called **active acquired immunity.** When IgG antibodies are transferred to the fetus in utero, **passive acquired immunity** results because the fetus does not produce the antibodies itself. IgG is very active against bacterial toxins.

Because the maternal immunoglobin is transferred primarily during the third trimester, preterm infants (especially those born prior to 34 weeks) may be more susceptible to infection. In general newborns have maternally induced immunity to tetanus, diphtheria, smallpox, measles, mumps, poliomyelitis, and a variety of other bacterial and viral diseases. The period of resistance varies: Immunity against common viral infections such as measles may last 4 to 8 months, whereas immunity to certain bacteria may disappear within 4 to 8 weeks.

The normal newborn does produce antibodies in response to an antigen, but not as effectively as an older child would. It is customary to begin immunization at 2 months of age so the infant can develop active acquired immunity.

IgM immunoglobulins are produced in response to blood group antigens, gram-negative enteric organisms, and some viruses in the expectant mother. Because IgM does not normally cross the placenta, most or all is produced by the fetus beginning at 10 to 15 weeks' gestation. Elevated levels of IgM at birth may indicate placental leaks or, more commonly, fetal antigenic stimulation in utero. Consequently, elevations suggest that the infant was exposed to an intrauterine infection such as syphilis or a TORCH (toxoplasmosis, rubella, cytomegalovirus, herpes virus hominis type 2) infection. (For in-depth discussion see Table 32–6.) The lack of available maternal IgM in the newborn also accounts for the infant's susceptibility to gram-negative enteric organisms such as *Escherichia coli.*

The functions of IgA immunoglobins are not fully understood. IgA appears to provide protection mainly on secreting surfaces such as the respiratory tract, gastrointestinal tract, and eyes. Serum IgA does not cross the placenta and is not normally produced by the fetus in utero. Unlike the other immunoglobins, IgA is not affected by gastric action. Colostrum, the forerunner of breast milk, is very high in the secretory form of IgA. Consequently, it may be of significance in providing some passive immunity to the infant of a breastfeeding mother. Newborns begin to produce secretory IgA in their intestinal mucosa at about 4 weeks after birth.

NEUROLOGIC AND SENSORY-PERCEPTUAL ADAPTATIONS

The newborn's brain is about one-quarter the size of an adult's, and myelination of nerve fibers is incomplete. Unlike the cardiovascular or respiratory systems, which undergo tremendous changes at birth, the nervous system is minimally influenced by the actual birth process.

Because many biochemical and histologic changes have yet to occur in the newborn's brain, the postnatal period is considered a time of risk in regard to the development of the brain and nervous system. For neurologic development—including development of intellect—to proceed, the brain and other nervous system structures must mature in an orderly, unhampered fashion. For discussion of cranial nerves see Chapter 28.

Intrauterine Factors Influencing Newborn Behavior

Newborns respond to and interact with the environment in a predictable pattern of behavior that is somewhat shaped by their intrauterine experience. This intrauterine experience is affected by intrinsic factors such as maternal nutrition and external factors such as the mother's physical environment. Depending on the newborn's intrauterine experience and individual temperament, newborn behavioral responses to various stresses vary from dealing quietly with the stimulation to becoming overreactive and tense; or an individual may exhibit a combination of the two.

Brazelton and colleagues (1977) found a positive association between newborn behavior and nutritional status of the pregnant woman. Newborns with higher birth weight attended to and responded to visual and auditory cues and exhibited more mature motor activity than newborns with low birth weight.

Factors such as exposure to intense auditory stimuli in utero can eventually be manifested in the behavior of the newborn. For example, the fetal heart rate initially increases when the pregnant woman is exposed to an auditory stimuli, but repetition of the stimuli leads to decreased FHR. Thus the newborn who was exposed to intense noise during fetal life is significantly less reactive to loud sounds postnatally.

Characteristics of Newborn Neurologic Function

Partially flexed extremities with the legs near the abdomen is the usual position of the normal newborn. When awake, the newborn may exhibit purposeless, uncoordinated bilateral movements of the extremities. The organization and intensity of the newborn's motor activity are influenced by a number of factors, including the following (Brazelton 1984): (1) sleep-wake states; (2) presence of environmental stimuli such as heat, light, cold, and noise; (3) conditions causing a chemical imbalance, such as hypoglycemia; (4) hydration status; (5) state of health; and (6) recovery from the stress of labor and birth.

Eye movements are observable during the first few days of life. An alert neonate is able to fixate on faces and geometric objects or patterns such as black and white stripes. If a bright light shines in the newborn's eyes, the blinking reflex is elicited.

The cry of the newborn should be lusty and vigorous. High-pitched cries, weak cries, or no cries are all causes for concern.

Growth of the newborn's body progresses in a cephalocaudal (head-to-toe), proximal-distal fashion. The newborn is somewhat hypertonic; that is, there is resistance to extending the elbow and knee joints. Muscle tone should be symmetric. Diminished muscle tone and flaccidity may indicate neurologic dysfunction.

Specific symmetric deep tendon reflexes can be elicited in the newborn. The knee jerk is brisk; a normal ankle clonus may involve three or four beats. Plantar flexion is present. Other reflexes, including the Moro, grasping, rooting, Babinski, and sucking reflexes are characteristics of neurologic integrity. (For further discussion see Chapter 28.)

Performance of complex behavioral patterns reflects the newborn's neurologic maturation and integration. The newborn who can bring a hand to the mouth is demonstrating motor coordination as well as a self-quieting technique, thus increasing the complexity of the behavioral response. Neonates also possess complex organized defensive motor patterns as exhibited by the ability to remove an obstruction, such as a cloth across the face.

Periods of Reactivity

The baby usually shows a predictable pattern of behavior during the first several hours after birth, characterized by two **periods of reactivity** separated by a sleep phase.

First Period of Reactivity

This phase lasts approximately 30 minutes after birth. During this phase the newborn is awake and active and may appear hungry and have a strong sucking reflex. This is a natural opportunity to initiate breastfeeding if the mother has chosen it (Figure 27–13). Bursts of random, diffuse movements alternating with relative immobility may occur. Respirations are rapid, as high as 80 breaths/minute, and there may be retraction of the chest, transient flaring of the nares, and grunting. The heart rate is rapid, and rhythm may be irregular. Bowel sounds are usually absent.

Period of Inactivity to Sleep Phase

After approximately half an hour, the newborn's activity gradually diminishes, and the heart rate and respirations decrease as the newborn enters the sleep phase. The sleep phase may last from a few minutes to 2–4 hours. During this period the newborn will be difficult to awaken and will show no interest in sucking. Bowel sounds become audible, and cardiac and respiratory rates return to baseline values.

Second Period of Reactivity

The newborn is again awake and alert. This phase lasts 4–6 hours in the normal newborn. Physiologic responses

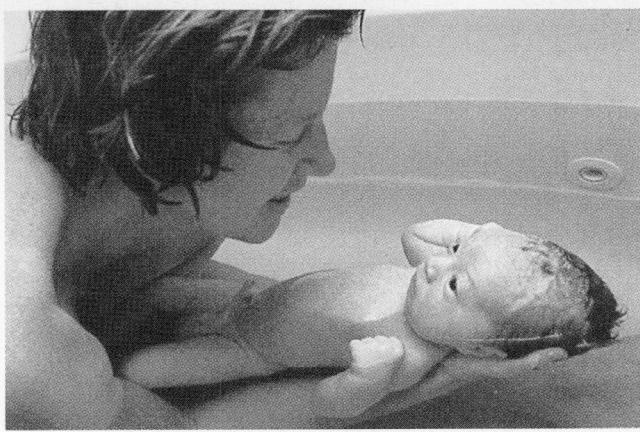

FIGURE 27-13 Mother and baby gaze at each other. This quiet alert state is the optimal state for interaction.

are variable during this stage. The heart and respiratory rates increase; however, the nurse must be alert for apneic periods, which may cause a drop in the heart rate. The newborn is stimulated to continue breathing during such times. The newborn may develop rapid color changes and become mildly cyanotic or mottled during these fluctuations. Production of respiratory and gastric mucus increases, and the newborn responds by gagging, choking, and regurgitating.

Continued close observation and intervention may be required to maintain a clear airway during this period of reactivity. The gastrointestinal tract becomes more active. The first meconium stool is frequently passed during this second active stage, and the initial voiding may also occur at this time. The newborn will indicate readiness for feeding by such behaviors as sucking, rooting, and swallowing. If feeding was not initiated in the first period of reactivity, it is done at this time. See Chapter 30 for further discussion of this first feeding.

Behavioral States of the Newborn

The behavior of the newborn can be divided into two categories: the sleep state and the alert state (Brazelton 1984). These postnatal behavioral states are similar to those that have been identified during pregnancy. Subcategories are identified under each major category.

Sleep States

The sleep states in the newborn are as follows:

1. *Deep or quiet sleep.* Deep sleep is characterized by closed eyes with no eye movements, regular even breathing, and jerky motion or startles at regular intervals. Behavioral responses to external stimuli are likely to be delayed. Startles are rapidly suppressed, and changes in state are not likely to occur.

Heart rate may range from 100 to 120 beats per minute.

2. *Active REM.* Irregular respirations, eyes closed with REM, irregular sucking motions, minimal activity, and irregular but smooth movement of the extremities can be observed in active REM sleep. Environmental and internal stimuli initiate a startle reaction and a change of state.

Sleep cycles in the newborn have been recognized and defined according to duration. The length of the cycle depends on the age of the newborn. At term REM active sleep and quiet sleep occur in intervals of 45 to 50 minutes. About 45% to 50% of the total sleep of the neonate is active sleep, 35% to 45% is quiet (deep) sleep, and 10% of sleep is transitional between these two periods. It is hypothesized that REM sleep stimulates the growth of the neural system. Over a period of time the newborn's sleep-wake patterns become diurnal; that is, the newborn sleeps at night and stays awake during the day. (See Chapter 28 for in-depth discussion of assessment of neonatal states.)

Alert States

Periods of alertness tend to be short the first 2 days after birth to allow the baby to recover from the birth process. Subsequently, alert states are of choice or of necessity (Brazelton 1984). Increasing choice of wakefulness by the newborn indicates a maturing capacity to achieve and maintain consciousness. Heat, cold, and hunger are but a few of the stimuli that can cause wakefulness by necessity. Once the disturbing stimuli are removed, sleep tends to recur.

The following are subcategories of the alert state (Brazelton 1984):

1. *Drowsy or semidozing.* The behaviors common to the drowsy state are open or closed eyes, fluttering eyelids, semidozing appearance, and slow, regular movements of the extremities. Mild startles may be noted from time to time. Although the reaction to a sensory stimulus is delayed, a change of state often results.

2. *Wide awake.* In the wide awake state, the newborn is alert and follows and fixates on attractive objects, faces, or auditory stimuli. Motor activity is minimal, and the response to external stimuli is delayed.

3. *Active awake.* The eyes are open, and motor activity is quite intense, with thrusting movements of the extremities in the active awake state. Environmental stimuli increase startles or motor activity, but discrete reactions are difficult to distinguish because of generalized high activity level.

4. *Crying.* Intense crying is accompanied by jerky motor movements. Crying serves several purposes for

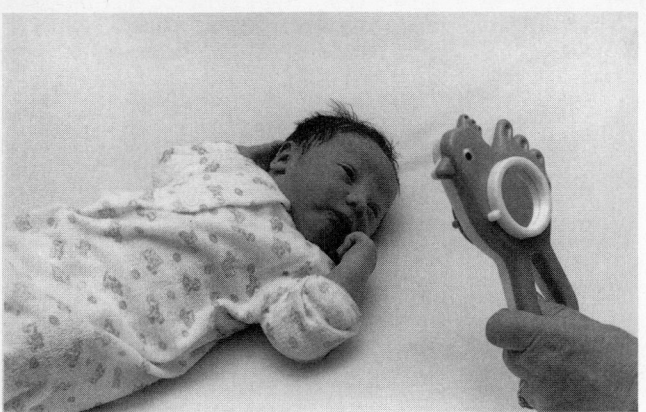

FIGURE 27-14   Head turning to follow an object.

the newborn. It may be used as a distraction from disturbing stimuli such as hunger and pain. Fussiness often allows the newborn to discharge energy and reorganize behavior. Most important, crying elicits an appropriate response of help from the parents.

Behavioral and Sensory Capacities of the Newborn

Habituation is the newborn's ability to process and respond to complex visual and auditory stimulation. For example, when a bright light is flashed into the newborn's eyes, the initial response is blinking, constriction of the pupil, and perhaps a slight startle reaction. However, with repeated stimulation the newborn's response repertoire gradually diminishes and disappears. The capacity to ignore repetitious disturbing stimuli is a neonatal defense mechanism readily apparent in the noisy, well-lighted nursery.

Orientation is the newborn's ability to be alert to, to follow, and to fixate on complex visual stimuli that have a particular appeal and attraction. The newborn prefers the human face and eyes and bright shiny objects. As the face or object is brought into the line of vision, the neonate responds with bright, wide eyes, still limbs, and fixed staring. This intense visual involvement may last several minutes, during which time the newborn is able to follow the stimulus from side to side. Figure 27–14 illustrates this response. The newborn uses this sensory capacity to become familiar with family, friends, and surroundings.

Self-quieting ability refers to newborns' ability to use their own resources to quiet and comfort themselves. Their repertoire includes hand-to-mouth movements, sucking on a fist or tongue, and attending to external stimuli. Neurologically impaired newborns are unable to use self-quieting activities and require more frequent comforting from care givers when stimulated. For example, drug-positive newborns often exhibit abnormal sleep and feeding patterns and irritability (Taeusch et al 1991).

Auditory Capacity

The newborn responds to auditory stimulation with a definite, organized behavior repertoire. The stimulus used to assess auditory response should be selected to match the state of the newborn. A rattle is appropriate for light sleep, a voice for an awake state, and a clap for deep sleep. As the neonate hears the sound, the cardiac rate rises, and a minimal startle reflex may be seen. If the sound is appealing, the newborn will become alert and search for the site of the auditory stimulus.

Olfactory Capacity

Newborns are apparently able to select people by smell. In one study newborns were able to distinguish their mothers' breast pads from those of other mothers at just 1 week postnatally (Brazelton 1984).

Taste and Sucking

The newborn responds differently to varying tastes. Sugar, for example, increases sucking. Sucking pattern variations also exist in newborns fed with a rubber nipple versus the breast. When breastfeeding, the newborn sucks in bursts with frequent regular pauses. The bottle-fed newborn tends to suck at a regular rate with infrequent pauses.

When awake and hungry, the newborn displays rapid searching motions in response to the rooting reflex. Once feeding begins, the newborn establishes a sucking pattern according to the method of feeding. Finger sucking is not only present postnatally, but in utero. The newborn frequently uses nonnutritive sucking as a self-quieting activity, which assists in the development of self-regulation. Nonnutritive sucking with a pacifier should not be discouraged if the infant is bottle-fed. For breastfed infants pacifiers should be offered only after breastfeeding is well established. If the pacifier is offered too soon, a phenomenon called "nipple confusion" may occur in which the breastfed infant has difficulty learning to suck from the breast. (See Chapter 30 for a more in-depth discussion.)

Tactile Capacity

The newborn is very sensitive to being touched, cuddled, and held. Often a mother's first response to an upset or crying newborn is touching or holding. Swaddling, placing a hand on the abdomen, or holding the arms to prevent a startle reflex are other methods of soothing the newborn. The settled newborn is then able to attend to and interact with the environment.

Newborn respiration is initiated primarily by chemical and mechanical events in association with thermal and sensory stimulation.

The production of surfactant is crucial to keeping the lungs expanded during expiration by reducing alveolar surface tension.

The newborn is an obligatory nose breather. Respirations move from being primarily shallow, irregular, and diaphragmatic to synchronous abdominal and chest breathing. Normal respiratory rate is 30–60/minute.

Periodic breathing is normal, and newborn sleep states affect breathing patterns.

The status of the cardiopulmonary system may be measured by evaluating the heart rate, blood pressure, and presence or absence of murmurs. The normal heart rate is 120–160 bpm.

Oxygen transport in the newborn is significantly affected by the presence of greater amounts of HbF (fetal hemoglobin) than HbA (adult hemoglobin). HbF holds oxygen more efficiently but releases it to the body tissues only at low PO_2 levels.

Blood values in the newborn are modified by several factors such as site of the blood sample, gestational age, prenatal and/or perinatal hemorrhage, and the timing of the clamping of the umbilical cord.

Blood glucose levels should reach 60–70 mg/dL by the third postnatal day.

The newborn is considered to have established thermoregulation when oxygen consumption and metabolic activity are minimal.

Evaporation is the primary heat loss mechanism in newborns who are wet from amniotic fluid or a bath. In addition, excessive heat loss occurs from radiation and convection because of the newborn's larger surface area compared to weight and from thermal conduction because of the marked difference between core temperature and skin temperature.

The primary source of heat in the cold-stressed newborn is brown adipose tissue.

The normal newborn possesses the ability to digest and absorb nutrients necessary for newborn growth and development.

The newborn's liver plays a crucial role in iron storage, carbohydrate metabolism, conjugation of bilirubin, and coagulation.

The newborn's stools change from meconium (thick, tarry, black) to transitional stools (thinner, brown to green) and then to the distinct forms for either breastfed newborns (yellow-gold, soft, or mushy) or bottle-fed newborns (pale yellow, formed, and pasty). Most newborns pass their first stool within 24 hours of birth.

The newborn's kidneys are characterized by a decreased rate of glomerular flow, limited tubular reabsorption, limited excretion of solutes, and limited ability to concentrate urine. Most newborns void within 24 hours of birth.

The immune system in the newborn is not fully activated until sometime after birth, but the newborn does possess some immunologic abilities.

Neurologic and sensory-perceptual functioning in the newborn is evident from the newborn's interaction with the environment, presence of synchronized motor activity, and well-developed sensory capacities.

The first period of reactivity lasts for 30 minutes after birth. The newborn is alert and hungry at this time, making this a natural opportunity to promote attachment.

The second period of reactivity requires close monitoring by the nurse because apnea, decreased heart rate, gagging, choking, and regurgitation are likely to occur and require nursing intervention.

Behavioral states in the newborn can be divided into sleep states and alert states.

REFERENCES

Blackburn ST: Renal function in the neonate. *J Perinat Neonatal Nurs* 1994; 8(1):37.

Blackburn ST, Loper DL: *Maternal, Fetal, and Neonatal Physiology: A Clinical Perspective*. Philadelphia: WB Saunders, 1992.

Brazelton TB: *Neonatal Behavioral Assessment Scale*, 2nd ed. London: Heineman, 1984.

Brazelton TB et al: The behavior of nutritionally deprived Guatemalan neonates. *Dev Med Child Neurol* 1977; 19:364.

Cunningham FG, MacDonald PC, Gant NG: *Williams Obstetrics*, 19th ed. Norwalk, CT: Appleton & Lange, 1993.

Eden RD, Boehm FH (editors): *Assessment and Care of the Fetus: Physiological, Clinical, and Medicolegal Principles*. Norwalk, CT: Appleton & Lange, 1990.

Fanaroff AA, Martin RJ: *Neonatal-Perinatal Medicine*, 5th ed. St. Louis: Mosby, 1992.

Fletcher ME: Physical assessment and classification. In: *Neonatology: Pathophysiology and Management of the Newborn*, 4th ed. Avery GB, Fletcher M, MacDonald MG (editors). Philadelphia: Lippincott, 1994.

Hey E: Thermoregulation. In: *Neonatology: Pathophysiology and Management of the Newborn*, 4th ed. Avery GB, Fletcher M, MacDonald MG (editors). Philadelphia: Lippincott, 1994.

James LS, Adamsons K: The neonate and resuscitation. In: *Danforth's Obstetrics and Gynecology*, 7th ed. Scott JR et al (editors). Philadelphia: Lippincott, 1994.

Long WA: *Fetal and Neonatal Cardiology*. Philadelphia: WB Saunders, 1990.

Maisels MJ: Jaundice. In: *Neonatology: Pathophysiology and Management of the Newborn*, 4th ed. Avery GB, Fletcher M, MacDonald MG (editors). Philadelphia: Lippincott, 1994.

Nelson N: Physiology of transitions. In: *Neonatology: Pathophysiology and Management of the Newborn*, 4th ed. Avery GB, Fletcher M, MacDonald MG (editors). Philadelphia: Lippincott, 1994.

Newman TB, Maisels MJ: Evaluation and treatment of jaundice in the term newborn: A kinder, gentler approach. *Pediatrics* 1992; 89(5):809.

Polin RA, Fox WW: *Fetal and Neonatal Physiology*. Philadelphia: WB Saunders, 1992.

Salariya EM, Robertson CM: The development of a neonatal stool colour comparator. *Midwifery* 1993; 9:35.

Taeusch HW, Ballard RA, Avery ME: *Schaffer and Avery's Diseases of the Newborn*, 6th ed. Philadelphia: WB Saunders, 1991.

Wilkerson NN: A comprehensive look at hyperbilirubinemia. *MCN* 1988; 13:360.

CHAPTER 28

NURSING ASSESSMENT OF THE NEWBORN

*S*omething very special occurs within the first hour after birth. If the environment is quiet, the birthing without complications, the lights lowered, the handling diminished, newborn infants—aside from all the physiological adaptations they must make—begin in a uniquely human way to adapt to the new experience of being in the world.

~THE AMAZING NEWBORN~

OBJECTIVES

Delineate the normal physical and behavioral characteristics of the newborn.

Summarize the components of a complete newborn assessment and the significance of normal variations and abnormal findings.

Explain the various components of the gestational age assessment.

Discuss the neurologic and neuromuscular characteristics of the newborn and the reflexes that may be present at birth.

Describe the categories of the newborn behavioral assessment.

nlike adults, newborns communicate needs primarily by behavior. Because nurses are the most consistent observers of the newborn, they must be able to interpret this behavior to gain information about the newborn's condition and to respond with appropriate nursing interventions. This chapter focuses on the assessment of the newborn and interpretation of findings.

Assessment of the newborn is a continuous process used to evaluate development and adjustments to extrauterine life. In the birthing area, Apgar scoring and careful observation of the newborn form the basis of the assessment and are correlated with information such as the following:

- Maternal prenatal care history
- Birthing history
- Maternal analgesia and anesthesia
- Complications of labor or birth
- Treatment instituted in the birthing room, in conjunction with determination of clinical gestational age
- Consideration of the newborn's classification by weight and gestational age and neonatal mortality risk
- Physical examination of the newborn

The nurse incorporates data from these sources with the assessment findings during the first 1 to 4 hours after birth to formulate a plan for nursing intervention.

The various newborn assessments and the data obtained from them are only as effective as the degree to which the findings are shared with the parents. The parents must be included in the assessment process from the moment of their child's birth. The Apgar score and its meaning should be explained immediately to the family. As soon as possible the parents should be a part of the physical and behavioral assessments as well.

The nurse can encourage the parents to identify the unique behavioral characteristics of their newborn and to learn nurturing activities. Attachment is promoted when parents are allowed to explore their newborn in private, identifying individual physical and behavioral characteristics. The nurse's supportive responses to the parents' questions and observations are essential throughout the assessment process.

TIMING OF NEWBORN ASSESSMENTS

The first 24 hours of life are significant because during this period the newborn makes the critical transition from intrauterine to extrauterine life. The risk of mortal-

ity and morbidity is statistically high during this period. Assessment of the newborn is essential to ensure that the transition is proceeding successfully.

There are three major time frames for assessments of newborns while they are in the birth facility. The first assessment is done in the birthing area immediately after birth to determine the need for resuscitation or other interventions. The newborn who is stable can stay with the family after birth to initiate early attachment. The newborn who has complications is usually taken to the nursery for further evaluation and intervention.

A second assessment is done in the first 1 to 4 hours after birth as part of the routine admission procedures. During this assessment the nurse carries out a brief physical examination to evaluate the newborn's adaptation to extrauterine life and to estimate gestational age. Any problems that place the newborn at risk are assessed further during this time.

Prior to discharge, a certified nurse-midwife/physician/nurse practitioner does a complete physical examination to detect any emerging or potential problems. A general assessment is also done at this time (Table 28–1).

This chapter presents the procedures for estimating gestational age and performing the complete physical examination and behavioral assessment. Chapter 20 discusses the immediate postbirth assessment. Chapter 29 describes the brief assessment performed during the first 4 hours of life.

ESTIMATION OF GESTATIONAL AGE

The nurse must establish the newborn's gestational age in the first 4 hours after birth so that careful attention can be given to age-related problems. Traditionally, a newborn's

TABLE 28-1	Timing and Types of Newborn Assessments

Assess immediately after birth: need for resuscitation or if newborn is stable and can be placed with parents to initiate early attachment/bonding

Assessments within 1 to 4 hours after birth:
    Progress of newborn's adaptation to extrauterine life
    Determination of gestational age
    Ongoing assessment for high-risk problems

Assessment procedures within first 24 hours or prior to discharge:
    Complete physical examination (Depending on agency protocol, the nurse may complete some components independently with the certified nurse-midwife/physician/nurse practitioner completing the exam prior to discharge.)
    Nutritional status and ability to bottle- or breastfeed satisfactorily.
    Behavioral state organization abilities

NEWBORN MATURITY RATING & CLASSIFICATION

ESTIMATION OF GESTATIONAL AGE BY MATURITY RATING
Symbols: X - 1st Exam   O - 2nd Exam

NEUROMUSCULAR MATURITY

	−1	0	1	2	3	4	5
Posture							
Square Window (wrist)	>90°	90°	60°	45°	30°	0°	
Arm Recoil		180°	140°–180°	110°–140°	90°–110°	<90°	
Popliteal Angle	180°	160°	140°	120°	100°	90°	<90°
Scarf Sign							
Heel to Ear							

PHYSICAL MATURITY

Skin	sticky friable transparent	gelatinous red, translucent	smooth pink, visible veins	superficial peeling &/or rash, few veins	cracking pale areas rare veins	parchment deep cracking no vessels	leathery cracked wrinkled
Lanugo	none	sparse	abundant	thinning	bald areas	mostly bald	
Plantar Surface	heel-toe 40–50mm:−1 <40mm:−2	>50mm no crease	faint red marks	anterior transverse crease only	creases ant. 2/3	creases over entire sole	
Breast	imperceptible	barely perceptible	flat areola no bud	stippled areola 1–2mm bud	raised areola 3–4mm bud	full areola 5–10mm bud	
Eye/Ear	lids fused loosely:−1 tightly:−2	lids open pinna flat stays folded	sl. curved pinna; soft; slow recoil	well curved pinna; soft but ready recoil	formed & firm instant recoil	thick cartilage ear stiff	
Genitals male	scrotum flat, smooth	scrotum empty faint rugae	testes in upper canal rare rugae	testes descending few rugae	testes down good rugae	testes pendulous deep rugae	
Genitals female	clitoris prominent labia flat	prominent clitoris small labia minora	prominent clitoris enlarging minora	majora & minora equally prominent	majora large minora small	majora cover clitoris & minora	

Gestation by Dates _____ wks

Birth Date _____ Hour _____ am/pm

APGAR _____ 1 min _____ 5 min

MATURITY RATING

score	weeks
−10	20
−5	22
0	24
5	26
10	28
15	30
20	32
25	34
30	36
35	38
40	40
45	42
50	44

SCORING SECTION

	1st Exam = X	2nd Exam = 0
Estimating Gest Age by Maturity Rating	_____Weeks	_____Weeks
Time of Exam	Date _____ Hour_____ am/pm	Date _____ Hour_____ am/pm
Age at Exam	_____ Hours	_____ Hours
Signature of Examiner	_____ M.D.	_____ M.D.

FIGURE 28-1   Newborn maturity rating and classification. If a 1-hour-old newborn is given a score of 3 for each of the physical characteristics and neuromuscular assessments, the newborn's total score would be 36. A total score of 36 correlates with 38+ weeks' gestation. SOURCE: Ballard JL et al: New Ballard score, expanded to include extremely premature infants. *J Pediatr* 1991; 119:417.

gestational age was determined from the date of the pregnant woman's last menstrual period. This method was accurate only 75% to 85% of the time. Because of the problems that develop with the newborn who is preterm or whose weight is inappropriate for gestational age, a more accurate system was developed to evaluate the newborn. Once learned, the procedure can be done in a few minutes. *It is essential that the nurse wear gloves when assessing the newborn in these early hours after birth prior to the first bath.*

Clinical **gestational age assessment tools** have two components: external physical characteristics and neurologic and/or neuromuscular development evaluations. Physical characteristics generally include sole creases, amount of breast tissue, amount of lanugo, cartilaginous development of the ear, testicular descent, and scrotal rugae or labial development. These objective clinical criteria are not influenced by labor and birth and do not change significantly within the first 24 hours after birth.

During the first 24 hours of life the newborn's nervous system is unstable; thus neurologic evaluation findings based on reflexes or assessments dependent on the higher brain centers may not be reliable. If the neurologic findings drastically deviate from the gestational age derived by evaluation of the external characteristics, a second assessment is done in 24 hours.

The neurologic components (excluding reflexes) can aid in assessing neonates of less than 34 weeks' gestation. Between 26 and 34 weeks neurologic changes are significant, whereas significant physical changes are less evident. The important neurologic changes consist of replacement of extensor tone by flexor tone in a *caudocephalad* (tail to head) progression. Neurologic examination facilitates assessment of functional or physiologic maturation in addition to physical development.

Of the gestational assessment aids Dubowitz and Dubowitz's (1977) tool was the first thoroughly documented and validated way to assess intrauterine growth alterations and preterm neonates.

Ballard's (1979) *estimation of gestational age* by maturity rating is a simplified version of the Dubowitz tool. The Ballard tool omits some of the neuromuscular tone assessments, such as head lag, ventral suspension (which is difficult to assess in very ill newborns or those on respirators), and leg recoil. The scoring method of Ballard's tool is much like that of the Dubowitz tool; each physical and neuromuscular finding is given a value, and the total score is matched to a gestational age (Figure 28–1). The maximum score on the Ballard's tool is 50, which corresponds to a gestational age of 44 weeks.

For example, upon completing a gestational assessment of a 1-hour-old newborn, the nurse gives a score of 3 to all the physical characteristics, for a total of 18, and gives a score of 3 to all the neuromuscular assessments, for a total neurologic score of 18. The physical characteristics score of 18 is added to the neurologic score of 18 for a total score of 36, which correlates with 38+ weeks' ges-

tation. Because all newborns vary slightly in the development of physical characteristics and maturation of neurologic function, scores will usually vary instead of all being 3, as in the example.

Both of these tools have been shown to lose accuracy when newborns of fewer than 28 weeks' or more than 43 weeks' gestation are assessed. Both Ballard and Dubowitz tended to overestimate the gestational age of newborns weighing less than 1500 g (Sanders et al 1991). In 1988 Ballard added criteria for more accurate assessment of the gestational age of newborns 20–28 weeks old and less than 1500 g. Ballard and colleagues (1991) suggest that the assessment be made within 12 hours of birth to optimize accuracy, especially in infants of less than 26 weeks' gestational age.

In carrying out gestational age assessments, the nurse keeps in mind that some maternal conditions, such as pregnancy-induced hypertension (PIH), diabetes, and maternal analgesia and anesthesia, may affect certain gestational assessment components and warrant further study. Maternal diabetes, although it appears to accelerate fetal physical growth, seems to retard maturation. Maternal hypertensive states, which retard fetal physical growth, seem to speed maturation.

Newborns of women with PIH have a poor correlation with the criteria involving active muscle tone and edema. Maternal analgesia and anesthesia may cause the baby to have respiratory depression. Babies with respiratory distress syndrome (RDS) tend to be flaccid and edematous and to assume a "froglike" posture. These characteristics affect the scoring of the neuromuscular components of the assessment tool used.

Assessment of Physical Characteristics

The nurse first evaluates observable characteristics without disturbing the baby. Selected physical characteristics common to both gestational assessment tools are presented here in the order in which they might be evaluated most effectively:

1. *Resting posture*, although a neuromuscular component, should be assessed as the baby lies undisturbed on a flat surface (Figure 28–2).

2. *Skin* in the preterm newborn appears thin and transparent, with veins prominent over the abdomen early in gestation. As term approaches, the skin appears opaque because of increased subcutaneous tissue. Disappearance of the protective vernix caseosa promotes skin desquamation and is commonly seen in postmature infants (infants of more than 42 weeks' gestational age and showing signs of placental insufficiency; see Chapter 31).

3. *Lanugo*, a fine hair covering, decreases as gestational age increases. The amount of lanugo is greatest at 28 to 30 weeks and then disappears, first from the face, then from the trunk and extremities.

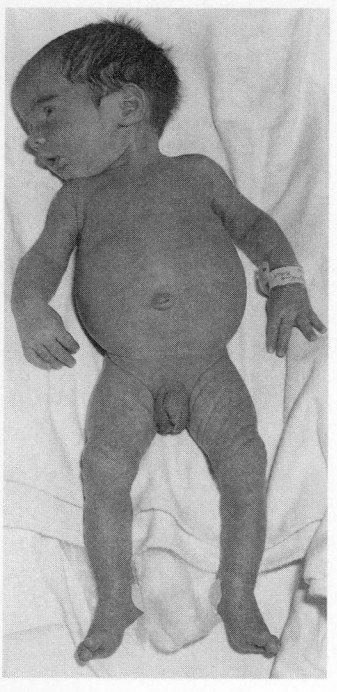
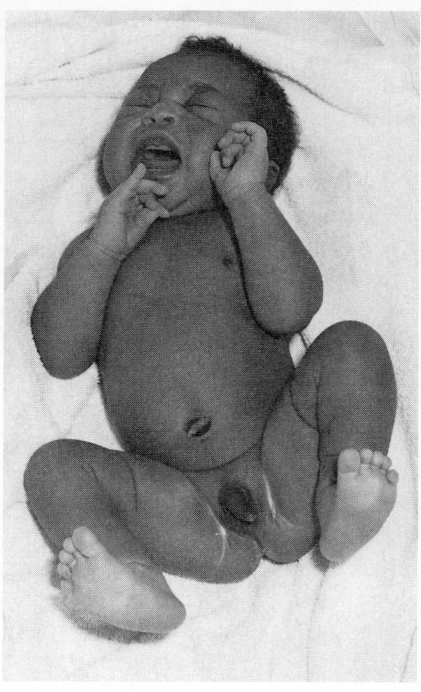
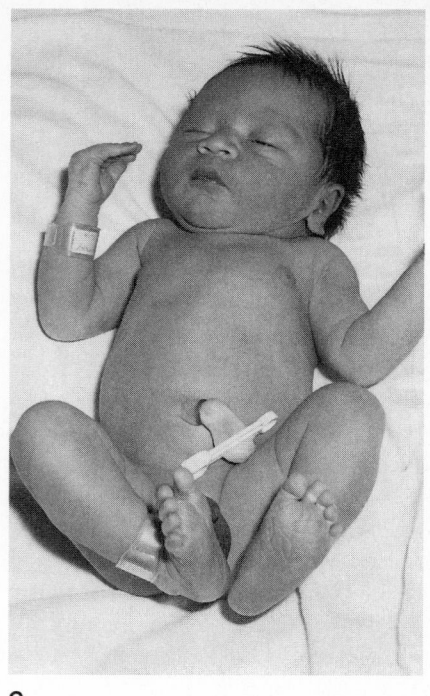

A   **B**   **C**

FIGURE 28-2   Resting posture. *A* Infant exhibits beginning of flexion of the thigh. The gestational age is approximately 31 weeks. Note the extension of the upper extremities. *B* Infant exhibits stronger flexion of the arms, hips, and thighs. The gestational age is approximately 35 weeks. *C* The full-term

infant exhibits hypertonic flexion of all extremities. SOURCE: Dubowitz L, Dubowitz V: *The Gestational Age of the Newborn.* Menlo Park, CA: Addison-Wesley, 1977. Reprinted by permission of V Dubowitz, MD, Hammersmith Hospital, London, England.

4. *Sole (plantar) creases* are reliable indicators of gestational age in the first 12 hours of life. After this the skin of the foot begins drying, and superficial creases appear. Development of sole creases begins at the top (anterior) portion of the sole and, as gestation progresses, proceeds to the heel (Figure 28–3). In the postterm baby deep creases line the entire sole, and peeling may also occur. Plantar creases vary with race. In newborns of African descent sole creases may be less developed at term.

5. The *areola* is inspected and the *breast bud tissue* is gently palpated by application of the forefinger and middle finger to the breast area and is measured in centimeters or millimeters (Figure 28–4). At term gestation the tissue will measure between 0.5 and 1 cm (5 to 10 mm). During the assessment the nipple should not be grasped firmly because skin and subcutaneous tissue will prevent accurate estimation of size. The nurse may also cause trauma to the breast tissue if this procedure is not done gently.

    As gestation progresses, the breast tissue mass and areola enlarge. However, a large breast tissue mass can occur as a result of conditions other than advanced gestational age or the effects of maternal hormones on the baby. The infant of a diabetic

mother tends to be large for gestational age (LGA), and the accelerated development of breast tissue is a reflection of subcutaneous fat deposits. Small-for-gestational-age (SGA) term or postterm newborns may have used subcutaneous fat (which would have been deposited as breast tissue) to survive in utero; as a result their lack of breast tissue may indicate a gestational age of 34 to 35 weeks, even though other factors indicate a *term* or *postterm* neonate.

6. *Ear form and cartilage distribution* develop with gestational age. The cartilage gives the ear its shape and substance (Figure 28–5). In a newborn of less than 34 weeks' gestation the ear is relatively shapeless and flat; it has little cartilage, so the ear folds over on itself and remains folded. By approximately 36 weeks' gestation some cartilage and slight incurving of the upper pinna are present, and the pinna springs back slowly when folded. (This response is tested by holding the top and bottom of the pinna together with the forefinger and thumb and then releasing it, or by folding the pinna of the ear forward against the side of the head and releasing it, and observing the response.) By term the newborn's pinna is firm, stands away from the head, and springs back quickly from the folding.

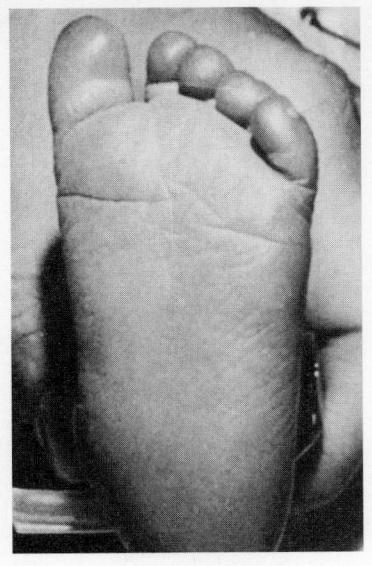

A

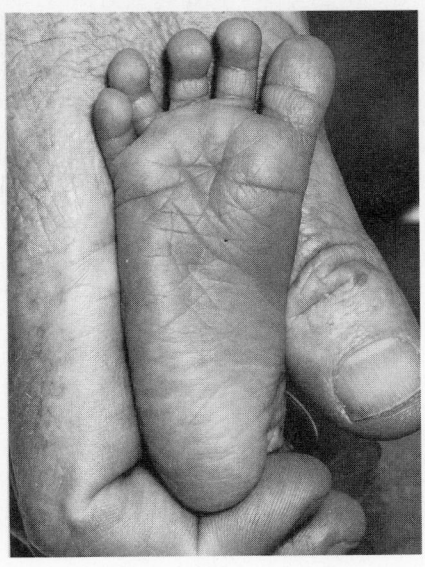

B

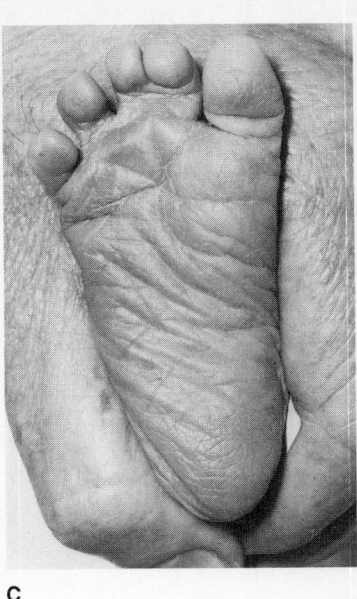

C

FIGURE 28-3 Sole creases. *A* Infant has a few sole creases on the anterior portion of the foot. Note the slick heel. The gestational age is approximately 35 weeks. *B* Infant has a deeper network of sole creases on the anterior two-thirds of the sole. Note the slick heel. The gestational age is approximately 37 weeks. *C* The full-term infant has deep sole creases down to and including the heel as the skin loses fluid and dries after birth. Sole (plantar) creases can be seen even in preterm newborns. SOURCE: Dubowitz L, Dubowitz V: *Gestational Age of the Newborn.* Menlo Park, CA: Addison-Wesley, 1977. Reprinted by permission of V Dubowitz, MD, Hammersmith Hospital, London, England.

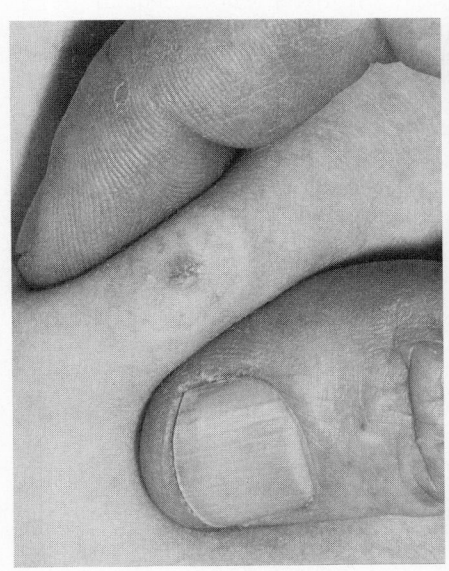

A

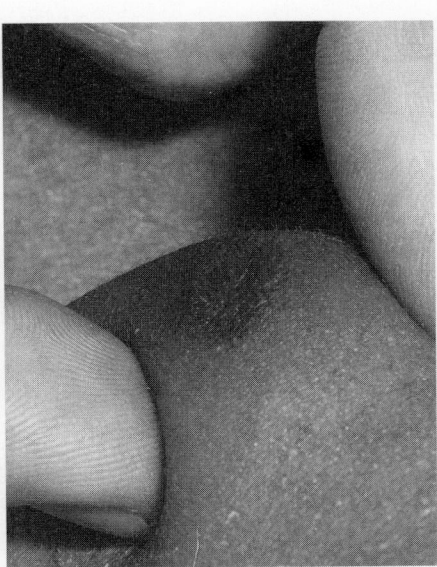

B

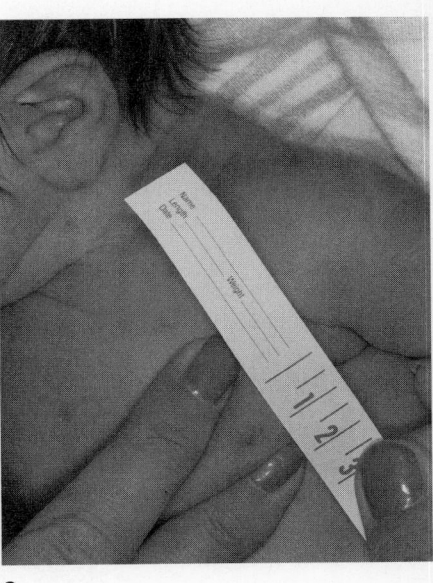

C

FIGURE 28-4 Breast tissue. *A* Newborn has a visible raised area. On palpation the area is 4 mm. The gestational age is 38 weeks. *B* Newborn has 10 mm breast tissue area. The gestational age is 40 to 44 weeks. *C* Gently compress the tissue between the middle and index fingers, and measure the tissue in centimeters or millimeters. Absence of or decreased breast tissue often indicates premature or SGA newborn. SOURCE: Dubowitz L, Dubowitz V: *Gestational Age of the Newborn.* Menlo Park, CA: Addison-Wesley, 1977. Reprinted by permission of V Dubowitz, MD, Hammersmith Hospital, London, England.

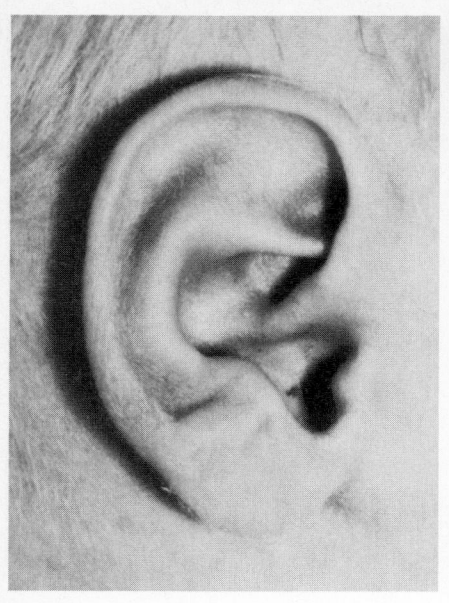

A

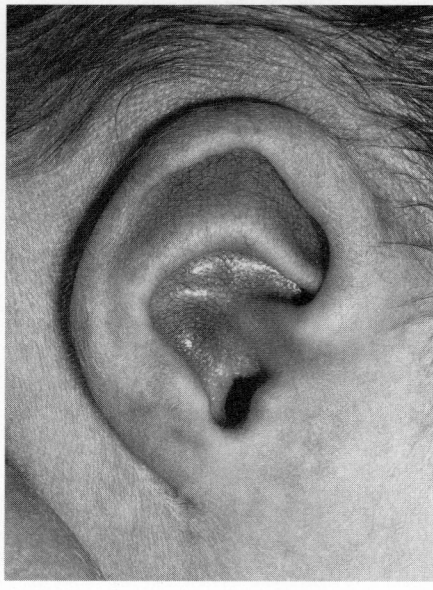

B

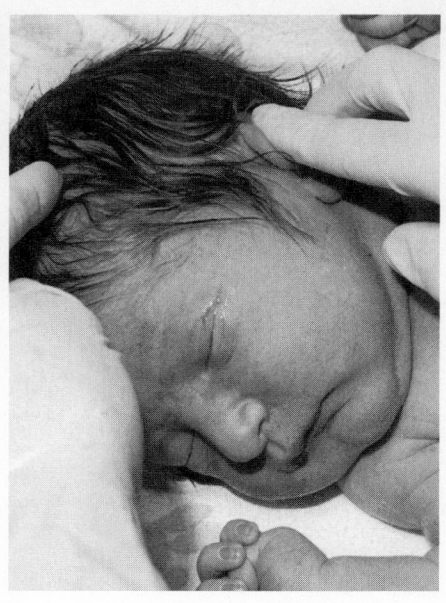

C

FIGURE 28-5   Ear form and cartilage. *A* The ear of the infant at approximately 36 weeks' gestation shows incurving of the upper two-thirds of the pinna. *B* Infant at term shows well-defined incurving of the entire pinna. *C* If the auricle stays in the position in which it is pressed or returns slowly to its origi-nal position, it usually means the gestational age is less than 38 weeks. SOURCE: *A* and *C*; Dubowitz L, Dubowitz V: *Gesta-tional Age of the Newborn.* Menlo Park, CA: Addison-Wesley, 1977. Reprinted by permission of V Dubowitz, MD, Hammer-smith Hospital, London, England.

7. *Male genitals* are evaluated for size of the scrotal sac, the presence of rugae, and descent of the testes (Figure 28–6). Prior to 36 weeks the small scrotum has few rugae, and the testes are palpable in the inguinal canal. By 36 to 38 weeks the testes are in the upper scrotum, and rugae have developed over the anterior portion of the scrotum. By term the testes are generally in the lower scrotum, which is pendulous and covered with rugae.

8. The appearance of the *female genitals* depends in part on subcutaneous fat deposition and therefore relates to fetal nutritional status (Figure 28–7). The clitoris varies in size and occasionally is so large that it is difficult to identify the sex of the newborn. This may be caused by adrenogenital syndrome, which causes the adrenals to secrete excessive amounts of androgen and other hormones. At 30 to 32 weeks' gestation the clitoris is prominent, and the labia

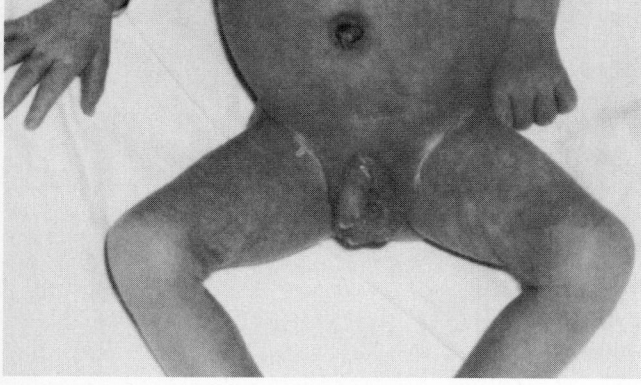

A

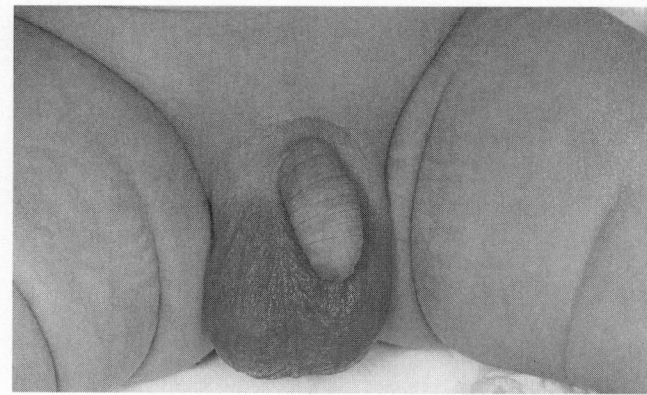

B

FIGURE 28-6   Male genitals. *A* Preterm infant's testes are not within the scrotum. The scrotal surface has few rugae. *B* Term infant's testes are generally fully descended. The entire surface of the scrotum is covered by rugae.

SOURCE: Dubowitz L, Dubowitz V: *Gestational Age of the Newborn.* Menlo Park, CA: Addison-Wesley, 1977. Reprinted by permission of V Dubowitz, MD, Hammersmith Hospital, London, England.

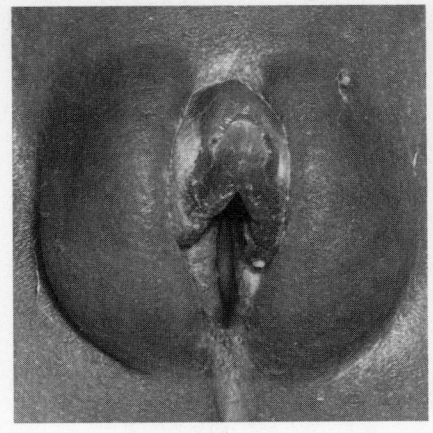
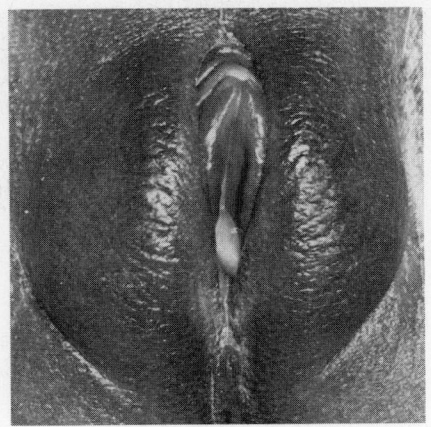
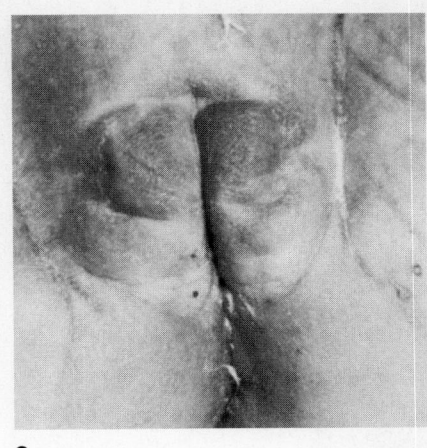

A   **B**   **C**

FIGURE 28-7   Female genitals. *A* Infant has a prominent clitoris. The labia majora are widely separated, and the labia minora, viewed laterally, would protrude beyond the labia majora. The gestational age is 30–36 weeks. *B* The clitoris is still visible. The labia minora are now covered by the larger labia majora. The gestational age is 36–40 weeks. *C* The term infant has well-developed, large labia majora that cover both clitoris and labia minora. SOURCE: Dubowitz L, Dubowitz V: *Gestational Age of the Newborn.* Menlo Park, CA: Addison-Wesley, 1977. Reprinted by permission of V Dubowitz, MD, Hammersmith Hospital, London, England.

majora are small and widely separated. As gestational age increases, the labia majora increase in size. At 36 to 40 weeks they nearly cover the clitoris. At 40 weeks and beyond the labia majora cover the labia minora and clitoris.

In the full-term female newborn some tissue may protrude from the floor of the vagina. This tissue, the hymenal tag, is a normal segment of the hymen and disappears in several weeks.

Other physical characteristics assessed by some gestational age scoring tools include the following:

1. *Vernix* covers the preterm newborn. The postterm newborn has no vernix. After noting vernix distribution, the birthing area nurse (wearing gloves) dries the newborn to prevent evaporative heat loss, thus disturbing the vernix and potentially altering this gestational age criterion. The birthing area nurse must communicate to the neonatal nurse the amount of vernix and the areas of vernix coverage.

2. *Hair* of the preterm newborn has the consistency of matted wool or fur and lies in bunches rather than in the silky, single strands of the term newborn's hair.

3. *Skull firmness* increases as the fetus matures. In a term newborn the bones are hard, and the sutures are not easily displaced. The nurse should not attempt to displace the sutures forcibly.

4. *Nails* appear and cover the nail bed at about 20 weeks' gestation. Nails extending beyond the fingertips may indicate a postterm newborn.

Assessment of Neuromuscular Maturity Characteristics

The central nervous system of the human fetus matures at a fairly constant rate. Specific neurologic parameters have been correlated with gestational age. In particular, tests have been designed to evaluate neurologic status as manifested by development of neuromuscular tone. In the fetus, neuromuscular tone develops from the lower to the upper extremities. The neurologic evaluation requires more manipulation and disturbances than the physical evaluation of the newborn.

The neuromuscular evaluation (see Figure 28–1) is best performed when the infant has stabilized. The following characteristics are evaluated:

1. The *square window sign* is elicited by flexing the baby's hand toward the ventral forearm until resistance is felt. The angle formed at the wrist is measured (Figure 28–8).

2. *Recoil* is a test of flexion development. Because flexion first develops in the lower extremities, recoil is first tested in the legs. The newborn is placed on its back on a flat surface. With a hand on the newborn's knees and while manipulating the hip joint, the nurse places the baby's legs in flexion, then extends them parallel to each other and flat on the surface. The response to this maneuver is recoil of the newborn's legs. According to gestational age, they may not move, or they may return slowly or quickly to the flexed position. Preterm infants have less muscle tone than term infants, so preterm infants have less recoil.

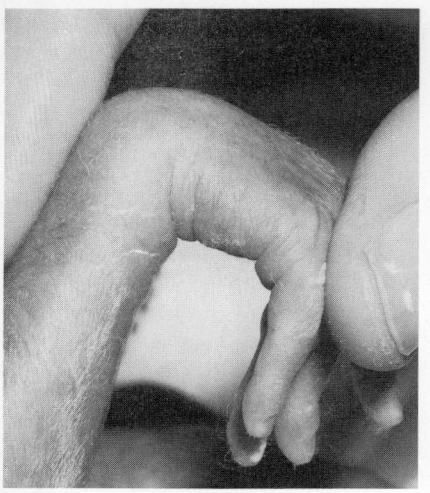

A

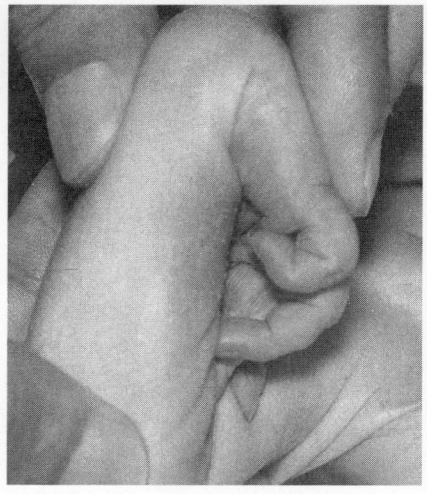

B

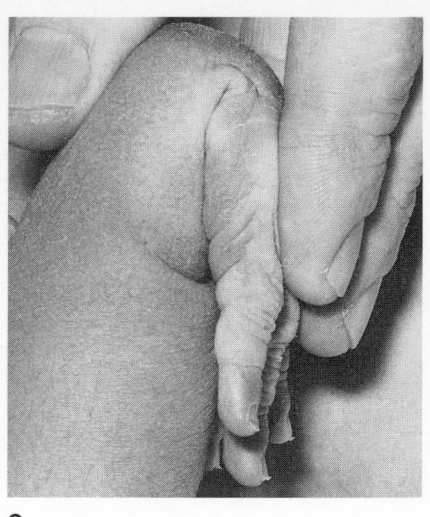

C

FIGURE 28-8 Square window sign. *A* This angle is 90 degrees and suggests an immature newborn of 28 to 32 weeks' gestation. *B* A 30-degree angle is commonly found from 38 to 40 weeks' gestation. *C* A 0-degree angle occurs from 40 to 42 weeks.

SOURCE: Dubowitz L, Dubowitz V: *Gestational Age of the Newborn*. Menlo Park, CA: Addison-Wesley, 1977. Reprinted by permission of V Dubowitz, MD, Hammersmith Hospital, London, England.

Arm recoil is tested by flexion at the elbow and extension of the arms at the newborn's side. While the baby is in the supine position, the nurse completely flexes both elbows, holds them in this position for 5 seconds, extends the arms at the baby's side, and releases them. Upon release, the elbows of a full-term newborn form an angle of less than 90 degrees and rapidly recoil back to flexed position. The elbows of preterm newborns have slower recoil time and form a greater than 90-degree angle. Arm recoil is also slower in healthy but fatigued newborns after birth;

therefore arm recoil is best elicited after the first hour of birth when the baby has had time to recover from the stress of birth. The deep sleep state also decreases the arm recoil response. Assessment of arm recoil should be bilateral in order to rule out brachial palsy.

3. The *popliteal angle* (degree of knee flexion) is determined with the newborn flat on its back. The thigh is flexed on the abdomen/chest, and the nurse places the index finger of the other hand behind the new-

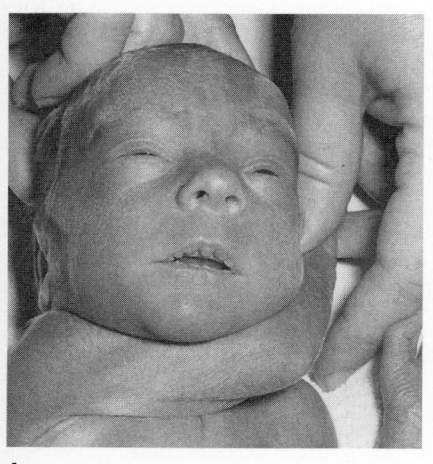

A

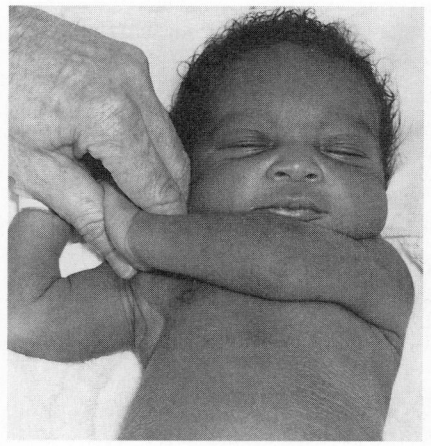

B

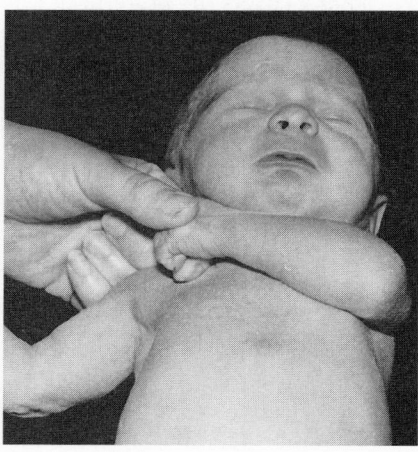

C

FIGURE 28-9 Scarf sign. *A* No resistance is noted until after 30 weeks' gestation. The elbow can be readily moved past the midline. *B* The elbow is at midline at 36 to 40 weeks' gestation. *C* Beyond 40 weeks' gestation the elbow will not reach

the midline. SOURCE: Dubowitz L, Dubowitz V: *Gestational Age of the Newborn*. Menlo Park, CA: Addison-Wesley, 1977. Reprinted by permission of V Dubowitz, MD, Hammersmith Hospital, London, England.

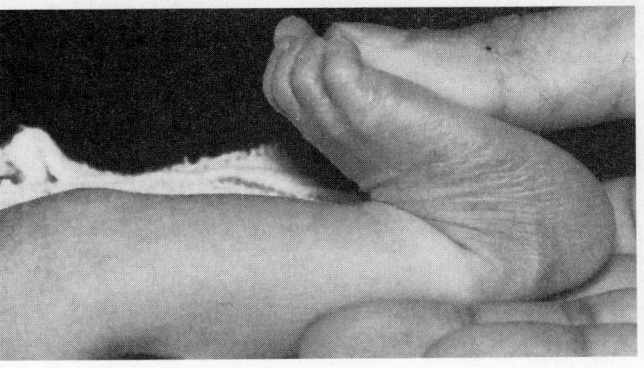

A

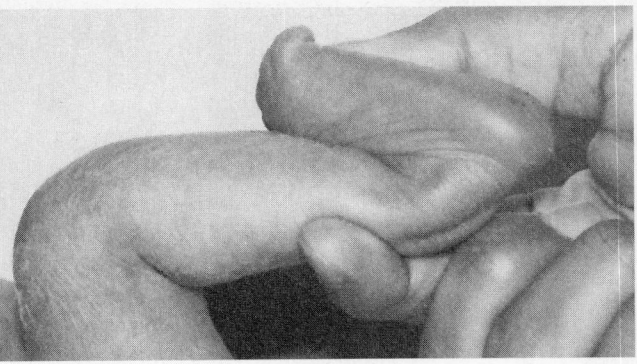

B

FIGURE 28-10 Ankle dorsiflexion. *A* A 45-degree angle indicates 32 to 36 weeks' gestation. A 20-degree angle indicates 36 to 40 weeks' gestation. *B* A 0-degree angle is common at 40 weeks or more gestational age.

SOURCE: Dubowitz L, Dubowitz V: *Gestational Age of the Newborn.* Menlo Park, CA: Addison-Wesley, 1977. Reprinted by permission of V Dubowitz, MD, Hammersmith Hospital, London, England.

born's ankle to extend the lower leg until resistance is met. The angle formed is then measured. Results vary from no resistance in the very immature infant to an 80-degree angle in the term infant.

4. The *scarf sign* is elicited by placing the newborn supine and drawing an arm across the chest toward the newborn's opposite shoulder until resistance is met. The location of the elbow is then noted in relation to the midline of the chest (Figure 28-9).

5. The *heel-to-ear extension* is performed by placing the newborn in a supine position and then gently drawing the foot toward the ear on the same side until resistance is felt. The nurse should allow the knee to bend during the test. It is important to hold the buttocks down to keep from rolling the baby. Both the proximity of foot to ear and degree of knee extension are assessed. A preterm, immature newborn's leg will remain straight, and its foot will go to the ear or beyond. With advancing gestational age the newborn demonstrates increasing resistance to this maneuver. Maneuvers involving the lower extremities of newborns who had frank breech presentation should be delayed to allow for resolution of leg positioning (Ballard et al 1979).

6. *Ankle dorsiflexion* is determined by flexing the ankle on the shin. The examiner uses a thumb to push on the sole of the newborn's foot while the fingers support the back of the leg. Then the angle formed by the foot and the interior leg is measured (Figure 28-10). This sign can be influenced by intrauterine position and congenital deformities.

7. *Head lag* (neck flexors) is measured by pulling the baby to a sitting position and noting the degree of head lag. Total lag is common in infants up to 34 weeks' gestation, whereas the postmature newborn (42+ weeks) will hold the head in front of the body

line. Full-term newborns are able to support their heads momentarily.

8. *Ventral suspension* (horizontal position) is evaluated by holding the newborn prone on the examiner's hand. The position of head and back and degree of flexion in the arms and legs are then noted. Some flexion of arms and legs indicates 36 to 38 weeks' gestation; fully flexed extremities, with head and back even, are characteristic of a term newborn.

9. *Major reflexes* such as sucking, rooting, grasping, Moro, tonic neck, Babinski, and others are also evaluated during the newborn exam.

A supplementary method for estimating gestational age (done by the physician or NP) is to view the vascular network of the cornea with an ophthalmoscope. The amount of vascularity present over the surface of the lens has excellent correlation with infants of 27 through 34 weeks' gestational age. In babies of less than 27 weeks' gestation, the cornea is cloudy, and the vascular network is not visible; after 34 weeks' gestation the vascular network has generally disappeared completely.

When the gestational age determination and birth weight are considered together, the newborn can be identified as one whose *growth is below the 10th percentile or small for gestational age (SGA); appropriate for gestational age (AGA); or above the 90th percentile or large for gestational age (LGA)* (Figure 28-11). This determination enables the nurse to anticipate possible physiologic problems. This information is used in conjunction with a complete physical examination to establish a plan of care appropriate for the individual newborn. For example, an SGA newborn often requires frequent glucose monitoring and early feedings. See Chapter 31 for discussion of these categories and their potential problems.

The nurse also plots the gestational age against the newborn's length, head circumference, and weight on the

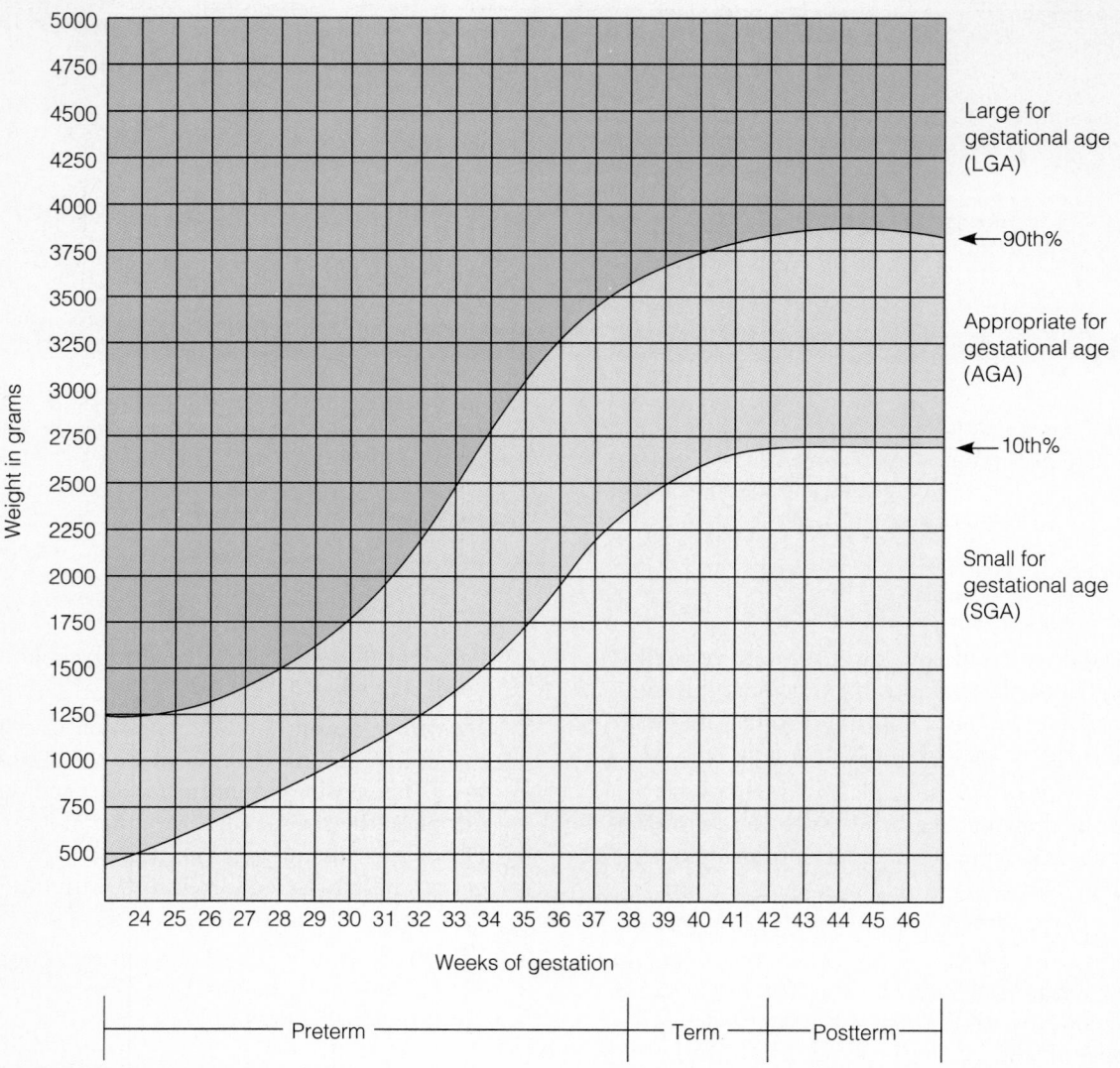

FIGURE 28-11   Classification of newborns by birth weight and gestational age. The newborns' birth weight and gestational age are placed on the graph. The newborn is then classified as large for gestational age (LGA), appropriate for gestational age (AGA), or small for gestational age (SGA).
SOURCE: Battaglia FC, Lubchenco LO: A practical classification of newborn infants by weight and gestational age. *J Pediatr* 1967; 71:161.

appropriate growth chart to determine if these measurements fall within the average range—the 10th to 90th percentile for the corresponding gestational age (Figure 28–12). These correlations further document the level of maturity and appropriate category for the newborn. The comparison of the infant's weight/length ratio further facilitates identification of SGA infants as being symmetrically or asymmetrically growth retarded. See Chapter 31 for further discussion.

PHYSICAL ASSESSMENT

After the initial determination of gestational age and related potential problems, a more extensive physical assessment is done. The nurse should choose a warm, well-lighted area that is free of drafts. Completing the physical assessment in the presence of the parents provides an op-

portunity to acquaint them with their unique newborn. The examination is performed in a systematic, head-to-toe manner, and all findings are recorded. When assessing the physical and neurologic status of the newborn, the nurse should first consider general appearance and then proceed to specific areas.

The Newborn Physical Assessment Guide on pages 840–854 outlines how to systematically assess the newborn. Normal findings, alterations, and related causes are presented and correlated with suggested nursing responses. The findings are typical for a full-term newborn.

General Appearance

The newborn's head is disproportionately large for the body. The center of the baby's body is the umbilicus rather than the symphysis pubis, as in the adult. The body

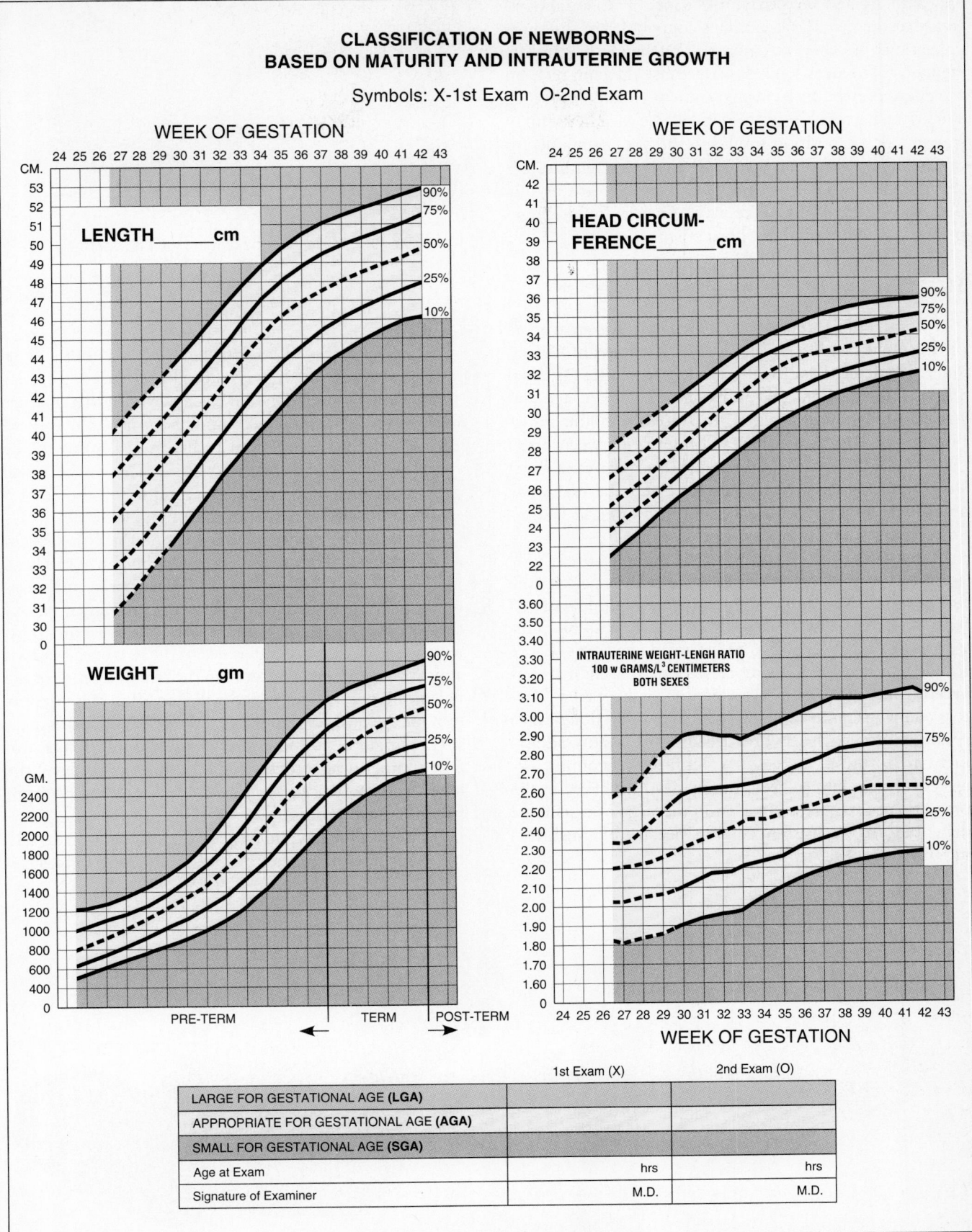

FIGURE 28-12 Classification of newborns based on maturity and intrauterine growth. SOURCES: Adapted from Lubchenco LO, Hansman C, Boyd E: *Pediatrics* 1966; 37:403; Battaglia FC, Lubchenco LO: A practical classification of newborn infants by weight and gestational age. *J Pediatr* 1967; 71:159.

appears long and the extremities short. The flexed position that the newborn maintains contributes to the short appearance of the extremities. The hands are tightly clenched. The neck looks short because the chin rests on the chest. Newborns have a prominent abdomen, sloping shoulders, narrow hips, and rounded chests. They tend to stay in a flexed position similar to the one maintained in utero and will offer resistance when the extremities are straightened. After a breech birth, the feet are usually dorsiflexed, and it may take several weeks for the newborn to assume typical newborn posture.

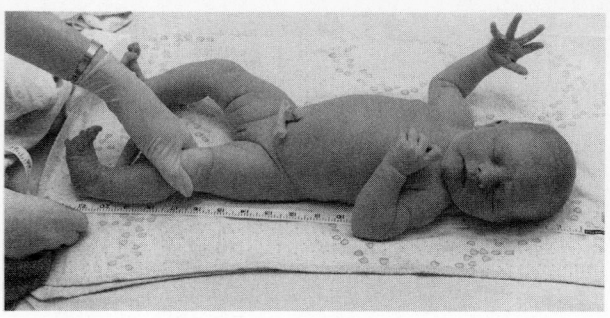

FIGURE 28-13   Measuring the length of the newborn.

Weight and Measurements

The normal full-term Caucasian newborn has an average birth weight of 3405 g (7 lb, 8 oz). Newborns of African and Asian descent are usually somewhat smaller (Yip et al 1991). Other factors that influence weight are age and size of parents, health of mother (smoking and malnutrition decrease birth weight), and interval between pregnancies (if too close together, such as every year, birth weight also tends to be decreased). After the first week and for the first 6 months, the newborn's weight will increase about 198 g (7 oz) weekly.

Approximately 70% to 75% of the newborn's body weight is water. During the initial newborn period (the first 3 or 4 days), there is a physiologic weight loss of 5% to 10% for term newborns because of fluid shifts. This weight loss may reach 15% for preterm newborns. Large babies may tend to lose more weight. If weight loss is greater than 10%, clinical reappraisal is necessary. Factors contributing to weight loss include small fluid intake resulting from delayed breastfeeding or a slow adjustment to formula, increased volume of meconium excreted, and urination. Weight loss may be marked in the presence of temperature elevation (because of associated dehydration) or consistent chilling (because of nonshivering thermogenesis).

The length of the normal newborn is difficult to measure because the legs are flexed and tensed. To measure length, the nurse should place newborns flat on their backs with legs extended as much as possible (Figure 28-13). The average length is 50 cm (20 in), with the range being 45 to 55 cm (18 to 22 in). The newborn will grow approximately an inch a month for the next 6 months. This is the period of most rapid growth.

At birth the newborn's head is one-third the size of an adult's head. The circumference of the newborn's head is 32 to 37 cm (12.5 to 14.5 in). For accurate measurement, the tape is placed over the most prominent part of the occiput and brought to just above the eyebrows (Figure 28-14A). The circumference of the newborn's head is approximately 2 cm greater than the circumference of the newborn's chest at birth and will remain in this proportion for the next few months. (Factors that alter this measurement are discussed under Head section.) It is best to take another head circumference on the second day if the newborn experienced significant head molding or caput from the birth process.

The average circumference of the chest at birth is 32 cm (12.5 in) and ranges from 30–35 cm. Chest measure-

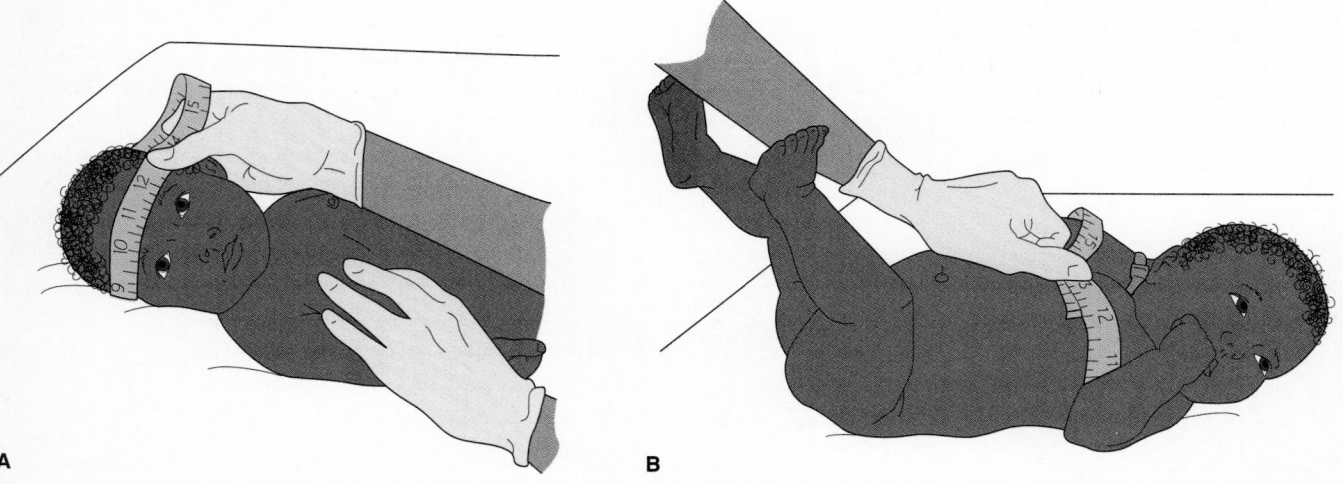

A   B

FIGURE 28-14   *A* Measuring the head circumference of the newborn. *B* Measuring the chest circumference of the newborn.

TABLE 28-2   Newborn Measurements

Weight

Average: 3405 g (7 lb, 8 oz)

Range: 2500–4000 g (5 lb, 8 oz–8 lb, 13 oz)

Weight is influenced by racial origin and maternal age and size.

Physiologic weight loss: 5%–10% for term newborns, up to 15% for preterm newborns

Growth: 198 g (7 oz) per week for first 6 months

Length

Average: 50 cm (20 in)

Range: 45–55 cm (18–22 in)

Growth: 2.5 cm (1 in) per month for first 6 months

Head Circumference

32–37 cm (12.5–14.5 in)

Approximately 2 cm larger than chest circumference

Chest Circumference

Average: 32 cm (12.5 in)

Range: 30–35 cm (12–14 in)

ments should be taken with the tape measure at the lower edge of the scapulas and brought around anteriorly directly over the nipple line (Figure 28–14*B* and Table 28–2). The abdominal circumference or girth may also be measured at this time by placing the tape around the newborn's abdomen at the level of the umbilicus, with the bottom edge of the tape at the top edge of the umbilicus.

Temperature

Initial assessment of the newborn's temperature is critical. In utero the temperature of the fetus is about the same as or slightly higher than the expectant mother's. When babies enter the outside world, their temperatures can suddenly drop as a result of exposure to cold drafts and the skin's heat loss mechanisms.

If no heat conservation measures are started, the normal term newborn's deep body temperature falls 0.1 C (0.2 F) per minute; skin temperature lowers 0.3 C (0.5 F) per minute. Marked decrease in skin temperature occurs within 10 minutes after exposure to room air. The temperature should stabilize within 8 to 12 hours. Temperature should be monitored when the newborn is admitted to the nursery and at least every 30 minutes until the newborn's status has remained stable for 2 hours. After that the nurse should assess temperature at least once every 8 hours or according to institutional policy (AAP 1992). (See Chapter 27 for a discussion of the physiology of temperature regulation.)

Body temperature can be assessed by the axillary skin method, a continuous skin probe, the rectal route, or using a tympanic thermometer. Axillary temperature reflects body temperature and the body's compensatory response to the thermal environment. Axillary temperatures are the preferred method and are considered to be a

Thermal imbalance may occur in the normal newborn during the transition from intrauterine to extrauterine life. Challenges to the newborn's thermoregulatory system can result in hypoglycemia, metabolic acidosis, and other problems. The normal newborn combats heat loss through nonshivering thermogenesis (NST), which combines several metabolic processes to maintain core body temperature. Shunting of up to 25% of cardiac output through the newborn's brown adipose tissue (BAT) partially assists with nonshivering thermogenesis. This tissue is located in the axillae, around the kidney, and in other areas of the body.

Jane Bliss-Holtz suggested that during NST the axillary temperature becomes elevated. She designed a study to determine the thermoregulatory state in full-term infants by comparing axillary and tympanic temperatures taken in the first 4 hours after birth. The purpose of the study was to ascertain if the relationship between axillary and tympanic temperatures could determine thermoregulatory status and could predict decreases in core or tympanic temperature.

The three thermoregulatory states included: thermoneutral with axillary and core temperatures in normal range; thermally compensated with axillary temperature increased and core temperature within normal limits; and thermally decompensated with core temperature below normal limits. The thermally decompensated state occurs when activation of BAT fails or when the NST mechanism becomes overwhelmed.

Data collection consisted of obtaining nine sets of temperature measurements for each of 24 male and 21 female newborns. Data collection started 10 minutes after birth, then occurred every 20 minutes for 2 hours, followed by every hour for 2 hours. Results identified 32 episodes of decreased tympanic temperature. In 24 of the episodes when the tympanic temperature fell below 98.3 F, the axillary temperature rose either at that reading or the previous reading. Twenty-five of the 32 episodes could have resulted from a preceding procedure such as bathing or transfer to an open crib. These procedures could have affected the baby's thermal environment.

Clinical Application of Study

Although this study is somewhat difficult to read in terms of both depth of information given and explanation of results, it did predict thermal decompensation with a preceding increase in axillary temperature. The study also supports the practice of obtaining both core and axillary temperature to validate thermal environmental adequacy.

SOURCE: Bliss-Holtz: Determination of thermoregulatory state in full-term infants. *Nurs Res* 42(4):204.

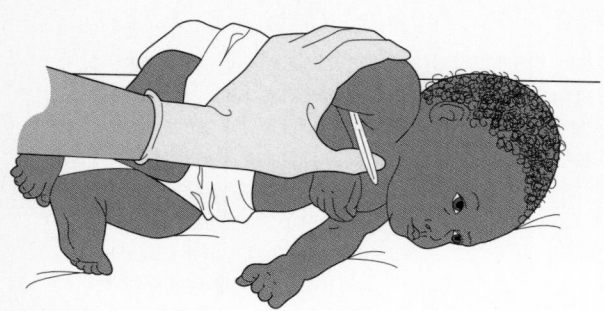

FIGURE 28-15 Axillary temperature measurement. The axillary temperature should be taken for 3 minutes. The newborn's arm should be tightly but gently pressed against the thermometer and the newborn's side as illustrated.

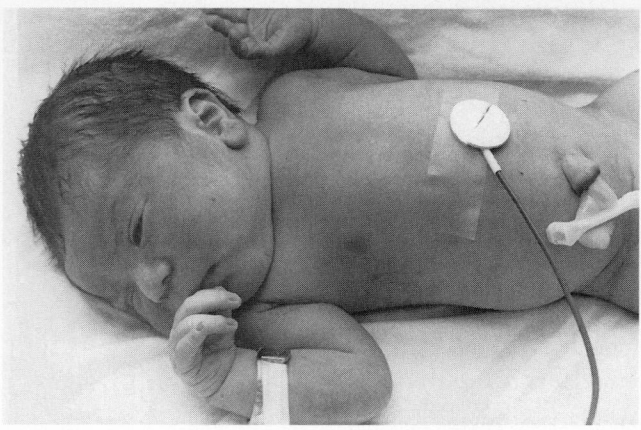

FIGURE 28-16 Temperature monitoring for the newborn. A skin thermal sensor is placed on the newborn's abdomen, upper thigh, or arm and secured with porous tape or a foil-covered foam pad.

close estimation of the rectal temperature. In preterm and term newborns there is less than 0.1 C (0.2 F) difference between the axillary and rectal route. If the axillary method is used, the thermometer must remain in place at least 3 minutes unless an electronic thermometer is used (Figure 28–15). Normal axillary temperature ranges from 36.4 C–37.2 C (97.5 F–99 F). Keep in mind that axillary temperatures can be misleading because the friction caused by apposition of the inner arm skin and upper chest wall and the nearness of brown fat to the probe may elevate the temperature.

The best measure of skin temperature is by means of continuous skin probe rather than axillary temperature, especially for small newborns or newborns maintained in incubators or under radiant warmers. Normal skin temperature is 36 C to 36.5 C (96.8 F to 97.7 F). Skin temperature assessment allows time for initiation of interventions prior to a more serious fall in core temperature (Figure 28–16).

Rectal temperature is assumed to be the closest approximation to core temperature, but this depends on the depth of the thermometer insertion. Normal rectal temperature is 36.6 C to 37.2 C (97.8 F to 99 F). The rectal route is not recommended as a routine method because it may predispose to rectal mucosal irritation and increase chances of perforation. If the temperature must be taken rectally, the nurse inserts the lubricated thermometer to a depth of no greater than 0.5 in (1.27 cm) into the rectum and continuously holds it in the rectum while stabilizing the infant's lower extremities.

Some institutions are now using tympanic thermometers. These are portable sensor probes with disposable covers that are placed in the auditory canal. The probe uses infrared technology to measure the temperature of the internal carotid artery blood flow within several seconds. Early research findings indicate that tympanic temperatures are as accurate an estimation of body temperature in the newborn as axillary temperatures (Weiss 1991).

Temperature instability, a deviation of more than 1 C (2 F) from one reading to the next, or a subnormal temperature may indicate an infection. In contrast with an elevated temperature in older children, an increased temperature in a newborn may indicate reactions to too much covering, too hot a room, or dehydration. Dehydration, which tends to increase body temperature, occurs in newborns whose feedings have been delayed for any reason. Newborns respond to overheating (temperature greater than 37.5 C or 99.5 F) by increased restlessness and eventually by perspiration. The perspiration is initially seen on the head and face, then on the chest. Many newborns initially cannot perspire, but increase respirations and heart rate, which increases oxygen consumption.

Skin Characteristics

Although the newborn's skin color varies with genetic background, all healthy newborns have a pink tinge to their skin. The ruddy hue results from increased red blood cell concentrations in the blood vessels and from limited subcutaneous fat deposits.

Skin pigmentation is slight in the newborn period, so color changes may be seen even in darker skinned babies. A newborn who is cyanotic at rest and pink only with crying may have choanal atresia (congenital blockage of the passageway between the nose and pharynx). If crying increases the cyanosis, heart or lung problems may be sus-

---

Critical Thinking Question

How do you differentiate between central cyanosis and peripheral cyanosis?

pected. Very pale newborns may be anemic or have hypovolemia (low BP) and are evaluated for these problems.

Acrocyanosis

pected. Very pale newborns may be anemic or have hypovolemia (low BP) and are evaluated for these problems.
Acrocyanosis (bluish discoloration of the hands and feet) may be present in the first 2 to 6 hours after birth (Figure 28–17). This condition is due to poor peripheral circulation, which results in vasomotor instability and capillary stasis, especially when the baby is exposed to cold. If the central circulation is adequate, the blood supply should return quickly to the extremity after the skin is blanched with a finger. Blue hands and nails are a poor indicator of oxygenation in a newborn. The face and mucous membranes should be assessed for pinkness reflecting adequate oxygenation.

Mottling (lacy pattern of dilated blood vessels under the skin) occurs as a result of general circulation fluctuations. It may last several hours to several weeks or may come and go periodically (Hoekelman et al 1992). Mottling may be related to chilling or prolonged apnea.

Harlequin Sign

Harlequin sign (clown) color change is occasionally noted: A deep color develops over one side of the newborn's body while the other side remains pale, so that the skin resembles a clown's suit. This color change results from a vasomotor disturbance in which blood vessels on one side dilate while the vessels on the other side constrict. It usually lasts from 1 to 20 minutes. Affected neonates may have single or multiple episodes, but they are transient and not of clinical significance.

Jaundice

Jaundice is first detectable on the face (where skin overlies cartilage) and the mucous membranes of the mouth as well as the sclera. It is evaluated by blanching the tip of the nose, the forehead, or the gum line. This procedure must be carried out in appropriate lighting. If jaundice is present, the area will appear yellowish immediately after blanching. Evaluation and determination of the cause of jaundice must be initiated immediately to prevent possibly serious sequelae. The jaundice may be related to breastfeeding (small incidence), hematomas, immature liver function, or bruises from forceps or it may be caused by blood incompatibility, oxytocin (Pitocin) augmentation or induction, or severe hemolytic process. Any jaundice noted before 24 hours of age should be reported to the physician or nurse practitioner. For a detailed discussion of the causes and assessment of jaundice see Chapter 32.

Erythema Toxicum

Erythema toxicum is a perifollicular erupton of lesions that are firm, vary in size from 1 to 3 mm, and consist of a white or pale yellow papule or pustule with an erythematous base. It is often called "newborn rash" or "flea bite" dermatitis. The rash may appear suddenly, usually over the trunk and diaper area, and is frequently widespread (Figure 28–18). The lesions do not appear on the palms of the hands or the soles of the feet. The peak incidence is at 24–48 hours of life. The condition rarely presents at birth or after 5 days of life (Hoekelman et al 1992). The cause is unknown and no treatment is necessary. Some clinicians feel it may be caused by irritation from clothing. The lesions disappear in a few hours or days. Should a maculopapular rash (eruption consisting of both macules and papules) appear, a smear of the aspirated papule will show numerous eosinophils on staining; no bacteria will be cultured if it is erythema toxicum.

Skin Turgor

Skin turgor is assessed to determine hydration status, the need to initiate early feedings, and the presence of any infectious processes. The usual place to assess skin turgor is over the abdomen or the thigh. Skin should be elastic and should return rapidly to its original shape.

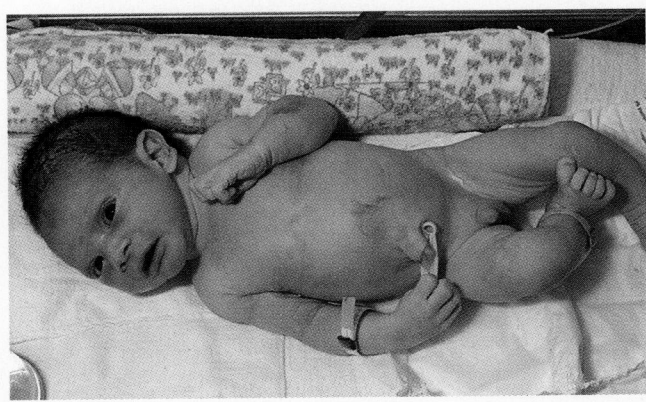

FIGURE 28-17   Acrocyanosis.

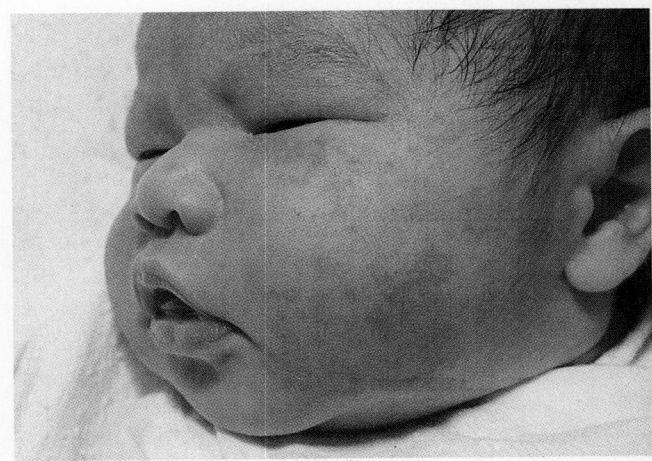

FIGURE 28-18   Erythema toxicum.

Vernix Caseosa

Vernix caseosa, a whitish cheeselike substance, covers the fetus while in utero and lubricates the skin of the newborn. The skin of the term or postterm newborn has less vernix and is frequently dry; peeling is common, especially on the hands and feet.

Milia

Milia, which are exposed sebaceous glands, appear as raised white spots on the face, especially across the nose (Figure 28–19). No treatment is necessary because they will clear up spontaneously within the first month (Hoekelman et al 1992). Infants of African heritage have a similar condition called transient neonatal pustular melanosis (Tauesch et al 1991).

Forceps or Vacuum Extractor Marks

Forceps marks may be present after a difficult forceps birth. The newborn may have reddened areas over the cheeks and jaws. It is important to reassure the parents that these will disappear, usually within 1 or 2 days. Transient facial paralysis resulting from the forceps pressure is a rare complication. Suction marks on the vertex of the scalp are often seen when vacuum extractors are used to assist with the birth. These are benign and do not indicate any underlying brain lesions (Hoekelman et al 1992).

Birthmarks

Telangiectatic Nevi

Telangiectatic nevi (stork bites) appear as pale pink or red spots and are frequently found on the eyelids, nose, lower occipital bone, and nape of the neck (Figure 28–20). These lesions are common in light-complexioned newborns and are more noticeable during periods of crying. These areas have no clinical significance and usually fade by the second birthday.

Mongolian Spots

Mongolian spots are macular areas of bluish-black or gray-blue pigmentation found on the dorsal area and the buttocks (Figure 28–21). They are common in newborns of Asian and African descent and other dark-skinned races. They gradually fade during the first or second year of life. They may be mistaken for bruises and should be documented in the newborn's chart.

Nevus Flammeus

Nevus flammeus (port wine stain) is a capillary angioma directly below the epidermis. It is a nonelevated, sharply demarcated, red to purple area of dense capillaries (Figure 28–22). In infants of African descent it may appear as a purple-black stain. The size and shape varies,

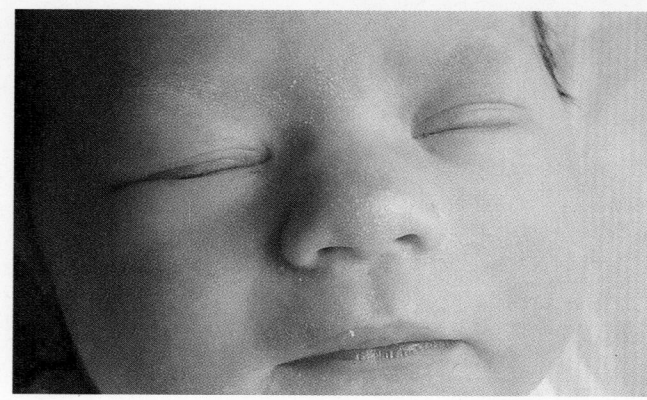

FIGURE 28-19   Facial milia.

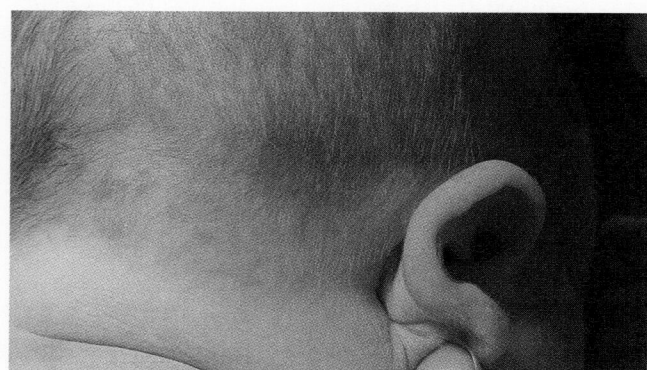

FIGURE 28-20   Stork bites.

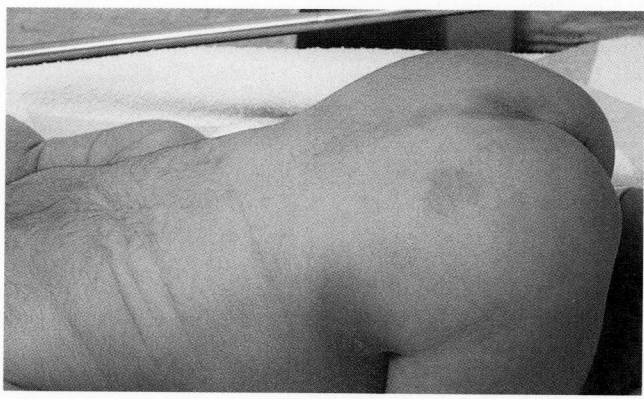

FIGURE 28-21   Mongolian spots.

but it commonly appears on the face. It does not grow in size, does not fade with time, and does not blanch as a rule. The birthmark may be concealed by using an opaque cosmetic cream. If convulsions and other neurologic problems accompany the nevus flammeus, it is suggestive of Sturge-Weber syndrome with involvement of the fifth cranial nerve (the ophthalmic branch of the trigeminal nerve).

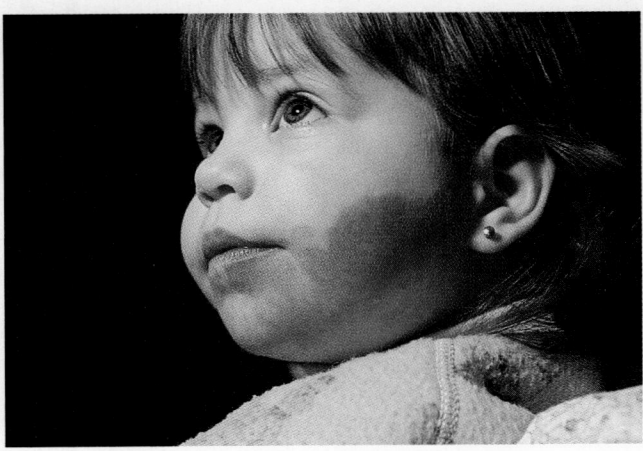

FIGURE 28-22   Port wine stain.

Nevus Vasculosus

Nevus vasculosus (strawberry mark) is a capillary hemangioma. It consists of newly formed and enlarged capillaries in the dermal and subdermal layers. It is a raised, clearly delineated, dark red, rough-surfaced birthmark commonly found in the head region. Such marks usually grow (often rapidly) for several months, and become fixed in size by 8 months. They then begin to shrink and start to resolve spontaneously several weeks to months after peak growth is reached. About 90% of cases resolve by the time the child is 9 years old (Hoekelman et al 1992). Parents can be told that resolution is heralded by a pale purple or gray spot on the surface of the hemangioma. The best cosmetic effect is achieved when the lesions are allowed to resolve spontaneously.

Birthmarks are frequently a cause of concern for the parents. The mother may be especially anxious, fearing that she is to blame. ("Is my baby marked because of something I did?") Guilt feelings are common in the presence of misconceptions about the cause. Birthmarks should be identified and explained to the parents. By providing appropriate information about the cause and course of birthmarks, the nurse frequently relieves the fears and anxieties of the family. The nurse should note any bruises, abrasions, or birthmarks seen upon admission to the nursery.

Head

General Appearance

The newborn's head is large (approximately one-fourth of the body size), with soft, pliable skull bones. The head may appear asymmetric in the newborn of a vertex delivery. This asymmetry, called **molding**, is caused by overriding of the cranial bones during labor and birth (Figure 28-23). The degree of molding varies with the amount and length of pressure exerted on the head. Within a few days after birth, the overriding usually diminishes, and the suture lines become palpable. Because head measurements are affected by molding, a second measurement is indicated a few days after birth. The heads of breechborn newborns and those born by elective cesarean birth are characteristically round and well shaped because pressure was not exerted on them during birth. Any extreme differences in head size may indicate microcephaly or hydrocephalus. Variations in the shape, size, or appearance of the head may be due to *craniostenosis* (premature closure of the cranial sutures), which is corrected through surgery to allow brain growth, or *plagiocephaly* (asymmetry caused by pressure on the fetal head during gestation).

Two *fontanelles* ("soft spots") may be palpated on the newborn's head. Fontanelles, which are openings at the juncture of the cranial bones, can be measured with the fingers. Accurate measurement necessitates that the examiner's finger be measured in centimeters. The assessment should be carried out with the newborn in sitting position and not crying. The diamond-shaped *anterior fontanelle* is 3 to 4 cm long by 2 to 3 cm wide. It is located at the juncture of the frontal and parietal bones. The *posterior fontanelle*, smaller and triangular, is formed by the parietal bones and the occipital bone and is 0.5 cm by 1 cm. Newborns of African descent have been found to have larger anterior and posterior fontanelles than Caucasian newborns (Faix 1982). The fontanelles will be smaller immediately after birth than several days later because of molding. The anterior fontanelle closes within 18 months, whereas the posterior fontanelle closes within 8 to 12 weeks.

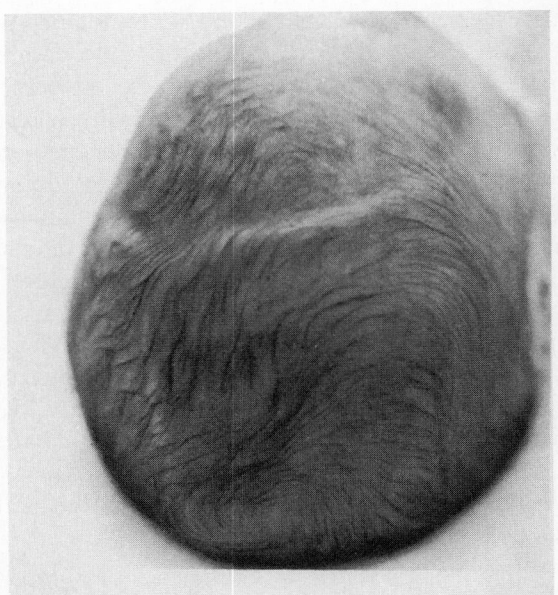

FIGURE 28-23   Overlapped cranial bones produce a visible ridge in a small premature infant. Easily visible overlapping does not occur often in term infants. SOURCE: Korones SB: *High-Risk Newborn Infants,* 4th ed. St Louis: Mosby, 1986.

The fontanelles are a useful indicator of the newborn's condition. The anterior fontanelle may swell when the newborn cries or passes a stool or may pulsate with the heartbeat, which is normal. A bulging fontanelle usually signifies increased intracranial pressure, and a depressed fontanelle indicates dehydration.

The sutures between the cranial bones should be palpated for amount of overlap. In growth-retarded newborns the sutures may be wider than normal, and the fontanelles may also be larger due to impaired fetal growth of the cranial bones. In addition to being inspected for degree of molding and size, the head should be evaluated for soft tissue edema and bruising.

Cephalhematoma

Cephalhematoma is a collection of blood resulting from ruptured blood vessels between the surface of a cranial bone (usually parietal) and the periosteal membrane (Figure 28–24). The scalp in these areas feels loose and slightly edematous. These areas emerge as defined hematomas between the first and second day. Although external pressure may cause the mass to fluctuate, it does not increase in size when the newborn cries. Cephalhematomas may be unilateral or bilateral and do not cross suture lines. They are relatively common in vertex births and may disappear within 2 to 3 weeks or slowly over subsequent months. Cephalhematoma may be a cause of physiologic jaundice because of the extra red blood cells being destroyed within it.

Caput Succedaneum

Caput succedaneum is a localized, easily identifiable soft area of the scalp, generally resulting from a long and difficult labor or vacuum extraction. The sustained pressure of the presenting part against the cervix results in compression of local blood vessels, and venous return is slowed. This causes an increase in tissue fluids, an edematous swelling, and occasional bleeding under the periosteum. The caput may vary from a small area to a large area covering a severely elongated head. The fluid in the caput is reabsorbed within 12 hours to a few days after birth. Caputs resulting from vacuum extractors are sharply outlined, circular areas up to 2 cm thick. They disappear more slowly than naturally occurring edema. It is possible to distinguish between a cephalhematoma and a caput because the caput overrides suture lines (Figure 28–25), whereas the cephalhematoma, because of its location, never crosses a suture line (Table 28–3). Caput succedaneum is present at birth, whereas cephalhematoma generally is not.

Face

The newborn's face is well designed to help the infant suckle. Sucking (fat) pads are located in the cheeks, and a labial tubercle (sucking callus) is frequently found in the

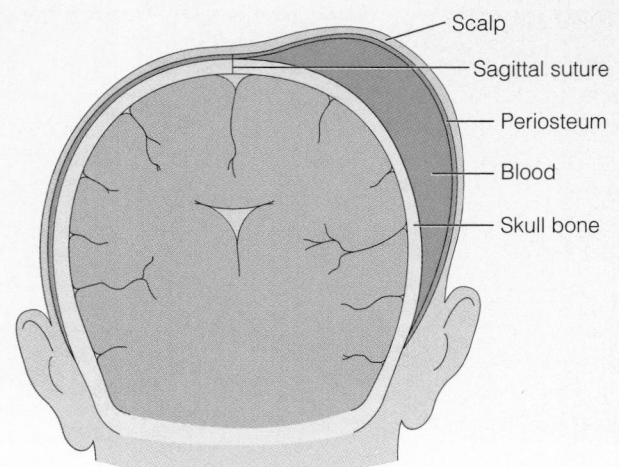

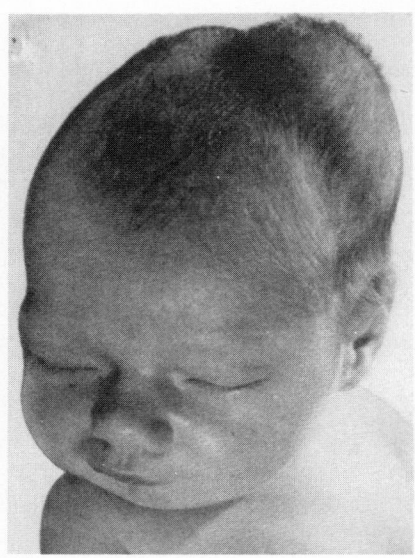

FIGURE 28-24 Cephalhematoma is a collection of blood between the surface of a cranial bone and the periosteal membrane. This is a cephalhematoma over the left parietal bone. SOURCE: Photo reproduced with permission from Porter EL, Craig JM: *Pathology of the Fetus and Infant,* 3rd ed. Chicago: Year Book Medical Publishers, 1975.

center of the upper lip. The chin is recessed, and the nose is flattened. The lips are sensitive to touch, and the sucking reflex is easily initiated.

Symmetry of the eyes, nose, and ears is evaluated. See the Newborn Physical Assessment Guide for deviations in symmetry and variations in size, shape, and spacing of facial features. Facial movement symmetry should be assessed to determine the presence of facial palsy.

Facial paralysis appears when the newborn cries; the affected side is immobile, and the palpebral (eyelid) fissure widens (Figure 28–26). Paralysis may result from forceps-assisted birth or pressure on the facial nerve from the maternal pelvis during birth. Facial paralysis usually

Labels in figure: Scalp, Sagittal suture, Periosteum, Blood, Skull bone

TABLE 28-3 Comparison of Cephalhematoma and Caput Succedaneum

Cephalhematoma

Collection of blood between cranial (usually parietal) bone and periosteal membrane

Does not cross suture lines

Does not increase in size with crying

Appears on first and second day

Disappears after 2 to 3 weeks or may take months

Caput Succedaneum

Collection of fluid, edematous swelling of the scalp

Crosses suture lines

Present at birth or shortly thereafter

Reabsorbed within 12 hours or a few days after birth

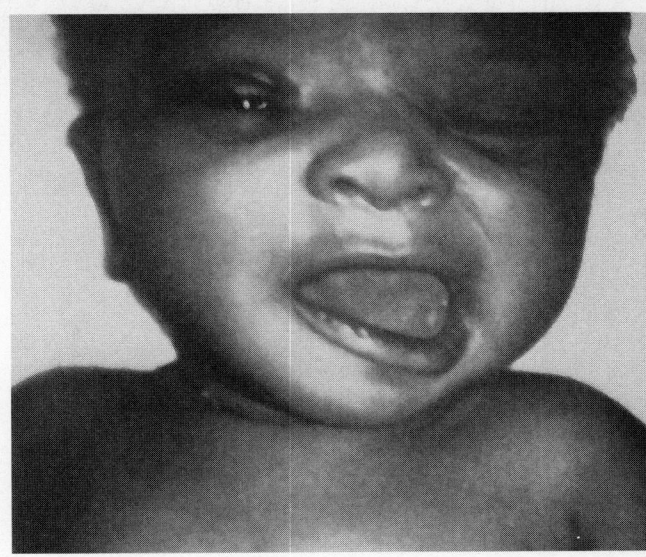

FIGURE 28-26   Paralysis of the right side of the face from an injury to the right facial nerve. SOURCE: Potter EL, Craig JM: *Pathology of the Fetus and Infant,* 3rd ed. Chicago: Year Book Medical Publishers, 1975. Courtesy Dr Ralph Platow.

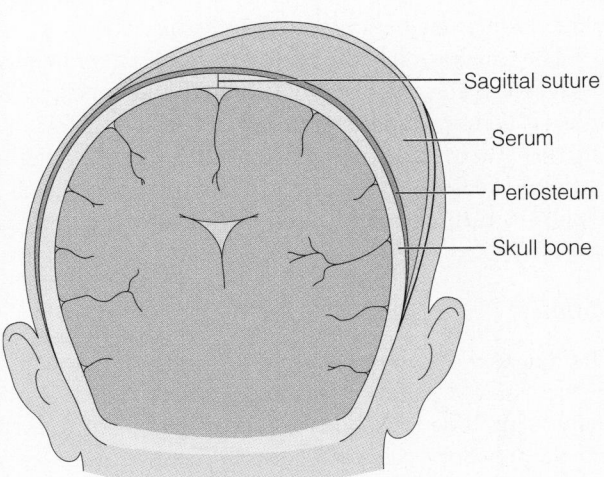

- Sagittal suture
- Serum
- Periosteum
- Skull bone

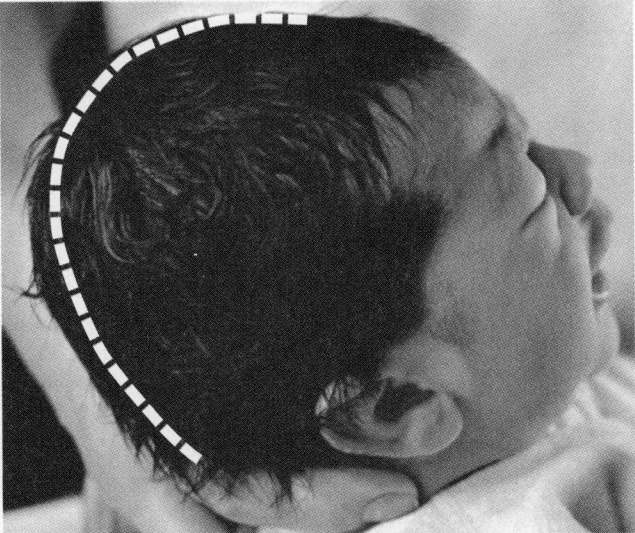

FIGURE 28-25   Caput succedaneum is a collection of fluid (serum) under the scalp. SOURCE: Photo courtesy Mead Johnson Laboratories, Evansville, IN.

disappears within a few days to 3 weeks, although in some cases it may be permanent.

Eyes

The eyes of newborns of Northern European descent are a blue or slate blue-gray. Scleral color tends to be white to bluish-white because of its relative thinness. A blue sclera is associated with osteogenesis imperfecta (Tappero & Honeyfield 1993). The infant's eye color is usually established at approximately 3 months, but it may change any time up to 1 year. Dark-skinned neonates tend to have dark eyes at birth.

The eyes should be checked for size, equality of pupil size, reaction of pupils to light, blink reflex to light, and edema and inflammation of the eyelids. The eyelids can be edematous during the first few days of life because of the pressure associated with birth. Erythromycin and tetracycline are now frequently used prophylactically instead of silver nitrate and usually don't cause chemical irritation of the eye. The instillation of silver nitrate drops in the newborn's eyes may cause edema and **chemical conjunctivitis,** which may appear a few hours after instillation and disappear in 1 to 2 days. If infectious conjunctivitis exists, the newborn has the same purulent (greenish-yellow) discharge as in chemical conjunctivitis, but it is caused by gonococcus, *Chlamydia,* staphylococci, or a variety of gram-negative bacteria and requires treatment with ophthalmic antibiotics. Onset is usually after the second day. Edema of the orbits or eyelids may persist for several days until the newborn's kidneys can evacuate the fluid.

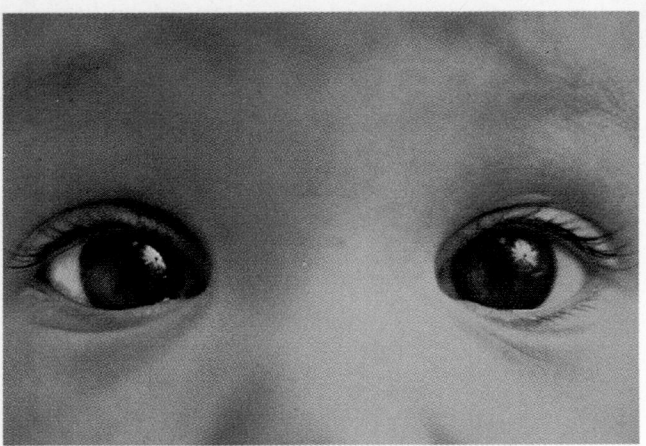

FIGURE 28-27 Transient strabismus may be present in the newborn due to poor neuromuscular control. SOURCE: Courtesy Mead Johnson Laboratories, Evansville, IN.

Small **subconjunctival hemorrhages** appear in about 10% of newborns and are commonly found on the sclera. These hemorrhages are caused by the changes in vascular tension or ocular pressure during birth. They will remain for a few weeks and are of no pathologic significance. Parents need reassurance that the infant is not bleeding from within the eye and that vision will not be impaired.

The newborn may demonstrate transient strabismus (pseudostrabismus) or squinting caused by neuromuscular control of eye muscles (Figure 28–27). It gradually regresses in 3 to 4 months. The "doll's eye" phenomenon is also present for about 10 days after birth. As the newborn's head position is changed to the left and then to the right, the eyes move to the opposite direction. This results from underdeveloped integration of head-eye coordination.

The nurse should observe the newborn's pupils for opacities or whiteness and for the absence of a normal red retinal reflex. Red retinal reflex is a red-orange flash of color observed when an ophthalmoscope light reflects off the retina. In a newborn with dark skin color the retina may appear paler or more grayish. Absence of red reflex occurs with cataracts. Congenital cataracts should be suspected in infants of mothers with a prenatal history of rubella, cytomegalic inclusion disease, or syphilis.

The cry of the newborn is commonly tearless because the lacrimal structures are immature at birth and are not usually fully functional until the second month of life. Some babies may produce tears during the newborn period. Poor oculomotor coordination and absence of accommodation limit visual abilities, but the newborn does have peripheral vision and can fixate on near objects (10 to 20 in) in front of their faces for short periods, can accommodate to large objects (3 in tall by 3 in wide), and can seek out high-contrast geometric shapes (Ludington-

Hoe & Golani 1988). The newborn can perceive faces, shapes, and colors and begins to show visual preferences early. Visual acuity has been reported to be 20/100 and 20/400 (Steinkuller 1988). The newborn blinks in response to bright lights, to a tap on the bridge of the nose (glabellar reflex), or to a light touch on the eyelids. Pupillary light reflex is also present. Examination of the eye is best accomplished by rocking the newborn from an upright position to the horizontal a few times or by other methods such as diminishing overhead lights that will elicit an opened-eye response.

Nose

The newborn's nose is small and narrow. Infants are characteristically nose breathers for the first few months of life. The newborn generally removes obstructions by sneezing. Nasal patency is assured if the baby breathes easily with mouth closed. If respiratory difficulty occurs, the nurse checks for *choanal atresia* (congenital blockage of the passageway between nose and pharynx).

The newborn has the ability to smell after the nasal passages are cleared of amniotic fluid and mucus. This ability is demonstrated by the search for milk. Newborns will turn their heads toward the milk source, whether bottle or breast. Newborns react to strong odors such as alcohol by turning their heads away or blinking (Sullivan et al 1991).

Mouth

The lips of the newborn should be pink, and a touch on the lips should produce sucking motions. Saliva is normally scant. The taste buds are developed prior to birth, and the newborn can easily discriminate between sweet and bitter.

The easiest way to examine the mouth completely is to stimulate infants gently to cry by depressing their tongue, thereby causing them to open the mouth fully. It is extremely important to observe the entire mouth to look for a cleft palate, which can be present even in the absence of a cleft lip. The examiner moves a gloved index finger along the hard and soft palate to feel for any openings (Figure 28–28). Glove powder should always be removed before examining the newborn's mouth.

Occasionally, an examination of the gums will reveal *precocious teeth* on the lower central incisor. If they appear loose, they should be removed to prevent aspiration. Gray-white lesions (*inclusion cysts*) on the gums may be confused with teeth. On the hard palate and gum margins **Epstein's pearls,** small glistening white specks (keratin-containing cysts) that feel hard to the touch are often present. These usually disappear in a few weeks and are of no significance. **Thrush** may appear as white patches that look like milk curds adhering to the mucous membranes and cause bleeding when removed. Thrush is caused by *Candida albicans*, often acquired from an infected vaginal tract during birth or if the mother uses poor hand wash-

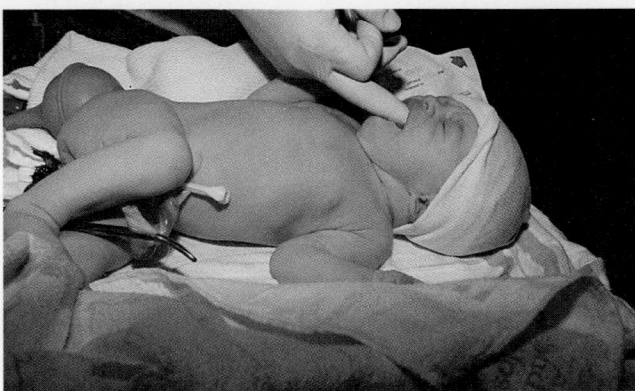

FIGURE 28-28 The nurse inserts the index finger into the newborn's mouth and feels for any openings along the hard and soft palates. Note gloves are worn to examine the palate.

ing when handling her newborn. Thrush is treated with a preparation of nystatin (Mycostatin).

A newborn who is *tongue-tied* has a ridge of frenulum tissue attached to the underside of the tongue at varying lengths from its base, causing a heart shape at the tip of the tongue. "Clipping the tongue," or cutting the ridge of tissue, is not recommended. This ridge does not affect speech or eating, but cutting does create an entry for infection.

Transient nerve paralysis resulting from birth trauma may be manifested by asymmetric mouth movements when the newborn cries or by difficulty with sucking and feeding.

Ears

The ears of the newborn should be soft and pliable and should recoil readily when folded and released. In the normal newborn the top of the ear (pinna) should be parallel to the outer and inner canthus of the eye. The ears should be inspected for shape, size, position, and firmness of ear cartilage. *Low-set ears* are characteristic of many syndromes and may indicate chromosomal abnormalities (especially trisomies 13 and 18), mental retardation, and/or internal organ abnormalities, especially bilateral renal agenesis as a result of embryologic developmental deviations (Figure 28–29). A *preauricular skin tag* may be present just in front of the ear. Preauricular tags are ligated at the base and allowed to slough off.

Visualization of the tympanic membranes is not usually done soon after birth because blood and vernix block the ear canal.

Following the first cry, the newborn's hearing becomes acute as mucus from the middle ear is absorbed, and the eustachian tube is aerated. Risk factors (AAP 1992) associated with potential hearing loss include the following:

- The presence of hearing loss in any family member prior to the age of 50 years
- Serum bilirubin level greater than 20 mg/dL for the full-term newborn or hyperbilirubinemia with a level exceeding indications for exchange transfusion due to toxic drugs
- Suspected maternal rubella infection during pregnancy, resulting in congenital rubella syndrome
- Congenital infection with herpes, cytomegalovirus, toxoplasmosis, or syphilis
- Bacterial meningitis
- Congenital defects of the ear, nose, or throat
- Small neonatal size, particularly less than 1500 g at birth
- Perinatal asphyxia

The newborn's hearing is evaluated by response to loud or moderately loud noises unaccompanied by vibrations. The sleeping newborn should stir or awaken in response to the nearby sounds. (This is not a very accurate test, but it may help to alert the examiner to possible problems.) The newborn can discriminate the individual characteristics of the human voice and is especially sensitive to sound levels within the normal conversation range (Querleu et al 1989). The newborn in a noisy nursery may be able to habituate to the sounds and not stir unless the sound is sudden or much louder.

Neck

A short neck, creased with skin folds, is characteristic of the normal newborn. Because muscle tone is not well developed, the neck cannot support the full weight of the head, which rotates freely. The head lags considerably when the newborn is pulled up from a supine to a sitting

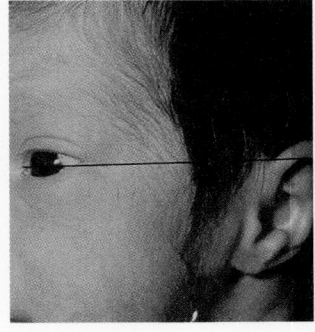 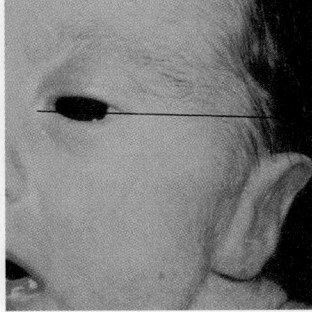

A   B

FIGURE 28-29 The position of the external ear may be assessed by drawing a line across the inner and outer canthus of the eye to the insertion of the ear. *A* Normal position. *B* True low-set position. SOURCE: Courtesy Mead Johnson Laboratories, Evansville, IN.

position, but the prone newborn is able to raise the head slightly. The neck is palpated for masses and presence of lymph nodes and is inspected for webbing. Adequacy of range of motion and neck muscle function is determined by fully extending the head in all directions. Injury to the sternocleidomastoid muscle (congenital torticollis) must be considered in the presence of neck rigidity.

The clavicles are evaluated for evidence of fractures, which occasionally occur during difficult births or in neonates with broad shoulders. The normal clavicle is straight. If fractured, a lump and a grating sensation (crepitus) during movements may be palpated along the course of the side of the break. The Moro reflex (see Assessment of Neurologic Status) is also elicited to evaluate bilateral equal movement of the arms. If the clavicle is fractured, this response will be demonstrated only on the unaffected side.

Chest

The thorax is cylindrical and symmetric at birth, and the ribs are flexible. The general appearance of the chest should be assessed. A protrusion at the lower end of the sternum, called the *xiphoid cartilage*, is frequently seen. It is under the skin and will become less apparent after several weeks as the infant accumulates adipose tissue.

Engorged breasts occur frequently in both male and female newborns. This condition, which occurs by the third day, is a result of maternal hormonal influences and may last up to 2 weeks (Figure 28–30). A whitish secretion from the nipples may also be noted. The infant's breast should not be massaged or squeezed because this practice may cause a breast abscess. Extra or *supernumerary nipples* are occasionally noted below and medial to the true nipples. These harmless pink or brown (in darker skinned newborns) spots vary in size and do not contain glandular tissue. Accessory nipples can be differentiated from a pigmented nevi (mole) by placing the fingertips alongside the accessory nipple and pulling the adjacent tissue laterally. The accessory nipple will appear dimpled. At puberty the accessory nipple may darken.

Cry

The newborn's cry should be strong, lusty, and of medium pitch. A high-pitched, shrill cry is abnormal and may indicate neurologic disorders or hypoglycemia. Periods of crying vary in length after consoling measures are used. Babies' cries are an important method of communication and alert care givers to changes in their condition and needs.

Respiration

Normal breathing for a term newborn is 30 to 60 respirations per minute and predominantly diaphragmatic, with associated rising and falling of the abdomen during inspi-

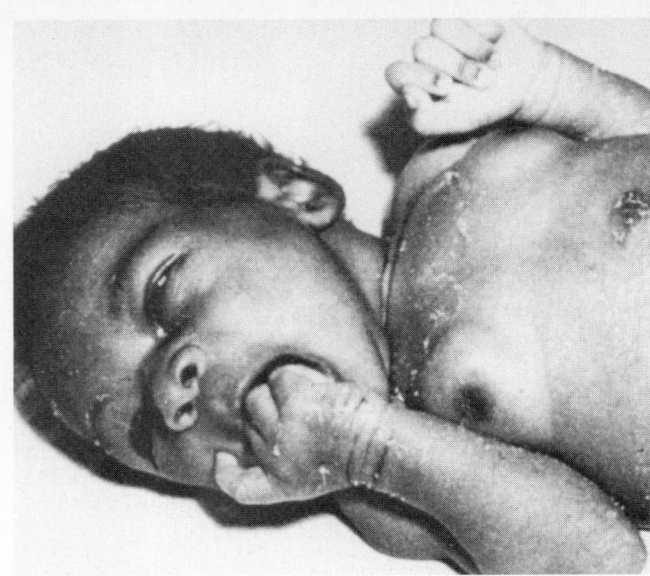

FIGURE 28-30   Breast hypertrophy. SOURCE: Korones SB: *High-Risk Newborn Infants,* 4th ed. St Louis: Mosby, 1986.

ration and expiration. Any signs of respiratory distress, nasal flaring, intercostal or xiphoid retractions, expiratory grunting or sigh, seesaw respirations, or tachypnea (sustained or greater than 60 respirations per minute) should be noted. Hyperexpansion (chest appears high) or hypoexpansion (chest appears low) of the anteroposterior diameter of the chest should also be noted. Both the anterior and posterior chest are auscultated. Some breath sounds are heard better when the newborn is crying, but localization and identification of breath sounds are difficult in the newborn. Upper airway noises and bowel sounds may also be heard over the chest wall and make auscultation difficult. Because sounds may be transmitted from the unaffected lung to the affected lung, the absence of breath sounds may not be diagnosed. Air entry may be noisy in the first couple of hours until lung fluid resolves, especially in cesarean births. Brief periods of apnea (episodic breathing) occur, but no color or heart rate changes occur in healthy, full-term newborns.

TEACHING MOMENT

Vital sign assessments are most accurate if the newborn is at rest, so measure pulse and respirations first if the baby is quiet. To soothe a crying baby, try placing your moistened gloved finger in the baby's mouth, and then complete your assessment while the baby suckles.

Heart

Heart rates can be as rapid as 180 beats per minute in newborns and fluctuate a great deal, especially if the baby moves or is startled. Normal range is 120–160 beats per minute. Auscultation provides the nurse with valuable assessment data. The heart is examined for rate and rhythm, position of the apical impulse, and heart sound intensity. Dysrhythmias should be reassessed by the physician.

The pulse rate is variable and is influenced by physical activity, crying, state of wakefulness, and body temperature. Auscultation is performed over the entire heart region (precordium), below the left axilla, and below the scapula. Apical pulse rates are obtained by auscultation for a full minute, preferably when the newborn is asleep.

The placement of the heart in the chest should be determined when the newborn is in a quiet state. The heart is relatively large at birth and is located high in the chest, with its apex somewhere between the fourth and fifth intercostal spaces.

A shift of heart tones in the mediastinal area to either side may indicate pneumothorax, dextrocardia (heart placement on the right side of the chest), or a diaphragmatic hernia. The experienced nurse can diagnose these and many other problems early with a stethoscope. Normally, the heartbeat has a "toc tic" sound. A slur or slushing sound (usually after the first sound) may indicate a *murmur*. Although 90% of all murmurs are transient and are considered normal, they should be observed closely by a physician. Many murmurs are related to a patent ductus arteriosus, which closes in about 1 to 2 days.

In newborns, a low-pitched, musical murmur heard just to the right of the apex of the heart is fairly common. Occasionally, significant murmurs will be heard, including the murmur of a patent ductus arteriosus, aortic or pulmonary stenosis, or small ventricular septal defect. See Chapter 31 for a discussion of congenital heart defects.

Peripheral pulses (brachial, femoral, pedal) are also evaluated to detect any lags or unusual characteristics. Brachial pulses are palpated bilaterally for equality and compared with the femoral pulses. Femoral pulses are palpated by applying gentle pressure with the middle finger over the femoral canal (Figure 28–31). Decreased or absent femoral pulses indicate coarctation of the aorta and require additional investigation. A wide difference in blood pressure between the upper and lower extremities also indicates coarctation. The measurement of blood pressure is best accomplished by using the Doppler technique or a 1- to 2-inch cuff and a stethoscope over the brachial artery (Figure 28–32). If a Dinemap or Doppler device is used, the newborn's extremities must be immobilized during the assessment, and the cuff should cover two-thirds of the upper arm or upper leg. Movement, crying, and inappropriate cuff size can give inaccurate measurements of the blood pressure.

Blood pressure may not be measured routinely on healthy newborns but is a routine measurement on newborns who are having distress, are premature, or are suspected of cardiac anomaly (Taeusch et al 1991). If cardiac anomaly is suspected, blood pressure is palpated in all

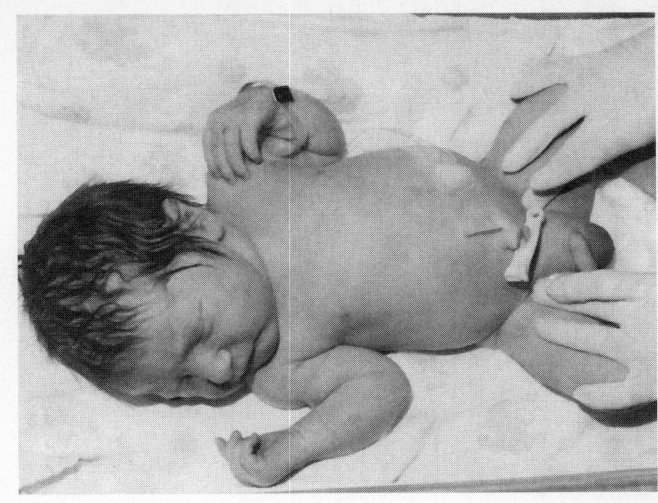

A

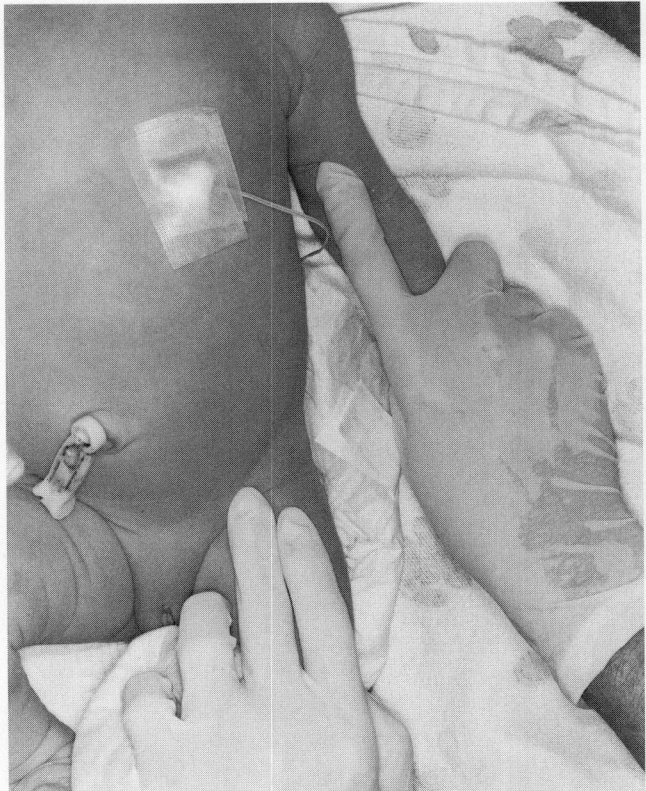

B

FIGURE 28-31 *A* Bilaterally palpate the femoral arteries for rate and intensity of the pulses. Press fingertip gently at the groin as shown. *B* Compare the femoral pulses to the brachial pulses by palpating the pulses simultaneously for comparison of rate and intensity.

four extremities (Table 28–4). Blood pressure is usually 80–60/45–40 mm Hg at birth, and by the tenth day of life it rises to 100/50 mm Hg.

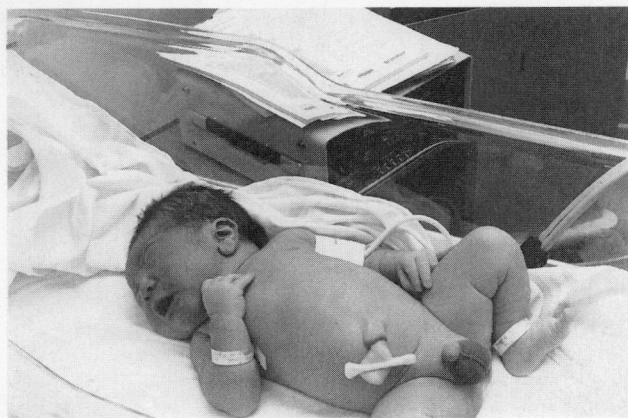

FIGURE 28-32 Blood pressure measurement using the Dinemapp and Doppler devices. The cuff can be applied to either the neonate's upper arm or thigh.

Abdomen

The nurse can learn a great deal about the newborn's abdomen without disturbing the infant. It should be cylindrical, protrude slightly, and move with respiration. A certain amount of laxness of the abdominal muscles is normal. A scaphoid (hollow-shaped) appearance suggests the absence of abdominal contents. No cyanosis should be present, and few if any blood vessels should be apparent to the eye. There should be no gross distention or bulging. The more distended the abdomen, the tighter the skin becomes, and engorged vessels appear. Distention is the first sign of many of the abnormalities found in the gastrointestinal tract.

TABLE 28-4 Newborn Vital Signs

Pulse
120–160 bpm
During sleep as low as 100 bpm; if crying, up to 180 bpm
Apical pulse counted for 1 full minute

Respirations
30–60 respirations/minute
Predominantly diaphragmatic but synchronous with abdominal movements
Respirations are counted for 1 full minute

Blood Pressure
80–60/45–40 mm Hg at birth
100/50 mm Hg at day 10

Temperature
Normal range: 36.5–37.5 C (97.7–99.4 F)
Axillary: 36.4–37.2 C (97.5–99 F)
Skin: 36–36.5 C (96.8–97.7 F)
Rectal: 36.6–37.2 C (97.8–99 F)

Before palpation of the abdomen, the presence or absence of bowel sounds should be auscultated in all four quadrants. Bowel sounds should be present by 1 hour after birth. Palpation can cause a transient decrease in bowel sound intensity.

Abdominal palpation should be done systematically. The nurse palpates each of the four abdominal quadrants, moving in a clockwise direction, checking for softness, tenderness, and the presence of masses. When palpating the abdomen, the nurse may feel for the liver. The newborn's liver is large in proportion to the rest of the body and can usually be felt between 1 and 2 cm below the right costal margin. Depending on institutional protocol, palpation of the kidney may be done by the staff nurse. Kidneys are more difficult to feel, but examination is easier if done within 4 to 6 hours after birth, before the intestines become distended with air and feedings are initiated. By placing a finger at the posterior flank and pushing upward while pressing downward with the opposite hand, each kidney may be palpated as a firm oval mass between the examiner's finger and hand. The lower pole of the kidney is usually found 1 to 2 cm above the umbilicus. The spleen tip may be palpated in the lateral aspect of the left upper quadrant in the normal newborn.

Umbilical Cord

Initially, the umbilical cord is white and gelatinous in appearance, with the two umbilical arteries and one umbilical vein readily apparent. Because a single umbilical artery is frequently associated with congenital anomalies, the vessels should be counted as part of the newborn assessment. The cord begins drying within 1 or 2 hours after birth and is shriveled and blackened by the second or third day. Within 7 to 10 days it sloughs off, although a granulated area may remain for a few days longer.

Cord bleeding is abnormal and may result because the cord was inadvertently pulled or because the cord clamp was loosened. Foul-smelling drainage is also abnormal and is generally caused by infection, which requires immediate treatment to prevent septicemia. If the neonate has a patent urachus (abnormal connection between the umbilicus and bladder), moistness or draining urine may be apparent at the base of the cord.

Serous or serosanguineous drainage that continues after the cord falls off may indicate a granuloma. It appears as a small, red button deep in the umbilicus. Treatment involves cauterization by a physician with a silver nitrate stick.

Genitals

Female Infants

The labia majora, labia minora, and clitoris are examined, and the nurse notes the size of each as appropriate for gestational age. A vaginal tag or hymenal tag is often evident and will usually disappear in a few weeks. During the first week of life the newborn may have a vaginal discharge composed of thick whitish mucus. This discharge, which can become tinged with blood, is referred to as **pseudomenstruation** and is caused by the withdrawal of maternal hormones. Smegma, a white cheeselike substance, is often present between the labia. Removing it may traumatize tender tissue.

Male Infants

The penis is inspected to determine whether the urinary orifice is correctly positioned. *Hypospadias* occurs when the urinary meatus is located on the ventral surface of the penis. It occurs most commonly among Caucasians in the United States. *Phimosis* is a condition occurring in newborn males in which the opening of the foreskin (prepuce) is small, and the foreskin cannot be pulled back over the glans at all. This condition may interfere with urination, so the adequacy of the urinary stream should be evaluated.

The scrotum is inspected for size and symmetry and should be palpated to verify the presence of both testes and to rule out cryptorchidism (failure of testes to descend). The testes are palpated separately between the thumb and forefinger, with the thumb and forefinger of the other hand placed together over the inguinal canal.

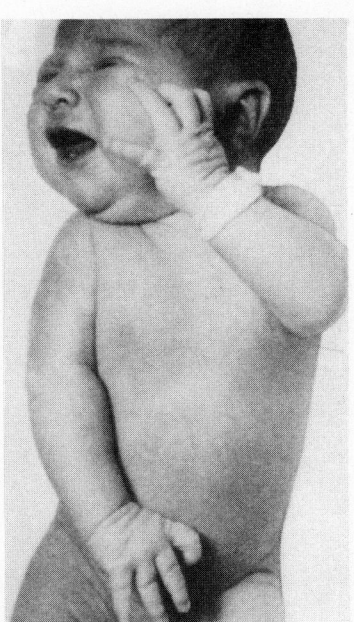

FIGURE 28-33   Right Erb palsy resulting from injury to the fifth and sixth cervical roots of brachial plexus. SOURCE: Potter EL, Craig JM: *Pathology of the Fetus and Infant,* 3rd ed. Chicago: Year Book Medical Publishers, 1975. Reproduced with permission.

Scrotal edema and discoloration are common in breech births. *Hydrocele* (a collection of fluid surrounding the testes in the scrotum) is common in newborns and should be identified. It usually resolves without intervention.

Anus

The anal area is inspected to verify that it is patent and has no fissure. Imperforate anus and rectal atresia may be ruled out by a digital examination. The passage of the first meconium stool is also noted. Atresia of the gastrointestinal tract or meconium ileus with resultant obstruction must be considered if the newborn does not pass meconium in the first 24 hours of life.

Extremities

Extremities are examined for gross deformities, extra digits or webbing, clubfoot, and range of motion. Normal newborn extremities appear short, are generally flexible, and move symmetrically.

Arms and Hands

Nails extend beyond the fingertips in term newborns. Fingers and toes should be counted. *Polydactyly* is the presence of extra digits on either the hands or the feet. *Syndactyly* refers to fusion (webbing) of fingers or toes. Hands should be inspected for normal palmar creases. A single palmar crease, called *simian line* (see also Figure 7–20), is frequently present in children with Down syndrome.

Brachial palsy, which is partial or complete paralysis of portions of the arm, results from trauma to the brachial plexus during a difficult birth. It occurs most commonly when strong traction is exerted on the head of the newborn in an attempt to deliver a shoulder lodged behind the symphysis pubis in the presence of shoulder dystocia. Brachial palsy may also occur during a breech birth if an arm becomes trapped over the head and traction is exerted.

The portion of the arm affected is determined by the nerves damaged. **Erb-Duchenne paralysis** involves damage to the upper arm (fifth and sixth cervical nerves) and is the most common type. Injury to the eighth cervical and first thoracic nerve roots and the lower portion of the plexus produces the relatively rare *lower arm injury*. The *whole arm type* results from damage to the entire plexus.

With Erb-Duchenne paralysis (Erb palsy) the newborn's arm lies limply at the side (Figure 28–33). The elbow is held in extension, with the forearm pronated. The newborn is unable to elevate the arm, and therefore the Moro reflex cannot be elicited on the affected side. When lower arm injury occurs, paralysis of the hand and wrist results; complete paralysis of the limb occurs with the whole arm type.

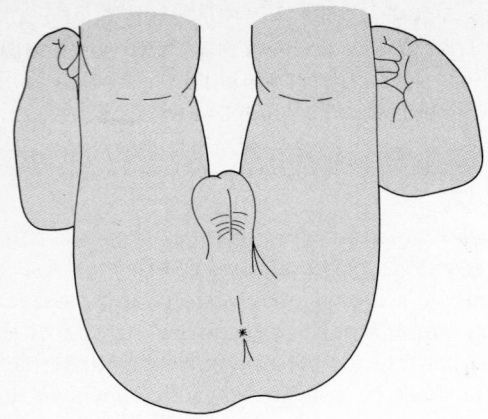

A

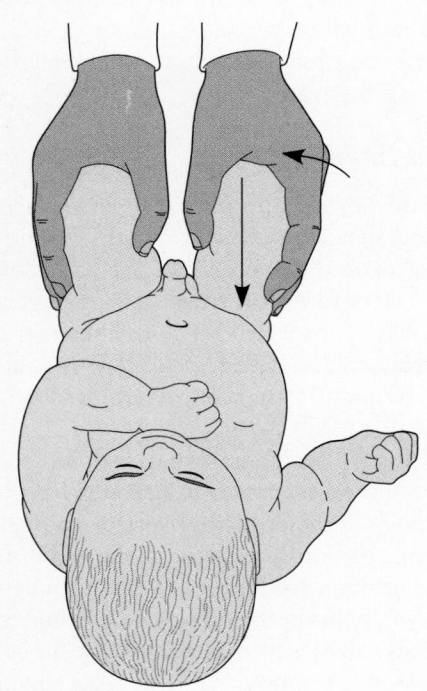

Treatment involves passive range-of-motion exercises to prevent muscle contractures and to restore function. The nurse should carefully instruct the parents in the correct method of performing the exercises and supervise practice sessions. In more severe cases splinting of the arm is indicated until the edema decreases. The arm is held in a position of abduction and external rotation with the elbow flexed 90 degrees. The "Statue of Liberty" splint is commonly used, although similar results are obtained by attaching a strip of muslin to the head of the crib and tying the other end around the wrist, thereby holding the arm up.

Prognosis is related to the degree of nerve damage resulting from trauma and hemorrhage within the nerve sheath. Complete recovery occurs within a few months with minimal trauma. Moderate trauma may result in some partial paralysis. Recovery is unlikely with severe trauma, and muscle wasting may develop. A pilonidal dimple should be examined to ascertain that there is no connection to the spinal canal.

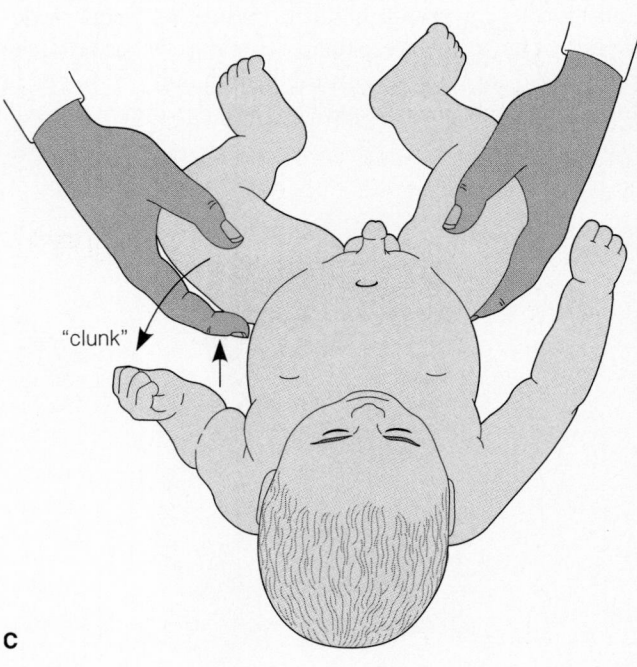

"clunk"

C

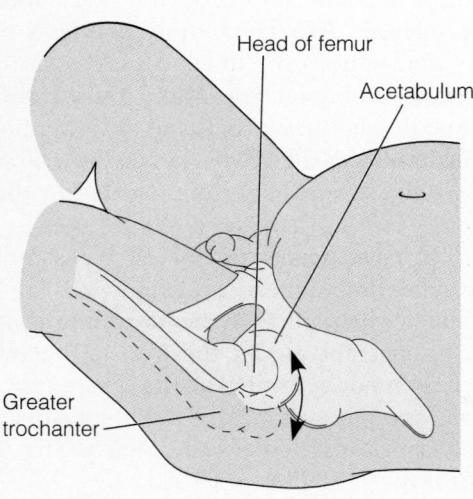

Head of femur

Acetabulum

Greater trochanter

B

FIGURE 28-34 *A* Congenitally dislocated right hip in a young infant as seen on gross inspection. *B* Barlow's (dislocation) maneuver. Baby's thigh is grasped and adducted with gentle downward pressure. Dislocation is palpable as femoral head slips out of acetabulum. *C* Ortolani's maneuver puts downward pressure on the hip and then inward rotation. If the hip is dislocated, this will force the femoral head over the acetabular rim with a noticeable "clunk."

Legs and Feet

The legs of the newborn should be of equal length, with symmetric skin folds. However, they may assume a "fetal posture" secondary to position in utero, and it may take several days for the legs to relax into normal position.

To evaluate for hip dislocation or hip instability, Ortolani's and Barlow's maneuvers are performed. Ortolani's maneuver is a test for hip dislocation. It is performed with the infant relaxed and quiet on a firm surface, with hips and knees flexed at a 90-degree angle. The nurse grasps the infant's thigh with the middle finger over the greater trochanter and lifts the thigh to bring the femoral head from its posterior position toward the acetabulum. With gentle abduction of the thigh the femoral head is returned to the acetabulum. Simultaneously, the examiner feels a sense of reduction or a "clunk" as the femoral returns. This reduction is audible. Barlow's maneuver is the opposite of Ortolani's maneuver and is used to evaluate whether the femoral head can be moved out of the acetabulum. The infant's thigh is again grasped and adducted, and gentle downward pressure is applied. Dislocation is felt as the femoral head slips out of the acetabulum. The femoral head is then returned to the acetabulum using Ortolani's maneuver, confirming the diagnosis of an unstable or dislocatable hip (Figure 28–34).

The feet are then examined for evidence of a talipes deformity (clubfoot). Intrauterine position frequently causes the feet to appear to turn inward (Figure 28–35); this is termed a "positional" clubfoot. If the feet can easily be returned to midline by manipulation, no treatment is indicated. Range-of-motion exercises can be taught to the family. Further investigation is indicated when the foot will not turn to the midline position or align readily. This is considered the most common and severe type of "true clubfoot" or *talipes equinovarus.*

Back

With the baby prone, the nurse examines the back. The spine should appear straight and flat because the lumbar and sacral curves do not develop until the infant begins to sit. The base of the spine is then examined for a dermal sinus. The nevus pilosus ("hairy nevus") is only occasionally found at the base of the spine in newborns, but it is significant because it is frequently associated with spina bifida.

Assessment of Neurologic Status

The neurologic examination should begin with a period of observation, noting the general physical characteristics and behavior of the newborn. Important behaviors to assess are the *state of alertness, resting posture, cry,* and *quality of muscle tone* and *motor activity.*

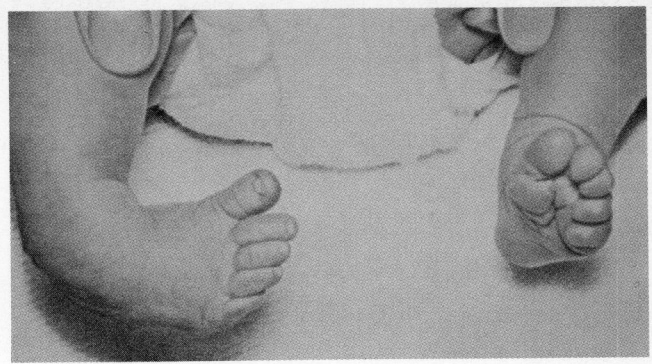

A

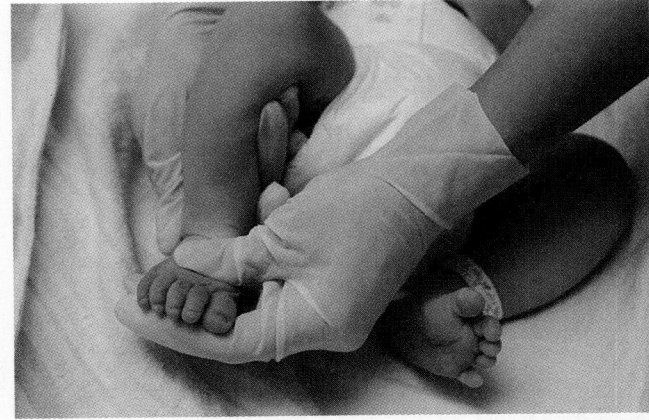

B

FIGURE 28-35 *A* Unilateral talipes equinovarus (clubfoot). *B* To determine the presence of clubfoot, the nurse moves the foot to the midline. Resistance indicates true clubfoot.

The usual position of the newborn is with partially flexed extremities with the legs abducted to the abdomen. When awake, the newborn may exhibit purposeless, uncoordinated bilateral movements of the extremities. If these movements are absent, minimal, or obviously asymmetric, neurologic dysfunction should be suspected. Eye movements are observable during the first few days of life. An alert neonate is able to fixate on faces and brightly colored objects. If a bright light shines in the newborn's eyes, the blinking response is elicited.

Muscle tone is evaluated with the head of the newborn in a neutral position as various parts of the body are passively moved. The newborn is somewhat hypertonic; that is, there is resistance to extending the elbow and knee. Muscle tone should be symmetric. Diminished muscle tone and flaccidity require further evaluation.

Tremors are common in the full-term newborn and must be evaluated to differentiate them from a convulsion. A fine jumping of the muscle is likely to be a central nervous system disorder and requires further evaluation. Newborn tremors may also be related to hypoglycemia or hypocalcemia. Neonatal seizures may consist of no more than chewing or swallowing movements, deviations of

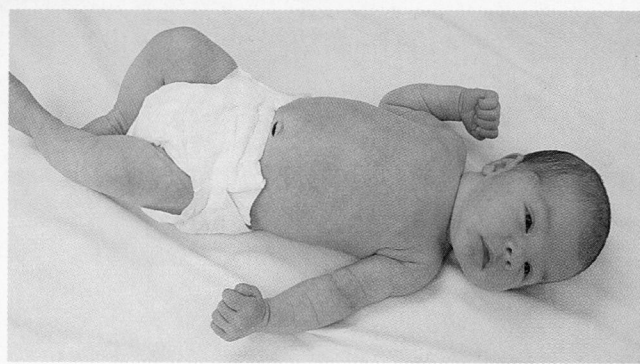

FIGURE 28-36   Tonic neck reflex.

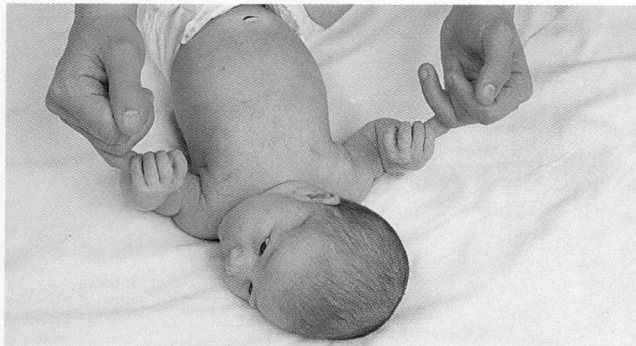

FIGURE 28-37   Grasping reflex.

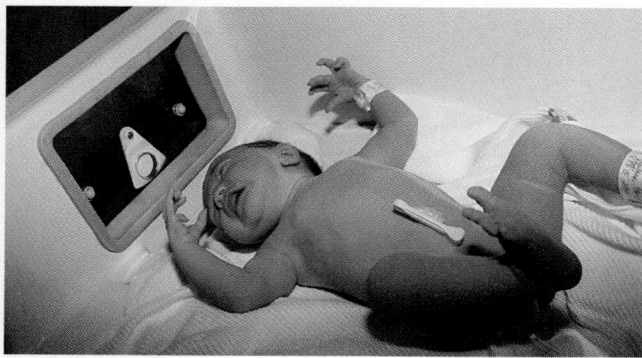

FIGURE 28-38   Moro reflex.

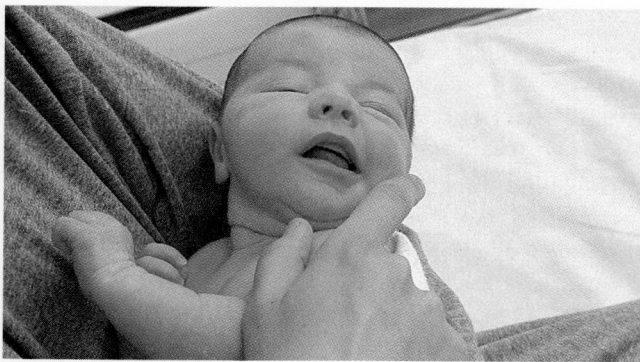

FIGURE 28-39   Rooting reflex.

the eyes, rigidity, or flaccidity because of central nervous system immaturity.

Specific deep tendon reflexes can be elicited in the neonate but have limited value unless they are obviously asymmetric. The knee jerk is brisk; a normal ankle clonus may involve three or four beats. Plantar flexion is present.

The central nervous system of the newborn is immature and characterized by a variety of reflexes. Because the newborn's movements are uncoordinated, methods of communication are limited, and control of bodily functions is drastically limited, the reflexes serve a variety of purposes. Some are protective (blink, gag, sneeze); some aid in feeding (rooting, sucking) and may not be very active if the infant has eaten recently; some stimulate human interaction (grasping). Neonatal reflexes and general neurologic activity should be carefully assessed.

The most common reflexes found in the normal newborn are the following:

- The **tonic neck reflex** (*fencer position*) is elicited when the newborn is supine and the head is turned to one side. In response the extremities on the same side straighten, whereas on the opposite side they flex (Figure 28–36). This reflex may not be seen during the early newborn period, but once it appears, it persists until about the third month.

- The **grasping reflex** is elicited by stimulating the newborn's palm with a finger or object. The newborn will grasp and hold the object or finger firmly enough to be lifted momentarily from the crib (Figure 28–37).

- The **Moro reflex** is elicited when the newborn is startled by a loud noise or is lifted slightly above the crib and then suddenly lowered. In response the newborn straightens arms and hands outward while the knees flex. Slowly, the arms return to the chest, as in an embrace. The fingers spread, forming a C, and the infant may cry (Figure 28–38). This reflex may persist until about 6 months of age.

- The **rooting reflex** is elicited when the side of the newborn's mouth or cheek is touched. In response the newborn turns toward that side and opens the lips to suck (Figure 28–39).

- The **sucking reflex** is elicited when an object is placed in the newborn's mouth or anything touches the lips. Newborns suck even while sleeping; this is called nonnutritive sucking, and it can have a quieting effect on the baby.

- The **Babinski reflex** or fanning and hyperextension of all toes occurs when the lateral aspect of the sole is stroked from the heel upward across the ball of the foot. In adults the toes flex.

- **Trunk incurvation (Galant reflex)** is seen when the newborn is prone. Stroking the spine causes the pelvis to turn to the stimulated side.

In addition to these reflexes newborns can *blink, yawn, cough, sneeze,* and *draw back from pain* (protective reflexes). They can even move a little on their own. When placed on their stomachs, they push up and try to crawl (*prone crawl*). When held upright with one foot touching a flat surface, the newborn puts one foot in front of the other and "walks" (*stepping reflex*) (Figure 28–40). This reflex is more pronounced at birth and is lost in 4 to 5 months. Table 28–5 summarizes the stimulus for and response of the common newborn reflexes.

Brazelton (1984) recommends the following steps as a means of assessing central nervous system integration:

1. Insert a gloved finger into the newborn's mouth to elicit a sucking reflex.

2. As soon as the newborn is sucking vigorously, assess hearing and vision responses by noting sucking changes in the presence of a light, a rattle, and a voice.

3. The newborn should respond with a brief cessation of sucking followed by continuous sucking with repeated stimulation.

This examination demonstrates auditory and visual integrity as well as complex behavioral interactions.

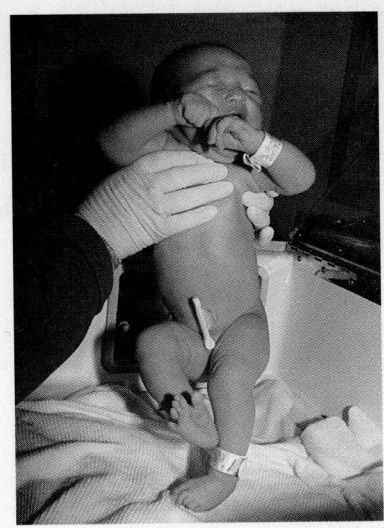

FIGURE 28-40   The stepping reflex disappears after 4 to 5 months.

NEWBORN PHYSICAL ASSESSMENT

Following is a guide for systematically assessing the newborn. Normal findings, alterations, and related causes are presented in correlation with suggested nursing responses. The findings are typical for a full-term newborn.

TABLE 28-5   Common Reflexes of the Newborn

Reflex Name	Evoking Stimulus	Response
Blinking reflex	Light flash	Eyelids close.
Pupillary reflex	Light flash	Pupil constricts.
Rooting reflex	Light touch of finger on cheek close to mouth	Head rotates toward stimulation; mouth opens and attempts to suck finger. Disappears by about 4 months of age.
Sucking reflex	Finger (or nipple) inserted into mouth	Rhythmic sucking occurs.
Moro reflex	Infant lying on back: slightly raised head suddenly released; infant held horizontally, lowered quickly about 6 in, and stopped abruptly	Arms are extended, head is thrown back, fingers are spread wide; arms are then brought back to center convulsively with hands clenched; spine and lower extremities are extended. Disappears by about 6 months of age.
Startle reflex	Loud noise	Similar to Moro reflex flexion in arms; fists are clenched.
Grasping reflex	Finger placed in palm of hand	Infant's fingers close around and grasp object.
Tonic neck reflex	Head turned to one side while infant lies on back	Arm and leg are extended on the side the infant faces. Opposite arm and leg are flexed.
Abdominal reflex	Tactile stimulation or tickling	Abdominal muscles contract.
Withdrawal reflex	Slight pinprick to the sole of the infant's foot	Leg flexes.
Walking reflex	Infant supported in an upright position with feet lightly touching a flat surface	Rhythmic stepping movement. Disappears at about 4 months of age.
Babinski reflex	Gentle stroking on the sole of each foot	Fanning and extension of the toes (adults respond to this stimulation with flexion of toes).
Plantar, or toe-grasping, reflex	Pressure applied with the finger against the balls of the infant's feet	A plantar flexion of all toes. Disappears by the end of the first year of life.

SOURCE: Adapted from Mott SR, James SR, Sperhac AM: *Nursing Care of Children and Families: A Holistic Approach,* 2nd ed. Menlo Park, CA: Addison-Wesley Nursing, 1990.

Assessment and Normal Findings	Alterations and Possible Causes*	Nursing Responses to Data†

Vital Signs

Blood pressure (BP):

At birth: 80–60/45–40 mm Hg
Day 10: 100/50 mm Hg (may be unable to measure diastolic pressure with standard sphygmomanometer)

Low BP (hypovolemia, shock)

Monitor BP in all cases of distress, prematurity, or suspected anomaly.

Low BP: Refer to physician immediately so measures to improve circulation are begun.

Pulse:

120–160 bpm (if asleep 100 bpm; if crying, up to 180 bpm)

Weak pulse (decreased cardiac output)

Bradycardia (severe asphyxia, arrhythmia)

Tachycardia (over 160 bpm at rest) (infection, central nervous system problems, arrhythmia)

Assess skin perfusion by blanching (capillary refill test).

Correlate finding with BP assessments; refer to physician.

Carry out neurologic and thermoregulation assessments.

Respirations

30–60 breaths/minute
Synchronization of chest and abdominal movements
Diaphragmatic and abdominal breathing

Tachypnea (pneumonia, respiratory distress syndrome [RDS])
Rapid, shallow breathing (hypermagnesemia due to large doses given to mothers with PIH)
Respirations below 30 breaths/minute (maternal anesthesia or analgesia)

Identify sleep-wake state; correlate with respiratory pattern.
Evaluate for all signs of respiratory distress; report findings to physician.

Transient tachypnea

Expiratory grunting, subcostal and substernal retractions; flaring of nares (respiratory distress); apnea (cold stress, respiratory disorder)

Evaluate for cold stress.
Report findings to physician/nurse practitioner.

Crying:

Strong and lusty
Moderate tone and pitch
Cries vary in length from 3 to 7 minutes after consoling measures are used

High pitched, shrill (neurologic disorder, hypoglycemia)
Weak or absent (CNS disorder, laryngeal problem)

Discuss newborn's use of cry for communication.
Assess and record abnormal cries.
Reduce environmental noises.

Temperature:

Axilla 36.4–37.2 C (97.5–99 F)
Rectal 36.6–37.2 C (97.8–99 F); 36.8 C (98.8 F) desired
Heavier neonates tend to have higher body temperatures

Elevated temperature (room too warm, too much clothing or covers, dehydration, sepsis, brain damage)
Subnormal temperature (brain stem involvement, cold, sepsis)
Swings of more than 2 F from one reading to next or subnormal temperature (infection)

Notify physician of elevation or drop.
Counsel parents on possible causes of elevated or low temperatures, appropriate home-care measures, when to call physician.
Teach parents how to take rectal and/or axillary temperature; assess parents' information regarding use of thermometer; provide teaching as needed.

Weight

2500–4000 g (5–8.75 lb)

< 2748 g (< 6 lb) = SGA or preterm infant
> 4050 g (> 9 lb) = LGA or infants of diabetic mothers

Plot weight and gestational age on growth chart to identify high-risk infants.
Ascertain body build of parents.
Counsel parents regarding appropriate caloric intake.

*Possible causes of alterations are placed in parentheses.

†This column provides guidelines for further assessment and initial nursing interventions.

Assessment and Normal Findings	Alterations and Possible Causes*	Nursing Responses to Data †
Within first 3 to 4 days, normal weight loss of 5%–10% Large babies tend to lose more due to greater fluid loss in proportion to birth weight except infants of diabetic mother	Loss greater than 15% (small fluid intake, loss of meconium and urine, feeding difficulties)	Notify physician of net losses or gains. Calculate fluid intake and losses from all sources (insensible water loss, radiant warmers, and phototherapy lights).
Length: 45–55 cm (18–22 in) Grows 10 cm (3 in) during first 3 months	Less than 45 cm (congenital dwarf) Short/long bones proximally (achondroplasia) Short/long bones distally (Ellis-Van Creveld syndrome)	Assess for other signs of dwarfism. Determine other signs of skeletal system adequacy. Plot progress at subsequent well-baby visits.
Posture Body usually flexed, hands may be tightly clenched, neck appears short as chin rests on chest In breech births feet are usually dorsiflexed	Only extension noted, inability to move from midline (trauma, hypoxia, immaturity) Constant motion (maternal caffeine intake)	Record spontaneity of motor activity and symmetry of movements. If parents express concern about newborn's movement patterns, reassure and evaluate further if appropriate.
Skin *Color* Color consistent with genetic background Newborns of European descent: pink-tinged or ruddy color over face, trunk, extremities Newborns of African or Native American descent: pale pink with yellow or red tinge Newborns of Asian descent: pink or rosy red to yellow tinge Common variations: acrocyanosis, circumoral cyanosis, or harlequin color change	Pallor of face, conjunctiva (anemia, hypothermia, anoxia) Beefy red (hypoglycemia, immature vasomotor reflexes, polycythemia)	Discuss with parents common skin color variations to allay fears. Document extent and time of occurrence of color change.
	Meconium staining (fetal distress) Jaundice (hemolytic reaction from blood incompatibility within first 24 hours, sepsis)	Obtain Hb and hematocrit values; obtain bilirubin levels. Assess for respiratory difficulty. Differentiate between physiologic and pathologic jaundice. Assess degree of (central or peripheral) cyanosis and possible causes; refer to physician.
Mottled when undressed	Cyanosis (choanal atresia, CNS damage or trauma, respiratory or cardiac problem, cold stress)	
Minor bruising over buttocks in breech presentation and over eyes and forehead in facial presentations		Discuss with parents cause and course of minor bruising related to labor and birth.

*Possible causes of alterations are placed in parentheses.

†This column provides guidelines for further assessment and initial nursing interventions.

Assessment and Normal Findings	Alterations and Possible Causes*	Nursing Responses to Data†
Texture:		
Smooth, soft, flexible; may have dry, peeling hands and feet	Generalized cracked or peeling skin (SGA or postterm; blood incompatibility; metabolic, kidney dysfunction)	Report to physician.
	Seborrhea-dermatitis (cradle cap)	Instruct parents to shampoo the scalp and anterior fontanelle areas daily with soap; rinse well; avoid use of oil.
	Absence of vernix (postmature)	
	Yellow vernix (bilirubin staining)	
Turgor:		
Elastic, returns to normal shape after pinching	Maintains tent shape (dehydration)	Assess for other signs and symptoms of dehydration.
Pigmentation:		
Clear; milia across bridge of nose, forehead, or chin will disappear within a few weeks		Advise parents not to pinch or prick these pimplelike areas.
Café-au-lait spots (one or two)	Six or more (neurologic disorder such as Von Recklinghausen disease, cutaneous neuro-fibromatosis)	If there are six or more café-au-lait spots, refer for genetic and neurologic consult.
Mongolian spots common over dorsal area and buttocks in dark-skinned infants		Assure parents of normalcy of this pigmentation; it will fade in first year or two.
Erythema toxicum	Impetigo (group A β-hemolytic streptococcus or *Staphylococcus aureus* infection)	If impetigo occurs, instruct parents about hand washing and linen precautions during home care.
Telangiectatic nevi	Hemangiomas:	Collaborate with physician.
	Nevus flammeus (port wine stain)	Counsel parents about birthmark's progression to allay misconceptions.
	Nevus fascularis (strawberry hemangioma)	
	Cavernous hemangiomas	Record size and shape of hemangiomas.
		Refer for follow-up at well-baby clinic.
Rashes	Rashes (infection)	Assess location and type of rash (macular, papular, vesicular).
		Obtain history of onset, prenatal history, and related signs and symptoms.
Petechiae of head or neck (breech presentation, cord around neck)	Generalized petechiae (clotting abnormalities)	Determine cause; advise parents if further health care is needed.
Head		
General appearance, size, movement	Asymmetric, flattened occiput on either side of the head (plagiocephaly)	Instruct parents to change infant's sleeping positions frequently.
Round, symmetric, and moves easily from left to right and up and down; soft and pliable	Head held at angle (torticollis)	
	Unable to move head side to side (neurologic trauma)	Determine adequacy of all neurologic signs.

*Possible causes of alterations are placed in parentheses.

†This column provides guidelines for further assessment and initial nursing interventions.

Assessment and Normal Findings	Alterations and Possible Causes*	Nursing Responses to Data†
Circumference: 32–37 cm (12.5–14.5 in); 2 cm greater than chest circumference Head one-fourth of body size	Extreme differences in size may be microencephaly (Cornelia de Lange syndrome, cytomegalic inclusion disease [CID]), rubella, toxoplasmosis, chromosome abnormalities), hydrocephalus (meningomyelocele, achondroplasia), anencephaly (neural tube defect) Head is 3 cm or more larger than chest circumference (preterm, hydrocephalus)	Measure circumference from occiput to frontal area using metal or paper tape. Measure chest circumference using metal or paper tape and compare to head circumference. Record measurements on growth chart. Reevaluate at well-baby visits.
Common variations: Molding Breech and cesarean newborns' heads are round and well shaped	Cephalhematoma (trauma during birth persists up to 3 weeks) Caput succedaneum (long labor and birth; disappears in 1 week)	Evaluate neurologic response. Observe for hyperbilirubenimia. Reassure parents regarding common manifestations due to birth process and when they should disappear.
Fontanelles: Palpation of juncture of cranial bones Anterior fontanelle: 3–4 cm long by 2–3 cm wide, diamond shaped	Overlapping of anterior fontanelle (malnourished or preterm newborn)	Discuss normal closure times with parents and care of "soft spots" to allay misconceptions.
Posterior fontanelle: 1–2 cm at birth, triangle shaped	Premature closure of sutures (craniostenosis) Late closure (hydrocephalus)	Refer to physician. Observe for signs and symptoms of hydrocephalus. Refer to physician.
Slight pulsation	Moderate to severe pulsation (vascular problems)	
Moderate bulging noted with crying, stooling, or pulsations with heartbeat	Bulging (increased intracranial pressure, meningitis) Sunken (dehydration)	Evaluate hydration status. Evaluate neurologic status. Report to physician.
Hair *Texture:* Smooth with fine texture variations (Note: Variations depend on ethnic background.)	Coarse, brittle, dry hair (hypothyroidism) White forelock (Waardenburg syndrome)	Instruct parents regarding routine care of hair and scalp.
Distribution: Scalp hair high over eyebrows (Spanish-Mexican hairline begins mid-forehead and extends down back of neck.)	Low forehead and posterior hairlines may indicate chromosomal disorders.	Assess for other signs of chromosomal aberrations. Refer to physician.
Face Symmetric movement of all facial features, normal hairline, eyebrows and eyelashes present		Assess and record symmetry of all parts, shape, regularity of features, sameness or differences in features.

*Possible causes of alterations are placed in parentheses.

†This column provides guidelines for further assessment and initial nursing interventions.

Assessment and Normal Findings	Alterations and Possible Causes*	Nursing Responses to Data†
Spacing of features:		
Eyes at same level, nostrils equal size, cheeks full, and sucking pads present	Eyes wide apart—ocular hypertelorism (Apert syndrome, cri-du-chat, Turner syndrome)	Observe for other signs and symptoms indicative of disease states or chromosomal aberrations.
Lips equal on both sides of midline	Abnormal face (Down syndrome, cretinism, gargoylism)	
Chin recedes when compared to other bones of face	Abnormally small jaw—micrognathia (Pierre Robin syndrome, Treacher Collins syndrome)	Maintain airway; do not position supine. Initiate surgical consultation and referral.
Movement:		
Makes facial grimaces	Inability to suck, grimace, and close eyelids (cranial nerve injury)	Initiate neurologic assessment and consultation.
Symmetric when resting and crying	Asymmetry (paralysis of facial cranial nerve)	Assess and record symmetry of all parts, shape, regularity of features, and sameness or differences in features.
Eyes		
General placement and appearance:		
Bright and clear; even placement; slight nystagmus (involuntary cyclical eye movements)	Gross nystagmus (damage to third, fourth, and sixth cranial nerves)	
Concomitant strabismus	Constant and fixed strabismus	Reassure parents that strabismus is considered normal up to 6 months.
Move in all directions		
Blue- or slate-blue gray	Lack of pigmentation (albinism) Brushfield spots may indicate Down syndrome (a light or white speckling of the outer two-thirds of the iris)	Discuss with parents any necessary eye precautions. Assess for other signs of Down syndrome.
Brown color at birth in dark-skinned infants		Discuss with parents that permanent eye color is usually established by 3 months of age.
Eyelids:		
Position: above pupils but within iris, no drooping	Elevation or retraction of upper lid (hyperthyroidism)	Assess for signs of hydrocephalus and hyperthyroidism.
	"Sunset sign" lid retraction and downward gaze (hydrocephalus), ptosis (congenital or paralysis of oculomotor muscle)	Evaluate interference with vision in subsequent well-baby visits.
Eyes on parallel plane Epicanthal folds in Asian and 20% of newborns of Northern European descent	Upward slant in non-Asians (Down syndrome) Epicanthal folds (Down syndrome, cri-du-chat syndrome)	Assess for other signs of Down syndrome.
Movement:		
Blink reflex in response to light stimulus Eyes open wide in dimly lit room	Blink absent (CNS injury)	Evaluate neurologic status. Refer to physician.

*Possible causes of alterations are placed in parentheses.

†This column provides guidelines for further assessment and initial nursing interventions.

Assessment and Normal Findings	Alterations and Possible Causes*	Nursing Responses to Data†
Inspection: Edematous for first few days of life, resulting from birth and instillation of silver nitrate (chemical conjunctivitis); no lumps or redness	Purulent drainage (infection); infectious conjunctivitis (gonococcus, chlamydia, staphylococcus, or gram-negative organisms) Marginal blepharitis (lid edges red, crusted, scaly)	Initiate good hand washing. Refer to physician. Evaluate infant for seborrheic dermatitis; scales can be removed easily.
Cornea: Clear Corneal reflex present	Ulceration (herpes infection); large cornea or corneas of unequal size (congenital glaucoma) Clouding, opacity of lens (cataract)	Refer to ophthalmologist. Assess for other manifestations of congenital herpes; institute nursing care measures.
Sclera: May appear bluish in newborn, then white; slightly brownish color frequent in newborns of African descent	True blue sclera (osteogenesis imperfecta)	Refer to physician.
Pupils: Pupils equal in size, round, and react to light by accommodation	Anisocoria—unequal pupils (CNS damage) Dilation or constriction (intracranial damage, retinoblastoma, glaucoma) Pupils nonreactive to light or accommodation (brain injury)	Refer for neurologic examination.
Slight nystagmus in newborn who has not learned to focus Pupil light reflex demonstrated at birth or by 3 weeks of age	Nystagmus (labyrinthine disturbance, CNS disorder)	
Conjunctiva: Chemical conjunctivitis Subconjunctival hemorrhage	Pale color (anemia)	Obtain hematocrit and hemoglobin. Reassure parents that chemical conjunctivitis will subside in 1 to 2 days and subconjunctival hemorrhage disappears in a few weeks.
Palpebral conjunctiva (red but not hyperemic)	Inflammation or edema (infection, blocked tear duct)	
Vision: 20/150 Tracks moving object to midline Fixed focus on objects at a distance of about 10–20 in; may be difficult to evaluate in newborn Prefers faces, geometric designs, and black and white to colors	Cataracts (congenital infection)	Record any questions about visual acuity, and initiate follow-up evaluation at first well-baby checkup.

*Possible causes of alterations are placed in parentheses.

†This column provides guidelines for further assessment and initial nursing interventions.

Assessment and Normal Findings	Alterations and Possible Causes*	Nursing Responses to Data†
Lashes and lacrimal glands:		
Presence of lashes (lashes may be absent in preterm newborns)	No lashes on inner two-thirds of lid (Treacher Collins syndrome); bushy lashes (Hurler syndrome); long lashes (Cornelia de Lange syndrome)	
Cry commonly tearless	Excessive tearing (plugged lacrimal duct, natal narcotic withdrawal), glaucoma	Demonstrate to parents how to milk blocked tear duct. Refer to ophthalmologist if tearing is excessive before third month of life.
Nose		
Appearance of external nasal aspects:		
May appear flattened as a result of birth process	Continued flat or broad bridge of nose (Down syndrome)	Arrange consultation with specialist.
Small and narrow in midline, even placement in relationship to eyes and mouth	Low bridge of nose, beaklike nose (Apert syndrome, Treacher Collins syndrome) Upturned (Cornelia de Lange syndrome)	Initiate evaluation of chromosomal abnormalities.
Patent nares bilaterally (nose breathers)	Blockage of nares (mucus and/or secretions), choanal atresia	Inspect for obstruction of nares.
Sneezing common to clear nasal passages	Flaring nares (respiratory distress)	Maintain oral airway until surgical correction is made.
Responds to odors, may smell breast milk	No response to stimulating odors	Inspect for obstruction of nares.
Mouth		
Function of facial, hypoglossal, glossopharyngeal, and vagus nerves:		
Symmetry of movement and strength	Mouth draws to one side (transient seventh cranial nerve paralysis due to pressure in utero or trauma during birth, congenital paralysis)	Initiate neurologic consultation. Administer eye care if eye on affected side of face is unable to close.
	Fishlike shape (Treacher Collins syndrome)	
Presence of gag, swallowing, coordinated with sucking reflexes Adequate salivation	Suppressed or absent reflexes	Evaluate other neurologic functions of these nerves.
Palate (soft and hard):		
Hard palate dome shaped Uvula midline with symmetrical movement of soft palate	High-steepled palate (Treacher Collins syndrome), bivid uvula (congenital anomaly)	Assess for other congenital anomalies.
Palate intact, sucks well when stimulated	Clefts in either hard or soft palate (polygenic disorder)	Initiate a surgical consultation referral.

*Possible causes of alterations are placed in parentheses.

†This column provides guidelines for further assessment and initial nursing interventions.

Assessment and Normal Findings	Alterations and Possible Causes*	Nursing Responses to Data†
Epithelial (Epstein's) pearls appear on mucosa		Assure parents that these are normal and will disappear at 2 or 3 months of age.
Esophagus patent, some drooling common in newborn	Excessive drooling or bubbling (esophageal atresia)	Test for patency of esophagus.
Tongue:		
Free moving in all directions, midline	Lack of movement or asymmetric movement (neurologic damage) Tongue-tied Deviations from midline (cranial nerve damage)	Further assess neurologic functions. Test reflex elevation of tongue when depressed with tongue blade. Check for signs or weakness or deviation.
Pink color, smooth to rough texture, non-coated	White cheesy coating (thrush) Tongue has deep ridges	Differentiate between thrush and milk curds. Reassure parents that tongue pattern may change from day to day.
Tongue proportional to mouth	Large tongue with short frenulum (cretinism, Down syndrome, other syndromes)	Evaluate in well-baby clinic to assess development delays. Initiate referrals.
Ears		
External ear:		
Without lesions, cysts, or nodules	Nodules, cysts, or sinus tracts in front of ear Adherent earlobes Low set	Evaluate characteristics of lesions. Counsel parents to clean external ear with washcloth only; discourage use of cotton-tip applicators.
	Preauricular skin tags	Refer to physician for ligation.
Hearing:		
Eustachian tubes are cleared with first cry Absence of all risk factors	Presence of one or more risk factors	Assess history of risk factors for hearing loss.
Attends to sounds; sudden or loud noise elicits Moro reflex	No response to sound stimuli (deafness)	Test for Moro reflex.
Neck		
Appearance:		
Short, straight, creased with skin folds	Abnormally short neck (Turner syndrome) Arching or inability to flex neck (meningitis, congenital anomaly)	Report findings to physician.
Posterior neck lacks loose extra folds of skin	Webbing of neck (Turner syndrome, Down syndrome, trisomy 18)	Assess for other signs of the syndromes.
Clavicles:		
Straight and intact	Knot or lump on clavicle (fracture during difficult birth)	Obtain detailed labor and birth history; apply figure-8 bandage.

*Possible causes of alterations are placed in parentheses.

†This column provides guidelines for further assessment and initial nursing interventions.

Assessment and Normal Findings	Alterations and Possible Causes*	Nursing Responses to Data†
Moro reflex elicitable	Unilateral Moro reflex response on unaffected side (fracture of clavicle, brachial palsy, Erb-Duchenne paralysis)	Collaborate with physician.
Symmetric shoulders	Hypoplasia	

Chest

Appearance and size:

Circumference: 32.5 cm, 1–2 cm less than head		Measure at level of nipples after exhalation.
Wider than it is long		
Normal shape without depressed or prominent sternum	Funnel chest (congenital or associated with Marfan syndrome)	Determine adequacy of other respiratory and circulatory signs.
Lower end of sternum (xiphoid cartilage) may be protruding; is less apparent after several weeks	Continued protrusion of xiphoid cartilage (Marfan syndrome, "pigeon chest")	Assess for other signs and symptoms of various syndromes.
Sternum 8 cm long	Barrel chest	

Expansion and retraction:

Bilateral expansion	Unequal chest expansion (pneumonia, pneumothorax, respiratory distress)	Assess respiratory effort regularity, flaring of nares, difficulty on both inspiration and expiration.
No intercostal, subcostal, or supracostal retractions	Retractions (respiratory distress)	Record and consult physician.
	See saw respirations (respiratory distress)	

Auscultation:

Breath sounds are louder in infants	Decreased breath sounds (decreased respiratory activity, atelectasis, pneumothorax)	Perform assessment and report to physician any positive findings.
Chest and axilla clear on crying	Increased breath sounds (resolving pneumonia or in cesarean births)	
Bronchial breath sounds (heard where trachea and bronchi closest to chest wall, above sternum and between scapulae):		
Bronchial sounds bilaterally	Adventitious or abnormal sounds (respiratory disease or distress)	Evaluate color for pallor or cyanosis.
Air entry clear		Report to physician.
Rales may indicate normal newborn atelectasis		
Cough reflex absent at birth, appears in 2 or more days		

Breasts:

Flat with symmetric nipples	Lack of breast tissue (preterm or SGA)	Evaluate for infection.
Breast tissue diameter 5 cm or more at term	Discharge	
Distance between nipples 8 cm	Enlargement	
Breast engorgement occurs on third day of life; liquid discharge may be expressed in term newborns	Breast abscesses	Reassure parents of normality of breast engorgement.

*Possible causes of alterations are placed in parentheses.

†This column provides guidelines for further assessment and initial nursing interventions.

Assessment and Normal Findings	Alterations and Possible Causes*	Nursing Responses to Data†
Nipples	Supernumerary nipples Dark-colored nipples	No intervention is necessary.

Heart

Auscultation:

Location: lies horizontally, with left border extending to left of midclavicle Regular rhythm and rate	Arrhythmia (anoxia), tachycardia, bradycardia	Refer all arrhythmia and gallop rhythms. Initiate cardiac evaluation.
Determination of point of maximal impulse (PMI) Usually lateral to midclavicular line at third or fourth intercostal space	Malpositioning (enlargement, abnormal placement, pneumothorax, dextrocardia, diaphragmatic hernia)	
Functional murmurs No thrills	Location of murmurs (possible congenital cardiac anomaly)	Evaluate murmur: location, timing, and duration; observe for accompanying cardiac pathology symptoms; ascertain family history.
Horizontal groove at diaphragm shows flaring of rib cage to mild degree	Marked rib flaring (vitamin D deficiency) Inadequacy of respiratory movement	Initiate cardiopulmonary evaluation; assess pulses and blood pressures in all four extremities for equality and quality.

Abdomen

Appearance:

Cylindrical with some protrusion, appears large in relation to pelvis, some laxness of abdominal muscles No cyanosis, few vessels seen Diastasis recti—common in infants of African descent	Distention, shiny abdomen with engorged vessels (gastrointestinal abnormalities, infection, congenital megacolon) Scaphoid abdominal appearance (diaphragmatic hernia) Increased or decreased peristalsis (duodenal stenosis, small bowel obstruction) Localized flank bulging (enlarged kidneys, ascites, or absent abdominal muscles)	Examine abdomen thoroughly for mass or organomegaly. Measure abdominal girth. Report deviations of abdominal size. Assess other signs and symptoms of obstruction. Refer to physician.

Umbilicus:

No protrusion of umbilicus (protrusion of umbilicus common in infants of African descent) Bluish-white color Cutis navel (umbilical cord projects), granulation tissue present in navel	Umbilical hernia Patent urachus (congenital malformation) Omphalocele Gastroschisis Redness or exudate around cord (infection) Yellow discoloration (hemolytic disease, meconium staining)	Measure umbilical hernia by palpating the opening and record; it should close by 1 year of age; if not, refer to physician. Cover omphalocele with sterile, moist dressing. Instruct parents on cord care and hygiene.
Two arteries and one vein apparent Begins drying 1 to 2 hours after birth No bleeding	Single umbilical artery (congenital anomalies) Discharge or oozing of blood from the cord	Refer anomalies to physician.

*Possible causes of alterations are placed in parentheses.

†This column provides guidelines for further assessment and initial nursing interventions.

Assessment and Normal Findings	Alterations and Possible Causes*	Nursing Responses to Data†
Auscultation and percussion Soft bowel sounds heard shortly after birth every 10–30 seconds	Bowel sounds in chest (diaphragmatic hernia) Absence of bowel sounds Hyperperistalsis (intestinal obstruction)	Collaborate with physician. Assess for other signs of dehydration and/or infection.
Femoral pulses: Palpable, equal, bilateral	Absent or diminished femoral pulses (coarctation of aorta)	Monitor blood pressure in upper and lower extremities.
Inguinal area: No bulges along inguinal area No inguinal lymph nodes felt	Inguinal hernia	Initiate referral. Continue follow-up in well-baby clinic.
Bladder: Percusses 1–4 cm above symphysis Emptied about 3 hours after birth; if not, at time of birth Urine—inoffensive, mild odor	Failure to void within 24–48 hours after birth Exposure of bladder mucosa (exstrophy of bladder) Foul odor (infection)	Check if baby voided at birth. Obtain urine specimen if infection is suspected. Consult with clinician.
Genitals Gender clearly delineated	Ambiguous genitals	Refer for genetic consultation.
Male: *Penis:* Slender in appearance, about 2.5 cm long, 1 cm wide at birth Normal urinary orifice, urethral meatus at tip of penis Noninflamed urethral opening	Micropenis (congenital anomaly) Meatal atresia Hypospadias, epispadias Urethritis (infection)	Observe and record first voiding. Collaborate with physician in presence of abnormality. Delay circumcision. Palpate for enlarged inguinal lymph nodes and record painful urination.
Foreskin adheres to glans	Ulceration of meatal opening (infection, inflammation)	Evaluate whether ulcer is due to diaper rash; counsel regarding care.
Uncircumcised foreskin tight for 2 to 3 months Circumcised Erectile tissue present	Phimosis—if still tight after 3 months	Instruct parents on how to care for uncircumcised penis. Teach parents how to care for circumcision.
Scrotum: Skin loose and hanging or tight and small; extensive rugae and normal size Normal skin color Scrotal discoloration common in breech	Large scrotum containing fluid (hydrocele) Red, shiny scrotal skin (orchitis) Minimal rugae, small scrotum	Shine a light through scrotum (transilluminate) to verify diagnosis. Assess for prematurity.

*Possible causes of alterations are placed in parentheses.

†This column provides guidelines for further assessment and initial nursing interventions.

Assessment and Normal Findings	Alterations and Possible Causes*	Nursing Responses to Data†
Testes:		
Descended by birth; not consistently found in scrotum	Undescended testes (cryptorchidism)	If testes cannot be felt in scrotum, gently palpate femoral, inguinal, perineal, and abdominal areas for presence.
Testes size 1.5–2 cm at birth	Enlarged testes (tumor) Small testes (Klinefelter syndrome or adrenal hyperplasia)	Refer and collaborate with physician for further diagnostic studies.
Female		
Mons:		
Normal skin color, area pigmented in dark-skinned infants Labia majora cover labia minora in term and postterm newborns; symmetric size appropriate for gestational age	Hematoma, lesions (trauma) Labia minora prominent	Evaluate for recent trauma. Assess for prematurity.
Clitoris:		
Normally large in newborn Edema and bruising in breech birth	Hypertrophy (hermaphroditism)	Refer for genetic workup.
Vagina:		
Urinary meatus and vaginal orifice visible (0.5 cm circumference) Vaginal tag or hymenal tag disappears in a few weeks	Inflammation; erythema and discharge (urethritis) Congenital absence of vagina	Collect urine specimen for laboratory examination. Refer to physician.
Discharge; smegma under labia	Foul-smelling discharge (infection)	Collect data and further evaluate reason for discharge.
Bloody or mucoid discharge	Excessive vaginal bleeding (blood coagulation defect)	
Buttocks and Anus		
Buttocks symmetric	Pilonidal dimple	Examine for possible sinus. Instruct parents about cleansing this area.
Anus patent and passage of meconium within 24–48 hours after birth	Imperforate anus, rectal atresia (congenital gastrointestinal defect)	Evaluate extent of problems. Initiate surgical consultation. Perform digital examination to ascertain patency if patency uncertain.
No fissures, tears, or skin tags	Fissures	
Extremities and Trunk		
Short and generally flexed, extremities move symmetrically through range of motion but lack full extension	Unilateral or absence of movement (spinal cord involvement) Fetal position continued or limp (anoxia, CNS problems, hypoglycemia)	Review birth record to assess possible cause.

*Possible causes of alterations are placed in parentheses.

†This column provides guidelines for further assessment and initial nursing interventions.

Assessment and Normal Findings	Alterations and Possible Causes*	Nursing Responses to Data†
All joints move spontaneously; good muscle tone, of flexor type, birth to 2 months	Spasticity when infant begins using extensors (cerebral palsy, lack of muscle tone, "floppy baby" syndrome) Hypotonia (Down syndrome)	Collaborate with physician.
Arms: Equal in length Bilateral movement Flexed when quiet	Brachial palsy (difficult birth) Erb-Duchenne paralysis Muscle weakness, fractured clavicle Absence of limb or change of size (phocomelia, amelia)	Report to clinician.
Hands: Normal number of fingers	Polydactyly (Ellis-Van Creveld syndrome) Syndactyly—one limb (developmental anomaly) Syndactyly—both limbs (genetic component)	Report to clinician.
Normal palmar crease Normal size hands	Simian line on palm (Down syndrome) Short fingers and broad hand (Hurler syndrome)	Refer for genetic workup.
Nails present and extend beyond fingertips in term newborn	Cyanosis and clubbing (cardiac anomalies) Nails long or yellow stained (postterm)	Evaluate for history of distress in utero.
Spine: C-shaped spine Flat and straight when prone Slight lumbar lordosis Easily flexed and intact when palpated At least half of back devoid of lanugo Full-term infant in ventral suspension should hold head at 45-degree angle, back straight	Spina bifida occulta (nevus pilosus) Dermal sinus Myelomeningocele Head lag, limp, floppy trunk (neurologic problems)	Evaluate extent of neurologic damage; initiate care of spinal opening.
Hips: No sign of instability	Sensation of abnormal movement, jerk, or snap of hip dislocation	Examine all newborn infants for dislocated hip prior to discharge from birthing center.
Hips abduct to more than 60 degrees		If this is suspected, refer to orthopedist for further evaluation. Reassess at well-baby visits.
Inguinal and buttock skin creases: Symmetric inguinal and buttock creases	Asymmetry (dislocated hips)	Refer to orthopedist for evaluation. Counsel parents regarding symptoms of concern, and discuss therapy.

*Possible causes of alterations are placed in parentheses.

†This column provides guidelines for further assessment and initial nursing interventions.

Assessment and Normal Findings	Alterations and Possible Causes*	Nursing Responses to Data†
Legs: Legs equal in length Legs shorter than arms at birth	Shortened leg (dislocated hips) Lack of leg movement (fractures, spinal defects)	Refer to orthopedist for evaluation. Counsel parents regarding symptoms of concern, and discuss therapy.
Feet: Foot is in straight line Positional clubfoot—based on position in utero Fat pads and creases on soles of feet	Talipes equinovarus (true clubfoot) Incomplete sole creases in 1st 24 hours of life (premature)	Discuss differences between positional and true clubfoot with parents. Teach parents passive manipulation of foot. Refer to orthopedist if not corrected by 3 months of age.
Talipes planus (flat feet) normal under 3 years of age		Reassure parents that flat feet are normal in infants.
Neuromuscular *Motor function:* Symmetric movement and strength in all extremities	Limp, flaccid, or hypertonic (CNS disorders, infection, dehydration, fracture)	Appraise newborn's posture and motor functions by observing activities and motor characteristics.
May be jerky or have brief twitchings	Tremors (hypoglycemia, hypocalcemia, infection, neurologic damage)	Evaluate electrolyte imbalance, hypoglycemia, and neurologic functioning.
Head lag not over 45 degrees	Delayed or abnormal development (preterm, neurologic involvement)	
Neck control adequate to maintain head erect briefly	Asymmetry of tone or strength (neurologic damage)	Refer for genetic evaluation.
Reflexes *Blink:* Stimulated by flash of light; response is closure of eyelids	Lack of blink response (damage to cranial nerve, CNS injury)	Assess neurologic status.
Pupillary reflex: Stimulated by flash of light; response is constriction of pupil	Lack of reflex (damage to cranial nerve, CNS injury)	
Moro: Response to sudden movement or loud noise should be one of symmetric extension and abduction of arms with fingers extended; then return to normal relaxed flexion Infant lying on back: slightly raised head suddenly released; infant held horizontally, lowered quickly about 6 in, and stopped abruptly Fingers form a C Present at birth; disappears by 6 months of age	Asymmetry of body response (fractured clavicle, injury to brachial plexus) Consistent absence (brain damage)	Discuss normality of this reflex in response to loud noises and/or sudden movements. Absence of reflex requires neurologic evaluation.

*Possible causes of alterations are placed in parentheses.

†This column provides guidelines for further assessment and initial nursing interventions.

Assessment and Normal Findings	Alterations and Possible Causes*	Nursing Responses to Data†
Rooting and sucking: Turns in direction of stimulus to cheek or mouth; opens mouth and begins to suck rhythmically when finger or nipple is inserted into mouth; difficult to elicit after feeding; disappears by 4 to 7 months of age Sucking is adequate for nutritional intake and meeting oral stimulation needs; disappears by 12 months	Poor sucking or easily fatigable (preterm, breastfed infants of barbiturate-addicted mothers, possible cardiac problem) Absence of response (preterm, neurologic involvement, depressed newborns)	Evaluate strength and coordination of sucking. Observe newborn during feeding, and counsel parents about mutuality of feeding experience and newborn's responses.
Palmar grasp: Fingers grasp adult finger when palm is stimulated and hold momentarily; lessens at 3 to 4 months of age	Asymmetry of response (neurologic problems)	Evaluate other reflexes and general neurologic functioning.
Plantar grasp: Toes curl downward when sole of foot is stimulated; lessens by 8 months	Absent (defects of lower spinal column)	Assess for other lower extremity neurologic problems.
Stepping: When held upright and one foot touching a flat surface, will step alternately; disappears at 4 to 5 months of age	Asymmetry of stepping (neurologic abnormality)	Evaluate muscle tone and function on each side of body. Refer to specialist.
Babinski: Fanning and extension of all toes when one side of sole is stroked from heel upward across ball of foot; disappears at about 12 months	Absence of response (low spinal cord defects)	Refer for further neurologic evaluation.
Tonic neck: Fencer position—when head is turned to one side, extremities on same side extend and on opposite side flex; this reflex may not be evident during early neonatal period; disappears at 3 to 4 months of age Response often more dominant in leg than in arm	Absent after 1 month of age or persistent asymmetry (cerebral lesion)	Assess neurologic functioning.
Prone crawl: While on abdomen, neonate pushes up and tries to crawl	Absence or variance of response (preterm, weak, or depressed newborns)	Evaluate motor functioning. Refer to specialist.
Trunk incurvation (Galant): In prone position stroking of spine causes pelvis to turn to stimulated side	Failure to rotate to stimulated side (neurologic damage)	

*Possible causes of alterations are placed in parentheses.

†This column provides guidelines for further assessment and initial nursing interventions.

Newborn Behavioral Assessment

Two conflicting forces influence parents' perceptions of their newborn. One is the parents' preconceptions, based on hopes and fears, of what their newborn will be like. The other is their initial reaction to their baby's temperament, behaviors, and physical appearance. Nurses can assist parents in identifying their baby's specific behaviors.

One of the newborn's first responses is to move into a quiet but alert state of consciousness. The baby is still; his body molds to yours; his hands touch your skin; his eyes open wide and are bright and shiny. He looks directly at you.

This special alert state, this innate ability to communicate, may be the initial preparation for becoming attached to other human beings. One feels awed by the intensity and appealing power of this little bud of humanity meeting the world for the first time.

~ The Amazing Newborn ~

Brazelton's neonatal behavioral assessment scale provides valuable guidelines for assessing the newborn's state changes, temperament, and individual behavior patterns. It furnishes a means by which the health care provider, in conjunction with the parents (primary care givers), can identify and understand the individual newborn's states and capabilities. Families learn which responses, interventions, or activities best meet the special needs of their newborn, and this understanding fosters positive attachment experiences.

The assessment tool attempts to identify the newborn's repertoire of behavioral responses to the environment and also documents the newborn's neurologic adequacy and capabilities. The examination usually takes 20 to 30 minutes and involves about 30 tests. Some items are scored according to the newborn's response to specific stimuli. Others, such as consolability and alertness, are scored as a result of continuous behavioral observations throughout the assessment. For a complete discussion of all test items and maneuvers, see Brazelton (1973). The entire tool is not routinely used in clinical practice.

Because the first few days after birth are a period of behavioral disorganization, the complete assessment should be done on the third day after birth. Every effort should be made to elicit the best response. This may be accomplished by repeating tests at different times or by testing during situations that facilitate the best possible response, such as when parents are holding, cuddling, rocking, and singing to their baby.

The assessment of the newborn should be carried out initially in a quiet, dimly or softly lit room, if possible. The newborn's state of consciousness should be determined because scoring and introduction of the test items are correlated with the sleep or awake state. The newborn's state depends on physiologic variables, such as the amount of time from the last feeding, positioning, envi-

Critical Thinking in Practice

Maria Reyes, a 19-year-old G2 now P2 mother, delivered a 40-week-old female neonate 24 hours ago. The newborn exam was normal. Mrs Reyes asks about the newborn's exam. She says she has noticed that the baby cries more than her first child and seems to require holding for longer periods of time after feeding before "quieting down." She is concerned that there is something she is doing wrong and wants to know when her newborn will start to act like her first baby. What should you discuss with her about newborn behavior?

Answers can be found in Appendix I.

ronmental temperature, and health status; presence of such external stimuli as noises and bright lights; and the sleep-wake cycle of the infant. An important characteristic of the neonatal period is the *pattern of states*, as well as the transitions from one state to another. The pattern of states is a predictor of the newborn's receptivity and ability to respond to stimuli in a cognitive manner. Babies learn best in a quiet, alert state and in an environment that is supportive and protective and that provides appropriate stimuli.

The nurse should observe the newborn's sleep-wake patterns (as discussed in Chapter 27) and the rapidity with which the newborn moves from one state to another, the newborn's ability to be consoled, and the newborn's ability to diminish the impact of disturbing stimuli. The following questions may provide the nurse with a framework for assessment:

- Does the newborn's response style and ability to adapt to stimuli indicate a need for parental interventions that will alert the newborn to the environment so that the baby can grow socially and cognitively?

- Are parental interventions necessary to lessen the outside stimuli, as in the case of the baby who responds to sensory input with intensity?

- Can the baby control the amount of sensory input to be dealt with?

The behaviors and the sleep-wake states in which they are assessed are categorized as follows:

- *Habituation.* The infant's ability to diminish or shut down innate responses to specific repeated stimuli, such as a rattle, bell, light, or pinprick to heel, is assessed.

- *Orientation to inanimate and animate visual and auditory assessment stimuli.* How often and where the newborn attends to auditory and visual stimuli are observed. The infant's orientation to the environment is determined by an ability to respond to cues given by others and by a natural ability to fix on and to follow a visual object horizontally and vertically. This capacity and parental appreciation of it are important for positive communication between infant and parents; the parents' visual (en face) and auditory (soft, continuous voice) presence stimulates their infant to orient to them. Inability or lack of response may indicate visual or auditory problems. It is important for parents to know that their newborn can turn to voices usually soon after birth or by 3 days of age and can become alert at different times with a varying degree of intensity in response to sounds.

- *Motor activity.* Several components are evaluated. Motor tone of the newborn is assessed in the most characteristic state of responsiveness. This summary assessment includes overall use of tone as the neonate responds to being handled—whether during spontaneous activity, prone placement, or horizontal holding—and overall assessment of body tone as the neonate reacts to all stimuli.

- *Variations.* Frequency of alert states, state changes, color changes (throughout all states as examination progresses), activity, and peaks of excitement are assessed.

- *Self-quieting activity.* Assessment is based on how often, how quickly, and how effectively newborns can use their resources to quiet and console themselves when upset or distressed. Considered in this assessment are such self-consolatory activities as putting hand to mouth, sucking on a fist or the tongue, and attuning to an object or sound. The newborn's need for outside consolation must also be considered—for example, seeing a face; being rocked, held, or dressed; using a pacifier; and being swaddled.

- *Cuddliness or social behaviors.* This area encompasses the infant's need for and response to being held. Also considered is how often the newborn smiles. These behaviors influence the parents' self-esteem and feelings of acceptance or rejection. Cuddling also appears to be an indicator of personality. Cuddlers appear to enjoy, accept, and seek physical contact; are easier to placate; sleep more; and form earlier and more intense attachments. Noncuddlers are active, restless, have accelerated motor development, and are intolerant of physical restraint. Smiling, even as a grimace reflex, greatly influences parent-infant feedback. Parents identify this response as positive.

REFERENCES

AAP Committee on Fetus and Newborn and ACOG Committee on Obstetrics: *Guidelines for Perinatal Care.* Evanston, IL: American Academy of Pediatrics, 1992.

Ballard JL et al: New Ballard score, expanded to include extremely premature infants. *J Pediatr* 1991; 119:417.

Ballard JL et al: A simplified score for assessment of fetal maturation of newly born infants. *J Pediatr* November 1979; 95:769.

Brazelton T: *The Neonatal Behavioral Assessment Scale*. Philadelphia: Lippincott, 1973.

Brazelton T: Neonatal behavior and its significance. In: *Schaffer's Diseases of the Newborn*. Avery ME, Taeusch HW (editors). Philadelphia: WB Saunders, 1984.

Dubowitz L, Dubowitz V: *Gestational Age of the Newborn*. Menlo Park, CA: Addison-Wesley, 1977.

Faix RG: Fontanelle size in Black and White term infants. *J Pediatr* 1982; 100:304.

Hoekelman RA et al: *Primary Pediatric Care*, 2nd ed. St Louis: Mosby, 1992.

Ludington-Hoe SM, Golani S: *How To Have a Smarter Baby*. New York: Bantam, 1988.

Querleu D et al: Hearing by the human fetus? *Semin Perinatol* October 1989; 13:409.

Sanders M et al: Gestational age assessment in preterm neonates weighing less than 1500 grams. *Pediatrics* 1991; 88:542.

Steinkuller PG: Best methods for visual assessment in children. Paper presented at the Cullen Course, Baylor College of Medicine, Dallas, March 1988.

Sullivan RM et al: Olfactory classical conditioning in neonates. *Pediatrics* 1991; 87:511.

Taeusch HW, Ballard RA, Avery ME: *Schaffer and Avery's Diseases of the Newborn*, 6th ed. Philadelphia: WB Saunders, 1991.

Tappero EP, Honeyfield ME: *Physical Assessment of the Newborn*. Petaluma, CA: NICU Ink, 1993.

Weiss M: Tympanic thermometry for full-term and preterm neonates. *Clin Pediatr* 1991; 30(suppl):42.

Yip R, Li Z, Chong W-H: Race and birth weight: The Chinese example. *Pediatrics* 1991; 87(5):688.

CHAPTER 29

THE NORMAL NEWBORN: NEEDS AND CARE

*T*his moment of meeting seemed to be a birthtime for both of us; her first and my second life. Nothing, I knew, could ever be the same again.

~LAURIE LEE, *TWO WOMEN*~

KEY TERMS

Circumcision

Newborn screening tests

Parent-newborn attachment

OBJECTIVES

Summarize the essential areas of information to be obtained about a newborn's birth experience and immediate postnatal period.

Explain the physiologic and behavioral responses of newborns and possible interventions needed.

Discuss the major nursing considerations and activities to be carried out during the first 4 hours after birth (admission and transitional period) and subsequent daily care.

Identify activities that should be included in a daily care plan for a normal newborn.

Determine common concerns of families regarding their newborns.

Describe topics and related content to be included in parent education on newborn and infant care.

Identify opportunities to individualize parent teaching and enhance each parent's abilities and confidence while providing infant care in the birthing unit.

Delineate information to be included in discharge planning with the newborn's family.

At the moment of birth numerous physiologic adaptations begin to take place in the newborn's body. Because of these dramatic changes, newborns require close observation to determine how smoothly they are making the transition to extrauterine life. Newborns also require special care that enhances their chances of making the transition successfully.

The two broad goals of nursing care during this period are to promote the physical well-being of the newborn and to enhance the establishment of a well-functioning family unit. The first goal is met by providing comprehensive care to newborns while they are in the mother-baby unit. The second goal is met by teaching family members how to care for their new baby and by supporting their parenting efforts so that they feel confident and competent.

Thus the nurse must be knowledgeable about family adjustments that need to be made, as well as the health care needs of the newborn. It is important that the family return home with the positive feeling that they have the support, information, and skills to care for their newborn. Equally important is the need for each member of the family to begin a unique relationship with the newborn. The cultural and social expectations of individual families and communities affect the way normal newborn care is carried out.

The previous two chapters have presented an informational database regarding the physiologic and behavioral changes occurring in the newborn and the pertinent nursing assessments that are needed. This chapter discusses nursing care during the newborn period. The Newborn Critical Pathway starts on page 860.

NURSING DIAGNOSIS DURING ADMISSION AND FIRST 4 HOURS

Nursing diagnoses are based on an analysis of the assessment findings. Physiologic alterations of the newborn form the basis of many nursing diagnoses, as does the family's incorporation of them in caring for their new baby. Nursing diagnoses that may apply to the newborn include the following:

- Ineffective airway clearance related to presence of mucus and retained lung fluid

- Risk for altered body temperature related to evaporative, radiant, conductive, and convective heat losses

- Altered nutrition: Less than body requirements related to limited fluid intake

- Altered peripheral tissue perfusion related to decreased thermoregulation

- Pain related to vitamin K injection or heel sticks for glucose or hematocrit

Many of these nursing diagnoses and associated interventions must be identified and implemented very quickly during this period. As discussed in Chapter 27, the newborn's physiologic adaptation to extrauterine life occurs rapidly. All the body systems are affected. Thus the newborn requires close monitoring during the first few hours of life so that any deviation from normal can be identified immediately and appropriate interventions made.

During the assessment in the first 4 hours after birth the nurse focuses on the newborn's physiologic adaptations. A complete physical examination is done later by the physician or nurse practitioner, usually within the first 24 hours of life or just prior to discharge (see Chapter 28 and Table 28–1).

Critical Thinking Question

Which critical perinatal and neonatal assessments have the most significant impact on the newborn's care during the first 4 hours after birth?

NURSING PLAN AND IMPLEMENTATION DURING ADMISSION AND FIRST 4 HOURS

The nurse initiates newborn admission procedures and evaluates the newborn's need to remain under observation. The nurse also monitors the newborn's ability to maintain a clear airway and stable vital signs, maintain body temperature, demonstrate normal neurologic status and no observable complications, and tolerate the first feeding. If these criteria are met, it indicates a successful beginning adaptation to extrauterine life, and the baby is moved to a regular nursery or back to the mother's room. This transfer usually takes place between 2 and 6 hours after birth.

Initiation of Admission Procedures

After birth the baby is formally admitted to the health care facility. The admission procedures include an assessment to ensure that the newborn's adaptation to extrauterine life is proceeding normally. Several interventions to promote successful adaptation are also included (see Essential Precautions in Practice: During Newborn Care on page 862).

If the initial assessment indicates that the newborn is not at risk physiologically, many of the routine admission

NEWBORN CRITICAL PATHWAY

Category	First 4 Hours	4–8 Hours Past Birth	8–24 Hours Past Birth
Referral	Review labor/birth record Review transitional nursing record Check ID bands	Check ID bands Transfer to mother/baby care at 4 hours of age Circumcision permit signed	Check ID bands q shift
Assessments	Continue assessments begun first hour after birth Vital signs: T, P, R, B/P q1h × 4 (skin temp 97.8–98.6 F, resp may be irregular but within 30–60 per min) Newborn assessments include: • Respiratory status with resp distress scale × 1 then prn If resp distress, assess q5–15min • Cord—bluish white color, clamp in place • Skin, mucus membranes, extremities—color (trunk pinkish with slight acrocyanosis of hands and feet) • Wt (5 lb 8 oz–8 lb 13 oz), Length (18–22 in), HC (12.5–14.5 in), CC (32.5 cm, 1–2 cm less than head) • Extremity movement—may be jerky or brief twitches • GA classification—Term AGA • Anomalies (cong. anomalies can interfere with normal extrauterine adaptation)	Assess newborn's progress thru periods of reactivity Vital signs: T, P, R, B/P q4h Newborn assessments include: • Skin color q4h (circulatory system stabilizing, acrocyanosis decreased) • Eyes for drainage, redness, hemorrhage • Ausculate lungs q4h (noisy wet resp normal) • Increased mucus production (normal in 2nd period of reactivity) • Check apical pulse q4h • Umbilical cord base for redness, drainage, foul odor, drying. Clamp remains in place. • Extremity movement q4h • Check for expected reflexes (suck, rooting, Moro, grasp, blink, yawn, sneeze, tonic neck, Babinski) • Note common normal variations • Assess suck and swallow during feeding • Note behavioral characteristics • Temp before and after admission bath	VS q4h–range: T, 97.5–99 F; P, 120–160; R, 30–60; B/P, 60–80/45–40 mm Hg Continue newborn assessments: • Skin color q4h • Signs of drying or infection in cord area • Check cord clamp in place until removed before discharge • Check circ for bleeding after procedure, then q30min × 2, then at least q4h
Teaching/ psychosocial	Admission activities performed at mother's bedside if possible Teach parents use of bulb syringe, signs of choking, positioning, and when to call for assistance Teach reasons for radiant warmer use and the need to wrap baby in warmed blankets when out of warmer	Reinforce teaching about choking, bulb syringe, positioning, maintaining warmth by use of blankets and clothing Teach infant positioning to facilitate breathing and digestion Teach new parents holding and feeding skills Teach parents soothing/calming techniques	Teach parents re: diapering, normal void and stool patterns, bathing, nail and cord care, circumcision/uncircumcised penis care, rashes, jaundice, sleep/wake cycles and soothing activities, taking temperatures and reading thermometer Explain S&S of illness and when to call health care provider No tub bath until cord falls off
Therapeutic nursing interventions and reports	Place under radiant warmer Put hat on newborn (decreases convection heat loss) Suction nares/mouth with bulb syringe prn Keep bulb syringe in crib Obtain lab tests: blood type, Rh, Coombs on cord blood as needed; glucose, HSV culture if hx of maternal or paternal HSV	Keep under radiant warmer as needed Bathe infant if temp > 97.8 F Position on side Suction nares (esp during 2nd period of reactivity) Obtain peripheral Hct per protocol Cord care per protocol (alcohol or triple dye prn) Fold diaper below cord (for plastic diapers, turn plastic layer away from skin)	Check for hearing test results Weigh before discharge Cord care q shift DC cord clamp before discharge Perform newborn screening blood tests before discharge Circumcision care: position on side, change dressing when soiled
Activity and comfort	Place under radiant warmer or wrap in prewarmed blankets until stable Soothe baby as needed with voice and/or touch	Leave in warmer until stable then swaddle Position on side or abd after each feeding	Place in open crib Swaddle and allow movement of extremities in blanket
Nutrition	Assist newborn to breastfeed as soon as mother/baby condition allows Initiate bottle feeding within first hour Gavage feed if necessary to prevent hypoglycemia Supplement breast only when medically indicated or per agency policy	Breastfeed at least q3–4h or on demand Bottle feed q3–6h or on demand Determine readiness to feed and feeding tolerance	Continue breast/bottle feeding pattern Assess feeding tolerance q4h Discuss normal feeding requirements, signs of hunger and satiation, handling feeding problems, and when to seek help

Category	First 4 Hours _continued_	4–8 Hours _continued_	8–24 Hours Past Birth _continued_
Elimination	Note first void and stool if not done at birth	Note all voids and color of stools q4h	Evaluate all voids and color of stools q8h
Medication	Prophylactic ophthalmic ointment OU after baby makes eye contact with parents within 1 h after birth Administer vitamin K injection, 1 mg IM per agency protocol	Hepatitis B if ordered by Dr or consent signed by parent	Hepatitis B vaccine before discharge
Discharge planning/ home care	Hepatitis B form signed Hearing and screen consent signed Plan discharge call with parent/guardian in 24 hours to 2 days Assess parents discharge plans and support systems	Review/reinforce teaching with mother and significant other	Initial newborn screening tests (hearing, blood tests ie, PKU) before discharge Bath and feeding classes, videos, or written information given Give written copy of discharge instructions Set up appointment for follow-up PKU test Discuss infant safety needs Have car seat available before discharge All discharge referrals made Give Hepatitis B vaccine as ordered
Family involvement	Facilitate early investigation of baby's physical characteristics (maintain temp during unwrapping), hold infant en face Dim lights to help infant keep eyes open Provide uninterrupted time with family	Assess parents knowledge of newborn behaviors, such as alertness, suck and rooting behavior, and attention to human voice	Assess Mother-baby bonding/interaction Incorporate father and sibs into care Enhance parent-infant interaction by sharing characteristics & behavioral assessment Support positive parenting behaviors Identify community referral needs and refer to community agencies

procedures are performed in the presence of the parents in the birthing area. The care measures indicated by the assessment findings may be performed by the nurse or by the parents under the guidance of the nurse in an effort to educate and support the family. Other interventions may be delayed if the newborn is transferred to an observational nursery.

The nurse responsible for the newborn first checks and confirms the newborn's identification with the mother's identification and then obtains and records all significant information. The essential data to be recorded as part of the newborn's chart include the following:

1. _Condition of the newborn._ Pertinent information includes the newborn's Apgar scores at 1 and 5 minutes, resuscitative measures required in the birthing area, vital signs, voidings, and passing of meconium. Complications to be noted are excessive mucus, delayed spontaneous respirations or responsiveness, abnormal number of cord vessels, and obvious physical abnormalities.

2. _Labor and birth record._ A copy of the labor and birth record should be placed in the newborn's chart. The record contains all the significant data about the birth, for example, duration, course, and status of mother and fetus throughout labor and birth and

any analgesia or anesthesia administered to the mother. Particular care is taken to note any variation or difficulties such as prolonged rupture of membranes, abnormal fetal position, meconium-stained amniotic fluid, signs of fetal distress during labor, nuchal cord (cord around the newborn's neck at birth), precipitous birth, use of forceps, and maternal analgesia and anesthesia received within 1 hour of birth.

3. _Antepartal history._ Any maternal problems that may have compromised the fetus in utero, such as PIH, spotting, illness, recent infections, rubella status, serology results, hepatitis B screen results, exposure to Group B streptococci, or a history of maternal substance abuse, are of immediate concern in newborn assessment (American Academy of Pediatrics 1992). Information about maternal age, estimated date of birth (EDB), previous pregnancies, and presence of any congenital anomalies is also included.

4. _Parent-newborn interaction information._ Parental interactions with their newborn and their desires regarding care, such as rooming-in, circumcision, and type of feeding, are noted. Information about other children in the home, available support systems, and interactional patterns within each family unit assists in providing comprehensive care.

TABLE 29-1	Signs of Newborn Transition

Normal findings for the newborn during the first few days of life include the following:
Pulse: 120–160 beats/minute
   During sleep as low as 100 beats/minute
   If crying, up to 180 beats/minute
   Apical pulse is counted for 1 full minute because rate may fluctuate.
Respirations: 30–60 respirations/minute
   Predominantly diaphragmatic but synchronous with abdominal movements
   Brief periods of apnea (5–10 seconds) with no color or heart rate changes
Temperature: axillary: 36.4–37 C (97.5–99 F)
   Skin: 36–36.5 C (96.8–97.7 F)
Blood pressure: 80–60/45–40 mm Hg at birth; 100/50 mm Hg at day 10
Chemstrip: greater than 40 mg%
Hematocrit: less than 65%–70% central venous sample

Three routine measurements are length, circumference of the head, and circumference of the chest. In some facilities abdominal girth may also be measured. The nurse rapidly assesses the baby's color, muscle tone, alertness, and general state. Remember that the first period of reactivity may have concluded, and the baby may be in the sleep-inactive phase, which makes the infant hard to arouse. Basic assessments for estimating gestational age are done, and the physical assessment is completed. (For more discussion of the process of newborn assessment see Chapter 28).

In addition to obtaining vital signs, the nurse may perform a hematocrit and blood glucose evaluation on all newborns or as clinically indicated (such as for small-for-gestational-age [SGA] or large-for-gestational-age [LGA] infants or if the newborn is jittery). These proce-

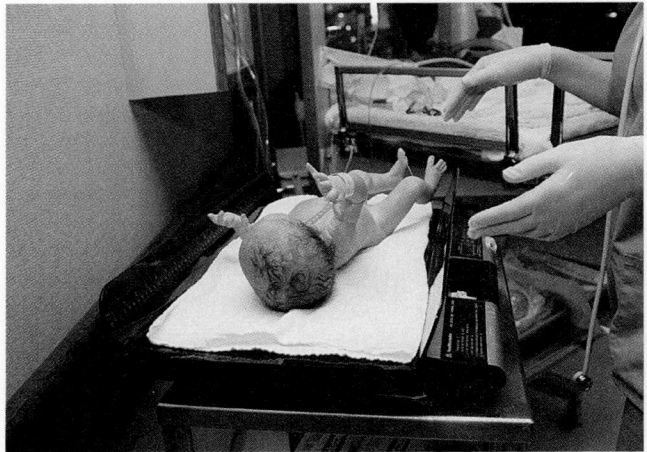

FIGURE 29-1   Weighing a newborn. The scale is balanced before each weighing, with the protective pad in place. The care giver's hand is poised above the infant as a safety measure.

As discussed in Chapter 27 the newborn's physiologic adaptations to extrauterine life occur rapidly. All the body systems are affected. The nurse must be able to monitor the newborn's physiologic adaptation and behavior during the transitional periods of the first few hours of life so that any deviation from normal can be identified immediately (Table 29–1).

As part of the admission procedure, the newborn is weighed and measured in both grams and pounds; parents understand weights best when stated in pounds and ounces (Figure 29–1). The scales are cleaned and covered each time a newborn is weighed to prevent cross-infection and heat loss from conduction.

The newborn is then measured, and the measurements are recorded in both centimeters and inches.

dures may be done on admission or within the first 4 hours after birth (American Academy of Pediatrics 1992) (see Procedure 32–1).

Maintenance of a Clear Airway and Stable Vital Signs

The nurse positions the newborn on his or her side. If necessary, a bulb syringe or DeLee wall suction (Procedure 23–1) is used to remove mucus from the nasal passages and oral cavity. A DeLee catheter attached to suction may be used to remove mucus from the stomach to help prevent possible aspiration. This procedure also ensures that the esophagus is patent prior to the newborn's first feeding. Gastric suctioning can cause vagal nerve stimulation, which may result in bradycardia and apnea in the unstabilized newborn.

In the absence of any newborn distress, the nurse continues with the admission by taking the newborn's vital signs. The initial temperature is taken by the axillary method. A wider range of normal for axillary temperature is being recommended (Merestein & Gardner 1992). This range is 36.4–37.2 C (97.5–99 F).

Once the initial temperature is taken, the core temperature is monitored either by obtaining axillary temperatures at intervals or by placing a skin sensor on the newborn for continuous reading. The usual skin sensor placement site is on the newborn's abdomen, but placement on the upper thigh or arm can give a reading closely correlated with the mean body temperature. The vital signs for a healthy term newborn should be monitored at least every 30 minutes until the newborn's condition has remained stable for 2 hours (American Academy of Pediatrics 1992). The newborn's respirations may be irregular and still be normal. Brief periods of apnea, lasting only 5–10 seconds with no color or heart rate changes, are considered normal. The normal pulse range is 120–160 beats per minute, and the normal respiratory range is 30–60 respirations per minute.

Maintenance of a Neutral Thermal Environment

A neutral thermal environment is essential to minimize the newborn's need for increased oxygen consumption and use of calories to maintain body heat in the optimal range of 36.4–37.2 C (97.5–99 F). If the newborn becomes hypothermic, the body's response can lead to metabolic acidosis, hypoxia, and shock.

A neutral thermal environment is best achieved by performing the assessment and interventions with a newborn unclothed and under a radiant warmer. The thermostat of the radiant warmer is controlled by the thermal skin sensor taped to the newborn's abdomen, upper thigh, or arm. The sensor indicates when the newborn's temperature exceeds or falls below the acceptable temperature range. The nurse should be aware that leaning over the newborn may block the radiant heat waves from reaching the newborn.

It is common practice in some institutions to cover the neonate's head with a stockinette or knit cap to prevent further heat loss in addition to placing the baby under a radiant warmer. Ruchala (1985) compared axillary temperatures of newborns whose heads were covered and those remaining uncovered. The study failed to demonstrate a significant difference 2 hours after birth, which raised the question of whether heat can more effectively be retained by using a head covering while the newborn is outside the radiant warmer but not when the newborn is under the radiant warmer (to avoid a barrier effect). This led to the practice of covering the head after birth.

When the newborn's temperature is normal and vital signs are stable (about 2 to 4 hours after birth), the baby may be given a sponge bath. However, this admission bath may be postponed for some hours if the newborn's condition dictates or the parents wish to give the first bath. The baby is bathed while still under the radiant warmer. This may be done in the parents' room. Bathing the newborn offers an excellent opportunity for teaching and welcoming parent involvement in the care of their baby.

The temperature is rechecked after the bath, and if it is stable, the newborn is dressed, wrapped, and placed in an open crib at room temperature. If the baby's axillary temperature is below 36.4 C (97.5 F), the baby is returned to the radiant warmer. The rewarming process should be gradual to prevent the possibility of hyperthermia. Slow rewarming is accomplished by maintaining the ambient temperature 1.5 C (3 F) higher than the infant's current skin temperature (Neonatal Thermoregulation 1990). When this new skin temperature is reached, the control point of the heater can be set another 1.5 C higher until the desired skin temperature is reached. Once the newborn is rewarmed, the nurse implements measures to prevent further neonatal heat loss, such as keeping the newborn dry, double-wrapped with hat on and away from cool surfaces or use of cool instruments. The newborn is also protected from drafts, open windows or doors, or air conditioners. Blankets and clothing are stored in a warm place. See Temperature Regulation in Chapter 27 and Procedure 29–1 on page 864.

Prevention of Complications of Hemorrhagic Disease of Newborn

A prophylactic injection of vitamin K_1 (AquaMEPHYTON) is given to prevent hemorrhage, which can occur due to low prothrombin levels in the first few days of life (see the Drug Guide: Vitamin K_1, Phytonadione [AquaMEPHYTON] on page 865). The potential for

Nursing Action	Rationale
Objective: Prepare warming equipment	
Prewarm incubator or radiant warmer. Have warmed towels/lightweight blankets available.	*Change from warm, moist intrauterine environment to cool, dry, drafty environment stresses the immature thermoregulation mechanisms of newborn.*
Maintain birthing room at 22 C (71 F) with relative humidity of 60% to 65%.	
Objective: Establish a stable temperature after birth	
Wipe newborn free of blood and excessive vernix, especially from the head, with prewarmed towels.	*Prevents loss of body heat from large surface area through evaporation*
Place newborn under radiant warmer.	*Creates a heat-gaining environment*
Wrap newborn in prewarmed blanket and transfer to mother.	*Reduces convective heat loss* *Facilitates immediate maternal-infant contact without compromising infant thermoregulation*
Place skin to skin with mother under warmed blanket.	*Skin-to-skin contact with mother or father acts to maintain newborn's temperature.*
Objective: Maintain stable infant temperature	
Diaper newborn and place hat on head. Place newborn uncovered (except for diaper and hat) under radiant warmer.	*Radiant heat warms outer surface skin, so skin needs to be exposed.*
Tape servocontrol probe on infant's anterior abdominal wall (metal side next to skin), and cover with aluminum heat deflector patch	*Aluminum cover prevents heating of probe directly and overheating of infant. Turn heater to servocontrol mode with abdominal skin temperature maintained at 36.5–37 C.*
Monitor infant's axillary and skin probe temperature per institution protocol.	*Rechecking temperature ensures that it is within desired range. Temperature indicator on the radiant warmer continually displays baby's probe temperature, so nurse checks baby's axillary temperature to ensure that the machine accurately reports baby's temperature.*
Once infant's temperature reaches 37 C (98.6 F), remove infant from radiant warmer. Dress infant in T-shirt, diaper, and stocking hat. Then wrap in two blankets (called double wrap). Place infant in open crib. Recheck axillary temperature in 1 hour.	*It is important to monitor infant's ability to maintain own thermoregulation.*
Objective: Rewarm infant gradually if temperature < 36.1 C (97 F).	
Assess temperature frequently. Check axillary temperature per hospital routine, usually every 2 to 4 hours.	*Early detection of hypothermia, which predisposes infant to cold stress*
Place unclothed infant with diaper under radiant warmer with servocontrol probe on abdomen.	*Rapid heating leads to hyperthermia.*
Gradually rewarm infant back to normal temperature.	*Hyperthermia caused by too rapid warming is associated with apnea, increased insensible water loss, and increased metabolic rate.*
Recheck temperature in 30 minutes, then hourly.	
Once infant's temperature reaches 37 C (98.6 F), remove from heater, dress, double wrap with hat on, and place in open crib. Recheck temperature in 1 hour.	
Objective: Prevent drops in baby's temperature.	
Keep infant clothing and bedding dry.	*Prevents heat loss by conduction, convection, radiation, and evaporation.*
Double-wrap with hat on.	
Use radiant warmer during procedures.	
Reduce exposure to drafts.	
Warm objects coming in contact with infant (eg, stethoscopes).	
Encourage mother to snuggle with infant under blankets or breastfeed with hat and light cover on infant.	

VITAMIN K₁ PHYTONADIONE (AQUAMEPHYTON)

Overview of Neonatal Action

Phytonadione is used in prophylaxis and treatment of hemorrhagic disease of the newborn. It promotes liver formation of the clotting factors II, VII, IX, and X. At birth the neonate does not have the bacteria in the colon that are necessary for synthesizing fat-soluble vitamin K₁, therefore the newborn may have decreased levels of prothrombin during the first 5–8 days of life reflected by a prolongation of prothrombin time.

Route, Dosage, Frequency

Intramuscular injection is given in the vastus lateralis thigh muscle. A one-time only prophylactic dose of 0.5–1 mg IM is given in the birthing area or upon admission to the newborn nursery. A one-time dose of 2 mg is given if the route of administration is by mouth. If the mother received anticoagulants during pregnancy, an additional dose may be ordered by the physician and is given at 6–8 hours post first injection.

Neonatal Side Effects

Pain and edema may occur at injection site. Possible allergic reactions such as rash and urticaria.

Nursing Considerations

Observe for bleeding (usually occurs on second or third day). Bleeding may be seen as generalized ecchymoses or bleeding from umbilical cord, circumcision site, nose, or gastrointestinal tract. Results of serial PT and PTT should be assessed.

Observe for jaundice and kernicterus, especially in preterm infants.

Observe for signs of local inflammation.

Protect drug from light.

Give vitamin K₁ before circumcision procedure.

---

hemorrhage is considered to result from the absence of gut bacterial flora, which influences the production of vitamin K in the newborn. (See Chapter 32 for further discussion.) Controversy exists over whether the administration of vitamin K may predispose the newborn to significant hyperbilirubinemia. However, Cunningham et al (1993) indicate there is no evidence to support this concern as long as a standard dose of 1 mg is given. Some people have questioned the need to give vitamin K to newborns who have had a nontraumatic birth.

A study by Von Kries (1988) looked at replacing parenteral vitamin K with oral vitamin K to avoid injecting the infant. The study demonstrated a considerably higher level of vitamin K present after intramuscular administration than after oral administration. Thus parenteral vitamin K prophylaxis is a safer means of providing infants with a high vitamin K load. Parents may request that vitamin K be given orally. To ensure an adequate dose, 2 mg (twice the usual IM dosage) is given by mouth.

Vitamin K injection is given intramuscularly in the middle one-third of the vastus lateralis muscle located in the lateral aspect of the thigh (Figure 29–2). Before injecting, the nurse must clean the newborn's skin site for the injection thoroughly with a small alcohol swab. The nurse uses a 25-gauge, ⅝ inch needle for the injection. An alternative site is the rectus femoris muscle in the anterior aspect of the thigh. However, this site is near the sciatic nerve and femoral artery and should be used with caution (Figure 29–3). Remember that vitamin K₁ needs to be protected from the light.

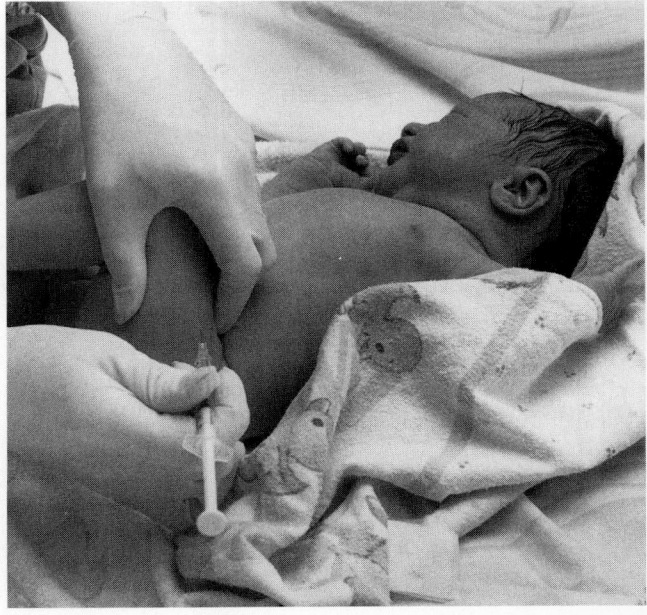

FIGURE 29-2   Procedure for vitamin K injection. Cleanse area thoroughly with alcohol swab and allow skin to dry. Bunch the tissue of the upper thigh (vastus lateralis muscle) and quickly insert a 25-gauge ⅝ inch needle at a 90-degree angle to the thigh. Aspirate, then slowly inject the solution to distribute the medication evenly and minimize the baby's discomfort. Remove the needle and massage the site with an alcohol swab.

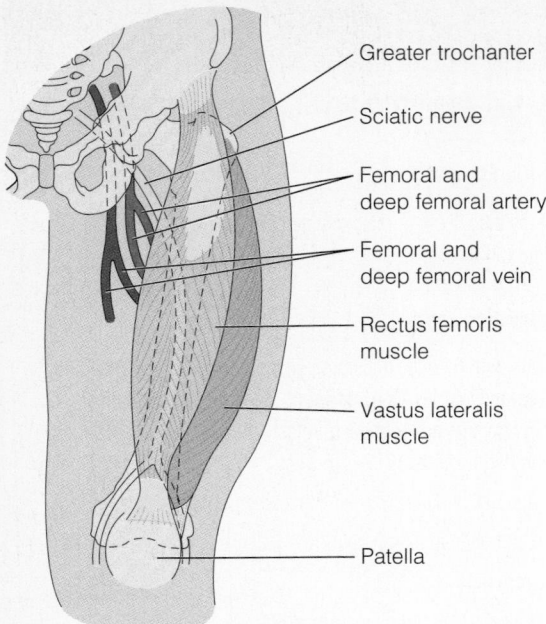

Greater trochanter

Sciatic nerve

Femoral and
deep femoral artery

Femoral and
deep femoral vein

Rectus femoris
muscle

Vastus lateralis
muscle

Patella

FIGURE 29-3 Injection sites. The middle third of the vastus lateralis muscle is the preferred site for intramuscular injection in the newborn. The middle third of the rectus femoris is an alternate site, but its proximity to major vessels and the sciatic nerve necessitates caution in using this site for injection.

Prevention of Eye Infection

The nurse is also responsible for giving the legally required prophylactic eye treatment for *Neisseria gonorrhoea*, which may have infected the newborn of an infected mother during the birth process. In the past the drug of choice was 1% silver nitrate solution. Now other ophthalmic ointments are used instead of silver nitrate. Erythromycin (Ilotycin Ophthalmic) (see the Drug Guide: Erythromycin [Ilotycin Ophthalmic]), tetracycline, or penicillin all are also effective against chlamydia, which has a higher incidence than gonorrhea. A recent study showed erythromycin or tetracycline wasn't any more effective against *Chlamydia trachomatis* than silver nitrate (Zanoni et al 1992). Bell and associates (1993) showed that either one of the possible eye prophylaxis medications or no prophylaxis at all is reasonable for newborns born to women who received prenatal care and didn't have any sexually transmitted infection during pregnancy.

The eyes should be treated within the first few hours after birth. Successful eye prophylaxis requires that the medication be instilled into the lower conjunctival sac (Figure 29–4). It may be delayed up to a few hours after birth to allow eye contact during parent-newborn bonding (American Academy of Pediatrics 1992) (Procedure 29–2).

The eye prophylaxis medication can cause chemical conjunctivitis, which gives the newborn some discomfort and may interfere with the baby's ability to focus on the parents' faces. The resulting edema, inflammation, and

---

DRUG GUIDE

ERYTHROMYCIN OPHTHALMIC OINTMENT (ILOTYCIN OPHTHALMIC)

Overview of Neonatal Action

Erythromycin (Ilotycin Ophthalmic) is used as prophylactic treatment of ophthalmia neonatorum, which is caused by the bacteria *Neisseria gonorrhoeae*. Preventive treatment of gonorrhea in the newborn is required by law. Erythromycin is also effective against ophthalmic chlamydial infections. It is either bacteriostatic or bactericidal, depending on the organisms involved and the concentration of drug.

Route, Dosage, Frequency

Ophthalmic ointment (0.5%) is instilled as a narrow ribbon or strand, 1/4 inch long, along the lower conjunctival surface of each eye, starting at the inner canthus. It is instilled only once in each eye. Administration may be done in the birthing area or later in the nursery so that eye contact is facilitated and the bonding process immediately after birth is not interrupted. After administration gently close eye and manipulate to ensure spread of ointment (Milan & McFeely 1990; Pawlak & Tabor-Herfert 1990).

Neonatal Side Effects

Sensitivity reaction; may interfere with ability to focus and may cause edema and inflammation. Side effects usually disappear in 24–48 hours.

Nursing Considerations

Wash hands immediately prior to instillation to prevent introduction of bacteria.

Do not irrigate the eyes after instillation. Use new tube or single-use container for ophthalmic ointment administration shortly after birth. May wipe away excess after 1 minute.

Observe for hypersensitivity.

Teach parents about need for eye prophylaxis. Educate them regarding side effects and signs that need to be reported to the health care provider.

discharge may cause concern if the parents have not been given information that the side effects will clear in 24 to 48 hours and that this prophylactic eye treatment is necessary for the newborn's well-being.

Early Assessment of Neonatal Distress

During the first 24 hours of life, nurses are constantly alert for signs of distress that signify maladaptation to extrauterine life whether newborns are with them or the parents. Parents must be assured that the nursing staff is available to them immediately should the baby develop distress (Table 29–2). Extra care must be taken to teach them how to maintain their newborn's temperature, recognize the hallmarks of newborn distress, and respond immediately to signs of respiratory problems. The parents should be taught to observe their infant for changes in color or activity, rapid breathing with chest retractions, or facial grimacing. Their interventions should include nasal and oral suctioning with a bulb syringe, positioning, and vigorous fingertip stroking of the newborn's spine to stimulate respiratory activity if necessary.

Initiation of First Feeding

The timing of the first feeding varies, depending on whether the newborn is to be breastfed or bottle-fed or there were any complications during pregnancy or birth (IDM, IUGR, and so forth). Mothers who choose to

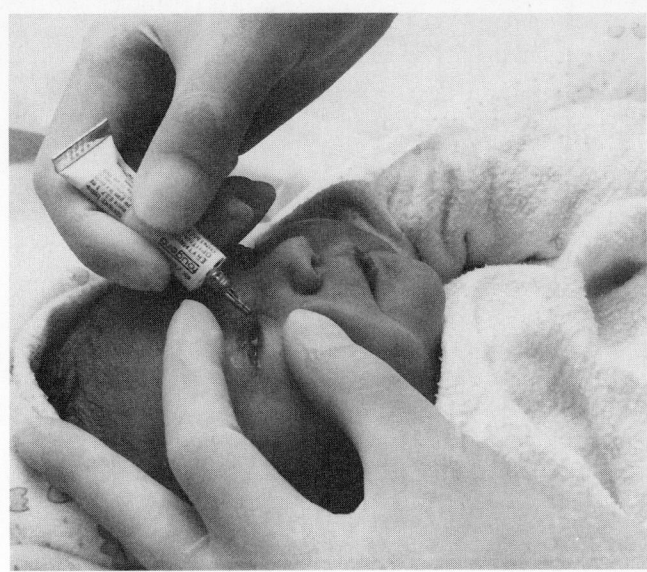

FIGURE 29-4 Ophthalmic ointment. Retract lower eyelid outward to instill a ¼ inch strand of ointment from a single-dose ampule along the lower conjunctival surface.

breastfeed their newborns may seek to put their baby to breast while in the birthing area. This practice should be encouraged because successful, long-term breastfeeding during infancy appears to be related to beginning breastfeedings in the first few hours of life. Bottlefed newborns usually begin the first feedings by 5 hours of age, during

---

PROCEDURE 29-2
INSTILLATION OF OPHTHALMIC ILOTYCIN OINTMENT

Nursing Action	Rationale
Objective: Provide newborn prophylactic eye care	
Wash hands and put on gloves prior to instillation.	Prevents introduction of bacteria.
Clean infant's eyes of any drainage.	Removal of exudate allows instillation and absorption of ointment.
Retract lower eyelid outward with forefinger to allow instillation of 1/4 inch long strand of ointment along lower conjunctival surface, starting at inner canthus.	Maximizes absorption of ointment.
Repeat process on other eye.	
Instill only a single dose per eye.	Prophylaxis requires only a single dose.
Excess ointment may be wiped away after 1 minute (American Academy of Pediatrics 1992).	
Do not irrigate eyes.	Irrigation will remove ointment.
Assess for sensitivity reaction such as edema, inflammation, drainage.	May interfere with ability to focus and the bonding process.
Inform parents about rationale for eye prophylaxis, that instillation can be done in the birthing area or admission nursery, it may interfere with newborn's ability to focus on parents' faces, and that there may be temporary side effects.	Preventive treatment of gonorrhea and chlamydia infection, which can cause blindness. Required by law. Side effects usually disappear in 24 to 48 hours.
Objective: Record completion of procedure	
Document the instillation of the prophylaxis eye medication.	Provides a permanent record to meet the legal requirements.

TABLE 29-2	Signs of Neonatal Distress

Increased rate (more than 60/minute) or difficult respirations

Sternal retractions

Nasal flaring

Grunting

Excessive mucus

Facial grimacing

Cyanosis (central: skin, lips, tongue)

Abdominal distention or mass

Vomiting of bile-stained material

Absence of meconium elimination within 24 hours of birth

Absence of urine elimination within 24 hours of birth

Jaundice of the skin within 24 hours of birth or due to hemolytic process

Temperature instability (hypothermia or hyperthermia)

Jitteriness or glucose less than 40 mg%

SOURCE: Adapted from Tappero EP, Honeyfield ME: *Physical Assessment of the Newborn.* Petaluma, CA: NICU Ink, 1993.

the second period of reactivity, when they awaken and appear hungry.

Signs indicating newborn readiness for the first feeding are active bowel sounds, absence of abdominal distention, and a lusty cry that quiets with rooting and sucking behaviors when a stimulus is placed near the lips.

Facilitation of Parent-Newborn Attachment

Eye-to-eye contact between the parents and their newborn is extremely important during the early hours after birth, when the newborn is in the first period of reactivity. The newborn is alert during this time, the eyes are wide open, and often direct eye contact is made with human faces within optimal range for visual acuity (7 to 8 in). It is theorized that this eye contact is an important foundation in establishing attachment in human relationships (Klaus & Klaus 1985). Consequently, the prophylactic eye medication is often delayed up to 1 hour to provide an opportunity for this period of eye contact between parents and their newborn, thus facilitating the attachment process (American Academy of Pediatrics 1992).

NURSING DIAGNOSIS FOR DAILY NEWBORN CARE

Possible nursing diagnoses during daily care of the newborn include the following:

- Altered peripheral tissue perfusion related to transition to extrauterine environment
- Risk for ineffective breathing pattern related to periodic breathing

- Altered nutrition: Less than body requirements related to limited nutritional/fluid intake and increased caloric expenditure
- Altered urinary elimination related to meatal edema secondary to circumcision
- Altered bowel elimination related to immature gastrointestinal system or delayed passage of meconium
- Risk for infection related to umbilical cord healing, circumcision site, or immature immune system

Possible nursing diagnoses of the newborn's family during the first few days of the newborn's life include the following:

- Knowledge deficit related to lack of information about male circumcision or pros and cons of breast-feeding and bottle-feeding
- Risk for altered parenting related to lack of experience with infant care or transition to parental role
- Altered family processes related to integration of newborn into family unit or demands of newborn feeding schedule

NURSING PLAN AND IMPLEMENTATION OF DAILY NEWBORN CARE

Maintenance of Cardiopulmonary Function

Vital signs are taken every 6 to 8 hours or more, depending on the newborn's status. The newborn should be placed in a propped, side-lying position when left unattended to prevent aspiration and facilitate drainage of mucus (Infant Sleep Positioning and SIDS Position Statement 1992). A bulb syringe is kept within easy reach should the baby need oral-nasal suctioning. If the newborn has respiratory difficulty, the airway is cleared. Vigorous fingertip stroking of the baby's spine will frequently stimulate respiratory activity. A cardiorespiratory monitor can be used on newborns who are not being observed at all times and are at risk for decreased respiratory or cardiac function. Indicators of risk are pallor, cyanosis, ruddy color, apnea, or other signs of instability, and changes in skin color may indicate the need for closer assessment of temperature, cardiopulmonary status, hematocrit, and bilirubin levels.

Maintenance of Neutral Thermal Environment

Every effort is made to maintain the newborn's temperature within the normal range. The nurse must make certain the newborn is undressed and exposed to the air as little as possible. A stockinette or knit head covering should be used for the small newborn who has less subcutaneous fat to act as insulation in maintaining body heat. The ambient temperature of the room where the newborn is kept should be monitored routinely and kept at approximately 32.5–33.9 C (90.5–93.1 F) for large babies and 35.4 ± 0.5 C for smaller babies (Merenstein & Gardner 1992). Parents may be advised to dress the newborn in one more layer of clothing than is necessary for an adult to maintain thermal comfort.

A newborn whose temperature falls below optimal levels will use calories to maintain body heat rather than for growth. Chilling also decreases the affinity of serum albumin for bilirubin, thereby increasing the likelihood of newborn jaundice. It also increases oxygen use and may cause respiratory distress.

A newborn who is overheated will increase activity and respiratory rate in an attempt to cool the body. Both measures deplete caloric reserves. In addition, the increased respiratory rate leads to increased insensible fluid loss.

Promotion of Adequate Hydration and Nutrition

Newborn nutrition is addressed in depth in Chapter 30. The nurse records the newborn's caloric and fluid intakes. Adequate hydration is enhanced by maintaining a neutral thermal environment and by offering early and frequent feedings. Early feedings promote gastric emptying and increase peristalsis, thereby decreasing the degree of hyperbilirubinemia by decreasing the amount of time fecal material is in contact with the enzyme beta-glucuronidase in the small intestine. This enzyme acts to free the bilirubin from the stool, allowing bilirubin to be reabsorbed into the vascular system. Voiding and stooling patterns are recorded. If 24 hours have passed and the first voiding and passage of stool has not occurred, the nurse continues the normal observation routine while assessing for abdominal distention, status of bowel sounds, hydration, fluid intake, and temperature stability.

The newborn should be weighed at the same time each day for accurate comparisons. A weight loss of up to 10% for term newborns is considered within normal limits during the first week of life. This is the result of limited intake, loss of excess extracellular fluid, and passage of meconium. Parents should be told about the expected weight loss, the reason for it, and the expectations for regaining the birth weight. Birth weight should be regained by 2 weeks if feedings are adequate.

Excessive handling of the newborn can cause an increase in the newborn's metabolic rate and caloric use. The nurse should be alert to the baby's subtle cues of fatigue. These include turning the head away from eye contact, decrease in muscle tension and activity in the extremities and neck, and loss of eye contact, which may be manifested by fluttering or closing the eyelids. The nurse quickly ceases stimulation when signs of fatigue appear. The nurse's care should demonstrate to the parents the need for awareness of newborn cues and the use of periods of alertness in the baby for contact and stimulation. The nurse is also responsible for assessing the woman's comfort and latching-on techniques in breastfeeding or bottle-feeding.

Prevention of Complications and Promotion of Safety

Newborns are at continued risk for the complications of hemorrhage, late-onset cardiac symptoms, and infection. Pallor may be an early sign of hemorrhage and must be reported to the physician. The newborn is placed on a cardiorespiratory monitor to permit continuous assessment if severe bleeding occurs. Several newborn conditions put the newborn at risk for bleeding. This is especially true following a circumcision procedure (discussed later in this chapter.)

The circumcision is assessed for signs of hemorrhage and infection. The first voiding after a circumcision is also a significant assessment in order to evaluate for possible urinary obstruction due to trauma and edema. Vaseline gauze is applied to the circumcision site to prevent bleeding and allow the gauze to be removed and replaced if it gets soiled.

The umbilical cord is assessed for signs of bleeding or infection, such as oozing and foul smell. Triple dye is usually applied to the normal newborn's cord. Then the nurse is responsible for giving cord care with alcohol each time the diaper is changed.

Cyanosis that is not relieved by oxygen administration requires emergency intervention, may indicate a congenital cardiac condition or shock, and requires ongoing assessment.

Infection in the nursery is best prevented by requiring that all personnel having direct contact with newborns scrub for 2–3 minutes from fingertips to and including elbows at the beginning of each shift. The hands must be washed with soap and rubbed vigorously for 15 seconds (Neonatal Skin Care 1992) before and after contact with every newborn or after touching any soiled surface such as the floor or one's hair or face. Parents are often instructed to use an antiseptic hand cleaner before touching the baby. Anyone with an infection should refrain from working with newborns until the infection has cleared. Some agencies ask family members to wear a gown (preferably disposable) over their street clothes. Parents need to be taught that everyone handling the baby should *always* wash their hands before doing so, even after the baby is home.

Safety of the newborn is provided through a variety of nursing interventions and institutional security measures. It is essential to verify the identity of the newborn by seeing and comparing the numbers and names on the identification bracelets of mother and newborn before giving a baby to a parent and to follow institutional policies for identification of all nursery personnel. Other safety issues are specifically covered later in the sections on positioning and handling, bathing, nail care, circumcision, and safety considerations for discharge.

Critical Thinking Question

What factors should you consider when providing parents with information about their baby's care needs?

Enhancement of Parent-Newborn Attachment and Parental Knowledge of Newborn Care

Parent-newborn attachment is promoted by encouraging all family members to be involved with the new member of the family. Some specific interventions are examined in Chapters 23 and 34; for more detailed discussion see Chapter 35.

To meet parent needs for information, the nurse who is responsible for the daily care of the mother and newborn should assume the primary responsibility for education. Nearly every contact with the parents presents an opportunity for sharing information that can facilitate their sense of competence in newborn care. The nurse also needs to recognize and respect the fact that there are many good ways to provide safe care. The parents' methods of giving care should be reinforced rather than contradicted, unless their care methods are harmful to the newborn. The nurse also needs to be sensitive to the cultural beliefs and values of the family (Table 29–3).

The information that follows is provided to increase the nurse's knowledge of newborn care and can also be used to meet parents' needs for information. Parents may be familiar with handling and caring for infants, or this may be their first time to interact with a newborn. If they are new parents, the sensitive nurse gently teaches them by example and provides instructions geared to their needs and previous knowledge about the various aspects of newborn care.

The length of stay in the birthing unit for mother and baby after birth is often 24 hours or less. One proposal to deal with early discharge is for labor and delivery nurses to start newborn care by assessing vital signs and administering vitamin K and eye prophylaxis. Then admission nursery care is viewed as a continuation of newborn care, and time spent during this period is cut in half. This approach to newborn care also provides for earlier identification of those newborns in need of more aggressive intervention (McGregor 1994). The challenge for the nurse is to use every opportunity to teach, guide, and support individual parents, fostering their own capabilities and confidence in caring for their newborn.

TABLE 29-3	Examples of Some Cultural Beliefs and Practices Regarding Baby Care

Umbilical Cord

People of Hispanic or Filipino cultural background may use an abdominal binder or bellyband to protect against dirt, injury, and umbilical hernia. They may also apply oils to the stump of the cord or tape metal to the umbilicus to ward off evil spirits.

People of northern European ancestry may expect a sterile cutting of the cord at birth. They may allow the stump to air dry and discard the cord once it falls off.

Mother-Infant Contact

People of Asian ancestry may pick up the baby as soon as it cries, or they may carry the baby at all times.

Some Native Americans, notably the Navajos, may use cradle boards.

Feeding

Some people of Asian heritage may breastfeed their babies for the first 1 to 2 years of life.

People of Iranian heritage may breastfeed female babies longer than males.

Some people of African ancestry may wean their babies after they begin to walk.

Circumcision

People of Muslim and Jewish ancestry practice circumcision as a religious ritual (Hutchinson & Baqi-Aziz 1994).

Many natives of Africa and Australia practice circumcision as a puberty rite.

Most Native Americans and people of Asian and Hispanic cultures rarely perform circumcision.

Only 15% of the world's male population is circumcised.

Health/Illness

Some people from Hispanic cultural backgrounds may believe that touching the face or head of an infant when admiring it will ward off the "evil eye." They may also neglect to cut the baby's nails to avoid nearsightedness and instead put mittens on the baby's hands to prevent scratching. They also may believe that fat babies are healthy.

Some people of Asian heritage may not allow anyone to touch the baby's head without asking permission.

Some Orthodox Jews believe that saying the baby's name before the formal naming ceremony will harm the baby.

Some people of Vietnamese ancestry believe that cutting a baby's hair or nails will cause illness.

NOTE: The above are meant only as examples of some of the behaviors that may be found within certain cultures. Not all members of a culture will practice the behaviors described.

SOURCE: Adapted from Andrews NM: Transcultural perspectives in the nursing care of children and adolescents. In: *Transcultural Concepts in Nursing Care.* Boyle JS, Andrews NM (editors). Philadelphia: Lippincott, 1989; Riordan J, Auerbach KG: *Breastfeeding and Human Lactation.* Boston: Jones & Bartlett, 1993.

The nurse observes how parents interact with their infant during feeding and care-giving activities. Rooming-in, even for a short time, offers opportunities for the nurse to provide information and evaluate whether the parents are comfortable with changing diapers and wrapping, handling, and feeding their newborn. Do both parents get involved in the infant's care? Is the mother depending on someone else to help her at home? Does the mother give excuses for not wanting to be involved in her baby's care? ("I am too tired," "My stitches hurt," or "I will learn later.") All these considerations need to be taken into account when evaluating the educational needs of the parents.

Several methods may be used to teach parents about newborn care. Daily child care classes are a nonthreaten-

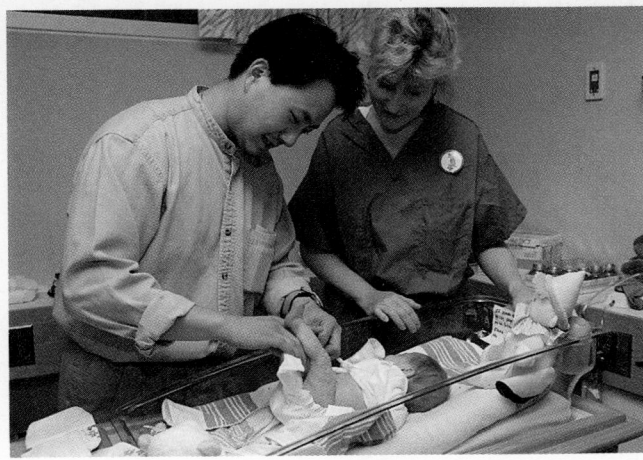

FIGURE 29-5 Individualizing parent education. Father returns demonstration of diapering his son.

Early birthing center discharge influences the amount and type of postpartum education that new mothers receive from health care providers. Little research has been reported regarding what knowledge the mother actually acquires during the early postpartum period. Judith Maloni formulated a study to identify (1) the specific knowledge acquired about the infant in the first 14 days postpartum, (2) daily patterns of acquisition, and (3) sources of knowledge for the new mother. Dr Maloni specifically wanted to examine caretaking knowledge and personal knowledge or information about newborn needs and characteristics.

The author used a random number table to select a convenience sample from healthy primiparas who had delivered within the previous 24 hours. The sample of 33 mothers consisted of primarily Caucasian, middle- to upper-middle-class women with a mean of 15.4 years of education. The mothers maintained a daily diary in which they responded to open-ended questions or statements about learning to care for their baby, learning about their baby as a person, and sources of information.

Data analysis included both category and subcategory development through identifying and grouping codes. The caretaking category included such items as cord and genital care, feeding, and comfort. The personal knowledge category contained physical characteristics, activity, and psychologic needs. Every subcategory was then quantified to produce a daily knowledge score for each. Results showed specific patterns of caretaking skill development. For example, the typical mother learned the most about feeding her infant in the first 6 days. In terms of personal knowledge acquisition, mothers learned more about their infant's activity patterns on the 2nd through the 13th days. The mothers learned more about their infants as people than about how to care for them during the 2-week period ($t[32] = -3.83$, $p < .001$). Mothers perceived that their most important source of information was themselves as they interacted with the newborn. Other, less commonly noted sources included nurses, physicians, and printed materials.

Clinical Application of Study

In the qualitative section of the study it is not clear whether new categories could have emerged because preestablished coding rules were used. As the author notes, parent education classes should teach the new mother how to identify her infant's behavioral cues, inform the parents about other sources of information, and continue to focus on how to care for the newborn.

SOURCE: Maloni J: The content and sources of maternal knowledge about the infant. *Maternal-Child Nursing Journal* 1994; *22*(4):111.

ing way to convey general information. Individual instruction is helpful to answer specific questions or to clarify an item that may have been confusing in class (Figure 29–5). See Teaching Guide: What To Tell Parents About Daily Infant Care on page 872. Including mother-baby couplet care and home care instruction on the night shift assists with education needs for early discharge parents.

Discharge teaching is necessary to verify the parents' knowledge when they leave the birthing unit. Follow-up calls or visits after discharge lend added support by providing another opportunity for parents to have their questions answered.

> With the new life come new rhythms. Or perhaps I should say no rhythms. The day is divided into phone calls, meals eaten on the run, visitors who've come to see the baby, trips from hospital to home to walk the dog.
>
> The new life brings new thoughts, new perceptions of the world. Why don't men take paternity leave? Why is time off, if any, basically reserved for women? Why don't we take a month off. In those first few chaotic days, filled with ecstasy and fear, the family needs to be together. Being together in times of joy and sadness is what a family is. A month's distance from the office grind, from the bottom line could not help but create a healthier world.
> ~DENNIS DONZIGER, *DADDY*~

Positioning and Handling

Methods of positioning and handling the newborn are demonstrated to parents as needed. As the family provides care, the nurse can enhance parental confidence by giving them positive feedback. If the family encounters problems, the nurse can express confidence in their abilities to master the new skill or information, suggest alternatives, and serve as a role model.

How to pick up a newborn is one of the first concerns of anyone who has not had experience. The newborn is easily picked up by sliding one hand under the neck and shoulders and the other hand under the buttocks or between the legs, then gently lifting the newborn. This

WHAT TO TELL PARENTS ABOUT DAILY INFANT CARE

Assessment   The nurse determines parents' prior knowledge and experience with newborns and any concerns they may have about caring for their baby.

Nursing Diagnosis   The key nursing diagnoses would be: Knowledge deficit related to lack of information about ongoing newborn daily care needs and Altered parenting related to integration of new family member.

Nursing Plan and Implementation   The teaching plan will include information about sponge and tub baths, umbilical cord care, care of circumcised and uncircumcised infant, feeding techniques, positioning, elimination patterns, use of bulb syringe, signs and symptoms of illness, expected sleep patterns, comfort measures, and attachment behaviors.

Demonstration of bath, cord care, use of bulb syringe, thermometer, and comfort measures

Parent Goals   At the completion of the class the parents will be able to:

1. Demonstrate safe techniques of caring for their newborn, especially in use of bulb syringe, thermometer, cord cleaning, and comforting measures.

2. List signs and symptoms of illness.

3. Describe infant's sleep patterns and attachment behaviors.

4. Demonstrate an emerging comfort level and confidence in their ability to care for their infant.

Teaching Plan

Content   Demonstrate sponge and tub bathing techniques, emphasizing safety and timing of cord separation. Demonstrate cord care to be carried out at home—Teaching Guide: What To Tell Families About Home Cord Care for specific techniques.

Discuss care required for circumcised and uncircumcised infants.

Discuss the signs of illness (see Table 29–1) and demonstrate use of thermometer and bulb syringe.

Discuss normal newborn eating, sleep, and elimination patterns and behavioral characteristics.

Demonstrate comfort measures for newborns.

Evaluation   Parents are able to describe general newborn care. Parents demonstrate use of bulb syringe, taking temperature, umbilical cord care, and care of circumcision (if appropriate) to primary nurse prior to discharge from birthing center.

Teaching Method   Discussion and demonstration. Stress basic useful information that new parents need. Avoid patronizing tone. Provide opportunities for parents to practice.

Demonstration, discussion

Discussion, handouts, pamphlets and posters are helpful, as are videos.

Discussion, demonstration, and return demonstration.

Provide positive feedback to build confidence.

---

technique provides security and support for the head (which the baby is unable to support until 3 or 4 months of age).

After the baby is out of the crib, one of the following three holds may be used (Figure 29–6). The *cradle hold* is frequently used during feeding. It provides a sense of warmth and closeness, permits eye contact, frees one of the nurse's or parent's hands, and provides security because the cradling protects the newborn's body. Extra security is provided by gripping the thigh with the hand while the arm supports the newborn's body. The *upright position* provides security and a sense of closeness and is a good position for burping. One hand should support the neck and shoulders while the other hand holds the buttocks or is placed between the newborn's legs. The *football hold* frees one of the care giver's hands and permits eye contact. This hold is ideal for shampooing, carrying, or breastfeeding. It frees the care giver to talk on the telephone or answer the door at home or do the myriad tasks that await attention.

TEACHING MOMENT

You'll find that left-handed people tend to hold the baby over their right shoulder, and right-handed people do the opposite. This keeps the dominant hand free. However, most health personnel wear their name tags on the left side. To avoid scratching the baby's face, wear your name tag on the same side as your dominant hand.

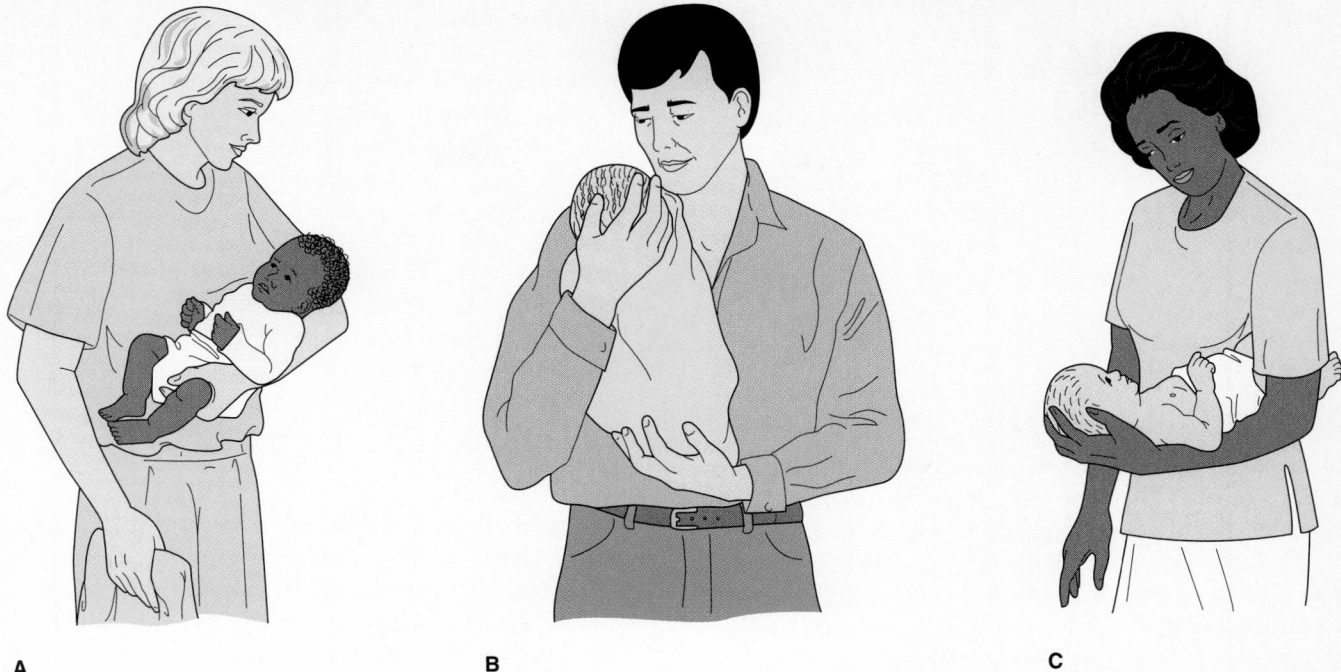

FIGURE 29-6   Various positions for holding an infant. *A* Cradle hold. *B* Upright position. *C* Football hold.

The newborn infant is most frequently positioned on the side with a rolled blanket or cloth diaper behind the back for support to prevent rolling back (Figure 29–7). A side-lying position aids drainage of mucus and allows air to circulate around the cord. It is also more comfortable for the newly circumcised male. After feeding, the newborn is placed on the right side to aid digestion and to prevent aspiration of regurgitated food; this position makes it easier to expel air bubbles from the stomach.

In the Japanese culture, babies are traditionally laid on their backs so they won't suffocate. A firm, flat mattress without pillows should be provided for the newborn in this case. Recent studies have shown an increased incidence of Sudden Infant Death Syndrome (SIDS) in infants who sleep on their stomachs. There is no evidence that sleeping on the back or side is harmful to healthy infants. There are still certain infants who may need to be placed on their stomachs, including:

*   Premature infants with respiratory distress (severe breathing problems)
*   Infants with symptoms of gastroesophageal reflux (severe spitting up)
*   Infants with certain upper airway abnormalities

There may be other valid reasons for infants to be placed on their stomachs for sleep. Parents should discuss their individual circumstances with their pediatrician. Although the risk of SIDS for infants who sleep on their stomachs may be higher than for those who sleep on their sides or backs, the actual risk of SIDS when placing infants on their stomachs is still extremely low (Infant Sleep Position and SIDS Position Statement 1992).

The baby's position should be changed periodically during the early months of life because neonatal skull bones are soft, and permanently flattened areas may develop if the newborn consistently lies in one position.

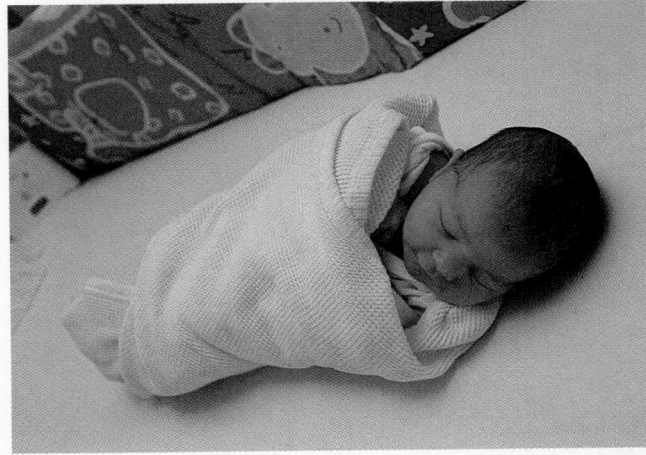

FIGURE 29-7   The most common sleeping position of the newborn is on the side. A rolled blanket may be placed behind the back to provide additional support.

CRITICAL THINKING IN PRACTICE

A mother calls you to her room. She sounds frightened and says her baby can't breathe. You find the mother cradling her infant in her arms. The infant is mildly cyanotic, waving her arms, and has mucus coming from her nose and mouth. What would you do?

Answers can be found in Appendix I.

Nasal and Oral Suctioning

Most babies are obligatory nose breathers for the first months of life. They generally maintain air passage patency by coughing or sneezing. During the first few days of life, however, the newborn has increased mucus, and gentle suctioning with a bulb syringe may be indicated. The nurse can demonstrate the use of the bulb syringe in the nose and mouth and have the parents do a return demonstration. The parents should repeat this demonstration before discharge so they will feel more confident and comfortable with the procedure. Care should be taken to apply only gentle suction so nasal bleeding does not occur.

To suction the newborn, the bulb syringe is compressed. Then the tip is placed in the nostril and the bulb is permitted to reexpand slowly as the nurse or parent releases the compression on the bulb (Figure 29–8). The bulb syringe is removed from the nostril, and drainage is then compressed out of the bulb onto a tissue. The bulb syringe may also be used in the mouth if the newborn is spitting up and unable to handle the excess secretions. The bulb is compressed; the tip of the bulb syringe is placed about 1 in to one side of the newborn's mouth; and

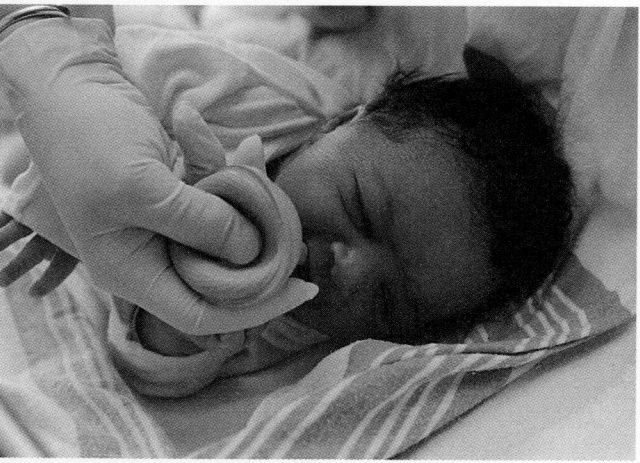

FIGURE 29-8   Nasal and oral suctioning. The bulb is compressed; then the tip is placed in either the mouth or nose, and the bulb is released.

compression is released. This draws up the excess secretions. The procedure is repeated on the other side of the mouth. The roof of the mouth and back of the throat are avoided because suction in this area might stimulate the gag reflex. The bulb syringe should be washed in warm, soapy water and rinsed in warm water daily and as needed after use. A bulb syringe should always be kept near the newborn. New parents and nurses who are inexperienced with babies may fear that the baby will choke and may be relieved if they know how to take action if such an event occurs. They should be advised to turn the newborn's head to the side or down as soon as there is any indication of gagging or vomiting and to use the bulb syringe as needed.

Bathing

An actual bath demonstration is the best way for the nurse to provide information to parents. Because excess bathing and use of soap will dry out the baby's sensitive skin, bathing should be done every other day or twice a week. Sponge baths are recommended for the first 2 weeks or until the umbilical cord completely falls off and has healed. Some agencies use a tub bath for the bath demonstration and apply alcohol to the cord after the bath to facilitate drying.

Supplies can be kept in a plastic bag or some type of container to avoid hunting for them each time. At home the family may want to use a small plastic tub, a clean kitchen or bathroom sink, or a large bowl as the baby's tub. Expensive baby tubs are not necessary, but some parents may prefer to purchase them (Table 29–4).

Before starting, if no one else is at home, the parent may want to take the phone off the hook and put a sign on the door to prevent being disturbed. Having someone home during the first few baths will be helpful because that person can get forgotten items, attend to interruptions, and provide moral support. The room should be warm and free of drafts.

Sponge Bath   After the supplies are gathered, the tub (or any of the containers mentioned) is filled with water that is warm to the touch. The water temperature is tested with an elbow or forearm. Families may also choose to purchase a thermometer to help them determine when the bath water is at approximately 37.8 C (100 F) and safe to use. Soap should not be added to the water. The newborn should be wrapped in a blanket, with a T-shirt and diaper on to keep him or her warm and secure.

To start the bath, the adult wraps a washcloth once around the index finger. The baby's eyes are gently wiped from inner to outer corner. This direction prevents the potential for clogging the tear duct at the inner corner, where the eye naturally drains. A different portion of the washcloth is used for each eye to prevent cross-contamination. Cotton balls can also be used for this purpose, using a new one for each eye. Some swelling and drainage

TABLE 29-4	Bath Supplies	
Washcloths (2)	Petroleum jelly or A and D ointment
Towels (2)	Rubbing alcohol
Blankets (2)	Cotton balls
Unperfumed mild soap (eg, Castile, Neutrogena)	Diapers
Shampoo	Clean clothes

may be common the first few days after birth, usually due to the eye prophylaxis used.

The ears are washed next by wrapping the washcloth once around an index finger and gently cleaning the external ear and behind the ear. Cotton swabs are never used in the ear canal because it is possible to put the swab too far into the ear and damage the eardrum. In addition the swab may pack any discharge farther down into the ear canal.

The remainder of the baby's face is then wiped with the soap-free washcloth. Many babies start to cry at this point. The face should be washed every day and the mouth and chin wiped off after each feeding.

The neck is washed carefully but thoroughly with the washcloth. Soap may now be used. Formula or breast milk and lint collect in the skin folds of the neck, so it may be helpful to sit the baby up, supporting the neck and shoulders with one hand while washing the neck with the other hand.

The blanket is now unwrapped and the T-shirt is removed. The chest, back, and arms are wet with the washcloth. The care giver may then lather his or her hands with soap and wash the baby's chest, back, and arms. Wetting the cord is avoided, if possible, because it delays drying. Soap is rinsed off with the wet washcloth, and the upper part of the body is dried with a towel or blanket. The newborn's upper body is then wrapped with a dry clean blanket to prevent a chill.

Next the newborn's legs are unwrapped, wet with the washcloth, lathered, rinsed, and well dried. If the infant has dry skin, a *small* amount of unscented lotion or ointment (petroleum jelly or A and D ointment) may be used. Ointments are thought to be better than lotions for dry, cracked feet and hands. Baby oil is not recommended because it clogs skin pores. Powders are not currently recommended. Some believe they aggravate dry skin, and others avoid powders because of the possible danger of inhalation. Parents should be warned that baby powder can cause serious respiratory problems if inhaled. If parents want to use powder, advise them to select one that is talc free. The powder should be shaken into the hand and then placed on the newborn rather than shaking the powder directly over the baby.

The genital area is cleaned daily with soap and water and with water after each wet or dirty diaper. Females are washed from the *front* of the genital area toward the rectum to avoid fecal contamination of the urethra and thus to the bladder. Newborn females often have a thick, white mucous discharge or a slight bloody discharge from their vagina. This discharge is normal for the first 1 to 2 weeks and should be wiped off gently with a damp cloth at diaper changes.

Parents of uncircumcised newborn males should clean the small exposed area of the glans daily. Even minimal retraction of the foreskin is not advised. For in-depth discussion of care of uncircumcised boys, see Circumcision: Nurses Role later in this chapter.

Newborn males who have been circumcised also need daily gentle cleaning. A very wet washcloth is rubbed over a bar of soap. The washcloth is squeezed above the baby's penis, letting the soapy water run over the circumcision site. The area is rinsed off with plain warm water and lightly patted dry. A small amount of petroleum jelly, A and D ointment, or bactericidal ointment may be put on the circumcised area, but excessive amounts may block the meatus and should be avoided. If a Plastibell is in place, no ointment should be put on the penis. The Plastibell usually falls off within 5 to 8 days. If it doesn't, the family needs to call the health care provider.

It is important to cleanse the diaper area with each diaper change in order to prevent diaper rash. Although this cleansing is done on a routine basis, a diaper rash may occasionally occur.

Baby powder (or cornstarch) is not recommended for diaper rash. Baby powder may cake with urine and irritate the perineal area. Cornstarch may promote fungal infection. Ointments that provide a barrier, such as zinc oxide, A and D ointment, or petroleum jelly, are more effective for diaper rash. It is important to cleanse the diaper area before applying these products. If the ointment does not help the rash, parents using disposable diapers should try another brand of diaper. If cloth diapers are used, using a different detergent or fabric softener and/or hanging them in the sun to dry may alleviate the problem. If the rash persists, parents should discuss the problem with a

CRITICAL THINKING IN PRACTICE

You are caring for a new mother who had her first child, a daughter, about 4 hours ago. She appears visibly upset when changing her infant's diaper and says she thinks something is wrong because her daughter has tissue protruding from her vagina and some blood in her diaper. What would you do?

Answers can be found in Appendix I.

nurse practitioner or physician because it may be due to a yeast or fungal infection.

The umbilical cord should be kept clean and dry. The close proximity of the umbilical vessels makes the cord a common portal for infection. Various preparations such as triple dye, alcohol, hexachlorophene, Betadine, and Bacitracin are used for newborn cord care in nurseries to promote drying and provide a bactericidal effect. Triple dye may be used and seems to be a highly effective

antistaphylococcal agent (Coen & Koeffler 1987). At discharge most parents are advised to clean the area around the cord with a cotton ball and alcohol two to three times a day until the cord is completely gone and the stump is healed. The cord stump generally falls off in 7 to 14 days. The diaper should be folded down to allow air to circulate around the cord. The care provider should be consulted if redness appears around the umbilicus, bright red bleeding or puslike drainage occurs, if it has a foul odor,

---

TEACHING GUIDE

WHAT TO TELL FAMILIES ABOUT HOME CORD CARE

Assessment   The nurse focuses on the family's previous experience with newborns and their understanding of what the umbilical cord is and what naturally happens during the first few weeks after birth.

Nursing Diagnosis   The essential nursing diagnoses would probably be: Knowledge deficit related to lack of information about home care of the umbilical cord and Risk for infection related to contamination of umbilical cord.

Nursing Plan and Implementation   The teaching plan will include information about the need for daily cleansing, expected changes in the

umbilical cord, and demonstration of actual procedure for care of the umbilical cord.

Parent Goals   At the completion of the teaching session the parents will be able to:

1. State the normal changes in the umbilical cord.
2. List the signs of infection of the cord.
3. Demonstrate proper cord care.

Teaching Plan

Content   Clean the cord and skin around base of cord with a cotton ball or cotton-tipped swab using a cotton ball wet with 70% isopropyl alcohol. Lift the cord stump and wipe around the cord. Start at the top and wipe around halfway; then rotate cotton ball and start at the top again and wipe around the other half of the cord. Swabbing around the base of the cord cleans away drainage, and bacteria grows on dried drainage. Cord care should be done at least two to three times a day, or it could be done with each diaper change. The newborn may cry when the cold alcohol touches the abdomen; however, cord care is not painful because there are no nerve ends in the cord. No tub baths are given until the cord falls off in 7–14 days.
Fold diapers below umbilical cord to air-dry the cord. Contact with wet or soiled diapers slows the drying process and increases the possibility of infection.
Check cord each day for any odor, oozing of yellow puslike material, or reddened areas around the cord. Area around cord may also be tender. Report to health care provider any signs of infection.
Normal changes in cord: Cord should look dark and dry up before falling off. A little drop of blood may appear on the diaper as the cord is about to fall off. Never pull the cord or attempt to loosen it.

Teaching Method   Discussion: Use of poster showing cleaning techniques, position of diapers, and colored pictures of signs of infection. Demonstration of cord cleaning.

Evaluation   The nurse presented the information and demonstrated the proper procedure for cord care. Parents were able to identify the signs of infection and normal changes seen in the cord prior to its falling off and carried out proper cord care procedure before their newborn's discharge.

or the area remains unhealed 2 to 3 days after the cord stump has sloughed off. See Teaching Guide: What To Tell Families About Home Cord Care.

The last step in bathing is washing the infant's hair (some suggest doing this step first). The newborn is swaddled in a dry blanket, leaving only the head exposed, and held in the football hold with the head tilted slightly downward to prevent water running in the eyes. Water should be brought to the head by a cupped hand. The hair is moistened and lathered with a small amount of shampoo. A *very* soft brush may be used to massage the shampoo over the entire head. The brush may be used over the soft spots. Frequently, a disposable soapless scrub brush is used because the bristles are soft and pliable. The hair is then rinsed and toweled dry. To assist in preventing cradle cap, the infant's hair should be brushed every day and the hair washed during baths. Oils or lotions are not used on the newborn's head unless there is evidence of cradle cap. Moistening the scaly area with lotion or mineral oil half an hour or more before shampooing softens the crusts or scales and facilitates their removal with a soft brush during the shampoo.

Tub Bath   The baby may be put in a tub after the cord has fallen off and the circumcision site is healed (approximately 2 weeks) (Figure 29–9). Newborns usually enjoy a tub bath more than a sponge bath, although some cry during either type.

Only 3 or 4 inches of water are needed in the tub. To prevent slipping, a washcloth is placed in the bottom of the tub or sink, or the newborn can be brought into a tub with the parent.

The face is washed in the same manner as for a sponge bath. The parent then places the newborn in the tub, using the cradle hold and grasping the distal thigh. The neck is supported by the parent's elbow in the cradle position. An alternative hold is to support the newborn's head and neck with the forearm while grasping the distal shoulder and arm.

Because wet newborns are slippery, some parents have found that pulling a cotton sock (with holes cut out for the fingers) over the arm will prevent slipping.

The newborn's body may be washed with a soapy washcloth or hand. To wash the back, the adult places his or her noncradling hand on the newborn's chest with the thumb under the newborn's arm closest to the parent. Gently tipping the baby forward onto the supporting hand frees the cradling arm to wash the back of the baby. After the bath the baby is lifted out of the tub in the cradle position, dried well, and wrapped in a dry blanket. The hair can then be washed in the same way as for a sponge bath.

Nail Care

The nails of the newborn are seldom cut in the birthing unit. During the first days of life, the nails may adhere to the skin of the fingers, and cutting is contraindicated. Within a week the nails separate from the skin and fre-

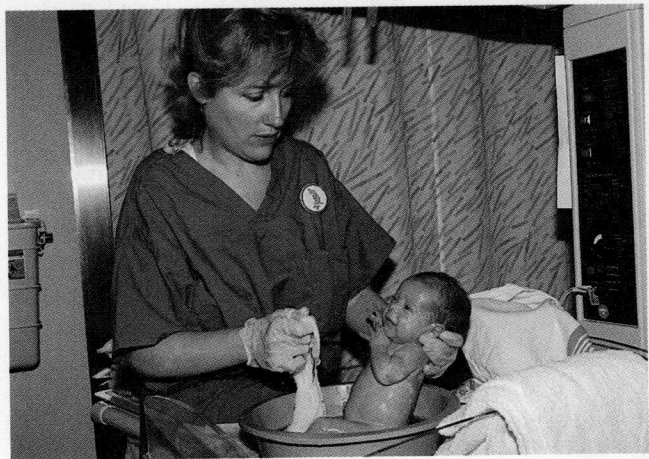

FIGURE 29-9   When bathing an infant in a tub, it is important to support the head and to hold onto a limb gently but firmly. Wet babies are very slippery.

quently break off. If the nails are long or if infants are scratching themselves, the nails may be trimmed. This is most easily done while babies sleep. Nails should be cut straight across using adult cuticle scissors or blunt-ended infant cuticle scissors.

Wrapping the Newborn

Wrapping (swaddling) helps the newborn maintain body temperature, provides a feeling of closeness and security, and may be effective in quieting a crying baby. When wrapping, a blanket is placed on the crib (or secure surface) in the shape of a diamond. The top corner of the blanket is folded down slightly, and the baby's body is placed with the head at the upper edge of the blanket. The right corner of the blanket is wrapped around the infant and tucked under the left side (not too tightly—newborns need a little room to move). The bottom corner is then pulled up to the chest, and the left corner is wrapped around the baby's right side (Figure 29–10).

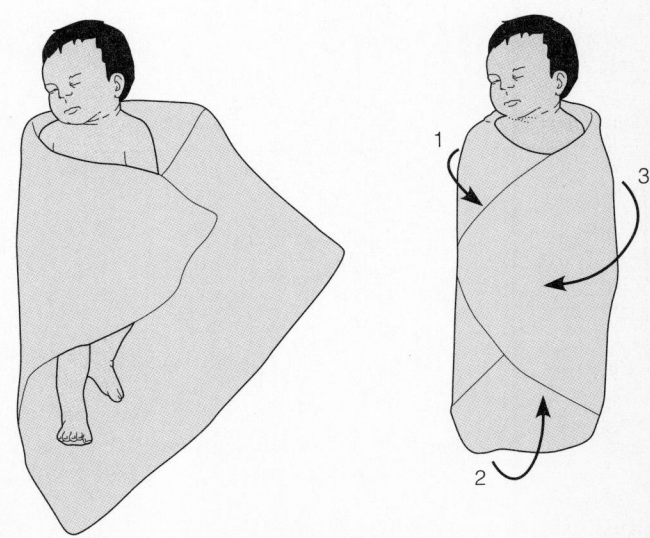

FIGURE 29-10   Steps used for wrapping a baby.

This wrapping technique can be shared with a new mother so she will feel more skilled in handling her baby.

Dressing the Newborn

Newborns need to wear a T-shirt, diaper (diaper cover or plastic pants if using cloth diapers), and a sleeper. On a fairly cool day they should also be wrapped in a light blanket while being fed. The newborn infant may be covered with a blanket in air-conditioned buildings. The blanket should be unwrapped or removed when inside a warm building.

At home the amount of clothing the newborn wears is determined by the temperature. Families who maintain the home at 60–65 F should dress the infant more warmly than those who maintain the temperature at 70–75 F.

Newborns should wear head coverings outdoors to protect their sensitive ears from drafts. The blanket can be wrapped around the infant, leaving one corner free to place over the head while outdoors or in crowds for added protection. Families must also be advised of the ease with which a baby's skin can burn when exposed to the sun. To prevent sunburn, the baby should remain shaded, wear a light layer of clothing, or be protected with a sunscreen product.

TEACHING MOMENT

You may be surprised by the difficulty you encounter when attempting to put a T-shirt on a newborn. This is most easily done by placing your fingers through the sleeve, grasping the infant's hand, and drawing it back through the sleeve. This technique keeps the baby from grasping the fabric.

Diaper shapes vary and are subject to personal preference (Figure 29–11). Prefolded and disposable diapers are usually rectangular. Cloth diapers may also be triangular or kite-folded.

TEACHING MOMENT

When you talk to parents about cloth diapers, advise them to put the extra cloth in the front for boys and in the back for girls to give extra absorbency.

Baby clothing should be laundered separately using a mild soap or detergent. Diapers may be presoaked before washing. All clothing should be rinsed twice to remove soap and residue and to decrease the possibility of rash. Some babies may not tolerate clothing treated with fabric softeners added to the washer or softener sheets added to the dryer.

Temperature Assessment

The nurse shows the parents how to take the newborn's axillary temperature. A return demonstration is an effective way to evaluate their understanding. The different types of thermometers are discussed with parents. It is important that parents understand the differences and how to select the appropriate one. Other general instructions include how to shake the mercury down (the mercury needs to be below 94 F on the thermometer) and how to read the thermometer. Parents should be discouraged from taking the temperature rectally because this method can be both irritating and unsafe for the baby.

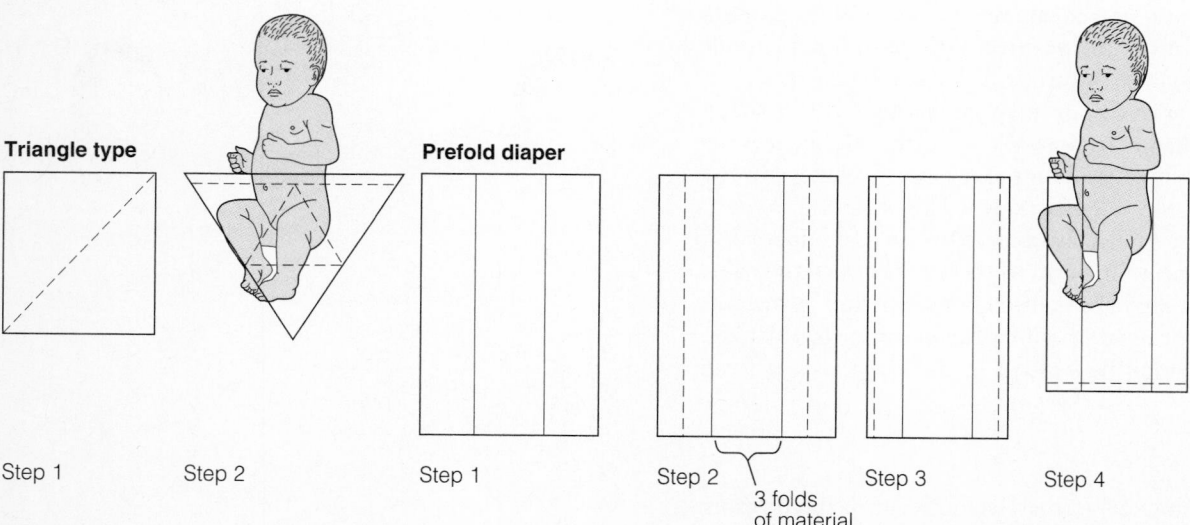

Triangle type   Step 1   Step 2   **Prefold diaper**   Step 1   Step 2   3 folds of material   Step 3   Step 4

FIGURE 29-11   Two basic cloth diaper shapes. Dotted lines indicate folds.

When taken properly, axillary temperatures are an accurate and comfortable method to measure the baby's temperature.

To take an axillary temperature, the thermometer is placed under one of the infant's arms, making sure that the bulb of the thermometer is underneath the armpit. It is held in place *3 to 4 minutes*. It is important to hold the baby's arm still because friction between the arm and chest creates heat and can make the thermometer record an inaccurate temperature.

A parent needs to take the newborn's temperature only when signs of illness are present. When parents find their newborn has a fever, they may expect to give an antipyretic such as Tylenol (acetaminophen), following closely the dosage on the label. Parents are advised to call their physician or pediatric nurse practitioner immediately if any of the signs listed in Table 29–5 occur. Parents should also check with their clinician for advice about over-the-counter medications they should have in the medicine cabinet. All parents should be advised to avoid giving any form of aspirin to their infants for any illness that may be viral. Use of aspirin in viral illnesses has been linked to Reye syndrome in children.

Flu, colds, teething, constipation, diarrhea, and other common ailments and their management should be discussed with their clinician before they occur. When analgesic and/or antipyretic medication is needed, clinicians frequently advise acetaminophen drops.

Stools and Urine

The appearance and frequency of a newborn's stools can cause concern for parents. The nurse prepares them by discussing and showing pictures of meconium stools and transitional stools and by describing the difference between breast milk and formula stools (see also Figure 27–12). Although all babies develop their own stooling patterns, parents can be given an idea of what to expect. They should be told the following:

- Breastfed newborns may have six to ten small, semiliquid, yellow stools per day by the third or fourth day because milk production is now established, unless the mother is having problems with her milk supply. Once breastfeeding is well established, usually by 1 month, the newborn may have only one stool every few days because of the increased digestibility of breast milk or still may have several daily. Constipation is unlikely to occur in newborns receiving only breast milk. Infrequent stooling in the first few weeks may be indicative of inadequate milk intake (Neifert 1989).

- Formula-fed babies may have only one or two stools a day; they are more formed and yellow or yellow-brown.

The parents may also be shown pictures of a constipated stool (small, pelletlike) and diarrhea (loose, green,

| TABLE 29-5 | When Parents Should Call Their Health Care Provider |

Temperature above 38.4 C (101 F) rectally or 38 C (100.4 F) axillary or below 36.1 C (97 F) rectally or 36.6 C (97.8 F) axillary

Continual rise in temperature

More than one episode of forceful vomiting or frequent vomiting over a 6-hour period

Refusal of two feedings in a row

Lethargy (listlessness), difficulty in awakening baby

Cyanosis with or without a feeding

Absence of breathing longer than 15 seconds

Inconsolable infant (quieting techniques are not effective) or continuous high-pitched cry

Discharge or bleeding from umbilical cord, circumcision, or any opening (except vaginal mucus or pseudomenstruation)

Two consecutive green, watery stools

No wet diapers for 18 to 24 hours or fewer than six to eight wet diapers per day

Development of eye drainage

or perhaps blood tinged). Families should understand that a green color is common in transitional stools so they don't confuse transitional stools with diarrhea the first week of a newborn's life.

Constipation may be an indication that the newborn needs additional fluid intake. Parents may try offering additional water in an attempt to reverse the constipation.

Babies normally void (urinate) five to eight times per day. Less than six to eight wet diapers a day may indicate the newborn needs more fluids. Frequency of voiding is easy to assess with cloth diapers. Parents who use the newer superabsorbent disposable diapers may have difficulty determining voiding patterns.

TEACHING MOMENT

Because baby boys often void into the air when the diaper is removed, you can avoid an unanticipated shower by having a dry diaper ready before removing the wet one.

Sleep and Activity

Perhaps nothing is more individual to each baby than the sleep-activity cycle. It is important for the nurse to recognize the individual variations of each newborn and to assist parents as they develop sensitivity to their infant's communication signals and rhythms of activity and sleep (Table 29–6).

The newborn demonstrates several different sleep-wake states (see Chapter 27) after the initial periods of reactivity described earlier. It is not uncommon for a baby

TABLE 29-6   Infant State* Chart (Sleep and Awake States)

Sleep States	**Characteristics of State**					
	Body Activity	Eye Movement	Facial Movement	Breathing Pattern	Level of Response	Implications for Care Giving
Deep sleep	Nearly still except for occasional startle or twitch	None	Without facial movements, except for occasional sucking movement at regular intervals	Smooth and regular	Only very intense and disturbing stimuli will arouse infants.	Care givers trying to feed infant in deep sleep will probably find the experience frustrating. Infants will be unresponsive, even if care givers use disturbing stimuli (flicking feet) to arouse infants. Infants may arouse only briefly and then become unresponsive as they return to deep sleep. If care givers wait until infants move to a higher, more responsive state, feeding or care giving will be much more pleasant.
Light sleep	Some body movements	Rapid eye movement (REM): fluttering of eyes beneath closed eyelids	May smile and make brief fussy or crying sounds	Irregular	Infants are more responsive to internal and external stimuli. When these stimuli occur, infants may remain in light sleep or move to drowsy state.	Light sleep makes up the highest proportion of newborn sleep and usually precedes awakening. Care givers who are not aware that the brief fussy or crying sounds made during this state occur normally may think it is time for feeding and may try to feed infants before they are ready to eat.
Drowsy	Activity level variable, with mild startles interspersed from time to time; movements usually smooth	Eyes open and close occasionally; are heavy-lidded with dull, glazed appearance	May have some facial movements; often are none and the face appears still	Irregular	Infants react to sensory stimuli although responses are delayed. State change after stimulation frequently noted.	From the drowsy state infants may return to sleep or awaken further. In order to wake them, care givers can provide something for infants to see, hear, or suck. This may arouse them to a quiet alert state, a more responsive state. Infants left alone without stimuli may return to a sleep state.
Quiet alert	Minimal	Brightening and widening of eyes	Faces have bright, shining, sparkling looks	Regular	Infants attend most to environment, focusing attention on any stimuli that are present.	Infants in this state provide much pleasure and positive feedback for care givers. Providing something for infants to see, hear, or suck will often maintain a quiet alert state in the first few hours after birth. Most newborns commonly experience a period of intense alertness before going into a long sleeping period.
Active alert	Much body activity; may have periods of fussiness	Eyes open with less brightening	Much facial movement; faces not as bright as in alert state	Irregular	Infants are increasingly sensitive to disturbing stimuli (hunger, fatigue, noise, excessive handling).	Care givers may intervene at this stage to console and to bring infants to a lower state.
Crying	Increased motor activity with color changes	Eyes may be tightly closed or open	Grimaces	More irregular	Infants are extremely responsive to unpleasant external or internal stimuli.	Crying is the infant's communication signal. It is a response to unpleasant stimuli from the environment or from within infants (fatigue, hunger, discomfort). Crying tells us infants have been reached. Sometimes infants can console themselves and return to lower states. At other times they need help from care givers.

*State is a group of characteristics that regularly occur together: body activity, eye movements, facial movements, breathing pattern, and level of response to external stimuli (eg, handling) and internal stimuli (eg, hunger).

SOURCE: Blackburn S, Kang R: Early Parent-Infant Relationships, 2nd ed, module 3, series 1. *The First Six Hours After Birth.* White Plains, NY: March of Dimes Birth Defects Foundation, 1991. Reprinted with permission of the copyright holder.

to sleep almost continuously for the first 2 to 3 days following birth, awakening only for feedings every 3 or 4 hours. Some newborns bypass this stage of deep sleep and may require only 12 to 16 hours of sleep. The parents need to know that this is normal.

Quiet sleep is characterized by regular breathing and no movement except for sudden body jerks. During this sleep state, normal household noise will not awaken the infant. In the *active sleep state*, the newborn has irregular breathing and fine muscular twitching. Newborns may cry out during sleep, but this does not mean they are uncomfortable or awake. Unusual household noise may awaken infants more easily in this state; however, they quickly go back to sleep.

Quiet alert is a state in which newborns are quietly involved with the environment. They watch a moving mobile, smile, and as they become older, discover and play with their hands and feet. When infants become uncomfortable due to wet diapers, hunger, or cold, they enter the *active awake and crying state*. In this state the cause of the crying should be identified and eliminated. Sometimes parents are frustrated as they try to identify the external or internal stimuli that are causing the angry, hurt crying. Parents need to be told that the baby's state may be changed from crying to quiet alert by moving the baby toward an upright position where scanning and exploration are possible (Klaus & Klaus 1985).

Crying

For the newborn crying is the only means of expressing needs vocally. Parents and care givers learn to distinguish different tones and qualities of the newborn's cry. The amount of crying is highly individual. Some will cry as little as 15–30 minutes in 24 hours or as long as 2 hours every 24 hours. When crying continues after causes such as discomfort or hunger are eliminated, the newborn may be comforted by swaddling or by rocking and other reassuring activities. There is some indication that infants who are held more tend to be calmer and cry less when not being held. Some parents may be afraid that holding the baby may "spoil" the baby and will need reassurance and information. Excessive crying should be noted and assessed, taking other factors into consideration. After the first 2 or 3 days newborns settle into individual patterns.

Circumcision

Circumcision is a surgical procedure in which the prepuce, an epithelial layer covering the penis, is separated from the glans penis and excised. This permits exposure of the glans for easier cleaning.

The parents make the decision about circumcision for their newborn male child. In most cases the choice is based on cultural, social, and family tradition. To ensure informed consent, parents should be informed about possible long-term medical effects of circumcision and noncircumcision during the prenatal period.

TO CIRCUMCISE OR NOT TO CIRCUMCISE?

Circumcision is the most frequently performed surgical procedure in the United States. Circumcisions are carried out on anywhere from 30% of males born in alternative birth settings to 80% to 90% of those born in traditional hospital settings. This surgical procedure continues in spite of the American Academy of Pediatrics Committee on Fetus and Newborn (1989, p 390) statement "that newborn circumcision has potential medical benefits and advantages as well as disadvantages and risks. When circumcision is being considered the benefits and risks should be explained to the parents and informed consent obtained."

What then motivates parents to have their male newborns circumcised? Various reasons have been given for the circumcision, including traditional practice (It's always been done—why question it?); wanting the child to have a similar appearance to the father or male siblings; rites of passage into manhood (religious and cultural rites); desire to conform to the dominant culture; sexual adequacy and cosmetic appearance; and hygiene. Opponents provide equally strong rationale and cultural data for not carrying out this procedure. It is important for nurses to identify and acknowledge the sociocultural motivating factors involved in the decision to circumcise or not to circumcise.

The current controversy over the continuation of the practice of circumcision raises important issues and concerns of parents.

- When is the optimal time for providing parents information about the circumcision procedure?

- What information should be provided to facilitate an informed choice?

- How do sociocultural factors influence the continued practice of circumcision?

- How does the health professional's ethnocentrism affect the information provided parents and willingness to use pain relief measures?

- Does the child have a right to freedom from pain (if circumcision is done without anesthesia)?

Current Recommendations Recommendations regarding circumcision have varied in the past. Before about 1980, circumcision was recommended by the American Academy of Pediatrics; then from 1980 to 1988 it was no longer recommended. Cultural practices, social customs, parental wishes, and (sometimes) lack of knowledge regarding the procedure result in many families choosing to have the male newborn circumcised. In 1989 the American Academy of Pediatrics wrote a position paper again recommending circumcision and cited the following medical reasons:

- It helps prevent phimosis (stenosis of the preputial space) and inflammation of the glans penis and foreskin.

- The incidence of penile cancer is lower in circumcised men in the United States.

- There is a decreased incidence of urinary tract infection in children under 1 year of age.

Circumcision should still be considered an elective procedure, but the procedure should not be performed if the newborn is premature or compromised, has a known bleeding problem, or is born with a genitourinary defect such as hypospadias or epispadias, which may necessitate the use of the foreskin in future surgical repairs (Cunningham et al 1993).

Circumcision was originally a religious rite practiced by Jews and Moslems. The practice gained widespread cultural acceptance in the United States but is done infrequently in many European countries. Many parents choose circumcision because they want the male child to have a similar physical appearance to the father or the majority of other children, or they may feel that it is expected by society (Chessare 1992).

Another frequently cited reason for circumcising newborn males is to prevent the need for anesthesia, hospitalization, pain, and trauma should the procedure be needed later in life. Cunningham and colleagues (1993) noted that only 5% to 10% of males are estimated to be in this category.

Nurse's Role The nurse plays an essential role in providing parents with current information about circumcision. Nurses can facilitate parental informed consent because of their knowledge of the medical, social, and psychologic aspects of newborn circumcision. A well-informed nurse can allay parents' anxiety by sharing information and allowing them to express their concerns. Parents must be informed about potential risks and outcomes of circumcision. Hemorrhage, infection, difficulty in voiding, separation of the edges of the circumcision, discomfort, and restlessness are early potential problems. Later there is the risk that the glans and urethral meatus can become irritated and inflamed from contact with ammonia from urine. Ulcerations and progressive stenosis may develop. Adhesions, entrapment of the penis, and damage to the urethra are all potential complications that could require surgical correction (Wiswell 1992).

Parents who are doubtful about their ability to use good hygienic practices in caring for their uncircumcised male infant and child require information from the nurse. They should be told that the foreskin and glans are two similar layers of cells that separate from each other. The separation process begins prenatally and is normally completed at between 3 and 5 years of age. In the process of separation, sterile sloughed cells build up between the layers (Lund 1990). This buildup looks similar to the smegma secreted after puberty, and it is harmless. Occasionally during the daily bath, the parents can gently test

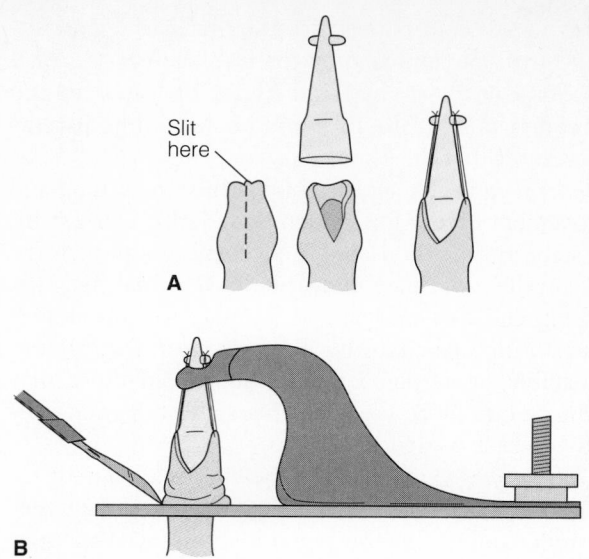

FIGURE 29-12 Circumcision using the Yellen or Gumco clamp. *A* The prepuce is drawn over the cone. *B* The clamp is applied. Pressure is maintained for three to four minutes. Then the excess prepuce is cut away.

for retraction. If retraction has occurred, daily gentle washing of the glans with soap and water is sufficient to maintain adequate cleanliness. The child should be taught to incorporate this practice into his daily self-care activities.

If circumcision is desired, the procedure should be performed after the newborn is well stabilized and has received his initial physical examination by a physician. The parents may also choose to have the circumcision done after discharge. However, they need to be advised that if the baby is older than 1 month, the current practice is to hospitalize him for the procedure.

The nurse's responsibilities during a circumcision are to determine if the parents have any further questions about the procedure and to ensure that the circumcision permit is signed. The nurse gathers the equipment and prepares the newborn by removing the diaper and placing him on a circumcision board or some other type of restraint. In the Jewish ceremonies the infant is held by the parent and given wine before the procedure.

There are a variety of techniques for circumcision (Figures 29–12, 29–13), and all produce minimal bleeding. During the procedure the nurse assesses the newborn's response. One consideration is pain experienced by the newborn. Some physicians use local anesthesia for this procedure. The American Academy of Pediatrics Committee on the Fetus and Newborn and Committee on Drugs (1987) have published a policy statement endorsing the administration of local or systemic anesthesia to infants undergoing surgical procedures. A dorsal penile nerve block (DPNB) using 1% lidocaine (Xylocaine)

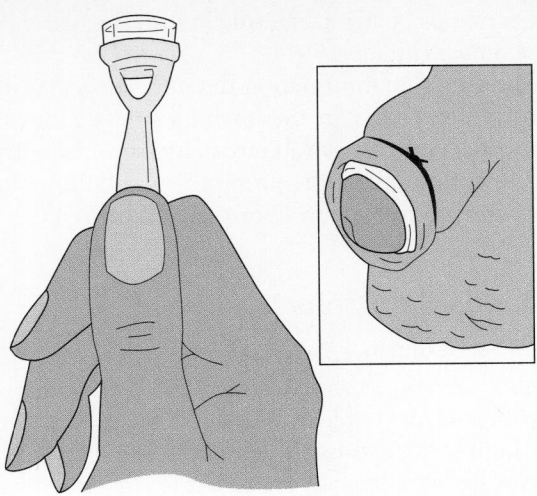

FIGURE 29-13   Circumcision using the Plastibell. The bell is fitted over the glans. A suture is tied around the bell's rim, and the excess prepuce is cut away. The plastic rim remains in place for 3–4 days until healing takes place. The bell may be allowed to fall off or removed if still in place after 8 days.

or chloroprocaine (Nesacaine) without epinephrine significantly minimizes the pain and the shifts in behavioral patterns such as crying, irritability, and erratic sleep cycles (Schoen & Fischell 1991). Other studies are investigating the use of topical anesthetic (30% lidocaine cream) applied 20 minutes prior to prepuce removal, acetaminophen, and cryoanalgesia (Weatherstone et al 1993; Wiswell 1992). Wellington and Rieder (1993) found that many physicians continue not to employ analgesics or use analgesics of questionable efficacy when performing newborn circumcisions.

The nurse can provide comfort measures such as lightly stroking the baby's head, providing a pacifier, and talking to him. Following the circumcision he should be held and comforted by a family member or the nurse. The nurse must be alert to any cues that these measures are overstimulating the newborn instead of comforting him. Such cues are turning away of the head, increased generalized body movement, skin color changes, hyperalertness, and hiccoughing.

After the circumcision, A and D ointment is placed on the penis to keep the diaper from adhering to the site in all procedures except those using the Plastibell. New ointment is applied with each diaper change or at least four to five times a day for at least 24 to 48 hours. Petroleum jelly or an antibiotic ointment may be used instead of A and D ointment.

The baby's voiding is assessed for amount, adequacy of stream, and presence of blood. If bleeding does occur, light pressure is applied intermittently to the site with a sterile gauze pad, and the physician is notified. The newborn may cry when he voids after circumcision. He should be positioned on his side with the diaper fastened

loosely to prevent undue pressure. He may remain fussy for several hours and be less interested in feedings.

The parents should be instructed to squeeze water gently over the penis and pat it dry after each diaper change. The diaper is loosely fastened for 2 to 3 days because the glans remains tender for this length of time.

Before discharge, the parents should be instructed to observe the penis for bleeding or possible signs of infection. A whitish yellow exudate that adheres to the glans is granulation tissue. It is normal and not indicative of an infection. The exudate may be noted for about 2 or 3 days and should not be removed.

If the Plastibell is used, parents are informed that it can remain in place for up to 8 days and then falls off. If it is still in place after 8 days, it may require manual removal by the clinician.

NURSING DIAGNOSIS FOR DISCHARGE

Nursing diagnoses that may apply to the newborn in preparation for discharge include the following:

- Impaired skin integrity related to moist umbilical cord or recent circumcision
- Risk for infection related to immunologic immaturity

Nursing diagnoses that may apply to the family at this time include the following:

- Risk for altered parenting related to transition to the role of parent
- Knowledge deficit related to lack of information about car seat requirements
- Knowledge deficit related to lack of information about infant health promotion needs
- Altered family processes related to the need to integrate the newborn into the family unit

Critical Thinking Question

What behaviors would you consider indicative of new parents' readiness for discharge and for the integration of the baby into the family?

NURSING PLAN AND IMPLEMENTATION FOR DISCHARGE

The nurse can do much to assist parents in feeling comfortable with newborn care before the family is sent home with their new baby. By discussing with parents how to meet their newborns' needs, ensure her or his safety, and appreciate the newborn's unique characteristics and behaviors, the nurse can get the new family off to a good

Dear Parents:

I come to you a small, immature being with my own style and personality. I am yours for only a short time; enjoy me.

1. Please take time to find out who I am, how I differ from you and how much I can bring you joy.

2. Please feed me when I am hungry. I never knew hunger in the womb, and clocks and time mean little to me.

3. Please hold, cuddle, kiss, touch, stroke, and croon to me. I was always held closely in the womb and was never alone before.

4. Please don't be disappointed when I am not the perfect baby that you expected, nor disappointed with yourselves that you are not the perfect parents.

5. Please don't expect too much from me as your newborn baby, or too much from yourself as a parent. Give us both six weeks as a birthday present—six weeks for me to grow, develop, mature and become more stable and predictable, and six weeks for you to rest and relax and allow your body to get back to normal.

6. Please forgive me if I cry a lot. Bear with me and in a short time, as I mature, I will spend less and less time crying and more time socializing.

7. Please watch me carefully and I can tell you the things that soothe, console and please me. I am not a tyrant who was sent to make your life miserable, but the only way I can tell you that I am not happy is with my cry.

8. Please remember that I am resilient and can withstand the many natural mistakes you will make with me. As long as you make them with love, you cannot ruin me.

9. Please take care of yourself and eat a balanced diet, rest and exercise so that when we are together, you have the health and strength to take care of me.

10. Please take care of your relationship with others. Relationships that are good for you, support both you and me.

Although I may have turned your life upside down, please realize that things will be back to normal before long.

Thank you,

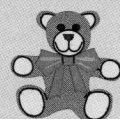 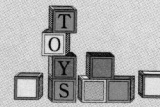

Your Loving Child

FIGURE 29-14 A letter from your baby.

start. The nurse also plays a vital role in fostering parent-infant attachment (Figure 29–14).

In addition to the information the nurse provides to parents during their stay in the birthing site, the nurse should provide information about safety, the newborn screening and immunization program, and follow-up care before the mother and newborn are discharged.

Safety Considerations

Nurses can be excellent role models for parents in the area of safety. Newborns should always be positioned on the side with a blanket rolled up behind them. Correct use of the bulb syringe must be demonstrated. The baby should never be left alone anywhere but in the crib. The mother is reminded that while she and the newborn are together in the birthing unit, she should never leave the baby alone because newborns spit up frequently the first day or 2 after birth.

Individual birthing units should practice safety measures to prevent infant abduction and provide teaching and information to parents regarding their role in this area. Accidents are the number one cause of death in children, with car accidents causing the most deaths, followed by poisonings. Half the children killed or injured in automobile accidents could have been protected by the use of a federally approved car seat. Newborns should go home from the birthing unit in a car seat adapted to fit newborns (Figure 29–15). The seat should be positioned to face the rear of the car until the baby is a year old or weighs 20 pounds (9.09 kg). At this time the child's bone structure is adequately mineralized and better able to withstand a forward impact in a five-point harness restraint belt. In many states the use of car seats for children up to the age of 4 is mandatory.

Newborns do not need pillows or stuffed animals in the crib while they sleep; these items could cause suffocation. Mattresses should fit snugly in a crib to prevent entrapment and suffocation, and the crib should be inspected regularly to determine whether it is in safe working order. Crib slats should be no more than 2⅜ inches apart. Parents can be encouraged to attend infant cardiopulmonary resuscitation (CPR) classes, especially if there is a history of SIDS or the infant requires special care.

Newborn Screening and Immunization Program

Before the newborn and mother are discharged from the birthing unit, parents are informed about the normal screening tests for newborns and should be told when to return to the birthing center or clinic if further tests are needed. **Newborn screening tests** detect disorders that cause mental retardation, physical handicaps, or death if left undiscovered. Inborn errors of metabolism can usually be detected within 1 to 2 weeks after birth and im-

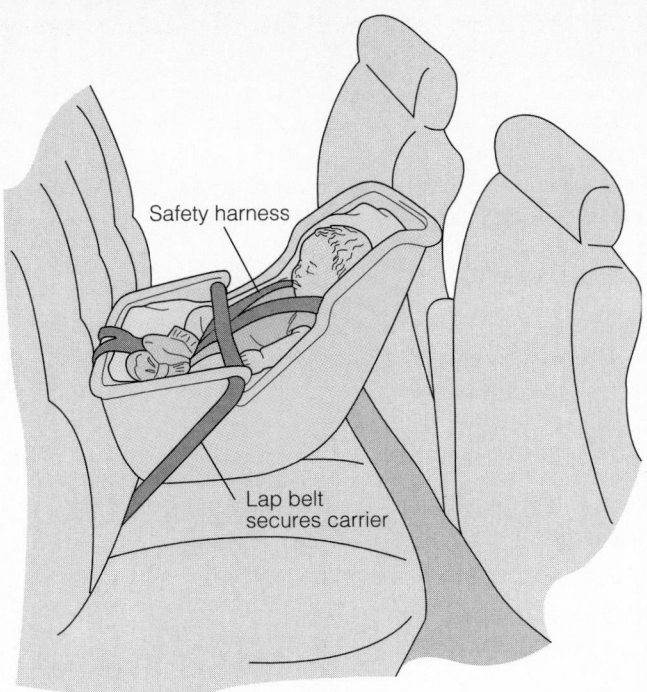

FIGURE 29-15 Infant car restraint. Infant car restraint for use from birth to about 12 months of age. SOURCE: Mott SR, James SB, Sperhac AM: *Nursing Care of Children and Families,* 2nd ed. Redwood City, CA: Addison-Wesley Nursing, 1990, p 530.

portant treatment begun before any damage has occurred. The disorders that can be identified from several drops of blood obtained by a heel stick on the second or third day are galactosemia, homocystinuria, hypothyroidism, maple syrup urine disease, phenylketonuria (PKU), and sickle cell anemia. Parents should be instructed that a second blood specimen will be required after 7 to 14 days (American Academy of Pediatrics Committee on Genetics 1992). In some states the second blood specimen is not recommended if the first specimen is obtained after 48 hours of age. It must be clarified that an abnormal test result is not diagnostic. More definitive tests must be performed to verify the results.

If additional tests are positive, treatment is initiated. These conditions may be treated by dietary means or by administration of the missing hormones. The inborn conditions cannot be cured, but they can be treated. Although they are not contagious, they may be inherited (see also Chapters 7 and 31).

Immunization programs against the hepatitis B virus during the newborn period and infancy are in place in many states, at least 20 countries, and high-incidence areas such as Alaska and American Samoa (Freij & Sever 1994). Universal hepatitis B vaccination for all infants, regardless of maternal HBsAg status, is currently recommended by the CDC and American Academy of Pediatrics. The current recommendation is that newborns receive the first vaccine dose within 12 hours of birth (0.5 mL of either vaccine preparation) and then a second dose

at 1 month of age and the last dose at 6 months of age (Freij & Sever 1994). See the Drug Guide: Recombinant Hepatitis B Vaccines on page 886. Parents need to be advised if their birthing center is doing newborn hepatitis vaccination so that an adequate follow-up program can be set in motion (Freed et al 1994).

Early discharge has impacted both the timing of newborn metabolic screening tests and the acquisition of subsequent immunization. For example, the accuracy of the test for PKU is directly related to the newborn's age. The likelihood of detecting PKU increases as the infant grows older, with the infant needing to be at least 24 hours old for a valid test (Coody et al 1993).

Follow-Up Care

Each newborn will have variations in normal physiologic responses and growth and development patterns. Parents need to learn how to interpret these changes in their child. To assist parents in caring for their newborn at home, some physicians encourage pediatric prenatal visits so that this contact is established before the birth. Public health nurses have long been involved in newborn care and parent education. Birthing units are now expanding their primary care functions to the new family to include one home visit by the primary nurse who cared for the family in the birthing unit. Some institutions have initiated postpartum visits (PPV) as a solution to early discharge problems for parents where a home visit is not an option. The PPV program offers parents a return visit to the birthing unit within 48–72 hours after discharge at no additional charge (Weinberg 1994). Physical exams of mother and baby are completed, teaching and emotional support provided, and, if necessary, referrals are made during this visit. Both parents have an opportunity to share how the family is managing at home. A follow-up telephone call is made 2 weeks later. Two benefits of this program are it facilitates breastfeeding and provides early intervention if problems such as increasing newborn jaundice and puerperal and wound infections occur (Weinberg 1994). The birthing unit and nursery staffs may also make themselves available as a 24-hour telephone resource for the new family that needs additional support and consultation during the first few days at home with their newborn.

Routine well-baby visits should be scheduled with the clinic, pediatric nurse practitioner, or physician. A recent study conducted with a poor and low-income patient population identified the following predictors of nonattendance at the first newborn health visit: a multiparous mother, no telephone in the home, and an unmarried teenage mother (Specht & Bourquet 1994). Although these predictors are easily identified from the baby's record, successful, cost-effective interventions will be more difficult to come by. An assessment of the adequacy of social environment and parenting skills should play an important part in the early discharge decision-making process (Britton et al 1994).

RECOMBINANT HEPATITIS B VACCINES

Overview of Neonatal Action

Recombinant Hepatitis B vaccines is used as a prophylactic treatment against all subtypes of hepatitis B virus. It provides passive immunization for newborns of HBsAg-negative and HBsAg-positive mothers. Hepatitis B can be transmitted across the placenta, but most newborns are infected during birth. It is produced from baker's yeast and plasmid containing the HBsAg gene.

Hepatitis B vaccine contains more than 95% HBsAg protein and is an inactivated (noninfective) product. Universal immunization is recommended.

Infants of HBsAg-positive mothers should concurrently receive 0.5 mL of hepatitis B immunoglobulin (HBIG) prophylaxis.

Route, Dosage, Frequency

The first dose of 0.5 mL (10 μg) is given intramuscularly into the anterolateral thigh within 12 hours of birth for infants born to HBsAg-positive mothers. The second dose of vaccine is given at 1 month of age and followed by a final dose at 6 months of age.

Infants born to HBsAg-negative mothers receive their first dose of vaccine at birth, the second dose at 1–2 months, and the third dose at 6–18 months (American Academy of Pediatrics 1992).

Infants whose mother's HBsAg status is unknown receive the same doses of vaccine as infants born to HBsAg-positive mothers.

Neonatal Side Effects

The only common side effect is soreness at the injection site. Occasionally, there is erythema, swelling, warmth, and induration at the injection site or a low-grade fever.

Nursing Considerations

Delay administration during active infection; the vaccine will not prevent infection during its incubation period.

The vaccine should be used as supplied. Do not dilute.

Do not inject intravenously or interdermally.

Monitor for adverse reactions. Monitor temperature closely.

Have epinephrine available to treat possible allergic reactions.

Responsiveness to the vaccine is age dependent. Preterm infants weighing less than 1000 g have lower seroconversion rates. Consider delaying the first dose until the infant is term PCA (postconceptual age) or use a four-dose schedule.

The family should be taught all necessary care-giving methods before discharge. A checklist may be helpful to see if the teaching has been completed. The nurse needs to review all areas for understanding or any outstanding questions with the mother and dad, without rushing, taking time to answer all queries. The family should have the certified nurse-midwife/nurse practitioner/physician's phone number, address, and any specific instructions. Having the birthing unit or nursery phone number is also reassuring to a newborn's family. They are encouraged to call with questions.

Documentation

The final step of discharge planning is documentation. Any concerns of the parents or nurse are noted. The nurse records which demonstrations and/or classes the woman and/or partner attended and their expressed understanding of the instructions given to them.

One method of documenting health teaching during the hospital stay is to use a multiple-copy teaching checklist that is dated and initialed by the nurse after completion of each topic. Parents sign the sheet, acknowledging their understanding of the material, and are given a copy upon discharge (Figure 29–16).

Education is a wonderful aspect of family-centered maternity care. The nurse who takes the time to get the family off to a good start can feel the satisfaction that optimal care is being provided.

EVALUATION

When evaluating the nursing care provided during the newborn period, the following outcomes may be anticipated:

- The newborn baby's adaptation to extrauterine life is supported and complete.

- The baby's physiologic and psychologic integrity is supported.

- The newborn feeding pattern will be satisfactorily established.

- The parents demonstrate safe techniques for caring for their baby.

- The parents express understanding of the bonding process and display attachment behaviors.

- The parents verbalize developmentally appropriate behavioral expectations of and follow-up care for their newborn.

DATE AND TIME OF BIRTH _____

TOPICS:	TIME & DATE	INT.	COMMENTS:
I. PHYSICIAN INSTRUCTION BOOKLET			
II. INITIAL M/B CONTACT ON MATERNITY			
A. Orient to Mother/Baby			
B. Permits (PKU, Circ)			
C. Diapering & wrapping			
D. Crying			
E. Positioning in crib			
F. Bulb syringe			
G. Regurgitation			
III. BREASTFEEDING			
A. Mechanics & position			
B. Length of feeding			
C. Rooting reflex			
D. New bottle pc			
E. Expression/pump			
F. Burping			
G. Formula & preparation			
IV. BOTTLE FEEDING			
A. Mechanics			
B. Rooting reflex			
C. New bottle each feeding			
D. Propping			
E. Amount & time			
F. Burping			
G. Formula & preparation			
V. NEWBORN CHARACTERISTICS			
A. Rash, milia			
B. Vag. discharge			
C. Jaundice (Handout)			
D. Molding			
E. Coloring			
F. Vision & hearing			
VI. BATH DEMONSTRATION			
A. Cord care			
B. Genital care			
C. Circumcision care			
D. Support & safety			
VII. DISCHARGE INSTRUCTIONS			
A. Normal void & stool			
B. Constipation			
C. Car seats			
D. When to call Doctor			
E. Choking baby			
F. Use of thermometer			
G. Safety			
H. PKU			

   I. Referral   YES ___ NO ___

Parent's Signature _____ Comments: _____

Witness to Signature _____

FIGURE 29-16   Infant teaching checklist. Sections I and II are completed upon initial contact. Sections III and IV are completed by 4 hours from initial contact. Section V is completed by 12 hours from initial contact. Sections VI and VII are completed by the time of discharge. SOURCE: Adapted from Memorial Hospital, Colorado Springs.

The overall goal of newborn nursing care is to provide comprehensive care while promoting the establishment of a well-functioning family unit.

The period immediately following birth, during which adaptation to extrauterine life occurs, requires close monitoring to identify any deviations from normal.

Nursing goals during the first 4 hours after birth (admission period) are to maintain a clear airway, maintain a neutral thermal environment, prevent hemorrhage and infection, initiate oral feedings, and facilitate attachment.

The newborn is routinely given prophylactic vitamin K to prevent possible hemorrhagic disease of the newborn.

Prophylactic eye treatment for *Neisseria gonorrhoeae* is legally required on all newborns.

Nursing goals in daily newborn care include maintenance of cardiopulmonary function, maintenance of neutral thermal environment, promotion of adequate hydration and nutrition, prevention of complications, promotion of safety, and enhancement of attachment and family knowledge of child care.

Essential daily care includes assessments of the vital signs, weight, overall color, intake, output, umbilical cord and circumcision, newborn nutrition, parent education, and attachment.

The clinician should be notified if there is evidence of bright red bleeding or puslike drainage near the cord stump or if the umbilicus remains unhealed.

Following a circumcision, the newborn must be observed closely for signs of bleeding, inability to void, and signs of infection.

Signs of illness in newborns include temperature above 38.4 C (101 F) or below 36.1 C (97 F), more than one episode of forceful vomiting, refusal of two feedings in a row, lethargy, cyanosis with or without a feeding, and absence of breathing for longer than 15 seconds.

Newborn screening for galactosemia, homocystinuria, hypothyroidism, maple syrup urine disease, phenylketonuria, and sickle cell anemia is done on all newborns in the first 1 to 3 days. A second blood specimen may be drawn after 7 to 14 days.

REFERENCES

American Academy of Pediatrics. *Guidelines for Perinatal Care*, 3rd ed. Chicago: American Academy of Pediatrics, 1992.

American Academy of Pediatrics Committee on Fetus and Newborn: Report of the Ad Hoc Task Force on Circumcision. *Pediatrics* 1989; 84:388.

American Academy of Pediatrics Committee on Fetus and Newborn and Committee on Drugs: Neonatal anesthesia. *Pediatrics* 1987; 80:446.

American Academy of Pediatrics Committee on Genetics: Issues in newborn screening. *Pediatrics* 1992; 89:345.

Andrews NM: Transcultural perspectives in the nursing care of children and adolescents. In: *Transcultural Concepts in Nursing Care.* Boyle JS, Andrews NM (editors). Philadelphia: Lippincott, 1989.

Bell TA et al: Randomized trial of silver nitrate, erythromycin, and no eye prophylaxis for the prevention of conjunctivitis among newborns not at risk for gonococcal ophthalmitis. *Pediatrics* 1993; 92(6):755.

Britton JR et al: Early discharge of the term newborn: A continued dilemma. *Pediatrics* 1994; 94(3):291.

Chessare JB: Circumcision: Is the risk of urinary tract infection really the pivotal issue? *Clin Pediatr* February 1992; 100.

Coen RW, Koeffler H: *Primary Care of the Newborn.* Boston: Little, Brown, 1987.

Coody D et al: Early hospital discharge and the timing of newborn metabolic screening. *Clin Pediatr* August 1993; 463.

Cunningham FG, MacDonald PC, Gant NG: *Williams Obstetrics*, 18th ed. Norwalk, CT: Appleton & Lange, 1993.

Freed GL et al: Universal hepatitis B immunization of infants: Reactions of pediatricians and family physicians over time. *Pediatrics* 1994; 93(5):747.

Freij BJ, Sever JL: Chronic infections. In: *Neonatalogy: Pathophysiology and Management of the Newborn*, 14th ed. Avery GB, Fletcher MA, MacDonald MG (editors). Philadelphia: Lippincott, 1994.

Hutchinson MK, Baqi-Aziz M: Nursing care of the childbearing Muslim family. *JOGNN* 1994; 23(9):767.

Infant Sleep Positioning and SIDS Position Statement. Evanston, IL: American Academy of Pediatrics, 1992.

Klaus M, Klaus P: *The Amazing Newborn.* Menlo Park, CA: Addison-Wesley, 1985.

Lund MM: Perspectives on newborn male circumcision. *Neonatal Network* 1990; 9(3):7.

McGregor LA: Short, shorter, shortest: Improving the hospital stay for mothers and newborns. *MCN* 1994; 19(2):91.

Merestein GB, Gardner SL: *Handbook of Neonatal Intensive Care*, 3rd ed. St Louis: Mosby, 1992.

Milan EM, McFeely EJ: *Memory Bank for Neonatal Drugs.* Baltimore: Williams & Wilkins, 1990.

Neifert M: *Breastfeeding Standards of Care for Low Risk Infants.* Denver: Presbyterian/St Luke's Medical Center, 1989.

Neonatal Skin Care. *NAACOG-OGN Nursing Practice Resource.* January 1992.

Neonatal Thermoregulation. *NAACOG-OGN Nursing Practice Resource.* February 1990.

Pawlak RP, Tabor Herfert LA: *Drug Administration in the NICU: A Handbook for Nurses*, 2nd ed. Petaluma, CA: Neonatal Network, 1990.

Riordan J, Auerbach KG: *Breastfeeding and Human Lactation.* Boston: Jones & Bartlett, 1993.

Ruchala P: The effect of wearing head covering on the axillary temperature of infants. *MCN* July/August 1985; 10:240.

Schoen EJ, Fischell AA: Pain in neonatal circumcision. *Clin Pediatr* 1991; 30(7):429.

Specht EM, Bourquet CC: Predictors of nonattendance at the first newborn health supervision visit. *Clin Pediatr* May 1994; 273.

Tappero EP, Honeyfield ME: *Physical Assessment of the Newborn.* Petaluma, CA: NICU Ink, 1993.

Von Kries R: Vitamin K prophylaxis: Oral or parenteral. *Am J Dis Child* 1988; 142:14.

Weatherstone KB et al: Safety and efficacy of a topical anesthetic for neonatal circumcision. *Pediatrics* 1993; 92(5):710.

Weinberg SH: An alternative to meet the needs of early discharge: The tender beginnings postpartum visit. *MCN* 1994; 19(6):339.

Wellington N, Rieder MJ: Attitudes and practice regarding analgesia for newborn circumcision. *Pediatrics* 1993; 92:541.

Wiswell TE: Circumcision: An update. *Curr Probl Pediatr* 1992; 22(10):424.

Zanoni D, Isenberg SJ, Apt L: A comparison of silver nitrate with erythromycin for prophylaxis against ophthalmia neonatorum. *Clin Pediatr* May 1992; 295.

CHAPTER 30

NEWBORN NUTRITION

I had been told that most babies ate every three or four hours and slept the rest of the time. Not mine! She wanted to nurse every two hours, and sometimes more often than that. Sometimes she would sleep for an hour, sometimes for fifteen minutes. I loved her, but I also felt consumed by her needs. It was hard to adjust to the fact that I couldn't get anything finished, whether it was an article I was reading or folding the laundry. At the end of the day I would realize I hadn't accomplished anything. Once I accepted the fact that I was not going to function at my old efficient rate (at least for a while) and stopped feeling guilty about what I wasn't getting done, I felt free to enjoy the time I was spending with my baby.

~The New Our Bodies, Ourselves~

KEY TERMS

Alveoli

Colostrum

Foremilk

Hindmilk

La Leche League

Let-down reflex

Mature milk

Milk/plasma ratio

Oxytocin

Prolactin

Transitional milk

Weaning

OBJECTIVES

Compare the nutritional value and composition of breast milk and formula preparations.

Identify the benefits of breastfeeding for both mother and infant.

Develop guidelines for helping both breastfeeding and bottle-feeding mothers to feed their infants successfully.

Delineate nursing responsibilities for client education about problems the breastfeeding mother may encounter at home.

Describe an appropriate process for weaning an infant from breastfeeding.

Incorporate knowledge of newborn nutrition and normal growth patterns into parent education and infant assessment.

Recognize the influence of cultural values on infant care, especially feeding practices.

$\mathscr{F}$eeding their newborn is an exciting, satisfying, and often worrisome task for parents. Meeting this essential need of their new child helps parents strengthen their attachment to their baby and fosters their self-images as nurturers and providers. Whether a woman chooses to breastfeed or bottle-feed, she can be reassured that she can adequately meet her infant's needs. Questions about feeding may arise, however, and the nurse works with the woman to help her develop skill in her chosen method. In every interaction it is the nurse's responsibility to support the parents and promote the family's sense of confidence.

NUTRITIONAL NEEDS OF THE NEWBORN

The newborn's diet must supply nutrients to meet the rapid rate of physical and mental growth and development. A neonatal diet should provide adequate calories and include protein, carbohydrate, fat, water, vitamins, and minerals. The recommended dietary allowances (RDAs) for birth through the first 6 months are listed in Table 30–1.

The calories (105–110 kcal/kg/day or 50–55 kcal/lb/day) in the newborn's diet are divided among protein, carbohydrate, and fat. Protein is needed for rapid cellular growth and maintenance. Carbohydrates provide energy. The fat portion of the diet provides calories, regulates fluid and electrolyte balance, and is necessary for the normal development of the neonatal brain and neurologic system.

Water requirements are high (140–160 mL/kg/day or 64–73 mL/lb/day) because of the newborn's inability to concentrate urine. Fluid needs are further increased in illness or hot weather.

The iron needs of the infant will be affected by accumulation of iron stores during the fetal life and by the mother's iron and other food intake if she is breastfeeding. Ascorbic acid (usually in the form of fruit juices) and meat, poultry, and fish are known to enhance absorption of iron in the mother just as it does later in the infant. Adequate minerals and vitamins are needed by the newborn to prevent deficiency states such as scurvy, cheilosis, and pellagra.

Animals' growth rates vary according to the composition of their milk. Human milk contains the lowest concentration of protein of any mammal's, so human infants grow the slowest. Infants who are formula fed gain weight faster than breastfed infants because of the differences in composition between the foods and also because larger volumes of formula than breast milk are needed to obtain the same nutrients. (Because breast milk is digested more easily than formula, the nutrients are more readily available.) Bottle-fed infants tend to regain their birth weight by 10 days after birth (Pipes 1989) and may gain as much as 30 g (1 oz) per day up to 6 months of age. Healthy breastfed babies, however, tend to regain their birth weight about 14 days after birth and gain approximately 15 g (0.5 oz) per day in the first 6 months of life (Sawley 1989). Formula-fed infants generally double their weight in 3.5 to 4 months, whereas nursing infants double their weight at about 5 months of age. Substituting milk from other species in a baby's diet creates difficulties because the infant does not receive the nutrients specific to his or her own needs. Human milk is the perfect food for human infants.

Breast Milk

The composition of human milk varies with the stage of lactation, the time of day, the time during the feeding, maternal nutrition, and gestational age of the newborn at birth. During the establishment of lactation there are three stages of human milk: colostrum, transitional milk, and mature milk.

Colostrum is a yellowish or creamy-appearing fluid that is thicker than later milk and contains more protein,

---

TABLE 30–1 Recommended Dietary Allowances for the Normal Newborn

Daily Requirements, Birth–6 Months		
Calories	108	kcal/kg
Protein	2.2	g/kg
Fat	30–35%	total kcal
Carbohydrate	50–55%	total kcal
Water	1.5	ml/kcal
Calcium	400	mg
Phosphorous	300	mg
Magnesium	40	mg
Iron	6	mg
Zinc	5	mg
Iodine	40	μg
Selenium	10	μg
Vitamins		
A	420	μg
B_6	0.3	mg
B_{12}	0.3	μg
D	400	IU
E	3	mg
K	5	μg
C	30	mg
Thiamine	0.3	mg
Riboflavin	0.4	mg
Niacin	5	mg
Folate	25	μg

NOTE: The allowances, expressed as average daily intakes, are intended to provide for individual variations among normal persons in the United States under usual environmental stresses.

SOURCE: Food and Nutrition Board, National Academy of Sciences—National Research Council: *Recommended Dietary Allowances*, 10th ed. Washington, DC, 1989.

fat-soluble vitamins, and minerals. It also contains high levels of immunoglobulins (antibodies, such as IgA), which are a source of passive immunity for the newborn. Colostrum production begins early in pregnancy and may last for several days after birth. However, in most cases colostrum is replaced by transitional milk within 2 to 4 days after birth. Even though only small amounts of colostrum are produced, it is invaluable for the newborn.

Transitional milk is produced from the end of colostrum production and approximately 2 weeks postpartum. This milk contains elevated levels of fat, lactose, water-soluble vitamins, and more calories than colostrum contains.

The final milk produced, **mature milk,** contains about 10% solids (carbohydrates, proteins, fats) for energy and growth; the rest is water, which is vital for maintaining hydration. The composition of mature milk varies according to the time during the feeding. **Foremilk** is the milk obtained at the beginning of the feeding. It is high in water content and contains vitamins and protein. **Hindmilk** is released after the initial let-down, or release of milk, and has higher fat concentration.

Although mature milk appears similar to skim milk and may cause mothers to question whether their milk is "rich enough," mature breast milk provides 20 kcal/oz, as do most prepared formulas. However, the percentage of calories derived from protein is lower in breast milk than in formulas, and a greater proportion of calories is derived from fat (Riordan & Auerbach 1993). The nitrogen wastes produced by protein metabolism are, therefore, lessened in the breastfed newborn, and this has a positive effect on the infant's immature renal system.

The American Academy of Pediatrics Committee on Nutrition (1992) recommended breast milk as the optimal food for the first 6 to 12 months of life. Breastfeeding provides newborns and infants with immunologic, nutritional, and psychosocial advantages.

Immunologic Advantages

Immunologic advantages include varying degrees of protection from respiratory and gastrointestinal infections, otitis media, meningitis, sepsis, and allergies. This protection has a positive effect on the breastfed baby's health in the newborn period. All newborn babies' immunoglobulins are active by 18 months of age. In 1981 it was estimated that if breastfeeding were universal, 5000 lives would be saved in the United States annually (Riordan & Auerbach 1993).

Secretory IgA, an immunoglobulin present in colostrum and breast milk, has antiviral, antibacterial, and antigenic-inhibiting properties. It is theorized that the infant's immature intestine allows antigenic macromolecules, such as those found in cow's milk, to cross the mucosa of the small intestine. Secretory IgA plays a role in decreasing the permeability of the intestine to these macromolecules. Other components of colostrum and breast milk that act to inhibit the growth of bacteria and/or viruses are *Lactobacillus bifidus*, lysozymes, lactoperoxidase, lactoferrin, transferrin, and various immunoglobulins. Immunoglobulins to the poliomyelitis virus are also present in the breast milk of mothers who have immunity to this virus. Because the presence of these immunoglobulins may inhibit the desired intestinal infection and immune response of the infant, some clinics suggest that breastfeedings be withheld for 30 to 60 minutes following the administration of the Sabin oral polio vaccine. In addition to its immunologic properties, breast milk is known to be nonallergenic and is not affected by unsafe water or insect-carried disease (Lawrence 1994).

Nutritional Advantages

Breast milk is composed of lactose, lipids, polyunsaturated fatty acids, and amino acids, especially taurine, and has a whey:casein protein ratio that facilitates its digestion, absorption, and full use compared to formulas (Worthington-Roberts & Williams 1993). Some researchers feel the high concentration of cholesterol and the balance of amino acids in breast milk make it the best food for myelination and neurologic development. High cholesterol levels in breast milk may stimulate the production of enzymes that lead to more efficient metabolism of cholesterol, thereby reducing its harmful long-term effects on the cardiovascular system (Worthington-Roberts & Williams 1993).

Another reason human milk is considered the ideal first food is that its composition varies according to gestational age and stage of lactation. For example, the milk of a preterm mother has more long chain polyunsaturated fatty acids (LC-PUFA) than mothers of full-term babies. LC-PUFA are essential for brain growth (Hamosh 1994), and preterm infants are born with very low LC-PUFA reserves.

Breast milk provides newborns with minerals in more appropriate doses than do formulas (Worthington-Roberts & Williams 1993). The iron found in breast milk, even though much lower in concentration than that of prepared formulas, is much more readily and fully absorbed and appears sufficient to meet the infant's iron needs for the first 4 to 6 months. The American Academy of Pediatrics Committee on Nutrition (1992) states that there is generally no need to give supplemental iron to full-term breastfed newborns before the age of 4–6 months. Supplemental iron may decrease the ability of breast milk to protect the newborn by interfering with lactoferrin, an iron-binding protein that enhances the absorption of iron and has anti-infective properties.

Another advantage of breast milk is that all its components are delivered to the infant in an unchanged form, and vitamins are not long through processing and heating. If the breastfeeding mother is taking daily multivitamins and her diet is adequate, the only supplements the infant will need until the age of 6 months are vitamin D and fluoride (American Academy of Pediatrics Committee on Nutrition 1992). If the mother's diet or vitamin intake is inadequate or questionable, care givers may choose to prescribe additional vitamins for the infant.

Psychosocial Advantages

Psychophysiologic reactions during nursing have been shown to affect maternal-infant attachment. The mother's level of oxytocin generally increases with breast-feeding, and studies indicate that this hormonal change coincides with more even mood responses and increased feelings of maternal well-being (Lawrence 1994). In addition, research demonstrates that female rats fail to care for young when the effects of oxytocin are inhibited. Conversely, the administration of oxytocin (following estrogen priming) induces maternal behavior in virgin rats (Pederson et al 1992).

Breastfeeding enhances attachment by providing the opportunity for frequent, direct skin contact between the newborn and the mother. The newborn's sense of touch is highly developed at birth and is a primary means of communication. The tactile stimulation associated with breastfeeding can communicate warmth, closeness, and comfort. The increased closeness provides both newborn and mother with the opportunity to learn each other's behavioral cues and needs. The mother's sense of accomplishment in being able to satisfy her baby's needs for nourishment and comfort is enhanced when the newborn suckles vigorously and is satiated and calmed by the breastfeeding. Some mothers prefer breastfeeding as a means of extending the close, unique, nourishing relationship between mother and baby that existed prior to birth. As Lawrence (1994, p 60) states, there are psychologic advantages for the baby as well as the mother: "A good experience with breastfeeding can ensure an intense interaction and synchronous response of giving and taking and this is the essence of the infant's beginning to create a secure world for himself."

In the event of a twin birth, breastfeeding not only is possible but also enhances the mother's individualization and attachment to each newborn. The fantasized single baby is replaced more readily with the reality of two individual babies when the mother has close and frequent contact with each (Sollid et al 1989). Fathers can also be encouraged to be a part of the feeding experience by offering fresh pumped or thawed (frozen) breast milk to the baby at one or more feeding daily.

Contraindications and Disadvantages

There are some medical contraindications to breastfeeding. A mother with a diagnosis of breast cancer should not breastfeed so that she may begin treatment immediately. With regard to AIDS, the CDC recommend counseling the mother against breastfeeding except in a country where the risk of neonatal death from diarrhea and

RESEARCH IN PRACTICE

Two types of jaundice occur in otherwise healthy newborns: exaggerated physiologic jaundice or breast milk jaundice. Exaggerated physiologic jaundice develops by the third or fourth day after birth and is characterized by bilirubin levels of 10 mg/dL or higher. Some have suggested that this problem may be a form of breast milk jaundice. In breast milk jaundice bilirubin levels start to rise between the fourth and seventh days, peak around day 14 at 15 to 25 mg/dL, remain stable for 2 weeks, and return to normal between weeks 4 and 16. Linda Brown and her colleagues examined the incidence and pattern of jaundice in the first month of life of otherwise healthy breastfed babies.

One hundred fifty-five White, healthy, full-term infants who had been breastfed for 1 month comprised the sample for this study. The authors measured bilirubin with a noninvasive transcutaneous bilirubinometer (TcB). Since a pilot test showed some discrepancy between the two meters used, each infant was followed with the same meter. Bilirubin levels were obtained on days 2, 3, 5, 7, 9, 11, and 13 after birth. When a bilirubin level of ≥10 mg/dL was measured, the screening nurse notified the attending pediatrician in the mother's presence. If a baby's reading was ≥10 mg/dL on day 13, the investigators continued to monitor the infant's TcB every other day until the bilirubin level dropped below 10 mg/dL.

Results of the study showed that 25.8% of the newborns reached bilirubin levels high enough to be considered jaundiced (≥10 mg/dL) by day 2. By day 3, 49.7% of the infants demonstrated jaundice. After that peak on day 3 the percentage of jaundiced infants declined at a steady rate so that only 10.3% were jaundiced at day 13 and only 2.6% at day 19. The peak bilirubin levels of those infants who were still jaundiced at day 13 had occurred by day 3. This pattern indicated that TcB readings do not differentiate between exaggerated physiologic and breast milk jaundice. Infants with low TcB readings on days 2, 3, and 5 never developed an elevated bilirubin level. Other results of this study indicated that infants with siblings who had exhibited neonatal jaundice were more likely to develop jaundice than those infants whose siblings had not developed jaundice.

Clinical Application of Study

The authors note that early elevated bilirubin readings may be determined by TcB monitoring before discharge in order to identify those infants at risk for developing jaundice. Mothers with babies at risk should receive special information regarding breastfeeding and jaundice and could return the infant in 1 week postpartum for further bilirubin testing.

SOURCE: Brown L et al: Incidence and pattern of jaundice in healthy breast-fed infants during the first months of life. *Nurs Res* 1993; 42(2):106.

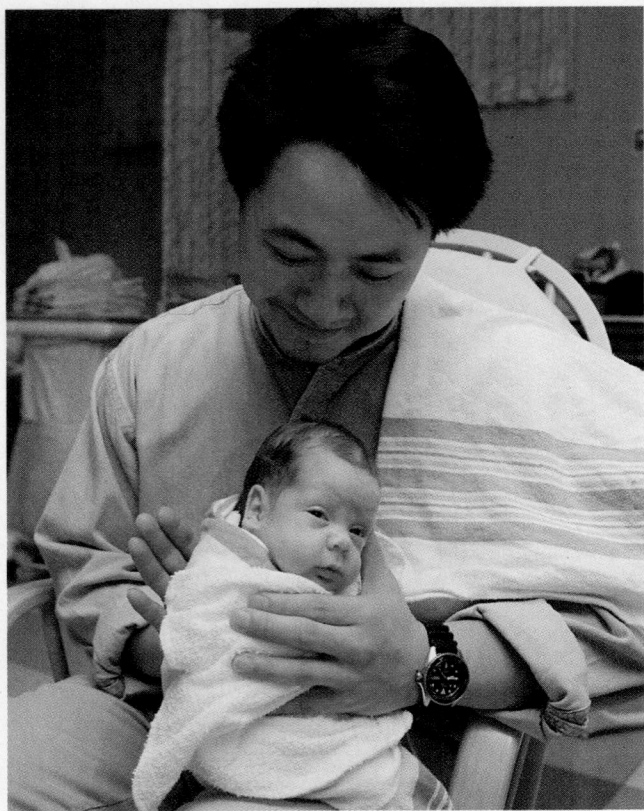

FIGURE 30-1   A father can nurture his baby in many ways.

other disease (excluding AIDS) is 50% or greater (Lawrence 1994). Breastfeeding is also contraindicated for the infant suffering from galactosemia (Eggert & Rayburn 1994).

Maternal medications may preclude breastfeeding, as discussed in Chapters 18 and 31. One drug of particular note is cocaine, which, because of its high lipid solubility, passes easily into breast milk and is harmful to the breastfeeding infant. In terms of newborn illnesses management of jaundice in particular may include suspension of breastfeeding (see Chapter 32).

The disadvantages of breastfeeding include factors that the mother may perceive as inconvenient. In the dominant Western culture, where women are actively pursuing activities outside the home, being "tied down" to an infant for 9 to 12 feedings every day may be considered inconvenient and stressful. Another often cited disadvantage of breastfeeding is exclusion of the father from the nurturing involved in feeding the infant. Our society fails to acknowledge that both parents cannot do all things equally well. Of course only the mother is biologically capable of feeding. As Lawrence (1994) contends, nurturing encompasses more than just feeding, and the father can comfort and attend to the baby in many other ways (Figure 30–1).

Opinion varies as to the advisability of continuing breastfeeding in the event of another pregnancy. Some feel the nutritional demands on the pregnant mother are too great and advocate gradual weaning. Others suggest that with adequate rest, a proper diet, and strong emotional support continued breastfeeding during pregnancy is a valid choice. The practice of nursing one infant throughout pregnancy and then breastfeeding both infants after birth is called *tandem nursing* (Lawrence 1994). When pregnancy occurs, the decision of how to handle nursing is best made on an individual basis after considering maternal health and motivation and the age of the first child.

Even though many mothers obtain information about breastfeeding from written sources, family and friends, and the **La Leche League** (an international breastfeeding support and information group), the nurse needs to be a ready source of information, encouragement, and support as well. The nurse can be helpful when parents are deciding whether to breastfeed, after birth when breastfeedings are just being established, and after the family returns home.

Formula Feeding

Commercially prepared milk formulas differ from breast milk in their concentrations of amino acids: Formulas contain more tyrosine and phenylalanine and less taurine than does breast milk. Formulas also contain mostly saturated fatty acids, whereas breast milk is higher in unsaturated fatty acids, long chain fats, and cholesterol. Calcium, sodium, and chloride concentrations are higher in some commercially made formulas. If formula is prepared improperly (such as by adding excessive powder), the excess salts (ie, sodium) may be detrimental to the newborn's immature kidneys. This high solute load may also lead to thirst in the formula-fed infant, causing overfeeding and possible obesity. If formula is overdiluted, the infant will not receive adequate nutrients.

Another potential problem with formulas is an allergic reaction in the newborn. The small intestine of the infant is permeable to macromolecules such as those found in cow's milk and mild-based formulas. The introduction of foreign proteins in formula may cause an allergic reaction, with signs such as vomiting, colic, diarrhea, colitis, reluctance to feed, and eczema (Table 30–2).

Clinicians recommend that parents who are bottle feeding use iron-fortified formulas or supplements because iron deficiency anemia is still prevalent. The RDA for iron is 6 mg per day from birth to 6 months and 10 mg per day from 6 to 12 months. However, the nurse must be aware that too much iron in the form of iron-fortified cereal may interfere with the infant's natural ability to defend against disease (Winick 1989). Parents also need to be informed about the constipation that sometimes results from iron-enriched formula and about various methods of alleviating the constipation. Opinion varies about the use of vitamin supplements for newborns, but it is generally agreed that commercially prepared formulas

| TABLE 30-2 | Comparison of Breastfeeding and Bottle-Feeding |

Breast	**Bottle (Feeding Iron-Enriched Formula)**
Nutrition	
Breast milk is species specific (ie, perfect balance of proteins, carbohydrates, fats, vitamins, and minerals for human infants).	Formula is as close to human milk as possible, but nutrients are not as efficiently utilized.
Breast milk contains higher levels of lactose, cystine, and cholesterol, which are necessary for brain and nerve growth.	Nutritional adequacy depends on proper preparation (overdilution results in decreased nutrients delivered to infant).
Proteins are easily digested and fats are well absorbed.	Some babies cannot tolerate the fats or carbohydrates found in regular formula. Companies are offering alternative formulas.
Composition varies according to gestational age and stage of lactation, thereby meeting the changing nutritional requirements of individual infants as they grow.	
Infants determine the volume of milk consumed.	Pediatrician or care giver determines the volume consumed. Overfeeding may occur if care giver is determined that baby will empty bottle.
Frequency of feeding is determined by infant cues rather than by time schedule.	Feeding commonly occurs according to a preset schedule.
Anti-Infective and Antiallergic Properties	
Breast milk contains immunoglobulins, enzymes, and leukocytes that protect against pathogens.	Formula is linked to an increased number of GI and respiratory infections.
Bacteriostatic properties permit storage at room temperature up to 6 hours, in refrigerator for 24 hours, and freezing for 6 months.	Potential for bacterial contamination exists during preparation and storage.
Breast milk decreases the incidence of allergy by eliminating exposure to potential antigens (cow and soy protein).	Some babies are allergic to cow or soy protein. Formula companies are offering alternative formulas suitable for babies who develop allergies.
Psychosocial Aspects	
Skin-to-skin contact enhances closeness.	Bottle-feeding can provide an opportunity for positive parent-infant interaction.
Hormones of lactation promote maternal feelings and sense of well-being.	
The value system of an industrial society can create barriers to successful breastfeeding: Mother may feel ashamed or embarrassed. Breastfeeding after return to work may be difficult.	
Father is not able to breastfeed, but he can feed expressed breast milk from a bottle and nurture the infant in ways other than feeding.	Father can feed the baby.
Cost	
Healthy diet for mother.	Formula is a major expense.
Optional, but recommended, items include nursing pads, nursing bras.	Bottles or disposable nursers with plastic liners, nipples, and nipple caps must be purchased.
A breast pump may be needed.	A refrigeration system is necessary if mixing formula for more than one feeding at a time or using large containers of ready-to-feed formula.
Convenience	
The milk is always the perfect temperature.	
No preparation time is needed.	Varying amounts of time are involved in formula preparation.
The mother must be available to feed or provide expressed milk to be given in her absence.	Anyone can feed the baby.
If she misses a feeding, the mother must express milk to maintain lactation.	
The mother may experience slight discomfort in the early days of lactation.	
Maternal medication may interrupt breastfeeding.	

adequately meet the needs of the healthy newborn and infant.

Many companies make enriched formulas that are similar to breast milk. These formulas all have sufficient levels of carbohydrate, protein, fat, vitamins, and minerals to meet the newborn's nutritional needs.

Formula companies offer a variety of products for infants suffering from metabolic disorders or allergy to cow's milk. For many years soy protein was substituted for bovine protein in formula given to babies exhibiting signs of allergy. However, reports of allergic reaction to soy protein are prompting formula companies to create a nonantigenic substitute for cow's milk protein. Casein hydrolysate is essentially a "predigested" protein that presents protein fragments too small to be recognized by the infant's immune system as an antigen, thereby decreasing the baby's allergic response (Mead Johnson Nutritionals 1993). Corn syrup products and corn, soy, and coconut oils serve as substitute carbohydrate and fat sources for babies with carbohydrate intolerance or fat malabsorption.

In its 1992 position paper on nutrition, the American Academy of Pediatrics recommended that infants be given breast milk or iron-fortified formula rather than whole milk until 1 year of age. Neither unmodified cow's milk nor skim milk is an acceptable alternative for newborn feeding. The protein content in cow's milk is too high (50% to 75% more than human milk), is poorly digested, and may cause bleeding of the gastrointestinal tract. It also has higher levels of calcium, phosphorus, sodium, and potassium, which increase the renal solute load and result in greater obligatory water loss. Unmodified cow's milk is also inadequate in vitamins. Skim milk lacks adequate calories, fat content, and essential fatty acids necessary for proper development of the neonate's neurologic system. Nutritionists advise against use of unmodified cow's milk, cow's milk with decreased fat content, or skim milk for children under 2 years of age.

NEWBORN FEEDING

Initial Feeding

Assessment of the newborn's physiologic status is of primary and ongoing concern to the nurse throughout the first feeding. Extreme fatigue coupled with rapid respiration, circumoral cyanosis, and diaphoresis of the head and face may indicate cardiovascular complications and should be assessed further. The initial feeding also requires assessment of the infant for the congenital anomalies tracheoesophageal fistula and esophageal atresia (Chapter 31). Findings associated with esophageal anomalies include maternal polyhydramnios and increased oral mucus in the infant. In cases of esophageal atresia the feeding is taken well initially, but as the esophageal pouch fills, the feeding is quickly regurgitated unchanged by stomach contents. If a fistula is present, the infant gags, chokes, regurgitates mucus, and may become cyanotic as fluid passes through the fistula into the lungs.

Because colostrum is not irritating if aspirated (which may occur because of the newborn's initially uncoordinated sucking and swallowing abilities) and is readily absorbed by the respiratory system, breastfeeding can usually begin immediately after birth. Contraindications to immediate nursing include heavy sedation of the mother and physical compromise of either mother or baby.

Many institutions offer the newborn who is to be formula fed a few milliliters of sterile water or 5% dextrose 1 to 4 hours after birth. There is no current evidence to support this practice because it is the aspirated gastric contents with acid that are harmful and not the type of feeding (Fletcher 1994). The first feeding provides an opportunity for the nurse to assess the effectiveness of the newborn's suck, swallow, and gag reflexes.

The time of the first feeding for all newborns should be determined by their physiologic and behavioral cues. Bottle-feeding newborns are offered formula as soon as they show an interest an ability to suck and swallow. The mother who plans to breastfeed should be encouraged to nurse her newborn immediately following birth, allowing the baby to nurse to satiety. Throughout the first 2 hours after birth, especially during the first 20–30 minutes, the infant is usually alert and ready to nurse. However, newborn suckling patterns vary, and although many babies are eager to suckle at this time, many will simply lick or nuzzle the nipple. This behavior is beneficial because the licking stimulates the release of oxytocin, which aids uterine involution and lactation (let-down). The mother should be encouraged to interpret this as a positive breastfeeding interaction (Riordan & Auerbach 1993).

Early feedings are of great benefit to the breastfeeding pair because oxytocin helps expel the placenta and prevent excessive maternal blood loss; the infant receives the immunologic protection of colostrum; the infant's peristalsis is stimulated, facilitating elimination of the byproducts of bilirubin conjugation, which decreases the risk of jaundice; lactation is accelerated; and maternal-infant attachment is enhanced (Riordan & Auerbach 1993).

It is not unusual for the newborn to regurgitate some mucus, water, or colostrum following a feeding, even if it was taken without difficulty. Consequently, the newborn is observed closely and positioned on the right side after a feeding to aid drainage and facilitate gastric emptying.

Establishing a Feeding Pattern

In the past it was typical to establish artificial, every 3- to 4-hour schedules for feedings after the initial feeding. This scheduling failed to recognize the individual needs of the newborn infant and presented difficulties for the new mother just establishing lactation. Breast milk is rapidly digested by the newborn, who will nurse eight to ten times in a 24-hour period. After the initial period of alertness and eagerness to suckle, the infant progresses to light sleep, then deep sleep, followed by increased wakefulness and interest in nursing. As wakefulness and interest in nursing increase, the infant will often cluster five to ten feeding episodes over 2 to 3 hours, followed by a 4- to 5-hour deep sleep. After this cluster of minifeeds and deep sleep, the infant will feed frequently, but at more regular intervals (Riordan & Auerbach 1993).

Research suggests that maternal medication received during labor may affect newborn feeding behavior by delaying early cluster feedings that usually occur in the initial 1 to 2 days after birth. Delays in normal feeding patterns depend on the specific drug and its half-life. Newborns whose mothers received epidural analgesia have been noted to be irritable and demonstrate reduced motor organization, poor self-quieting skills, and decreased visual skills and alertness (Riordan & Auerbach 1993).

Rooming-in permits the mother to learn about and respond to her infant's early feeding cues. Early cues that indicate a newborn is interested in feeding include hand-to-mouth or hand-passing-mouth motion, whimpering, sucking, and rooting (Mulford 1992). Crying is a late sign of hunger. When rooming-in is not available, a supportive nursing staff and flexible nursery policies will allow

TABLE 30-3	Infant Feeding Behaviors		
Age	**Hunger Behavior**	**Feeding Behavior**	**Satiety Behavior**
Birth to 13 weeks (0–3 months)	Cries; hands fisted; body tense	Rooting reflex; medial lip closure; strong suck reflex; suck-swallow pattern; tongue thrust and retraction; palmomental reflex, gags easily, needs burping	Withdraws head from nipple; falls asleep; hands relaxed; relief of body tension
14–24 weeks (4–6 months)	Eagerly anticipates; grasps and draws bottle or breast to mouth; reaches with open mouth	Aware of hands; generalized reaching; intentional hand to mouth; tongue elevation; lips purse at corners—pucker; shifts food in mouth—prechewing; tongue protrudes in anticipation of nipple; tongue holds nipple firm; tongue projection strong; suck strength increases; coughs and chokes easily; preference for tastes	Tosses head back; fusses or cries; covers mouth with hands; ejects food; distracted by surroundings

SOURCE: Mott S et al: *Nursing Care of Children and Families,* 2nd ed. Redwood City, CA: Addison-Wesley Nursing, 1990, p 155.

the mother to feed her infant on cue. It is very frustrating to a new mother to attempt to feed a newborn who is sound asleep because he or she is either not hungry or exhausted from crying. Table 30–3 can be used to help parents identify their baby's cues for hunger and satiation.

Contrary to popular belief, taking the newborn to a central nursery during the night does not necessarily improve the mother's sleep. In Keefe's (1988) study, mothers whose babies roomed in at night reported sleeping better than those whose babies were in the nursery. Sleeping medication did not significantly improve the mothers' sleep. Research also indicates that babies experience more REM sleep and cry less when rooming-in with the mother at night. Although our society accepts crying as normal and healthy behavior for newborns, it may actually delay the transition to extrauterine life. Crying involves a Valsalva maneuver that results in increased pulmonary vascular pressure, which may cause unoxygenated blood to be shunted into systemic circulation through the foramen ovale and ductus arteriosus. Therefore, it may be advantageous for the baby to be in the room with the mother because she will respond to the baby's needs more quickly than the nursery staff may be able to, resulting in less infant crying.

Formula-fed newborns may awaken for feedings every 2 to 5 hours but are frequently satisfied with feedings every 3 to 4 hours. Because formula is digested more slowly, the bottle-fed infant may go longer between feedings but should not go longer than 4 hours. Babies may begin skipping the night feeding at about 8 to 12 weeks of age (Riordan & Auerbach 1993). This is very individualized, depending on the infant's size and development.

Both breastfed and bottle-fed infants experience growth spurts at certain times and required increased feeding. The mother of a breastfed infant will meet these increased demands by nursing more frequently to increase her milk supply. It will take about 24 hours for the milk supply to increase adequately to meet the new demand (Lawrence 1994). A slight increase in the amount of formula given at each feeding will meet the needs of the formula-fed infant.

Providing nourishment for her newborn is a major concern for the new mother. Her feelings of success or failure may influence her self-concept as she assumes her maternal role. With proper instruction, support, and encouragement from health care providers, feeding becomes a source of pleasure and satisfaction to both parents and infant.

PROMOTION OF SUCCESSFUL INFANT FEEDING

Parents may see the task of feeding their baby as the center of their relationship with the new family member. Whether the mother has chosen to bottle-feed or breast-feed, the nurse can help the mother have a successful experience while in the hospital and during the early days at home. Feeding and caring for newborns may be routine tasks for the nurse, but the success or nonsuccess that a mother achieves the first few times may determine her feelings about herself as an adequate mother.

The newborn's response to caring is an expression of personality. A parent may interpret the newborn's behavior as rejection, which may alter the parent-child relationship. A parent may also interpret the sleepy infant's refusal to suck or inability to retain formula as evidence of his or her incompetence as a parent. The breastfeeding mother may deduce that the newborn does not like her if the baby fails to take her nipple readily. Conversely, infants pick up messages from the muscular tension of those holding them.

A nurse who is sensitive to the needs of the mother can form with her a relationship that permits sharing of knowledge about techniques and emotions connected with feeding. Breastfeeding women frequently express disappointment in the help given to them by birthing unit or hospital nurses, saying they would like more encouragement, support, and practical information about feeding their newborns, especially in the case of early discharge (Renfrew et al 1990). This desire and need also apply to nonnursing mothers. Consistency in teaching by nursing personnel is paramount. A new mother becomes very frustrated if she is shown a number of different methods of feeding her newborn.

The decision by the mother about whether to breast-feed or bottle-feed is usually made by the sixth month of pregnancy and often even before conception. The final decision, however, may not be made until the mother's admission to the birth center. The decision is frequently influenced by relatives, especially the baby's father and maternal grandmother (Littman et al 1994), and by friends and social customs, rather than being based on knowledge about the nutritional and psychologic needs of herself and her newborn.

It is the health care provider's responsibility to provide the parents with accurate information regarding the distinct advantages of breastfeeding to the mother and infant. Many mothers who chose to bottle-feed admit they could have been persuaded to breastfeed if someone had cared enough to tell them how important it is. Parents have a right to hear about the data so they can make their own informed choice (Lawrence 1994). However, as Lawrence (1994, p 212) points out, a sense of balance must be maintained. "It is necessary to appreciate that there are normal women who cannot or will not nurse their babies. Their babies will survive and grow normally." Once an *informed* choice has been made, the nurse's primary responsibility is to support the family's decision and to help the family achieve a positive result. No woman should be made to feel inadequate or superior because of her choice in feeding because positive bonds in parent-child relationships may be developed with either breastfeeding or bottle-feeding.

Preparing To Feed

It is important to teach the mother comfortable positions for feeding her infant and to coach the parents in their responses to their newborn's cues as needed. Before feeding, the mother should be made as comfortable as possi-

ble. Preparations may include voiding, washing her hands, and assuming a position of comfort.

The woman who has had a cesarean birth needs support so that the infant does not rest on her abdomen for long periods of time. When she is breastfeeding, she may be more comfortable lying on her side with a pillow behind her back and one between her legs. The nurse can position the newborn next to the woman's breast and place a rolled towel or small pillow behind the infant for support. The mother will initially need assistance turning from side to side and burping the newborn. She may prefer to breastfeed sitting up with a pillow on her lap and the infant resting on the pillow rather than directly on her abdomen. It may be helpful to place a rolled pillow under the arm supporting the infant's head. An alternative position that avoids pressure on the incision while allowing for maximum visualization of the infant's face is the football hold. See Figure 30–2 for a variety of breastfeeding positions. Bottle-feeding mothers who have undergone cesarean birth frequently use the sitting position also. If incisional pain makes this position difficult, the bottle-feeding mother may also find it helpful to assume the side-lying position. The infant can be positioned in a semisitting position against a pillow close to the mother.

Depending on the newborn's level of hunger, the parents may want to use the time before feeding to get acquainted with their infant. The presence of the nurse during part of this time to answer questions and provide reinforcement of parenting skills will be helpful for the family.

For the sleepy baby a period of playful activity—such as gently rubbing the feet and hands or adjusting clothing and loosening coverings to expose the infant to room air—may increase alertness so that, when the feeding is initiated, the infant is ready and sucks eagerly. If an infant is overly hungry and upset, talking quietly and rocking gently may provide the baby with an opportunity to calm down so that he or she can find and grasp the nipple effectively. After the feeding, when the infant is satisfied and asleep, parents may explore the characteristics unique to their newborn. Routines must be flexible enough to allow this time for the family. Rooming-in offers spontaneous, frequent encounters for the family and provides opportunities to practice handling skills, thereby increasing confidence in care after discharge. It also encourages feeding in response to cues from the baby, rather than feeding by a fixed schedule.

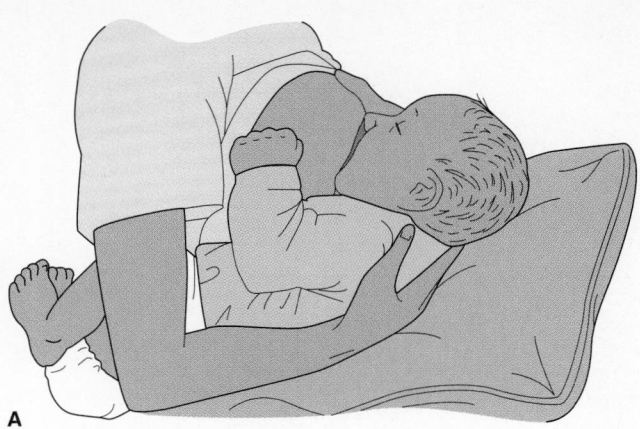

A

- Hold the baby's back and shoulders in the palm of your hand.
- Tuck the baby up under your arm, lining up the baby's lips with your nipple.
- Support the breast to guide it into the baby's mouth.
- Hold your breast until the baby nurses easily.

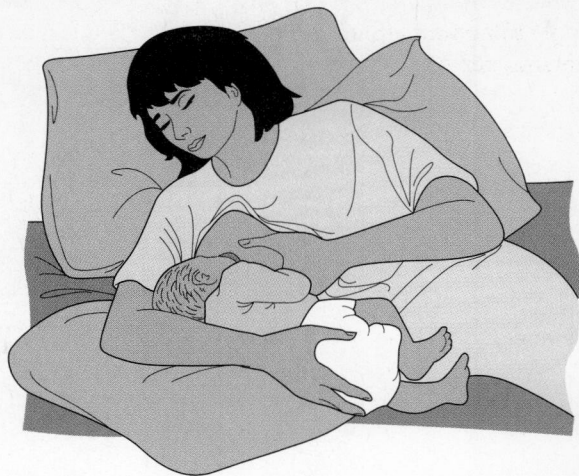

B

- Lie on your side with a pillow at your back and lay the baby so you are facing each other.
- To start, prop yourself up on your elbow and support your breast with the opposite hand.
- Pull the baby close to you, lining up the baby's mouth with your nipple.
- Lie back down once the baby is nursing well.

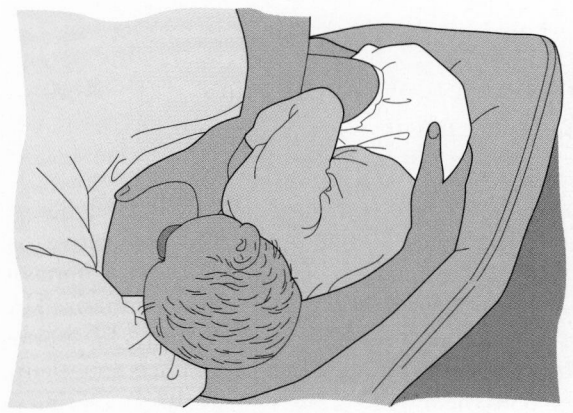

C

- Cradle the baby in the arm closest to the breast, with the baby's head in the crook of the arm.
- Have the baby's body facing you, tummy-to-tummy.
- Use your opposite hand to support the breast.

FIGURE 30-2 Four common breastfeeding positions. *A* Football hold. *B* Lying down. *C* Cradling. *D* Across the lap. SOURCE: *Breastfeeding: A Special Relationship.* Eagle Video Productions, Raleigh, NC. Copyright Lactation Consultants of NC.

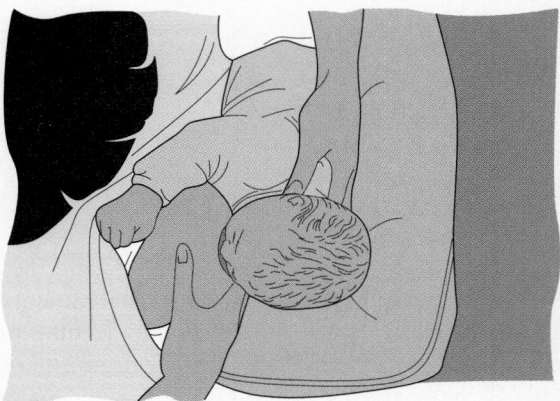

D

- Lay your baby on pillows across your lap.
- Turn the baby facing you.
- Reach across your lap to support the baby's back and shoulders with the palm of your hand.
- Support your breast from underneath to guide it into the baby's mouth.

Cultural Considerations in Infant Feeding

It is important for the nurse to understand how culture and society influence infant feeding. In an industrial society in which mothers pursue activities outside the home and infants go to day care, breastfeeding can be especially challenging. As Lawrence (1994, p 212) states, "The fact that the mother is committed to the infant for 6–12 feed-

ings a day for months is overwhelming to a woman who has been free and independent." Motherhood itself changes the woman's life-style. Perceptions of the mother's role and of breastfeeding as a biologic act also influence the mother's comfort with breastfeeding. In Western cultures the biologic uses of breasts have been downplayed, and the breasts are regarded as sex objects. Some mothers identify shame, modesty, and embarrassment as reasons they chose not to breastfeed. The

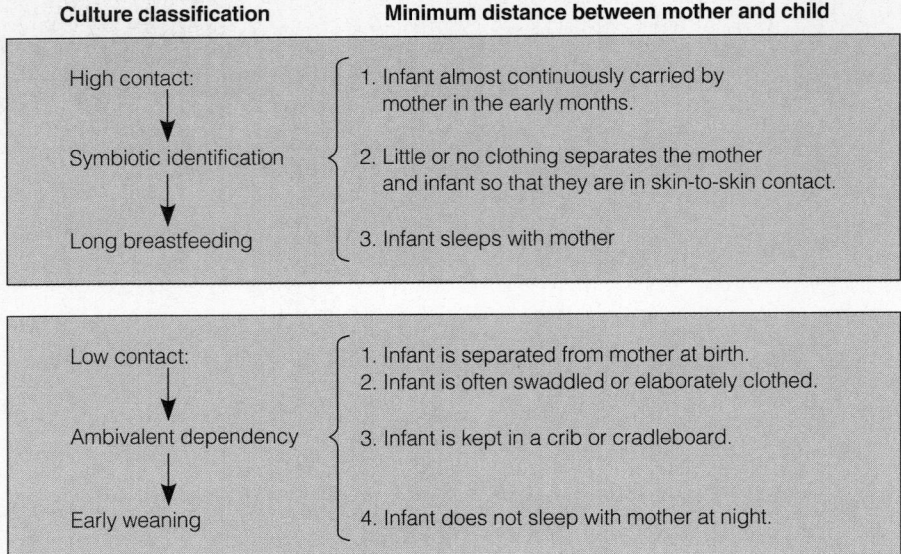

Culture classification	Minimum distance between mother and child
High contact: ↓ Symbiotic identification ↓ Long breastfeeding	1. Infant almost continuously carried by mother in the early months. 2. Little or no clothing separates the mother and infant so that they are in skin-to-skin contact. 3. Infant sleeps with mother
Low contact: ↓ Ambivalent dependency ↓ Early weaning	1. Infant is separated from mother at birth. 2. Infant is often swaddled or elaborately clothed. 3. Infant is kept in a crib or cradleboard. 4. Infant does not sleep with mother at night.

FIGURE 30-3 Culturally determined mother-child body interaction and implications for breastfeeding practices. The amount of contact and degree of closeness between mother and infant is often culturally determined and may influence how long the mother will breastfeed. SOURCE: Lawrence RA: *Breastfeeding: A Guide for the Medical Profession,* 4th ed. St Louis: Mosby, 1994, p 185.

amount of body contact considered acceptable also influences parental behaviors (Figure 30–3). North American and European societies sometimes consider it indecent to expose the breast, believe that too much handling spoils children, and regard weaning as a sign of infant development (Lawrence 1994).

Not only does the nurse need to understand the impact of the culture on the infant feeding method, but also its effects on the idiosyncrasies of specific feeding practices. For example, in many cultures (Mexican American, Navajo, Filipino, and Vietnamese) and in some countries (Guinea, Pakistan) colostrum is not offered to the newborn (Gunnlaugsson et al 1994). Breastfeeding begins only after the milk flow is established. In some Asian cultures the newborn is given boiled water until the mother's milk flows. The newborn is fed on demand and cries are responded to immediately. If the crying continues, evil spirits may be blamed, and a priest's blessing may be sought. Although many of the Hmong women of Laos combine breastfeeding with some bottle-feeding, they find expressing their milk or pumping their breasts unacceptable. Thus other methods of providing relief should be suggested if breast engorgement develops (LaDu 1985). Most Muslim mothers breastfeed because the Qur'an encourages it until the child is 2 years old (Hutchinson & Baqi-Aziz 1994).

When faced with an infant care practice different from the ones to which they are accustomed, nurses need to evaluate the effect of the practice. Just because a practice is different does not mean it is inferior. The nurse should intervene only if the practice is actually harmful to the mother or baby.

Physiology of the Breasts and Lactation

The female breast is divided into 15 to 24 lobes, separated from one another by fat and connective tissue. These lobes are subdivided into lobules, composed of small units called **alveoli** where milk is synthesized by the alveolar secretory epithelium. The lobules have a system of lactiferous ductiles that join larger ducts and eventually open onto the nipple surface (Figure 30–4). During pregnancy increased levels of estrogen stimulate breast duct proliferation and development, and elevated progesterone levels promote the development of lobules and alveoli in preparation for lactation.

Birth results in a rapid drop in estrogen and progesterone with a concomitant increase in the secretion of **prolactin** by the anterior pituitary. This hormone promotes milk production by stimulating the alveolar cells of the breasts. Prolactin levels rise in response to the infant suckling. A mother who smokes cigarettes will have lower prolactin levels than one who does not (Baron et al 1986).

The newborn's suckling also stimulates the release of **oxytocin** from the pituitary. This hormone increases the contractility of the myoepithelial cells lining the walls of the mammary ducts, and a flow of milk results. This is called the **let-down reflex** or milk injection. Mothers have described the let-down reflex as a prickling or tingling sensation during which they feel the milk coming down. Other signs of let-down include increased uterine cramps and increased lochia (during the early postpartum period), milk leaking from the other breast, and a feeling

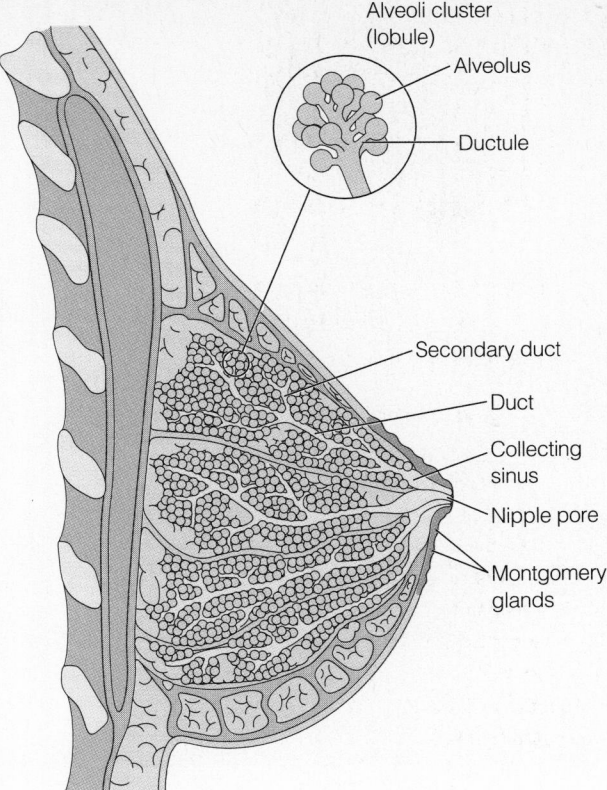

FIGURE 30-4 Structure of the human breast during lactation.

Alveoli cluster (lobule)
Alveolus
Ductule
Secondary duct
Duct
Collecting sinus
Nipple pore
Montgomery glands

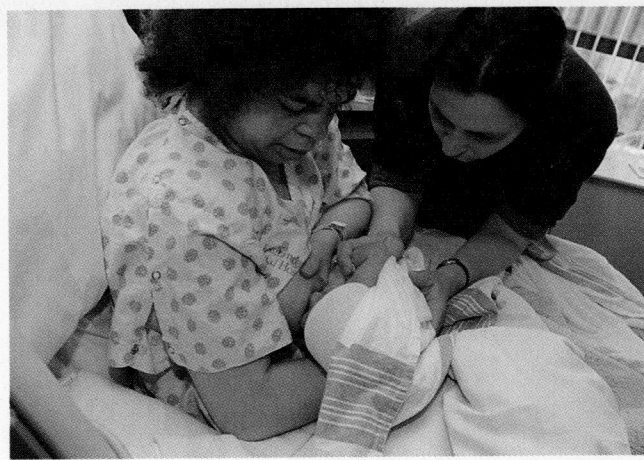

FIGURE 30-5 For many mothers, the nurse's support and knowledge are instrumental in establishing successful breast-feeding.

of relaxation. It is not unusual for the breasts to leak some milk prior to feeding.

The let-down reflex can be stimulated by the new-born's suckling, presence, or cry, or even by maternal thoughts about her baby. It may also occur during sexual orgasm because oxytocin is released. Conversely, the mother's lack of self-confidence, fear of, embarrassment about, or pain connected with breastfeeding may prevent the milk from being ejected into the duct system. Milk production is decreased with repeated inhibition of the milk ejection reflex. Failure to empty the breasts frequently and completely also decreases production because as milk accumulates and is not withdrawn, the buildup of pressure in the alveoli suppresses secretion.

Once lactation is well established, prolactin production decreases. Oxytocin and suckling continue to be the facilitators of milk production.

Client Teaching for Breastfeeding

Breastfeeding Process

The nurse caring for the breastfeeding mother should help the woman achieve independence and success in her feeding efforts (Figure 30–5). Prepared with a knowledge of the anatomy and physiology of the breast and lactation, the components and positive effects of breast milk, and

the techniques of breastfeeding, the nurse can help the woman and her family use their own resources to achieve a successful experience. The objectives of breastfeeding are (1) to provide adequate nutrition, (2) to facilitate maternal-infant attachment, and (3) to prevent trauma to the nipples. All instructions are aimed toward these goals. When assisting the mother with breastfeeding, the nurse should use disposable gloves. (See Essential Precautions in Practice: During Breastfeeding.)

To facilitate successful breastfeeding, the nurse should arrange for privacy, help the mother find a comfortable position, and help position the baby comfortably close to her. The mother should support her breast with

ESSENTIAL PRECAUTIONS IN PRACTICE

DURING BREASTFEEDING

Examples of times when disposable gloves should be worn include the following:

- Assisting the mother to breastfeed the newborn immediately after birth
- Handling breast milk for breast milk banking
- Assisting with manual expression of breast milk
- Handling used breastfeeding pads

Excellent handwashing is essential when assisting a breastfeeding mother.

REMEMBER to wash your hands prior to putting the disposable gloves on and AGAIN immediately after you remove the gloves.

For further information consult OSHA and CDC guidelines.

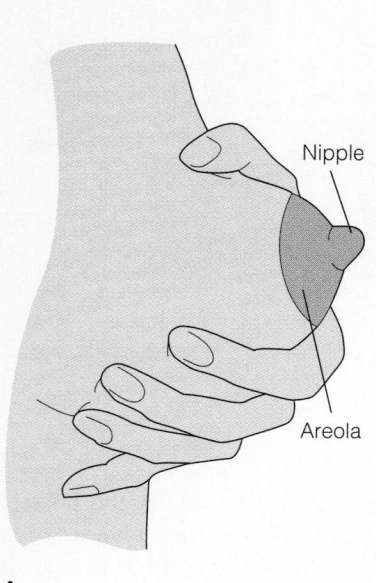

Nipple

Areola

A

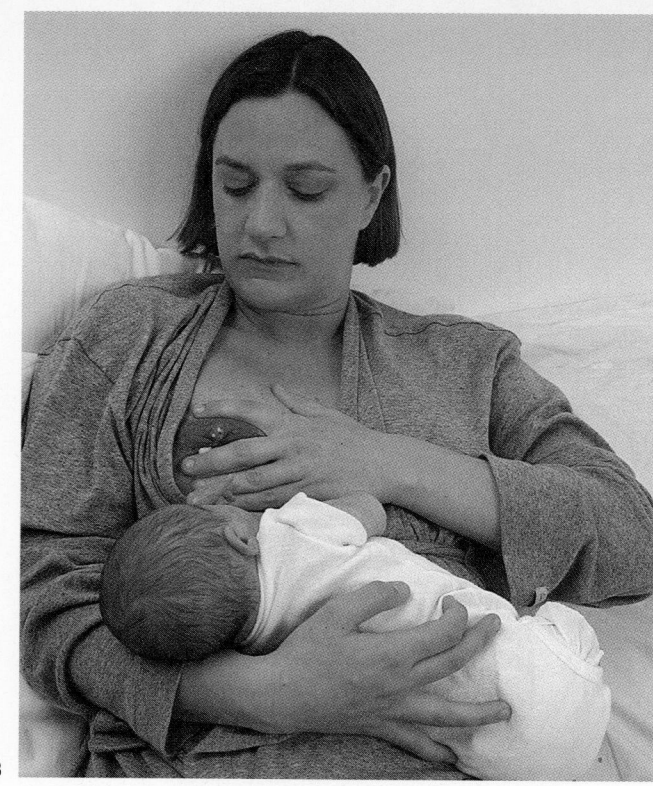

B

FIGURE 30-6   *A* C-hold. (Courtesy Childbirth Graphics Ltd., Rochester, NY) *B* Scissors hold.

her hand, using either the C-hold or the scissors hold. The C-hold is accomplished by placing her thumb well above the areola and the rest of her fingers below the areola and under the breast. The mother may also use the scissors hold, placing her index finger above the areola and her other three fingers below the areola and under the breast. Either method of presenting the breast to the infant is acceptable as long as the hands are well away from the nipple so as not to interfere with the baby's latching to the breast (Lawrence 1994) (Figure 30-6).

The mother should position the baby so that his or her nose is at the level of the nipple. She then lightly tickles the baby's lower lip with her nipple until the baby opens his or her mouth wide. When the baby's mouth is open wide, the mother brings the baby to the breast. The baby needs to take the whole nipple into the mouth so that the gums are on the areola. This allows the jaws to compress the milk ducts directly beneath the areola when the baby suckles (Figure 30–7). The baby's nose and chin should touch the breast. If the breast occludes the baby's airway, simply lifting up on the breast will usually clear the nares. The baby's lips should be relaxed and flanged outward with the tongue over the lower gum. At this point the baby should be facing the mother (tummy to tummy or chest to chest) with the ear, shoulder, and hip aligned (Figure 30–8).

Riordan and Auerbach (1993) state that during these early feedings the infant should be offered both breasts at

each feeding to stimulate the supply-demand response. In some cases the neonate will suckle only one breast well before falling asleep. As long as each breast is offered frequently (at least every 2 hours), single-breast feeds of whatever duration the baby wishes are an appropriate option until the baby shows a desire for both breasts (Woolridge & Baum 1993).

Suggest that the mother feed until she becomes relaxed to the point of sleepiness—a delightful side effect of oxytocin secretion (Mulford 1990)—or until she notes cues from the infant suggesting satiety (suckling activity ceases or the baby falls asleep). The length of the feedings is up to her; she need not watch a clock. Recent literature suggests that imposing time limits for breastfeeding does not prevent nipple soreness and in fact interferes with successful feeding. For example, the length of nursing time necessary to stimulate the milk ejection reflex varies with the individual. If the mother feeds according to the clock and disengages the baby prior to let-down, the baby will not get the hindmilk. Because the hindmilk is higher in fat and calories than the foremilk, the baby will be less satisfied, will need to nurse again sooner, and will gain less weight. The mother should be taught to feed in response to the cues from her baby and her body, not in accordance with an arbitrary time schedule. If the mother wishes to end the feeding before the infant falls asleep or detaches himself or herself, she should break the suction by gently inserting her finger between the baby's gums.

Breastfeeding Assessment

During the birthing unit stay the nurse must carefully monitor the progress of the breastfeeding pair. A systematic assessment of several breastfeeding episodes provides the opportunity to teach the new mother about the lactation and breastfeeding process, provide anticipatory guidance, and evaluate the need for follow-up care after discharge. Criteria for evaluation of a breastfeeding session include maternal and infant cues, latch-on, position, let-down, nipple condition, infant response, and maternal response. The literature provides various tools to guide the assessment and documentation of the breastfeeding efforts. The Mother-Baby Breastfeeding Assessment Tool developed by Chris Mulford is one example (Figure 30–9).

Leaking

Initially, more milk is produced than the infant requires. During the first few weeks, infant needs and maternal responses are not yet well attuned, daily variabilities of feeding frequency and duration are greatest, and most women experience breast leaking. Stimuli that result in let-down or leaking breast milk include hearing a baby cry and thinking about her baby. The mother should be forewarned of this and use breast pads in her bra to absorb the secretions. She should be cautioned to remove wet pads frequently to avoid irritation or infection of the nipples. (Breast pads with plastic liners interfere with air circulation; the plastic should be removed before using them.) The mother may also be taught to stop leakage by applying direct pressure to the breast with her hand or

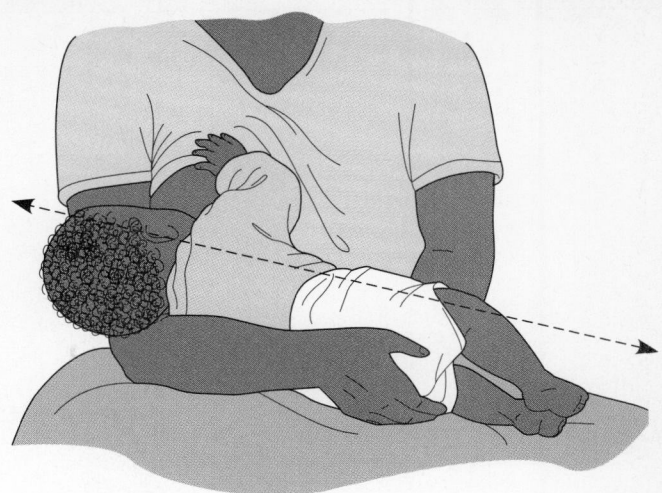

FIGURE 30-8 Infant in good breastfeeding position: tummy-to-tummy; ear, shoulder, and hip aligned. SOURCE: Adapted from Riordan J, Auerbach K: *Breastfeeding and Lactation*. Boston: Jones & Bartlett, 1993, p 248.

forearm once breastfeeding patterns are well established, usually after the first month.

Supplementary Feedings

Using supplementary bottle feedings for the breastfeeding infant may weaken or confuse the suckling reflex or decrease the infant's interest in nursing. To grasp the mother's nipple, the newborn has to open her or his mouth wider than needed to grasp a bottle nipple. The shape of the mouth and lips and the sucking mechanism are also different for sucking the breast and the bottle nipple. While suckling at the breast, the infant's tongue moves in a peristaltic manner from front to back, squeezing the milk from the nipple. While sucking on a rubber nipple, the tongue pushes forward against the nipple to control the milk flow. Some breastfeeding babies who are given supplementary bottles cannot adjust to these different techniques and push the mother's nipple out of their mouth in subsequent breastfeeding attempts. This can be frustrating for both mother and baby. Breastfeeding mothers should avoid introducing bottles until breastfeeding is well established.

Parents are often concerned because they have no visual assurance of the amount of breast milk consumed. The mother should be taught the signs of milk transfer to the infant (ie, audible swallowing, milk appearing in the baby's mouth, her breasts feeling soft after feeding, milk leaking from the opposite breast) (Mulford 1992). In addition, if the infant gains weight and has six or more wet diapers without supplemental feedings of water or formula, he or she is receiving adequate amounts of milk. Parents should know that, because breast milk is more easily digested than formulas, the breastfed infant

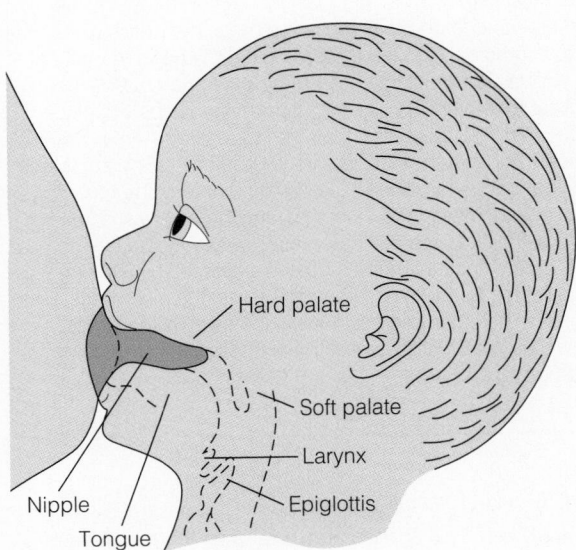

FIGURE 30-7 Baby properly positioned at the breast with good latch-on. Nose is near the breast, gums are on the areola, lips are flanged out, tongue is over the bottom gum. SOURCE: Adapted from Lawrence RA: *Breastfeeding: A Guide for Medical Profession,* 4th ed. St Louis: Mosby, 1994, p 219.

Using the MBA Scoring System

Steps/Points   What to look for criteria

1. Signaling

   1   Mother watches and listens for baby's cues. She may hold, stroke, rock, talk to baby. She stimulates baby if he is sleepy, calms baby if he is fussy.

   1   Baby gives readiness cues; stirring, alertness, rooting, sucking, hand-to-mouth, vocal cues, cry.

2. Positioning

   1   Mother holds baby in good alignment within latch-on range of nipple. Baby's body is slightly flexed, entire ventral surface facing mother's body. Baby's head and shoulders are supported.

   1   Baby roots well at breast, opens mouth wide, tongue cupped and covering lower gum.

3. Fixing

   1   Mother holds her breast to assist baby as needed, brings baby in close when his mouth is wide open. She may express drops of milk.

   1   Baby latches on, takes all of nipple and about 2 cm (1 inch) of areola into mouth, then suckles, demonstrating a recurrent burst-pause sucking pattern.

4. Milk Transfer

   1   Mother reports feeling any of the following: thirst, uterine cramps, increased lochia, breast ache or tingling, relaxation, sleepiness. Milk leaks from opposite breast.

   1   Baby swallows audibly; milk is observed in baby's mouth; baby may spit up milk when burping. Rapid "call-up sucking" rate (two sucks/second) changes to "nutritive sucking" rate of about 1 suck/second.

5. Ending

   1   Mother's breasts are comfortable; she lets baby suckle until he is finished. After nursing, her breasts feel softer; she has no lumps, engorgement, or nipple soreness.

   1   Baby releases breast spontaneously, appears satiated. Baby does not root when stimulated. Baby's face, arms, and hands are relaxed; baby may fall asleep.

   ___
   10

This is an assessment method for rating the progress of a mother and baby who are *learning* to breastfeed.

For every step, each person—both mother and baby—should receive a "+" before either one can be scored on the following step. If the observer does not observe any of the designated indicators, score "0" for that person on that step.

If help is needed at any step for either the mother or the baby, check "Help" for that step. This notation will not change the total score for mother and baby.

A

---

becomes hungry sooner. Thus the frequency of breast-feeding will be greater. The parents may also expect the infant to demand more frequent nursing during growth spurts, such as 10 days to 2 weeks, 5 to 6 weeks, and 2½ to 3 months (Bear & Tigges 1993).

Critical Thinking Question

Mathew and Bhatia (1989) showed that breastfed infants have a prolonged inspiration and shortened expiration during feeding. Bottle-fed infants have prolonged expirations and shortened inspirations as they feed. How do you think these differences influence the practice of supplementing the breastfeeding newborn with formula or water from a bottle?

	M	B	HELP
Signaling	+	+	
Positioning	+	+	✓
Fixing	+		✓
Milk transfer			
Ending			

TOTAL SCORE   _5 w/help_

Example: A mother in hospital calls the nurse into her room 12 hours after birth. Her baby has begun to suck her fists; the mother has picked up her baby, but is unsure what to do next. The nurse helps her position the baby comfortably in the football hold and shows her how to express drops of milk. The baby licks and nuzzles the breast for several minutes, getting many drops of colostrum into her mouth and on her face. Each time she opens her mouth wide, the mother, with the nurse assisting, brings her closer, aiming the nipple at the roof of her mouth. When this happens, the baby gives a few sucks, then pauses, relaxes, closes her eyes and lets go. After each encounter, the mother wakens her by stroking and talking to her; then, when she roots, the mother tries again to help her baby fix. Finally the baby is too sleepy to waken. The mother settles back and relaxes, cuddling the baby in her arms.

B

FIGURE 30-9   Mother-Baby Breastfeeding Assessment Tool (MBA). *A (at left)* This assessment tool rates the progress of a mother and baby who are learning to breastfeed. Both are rated on each of the five steps and given a score of 1 for each behavior they display. The total possible score on this assessment tool is 10. *B* A sample mother-baby assessment using a grid for the MBA scoring system. SOURCE: Mulford C: The mother-baby assessment (MBA): An "Apgar score" for breast-feeding. *J Hum Lact* August 1992; p 81, 82.

Expression of Milk

If the mother who desires to breastfeed is unable to nurse her baby for medical or workplace reasons, she must be taught other means of stimulating milk production and removing milk from her breasts. She may express the milk either manually or with a breast pump. The choice of method may depend on the mother's physiologic capabilities to produce the desired amount of milk and her personal preference. During the early postpartum period, if the baby can't nurse at the breast (as in the case of some premature or sick infants), the mother needs frequent breast stimulation to establish and increase her milk supply to prepare for later breastfeeding (Lawrence 1994). She should use an electric breast pump at least eight times in each 24-hour period (Riordan & Auerbach 1993). Research has shown that a pulsatile electric pump and double setup (allowing both breasts to be stimulated simultaneously) results in higher prolactin levels and a greater volume of milk than does manual expression (Zinaman et al 1992) (Figure 30–10). After lactation is established, milk expression may be accomplished by the method that the mother finds most effective and convenient.

To express her milk manually, the woman washes her hands, then massages her breast to stimulate let-down. To massage her breast, the woman grasps the breast with both hands at the base of the breast near the chest wall. Using the palms of her hands, she firmly slides her hands toward her nipple. She repeats this process several times. Then she is ready to begin hand expression. The woman generally uses her left hand for her right breast and right hand for her left breast. However, some women find it preferable to use the hand on the same side as the breast. The nurse should encourage the woman to use the method she finds most effective. She grasps the areola with her thumb on the top and her first two fingers on the lower portion (Figure 30–11). Without allowing her fingers to slide on her skin, she pushes inward toward the

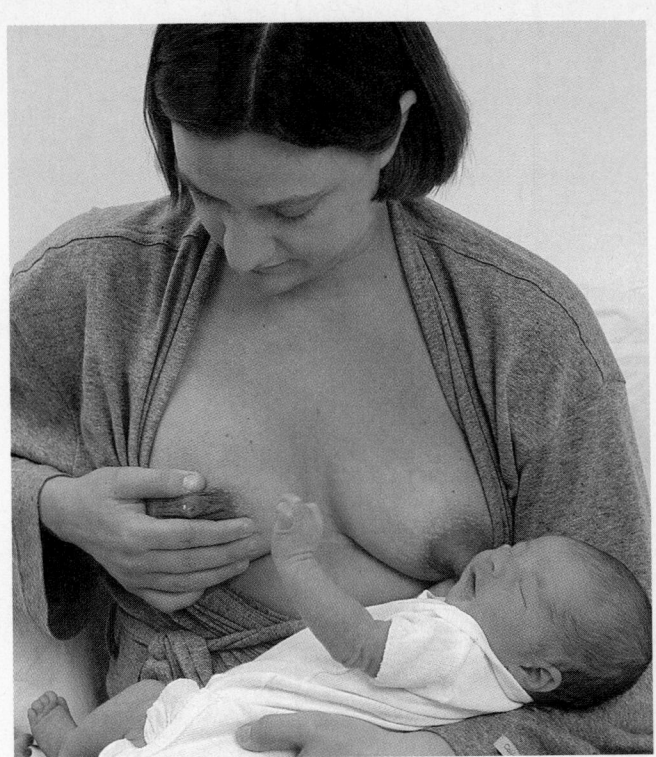

FIGURE 30-11 Hand position for manual expression of milk.

chest and then squeezes her fingers together while pulling forward on the areola. She can use a container to catch any fluid that is squeezed out. She then repositions her hand by rotating it slightly so that she can repeat the process. She continues to reposition her hand and repeat the process to empty all the milk sinuses.

Breast pumps use suction to express the milk. Some have collection systems to conveniently store the milk. Hand pumps are portable and inexpensive. Battery-operated pumps are more efficient than hand pumps but are also more expensive. Electric pumps are the most efficient but are bulky and expensive; however, they may be rented in many areas. Many agencies have a variety of pumps available and provide instruction on correct use (Figure 30–12). Videotapes or photographs are also useful in demonstrating the process to new mothers. (Table 30–4.)

Storing Breast Milk

Breast milk has bacteriostatic qualities because of the presence of IgA and IgG antibodies, which retard bacterial growth. It may be stored for up to 6 hours at room temperature or up to 5 days in a refrigerator. If breast milk is to be refrigerated and then fed to the infant, it should be stored in clean plastic containers because the white blood cells will adhere to glass, and their protective effect will be lost. Breast milk may be frozen in either glass or plastic because freezing destroys the white blood

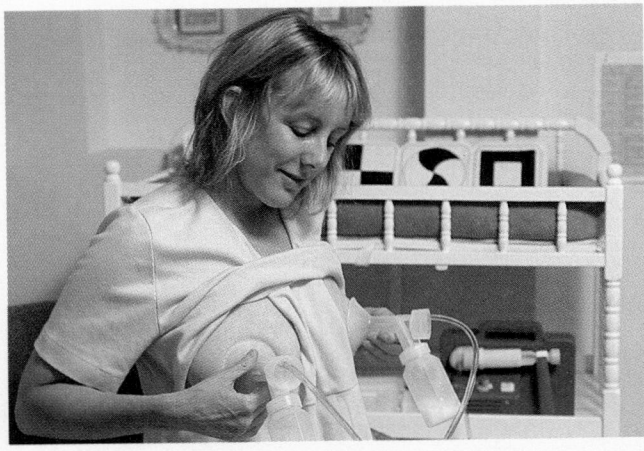

FIGURE 30-10 Mother using electric breast pump and double setup.

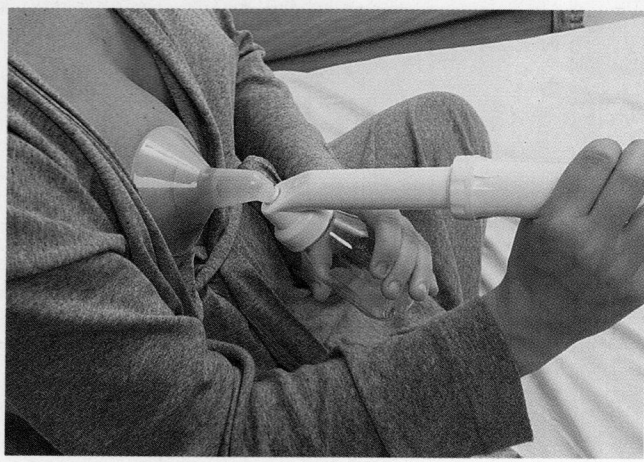

FIGURE 30-12 A mother expresses milk with her Kaneson hand pump.

cells anyway. Breast milk may be stored in a freezer compartment inside the refrigerator for up to 2 weeks, in a self-contained freezer unit of a refrigerator up to 1 month, and in a separate deep freeze unit at 0 degrees up to 6 months. Frozen breast milk can be thawed by running warm water over the container. The container should then be shaken well to return to suspension the fat molecules that separate during freezing.

External Supports

Childbirth and the beginning of motherhood are a critical time in a woman's life. So physical, psychologic, and social supports are of paramount importance. The father or other partner is the most important support person, and the baby can also provide some support in the form of positive feedback. However, with the evolution of an industrial society and the resulting nuclear family, more ex-

---

TABLE 30-4	Recommendations for the Nursing Mother Who Uses a Pump

General Pumping Recommendations

1. Read the instructions on the use and cleaning of a pump before expressing milk with any product.

2. Hands should be washed before each pumping session.

3. Frequency: For occasional pumping, pump during, after, or between feedings, whichever gives the best results. Most mothers tend to express more milk in the morning. For working mothers pumping should occur on a regular basis for the number of nursings that are missed. For premature or ill babies who are not at breast the number of pumpings should total eight or more in 24 hours. Initiation of pumping should be delayed no longer than 6 hours following birth unless medically indicated. This assures appropriate development and sensitivity of prolactin receptors. More frequent pumping will avoid the buildup of excessive back pressure of milk during engorgement.

4. Duration: With single-sided pumping optimal duration is 10 to 15 minutes with an electric pump and 10 to 20 minutes with a manual pump. If double pumping with an electric or two battery-operated pumps, 7 to 15 minutes is optimal. Encourage mothers to tailor these times to their own situation.

5. Technique:
   • Elicit the milk ejection reflex before using any pump.
   • Use only as much suction as is needed to maintain milk flow.
   • Massage the breast in quadrants during pumping to increase intramammary pressure.
   • Allow enough time for pumping to avoid anxiety.
   • Use inserts or different flanges if needed to obtain the best fit between pump and breast.
   • Avoid long periods of uninterrupted vacuum.
   • Stop pumping when the milk flow is minimal or has ceased.

Recommendations for Specific Types of Pumps

1. Avoid pumps that use rubber bulbs to generate vacuum.

2. Cylinder pumps:
   • When "O" rings are used, they must be in place for proper suction.
   • Gaskets must be removed *after each use* for cleaning to avoid harboring bacteria in the pump.
   • The gasket on the inner cylinder may be rolled back and forth to restore it to its original shape.
   • The pump stroke may need to be shortened as the outer cylinder fills with milk.
   • The user may need to empty the outer cylinder once or twice during pumping.
   • Hand position should be palm up with the elbow held close to the body.

3. Battery-operated pumps:
   • Use alkaline batteries.
   • Replace batteries when cycles per minute decrease.
   • Interrupt vacuum frequently to avoid nipple pain and damage.
   • Use an AC adapter when possible, especially if the pump generates fewer than six cycles per minute.
   • Consider renting an electric pump for pumping that will continue for longer than 1 or 2 months.
   • Use two pumps simultaneously if pumping time is limited or to increase the quantity of milk obtained.
   • Choose a pump in which the vacuum can be regulated.
   • Massage the breast by quadrants during pumping.

4. Semiautomatic pumps:
   • Vacuum may be easier to control if the mother does not lift her finger completely off the hole but rolls it back and forth rhythmically so that the vacuum is efficient but not painful.

5. Automatic electric pumps:
   • Use the lowest pressure setting that is efficient.
   • Use a double setup (simultaneous pumping) when time is limited to increase the milk supply and for prematurity, maternal or infant illness, or other special situations.

SOURCE: Riordan J, Auerbach K: *Breastfeeding and Human Lactation.* Boston: Jones & Bartlett, 1993, p 283.

tensive family support systems have diminished. Mothers, sisters, and other females who could mentor and care for the new mother are frequently not available. As evidenced by the frequent discontinuation of breastfeeding in the early postpartum weeks, there is a need for assistance and follow-up in this area. Also, in an industrialized society where women work outside the home and early weaning is commonplace, ongoing support is necessary (Fendrick et al 1994; Lawrence 1994).

Nurses, dietitians, childbirth educators, certified nurse-midwives, lactation consultants, mother-to-mother support groups, and physicians must collaborate to provide consistent, timely information and support and to attend to the new mother's special needs. Breastfeeding mothers who work outside the home and who receive support for their decision tend to breastfeed their infants for longer periods of time (Fendrick et al 1994).

La Leche League International is an organized group of volunteers who work to provide education about breastfeeding and assistance to women who are breastfeeding. Organized as small, neighborhood-based groups, it sponsors activities, has printed material available, has electric breast pumps available for rental, offers one-to-one counseling to mothers with questions or problems, and provides group support to breastfeeding mothers.

Lactation consultants offer a wide range of services through private practice and health care facilities. There is a variety of lactation education programs available with differing prerequisites and objectives. Numerous books, pamphlets, and educational videos are available to help the breastfeeding mother. The mother needs the support of all family members, her certified nurse-midwife/physician, pediatrician or certified nurse-practitioner, and all nursing personnel because it is often the attitudes of these people that ultimately lead the woman to success or failure at breastfeeding her baby.

Drugs and Breastfeeding

As Riordan and Auerbach (1993) point out, there are three "knows" about drugs and human milk. First, most drugs pass into breast milk. Second, almost all medications appear in only small amounts in human milk—usually less than 1% of the maternal dosage. Third, very few drugs are contraindicated for breastfeeding women. Concerns about the consequences of the presence of drugs in breast milk focus on the effect on the infant and on the milk volume.

Characteristics of the drug that influence its passage into breast milk include the following:

1. *Degree of protein binding.* Unbound drugs are most likely to enter the breast milk.

2. *Degree of ionization.* Drugs tend to cross into breast milk in un-ionized form.

3. *Molecular weight.* Drugs with a molecular weight greater than 200 will not cross into breast milk.

4. *Degree of solubility in fat and water.* Alveolar epithelium is a lipid barrier with water-filled pores, but colostrum makes epithelium more permeable to lipid-soluble drugs.

5. *Mechanism of transport.* Drugs enter breast milk by active transport, simple diffusion, or carrier-mediated diffusion.

6. *The pH.* Breast milk, which is acidic, attracts drugs that are weak bases.

7. *Half-life.* Rates of absorption, metabolism, and excretion determine a drug's half-life, or how fast it leaves the body. The longer the half-life, the greater the risk of accumulation in tissues.

8. *Milk/plasma ratio.* The higher the **milk/plasma ratio,** the higher the drug concentration in the breast milk compared to the drug concentration in the plasma. An M/P ratio of 1.0 indicates that the milk and plasma contain equal concentrations of the drug. An M/P ratio of less than 1.0 indicates that the concentration of the drug in the milk is lower than its plasma concentration, whereas an M/P ratio greater than 1.0 indicates the drug's concentration in milk is greater than in plasma.

Other variables that affect the passage of drugs into breast milk include the amount of the drug taken, the frequency and route of administration, and the timing of the dose in relationship to infant feeding. The drug's effects are influenced by the infant's age, the feeding frequency, the volume of milk taken, and the degree of absorption through the gastrointestinal tract.

Four adjustments should be made when administering drugs to a nursing mother to decrease the effects on the infant (Lawrence 1994):

1. Long-acting forms of drugs should be avoided. The infant may have difficulty metabolizing and excreting them, and accumulation may be a problem.

TABLE 30-5   Breastfeeding Problems and Remedies

Nipples Not Graspable

Flat or inverted nipples

- Use Hoffman technique to break adhesions.
- Wear milk cups to encourage nipples to protrude.
- Use nipple tug and roll to increase protractility.
- Form the nipple prior to nursing by hand shaping, ice, wearing milk cups a half-hour before feeding.
- As a last resort, use nipple shield for first few minutes of feeding to draw out nipple; then place baby on breast.

Engorged breasts

- Treat engorgement by relieving fullness with hand expression of milk prior to nursing and instituting frequent feeding so nipple is more prominent.

Large breasts

- Support breast with opposite hand, or use rolled towel under breast to bring nipple to the level of baby's mouth.
- Use C-hold to make nipple accessible to baby.

Engorgement

Missed or infrequent feedings

- Nurse frequently (every $1\frac{1}{2}$ hours).
- Massage and hand express or pump to empty breasts completely when feedings are missed or when a full feeling develops in breasts and baby is not available or willing to nurse.

Breasts not emptied at feedings

- Nurse long enough to empty breasts (10–15 minutes on each side at each feeding).
- If baby will not nurse long enough to empty breasts, hand express or pump after feeding.

Inadequate let-down

- Use relaxation techniques, massage, and warm or cool compresses before nursing.
- Relax in warm shower with water running from back over shoulders and breasts, hand expressing to relieve fullness.
- If due to anxiety, try to eliminate the source of tension.

Baby sleepy or not eager to nurse

- Use rousing techniques (eg, hold baby upright, unwrap blanket, change diaper).
- Pre-express milk onto nipple or baby's lips to entice baby.
- Avoid use of bottles of water or formula; these will decrease baby's willingness to suckle.

Inadequate Let-Down

Let-down not well established

- Give the baby ample time at the breast (at least 15 minutes per side) to allow for let-down and complete emptying.
- Nurse in a quiet spot away from distractions.
- Massage breasts before nursing.
- Drink juice, water, tea (no caffeine) before and during nursing.
- Condition let-down by setting up a routine for beginning feedings.
- Use relaxation and breathing techniques.
- Stimulate the nipple manually before nursing.
- Concentrate thought on the baby and milk flow; turn on a faucet so that the sound of running water helps stimulate let-down.
- Use synthetic oxytocin nasal spray several times during a feeding. (This should condition let-down within 24 hours. Then it is no longer needed. Spray must be prescribed by a doctor.)

Mother overtired or overextended

- Nap or rest when the baby rests.
- Lie down to nurse.
- Nurse the baby in bed at night.
- Simplify daily chores; set priorities.

Mother tense, pressured

- Identify the causes of tensions and eliminate or minimize them.
- Decrease fatigue.

Mother caught in cycle of little milk, worry, less milk

- Try all the actions above.
- Develop confidence in mothering skills. (A home visit by a counselor may help.)

Cracked Nipples

All causes of sore nipples carried to extreme

- Refer to all actions for sore nipples.
- Consult doctor about using aspirin, Tylenol, or other painkiller.
- Improve nutritional status, increasing protein, vitamin C, zinc.

Local infection (baby with staph or other organism may have infected mother's nipples)

- Refer to physician.

Plugged Ducts

Poor positioning

- Try a variety of positions for complete emptying.

Incomplete emptying of breast

- Nurse at least 10 minutes per side after let-down.
- Alternate nursing positions.
- If baby does not empty breasts, pump or express milk after feedings.

External pressure on breast

- Use larger size bras, insert bra extender, or go braless.
- Use nursing bra instead of pulling up conventional bra to nurse to avoid pressure on ducts.
- Avoid bunching up sweater or nightgown under arm during nursing.

Sore Nipples

Poor positioning

- Alternate nursing positions throughout the day.
- Bring the baby close to nurse so the baby does not pull on the breast.
- Place the nipple and some of the areola in the baby's mouth.
- Check to ensure the baby is put on and off the breast properly.
- Check to ensure the nipple is back far enough in the baby's mouth.
- Hold the baby closely during nursing so the nipple is not constantly being pulled.

Baby chewing or nuzzling onto nipple

- Form the nipple for the baby.
- Set up a pattern of getting the baby onto the breast using the rooting reflex.

Baby nursing on end of nipple

- Ensure the nipple is way back in the baby's mouth by getting the baby properly onto the breast.
- Check for an inverted nipple.
- Check for engorgement.

Baby chewing his or her way off the nipple (nipple being pulled out of baby's mouth at end of feeding)

- Remove the baby from the breast by placing a finger between the baby's gums to ensure suction is broken.
- End feeding when the baby's suckling slows, before he or she has a chance to chew on the nipple.

| **TABLE 30-5** | continued |

Sore Nipples (cont)

Baby overly eager to nurse

- Nurse more often.
- Pre-express milk to hasten let-down, avoiding vigorous suckling.

Dry colostrum or milk causing nipple to stick to bra or breast pads

- Moisten bra or pads before taking off so as not to remove keratin.

Nipples not allowed to dry

- Remove plastic liners from milk pads.
- Air dry breast completely after nursing.
- Change milk pads frequently.

Improper use of breast shield

- Use shield only to draw out nipple; then have the baby nurse on the breast.
- Cut tip of shield back bit by bit and eventually discard.

Nipple skin not resistant to stress

- Improve diet, especially adding fresh fruits and vegetables and vitamin supplements.
- Eliminate or decrease use of sugary foods, alcohol, caffeine, cigarettes.
- Check use of cleansing or drying agents.

Natural oils removed or keratin layers broken down by drying agents (soap, alcohol, shampoo, deodorant)

- Eliminate irritants.
- Wash breasts with water only.

SOURCE: Adapted from Lauwers J, Woessner C: *Counseling the Nursing Mother: A Reference Handbook for Health Care Providers and Lay Counselors*, 2nd ed. Garden City Park, NY: Avery, 1990, pp 385–397.

2. Absorption rates and peak blood levels should be considered in scheduling the administration of the drugs. Less of the drug crosses into the milk if the medication is given immediately after the woman has nursed her baby.

3. The infant should be closely observed for any signs of drug reaction, including rash, fussiness, lethargy, or changes in sleeping habits or feeding pattern.

4. Whenever alternatives are available, the drug that shows the least tendency to pass into breast milk should be selected.

The mother should be given information about the potential of most drugs to cross into breast milk (American Academy of Pediatrics Committee on Drugs 1994). She should also be advised to tell any physician who may prescribe medications for her that she is breastfeeding.

The effect of maternal medication on milk volume is also a concern for the breastfeeding mother. Barbiturates, antihistamines, diuretics, ergot alkaloids (Parlodel), and oral contraceptives high in estrogen generally decrease milk output. Some psychotherapeutic drugs increase the milk supply (Riordan & Auerbach 1993).

In counseling the nursing mother, the health care provider should weigh the benefits of the medication against the possible risk to the infant and its possible effects on the breastfeeding process. The potential risk to the infant must also be weighed against the effect of interrupting breastfeeding.

Selected Potential Problems in Breastfeeding

Many of the "problems" of breastfeeding are normal phenomena that are perceived as problems or become problems due to mismanagement. Because mothers are discharged from the hospital before breastfeeding is well established, they are frequently alone when they encounter many changes in the breastfeeding process. Many women stop nursing if the situations they encounter seem problematic. Nurses can offer anticipatory guidance regarding common breastfeeding phenomena and provide resources for the woman's use after discharge. A summary of potential problems, their causes, and appropriate interventions is provided in Table 30–5, and these are described in more detail in the following sections.

Flat or Inverted Nipples   If the mother does not have a prominent nipple or if she has an inverted nipple, she may try rolling the nipple between her thumb and forefinger or stretching it by pressing inward and outward around the nipple prior to feeding (Hoffman's technique). Breast shells, or milk cups, are hard, formed plastic that fits over the nipple, causing it to protrude (Figure 30–13). The mother wears the shells prenatally and between feedings so that the nipple is more prominent at the beginning of the feeding. Use of an electric breast pump will quickly stimulate the nipple to become more prominent, and when a few drops of colostrum are expressed, the infant becomes more eager to latch on.

The use of a traditional red rubber nipple shield after the baby's birth to correct nipple position may reduce the transfer of milk from the breast to the infant by 58% while increasing the infant's suck effort and rate, thereby increasing the time the baby needs to rest during the feeding. New thin latex shields do not affect sucking patterns, but they reduce milk transfer by 22% (Lawrence 1994). A shield should be used as a last resort and preferably after consultation with a lactation expert. Any rubber or artificial nipple is more pliable than the breast and thus allows more milk to pass through it per suck. As a result of the different milking actions required, the infant may experience "nipple confusion" and refuse the breast when it is offered again (Lawrence 1994).

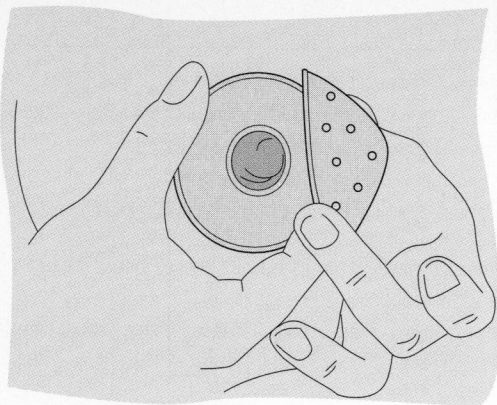

FIGURE 30-13   Breast shells can help correct flat or inverted nipples. SOURCE: Courtesy Medela, Inc: *Breastfeeding Information Guide.* McHenry, IL, p 5.

Breast Engorgement   A distinction should be made between breast fullness and engorgement. All lactating women experience a transient fullness at first. This is caused by venous congestion and later by accumulating milk. However, this generally lasts only 24 hours, the breasts remain soft enough for the newborn to suckle, and there is no pain. Engorged breasts are hard, painful, and appear taut and shiny. In this case nursing is difficult for the infant and painful for the mother. Engorgement occurs when breastfeeding is delayed or restricted in duration or frequency.

The infant should suckle for an average of 15 minutes per feeding and should feed at least eight times in 24 hours (Riordan & Auerbach 1993). If the baby is unable to nurse more frequently, the mother may express some milk manually or with a pump, being careful not to traumatize the breast tissue. Warm or cool compresses before nursing stimulate let-down and soften the breast so that the infant can more easily grasp the areola. The mother should be encouraged to wear a well-fitting nursing bra 24 hours a day. The bra supports the breasts and prevents further discomfort from tension and pulling on the Cooper's ligament. Analgesics such as acetaminophen or aspirin, alone or in combination with codeine, are appropriate, especially if taken just prior to nursing. The pain will be relieved, but the medication will not reach the milk for at least 30 minutes (Lawrence 1994). An additional relief measure may include cultivated South African cabbage leaves, which have proven successful when placed on engorged breasts. Nikodem and colleagues (1993), using a small sample of breastfeeding women, found that cabbage leaves helped with breast engorgement, enabling the women to continue breastfeeding exclusively for a longer time.

Nipple Soreness   The mother should be made aware that often some discomfort occurs initially with breast-feeding, peaking between the third and sixth days, and then receding (Riordan & Auerbach 1993). The discomfort normally results from the negative pressure on the relatively empty ductules in the breast and the stretching of the nipple. The infant should not be switched to bottle-feeding or have feedings delayed. These measures will only cause engorgement and more soreness. Discomfort that lasts throughout the feeding or past the first week demands attention.

The baby's position at the breast is one of the most critical factors in nipple soreness. The mother's hand should be off the areola, and the baby should be facing the mother's chest with ear, shoulder, and hip aligned (see Figure 30–8).

Because the area of greatest stress to the nipple is in line with the newborn's chin and nose, nipple soreness may be decreased by encouraging the mother to rotate positions when feeding the infant. (Figure 30–2 illustrates four common breastfeeding positions.) Changing position alters the focus of greatest stress and promotes more complete breast emptying.

Nipple soreness may also develop if the infant has faulty sucking habits. Nipples may be bruised, scabbed, or blistered from the nipple entering the baby's mouth at an upward angle and rubbing against the roof of the mouth (Lawrence 1994). Soreness may also develop due to continuous negative pressure if the infant falls asleep with the breast in his or her mouth (Ziemer et al 1990).

Nipples may be chewed if they are improperly positioned, leading to cracking or tenderness at or near the base. In these cases the baby's jaws close only on the nipple instead of the areola, or the baby's mouth is not opened wide enough, or the infant's mouth has slipped down to the nipple from the areola as a result of engorgement. Soreness on the underside of the nipple is caused by the infant nursing with her or his bottom lip tucked in rather than out, causing a friction burn. Vigorous sucking produces little milk because the milk sinuses under the areola are not compressed. This results in a frustrated infant and marked soreness for the mother. The problem is overcome by positioning the infant with as much areola as possible in his or her mouth and rotating the baby's positions at the breast.

Nipple soreness is especially pronounced during the first few minutes of the feeding. If the mother is not expecting this, she may become discouraged and quickly stop. The let-down reflex may take a few minutes to activate, and it may not occur if the mother stops nursing too quickly. The problem is compounded if the infant is unsatisfied, and the possibility of breast engorgement increases.

Because nipple soreness can also result from an overeager infant, the mother may find it helpful to nurse more frequently. This helps ease the vigorous sucking of a ravenous infant. The woman can also apply ice to her nipples and areola for a few minutes prior to feeding.

This promotes nipple erectness and numbs the tissue to ease the initial discomfort.

To prevent excoriation and skin breakdown, the nipples and areola should be washed with water and then allowed to dry thoroughly. Drying may be accomplished by leaving the bra flaps down for several minutes after feeding or by exposing the nipples to sunlight or ultraviolet light for 30 seconds at first and gradually increasing to 3 minutes. Drying the nipples with a hair dryer on low heat setting also facilitates drying and promotes healing, especially if breast milk is allowed to dry on the nipples (Lawrence 1994).

The use of substances such as lanolin, Massé breast cream, Eucerin cream, or A and D ointment on the nipples between feedings should be discouraged. These preparations may cause allergic reactions, or irritation may be increased if the substance needs to be washed off prior to nursing. The substance may contain irritants that plug sebaceous and Montgomery glands of the areola and nipple. Environmental conditions also affect how ointments act; for example, in high humidity areas greasy, moisture-sealing ointments aggravate the skin. In very dry environments creams may well be appropriate. Lanolin is most hazardous to women with wool allergy (Lawrence 1994). Lansinoh is a purified, alcohol-free, and "allergen-free" ointment that is considered safe if an ointment is indicated.

Alternatively, rapid healing has been demonstrated by the application of breast milk, which is then allowed to dry on the nipples (Renfrew et al 1990). Breast milk is high in fat, fights infection, and will not irritate the nipples. An obvious advantage is that it is readily available at no cost to the mother.

If the woman finds that her bra or clothing rubs against her nipples and adds to her discomfort, she may insert shields into her bra to prevent this. Both Medela shells and Woolrich shields, for example, relieve friction and promote air circulation. If a woman uses breast pads inside her bra to keep milk from leaking onto her clothes, the pads should be changed frequently so the nipples remain dry.

Older remedies for nipple soreness are receiving renewed acceptance. For instance, tea bags may be moistened in warm water and applied to the nipples. The tannic acid seems to help toughen the nipples, and the warmth is soothing and promotes healing. However, tannic acid can cause drying and cracking and so is not appropriate in all situations (Lawrence 1994).

Nipple dermatitis causes swollen, erythematous, burning nipples. It is most commonly caused by thrush or by allergic response to breast creams. If the nipple soreness has a sudden onset, accompanied by burning or itching, shooting pains through the breast, and a deep pink coloration of the nipple, it may be caused by a thrush infection transmitted from the infant. White patches or streaks in the infant's mouth indicate a need for treatment of the mouth and nipple infection. The disease can be treated with a variety of antifungal preparations and does not preclude breastfeeding.

Cracked Nipples   Nipple soreness is frequently coupled with cracked nipples. Whenever a breastfeeding mother complains of soreness, the nipples must be carefully examined for fissures or cracks, and the mother should be observed during breastfeeding to see whether the infant is correctly positioned at the breast and latched onto the nipple. If the positioning is correct but cracks exist, further interventions are necessary. The mother's first reaction may be to cease nursing on the sore breast, but this may aggravate the problem if engorgement and plugged ducts result. All the interventions described for sore nipples may be used. It may also help the mother to begin nursing sessions using the breast that is less sore. This allows the let-down reflex to occur in the affected breast, and the infant does more vigorous sucking on the less tender breast, which decreases trauma to the cracked nipple. With severe cases, the temporary use of a nipple shield for nursing may be appropriate. For the mother's comfort analgesics may be taken after nursing.

Plugged Ducts   Some mothers experience plugging of one or more ducts, especially in conjunction with or following engorgement. This is often referred to as caked breasts. Manifested as an area of tenderness or "lumpiness" in an otherwise well woman, plugging may be relieved by the use of heat and massage. The mother can be encouraged to massage her breasts from her chest wall forward to the nipple while standing in a warm shower or following the application of hot packs to the breast (Riordan & Auerbach 1993). She should then nurse her infant, starting on the unaffected breast if the plugged breast is tender. Frequent nursing and trying a variety of positions to ensure complete emptying will help prevent the problem. In cases of repeatedly plugged ducts or caked breasts, it may be necessary for the mother to limit her fat intake to polyunsaturated fats and to add lecithin to her diet (Lawrence 1994).

Breastfeeding and the Working Mother

A 1992 study estimated that 57.8% of working women will have children who are between 6 months and 3 years of age (Ross Laboratories 1993). Women work because today's economy demands it and because often our society does not perceive childrearing as productive. The employer, by virtue of maternity leave policy, determines how long the mother is home with her new baby. The best preparation for maintaining lactation after return to work is frequent, unlimited breastfeeding and enjoying the baby. Even when planned, the first day back to work may be fraught with emotional and physical distresses (Riordan & Auerbach 1993). Anticipatory guidance from the nurse may facilitate the transition from maternity leave to work.

The earlier the breastfeeding mother returns to work, the more often she will need to pump her breasts to express the breast milk (Riordan & Auerbach 1993). Because milk production follows the principle of supply and demand, if breasts are not pumped, the milk supply will decrease. An electric breast pump and double collection system are considered the optimal means of milk expression. But this is not the only method; mechanical means may not suit some women (Neifert 1989).

Sometimes a mother has a flexible schedule and can return home to nurse at lunchtime or have the baby brought to her. If this is not possible, the infant may be fed expressed milk. For proper storage of breast milk, see Storing Breast Milk earlier in this chapter. While the mother is absent, the infant can be bottle-fed or spoon-fed. If the baby is 3 months or older, cup-feeding is an option. The mother should wait until lactation is well established before introducing the bottle. Most babies will adjust to the bottle within 7–10 days (Riordan & Auerbach 1993).

To maintain an adequate milk supply, the working mother must pay special attention to her fluid intake. She can ensure an adequate intake by drinking extra fluid at each break whenever possible during the day. In addition it is helpful to nurse more on weekends, to nurse during the night, to eat a nutritionally sound diet, and to continue manual expression or pumping when not nursing (Neifert 1989).

Night nursing presents a dilemma in that it may help a working mother maintain her milk supply but may also contribute to fatigue. Some women choose to have the infant sleep with them so that breastfeeding is more easily accomplished. If a woman finds it difficult to sleep soundly when the infant is in the same bed, she might put the crib in her room. Another alternative is to limit breastfeeding to the morning and evening, with supplemental feeding at other times. Pinella and Birch (1993) studied how the use of focal feeds (feeding between 10 PM to midnight) and the teaching of parents how to help their babies develop self-soothing activities can help with sleeping for longer intervals at night.

Weaning

The decision to wean the baby from the breast may be made for a variety of reasons, including family or cultural pressures, change in the home situation, pressure from the woman's partner, or a personal opinion about when **weaning** should occur (Weigley 1990). For the woman who is comfortable with breastfeeding and well-informed about the process the appropriate time to wean her infant will become evident if she is sensitive to the child's cues. Often weaning falls between periods of great developmental activity for the child. Thus weaning commonly occurs at 8 to 9 months, 12 to 14 months, 18 months, 2 years, or 3 years of age. Within our society, however, weaning commonly occurs before the child is 9 months old, although it may occur any time from soon after birth to 4 years of age (Barness 1990).

If weaning is timed to respond to the child's cues and if the mother is comfortable with the timing, it can be accomplished with less difficulty than if the process is begun before both mother and child are ready emotionally. Nevertheless, weaning is a time of emotional separation for mother and baby; it may be difficult for them to give up the closeness of their nursing sessions. The nurse who is understanding about this possibility can help the mother see that her infant is growing up and plan other comforting, consoling, and play activities to replace breastfeedings. A gradual approach is the easiest and most comforting way to wean the child from breastfeeding. Other activities can enhance the parent-infant attachment process.

During weaning the mother should substitute one cup-feeding or bottle-feeding for one breastfeeding session over several days to a week so that her breasts gradually produce less milk. Eliminating the breastfeedings associated with meals first facilitates the mother's ability to wean the infant as satiation with food lessens the desire for milk. Over a period of several weeks she should substitute more cup-feedings or bottle-feedings for breastfeedings. Many mothers continue to nurse once a day in the early morning or late evening for several months until the milk supply is gone. The slow method of weaning prevents breast engorgement, allows infants to alter their eating methods at their own rates, and allows time for psychologic adjustment.

Client Teaching for Bottle-Feeding

With the great emphasis placed on successful breastfeeding, the teaching needs of the bottle-feeding new mother may be overlooked. If she has had only limited experience in feeding infants, she may need some guidelines to feed her newborn successfully. The following important principles should be included in the teaching provided:

1. Bottles should always be held, not propped. Positional otitis media may develop when the infant is fed horizontally because milk and nasal mucus may occlude the eustachian tube. Holding the infant provides social and close physical contact for the baby and an opportunity for parent-infant interaction and bonding (Figure 30–14).

2. The nipple should have a hole big enough to allow milk to flow in drops when the bottle is inverted. Too large an opening may cause overfeeding or regurgitation because of rapid feeding. If feeding is too fast, the nipple should be changed, and the infant should be helped to eat more slowly by stopping the feeding frequently for burping and cuddling.

3. The nipple should be pointed directly into the mouth, not toward the palate or tongue, and should

be on top of the tongue. The nipple should be full of liquid at all times to avoid ingestion of air, which decreases the amount of feeding and increases discomfort.

4. The infant should be burped at intervals, preferably at the middle and end of the feeding. The infant who seems to swallow a great deal of air while sucking may need more frequent burping. If the infant has cried before being fed, air may have been swallowed, and the infant should be burped before beginning to feed or after taking just enough to calm down. Burping is done by holding the infant upright on the shoulder or by holding the infant in a sitting position on the feeder's lap with chin and chest supported on one hand. The back is then gently patted or stroked with the other hand. Too frequent burping may confuse a newborn who is attempting to coordinate sucking, swallowing, and breathing simultaneously.

5. Newborns frequently regurgitate small amounts of feedings. This may look like a large amount to the inexperienced parent, however, and she or he may require reassurance that this is normal. Initially, it may be due to excessive mucus and gastric irritation from foreign substances such as aspirated blood in the stomach from birth. Later, regurgitation may result when the infant feeds too rapidly and swallows air. It may also occur when the infant is overfed and the cardiac sphincter allows the excess to be regurgitated. Because this is such a common occurrence, experienced parents and nurses generally keep a "burp cloth" available. Although regurgitation is normal, vomiting or a forceful expulsion of fluid is not. When forceful expulsion occurs, further evaluation may be indicated, especially if other symptoms are present.

6. A fat baby is not necessarily a healthy one. Parents should be encouraged to avoid overfeeding or feeding infants every time they cry. Infants should be encouraged but not forced to feed and should be allowed to set their own pace once feedings are established. Parents sometimes set artificial goals— "The baby must take all 5 ounces"—and tend to keep feeding the child until those goals are met, even though the infant may not be hungry. Overfeeding results in infant obesity. During early feedings, however, the infant may need simple tactile stimulation—such as gently rubbing feet and hands, adjusting clothing, and loosening coverings—to maintain adequate sucking for a sufficient time to complete a full feeding.

Formula preparation and sterilization techniques are always important to discuss with families. Cleanliness is essential, but sterilization is necessary only if the water source is questionable (Procedure 30–1: Methods of Bottle Sterilization). Bottles may be effectively prepared in

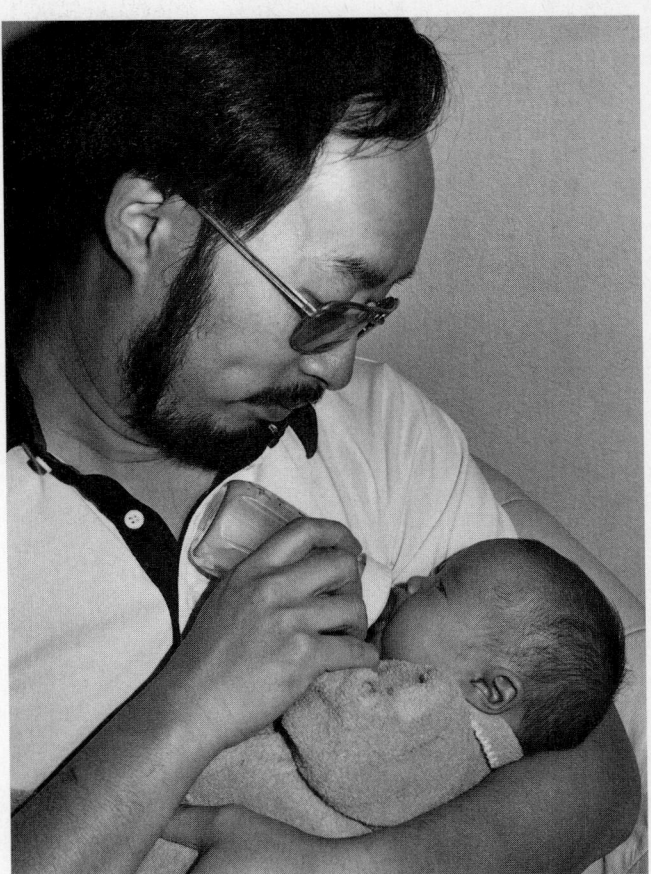

FIGURE 30-14   An infant is supported comfortably during bottle-feeding.

dishwashers or washed thoroughly in warm soapy water and rinsed well. Nipples may be weakened by the temperature of dishwashers and therefore should be washed thoroughly by hand and rinsed well. Tap water, if from an uncontaminated source, may be used for mixing powdered formulas, which are less expensive than the concentrated or ready-to-use prepared formulas. Honey should not be used as a "sugar source" because of the danger of infant botulism (Mott et al 1990).

Bottles may be prepared individually, or up to one day's supply of formula may be prepared at one time. Extra bottles are stored in the refrigerator and should be warmed slightly before feeding. Ready-to-use disposable bottles of formula are very convenient but are also expensive (Table 30–6 on page 915).

NUTRITIONAL ASSESSMENT OF THE INFANT

During the early months of life the food offered to and consumed by infants will be instrumental to their proper growth and development. The infant's nutritional status is assessed at each well-baby visit. Assessment should include four components:

Terminal Sterilization

Advantages

1. Safest, most efficient method
2. More easily learned

Disadvantages

1. Prolonged cooling period (1 hour)
2. Not suitable for disposable bottles

Aseptic Method of Sterilization

Advantages

1. May be modified for use with disposable bottles

Disadvantages

1. Difficult to learn
2. Contamination more likely

Procedure

1. Assemble equipment and wash hands.
2. Thoroughly wash bottles, caps, and nipples in warm soapy water; squeeze some water through holes to rid them of accumulated milk; rinse well.
3. Wash the lid of the formula can (if using a liquid) and prepare formula according to directions.
4. Fill the bottles with the desired amount of formula, and loosely apply the nipples and caps; one or two bottles of water may be prepared at the same time.
5. Place the prepared bottles in a large kettle or bottle sterilizer and add the appropriate amount of water (as specified on the sterilizer or 2–3 inches if a kettle is used).
6. Cover the sterilizer, bring the water to a gentle boil, and boil for 25 minutes at 212 F.
7. Remove from heat, but let the bottles remain in the sterilizer with the lid on until the sides of the pan are cool to the touch.
8. Remove the bottles, tighten the lids, and refrigerate until needed.

Procedure

1. Same as steps 1 and 2 of terminal method.
2. Place all equipment needed (bottles, nipples, caps, can opener, tongs, measuring pitcher, and spoon) in a large kettle or sterilizer, cover with water, and boil for 5 minutes.
3. In another pan, boil for 5 minutes the amount of water necessary to make the formula.
4. Drain the water from the sterilizer pan and let the equipment cool 1 hour.
5. Remove the measuring pitcher, being certain to touch only the handle.
6. Use the sterilized can opener to open a can of formula after first washing the lid with soapy water and rinsing well. Pour the formula into the prepared measuring pitcher, add the correct amount of boiled water, and mix with the prepared spoon.
7. Use tongs to remove the bottles from the sterilizer and fill them with the desired amount of formula. (One or two bottles of water may also be prepared by boiling enough additional water.)
8. Use the tongs to set the nipples on the bottles; then apply the caps, touching only the edges.
9. Refrigerate until needed.

To modify for disposable bottles:
Complete all steps as directed except *do not boil the bottles* with the other equipment and allow the water to cool for 15–20 minutes before preparing the formula. (The plastic bag may melt if the formula is too hot.)

Dishwasher Sterilization

Advantages

1. Easy

Disadvantages

1. May not have access to dishwasher
2. Hot water tank needs to be set at 120 F or medium heat setting

Procedure

1. Place bottles, caps into dishwasher rack.
2. Wash on hot water cycle; then machine dry.
3. Spoon dry formula powder into bottles, cap with nipples, invert, and store at room temperature. Add tap water at time of feeding.
4. If liquid formula is used, add unboiled tap water to the liquid formula after dishwasher sterilization of bottles; refrigerate filled, capped bottles until needed.
5. Clean nipples separately with hot, soapy water; rinse thoroughly; then boil for 5 minutes. Cool for 1 hour. Nipples become softened if sterilized in dishwater.
6. Sterilize disposable bottles in the top rack of dishwasher; clean nipples as in step 5 above.

- Nutritional history from the parent
- Weight gain since the last visit
- Growth chart percentiles
- Physical examination

The nutritional history reports the type, amount, and frequency of milk and supplemental foods, vitamins, and minerals being given to the infant on a daily basis. If the baby is taking formula, the history also includes how the formula is mixed (checking for under- or over-dilution) and stored. The healthy formula-fed infant should generally gain 30 g (1 oz) per day for the first 6 months of life and 15 g (0.5 oz) per day for the second 6 months. Individual charts show the infant's growth with respect to height, weight, and head circumference. The important consideration is that infants continue to grow at their own individual rates.

For the breastfeeding mother who is concerned about whether her infant is getting adequate nutrition the nurse can recommend looking for an appearance of weight gain and counting the number of wet diapers in a 24-hour period. Approximately six wet diapers or more in a day indicate adequate nutrition is being attained in the totally breastfed infant. If additional water is ingested, the diaper count should be higher. The presence of urine can most accurately be assessed when the diaper is free of feces. This is most likely prior to feedings. The gastrocolic reflex often stimulates stooling following a feeding. For the anxious parent another means of reassurance of adequate intake and output is to keep a record of the frequency and duration of feedings and the exact number of wet and/or soiled diapers. Keeping a record tends to give the worried parent a sense of control and a tangible indication on which to rule out or base concern (Table 30–7).

The physical examination will help identify any nutritional disorders. Iron deficiency should be suspected in a pale, diaphoretic, irritable infant who is obese.

TABLE 30-6   Formula Preparation

Ready to Feed (20 kcal/oz (available in 32 oz cans or 4 oz bottles):

Use within 30 minutes to 1 hour once opened.

Do not dilute. Use directly from can, no mixing required.

Just add clean nipple to bottle.

Most expensive type of formula preparation.

Formula Concentrate (available in 13 oz cans):

Mix equal amounts of concentrate and water from uncontaminated source. This provides a 20 kcal/30 mL (1 oz) dilution. For example, for a 4 oz feeding mix 2 oz of formula concentrate with 2 oz water.

Wash punch-type can opener and top of formula can before opening.

Prepare a single feeding by measuring water and liquid directly into nursing bottle.

Cover opened concentrate formula cans with foil or plastic wrap and refrigerate until next bottle is made up.

Powdered Formula (52 scoops per can):

Mix one unpacked level scoop of powdered formula with each 60 mL (2 oz) of warm water.

Always pour water into bottle first; then add powder and stir well.

Make sure the powder and water are well mixed to ensure the formula composition is 20 kcal/30 mL (1 oz).

After opening, keep can tightly covered and use contents within 1 month to assure freshness.

Least expensive type.

TABLE 30-7   Successful Breastfeeding Evaluation

Babies are probably getting enough milk if:

They are nursing at least eight times in 24 hours.

In a quiet room, their mothers can hear them swallow while nursing.

Their mothers' breasts appear to soften after nursing.

The number of wet diapers increases by the fourth or fifth day after birth, or there are at least six to eight wet diapers every 24 hours after day 5.

The baby's stools are yellow or are beginning to lighten in color by the fourth or fifth day after birth.

Offering a supplemental bottle is not a reliable indicator because most babies will take a few ounces even if they are getting enough breast milk (Huggins 1990).

By calculating the nutritional needs of infants the nurse can recommend a diet that supplies appropriate nutrition for infant growth and development. The assessment is especially helpful in counseling mothers of infants under 6 months of age in view of the tendency to add too many supplemental foods or offer too much formula to infants of this age. Clinicians generally advise that an infant not be given more than 32 oz of formula in 1 day. If additional calories are needed, supplemental foods should be added to the diet. Conversely, if the caloric intake is adequate or excessive, formula alone gives the infant enough calories, and introduction of solid foods can be delayed.

When an infant's caloric intake and weight gain are found to be excessive, clinicians do not advise putting the infant on a weight reduction diet because tissue growth is rapid during this period and must be supported. The appropriate advice is to provide a maintenance caloric intake as a means of allowing the infant to maintain weight while maturing and growing in length.

Nutritional intake can be assessed by comparing the infant's dietary intake with the desired caloric intake, weight, and age. Most commercial formulas prescribed for the normal healthy newborn contain 20 kcal per 30 mL (1 oz). If the infant is eating solids, the caloric value of those foods must be determined and included in the calculations of nutritional intake. With knowledge of the number of calories needed by the infant according to weight [108 kcal/kg/day (55 kcal/lb/day)], the nurse can counsel the parents about how many ounces per day the infant needs to meet caloric requirements. The following example shows the effectiveness of these assessments and interventions.

Jamie, age 1 week, is visited at home by the nurse associated with a health maintenance organization. Jamie is Mrs Adams's first child, and Mrs Adams is concerned about whether she is getting adequate nourishment. Jamie weighed 7 lb at birth and has regained her birth weight after an 11 oz (10%) loss. Mrs Adams reports that Jamie takes 3 oz of formula every 3 hours, does not spit up any formula, and has eight to ten wet diapers a day

with one to two soft bowel movements per day. Jamie is a contented baby who sleeps between feedings.

Based on requirements of 108 kcal/kg/day, the nurse calculates 1-week-old Jamie's dietary needs as follows:

- Jamie's weight = 7 lb. Converting weight into kg (2.2 lb/kg), Jamie weighs 3.2 kg.

- Jamie's 24-hour caloric need = 3.2 kg (Jamie's weight) × 108 kcal/kg/day = 346 kcal/day.

- Amount of formula (at 20 kcal/oz) needed in 24 hours = 17 oz.

- Jamie's 24-hour intake = 24 oz (3 oz every 3 hours) × 20 kcal/oz = 480 kcal.

The nurse makes the following nursing diagnoses:

- Knowledge deficit related to lack of information about assessing adequacy of food intake

- Altered nutrition: More than body requirement related to formula intake that is greater than necessary to meet Jamie's growth needs

The nursing plan outlines the following actions:

- Discuss Jamie's feeding cues with Mrs Adams. How does Mrs Adams decide when to feed Jamie? Is she feeding in response to Jamie or in response to a time schedule? Explain that infants have a need for nonnutritive sucking that can be met with a pacifier.

- Explain normal infant sleep-wake cycles and how babies can self-regulate in phases of light sleep, although they may make stirring noises.

- Explain that Jamie is ingesting more calories than necessary, and point out the need to reduce her intake by approximately 7 oz/day. Mrs Adams can accomplish this by feeding Jamie a little less frequently and feeding slightly less formula (approximately 0.5 oz or less) each feeding. Giving Jamie 75 mL (2.5 oz) at each of seven feedings provides 350 cal/day. Teach Mrs Adams to feed Jamie in response to feeding cues such as rooting and hand-to-mouth activity. When Jamie has taken 75–90 mL (2.5–3 oz) of formula, substitute a pacifier to provide nonnutritive sucking. Explain that if Jamie takes 2.5–3 oz and seems to want to eat again before 3–4 hours, Mrs Adams should try other comfort measures, such as changing Jamie's diaper, rocking her, giving her a pacifier, or putting her in a swing, before resorting to feeding.

- Discuss with Mrs Adams the behaviors that indicate satiation. These include minimal sucking with release of the nipple and falling asleep with hands and body relaxed. She should not attempt to force the remaining milk, if any, but should discard it because of the potential for bacterial growth even if refrigerated.

- Formula amounts can be increased gradually to meet Jamie's changing caloric needs and growth without excessive caloric intake. Once Jamie is ingesting 32 oz a day, the addition of solid foods can be considered after discussion with the health provider.

- Explore alternative methods for providing comfort to a newborn.

On a follow-up well-baby visit, Jamie is weighed and is gaining 30 g (1 oz) per day. Jamie continues to have approximately eight to ten wet diapers a day and is alert and responsive.

KEY CONCEPTS

The RDA for calories for the newborn is 105–110 kcal/kg/day (50–55 kcal/lb/day).

The nurse must monitor the first feeding because this is when the newborn may initially manifest signs of cardiac complications or anomalies of the upper GI tract.

Breast milk is the optimal food for the first year of life.

Commercially prepared formulas (unless otherwise noted) provide 20 kcal/30 mL (1 oz). The composition of breast milk varies in response to a wide variety of factors, but the average calorie content is 20 kcal/oz. Breast milk is more easily digested than formula; therefore nutrients and calories in breast milk are utilized more efficiently.

Formula-fed infants regain their birth weight by approximately 10 days of age, then gain 30 g (1 oz) per day for the first 6 months and 15 g (0.5 oz) per day for the second 6 months. Birth weight is doubled at 3.5–4 months of age. Healthy breastfed babies regain their birth weight by about 14 days of age, then gain approximately 15 g (0.5 oz) per day in the first 6 months of life. Birth weight is doubled at approximately 5 months of age.

Nurses must recognize that cultural values influence infant feeding practices, be sensitive to ethnic backgrounds of minority populations, and understand that the dominant culture in any society defines "normal" maternal-infant feeding interaction.

The nurse is obligated to provide parents with accurate, current, and comprehensive information concerning methods of infant feeding. Once the mother has made an *informed* decision, the nurse must support her choice.

Most maternal medications are transmitted through breast milk. The effects on the infant and lactation depend on a variety of factors, including route of administration, timing of the dose with respect to feeding time, and multiple properties of the medication.

Breastfed infants are getting adequate nutrition if they are gaining weight and have at least six wet diapers a day when not receiving water supplements.

Breastfeeding mothers should be encouraged to ensure that the infant is correctly positioned at the breast, with a large portion of areola in the mouth and not under the tongue. The mother is advised to rotate the baby's position periodically to ensure that all ducts are emptied.

Formula-fed infants need no vitamins or mineral supplements other than iron, if it is not already in the formula, and fluoride, if it is not in the water.

The bottle-feeding mother may need help feeding and burping her infant. She will also benefit from information about feeding schedules and types of formula.

The use of skim milk, cow's milk with lowered fat content, or unmodified cow's milk is not recommended for children under 2 years old.

Nutritional assessment of the infant includes nutritional history from the parent, measurement of weight gain, determination of growth chart percentiles, and physical examination.

REFERENCES

American Academy of Pediatrics, Committee on Drugs: The transfer of drugs and other chemicals into human milk. *Pediatrics* 1994; 93(1):137.

American Academy of Pediatrics, Committee on Nutrition: Follow-up of weaning formulas. *Pediatrics* 1992; 89:1105.

Barness LA: Bases of weaning recommendations. *J Pediatr* 1990; 117:S84.

Baron JA et al: Cigarette smoking and prolactin in women. *Brit Med J* 1986; 293:482.

Bear K, Tigges BB: Management strategies for promoting successful breastfeeding. *Nurse Pract* 1993; 18(6):50.

Eggert JV, Rayburn WF: Nutrition and lactation. In: *Gynecology and Obstetrics*, vol 2. Sciarra JJ (editor). Philadelphia: HarperCollins, 1994.

Fendrick SM, Major AL, Brown FR: Nursing mothers service: A community breast-feeding program. *Pediatr Nurs* 1994; 20(3):241.

Fletcher AB: Nutrition. In: *Neonatology: Pathophysiology and Management of the Newborn*, 4th ed. Avery GB et al (editors). Philadelphia: Lippincott, 1994.

Food and Nutrition Board, National Academy of Sciences—National Research Council: *Recommended Dietary Allowances*, 10th ed. Washington, DC, 1989.

Gunnlaugsson G, da Silva MC, Smedman L: Age at breast feeding start and postneonatal growth and survival. *Arch Dis Child* 1994; 69:134.

Hamosh M: Digestion in the preterm infant: The effects of human milk. *Semin Perinatol* 1994; 18(6):485.

Huggins K: *The Nursing Mother's Companion*. Boston: Harvard Common Press, 1990.

Hutchinson MK, Baqi-Aziz M: Nursing care of the childbearing Muslim family. *JOGNN* 1994; 23(9):767.

Keefe M: The impact of rooming-in on maternal sleep at night. *JOGNN* 1988; 17(2):122.

LaDu EB: Childbirth care for Hmong families. *MCN* November/December 1985; 10:382.

Lawrence RA: *Breastfeeding: A Guide for the Medical Profession*, 4th ed. St Louis: Mosby, 1994.

Littman H, VanderBrug Medendorp S, Goldfarb J: The decision to breastfeed. *Clin Pediatr* 1994; 214.

Mathew OP, Bhatia J: Sucking and breathing patterns during breast- and bottle-feeding in term neonates. *Am J Dis Child* 1989; 143:588.

Mead Johnson Nutritionals: *Infant Formula Product Advisor.* Evansville, IN: Mead Johnson, 1993.

Mott SR, James SR, Sperhac AM: *Nursing Care of Children and Families*, 2nd ed. Redwood City, CA: Addison-Wesley Nursing, 1990.

Mulford C: Subtle signs and symptoms of the milk ejection reflex. *J Hum Lact* 1990; 6:177.

Mulford C: The mother-baby assessment (MBA): An "Apgar score" for breastfeeding. *J Hum Lact* 1992; 8:79.

Neifert M: *Breastfeeding Standards of Care for Low Risk Infants.* Denver: St Luke's Hospital, 1989.

Nikodem VC et al: Do cabbage leaves prevent breast engorgement? A randomized, controlled study. *Birth* 1993; 20(2):61.

Pedersen CA et al: Oxytocin activation of maternal behavior in the rat. *Ann NY Acad Sci* 1992; 652:58.

Pinilla T, Birch LL: Help me make it through the night: Behavioral entrainment of breast-fed infants' sleep patterns. *Pediatrics* 1993; 91(2):436.

Pipes P: *Nutrition in Infancy and Childhood*, 4th ed. St Louis: Mosby, 1989.

Renfrew M, Fisher C, Arms S: *Breastfeeding: Getting Breastfeeding Right for You.* Berkeley, CA: Celestial Arts, 1990.

Riordan J, Auerbach K: *Breastfeeding and Human Lactation.* Boston: Jones & Bartlett, 1993.

Ross Laboratories: *National Mothers' Survey.* Columbus, OH: Ross Laboratories, 1993.

Sawley L: Infant feeding. *Nursing* 1989; 13:69.

Sollid DT et al: Breastfeeding multiples. *J Perinatal Neonatal Nurs* 1989; 3(1):46.

Weigley ES: Changing patterns in offering solids to infants. *Pediatr Nurs* 1990; 16(5):439.

Winick M: *Nutrition, Pregnancy, and Early Infancy.* Baltimore: Williams & Wilkins, 1989.

Woolridge MW, Baum JD: Recent advances in breast feeding. *Acta Paediatr Japonica* 1993; 35:12.

Worthington-Roberts B, Williams SR: *Nutrition in Pregnancy and Lactation*, 5th ed. St Louis: Mosby, 1993.

Ziemer MM et al: Methods to prevent and manage nipple pain in breastfeeding women. *West J Nurs Res* 1990; 12(6):732.

Zinaman MJ et al: Acute prolactin, oxytocin responses and milk yield to infant sucking and artificial methods of expression in lactating women. *Pediatrics* 1992; 89:437.

CHAPTER 31

THE NEWBORN AT RISK: CONDITIONS PRESENT AT BIRTH

he rhythmic tides of her sleeping and feeding spaciously measured her days and nights. Her frail absorption was a commanding presence, her helplessness strong as a rock.

~LAURIE LEE, *TWO WOMEN*~

KEY TERMS

Drug-dependent infants

Fetal alcohol effects (FAE)

Fetal alcohol syndrome (FAS)

Grief work

Inborn errors of metabolism

Infant of diabetic mother (IDM)

Intrauterine growth restriction (IUGR)

Large for gestational age (LGA)

Neonatal mortality risk

Phenylketonuria (PKU)

Postterm newborn

Postmaturity

Preterm infant

Small for gestational age (SGA)

OBJECTIVES

Identify factors which help identify an at-risk newborn.

Compare the underlying etiologies of the similar physiologic complications of small-for-gestational-age (SGA) newborns and preterm appropriate-for-gestational-age (Pr AGA) newborns.

Describe the impact of maternal diabetes mellitus on the newborn.

Compare the characteristics and potential complications of the postterm newborn and the newborn with postmaturity syndrome.

Discuss the physiologic characteristics of the preterm newborn that predispose each body system to various complications.

Identify the data used in developing the nursing diagnoses required to plan interventions for the care of the Pr AGA newborn.

Explain the special care needed by alcohol- or drug-exposed newborns.

Relate the consequences of maternal AIDS to the management of the infant in the neonatal period.

Identify the nursing assessments that would make the nurse suspect a congenital cardiac defect during the early newborn period.

Discuss the nursing assessments of and initial interventions for selected congenital anomalies.

Explain the special care needed by newborns with inborn errors of metabolism.

Delineate interventions to facilitate parental attachment with the at-risk newborn.

Identify the nursing actions necessary to support family members dealing with the birth of an at-risk infant.

*W*ithin the past three decades the field of neonatology has expanded greatly. Many levels of nursery care have evolved in response to increasing knowledge about the newborn: special care; transitional care; low-, medium-, and high-risk care. The nurse is an important care giver in all these settings. As a member of the multidisciplinary health care team, the nurse contributes to the high-touch care necessary in today's high-tech perinatal environment.

Although a high level of newborn care is available, a variety of other factors influences the outcomes of these at-risk infants, including the following:

- Birth weight
- Gestational age
- Type and length of newborn illness
- Environmental and maternal factors
- Maternal-infant separation

IDENTIFICATION OF AT-RISK NEWBORNS

An at-risk infant is one who is susceptible to illness (morbidity) or even death (mortality) because of dysmaturity, immaturity, physical disorders, or complications during or after birth. In most cases the infant is the product of pregnancy involving one or more predictable risk factors, including the following:

- Low socioeconomic level of the mother
- Exposure to environmental dangers such as toxic chemicals
- Preexisting maternal conditions such as heart disease, diabetes, hypertension, and renal disease
- Maternal factors such as age or parity
- Medical conditions related to pregnancy such as prenatal maternal infection
- Pregnancy complications such as abruptio placentae

Various risk factors and their specific effects on the pregnancy outcome are listed in Table 14–2).

Because these factors and the perinatal risks associated with them are known, the birth of at-risk newborns can often be anticipated and prepared for through adequate prenatal care. The pregnancy can be closely monitored, treatment can be instituted as necessary, and arrangements can be made for birth to occur at a facility with appropriate equipment and personnel to care for both mother and infant.

Identification of at-risk infants cannot always be made before labor because the course of labor and birth or how the infant will withstand the stress of labor is not known prior to the actual birth process. Thus during labor, electronic fetal heart monitoring or continuous fetoscope monitoring by the nurse has played a significant role in detecting fetuses in distress.

Immediately after birth the Apgar score is a useful tool in identifying the at-risk newborn, but it is difficult to predict long-term outcome based solely on Apgar scores. In general the lower the Apgar score at 5 minutes after birth, the higher the incidence of neurologic abnormalities seen at 1 year of age. Neurologic abnormalities also increase significantly as birth weight decreases.

The newborn classification and neonatal mortality risk chart is another useful tool in identifying newborns at risk (Figure 31–1). Before this classification tool was developed, birth weight of less than 2500 g was the sole criterion for determination of immaturity. It was eventually recognized that an infant could weigh more than 2500 g but still be immature. Conversely, an infant weighing less than 2500 g might be functionally mature at term or beyond. Thus birth weight and gestational age together became the criteria used to assess neonatal maturity and mortality risk.

According to the newborn classification and neonatal mortality risk chart, gestation is divided as follows:

- Preterm = 0–37 (completed) weeks
- Term = 38–41 (completed) weeks
- Postterm = greater than 42 weeks

As shown in Figure 31–1, large-for-gestational-age (LGA) infants are those above the curved line labeled 90th percentile. Appropriate-for-gestational-age (AGA) infants are those between the lines labeled 10th percentile and 90th percentile. Small-for-gestational-age (SGA) infants are those below the curved line labeled 10th percentile. A newborn is assigned to a category depending on birth weight and gestational age. For example, a newborn classified as Pr SGA is preterm and small for gestational age. The full-term newborn whose weight is appropriate for gestational age is classified F AGA.

Neonatal mortality risk is the chance of death within the newborn period, that is, within the first 28 days of life. As indicated in Figure 31–1, the neonatal mortality risk decreases as both gestational age and birth weight increase. Infants who are preterm and small for gestational age have the highest neonatal mortality risk. The mortality for LGA infants has decreased at most perinatal centers because of improved management of diabetes in pregnancy and increased recognition of potential complications of LGA infants.

Newborn morbidity can be anticipated based on birth weight and gestational age. In Figure 31–2 the infant's birth weight is located in the vertical column, and the gestational age in weeks is found horizontally. The area where the two meet on the graph identifies commonly occurring problems. This tool assists in determin-

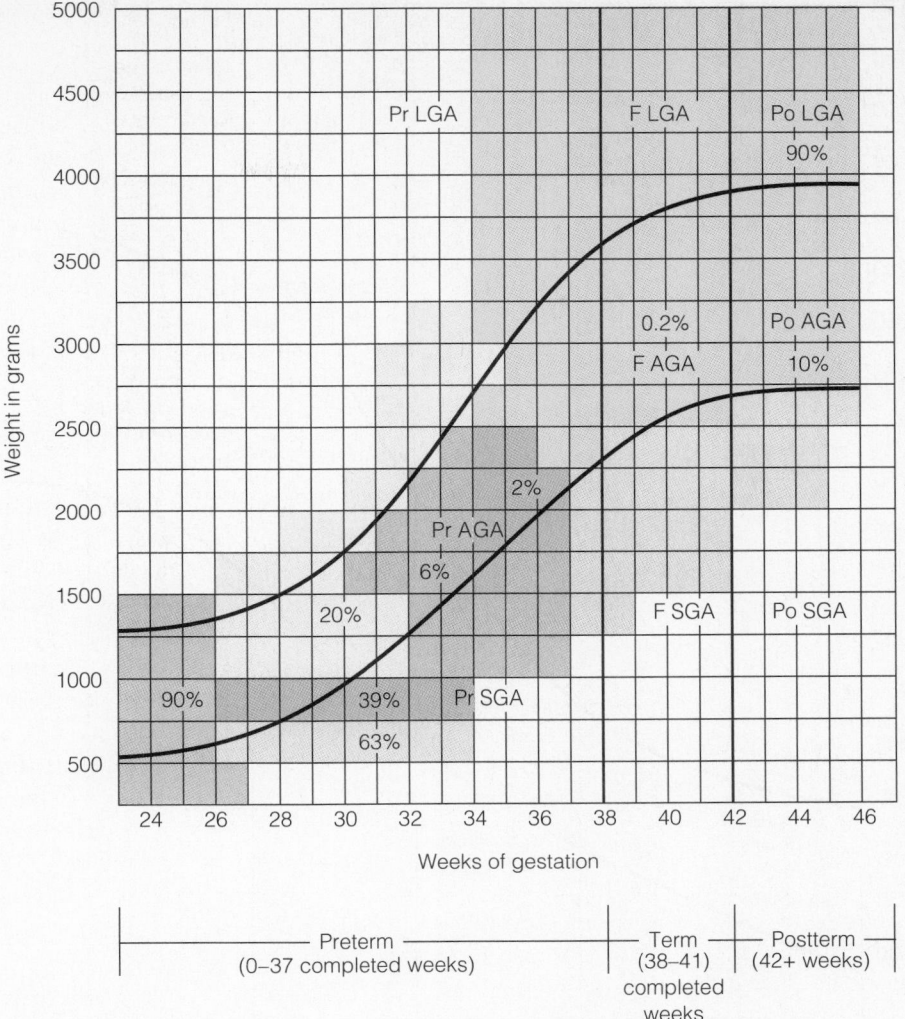

FIGURE 31-1 Newborn classification and neonatal mortality risk chart. Infants are classified according to weight as small for gestational age (SGA), appropriate for gestational age (AGA), or large for gestational age (LGA) and by weeks of newborn as preterm (Pr), term (F), or postterm (Po). Corresponding neonatal mortality risks are indicated by the percentages in the various colored regions. SOURCE: Koops BL, Morgan LP, Battaglia FC: Neonatal mortality risk in relationship to birth weight and gestational age. *J Pediatr* 1982; 101(6):969.

ing the needs of particular infants for special observation and care. For example, an infant of 2000 g at 40 weeks' gestation should be carefully assessed for evidence of fetal distress, hypoglycemia, congenital anomalies, congenital infection, and polycythemia.

Identification of the nursing care needs of the at-risk newborn depends on minute-to-minute observations of the changes in the newborn's physiologic status. It is essential to a baby's survival that the nurse understand the basic physiologic principles that guide nursing management of the at-risk newborn. The organization of nursing care must be directed toward the following:

- Decreasing physiologically stressful situations
- Constantly observing for subtle signs of change in clinical condition
- Interpreting laboratory data and coordinating interventions

- Conserving the infant's energy, especially in frail, debilitated newborns
- Providing for developmental stimulation and sleep cycle
- Assisting the family in developing attachment behaviors
- Involving the family in the planning and provision of care

CARE OF THE SMALL-FOR-GESTATIONAL-AGE NEWBORN

A **small-for-gestational-age (SGA)** newborn is any newborn who at birth is at or below the tenth percentile for weight (intrauterine growth curves) on the newborn

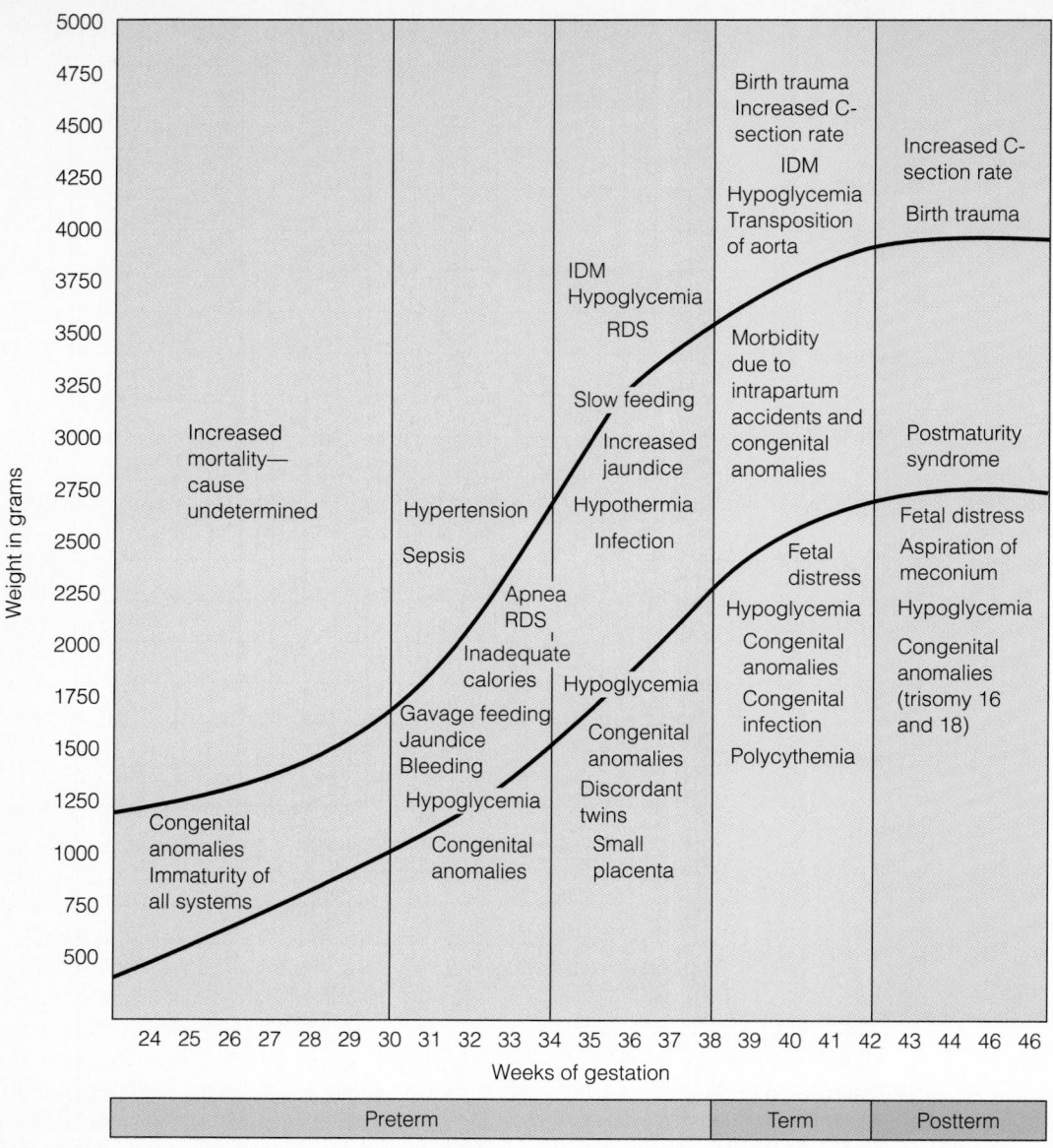

FIGURE 31-2 Neonatal morbidity by birth weight and gestational age.
SOURCE: Lubchenco LO: *The High Risk Infant*. Philadelphia: WB Saunders, 1976, p 122.

classification chart (Figure 31–1). It should be noted that intrauterine growth charts are influenced by altitude and ethnicity. There is a high correlation between increase in altitude and decrease in birth weight (Nagey & Viscardi 1993). When assigning SGA classification to a newborn, birth weight charts should be based on the local population into which the newborn is born (Creasy & Resnik 1994). An SGA newborn may be preterm, term, or postterm. Other terms used to designate an undergrown newborn include **intrauterine growth restriction (IUGR),** which describes the pregnancy circumstance of advanced gestation and limited fetal growth (Cunningham 1993) and *dysmature*. We use SGA and IUGR interchangeably.

Small-for-gestational-age infants have a fivefold greater incidence of perinatal asphyxia and an eightfold

higher perinatal mortality than AGA infants (Palo 1992). The incidences of polycythemia and hypoglycemia are also increased in this group of infants.

Factors Contributing to IUGR

IUGR may be caused by maternal, placental, or fetal factors and may not be apparent antenatally. Intrauterine growth is linear in the normal pregnancy from approximately 28 to 38 weeks' gestation. After 38 weeks, growth is variable, depending on the genetic growth potential of the fetus and placental function. The most common factors affecting growth restriction are the following:

- *Genetics*. Genetic size predisposition is correlated with the parents' stature. Small parents are likely to have small infants. These infants are proportionately SGA.

- *Malnutrition.* Maternal nutrition has not been found to influence the birth weight of the newborn significantly unless starvation occurs during the last trimester of pregnancy. Before the third trimester the nutritional supply far exceeds the needs of the fetus.

- *Vascular complications.* Complications related to pregnancy-induced hypertension (PIH), chronic hypertensive vascular disease, and advanced diabetes mellitus cause diminished blood flow to the uterus.

- *Maternal disease.* Maternal heart disease, substance abuse (drugs and alcohol), sickle-cell anemia, phenylketonuria (PKU), and asymptomatic pyelonephritis affect IUGR.

- *Maternal factors.* Primiparity, grand multiparity, smoking, lack of prenatal care, age extremes (under 16 or over 40), and low socioeconomic status (which can result in inadequate health care, inadequate education, and inadequate living conditions) affect IUGR (Wen et al 1990).

- *Environmental factors.* High altitude, x-rays, excessive exercise, hyperthermia, and maternal use of drugs, such as antimetabolics, anticonvulsants, and trimethadione, which have teratogenic effects, affect IUGR (Cunningham 1993).

- *Placental factors.* Placental conditions such as small placenta, infarcted areas, abnormal cord insertions, placenta previa, or thrombosis may affect circulation to the fetus, which becomes more deficient with increasing gestational age (Harrington & Campbell 1993).

- *Fetal factors.* Congenital infections (rubella, toxoplasmosis, syphilis, cytomegalic inclusion disease) or malformations, multiple pregnancy (twins or triplets), discordant twins, sex of the fetus (females tend to be smaller), chromosomal syndromes, and inborn errors of metabolism can predispose a fetus to IUGR (Creasy & Resnik 1994).

Antenatal identification of fetuses with IUGR is the first step in the detection of common disorders of the SGA newborn. The perinatal history of maternal conditions, early serial ultrasound measurements, Doppler velocimetry, examination of the placenta (by pathology), and the physical and neurologic assessment of the newborn are also important (Witter 1993).

Patterns of IUGR

Intrauterine growth occurs by an increase in cell number and by an increase in cell size. If insult occurs early during the critical period of organ development in the fetus, fewer new cells are formed, organs are small, and organ weight is subnormal. Growth failure that begins later in pregnancy does not affect the total number of cells, but only their size. The organs are normal, but their size is diminished.

Two clinical pictures of SGA newborns have been described. These clinical presentations are classified as either *symmetric* (proportional) IUGR or *asymmetric* (disproportional) IUGR.

Symmetric IUGR is caused by long-term maternal conditions (such as chronic hypertension, severe malnutrition, chronic intrauterine infection, substance abuse, and anemia) or fetal genetic abnormalities (Creasy & Resnik 1994). Symmetric IUGR can be noted by ultrasound in the first half of the second trimester. In symmetric IUGR there is chronic prolonged restriction of growth in size of organs, body weight, body length, and, in severe cases, head circumference.

Asymmetric IUGR is associated with an acute compromise of uteroplacental blood flow. Some associated causes are placental infarcts, pregnancy-induced hypertension (PIH), and poor weight gain in pregnancy. The growth restriction is usually not evident before the third trimester because, although weight is decreased, length and head circumference remain appropriate for that gestational age. After 36 weeks' gestation, the abdominal circumference of a normal fetus becomes larger than the head circumference. In asymmetric IUGR the head circumference remains larger than the abdominal circumference. Thus measuring only the biparietal diameter on ultrasound will not reveal asymmetric IUGR. An early indicator of asymmetric SGA is a decrease in the growth rate of the abdominal circumference, reflecting subnormal liver growth and a paucity of subcutaneous fat (Creasy & Resnik 1994). Birth weight is reduced below the 10th percentile, whereas head circumference and/or length may be between the 10th and 90th percentiles.

Asymmetric SGA newborns are particularly at risk for perinatal asphyxia, pulmonary hemorrhage, hypocalcemia, and hypoglycemia in the newborn period. Despite growth restriction, physiologic maturity develops according to gestational age. Therefore the SGA newborn may be more physiologically mature than the preterm AGA newborn and less predisposed to complications of prematurity such as respiratory distress syndrome and hyperbilirubinemia. The SGA newborn's chances for survival are better because of organ maturity, although this newborn still faces many other potential difficulties in the newborn period and beyond.

Common Complications of the SGA Newborn

The complications occurring most frequently in the SGA newborn include the following:

- *Perinatal asphyxia.* The SGA infant suffers chronic hypoxia in utero, which leaves little reserve to withstand the demands of normal labor and birth. Cesarean birth may be necessary. Thus intrauterine asphyxia occurs with its potential systemic problems.

- *Aspiration syndrome.* In utero hypoxia can cause the fetus to gasp during birth, resulting in aspiration of amniotic fluid into the lower airways. It can also lead to relaxation of the anal sphincter and passage of meconium. This results in aspiration of the meconium in utero or with the first breaths after birth.

- *Heat loss.* Diminished subcutaneous fat (used for survival in utero), depletion of brown fat in utero, and a large surface area decrease the IUGR newborn's ability to conserve heat. The effect of surface area is diminished somewhat because of the flexed position assumed by the term SGA newborn.

- *Hypoglycemia.* An increase in metabolic rate in response to heat loss and poor hepatic glycogen stores cause hypoglycemia. In addition the infant is compromised by inadequate supplies of enzymes to activate gluconeogenesis (conversion of non-glucogen sources such as fatty acids and proteins to glucose).

- *Hypocalcemia.* Decreased calcium levels occur secondary to birth asphyxia and preterm birth.

- *Polycythemia.* The number of red blood cells is increased in the SGA newborn. This finding is considered a physiologic response to in utero chronic hypoxic stress.

Newborns who have significant IUGR tend to have a poor prognosis, especially when born before 37 weeks' gestation. Factors contributing to poor outcome for these infants are as follows:

- *Congenital malformations.* Congenital malformations occur 10 to 20 times more frequently in SGA infants than in AGA infants. The more severe the IUGR, the greater the chance for malformation as a result of impaired mitotic activity and hypoplastic cells.

- *Intrauterine infection.* When fetuses are exposed to intrauterine infections such as rubella and cytomegalovirus, they are profoundly affected by direct invasion of the brain and other vital organs.

- *Continued growth difficulties.* It is generally agreed that SGA newborns tend to be shorter than newborns of the same gestational age (Paz et al 1993). Asymmetric IUGR infants can be expected to catch up in weight to normal growth infants by 3 to 6 months of age. Symmetric SGA infants reportedly have varied growth potential but tend not to catch up to their peers (Warshaw 1994b).

- *Learning difficulties.* Often SGA newborns exhibit poor brain development and subsequent failure to catch up, and learning disabilities are not uncommon. The disabilities are characterized by hyperactivity, short attention span, and poor fine motor coordination (reading, writing, and drawing) (Witter 1993). Poor scholastic performance is also a common problem (Creasy & Resnik 1994). Some hearing loss and speech defects also occur.

Studies have determined that the quality of the home environment of an SGA infant predicts developmental outcome better than any single biologic risk factor (Watt 1989).

Medical Therapy

The goal of medical therapy for SGA infants is early recognition and implementation of medical management of the potential problems.

APPLYING THE NURSING PROCESS

Nursing Assessment

The nurse is responsible for assessing gestational age and identifying signs of potential complications associated with SGA infants.

All body parts of the symmetric IUGR infant are in proportion, but they are below normal size for the baby's gestational age. Therefore the head does not appear overly large or the length excessive in relation to the other body parts. These newborns are generally vigorous.

The asymmetric IUGR infant may appear long, thin, and emaciated, with loss of subcutaneous fat tissue and muscle mass (Figure 31–3). The baby may have loose skin folds; dry, desquamating skin; and a thin and often meconium-stained cord. The head appears relatively large (although it approaches normal size) because the chest size and abdominal girth are decreased. The baby may have a vigorous cry and appear alert and wide-eyed.

Nursing Diagnosis

Nursing diagnoses that may apply are included in the Nursing Care Plan: Small-for-Gestational-Age Newborn on page 926.

Nursing Plan and Implementation

Hypoglycemia, the most common metabolic complication of IUGR, can produce CNS abnormalities and mental retardation. Conditions such as asphyxia, hyperviscosity, and cold stress may also affect the baby's outcome. Meticulous attention to physiologic parameters is essen-

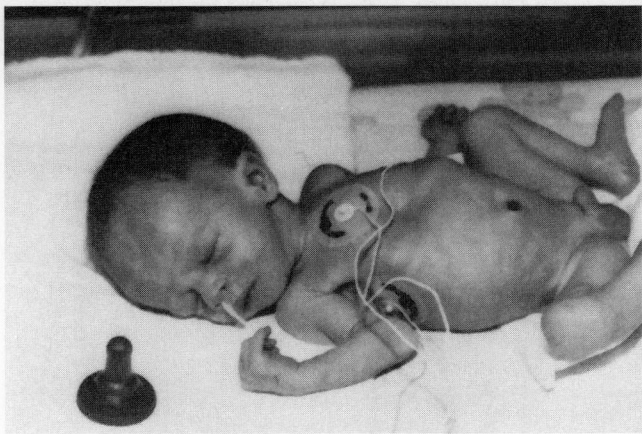

FIGURE 31-3 The infant with asymmetric IUGR appears long, thin, and emaciated. The gestational age of the infant shown here is 41 weeks. He weighed approximately 1560 g at birth.

tial for immediate nursing management and reduction of long-term disorders (see the Nursing Care Plan: Small-for-Gestational-Age Newborn on page 926).

Home Care

The long-term needs of the SGA newborn include careful follow-up evaluation of patterns of growth and possible disabilities that may later interfere with learning or motor functioning. Long-term follow-up care is especially necessary for those infants with congenital malformations, congenital infections, and obvious sequelae from physiologic problems. In addition the parents of the IUGR baby need support because a positive atmosphere can enhance the baby's growth potential and the child's ultimate outcome.

Evaluation

Anticipated outcomes of nursing care include:

*   The SGA newborn is free from respiratory compromise.

*   The SGA newborn maintains a stable temperature and glucose hemostasis.

*   The SGA newborn gains weight and takes nipple or bottle feedings without physiologic distress or fatigue.

*   The parents verbalize their concerns surrounding their baby's health problems and understand the rationale behind management of their newborn.

CARE OF THE LARGE-FOR-GESTATIONAL-AGE NEWBORN

A **large-for-gestational-age (LGA)** neonate is one whose birth weight is at or above the 90th percentile on the intrauterine growth curve (at any week of gestation). The classification of LGA may vary, depending on the intrauterine growth curve chart used; therefore the chart used should correlate with the characteristics of the client population (ACOG technical bulletin #159 1992; Harrington & Campbell 1993). Some LGA newborns have been incorrectly categorized as LGA because of miscalculation of the date of conception due to postconceptional bleeding. Careful gestational age assessment is therefore essential to identify the potential needs and problems of such infants.

The best known condition associated with excessive fetal growth is maternal diabetes (White's classes A–C; see Table 18–2). However, only a small fraction of LGA newborns are born to diabetic mothers. The cause of the majority of cases of LGA infants is unclear, but certain factors or situations have been found to correlate with their births:

*   Genetic predisposition is correlated proportionally to the mother's prepregnancy weight and to weight gain during pregnancy. Large parents tend to have large infants.

*   Multiparous women have two to three times the number of LGA infants as primigravidas (ACOG technical bulletin #159 1992).

*   Male infants are typically larger than female infants.

*   Infants with erythroblastosis fetalis, Beckwith-Wiedemann syndrome (a genetic condition associated with macroglossia, omphalocele, and newborn hypoglycemia and hyperinsulinemia), or transposition of the great vessels are usually LGA.

The increase in the LGA infant's body size is characteristically proportional, although head circumference and body length are in the upper limits of intrauterine growth. The exception to this rule is the infant of the diabetic mother, whose body weight increases, but whose length and head circumference may be in the normal range. Macrosomic infants are less competent motorically and have more difficulty in behavioral state regulation. LGA infants tend to be more difficult to arouse and may have problems maintaining a quiet alert state. They may also have feeding difficulties (Pressler 1991).

Common Complications of the LGA Newborn

Common disorders of the LGA infant include:

*   *Birth trauma because of cephalopelvic disproportion (CPD). Often these newborns have a biparietal*

Text continues on page 929

SMALL-FOR-GESTATIONAL-AGE NEWBORN

Nursing Assessment

Nursing History

1. Maternal factors:
   a. Vascular: PIH, chronic hypertension, advanced diabetes
   b. Preexisting diseases: heart disease, alcoholism, narcotic addiction, sickle cell anemia, phenylketonuria (PKU)
   c. Primiparity, smoking, lack of prenatal care, low socioeconomic level, very young or old
2. Environmental factors: high altitude, x-rays, maternal drug use (antimetabolites, anticonvulsants)
3. Placental factors: infarcts, placenta previa
4. Fetal factors:
   a. Congenital infections
   b. Multiple fetus
   c. Inborn errors of metabolism
   d. Chromosomal syndrome

Physical Examination

1. Large-appearing head in proportion to chest and abdomen (asymmetrical SGA)
2. Loose, dry skin
3. Scarcity of subcutaneous fat, with emaciated appearance
4. Long, thin appearance
5. Sunken abdomen
6. Sparse scalp hair
7. Anterior fontanelle may be depressed.
8. May have vigorous cry and appear alert.
9. Birth weight below tenth percentile

Diagnostic Studies

1. Blood glucose and Dextrostix/Chemstrip
2. Hematocrit
3. Total bilirubin level
4. Calcium levels
5. Chest x-ray

NURSING DIAGNOSIS: Impaired gas exchange related to aspiration of meconium

EXPECTED OUTCOME: Newborn will show no signs of meconium aspiration.

Nursing Interventions	Rationale
Auscultate breath sounds every 4 hours. Suction endotracheal tube every 3–4 hours. Give oxygen prior to suction as needed. Ensure chest physiotherapy is done as indicated.	*In utero, hypoxia causes relaxation of the anal sphincter with passage of meconium into the amniotic fluid and reflex gasping of meconium. Periodic suctioning maintains airway patency.*
Observe for worsening signs of respiratory distress such as generalized cyanosis; worsening retractions, grunting, and nasal flaring, evidenced by Silverman-Andersen respiratory index (see Chapter 32); sustained tachypnea; apnea episodes; inequality of breath sounds; presence of rales and rhonchi.	
Administer oxygen per order for relief of respiratory distress signs (Chapter 32) for nursing care and treatment of meconium aspiration, infant resuscitation). Implement treatment plan for respiratory distress.	
Monitor blood glucose levels every 8 hours until stable or by Dextrostix/Chemstrip within 1–2 hours after birth and frequently for 2–3 days.	*Respiratory distress increases consumption of glucose.*

OUTCOME MET IF:

- Newborn's respiratory rate is 30–60/minute
- Newborn shows no signs of apnea, intermittent cyanosis, sternal retractions, grunting, nasal flaring, or rales or rhonchi.
- Newborn's blood glucose levels >40 mg/dL.

NURSING DIAGNOSIS: Hyperthermia related to decreased subcutaneous fat

EXPECTED OUTCOME: Newborn will maintain temperature.

Nursing Interventions	Rationale
Provide neutral thermal environment range for newborn based on postnatal weight.	*Neutral thermal environment charts used for preterm babies must be altered for SGA newborns.*
Use skin probe to maintain skin temperature at 36.1–36.7 C.	*Diminished subcutaneous fat and a large body surface compared to body weight predispose SGA baby to thermoregulation problems.*
Obtain axillary temperatures and compare to registered skin probe temperature every 2–3 hours and PRN. If discrepancy exists, evaluate potential cause.	*Discrepancies between axillary temperature and skin probe temperature may be due to mechanical causes or the burning of brown fat.*
Adjust and monitor incubator or radiant warmer to maintain skin temperature.	

SMALL-FOR-GESTATIONAL-AGE NEWBORN *continued*

Nursing Interventions	Rationale
Minimize heat losses and prevent cold stress by 1. Warming and humidifying oxygen (Avoid blowing it over the face in order not to increase oxygen consumption) 2. Keeping skin dry 3. Keeping incubators, radiant warmers, and cribs away from windows and cold external walls and out of drafts 4. Avoiding placing infant on cold surfaces such as metal treatment tables, cold x-ray plates 5. Padding cold surfaces with diapers and using radiant warmers during procedures 6. Warming blood for exchange transfusions	*SGA infant has increased heat loss due to decreased available brown fat stores for heat production and less fat insulation.*
Monitor for signs and symptoms of cold stress: decreased temperatures, lethargy, pallor (for further discussion, see Chapter 32).	*Cold stress increases oxygen requirements.*

OUTCOME MET IF:
- Newborn's skin temperature is maintained between 36.1 and 36.7 C.
- Newborn shows no signs of lethargy, pallor, or cyanosis.

NURSING DIAGNOSIS: Risk for injury to tissues related to decreased glycogen stores and impaired gluconeogenesis

EXPECTED OUTCOME: Newborn will maintain blood glucose levels.

Nursing Interventions	Rationale
Monitor blood glucose per SGA protocol and report values <40 mg/dL.	*Combined with depletion of glycogen stores, impaired gluconeogenesis predisposes SGA infants to profound hypoglycemia within first 2 days of life.*
Observe, record, and report signs of hypoglycemia: cyanosis, lethargy, jitteriness, seizure activity, and apnea.	*Hypoglycemia causes CNS irritability.*
Notify physician if values are low. Monitor vital signs every 2 hours prn.	
Initiate feeding schedule for SGA newborns per agency protocol. Continue to monitor blood glucose.	*Frequent monitoring of blood glucose assists in identifying decreasing glucose levels.*
Provide glucose intake either through early enteral feeding (before 4 hours of age) or by IV per physician order. (See further discussion on p 1017.)	*Provision of glucose through early feedings or IV maintains needed glucose levels. Decreasing glucose is reflected in lethargy, decreased appetite.*
Record I & O, monitor IV rate and site hourly.	

OUTCOME MET IF:
- Newborn's blood glucose is greater than 40 mg/dL.
- Newborn shown no signs of cyanosis, lethargy, jitteriness, seizure activity, or apnea.

NURSING DIAGNOSIS: Altered nutrition: Less than body requirements related to SGA's increased metabolic rate

EXPECTED OUTCOME: Newborn maintains or gains weight.

Nursing Interventions	Rationale
Initiate test water feeding at 1 hour of age, followed by early formula feeding every 2–3 hours.	*Sterile water is desirable for first feeding because it causes fewer pulmonary complications if aspirated.*
Supplement oral feedings with intravenous intake per physician order.	*SGA newborns require more calories/kg for growth because of increased metabolic activity and oxygen consumption secondary to increased percentage of body weight made up by visceral organs.*
Monitor I & O every 4 hours or more frequently.	
Use concentrated formulas that supply more calories in less volume, such as Similac 24.	*Small, frequent feedings of high-calorie formula are used because of limited gastric capacity and decreased gastric emptying.*
Promote growth by providing caloric intake of 120 kcal/kg/day in small amounts. Monitor and record signs of respiratory distress or fatigue occurring during feedings.	

SMALL-FOR-GESTATIONAL-AGE NEWBORN *continued*

Nursing Interventions	Rationale
Supplement gavage, bottle-, or breastfeedings with intravenous therapy per physician order until oral intake is sufficient to support growth.	*Adequate nutritional intake promotes growth and prevents such complications as metabolic catabolism and hypoglycemia.*
Begin bottle- or breastfeeding slowly, such as once per day, then once per shift, then every other feeding.	*Gavage feedings require less energy expenditure on the part of the newborn.*
Monitor daily weight with anticipation of small amount of weight loss when bottle- or breastfeedings start.	*Bottle- or breastfeeding entail active rather than passive intake of nutrition and require energy expenditure, burning of calories, and potential weight loss.*

OUTCOME MET IF:
- Newborn does not lose more than 2% of body weight per day.
- Newborn receives and tolerates 120 kcal/kg/day.
- Newborn takes formula without tiring.

NURSING DIAGNOSIS: Risk for altered tissue perfusion related to increased blood viscosity

EXPECTED OUTCOME: Newborn will show no signs of complications from increased blood viscosity.

Nursing Interventions	Rationale
Obtain central hematocrit on admission.	Polycythemia *is defined as a central venous hematocrit above 65–70% in the first week of life. Hyperviscosity is resultant thickness and decreased deformability of red-cell-rich blood so that its ability to perfuse the tissues is disturbed. Exact etiology of polycythemia in SGA is not known but is thought to be a physiologic response to chronic hypoxia with increased erythropoietin production.*
Monitor, record, and report symptoms, including: 1. Decrease in peripheral pulses, discoloration of extremity, alteration in activity or neurologic depression, renal vein thrombosis with decreased urine output, hematuria, or proteinuria in thromboembolic conditions 2. Tachycardia or congestive heart failure 3. Respiratory distress syndrome, cyanosis, tachypnea, increased oxygen need, labored respirations, or hemorrhage in respiratory system	
Watch for other signs of increased hematocrit, such as hyperbilirubinemia. Monitor bilirubin levels every 8 hours.	*As the increased red blood cells begin to break down, hyperbilirubinemia may present.*
Assist with partial plasma exchange.	*Partial plasma exchange decreases blood volume and blood viscosity to less than 60%.*

OUTCOME MET IF:
- Newborn's hemoglobin is less than 22 g/dL.
- Newborn's hematocrit is less than 65%.
- Newborn shows no sign of cyanosis, tachypnea, labored respirations, or hyperbilirubinemia.

NURSING DIAGNOSIS: Risk for altered parenting related to prolonged separation of newborn from parents secondary to illness

EXPECTED OUTCOME: Parents will demonstrate evidence of positive physical and social interaction with newborn.

Nursing Interventions	Rationale
Include parents in determining infant's plan of care, and encourage their participation. Encourage parents to visit frequently. Provide opportunities for parents to touch, hold, talk to, and care for their infant. Determine the type and amount of appropriate sensory stimulation, and implement sensory stimulation program.	*Parent-infant bonding begins in the first few hours or days following the birth of an infant. SGA infants experience prolonged periods of separation from their parents, which necessitates intervention to ensure parent-infant bonding. Emotional support of the psychologic well-being of the family, including positive parent-infant bonding and sensory stimulation of the infant, is important.*

OUTCOME MET IF:
- Parents demonstrate two or more of the following physical interactions: good eye contact, touching baby, holding baby close, attempting to comfort baby, kissing baby.
- Parents demonstrate two or more of the following social interactions: calling baby by name, making positive comments about baby, asking questions about baby, asking questions about newborn care, talking to baby.

SMALL-FOR-GESTATIONAL-AGE NEWBORN continued

NURSING DIAGNOSIS: Knowledge deficit related to lack of information about care of newborn at home

EXPECTED OUTCOME: Parents will be able to manage newborn care at home.

Nursing Interventions	Rationale
Prepare for discharge by instructing parents in such areas as feeding techniques, formula preparation (including bottle sterilization), and breastfeeding; bathing, diapering, hygiene; temperature monitoring; administration of vitamins; sibling ri~alry; care of complications and preventing exposure to infections; normal elimination patterns, expected weight gain patterns, normal reflexes and activity, and how to promote normal growth and development without being overprotective; returning for continued medical care; and availability of community resources if indicated.	*Parents should receive the same postpartum teaching as any parent taking a new infant home. Parents need to understand the changes to expect in color of the infant's stool and number of bowel movements, plus odor from bottle- or breast-feeding, to avoid unnecessary concern. Preterm infants usually do not require referral to community agencies unless there is a specific problem requiring assistance. Infants with congenital abnormalities, feeding problems, or resolving complications with infections or mothers unable to cope with defective infants may require referral to community resources.*

OUTCOME MET IF: • Parents verbalize/demonstrate ability to care for newborn at home, when to return for follow-up visits, what signs and symptoms to report to health care provider, and available community resources.

Essential Nursing Activities to Achieve Outcomes

Maternal Assessment

1. Conduct accurate maternal history and exam to identify potential for SGA baby.
2. Note any factors contributing to SGA:
   a. Malnutrition (mainly in last trimester)
   b. Vascular complications such as PIH or diabetes
   c. Maternal disease such as heart disease, PKU
   d. Maternal factors such as smoking, substance abuse, poor living conditions
   e. Environmental factors such as high altitude, x-rays
   f. Placental factors such as placenta previa, abnormal cord insertion
   g. Fetal factors such as congenital infections, multiple pregnancy, inborn errors of metabolism.
1. Conduct antepartal testing to assess for fetal well-being and placental reserve: NST, CST, BPP.
2. Assess maternal-infant interaction.

Newborn Assessment

1. Estimate gestational age to determine SGA (IUGR) status.
2. Determine if IUGR is symmetric (chronic, longterm) or asymmetric (acute).

3. Assess for potential complications of
   a. Perinatal asphyxia
   b. Aspiration syndrome
   c. Hypothermia
   d. Hypoglycemia
   e. Hypocalcemia
   f. Polycythemia
4. Assess breath sounds every 4 hours.
5. Assess for cyanosis, grunting, nasal flaring.
6. Maintain skin temperature at 36.1–36.7 C.
7. Monitor blood glucose per SGA protocol. Glucose levels should be >40 mg/dL.
8. Assess I & O.
9. Assess feeding tolerance.
10. Assess for signs of jaundice.
11. Assess blood work: hematocrit <65%; hemoglobin <22 g/dL; bilirubin <12 mg/dL.
12. Weigh daily.

---

diameter greater than 10 cm (4 in) or are associated with a maternal fundal height measurement greater than 42 cm (16 in) without the presence of hydramnios. Because of their excessive size, there are more breech presentations and shoulder dystocias. These complications may result in asphyxia, fractured clavicles, brachial plexus palsy, facial paralysis, phrenic nerve palsy, depressed skull fractures, hematomas, and bleeding due to birth trauma.

• *Increased incidence of cesarean births and oxytocin-induced births due to fetal size.* These births are accompanied by all the risk factors associated with cesarean births (ACOG technical bulletin #159 1992).

• *Hypoglycemia, polycythemia, and hyperviscosity.* These disorders are most often seen in infants of diabetic mothers and infants with erythroblastosis fetalis or Beckwith-Wiedemann syndrome.

Nursing Care

The perinatal history, in conjunction with ultrasonic measurement of fetal skull and gestational age testing, is important in identifying an at-risk LGA newborn. Nursing care is directed toward early identification and immediate treatment of the common disorders. Essential components of the nursing assessment are monitoring vital signs, screening for hypoglycemia and polycythemia, and observing for signs and symptoms related to birth trauma. Parental concerns about the visual signs of birth trauma need to be addressed (Pressler 1991), as does the potential for continuation of the overweight pattern. The nurse needs to help parents learn to arouse and console their newborn and to facilitate nutritional intake and attachment behaviors. Mothers of LGA infants with bruising of the face and/or head may be reluctant to interact with their infant because they fear increasing the bruising or causing their infants pain (Pressler 1991). The nursing care involved in the complications associated with LGA newborns is the same as the care needed by the infant with a diabetic mother and is discussed next.

CARE OF THE INFANT OF A DIABETIC MOTHER

Infants of diabetic mothers (IDMs) are considered at risk and require close observation the first few hours to the first few days of life. Mothers with severe diabetes or diabetes of long duration (type I or White's classes D–F, associated with vascular complications; see Table 18–2) may give birth to SGA infants. The typical IDM (Type I or White's classes A and C), however, is LGA. These infants are fat, macrosomic, and ruddy in color (Figure 31–4). The umbilical cord and placenta are also large.

IDMs have decreased total body water, particularly in the extracellular spaces, and are therefore not edematous. Their excessive weight is due to increased weight of the visceral organs, cardiomegaly (hypertrophy), and increased body fat. The only organ not affected is the brain (Ogata 1994).

The excessive fetal growth of the IDM is caused by exposure to high levels of maternal glucose, which readily crosses the placenta. The fetus responds to these high glucose levels with increased insulin production and hyperplasia of the pancreatic beta cells. The main action of insulin is to facilitate the entry of glucose into muscle and fat cells in a function similar to a cellular growth hormone. Once in the cells, glucose is converted to glycogen and stored. Insulin also inhibits the breakdown of fat to free fatty acids, thereby maintaining lipid synthesis; increases the uptake of amino acids; and promotes protein synthesis. Insulin is an important regulator of fetal metabolism and has a "growth hormone" effect that results in increased linear growth (Warshaw 1994a). There has been an association between IDM and childhood obesity (Hod & Diamant 1992).

Common Complications of the IDM

Although IDMs are usually large, they are immature in physiologic functions and exhibit many of the problems of the preterm (premature) infant. The complications most often seen in an IDM are the following:

- *Hypoglycemia*. After birth the most common problem of an IDM is hypoglycemia. Even though the high maternal blood sugar supply is lost, this newborn continues to produce high levels of insulin, which deplete the infant's blood glucose within hours after birth. IDMs also have less ability to release glucagon and catecholamines, which normally stimulate glucagon breakdown and glucose release. The incidence of hypoglycemia in IDMs is around 20% (Cordero & Landon 1993). Incidence of hypoglycemia varies according to the degree of success in controlling the maternal diabetes, the maternal blood sugar level at the time of birth, the length of labor, the class of maternal diabetes, and early versus late feedings of the newborn.

- *Hypocalcemia*. This complication may be due to the increased incidence of prematurity and to the stresses of difficult pregnancy, labor, and birth, which predispose any infant to hypocalcemia. Diabetic women tend to have higher calcium levels at term, which causes secondary hypoparathyroidism in their infants (Ogata 1994). Other factors may include vitamin D antagonism, which results from elevated corticol levels, hypophosphatemia from tissue catabolism, and decreased serum magnesium levels.

- *Hyperbilirubinemia*. This condition may be seen at 48 to 72 hours after birth. It may be caused by slightly decreased extracellular fluid volume, which increases the hematocrit level, and the presence of hepatic immaturity (Warshaw 1994a). Enclosed hemorrhages resulting from complicated vaginal birth may also cause hyperbilirubinemia. There may also be an increase in the rate of bilirubin production in the presence of polycythemia.

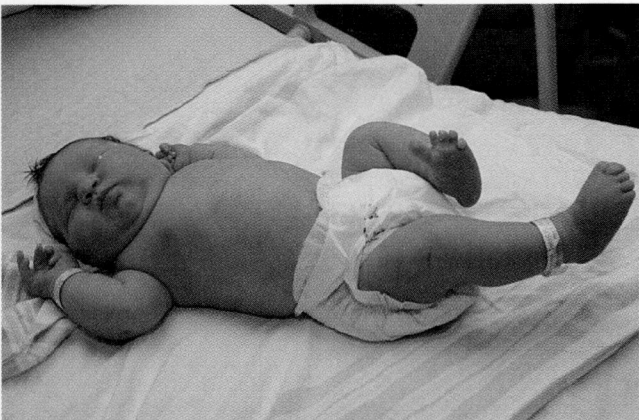

FIGURE 31-4 Macrosomic infant of a diabetic mother. X-ray examination of these infants often reveal caudal regression of the spine.

- *Birth trauma.* Because most IDMs are LGA, trauma may occur during labor and birth.

- *Polycythemia.* This condition may be caused by the decreased extracellular fluid volume in IDMs. (See the discussion in Chapter 32.) Fetal hyperglycemia and hyperinsulinism results in increased oxygen consumption, leading to fetal hypoxia (Warshaw 1994a). Recent research has focused on the ability of hemoglobin A_{1c} to bind to oxygen, which decreases the oxygen available to the fetal tissues. This tissue hypoxia stimulates increased erythropoietin production, which increases the hematocrit level.

- *Respiratory distress syndrome (RDS).* This complication occurs especially in newborns of White's classes A–C diabetic mothers. It has been demonstrated that insulin antagonizes the cortisol-induced stimulation of lecithin synthesis that is necessary for lung maturation. Therefore IDMs may have lungs that are less mature than expected for their gestational age. There is also a decrease in the phospholipid PG that stabilizes surfactant, thus increasing the incidence of RDS. RDS does not appear to be a problem for infants born to diabetic mothers in White's classes D–F; instead the stresses of poor uterine blood supply may lead to increased production of steroids, which accelerates lung maturation.

- *Congenital birth defects.* Congenital anomalies that may occur in IDMs are transposition of the great vessels, ventricular septal defect, patent ductus arteriosus, small left colon syndrome, and sacral agenesis (caudal regression) (Cordero & Landon 1993). Early and careful control of maternal glucose prior to and during pregnancy decreases the risk of birth defects (Wyse et al 1994).

Medical Therapy

The goal of medical therapy is the early detection of and intervention in the problems associated with infants born to diabetic mothers. Prenatal management is directed toward control of maternal hyperglycemia, which minimizes the common complications of IDMs: pulmonary problems, macrosomia, polycythemia, and hypoglycemia.

Because the onset of hypoglycemia occurs between 1 and 3 hours after birth in IDMs (with a spontaneous rise to normal levels by 4 to 6 hours), blood glucose determinations should be done on cord blood hourly during the first 4 hours after birth and then at 4-hour intervals until the risk period (about 24 hours) has passed (Ogata 1994).

IDMs whose serum glucose falls below 40 mg/dL should have early feedings with formula or breast milk (colostrum). The infant may need to be gavage fed if lethargic. If normal glucose levels cannot be maintained with oral feeding or if seizures occur, an intravenous infusion of glucose will be necessary. The rate of 4–6 mg/kg/minute usually maintains normoglycemia in the

IDM (Ogata 1994). Once the blood glucose has been stable for 24 hours, the infusion rate can be decreased as oral feedings are increased. The newborn's blood glucose levels must be carefully monitored. Dextrose (25%–50%) as a rapid infusion is contraindicated because it may lead to severe rebound hypoglycemia following an initial brief increase in glucose level.

APPLYING THE NURSING PROCESS

Nursing Assessment

In caring for the IDM, the nurse assesses signs of respiratory distress, hyperbilirubinemia, birth trauma, and congenital anomalies. Close and ongoing nursing assessments and care are essential in decreasing the potential harmful effects of the problems associated with IDMs.

Critical Thinking Question

What information would you provide to a diabetic woman prior to conception that could decrease the possible complications for her baby?

Nursing Diagnosis

Nursing diagnoses that may apply to IDMs include the following:

- Altered nutrition: Less than body requirements related to increased glucose metabolism secondary to hyperinsulinemia

- Impaired gas exchange related to respiratory distress secondary to impaired production of surfactant

- Ineffective family coping: Compromised, related to the illness of the baby

TEACHING MOMENT

Don't be lulled into thinking that a big baby is a mature baby. In almost every case, because of his or her large size, the infant of a diabetic mother (class A, B, or C) will appear older than gestational age scoring indicates. You must consider both the gestational age and whether the baby is AGA or LGA in planning and providing safe care.

Nursing Care

Nursing care of the IDM is directed toward early detection and ongoing monitoring of hypoglycemia (by doing glucose tests) and polycythemia (by obtaining central hematocrits), respiratory distress, and hyperbilirubinemia. For specific nursing interventions for respiratory distress syndrome, hypoglycemia, hyperbilirubinemia, and polycythemia see Chapter 32.

The nurse educates parents about prevention of macrosomia and resultant fetal newborn problems and institutes early and ongoing diabetic control. Parents are advised that with early identification and care, most IDMs' newborn problems have no significant sequelae.

Evaluation

Anticipated outcomes of nursing care include:

- The IDM's respiratory and metabolic alteration problems are minimized.

- The parents understand the cause of the baby's health problems and preventative steps they can initiate to decrease the impact of maternal diabetes on subsequent fetuses.

- The parents verbalize their concerns surrounding their baby's health problems and understand the rationale behind management of their newborn.

CARE OF THE POSTTERM NEWBORN

The **postterm newborn** is any newborn born after 42 weeks' gestation. In the past the terms *postterm* and *postmature* were used interchangeably. The term **postmaturity** is now used only when the infant is born after 42 weeks of gestation and also demonstrates characteristics of the *postmaturity syndrome*. Postterm or prolonged pregnancy occurs in approximately 3% to 12% of all pregnancies (Spellacy 1994).

The cause of postterm pregnancy is not completely understood, but several factors are known to be associated with it, including primiparity, high multiparity (five or more pregnancies), and a history of prolonged pregnancies. Many pregnancies classified as prolonged are thought to be a result of inaccurate estimation of the estimated date of birth (EDB) (Spellacy 1994). The causes of most true postterm gestations are unknown. A positive correlation exists between postterm pregnancy and Australian, Greek, and Italian ethnic groups (Iams & Zuspan 1990).

Most babies born as a result of prolonged pregnancy are of normal size and health; some keep on growing and are over 4000 g at birth, which supports the premise that the postterm fetus can remain well nourished (Harrington & Campbell 1993). Intrapartal problems for these healthy but large fetuses are cephalopelvic disproportion (CPD) and shoulder dystocia. At birth about 5% of postterm newborns show signs of postmaturity syndrome (Iams & Zuspan 1990). The major portion of the following discussion will address the fetus who is not tolerating the prolonged pregnancy, is suffering from uteroplacental compromise to blood flow and resultant hypoxia, and is therefore considered to have postmaturity syndrome.

Common Complications of the Newborn with Postmaturity Syndrome

The truly postmature newborn is at high risk for morbidity and has a mortality rate two to three times higher than that of term infants. Although today the percentages are extremely low, the majority of postmature fetal deaths occur during labor because by that time the fetus has used up necessary reserves. Because of decreased placental function, oxygenation and nutrition transport are impaired, leaving the fetus prone to hypoglycemia and asphyxia when the stresses of labor begin. These infants often do not tolerate labor and are delivered by cesarean section. The following are other common disorders of the postmature newborn:

- Hypoglycemia, from nutritional deprivation and resultant depleted glycogen stores.

- Meconium aspiration in response to in utero hypoxia (In the presence of oligohydramnios the danger of aspirating thick meconium is increased. Severe meconium aspiration syndrome increases the baby's chance of developing persistent pulmonary hypertension, pneumothorax, and pneumonia) (see Chapter 32).

- Polycythemia due to increased production of red blood cells (RBCs) in response to hypoxia

- Congenital anomalies of unknown cause

- Seizures because of hypoxic insult

- Cold stress because of loss or poor development of subcutaneous fat

The long-term effects of postmaturity syndrome are unclear. At present studies do not agree on the effect of postmaturity syndrome on weight gain and IQ scores.

Just prolonged pregnancy itself is not responsible for the postmaturity syndrome. The characteristics of the postmature newborn are primarily caused by a combination of placental aging and subsequent insufficiency and continued exposure to amniotic fluid (Resnik 1994).

Medical Therapy

The goal of medical therapy is identification and management of the postmature newborn's potential problems. Antenatal management is directed at differentiating the fetus who has postmaturity syndrome from the fetus who is large, well-nourished, and equally alert and who is tolerating the prolonged (postterm) pregnancy.

Antenatal tests that can be done to evaluate fetal status and determine obstetric management include fetal ultrasound, assessment of amniotic fluid volume, fetal biophysical profile (refer to Chapter 20), measurement of serum placental hormones such as human chorionic gonadotropin (hCG) and human placental lactogen (hPL), and the nonstress test (NST) and contraction stress test (CST). These tests and their use in postterm pregnancy are discussed in more depth in Chapter 25.

If the amniotic fluid is meconium stained, the baby's nose and mouth should be suctioned by the clinician prior to birth of the chest and trunk and before the baby takes its first breath to minimize the chance of meconium aspiration syndrome. In some cases direct suctioning of the trachea is needed. For detailed discussion of medical management and nursing assessments and care of this condition see Chapter 32.

Hypoglycemia is monitored by serial glucose determinations. The baby may be placed on glucose infusions or given early feedings if respiratory distress is not present; but these measures must be instituted with caution because of the frequency of asphyxia in the first 24 hours (Cunningham 1993). Postmature newborns are often voracious eaters.

As with SGA infants, peripheral and central hematocrits are tested to assess the presence of polycythemia. A partial exchange transfusion may be necessary to prevent polycythemia and adverse sequelae such as hyperviscosity. Oxygen is provided for respiratory distress. Also, temperature instability and excessive body heat loss can take place (Cunningham 1993). See Chapter 29 for thermoregulation techniques.

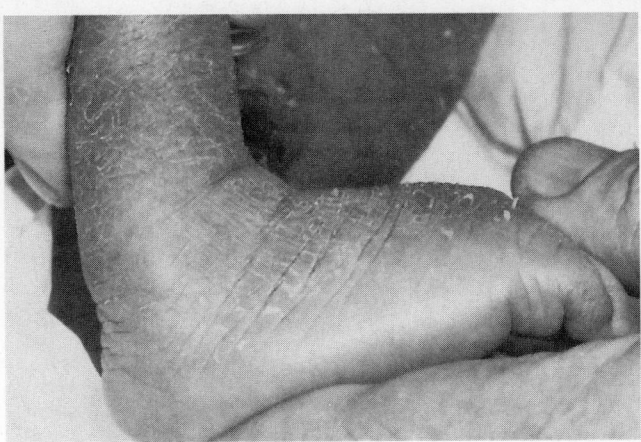

FIGURE 31-5 Postterm infant demonstrates deep cracking and peeling of skin. SOURCE: Dubowitz L, Dubowitz V: *The Gestational Age of the Newborn.* Menlo Park, CA: Addison-Wesley, 1977. Reprinted by permission of V Dubowitz, MD, Hammersmith Hospital, London, England.

meconium was a single recent event or a chronic problem. Green coloring indicates a more recent event.

Nursing Diagnosis

Nursing diagnoses that may apply to the postmature newborn include the following:

- Hypothermia related to decreased liver glycogen and brown fat stores

- Altered nutrition: Less than body requirements related to increased use of glucose secondary to stress in utero and decreased placental perfusion

- Impaired gas exchange in the lungs and at the cellular level related to airway obstruction from meconium aspiration

Nursing Plan and Implementation
Promotion of Physical Well-Being

Nursing interventions are primarily supportive measures. They include the following:

- Observation of cardiopulmonary status because the stresses of labor are poorly tolerated and severe asphyxia can occur at birth

- Provision of warmth to counterbalance the infant's poor response to cold stress and decreased liver glycogen and brown fat stores

- Frequent monitoring of blood glucose and initiation of early feeding (at 1 or 2 hours of age) or intravenous glucose per physician order

- Observation for the common disorders identified earlier and institution of nursing care and medical management as ordered

> APPLYING THE NURSING PROCESS

Nursing Assessment

The newborn with postmaturity syndrome appears alert. This wide-eyed, alert appearance is not necessarily a positive sign because it may indicate chronic intrauterine hypoxia.

The infant has dry, cracking, parchmentlike skin without vernix or lanugo (Figure 31–5). Fingernails are long, and scalp hair is profuse. The infant's body appears long and thin. The wasting involves depletion of previously stored subcutaneous tissue, causing the skin to be loose. Fat layers are almost nonexistent.

Postmature newborns frequently have meconium staining, which colors the nails, skin, and umbilical cord. The varying shades (yellow to green) of meconium staining can give some clue about whether the expulsion of

Provision of Emotional Support to the Parents

The nurse encourages parents to express their feelings and fears regarding the newborn's condition and potential long-term problems. The nurse gives careful explanations of procedures and includes the parents in development of care plans for their baby and encourages follow-up care as needed.

Evaluation

Anticipated outcomes of nursing care include:

- The postterm newborn establishes effective respiratory function.
- The postmature baby is free of metabolic alterations (hypoglycemia) and maintains a stable temperature.

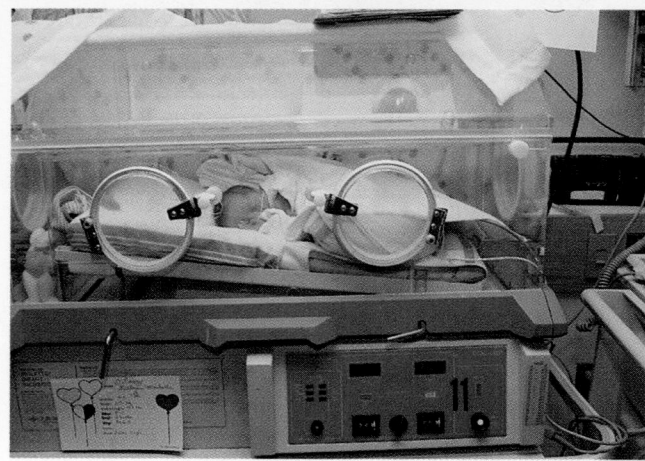

FIGURE 31-6 Preterm infant.

CARE OF THE PRETERM (PREMATURE) NEWBORN

A **preterm infant** is any infant born before the end of 37 completed weeks' gestation. The length of gestation and thus the level of maturity vary even in the "premature" population. Figure 31–6 shows a preterm newborn.

The incidence of preterm births in the United States ranges from 7% of White newborns to 14% to 15% of non-Whites. A higher incidence of prematurity is also seen in single women and adolescents. Prematurity and low birth weight are two common outcomes of pregnancy in young mothers.

The causes of preterm labor are poorly understood, but more and more of the factors that influence preterm labor and birth are being identified. (See Chapter 19 for a discussion of preterm labor and birth.) With the help of modern technology some babies under 500 g and between 23 and 26 weeks' gestation are surviving, but not without significant morbidity.

Physiologic Considerations

The major problem of the preterm newborn is variable immaturity of all systems. The degree of immaturity depends on the length of gestation. For example, newborns of 32 weeks' gestation can be expected to exhibit more immaturity than newborns of 36 weeks' gestation. The degree of immaturity also presents problems of management because maintenance of the preterm newborn falls within narrow physiologic parameters. Improper physiologic management (or lack of management) adds stress and feeds the vicious cycle of physiologic deterioration. "Catch-up care" is not always possible if ground is lost in initial management.

The preterm newborn must traverse the same complex, interconnected pathways from intrauterine to extrauterine life as the term newborn. Because of immaturity, the preterm newborn is ill equipped to make this transition smoothly. This section addresses the physiologic and nutritional factors associated with prematurity.

Respiratory and Cardiac Physiology and Considerations

The preterm newborn is at risk for respiratory problems because the lungs are not fully mature and ready to take over the process of oxygen and carbon dioxide exchange until 37 to 38 weeks' gestation. The most critical influencing factor in the development of respiratory distress is the preterm infant's inability to produce adequate amounts of surfactant. (See Chapter 27 for discussion of respiratory adaptation and development.) When surfactant is decreased, compliance (ability of the lung to fill with air easily) is also lessened, and the inspiratory pressure needed to expand the lungs with air increases. The collapsed (or atelectatic) alveoli will not facilitate an exchange of oxygen and carbon dioxide, resulting in hypoxia, inefficient pulmonary blood flow, and depletion of the preterm newborn's available energy.

Besides adequate surfactant production, alveolar sacs must be present in sufficient number to provide the surface area needed to accomplish oxygen and carbon dioxide exchange. The term infant has about 20 million alveoli; the 8-year-old child has 300 million to 400 million (Whitsett et al 1994).

Lung development begins at around 24 days of fetal life, when the primitive lung bud appears (Figure 31–7). The primitive lung bud branches at about 26 to 28 days to form the major right and left bronchi. Growth and branching continue throughout gestation, forming terminal bronchioles to respiratory bronchioles, from which arise alveolar ducts. The alveolar ducts are differentiated by approximately 24 weeks' gestation and give rise to

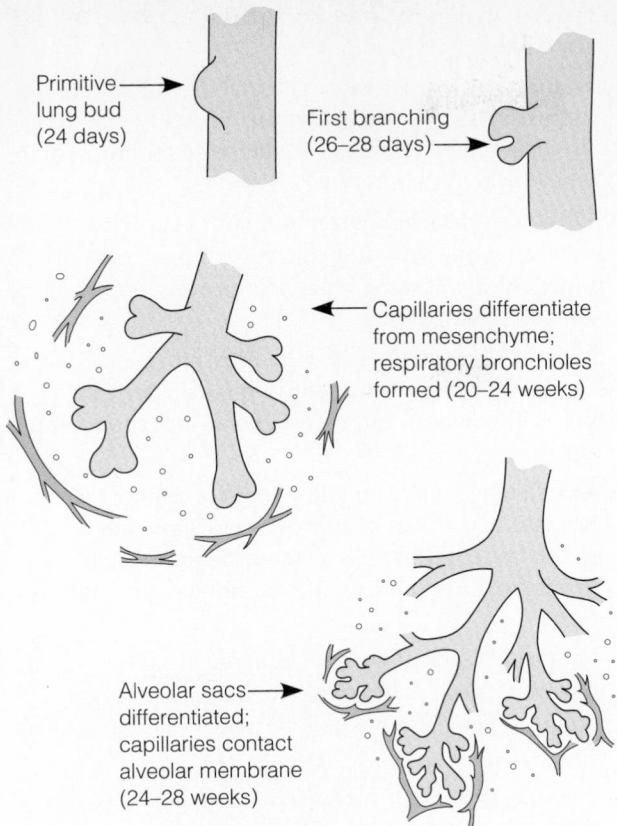

Primitive
lung bud
(24 days)

First branching
(26–28 days)

Capillaries differentiate
from mesenchyme;
respiratory bronchioles
formed (20–24 weeks)

Alveolar sacs
differentiated;
capillaries contact
alveolar membrane
(24–28 weeks)

FIGURE 31-7 Development of primitive lung bud and subsequent branching into surrounding mesenchyme. SOURCE: Korones SB: *High Risk Newborn Infants,* 3rd ed. St Louis: Mosby, 1986.

thin-walled terminal air sacs. From 24 weeks until birth growth and development of these terminal air sacs or premature alveoli are continuous. At about 24 to 26 weeks' gestation, the surface area available for gas exchange is very limited (because of inadequate number and size of alveoli), and inadequate surfactant is produced, making survival at this time less likely.

By 27 to 28 weeks, more alveolar sacs have developed, and more capillaries are in contact with the alveolar membrane. This allows some exchange of oxygen from the alveoli to the capillaries and carbon dioxide from the capillaries to the alveoli. Surfactant production at this time is unstable and inadequate, but with respiratory assistance and surfactant administration, survival is possible. The newborn is at risk, however, for many complications, such as RDS, hypoxemia, acidemia, intraventricular hemorrhage, cold stress, and metabolic imbalances, any one of which may compromise ultimate survival.

Between 29 and 30 weeks, additional differentiation of the alveolar sacs occurs, and additional surfactant is released. After 30 weeks' gestation, growth of new primitive alveoli is rapid, and by 36 weeks mature alveoli are present. Also by this time surfactant production increases rapidly as the second pathway of surfactant production begins optimal functioning. If the fetus is unstressed and

without iatrogenic complications, adequate amounts of surfactant should be produced for lung expansion and gas exchange at this time. In the presence of asphyxia, hypoxemia, acidemia, or cold stress, surfactant production is impaired, resulting in increased chances of respiratory distress. The more immature the infant, the more devastating the physiologic complications.

In the preterm infant the muscular coat of the pulmonary arterioles is incompletely developed. This muscular development occurs late in gestation; therefore the more premature the infant, the less muscular the pulmonary arterioles (Whitsett et al 1994). Because of decreased pulmonary arteriole musculature, vasoconstriction is not effective in response to decreased oxygen levels. Therefore, the healthy preterm infant has a lower pulmonary vascular resistance than a full-term infant. This lowered resistance leads to increased left-to-right shunting through the ductus arteriosus, which steps up the blood flow back into the lungs. The preterm infant who develops respiratory distress and its complications (acidemia and hypoxemia) is at greater risk for increasing pulmonary vascular resistance because decreased PO_2 triggers vasoconstriction. Increased resistance decreases blood flow through the lungs, causing additional hypoxemia and acidemia. The ductus arteriosus usually responds to increasing oxygen levels by vasoconstriction; in the preterm infant, who has higher susceptibility to hypoxia, the ductus may remain open. A patent ductus increases the blood volume to the lungs, causing pulmonary congestion, increased respiratory effort, and higher oxygen use.

Thermoregulation and Considerations

Maintaining a normal body temperature in the preterm infant presents a nursing challenge. Heat loss is a major problem that the nurse can do much to prevent. Two limiting factors in heat production, however, are the availability of glycogen in the liver (glycogen stores are primarily laid down during the third trimester) and the amount of brown fat available for metabolism (the preterm infant does not have a full supply of brown fat). If the baby is chilled after birth, both glycogen and brown fat stores are metabolized rapidly for heat production, leaving the newborn with no reserves in the event of future stress. Because the muscle mass is small in preterm infants and muscular activity is diminished (they are unable to shiver), little heat is produced.

Heat loss occurs as a result of five physiologic and anatomic factors:

1. The preterm baby has a high ratio of body surface to body weight. This means that the baby's ability to produce heat (based on body weight) is much less than the potential for losing heat (based on surface area). The loss of heat in a preterm infant weighing 1500 g is five times greater per unit of body weight than in an adult.

2. The preterm baby has very little subcutaneous fat, which is the human body's insulation. Without adequate insulation, heat is easily conducted from the core of the body (water temperature) to the surface of the body (cooler temperature). Heat is lost from the body as the blood vessels, which lie close to the skin surface in the preterm infant, transport blood from the body core to the subcutaneous tissues.

3. The preterm baby has thinner, more permeable skin than the term infant. This increased permeability contributes to a greater insensible water loss as well as heat loss.

4. The posture of the preterm baby is another important factor influencing heat loss. Flexion of the extremities decreases the amount of surface area exposed to the environment. Extension increases the surface area exposed to the environment and thus increases heat loss. The gestational age of the infant influences the amount of flexion, from completely hypotonic and extended at 28 weeks to strong flexion displayed by 36 weeks.

5. The preterm baby has a decreased ability to vasoconstrict superficial blood vessels and conserve heat in the body core.

In summary, the more premature the baby, the less able he or she is to maintain heat balance. Preventing heat loss by providing a neutral thermal environment is one of the most important considerations in nursing management of the preterm infant. Cold stress, with its accompanying severe complications, can be prevented (see Chapter 32).

Gastrointestinal Physiology and Considerations

The basic structure of the gastrointestinal tract is formed early in gestation, so even the very premature newborn is able to take in some nourishment. However, the digestive and absorptive processes are not fully functional until later in gestation. The reflexes that control food ingestion are also immature until late.

As a result of these immaturities the preterm newborn has the following ingestion, digestion, and absorption problems:

- There is marked danger of aspiration and its associated complications because of the infant's poorly developed gag reflex, incompetent esophageal cardiac sphincter, and poor sucking and swallowing reflexes.

- Small stomach capacity limits the amount of fluid that can be introduced to meet the infant's high caloric needs.

- Limited ability exists to convert certain essential amino acids to nonessential amino acids. (Certain amino acids, such as histidine, taurine, and cysteine, are essential to the preterm infant but not to the term infant.)

- Kidney immaturity causes an inability to handle the increased osmolarity of formula protein. The preterm infant requires a higher concentration of whey protein than casein.

- Difficulty absorbing saturated fats occurs because of decreased bile salts and pancreatic lipase. Severe illness of the newborn may also prevent intake of adequate nutrients.

- Lactose digestion may not be fully functional during the first few days of a preterm infant's life. The preterm newborn can digest and absorb most simple sugars.

- Deficiency of calcium and phosphorus may exist because two-thirds of these minerals are deposited in the last trimester. As a result the preterm infant is prone to rickets and significant bone demineralization.

- Fatigue associated with sucking may lead to increased basal metabolic rate, increased oxygen requirements, and possible necrotizing enterocolitis (NEC).

- There is feeding intolerance and NEC due to diminished blood flow to the intestinal tract because of shock or prolonged hypoxia at birth.

Renal Physiology and Considerations

The kidneys of the preterm infant are immature in comparison with those of the full-term infant, which poses clinical problems in the management of fluid and electrolyte balance. Specific characteristics of the preterm infant include the following:

- The glomerular filtration rate (GFR) is lower due to decreased renal blood flow. The GFR is directly related to lower gestational age, so the more preterm the newborn, the lower the GFR. The GFR is also decreased in the presence of diseases or conditions that decrease the renal blood flow and/or oxygen content, such as severe respiratory distress and perinatal asphyxia. Anuria and/or oliguria may be observed in the preterm infant after severe asphyxia with associated hypotension.

- The preterm infant's kidneys are limited in their ability to concentrate urine or to excrete excess amounts of fluid. This means that if excess fluid is administered, the infant is at risk for fluid retention and overhydration. If too little is administered, the infant will become dehydrated because of the inability to retain adequate fluid.

- The kidneys of the preterm infant begin excreting glucose at a lower serum glucose level than those of the term infant. Therefore glycosuria with hyperglycemia is common.

- The buffering capacity of the kidney is reduced, predisposing the infant to metabolic acidosis. Bicarbonate is excreted at a lower serum level, and excretion of acid is accomplished more slowly. Therefore after periods of hypoxia or insult the preterm infant's kidneys require a longer time to excrete the lactic acid that accumulates. Sodium bicarbonate is frequently required to treat the metabolic acidosis.

- The immaturity of the renal system affects the preterm infant's ability to excrete drugs. Because excretion time is longer, many drugs are given over longer intervals (for example, every 12 hours instead of every 8 hours). Urine output must be carefully monitored when the infant is receiving nephrotoxic drugs such as gentamicin and nafcillin. In the event of poor urine output, drugs can become toxic in the infant much more quickly than in the adult.

Hepatic Physiology and Considerations

Immaturity of the preterm newborn's liver predisposes the infant to several problems. First, glycogen is stored in the liver throughout gestation, reaching approximately 5% of the weight of the liver by term (Kliegman 1993). After birth the glycogen stores are rapidly used for energy. Glycogen deposits are affected by asphyxia in utero and after birth by both asphyxia and cold stress. The baby born preterm has decreased glycogen stores at birth and frequently experiences stress, which uses up the glycogen rapidly. Therefore the preterm newborn is at high risk for hypoglycemia and its complications.

Iron is also stored in the liver, and the amount greatly increases during the last trimester of pregnancy. Therefore the preterm newborn is born with low iron stores. If subject to hemorrhage, rapid growth, and excess blood sampling, the preterm infant is likely to become iron depleted more quickly than the term infant. Many preterm babies require transfusions of packed cells to replace the blood withdrawn by frequent blood sampling.

Conjugation of bilirubin in the liver is also impaired in the preterm infant. Thus bilirubin levels increase more rapidly and to a higher level than in the full-term infant. Early clinical assessment of jaundice at nontoxic bilirubin levels is more difficult in preterm newborns because they lack subcutaneous fat.

Immunologic Physiology and Considerations

The preterm infant is at a much greater risk for infection than the term infant. This increased susceptibility is partially attributable to an underdeveloped cellular immune system but may also be the result of an infection acquired in utero, which precipitates preterm labor and birth.

In utero the fetus receives passive immunity against a variety of infections from maternal IgC immunoglobulins, which cross the placenta (see Chapter 27). Because most of this immunity is acquired in the last trimester of pregnancy, the preterm infant has few antibodies at birth. These provide less protection and become depleted earlier than in a full-term infant. This may be a contributing factor in the higher incidence of recurrent infection during the first year of life as well as in the immediate neonatal period.

The other immunoglobulin significant for the preterm infant is secretory IgA, which does not cross the placenta but is found in breast milk in significant concentrations. Breast milk's secretory IgA provides immunity to the mucosal surfaces of the gastrointestinal tract, protecting the newborn from enteric infections such as those caused by *Escherichia coli* and *Shigella*. Ill preterm infants may be unable to have breast milk and thus are at risk for enteric infections.

Another altered defense against infection in the preterm infant is the skin surface. In very small infants the skin is easily excoriated, and this factor, coupled with many invasive procedures, places the infant at great risk for nosocomial infections. It is vital to use good hand-washing techniques in the care of these infants to prevent unnecessary infection.

Hematologic Physiology and Considerations

The normal cord hemoglobin in an infant of 34 weeks' gestation is approximately 16.8 g/dL, and total blood volume ranges from 89 mL/kg to 105 mL/kg (Blanchette et al 1994). Because of the small total blood volume, any blood loss is highly significant to the preterm infant. For this reason all blood taken for sampling must be recorded. When the infant has lost 10% of total blood volume, clinical status is assessed, and a decision is made whether or not to replace the lost blood volume.

Central Nervous System Physiology and Considerations

After the general shape of the brain is formed during the first 6 weeks of gestation, the human nervous system begins a complex evolution that continues into adult life. Between the second and fourth months of gestation there is proliferation of the brain's total complement of neurons and migration of these neurons to specific sites throughout the central nervous system. Organization of the neurons that establish the nerve impulse pathways occurs from the sixth month of gestation to several years after birth. The final step in neurologic development is the covering of these nerves with myelin. Myelination begins in the second trimester of gestation and continues into adult life (Volpe 1995).

Because the period of most rapid brain growth and development occurs during the third trimester of pregnancy, the closer to term an infant is born, the better the neurologic prognosis. A common interruption of neurologic development in the preterm infant is caused by intraventricular hemorrhage (IVH). (This is discussed in more detail later in this chapter.)

Reactivity Periods and Behavioral States

The newborn infant's response to extrauterine life is characterized by two periods of reactivity, as discussed in Chapter 27. Because of the immaturity of all systems in comparison to those of the full-term newborn, the preterm infant's periods of reactivity are delayed. In the very ill infant these periods of reactivity may not be observed at all because the infant may be hypotonic and unreactive for several days after birth.

As the preterm newborn grows and the condition stabilizes, identifying behavioral states and traits unique to each infant becomes increasingly possible. This is a very important part of nursing management of the high-risk infant because it facilitates parental knowledge of their infant's cues for interaction.

In general, stable preterm infants do not demonstrate the same behavioral states as term infants. Preterm infants are more disorganized in their sleep-wake cycles and are unable to attend as well to the human face and objects in the environment. Neurologically, their responses are weaker (sucking, muscle tone, states of arousal) than full-term infants' responses.

By observing each infant's patterns of behavior and responses, especially the sleep-wake states, the nurse can teach parents optimal times for interacting with their infant. The parents and nurse can plan nursing care around the times when the infant is alert and best able to attend. In addition, the more knowledge parents have about the meaning of their infant's responses and behaviors, the better prepared they will be to meet their newborn's needs and to form a positive attachment with their child.

Management of Nutrition and Fluid Requirements

Providing adequate nutrition and fluids for the preterm infant is a major concern of the health care team. Early feedings are extremely valuable in maintaining normal metabolism and lowering the possibility of such complications as hypoglycemia, hyperbilirubinemia, hyperkalemia, and azotemia. However, the preterm newborn is at risk for complications that may develop because of immaturity of the digestive system.

Nutritional Requirements

Oral (enteral) caloric intake necessary for growth in an uncompromised healthy preterm infant is 110 to 130 kcal/kg/day (Bernbaum 1994). In addition to these relatively high caloric needs, the preterm infant requires more protein (3 g/kg/day, as opposed to 2.0 to 2.5 g/kg/day for the full-term infant) (Fletcher 1994). To meet these needs, many institutions use breast milk or special preterm formulas.

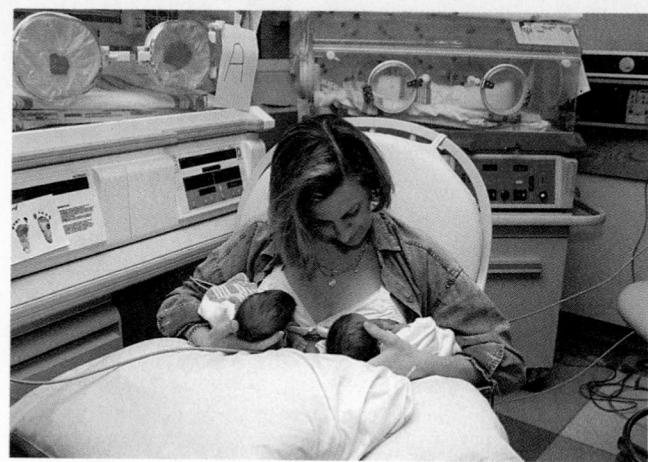

FIGURE 31–8 Mother visits intensive care unit to breastfeed her preterm twin infants.

Besides breast milk's many benefits for the infant, it allows the mother to actively contribute to the infant's well-being (Figure 31–8). The nurse should encourage mothers to breastfeed if they choose to do so. It is important for the nurse to be aware of the advantages of breastfeeding as well as the possible disadvantages if breast milk is the sole source of food for the preterm infant. See Chapter 30 for a detailed discussion of the advantages and disadvantages of breastfeeding.

Whether breast milk or formula is used, feeding regimens are established based on the infant's weight and estimated stomach capacity (Table 31–1). Initial formula feedings may be diluted to 12 cal/oz and gradually increased, as the infant tolerates them, to 24 cal/oz. In many institutions it is necessary to supplement the oral feedings with parenteral fluids to maintain adequate hydration and caloric intake until the baby is on full oral feeds.

In addition to a higher calorie and higher protein formula, preterm infants should receive supplemental multivitamins, including vitamin E. The requirement for vitamin E is increased by a diet high in polyunsaturated fats (which preterm infants tolerate best). Preterm infants fed iron-fortified formulas have higher red cell hemolysis and lower vitamin E concentrations and thus require additional vitamin E (Fletcher 1994).

Rickets and significant bone demineralization have been documented in very-low-birth-weight infants and otherwise healthy preterm infants. Preterm infant formulas have increased concentrations of calcium and phosphorus. If these specially designed preterm formulas are not used, oral supplements are recommended. In addition to calcium and phosphorus supplementation vitamin D should be supplemented to facilitate retention of calcium and increase bone densities. Preterm formulas also need to contain medium-chain triglycerides (MCT) and additional amino acids such as cysteine.

TABLE 31-1   Oral Feeding Schedule for the Low-Birth-Weight Infant

Time	Substance*	≤ 1000 g		1001–1500 g		1501–2000 g		> 2000 g	
		Amount	Frequency	Amount	Frequency	Amount	Frequency	Amount	Frequency
First feeding	½-strength human milk or ¼-strength formula	1–2 mL/kg	1–2 hours	2–3 mL/kg	2 hours	3–4 mL/kg	2–3 hours	10 mL/kg (full strength)	3 hours
Subsequent feedings, 12–72 hours	Formula or ½ to full-strength human milk	Increase 1 mL† every other feeding to maximum of 5 mL	2 hours	Increase 1 mL† every other feeding to maximum of 10 mL	2 hours	Increase 2 mL every other feeding to maximum of 15 mL	2–3 hours	Increase 5 mL every other feeding to maximum of 20 mL	3 hours
Final feeding schedule	Full-strength formula or human milk	10–15 mL	2 hours	20–28 mL	2–3 hours	28–37 mL	3 hours	37–50 mL, then *ad libitum*	3–4 hours
Total time to full oral feeds		10–14/day or more for infants <750 g		7–10/day		5–7/day		3–5/day	

*Supplemental IV fluids should be given to fulfill requirements of 140–160 mL/kg (urine specific gravities 1.008–1.010) and caloric requirements of 90–130 cal/kg.

†Strength should alternately be increased with volume.

Source: Modified from Avery GB, Fletcher MA, MacDonald MG (editors): *Neonatology: Pathophysiology and Management of the Newborn,* 4th ed. Philadelphia: Lippincott, 1994, p 334.

Types and Methods of Feeding for Preterm Newborns

Methods of Feeding   The preterm infant is fed by various methods, depending on the infant's gestational age, health and physical condition, and neurologic status. The three most common oral feeding methods are nipple, breast, and gavage feeding.

Nipple Feeding   Preterm infants who have a coordinated suck and swallow reflex and those showing continued weight gain (20–30 g/day) may be fed by nipple. To avoid excessive expenditure of energy, a soft, smaller nipple is usually used.

The feeding should take no longer than 15 to 20 minutes. A premature infant nipple or regular-sized nipple may be used, depending on the infant's strength and ability (nippling requires more energy than other methods). The infant is fed in a semisitting position and burped gently after each half ounce or ounce. Babies who are progressing from gavage feedings to bottle-feeding should start with one session of bottle-feeding a day and slowly increase the number of times a day a bottle is given until the baby tolerates all feedings from a bottle.

The infant's ability to suck is assessed. Sucking may be affected by age, asphyxia, sepsis, intraventricular hemorrhage, or other neurologic insult. Before initiating nip-

ple feeding, observe the infant for any signs of stress, such as tachypnea (more than 60 respirations/minute), respiratory distress, or hypothermia, which may increase the risk of aspiration. During the feeding the infant should be observed for signs of difficulty with feeding (tachypnea, cyanosis, bradycardia, lethargy, and uncoordinated suck and swallow). After the feeding, the infant is gently burped and positioned on the right side or abdomen.

Breastfeeding   Mothers who wish to breastfeed their preterm infants should be given the opportunity to put the infant to breast as soon as the infant has demonstrated a coordinated suck and swallow reflex, is showing consistent weight gain, and can control body temperature outside of the isolette, regardless of weight. Delaying transition from bottle to breast results in the infant developing a sucking mechanism specific to the artificial nipple that impedes subsequent transfer to the breast (Auerbach & Walker 1994).

Even if the infant can't be put to the breast, mothers can pump their breasts, and the breast milk can be given via gavage. Use of the double pumping system produces higher levels of prolactin than sequential pumping of the breasts. Lactaids can also be used as adjuncts to the mother's breast milk to increase the amount of fluid the infant receives without becoming tired (Auerbach & Walker 1994). Studies have shown that preterm infants tolerate breastfeeding with higher transcutaneous oxygen pressure and better maintenance of body temperature than during bottle-feeding (Meier 1988).

The infant is placed at the mother's breast. It has been suggested that the football hold is a convenient position for preterm babies. Feeding time may take up to 45 minutes, and babies should be burped as they alternate breasts.

Nursing responsibilities are the same as with an infant who is bottle-feeding. In addition the nurse coordinates a flexible feeding schedule so babies can nurse during alert times and be allowed to set their own pace. A similar regimen should be used for the baby who is progressing from gavage feeding to breastfeeding. The baby should begin with one feeding at the breast and then gradually increase the number of times during the day that the baby breastfeeds.

Gavage Feeding The gavage feeding method is used with preterm infants who lack or have a poorly coordinated suck and swallow reflex or are ill. Gavage feeding may be used as an adjunct to nipple feeding if the infant tires easily or as an alternative if an infant is losing weight because of the energy expenditure required for nippling. Gavage feedings are administered by either the nasogastric or orogastric route and by intermittent bolus or continuous drip method. See Procedure 31–1 for a description of this method of feeding and associated nursing care.

Transpyloric Feeding An alternative method of feeding is transpyloric feeding. This feeding method should be used only in specially equipped and staffed high-risk nurseries because it can perforate the stomach or intestines. Preterm infants who cannot tolerate any oral (enteral) feedings may be given nutrition by total parenteral nutrition (hyperalimentation).

Transpyloric, nasojejunal, or nasoduodenal feeding involves a continuous infusion of formula into the duodenum or jejunum of the baby to prevent vomiting. An indwelling feeding tube is passed through the nostril, into the stomach, past the pylorus, and into the small intestine. Tube placement is confirmed by x-ray examination. A constant infusion pump is used to administer small amounts of formula continuously. The tube is left in place and changed every 3 days.

Although this feeding method has advantages (for example, decreased risk of aspiration), it poses risks of stomach and intestinal perforation and accidental bolus infusion by the pump. Because of a possible link between jejunal feedings and NEC, this method is often not recommended for newborns weighing less than 2000 g. Formula bypasses the digestive activity of the stomach. The transpyloric method is never used in some centers, where the risks are believed to outweigh the benefits.

The nurse assists with the passing of the tube, observing the infant's vital signs and watching for any intolerance of the procedure. After the transpyloric feedings have begun, the nurse does the following:

- Observes and records infusion rate hourly to make sure the correct amount is infusing
- Changes the infusion setup every 8 hours to decrease the chances of bacterial growth in the formula
- Ensures that no more than 3 hours' worth of formula is hung at one time to prevent "dumping" of excess formula
- Checks all stools for blood and glucose (signs of necrotizing enterocolitis)
- Measures abdominal girth and compares it with previous measurements (signs of paralytic ileus, distention, or NEC)

Total Parenteral Nutrition Total parenteral nutrition (TPN) is used in situations that contraindicate feeding the infant through the gastrointestinal tract. Contraindications include gastrointestinal anomalies requiring surgical intervention, necrotizing enterocolitis, intolerance of feedings, and extreme prematurity.

The TPN method provides complete nutrition to the infant intravenously. TPN includes use of hyperalimentation and intralipids. Hyperalimentation gives calories, vitamins, minerals, protein, and glucose. Intralipids must also be administered to provide essential fatty acids. Hyperalimentation may be infused through either a central or a peripheral line. Intralipids may also be infused peripherally or centrally; if added as a piggyback to the hyperalimentation, they must be piggybacked as close to the infusion site as possible and not through the filter.

The nurse needs to monitor serum glucose levels carefully during TPN. Urine is checked for protein, sugar, and specific gravity at least every 8 hours. The intravenous rate is monitored hourly to maintain accurate intake. The rate should not be increased to "catch up" if behind. The intravenous site should be observed hourly for signs of infiltration—hyperalimentation is extremely caustic and causes severe tissue destruction if it infiltrates. Intake and output are carefully monitored (hyperglycemia causing an osmotic diuresis can lead to dehydration). The nurse observes for signs of reaction to intralipids (eg, dyspnea, vomiting, elevated temperature, or cyanosis).

Fluid Requirements

Calculation of fluid requirements takes into account the infant's weight and postnatal age. Recommendations for fluid therapy in the preterm infant are approximately 80–100 mL/kg/day for day 1, 100–120 mL/kg/day for day 2, and 120–150 mL/kg/day by day 3 of life. These amounts may be increased up to 200 mL/kg/day if the infant is very small, receiving phototherapy, or under a radiant warmer. The infant may need less fluid if a heat shield is used, the environment is more humid, or humidified oxygen is being provided.

Nutritional intake is considered adequate when there is consistent weight gain of 20–30 g per day. Initially, no

Text continues on page 943

Nursing Action

Objective: Prepare for smooth accomplishment of the procedure.

Gather necessary equipment, including:

1. No. 5 or no. 8 Fr. feeding tube
2. 10–30 mL syringe
3. ¼ in paper tape
4. Stethoscope
5. Appropriate formula
6. Small cup of sterile water

Explain procedure to parents.

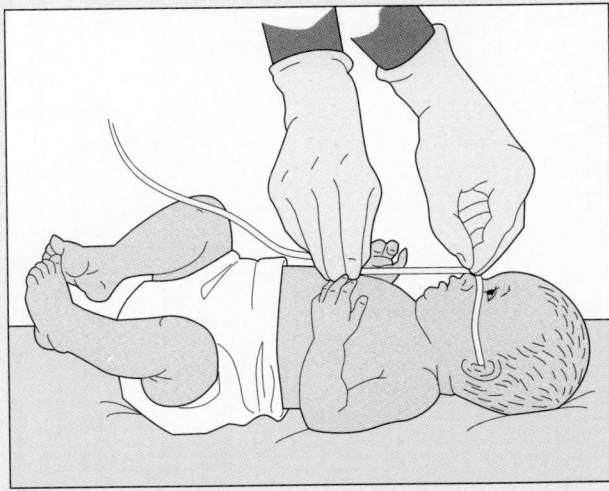

FIGURE 31-9 Measuring gavage tube length.

Objective: Insert tube accurately into stomach.

Position infant on back or side with head of bed elevated.

Take tube from package, measure the distance from the tip of the ear to the nose to the xiphoid process, and mark the point with a small piece of paper tape (Figure 31–9).

If inserting tube nasally, lubricate tip in cup of sterile water. Shake excess drops to prevent aspiration.

Stabilize infant's head with one hand, and pass the tube via the mouth (or nose) into the stomach, to the point previously marked. If the infant begins coughing or choking or becomes cyanotic or aphonic, remove the tube immediately.

If no respiratory distress is apparent, lightly tape tube in position, draw up 0.5–1.0 mL of air in syringe, and connect it to tubing. Place stethoscope over the epigastrium and briskly inject the air (Figure 31–10).

Rationale

Considerations in choosing size of catheter include size of the infant, area of insertion (oral or nasal), and rate of flow desired. The very small infant (less than 1600 g) requires a 5 Fr. feeding tube; an infant greater than 1600 g may tolerate a larger tube. Orogastric insertion is preferred over nasogastric insertion because most infants are obligatory nose breathers. If nasogastric insertion is used, a 5 Fr. Catheter should be used to minimize airway obstruction. The size of the catheter will influence the rate of flow. The syringe is used to aspirate stomach contents prior to feeding, to inject air into the stomach for testing tube placement, and for holding measured amount of formula during feeding. Tape is used to mark tube for insertion depth as well as for securing tube during feeding. Stethoscope is needed to auscultate rush of air into stomach when testing tube placement.

Sterile water may be used to lubricate feeding tube when inserted nasally. With oral insertion there are enough secretions in the mouth to lubricate the tube adequately.

The cup of sterile water may also be used to test for placement by placing the end of the tube into the water to check for air bubbles from the lungs. However, this test may not be accurate because air may also be present in the stomach.

This position allows easy passage of the tube.

This measuring technique ensures enough tubing to enter stomach.

Water should be used, as opposed to an oil-based lubricant, in case the tube is inadvertently passed into a lung.

Any signs of respiratory distress signal likelihood that tube has entered trachea. Orogastric insertion is less likely than nasogastric insertion to result in passage into the trachea.

Nurse should hear a sudden rush of air as it enters stomach.

Nursing Action	Rationale

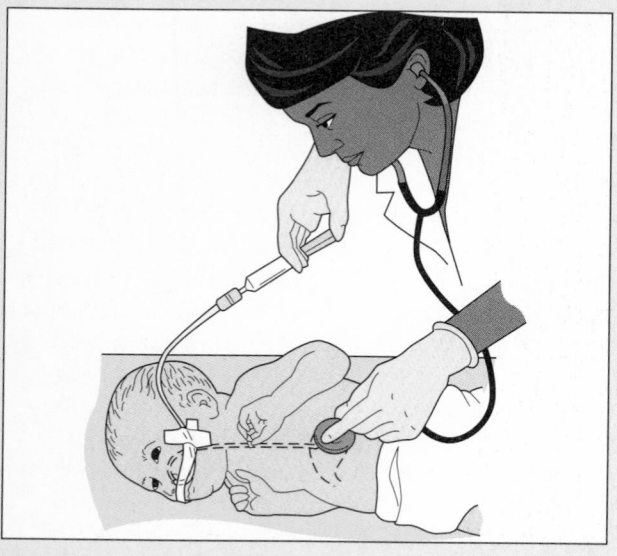

FIGURE 31-10   Auscultation for placement of gavage tube.

Aspirate stomach contents with syringe, and note amount, color, and consistency. Return residual to stomach unless otherwise ordered to discard it.

Residual formula should be evaluated as part of the assessment of infant's tolerance of gavage feeding. It is not discarded, unless particularly large in volume or mucoid in nature, because of the potential for causing an electrolyte imbalance.

If only a clear fluid or mucus is found upon aspiration and if any question exists as to whether the tube is in the stomach, the aspirate can be tested for pH.

Stomach aspirate tests in the 1–3 range for pH.

Objective: Introduce formula into stomach without complication.

Hold infant for feeding, or position on right side if infant cannot be held.

Positioning on side decreases the risk of aspiration in case of emesis during feeding.

Separate syringe from tube, remove plunger from barrel, reconnect barrel to tube, and pour formula into syringe.

Feeding should be allowed to flow in by gravity. It should not be pushed in under pressure with a syringe.

Elevate syringe 6–8 inches over infant's head. Allow formula to flow at slow, even rate.

Raising column of fluid increases force of gravity. Nurse may need to initiate flow of formula by inserting plunger of syringe into barrel just until formula is seen to enter feeding tube. Rate should be regulated to prevent sudden stomach distention, with possibility of vomiting and aspiration.

Continue adding formula to syringe until desired volume has been absorbed. Then clear tubing with 2–3 mL sterile water or air.

Clearing tube ensures that infant receives all of formula. It is especially important to clear tube if it is going to be left in place because this decreases risk of clogging and bacterial growth in tube.

Remove tube by loosening tape, folding the tube over on itself, and quickly withdrawing it in one smooth motion. If tube is to be left in, position it so that infant is unable to remove it.

Folding tube over on itself minimizes potential for aspiration of fluid, which would otherwise flow from tubing as it passes epiglottis. A tube left in place should be replaced at least every 24 hours.

Nursing Action	Rationale
Objective: Maximize feeding pleasure of infant.	Feeding time is important to infant's tactile sensory input.
Whenever possible, hold infant during gavage feeding. If it is too awkward to hold infant during feeding, be sure to take time for holding afterward.	
Offer a pacifier to infant during feeding.	Infants fed for long periods by gavage can lose their sucking reflex. Sucking during feeding comforts and relaxes infant, making formula flow more easily. One study showed that infants allowed to suck during feedings were able to nipple sooner and were discharged earlier than a control group of infants who did not suck during tube feedings.

weight gain may be noted for several days, but total weight loss should not exceed 15% of the total birth weight or more than 1% to 2% per day. Some institutions add the criteria of head circumference growth and increase in body length of 1 cm/week once the newborn is stable.

Common Complications of Preterm Newborns and Their Medical Management

The goals of medical therapy are to meet the growth and development needs of the preterm newborn and to anticipate and manage the complications associated with prematurity. Complications associated with prematurity that require medical intervention are respiratory distress syndrome (RDS), patent ductus arteriosus (PDA), apnea, and intraventricular hemorrhage (IVH). Long-term problems include retinopathy of prematurity (ROP), and bronchopulmonary dysplasia (BPD).

An in-depth discussion of RDS and BPD, including pathophysiology, medical management, and nursing care, is contained in Chapter 32. Patent ductus arteriosus, apnea, intraventricular hemorrhage, retinopathy of prematurity, and other complications are discussed below.

Patent Ductus Arteriosus

Spontaneous closure of the connection between the aorta and pulmonary artery is often delayed in preterm infants. The incidence of symptomatic patent ductus arteriosus is related to birth weight in preterm infants and has been shown to decrease with increase in birth weight.

Symptomatic PDA is often seen around the third day of life when the premature infant is recovering from RDS. Initially, when the preterm newborn is hypoxic secondary to RDS, the pulmonary vascular resistance (PVR) can be higher than the systemic vascular resistance, and right-to-left shunting through the ductus will occur. However, as the RDS improves and adequate oxygenation is maintained, the lungs open up, and more blood flows into them, leading to ventricular volume overload, pulmonary edema, and congestive failure (Flanagan & Fyler 1994). Oxygenation is again compromised, and ventilator requirements will increase, leading to the possibility of long-term pulmonary sequelae.

Ductal patency with left-to-right shunting is manifested with a continuous or systolic murmur, active precordium (visible heart pulsation), bounding pulses (increased pulse pressure), tachycardia, tachypnea, hepatomegaly, and pulmonary edema. These problems lead to signs of respiratory distress and continued oxygen and ventilator requirements. Chest radiographs reveal cardiomegaly with increased pulmonary vascularity. Patency of the ductus arteriosus can be determined by aortic contrast echocardiography.

The goal of medical therapy is to achieve ductal closure. Early identification of symptomatic infants and prompt medical intervention will minimize long-term complications. Three methods are currently used, separately or in combination, to effect closure:

1. *Medical therapy.* Initial medical management consists of providing adequate respiratory support, maintaining a relatively high hematocrit (greater than 40%), restricting fluids, and using diuretics (to decrease pulmonary edema) and perhaps digoxin while

waiting for spontaneous closure of the ductus to occur.

2. *Pharmacologic therapy.* Administration of prostaglandin synthetase inhibitors such as indomethacin impairs synthesis of the E series prostaglandins responsible for dilatation of the ductus and can cause ductal closure. Indomethacin is effective, but it is not without side effects and must be used cautiously. Side effects include decreased platelet aggregation, association with intracranial bleeding, gastrointestinal hemorrhage, and transient renal dysfunction. BUN and creatinine levels should be monitored. In the event of decreased renal function, monitor aminoglycoside levels. Indomethacin treatment produces closure in about 85% of babies (Flanagan & Fyler 1994).

3. *Surgical therapy.* The ductus may be surgically ligated.

Patent ductus arteriosus will often prolong the course of illness in a preterm newborn and lead to chronic pulmonary dysfunction. Early identification is essential for prompt treatment to minimize the complications that may have long-term effects.

Apnea

Apnea of prematurity refers to cessation of breathing for 20 seconds or longer or for less than 20 seconds when associated with cyanosis, bradycardia, and/or limpness (Grisemer 1990). Apnea is a common problem in the preterm infant (of less than 37 weeks' gestation) and is thought to be primarily a result of neuronal immaturity, a factor that contributes to the preterm infant's irregular breathing patterns. The immaturity of the preterm's CNS increases the baby's vulnerability to any adverse factors affecting nerve cell metabolism. This may be particularly problematic for the respiratory neurons in the brain stem. Factors that adversely affect brain nerve cells include hypoxia, acidosis, edema, intracranial bleeding, hyperbilirubinemia, hypoglycemia, hypocalcemia, and sepsis.

Nursing Care Apneic onset is often insidious; cardiorespiratory monitoring allows for early recognition and intervention, thus decreasing the need for resuscitative efforts. The nurse checks during each shift to make sure alarms are set and working properly. Apnea may occur during feeding, suctioning, or while stooling. However, there may be no observable activity related to apnea. All episodes of apnea are documented. The documentation includes activity at the time of apnea, length of episode, along with any bradycardia, color change, or desaturation on pulse-oximeter associated with apneic episodes, and treatment required to bring the baby out of the apneic spell. These data are useful in determining etiology and possible treatment.

The nurse needs to make careful observations and quickly assess the need for intervention. The intervention required depends on the severity of the apneic episode and the baby's response. If an apneic episode occurs the nurse may do the following:

1. Observe the infant briefly to see if treatment is necessary or if the infant is having periodic breathing and begins to breathe spontaneously.

2. Begin stimulation by gently rubbing the soles of the feet, the ankles, and the infant's back. Rubbing bony prominences is uncomfortable to the infant and therefore more stimulating than rubbing other areas of the body.

3. Suction nasopharynx and oropharynx, provide additional oxygen, and prepare for bag and mask ventilation if the infant is dusky, cyanotic, or bradycardic. Obstruction of the airway by mucus or formula may result in apnea and bradycardia. Clearing the airway while providing increased oxygen concentration and stimulation may resolve apneic episodes. If the infant does not respond, bag and mask ventilation may be required to relieve cyanosis and return heart rate to normal.

4. Administer oxygen and warm humidified air per physician order to control dyspnea and cyanosis. Increased oxygen may alleviate episodes of apnea and bradycardia. Monitor and record the oxygen concentration every 2 hours.

5. Prepare for a sepsis workup if the infant is not already on antibiotics.

6. Prepare for mechanical assistance of respirations. Use of nasal CPAP (continuous positive airway pressure) or intubation and use of the ventilator may be necessary if the infant has frequent apneic episodes that require bag and mask ventilation. Ventilatory assistance may be necessary to prevent possible sequelae of frequent apneic spells with resulting hypoxemia.

7. Report and assess variations in blood gases and laboratory reports. Apnea is associated with elevated $PaCO_2$, decreased PaO_2, and electrolyte imbalances.

8. Maintain thermal neutrality. Temperature instability may precipitate apnea.

9. Use methylxanthine drugs (aminophylline, theophylline, or caffeine) to treat apnea of prematurity. Advantages of caffeine over theophylline include a larger therapeutic index, once-daily administration, a small fluctuation in plasma concentrations, a potent central respirogenic effect, and fewer peripheral adverse effects (Martin 1993).

The general care given an apneic baby should include gentle handling to prevent unnecessary stress. Keeping the airway clear is very important, but nasopharyngeal suctioning should be done gently and only as necessary because it can cause apnea. Use of indwelling oro-gastric or nasogastric tubes may be preferred to intermittent passage of feeding tubes. The nurse provides IV fluids as ordered to maintain adequate fluid and electrolyte balance. Severe apnea may preclude oral feeding for a time, and the infant may require nutritional maintenance with intravenous therapy. Adequate nutrition prevents catabolism of body tissues as well as biochemical aberrations such as hypoglycemia, hyperglycemia, acidosis, or electrolyte imbalance. Following feedings, the baby should be positioned prone or supported on the right side with the head of the bed elevated.

Intraventricular Hemorrhage

Intraventricular hemorrhage (IVH) is the most common type of intracranial hemorrhage in the small preterm infant. Those most susceptible to IVH are infants weighing less than 1500 g or of less than 34 weeks' gestation. The incidence of intracranial hemorrhage in these newborns is about 50% (Bernbaum 1994).

An IVH frequently occurs after an insult to the infant that results in hypoxia such as respiratory distress, birth trauma, and birth asphyxia, with the more immature infants being at higher risk for these complications.

The most common site of hemorrhage is in the periventricular subependymal germinal matrix, where there is a rich blood supply and the capillary walls are thin and fragile. The matrix provides little supportive tissue for the fragile blood vessels. Before 32 weeks' gestation an infant is much more susceptible to hemorrhage of these tiny vessels because they are vulnerable to hypoxic events that damage vessel walls and cause them to rupture. Computerized axial tomography (CT) or serial head ultrasound scanning can be used to identify both the site and the extent of hemorrhage.

The clinical signs observed in an infant with IVH are variable. The infant may suddenly "crash" (characterized by pallor and shocklike appearance) and die or may show very subtle or no signs at all. The most common manifestations are neurologic signs, hypotonia, lethargy, temperature instability, nystagmus, bulging fontanelle, falling hematocrit, apnea, bradycardia, hypotension, and a worsening in the respiratory condition (increasing hypoxia) with metabolic acidosis. Seizures may occur, and decerebrate posturing may be observed.

Prenatal interventions include prevention of premature birth and maternal transport to a tertiary care center. Administration of phenobarbital and vitamin K to the mother is being studied for their preventive effect. Postnatal preventive interventions include careful resuscitation, correction or prevention of major hemodynamic disturbances, and correction of coagulation abnormalities. Potential postnatal preventive pharmacologic interventions include phenobarbital to control seizures, indomethacin to control the hemodynamics resulting from PDA, and vitamin E for its antioxidant abilities (Volpe 1995).

The outcome for the infant depends on the size of the intracerebral bleed and the gestational age of the infant. The most severe hemorrhages may cause motor deficits, posthemorrhagic hydrocephalus, hearing loss, and blindness. Less severe bleeds may have no observable effects (Bernbaum 1994).

Nursing Care   Vital signs, fontanelle tenseness, seizure activity, hematocrit, blood pressure, and changes in muscle tone or activity should be monitored closely. The nurse prepares the infant and assists with lumbar puncture for spinal fluid analysis. While administering replacement whole blood or albumin, the nurse monitors blood pressure. Thermal neutrality must be maintained. After a suspected bleed, the occipital frontal circumference is checked closely because hydrocephalus may occur. The nurse also monitors for signs of increased intracranial pressure (apnea, bradycardia, hypotension). The treatment of infants with severe hemorrhagic-intracerebral involvement brings up complex ethical issues for parents and health care providers such as quality of life and allocation of limited resources.

In caring for the infant with an IVH, the nurse provides continuing support for the parents, identifying their level of understanding and facilitating interdisciplinary communication with them.

Long-Term Needs and Outcome

The care of the preterm infant and the family does not stop on discharge from the nursery. Follow-up care is extremely important because many developmental problems are not noted until the infant is older and begins to demonstrate motor delays or sensory disability.

Within the first year of life, low-birth-weight preterm infants face higher mortality than term infants. Causes of death include sudden infant death syndrome (SIDS) (which occurs about five times more frequently in the preterm infant), respiratory infections, and neurologic defects. Morbidity is also much higher among preterm infants, with those weighing less than 1500 g at highest risk for long-term complications.

The most common long-term problems observed in preterm infants include retinopathy of prematurity and auditory, speech, and neurologic defects.

Retinopathy of Prematurity   Premature newborns are particularly susceptible to characteristic retinal changes known as retinopathy of prematurity (ROP). This disease has previously been referred to as retrolental fibroplasia (RLF).

Until recently, ROP was thought to be exclusively the result of excessive use of oxygen in the treatment of premature infants. However, ROP has also occurred in premature infants who never received oxygen, in full-term infants with cyanotic congenital heart disease, and in certain other congenital anomalies. The disease is now viewed as multifactorial in origin. Increased survival of very-low-birth-weight (VLBW) infants may be the most important factor in the increased incidence of ROP. In those with birth weights below 900 g the incidence can be as high as 90% (Bowen & Tasman 1993).

An international classification system for ROP has been developed to describe the disease and the extent of retinal changes (Committee for the Classification of Retinopathy of Prematurity 1984).

The fetal retina is unique in that its vascularization does not begin until the fourth month of gestation, with the temporal peripheral area of retinal vasculature lagging in development. Vascularization is not completed until term. Consequently, the immature vascular system is susceptible to damage in the preterm neonate and occasionally in the term neonate. The fragile vessels often rupture to produce retinal and vitreous hemorrhage. Scar tissue forms and traction may occur, leading to retinal detachment and subsequent blindness.

The goal of management is early identification and in some institutions antioxidant therapy with vitamin E supplementation. An initial fundal examination with an indirect ophthalmoscope should be performed between 5 and 7 weeks of age, then every 2 weeks until disease regression starts. The American Academy of Pediatrics Committee on Fetus and Newborn (1992) recommends eye examinations for all infants of less than 35 weeks' gestation; all infants who weigh less than 1800 g and received oxygen therapy; and all infants weighing less than 1300 g or born before 30 weeks' gestation, whether they received oxygen or not. Frequency of repeat examinations depends on the rapidity of progression or the severity of the disease. Follow-up exams for mild or regressed disease should be given every 3 to 6 months until there is no evidence of ocular changes and then yearly for life. In cases of scarring or cicatrical disease, long-term care requires an intensive rehabilitation follow-up program (Bowen & Tasman 1993).

Treatment of the acute stages of ROP with laser or cryotherapy is an option. Cryotherapy obliterates the neovascularization (new vessel formation) and reduces the traction that causes retinal detachment. Because most acute cases of ROP regress spontaneously with no long-term visual impairment, the possibility of regression must be weighed against the risk of an unfavorable outcome.

For infants with bilateral traction and retinal detachment surgical vitrectomy and scleral buckling have been used experimentally. Because they are experimental, further follow-up is required for evaluation.

Nursing Care Nursing care for the visually impaired infant must concentrate on parental support and education. When the crisis of premature birth is quickly followed by the devastating news of suspected visual impairment or blindness, the parents will need extensive support by all members of the management team. The parents again experience overwhelming anxiety and uncertainty about their infant's future abilities.

Premature infants with blindness due to ROP may be at increased risk of cognitive and emotional problems. The evidence suggests that this increased risk may be due to environmental factors rather than to inherent intellectual or neurologic factors. Isolation, overprotectiveness, understimulation, and parental despair or emotional withdrawal may accentuate the problems of blindness (Teplin 1983). Figure 31–11 demonstrates the "vicious cycle" leading to emotional and developmental problems that may arise when the problems of parental attachment to a premature infant are compounded by the news of visual impairment.

Nurses can prevent the development of this cycle by helping parents develop appropriate attachment behaviors. Parents can be assured that their infant will be able to recognize them by voice and touch. They must also be told that visually impaired infants may not show recognition or feeling by changes in facial expressions. They will need to look for other cues or body language that their infant uses for self-expression.

In caring for the infant, the nurse can model specific developmental intervention activities and give the parents information on normal developmental milestones. Because the visually impaired child uses the other senses for exploration, parents can be taught specific activities to enhance their child's learning.

Prior to discharge the management team should provide detailed information about and contacts with available community services and resource groups. Community agencies can provide support and direction for the parents as their child grows and new problems are encountered.

Auditory Defects Preterm infants have a 1% to 4% incidence of moderate to profound hearing loss and should have a formal audiologic exam prior to discharge and at 3–6 months (corrected age). The brain stem auditory evoked response (BAER) is the best test, and any infant with abnormal results on the BAER should be referred to speech and language specialists (Hulseman & Norman 1992). Those at increased risk include infants with congenital viral infections, hyperbilirubinemia, perinatal asphyxia, and birth trauma. Damage from ototoxic drugs such as gentamicin and furosemide (Lasix) is variable and related to multiple factors, including renal function, age, duration of treatment, and concomitant administration of other ototoxic agents.

Speech Defects The most frequently observed speech defects involve delayed development of receptive and expressive ability that may persist into the school-age years.

Neurologic Defects The most common neurologic defects include cerebral palsy, hydrocephalus, seizure disorders, lower IQ scores, and learning disabilities. However, the socioeconomic climate and family support systems have been shown to be important factors

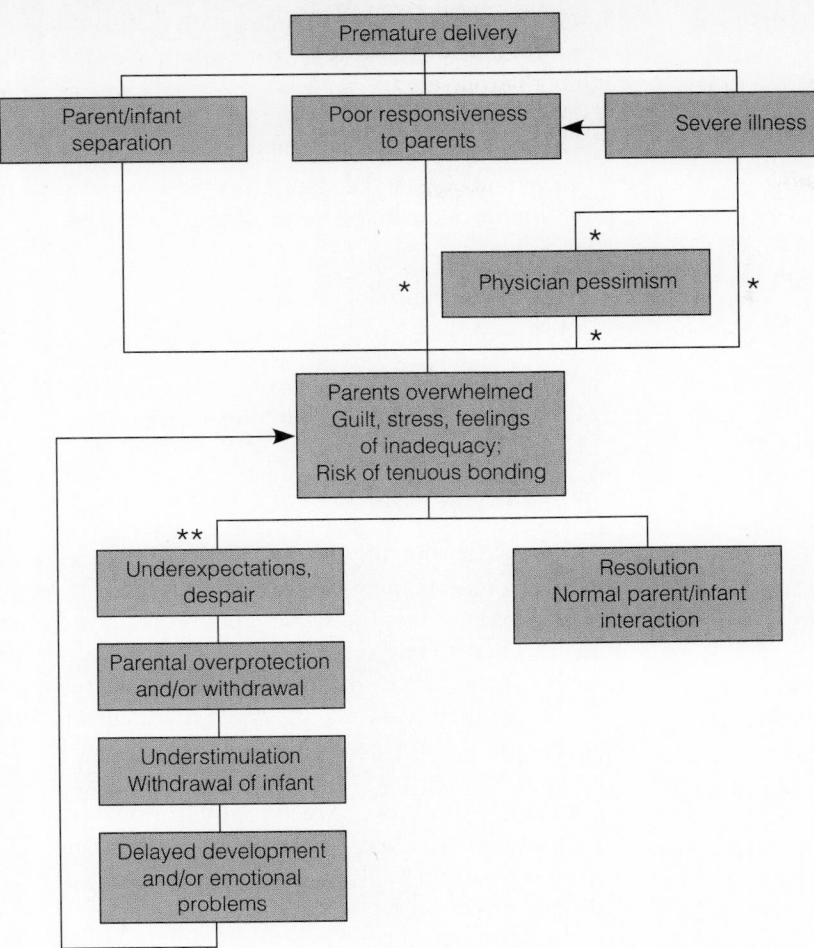

FIGURE 31-11 Suggested causes and outcomes of altered parental attachment to premature infants with blindness due to ROP. A single asterisk indicates factors affecting attachment in all premature babies that are exacerbated by discovery of blindness. A double asterisk indicates onset of "vicious cycle" leading to emotional/developmental problems (pseudoretardation). SOURCE: Teplin SW: Development of blind infants and children with retrolental fibroplasia: Implications for physicians. *Pediatrics* 1983; 71:6.

influencing the child's ultimate school performance in the absence of major neurologic defects. Families can be reminded that risk does not equal injury, injury does not equal damage, and description of damage does not allow a precise prediction about recovery or outcome.

When evaluating an infant's abilities and disabilities, it is important for parents to understand that the developmental level cannot be evaluated based on chronologic age. Developmental progress must be evaluated from the expected date of birth, not from the actual date of birth. In addition the parents need the consistent support of health care professionals in the long-term management of their infant. Many new and ongoing concerns arise as the high-risk infant grows and develops; the goal is to promote the highest quality of life possible.

APPLYING THE NURSING PROCESS

Nursing Assessment

Accurate assessment of the physical characteristics and gestational age of the preterm newborn is imperative to anticipate the special needs and problems of this baby.

Physical characteristics vary greatly, depending on the gestational age, but the following characteristics are frequently present:

- *Color.* Usually pink or ruddy but may be acrocyanotic (Cyanosis, jaundice, or pallor are abnormal and should be noted.)
- *Skin.* Reddened, translucent, blood vessels readily apparent, lack of subcutaneous fat
- *Lanugo.* Plentiful, widely distributed
- *Head size.* Appears large in relation to body
- *Skull.* Bones pliable, fontanelle smooth and flat
- *Ears.* Minimal cartilage, pliable, folded over
- *Nails.* Soft, short
- *Genitals.* Small; testes may not be descended
- *Resting position.* Flaccid, froglike
- *Cry.* Weak, feeble
- *Reflexes.* Poor suck, swallow, and gag
- *Activity.* Jerky, generalized movements (Seizure activity is abnormal.)

Determination of gestational age in preterm newborns requires knowledge and experience in administering gestational assessment tools. The tool used should be

Nursing Diagnosis

Nursing diagnoses that may apply to the preterm newborn include the following:

- Impaired gas exchange related to immature pulmonary vasculature

- Ineffective breathing pattern: apnea related to immature central nervous system

- Altered nutrition: Less than body requirements related to weak suck and swallow reflexes and decreased ability to absorb nutrients

- Fluid volume deficit related to high insensible water losses and inability of kidneys to concentrate urine

- Altered metabolic processes related to cold stress

Nursing diagnoses that may apply to the family of the preterm newborn include the following:

- Ineffective family coping related to anger/guilt at having delivered a premature baby

- Grieving related to actual or perceived loss of a normal newborn

- Grieving related to anticipated loss

Nursing Plan and Implementation

Maintenance of Respiratory Function

There is increased danger of respiratory obstruction in preterm newborns because their bronchi and trachea are so narrow that mucus can obstruct the airway. The nurse needs to use suctioning judiciously to maintain airway patency.

Positioning of the newborn can also affect respiratory function. If the baby is in the supine position, the nurse should slightly elevate the infant's head to maintain the airway. Because the newborn has weak neck muscles and cannot control head movement, the nurse should ensure by using a small roll under the shoulders that this head position is maintained. The nurse should avoid placing the infant in the supine position because the newborn has difficulty raising the chest because of weak chest and abdominal muscles. The prone position splints the chest wall and decreases the amount of respiratory effort used to move the chest wall. The prone position therefore facilitates chest expansion and improves air entry and oxygenation. Weak or absent cough or gag reflexes increase the chance of aspiration in the premature newborn. The nurse should ensure that the infant's position facilitates drainage of mucus or regurgitated formula.

The nurse monitors heart and respiratory rates with cardiorespiratory monitors and observes the newborn to identify alterations in cardiopulmonary status. Nursery nurses must be alert to signs of respiratory distress, including the following:

- Cyanosis (serious sign when generalized)

- Tachypnea (sustained respiratory rate greater than 60/minute after first 4 hours of life)

- Retractions

- Expiratory grunting

- Flaring nostrils

- Apneic episodes

- Presence of rales or rhonchi on auscultation

- Diminished air entry

- Fatigue

The nurse who observes any of these alterations records and reports them for further evaluation. If respiratory distress occurs, the nurse administers oxygen per physician order to relieve hypoxemia. If hypoxemia is not treated immediately, it may result in patent ductus arteriosus or metabolic acidosis. If oxygen is administered to the newborn, the nurse monitors the oxygen concentration with devices such as the transcutaneous oxygen monitor ($tcPO_2$) or the pulse-oximeter. Monitoring of oxygen concentration in the baby's blood is essential because hyperoxemia may lead to blindness (see Retinopathy of Prematurity earlier in this chapter).

The nurse also needs to consider respiratory function during feeding. To prevent aspiration, increased energy expenditure, and increased oxygen consumption, the nurse needs to ensure that the infant's gag and suck reflexes are intact before initiating oral feedings.

Maintenance of Neutral Thermal Environment

Provision of a neutral thermal environment minimizes the oxygen consumption required to maintain a normal core temperature; it also prevents cold stress and facilitates growth by decreasing the calories needed to maintain body temperature. The preterm infant's immature central nervous system provides poor temperature control, and stores of brown fat are decreased. A small infant (<1200 g) can lose 80 kcal/kg/day through its attempts to increase body temperature.

To minimize heat loss and the effects of temperature instability, the nurse should do the following:

1. Warm and humidify oxygen without blowing it over the infant's face to minimize convective heat loss and increase oxygen consumption.

2. Place the baby in a double-walled incubator, and use a heat shield over small preterm infants.

3. Avoid placing the baby on cold surfaces such as metal treatment tables and cold x-ray plates; pad cold surfaces with diapers and use radiant warmers

during procedures; and warm hands before handling the baby to prevent heat transfer via conduction.

4. Warm the blood before administration.

5. Keep the skin dry, and place a cap on the baby's head to prevent heat loss via evaporation. (The head makes up 25% of the total body size.)

6. Keep radiant warmers and cribs away from windows and cold external walls and out of drafts to prevent heat loss by radiation.

7. Use a skin probe to monitor the baby's skin temperature. Correlate ambient temperatures with the skin probe in the incubator. The temperature should be 36–37 C (96.8–97.7 F). Temperature fluctuations indicate hypothermia or hyperthermia.

8. Warm formula or stored breast milk before feeding.

The nurse begins the weaning to a crib process when the premature infant is medically stable, doesn't require assisted ventilation, weighs approximately 1500 g, has 5 days of consistent weight gain, is taking oral feedings, and apnea and bradycardia episodes have stabilized. Once preterm infants are medically stable, they should be clothed with a double-thickness cap, cotton shirt, and diaper (Medoff-Cooper 1994).

Maintenance of Fluid and Electrolyte Status

Hydration is maintained by providing adequate intake based on the newborn's weight, gestational age, chronologic age, and volume of sensible and insensible water losses. Adequate fluid intake should provide sufficient water to compensate for increased insensible losses and to provide the amount needed for renal excretion of metabolic products. Insensible water losses can be minimized by providing a high ambient humidity, humidifying oxygen, using heat shields, covering the skin with plastic wrap, and placing the infant in a double-walled incubator.

The nurse evaluates the baby's hydration status by assessing and recording signs of dehydration. Signs of dehydration include the following:

- Sunken fontanelle
- Loss of weight
- Poor skin turgor (Skin returns to position slowly when squeezed gently.)
- Dry oral mucous membranes
- Decreased urine output
- Increased urine specific gravity (>1.013)

The nurse must also identify signs of overhydration by observing the newborn for edema or excessive weight gain and by comparing urine output with fluid intake.

The preterm infant should be weighed at least once daily at the same time each day. Weight change is one of the most sensitive indicators of fluid balance. Weighing diapers is also important to accurate input and output measurement. A comparison on intake and output measurements over an 8-hour or 24-hour period provides important information about renal function and fluid balance. Assessment of patterns and whether they show a net gain or loss over several days is also essential to fluid management. Blood serum levels and pH should be monitored to evaluate for electrolyte imbalances.

Accurate hourly intake calculations should be maintained when administering intravenous fluids. Because the preterm infant is unable to excrete excess fluid, it is important to maintain the correct amount of intravenous fluid to prevent fluid overload. This can be accomplished by using neonatal or pediatric infusion pumps. To prevent electrolyte imbalance and dehydration, care must be taken to give the correct IV solutions and volumes and concentrations of formulas. Urine specific gravity and pH are obtained periodically. Urine osmolality provides an indication of hydration, although this factor must be correlated with other assessments (for example, serum sodium). Hydration is considered adequate when the urine output is 1 to 3 mL/kg/hour.

Provision of Adequate Nutrition and Prevention of Fatigue During Feeding

The feeding method depends on the preterm newborn's feeding abilities and health status (see Methods of Feeding earlier in this chapter). Both nipple and gavage methods are initially supplemented with intravenous therapy until oral intake is sufficient to support growth (110 to 130 kcal/kg/day). The first feedings are small amounts given every 2–3 hours. These small amounts are increased slowly by 1–2 mL. Formula or breast milk (with or without fortifiers to increase caloric content) is incorporated into the feedings slowly; initially, it may be at quarter-strength, then half-strength, and so on. This is done to avoid overtaxing the digestive capacity of the preterm newborn. The nurse should carefully watch for any signs of feeding intolerance, including the following:

- Increasing gastric residuals
- Abdominal distention (measured routinely before feedings)
- Guaiac-positive stools (occult blood in stools)
- Presence of glucose in stools
- Vomiting
- Diarrhea

The nurse also must be watchful for any signs of respiratory distress or fatigue during feedings. Before each feeding, the nurse measures abdominal girth and auscultates the abdomen to determine the presence and quality of bowel sounds. Such assessments promote early detection of abdominal distention and decreased peristaltic activity, which may indicate necrotizing enterocolitis (NEC) or paralytic ileus. The nurse also checks for residual formula in the stomach prior to feeding. This is done when the newborn is fed by gavage or in the presence of abdominal distention in a nipple-fed newborn. The presence of residual formula may indicate intolerance to the type or amount of feeding or the increase in amount of feeding. Residual formula is usually readministered because digestive processes have already been initiated.

Preterm newborns who are ill or fatigue easily with nipple feedings are usually fed by gavage or transpyloric feeding. The infant is essentially passive with these methods, thus conserving energy and calories. As the baby matures, gavage feedings are replaced with nipple feedings to assist in strengthening the sucking reflex and meeting oral and emotional needs. Nurses are key in the decision of when preterm infants are ready to start a nippling program. Factors used to indicate readiness are a strong gag reflex, presence of nonnutritive sucking, rooting behavior, gestational age of 34 weeks or more, and weight over 1500 g. A recent study has raised questions about using hunger cues such as crying to initiate feeding because both low-birth-weight and preterm infants nipple-feed more effectively in a quiet state (Kinneer & Beachy 1994). The nurse establishes a nipple-feeding program that is begun and progresses slowly, such as one nipple feeding per day, then one nipple feeding per shift, and then a nipple feeding every other feeding. Daily weights are monitored because often there is a small weight loss when nipple feedings are started. After feedings the baby is placed on the right side (with support to maintain this position) or on the abdomen. These positions enhance gastric emptying and decrease the chance of aspiration if regurgitation occurs. Gastroesophageal reflux is *not* uncommon in preterm newborns.

The nurse involves the parents in feeding their preterm baby. This is essential to the development of attachment between parents and infant. In addition such involvement increases parental knowledge about the care of their infant and helps them cope with the situation.

Prevention of Infection

The nurse is responsible for minimizing the preterm newborn's exposure to pathogenic organisms. The preterm newborn is susceptible to infection because of an immature immune system and thin, permeable skin. Invasive procedures, techniques such as umbilical catheterization and mechanical ventilation, and prolonged hospitalization place the infant at greater risk for infection.

Strict hand washing, reverse isolation, and using separate equipment for each infant help minimize exposure of the preterm newborn to infectious agents. Many intensive care nurseries require staff to scrub 2 to 3 minutes using iodined antibacterial solutions, which inhibit the growth of gram-positive cocci and gram-negative rod organisms. Other specific nursing interventions include limiting visitors; requiring visitors to wash their hands; and maintaining strict aseptic practices when changing intravenous tubing and solutions (IV solutions and tubing

should be changed every 24 hours), administering parenteral fluids, and assisting with sterile procedures. If infection is detected, the infant is placed in an incubator or isolation room. Incubators and radiant warmers should be changed weekly. Pressure area breakdown is prevented by changing the baby's position, doing range-of-motion exercises, or using a sheepskin or a water bed. To avoid skin tears, a protective transparent covering can be applied over vulnerable joints (*Neonatal Skin Care* 1992). There should be minimal use or avoidance of chemical skin preps and tape, which may cause skin trauma.

If infection (sepsis) occurs in the preterm newborn, the nurse may be the first to identify the associated subtle clinical signs. The nurse informs the clinician of the findings immediately and implements the treatment plan per clinician orders in the presence of infection. For specific nursing care required for the newborn with an infection, see Chapter 32.

Promotion of Parent-Infant Attachment

Preterm newborns can be separated from their parents for prolonged periods after illness or complications that are detected in the first few hours or days following birth. The resultant interruption in parent-newborn bonding necessitates intervention to ensure successful attachment of parent and infant.

Nurses should take measures to promote positive parental feelings toward the newborn. Photographs of the baby are given to parents to have at home or to the mother if she is in a different hospital or too ill to come to the nursery and visit. The infant's first name is placed on the incubator as soon as it is known to help the parents feel that their infant is a unique and special person. A weekly card with the baby's footprint, weight, and length is also sent to promote bonding. The telephone number of the nursery or intensive care unit and names of staff members are given to parents so they have access to information about their baby at any time of the day or night. Equipment and therapies are explained to parents, and the explanations are repeated as often as necessary to familiarize them with the treatment and decrease their anxiety.

Parents are included in determining the baby's plan of care. Early involvement in the care and decisions regarding their baby provides parents with realistic expectations for their baby. Bonding is influenced by the individual personality characteristics of the infant and the parents; these contribute to the interactive process. Information is another important variable. Parents need education to develop care-giving skills and to understand the premature infant's behavioral characteristics (Haut et al 1994). Their daily participation (if possible) is encouraged, as are early and frequent visits. The nurse provides opportunities for the parents to touch, hold, talk to, and care for the baby. Skin-to-skin (kangaroo) holding has been shown to help parents feel close to their small intu-

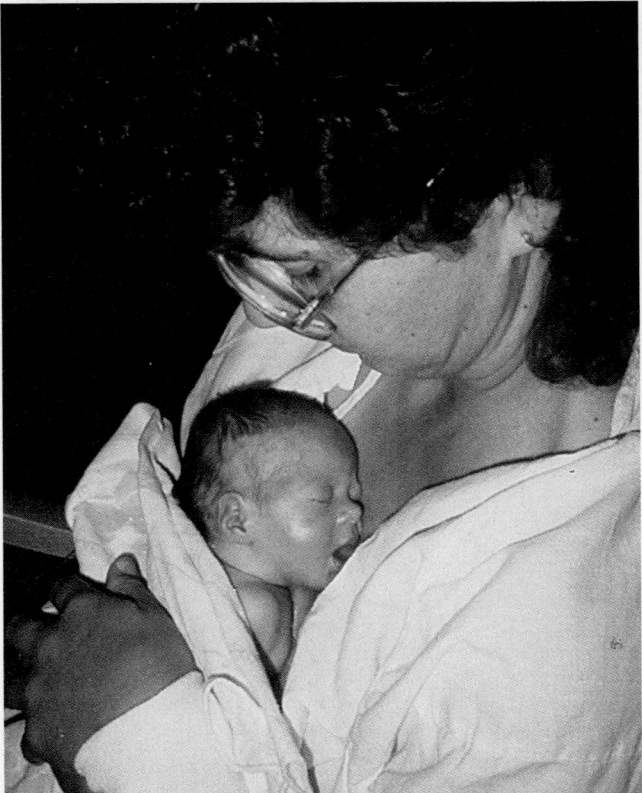

FIGURE 31-12   Kangaroo (skin to skin) care facilitates a closeness and attachment between parents and their premature infant. SOURCE: Courtesy of Kadlac Medical Center Kangaroo Care Study and Carol Thompson, RNC, BSN, NNP.

bated or nonintubated infants even with parents at risk for attachment difficulties (Gale et al 1993) (Figure 31–12).

Some parents may progress easily to touching and cuddling their infant; others will not. Parents need to know that their apprehension is normal and the progression of acquaintanceship is slow. Rooming-in can provide another opportunity for the stable preterm infant and family to get acquainted. It offers an environment that is more private but where help is readily available (Cusson & Lee 1994). Parents are started with simple tasks, based on the nurse's assessment of their skill and coping abilities. Early success in performing simple tasks builds parents' confidence in their caretaking abilities.

Promotion of Developmentally Supportive Care

Prolonged separation and the neonatal intensive care unit (NICU) environment necessitate individualized baby sensory stimulation programs. The nurse plays a key role in determining the appropriate type and amount of sensory (visual, tactile, and auditory) stimulation.

Research into the unique behavioral characteristics of the preterm infant highlights many responses that

RESEARCH IN PRACTICE

A technique for holding babies known as kangaroo care (KC) promotes closeness between the mother and her premature infant. The technique involves the mother holding the diaper-clad infant upright between her bare breasts for skin-to-skin contact. Susan Ludington-Hoe and her colleagues conducted a clinical trial involving preterm infants in open-air cribs who received kangaroo care. The investigators wanted to establish KC as a nursing intervention.

The study was conducted during three time periods over the course of 1 day. The infants were monitored for heart rate, respiratory rate, oxygen saturation, skin temperature, and state of arousal. The time periods usually lasted from one feeding to the next and consisted of a pretest time, a treatment period, and a posttest interval. The sample of 11 KC and 13 control preterm infants had all been born at 31 to 36 weeks' gestation and had 5-minute Apgar scores ranging from 8 to 10. The average birth weight of the treatment group was 1876 g, and the control group had an average of 2006 g. During the pre- and posttest times the infants from both groups were in their open-air cribs on their right sides.

Data from the study were analyzed using a two-factor repeated analysis of variance. The researchers found statistically significant increases in average heart rate and average skin temperature in the group receiving KC. The infants had virtually no periodic breathing during KC, although this type of breathing was common in both groups while in the crib. Another important difference concerned quiet regular sleep: The infants receiving KC spent 19% of the time in this deep sleep state during KC compared to 9.5% during pre- and 7% during posttreatment. The control group did not experience any changes in quiet regular sleep.

Because of the positive results from this study, the authors began a pilot study of six incubator care infants. These infants were younger (32–33 weeks' gestation), sicker, and smaller. The authors included descriptive results showing increased mean heart rate, increased mean skin temperature, and decreased mean respiratory rate during KC.

Clinical Application of Study

The control and treatment groups of this study had small numbers for an analysis of variance; also, the authors might have included ANOVA tables for their readers. The study provides guidelines for incorporating kangaroo care into a neonatal unit and suggests conditions that might contraindicate its use. The researchers note that KC can be safely advocated for open-air crib infants.

SOURCE: Ludington-Hoe S et al: Kangaroo care: Research results, and practice implications and guidelines. *Neonatal Network* 1994; 13(1):19.

reflect disorganization of the autonomic system. This work suggests that some preterm infants are not developmentally able to deal with more than one sensory input at a time. The assessment of preterm infant behavior (APIB) scale (Als et al 1982) identifies the individual preterm newborn behaviors according to five areas of development. The infant's physiologic and behavioral subsystems are autonomic, motor control, state differentiation, attention maintenance and social interaction, and finally overall system regulation or self-regulation. Integration of these subsystems improves with increasing gestational and postconceptual age. If the premature infant's self-regulatory capacity is exceeded and the infant is not able to return to previously integrated subsystem functioning, maladaptive behaviors may result when the infant is confronted with environmental demands. The baby's behavioral reactions to stimulation are observed, and developmental interventions are then based on reducing detrimental environmental stimuli to the lowest possible level and providing appropriate opportunities for development.

The NICU environment contains many detrimental stimuli that the nurse can help reduce. Noise levels can be lowered by responding to and silencing alarms quickly and keeping conversations away from the baby's bedside. Bright lights can be modified by shielding the baby's eyes with blankets over the top portion of the incubator. Dimming the lights may encourage infants to open their eyes and be more responsive to their parents (Cusson & Lee 1994). Nursing care should be planned to decrease the number of times the baby is disturbed. Signs (ie, "Quiet Please") can be placed near the bedside to allow the baby some periods of uninterrupted sleep (NANN Practice Committee 1993). Some other suggested developmentally supportive interventions include the following:

- Facilitate handling by using containment measures when turning or moving the infant or doing procedures such as suctioning. Containment is accomplished by using your hands to hold the infant's arms and legs, flexed, close to the midline of the body. This helps stabilize the infant's motor and physiologic subsystems during stressful activities.

- Touch the infant gently and avoid sudden postural changes.

- Facilitate self-consoling and/or soothing activities such as placing blanket rolls or approved manufactured devices next to the infant's sides and against the feet to provide "nesting." Swaddle the infant to maintain extremities in a flexed position while ensuring that the hands can reach the face. This permits the infant to use hand-to-mouth activities, which can be consoling (Figure 31–13).

- Simulate the kinesthetic advantages of the intrauterine environment by using sheepskin and approved waterbeds. Waterbed use by infants has been reported to improve sleep and decrease motor activity as well as leading to more mature motor behavior, fewer state changes, and a decreased heart rate.

- Provide opportunities for nonnutritive sucking with a pacifier. This improves transcutaneous oxygen saturation; decreases body movement; improves sleep, especially after feedings; and increases weight gain.

- Provide objects for the infant to grasp (eg, a piece of blanket, oxygen tubing, or a finger) during care giving. Grasping may comfort the baby.

Teaching the parents to read behavioral cues will help them move at their infant's pace when providing stimulation. Parents are ideally equipped to meet the baby's need for stimulation. Stroking, rocking, cuddling, quiet singing, and talking to the baby can all be an integral part of the baby's care. Visual stimulation in the form of en face interaction with the care givers and mobiles is also important.

Preparation for Home Care

Parents are often anxious when their premature infant is transferred out of the NICU or is discharged home. Parents of preterm babies should receive the same postpartal teaching as any parent taking a new infant home. In preparing for discharge, parents are encouraged to spend time caring directly for their baby. This familiarizes them with their baby's behavior patterns and helps them establish realistic expectations about the infant.

Discharge instruction includes breast- and bottle-feeding techniques, formula preparation (including bottle sterilization), and vitamin administration. Mothers of preterm babies desiring to breastfeed are taught to pump their breasts to keep the milk flowing and provide milk

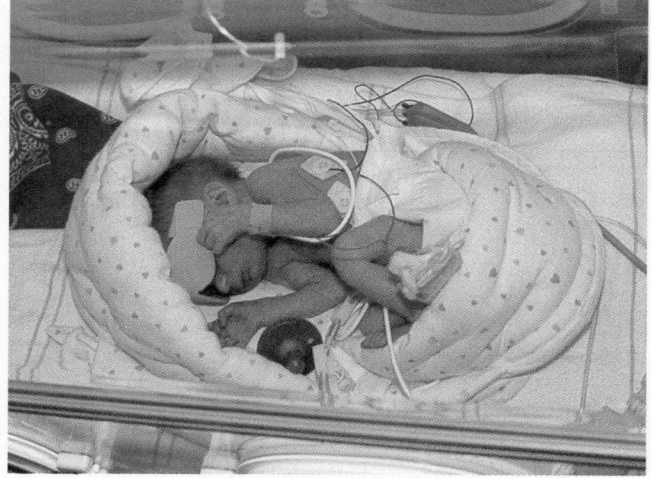

FIGURE 31-13 Infant is "nested." Hand to mouth behavior facilitates self-consoling/soothing activities. SOURCE: Courtesy of Theresa Kledzik, RN, Developmental Nurse, Memorial Hospital.

even before discharge. Information on bathing, diapering, hygiene, and normal elimination patterns is given. Parents should be told to expect changes in the color of the baby's stool, number of bowel movements, and timing of elimination when the infant is switched from bottle- to breastfeeding. This information can prevent unnecessary concern by the parents. Normal growth and development patterns, reflexes, and activity for preterm infants are discussed. Emphasis should be placed on bonding behaviors and dealing with newborn crying. Care of the preterm infant with complications, prevention of infections, signs of a sick baby, and the need for continued medical follow-up are emphasized.

Families with preterm infants usually do not need to be referred to community agencies, such as visiting nurse assistance. Referral may be necessary if the infant has severe congenital abnormalities, feeding problems, or complications with infections or respiratory problems or if the parents seem unable to cope with an at-risk baby. Parents should be taught CPR, the use of apnea monitors (if required at home), and the importance of follow-up eye, ear, and Denver II examinations. Parents of preterm infants can benefit from meeting with others in a similar situation to share common experiences and concerns. Nurses should refer parents to support groups sponsored by the hospital or by others in the community.

Evaluation

Anticipated outcomes of nursing care include:

- The preterm newborn is free of respiratory distress and establishes effective respiratory function.

- The preterm newborn gains weight and shows no signs of fatigue and/or aspiration during feedings.

- The parents are able to verbalize their anger, anxieties, and guilt feelings about the birth of a preterm baby and show attachment behavior such as frequent visits and growing confidence in their participatory care activities.

Critical Thinking Question

What ethical issues arise from the birth and survival of increasing numbers of very-low-birth-weight infants?

CARE OF THE INFANT OF A SUBSTANCE-ABUSING MOTHER

An infant of a substance-abusing mother (ISAM) was formerly called an infant of an addicted mother. The newborn of an alcoholic or drug-addicted woman may also be alcohol or drug dependent. After birth, when an infant's connection with the maternal blood supply is severed, the baby may suffer withdrawal. In addition the drugs the mother ingested may be teratogenic, resulting in congenital anomalies.

Alcohol Dependency

Infants born to alcohol-dependent mothers can suffer long-term complications in addition to suffering withdrawal symptoms.

The **fetal alcohol syndrome (FAS)** includes a series of malformations frequently found in infants born to women who have been severe alcoholics (Volpe 1995). It has been estimated that complete FAS syndrome occurs in the range of 0.3 to 1.9 live births per 1000 (Coles 1993; Committee on Substance Abuse and Committee on Children with Disabilities 1993). FAS rates among American Indians and Alaska natives are estimated at 1.3 to 10.3 per 1000 live births because of increased alcohol consumption in these populations (Duimstra et al 1993). **Fetal alcohol effects (FAE),** or alcohol-related birth defects (ARBD), are less severe effects of maternal alcohol use during pregnancy and include mild to moderate cognitive problems and physical growth retardation.

Controversy surrounds the exact cause of FAS. Although it is known that ethanol freely crosses the placenta to the fetus, it is still not known whether the alcohol alone or the breakdown products of alcohol causes the damage. For in-depth discussion of alcohol abuse in pregnancy see Chapter 18. The effects of other substances often combined with alcohol, such as nicotine, diazepam (Valium), marijuana, and caffeine, as well as poor diet, enhance the likelihood of FAS.

Long-Term Complications for the Infant with FAS

The long-term prognosis for the FAS newborn is less than favorable. Most infants with FAS are growth deficient at birth, and few infants have demonstrated postnatal catchup growth (Krishna & Phillips 1994). In fact most FAS infants are evaluated for failure to thrive. Decreased adipose tissue is a constant problem in individuals with FAS.

Feeding problems are frequently present during infancy and preschool years. These infants have a delay in the normal progression of oral feeding development but have a normal progression of oral motor function. Many FAS infants nurse poorly and have persistent vomiting until 6 to 7 months of age. They have difficulty adjusting to solid foods and show little spontaneous interest in food.

The brain is the organ most sensitive to damage from alcohol in the fetus (Volpe 1995). Central nervous system dysfunctions are the most common and serious problem associated with FAS. Most children exhibiting FAS are mildly to severely mentally retarded. The more dysmorphic (abnormal) the facial features, the lower the IQ scores. However, cases of infants of chronic alcoholics in whom neurologic disturbance appeared to be the only apparent abnormality are well documented (Volpe 1995). Providing a better environment for infants with FAS has been found to have no remarkable influence on IQ, which indicates that the brain damage occurred prenatally (Spohr et al 1993). These children are often hyperactive and show a high incidence of speech and language abnormalities indicative of CNS disorders.

Medical Therapy

Prevention of alcohol-induced complications is the foremost goal of medical therapy. This can be accomplished by educating the pregnant woman about the risks of alcohol ingestion and having the woman eliminate, or at least significantly reduce, her alcohol intake. Reducing alcohol intake during midpregnancy can prevent growth retardation, although malformations may still occur. The best advice is to drink no alcohol at all during pregnancy. The medical goal during the newborn period is managing CNS dysfunction and withdrawal. Seizures are treated with phenobarbital or diazepam.

APPLYING THE NURSING PROCESS

Nursing Assessment

Newborns with FAS show the following characteristics:

- *Abnormal structural development and CNS dysfunction.* This may include mental retardation, microcephaly, and hyperactivity.
- *Growth deficiencies.* Infants with FAS are often IUGR with weight, length, and head circumference being affected. These infants continue to show a persistent postnatal growth deficiency with weight being more affected than linear growth.
- *Distinctive facial abnormalities.* These include short palebral fissures, midfacial and maxillary hypoplasia, micrognathia (abnormally small lower jaw), hypoplastic upper lip, and diminished or absent philtrum (groove on upper lip).
- *Associated anomalies.* Abnormalities affecting cardiac (primarily septal and valvular defects), ocular, renal, and skeletal (especially involving joints such as congenital dislocated hips) systems are often noted.

Withdrawal symptoms of the alcohol-dependent newborn have been documented in children with normal facial features as well as in those with the typical features of FAS. These symptoms include tremors, seizures, sleeplessness, inconsolable crying, abnormal reflexes, hyperactivity with little ability to maintain alertness and attentiveness to environment, abdominal distention, and exaggerated mouthing behaviors such as hyperactive rooting and increased nonnutritive sucking.

Signs and symptoms of withdrawal often appear within 6 to 12 hours and at least within the first 3 days of life. Seizures after the newborn period are rare. Alcohol dependence in the infant is physiologic, not psychologic.

Nursing Diagnosis

Nursing diagnoses that may apply to the FAS newborn include the following:

- Altered nutrition: Less than body requirements related to decreased food intake and hyperirritability
- Risk for injury related to seizure activity secondary to CNS dysfunction or chemical dependence
- Ineffective family coping related to dysfunctional family dynamics and substance-dependent mother

Nursing Plan and Implementation

Promotion of Physical Well-Being

The nurse's awareness of the signs and symptoms of fetal alcohol syndrome is important in structuring and guiding nursing care. Nursing care of the FAS newborn is aimed at avoiding heat loss, protecting the infant from injury during seizures, administering medications such as phenobarbital or diazepam to limit convulsions, monitoring intravenous fluid therapy, and reducing environmental stimuli. The FAS baby is most comfortable in a quiet, dimly lit environment. Because of feeding problems, these infants require extra time and patience during feedings.

Mothers should be informed that breastfeeding is not contraindicated but that excessive alcohol consumption may intoxicate the newborn and inhibit the let-down reflex. The nurse should monitor the newborn's vital signs closely and observe for evidence of seizure activity and respiratory distress.

Promotion of Family Adaptation

Infants affected by maternal alcohol abuse are also at risk psychologically. Restlessness, sleeplessness, agitation, resistance to cuddling or holding, and frequent crying can be frustrating to parents as their efforts to relieve the distress are unrewarded. Feeding dysfunction can also result in frustrations for the care giver and digestive upsets for the infant. Frustration may cause the parents to punish the baby or result in the unconscious desire to "stay away from the infant." Either outcome may create an unstable family environment and result in the infant's failure to thrive.

The nurse should focus on providing support for the parents and reinforcing positive parenting activity. Prior to discharge, parents should be given opportunities to provide baby care so that they can feel confident in their interpretations of their baby's cues and their ability to meet the baby's needs. Referring the family to social services and visiting nurse or public health nurse associations is essential for the well-being of the infant. Follow-up care and teaching can strengthen the parents' skills and coping abilities and help them create a stable, healthy environment for their family.

Evaluation

Anticipated outcomes of nursing care include:

- The FAS newborn is able to tolerate feedings and gain weight.

- The FAS infant's hyperirritability and/or seizures are controlled, and the baby has suffered no physical injuries.

- The parents are able to identify and meet the special needs of their newborn and accept outside assistance as needed.

Drug Dependency

Drug-dependent infants are predisposed to a number of problems. Almost all narcotic drugs cross the placenta and enter the fetal circulation, so the fetus can develop problems in utero and/or soon after birth.

The greatest risks to the fetus of the drug-dependent mother are listed below:

- *Intrauterine asphyxia.* Often a direct result of fetal withdrawal secondary to maternal withdrawal, fetal withdrawal is accompanied by hyperactivity with increased oxygen consumption. If not adequately compensated, this can lead to fetal asphyxia. Moreover, narcotic-addicted women tend to have a higher incidence of PIH, abruptio placentae, and placenta previa, resulting in placental insufficiency and fetal asphyxia.

- *Intrauterine infection.* Sexually transmitted diseases and hepatitis are often connected with the pregnant addict's life-style. Such infections can involve the fetus.

- *Alterations in birth weight.* These may depend on the type of drug the mother uses. Women using predominantly heroin have infants of lower birth weight who are SGA. Women maintained on methadone have higher-birth-weight infants, some of whom are LGA.

- *Low Apgar scores.* These may be related to the intrauterine asphyxia or the medication the woman received during labor. The use of a narcotic antagonist (nalorphine or naloxone) to reverse respiratory depression is contraindicated because it may precipitate acute withdrawal in the infant.

Patterns of abuse of alcohol, marijuana, and heroin in childbearing women have changed very little in the past few years, but the incidence of cocaine (especially "crack") use has recently risen dramatically. (See Chapter 18 for more discussion of maternal substance abuse.) Marijuana, alcohol, and nicotine are sometimes used in conjunction with cocaine. Therefore the effects of secondary drugs on the newborn must also be taken into consideration.

Common Complications of the Drug-Addicted Newborn

The newborn of a woman who abused drugs during her pregnancy is predisposed to the following problems:

- *Respiratory distress.* The heroin-addicted newborn frequently suffers respiratory stress, mainly meconium-aspiration pneumonia and transient tachypnea. Meconium aspiration is usually secondary to increased oxygen consumption and activity experienced by the fetus during intrauterine withdrawal. Transient tachypnea may develop secondary to the inhibitory effects of narcotics on the reflex responsible for clearing the lungs. Respiratory distress syndrome occurs less in heroin-addicted newborns even in the presence of prematurity because they have tissue-oxygen unloading capabilities comparable to those of a 6-week-old term infant. In addition heroin stimulates production of glucocorticoids via the anterior pituitary gland. Cocaine-exposed infants have increased incidence of apnea.

- *Jaundice.* Newborns of methadone-addicted women may develop jaundice due to prematurity. Heroin and cocaine contribute to early maturity of the liver, leading to a lower incidence of hyperbilirubinemia for these groups of babies (Wennberg et al 1994).

- *Congenital anomalies and growth retardation.* The incidence of anomalies of the genitourinary and cardiovascular systems is slightly increased in infants of heroin- and cocaine-addicted mothers. Infants of cocaine-addicted mothers exhibit congenital malformations involving bony skull defects such as microencephaly and symmetric intrauterine growth retardation (Jhaveri et al 1993).

- *Behavioral abnormalities.* Babies exposed to cocaine have poor state organization. They exhibit decreased interactive behaviors when tested with the Brazelton Neonatal Behavioral Assessment Scale (Frank et al 1993). These infants also have difficulty moving through the various sleep and awake states and have problems attending to and actively engaging in auditory and visual stimuli.

- *Withdrawal.* The most significant postnatal problem of the drug-addicted newborn is that of narcotic withdrawal (usually from heroin or methadone). The onset of the withdrawal manifestations usually occurs within the first 72 hours after birth. For heroin-addicted newborns, a majority of withdrawal symptoms are seen within the first 24 to 48 hours. For newborns exposed to barbiturates, symptoms may be delayed for several days. Withdrawal for cocaine-addicted infants may occur 4 to 5 days after birth. For methadone-addicted infants, withdrawal symptoms may appear immediately after birth or within the first 48 hours of life (Frank et al 1993). In most cases the withdrawal manifestations peak in the newborn about the third day and subside by the fifth to seventh day. See Nursing Assessment below for a discussion of withdrawal symptoms.

Long-Term Complications

During the first 2 years of life, many cocaine-exposed infants demonstrate deviant psychologic behavior. This is attributed to the irreversible damage to dopamine neurons caused by long-term administration of cocaine. The damage is manifested by susceptibility to behavior lability and the inability to express strong feelings such as pleasure, anger, or distress or even a strong reaction to being separated from their parents. Cocaine-exposed infants are at higher risk for motor development problems, delays in expressive language skills, and feeding difficulties because of swallowing problems.

Infants of drug-addicted mothers often demonstrate a higher incidence of gastrointestinal and respiratory illnesses; it is believed these are related not to narcotic addiction but to the mothers' lack of education regarding proper infant care, feeding, and hygiene.

Another important long-term complication is the high (15–20 per 1000 births) rate of sudden infant death syndrome (SIDS) for heroin- or methadone-exposed infants when compared to those in the general population (Frank et al 1993). Some studies have shown that infants of cocaine-addicted mothers have a SIDS rate of 8.5 per 1000 births and suggest that the rate may be even higher in those infants who have moderate to severe postnatal withdrawal.

After birth the infant born to a drug-dependent mother may also be subject to neglect and/or abuse (Scherling 1994).

Medical Therapy

The goal of medical therapy is prevention through prenatal management (see Chapter 18) and pharmacologic management of newborn narcotic withdrawal. For optimal fetal and newborn outcome, the narcotic-addicted woman should receive complete prenatal care as early as possible. She should be started on a methadone program with a reduction in dosage to 20 mg or less, if possible. The aim of methadone maintenance during pregnancy is the prevention of heroin use. The dose of methadone used for maintenance should be sufficient to ensure this goal even if the dose is greater than 20 mg. It is not recommended that the woman be withdrawn completely from narcotics while pregnant because this induces fetal withdrawal with poor newborn outcomes.

Newborn treatment may include management of newborn complications; serologic tests for syphilis, HIV, and hepatitis B; drug screen and meconium analysis for cocaine; and social service referral (Ryan et al 1994). About 50% of newborns of addicted mothers experience withdrawal symptoms severe enough to require treatment. Drugs to control withdrawal symptoms are phenobarbital or paregoric. Nutritional support is important in light of the increase in energy expenditure that withdrawal may entail. In 1989, the American Academy of Pediatrics recommended use of a formula that supplies 24 cal/oz (30 mL) to provide 150 to 250 kcal/kg/day if the infant has diarrhea and vomiting or if the infant is excessively active (Angelini & Knapp 1991).

Nursing Assessment

Early identification of the newborn needing medical or pharmacologic interventions decreases the incidence of mortality and morbidity. During the newborn period nursing assessment focuses on the following:

- Discovering the mother's last drug intake and dosage level. This is accomplished through the prenatal history and laboratory tests. Women may be reluctant to disclose this information; therefore a nonjudgmental interview technique is essential.

- Assessing for congenital malformations and the complications related to intrauterine withdrawal such as SGA, intrauterine asphyxia, meconium aspiration, and prematurity. For nursing care of SGA newborns see Care of the SGA Newborn earlier in this chapter; for nursing care of premature newborns see Care of the Preterm (Premature) Newborn earlier in this chapter; for nursing care of the infant who suffered intrauterine asphyxia, see Chapter 32.

- Identifying the signs and symptoms of newborn withdrawal or newborn abstinence syndrome. Signs and symptoms of newborn withdrawal can be classified in five groups:

1. Central nervous system signs
   a. Hyperactivity
   b. Hyperirritability (persistent high-pitched cry)
   c. Increased muscle tone
   d. Exaggerated reflexes

e. Tremors, seizures

f. Sneezing, hiccups, yawning

g. Short, unquiet sleep

h. Fever

2. Respiratory signs

   a. Tachypnea

   b. Excessive secretions

3. Gastrointestinal signs

   a. Disorganized, vigorous suck

   b. Vomiting

   c. Drooling

   d. Sensitive gag reflex

   e. Hyperphagia

   f. Diarrhea

   g. Abdominal cramping

4. Vasomotor signs

   a. Stuffy nose, yawning, sneezing

   b. Flushing

   c. Sweating

   d. Sudden, circumoral pallor

5. Cutaneous signs

   a. Excoriated buttocks, knees, elbows

   b. Facial scratches

   c. Pressure point abrasions

Although many of the signs and symptoms of narcotic withdrawal are similar to those seen with hypoglycemia and hypocalcemia, glucose and calcium values are reported to be within normal limits for this group of infants.

The severity of withdrawal can be assessed by a scoring system based on clinical manifestations. It evaluates the infant on potentially life-threatening signs such as vomiting, diarrhea, weight loss, irritability, tremors, and tachypnea (Table 31–2). Drugs are used to treat severe clinical signs.

Nursing Diagnosis

Nursing diagnoses that may apply to drug-dependent mothers include the following:

- Altered nutrition and fluid intake: Less than body requirements related to vomiting and diarrhea, uncoordinated suck and swallow reflex, hypertonia secondary to withdrawal

- Impaired skin integrity related to constant activity

- Altered parenting related to hyperirritable behavior of the infant

- Ineffective family coping related to drug abuse, poverty, and lack of education

Nursing Plan and Implementation

Promotion of Physical Well-Being

Care of the drug-dependent newborn is based on reducing withdrawal symptoms and promoting adequate respiration, temperature, and nutrition. See the Nursing Care Plan: Newborn of a Substance-Abusing Mother on page 958 for specific nursing care measures. Some general nursery care measures include the following:

- Temperature regulation

- Careful monitoring of pulse and respirations every 15 minutes until stable; stimulation if apnea occurs

- Small frequent feedings, especially in the presence of vomiting, regurgitation, and diarrhea

- Intravenous therapy as needed

- Medications as ordered, such as phenobarbital, paregoric, chlorpromazine hydrochloride (Thorazine), or laudanum. Methadone should not be given because of possible newborn addiction to it.

Text continues on page 960

| TABLE 31-2 | Assessment of the Clinical Severity of Neonatal Narcotic Withdrawal |

Symptom	Mild	Moderate	Severe
Vomiting	Spitting up	Extensive vomiting for three successive feedings	Vomiting associated with imbalance of serum electrolytes
Diarrhea	Watery stools < four times per day	Watery stools five to six times per day for 3 days; no electrolyte imbalance	Diarrhea associated with imbalance of serum electrolytes
Weight loss	<10% of birth weight	10%–15% of birth weight	>15%
Irritability	Minimal	Marked but relieved by cuddling or feeding	Unrelieved by cuddling or feeding
Tremors or twitching	Mild tremors when stimulated	Marked tremors or twitching when stimulated	Convulsions
Tachypnea	60–80 breaths/minute	80–100 breaths/minute	>100 breaths/minute; associated with respiratory alkalosis

Source: Ostrea EM, Chavez CJ, Stryker JS: *The Care of the Drug Dependent Woman and Her Infant.* Lansing, MI: Michigan Department of Public Health, 1978, p 33.

NURSING CARE PLAN

NEWBORN OF A SUBSTANCE-ABUSING MOTHER

Nursing Assessment

Nursing History

1. Type and amount of drug(s) consumed by the mother during each month of pregnancy
2. Type and amount of prenatal care received
3. Prior history of addiction and treatment
4. Maternal disease/infection such as placenta previa, hypertension, bacterial and TORCH infections, HIV seropositive, and sexually transmitted infections
5. Preterm labor and birth

Physical Examination

Withdrawal symptoms: hyperactivity, jitteriness, irritability, shrill high-pitched cry, vomiting, diarrhea, weak suck, stuffy nose, frequent sneezing, yawning, tachycardia, hypertension, apnea. Cocaine withdrawal pattern may be unpredictable or may be asymptomatic with only subtle behavioral state organization problems. Disturbed sleep-wake cycle and rhythm at 24–28 hours.

Diagnostic Studies

1. Toxicology screen: Identify drug(s) and drug levels in mother and infant blood and urine.
2. Serum electrolyte (Na, K, Ca): Detect losses from vomiting, diarrhea; detect causes of neurologic symptoms or seizures.
3. Glucose
4. Serial capillary gases
5. CBC and blood culture: Detect sepsis.
6. Urine specific gravity: May be high due to dehydration.

NURSING DIAGNOSIS: Sleep pattern disturbance related to CNS excitation secondary to drug withdrawal

EXPECTED OUTCOME: Newborn will be free of signs and symptoms of withdrawal.

Nursing Interventions	Rationale
Assess for withdrawal symptoms, including frequent sneezing and yawning, restlessness, high-pitched shrill cry, hypertonicity, vomiting or diarrhea, wakefulness.	Most addicted newborns will show symptoms of withdrawal as early as 12 hours after birth. These begin with jitteriness, hyperactivity, and wakefulness and progress to GI symptoms and seizures. Early identification allows for early intervention and prevention of complications.
Provide calming techniques, including: Swaddling infant tightly in side-lying or prone position with small pillow supporting back.	Positioning provides for rest, discourages hyperactivity, and increases comfort while reducing stimuli.
Provide quiet, dim environment for rest.	Quiet environment decreases external stimuli and therefore infant's irritability.
Hold, rock, and cuddle infant. Use touching, patting, smiling, and talking. Use infant snuggles for closeness.	Holding infant as often as possible promotes comfort, and cuddling quiets and comforts infant. These activities promote close contact.
Provide pacifier or position baby so that baby can get hand to mouth.	Hand-to-mouth activity or pacifier satisfies increased need to suck during withdrawal.
Schedule tests or treatments to avoid stress.	Planned care allows for maximum rest and reduces external stimuli.
Administer medications for withdrawal as ordered, such as paregoric, chlorpromazine, Valium, phenobarbital; observe for effectiveness and side effects.	Pharmacologic agents alleviate withdrawal symptoms.

OUTCOME MET IF:
- Newborn is free from jitteriness, vomiting, diarrhea, and wakefulness.
- Newborn has normal sleep-wake behavior.

NURSING DIAGNOSIS: Altered nutrition: Less than body requirements related to withdrawal symptoms

EXPECTED OUTCOME: Newborn gains and/or maintains weight.

Nursing Interventions	Rationale
Assess for increased nutritional needs because of gestational age, weight, uncoordinated suck and swallow, vomiting, diarrhea, and regurgitation.	Infants of drug-addicted mothers tend to be SGA and premature. CNS stimulation causes hyperactivity, leading to poor feeding, GI hypermotility, and irritation, leading to inability to retain or absorb nutrients.
Provide appropriate nutrition: Initiate IV feedings until stable.	Oral feeding of an irritable infant with possible seizures may foster aspiration.
Supplement oral or gavage feedings with intravenous intake per orders.	SGA infants need 110–120 kcal/kg/day for optimal nutrition.
Give small, frequent feedings of high-calorie formula (may start feedings at one-half strength every 3 hours).	Smaller feedings facilitate nutritional intake.

NEWBORN OF A SUBSTANCE-ABUSING MOTHER *continued*

Nursing Interventions	Rationale
Check for residuals after oral or gavage feedings; reduce feeding volume if residuals are high. As hyperactivity decreases, increase feedings as tolerated.	*Prevents vomiting from overeeding while still providing IV fluids according to infant's tolerance.*
Place on right side with back support or on abdomen after feedings.	*Positioning decreases vomiting, regurgitation, and distention.*

OUTCOME MET IF:
- Newborn does not lose more than 2% per day of body weight.
- Newborn has vigorous suck reflex.
- Newborn tolerates feedings without vomiting, fatigue, or aspiration.

NURSING DIAGNOSIS: Knowledge deficit related to lack of information about infant care

EXPECTED OUTCOME: Mother/family will be able to manage newborn care at home.

Nursing Interventions	Rationale
Identify mother's/family's knowledge needs and readiness for learning.	*Assessment provides information regarding mother's/family's ability to care for infant.*
Provide information including:	
1. Signs and symptoms of baby's withdrawal, current condition, and rationale for treatment	*Helps the mother/family to understand baby's behavior and how to care for the baby's symptoms.*
2. Newborn capabilities and developmental behaviors	*Assists mother/family to be realistic about infant's progress.*
3. Newborn's need for appropriate stimulation as well as rest, depending on cues	*Mother/family needs to adjust infant interaction based on infant's cues.*
4. Physical care needs such as feeding, bathing, clothing, and holding	*This information helps mother/family provide for safe infant care.*
Encourage and support positive mothering/parenting behaviors with infant.	*Increases mother's/family's feelings of competence in parenting abilities.*

OUTCOME MET IF:
- Mother/family verbalizes understanding of signs and symptoms to report to health care provider; schedule for follow-up appointments; importance of keeping appointments; available community resources; and the newborn's need for stimulation and rest periods.
- Mother/family demonstrates ability to feed, bathe, clothe, and hold newborn and to pick up on the baby's behavioral cues.

Essential Nursing Activities to Achieve Outcomes

Maternal Assessments

1. Identify woman at risk for drug abuse.
2. Obtain information regarding drug usage in a nonjudgmental manner from all clients admitted to birthing unit:
   - Prior drug use
   - Prior history of addiction
   - Type and amount of drug usage
   - Last drug intake (amount, type, time)
3. Gather the prenatal history:
   - Number of visits
   - HIV, Herpes, TORCH
   - Hypertension
   - Preterm labor
   - PROM
   - Placenta previa
   - Abruptio placentae
4. Assess parent-infant bonding and attachment.
5. Assess support systems.
6. Assess knowledge of community resources.

Newborn Assessments

1. Identify early those newborns needing medical or pharmacological intervention.
2. Complete gestational age assessment on admission to nursery.
3. If newborn is identified as SGA or IUGR, observe for common problems:
   - Hypoglycemia
   - Hypothermia
   - RDS
4. Assess for congenital anomalies.
5. Assess for signs and symptoms of withdrawal:
   - CNS signs
   - Respiratory signs
   - Gastrointestinal signs
   - Vasomotor signs
   - Cutaneous signs
6. Observe baby for normal sleep-wake behavior.
7. Assess I & O: six to eight wet diapers per 24 hours.

Interventions

1. Monitor pulse and respiration every 15 minutes until stable.
2. Stimulate if apnea occurs.
3. Maintain an adequate skin temperature: 36.1–36.7 C (97–98 F).
4. Provide small, frequent feedings.
5. Maintain adequate fluid intake.
6. Administer IV therapy as ordered.
7. Administer meds per physician order.
8. Position on the right side to prevent aspiration.
9. Swaddle to minimize injury.
10. Weigh daily.
11. Record all assessment data accurately.

- Proper positioning on the right side to avoid possible aspirations of vomitus or secretions
- Frequency of diarrhea and vomiting noted and infant weighed every 8 hours during withdrawal (Ostrea 1993)
- Observation for problems of SGA or LGA newborns
- Swaddling with hands near mouth to minimize injury and achieve more organized behavioral state
- Placing newborn in quiet, dimly lit area of nursery

Critical Thinking Question

What issues need to be addressed to meet the needs of babies of substance-abusing mothers?

Home Care   Parents should be prepared for what they can expect for the first few months at home. At the time of discharge the mother should be instructed to anticipate mild jitteriness and irritability in the newborn, which may persist from 8 to 16 weeks, depending on the initial severity of the withdrawal. The nurse should help the mother learn feeding techniques and comforting measures. In one study substance-abusing mothers tended to become frustrated with their failure to engage their unresponsive infants and detach emotionally from them or to overstimulate their infants (Brooks-Gunn et al 1994). Parents are to be counseled regarding available resources, such as support groups, and signs and symptoms that indicate the need for further care. Ongoing evaluation is necessary because of the potential for long-term problems.

Evaluation

Anticipated outcomes of nursing care include:

- The newborn tolerates feedings, gains weight, and has a decreased number of stools.
- The parents learn ways to comfort their newborn.
- The parents are able to cope with their frustrations and begin to use outside resources as needed.

CARE OF THE NEWBORN AT RISK FOR AIDS

An increasing number of newborns are being born infected with HIV or at risk for acquiring it in the newborn period or early infancy. Transmission during the perinatal and newborn periods can occur across the placenta or through breast milk and/or contaminated blood. Ongo-ing prospective studies indicate maternal to newborn vertical transmission rates of about 30%–40%. Vertical transmission can be decreased to about 8% in mothers taking AZT during gestation (Kinsey 1994). For discussion of maternal and fetal AIDS characteristics see Chapter 18.

Early identification of babies with or at risk for AIDS is essential during the newborn period. The currently available HIV serologic tests (ELISA and Western blot test) cannot distinguish between maternal and infant antibodies; therefore they are inappropriate for infants up to 15 months of age. It may take up to 15 months for infected infants to form their own antibodies to HIV (Kellinger 1994). In infants under 15 months, HIV culture or viral p24 antigen detection can be used for diagnosing congenital AIDS. New diagnostic tests that detect the infant's specific antibody (IgG or IgM) response to HIV or tests for viral DNA may become generally available in the future (Kellinger 1994). Opportunistic diseases such as gram-negative sepsis and problems associated with prematurity are the primary causes of mortality in HIV-infected babies.

APPLYING THE NURSING PROCESS

Nursing Assessment

Many newborns with AIDS are premature and/or SGA and show failure to thrive during the newborn and infant periods. They can show signs and symptoms of disease within days of birth. Signs that may be seen in the newborn period include failure to thrive, enlarged spleen and liver, swollen glands, interstitial pneumonia (rarely seen in adults), recurrent gastrointestinal problems (diarrhea and weight loss), urinary system infections, persistent or recurrent oral candidiasis, evidence of Epstein-Barr virus, developmental delays or failure to reach developmental milestones, and neurologic deficits (Kellinger 1994; Scott & Parks 1994). Some cranial and facial stigmas have been associated with AIDS contracted in utero. However, these findings do not establish a diagnosis of HIV infection at birth (Yogev & Conner 1992).

Nursing Diagnosis

Nursing diagnoses that may apply to the infant at risk for AIDS include the following:

- Altered nutrition: Less than body requirements related to formula intolerance and inadequate intake
- Impaired skin integrity related to chronic diarrhea
- Risk for infection related to immunosuppression secondary to AIDS

Resuscitation	For suctioning use a bulb syringe, mucus extractor, or meconium aspirator with wall suction on low setting.
Admission care	To remove blood from baby's skin, give warm water, mild soap bath using gloves as soon as possible after admission.
Hand washing	Thorough hand washing is indicated before and after caring for infant. Hands must be washed immediately if contaminated with blood or body fluids. Wash hands after removal of gloves.
Gowns	Long-sleeved gowns are indicated when at bedside.
Gloves	Gloves are indicated when touching blood or body fluids. Gloves should also be worn when handling newborns before and during their initial baths, cord care, eye prophylactics, and vitamin K administration.
Mask	Not routinely needed. Masks are indicated if mouth is likely to come in contact with body fluids (eg, when caring for intubated or coughing infant who has copious secretions) or if care giver feels she or he is infectious, thereby posing risk to infant.
Goggles	Not routinely needed. Goggles are indicated if eyes are likely to come in contact with body fluids (eg, when caring for intubated or coughing infant who has copious secretions). If glasses are worn, goggles are not necessary.

Needles and syringes	Care should be taken to avoid needle stick injuries. Used needles should not be recapped or bent; they should be placed in a prominently labeled, puncture-resistant plastic container designed specifically for such disposal and belonging specifically to that baby. After the newborn is discharged the container is discarded.
Specimens	Blood and other specimens should be double-bagged and/or sealed in an impervious container and labeled "blood/body fluids precautions."
Equipment and linen	Articles contaminated with blood or body fluids should be discarded or bagged according to isolation protocol or institution and labeled "blood/body fluids precautions" before being sent for decontamination and reprocessing.
Body fluid spills	Blood and body fluids should be cleaned promptly with a solution of 5.25% sodium hypochlorite (household bleach) diluted 1:10 with water.
Education and support	Provide education and psychologic support for family and staff. Care givers who avoid contact with baby at risk or who overdress in unnecessary isolation garb subtly exacerbate an already difficult family situation. Information resources include the National AIDS Hotline (1-800-342-2437).
Exempted personnel	Immunologically compromised staff (pregnant women may be included in this group) and possibly infectious staff members should not care for these infants.

Sources: Adapted from Mendez H, Jule JE: Care of the infant born exposed to HIV. *Obstet Gynecol Clin North Am* 1990; 17(3):637; Berry RK: Home care of the child with AIDS. *Pediatr Nurs* July/August 1988; 14(4):341.

- Impaired physical mobility related to decreased neuromuscular development
- Altered growth and development related to lack of attachment and stimulation
- Altered parenting related to diagnosis of AIDS
- Ineffective family coping related to diagnosis of AIDS

Nursing Plan and Implementation

Nursing care of the newborn at risk for AIDS calls for all the normal care required for any newborn in an NICU. In addition the nurse must include care for a newborn suspected of having a blood-borne infection, as with hepatitis B. Universal precautions should be used when caring for the newborn immediately after birth and when obtaining blood samples via vein puncture or heel stick. (The blood of *all* newborns must be considered potentially infectious because the status of the infant's blood is often not known until after the infant is discharged, and there is a window of time before seroconversion occurs during which the baby is still considered infectious.) See Table 31–3. Nursing care involves providing for comfort; keeping the newborn well nourished and protected from opportunistic infections; and facilitating growth, development, and attachment. See the Nursing Care Plan: Newborn at Risk for AIDS on page 962 for specific nursing care measures.

Home Care

Hand washing is crucial when caring for newborns at risk for AIDS. Parents should be taught proper hand-washing technique. Nutrition is essential because failure to thrive and weight loss are common. Small frequent feedings and food supplementation are helpful. The nurse should discuss sanitary formula preparation with parents. The baby should not be put to bed with juice or formula because of potential bacteria growth.

Parents need to be alert to the signs of feeding intolerance such as increasing regurgitation, abdominal distention, and loose stools. The newborn should be weighed three times a week.

Prompt diaper changing and perineal care can prevent or minimize diaper rash and promote comfort. The diaper-changing area in the home should be separate from the food preparation and serving areas. Disposable diapers are recommended over cloth diapers. The diapers are to be placed in plastic bags, sealed, and placed in the garbage can daily. Even though the American Academy of Pediatrics doesn't require gloves to be worn during routine diaper changes (American Academy of Pediatrics Committee on Fetus and Newborn 1992), most institutions recommend that their care givers wear gloves during all diaper changes and examination of babies. Disposable gloves are worn when changing diapers or cleaning the diaper area, especially in the presence of diarrhea, because blood may be in the stool (Mendez & Jule 1990). Good skin care is essential to prevent skin rashes.

Text continues on page 964

NEWBORN AT RISK FOR AIDS

Nursing Assessment

Nursing History

1. Maternal history of drug abuse or needle sharing
2. Sexual partner or partners of the mother with a positive HIV antibody test or ELISA test

Physical Examination

1. Complete physical examination. Findings may vary, depending on type of opportunistic infection present.

Diagnostic Studies

1. ELISA test detects HIV antibody.
2. Viral antigen detection—quantitative assessment of p24 (HIV protein).

NURSING DIAGNOSIS: Risk for infection related to perinatal exposure and immunoregulation suppression

EXPECTED OUTCOME: Infant will not develop infection while in birthing area.

Nursing Interventions	Rationale
Assess infant for signs of ongoing infection such as: • Failure to thrive • Weight loss over 10% at time of diagnosis • Temperature instability • More than three diarrhea episodes a day • Hepatosplenomegaly—palpate once a day for continued enlargement • Lethargy	Signs and symptoms of infection and inflammation may persist prior to definite AIDS diagnosis. Decreased activity and lethargy can indicate sepsis.
Assess for opportunistic diseases such as: • Herpes simplex lasting more than 1 month • Cytomegalovirus disease • Lymphoid interstitial pneumonia • Viral, fungal, or protozoal infections	Opportunistic infections occur because of immune system suppression.
Maintain universal precautions—especially until baby has had first bath—when changing diapers, drawing blood or doing heel sticks, and suctioning newborn.	Universal precautions protect care givers from newborn's body secretions. Also newborn is protected from other infectious agents.
Newborn should not receive any injections, have blood drawn, or have eye treatments until after initial bath with soap and water.	Removal of maternal secretions before injections or eye treatment prevents spread of HIV disease to newborn who may not already have been infected.

OUTCOME MET IF: • Newborn shows no signs of failure to thrive, weight loss, temperature instability, diarrhea, hepatosplenomegaly, lethargy, respiratory difficulties, skin lesions, or general lymphadenopathy.

NURSING DIAGNOSIS: Altered nutrition: Less than body requirements related to formula intolerance and inadequate intake

EXPECTED OUTCOME: Baby will not lose weight.

Nursing Interventions	Rationale
Assess for residuals and abdominal distention (abdominal girth measurements) prior to each feeding. Obtain accurate I & O (weigh diapers).	Feeding intolerance causes gastric residuals, increasing abdominal girth and dehydration.
Provide small frequent feedings.	
Monitor stools for amount, type, consistency, and any change in pattern. Check stools for occult blood and reducing substances.	Loose stools and presence of reducing substances may indicate feeding intolerance. Occult blood indicates irritation or ulceration of bowel mucosa.

OUTCOME MET IF: • Newborn has steady weight gain.
• Newborn follows normal growth curve.

NEWBORN AT RISK FOR AIDS *continued*

NURSING DIAGNOSIS: Risk for impaired skin integrity related to diarrhea

EXPECTED OUTCOME: The infant will have no skin breakdown.

Nursing Interventions	Rationale
Assess skin for breakdown or rashes.	*Infant with AIDS may have recurrent diarrhea and skin rashes caused by* Candida albicans.
Provide meticulous and frequent skin care, especially after voiding or stooling.	
Instruct parents/care givers of need after discharge for frequent position changes, thorough skin cleansing with each diaper change, and to report any signs and symptoms of rash or skin breakdown to health care provider.	

OUTCOME MET IF:
- Infant has no skin breakdown.
- Mother/family verbalizes understanding of need to thoroughly cleanse skin after voiding and/or stooling and need to report signs and symptoms of skin breakdown and/or rash to health care provider.

NURSING DIAGNOSIS: Altered parenting related to diagnosis of AIDS and fear of future outcome

EXPECTED OUTCOME: Parents will express fears and begin to bond with their infant.

Nursing Interventions	Rationale
Assess cause of parental fear by: 1. Providing time for expression of concerns 2. Determining parental understanding of AIDS	*Lack of information and distorted perception of AIDS may increase parents' fears.*
Provide information about cause of AIDS, signs of HIV in infants, current and experimental treatment modalities, support groups, and community resources.	*Accurate information about AIDS reduces fear. Access to community services and participation in support groups provide assistance with coping with a potentially critically ill child.*

OUTCOME MET IF:
- Mother/family demonstrates two or more of the following physical interactions: good eye contact, touching baby, holding baby close, attempting to comfort baby, and kissing baby.
- Mother/family demonstrates two or more of the following social interactions: calling baby by name, making positive comments about baby, asking questions about baby, asking questions about baby care, visiting baby frequently, talking to baby.
- Mother/family verbalizes reduced anxiety and fear.

Essential Nursing Activities to Achieve Outcomes

Newborn Assessments

1. Assess for signs and symptoms of infection, including weight loss, anemia, temperature instability, lethargy, respiratory difficulties, diarrhea, hepatosplenomegaly, and general lymphadenopathy.
2. Assess for CMV, *Herpes simplex,* and *Candida albicans.*
3. Assess skin for general skin rashes and diaper rash.
4. Assess nutritional status, including weight gain, % of weight loss, and feeding tolerance.
5. Assess parent-infant interaction, parental support system, and parental knowledge level.

Interventions

1. Take vital signs every 4 hours.
2. Change diapers frequently.
3. Give meticulous skin care after each voiding and stooling.
4. Maintain universal precautions:
   - Frequent hand washing
   - Gloves utilized in handling newborn at all times until after initial bath, then whenever changing diapers or obtaining blood specimens
5. Provide frequent, small feedings.
6. Instruct woman/family on newborn health needs:
   - Need for frequent diaper changes and meticulous skin care
   - Signs and symptoms of infection to report to health care provider
   - Importance of keeping scheduled follow-up appointments
7. Provide emotional support to mother/family if breastfeeding had been desired because mother unable to breastfeed if HIV positive.
8. Provide list of contact persons for available community resources.

The baby should have his or her own skin care items, towels, and washcloths. Most clothing and linens can be washed with other household laundry. Linen that is visibly soiled with blood or body fluids should be kept separate and washed separately in hot sudsy water with household bleach. Diaper-changing areas should be cleaned with a 1:10 dilution of household bleach after each diaper change. Toys should be kept as clean as possible, and they should not be shared with other children. Toys should be checked for sharp edges to prevent scratches.

Parents should be instructed on what signs of infection to be alerted to and when to call their health care provider. The inability to feed without pain may indicate esophageal yeast. Topical mycostatin or Desitin ointment is used for diaper rashes and oral mycostatin for oral thrush. If diarrhea occurs, the baby requires frequent perineal care and fluid replacements. Antidiarrheal medications are often ineffective. Irritability may be the first sign of fever. Rectal temperatures should be avoided because they may stimulate diarrhea. Tepid water sponging, fluids, and antipyretics are of use in managing fever.

Parents and family members need to be reassured that there are no documented cases of people contracting AIDS from routine care of infected babies. Emotional support for the family is essential because of the stress and social isolation they may face. Because of these stresses, attachment may not occur and/or the infant may suffer from lack of sensory and tactile stimulation (Bastin et al 1992). Babies should be held for feedings because they will benefit from frequent, gentle touch. Auditory stimulation may also be provided using music or tapes of parents' voices. Families should be informed about support groups, available counseling, and information resources. Current therapeutic information regarding HIV disease is available to both health care providers and families through the AIDS Clinical Trials Information Service (1-800-TRIALS-A) (Kellinger 1994). The CDC recommends that HIV-infected women *not* breastfeed because HIV has been found to be transmitted via breast milk. Therefore if there is a viable alternative feeding method, it should be used (Sison & Sever 1992).

CRITICAL THINKING IN PRACTICE

Mrs Jean Corrigan, a 23-year-old G1P1, positive for HIV, has just given birth to a 7 lb 1 oz baby girl. As she watches you assessing her daughter in the birthing room, she asks why you are wearing gloves and whether her daughter will have to be in isolation. What will your response be?

Answers can be found in Appendix I.

Preventive care for at-risk and HIV-infected infants is the same as for other infants and includes routine immunizations except that the live polio vaccine should be avoided. At 1 month of age the baby's physical exam should include a developmental assessment; complete blood count, including differential blood count, CD4 count, and Ig (quantitative immunoglobulins); HIV test or PCR (polymerase chain reaction) test for HIV, if available, or p24 antigen test for HIV after 1 month of age; and #2 dose of hepatitis vaccine (Kellinger 1994). Pediatric HIV disease raises many health care issues for the family. The parents, depending on their health status, may or may not be able to care for their infant, and they must deal with many psychosocial and economic issues.

Evaluation

Anticipated outcomes of nursing care include:

- The parents are able to bond with their infant and have realistic expectations about the baby.
- Early identification and treatment of potential opportunistic infections are provided.
- The parents verbalize their concerns surrounding their baby's existing and potential health problems and accept outside assistance as needed.

CARE OF THE NEWBORN WITH CONGENITAL ANOMALIES

The birth of a baby with a congenital defect places both newborn and family at risk. Many congenital anomalies can be life-threatening if not corrected within hours after birth; others are very visible and cause the families emotional distress. When one congenital anomaly is found, health care providers should look for other ones, particularly in body systems that develop at the same time during gestation. Table 31–4 identifies some of the more common anomalies and their early management and nursing care in the newborn period.

CARE OF THE NEWBORN WITH CONGENITAL HEART DEFECT

The incidence of congenital heart defects is 4 to 5 per 1000 live births. They account for one-third of the deaths caused by congenital defects in the first year of life. Because accurate diagnosis and surgical treatment are now

Text continues on page 967

Congenital Anomaly	Nursing Assessments	Nursing Goals and Interventions
Congenital hydrocephalus	Enlarged head Enlarged or full fontanelles Split or widened sutures "Setting sun" eyes Head circumference > 90% on growth chart	Assess presence of hydrocephalus: Measure and plot occipital-frontal baseline measurements; then measure head circumference once a day. Check fontanelle for bulging and sutures for widening. Assist with head ultrasound and transillumination. Maintain skin integrity: Change position frequently. Clean skin creases after feeding or vomiting. Use sheepskin pillow under head. Postoperatively, position head off operative site. Watch for signs of infection.
Choanal atresia	Occlusion of posterior nares Cyanosis and retractions at rest Snorting respirations Difficulty breathing during feeding Obstruction by thick mucus	Assess patency of nares: Listen for breath sounds while holding baby's mouth closed and alternately compressing each nostril. Assist with passing feeding tube to confirm diagnosis. Maintain respiratory function: Assist with taping airway in mouth to prevent respiratory distress. Position with head elevated to improve air exchange.
Cleft lip	Unilateral or bilateral visible defect May involve external nares, nasal cartilage, nasal septum, and alveolar process Flattening or depression of midfacial contour	Provide nutrition: Feed with special nipple. Burp frequently (increased tendency to swallow air and reflex vomiting). Clean cleft with sterile water (to prevent crusting on cleft prior to repair). Support parental coping: Assist parents with grief over loss of idealized baby. Encourage verbalization of their feelings about visible defect. Provide role model in interacting with infant. (Parents internalize others' responses to their newborn.)

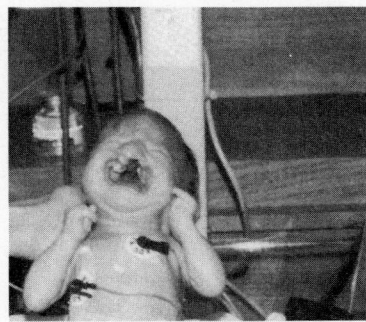

(At left) Unilateral cleft lip with cleft abnormality involving both hard and soft palates.

Cleft palate	Fissure connecting oral and nasal cavity May involve uvula and soft palate May extend forward to nostril involving hard palate and maxillary alveolar ridge Difficulty in sucking Expulsion of formula through nose	Prevent aspiration/infection: Place prone or in side-lying position to facilitate drainage. Suction nasopharyngeal cavity (to prevent aspiration or airway obstruction) During newborn period feed in upright position with head and chest tilted slightly backward (to aid swallowing and discourage aspiration). Provide nutrition: Feed with special nipple that fills cleft and allows sucking. Also decreases change of aspiration through nasal cavity. Clean mouth with water after feedings. Burp after each ounce (tend to swallow large amounts of air). Thicken formula to provide extra calories. Plot weight gain patterns to assess adequacy of diet. Provide parental support: Refer parents to community agencies and support groups. Encourage verbalization of frustrations because feeding process is long and frustrating. Praise all parental efforts. Encourage parents to seek prompt treatment for upper respiratory infection (URI) and teach them ways to decrease URI.
Tracheoesophageal fistula (type 3)	History of maternal hydramnios Excessive mucous secretions Constant drooling Abdominal distention beginning soon after birth Periodic choking and cyanotic episodes Immediate regurgitation of feeding Clinical symptoms of aspiration pneumonia (tachypnea, retractions, rhonchi, decreased breath sounds, cyanotic spells) Failure to pass nasogastric tube	Maintain respiratory status and prevent aspiration: Withhold feeding until esophageal patency is determined. Quickly assess patency before putting to breast in birth area. Place on low intermittent suction to control saliva and mucus (to prevent aspiration pneumonia). Place in warmed, humidified incubator (liquefies secretions, facilitating removal). Elevate head of bed 20–40 degrees (to prevent reflux of gastric juices). Keep quiet (crying causes air to pass through fistula and to distend intestines, causing respiratory embarrassment). Maintain fluid and electrolyte balance: Give fluids to replace esophageal drainage and maintain hydration. Provide parent education: Explain staged repair—provision of gastrostomy and ligation of fistula, then repair of atresia. Keep parents informed; clarify and reinforce physician's explanations regarding malformation, surgical repair, pre- and postoperative care, and prognosis (knowledge is ego strengthening).

Congenital Anomaly	Nursing Assessments	Nursing Goals and Interventions
Tracheoesophageal fistula (type 3) *continued*		Involve parents in care of infant and in planning for future; facilitate touch and eye contact (to dispel feelings of inadequacy, increase self-esteem and self-worth, and promote incorporation of infant into family).

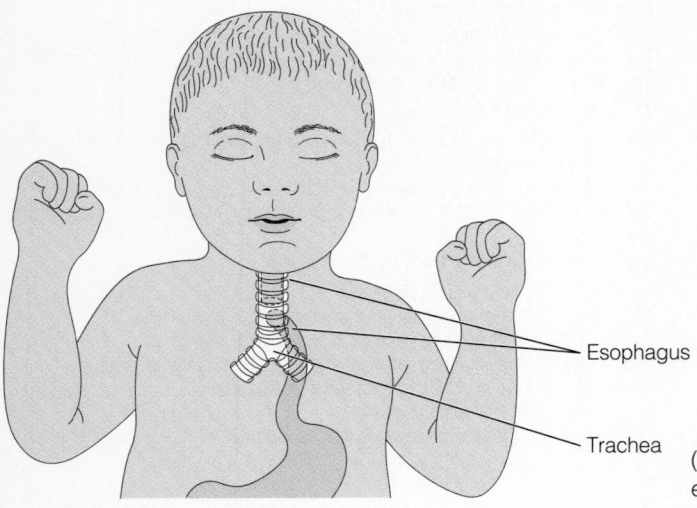

Esophagus

Trachea

(At left) The most frequently seen type of congenital tracheo-esophageal fistula and esophageal atresia.

| Diaphragmatic hernia | Difficulty initiating respirations
Gasping respirations with nasal flaring and chest retraction
Barrel chest and scaphoid abdomen
Asymmetric chest expansion
Breath sounds may be absent
Usually on left side
Heart sounds displaced to right
Spasmodic attacks of cyanosis and difficulty in feeding
Bowel sounds may be heard in thoracic cavity | Nurse should never ventilate with bag and mask O_2 because the stomach will inflate, further compressing the lungs.
Maintain respiratory status: Immediately administer oxygen.
Initiate gastric decompression.
Place in high semi-Fowler's position (to use gravity to keep abdominal organs' pressure off diaphragm).
Turn to affected side to allow unaffected lung expansion.
Carry out interventions to alleviate respiratory and metabolic acidosis.
Assess for increased secretions around suction tube (denotes possible obstruction).
Aspirate and irrigate tube with air or sterile water. |

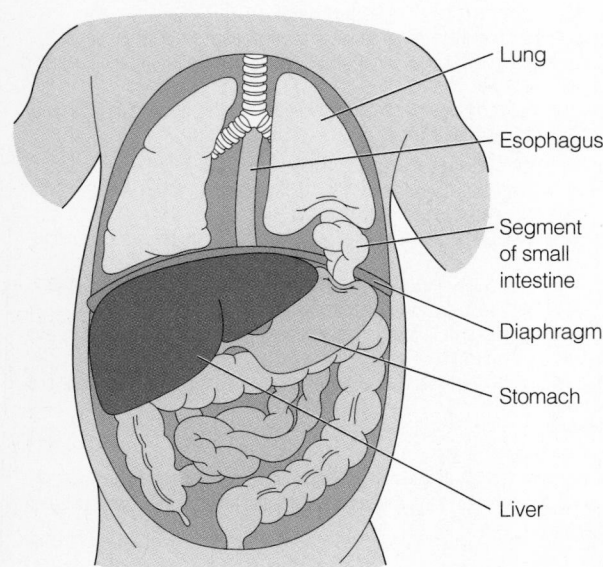

Lung

Esophagus

Segment of small intestine

Diaphragm

Stomach

Liver

(At left) Diaphragmatic hernia. Note compression of the lung by the intestine on the affected side.

| TABLE 31-4 | *continued* |

Congenital Anomaly	Nursing Assessments	Nursing Goals and Interventions
Myelomeningocele	Saclike cyst containing meninges, spinal cord, and nerve roots in thoracic and/or lumbar area	Prevent trauma and infection.
	Myelomeningocele directly connects to subarachnoid space so hydrocephalus often associated	Position on abdomen or on side and restrain (to prevent pressure and trauma to sac).
	No response or varying response to sensation below level of sac	Meticulously clean buttocks and genitals after each voiding and defecation (to prevent contamination of sac and decrease possibility of infection).
	May have constant dribbling of urine	May put protective covering over sac (to prevent rupture and drying).
	Incontinence or retention of stool	Observe sac for oozing of fluid or pus.
	Anal opening may be flaccid	Credé bladder (apply downward pressure on bladder with thumbs, moving urine toward the urethra) as ordered to prevent urinary stasis.
		Assess amount of sensation and movement below defect.
		Observe for complications:
		Obtain occipital-frontal circumference baseline measurements; then measure head circumference once a day (to detect hydrocephalus).
		Check fontanelle for bulging.

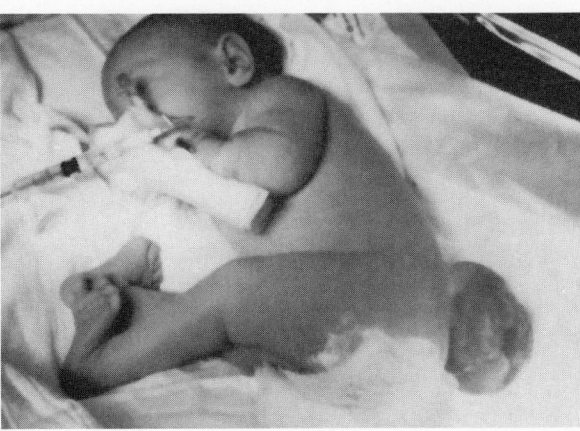

(At left) Newborn with lumbar myelomeningocele.
SOURCE: Courtesy Dr Paul Winchester.

Omphalocele	Herniation of abdominal contents into base of umbilical cord	Maintain hydration and temperature:
	May have an enclosed transparent sac covering	Provide D₅LR and albumin for hypovolemia.
		Place infant in sterile bag up to and covering defect.
		Cover sac with moistened sterile gauze, and place plastic wrap over dressing (to prevent rupture of sac and infection).
		Initiate gastric decompression by insertion of nasogastric tube attached to low suction (to prevent distention of lower bowel and impairment of blood flow).
		Prevent infection and trauma to defect.
		Position to prevent trauma to defect.
		Administer broad-spectrum antibiotics.
Imperforate anus, congenital dislocated hip, and clubfoot	See discussion in Chapter 28, Anus and Extremities	Identify defect and initiate appropriate referral early.

available, many such deaths can be prevented. It is now possible to do corrective surgery at an earlier age; for example, more than one-half of the children undergoing surgery are less than 1 year of age, and one-fourth are less than 1 month old (Benson 1989). It is crucial for the nurse to have comprehensive knowledge of congenital heart disease to detect deviations from normal and to initiate interventions. Table 31–5 presents the clinical manifestations and medical/surgical management of these cardiac defects.

Overview of Congenital Heart Defects

Factors that might influence development of congenital heart malformations can be classified as environmental or genetic. Infections of the pregnant woman, such as rubella, coxsackie B, and influenza, have been implicated. Thalidomide, steroids, alcohol, lithium, and some anticonvulsants have been shown to cause malformations of the heart. Seasonal spraying of pesticides has also been linked to an increase in congenital heart defects. Clinicians are also beginning to see cardiac defects in infants of mothers with phenylketonuria (PKU) who do not follow their diets.

Twelve percent of all infants with congenital heart disease were found to have chromosomal abnormalities (Lin & Garver 1988). Infants with Down syndrome and trisomy 13/15 and 16/18 frequently have heart lesions. Increased incidence and risk of recurrence of specific defects occur in families.

It is customary to describe congenital malformations of the heart as either *acyanotic*—those that do not present

Text continues on page 970

TABLE 31-5 Cardiac Defects of the Early Newborn Period

Congenital Heart Defect	Clinical Findings	Medical/Surgical Management
Acyanotic		
Patent ductus arteriosus (PDA) ↑ in females, maternal rubella, RDS, <1500 g preterm newborns, high-altitude births	Harsh grade 2–3 machinery murmur upper left sternal border (LSB) just beneath clavicle ↑ difference between systolic and diastolic pulse pressure Can lead to right heart failure and pulmonary congestion ↑ left atrial (LA) and left ventricular (LV) enlargement, dilated ascending aorta ↑ pulmonary vascularity	Indomethacin—0.2 mg/kg orally (prostaglandin inhibitor) Surgical ligation Use of O₂ therapy and blood transfusion to improve tissue oxygenation and perfusion Fluid restriction and diuretics

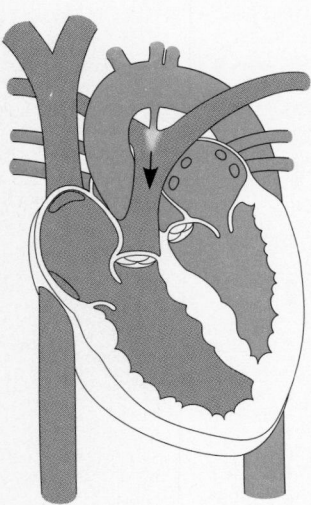

The patent ductus arteriosus is a vascular connection that, during fetal life, short-circuits the pulmonary vascular bed and directs blood from the pulmonary artery to the aorta. Post-natally, blood shunts through the ductus from the aorta to the pulmonary artery.

Congenital Heart Defect	Clinical Findings	Medical/Surgical Management
Atrial septal defect (ASD) ↑ in females and Down syndrome	Initially frequently asymptomatic Systolic murmur second left intercostal space (LICS) With large ASD, diastolic rumbling murmur lower left sternal (LLS) border Failure to thrive, upper respiratory infection (URI), poor exercise tolerance	Surgical closure with patch or suture
Ventricular septal defect (VSD) ↑ in males	Initially asymptomatic until end of first month or large enough to cause pulmonary edema Loud, blowing systolic murmur third–fourth intercostal space (ICS) pulmonary blood flow Right ventricular hypertrophy Rapid respirations, growth failure, feeding difficulties Congestive right heart failure at 6 weeks–2 months of age	Follow medically—some spontaneously close Use of lanoxin and diuretics in congestive heart failure (CHF) Surgical closure with Dacron patch
Coarctation of aorta Can be preductal or postductal	Absent or diminished femoral pulses Increased brachial pulses Late systolic murmur left intrascapular area Systolic BP in lower extremities Enlarged left ventricle Can present in CHF at 7–21 days of life	Surgical resection of narrowed portion of aorta

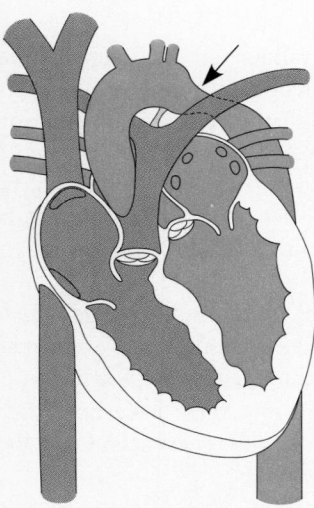

Coarctation of the aorta is characterized by a narrowed aortic lumen. The lesion produces an obstruction to the flow of blood through the aorta, causing an increased left ventricular pressure and work load.

TABLE 31-5   Cardiac Defects of the Early Newborn Period

Congenital Heart Defect	Clinical Findings	Medical/Surgical Management
Hypoplastic left heart syndrome	Normal at birth—cyanosis and shocklike congestive heart failure develop within a few hours to days Soft systolic murmur just left of the sternum Diminished pulses Aortic and/or mitral atresia Tiny, thick-walled left ventricle Large, dilated, hypertrophied right ventricle X-ray: cardiac enlargement and pulmonary venous congestion	Currently no effective corrective treatment

Cyanotic

Tetralogy of Fallot
   (Most common cyanotic heart defect)
   Pulmonary stenosis
   Ventricular septal defect (VSD)
   Overriding aorta
   Right ventricular hypertrophy
	May be cyanotic at birth or within first few months of life
	Harsh systolic murmur LSB
	Crying or feeding increases cyanosis and respiratory distress
	X-ray: boot-shaped appearance secondary to small pulmonary artery
	Right ventricular enlargement
		Prevention of dehydration, intercurrent infections
		Alleviation of paroxysmal dyspneic attacks
		Palliative surgery to increase blood flow to the lungs
		Corrective surgery—resection of pulmonic stenosis, closure of VSD with Dacron patch

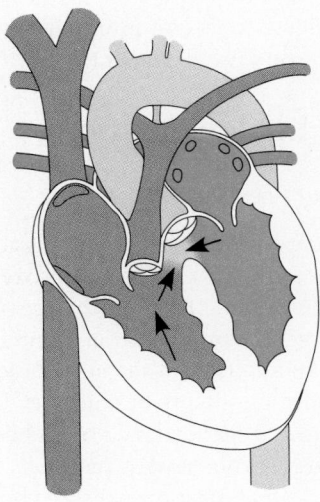

In tetralogy of Fallot, the severity of symptoms depends on the degree of pulmonary stenosis, the size of the ventricular septal defect, and the degree to which the aorta overrides the septal defect.

Transposition of great vessels (TGA) (↑ females, IDMs, LGAs)	Cyanosis at birth or within 3 days Possible pulmonic stenosis murmur Right ventricular hypertrophy Polycythemia "Egg on its side" x-ray	Prostaglandin E to vasodilate ductus to keep it open Initial surgery to create opening between right and left side of heart if none exists Total surgical repair—usually the arterial switch procedure

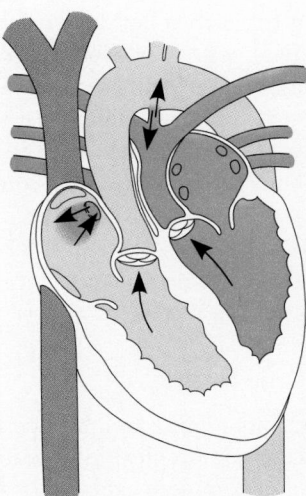

Complete transposition of great vessels is an embryologic defect caused by a straight division of the bulbar trunk without normal spiraling. As a result, the aorta originates from the right ventricle, and the pulmonary artery from the left ventricle. An abnormal communication between the two circulations must be present to sustain life.

SOURCE: All illustrations from *Congenital Heart Abnormalities.* Clinical Education Aid no 7, Ross Laboratories, Columbus, OH.

with cyanosis—or *cyanotic*—those that do present with cyanosis. If an opening exists between the right and left sides of the heart, blood will normally flow from the area of greater pressure (left side) to the area of lesser pressure (right side). This process is referred to as *left-to-right shunt*, and does not produce cyanosis because oxygenated blood is being pumped out to the systemic circulation. If pressure in the right side of the heart, due to obstruction of normal flow, exceeds that in the left side, unoxygenated blood will flow from the right side to the left side of the heart and out into the system. This *right-to-left shunt* causes cyanosis. If the opening is large, there may be a bidirectional shunt with mixing of blood in both sides of the heart, which also produces cyanosis.

The common cardiac defects seen in the first 6 days of life are left ventricular outflow obstructions (mitral stenosis, aortic stenosis, or atresia), hypoplastic left heart, coarctation of the aorta, patent ductus arteriosus (PDA, the most common defect), transposition of the great vessels, tetralogy of Fallot, and large ventricular septal defect or atrial septal defects. See also Table 31–5.

APPLYING THE NURSING PROCESS

Nursing Assessment

The primary goal of the neonatal nurse is early identification of cardiac defects and initiation of referral to the physician. The three most common manifestations of cardiac defect are cyanosis, detectable heart murmur, and congestive heart failure signs (tachycardia, tachypnea, diaphoresis, hepatomegaly, and cardiomegaly).

Nursing assessment of the following signs and symptoms assists in identifying the newborn with a cardiac problem:

1. *Tachypnea.* Reflects increased pulmonary blood flow
2. *Dyspnea.* Caused by increased pulmonary venous pressure and blood flow; can also cause chest retractions, wheezing
3. *Color.* Ashen, gray, or cyanotic because of decreased peripheral circulation or low oxygen saturation of the blood
4. *Difficulty in feeding.* Requires many rest periods before finishing even 1 or 2 oz
5. *Diaphoresis.* Beads of perspiration over the upper lip and forehead; may accompany feeding fatigue
6. *Stridor or choking spells*
7. *Failure to gain weight*
8. *Heart murmur.* May not be heard in left-to-right shunting defects because the pulmonary pressure in the newborn is greater than pressure in the left side of the heart in the early newborn period
9. *Hepatomegaly.* In right-sided heart failure caused by venous congestion in the liver
10. *Tachycardia.* Pulse over 160, may be as high as 200
11. *Cardiac enlargement*

Nursing Diagnosis

Nursing diagnoses that may apply to the newborn with cardiac defect and family include the following:

- Altered tissue perfusion related to decrease in circulating oxygen
- Ineffective breathing pattern related to fatigue
- Altered nutrition: Less than body requirements related to increased energy expenditure and fatigue
- Knowledge deficit related to lack of information about cardiac anomaly and implications for care

Nursing Plan and Implementation

Maintenance of Cardiopulmonary Status

When the baby has dyspnea or cyanosis, oxygen is to be given by an oxygen hood, tent, mask, cannula, or oxygen prongs. Mist is often ordered, and it requires the use of an oxygen hood or tent. Oxygen administration should always be accompanied by humidity, and the air should be warmed to decrease the drying effects of cold, dry oxygen. Vital signs are monitored for evidence of tachycardia, tachypnea, expiratory grunting, and retractions.

Although pain relief is an institution-specific choice, morphine sulfate, in a dose of 0.05 mg/kg of body weight, can be used if the infant is markedly irritable. Morphine is thought to decrease peripheral and pulmonary vascular resistance, which results in decreased tachypnea. However, fentanyl is becoming the pain relief drug of choice because it provides good pain control without the respiratory depression that may be seen with morphine sulfate. Also, infants in congestive heart failure are more comfortable in a semi-Fowler's position because the liver and spleen are frequently enlarged in babies with congenital heart disease.

The nurse administers a sedative as required for rest. Organizing nursing care is a key to decreasing energy requirements and providing periods of rest.

Family Education

After the baby is stabilized and gaining weight, decisions are made about ongoing care and surgical interventions. The parents need careful and complete explanations and the opportunity to take part in decision making. They also require ongoing emotional support. Families need genetic counseling regarding future conception with *any* baby born with a congenital abnormality.

Evaluation

Anticipated outcomes of nursing care include:

- The newborn's oxygen consumption and energy expenditure are minimal while at rest and during feedings.

- The newborn is protected from additional stresses such as infection, cold stress, and dehydration.

- The parents verbalize their concerns surrounding their baby's health maintenance and surgical intervention, and they understand the rationale for follow-up care.

CARE OF THE NEWBORN WITH INBORN ERRORS OF METABOLISM

Inborn errors of metabolism are a group of hereditary disorders that are transmitted by mutant genes. The mutant gene causes an enzyme defect that blocks a metabolic pathway and leads to an accumulation of metabolites that are toxic to the infant. Most of the disorders are transmitted by an autosomal recessive gene, requiring two heterozygous parents to produce a homozygous infant with the disorder. Heterozygous parents carrying some inborn errors of metabolism disorders can be identified by special tests, and some inborn errors of metabolism can be detected in utero.

Many inborn errors of metabolism are now detected neonatally through newborn screening programs. These programs test principally for disorders associated with mental retardation.

Phenylketonuria (PKU) is the most common of the group of metabolic errors known as amino acid disorders. Newborn screenings have set its incidence at about 1 in 12,000 live births worldwide and 1 in 15,000 live births in the United States (Seashore & Rinaldo 1993). The highest incidence is noted in White populations from northern Europe and the United States. It is rarely observed in people of African, Jewish, or Japanese descent.

Phenylalanine is an essential amino acid used by the body for growth, and in the normal individual any excess is converted to tyrosine. The newborn with PKU lacks this converting ability, which results in an accumulation of phenylalanine in the blood. Phenylalanine produces two abnormal metabolites, phenylpyruvic acid and phenylacetic acid, which are eliminated in the urine, producing a musty odor. Excessive accumulation of phenylalanine and its abnormal metabolites in the brain tissue leads to progressive mental retardation.

Maple syrup urine disease (MSUD) is an inborn error of metabolism and, when untreated, is a rapidly progressing and often fatal disease caused by an enzymatic defect in the metabolism of the branched chain amino acids leucine, isoleucine, and valine.

Homocystinuria is a disorder caused by a deficiency of the enzyme cystathionine B synthase, which blocks the normal conversion of methionine to cystine. High levels of serum methionine cause mental retardation, seizures, behavioral disorders, and early onset thrombosis (Wright et al 1992).

Galactosemia is an inborn error of carbohydrate metabolism in which the body is unable to use the sugars galactose and lactose. Enzyme pathways in liver cells normally convert galactose and lactose to glucose. In galactosemia, one step in that conversion pathway is absent, either because of the lack of the enzyme galactose 1-phosphate uridyl transferase or because of the lack of the enzyme galactokinase. High levels of unusable galactose circulate in the blood, causing cataracts, brain damage, and liver damage (Seashore & Rinaldo 1993).

Another disorder frequently included in mandatory newborn blood screening tests is *congenital hypothyroidism.* An inborn enzymatic defect, lack of maternal dietary iodine, or maternal ingestion of drugs that depress or destroy thyroid tissue can cause congenital hypothyroidism.

The incidence of metabolic errors is relatively low, but for affected infants and their families these disorders pose a threat to survival and frequently require lifelong treatment.

Medical Therapy

Identification via newborn screening and early medical intervention for inborn errors of metabolism has become more difficult with the advent of early discharge of newborns. In most states the Guthrie blood test for PKU is required for all newborns. The test, done before discharge, is a simple screening tool that uses a drop of blood collected from a heel stick and placed on filter paper. The Guthrie test should be done at least 24 hours, but preferably 72 hours, after the initiation of feedings containing the usual amounts of breast milk or formula. Phenylalanine is found in milk, so its metabolites begin to build up in the baby with PKU once milk feedings are initiated.

High-risk newborns should be receiving a 60% milk intake with no more than 40% of their total intake coming from nonprotein intravenous fluids. The PKU testing of high-risk newborns should be deferred for at least 48 hours after hyperalimentation is initiated. Hospitals and birthing centers frequently discharge mother and infant 24 to 48 hours after birth. It is vital that the parents understand the need for the screening procedure, and a follow-up check is necessary to confirm that the test was done.

Because it is possible to do the testing on an infant with PKU before the phenylalanine concentration rises and thus miss the diagnosis, some states routinely request a repeat test at 10 to 14 days. When the Guthrie blood test is performed early, during the first 3 to 4 days of life, a phenylalanine blood level of about 4 to 6 mg/dL is considered a presumptive positive; but only 1 in 20 to 30 infants with this level is a true positive (Seashore & Rinaldo 1993). Treatment involves stringent restriction of phenylalanine intake.

Some states simultaneously test all hospitalized newborns for MSUD, homocystinuria, and PKU during the first 3 to 4 days of life. Diagnosis of MSUD is made by analyzing blood levels of leucine, isoleucine, and valine. Confirmation of the diagnosis depends on blood assay for the enzyme oxidative decarboxylase. Dietary treatment prior to 12 days of life has been reported to result in normal intelligence (Kaplan et al 1991).

In several states newborn screening includes an enzyme assay for galactose 1-phosphate uridyl transferase; this test, however, does not detect galactosemia if it is caused by a deficiency of the enzyme galactokinase. There appear to be ethnic differences in age of onset of symptoms and in severity of course. Caucasians have more severe symptoms and earlier onset (3 to 14 days) than people of African descent (14 to 28 days) (Wright et al 1992). Treatment involves a galactose-free diet. Even with early treatment children may have learning disabilities, speech problems, and ovarian failure (Seashore & Rinaldo 1993).

For hypothyroidism, immediate and appropriate thyroid replacement therapy is established based on newborn screening and laboratory data. Frequently, premature infants of less than 30 weeks' gestation have low T_4 or thyroid-stimulating hormone (TSH) values when compared with normal values of term infants. This may reflect the premature infant's inability to bind thyroid. Management includes frequent laboratory monitoring and adjustment of thyroid medication to accommodate growth and development of the infant. With adequate treatment children remain free of symptoms, but if the condition is untreated, stunted growth and mental retardation occur.

APPLYING THE NURSING PROCESS

Nursing Assessment

The clinical picture of a PKU baby involves a normal-appearing newborn, most often with blond hair, blue eyes, and fair complexion. Decreased pigmentation may be related to the competition between phenylalanine and tyrosine for the available enzyme, tyrosinase. Tyrosine is needed for the formation of melanin pigment and the hormones epinephrine and thyroxin. Without treatment the infant fails to thrive and develops vomiting and eczematous rashes. By about 6 months of age the infant exhibits behavior indicative of mental retardation and other CNS involvement, including seizures and abnormal electroencephalogram (EEG) patterns.

Newborns with MSUD have feeding problems and neurologic signs (seizures, spasticity, opisthotonus) during the first week of life. A maple syrup odor of the urine is noted, and when ferric chloride is added to the urine, its color changes to gray-green.

Homocystinuria varies in its presentation, but the more common characteristics are skeletal abnormalities, dislocation of ocular lenses, intravascular thromboses, and mental retardation. Abnormalities occur because of the toxic effects of the accumulation of methionine and the metabolite homocystine in the blood.

Clinical manifestations of galactosemia include vomiting, diarrhea, failure to thrive (Wright et al 1992), hepatosplenomegaly, jaundice, and mental retardation. The condition is frequently associated with anemia, sepsis, and cataracts in the newborn period. Except for cataracts and mental retardation, those findings are reversible when galactose is excluded from the diet. Mental retardation can be prevented by early diagnosis and careful dietary management.

A large tongue, umbilical hernia, cool and mottled skin, low hairline, hypotonia, and large fontanelles are frequently associated with congenital hypothyroidism. Early symptoms include prolonged newborn jaundice, poor feeding, constipation, low-pitched cry, poor weight gain, inactivity, and delayed motor development.

Nursing Diagnosis

Nursing diagnoses that may apply to the newborn with an inborn error of metabolism include the following:

- Knowledge deficit related to parental lack of information about special dietary management required for inborn errors of metabolism
- Ineffective family coping related to parental guilt secondary to hereditary nature of disease

Nursing Plan and Implementation

Newborn Screening

Newborn screening for several inborn errors of metabolism is mandatory in many states. It is the nurse's responsibility to obtain the heel stick blood on the filter paper prior to discharge of the baby. The first filter paper test screens for PKU and other selected tests that are included in each state's mandated testing program (eg, homocystinuria, MSUD, galactosemia, sickle cell anemia, and cystic fibrosis). A second blood specimen is usually required 7 to 14 days after birth, but the nurse needs to remember that this second blood specimen test is only for PKU.

Some clinicians have the parents perform a diaper test for PKU. At about 6 weeks of age, the parent should take a freshly wet diaper and press the prepared test stick against the wet area. They note the color of the test stick, record the color on the prepared sheet, and mail the form back to the physician. A green color reaction is positive and indicates probable PKU.

Family Education—Dietary Management

Nursing responsibilities include prompt and appropriate dietary management of the newborn with an inborn error of metabolism. Once identified, an afflicted PKU infant can be treated by a special diet that limits ingestion of phenylalanine. Special formulas low in phenylalanine, such as Lofenalac, are available. Special food lists are helpful for parents of a PKU child. If treatment is begun before 3 months of age, CNS damage can be minimized.

Controversy exists about when, if ever, the special diet should be terminated. Because of the rigidity and severe limitations of the low-phenylalanine diet, many clinicians terminate the special diet at 6 years of age. Brain size does not dramatically increase after age 6, but myelination continues actively through adolescence and to some extent possibly through 40 years of age. Studies have shown loss of intellectual function some years after relaxation of dietary restriction (Wright et al 1992). Most centers now recommend keeping blood phenylalanine levels below 15 mg/dL, or even 10mg/dL, for life.

Female children with PKU are now living longer and may bear children. There is a 95% risk of producing a child with mental retardation if the mother with PKU is not on a low-phenylalanine diet during pregnancy. It is recommended that the woman reinstate her low-phenylalanine diet a few months before becoming pregnant (Wright et al 1992).

Dietary management of MSUD must be initiated immediately with a formula that is low in the branched chain amino acids, leucine, isoleucine, and valine, which must be continued indefinitely (American Academy of Pediatrics Committee on Pediatrics and Committee on Genetics 1989).

Infants with homocystinuria are managed on a diet that is low in methionine but supplemented with cystine and pyridoxine (vitamin B_6). Early diagnosis and careful management may prevent mental retardation.

Galactosemia is treated by the use of a galactose-free formula, such as Nutramigen (a protein hydrolysate process formula), a meat-base formula, or a soybean formula. As the infant grows, parents must be educated not only to avoid giving their child milk and milk products, but also to read all labels carefully and avoid any foods containing dry milk products.

Parent of affected newborns should be referred to support groups. The nurse should also ensure that parents are informed about centers that can provide them with information about biochemical genetics and dietary management.

Evaluation

Anticipated outcomes of nursing care include:

- The risk of inborn errors of metabolism is promptly identified, and early intervention is initiated.

- The parents verbalize their concerns about their baby's health problems, long-term care needs, and potential outcomes.

- The parents are aware of available community health resources and use them as indicated.

CARE OF THE FAMILY OF THE AT-RISK NEWBORN

The birth of a preterm or ill infant or an infant with a congenital anomaly is a serious crisis situation for a family. Acute grief reactions follow the loss of the perfect baby they have fantasized. In the case of a preterm birth, the mother is denied the last few weeks of pregnancy that seem to prepare her psychologically for the stress of birth and the attachment process. Attachment at this time is fragile, and interruption of the process by separation can affect the future mother-child relationship.

Feelings of guilt and failure often plague mothers of preterm newborns. They may ask themselves "Why did labor start? What did I do (or not do)?" A woman may have guilt fantasies and wonder "Was it because I had sexual intercourse with my husband (a week, 3 days, a day) ago?" "Was it because I carried three loads of wash up from the basement?" "Am I being punished for something done in the past—even in childhood?"

The birth of the newborn with an illness or congenital abnormalities also engenders feelings of guilt and failure. As in the birth of a preterm infant the woman may entertain ideas of personal guilt: "What did I do (or not do) to cause this?" "Am I being punished for something?"

Parental reactions and steps of attachment are altered by the birth of a preterm infant or one with an illness or a congenital anomaly. A variety of new feelings, reactions, and stresses must be recognized and dealt with before the family can work toward the establishment of a healthy parent-infant relationship.

Although reactions and steps of attachment are altered by the birth of these infants, a healthy parent-child relationship can occur. Kaplan and Mason (1974) have identified four psychologic tasks as essential for coping with the stress of an at-risk newborn and for providing a basis for the maternal-infant relationship:

1. Anticipatory grief as a psychologic preparation for possible loss of the child while still hoping for his or her survival

2. Acknowledgement of maternal failure to produce a term or perfect newborn expressed as anticipatory grief and depression and lasting until the chances of survival seem secure

3. Resumption of the process of relating to the infant, which was interrupted by the threat of nonsurvival (This task may be impaired by a continuous threat of death or abnormality, and the mother may be slow in her response of hope for the infant's survival.)

4. Understanding of the special needs and growth patterns of the at-risk newborn, which are temporary and yield to normal patterns

Most authorities agree that the birth of a preterm infant or a less-than-perfect infant does require major adjustments as the parents are forced to surrender the image of their ideal child they had nurtured for so long.

Solnit and Stark (1961) postulate that grief and mourning of the loss of the loved object—the idealized child—mark parental reactions to an infant with abnormalities. The parents must grieve the loss of the valued object—their wished-for perfect child. Simultaneously, they must adopt the imperfect child as the new love object. Parental responses to an infant with health problems may also be viewed as a five-staged process (Klaus & Kennell 1982):

1. *Shock* is felt at the reality of the birth of this baby. This stage may be characterized by forgetfulness, amnesia of the situation, and a feeling of desperation.

2. There is disbelief *(denial)* of the reality that the child is defective. This stage is exemplified by assertions that "It didn't really happen!" "There has been a mistake; it's someone else's baby."

3. *Depression* over the reality of the situation and a corresponding grief reaction follows acceptance of the situation. This stage is characterized by much crying and sadness. Anger about the reality of the situation may also occur at this stage. A projection of blame on others or on self and feelings of "not me" are characteristic of this stage.

4. Equilibrium and *acceptance* are characteristic of a decrease in the emotional reactions of the parents. This stage is variable and may be prolonged because of continuing threat to the infant's survival. Some parents experience chronic sorrow in relation to their child.

5. *Reorganization* of the family is necessary to deal with the child's problems. Mutual support of the parents facilitates this process, but the crisis of the situation may precipitate alienation between the mother and father.

These stages of parental adjustment are similar to the stage of grieving associated with death. Indeed, reorganization is necessary to deal with a crisis concerning an infant at risk.

In the birth of an infant with an anomaly or illness or a preterm infant the mourning process is necessary for attachment to the less-than-perfect baby. **Grief work,** the emotional reaction to significant loss, must occur before adequate attachment to the actual baby is possible. Parental detachment precedes parental attachment.

APPLYING THE NURSING PROCESS

Nursing Assessment

Development of a nurse-family relationship facilitates information gathering in areas of concern. A concurrent illness of the mother or other family members or other concurrent stress (lack of hospitalization insurance, loss of job, age of parents) may alter the family response to the baby. Feelings of apprehension, guilt, failure, and grief that are verbally or nonverbally expressed are important aspects of the nursing history. These observations enable all professionals to be aware of the parental state, coping behaviors, and readiness for attachment, bonding, and caretaking. Appropriate nursing observations during interviewing and relating to the family include:

1. *Level of understanding.* Observations concerning the ability to assimilate information given and to ask appropriate questions; the need for constant repetition of "the same" information

2. *Behavioral responses.* Appropriateness of behavior in relation to information given; lack of response; "flat" affect

3. *Difficulties with communication.* Deafness (reads lips only); blindness; dysphasia; understanding only a foreign language

4. *Paternal and maternal education level.* Parents unable to read or write; only eighth grade completed; mother an MD, RN, or PhD; and so on

Documentation of such information, obtained by the nurse through continuing contact and development of a therapeutic family relationship, enables all professionals to understand and use the nursing history in providing continuous individual care.

Visiting and care-giving patterns indicate the level or lack of parental attachment. A record of visits, caretaking procedures, affect (in relating to the newborn), and telephone calls from parents is essential. Serial observations, rather than just isolated instances of concern, must be obtained. Grant (1978) has developed a conceptual framework depicting adaptive and maladaptive responses to parenting of a preterm or less-than-perfect infant (Figure 31–14).

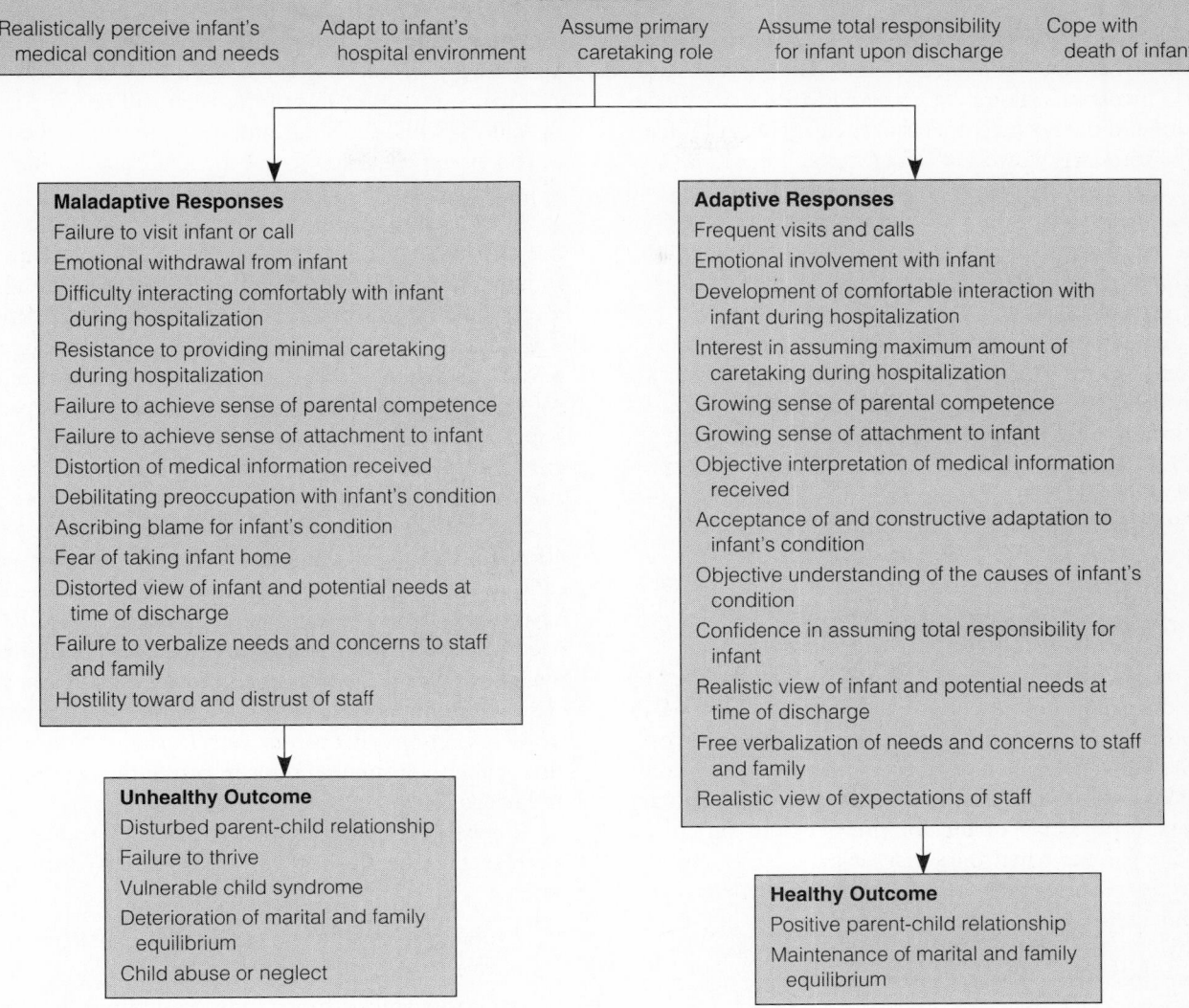

Parental Tasks				
Realistically perceive infant's medical condition and needs	Adapt to infant's hospital environment	Assume primary caretaking role	Assume total responsibility for infant upon discharge	Cope with death of infant

Maladaptive Responses

Failure to visit infant or call

Emotional withdrawal from infant

Difficulty interacting comfortably with infant during hospitalization

Resistance to providing minimal caretaking during hospitalization

Failure to achieve sense of parental competence

Failure to achieve sense of attachment to infant

Distortion of medical information received

Debilitating preoccupation with infant's condition

Ascribing blame for infant's condition

Fear of taking infant home

Distorted view of infant and potential needs at time of discharge

Failure to verbalize needs and concerns to staff and family

Hostility toward and distrust of staff

Adaptive Responses

Frequent visits and calls

Emotional involvement with infant

Development of comfortable interaction with infant during hospitalization

Interest in assuming maximum amount of caretaking during hospitalization

Growing sense of parental competence

Growing sense of attachment to infant

Objective interpretation of medical information received

Acceptance of and constructive adaptation to infant's condition

Objective understanding of the causes of infant's condition

Confidence in assuming total responsibility for infant

Realistic view of infant and potential needs at time of discharge

Free verbalization of needs and concerns to staff and family

Realistic view of expectations of staff

Unhealthy Outcome

Disturbed parent-child relationship

Failure to thrive

Vulnerable child syndrome

Deterioration of marital and family equilibrium

Child abuse or neglect

Healthy Outcome

Positive parent-child relationship

Maintenance of marital and family equilibrium

FIGURE 31-14   Maladaptive and adaptive parental responses during crisis period, showing unhealthy and healthy outcomes. SOURCE: Grant P: Psychological needs of families of high-risk infants. *Fam Commun Health* 1978; 11:93. By permission of Aspen Systems Corporation.

If a pattern of distancing behaviors evolves, appropriate intervention should be instituted. Follow-up studies have found that a statistically significant number of preterm, sick, and congenitally defective infants suffers from failure to thrive, battering, or other disorders of parenting. Early detection and intervention will prevent these aberrations in parenting behaviors from leading to irreparable damage or death.

Nursing Diagnosis

Nursing diagnoses that may apply to the family of a newborn at risk include the following:

- Grief related to loss of idealized newborn

- Fear related to emotional involvement with an at-risk newborn

- Altered parenting related to impaired bonding secondary to feelings of inadequacy about caretaking activities

Nursing Plan and Implementation

Preparation of Parents for Initial Visit with Newborn

Before parents see their child, the nurse must prepare them for the visit. It is important that a positive, realistic attitude regarding the infant, rather than a pessimistic one, be presented to the parents. An overly negative, fatalistic attitude further alienates the parents from their infant and retards attachment behaviors. In this case, instead of allowing attachment and bonding to develop, the mother will begin the process of grieving for the loss of her infant. Once started, this process is very difficult to reverse.

In preparing parents for the first view of their infant, it is important for the professional to have looked at the baby. The parents should be prepared to see both the deviations and the normal aspects of their infant. All infants exhibit strengths as well as deficiencies. The nurse may say, "Your baby is small, about the length of my two hands. She weighs 2 lb 3 oz but is very active and cries when we disturb her. She is having some difficulty breathing but is breathing without assistance and in only 35% oxygen."

The equipment being used for the at-risk newborn and its purpose should be described before the parents enter the intensive care unit. Many NICUs have booklets for parents to read before entering the unit. Through explanations and pictures the parents can be better prepared to deal with the feelings they may experience when they see their infant for the first time.

Support of Parents During Their Initial Visit with the Newborn

Upon entering the unit, parents may be overwhelmed by the sounds of monitors, alarms, and respirators, as well as by the unfamiliar language and "foreign" atmosphere. It is more reassuring when parents are prepared and accompanied to the unit by the same person(s). The primary nurse and physician caring for the newborn should be with the parents when they first visit the baby. Parental reactions are varied, but there is usually an element of initial shock. Provision of chairs and time to regain composure will assist the parents. Slow, complete, and simple explanations—first about the infant and then about the equipment—allay fear and anxiety.

As parents attempt to deal with the initial stages of shock and grief, they may fail to grasp new information. The parents may need repeated explanations in order to accept the reality of the situation, procedures, equipment, and the infant's condition on subsequent visits.

Misconceptions about equipment and its placement on the infant and about its potential harm are common. Such statements as "Does the fluid go into the brain?" "Does the white wire on the abdomen go into the stomach?" and "Does the monitor make the baby's heart beat?" imply much fear for the infant's safety and misconception about the machines. These worries are easily overcome by simple explanations of all equipment being used.

Concern about the infant's physical appearance is common, yet may remain unvoiced. Parents may express such concerns as "He looks so small and red—like a drowned rat." "Why do her genitals look so abnormal?" "Will that awful looking mouth [cleft lip and palate] ever be normal?" Such questions need to be anticipated by the nurse and addressed. Use of pictures, such as of an infant after cleft lip repair, may be reassuring to doubting parents. Knowledge of the development of a "normal" preterm infant will allow the nurse to make reassuring statements such as "The baby's labia may look very abnormal to you, but they are normal for her maturity. As she grows, the outer lips of the labia will become larger, the clitoris will be covered, and the genitals will then look as you expect them to. Your baby is normal for her level of maturity."

The tone of the neonatal intensive care unit is set by the nursing staff. Development of a safe, trusting environment depends on viewing the parents as essential care givers, not as visitors or nuisances in the unit. Privacy when needed and easy access to staff and facilities are important in developing an open, comfortable environment. An uncrowded and welcoming atmosphere lets parents know "You are welcome here." However, even in crowded physical surroundings an attitude of openness and trust can be conveyed by the nursing staff.

A trusting relationship is essential for collaborative efforts in caring for the infant. Nurses must therapeutically use their own responses to relate on a one-to-one basis with the parents. Each individual has different needs, different ways of adapting to crisis, and different means of support. Professionals must use techniques that are real and spontaneous to them and avoid adopting words or actions that are foreign to them. Nurses must also gauge their interventions to match the parents' pace and needs.

Powell (1981) suggests several positive strategies that increase the effectiveness of nursing interventions with parents:

- Problem solve with the family rather than giving advice.
- View the baby as a total individual rather than emphasizing the problem.
- Observe the uniqueness of the newborn rather than stereotyping or labeling the newborn as slow, unmanageable, and so forth.
- Avoid labeling parents as inadequate, rejecting, or angry.
- Stress the baby's similarities to other babies.
- Stress the strengths and competence of the parents.
- Help parents realize that they are in charge of their children and themselves.
- Be aware of the needs of all members of the family, including siblings.

Maternal Support   It is essential that the mother be reunited with her infant as soon as possible after birth so that the following can occur:

1. She knows her infant is alive.
2. She knows what the infant's real problems are. Early acquaintance between mother and infant allows a realistic perspective of the baby's condition.

3. She can begin the grief work over the loss of the idealized child and begin the process of attachment to the actual child.

4. She can share the experience of the infant's problems with the father, who may have already seen and touched the infant.

Facilitation of Attachment If Neonatal Transport Occurs

Small hospitals may be unable to care for sick infants. Transport to a regional referral center may be necessary. These centers may be as far as 500 miles from the parents' community; it is therefore essential that the mother see and touch her infant before the infant is transported. Facilitation of this important contact may be the responsibility of the referring hospital staff as well as the transport team.

Bringing the mother to the nursery or taking the infant in a warmed transport incubator to the mother's bedside will allow her to see the infant before transportation to the center. When the infant reaches the referral center, a staff member should call the parents with information about the infant's condition during transport, safe arrival at the center, and present condition.

Support of parents, with explanations from the professional staff, is crucial. Occasionally, the mother may be unable to see the infant before transport, for example, if she is still under general anesthesia or experiencing complications such as shock, hemorrhage, or seizures. In these cases the infant should be photographed before transport. The picture should be given to the mother, along with an explanation of the infant's condition, problems, and a detailed description of the infant's characteristics, to facilitate the attachment process until the mother can visit. An additional photograph is also helpful for the father to share with siblings and/or the extended family. With the increased attention to improved fetal outcome, prenatal maternal transports, rather than neonatal transports, are occurring more frequently. This practice gives the mother of an at-risk infant the opportunity to visit and care for her infant during the early postpartal period.

Promotion of Touching

Parents visiting a small or sick infant may need several visits to become comfortable and confident in their abilities to touch the infant without injuring her or him. Barriers such as incubators, incisions, monitor electrodes, and tubes may delay the mother's confidence. Knowledge of this "normal" delay in touching behavior will enable the nurse to understand parental behavior.

Klaus and Kennell (1982) observed a significant difference in the amount of eye contact and touching behaviors of mothers of normal newborns and mothers of preterm infants. Whereas mothers of normal newborns

progress within minutes to palm contact of the infant's trunk, the mother of a preterm infant is slower to progress from fingertip to palm contact and from the extremities to the trunk. The progression to palm contact with the infant's trunk may take several visits to the nursery.

Through support, reassurance, and encouragement the nurse can facilitate the mother's positive feelings about her ability and her importance to her infant. Touching facilitates "getting to know" the infant and thus establishes a bond with the infant. Touching as well as seeing the infant helps the mother to realize the "normals" and potentials of her baby (Figure 31–15).

The nurse can also encourage parents to meet their newborn's need for stimulation. Stroking, rocking, cuddling, singing, and talking should be an integral part of the parents' caretaking responsibilities.

Facilitation of Parental Caretaking

Bonding can be facilitated by encouraging parents to visit and become involved in their baby's care (Figure 31–16). When visiting is impossible, the parents should feel free to phone whenever they wish to receive information about their baby. A warm receptive attitude on the part of the nurse is very supportive. Nurses can also facilitate parenting by personalizing a baby to the parents, by referring to the infant by name, or by relating personal behavioral characteristics to the parents. Remarks such as "Jenny loves her pacifier" help make the infant more individual and unique.

Caretaking may be delayed for the mother of a preterm, defective, or sick infant. The variety of equipment needed for life support is hardly conducive to anxiety-free caretaking by the parents. However, even the sickest infant may be cared for, if only in a small way, by the parents. As a facilitator of parental caretaking, the nurse should promote the parents' success. Demonstration and explanation, followed by support of the parents in initial caretaking behaviors, positively reinforce this behavior. Changing the infant's diaper, giving their infant skin care or oral care, or helping the nurse turn the infant may at first be anxiety provoking for the parents, but they will become more comfortable and confident in caretaking and receive satisfaction from the baby's reactions and their ability "to do something." Complimenting the parent's competence in caretaking also increases their self-esteem, which has received recent "blows" of guilt and failure. It is vitally important that the parents never be given a task if there is any possibility they will not be able to accomplish it.

Often mothers of high-risk infants have ambivalent feelings toward the nurse. As the mother watches the nurse competently perform the caretaking tasks, she feels both grateful for the nurse's abilities and expertise and jealous of the nurse's ability to care for her infant. These feelings may be acted out in criticism of the care being received by the infant, manipulation of staff, or personal

STAGE I: Touching
Uses fingertips
Uses whole hand
Strokes child
Holds and studies child "en face"
Spontaneously lowers crib rails to fondle, hold, or talk to child

↓

STAGE II: Caretaking
Provides clean clothing, toys, grooming aids
Performs activities of daily living (bathing, diapering, feeding, dressing)
Performs caretaking tasks with proficiency and expresses pleasure in meeting infant's needs
Able to comfort child when distressed or crying
Able to meet child's special health needs (suctioning, cleaning stoma sites, treatments)

↓

STAGE III: Identity
Brings linens from home
Takes photographs
Brings individualized toys
Can make personalized observations about child
Offers suggestions and makes demands for personalized care
Demonstrates "advocacy" behavior
Feels he or she can care for child better than anyone else
Demonstrates consistent visiting and/or calling pattern
Questions focus on total child, not only physiologic parameters

FIGURE 31-15   Stages of parenting behavior toward an infant in intensive care. SOURCE: Schraeder BD: Attachment and parenting despite lengthy intensive care. *MCN* January/February 1980; 5:38. Reprinted with permission of the American Journal of Nursing Company.

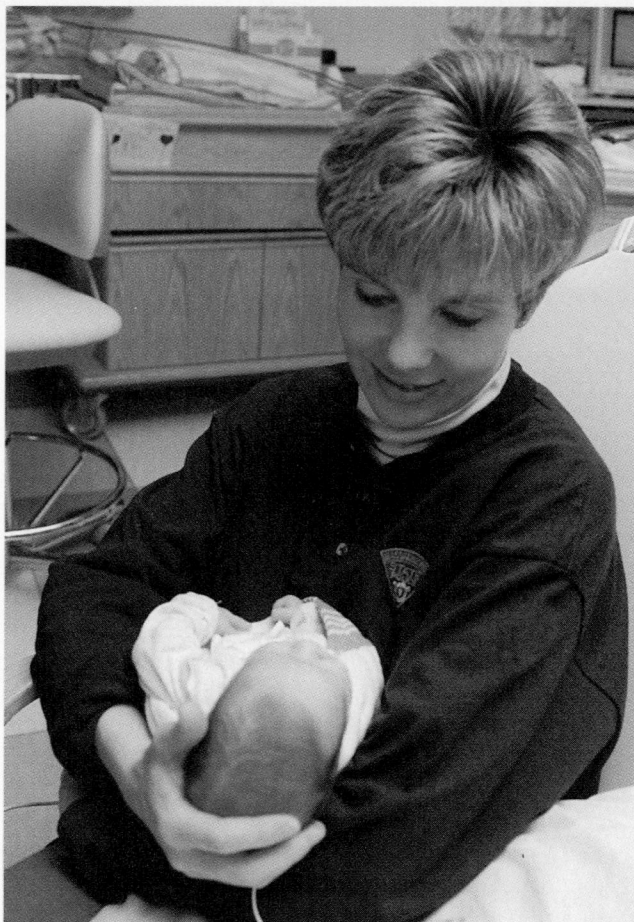

FIGURE 31-16   It is important that the parent of a high-risk infant be given the opportunity to get acquainted with her child. Physical contact is vital to the bonding process and should be encouraged whenever possible.

guilt. Instead of fostering (by silence) these inferiority feelings within mothers, nurses should recognize such feelings and intervene appropriately to enhance mother-infant attachment. The nurse needs to deal with ambivalent feelings that contribute to a competitive atmosphere. For example, the nurse should avoid making unfavorable comparisons between the baby's response to parental caretaking and the child's responses to the nurses. During a quiet time it may help for the nurse to encourage the parents to talk about their hopes and fears and to facilitate their involvement in parent groups (Mercer 1990).

Nurses who are understanding and secure will be able to support the parents' egos instead of collecting rewards for themselves. To reinforce positive parenting behaviors, professionals must first believe in the importance of the parents. The nurse can hardly convince doubting parents of their importance to the infant unless the nurse really believes it. Both attitudes and words must say: "You are a good mother/father. You have an important contribution to make to the care of your infant." Unless as much care is taken in facilitating parental attachment as in providing physiologic care, the outcome will not be a healthy family.

Verbalizations by the nurse that improve parental self-esteem are essential and easily shared. The nurse can point out that, in addition to physiologic use, breast milk is important because of the emotional investment of the mother. Pumping, storing, labeling, and delivering quantities of breast milk is time-consuming and a "labor of love" for mothers. Positive remarks regarding breast milk reinforce the maternal behavior of caretaking and providing for her infant: "Breast milk is something that only you can give your baby" or "You really have brought a lot of milk today" or "Look how rich this breast milk is" or "Even small amounts of milk are important, and look how rich it is."

If the infant begins to gain weight while being fed breast milk, it is important to point this out to the mother. Parents should also be advised that initial weight loss with beginning nipple feedings is common because of the increased energy expended when the infant begins active rather than passive nutritional intake.

Provision of care by the parents is appropriate even for very sick or defective infants who are likely to die. It has been found that detachment is easier after attachment because the parents are comforted by the knowledge that they did all they could for their child while he or she was alive.

Provision of Continuity in Information Giving

During crisis, maintenance of interpersonal relationships is difficult. Yet in a newborn intensive care area the parents are expected to relate to many different care providers. It is important that parents have as few professionals as possible relaying information to them. A primary nurse should coordinate and provide continuity in information giving to parents. Care providers are individuals and thus will use different terms, inflections, and attitudes. These subtle differences are monumental to parents and only confuse, confound, and produce anxiety (Bass 1991). The transfer of the baby from NICU to a step down unit is very anxiety producing for the parents because they must now deal with new health care givers. The nurse not only functions as a liaison between the parents and the wide variety of professionals interacting with the infant and parents, but also offers clarification, explanation, interpretation of information, and support to the parents.

Use of the Family's Support System

The parents should be encouraged to deal with the crisis with help from their support system. The support system attempts to meet the emotional needs and provide support for the family members in crisis and stress situations. Biologic kinship is not the only valid criterion for a support system; an emotional kinship is the most important factor. In our mobile society of isolated nuclear families, the support system may be a next-door neighbor, a best friend, or perhaps a school chum.

The nurse must search out the significant others in the lives of the parents and help them understand the problems so that they can be a constant parental support.

Facilitation of Family Adjustment

The impact of the crisis on the family is individual and varied. Information about the family's ability to adapt to the situation is obtained through the nurse-family relationship. The birth of the infant (normal newborn, preterm infant, infant with illness or congenital anomaly) should be viewed as it is defined by the family, and appropriate interventions can then be instituted.

Because the family is a unit composed of individuals who must deal with the situation, it is important to encourage open intrafamily communication. Keeping secrets should not be encouraged, especially between spouses, because secrets undermine the trust of their relationship. Well-meaning rationales such as "I want to protect her," "I don't want him to worry about it," and so on can be destructive to open communication and to the basic element of a relationship—trust.

The nurse should encourage open communication among family members, particularly between spouses. Open communication is especially important when the mother is hospitalized apart from the infant. The father is the first to visit the infant and relays information regarding the infant's care and condition to the mother. In this situation the mother has had minimal contact, if any, with her infant. Because of her anxiety and isolation, she may mistrust all those who provide information (the father, nurse, physician, or extended family) until she can see the infant for herself. This can put tremendous stress on the relationship between spouses. The parents (and family) should be given information together. This practice helps overcome misunderstandings and misinterpretations and promotes mutual "working through" of problems.

The entire family—siblings as well as extended relatives—should be encouraged to visit and receive information about the baby. Methods of intervention in assisting the family to cope with the situation include providing support, confronting the crisis, and helping the family understand the reality. Support, explanations, and the helping role must extend to the kin network, as well as to the nuclear family, in an attempt to aid them in communication and support ties with the nuclear family.

The needs of siblings should not be overlooked. They have been looking forward to the new baby, and they too suffer a degree of loss. Young children may react with hostility and older ones with shame at the birth of an infant with an anomaly. Both reactions make them feel guilty. Parents, preoccupied with working through their own feelings, often cannot give the other children the attention and support they need. Sometimes another child becomes the focus of family tension. Anxiety thus directed can take the form of finding fault or of overconcern. This is a form of denial; the parents cannot face the real worry—the infant at risk. After assessing the situation, the observant nurse could see that another family member or friend steps in and gives the needed support to the siblings of the affected baby.

Desires and needs of the individuals must be respected and facilitated; differences are tolerable and should be able to exist side by side. Eliciting the parents' feelings and the meaning of this experience to them is easily accomplished with the question: "How are you doing?" The emphasis is on *you*, and the interest must be sincere.

Families with children in the newborn intensive care unit become friends and support one another. To encourage the development of these friendships and to provide support, many units have established parent groups. The core of the groups consists of parents who previously have had an infant in the intensive care unit. Most groups make contact with families within a day or 2 of the infant's admission to the unit, either through phone calls or visits to the hospital. Early one-on-one parent contacts help families work through their feelings better than discussion groups. This personalized method gives the grieving parents an opportunity to express personal feelings about the pregnancy, labor, and delivery and their "different than expected" infant with others who have experienced the same feelings and with whom they can identify (Ladden & Damato 1992).

Provisions of Home Care Instruction

Predischarge planning begins once the infant's condition becomes stable and indications suggest the newborn will survive. Adequate predischarge teaching will help the parents transform their feelings of inadequacy and competition with the nurse into feelings of self-assurance and attachment. From the beginning the parents should be taught about their infant's special needs and growth patterns (Sudia Robinson 1991). This teaching and involvement is best facilitated by a nurse who has been familiar with the infant and his or her family over a period of time and who has developed a comfortable and supportive relationship with them.

The nurse's responsibility is to provide home care instructions in an optimal environment for parental learning. Learning should take place over time, to avoid the necessity of bombarding the parents with instructions in the day or hour before discharge. Parents often enjoy doing minimal caretaking tasks with gradual expansion of their role.

Many intensive care units provide facilities for parents to room in with their infants for a few days before discharge. This allows parents a degree of independence in the care of their infant with the security of nursing help nearby. This practice is particularly helpful for anxious parents, parents who have not had the opportunity to spend extended time with their infant, or parents who will be giving complex physical care at home, such as tracheostomy care.

The basic elements of home care instruction are as follows:

1. Teaching parents routine well-baby care, such as bathing, temperature taking, formula preparation, and breastfeeding.

2. Training parents to do special procedures as needed by the newborn, such as gavage or gastrostomy feedings, tracheostomy or enterostomy care, medication administration, cardiopulmonary resuscitation (CPR), and operation of an apnea monitor.

(Before discharge the parents should be as comfortable as possible with these tasks and should demonstrate independence. Written tools and instructions are useful for parents to refer to once they are home with the infant, but these should not replace participation in the infant's care.)

3. Referring parents to community health and support organizations. (The visiting nurses association, public health nurses, or social services can assist the parents in the stressful transition from hospital to home by providing the necessary home teaching and support. Some intensive care nurseries have their own parent support groups to help bridge the gap between hospital and home care. Parents can also find support from a variety of community support organizations, such as mothers of twins groups, trisomy 13 clubs, March of Dimes Birth Defects Foundation, handicapped children services, and teen mother and child programs. Each community has numerous agencies capable of assisting the family in adapting emotionally, physically, and financially to the chronically ill infant. The nurse should be familiar with community resources and help the parents identify which agencies may benefit them.)

4. Helping parents recognize the growth and development needs of their infant. (A developmental care program begun in the hospital can be continued at home, or parents may be referred to an infant development program in the community.)

5. Arranging medical follow-up care before discharge. (The infant may need to be followed up by a family pediatrician, a well-baby clinic, or a specialty clinic. The first appointment should be made before the infant is discharged from the hospital.)

6. Evaluating the need for special equipment for infant care (such as a respirator, oxygen, apnea monitor) in the home. (Any extra equipment or supplies should be placed in the home before the infant's discharge. The nurse can be instrumental in helping the parents assess the newborn's needs and coordinate services.)

Further evaluation after the infant has gone home is useful in determining whether the crisis has been resolved satisfactorily. The parents are usually given the intensive care nursery's telephone number to call for support and advice. The staff can follow up each family with visits or telephone calls at intervals for several weeks to assess and evaluate the infant's (and parents') progress.

Evaluation

Anticipated outcomes of nursing care include:

- The parents are able to verbalize their feelings of grief and loss.

- The parents verbalize their concerns about their

baby's health problems, care needs, and potential outcome.

- The parents are able to participate in their infant's care and show attachment behaviors.

CONSIDERATIONS FOR THE NURSE WHO WORKS WITH AT-RISK NEWBORNS

Support cannot be given unless it can be received. Working in an emotional environment of "lots of living and lots of dying" takes its toll on staff. Neonatal intensive care units are among the most stressful areas in health care for patients, families, and nurses. Nurses bear most of the stress and largely determine the atmosphere of the NICU. The nurse's ability to cope with stress is the key to creating an emotionally healthy environment and a positive working atmosphere. The emotional needs and feelings of the staff must be recognized and dealt with in order to enable them to support the parents. An environment of openness to feelings and support in dealing with their own human needs and emotions is essential for staff. As care givers, nurses may be unaware of their need to grieve for their own losses in the NICU. Nurses must also go through the grief work that parents experience. Techniques such as group meetings, individual support, and primary care nursing may assist in maintaining staff mental health.

The staff NICU nurses may never see the long-term results of the specialized, sensitive care they give to parents and their newborns. Their only immediate evidence of effective care may be the beginning of resolution of parental grief, discharge of a recovered thriving infant to the care of happy parents, and the beginning of reintegration of family life.

KEY CONCEPTS

Early identification of potential high-risk fetuses through assessment of prepregnant, prenatal, and intrapartal factors facilitates strategically timed nursing observations and interventions.

High-risk newborns, whether they are premature, SGA, LGA, postterm, or infants of a diabetic or substance-addicted mother, have many similar problems, although their problems are based on different physiologic processes.

Small-for-gestational-age newborns are associated with perinatal asphyxia and resulting aspiration syndrome, hypothermia, hypoglycemia, hypocalcemia, polycythemia, congenital anomalies, and intrauterine infections. Long-term problems include continued difficulties with growth and learning.

Large-for-gestational-age newborns are at risk for birth trauma as a result of cephalopelvic disproportion, hypoglycemia, polycythemia, and hyperviscosity.

Infants of diabetic mothers are at risk for hypoglycemia, hypocalcemia, hyperbilirubinemia, polycythemia, and respiratory distress due to delayed maturation of their lungs.

Postterm newborns often encounter intrapartal problems such as CPD (shoulder dystocia) and birth traumas, hypoglycemia, polycythemia, meconium aspiration, cold stress, and possible seizure activity. Long-term complications may involve poor weight gain and low IQ scores.

The common problems of the preterm newborn are results of the baby's immature body systems. Potential problem areas include respiratory distress (respiratory distress syndrome), patent ductus arteriosus, hypothermia and cold stress, feeding difficulties and necrotizing enterocolitis, marked insensible water loss and loss of buffering agents through the kidneys, infection, anemia of prematurity, apnea and intraventricular hemorrhage, retinopathy of prematurity, and behavioral state disorganization. Long-term needs and problems include bronchopulmonary dysplasia, speech defects, sensorineural hearing loss, and neurologic defects.

Newborns of alcohol-dependent mothers are at risk for physical characteristic alterations and the long-term complications of feeding problems; CNS dysfunction, including lower IQ, hyperactivity, and language abnormalities; and congenital anomalies.

Newborns born to drug-dependent mothers experience drug withdrawal as well as respiratory distress, jaundice, congenital anomalies, and behavioral abnormalities. With early recognition and intervention the potential long-term physiologic and emotional consequences of these difficulties can be avoided or at least lessened in severity.

Newborns born to mothers with AIDS require early recognition and treatment so that the physiologic and emotional consequences may be lessened in severity and CDC guidelines implemented.

Cardiac defects are a significant cause of morbidity and mortality in the newborn period. Early identification and nursing and medical care of newborns with cardiac defects are essential to the improved outcome of these infants. Care is directed toward lessening the work load of the heart and decreasing oxygen and energy consumption.

Inborn errors of metabolism such as galactosemia, PKU, homocystinuria, and maple syrup urine disease are usually included in a newborn screening program designed to prevent mental retardation through dietary management and medication.

The nursing care of the newborn with special problems involves the understanding of normal physiology, the pathophysiology of the disease process, clinical manifestations, and supportive or corrective therapies. Only with this theoretical background can the nurse make appropriate observations concerning responses to therapy and development of complications.

Newborns communicate needs only by their behavior; the nurse caring for newborns, through objective observations and evaluations, interprets this behavior to obtain meaningful information about the infant's condition.

The nurse is the facilitator of interdisciplinary communication with the parents, identifying their understanding of their infant's care and their needs for emotional support.

Parents of at-risk newborns need support from nurses and health care providers to understand the special needs of their baby and to feel comfortable in an overwhelmingly strange environment.

REFERENCES

ACOG technical bulletin #159: Fetal macrosomia. *Int J Gynecol Obstet* 1992; 39:341.

Als H et al: Assessment of preterm infant behavior (APIB). In: *Theory and Research in Behavioral Pediatrics*, vol 1. Fitzgerald Lester BM, Yogman MW (editors). New York: Plenum, 1982.

American Academy of Pediatrics Committee on Fetus and Newborn: *Guidelines for Perinatal Care*, 3rd ed. Elk Grove Village, IL: AAP, 1992.

American Academy of Pediatrics Committee of Pediatrics and Committee on Genetics: Newborn screening fact sheets. *Pediatrics* 1989; 83(3):449.

Angelini DJ, Knapp CM: Narcotic addiction in pregnancy. *Case Studies in Perinatal Nursing*. Rockville, MD: Aspen Publishers Inc, 1991.

Auerbach KG, Walker M: When the mother of a premature infant uses a breast pump: What every NICU nurse needs to know. *Neonatal Network* 1994; 13(4):23.

Bass LS: What do parents need when their infant is a patient in the NICU? *Neonatal Network* 1991; 10(4):25.

Bastin N et al: Postpartum care of the HIV-positive woman and her newborn, part 3. *JOGNN* 1992; 21(2):105.

Benson DW: Changing profile of congenital heart disease. *Pediatrics* 1989; 83(5):790.

Bernbaum JC: Medical care after discharge. In: *Neonatology: Pathophysiology and Management of the Newborn*, 4th ed. Avery GB, Fletcher M, MacDonald MG (editors). Philadelphia: Lippincott, 1994.

Blackburn ST, Loper DL: *Maternal, Fetal, and Neonatal Physiology: A Clinical Perspective*. Philadelphia: WB Saunders, 1992.

Blanchette V et al: Hematology. In: *Neonatology: Pathophysiology and Management of the Newborn*, 4th ed. Avery GB, Fletcher M, MacDonald MG (editors). Philadelphia: Lippincott, 1994.

Bowen FW, Tasman W: Retinopathy of prematurity. In: *Neonatology for the Clinician*. Pomerance JJ, Richardson CJ (editors). Norwalk, CT: Appleton & Lange, 1993.

Brooks-Gunn J, McCarton C, Hawley T: Effects of in utero drug exposure on children's development. *Arch Pediatr Adolesc Med* 1994; 148(1):33.

Coles CD: Impact of prenatal alcohol exposure on the newborn and the child. *Clin Obstet Gynecol* 1993; 36(2):255.

Committee for the Classification of Retinopathy of Prematurity: An international classification of retinopathy of prematurity. *Arch Ophthalmol* 1984; 102:1130.

Committee on Substance Abuse and Committee on Children with Disabilities: Fetal alcohol syndrome and fetal alcohol effects. *Pediatrics* 1993; 89(1):1004.

Cordero L, Landon MB: Infant of the diabetic mother. *Clin Perinatol* 1993; 20(3):635.

Creasy RK, Resnik R: Intrauterine growth restriction. In: *Maternal-Fetal Medicine: Principles and Practice*, 3rd ed. Creasy RK, Resnik R. Philadelphia: WB Saunders, 1994.

Cunningham MD: Special problems in the fetus and neonate. In: *Gellis & Kagan's Current Pediatric Therapy*, vol 14. Burg FD, Ingelfinger JR, Wald ER (editors). Philadelphia: WB Saunders, 1993.

Cusson RM, Lee AL: Parental interventions and the development of the preterm infant. *JOGNN* 1994; 23(1):60.

Duimstra C et al: A fetal alcohol syndrome surveillance pilot project in American Indian communities in the northern plains. *Pub Health Rep* 1993; 198(2):225.

Flanagan MF, Fyler DC: Cardiac disease. In: *Neonatology: Pathophysiology and Management of the Newborn*, 4th ed. Avery GB, Fletcher M, MacDonald MG (editors). Philadelphia: Lippincott, 1994.

Fletcher AB: Nutrition. In: *Neonatology: Pathophysiology and Management of the Newborn*, 4th ed. Avery GB, Fletcher M, MacDonald MG (editors). Philadelphia, Lippincott, 1994.

Frank DA, Bresnahan K, Zuckerman BS: Maternal cocaine use: Impact on child health and development. *Adv Pediatr* 1993; 40:65.

Gale G, Franck L, Lund C: Skin-to-skin (kangaroo) holding of the intubated premature infant. *Neonatal Network* 1993; 12(6):49.

Grant P: Psychological needs of families of high-risk infants. *Fam Commun Health* 1978; 11:93.

Grisemer AN: Apnea of prematurity: Current management and nursing implications. *Pediatr Nurs* 1990; 16(6):606.

Harrington K, Campbell S: Fetal size and growth. *Cur Op Obstet Gynecol* 1993; 5:186.

Haut C, Peddicord K, O'Brien E: Supporting parental bonding in the NICU: A care plan for nurses. *Neonatal Network* 1994; 13(8):19.

Hod M, Diamont YZ: The offspring of a diabetic mother: Short- and long-range implications. *Isr J Med Sci* 1992; 28:81.

Hulseman ML, Norman LA: The neonatal ICU graduate, part 1: Common problems. *Am Fam Phys* 1992; 45(3):1301.

Iams JD, Zuspan FP: *Manual of Obstetrics and Gynecology*, 2nd ed. St Louis: Mosby, 1990.

Jhaveri MK et al: Perinatal cocaine/crack exposure in infants: A different perspective. *Neonatal Int Care* May/June 1993; 18.

Kaplan DM, Mason EA: Maternal reactions to premature birth viewed as an acute emotional disorder. In: *Crisis Interventions*. Parad HJ (editor). New York: Family Services Association of America, 1974.

Kaplan P et al: Intellectual outcome in children with maple syrup urine disease. *J Pediatr* 1991; 119:46.

Kellinger KG: Providing primary care to the HIV-at-risk and infected child. *Nurse Pract* 1994; 19(8):48.

Kinneer MD, Beachy P: Nipple feeding premature infants in the neonatal intensive-care unit: Factors and decisions. *JOGNN* 1994; 23(2):105.

Kinsey KK: "But I know my man!" HIV/AIDS risk appraisals and heuristical reasoning patterns among childbearing women. *Holistic Nurs Pract* 1994; 8(2):79.

Klaus MH, Kennell JH: *Maternal-Infant Bonding*, 2nd ed. St Louis: Mosby, 1982.

Kliegman RM: Problems in metabolic adaptation: Glucose, calcium, and magnesium. In: *Care of the High-Risk Neonate*, 4th ed. Klaus MH, Fanaroff AA (editors). Philadelphia: WB Saunders, 1993.

Krishna A, Phillips LS: Fetal alcohol syndrome and insulinlike growth factors. *J Lab Clin Med* 1994; 124(2):149.

Ladden M, Damato E: Parenting and supportive programs. *NAACOG's Clin Issues Perinatal Women Health Nurs* 1992; 3(1):174.

Lin AE, Garver KL: Genetic counseling for congenital heart defects. *J Pediatr* 1988; 113(6):1105.

Martin GI: Infant apnea. In: *Neonatology for the Clinician.* Pomerance JJ, Richardson CJ (editors). Norwalk, CT: Appleton & Lange, 1993.

Medoff-Cooper B: Transition of the preterm infant to an open crib. *JOGNN* 1994; 23(4):329.

Meier P: Bottle and breast feeding: Effects on transcutaneous oxygen pressure and temperature in preterm infants. *Nurs Res* 1988; 37(1):36.

Mendez H, Jule JE: Care of the infant born exposed to human immunodeficiency virus. *Obstet Gynecol Clin North Am* 1990; 17(3):637.

Mercer R: *Parents at Risk.* New York: Springer, 1990.

NAACOG: *Neonatal Skin Care.* OGN nursing practice resource. Washington, DC, March 1985.

Nagey DA, Viscardi RM: Retarded intrauterine growth. In: *Neonatology for the Clinician.* Pomerance JJ, Richardson CJ (editors). Norwalk, CT: Appleton & Lange, 1993.

NANN Practice Committee: *Infant Developmental Care Guidelines.* Petaluma, CA: National Association of Neonatal Nurses, 1993.

Ogata ES: Carbohydrate homeostasis. In: *Neonatology: Pathophysiology and Management of the Newborn*, 4th ed. Avery GB, Fletcher M, MacDonald MG (editors). Philadelphia: Lippincott, 1994.

Ostrea EM: Infants of drug-dependent mothers. In: *Gellis & Kagan's Current Pediatric Therapy*, vol 14. Burg FD, Ingelfinger JR, Wald ER (editors). Philadelphia: WB Saunders, 1993.

Palo P: Significance of antenatal detection and the choice of the delivery place of severely small for gestational age fetuses. *Am J Perinatol* 1992; 9(3):135.

Paz I et al: Are children born small for gestational age at increased risk of short stature? *AJDC* 1993; 147(2):337.

Powell ML: *Assessment and Management of Developmental Changes and Problems in Children*, 2nd ed. St Louis: Mosby, 1981.

Pressler JL: Strategies useful in caring for macrosomic newborns. *J Pediatr Nurs* 1991; 6(3):149.

Resnik R: Post-term pregnancy. In: *Maternal Fetal Medicine: Principles and Practice*, 3rd ed. Creasy RK, Resnik R (editors). Philadelphia: WB Saunders, 1994.

Ryan RM et al: Meconium analysis for improved identification of infants exposed to cocaine in utero. *J Pediatr* 1994; 125(3):435.

Scherling D: Prenatal cocaine exposure and childhood psychopathology: A developmental analysis. *Am J Orthopsychiat* 1994; 64(1):9.

Scott GB, Parks WP: Pediatric AIDS. In: *Principles and Practice of Pediatrics*, 2nd ed. Oski FA et al (editors). Philadelphia: Lippincott, 1994.

Seashore MR, Rinaldo P: Metabolic disease of the neonate and young infant. *Sem Perinatol* 1993; 17(5):318.

Sison AV, Sever JL: HIV-1 infections in pregnancy and perinatal transmission of HIV-1: Current issues. *Pediatr AIDS and HIV Infect* 1992; 3(1):5.

Solnit A, Stark M: Mourning and the birth of a defective child. *Psychoanal Study Child* 1961; 16:505.

Spellacy WN: Postdate pregnancy. In: *Danforth's Obstetrics and Gynecology*, 7th ed. Scott JR et al (editors). Philadelphia: Lippincott, 1994.

Spohr HL, Willms J, Steinhausen HC: Prenatal alcohol exposure and long term developmental consequences. *Lancet* 1993; 341:907.

Sudia Robinson TM: Discharge teaching in the NICU. *Neonatal Network* 1991; 10(4):77.

Teplin SW: Development of blind infants and children with retrolental fibroplasia: Implications for physicians. *Pediatrics* 1983; 71:6.

Volpe JJ: *Neurology of the Newborn*, 3rd ed. Philadelphia: WB Saunders, 1995.

Warshaw JB: Infant of the diabetic mother. In: *Principles and Practice of Pediatrics*, 2nd ed. Oski FA et al (editors). Philadelphia: Lippincott, 1994a.

Warshaw JB: Intrauterine growth retardation. In: *Principles and Practice of Pediatrics*, 2nd ed. Oski et al (editors). Philadelphia: Lippincott, 1994b.

Watt J: The consequences of intrauterine growth retardation: What do we know? *Aust NZ Obstet Gynaecol* 1989; 29(3):279.

Wen SW et al: Intrauterine growth retardation and preterm delivery: Prenatal risk factors in an indigent population. *Am J Obstet Gynecol* 1990; 162:213.

Wennberg RP et al: Fetal cocaine exposure and neonatal bilirubinemia. *J Pediatr* 1994; 125(4):613.

Whitsett JA et al: Acute respiratory disorders. In: *Neonatology: Pathophysiology and Management of the Newborn*, 4th ed. Avery GB, Fletcher MA, MacDonald MG (editors). Philadelphia: Lippincott, 1994.

Witter FR: Perinatal mortality and intrauterine growth retardation. *Cur Op Obstet Gynecol* 1993; 5:56.

Wright L, Brown A, Davidson-Mundt A: Newborn screening: The miracle and the challenge. *J Pediatr Nurs* 1992; 17(1):26.

Wyse LJ, Jones M, Mandel F: Relationship of glycosylated hemoglobin, fetal macrosomia, and birthweight macrosomia. *J Perinatol* 1994; 11(4):260.

Yogev R, Conner E: *Management of HIV Infections in Infants and Children.* St Louis: Mosby-Year Book, 1992.

CHAPTER 32

THE NEWBORN AT RISK: BIRTH-RELATED STRESSORS

I watched her breathe every precious breath on the respirator. I saw her covered with wires and tubes. I kept watch. She was special to me and I would tell her over and over, "Daddy is here. Daddy loves you." The three days she lived were hell—not knowing if she would make it, uncertain about what plans we should make. Somehow I thought she would live; I was hopeful. When she died, at least I was there with her. The grief was unbearable. But there was also a sense of relief. The uncertainty, the waiting were finally over.

~ WHEN PREGNANCY FAILS ~

KEY TERMS

Bronchopulmonary dysplasia (BPD)

Cold stress

Erythroblastosis fetalis

Exchange transfusion

Hemolytic disease of the newborn

Hydrops fetalis

Hyperbilirubinemia

Hypocalcemia

Hypoglycemia

Jaundice

Kernicterus

Meconium aspiration syndrome (MAS)

Persistent pulmonary hypertension of the newborn (PPHN)

Phototherapy

Physiologic anemia

Pneumothorax

Polycythemia

Respiratory distress syndrome (RDS)

Sepsis neonatorum

OBJECTIVES

Discuss how to identify infants in need of resuscitation and the appropriate method of resuscitation based on the labor record and observable physiologic indicators.

Based on clinical manifestations, differentiate the various types of respiratory distress patterns (respiratory distress syndrome, transient tachypnea of the newborn, meconium aspiration syndrome, and persistent pulmonary hypertension) seen in newborns.

Apply the nursing process to caring for the infant with respiratory distress syndrome.

Correlate the clinical manifestations of bronchopulmonary dysplasia with the underlying disease process.

Discuss selected metabolic abnormalities (including cold stress, hypoglycemia, and hypocalcemia), their effects on the newborn, and their nursing implications.

Differentiate between physiologic and pathologic jaundice based on onset, cause, possible sequelae, and specific management.

Identify the nursing responsibilities in caring for the newborn receiving phototherapy or an exchange transfusion.

Explain the set of circumstances that must be present for the development of erythroblastosis and ABO incompatibility.

Summarize the nurse's role in the care of an infant with hemolytic disease.

Discuss selected hematologic problems such as anemia and polycythemia and the nursing implications associated with each one.

Describe the nursing assessment that would lead the nurse to suspect newborn sepsis.

Relate the consequences of selected maternally transmitted infections, such as maternal syphilis, gonorrhea, herpesvirus, or chlamydia, to the management of the infant in the neonatal period.

Identify the special initial and long-term needs of parents of at-risk infants.

arked homeostatic changes occur during the transition from fetal to newborn life. The most rapid anatomic and physiologic changes of this period occur in the cardiopulmonary system. Thus the major problems of the newborn are usually related to this system. These problems include asphyxia, respiratory distress syndrome, cold stress, jaundice, hemolytic disease, and anemia. Ideally, problems are anticipated and identified prenatally, and appropriate intervention measures are begun at or immediately after birth. See Essential Precautions in Practice: During Care of At-Risk Newborns.

CARE OF THE NEWBORN AT RISK DUE TO ASPHYXIA

Newborn asphyxia results from circulatory, respiratory, and biochemical factors. Circulatory patterns that accompany asphyxia are in effect a return to fetal-like circulatory patterns. They represent an inability to make the transition to extrauterine circulation. Failure of lung expansion and establishment of respiration rapidly produces hypoxia (decreased PaO_2), acidosis (decreased pH), and hypercarbia (increased PCO_2). These biochemical changes result in pulmonary vasoconstriction and high pulmonary vascular resistance, hypoperfusion of the lungs, and a large right-to-left shunt through the ductus arteriosus. As right atrial pressure exceeds left atrial pressure, the foramen ovale reopens, and blood flows from right to left.

Biochemical changes that occur in asphyxia contribute to these circulatory changes. The most serious biochemical abnormality is a change from aerobic to anaerobic metabolism when hypoxia is present. This change results in the accumulation of lactate and the development of metabolic acidosis, and, simultaneously, respiratory acidosis may also occur. In response to hypoxia and anaerobic metabolism, the amounts of free fatty acids (FFA) and glycerol in the blood increase. Glycogen stores are mobilized to provide a continuous glucose source for the brain. Rapid use of hepatic and cardiac stores of glycogen may occur during an asphyxial attack.

The newborn is supplied with protective mechanisms against hypoxic insults. These include a relatively immature brain and a resting metabolic rate lower than that observed in the adult; an ability to mobilize substances within the body for anaerobic metabolism and to use the energy more efficiently; and an intact circulatory system able to redistribute lactate and hydrogen ions in tissues still being perfused. Unfortunately, severe prolonged hypoxia will overcome these protective mechanisms, resulting in brain damage or death of the newborn.

The newborn who is apneic at birth requires immediate resuscitative efforts. The need for resuscitation can be anticipated if specific risk factors are present during the pregnancy or labor and birth period.

Risk Factors Predisposing to Asphyxia

Need for resuscitation may be anticipated in antepartal, intrapartal, or neonatal situations.

Antepartal risk factors for resuscitation include:

- Previous obstetric history of fetal or neonatal death; premature or intrauterine growth-retarded infant; history of large-for-gestational-age infant (infant weighing 10 lb or more)
- Maternal conditions that affect the placenta or fetus—pregnancy-induced hypertension (PIH), postterm (more than 42 weeks), preexisting hypertension, diabetes, infection, chronic renal disease, maternal obesity, and cardiac disease
- Maternal age—younger than 15 or over 35 years
- Isoimmunization
- Abruptio placentae or placenta previa
- Multiple gestation
- Abnormal presentation
- Prematurity
- Prolonged rupture of the membranes
- Hydramnios or oligohydramnios
- Abnormal estriol levels
- Less-than-mature L/S ratio
- Maternal drug usage (narcotic, barbiturate, tranquilizer, or alcohol)
- Anemia (hemoglobin less than 10 mg/dL)

Intrapartal risk factors for resuscitation are as follows:

- Abnormal labor pattern—dystocia, precipitous birth
- Meconium-stained amniotic fluid
- Fetal heart rate (FHR) patterns—tachycardia (greater than 160/minute without maternal temperature elevation); bradycardia (less than 120/minute, particularly associated with smooth baseline, an ominous sign); irregular rate; lack of baseline variability of FHR (smooth or fixed); lack of significant variability with fetal movement; ominous patterns (moderate to severe variable deceleration and late deceleration of any magnitude)
- Abnormal fetal presentation—breech, transverse lie, shoulder
- Prolapsed cord
- Abruptio placentae or placenta previa
- Indications for cesarean birth (see Chapter 26)

Neonatal risk factors for resuscitation include:

- Nonreassuring fetal heart rate pattern
- Difficult birth
- Fetal blood loss
- Apneic episode unresponsive to tactile stimulation
- Inadequate ventilation
- Prematurity
- Structural lung abnormality (congenital diaphragmatic hernia, lung hypoplasia)
- Cardiac arrest

Medical Therapy

The initial goal of medical management is to identify the fetus at risk for asphyxia so that resuscitative efforts can begin at birth.

Fetal biophysical assessment and monitoring fetal and maternal pH, blood gases, and fetal heart rates during the intrapartal period may help identify fetal distress. If fetal distress is present, appropriate measures can be taken to deliver the fetus immediately, before major damage occurs, and to treat the asphyxiated newborn.

The fetal biophysical profile includes tests for heart rate accelerations associated with fetal movement, sustained fetal breathing movements, fetal limb or trunk movements, extension and flexion movements, and measurement of amniotic fluid volume. Use of this testing procedure improves the ability to predict an abnormal perinatal outcome (see Chapter 20). Fetal scalp blood sampling may indicate asphyxic insult and related degree of fetal acidosis if considered in relation to stage of labor, uterine contractions, and nonreassuring FHR patterns. Normal fetal pH ranges from 7.30 to 7.35. The pH falls gradually during the first stage of labor. During the second stage and birth it decreases more drastically. The stress of labor causes an intermittent decrease in exchange of gases in the placental intervillous space, which causes a fall in pH and fetal acidosis. The acidosis is primarily metabolic rather than respiratory because exchange of CO_2 is more rapid than exchange of hydrogen ions in the placenta.

During labor a fetal pH of 7.25 or higher is considered normal. A pH value of 7.20–7.24 is considered preacidosis. A pH value of 7.20 or less is considered an ominous sign of fetal asphyxia (Jepson et al 1991). However, low fetal pH without associated hypoxia can be caused by maternal acidosis resulting from prolonged labor, dehydration, and maternal lactate production. Simultaneous testing of maternal venous pH and fetal pH may help rule out maternal acidosis as a contributing factor or to identify maternal alkalosis, which might result in a false normal fetal pH finding in the presence of fetal compromise.

Assessment of the newborn's need for resuscitation begins at the time of birth. The time of the first gasp, first cry, and onset of sustained respirations should be noted in order of occurrence. The Apgar score (see Chapter 23) may be helpful in determining the severity of neonatal depression but should not be used to determine the need for resuscitation of the newborn.

The treatment of fetal/neonatal asphyxia is resuscitation. The goal of resuscitation is to provide an adequate airway with expansion of the lungs, to decrease the P_{CO_2} and increase the P_{O_2}, to support adequate cardiac output, and to minimize oxygen consumption by reducing heat loss.

Initial resuscitative management of the newborn is extremely important. The baby should be kept in a level supine position with the neck in a neutral position prior to the first gasp. The oropharynx and nasopharynx must be suctioned immediately. Clearing the nasal and oral passages of fluid that may obstruct the airway establishes a patent airway. Suction is always performed before resuscitation so that mucus, blood, meconium, or formula is not aspirated into the lungs.

The infant is kept in a level position under a radiant heat source and is dried quickly with towels to maintain skin temperature at about 36.5 C (97.7 F). Drying is also a good stimulation to breathing. Heat loss through evaporation is tremendous during the first few minutes of life. The temperature of a wet 1500 g baby in a 16 C (62 F) room drops 1 C every 3 minutes. Hypothermia increases oxygen consumption. In an asphyxiated infant, it increases the hypoxic insult and may lead to severe acidosis and development of respiratory distress.

Breathing is established by employing the simplest form of resuscitative measures initially, with progression to more complicated methods as required. These are the following:

1. Provide simple stimulation by rubbing the back.
2. If respirations have not been initiated or are inadequate (gasping or occasional respirations), the lungs must be inflated with positive pressure. The mask is positioned securely on the face (over nose and mouth, avoiding the eyes) with the head in "sniffing" or neutral position (Figure 32–1). Hyperextension of the infant's neck will obstruct the trachea. An airtight connection is made between the baby's face and the mask (thus allowing the bag to inflate). The lungs are inflated rhythmically by squeezing the bag. Oxygen can be delivered at 100% with an anesthesia or Laerdal bag and adequate liter flow. The self-inflating bag delivers only 40% oxygen unless it has been adapted. In addition it may not be possible to maintain adequate inspiratory pressure with Ambu or Hope bags. In a crisis situation it is crucial that 100% O_2 be delivered with adequate pressure.
3. The rise and fall of the chest are observed for proper ventilation. Air entry and heart rate are checked by auscultation. Manual resuscitation is coordinated with any voluntary efforts. The rate of ventilation should be between 40 and 60 breaths per minute. Pressure should be adequate to move the chest wall. The pressure gauge (manonmeter) must be in place to avoid overdistention of the newborn's lungs and other problems such as pneumothorax or abdominal distension. In newborns with normal lungs, 15–25 cm H_2O may be adequate. If the newborn has lung disease, 20–40 cm H_2O may be necessary. If the newborn has not taken a first breath after birth, pressures of 30–40 cm H_2O may be transiently required to expand collapsed alveoli. If ventilation is adequate, the chest moves with each inspiration, bilateral breath sounds are audible, and the lips and mucous membranes become pink. If color and heart rate fail to respond to ventilatory efforts, poor or improper placement of an endotracheal tube may be the cause. If the baby is intubated properly, pneumothorax, diaphragmatic hernia, or hypoplastic lungs (Potter's syndrome) may exist. Distention of the stomach is controlled by inserting a nasogastric tube for decompression.
4. Endotracheal intubation (Figure 32–2) may be needed. However, most newborns except for very-

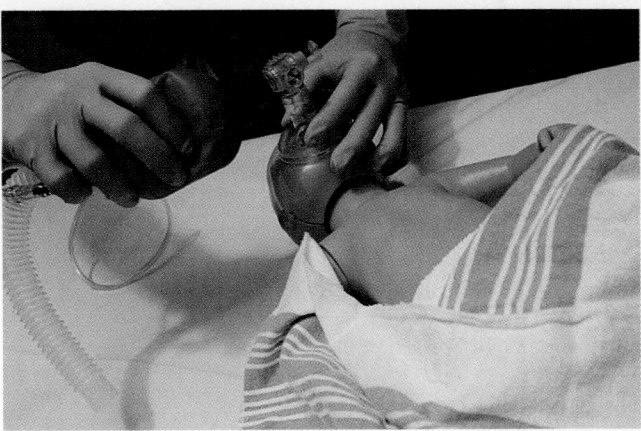

FIGURE 32-1 Demonstration of resuscitation of an infant with bag and mask. Note that the mask covers the nose and mouth, and the head is in a neutral position. The resuscitation bag is placed to the side of the baby so that chest movement can be seen.

low-birth-weight (VLBW) infants, can be resuscitated by bag and mask ventilation.

Once breathing has been established, the heart rate should increase to over 100 beats per minute. If the heart rate is less than 60 beats per minute or between 60 and 80 beats per minute and is not increasing despite 15 to 30 seconds of ventilation with 100% oxygen, external cardiac massage (chest compression) is begun. Chest compressions are started immediately if there is no detectable heartbeat.

1. The infant is positioned *properly* on a firm surface.
2. The resuscitator uses the two-fingers method (Figure 32–3) or may stand at the foot of the infant and place both thumbs over the lower third of the sternum (just below an imaginary line drawn between the nipples) with the fingers wrapped around and supporting the back.
3. The sternum is depressed approximately two-thirds of the distance to the vertebral column (1 to 2 cm or ½ to ¾ in) at a rate of 90 beats per minute (NRP Instructors Update 1993).
4. A 3:1 ratio of heartbeat to assisted ventilation is used.

Drugs that should be available in the birthing area include those needed in the treatment of shock, cardiac arrest, and narcosis. Oxygen, because of its effective use in ventilation, is the drug most often used.

If, after 30 seconds of ventilation and cardiac compression, the newborn has not responded with spontaneous respirations and a heart rate above 80 beats per minute, it is necessary to administer resuscitative medications. The most accessible route for administering

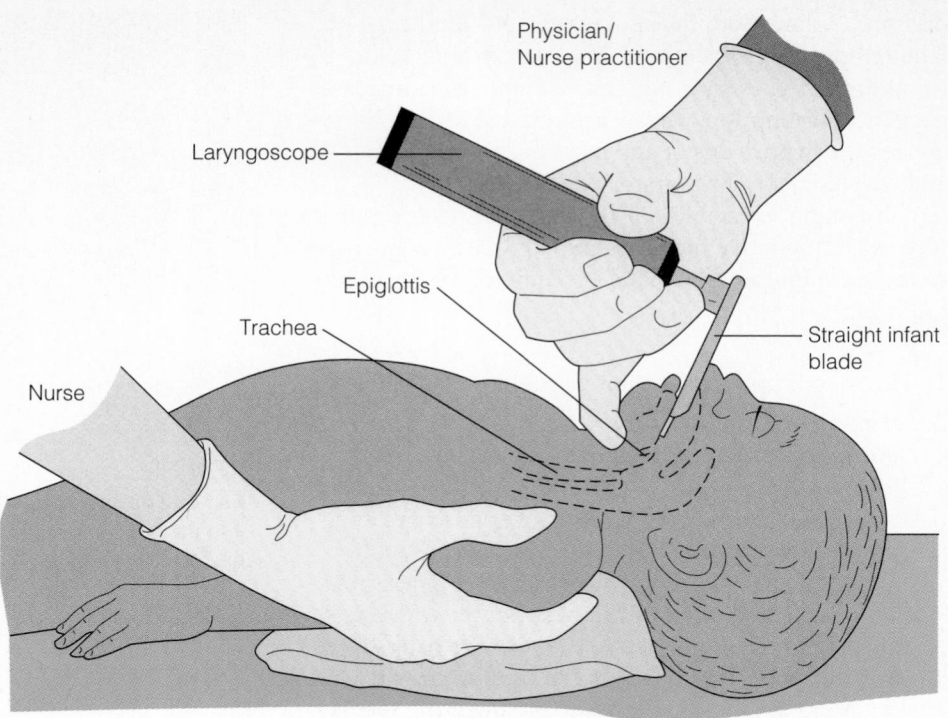

FIGURE 32-2 Endotracheal intubation is accomplished with the infant's head in the "sniffing" position. The clinician places the fifth finger under the chin to hold the tongue forward and inserts the laryngoscope blade. Once the blade is in position as shown, an endotracheal tube is inserted through the groove in the laryngoscope blade. The endotracheal tube is not seen in this illustration.

Physician/
Nurse practitioner

Laryngoscope

Epiglottis

Trachea

Straight infant blade

Nurse

medications is the umbilical vein. If bradycardia is present, epinephrine (0.1 to 0.3 mL/kg of 1:10,000 solution) is given through the umbilical vein catheter, the peripheral IV, or the endotracheal tube (if an IV has not yet been started). In a severely asphyxiated newborn, sodium bicarbonate (2 mEq/kg of 4.2% solution) is given slowly, at a rate of 1 mEq/kg/minute to correct metabolic acidosis, but only after adequate ventilation is established. Naloxone hydrochloride (0.1 mg/kg of 1 mg/mL solution), a narcotic antagonist, is used to reverse narcotic depression (Chameides 1990). See the Drug Guide: Sodium Bicarbonate and Drug Guide: Naloxone Hydrochloride (Narcan). Dextrose is given to prevent progression of hypoglycemia. A 10% dextrose in water intravenous solution is usually sufficient to prevent or treat hypoglycemia in the birthing area.

In the advent of shock (low blood pressure or poor peripheral perfusion), the baby may be given a volume

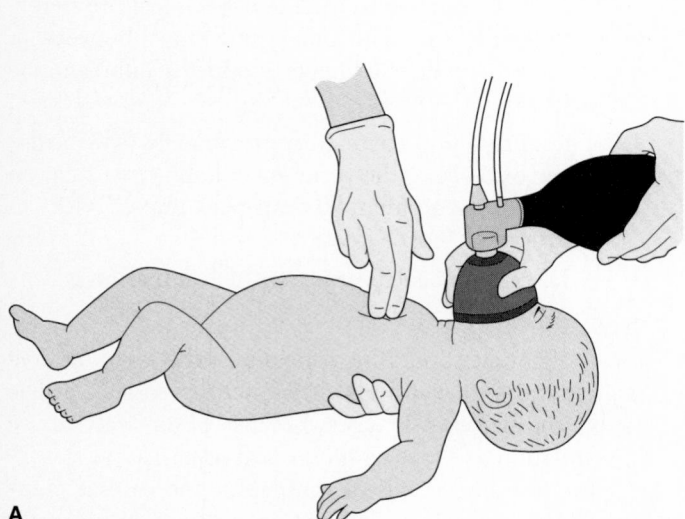

A

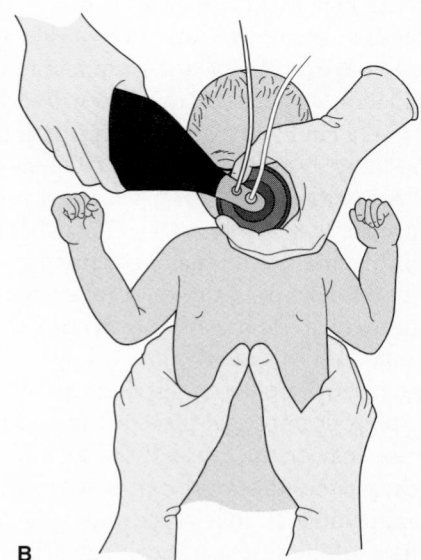

B

FIGURE 32-3 External cardiac massage. The lower third of the sternum is compressed with two fingertips or thumbs at a rate of 90 beats/minute. *A* The two-fingers method uses the tips of two fingers of one hand to compress the sternum and the other hand or a firm surface to support the infant's back. *B* The thumb method uses the fingers to support the infant's back and uses both thumbs to compress the sternum.

SODIUM BICARBONATE

Overview of Neonatal Action

Sodium bicarbonate is an alkalizing agent. It buffers an increase in hydrogen ions caused by accumulation of lactic acid from anaerobic metabolism occurring during hypoxemia. Sodium bicarbonate thereby raises the blood pH, reversing the metabolic acidosis. Sodium bicarbonate should be used to correct severe metabolic acidosis in asphyxiated newborns *only* once adequate ventilation has been established.

Note: Sodium bicarbonate dissociates in solution into sodium ion and carbonic acid, which can split into water and carbon dioxide. The carbon dioxide must be eliminated via the respiratory tract.

Route, Dosage, Frequency

For resuscitation and severe asphyxiation: intravenous slow push via umbilical vein catheter (infuse at rate no faster than 1 mEq/kg/minute). Dosage is 2 mEq/kg: 4 mL of 0.5 mEq/mL (4.2%) or 2 mL of 1 mEq/mL (8.4%). An 8.4% solution diluted at least 1:1 with sterile water to decrease the osmolarity. Can repeat every 15 minutes if needed for total of four doses. For marked metabolic acidosis: a pH of less than 7.05 and a base deficit of 15 mEq/L or more should be corrected using a 0.5 mEq/mL solution of sodium bicarbonate at a rate of 1 mEq/kg/minute or slower. Calculate total dosage by the following formula:

$$mEq = 0.3 \times \text{weight (kg)} \times \text{base deficit in mEq/L}$$

Neonatal Contraindications

Inadequate respiratory ventilation that causes a rise in Pco_2 and a decrease in pH

Presence of edema; metabolic or respiratory alkalosis; hypocalcemia, anuria, or oliguria

Neonatal Side Effects

Hypernatremia, hyperosmolarity, fluid overload

Intracranial hemorrhage (rapid infusion of bicarbonate increases serum osmolarity, causing a shift of interstitial fluid into the blood and capillary rupture)

Nursing Considerations

Assess for any contraindications.

Monitor intake and output rates.

Assess adequacy of ventilation by monitoring respiratory status, rate, and depth; ventilate as necessary.

Dilute bicarbonate prior to administration into umbilical vein catheter (for resuscitation) or peripheral IV to prevent sloughing of tissue.

Evaluate effectiveness of drug by monitoring arterial blood gases for Pco_2, bicarbonate concentration, and pH determination.

Incompatible with acidic solutions.

Administration with calcium creates precipitates.

NALOXONE HYDROCHLORIDE (NARCAN)

Overview of Neonatal Action

Naloxone hydrochloride (Narcan) is used to reverse respiratory depression due to acute narcotic toxicity. It displaces morphinelike drugs from receptor sites on the neurons; therefore the narcotics can no longer exert their depressive effects. Naloxone reverses narcotic-induced respiratory depression, analgesia, sedation, hypotension, and pupillary constriction.

Route, Dosage, Frequency

Intravenous dose is 0.1 to 0.2 mg/kg of 1.0 mg/mL or 0.25 mL/kg of 0.4 mg/mL concentration at birth, including premature infants. This drug is usually given through the umbilical vein or endotracheal tube, although naloxone can be given intramuscularly or subcutaneously. The use of neonatal naloxone (Narcan 0.02 mg/mL) is no longer recommended by the American Academy of Pediatrics Committee on Drugs because of the extremely small fluid volumes.

Reversal of drug depression occurs within 1 to 2 minutes. The duration of action is variable (minutes to hours) and depends on the amount of the drug present and the rate of excretion. Dose may be repeated in 5 minutes. If there is no improvement after two or three doses, discontinue naloxone administration. If initial reversal occurs, repeat dose as needed.

Neonatal Contraindications

Should not be administered to infants of narcotic-addicted mothers because it may precipitate acute withdrawal syndrome.

Respiratory depression resulting from nonmorphine drugs such as sedatives, hypnotics, anesthetics, or other nonnarcotic CNS depressants.

Neonatal Side Effects

Excessive doses may result in irritability, increased crying, and possible prolongation of partial thromboplastin time (PTT).

Tachycardia.

Nursing Considerations

Monitor respirations closely—rate and depth.

Assess for return of respiratory depression when naloxone effects wear off and effects of longer-acting narcotics reappear.

Have resuscitative equipment, O_2, and ventilatory equipment available.

Monitor bleeding studies.

Note that naloxone is incompatible with alkaline solutions.

expander such as 5% albumin or lactated Ringer's in a dose of 10 mL/kg. Whole blood, fresh frozen plasma, plasminate, and packed red blood cells can also be used for volume expansion and treatment of shock. In some instances of prolonged resuscitation associated with shock and poor response to resuscitation, Dopamine (5 μg/kg/minute) may be necessary (Osborne & Kassity 1993).

APPLYING THE NURSING PROCESS

Nursing Assessment

Communication between the obstetric office or clinic and the birthing area nurse facilitates the identification of newborns who may be in need of resuscitation. Upon arrival of the woman in the birthing area, the nurse should have the antepartal record and should note any contributory prenatal history factors and assess present fetal status. As labor progresses, nursing assessments include ongoing monitoring of fetal heartbeat and its response to contractions, assisting with fetal scalp blood sampling, and observing the presence of meconium in the amniotic fluid to identify fetal asphyxia. In addition, the nurse should alert the resuscitation team and the practitioner responsible for the care of the newborn of any potential high-risk laboring women.

Nursing Diagnosis

Nursing diagnoses that may apply to the newborn with asphyxia and the newborn's parents include the following:

- Ineffective breathing pattern related to lack of spontaneous respirations at birth secondary to in utero asphyxia

- Decreased cardiac output related to impaired oxygenation

- Ineffective parental coping related to baby's lack of spontaneous respirations at birth and fear of losing the baby

Nursing Plan and Implementation

Preparation of Resuscitation Equipment

Following identification of possible high-risk situations, the next step in effective resuscitation is assembling the necessary equipment and ensuring proper functioning (Table 32–1). It is desirable to provide for pH and blood gas determinations as well. Necessary equipment includes a radiant warmer that provides an overhead radiant heat source (a thermostatic mechanism that is taped to the infant's abdomen triggers the radiant warmer to turn on or off in order to maintain a level of thermoneutrality)

| TABLE 32-1 | Newborn Resuscitation Equipment |

Radiant warmer

Stethoscope

Bag (that can deliver 100% oxygen)

Mask (two mask sizes: one preterm and one newborn)

Tubing and pressure gauges for bag

Oxygen, flow meter, and provision for warmth and humidification

Suction equipment
  DeLee suction with mechanical suction apparatus
  Bulb syringe
  Suction catheters (Nos. 5, 6, and 8 Fr.)
  Meconium aspirator

Intubation equipment
  Magill forceps (if nasotracheal intubation is used at the institution)
  Endotracheal tubes (sizes 2.5, 3.0, 3.5, 4.0 mm, fitted with adapter)
  Wire stylets for tubes
  Laryngoscope handle with two blades (size 0 [premature]; size 1 [newborn])
  Four extra batteries
  Two extra bulbs

Nasogastric tube (for decompression of stomach)

Oral plastic airways (newborn and premature sizes)

K-Y lubricating jelly

Benzoin

Cotton applicators

Adhesive tape

Scissors

Safety pins (for attachments)

Syringes (tuberculin, 3, 5, and 10 mL)

Umbilical artery catheter tray (Nos. 3.5 and 5 Fr. catheters)

IV solution, tubing, needles, catheters, and IV pump

Drugs (solutions)
  Sodium bicarbonate (0.5 mEq/mL)
  Epinephrine (1:10,000 solution)
  Dextrose and water (D/W) (10% D/W for IV; hypoglycemia)
  Sterile water
  Narcan (1 mg/mL)
  Volume expanders (5% albumin, lactated Ringer's, normal saline)
  Normal saline (for suctioning)

Blood pressure cuff and gauge or pressure transducer

Doppler (to measure blood pressure)

EKG electrodes and heart rate monitor

Sterile gloves, masks, protective eye wear or face shields

and an open bed for easy access to the newborn. It is essential that the nurse keep the infant warm. The infant is dried quickly with warmed towels or blankets to prevent evaporative heat loss and is placed under the radiant warmer with servocontrol set at 36.5 C.

Resuscitative equipment in the birthing room must be sterilized after each use. In the high-risk nursery the need for resuscitation may occur at any time.

Equipment reliability must be maintained before an emergency arises. Inspect all equipment—bag and mask, pressure manometer, oxygen and flow meter, laryngoscope, and suction machine—for damaged or nonfunctioning parts before a birth or when setting up an admission bed. A systematic check of the emergency cart and equipment is a routine responsibility of each shift.

Provision and Documentation of Resuscitation

Training and knowledge about resuscitation are vital to personnel in the birth setting for both normal and high-risk births. Because resuscitation is at least a two-person effort, the nurse should call for assistance so that there is adequate staff available. The resuscitative efforts are recorded on the newborn's chart so that all members of the health care team will have access to this information.

Parent Education

Birthing room resuscitation is particularly distressing for the parents. If the need for resuscitation is anticipated, the parents should be assured that a team will be present at the birth to care specifically for their newborn. As soon as stabilization is accomplished, a member of the interdisciplinary team needs to discuss the baby's condition with the parents. The parents may have many fears about the reasons for resuscitation and the condition of their baby following the resuscitation.

Evaluation

Anticipated outcomes of nursing care include:

* The risk of asphyxia is promptly identified, and intervention is started early.

* The newborn's metabolic and physiologic processes are stabilized, and recovery proceeds without complications.

* The parents can describe the reason for resuscitation and what was done to resuscitate their newborn.

* The parents can verbalize their fears about the resuscitation process and potential implications for their baby's future.

CARE OF THE NEWBORN WITH RESPIRATORY DISTRESS

One of the severest conditions to which the newborn may fall victim is respiratory distress—an inappropriate respiratory adaptation to extrauterine life. The nursing care of a baby with respiratory distress requires understanding of the normal pulmonary and circulatory physiology (Chapter 27), the pathophysiology of the disease process, clinical manifestations, and supportive and corrective therapies. Only with this knowledge can the nurse make appropriate observations concerning responses to therapy and development of complications. Unlike the verbalizing adult client, the newborn communicates needs only by behavior. The neonatal nurse interprets this behavior as clues about the individual baby's condition.

Idiopathic Respiratory Distress Syndrome (Hyaline Membrane Disease)

Respiratory distress syndrome (RDS), also referred to as *hyaline membrane disease (HMD)*, is a complex disease that affects approximately 40,000 infants a year in the United States; these are primarily preterm infants (Nugent 1991). RDS accounts for approximately 7000 deaths per year in the United States alone or 20% of all newborn deaths (Glomella 1994). The syndrome occurs more frequently in premature White infants than in Black infants and almost twice as often in males as in females.

All the factors precipitating the pathologic changes of RDS have not been determined, but the main factors associated with its development are:

1. *Prematurity.* All preterm newborns—whether AGA, SGA, or LGA—and especially IDMs are at risk for RDS. The incidence of RDS increases with the degree of prematurity, with most deaths occurring in newborns weighing less than 1500 g. The maternal and fetal factors resulting in preterm labor and birth, complications of pregnancy, indications for cesarean birth, and familial tendency are all associated with RDS.

2. *Surfactant deficiency disease.* Normal pulmonary adaptation requires adequate surfactant, a lipoprotein that coats the inner surface of the alveoli. Surfactant provides alveolar stability by decreasing the alveoli's surface tension and tendency for collapse. In the normal or mature newborn lung, it is continuously synthesized, oxidized during breathing, and replenished. Adequate surfactant levels lead to better lung compliance and permit breathing with decreased work. Respiratory distress syndrome is due to alterations in surfactant quantity, composition, function, or production (Miller & Armstrong 1990).

Development of RDS indicates deficiency of surfactant activity. Upon expiration, alveolar instability increases atelectasis, which causes hypoxia and acidosis because of the lack of gas exchange. These conditions further inhibit surfactant production and cause pulmonary vasoconstriction. Thus the central pathophysiologic defect, lung instability due to abnormality in the surfactant system, leads to the biochemical problems of hypoxemia (decreased PO_2), hypercarbia (increased PCO_2), and acidemia (decreased pH), which further increase pulmonary vasoconstriction and hypoperfusion. The cycle of events of RDS leading to eventual respiratory failure is diagramed in Figure 32–4.

Because of these pathophysiologic conditions, the newborn must expend increasing amounts of energy to reopen the collapsed alveoli with every breath, so each breath becomes more difficult than the last. The progressive atelectasis with each expiration upsets the physiologic homeostasis of the pulmonary and cardiovascular systems and prevents adequate gaseous exchange. Lung

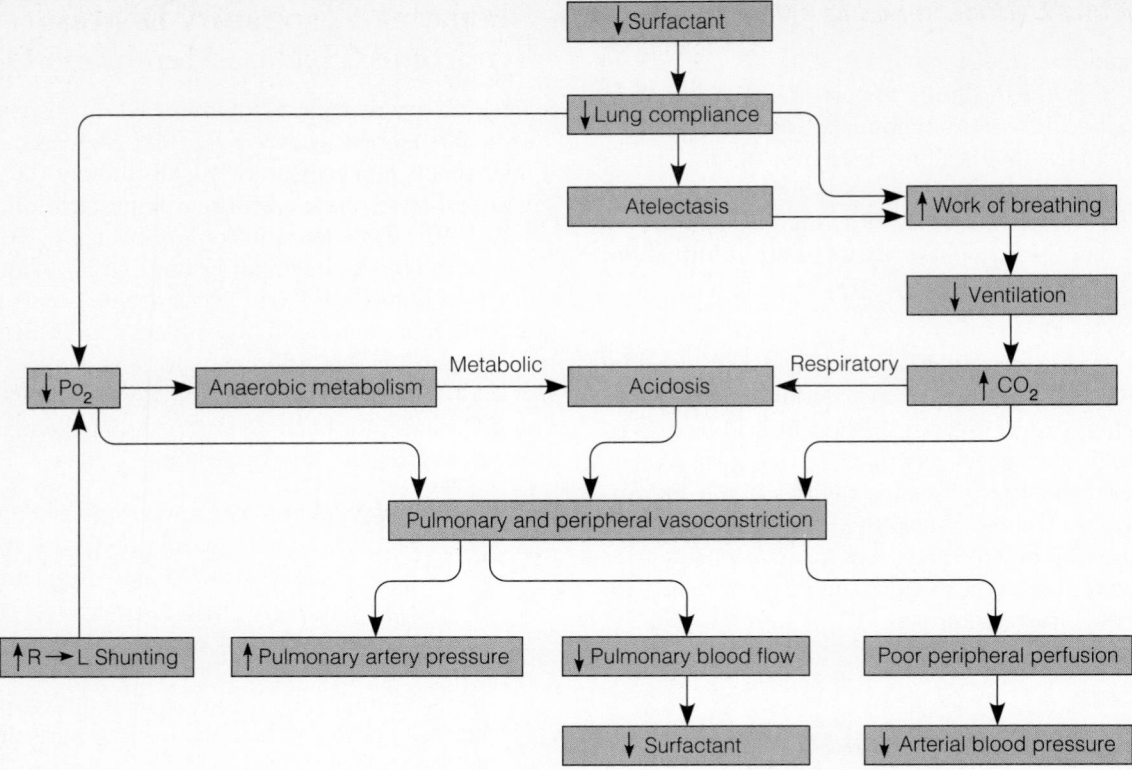

FIGURE 32-4 Cycle of events of RDS leading to eventual respiratory failure.
SOURCE: Modified from Gluck L, Kulovich MV: Fetal lung development.
Pediatr Clin North Am 1973; 20:375.

compliance decreases, and stiff lungs, which account for the difficulty of inflation, labored respirations, and the increased work of breathing, are the result.

The physiologic alterations of RDS produce the following complications:

1. *Hypoxia.* Hypoxia produces physiologic complications and consequences that increase the hypoxia and decrease pulmonary perfusion. As a result of hypoxia, the pulmonary vasculature constricts, pulmonary vascular resistance increases, and pulmonary blood flow is reduced. Increased pulmonary vascular resistance may precipitate a return to fetal circulation as the ductus opens and blood flow is shunted around the lungs. This increases the hypoxia and further decreases pulmonary perfusion. Hypoxia also causes impairment or absence of metabolic response to cold; reversion to anaerobic metabolism, resulting in lactate accumulation (acidosis); and impaired cardiac output, which decreases perfusion to vital organs.

2. *Respiratory acidosis.* Increased PCO_2 and decreased pH are results of alveolar hypoventilation. Carbon dioxide retention and the respiratory acidosis that results are the measure of ventilatory inadequacy, so that persistently rising PCO_2 and decrease in pH are

poor prognostic signs of pulmonary function and adequacy.

3. *Metabolic acidosis.* Decreased pH and decreased bicarbonate levels may be results of impaired delivery of oxygen at the cellular level. Because of the lack of oxygen, the newborn begins an anaerobic pathway of metabolism, with an increase in lactate levels and a resultant base deficit (loss of bicarbonate). As the lactate levels increase, the pH decreases, and the buffer base decreases in an attempt to maintain acid-base homeostasis.

The classic radiologic picture of RDS is diffuse reticulogranular density that occurs bilaterally, with portions of the air-filled tracheobronchial tree (air bronchogram) outlined by the opaque lungs. Opacification of the lungs on x-ray ("whiteout") may be due to massive atelectasis, diffuse alveolar infiltrate, or pulmonary edema. These conditions make the lungs difficult to inflate and thus lead to their opaque look on x-rays. The progression of x-ray findings parallels the pattern of resolution, which usually occurs in 4 to 7 days, and the time of surfactant reappearance, unless surfactant replacement therapy has been used. Echocardiography is a valuable tool in diagnosing vascular shunts that shunt blood either away from or toward the lungs.

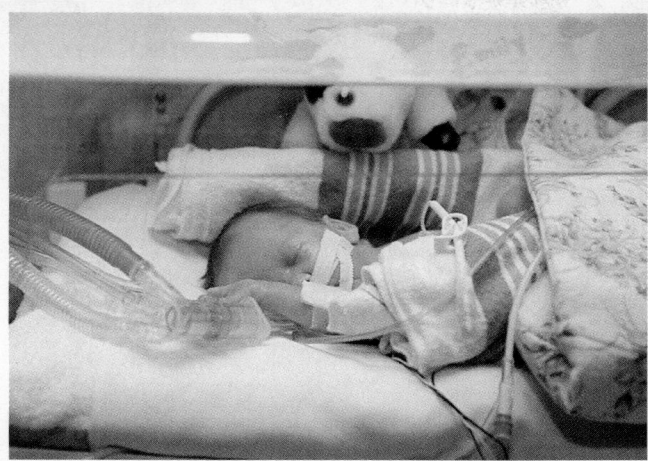

FIGURE 32-5   Infant on a respirator.

The clinical course for respiratory distress syndrome varies with the severity of the disease, size of the infant, presence of infection, degree of shunting of blood through a patent ductus arteriosus, and whether or not assisted ventilation was used.

Medical Therapy

The primary goal of prenatal medical management is the prevention of preterm birth through aggressive treatment of premature labor and possible administration of glucocorticoids to enhance fetal lung development (Moya & Gross 1993).

Supportive medical management consists of oxygenation, ventilatory therapy, transcutaneous oxygen and carbon dioxide monitoring, blood gas monitoring, correction of acid-base imbalance, environmental temperature regulation, adequate nutrition, and protection from infection. Ventilatory therapy is directed toward prevention of hypoventilation and hypoxia. Mild cases of RDS may require only increased humidified oxygen concentrations. Use of continuous positive airway pressure (CPAP) may be required in moderately afflicted infants. Babies with severe cases of RDS require mechanical ventilatory assistance from a respirator (Figure 32–5). Surfactant replacement therapy is now available for infants to decrease the severity of RDS in low-birth-weight newborns (Cotton 1994). Both artificial (Exosurf) and modified natural surfactant (Survanta) are available and have been widely studied. Delivery is through an endotracheal tube, and it may be given either in the delivery room or in the nursery after hospitalization and as indicated by the severity of respiratory distress syndrome. Repeated doses are often required. The most generally reported response to treatment is rapidly improved oxygenation and decreased need of ventilatory support (Cotton 1994). Extracorporeal membrane oxygenation (ECMO) and high-frequency ventilation have been tried when conventional ventilator therapy has not been successful (Nugent 1991). Both of these have specific protocols for eligibility for use and require specially trained nurses and respiratory therapists. In some institutions morphine or fentanyl is used for its analgesic and sedative effects. Sedation may be indicated for infants most likely to have air leak respiratory problems. Use of pancuronium for muscle relaxation in infants with RDS is controversial.

APPLYING THE NURSING PROCESS

Nursing Assessment

Characteristics of RDS the nurse should look for are increasing cyanosis, tachypnea, grunting respirations, nasal flaring, significant retractions, and apnea. Table 32–2 reviews clinical findings associated with respiratory distress in general. The Silverman-Andersen index (Figure 32–6) may be helpful in evaluating the signs of respiratory distress and can be done in the birthing area.

Nursing Diagnosis

Nursing diagnoses that may apply are included in the Nursing Care Plan: Newborn with Respiratory Distress Syndrome on page 996.

Nursing Plan and Implementation

Based on clinical parameters, the neonatal nurse implements therapeutic approaches to maintain physiologic homeostasis and provides supportive care to the newborn with RDS. See Nursing Care Plan: Newborn with Respiratory Distress Syndrome on page 996.

TEACHING MOMENT

In babies with respiratory distress syndrome who are on ventilators, increased urination (determined by weighing diapers) may be an early clue that the baby's condition is improving. As fluid moves out of the lungs into the bloodstream, alveoli open, and kidney perfusion increases, which results in increased voiding. At this point you must monitor chest expansion closely. If chest expansion is increasing, ventilator settings may have to be decreased. Too high a ventilator setting may "blow the lungs," resulting in pneumothorax.

Nursing interventions and criteria for instituting mechanical ventilatory assistance are done per institutional protocol. Methods of transcutaneous monitoring and

TABLE 32-2   Clinical Assessments Associated with Respiratory Distress

Clinical Picture	Significance
Skin Color	
Pallor or mottling	These represent poor peripheral circulation due to systemic hypotension and vasoconstriction and pooling of independent areas (usually in conjunction with severe hypoxia).
Cyanosis (bluish tint)	Depending on hemoglobin concentration, peripheral circulation, intensity and quality of viewing light, and acuity of observer's color vision, this is frankly visible in advanced hypoxia. Central cyanosis is most easily detected by examination of mucous membranes and tongue.
Jaundice (yellow discoloration of skin and mucous membranes due to presence of unconjugated [indirect] bilirubin)	Metabolic alterations (acidosis, hypercarbia, asphyxia) of respiratory distress predispose to dissociation of bilirubin from albumin-binding sites and deposition in the skin and central nervous system.
Edema (presents as slick, shiny skin)	This is characteristic of preterm infants because of low total protein concentration with decrease in colloidal osmotic pressure and transudation of fluid. Edema of hands and feet is frequently seen within first 24 hours and resolved by fifth day in infants with severe RDS.
Respiratory System	
Tachypnea (normal respiratory rate 30–60/minute, elevated respiratory rate 60+/minute)	Increased respiratory rate is the most frequent and easily detectable sign of respiratory distress after birth. This compensatory mechanism attempts to increase respiratory dead space to maintain alveolar ventilation and gas exchange in the face of an increase in mechanical resistance. As a decompensatory mechanism it increases work load and energy output by increasing respiratory rate, which causes increased metabolic demand for oxygen and thus increases alveolar ventilation of an already overstressed system. During shallow, rapid respirations, there is an increase in dead space ventilation, thus decreasing alveolar ventilation.
Apnea (episode of nonbreathing for more than 20 seconds; periodic breathing, a common "normal" occurrence in preterm infants, is defined as apnea of 5–10 seconds alternating with 10–15 seconds of ventilation)	This poor prognostic sign indicates cardiorespiratory disease, CNS disease, metabolic alterations, intracranial hemorrhage, sepsis, or immaturity. Physiologic alterations include decreased oxygen saturation, respiratory acidosis, and bradycardia.
Chest	Inspection of the thoracic cage includes shape, size, and symmetry of movement. Respiratory movements should be symmetrical and diaphragmatic; asymmetry reflects pathology (pneumothorax, diaphragmatic hernia). Increased anteroposterior diameter indicates air trapping (meconium aspiration syndrome).
Labored respirations (Silverman-Anderson chart in Figure 32–6 indicates severity of retractions, grunting, and nasal flaring, which are signs of labored respirations)	Indicates marked increase in the work of breathing.
Retractions (inward pulling of soft parts of the chest cage—suprasternal, substernal, intercostal, subcostal—at inspiration)	These reflect the significant increase in negative intrathoracic pressure necessary to inflate stiff, noncompliant lungs. Infants attempt to increase lung compliance by using accessory muscles. Lung expansion markedly decreases. Seesaw respirations are seen when the chest flattens with inspiration and the abdomen bulges. Retractions increase the work of breathing and O$_2$ need so that assisted ventilation may be necessary due to exhaustion.
Flaring nares (inspiratory dilation of nostrils)	This compensatory mechanism attempts to lessen the resistance of the narrow nasal passage.
Expiratory grunt (Valsalva maneuver in which the infant exhales against a closed glottis, thus producing an audible moan)	This increases transpulmonary pressure, which decreases or prevents atelectasis, thus improving oxygenation and alveolar ventilation. Intubation should not be attempted unless the infant's condition is rapidly deteriorating, because it prevents this maneuver and allows the alveoli to collapse (Lapido 1989).
Rhythmic body movement with labored respirations (chin tug, head bobbing, retractions of anal area)	This is a result of using abdominal and other respiratory accessory muscles during prolonged forced respirations.
Auscultation of chest reveals decreased air exchange with harsh breath sounds or fine inspiratory rales; rhonchi may be present	Decrease in breath sounds and distant quality may indicate interstitial or intrapleural air or fluid.
Cardiovascular System	
Continuous systolic murmur may be audible	Patent ductus arteriosus is a common occurrence with hypoxia, pulmonary vasoconstriction, right-to-left shunting, and congestive heart failure.
Heart rate usually within normal limits (fixed heart rate may occur with a rate of 110–120/minute)	A fixed heart rate indicates a decrease in vagal control.
Point of maximal impulse usually located at fourth to fifth intercostal space, left sternal border	Displacement may reflect dextrocardia, pneumothorax, or diaphragmatic hernia.
Hypothermia	This is inadequate functioning of metabolic processes that require oxygen to produce necessary body heat.
Muscle Tone	
Flaccid, hypotonic, unresponsive to stimuli	These may indicate deterioration in the newborn's condition and possible CNS damage due to hypoxia, acidemia, or hemorrhage.
Hypertonia and/or seizure activity	

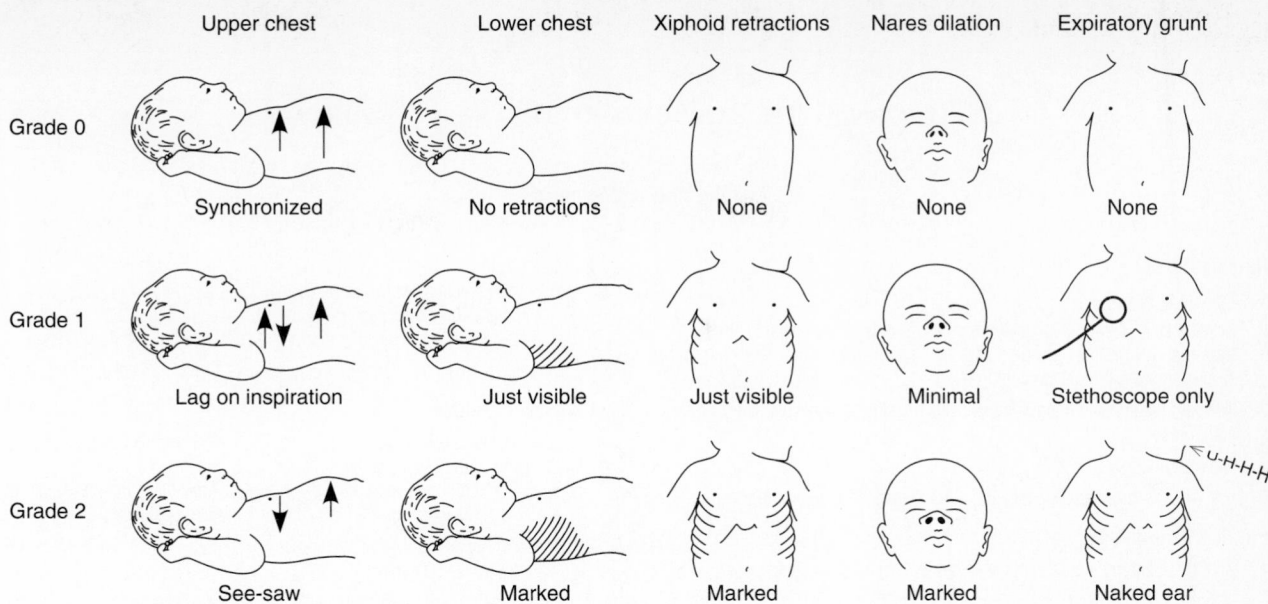

Upper chest | Lower chest | Xiphoid retractions | Nares dilation | Expiratory grunt

Grade 0
Synchronized — No retractions — None — None — None

Grade 1
Lag on inspiration — Just visible — Just visible — Minimal — Stethoscope only

Grade 2
See-saw — Marked — Marked — Marked — Naked ear

FIGURE 32-6 Evaluation of respiratory status using the Silverman-Andersen index. The baby's respiratory status is assessed. A grade of 0, 1, or 2 is determined for each area, and a total score is charted in the baby's record or on a copy of this tool and placed in the chart. SOURCE: Ross Laboratories, nursing inservice aid no 2, Columbus, OH; Silverman WA, Andersen DH: *Pediatrics* 1956; 17:1. Copyright 1956, American Academy of Pediatrics.

nursing interventions are included in Table 32–3 on page 1001. Ventilatory assistance with high-frequency ventilators is a new intervention that shows positive results.

The nursing care of infants on ventilators or with umbilical artery catheters is not discussed here. These infants have severe respiratory distress and are cared for in intensive care nurseries by nurses with advanced knowledge and training.

Evaluation

Anticipated outcomes of nursing care include:

- The risk of RDS is promptly identified, and early intervention is initiated.
- The newborn is free of respiratory distress and metabolic alterations.
- The parents verbalize their concerns about their baby's health problem/survival and understand the rationale behind management of their newborn.

Transient Tachypnea of the Newborn (Type II Respiratory Distress Syndrome or Retained Lung Fluid)

Some newborns, primarily AGA and near-term infants, develop progressive respiratory distress that clinically can resemble RDS. They may have had intrauterine or intra-partal asphyxia due to maternal oversedation, cesarean birth, maternal bleeding, prolapsed cord, breech birth, or maternal diabetes. Transient tachypnea of the newborn results from inadequate clearance of fluid from the lungs. Lung fluid clearance begins before labor and accelerates as labor proceeds. Fluid retained within the alveoli limits the amount of surface available for oxygen exchange. The newborn compensates to some degree by increasing the rate of breathing.

Usually little or no difficulty is experienced at the onset of breathing. However, shortly after admission to a nursery, expiratory grunting, flaring of the nares, and mild cyanosis may be noted in the newborn breathing room air. Tachypnea is usually present by 6 hours of age, with respiratory rates as high as 100 to 140 breaths per minute.

Medical Therapy

The goals of medical management are to identify the type of respiratory distress present and to start treatment.

Initial x-ray findings are sometimes identical to those showing RDS within the first 3 hours. However, radiographs of infants with transient tachypnea usually reveal a generalized overexpansion of the lungs (hyperaeration of alveoli), which is identifiable principally by flattened contours of the diaphragm. Dense streaks (increased vascularity) radiate from the hilar region and represent engorgement of the lymphatics, which clear alveolar fluid upon initiation of air breathing.

Ambient oxygen concentrations of 30–50% usually under an oxyhood may be required initially to correct the

Text continues on page 1000

NEWBORN WITH RESPIRATORY DISTRESS SYNDROME

Nursing Assessment

Nursing History

1. Preterm birth
2. Gestational history, including recent episodes of fetal or intrapartal stress (maternal hypotension, bleeding, maternal and resultant fetal oversedation), or severe fetal lung circulation compromise
3. Newborn history, including birth asphyxia resulting in acute hypoxia, and hypothermia
4. Familial tendency
5. Low Apgar score, requiring bag and mask resuscitation in birthing area

Physical Examination

1. At birth or within 2 hours, rapid development of signs of distress:
   a. Initially tachypnea (over 60 respirations/minute)
   b. Expiratory grunting (audible) or subcostal/intercostal retractions, followed by flaring of nares on inspiration
   c. Cyanosis and pallor
   d. Signs of increased air hunger (apneic spells, hypotonus), rhythmic movement of body and labored respirations, and chin tug

2. Auscultation:
   a. Initially breath sounds may be normal; then decreased air exchange occurs with harsh breath sounds and, upon deep inspiration, rales.
   b. Later a low-pitched systolic murmur indicates patent ductus arteriosus.

3. Increasing oxygen concentration requirements to maintain adequate Po_2 levels

Diagnostic Studies

1. Lung profile to determine lung maturity is done on amniotic fluid (for fetuses predisposed to RDS) as follows:
   - Lecithin/sphingomyelin ratio of 2:1 or more indicates pulmonary maturity.
   - Phosphatidylglycerol (PG): elevated at 35 weeks' gestation

2. Arterial blood gases (indicating respiratory failure): Pao_2 less than 50 mm Hg, and Pco_2 above 60 mm Hg

3. Potassium levels increase as potassium is released from injured alveolar cells.

4. X-ray: diffuse reticulogranular density bilaterally, with air-filled tracheobronchial tree outlined by opaque lungs (air bronchogram); atelectasis/hypoexpansion in severe cases

5. Clinical course worsens first 24–48 hours after birth and persists for more than 24 hours.

6. Dextrostix less than 40 mg %

NURSING DIAGNOSIS: Impaired gas exchange related to inadequate lung surfactant

EXPECTED OUTCOME: Newborn's oxygen requirement and work of breathing will diminish. Newborn's need for assisted ventilation will be noted early.

Nursing Interventions	Rationale
Determine baseline of respiratory effort and ventilatory adequacy: a. Observe chest wall movement. b. Assess skin, mucous membranes for color. c. Estimate degree and equality of air entry by auscultation, and assess arterial blood gases and pH.	*Alveoli of normal infant remain stable during expiration due to presence of surfactant. Alveoli of infant with RDS lack surfactant and collapse with expiration. Values used to determine adequate oxygenation: normal Pao2 50–70 mm Hg. Adequate ventilation: normal Paco2 35–45 mm Hg. Acid-base balance: normal pH 7.35–7.45.*
Maintain on respiratory and cardiac monitors: a. Note rates every 30–60 minutes or more often as indicated by the severity of infant's distress, such as grunting. b. Check and calibrate all monitoring and measuring devices every 8 hours. c. Calibrate oxygen devices to 21% and 100% O_2 concentrations.	*Alveolar atelectasis and intrapulmonary shunting results in poor gas exchange, hypoxemia, hypercarbia, and acid-base derangements.* *Grunting, a compensatory mechanism, increases transpulmonary pressure, overcomes high surface tension, forces and prevents atelectasis, and thus enables improved oxygenation and a rise in Pao2. It is the sound of the glottis closing to stop exhalation of air by forcing it against the vocal cords.*
Provide warmed air 31.7–33.9 C (89–93 F) and humidified (40–60%) oxygen.	*Humidified oxygen prevents mucosal dryness.*
Monitor oxygen concentrations at least every hour.	*Maintains a constant level.*
Administer oxygen by oxygen hood (a small, transparent head hood that contains an oxygen inlet and carbon dioxide outlet) (Figure 32–7).	*Provides a constant oxygen environment. Incubators are not recommended for long-term oxygen delivery because the concentration is difficult to regulate and fluctuates when portholes are opened for care giving.*
Avoid hood touching infant's face.	*Contact with infant's face may cause apnea by stimulating facial nerve.*
Maintain stable oxygen concentration by increasing or decreasing oxygen by 5–10% increments and then obtain arterial blood gases.	*Stable concentration of oxygen is necessary to maintain Pao2 within normal limits (50–70 mm Hg). Sudden increase or decrease in O2 concentration may result in disproportionate increase or decrease in Pao2 due to vasoconstriction in response to hypoxemia.*
Monitor: 1. Color (pink), cyanosis (central or acrocyanosis), duskiness, pallor.	*Observations of clinical conditions are taken serially for trends and changes.*
2. Respiratory effort (evaluation at rest), rate of respirations, patterns (apnea, periodic breathing), quality (easy, unlabored; abdominal, labored), auscultation (site of breath sounds—overall or part of lung fields—describe quality of breath sounds every 1–2 hours), accompanying sounds with respiratory effort (change from previous observations).	*Observations should be taken while infant is receiving oxygen and with any oxygen adjustment.*

NEWBORN WITH RESPIRATORY DISTRESS SYNDROME *continued*

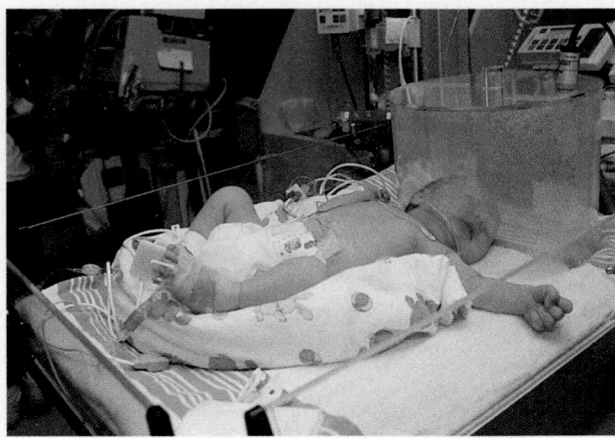

FIGURE 32-7   Infant in oxygen hood.

3. Activity—less active, flaccid, lethargic, unresponsive, increased activity, restless, irritable; inability to tolerate exertion, crying, sucking, or nursing care activity.

4. Circulatory response (evaluate at rest); rate, regularity, and rhythm of heart rate; periods of bradycardia; alterations of blood pressure.

Return O_2 concentration to previous levels if there is deterioration in newborn's condition or a drop below desired transcutaneous oxygen monitor (TCM) levels.

Any deterioration of clinical condition with oxygen adjustments (usually a decrease in ambient oxygen concentration) indicates inability of newborn to compensate for hypoxia.

Repeat arterial blood gases (keep Pao_2 50–70 mm Hg). Gases should be done within 15–20 minutes after any change in ambient O_2 concentration or after inspiratory or expiratory pressure changes.

Record and report clinical observations and action taken.

Maintain stable environment prior to collection of arterial blood gas sample:

1. Maintain constant O_2 concentration at least 15–30 minutes before sample.

2. Avoid any disturbances of infant 15 minutes before gases are drawn.

3. Do not suction.

Accurate arterial blood determinations are essential in management of any infant receiving oxygen because presence or absence of cyanosis is unreliable.
Crying or struggling may cause hyperventilation or breath holding and may increase shunting of blood.
If suction is absolutely necessary, delay blood sample.
Suctioning process may be associated with alterations in oxygenation, and blood gases may not reflect a steady state.

Maintain temperature of sample.

pH should be measured at body temperature.
Increased or decreased temperature will alter pH reading.

Provide arterial blood gas setup (a 3-mL syringe with heparinized solution and a heparinized tuberculin syringe) to obtain blood sample.

Use of temporal, radial, or brachial arteries takes skill, is time-consuming, and may have serious consequences; therefore most common technique for sampling is through umbilical artery catheter.

After blood sample is taken, recheck IV flow through line to assure patency and prevent establishment of clot.

Replace blood used to clear line.

Total blood volume of infant is small; blood removed to clear catheter must be returned to prevent hypovolemia, anemia.

Use heparanized flush solution before restarting IV solution to prevent clots in the line.

With transcutaneous Po_2 or pulse oximeter, monitor continuously or every hour and record. Calibrate sensor each shift, and rotate sensor position every 3–4 hours.

Transcutaneous monitors and pulse oximeter measure percentage of oxygen in inspired air and accuracy of readings. Rotating sensor prevents skin burns.
Transcutaneous electrode sites include chest, abdomen, and inner thigh. Oxygen diffuses through the skin from capillaries directly beneath the skin and can then be measured. Pulse oximeter is preferred because it doesn't produce heat.

Assess need for assisted ventilatory measures. Criteria for assisted ventilation:

1. Apnea

2. Hypoxia (Pao_2 <50 mm Hg)

3. Hypercarbia ($Paco_2$ >60 mm Hg)

4. Respiratory acidosis (pH <7.20)

Have ventilatory support equipment available.

Administer ventilator care per agency protocol.

Application of CPAP or PEEP produces the same stabilization force on alveoli as grunting does and produces same effect—improved oxygenation and rise in Pao_2.

Delivery of CPAP or PEEP can be done only by use of nasal prongs, nasopharyngeal or oral intubation.

NEWBORN WITH RESPIRATORY DISTRESS SYNDROME continued

OUTCOME MET IF:

- Newborn's respirations are 30–60/minute without apnea.
- Newborn shows no visible signs of retractions or nasal flaring.
- Newborn's Pao$_2$ is 50–70 mm Hg.
- Newborn's blood pH is 7.35–7.45.

NURSING DIAGNOSIS: Altered nutrition: Less than body requirements related to increased metabolic needs of stressed infant

EXPECTED OUTCOME: Newborn maintains normal glucose levels, follows normal weight curves, and is tolerating oral feedings.

Nursing Interventions	Rationale
Maintain IV rate at prescribed levels via infusion pump, usually 60–80 mL/kg/day.	This is the needed rate for initial fluid and caloric intake.
Maintain IV rate at prescribed level: a. Record type and amount of fluid infused hourly. Observe vital signs for signs of too-rapid infusion. b. Maintain normal urine output (1–3 mL/kg/hour). Maintain specific gravity of urine between 1.006 and 1.012. Take daily weights.	Fluids are provided to a sick newborn by intravenous route and are calculated to replace sensible and insensible water losses as well as evaporative losses due to tachypnea. Overload of circulatory system by too much or too rapid administration of fluid causes pulmonary edema and cardiac embarrassment that may be fatal.
Manage route of IV administration.	Greater nutritional fluid is required because of energy needed to cope with stress.
With umbilical catheter:	Stressed infants are predisposed to hypoglycemia because of increased metabolic demands as well as reduced glycogen stores and decreased ability to convert fat and protein to glucose.
Protect catheter from strain, tension, or dislodgement. Restrain as necessary. Keep catheter and stopcock on top of bed linens so they are easily visible.	
Observe for occlusion of vessels by clot and for vasospasm: discoloration of skin, discoloration of toes or feet (blanching or cyanosis).	Vasospasm in unwrapped foot will be relieved by treatment, and the discoloration will disappear and toes will be pink.
If discoloration occurs, contralateral foot may be wrapped with warm cloth, but this is controversial. Removal of catheter is preferred.	If discoloration persists, clot may be occluding vessel—catheter must be removed, or loss of extremity is possible.
Observe for signs of infection or sepsis: temperature instability, drainage, redness or foul odor from cord, lethargy, irritability, vomiting, poor feeding, hypotonia.	
Peripheral IV in scalp or extremity vein:	
Prepare equipment, insert IV in vein, and restrain infant.	
Place peripheral IV in vein (which doesn't pulsate).	If vessel chosen is an artery, it pulsates. Very small arteries may not pulsate, and arterial area will blanch if saline is infused.
	Ability to aspirate blood and/or easily inject small amount of saline indicates patent IV. Infiltration is evaluated by area of edema and redness about site, inability to obtain blood on aspiration, or difficulty in injecting solution.
Provide total parenteral nutrition (TNP) when indicated.	TPN is used as nutritional alternative if bowel sounds are not present and infant remains in acute distress.
Advance, based on tolerance, from intravenous to gastrointestinal feedings. Gavage or nipple feedings are used, and IV is used as supplement (discontinued when oral intake is sufficient) (see Procedure 31–1).	If IV discontinued before oral intake is established, baby will not receive adequate calories. Formula or breast milk stimulate GI hormones necessary for a functional absorptive GI tract. Avoid complications associated with nutrition by IV route only.
Provide adequate caloric intake: consider amount of intake, type of formula, route of administration, and need for supplementation of intake by other routes.	Calories are essential to prevent catabolism of body proteins, and metabolic acidosis due to starvation or inadequate caloric intake.
Monitor for hypocalcemia.	Hypocalcemia and hypoglycemia result from delayed or inadequate caloric intake and stress.
Monitor for hypoglycemia: Dextrose/chemstrip below 40 mg/dL, urine screening for glucose.	

OUTCOME MET IF:

- Newborn does not have >2%/day weight loss or a drop of more than 10–15% of birth weight.
- Newborn maintains >40 mg/dL of glucose level.
- Newborn progresses to and tolerates oral feedings.
- Newborn's urine output is 1–3 mL/kg/hour.

NEWBORN WITH RESPIRATORY DISTRESS SYNDROME *continued*

NURSING DIAGNOSIS: Risk for infection related to invasive procedures

EXPECTED OUTCOME: Newborn will be free of infection.

Nursing Interventions	Rationale
See section on sepsis nursing care.	*Decreased lung expansion predisposes to atelectasis and secondary superimposed infections.*
Provide for infection control by cleaning and replacing nebulizers/humidifiers at least every 24 hours.	*The warm, moist environment found in incubators and with oxygen equipment promotes growth of microorganisms.*
Use sterile tubing and replace every 24 hours. Use sterile distilled water.	

OUTCOME MET IF:
- Newborn maintains a stable temperature in the range of 36.5–37.5 C (97.7–99.4 F).
- Newborn maintains a stable BP with an average of 74/47 mm Hg in the term infant and 64/39 mm Hg in the premature.
- Newborn has no periods of apnea.
- Newborn has no pallor, duskiness, or cyanosis.

NURSING DIAGNOSIS: Ineffective thermoregulation related to increased respiratory effort secondary to RDS

EXPECTED OUTCOME: Newborn will maintain a stable temperature.

Nursing Interventions	Rationale
Observe infant for temperature instability and signs of increased oxygen consumption and metabolic acidosis.	*Cold stress increases oxygen consumption and promotes pulmonary vasoconstriction. This leads to hypoxis and acidosis, which further depress surfactant production.*
Maintain neutral thermal environment.	*Cold stress leads to chemical thermogenesis (burning brown fat to maintain body temperature), which increases oxygen needs in an already compromised infant.*
Use servocontrol to maintain constant temperature regulation.	
Warm all inspired gases. Place a thermometer in the oxygen hood and document the temperature of the delivered gas with vital signs.	*Cold air/oxygenation blown in face of newborn is source of cold stress and is stimulus for increased consumption of oxygen and glucose and increased metabolic rate.*
	Oxyhood and incubator temperature should be maintained in the infant's neutral thermal range.
Place thermometer in-line of ventilatory circuit and maintain inspired gas at 34–35 C.	
Use heat shields for small infants.	*Heat shields will prevent heat loss by convection and reduce insensible water losses.*

OUTCOME MET IF:
- Newborn's temperature remains stable within range of 36.5–37.5 C (97.7–99.4 F).
- Newborn maintains glucose levels greater than 40 mg/dL.
- No cyanosis, bradycardia, or apnea occurs.

NEWBORN WITH RESPIRATORY DISTRESS SYNDROME *continued*

Essential Nursing Activities to Achieve Outcomes

Newborn Assessments

Assess newborn every 1–2 hours or more frequently, depending on infant's distress.

1. Take vital signs:
   a. Respiratory rate of 30–60 breaths per minute without apnea.
   b. Temperature stable in range of 36.5–37.5 C (97.7–99.4 F).
   c. Pulse 120–160 bpm.
   d. Blood pressure: average reading term infant 74/47; preterm infant 64/39.
2. Inspect for color (cyanosis, pallor, duskiness).
3. Assess for respiratory effort (grunting, nasal flaring, retractions).
4. Assess for breath sounds.
5. Assess activity level and tolerance.
6. Assess need for assisted ventilatory measures.
7. Check oxygen concentration levels.
8. Assess I&O.
9. Check patency of IV lines.
10. Assess feeding tolerance.
11. Assess for signs of infection: temperature instability, lethargy, poor feeding, hypotonia.
12. Check blood work: Pao_2, Pco_2, pH, and hematocrit and hemoglobin.
13. Assess for hypocalcemia and hypoglycemia.

Family Assessments

1. Assess family knowledge level.
2. Assess family support systems.

Interventions

1. Administer humidified oxygen by designated route: oxygen hood, intubation, continuous positive airway pressure (CPAP).
2. Check and calibrate all monitoring and measuring devices.
3. Increase and decrease oxygen concentration by 5–10% increments based on Pao_2 levels.
4. Administer medication per physician order: antibiotics and diuretics.
5. Careful handwashing and attention to infection control.
6. Make time available for answering questions and emotional support for parents.
7. Record and report all clinical observations.

---

hypoxemia. Oxygen requirements usually decrease over the first 48 hours, unlike in infants with RDS, whose oxygen needs increase during this time.

The infant should be improving by 24 to 48 hours, except for modest O_2 dependence (less than 30%). The duration of the clinical course of transient tachypnea is approximately 72 hours. Mild respiratory and metabolic acidosis may be present at 2 to 6 hours.

Radiographs are usually normal within a week, and the infant is well within 2 to 5 days. If progressive deterioration occurs to the extent that assisted ventilation is required, a diagnosis of superimposed sepsis must be considered and treatment measures initiated.

Nursing Care

For nursing actions see the Nursing Care Plan: Newborn with Respiratory Distress Syndrome on page 996.

CARE OF NEWBORN WITH MECONIUM ASPIRATION SYNDROME

The presence of meconium in amniotic fluid indicates an asphyxial insult to the fetus before or during labor unless the baby is in breech position. The physiologic response to asphyxia is increased intestinal peristalsis, relaxation of the anal sphincter, and passage of meconium into the amniotic fluid.

Approximately 10% of all pregnancies will have meconium-stained fluid (Hudak & Jones 1990). This fluid may be aspirated into the tracheobronchial tree by the fetus in utero or during the first few breaths taken by the newborn. This aspiration is called **meconium aspira-**

CRITICAL THINKING IN PRACTICE

You are caring for baby girl Linn, who is a 39-week, AGA female born by repeat cesarean birth to a 34-year-old, G3 now P3 mother. Baby Linn's Apgar scores were 7 and 9 at 1 and 5 minutes. At 2 hours of age, an elevated respiratory rate of 70–80 and mild cyanosis were noted. She is now receiving 30% oxygen and has a respiratory rate of 100–120. The baby's clinical course, chest x-ray, and lab work are all consistent with transient tachypnea of the newborn. Her mother calls you to ask about her baby. She tells you that her last child was born at 30 weeks' gestation, had respiratory distress syndrome requiring ventilator support, and was hospitalized for 6 weeks. She asks you, "Is this the same respiratory distress?" What will you tell her?

Answers can be found in Appendix I.

TABLE 32-3 Transcutaneous Monitors

Type	Function and Rationale	Nursing Interventions
TcPo2 Measures oxygen diffusion across the skin Clark electrode is heated to 43 C (preterm) or 44 C (term) to warm the skin beneath the electrode and promote diffusion of oxygen across the skin surface. Po_2 is measured when oxygen diffuses across the capillary membrane, skin, and electrode membrane (Nugent 1991).	When transcutaneous monitors are properly calibrated and electrodes are appropriately positioned, they will provide reliable, continuous, noninvasive measurements of Po_2, Pco_2, and oxygen saturation. Readings vary when skin perfusion is decreased. Reliable as trend monitor. Frequent calibration necessary to overcome mechanical drift. Following membrane change, machine must "warm up" 1 hour prior to initial calibration; otherwise, after turning it on, it must equilibrate for 30 minutes prior to calibration. When placed on infant, values will be low until skin is heated; approximately 15 minutes required to stabilize. Second-degree burns are rare but can occur if electrodes remain in place too long. Decreased correlations noted with older infants (related to skin thickness); with infants with low cardiac output (decreased skin perfusion); and with hyperoxic infants. The adhesive that attaches the electrode may abrade the fragile skin of the preterm infant. May be used for both pre- and postductal monitoring of oxygenation for observations of shunting.	Use $TcPo_2$ to monitor trends of oxygenation with routine nursing care procedures. Clean electrode surface to remove electrolyte deposits; change solution and membrane once a week. Allow machine to stabilize before drawing arterial gases; note reading when gases are drawn, and use values to correlate. Ensure airtight seal between skin surface and electrode; place electrodes on clean, dry skin on upper chest, abdomen, or inner aspect of thigh; avoid bony prominences. Change skin site and recalibrate at least every 4 hours; inspect skin for burns; if burns occur, use lowest temperature setting and change position of electrode more frequently. Adhesive disks may be cut to a smaller size, or skin prep may be used under the adhesive circle only; allow membrane to touch skin surface at center.
Pulse Oximeter Monitors beat-to-beat arterial oxygen saturation. Microprocessor measures saturation by the absorption of red and infrared light as it passes through tissue. Changes in absorption related to blood pulsation through vessel determine saturation and pulse rate (Nugent 1991).	Calibration is automatic. Less dependent on perfusion than $TcPo_2$ and $TcPco_2$; however, functions poorly if peripheral perfusion is decreased due to low cardiac output. Much more rapid response time than $TcPo_2$—offers "real-time" readings. Can be located on extremity, digit, or palm of hand, leaving chest free; not affected by skin characteristics. Requires understanding of oxyhemoglobin dissociation curve. Pulse oximeter reading of 85% to 90% reflects clinically safe range of saturation. Extreme sensitivity to movement; decreases if average of 7th or 14th beat is selected rather than beat to beat. Poor correlation with extreme hyperoxia.	Understand and use oxyhemoglobin dissociation curve. Monitor readings and correlate with arterial blood gases. Use disposable cuffs (reusable cuffs allow too much ambient light to enter, and readings may be inaccurate).

tion syndrome (MAS). This syndrome primarily affects term, SGA, and postterm newborns and those who have experienced a long labor.

Presence of meconium in the lungs produces a ball-valve action (air is allowed in but not exhaled), so that alveoli overdistend; rupture with pneumomediastinum or pneumothorax is a common occurrence. The meconium also initiates a chemical pneumonitis in the lung with oxygen and carbon dioxide trapping and hyperinflation. Secondary bacterial pneumonias can occur. Clinical manifestations of MAS include (1) fetal hypoxia in utero a few days or a few minutes prior to birth indicated by a sudden increase in fetal activity followed by diminished activity, slowing of fetal heart rate or weak and irregular heartbeat, loss of beat-to-beat variability, and meconium staining of amniotic fluid and (2) presence of signs of distress at birth, such as pallor, cyanosis, apnea, slow heartbeat, and low Apgar scores (below 6) at 1 and 5 minutes. As victims of intrauterine asphyxia, meconium-stained newborns or newborns who have aspirated meconium are often depressed at birth and require resuscitation to establish adequate respiratory effort.

After the initial resuscitation, the severity of clinical symptoms correlates with the extent of aspiration. Many infants require mechanical ventilation at birth due to immediate signs of distress (generalized cyanosis, tachypnea, and severe retractions). An overdistended, barrel-shaped chest with increased anteroposterior diameter is common. Auscultation reveals diminished air movement with prominent rales and rhonchi. Abdominal palpation may reveal a displaced liver caused by diaphragmatic depression resulting from the overexpansion of the lungs. Yellowish staining of the skin, nails, and umbilical cord is usually present.

The chest x-ray film for newborns with MAS reveals nonuniform, coarse, patchy densities and hyperinflation (9- to 11-rib expansion). The densities are associated with focal areas of irregular aeration, some of which appear atelectatic or consolidated while others appear emphysemic. Evidence of pulmonary air leak is frequently present. These infants have serious biochemical alterations, which include (1) extreme metabolic acidosis resulting from the cardiopulmonary shunting and hypoperfusion; (2) extreme respiratory acidosis due to shunting and alveolar hypoventilation; and (3) extreme hypoxia, even in 100% O_2 concentrations and with ventilatory assistance. The extreme hypoxia is also caused by the cardiopulmonary shunting and resultant failure to oxygenate and can lead to persistent pulmonary hypertension of the newborn (PPHN).

Medical Therapy

The combined efforts of the obstetric and pediatric teams are needed to prevent MAS. The most effective form of preventive management is outlined as follows:

1. After the head of the newborn is born and the shoulders and chest are still in the birth canal, first the baby's oropharynx then the nasopharynx are suctioned. (The same procedure is followed with a cesarean birth.) To decrease the possibility of acquired immunodeficiency syndrome (AIDS) transmission, low pressure wall suction is used.

2. If the infant is vigorous and there is thick meconium in the amniotic fluid, the glottis is visualized, and meconium is suctioned from the trachea.

3. If the infant is vigorous and there is only thin meconium in the amniotic fluid, no subsequent special resuscitation is indicated.

4. For any depressed infant (heart rate less than 100 beats per minute or poor respiratory effort with meconium staining), the glottis is visualized and the trachea suctioned (Hudak & Jones 1990).

If the newborn's head is not adequately suctioned on the perineum, respiratory or resuscitative efforts will push meconium into the airway and into the lungs. Stimulation of the newborn should be avoided to minimize respiratory movements. Further resuscitative efforts are undertaken as indicated, following the same principles mentioned in medical therapy for asphyxia earlier in this chapter. Resuscitated newborns should be immediately transferred to the nursery for closer observation. An umbilical arterial line may be used for direct monitoring of arterial blood pressures; blood sampling for pH and blood gases; and infusion of intravenous fluids, blood, or medications.

Treatment usually involves delivery of high ambient oxygen concentrations and controlled ventilation. Low positive end-expiratory pressures (PEEP) are desired to avoid air leaks. Unfortunately, high pressures may be needed to cause sufficient expiratory expansion of obstructed terminal airways or to stabilize airways that are weakened by inflammation so that the most distal atelectic alveoli are ventilated.

Systemic blood pressure and pulmonary blood flow must be maintained. If pulmonary hypertension occurs as a result of this disorder, pulmonary vasodilators are often used to increase the pulmonary blood flow by overcoming the arterioles' vasoconstriction and pulmonary vasospasm, which has created a right-to-left cardiopulmonary shunt. Tolazoline must be used with extreme *caution* because dramatic falls in blood pressure can occur. Tolazoline is usually used in conjunction with dopamine or dobutamine and/or volume expanders to maintain systemic blood pressure.

Full-term newborns over 3.17 kg (7 lb) with respiratory failure who are not responding to ventilator therapy may require treatment with ECMO, a form of heart-lung bypass. This treatment has proven successful for newborns with meconium aspiration, pneumonia, and PPHN who are not responding to traditional treatment modalities (Krause & Younger 1992).

Treatment also includes chest physiotherapy (chest percussion, vibration, and drainage) to remove the debris. Prophylactic antibiotics are frequently given. Bicarbonate may be necessary for several days for severely ill newborns. Mortality in term or postterm infants is very high because the cycle of hypoxemia and acidemia is difficult to break.

APPLYING THE NURSING PROCESS

Nursing Assessment

During the intrapartal period, the nurse should observe for signs of fetal hypoxia and meconium staining of amniotic fluid. At birth the nurse assesses the newborn for signs of distress. During the ongoing assessment of the newborn, the nurse carefully observes for complications such as pulmonary air leaks; anoxic cerebral injury manifested by cerebral edema and/or convulsions; anoxic myocardial injury evidenced by congestive heart failure or cardiomegaly; disseminated intravascular coagulation (DIC) resulting from hypoxic hepatic damage with depression of liver-dependent clotting factors; anoxic renal damage demonstrated by hematuria, oliguria, or anuria; fluid overload; sepsis secondary to bacterial pneumonia; and any signs of intestinal necrosis from ischemia, including gastrointestinal obstruction or hemorrhage.

Nursing Diagnosis

Nursing diagnoses that may apply to the newborn with meconium aspiration syndrome and the infants' parents include the following:

- Impaired gas exchange related to aspiration of meconium and amniotic fluid during birth
- Altered nutrition: Less than body requirements related to respiratory distress and increased energy requirements
- Ineffective family coping related to life-threatening illness in a term newborn

Nursing Plan and Implementation

Initial interventions are aimed primarily at prevention of the aspiration by assisting with the removal of the meconium from the infant's oro- and nasopharynx prior to the first extrauterine breath.

When significant aspiration occurs, therapy is supportive with the primary goals of maintaining appropriate gas exchange and minimizing complications. Nursing interventions after resuscitation should include maintenance of adequate oxygenation and ventilation, temperature regulation, glucose strip test at 2 hours of age to check for hypoglycemia, observation of intravenous fluids, calculation of necessary fluids (which may be restricted in the first 48–72 hours due to cerebral edema), provision of caloric requirements, and monitoring of intravenous antibiotic administration.

Evaluation

Anticipated outcomes of nursing care include:

- The risk of MAS is promptly identified, and early intervention is initiated.
- The newborn is free of respiratory distress and metabolic alterations.
- The parents verbalize their concerns about their baby's health problem and survival and understand the rationale behind management of their newborn.

CARE OF THE NEWBORN WITH PERSISTENT PULMONARY HYPERTENSION

Persistent pulmonary hypertension of the newborn (PPHN) is a serious disorder that may affect near-term, term, or postterm newborns. It has been called persistent fetal circulation (PFC) because the problems that occur are a result of right-to-left (R–L) shunting of blood away from the lungs and through the fetal ductus arteriosus and patent foramen ovale.

The disease was originally described only in newborns who had suffered severe perinatal asphyxia. It has since been associated with several events causing hypoxemia and acidosis: postmaturity syndrome, RDS, MAS, intrapartal asphyxia, pneumonia, Group B streptococcal sepsis, and diaphragmatic hernia. Many fetuses have problems that compromise fetal oxygenation prior to the onset of labor.

During pregnancy, the fetal pulmonary vascular resistance (PVR) is high due to the low oxygen concentration of blood perfusing the lungs and the collapsed position of the lungs. After initiation of respiration at birth the cord is clamped, and systemic vascular resistance increases with the removal of the placental vascular bed. Expansion of the lungs opens the pulmonary circulation. The resulting decrease in the resistance of the pulmonary vasculature encourages flow of blood into the pulmonary vascular bed. With oxygenation of the blood, the pulmonary circulation dilates further, the ductus narrows, and within a very short time the adult circulatory pattern is established.

Depending on the cause, PPHN is classified as primary or secondary. Primary disease results from pulmonary vascular changes prior to birth, which cause abnormally high PVR. Small arteries develop in the lung periphery as alveolar development progresses. Alveolar hypoxia in utero, regardless of the cause, can stimulate precocious muscularization of these arteries. This early abnormal reconstruction of the arteries results in increased PVR, which interrupts the normal sequence of events that take place with the onset of respiration.

Secondary PPHN occurs when the initial sequences of respiration and change in circulation after birth are interrupted by events that increase the PVR. Hypoxemia and acidosis are the most potent stimulants of pulmonary vasoconstriction. The increased vascular resistance increases pulmonary artery pressure, hypoxemia, and R–L shunting of pulmonary blood across fetal shunts. Once this process has begun, it is self-perpetuating: Increasing PVR leads to R–L shunting across the ductus and/or foramen ovale, which leads to increasing hypoxemia, further increasing the PVR. The cycle is difficult to interrupt, and clinical deterioration is rapid (Mag-akat Angeles 1992).

Medical Therapy

The first goal of medical management is early diagnosis of this disorder to halt the progressive worsening of the R–L shunt. Certain diagnostic tests are often used to evaluate the increased PVR and shunting:

1. *Simultaneous preductal and postductal blood gases.* The ductus enters the aorta below the area of the right subclavian and carotid arteries. Thus, preductal blood samples will have a higher oxygen content than postductal samples in infants with significant R–L shunting. Simultaneous pre- and postductal

arterial blood gases demonstrates a 10% difference between the two PaO_2 values (>15 torr difference). Pre- and postductal transcutaneous monitors can also demonstrate ductal shunting.

2. *Hyperoxia-hyperventilation test.* Most PPHN infants have a "critical" PCO_2 level at which vasodilatation occurs. This PCO_2 level may be less than 20 torr in some infants. Once the critical PCO_2 is reached by manual hyperventilation, the resulting metabolic alkalosis causes pulmonary vasodilatation, which reverses the R–L shunt and improves oxygenation. A positive response to the hyperoxia-hyperventilation test is a rise in PaO_2 to greater than 100 torr with hyperventilation. The improved oxygenation can be noted clinically if the infant's mucus membranes turn pink. Arterial gases or transcutaneous monitoring can be used to document the increased PaO_2.

3. *Echocardiography.* This procedure will demonstrate R–L shunting and a prolonged ratio of right ventricular ejection period to right ventricular ejection time in infants with PPHN.

The goal of therapeutic intervention is to lower the PVR and reverse the process of shunting. Maintenance of tissue oxygenation in the presence of R–L shunting presents the greatest therapeutic challenge but is essential to minimize complications.

Initial therapeutic efforts are directed at relieving the precipitating factors, if identified, to reverse the hypertension. In addition ventilatory management is undertaken to decrease the PVR and increase oxygenation. Hyperventilation to achieve respiratory alkalosis (pH >7.55) will cause pulmonary vasodilatation, which increases oxygenation. To prevent respiratory interference and achieve hypocarbia, most infants require paralysis with a neuromuscular blocking agent such as pancuronium (Pavulon) or Fentanyl. Sodium bicarbonate infusion may also be used to achieve metabolic alkalosis. Either respiratory or metabolic alkalosis may decrease pulmonary vascular resistance.

If alkalosis alone does not lead to a decrease in the PVR, pharmacologic vasodilatation may be attempted by administration of intravenous tolazoline. Because tolazoline also induces systemic vasodilatation, dopamine and/or dobutamine may be required to maintain an adequate cardiac output to maintain the blood pressure.

Oxygenation, ventilation, and drug therapy efforts continue until the PaO_2 can be consistently maintained greater than 100 torr. When this level is achieved, reduction of ventilatory support must be made in extremely small increments with intensive surveillance to prevent excessive drops in oxygenation. Alkalosis and hyperoxia may have to be maintained for several days to avoid sudden return of hypoxemia and increased PVR. ECMO is also a therapeutic option for the newborn with PPHN who fails to respond to more conventional therapy.

Nursing Assessment

The nurse assesses for the onset of symptoms, which usually occur in the first 12 to 24 hours of life. Affected newborns exhibit signs of respiratory distress (grunting, nasal flaring, tachypnea), with increased anteroposterior diameter and cyanosis. They typically fail to respond to conventional methods of oxygenation and ventilation. There is significant unexplained hypoxemia in the absence of congenital heart disease. The chest radiograph might show no evidence of pulmonary parenchymal disease (depending on the underlying disease). The hypoxemia and cyanosis associated with PPHN are characteristic of extreme changeability. Marked, rapid changes in PaO_2 and color are seen with agitation, stimulation, or therapeutic intervention (suctioning).

Nursing Diagnosis

The following diagnoses may apply to a newborn with PPHN and the baby's parents:

- Altered oxygen and carbon dioxide exchange related to airway obstruction
- Altered cardiac output related to hypotension
- Ineffective family coping related to life-threatening illness in their full-term newborn

Nursing Plan and Implementation

Prevention of Complications

Infants with PPHN are critically ill and require experienced, skilled nurses to provide optimal care with minimal manipulation. Any disturbance may cause agitation, which leads to hypoxemia. Therefore goals and priorities of care must be established. If a paralyzing agent is used, nursing care includes monitoring the newborn's response to artificial oxygenation and mechanical ventilation. The nurse ensures that the oxygen is delivered in correct amounts and route and records the percentage of oxygen flow. The ventilator settings are checked frequently and recorded every 2 hours. The nurse carefully suctions the endotracheal tube as necessary while assessing the effect of the procedure on the baby's oxygenation and perfusion (see Procedure 32–1: Endotracheal Suctioning). The amount and type of secretions are noted. The nurse carefully assesses arterial blood gases and notifies the clinician if the results are out of the acceptable range. Transcutaneous monitoring is essential for identification of activities that may compromise the infant's status. (Nursing interventions required for transcutaneous monitoring are

Text continues on page 1007

Nursing Action	Rationale
Objective: Minimize potential for pulmonary infection through cross-contamination.	
Assess respiratory status to determine necessity for suctioning.	*Infant should be suctioned only as often as necessary to maintain patent airway and adequate oxygenation.*
Gather all necessary equipment: catheters, suction machine, disposable sterile suction tubing, saline (no preservatives), sterile syringe/needle, and gloves (not powdered). Ensure that gloves, catheters, and liquefying solutions are sterile.	*The healthy individual's lower respiratory tract is free of pathogenic organisms.*
Maintain sterile technique throughout entire suctioning procedure.	
Discard catheter, glove, and saline after each procedure.	*Once equipment is moistened and contaminated with body flora and mucus, it becomes a culture bed for noxious organism growth.*
Set wall suction for not more than 80 mm Hg.	*Mucosal hemorrhages and tissue invagination occur more frequently when higher pressure is used.*
Objective: Alleviate partial or total airway obstruction in support of cell oxygenation.	
Monitor transcutaneous readings during suctioning procedure and supplement with increased oxygen as needed.	*Suctioning physically removes oxygen from airways and mechanically occludes them, therefore diminishing the potential for oxygenation. It usually stimulates coughing and decreases the work of breathing, thereby increasing tissue demand for oxygen.*
Position and immobilize infant.	*Successfully suctioning an alert infant without restraint is difficult. An assistant should be employed to ensure effective, atraumatic suctioning in infants.*
Using sterile technique, don sterile gloves; hook up appropriate suction catheter; lubricate tip.	*Use a "whistle-tip" catheter for respiratory tract suctioning because it tends to be less traumatizing to tissues.*
	Catheter size should be no more than half the size of lumen to be suctioned in order to minimize hypoxemia due to airway obstruction.
Place sterile normal saline in a sterile specimen cup or unit dose plastic container.	*Prelubrication of the catheter is essential to minimize tissue trauma with subsequent obstructive edema.*
If infant is intubated:	
1. Disconnect source of oxygenation from newborn just prior to entry of suction catheter.	*Suction applied while entering airway increases removal of oxygen from airways.*
2. Assistant should stabilize endotracheal tube while suctioning.	*The tube can be easily dislodged during suctioning and increases potential for tissue invagination once the catheter tip passes end of tube. Passing the suction catheter more than 1 cm beyond the endotracheal tube risks damaging the carina and creating pneumothoraces (Figure 32–8).*
3. Insert catheter (without applied suction) into tube the distance from the proximal airway to no more than 1 cm below the end of the endotracheal tube. (This can be determined by noting centimeter markings on tube or by using calculations for oral-carinal distance.)	
NOTE: Measure the appropriate distance along the catheter according to weight. Add the length of the endotracheal tube (ET) that is sticking out of mouth. This is the maximum safe distance for insertion of suction catheter through ET tube.	

Nursing Action	Rationale

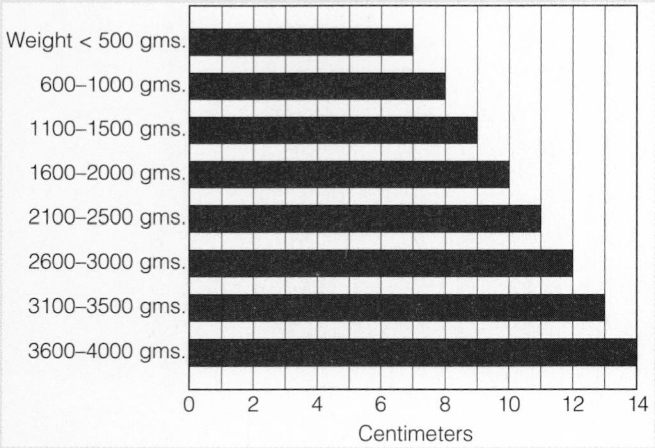

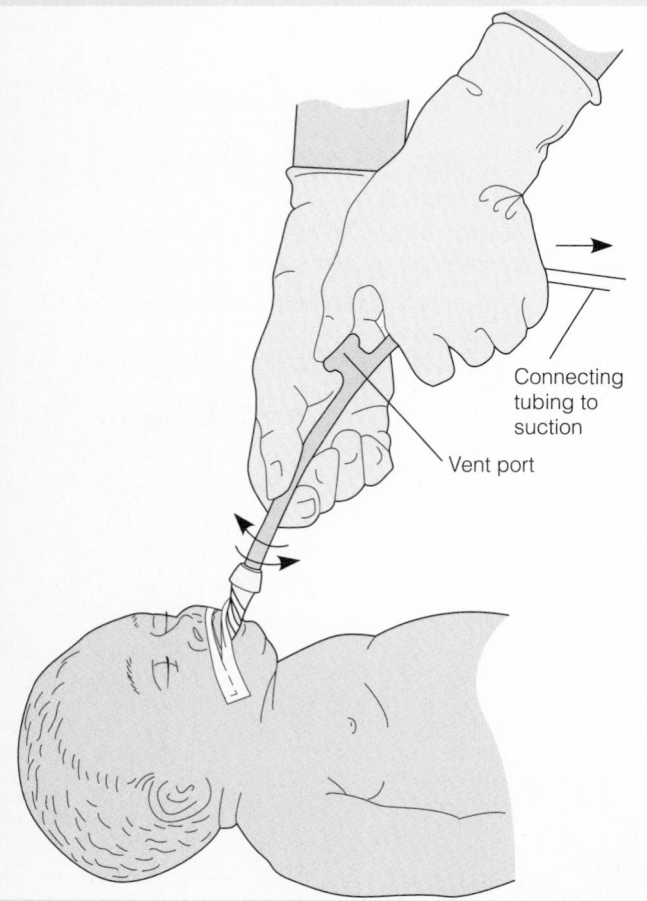

Weight	Centimeters
Weight < 500 gms.	
600–1000 gms.	
1100–1500 gms.	
1600–2000 gms.	
2100–2500 gms.	
2600–3000 gms.	
3100–3500 gms.	
3600–4000 gms.	

0 2 4 6 8 10 12 14
Centimeters

FIGURE 32-8   Safe length for endotracheal suctioning. SOURCE: Anderson D, Chandra R: Pneumothorax secondary to perforation of sequential bronchi by suction catheter. *J Ped Surg* 1976; 11:687.

4. Apply suction by placing thumb of assistive hand over vent port or Y-connector (Figure 32–9).

Placing thumb over venting device closes negative pressure system, which allows atmospheric pressure to push secretions and debris into catheter, facilitating their removal.

Connecting tubing to suction

Vent port

FIGURE 32-9   Suctioning of endotracheal tube. Sterile suctioning is done with the tubing encased in plastic wrap so that the tubing can be used many times without detaching it from the ventilation equipment.

Nursing Action	Rationale
5. Slowly withdraw catheter in a pill-rolling rotation.	*Rotating catheter in a slow, steady fashion maximizes catheter access to secretions while minimizing potential for tissue invagination.*
6. Clear catheter with sterile saline.	
7. After each suction attempt ventilate for a few breaths to reinflate atelectatic areas.	*Hypoxic insult with a drop in Pao2 occurs during suction efforts. Suction, the application of negative pressure to the airway, decreases the pulmonary compliance and tidal volume by 50%.* *Suction creates pulmonary atelectasis.*
8. If tenacious secretions are encountered, instill normal saline with syringe (needleless) into tube prior to suctioning.	*Instillation of normal saline liquefies and loosens secretions.*
If infant is not intubated: After having failed to get infant to cough voluntarily in effective manner, follow procedure for suctioning intubated infant with these exceptions:	*Suctioning to clear airways should be employed only when infant is unable to clear own airways effectively by use of cough reflex. It should be considered a last resort.*
1. Enter airway via nasopharynx, advancing catheter into trachea on inspiration.	*Inspiration opens glottis and tends to entrain catheter along with inspired air. Achieving coordination with inspiration is often quite easy with pediatric clients because they are frequently crying involuntarily during procedure. Instillation of liquefying agents directly into trachea in intubated infant is not possible. Indirect means must be used.*
2. Attempt to liquefy tenacious secretions by humidification via mist tent, face mask, or hand-held nebulizer.	
Objective: Minimize iatrogenic hypoxemia secondary to suctioning.	
Suction only when absolutely necessary.	*Always assess need for suctioning. There should never be standing orders such as "Suction every hour."*
Limit each catheter insertion to no more than 10 seconds. Reoxygenate newborn (monitoring transcutaneous readings) between each insertion and at conclusion of procedure.	*Limiting suction time and frequent oxygenation counterbalance the mechanical obstruction of airway and removal of available oxygen.*
Remove catheter with suction applied as soon as infant begins to cough.	*Holding catheter in airway while infant coughs can deprive infant of needed inspiratory volume at end of cough because of airway obstruction by catheter.*
During procedure assess infant for signs of bradycardia.	*Suctioning can cause vagal response in form of bradycardia, which, if unchecked, can lead to asystole.*
Objective: Record information on infant's record.	
Record infant's response during and after the procedure. Also record amount and type of secretions obtained.	*Provides record of infant's response to procedure.*

discussed in Table 32–3.) Continuous monitoring of vital signs and blood pressure is required, and careful inspection of the skin during positioning is necessary to avoid pressure necrosis.

Pharmacologic vasodilation may lead to precipitous central hypotension, which must be quickly identified and corrected. The infant is monitored for other side effects if tolazoline therapy is used (increased gastric secretion, gastrointestinal bleeding, and oliguria).

The potential for pneumothorax exists with aggressive ventilation. The nurse can best prevent complications by advanced preparation and close monitoring for signs of compromise. (See Pneumothorax later in this chapter for appropriate nursing interventions.)

Many infants suffering PPHN are born at or near term at a time when parents least expect problems—especially life-threatening problems—to occur. The magnitude of the infant's illness and the rapid deterioration may be overwhelming to parents. The nurse should assess their level of understanding and assist them by providing information about their baby's condition and therapies in easily understandable terms.

Attachment becomes difficult when the infant responds poorly to touching (as seen by decreased PaO_2). Parents can be encouraged to talk very softly to their infant because this will usually not compromise the baby's condition. Continuity of nursing care is helpful because it will be less threatening for the parents to relate to a smaller group of nurses.

Evaluation

Anticipated outcomes of nursing care include:

- The risks for development of persistent pulmonary hypertension (PPHN) are identified early, and immediate action is taken to minimize the development of sudden, severe illness.

- The newborn is free of respiratory distress and establishes effective respiratory function.

- The parents verbalize their concerns about their baby's illness and understand the rationale behind the management of their newborn.

CARE OF THE NEWBORN WITH COMPLICATIONS DUE TO RESPIRATORY THERAPY

Oxygen and mechanical ventilation, although required as therapeutic interventions to reduce hypoxia, hypercarbia, ischemia, and infarction to vital organs, may also have harmful effects. The concentrations of ambient oxygen administered to the newborn must be titrated according to oxygen tension within arterial blood. Pulmonary air leaks occur in approximately 15% of mechanically ventilated newborns. In many cases the air leaks are a consequence of injury due to the disease rather than the mechanical ventilation.

Pulmonary Interstitial Emphysema

Pulmonary interstitial emphysema (PIE) is the accumulation of air in lung tissues. Extra-alveolar air collections are most common with use of positive pressure ventilation. Air collections outside the lung are a function of

lung compliance and use of increased pressures to ventilate. Overdistention of alveoli may progress to PIE when rupture occurs and air escapes into the interstitial spaces. Air moves along perivascular spaces but not into the pleural space or mediastinum. As the air collections increase, blood vessels are constricted, and blood gas exchange is impaired. This condition is highly associated with subsequent bronchopulmonary dysplasia (BPD). It may also precede pneumothorax or pneumomediastinum.

Pneumothorax

Pneumothorax, a common complication of respiratory therapy, is an accumulation of air in the thoracic cavity between the parietal and visceral pleura. Pneumothorax occurs when alveoli are overdistended, usually by excessive intra-alveolar pressure and rupture; air then leaks into the thoracic cavity. Excessive intra-alveolar pressure is a result of stiff, noncompliant lungs and the use of assisted positive pressure ventilation with high inspiratory pressure. Meconium aspiration with subsequent obstruction of the airway and a ball-valve phenomenon produce poor lung compliance and trapping of air in the alveoli. Pneumothorax frequently develops as a complication.

Pneumothorax in the newborn causes several physiologic changes: collapse of the lung, compression of the heart and lungs and compromise of venous return to the right heart with mediastinal air, and development of tension in the pleural space. Symptoms of pneumothorax include a sudden, unexplained deterioration in the newborn's condition; decreased breath sounds; apnea; bradycardia; cyanosis; increased oxygen requirements; higher PCO_2; decrease in pH; mottled, asymmetric chest expansion; decreased arterial blood pressure; shocklike appearance; and a shift in the apical cardiac impulses to the side opposite the pneumothorax.

Transillumination of the chest is used for rapid evaluation of pneumothorax. Transillumination is the visualization of light through the air in the affected side (or sides, for bilateral pneumothorax) of the baby's chest. However, x-ray examination is the main method of diagnosing this complication. Follow-up radiographs should always be done to confirm the diagnosis and the extent of the pneumothorax.

Pneumothorax is a life-threatening situation for the neonate and demands immediate removal of the accumulated air. The air is aspirated with a syringe attached to an 18-gauge intercath or 23-gauge butterfly needle and inserted into the second or third intercostal space midclavicular line when the newborn is supine. This procedure is done only as an emergency measure and carries a risk of damaging the lung pleura with needle tracks as the air is evacuated and the collapsed lung reexpands. Only skilled and specifically trained personnel should do this procedure.

For complete resolution of the pneumothorax a No. 10 Fr. chest tube will be placed and connected to continuous negative pressure (10 to 15 cm H_2O) suction with an underwater seal.

Bronchopulmonary Dysplasia

Bronchopulmonary dysplasia (BPD), also called chronic lung disease of prematurity (CLD), most commonly occurs in very compromised low-birth-weight (LBW) infants who require oxygen therapy and assisted mechanical ventilation for the treatment of respiratory distress syndrome. The current diagnostic criterion of needing oxygen at 36 weeks' postconceptual age correlates with significant long-term pulmonary morbidity (Rozycki & Kirkpatrick 1993). It has also been associated with neonatal pneumonia, MAS, PPHN, congenital heart disease (PDA), and other congenital anomalies requiring high levels of ventilatory support. The incidence of BPD is generally reported at 20% of ventilated newborns, but wide variability exists between centers (Abman & Groothius 1994). The cause is multifactorial, and pulmonary immaturity, oxygen toxicity, barotrauma (leading to inflammatory changes and fluid leakage into the interstitial spaces), primary surfactant deficiency, patent ductus arteriosus, pulmonary edema, PIE, low-grade or asymptomatic pulmonary infection with ureaplasma urealyticum, and poor nutrition are all risk factors (Knoppert & Mackanjee 1994).

The process of BPD is one of continuous lung tissue injury and repair, delaying both lung and body growth. Northway and colleagues in 1967 described the pulmonary pathology of BPD as having four stages based on radiographic and clinical findings (Abman & Groothius 1994).

Stage 1 is clinically and radiographically indistinguishable from RDS. Lacking surfactant, the alveoli collapse; the resultant ischemia leads to necrosis of the surrounding tissue and capillaries. The sloughed necrotic material fills the terminal bronchioles, causing mucosal and ciliated cell damage.

In stage 2, severe lung disease, the radiographs progress to a characteristic "whiteout" with opacification of lung fields and indistinguishable cardiac borders. This clinical picture is similar to severe RDS with the complications of PDA and pulmonary edema.

During stage 3, or transition to chronic lung disease, regeneration begins in the lining cells of the bronchioles. Fibrous tissue forms as connective tissue cells proliferate. This leads to distortion and eventual rupture of the alveoli with small amounts of air being trapped in the interstitium. These emphysematous areas surrounded by collapsed alveoli are seen as small cystic light areas on x-ray films. PCO_2 increases despite adequate mechanical ventilation.

Stage 4 involves hypertrophy of the smooth muscles surrounding the bronchi and bronchioles, which leads to narrowing of the airways. During this period the mucus-producing cells also hypertrophy, and the increase in mucus production leads to further airway obstruction. Thick-

ening of the pulmonary arteries and capillary membranes leads to narrowing of these vessels, which causes pulmonary hypertension. Cor pulmonale with right ventricular hypertrophy and cardiomegaly may occur secondary to the pulmonary hypertension. Radiographs show enlargements of the emphysematous areas. In some, especially VLBW, infants only a diffuse haziness of the lung fields accompanied by prolonged oxygen requirements indicate the presence of bronchopulmonary dysplasia.

Medical Therapy

The goals of therapeutic intervention for the newborn with BPD are to provide adequate oxygenation and ventilation, prevent further lung damage, promote optimal nutrition, and give supportive care to ensure adequate rates of growth and development. New therapies, such as exogenous surfactant administration, high-frequency ventilation, and steroids (prenatal and postnatal) may have altered the severity of BPD; but chronic lung disease remains a major clinical problem.

Because of the chronic nature of this disease, therapeutic intervention must be individualized to meet the specific needs of the infant. Of prime importance is maintenance of adequate gas exchange. At each stage of BPD pulmonary pathologic changes interfere with adequate oxygenation and normal ventilation. Ventilatory assistance and increased ambient (environmental) oxygen must be regulated precisely by close monitoring of blood gases to prevent episodic hypoxemia or hyperoxemia and hypercarbia. Antibiotics are indicated for secondary infections. Diuretics and fluid restriction are frequently used to control pulmonary fluid retention and to improve lung function (Abman & Groothius 1994); electrolyte supplements are necessary to offset the results of chronic diuretic therapy. In addition bronchodilators are indicated to decrease airway resistance and to control bronchospasm. Serial echocardiography is used to monitor cardiac response to the chronic pulmonary disease.

APPLYING THE NURSING PROCESS

Nursing Assessment

At each stage of BPD, the infant exhibits recognizable clinical signs that reflect the pulmonary pathologic changes. Nursing assessment is based on a knowledge of these stages.

In stage 1, the infant exhibits typical signs of RDS with audible grunting, nasal flaring, and retractions. Due to the extensive alveolar damage the infant is hypoxic and requires supplemental oxygen and assisted ventilation.

During stage 2, when the cellular debris fills the lumens of the bronchi and bronchioles, the infant has increased pulmonary secretions that may interfere with extubation. With progression to stage 3, the alveoli rupture and the capillary membranes thicken. This leads to separation of the capillaries from the alveoli and impairment of oxygen and carbon dioxide exchange. The infant's oxygen dependency becomes apparent, and he or she begins to retain carbon dioxide, which prevents extubation. Lymphatic distortion leads to pulmonary interstitial fluid retention and evidence of diffuse rales with auscultation.

The hypertrophy of the bronchiolar smooth muscles characteristic of stage 4 increases the airway resistance and the risk of bronchospasm. During this stage, infants will manifest bronchospasm by intermittent wheezing respirations, cyanosis, and continued supplemental oxygen requirements. Marked carbon dioxide retention continues to be a problem, and ventilator dependency may result. Pulmonary fluid retention and mucus production will be manifested by audible rales and rhonchi, secretions, and chronic cough.

Nursing Diagnosis

Nursing diagnoses that may apply to a baby with BPD and the baby's parents include the following:

- Impaired gas exchange related to chronic retention of carbon dioxide and borderline oxygenation secondary to fibrosis of lungs
- Ineffective airway clearance related to chronic intubation and increased secretion secondary to BPD
- Ineffective parental coping related to prolonged hospitalization and decreased opportunities to hold the baby

Nursing Plan and Implementation

Maintenance of Oxygenation

The nurse observes carefully any changes in the newborn's oxygenation. Special attention must be given to maintaining the prescribed oxygen concentration during all activities, especially during periods of stress, such as when the infant is crying; when blood is drawn; while starting an IV; and during an LP, suctioning, chest physiotherapy (CPT), and feeding.

The current goal is to adjust the level of supplemental oxygen to consistently keep O_2 saturations between 92% and 96%, depending on the presence of associated clinical problems such as poor growth, recurrent bradycardia, and pulmonary hypertension (Abman & Groothius 1994). A decrease in the arterial oxygen levels will increase the risk of pulmonary hypertension or cor pulmonale (hypertrophy of the right ventricle of the heart). The nurse obtains blood gases based on the institution's chronic blood gas protocol—for example, every 3 days, 20 minutes after a permanent change in ambient oxygen concentration (FiO_2), or more frequently if the infant experiences increasing respiratory distress or increasing lethargy.

Postural drainage, CPT, and vibration followed by suctioning are carried out with close attention to the baby's tolerance. It is essential to time the care activities with rest periods to avoid fatiguing the infant. The nurse maintains the infant's body temperature because hypothermia or hyperthermia will increase oxygen consumption and may increase oxygen requirements. Positioning on the abdomen helps the baby maintain higher transcutaneous oxygen saturation ($TcPO_2$) and improved ventilation. Providing for adequate nutrition enhances formation of new alveoli and enlargement of the airway diameter.

Monitoring of Medications

Bronchodilators such as theophylline, albuterol, and terbutaline; diuretics; steroids; and electrolyte supplements may be used in the medical management of the BPD infant. Appropriate timing of administration is essential to maintain adequate blood levels. Many of the electrolyte and mineral side effects can be avoided by giving the diuretics every other day. Nephrocalcinosis still remains a problem with high doses of diuretics (Rozycki & Kirkpatrick 1993). The nurse must monitor the infant for toxic effects of the medication and adverse effects of the therapy (for example, electrolyte imbalance, such as hypokalemia, and fractures as a result of diuretic therapy).

Critical Thinking Question

Why is nutrition a critical therapy in BPD?

Provision of Adequate Nutrition

The nurse helps provide adequate nutrition and monitors the amount of calories the newborn ingests and the energy expended during the feeding process. If possible, at least 90 cal/kg/day should be given to the infant, with increases daily to at least 130 cal/kg/day and in some cases up to 200 cal/kg/day (Knoppert & Mackanjee 1994). The more severely ill the baby, the higher the caloric need in order to meet the greater expenditure of energy for survival and healing. As soon as tolerated, a 24 cal/oz formula for preterm infants is started, especially if the baby is on fluid restriction. More oxygen may be required during feeding, and the least energy-consuming feeding method should be used. If the feeding schedule is too stressful, smaller, more frequent feedings may be initiated (Chapter 31).

Providing adequate nutritional intake becomes a major nursing task. Infants with BPD frequently experience negative oral sensations due to suctioning and intubation. These can adversely affect their transition to nipple or spoon feeding. Positioning is often the key to adequate intake and decreasing gastroesophageal reflux (GER). In addition most infants receive numerous, possibly unpalatable, medications with meals. Attempts must be made to include pleasurable activities such as cuddling at

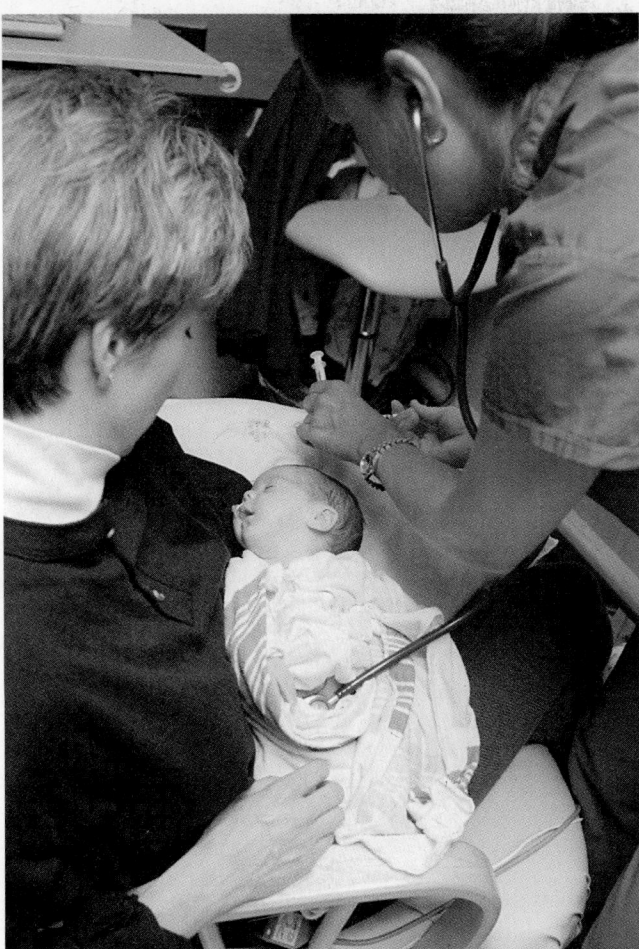

FIGURE 32-10   The baby with BPD has ongoing oxygen and nutritional needs as well as the need for gentle individualized care.

mealtime to develop positive associations with appropriate feeding behaviors (Figure 32–10).

Premature infants with BPD frequently require some type of feeding therapy to help them eat successfully (Kerwin et al 1994).

Prevention of Infection

Infants with BPD are very susceptible to infection; therefore it is important to discourage anyone with early signs of infectious disease from having contact with them. The infant's behavior and vital signs should be monitored for changes that might indicate early developing infection. Changes in color, quantity, or quality of pulmonary secretions are noted and reported. The frequency of CPT and suctioning may need to be increased.

Provision of Sensory Stimulation

Because BPD infants require prolonged hospitalization, the nurse should give special attention to formulating a program of early stimulation activities. Psychomotor delays are seen frequently in these infants and are most likely due in part to prolonged exposure to the hospital

environment. Because their tolerance level for activity is limited due to their illness, activities must be individualized for each baby. Families need to be included in the plans for their baby.

Home Care Preparation

The birth of a premature infant causes significant stress to the family. When the infant develops BPD and the family becomes aware of the implications of chronic illness and prolonged hospitalization, they may experience despair and find it difficult to cope with this added burden. The nurse can help the family cope by encouraging them to take an active role in their infant's daily activities. Their involvement will help dispel feelings of inadequacy and prepare them to perform the unique tasks necessary to meet their infant's needs.

With earlier discharges being encouraged, parents need to be able to demonstrate their ability to provide all the care their child will require at home before leaving the hospital. This may include feeding, adjusting O_2 support, O_2 saturation monitoring, suctioning and airway management, CPT, bathing, and giving medications. They also need to know when to call the home health nurse who is providing care. Parents should be taught how to assess the infant's respiratory condition and understand the BPD baseline respiratory pattern (frequency of respiration, rhythm, degree of retractions, and color of skin and mucous membranes) (Rozycki & Kirkpatrick 1993). Finally, parents must be taught to evaluate their infant's tolerance of activities and to recognize signs of distress due to poor oxygenation, inadequate ventilation, infection, fluid retention, and bronchospasm (Abman & Groothius 1994).

Evaluation

Anticipated outcomes of nursing care include:

- The parents understand the causes, risks, therapy options, and nursing care involved in the care of their newborn with BPD.

- The parents participate in their newborn's care and show attachment behaviors.

- The parents are able to cope with their frustrations and begin to use outside resources as needed.

CARE OF THE NEWBORN WITH COLD STRESS

Cold stress is excessive heat loss resulting in the use of compensatory mechanisms (such as increased respirations and nonshivering thermogenesis) to maintain core body temperature. Heat loss that results in cold stress

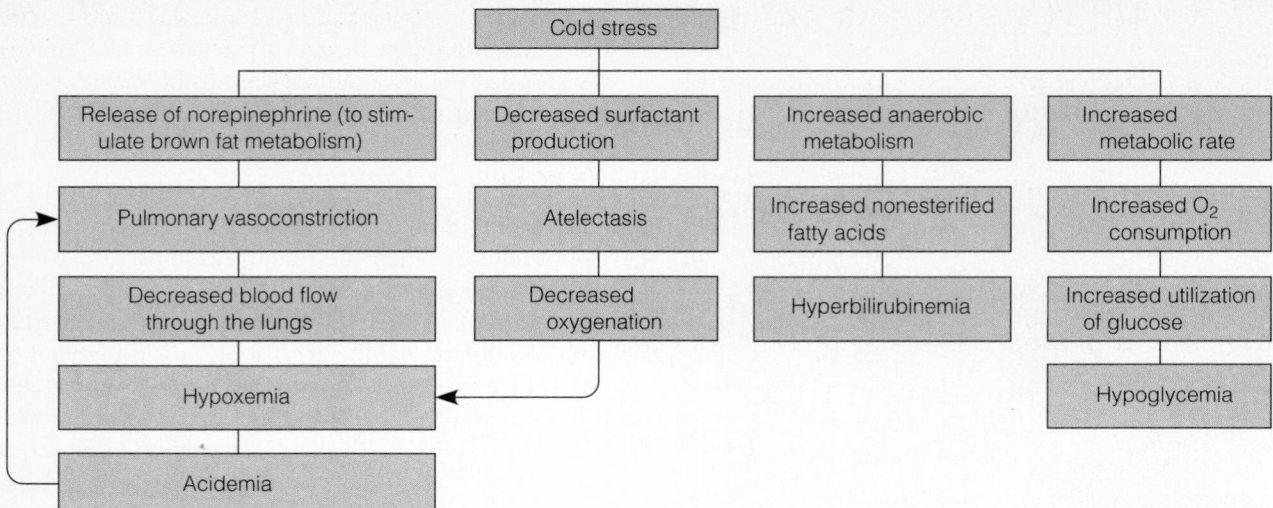

FIGURE 32-11 Cold stress chain of events. The hypothermic, or cold-stressed, newborn attempts to compensate by conserving heat and increasing heat production. These physiologic compensatory mechanisms initiate a series of metabolic events that result in hypoxemia and altered surfactant production, metabolic acidosis, hypoglycemia, and hyperbilirubinemia.

occurs in the newborn through the mechanisms of evaporation, convection, conduction, and radiation. (See Chapter 27 for a detailed discussion of thermoregulation.) Heat loss at birth that leads to cold stress can play a significant role in the severity of RDS and the ultimate outcome for the infant.

The amount of heat lost by an infant depends to a large extent on the actions of the nurse or care giver. Both preterm and SGA newborns are at risk for cold stress because they have decreased adipose tissue, brown fat stores, and glycogen available for metabolism.

As discussed in Chapter 27, the newborn infant's major source of heat production in nonshivering thermogenesis (NST) is brown fat metabolism. The ability of an infant to respond to cold stress by NST is impaired in the presence of several conditions:

- Hypoxemia (PO_2 less than 50 torr)
- Intracranial hemorrhage or any CNS abnormality
- Hypoglycemia (blood glucose < 40 mg/dL)

When these conditions occur, the infant's temperature should be monitored more closely and the neutral thermal environment conscientiously maintained. It is important for the nurse to recognize these conditions and treat them as soon as possible.

The metabolic consequences of cold stress can be devastating and potentially fatal to an infant. Oxygen requirements are raised, glucose use increases, acids are released into the bloodstream, and surfactant production decreases. The effects are graphically depicted in Figure 32–11.

Nursing Care

The nurse observes the baby for signs of cold stress. These include increased movements and respirations, decreased skin temperature and peripheral perfusion, development of hypoglycemia, and possibly development of metabolic acidosis.

Skin temperature assessments are used because initial response to cold stress is vasoconstriction, resulting in a decrease in skin temperature. Therefore, monitoring rectal temperature is not satisfactory. A decrease in rectal temperature means that the infant has long-standing cold stress with decompensation in the newborn's ability to maintain core body temperature.

If a decrease in skin temperature is noted, the nurse determines whether hypoglycemia is present. Hypoglycemia is a result of the metabolic effects of cold stress and is suggested by glucose strip values below 45 mg/mL, tremors, irritability or lethargy, apnea, or seizure activity.

If cold stress occurs, the following nursing interventions should be initiated:

- The newborn is warmed slowly because rapid temperature elevation may cause apnea.
- Skin temperature is monitored every 15 minutes to determine if the newborn's temperature is increasing.
- The newborn is placed and maintained in a neutral thermal environment.

The presence of anaerobic metabolism is assessed and interventions initiated for the resulting metabolic acidosis. Attempts to burn brown fat increase oxygen consumption, lactic acid levels, and metabolic acidosis. Hypoglycemia may be reversed by adequate glucose intake, as described in the following section.

Critical Thinking Question

Why are the physiologic alterations associated with cold stress potentially fatal for an infant?

CARE OF THE NEWBORN WITH HYPOGLYCEMIA

Hypoglycemia is the most common metabolic disorder occurring in IDM, SGA, and preterm AGA infants. The pathophysiology of hypoglycemia differs for each classification.

AGA preterm infants have not been in utero a sufficient time to store glycogen and fat. As a result they have a decreased ability to carry out gluconeogenesis. This situation is further aggravated by increased use of glucose by the tissues (especially the brain and heart) during stress and illness (chilling, asphyxia, sepsis, and RDS).

Infants of White's class A–C or type I diabetic mothers (women with diagnosed or gestational diabetes) have increased stores of glycogen and fat (Chapter 31). Circulating insulin and insulin responsiveness are also higher when compared with other newborns. Because the high glucose loads present in utero stop at birth, the newborn experiences rapid and profound hypoglycemia. The SGA infant has used up glycogen and fat stores because of intrauterine malnutrition and has a blunted hepatic enzymatic response with which to produce and use glucose. Any newborn who is stressed at birth (from asphyxia or cold) also quickly uses up available glucose stores and becomes hypoglycemic.

A recent study, reporting the incidence of hypoglycemia in AGA term newborns to be 7.9% after vaginal birth and 15.7% after cesarean section (without labor), suggests that epidural anesthesia may alter maternal-fetal glucose homeostasis, resulting in hypoglycemia (Cole & Peevy 1994).

Hypoglycemia is defined for all newborns as a blood glucose level below 40 mg/dL (Cornblath & Schwartz 1993). It may also be defined as a glucose oxidase reagent strip below 45 mg/dL, but only when corroborated with laboratory blood glucose (see Procedure 32–2: Glucose Chemstrip Test Using Accu-Check II Machine on page 1014). Glucose reagent strips should not be used by themselves to screen and diagnose hypoglycemia because their results depend on the baby's hematocrit, and there is a wide variance (5–15 mg/dL) when compared to laboratory determinations, especially with blood glucose values of less than 40–50 mg/dL (Cornblath & Schwartz 1993). Newer techniques such as using a glucose oxidase ana-

lyzer or an optical bedside glucose analyzer are more reliable for bedside screening but must also be validated with laboratory chemical analysis. A definitive diagnosis of hypoglycemia is made based on at least two successive values that are significantly low.

Medical Therapy

The goal of medical management includes early identification of hypoglycemia through observation and screening of newborns at risk. The baby may be asymptomatic, or any of the following may occur (Cornblath & Schwartz 1993):

- Lethargy, jitteriness
- Poor feeding
- Vomiting
- Pallor
- Apnea, irregular respirations, respiratory distress, cyanosis
- Hypotonia, possible loss of swallowing reflex
- Tremors, jerkiness, seizure activity
- High-pitched cry

Differential diagnosis of a newborn with nonspecific hypoglycemic symptoms includes determining if the newborn has any of the following:

- CNS disease
- Sepsis
- Metabolic aberrations
- Polycythemia
- Congenital heart disease
- Drug withdrawal
- Temperature instability
- Hypocalcemia

Aggressive treatment is recommended after a single low blood glucose value if the infant shows any of these symptoms. In high-risk infants, routine screening should be carried out at 2, 4, 6, 12, 24, and 48 hours of age or whenever any of the noted clinical manifestations appear.

Provision of adequate caloric intake is important. Early breast or formula feeding is one of the major preventive approaches. If early feeding or intravenous glucose is started to meet the recommended fluid and caloric needs, the blood glucose is likely to remain above the hypoglycemic level. During the first hours after birth, asymptomatic newborns may be given oral glucose, and then another plasma glucose measurement is obtained within 30–60 minutes after feeding. Intravenous infusions of a dextrose solution (5% to 10%) begun immediately after birth should prevent hypoglycemia. Plasma glucose levels are obtained when the parenteral infusion is started. However, in the very small AGA infant

Text continues on page 1016

Nursing Action	Rationale
Objective: Assemble equipment.	All necessary equipment must be ready to ensure that blood sample is collected at time and in manner necessary. Do not use needles because of danger of nicking periosteum. Warm heel for 5–10 seconds prior to heel stick with a warm wet wrap or specially designed chemical heat pad to facilitate blood flow.
Gather the following equipment:	
1. Lancet (do not use needles)	
2. Alcohol swabs	
3. 2 × 2 sterile gauze squares	
4. Small bandage	
5. Glucose strips and bottle	
6. Gloves	
Apply gloves.	To implement universal precautions and prevent nosocomial infections.
Objective: Prepare infant's heel for procedure.	
Select clear, previously unpunctured site. Clean site by rubbing vigorously with 70% isopropyl alcohol swab, followed by dry gauze square. Grasp lower leg and foot so as to impede venous return slightly.	Selection of previously unpunctured site minimizes risk of infection and excessive scar formation. Friction produces local heat, which aids vasodilation. Impeding venous return facilitates extraction of blood sample from puncture site.
Objective: Minimize trauma at puncture site.	
Blot site dry completely before lancing.	Alcohol is irritating to injured tissue and may also produce hemolysis.
With quick piercing motion puncture lateral heel with microlancet, being careful not to puncture too deeply (Figure 32–12). Toes are acceptable sites if necessary.	The lateral heel is the site of choice because it precludes damaging the posterior tibial nerve and artery, plantar artery, and important longitudinally oriented fat pad of the heel, which in later years could impede walking (Figure 32–13). This is especially important for infant undergoing multiple heel stick procedures. Optimal penetration is 4 mm.

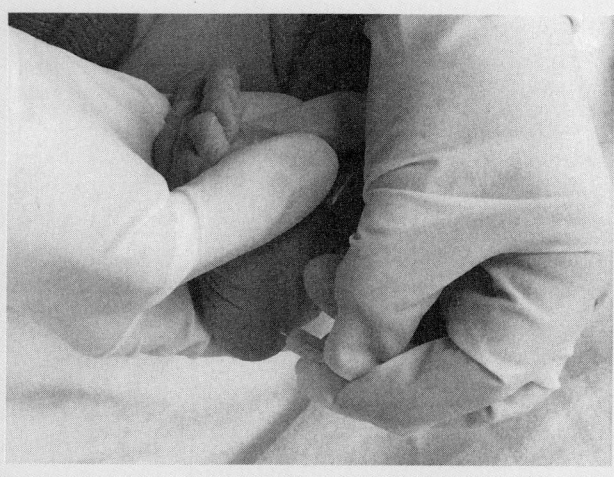

FIGURE 32-12 Glucose chemstrip test (heel stick).

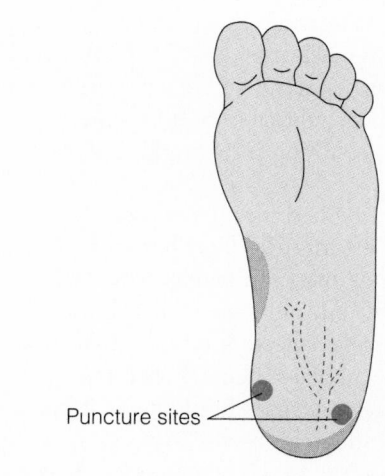

FIGURE 32-13 Potential sites for heel sticks. Avoid shaded areas in order to avoid injury to arteries and nerves in the foot.

Nursing Action	Rationale

Objective: Ensure accurate blood sampling.

After puncture is made, allow first drop of blood to touch both test pads on Chemstrip, making sure to cover both yellow and white squares completely (Figure 32–14).

If Dextrostix reagent strip was used, first drop of blood would be discarded.

Accuracy is best obtained if the first drop of blood is used and only the squares are covered with blood.

The first drop is usually discarded because it tends to be minutely diluted with tissue fluid from puncture.

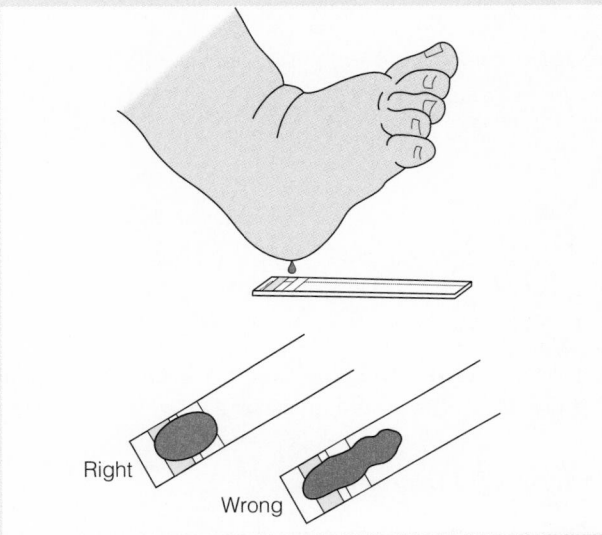

Right

Wrong

FIGURE 32-14   Application of drop of blood to glucose strip.

Objective: Read reagent strip via Accu-Check II machine.

Immediately press the TIME button. The meter will count to 60 but emit 3 high beeps on 57, 58, 59, then one low beep on 60. This is a warning to prepare for wiping the blood from the test strip. Wipe blood from test strips with clean dry cotton ball using moderate pressure when display reads 60. Do not leave any blood on test pad.

Machine will continue to count to 120 seconds. While meter is counting, turn test strip on side, with the test pads facing the on/off button, and insert the reacted test strip into the test strip adaptor. *The strip must be inserted before the display reads* 120.

When the display reads 120, a high beep will be emitted, followed by the blood sugar value on the display screen in mg/dL. Read the blood sugar value on the display screen.

  HHH = blood sugar > 500 mg/dL. Wait an additional minute, take the reacted test strip out of the meter, and compare it to the color chart on the side of the Chemstrip bG vial to estimate results up to 800 mg/dL.

  LLL = blood sugar is lower than the reading range of the instrument (less than 10 mg/dL). Values below 20 mg/dL have not been confirmed clinically.

For accurate results, directions must be followed closely, and reagent strips must be fresh. False low readings may be caused by the following:

1. *Timing*

2. *Blood left on test strip*

Nursing Action	Rationale
Objective: Prevent excessive bleeding. Apply folded gauze square to puncture site and secure firmly with bandage.	*A pressure dressing should be applied to puncture site to stop bleeding.*
Check puncture site frequently for first hour after sample.	*Active infants sometimes kick or rub their dressings off and can bleed profusely from puncture site, especially if bandage becomes moist or is rubbed excessively against crib sheet.*
Objective: Record findings on infant's record.	
Record test results. Report immediately any results under 45 mg/dL or over 175 mg/dL.	*Recording of infant's results assists in identifying possible complications.*

infusions of 10% dextrose solution may cause *hyperglycemia* to develop, requiring an alteration in the glucose concentration. Infants require 6 to 8 mg/kg/minute of glucose to maintain normal glucose concentrations (Cornblath & Schwartz 1993). Therefore an intravenous glucose solution should be calculated based on body weight of the infant, with blood glucose tests to determine adequacy of the infusion treatment (Sunnehag et al 1994).

A rapid infusion of 25% to 50% dextrose is *contraindicated* because it may lead to profound rebound hypoglycemia following an initial brief increase. In more severe cases of hypoglycemia, corticosteroids may be administered. It is thought that steroids enhance gluconeogenesis from noncarbohydrate protein sources (Cornblath & Schwartz 1993).

The prognosis for untreated hypoglycemia is poor. It may result in permanent, untreatable CNS damage or death.

APPLYING THE NURSING PROCESS

Nursing Assessment

The objective of assessment is to identify newborns at risk and to screen symptomatic infants. For newborns who are diagnosed as having hypoglycemia, assessment is ongoing with careful monitoring of glucose values. Glucose strips, urine dipsticks, and urine volume (monitor only if above 1 to 3 mL/kg/hour) are evaluated frequently for osmotic diuresis and glycosuria.

Nursing Diagnosis

Nursing diagnoses that may apply to the newborn with hypoglycemia include the following:

*   Altered nutrition: Less than body requirements related to increased glucose use secondary to physiologic stress
*   Ineffective breathing pattern related to tachypnea and apnea
*   Pain related to frequent heel sticks for glucose monitoring

Nursing Plan and Implementation

When caring for a preterm AGA infant, the nurse should monitor blood glucose levels using glucose strips or laboratory determinations every 4 to 8 hours for the first day of life and daily or as necessary thereafter. The IDM should be monitored hourly for the first several hours after birth because this is when precipitous falls in glucose are most likely. In the SGA newborn, symptoms usually appear between 24 and 72 hours of age; occasionally, they may begin as early as 3 hours of age. Infants who are below the tenth percentile on the intrauterine growth curve should have blood sugar assessments at least every 8 hours until 4 days of age or more frequently if any symptoms develop.

Calculation of glucose requirements and maintenance of intravenous glucose will be necessary for any symptomatic infant with low serum glucose levels. Careful attention to glucose monitoring is again required when the transition from intravenous to oral feedings is attempted. Titration of intravenous glucose may be required until the infant is able to take adequate amounts of formula or breast milk to maintain a normal blood sugar level. This titration is accomplished by decreasing the concentration of parenteral glucose gradually to 5%, then reducing the rate of infusion to 6 mg/kg/minute, then to 4 mg/kg/minute, and slowly discontinuing it over 4 to 6 hours.

The method of feeding greatly influences glucose and energy requirements. In addition the therapeutic nursing measure of nonnutritive sucking during gavage feedings has been reported to increase the baby's daily weight gain and lead to earlier bottle- or breastfeeding and discharge. *Nonnutritive sucking* may also lower activity levels, which allows newborns to conserve their energy stores. Activity can increase energy requirements; crying alone can double the baby's metabolic rate. Establishment and maintenance of a neutral thermal environment has a potent influence on the newborn's metabolism. The nurse pays careful attention to environmental conditions, physical activity, and organization of care and integrates these factors into delivery of nursing care. The nurse identifies any discrepancies between the baby's caloric requirements and received calories and weighs the newborn daily at consistent times, preferably before a feeding. Only then can findings of unusual weight losses or gains, as well as the pattern of weight gain, be considered reliable.

Evaluation

Anticipated outcomes of nursing care include:

- The risk of hypoglycemia is promptly identified, and intervention is started early.

- The newborn's metabolic and physiologic processes are stabilized, and recovery proceeds without sequelae.

CARE OF THE NEWBORN WITH HYPOCALCEMIA

Calcium is transported across the placenta in increasing amounts during the third trimester of pregnancy. This predisposes the infant who is born preterm to have lower serum calcium levels in the newborn period. This risk is increased in the presence of perinatal asphyxia, trauma,

RESEARCH IN PRACTICE

Investigators have conducted limited research on the physiologic responses of premature infants to pain. Bonnie Stevens and Celeste Johnston designed a study to evaluate how premature babies' behavioral states and the severity of their illnesses might influence their physiologic response to a heel stick procedure.

The authors collected data on 124 infants who exhibited the following characteristics: born at 32 to 34 weeks' gestation, 5 days or less since birth, no major congenital or neurologic abnormalities, and no need for surgery or a respirator. Data collected included heart rate, oxygen saturation, intracranial pressure (ICP), behavioral states, and physiologic stability score or severity of illness index. The researchers documented 89% interrater reliability for the behavioral state assessment using a random sample of 30 infants. They also established content, criterion, and construct validity for the Physiologic Stability Index (PSI) that they used.

Data were collected during four phases of a heel lance: (1) baseline, or first 60 seconds, (2) warming of heel, or second 60 seconds, (3) heel stick, or next 15 seconds, and (4) heel squeezing, or last 30 seconds. Results showed significant increases in the infants' maximun heart rate and ICP and decreases in minimum oxygen saturation during two (overlapping) periods: between baseline and stick, and between baseline and squeeze. However, a significant multivariate interaction effect of behavioral state by PSI group indicates that a combination of these two factors may impact physiologic measures not predictable when examining the factors separately. Specifically, a significant difference ($F[15.354] = 2.21$. $p < .01$) was found between the behavioral states and the physiologic responses. The significance resulted from differences in maximum heart rate between infants in quiet-sleep and quiet-awake or active-awake states and oxygen saturation variability between infants in quiet-awake and active-awake states.

Clinical Application of Study

The impact of the severity of a premature infant's illness on the baby's physiologic response to pain could not be determined by this study. However, the behavioral states of the babies studied did influence their physiologic responses. As the authors note, these premature babies are organized enough to feel and respond to a tissue-damaging stimulus.

SOURCE: Stevens B, Johnston C: Physiologic responses of premature infants to a painful stimulus. *Nurs Res* 1994; 43(4):226.

and hypotonia and with the use of bicarbonate in treating acidosis. IDMs, infants of mothers with hypoparathyroidism or chronic renal failure, and infants on furosemide therapy are also at higher risk for hypocalcemia. Low calcium levels are a common occurrence in the intrapartally asphyxiated newborn during the first 2–3 days of life because of a delay in oral feedings, which results in less intestinal absorption of calcium. Hypocalcemia is also associated with the practice of administering low-calcium or calcium-free intravenous therapy management and exchange transfusions. Late onset hypocalcemia can occur if the baby is fed formulas with an inappropriate calcium/phosphorus ratio.

Serum calcium levels should be monitored in at-risk newborns. Normal serum calcium levels range from 8.0 to 10.5 mg/dL. **Hypocalcemia** refers to serum calcium levels less than 6 mg/dL, less than 7 mg/dL with symptoms, or ionized calcium concentrations less than 3–3.5 mg/dL (Glomella 1994). Some institutions use ionized levels as high as 4 mg/dL as their diagnostic marker.

Medical Therapy

Identification of hypocalcemia by screening at-risk newborns is the first consideration of preventive management. Initial treatment of symptomatic hypocalcemia is intravenous therapy. Intravenous 10% calcium gluconate may be administered as a continuous infusion or in intermittent slow pushes. Intravenous push doses of calcium gluconate should not exceed 2 mL/kg at any one time. Doses may be repeated as necessary three or four times in 24 hours.

Maintenance calcium will be given either parenterally or orally. Oral calcium glubionate or calcium gluconate may be used for maintenance. Low-phosphorus milk may be used in the treatment of asymptomatic hypocalcemia.

Treatment for hypocalcemia is usually necessary for only 4 or 5 days unless other complications exist. Calcium levels should be monitored every 12 to 24 hours, and the dose should be tapered off gradually.

Nursing Care

Nursing assessment is aimed at identifying at-risk newborns, monitoring serum calcium levels, and closely observing for symptoms.

Schedules for screening serum calcium levels for various at-risk groups have been recommended and are as follows: IDMs at 6, 12, 24, and 48 hours of age; infants suffering from intrapartal asphyxia at 3, 6, and 12 hours of age; preterm newborns less than 1000 g at 6 hours; and preterm newborns between 1000 g and 1500 g at 12 hours of age. Healthy preterm newborns greater than

1500 g who are taking milk feedings need not be monitored.

The symptoms of hypocalcemia are nonspecific and are seen in conjunction with other disorders. The following signs and symptoms of acute hypocalcemia may be observed:

- Apnea
- Cyanotic episodes
- High-pitched cry
- Slight tremors of extremities, jitteriness, hyperreflexia
- Seizures (local or generalized)
- Abdominal distention
- Edema
- Arrhythmias
- Heightened sensitivity to sensory stimuli

The following signs and symptoms of chronic hypocalcemia may be observed:

- Apnea
- Bone demineralization and elevated alkaline phosphatase levels (rickets), resulting in rib and long bone fractures

The nurse must keep four precautions in mind when administering calcium gluconate intravenously:

1. When giving an intravenous push, calcium must be injected very slowly over a period of at least 10 minutes or no more than 1 mL per minute. The heart rate must be monitored, and if bradycardia or other cardiac arrhythmias occur, the infusion must be discontinued immediately.

2. When calcium is administered as a continuous drip, the heart rate must also be monitored constantly. The calcium infusion should be discontinued immediately if bradycardia develops.

3. The intravenous site must be observed closely for signs of infiltration because calcium is very damaging to the tissues. If extravasation at the infusion site occurs, necrosis and sloughing of the tissue are likely.

4. If the calcium is administered through an umbilical arterial catheter, the tip of the catheter should be far enough from the heart that calcium is not injected directly into the heart. If an umbilical venous catheter is used, the tip must be in the inferior vena cava to avoid necrosis of the liver.

Continued observation and monitoring of serum levels will be required during the transition from intravenous to oral maintenance therapy and again when calcium supplementation is tapered off.

CARE OF THE NEWBORN WITH JAUNDICE

The most common abnormal physical finding in newborns is **jaundice** (icterus neonatorium). Jaundice develops from the deposit of yellow pigment *bilirubin* in lipid tissues as described in Chapter 27. Fetal unconjugated bilirubin is normally cleared by the placenta in utero, so total bilirubin at birth is usually less than 3 mg/dL unless an abnormal hemolytic process has been present. Postnatally, the infant must conjugate bilirubin (convert a lipid-soluble pigment into a water-soluble pigment) in the liver.

The rate and amount of conjugation of bilirubin depend on the rate of hemolysis, the bilirubin load, the maturity of the liver, and the presence of albumin-binding sites. A normal, healthy, full-term infant's liver is usually mature enough and producing enough glucuronyl transferase that the total serum bilirubin concentration does not reach a *pathologic* level (above 12 mg/dL in the blood). However, *physiologic jaundice* remains a common problem for the term newborn and may require treatment with phototherapy. Physiologic jaundice is due to the shorter newborn red cell life span, slower uptake by the liver, a lack of intestinal bacteria, as well as poorly established hydration. Conjugation is also somewhat impaired in the newborn due to low levels of glucuronyl transferase in the liver and because a larger portion of bilirubin is also reabsorbed by the bowel and hydrolyzed back to unconjugated bilirubin. Physiologic jaundice differs from pathologic jaundice (described next), in which any one of a wide range of other pathologic processes intervenes to increase bilirubin levels. (See discussion of bilirubin conjugation pathway in Chapter 27.)

Pathophysiology

In pathologic jaundice, bilirubin reaches higher levels at specific times after birth than in physiologic jaundice, and the newborn is at increased risk for potential complications. One cause of this **hyperbilirubinemia,** or elevated bilirubin level, is an excess of RBCs to be broken down. This can occur due to enclosed hemorrhage, as in a cephalhematoma, extensive bruising, or polycythemia. Infections, both bacterial and viral, may produce hemolysis and can be associated with hyperbilirubinemia. Infectious processes, hypoxia, and acidosis may also decrease liver function, leading to hyperbilirubinemia. Neonatal hepatitis, atresia of the bile ducts, and gastrointestinal atresia all can alter bilirubin metabolism and excretion. Other causes of hyperbilirubinemia include hemolytic disease of the newborn, in which incompatibility in the Rh or ABO system leads to hemolysis of red cells and hyperbilirubinemia. Abnormal red cell shape is another hemolytic cause of hyperbilirubinemia because these cells may have abnormal, less deformable cell membranes and a shorter than normal life span. Other factors such as enzyme deficiency and drug effects may also produce hemolysis.

The bilirubin level at which an infant is harmed varies, but at that level the infant may suffer neurologic defects and possibly death. Although the exact mechanism of bilirubin-produced neuronal injury is uncertain, it is known that high concentrations of unconjugated bilirubin can be neurotoxic (Hansen 1994). Unconjugated bilirubin has a high affinity for extravascular tissue such as fatty tissue (subcutaneous tissue) and the brain. Thus bilirubin not bound to albumin can cross the blood-brain barrier. Various conditions decrease albumin binding, including hypothermia, hypoglycemia, asphyxia, and neonatal medications such as indomethacin. Maternal use of sulfa drugs or salicylates interferes with conjugation or with serum albumin–binding sites by competing with bilirubin for these sites.

Once the unconjugated bilirubin crosses the blood-brain barrier, it can damage cells of the CNS and produce kernicterus or bilirubin encephalopathy (Hansen 1994). **Kernicterus** (meaning "yellow nucleus") usually refers to the deposition of unconjugated bilirubin in the basal ganglia of the brain and to permanent neurological sequelae of untreated hyperbilirubinemia. The classic bilirubin encephalopathy of kernicterus most commonly found with Rh and ABO blood group incompatibility is virtually unknown today due to aggressive treatment with phototherapy and exchange transfusions.

Kernicterus, usually associated with unconjugated bilirubin levels of over 20 mg/dL in normal term infants and over 10 mg/dL in *sick* preterm newborns, has been noted at lower levels at autopsy in both types of babies. The risk of kernicterus at lowered bilirubin levels has been associated with asphyxia, acidosis, and low serum albumin levels. Current therapy can reduce the incidence of kernicterus encephalopathy but cannot distinguish all infants who are at risk. Complications associated with severe bilirubin encephalopathy include athetosis, hearing loss, limited upward gaze, and, in some, intellectual deficits (Shapiro 1994).

Causes of Hyperbilirubinemia

A primary cause of hyperbilirubinemia is **hemolytic disease of the newborn** secondary to Rh incompatibility or ABO incompatibility. Thus the pregnant woman who is Rh negative or who has blood type O should be asked about outcomes of any previous pregnancies and her history of blood transfusion. Prenatal amniocentesis with spectrophotographic examination may be indicated in some cases of Rh incompatibility. Cord blood from newborns is evaluated for bilirubin level, which normally does not exceed 5 mg/dL. Newborns of Rh negative and O blood type mothers are carefully assessed for blood type status, appearance of jaundice, and levels of serum bilirubin.

Isoimmune hemolytic disease, also known as **erythroblastosis fetalis,** occurs when an Rh− mother is pregnant with an Rh+ fetus and transplacental passage of maternal antibodies takes place. Maternal antibodies enter the fetal circulation, then attach to and destroy the fetal RBCs. The fetal system responds by increasing red blood cell production. Jaundice, anemia, and compensatory erythropoiesis result. There is a marked increase in immature red blood cells (erythroblasts), hence the designation erythroblastosis fetalis.

Hydrops fetalis occurs when markedly severe RBC destruction takes place and results in multiple organ system failure. Anemia is severe, and often cardiomegaly with severe cardiac decompensation and hepatosplenomegaly occur. Severe generalized massive edema (*anasarca*) and generalized fluid effusion into the pleural cavity (hydrothorax), pericardial sac, and peritoneal cavity (ascites) develop. Jaundice is not present until the newborn period because the bili pigments for the fetus are being excreted through the placenta into the maternal circulation. Severe anemia is also responsible for hemorrhage in pulmonary and other tissues. The hydropic hemolytic disease process is also characterized by hyperplasia of the adrenal cortex and pancreatic islets. Hyperplasia of the pancreatic islets predisposes the infant to neonatal hypoglycemia similar to that of IDMs. These infants also have increased bleeding tendencies due to associated thrombocytopenia and hypoxic damage to the capillaries. Hydrops is a frequent cause of intrauterine death among infants with Rh disease. In certain rare cases the grossly enlarged hydropic fetus and placenta may cause uterine rupture.

ABO incompatibility, more common but less severe than Rh disease, may result in jaundice, although it rarely results in hemolytic disease severe enough to be clinically diagnosed and treated. The most common incompatibility occurs when the mother is type O and the fetus is type A or B. It can also occur if the mother is type A and the fetus is B or if the mother is B and the fetus is type A. Hepatosplenomegaly may be found occasionally in newborns with ABO incompatibility, but hydrops fetalis and stillbirth are rare.

The best treatment for hemolytic disease is prevention. Prenatal identification of the fetus at risk for Rh or ABO incompatibility will allow prompt treatment. See Chapter 19 for discussion of in utero management of this condition.

Certain prenatal and perinatal factors predispose the newborn to hyperbilirubinemia. During pregnancy, maternal conditions that predispose to neonatal hyperbilirubinemia include hereditary spherocytosis, diabetes, intrauterine infections, gram-negative bacilli infections that stimulate production of maternal isoimmune antibodies, drug ingestion (such as sulfas, salicylates, novobiocin, and diazepam), oxytocin, hypothyroidism, and

excess doses of vitamin K. In addition, hepatitis from intrauterine infections or metabolic liver disease elevates the level of conjugated bilirubin. Newborns with congenital biliary duct atresia have a poor prognosis; about two-thirds have an inoperable lesion and die during the first 3 years of life.

The prognosis for a newborn with hyperbilirubinemia depends on the extent of the hemolytic process and the underlying cause. Severe hemolytic disease may result in fetal or early neonatal death from the effects of anemia—cardiac decompensation, edema, ascites, and hydrothorax. Hyperbilirubinemia may lead to kernicterus. The resultant neurologic damage may be responsible for cerebral palsy, mental retardation, sensory difficulties, or, to a lesser degree, perceptual impairment, delayed speech development, hyperactivity, muscle incoordination, or learning difficulties.

Medical Therapy

The goals of medical management are prompt identification of infants at risk for jaundice based on perinatal and neonatal history, laboratory tests to identify the cause of the jaundice, and prompt treatment to prevent the neurologic damage that can result from hyperbilirubinemia.

When one or more of the predisposing factors is present, laboratory determination should be made of the maternal and neonatal blood types for Rh or ABO incompatibility. Other necessary laboratory evaluations are Coombs' test, serum bilirubin levels (direct and total), hemoglobin, reticulocyte percentage, white cell count, and positive smear for cellular morphology.

Neonatal hyperbilirubinemia must be considered pathologic if any of the following criteria are met:

1. Clinically evident jaundice in the first 24 hours of life

2. Serum bilirubin concentration rising by more than 5 mg/dL per day

3. Total serum bilirubin concentrations exceeding 12.9 mg/dL in term infants or 15 mg/dL in preterm babies (because preterm newborns have less subcutaneous fat, bilirubin may reach higher levels before it is visible.)

4. Conjugated bilirubin concentrations greater than 2 mg/dL

5. Persistence of clinical jaundice beyond 7 days in term infants or beyond 14 days in preterm infants

Initial diagnostic procedures are aimed at differentiating jaundice resulting from increased bilirubin production, impaired conjugation or excretion, increased intestinal reabsorption, or a combination of these factors. The Coombs' test is performed to determine whether jaundice is due to Rh or ABO incompatibility.

If the hemolytic process is due to Rh sensitization, laboratory findings reveal the following: (1) an Rh positive newborn with a positive Coombs' test, (2) increased erythropoiesis with many immature circulating red blood cells (nucleated blastocysts), (3) anemia, in most cases, (4) elevated levels (5 mg/dL or more) of bilirubin in cord blood, and (5) a reduction in albumin-binding capacity. Maternal data may include an elevated anti-Rh titer and spectrophotometric evidence of fetal hemolytic process.

The indirect Coombs' test measures the amount of Rh positive antibodies in the mother's blood. Rh positive red blood cells are added to the maternal blood sample. If the mother's serum contains antibodies, the Rh positive red blood cells will agglutinate (clump) when rabbit immune antiglobulin is added, and the test results are labeled positive.

The direct Coombs' test reveals the presence of antibody-coated (sensitized) Rh positive red blood cells in the newborn. Rabbit immune antiglobulin is added to the specimen of neonatal blood cells. If the neonatal red blood cells agglutinate, they have been coated with maternal antibodies, and the rest result is positive.

If the hemolytic process is due to ABO incompatibility, laboratory findings reveal an increase in recticulocytes. The resulting anemia is usually not significant during the newborn period and is rare later on. The direct Coombs' test may be negative or mildly positive; the indirect Coombs' test may be strongly positive. Infants with a positive direct Coombs' test have increased incidence of jaundice with bilirubin levels in excess of 10 mg/dL. Increased numbers of spherocytes (spherical, plump, mature erythrocytes) are seen on a peripheral blood smear. Increased numbers of spherocytes are not seen on smears from Rh disease infants.

Regardless of the cause of hyperbilirubinemia, management of these infants is directed toward alleviating anemia, removing maternal antibodies and sensitized erythrocytes, increasing serum albumin levels, reducing serum bilirubin levels, and minimizing the consequences of hyperbilirubinemia. Early discharge of newborns from birthing centers has significantly influenced the diagnosis and management of neonatal jaundice, increasing the emphasis on outpatient and home care management (Gartner et al 1994).

Therapeutic methods of management of hyperbilirubinemia include phototherapy, exchange transfusion, infusion of albumin, and drug therapy. If hemolytic disease is present, it may be treated by phototherapy, exchange transfusion, and drug therapy. When determining the appropriate management of hyperbilirubinemia due to hemolytic disease, the three variables that must be taken into account are the newborn's (1) serum bilirubin level, (2) birth weight, and (3) age in hours. If a newborn has hemolysis with an unconjugated bilirubin level of 14 mg/dL, weighs less than 2500 g (birth weight), and is 24 hours old or less, an exchange transfusion may be the best management. However, if that same newborn is over 24 hours old, which is past the time where an increase in bilirubin would occur due to pathologic causes, pho-

totherapy may be the treatment of choice to prevent the possible complications of kernicterus. Ahlfors (1994) recommends using the bilirubin/albumin ratio to determine when an exchange transfusion therapy should be used. The ratio can quantify bilirubin-albumin binding and the unbound bilirubin concentration in the serum.

Phototherapy

Phototherapy is the exposure of the newborn to high-intensity light. It may be used alone or in conjunction with exchange transfusion to reduce serum bilirubin levels. Exposure of the newborn to high-intensity light (a bank of fluorescent light bulbs or bulbs in the blue-light spectrum) decreases serum bilirubin levels in the skin by facilitating biliary excretion of unconjugated bilirubin. This occurs when light absorbed by the tissue converts unconjugated bilirubin into two isomers called photobilirubin. The photobilirubin moves from the tissues to the blood by a diffusion mechanism. In the blood it is bound to albumin and transported to the liver. It moves into the bile and is excreted into the duodenum for removal with feces without requiring conjugation by the liver. In addition, the photodegradation products formed when light oxidizes bilirubin can be excreted in the urine. Phototherapy plays an important role in preventing a rise in bilirubin levels but does not alter the underlying cause of jaundice, and hemolysis may continue to produce anemia. Currently, there is no evidence that healthy term infants without a pathologic cause for the jaundice are at risk for brain damage, even at levels in the 20–24 mg/dL range (Newman & Maisels 1992).

It is generally accepted that phototherapy should be started at 4 to 5 mg/dL below the calculated exchange level for each infant. Sick newborns of less than 1000 g should have phototherapy instituted at a bilirubin concentration of 5 mg/dL. Many authors have recommended initiating phototherapy "prophylactically" in the first 24 hours of life in high-risk, very-low-birth-weight infants (Dennery et al 1995). Sick preterm infants who are at least 1500 g should have phototherapy instituted when the bilirubin level is 10 mg/dL. Any newborn with a bilirubin level of 20 mg/dL or above may need an exchange transfusion if illness or associated conditions are present (Dennery et al 1995) (Table 32–4).

An effective alternative method of delivering phototherapy to the term newborn is placing a fiberoptic blanket attached to a halogen light source around the trunk of the newborn (American Academy of Pediatrics 1994). The light stays on at all times, and the newborn is accessible for care, feeding, and diaper changes. The eyes are not covered. Fluid and weight loss are not complications of this system. Furthermore, it makes the infant accessible to the parents and is less alarming to parents than standard phototherapy (Tan 1994). The blanket is being used for home care by many institutions and pediatricians.

| TABLE 32-4 | Management of Jaundice in Low-Birth-Weight Infants |

	Indirect Bilirubin Concentrations					
Birth Weight	**5–6 mg/dL**	**7–9 mg/dL**	**10–12 mg/dL**	**12–15 mg/dL**	**15–20 mg/dL**	**>20 mg/dL**
≦1000 g	Phototherapy	⟶	Exchange transfusion*	⟶		
1001–1500 g	Observe and repeat BR	Phototherapy	⟶	Exchange transfusion	⟶	
1501–2000 g	Observe and repeat BR	⟶	Phototherapy	⟶	Exchange transfusion	⟶
>2000 g	Observe	Observe and repeat BR	Phototherapy (<2500 g)	Phototherapy (>2500 g)	⟶	Exchange transfusion

*Exchange if albumin binding is saturated or if serum indirect BR continues to rise. BR = bilirubin

SOURCE: Cashore W, Stern L: The management of hyperbilirubinemia. *Clin Perinatol* June 1984; 11(2):353.

Exchange Transfusion

Exchange transfusion is the withdrawal and replacement of the newborn's blood with donor blood. It is used to treat anemia with red blood cells that are not susceptible to maternal antibodies, remove sensitized red blood cells that would be lysed soon, remove serum bilirubin, and provide bilirubin-free albumin and increase the binding sites for bilirubin. In Rh incompatibility, fresh (under 2 days old) group O, Rh negative "low-titer" whole blood or washed packed red blood cells reconstituted with fresh frozen plasma is chosen. This type of blood contains no A or B antigens or Rh antigens; therefore the maternal antibodies still present in the newborn's blood will not cause hemolysis of the transfused blood. Packed cells are used if the infant is anemic. Citrate-phosphate-dextrose (CPD) blood is preferred because it presents less of an acid load to the infant.

In case of ABO incompatibility group O with Rh-specific cells and low titers of anti-A and anti-B donor blood is used, not the infant's blood type, because donor blood contains no antigens to further stimulate maternal antibodies. Every 4 to 8 hours after the transfusion, serum bilirubin determinations are made. Repeat exchange may be necessary if the bilirubin level exceeds 20 mg/dL or the exchange level for that infant. Daily hemoglobin estimates should be obtained until stable, and hemoglobin determinations done every 2 weeks for 2 months are valuable.

APPLYING THE NURSING PROCESS

Nursing Assessment

Assessment is aimed at identifying prenatal and perinatal factors that predispose to development of jaundice and identifying jaundice as soon as it is apparent. Clinically, ABO incompatibility presents as jaundice and occasion-

ally as hepatosplenomegaly. Hydrops is rare. Hemolytic disease of the newborn is suspected if the placenta is enlarged, if the newborn is edematous with pleural and pericardial effusion plus ascites, if pallor or jaundice is noted during the first 24 to 36 hours, if hemolytic anemia is diagnosed, or if the spleen and liver are enlarged. The nurse carefully notes changes in behavior and observes for evidence of bleeding. If laboratory tests indicate elevated bilirubin levels, the nurse checks the newborn for jaundice about every 2 hours and records observations.

To check for jaundice in lighter-skinned babies the nurse should blanch the skin over a bony prominence (forehead, nose, or sternum) by pressing firmly with the thumb. After pressure is released, if jaundice is present, the area appears yellow before normal color returns. The nurse should check oral mucosa and the posterior portion of the hard palate and conjunctival sacs for yellow pigmentation in darker-skinned babies. Assessment in daylight gives best results because pink walls and surroundings may mask yellowish tints, and yellow light makes differentiation of jaundice difficult. The time of onset of jaundice is recorded and reported. If jaundice appears, careful observation of the increase in depth of color and the infant's behavior is mandatory.

The newborn's behavior is assessed for neurologic signs of bilirubin encephalopathy, which are rare but may include hypotonia, diminished reflexes, lethargy, seizures, or opisthotonic posturing.

Nursing Diagnosis

Nursing diagnoses that may apply are included in the Nursing Care Plan: Newborn with Jaundice.

Nursing Plan and Implementation

Promotion of Effective Phototherapy and Exchange Transfusion

Ideally, the entire skin surface of the newborn is exposed to the light. Minimal covering may be applied over the

Text continues on page 1027

NEWBORN WITH JAUNDICE

Nursing Assessment

Nursing History

Maternal

1. ABO incompatibility and Rh negative status

2. Maternal disease such as diabetes; or presence of infection such as syphilis, cytomegalovirus, rubella, or toxoplasmosis; or presence of familiar blood dyscrasias such as spherocytosis or G-6-PD deficiency

3. Medications: Novobiocin, sulfonamides, and salicylates interfere with conjugation or compete for serum albumin-binding sites

4. Intrapartal stress

5. Number and outcome of previous pregnancies and the current health status of other children

6. Prior treatment with Rhogam

Paternal

1. Rh factor—negative or positive

Birth

1. Enlarged placenta (larger than one-seventh of newborn's weight)

2. Delayed clamping of umbilical cord

Newborn

1. Gestational age

2. Enclosed hemorrhage, hematoma, large bruises, or intracranial bleeding

3. Bacterial and/or viral infections (can affect liver and thus decrease glucuronyl transferase activity)

4. Polycythemia (central hematocrit of 65% or more)

5. Biliary atresia, cystic fibrosis

6. Congenital hypothyroidism

7. Conditions that decrease available albumin-binding sites:
   a. Fetal or neonatal asphyxia decreases binding affinity of bilirubin to albumin.
   b. Chilling and hypoglycemia create fatty acids to compete for binding sites.
   c. Preterm newborns tend to have lower serum albumin levels and therefore less albumin to bind to.

Physical Examination

1. Generalized edema with pleural and pericardial effusion

2. Pallor or jaundice noted in first 24–36 hours

3. May have enlargement of spleen or liver

4. Changes in behavior (lethargy, irritability), tremors

5. Dark, concentrated urine

6. Hypoactive bowel sounds

7. Hypotonia

8. Presence of hematomas or large bruises (assess for other signs of enclosed bleeding)

9. Excessive ecchymosis or petechiae

10. Meconium passage may be delayed

Diagnostic Studies

1. Coombs' test—direct on baby, indirect on mother's blood

2. Total bilirubin level

3. Indications for exchange transfusion: in ABO incompatibility, serum bilirubin levels >20 mg/dL (full-term) and 15 mg/dL (preterm); in Rh incompatibility, serum bilirubin >20 mg/dL (term), >15 mg/dL (large preterms), and >13 mg/dL (<1250 g preterms)

4. Total serum protein (provides measure of binding capacity)

5. CBC to assess anemia and polycythemia

6. Peripheral smear to evaluate red blood cells for immaturity or abnormality

7. Blood glucose

8. Reticulocyte count

9. Kleihauer-Betke test (detects fetomaternal hemorrhage)

10. Transcutaneous jaundice meter

NURSING DIAGNOSIS: Risk for injury related to predisposing factors associated with hyperbilirubinemia

EXPECTED OUTCOME: Newborns at risk for jaundice and with early signs of jaundice will be identified.

Nursing Interventions	Rationale
Evaluate baby's history for predisposing factors for hyperbilirubinemia.	*Early identification of risk factors enables the nurse to monitor babies for early signs of hyperbilirubinemia. Acidosis, hypoxia, hypothermia, and such increase the risk of hyperbilirubinemia at lower bilirubin levels.*
Observe color of amniotic fluid at time of rupture of membranes.	*Amber-colored amniotic fluid is indicative of hyperbilirubinemia.*
Assess baby for developing jaundice in daylight if possible.	*Early detection is affected by nursing environment. Artificial lights (with pink tint) may mask beginning of jaundice.*
1. Observe sclera.	*Most visible sign of hyperbilirubinemia is jaundice noted in skin, sclera, or oral musosa. In light-skinned babies, onset is first seen on face.*
2. Observe skin color and assess by blanching.	*Blanching the skin leaves a yellow color immediately after pressure is released.*
3. Check oral mucosa, posterior portion of hard palate, and conjunctival sacs for yellow pigmentation in dark-skinned newborns.	*Underlying pigment of dark-skinned people may normally appear yellow.*

OUTCOME MET IF:
- Bilirubin levels are <12 mg/dL.

NEWBORN WITH JAUNDICE *continued*

NURSING DIAGNOSIS: Risk for injury related to reabsorption of bilirubin secondary to decreased stooling

EXPECTED OUTCOME: Newborn is passing stools.

Nursing Interventions	Rationale
Initiate feedings as soon as possible, at least within 4–6 hours after birth or per protocol.	*Early feeding stimulates digestive enzymes involved in establishing gut bacterial flora and decreased enterohepatic circulation.*

OUTCOME MET IF:
- Newborn passes meconium stool within first 24 hours and continues stooling.
- Bowel sounds are auscultated in all four quadrants.
- Newborn starts feeding within 4–6 hours.

NURSING DIAGNOSIS: Fluid volume deficit secondary to phototherapy

EXPECTED OUTCOME: Newborn will be adequately hydrated.

Nursing Interventions	Rationale
Offer feedings every 2–4 hours. Do not skip feedings.	*Adequate hydration increases peristalsis and excretion of bilirubin.*
Provide 25% extra fluid intake. Offer water/formula between breast- or bottle-feedings.	*Replace fluid/calorie losses due to watery stools if under phototherapy.*
Assess for dehydration:	*Phototherapy treatment may cause liquid stools and increased insensible water loss, which increases risk of dehydration.*
1. Poor skin turgor	
2. Depressed fontanelles	
3. Sunken eyes	
4. Decreased urine output	
5. Weight loss	
6. Changes in electrolytes	
Weigh daily. Report signs of dehydration.	
Administer IV fluids. Monitor flow rates. Assess insertion site for signs of infection.	*IV fluids may be used if baby is dehydrated or in presence of other complications. IV may be started if exchange transfusion is to be done.*
Monitor I&O: Weigh diapers before discarding. Check specific gravity every 8 hours. Record urine color and frequency. Record quantity and characteristics of stools.	*Prevents fluid overload.*

OUTCOME MET IF:
- Newborn has good skin turgor.
- Newborn has clear amber urine of 1–3 mL/kg/hour.
- Newborn has six to eight wet diapers per day.
- Newborn maintains weight.

NURSING DIAGNOSIS: Risk for injury related to use of phototherapy

EXPECTED OUTCOME: Newborn will show no signs of injury from phototherapy.

Nursing Interventions	Rationale
Cover newborn's eyes with eye patches while under phototherapy lights. Cover testes/penis of male infants.	*Protects retina from damage due to high-intensity light, and testes from damage from heat.*
Make certain that eyelids are closed prior to applying eye patches. Ensure patches do not slip down over nose.	*Prevents corneal abrasions. Blocked nose causes upper airway obstruction and apnea.*
Remove newborn from under phototherapy and remove eye patches during feedings.	*Provides visual stimulation and facilitates attachment behaviors.*

NEWBORN WITH JAUNDICE continued

Nursing Interventions	Rationale
Inspect eyes every 8 hours for conjunctivitis, drainage, and corneal abrasions due to irritation from eye patches.	Prevents or facilitates prompt treatment of purulent conjunctivitis.
Administer thorough perianal cleansing with each stool or change of perianal protective covering.	Frequent stooling increases risk of skin breakdown. Prevents infection.
Provide minimal coverage of diaper area based on agency protocol.	Provides maximal exposure. Shielded areas become more jaundiced, so maximum exposure is essential.
If using paper face mask, remove nose strip.	Metal strip can burn baby's skin when heated by the lights.
Avoid the use of oily applications on the skin.	
Reposition baby every 2 hours.	Provides equal exposure of all skin areas and prevents pressure areas.
Observe for bronzing of skin.	Bronzing is related to use of phototherapy with increased direct bilirubin levels or liver damage; may last 2–4 months.
Place baby approximately 18 inches from light source.	Ensures correct exposure to the phototherapy lights.
Place Plexiglas shield between baby and light.	Decreases change of hyperthermia. Absorbs ultraviolet irradiation.
Monitor baby's skin and core temperature frequently until temperature is stable.	Hypothermia and hyperthermia are common complications of phototherapy. Hypothermia results from exposure to lights, subsequent radiation and convection losses.
Check axillary temperature with readings on servocontrolled unit on incubator.	Hyperthermia may result from the increased environmental heat.
Regulate incubator temperature as needed.	Additional heat from phototherapy lights frequently causes a rise in the baby's and the incubator's temperatures. Fluctuations in temperature may occur in response to radiation and convection.

OUTCOME MET IF:
- Newborn has no corneal irritation.
- Newborn maintains a stable temperature.
- Newborn has no skin breakdown.

NURSING DIAGNOSIS: Sensory/perceptual alterations related to neurologic damage secondary to kernicterus

EXPECTED OUTCOME: Newborn's neurologic status will be within normal limits.

Nursing Interventions	Rationale
Monitor any neurologic/behavioral changes in baby by taking vital signs every 2 hours. Report any changes promptly.	Baby may develop green, watery stools and green urine due to excretion of bilirubin byproducts.
Closely assess infant's daily patterns to detect notable changes in food ingestion, bowel and urine and sleeping and waking rhythms, irritability.	Changes in biologic rhythms caused by phototherapy are unclear and may indicate signs of worsening condition.
Report signs of worsening condition (kernicterus):	Deposition of bilirubin in brain leads to development of symptoms of kernicterus.
1. Hypotonia, lethargy, poor sucking reflex, hypertonicity	Note: Treatment may be more aggressive in presence of neonatal complications such as asphyxia, respiratory distress, metabolic acidosis, hypothermia, low serum protein, sepsis, signs of CNS deterioration (Maisels 1994).
2. Spasticity and opisthotonus	
3. Temperature instability	
4. Gradual appearance of extrapyramidal signs	
5. Impaired or absent hearing	
Monitor laboratory studies as indicated:	
1. Direct and indirect bilirubin	
2. CO_2	
3. Reticulocyte count	
4. Hematocrit and hemoglobin, total serum protein	

OUTCOME MET IF:
- Newborn shows no signs of hypotonia, hypertonicity, lethargy, or poor sucking reflex.

NEWBORN WITH JAUNDICE continued

NURSING DIAGNOSIS: Knowledge deficit related to lack of information about care of newborn with hyperbilirubinemia

EXPECTED OUTCOME: Parents understand the process and treatment of jaundice.

Nursing Interventions	Rationale
Provide explanation of: 1. Newborn's condition	*Parents may not understand what is happening or why.*
2. Signs of jaundice (example: yellow tinge to skin or sclera) and importance of reporting them to the health care team	*Parents know when to report recurrence of jaundice and importance of follow-up.*
3. Treatment modalities, causative and contributing factors of jaundice and hyperbilirubinemia	*Physician preference of treatment modalities may vary. Parents may not understand why their newborn is not receiving a treatment that another with the same condition is receiving.*
4. Reasons that mother may be asked to cease breastfeeding temporarily	*The etiology of breast milk jaundice remains uncertain. The serum bilirubin levels begin to fall within 48 hours after discontinuation of breastfeeding.* *Opinions of physicians vary regarding the need for discontinuing breastfeeding.*
5. Role of pumping. Help mother pump her breasts to maintain her milk supply. If breastfeeding is temporarily discontinued, assess mother's knowledge of pumping her breasts, and provide information and support as needed.	*Mother may need support and information to restart breastfeeding.*
6. Equipment being used and changes in bilirubin levels. Allow parents an opportunity to ask questions; reinforce or clarify information as needed.	

OUTCOME MET IF:
- Parents verbalize understanding of disease process, signs and symptoms of jaundice to report to health care provider, need for phototherapy, need for safety measures during phototherapy, and reasons for possible temporary cessation of breastfeeding.

NURSING DIAGNOSIS: Risk for altered parenting related to parenting a newborn with jaundice

EXPECTED OUTCOME: Parents will provide care and stimulation for their newborn.

Nursing Interventions	Rationale
Encourage parents to provide tactile stimulation during feeding and diaper changes.	*Newborn has normal needs for tactile stimulation.*
Provide cuddling and eye contact during feedings and talk to baby frequently.	*Provides comfort and decreases sensory deprivation.*
Encourage parents to come into nursery to bring baby to mother's room for feedings and to touch their baby. Provide opportunities for parents to express feelings.	*Presence of equipment may discourage parents from interacting with newborn.*

OUTCOME MET IF:
- Parents are involved in the care of their baby and the bonding process occurs.
- Parents demonstrate two or more physical interactions with baby: touch baby, hold baby close, attempt to comfort baby, kiss baby.
- Parents demonstrate two or more social interactions with baby: good eye contact, call baby by name, make positive comments about baby, ask questions about baby, ask questions about newborn care, and talk to baby.

Essential Nursing Activities to Achieve Outcomes

Immediately After the Birth

1. Identify newborns at risk: Evaluate maternal factors, birth factors, and neonatal factors.
2. Obtain blood work, including neonatal blood type and Rh (especially if mother type O or Rh−), glucose levels, direct Coomb's test, and CBC.
3. Assess for presence of hematomas or large bruises.

Ongoing Assessments

1. Observe newborn in daylight. Assess sclera, skin color by blanching and inspection, and oral mucosa in dark-skinned newborns.
2. Take vital signs every 2 hours.
3. Assess for jaundiced coloring, petechiae, pallor, hematoma, bruising, lethargy, poor sucking reflex, temperature instability, hypotonia, hypertonicity, adequate stooling and voiding, and seizures.

Interventions

1. Initiate feedings as soon as possible.
2. Continue feedings every 2–4 hours.
3. Frequent assessments for jaundice.

Photototherapy

1. Check light intensity with an irradiance meter.
2. Safety measures:
   a. Use eye patches while under lights; remove at least every 6 hours to inspect eyes for irritation.

2. Safety measures *continued:*
   b. Ensure maximum skin exposure with only genitals covered.
   c. Reposition every 2 hours to prevent pressure areas and maximize exposure.
   d. Monitor skin and core temperature to detect hypo- or hyperthermia.
   e. Monitor intake and output.
   f. Observe for signs and symptoms of dehydration.
   g. Note that the newborn requires additional fluids to compensate for increased water loss through skin and stools.
   h. Keep parents well informed; answer all questions.
   i. Accurately record all assessment data.

genitals and buttocks to expose maximum skin surface while still protecting the bedding from soiling. Phototherapy success is measured every 12 hours or daily by serum bilirubin levels. The lights must be turned off while drawing blood for serum bilirubin levels. Because it is not known if phototherapy injures the delicate eye structures, particularly the retina, the nurse applies eye patches over the newborn's closed eyes during exposure to phototherapy lights (Figure 32–15). Phototherapy is discontinued and the eye patches are removed at least once per shift to assess the eyes for the presence of conjunctivitis. Patches are also removed to allow eye contact during feeding (for social stimulation) or when parents are visiting (to promote parental attachment).

The irradiance level at the skin determines the effectiveness of the phototherapy. The desired level of irradiance is 5 to 6 microwatts per square centimeter per nonometer. Most phototherapy units will provide this

level of irradiance 42 to 45 cm below the lamps. Irradiance levels can be increased slightly as indicated. The nurse can use a photometer to measure and maintain desired levels.

The newborn's temperature is monitored to prevent hyperthermia or hypothermia. The newborn will require additional fluids to compensate for the increased water loss through the skin and loose stools. Loose stools and increased urine output are the results of increased bilirubin excretion. The infant is observed for signs of dehydration and perianal excoriation.

In light-skinned infants, a benign transient bronze discoloration of the skin may occur with phototherapy when the infant has elevated direct serum bilirubin levels or liver disease. As a side effect of phototherapy, some newborns develop a maculopapular rash. In addition to assessing the newborn's skin color for jaundice and bronzing, the nurse examines the skin for developing pressure areas. The newborn should be repositioned at least every 2 hours to permit the light to reach all skin surfaces, to prevent pressure areas, and to vary the stimulation to the infant. The nurse keeps track of the number of hours each lamp is used so that each can be replaced before its effectiveness is lost.

The nurse's responsibilities during exchange transfusion are to assemble equipment, prepare the baby, assist the physician during the procedure, and maintain a careful record of all events. After the procedure the nurse observes the newborn for complications from the transfusion and clinical signs of hyperbilirubinemia and neurologic damage (Procedure 32–3: Nursing Responsibilities During Exchange Transfusion on page 1028).

Provision of Parental Support for Phototherapy in the Birthing Room or at Home

The terms *jaundice, hyperbilirubinemia, exchange transfusion,* and *phototherapy* may sound frightening and threatening. Some parents may feel guilty about their baby's

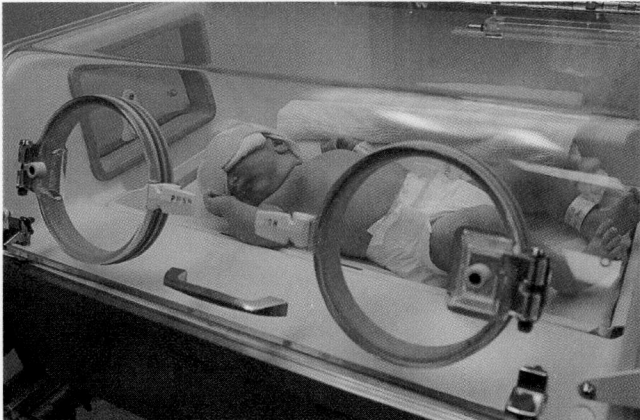

FIGURE 32-15 Infant receiving phototherapy. The phototherapy light is positioned over the incubator. Bilateral eye patches are always used during phototherapy to protect the baby's eyes.

Nursing Action	Rationale

Objective: Prepare infant.

1. Keep newborn NPO for 4 hours preceding exchange transfusion or aspirate stomach.

To decrease chance of regurgitation and aspiration by newborn.

2. Some physicians order salt-poor albumin (1 g/kg body weight) to be administered 1 hour before exchange transfusion.

To increase binding of bilirubin.
Do not give to severely anemic or edemic newborn or to newborn with congestive heart failure because of hazard of hypervolemia.

3. Assess vital signs.

To provide a baseline.

4. Position newborn in supine position, soft restraints; provide warmth under radiant warmer and have warm blankets available.

To provide maximum visualization, thermoregulation, and prevent chilling.

5. Clean abdomen with antiseptic solution.

To reduce number of bacteria present.

6. Attach monitor leads to infant.

To assess pulse and respiration.

Objective: Prepare equipment and assist with catheter placement.

1. Have resuscitation equipment available (oxygen, bag and mask, intubation equipment, suction, 10% glucose IV solution, sodium bicarbonate, epinephrine).

To provide life-support measures if necessary.

2. Obtain blood and check it with physician for type, Rh, and age.

To ensure using correct blood.

3. Attach blood tubing.

To allow infusion.

4. Apply blood warmer.

Blood temperature should be 37 C prior to procedure to reduce chill.

5. Open exchange transfusion and umbilical vein trays. Pour prep solution into basins.

To maintain sterility.

6. Prepare gown and gloves for physician.

Objective: Monitor infant status before and during procedure.

To recognize possible problems such as apnea, bradycardia, cardiac arrhythmia or arrest, and provide data on newborn's response to treatment.

Assess pulse, respirations, color, and activity state.

Objective: Record blood exchange and medications used.

1. Using blood exchange sheet, record time, amount of blood in, amount of blood out, medications and baby's response, and any other pertinent information.

Volume of donor blood given is 170 mL/kg of body weight. It replaces 85% of infant's own blood.

2. Inform physician when 100 mL of blood has been used.

Calcium gluconate may be given IV after each 100 mL of blood if indicated to decrease cardiac irritability.

*Exchange transfusion is a therapeutic procedure for hyperbilirubinemia of any etiology.

Nursing Action	Rationale
Objective: Assess newborn response after transfusion.	
After the exchange carefully monitor the following for 24–48 hours:	*To provide information on status of newborn and identify complications such as hypocalcemia, hyperkalemia, hypernatremia, hypoglycemia and acidosis, sepsis, shock, thrombus formation, thrombocytopenia, and transfusion mismatch reaction.*
1. Vital signs	
2. Neurologic signs (lethargy, increased irritability, jitteriness, convulsion)	
3. Amount and color of urine (hematuria)	
4. Presence of edema	
5. Signs of necrotizing enterocolitis	
6. Infection or hemorrhage at infusion site	
7. Signs of increasing jaundice	
8. Neurologic signs of kernicterus	
9. Calcium, glucose, and bilirubin levels	
10. Other complications such as hyper- or hypokalemia, septicemia, shock, and thrombosis	
Objective: Prepare blood samples.	
Label tubes and send to laboratory with appropriate laboratory slips.	*To ensure that baby receives correct blood if future exchange is necessary.*
Retype and cross-match two units of blood 2 hours postexchange.	*To provide for possible future exchange.*
Objective: Record information on infant's record.	
Record infant's response during and after the exchange procedure.	*To help identify possible complications.*

*Exchange transfusion is a therapeutic procedure for hyperbilirubinemia of any etiology.

condition and think they have caused the problem. Under stress, parents may not be able to understand the physician's first explanations. The nurse must expect that the parents will need explanations repeated and clarified and that they may need help voicing their questions and fears. Eye and tactile contact with the infant is encouraged. The nurse can coach parents when they visit with the baby. After the mother's discharge, parents are kept informed of their infant's condition and are encouraged to return to the hospital or telephone at any time so that they can be fully involved in the care of their infant. (See the Nursing Care Plan: Newborn with Jaundice on page 1023.)

While the mother is still hospitalized, phototherapy can also be carried out in the parents' room if the only problem is hyperbilirubinemia. The parent must be willing to keep the baby in the room for 24 hours a day, able to take emergency action as for choking if necessary, and complete instruction checklists. Some institutions re-

quire that parents sign a consent form. The nurse gives the instructions to the parents but also continues to monitor the infant's temperature, activity, intake and output, and positioning of eye patches at regular intervals (Table 32–5).

If the baby is to receive phototherapy at home, parents are taught to record the infant's temperature, weight, fluid intake and output, stools, and feedings and to use the phototherapy equipment. In addition, if phototherapy lights are being used, parents must agree that the baby will be exposed to the lights for long periods of time; that they will hold the baby for only short periods for feedings, comforting, and cleansing of the perineal area; and that the room temperature will be regulated to minimize heat loss. Fiberoptic phototherapy blankets eliminate the need for eye patches, decrease heat loss because the baby is clothed, and provide more opportunities for interaction between the baby and parents. The best

Explain and demonstrate the placement of eye patches and explain that they must be in place when the infant is under the lights.

Explain the clothing to be worn (diaper under lights, dress and wrap when away from the lights).

Explain the importance of taking the infant's temperature regularly.

Explain the importance of adequate fluid intake.

Explain the charting flow sheet (intake, output, eyes covered).

Explain how to position the lights at a proper distance.

Explain the need to keep the infant under phototherapy except during feeding and diaper changes.

method of home phototherapy depends on the cause of the hyperbilirubinemia and the rate of progression of the jaundice.

Evaluation

Anticipated outcomes of nursing care include:

- The risks for development of hyperbilirubinemia are identified, and action is taken to minimize the potential impact of hyperbilirubinemia.

- The baby will not have any corneal irritation or drainage, skin breakdown, or major fluctuations in temperature.

- Parents will understand the rationale for, goal of, and expected outcome of therapy. Parents verbalize their concerns about their baby's condition and identify how they can facilitate their baby's improvement.

CARE OF THE NEWBORN WITH HEMORRHAGIC DISEASE

Several transient coagulation mechanism deficiencies normally occur in the first several days of a newborn's life. Foremost among these is a slight decrease in the level of prothrombin, resulting in a prolonged clotting time during the initial week of life. Vitamin K is required for the liver to form prothrombin (factor II) and proconvertin (factor VII) for blood coagulation. Vitamin K, a fat-soluble vitamin, may be obtained from food, but it is usually synthesized by bacteria in the colon, and consequently a dietary source is unnecessary. However, intestinal flora are practically nonexistent in newborns, so they are unable to synthesize vitamin K.

Bleeding due to vitamin K deficiency generally occurs on the second or third day of life, but it may occur earlier in babies of mothers treated with phenytoin sodium (Dilantin) or phenobarbital. These drugs impair vitamin K activity, and bleeding may be seen at birth. Coumarin compounds are vitamin K antagonists that can cross the placenta. Thus the baby exposed to maternal coumarin can also manifest bleeding in the first 24 hours of life. Bleeding may also occur in babies receiving parenteral nutrition without adequate vitamin K additives (1 mg/week).

Bleeding from the nose, umbilical cord, circumcision site, gastrointestinal tract, and scalp, as well as generalized ecchymoses may be seen. Internal hemorrhage may occur.

This disorder can be completely prevented by the prophylactic use of an injection of vitamin K. A dose of 0.5–1 mg of AquaMEPHYTON is given as part of newborn care immediately following birth, and consequently the disease is rarely seen today (see Drug Guide, Chapter 29). Larger doses are contraindicated because they may result in the development of hyperbilirubinemia.

CARE OF THE NEWBORN WITH ANEMIA

Neonatal anemia is often difficult to recognize by clinical evaluation alone. The hemoglobin concentration in a full-term newborn is 15–20 g/dL, slightly higher than in premature infants, in whom the mean hemoglobin is 14–18 g/dL. Infants with hemoglobin values of less than 14 mg/dL (term) and 13 g/dL (preterm) are usually considered anemic. The most common causes of neonatal anemia are blood loss, hemolysis, and impaired red blood cell production.

Blood loss (hypovolemia) occurs in utero from placental bleeding (placenta previa or abruptio placentae). Intrapartal blood loss may be fetomaternal, fetofetal, or the result of umbilical cord bleeding. Birth trauma to abdominal organs or the cranium may produce significant blood loss, and cerebral bleeding may occur because of hypoxia.

Excessive hemolysis of red cells is usually a result of blood group incompatibilities but may be due to infections. The most common cause of impaired red cell production is a deficiency in G-6-PD, which is genetically transmitted. Anemia and jaundice are the presenting signs.

A condition known as **physiologic anemia** exists as a result of the normal gradual drop in hemoglobin for the first 6 to 12 weeks of life. Theoretically, the bone marrow stops production of red blood cells in response to the elevated oxygenation of extrauterine respirations. When the amount of hemoglobin becomes lower, reaching levels of 10 to 11 g/dL at about 6 to 12 weeks of age, the bone marrow begins production of RBCs again, and the anemia disappears.

Anemia in preterm newborns occurs earlier, and reversal by bone marrow is initiated at lower levels of hemoglobin (7 to 9 g/dL). The preterm baby's hemoglobin reaches a low sooner (4 to 8 weeks after birth) than does a term newborn's (6 to 12 weeks) because preterm red blood cell survival time is shorter than in the term newborn. This is due to two factors: The preterm infant's growth rate is relatively rapid, and a vitamin E deficiency is common in small preterm newborns.

Medical Therapy

The goal of management is early identification and correction of anemia. Hematologic problems can be anticipated based on the pregnancy history and clinical manifestations. The age at which anemia is first noted is also of diagnostic value.

Clinically, light-skinned anemic infants are very pale in the absence of other symptoms of shock and usually have abnormally low red blood cell counts. In *acute* blood loss symptoms of shock may be present, such as pallor, low arterial blood pressure, and a decreasing hematocrit value. The initial laboratory workup should include hemoglobin and hematocrit measurements, reticulocyte count, examination of peripheral blood smear, bilirubin determinations, direct Coombs' test of infant's blood, and examination of maternal blood smear for fetal erythrocytes (Kleihauer-Betke test). Medical management depends on the severity of the anemia and whether blood loss is acute or chronic. The baby should be placed on constant cardiac and respiratory monitoring. Mild or chronic anemia in an infant may be treated adequately with iron supplements alone or with iron-fortified formulas. Frequent determinations of hemoglobin, hematocrit, and bilirubin levels (in hemolytic disease) are essential. In severe cases of anemia, transfusions are the preferred method of treatment.

Nursing Care

The nurse assesses the newborn for symptoms of anemia (pallor). If the blood loss is acute, the baby may exhibit signs of shock (a capillary filling time greater than 3 seconds, decreased pulses, tachycardia, and low blood pressure). Continued observations will be necessary to identify physiologic anemia as the preterm newborn grows. Signs of compromise include poor weight gain, tachycardia, tachypnea, and apneic episodes. The nurse promptly reports any symptoms indicating anemia or shock. The amount of blood drawn for all laboratory tests is recorded so that total blood removed can be assessed and replaced by transfusion when necessary. If the newborn exhibits signs of shock, the nurse needs to notify the physician so that prompt treatment can occur.

CARE OF THE NEWBORN WITH POLYCYTHEMIA

Polycythemia is a condition in which blood volume and hematocrit values are increased. A common problem in nurseries, polycythemia affects 1.5% to 4% of newborns. It is observed more commonly in SGA and full-term infants than in preterm neonates. An infant is considered polycythemic when the central venous hematocrit value is greater than 65% or the venous hemoglobin level is greater than 22 g/dL during the first week of life (Blanchette et al 1994).

Several conditions predispose the newborn to polycythemia:

1. At the time of birth an excessive volume of placental blood may transfuse into the infant before the cord is clamped ("cord stripping"), or the infant may be placed or held lower than the placenta before the cord is clamped and cut, resulting in a blood volume increase.

2. During gestation or labor and birth, an increased amount of blood may cross the placenta to the infant (maternofetal transfusion), resulting in increased blood volume after birth.

3. A twin-to-twin transfusion may occur, in which one twin receives less blood and becomes anemic, and the other twin receives an excess amount of blood and becomes polycythemic.

4. Increased red blood cell production may occur in utero in response to chronic fetal distress in SGA, IDM, or postmature infants and secondary to conditions of PIH and placenta previa.

Other conditions that present with polycythemia are chromosomal anomalies such as trisomy 21, 18, and 13; endocrine disorders such as hypoglycemia and hypocalcemia; and births at altitudes over 5000 ft.

Medical Therapy

The goal of therapy is to reduce the central venous hematocrit to less than 60% in symptomatic infants. Treatment of asymptomatic infants is more controversial, but many authorities agree that these newborns benefit from prophylactic exchanges (Merestein & Gardner 1993). To decrease the red cell mass, the symptomatic infant receives a partial exchange transfusion in which blood is removed from the infant and replaced milliliter for milliliter with fresh plasma, 5% albumin, or normal saline (Merenstein & Gardner 1993). Supportive treatment of presenting symptoms is required until resolution, which usually occurs spontaneously following the partial exchange transfusion.

Nursing Care

The nurse assesses, records, and reports symptoms of polycythemia. The nurse also does an initial screening of the newborn's hematocrit on admission to the nursery. If a capillary hematocrit is done, warming the heel prior to obtaining the blood helps to decrease falsely high values. Peripheral venous hematocrit samples are usually obtained from the antecubital fossa.

Many infants are asymptomatic, but as symptoms develop, they are related to the increased blood volume, hyperviscocity (thickness) of the blood, and decreased deformability of red blood cells, all of which result in poor perfusion of tissues. The infants have a characteristic plethoric (ruddy) appearance. The most common symptoms observed include the following:

- Tachycardia and congestive heart failure due to the increased blood volume

- Respiratory distress with grunting, tachypnea, and cyanosis; increased oxygen need; or hemorrhage in respiratory system due to pulmonary venous congestion, edema, and hypoxemia

- Hyperbilirubinemia due to increased numbers of red blood cells breaking down

- Decrease in peripheral pulses, discoloration of extremities, renal vein thrombosis with decreased urine output, hematuria, or proteinuria due to thromboembolism

- Jitteriness, decreased activity and tone, seizures due to decreased perfusion of the brain and increased vascular resistance secondary to sluggish blood flow (This can result in neurologic or developmental problems.)

- Hypoglycemia due to IDM, SGA status, or the increased red cell mass

The nurse observes closely for signs of distress or change in vital signs during the partial exchange. The nurse assesses carefully for potential complications resulting from the exchange such as transfusion overload (which can result in congestive heart failure), irregular cardiac rhythm, bacterial infection, hypovolemia (because of decreased plasma volume), and anemia.

Parents need specific explanations about polycythemia and its treatment. The newborn needs to be reunited with the parents as soon after the exchange as the baby's status permits.

CARE OF THE NEWBORN WITH INFECTION

Newborns up to 1 month of age are particularly susceptible to infection, referred to as **sepsis neonatorum,** caused by organisms that do not cause significant disease in older children. Once any infection occurs in the newborn, it can spread rapidly through the bloodstream, regardless of its primary site. The incidence of primary neonatal sepsis is 1–10 per 1000 live births (0.1 to 1%) (Glomella 1994). Nosocomial infection frequency ranges from 0.6 to 1.7% in normal newborn infants and from 0.9 to 18.2% in infants in the NICU (Payne et al 1994).

One predisposing factor is prematurity. Prematurity and low birth weight are associated with nosocomial infection rates up to 15-fold higher than average (Payne et al 1994). The general debilitation and underlying illness often associated with prematurity necessitates invasive procedures such as umbilical catheterization, intubation, resuscitation, ventilatory support, monitoring, and parenteral alimentation (especially lipid emulsions); and prior broad-spectrum antibiotic therapy. However, even full-term infants are susceptible because their immunologic systems are immature. They lack the complex factors involved in effective phagocytosis and the ability to localize infection or to respond with a well-defined recognizable inflammatory response.

Most nosocomial infections in the NICU present as bacteremia/sepsis, urinary tract infections, meningitis, or pneumonia. Maternal antepartal infections such as rubella, toxoplasmosis, cytomegalic inclusion disease, and herpes may cause congenital infections and resulting disorders in the newborn. Intrapartal maternal infections, such as amnionitis and those resulting from premature rupture of membranes and precipitous birth, are sources of neonatal infection. (See Chapter 19 for more detailed information.) Passage through the birth canal and contact with the vaginal flora (β-hemolytic streptococci, herpes, listeria, and gonococci) expose the infant to infection (Table 32–6). With infection anywhere in the fetus or newborn, the adjacent tissues or organs are very easily penetrated, and the blood-brain barrier is ineffective. Septicemia is more common in males, except for those infections caused by group B β-hemolytic streptococcus.

Protection of the newborn from infections starts prenatally and continues throughout pregnancy and birth. Prenatal prevention should include maternal screening for sexually transmitted disease and monitoring of rubella titers in women who test negative. Intrapartally, sterile technique is essential, smears from genital lesions are taken, and placenta and amniotic fluid cultures are obtained if amnionitis is suspected. If genital herpes is present toward term, cesarean birth may be indicated. Local eye treatment with silver nitrate or an antibiotic ophthalmic ointment is given to all newborns to prevent damage from gonococcal infections.

At present gram-negative organisms (especially *Escherichia coli, Aerobacter, Proteus,* and *Klebsiella*) and the gram-positive organism β-hemolytic streptococcus are the most common causative agents. Pseudomonas is a common fomite contaminant of ventilatory support and oxygen therapy equipment. Gram-positive bacteria, especially coagulase-negative staphylococci, are common pathogens in nosocomial bacteremias, pneumonias, and

TABLE 32-6 Maternally Transmitted Newborn Infections

Infection	Nursing Assessment	Nursing Plan and Implementation
Group B Streptococcus 1% to 2% colonized with one in ten developing disease Early onset—usually within hours of birth or within first week Late onset—1 week to 3 months	Severe respiratory distress (grunting and cyanosis). May become apneic or demonstrate symptoms of shock. Meconium-stained amniotic fluid seen at birth.	Early assessment of clinical signs necessary. Assist with x-ray—shows aspiration pneumonia or hyaline membrane disease. Immediately obtain blood, gastric aspirate, external ear canal and nasopharynx cultures. Administer antibiotics, usually aqueous penicillin or ampicillin combined with gentamicin as soon as cultures are obtained. Early assessment and intervention are essential to survival. Initiate referral to evaluate for blindness, deafness, learning or behavioral problems.
Syphilis Spirochetes cross placenta after 16th–18th week of gestation	Check perinatal history for positive maternal serology. Assess infant for: 　Elevated cord serum IgM and FTA-ABS IgM 　Rhinitis (snuffles) 　Fissures on mouth corners and excoriated upper lip 　Red rash around mouth and anus 　Copper-colored rash over face, palms, and soles 　Irritability 　Generalized edema, particularly over joints; bone lesions; painful extremities 　Hepatosplenomegaly, jaundice 　Congenital cataracts 　SGA and failure to thrive	Initiate isolation techniques until infants have been on antibiotics for 48 hours. Administer penicillin. Provide emotional support for parents because of their feelings about mode of transmission and potential long-term sequelae.
Gonorrhea Approximately 30–35% of new-borns born vaginally to infected mothers acquire the infection.	Assess for: 　Ophthalmia neonatorum (conjunctivitis) 　Purulent discharge and corneal ulcerations 　Neonatal sepsis with temperature instability, poor feeding response, and/or hypotonia, jaundice	Administer 1% silver nitrate solution or ophthalmic antibiotic ointment (see Drug Guide: Erythromycin [Ilotycin] Ophthalmic Ointment in Chapter 29) or, in lieu of silver nitrate, penicillin. Initiate follow-up referral to evaluate any loss of vision.
Herpes Type 2 1 in 7500 births (Lott 1994). Usually transmitted during vaginal birth; a few cases of in utero transmission have been reported.	Small cluster vesicular skin lesions over all the body. Check perinatal history for active herpes genital lesions. Disseminated form—DIC, pneumonia, hepatitis with jaundice, he-patosplenomegaly, and neurologic abnormalities. Without skin lesions, assess for fever or subnormal temperature, respiratory congestion, tachypnea, and tachycardia.	Carry out careful hand washing and gown and glove isolation with linen precautions. Administer intravenous vidarabine (Vira A) or acyclovir (Zovirax). Initiate follow-up referral to evaluate potential sequelae of microcephaly, spasticity, seizures, deafness, or blindness. Encourage parental rooming-in and touching of their newborn. Show parents appropriate hand-washing procedures and precautions to be used at home if mother's lesions are active. Obtain throat, conjunctiva, cerebral spinal fluid (CSF), blood, urine, and lesion cultures to identify herpesvirus type 2 antibiotics in serum IgM fraction. Cultures positive in 24–48 hours.
Oral Candidal Infection (Thrush) Acquired during passage through birth canal.	Assess newborn's buccal mucosa, tongue, gums, and inside the cheeks for white plaques (seen 5 to 7 days of age). Check diaper area for bright red, well-demarcated eruptions. Assess for thrust periodically when newborn is on long-term antibiotic therapy.	Differentiate white plaque areas from milk curds by using cotton tip applicator (if it is thrush, removal of white areas causes raw, bleeding areas). Maintain cleanliness of hands, linen, clothing, diapers, and feeding apparatus. Instruct breastfeeding mothers on treating their nipples with nystatin. Administer gentian violet (1% to 2%) swabbed on oral lesions 1 hour after feeding or nystatin instilled in baby's oral cavity and on mucosa. Swab skin lesions with topical nystatin. Discuss with parents that gentian violet stains mouth and clothing. Avoid placing gentian violet on normal mucosa; it causes irritation.
Chlamydia Trachomatis Acquired during passage through birth canal	Assess for perinatal history of preterm birth. Symptomatic newborns present with pneumonia—conjunctivitis after 3–4 days. Chronic follicular conjunctivitis (corneal neovascularization and conjunctival scarring).	Instill ophthalmic erythromycin (see Drug Guide: Erythromycin [Ilotycin] Ophthalmic Ointment in Chapter 29). Initiate follow-up referral for eye complications and late development of pneumonia at 4–11 weeks postnatally.

urinary tract infections. Other gram-positive bacteria frequently isolated are enterococci and *Staphylococcus aureus*.

Medical Therapy

Infants with a history of possible exposure to infection in utero (for example, premature rupture of membranes [PROM] more than 24 hours before birth or questionable maternal history of infection) should have cultures taken as soon after birth as possible. Cultures are obtained before antibiotic therapy is begun.

1. Two blood cultures are obtained from different peripheral sites. They are taken from a peripheral rather than an umbilical vessel because catheters have yielded false positives resulting from contamination. The skin is prepared by cleaning with an antiseptic solution, such as one containing iodine, and allowed to dry; the specimen is obtained with a sterile needle/syringe.

2. Spinal fluid culture is done following a spinal tap.

3. Urine culture is best obtained from a specimen obtained by a suprapubic bladder aspiration.

4. Skin cultures are taken of any lesions or drainage from lesions or reddened areas.

5. Nasopharyngeal, tracheal, ear canal, gastric cultures, and (in some institutions) rectal cultures may be obtained at birth.

Other laboratory investigations include a complete blood count, chest x-ray examination, serology, and Gram stains of cerebrospinal fluid, urine, skin exudate, and umbilicus. White blood count (WBC) with differential may indicate the presence or absence of sepsis. A level of 30,000 WBC may be normal in the first 24 hours of life, while low WBC (less than 5000) may be indicative of sepsis. A low neutrophil count and high band (immature white cells) count indicate that an infection is present. Stomach aspirate should be sent for culture and smear if a gonococcal infection or amnionitis is suspected. Serum IgM levels are elevated (normal level less than 20 mg/dL) in response to transplacental infections. If available, counterimmuno-electrophoresis tests for specific bacterial antigens are done. Evidence of congenital infections may be seen on skull x-ray films for cerebral calcifications (cytomegalovirus, toxoplasmosis), on bone x-ray films (syphilis, cytomegalovirus), and in serum-specific IgM levels (rubella). Cytomegalovirus infection is best diagnosed by urine culture.

Critical Thinking Question

What is the danger in early or aggressive use of antibiotics to treat neonatal sepsis?

Because neonatal infection causes high mortality, therapy is instituted before results of the septic workup are obtained. A combination of two broad-spectrum antibiotics, such as ampicillin and gentamicin, is given in large doses until a culture with sensitivities is obtained.

After the pathogen and its sensitivities are determined, appropriate specific antibiotic therapy is begun. Combinations of penicillin or ampicillin and kanamycin have been used in the past, but new kanamycin-resistant enterobacteria and penicillin-resistant staphylococcus necessitate increasing use of gentamicin.

The possibility of rotating aminoglycosides has been suggested to prevent development of resistance. Use of cephalosporins and, in particular, cefotaxime has emerged as an alternative to aminoglycoside therapy in the treatment of neonatal infections. Duration of therapy varies from 7 to 14 days (Table 32–7). However, if cultures are negative and symptoms subside, antibiotics may be discontinued after 3 days. Supportive physiologic care may be required to maintain respiratory, hemodynamic, nutritional, and metabolic homeostasis.

APPLYING THE NURSING PROCESS

Nursing Assessment

Symptoms of infection are most often noticed by the nurse during daily care of the newborn rather than during the infant's sporadic contact with the physician. The infant may deteriorate rapidly in the first 24 hours after birth if β-hemolytic streptococcal infection is present, with signs and symptoms mimicking RDS. Or the onset of sepsis may be more gradual, with more subtle signs and symptoms. The most common symptoms observed include the following:

- Subtle behavioral changes—the infant "isn't doing well" and is often lethargic or irritable (especially after first 24 hours), hypotonic, and hypotensive. Color changes may include pallor, duskiness, cyanosis, or a "shocky" appearance. Skin is cool and clammy.

- Temperature instability, manifested most commonly by hypothermia (recognized by a decrease in skin temperature) or, rarely in newborns, hyperthermia (elevation of skin temperature) necessitates a corresponding increase or decrease in incubator temperature to maintain a neutral thermal environment.

- Feeding intolerance is evidenced by a decrease in total intake, abdominal distention, vomiting, poor sucking, lack of interest in feeding, and diarrhea.

- Hyperbilirubinemia is present.

- There is initially tachycardia, then spells of apnea/bradycardia.

TABLE 32-7 Neonatal Sepsis Antibiotic Therapy

Drug	Dose (mg/kg) Total Daily Dose	Schedule for Divided Doses	Route	Comments
Ampicillin	50–100 mg/kg	Every 12 hours* Every 8 hours†	IM or IV	Effective against gram-positive microorganisms and majority of *E coli* strains. Higher doses indicated for meningitis.
Cefotaxime	50–75 mg/kg 100–150 mg/kg/day	Every 12 hours* Every 8 hours†	IM or IV	Active against most major pathogens in infants; effective against aminoglycoside-resistant organisms; achieves CSF bactericidal activity; lack of ototoxicity and nephrotoxicity; wide therapeutic index (levels not required); resistant organisms can develop rapidly if used extensively; ineffective against pseudomonas, listeria.
Gentamicin	2.5 mg/kg 5.0–7.5 mg/kg/day	Every 12–24 hours* § Every 8–24 hours†	IM or IV	Effective against gram-negative rods and staphylococci; may be used instead of kanamycin against penicillin-resistant staphylococci and *E coli* strains and *Pseudomonas aeruginosa*. May cause ototoxicity and nephrotoxicity. Need to follow serum levels. Must never be given as IV push. Must be given over at least 30–60 minutes. In presence of oliguria or anuria, dose must be decreased or discontinued. In infants less than 1000 g or 29 weeks, lower dosage 2.5–3.0 mg/kg/day. Monitor serum levels before administration of second dose. Peak 5–10 µg/mL Trough 1–2 µg/mL
Methicillin	25–50 mg/dose 50–100 mg/kg/day	Every 12 hours* Every 6–8 hours†	IM or IV	Effective against penicillinase-resistant staphylococci.
Nafcillin	25–50 mg/kg 50–100 mg/kg/day	Every 8–12 hours* Every 6–8 hours†	IM or IV	Effective against penicillinase-resistant staphylococci.
Penicillin G (aqueous crystalline)	25,000–50,000 U/kg 50,000–125,000 U/kg/day	Every 12 hours* Every 8 hours†	IM or IV	Initial sepsis therapy effective against most gram-positive microorganisms except resistant staphylococci; can cause heart block in infants.
Vancomycin	10–15 mg/kg 30 mg/kg/day	Every 12–18 hours* § Every 8 hours†	IV	Effective for methicillin-resistant strains *(S epidermidis)*; must be administered by slow intravenous infusion to avoid prolonged cutaneous eruption. For smaller infants <1200 g; <29 weeks, smaller dosages and longer intervals between doses. Nephrotoxic, especially when given in combination with aminoglycosides. Peak 25–40 µg/mL Trough 5–10 µg/mL

* Up to seven days of age.

† Greater than seven days of age.

§ Dependent on GA.

Signs and symptoms may suggest CNS disease (jitteriness, tremors, seizure activity), respiratory system disease (tachypnea, labored respirations, apnea, cyanosis), hematologic disease (jaundice, petechial hemorrhages, hepatosplenomegaly), or gastrointestinal disease (diarrhea, vomiting, bile-stained aspirate, hepatomegaly). A differential diagnosis is necessary because of the similarity of symptoms to other more specific conditions.

Nursing Diagnosis

Nursing diagnoses that may apply to the infant with sepsis neonatorum and the family include the following:

- Risk of infection related to immature immunologic system

- Fluid volume deficit related to feeding intolerance

- Ineffective family coping related to present illness resulting in prolonged hospital stay for the newborn

Nursing Plan and Implementation

In the nursery, environmental control and prevention of acquired infection is the responsibility of the neonatal nurse. The nurse must promote strict hand-washing technique for all who enter the nursery, including nursing colleagues; physicians; laboratory, x-ray, and inhalation technicians; and parents. The nurse must be prepared to assist in the aseptic collection of specimens for laboratory investigations. Scrupulous care of equipment—changing and cleaning of incubators at least every 7 days, removal and sterilization of wet equipment every 24 hours, prevention of cross-use of linen and other equipment, periodic cleaning of sinkside equipment such as soap containers, and special care with the open radiant warmers—will prevent contamination or infection of debilitated, infection-prone newborns. An infected newborn can be effectively isolated in an incubator and receive close observation. Visiting of the nursery area by unnecessary personnel should be discouraged.

The nurse administers antibiotics as ordered by the clinician. It is the nurse's responsibility to be knowledgeable about the following:

- The proper dose to be administered, based on the weight of the newborn and desired peak and trough levels

- The appropriate route of administration because some antibiotics cannot be given intravenously

- The appropriate rate of administration

- Admixture incompatibilities because some antibiotics are precipitated by intravenous solutions or by other antibiotics
- Side effects and toxicity

Provision of Supportive Care

In addition to antibiotic therapy, physiologic supportive care is essential in caring for a septic infant. The nurse should do the following:

- Observe for resolution of symptoms or development of other symptoms of sepsis.
- Maintain a neutral thermal environment with accurate regulation of humidity and oxygen administration.
- Provide respiratory support: Administer oxygen and observe and monitor respiratory effort.
- Provide cardiovascular support: Observe and monitor pulse and blood pressure; observe for hyperbilirubinemia, anemia, and hemorrhagic symptoms.
- Provide adequate calories because oral feedings may be discontinued due to increased mucus, abdominal distention, vomiting, and aspiration.
- Provide fluids and electrolytes to maintain homeostasis. Monitor weight changes, urine output, and urine specific gravity.
- Observe for the development of hypoglycemia, hyperglycemia, acidosis, hyponatremia, and hypocalcemia.
- Detect and treat metabolic disturbances, a common occurrence.
- Cluster all nursing care as much as possible to allow the sick baby to preserve energy and heal more quickly.

Restriction of parent visits has not been shown to have any effect on the rate of infection and may indeed be harmful to the newborn's psychologic development. With instruction and guidance from the nurse, both parents should be allowed to handle the baby and participate in daily care. Support to the parents is crucial. They need to be informed of the newborn's prognosis as treatment continues and to be involved in care as much as possible. They also need to understand how infection is transmitted.

Evaluation

Anticipated outcomes of nursing care include:

- The risks for development of sepsis are identified early, and immediate action is taken to minimize the development of the illness.
- Appropriate use of aseptic technique protects the newborn from further exposure to illness.
- The baby's symptoms are relieved, and the infection is treated.

- The parents verbalize their concerns about their baby's illness and understand the rationale behind the management of their newborn.

CARE OF THE FAMILY OF A NEWBORN WITH A COMPLICATION

Adaptation of the Family

The birth of a baby with a problem or disorder is a traumatic event with the potential for either total disruption or growth of the involved family. Throughout the pregnancy both parents, together and separately, have felt excitement, experienced thoughts of acceptance, and pictured what their baby would look like. Both parents have wished for a perfect baby and feared a damaged, unhealthy one. Each parent and family member must accept and adjust when the fantasized fears become a reality.

Grieving for the loss of the hoped-for perfect child is necessary before the development of a positive relationship to the existing child can begin. Grief is expressed as shock and disbelief, denial of reality, anger toward self and others, guilt, blame, and concern for the future. Self-esteem and feelings of self-worth are jeopardized.

In some cases fear, separation, and grief begin during the birth, when the newborn requires immediate resuscitation or special treatment. Instead of being handed to its mother, the baby is given to a nurse or a pediatrician, who rushes it to a special care area. The joyful cries of "It's a boy!" or "It's a girl!" are absent; there is only the mother's pleading question, "What's wrong with my baby?" If no answer is given to the mother, she frequently fantasizes the worst and assumes that the baby is dead. It is extremely important for the mother's health and the mother-infant relationship that some immediate answer be given to the parents. Honest, simple, and positive facts can be shared: "Your baby is alive"; "Your baby is a girl"; "Your baby has a strong heartbeat but needs some help with breathing"; "Your baby is alive but needs some special care right now"; "The pediatrician is helping your baby now and will talk with you soon." The information that nurses share with parents must always be honest data that nurses can observe and document. Nurses should not make promises that they cannot fulfill and should refrain from offering empty reassurances that everything will be all right.

The period of waiting between suspicion and confirmation of abnormality or dysfunction is a very anxious one for parents because it is difficult, if not impossible, to begin attachment to the infant if the newborn's future is questionable. During the "not knowing period," parents need support and acknowledgement that this is an anxious time and must be kept informed about efforts to gather additional data and maintain the infant's livelihood. It is helpful to tell both parents about the problem at the same time with the baby present. An honest discussion of the problem and anticipatory management at the earliest possible time by health professionals help the parents (1) maintain trust in the physician and nurse, (2) appreciate the reality of the situation by dispelling fantasy and misconception, (3) begin the grieving process, and (4) mobilize internal and external support.

Nurses need to be aware that anger is a universal response and that it is best directed outward because holding it in check requires great energy, which is diverted away from grieving and physical recovery from pregnancy and giving birth. Anger may be directed unjustifiably at the physician and/or nurse, at the food, at nursing care, or at hospital regulations and routines. Anger with the baby is rarely demonstrated by parents and can precipitate guilt feelings.

A heightened concern for self may be misinterpreted by health professionals as rejection of the newborn. Both parents need time and understanding to deal with their own feelings before they can direct concern toward the baby. In a short span of time, the parent is confronted with the loss of the idealized child, the need to accept a child who deviates from normal, and a sense of personal failure. In addition the new mother may be suffering from fatigue and sleep deprivation from her pregnancy and labor and from discomforts arising from cesarean birth, episiotomy, inability to void, hemorrhoids, and afterpains. In the postpartal period concern for self and dependency are normal events.

In their sensitive and vulnerable state, parents are acutely perceptive of others' responses and reactions (particularly nonverbal) to the child. Parents can be expected to identify with the responses of others. Therefore it is imperative that medical and nursing staff be fully aware of their feelings and come to terms with those feelings so that they are comfortable and at ease with the baby and the grieving family.

Nurses may feel uncomfortable not knowing what to say to parents or may fear confronting their own feelings as well as those of the parents. Each nurse must work out personal reactions with instructors, peers, clergy, parents, or significant others. It is helpful to have a stockpile of therapeutic questions and statements to initiate meaningful dialogue with parents. Opening statements can be as follows: "You must be wondering what could have caused this"; "Are you thinking you (or someone else) may have done something?"; "How can I help?"; "Go ahead and cry. It's worth crying about"; or "Are you wondering how you are going to manage?" Avoid statements such as "It could have been worse"; "It's God's will"; "You have other children"; "You are still young and can have more"; and "I understand how you feel." *This* child is important *now*.

Some nurses find relief for themselves or a means of escape from painful circumstances by overzealous and unrealistic reassurance that "everything will be all right" and by avoidance of the newborn and family. Other medical and nursing staff take refuge in technical jargon and involvement in the technical aspects of the mother's care rather than taking time to talk about the situation. These approaches confuse the parents at a time when they need most to be understood and to understand.

Nurses show concern and support by planning time to spend with the parents, by being psychologically as well as physically present, by encouraging open discussion and grieving, by repetitious explanations (as necessary), by providing privacy as needed, and by encouraging contact with the newborn. Identification and clarification of feelings and fears decrease distortions in perception, thinking, and feeling. Nurses invest the baby with value in the eyes of the parents when they provide meticulous care to the newborn, talk and coo (especially in the face-to-face position) while holding or providing care to the newborn, refer to the child by gender or name, and relate the newborn's activities ("He took a whole ounce of formula"; "She burped so loud that . . ."; "He took hold of the blanket and just wouldn't let go"; "He voided all over the doctor"). Nurses should note the "normal" characteristics and capabilities of each newborn as well as the newborn's needs. The nurse should also learn the baby's name and refer to him or her by name.

Many physicians show parents "before" and "after" photographs of conditions requiring surgical intervention. Parents also may benefit from meeting other parents who have faced the same problem through a parental support group or organization that is specific to that problem. Specialists (plastic surgeons, perinatal clinic nurse specialists, neurosurgeons, orthopedists, oral surgeons, dentists, and rehabilitation therapists) can be reassuring and supportive of parents in their short- and long-term goals. However, these types of interventions must be carefully timed to the readiness of the parents.

Cues that the parents are ready to become involved with the child's care or planning for the future include their reference to the baby as "she" or "he" or by name and their questioning as to amount of feeding taken, appearance today, and the like.

Mothers may feel inadequate or guilty when they do not feel motherly toward their baby. One mother, looking at her child born with a severe cleft lip and palate, said, "God help me. I can't stand looking at her. I wish she wasn't mine. What a horrid thing to say, but I can't . . . I just can't." She could not bring herself to hold or touch the infant prior to cleft lip repair. She needed considerable assistance to talk of these feelings in a nonjudgmental and accepting atmosphere before she was able to hold the infant after surgery. She proceeded to learn to feed her daughter (whose cleft palate was not yet repaired) and become very "motherly" before the infant was discharged. Her husband, fortunately, facilitated the whole process by his continued love for and acceptance of his wife throughout the experience.

Occasionally, a mother may become overprotective and overoptimistic shortly after the baby's birth. The

WHEN THE NEWBORN ISN'T PERFECT

The issue of who is responsible and what should be done for a child with a congenital anomaly or severe handicap has recently become more complex. What is the impact on the child and the family at the time of the birth and in the future? How can we evaluate the distress the newborn with a severe disability is going through or will suffer during a lifetime?

Recently introduced legal terms are "wrongful life" and "wrongful birth" cases. A wrongful life case is a lawsuit brought by a child with a birth defect. It alleges that the physician failed to advise the parents of the risk of birth defects or failed to perform tests that would have indicated the presence or likelihood of birth defects. In addition the suit claims that because the child's parents were deprived of medical information to make an informed choice, the mother conceived and carried to term a child suffering from birth defects. A wrongful birth case is identical to a wrongful life case, but it is usually brought by the parents rather than the child. Courts have recognized wrongful birth cases over the past decade but have been perplexed by the wrongful life claims because of the view that the involved handicapped child is arguing that he or she would have been better off not being born rather than being born with a birth defect. The courts were unwilling to "weigh the value of life with impairments against the nonexistence of life itself." The courts are now addressing these cases with the focus on the child's right to be compensated for injuries caused by the physician's negligence. This dilemma has prompted philosophical, ethical, moral, legal, and economic questions. The questions and concerns that are being raised include the following:

- How does one measure the emotional impact of the birth of a severely disabled infant?

- Is not being born preferable to being born with a serious handicap or birth defect?

- Who or what determines quality of life?

- Is a certain quality of life guaranteed?

- What is the social and economic impact on the child and family over the lifetime of the child born with a birth defect or severe handicap?

- What constitutes a "defect"? Should we as a society reevaluate our insistence on "perfection" and widen our acceptance of "disability"?

nurse should accept her behavior but continue to remind her that it is okay and natural to feel disappointment, a sense of failure, helplessness, or anger. The overprotectiveness and overoptimism are defense mechanisms. To deny the negative feelings only entrenches them further, delays their resolution, and delays realistic planning.

Developmental Consequences

The baby who is born prematurely, is ill, or has a malformation or disorder is at risk in emotional and intellectual, as well as physical, development. The risk is directly proportional to the seriousness of the problem and the length of treatment. For example, resolution of a meconium plug syndrome during the expected hospital stay, allowing the infant to be discharged with the mother, is not expected to alter the child's developmental course. However, the physical appearance, immediate and repeated surgeries, and complex rehabilitation problems of exstrophy of the bladder or meningomyelocele preclude a normal developmental course for the child.

Medical, surgical, and technical advances in recent years have been responsible for salvaging increasing numbers of preterm and ill newborns. However, the necessary physical separation of family and infant and the tremendous emotional and financial burdens adversely affect the parent-child relationship. A considerable percentage of these children have been rescued only to be emotionally or physically battered by the parents. The most recent trend in many hospitals is to involve the parents with the neonate early, repeatedly, and over protracted periods of time. Early and continued involvement may only mean opportunities to look at or stroke the baby (Figure 32–16). Later, when the mother's and baby's conditions warrant it, the mother participates in her baby's care (to the extent she is willing) and in planning for the future. This type of involvement facilitates early bonding, attachment, and emotional investment. The parents need a sense of personal success, self-worth, self-esteem, and confidence from knowledge that they can cope with the situation. This atmosphere aids the baby as well—the child may escape battering and may instead be assisted toward self-actualization.

Mothers of newborns who are gravely ill are often unable to chance an emotional investment in their child. When their baby stabilizes, these mothers need assistance in perceiving the cues and hearing the words that indicate the baby is going to survive. They need time and support to establish a positive relationship with the newborn. A mother who is unable to develop maternal feelings may reject the baby or overcompensate because of underlying guilt feelings; in either case an unproductive relationship may develop. The child may then be further handicapped by inability to relate well to others and by seeing the world as unsatisfying and painful.

The parents must have a clear picture of the reality of the handicap and the types of developmental hurdles ahead. Unexpected behaviors and responses from the baby due to his or her defect or disorder can be upsetting and frightening. For example, parents find it difficult to cope with a baby's lack of motor or social responsiveness and tend to interpret the lack as a form of rejection. The parents may in return respond with rejection, and an unfortunate cycle is begun.

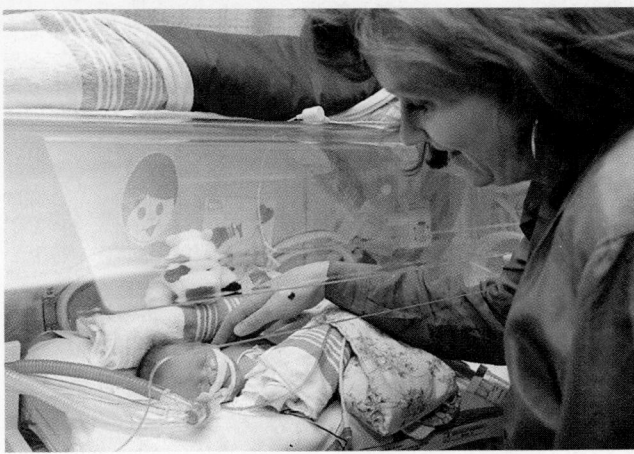

FIGURE 32-16 When parents participate in their baby's care, they tend to have realistic expectations of the child's long-term developmental needs.

The demands of care of the child and disputes regarding management or behavior stress family relationships. One or more members of the family may make a scapegoat of the child. Another may become the youngster's champion to the exclusion of others. One or the other spouse may feel pushed aside or denied attention and thus may withdraw or leave the family unit. Parents or siblings may feel that their own needs (schooling, material goods, freedom of movement) are being set aside while all assets (financial and other) go to support the one child's needs.

The entire multidisciplinary team may need to pool their resources and expertise to help parents of children born with problems or disorders so that both parents and children can thrive.

KEY CONCEPTS

The sick newborn—whether preterm, term, or postterm—must be managed with narrow physiologic parameters.

These parameters (respiratory, cardiovascular, and thermal regulation) will maintain physiologic homeostasis and prevent introduction of iatrogenic stress to the already stressed infant.

The nursing care of the newborn with special problems involves the understanding of normal physiology, the pathophysiology of the disease process, clinical manifestations, and supportive or corrective therapies. Only with this theoretical background can the newborn nurse make appropriate observations concerning responses to therapy and development of complications.

Asphyxia results in significant circulatory, respiratory, and biochemical changes in the newborn that make the suc-

cessful transition to extrauterine life difficult. Asphyxia requires early identification and resuscitative management.

Newborn conditions that commonly present with respiratory distress and require oxygen and ventilatory assistance are respiratory distress syndrome, transient tachypnea of the newborn, meconium aspiration syndrome, and persistent pulmonary hypertension.

Cold stress sets up the chain of physiologic events of hypoglycemia, pulmonary vasoconstriction, hyperbilirubinemia, respiratory distress, and metabolic acidosis.

Nurses are responsible for early detection and initiation of treatment for hypoglycemia. Nurses are essential in the initial screening and management of hypocalcemia.

Differentiation between pathologic and physiologic jaundice is the key to early and successful intervention.

Anemia (decreased amount of red blood cell volume) or polycythemia (excess amount) place the newborn at risk for alterations in blood flow and the oxygen-carrying capacity of the blood.

Nursing assessment of the septic newborn involves identification of very subtle clinical signs that are also seen in other clinical disease states.

The nurse is the facilitator for interdisciplinary communication with the parents, identifying their understanding of their infant's care and their needs for emotional support.

Parents of at-risk newborns need support from nurses and health care providers to understand the special needs of their baby and to feel comfortable in an overwhelmingly strange environment.

REFERENCES

Abman SH, Groothius JR: Pathophysiology and treatment of bronchopulmonary dysplasia: Current issues. *Pediatr Clin North Am* 1994; 41(2):277.

Ahlfors CE: Criteria for exchange transfusion in jaundiced newborns. *Pediatrics* 1994; 93(3):488.

American Academy of Pediatrics: Practice parameter: Management of hyperbilirubinemia in the healthy term newborn. *Pediatrics* 1994; 94(4):558.

Blanchette V et al: Hematology. In: *Neonatology-Pathophysiology and Management of the Newborn*, 4th ed. Avery GB et al (editors). Philadelphia: Lippincott, 1994.

Chameides L (editor): *Textbook of Neonatal Resuscitation*. Elk Grove Village, IL: American Heart Association and American Academy of Pediatrics, 1990.

Cole MD, Peevy K: Hypoglycemia in normal neonates appropriate for gestational age. *J Perinatol* 1994; 14(2):118.

Cornblath M, Schwartz R: Hypoglycemia in the neonate. *J Pediatr Endocrin* 1993; 6(2):113.

Cotton RB: A model of the effect of surfactant treatment on gas exchange in hyaline membrane disease. *Semin Perinatol* 1994; 18(1):19.

Dennery PA, Rhine WD, Stevenson DK: Neonatal jaundice: What now? *Clin Pediatr* February 1995:103.

Gartner LM, Catz CS, Yaffe SJ: Neonatal bilirubin workshop. *Pediatrics* 1994; 94(4):537.

Glomella TL: *Neonatology: Management, Procedures, On-Call Problems, Diseases and Drugs*, 3rd ed. Norwalk, CT: Appleton & Lange, 1994.

Hansen TWR: Bilirubin in the brain: Distribution and effects on neurophysiological and neurochemical processes. *Clin Pediatr* August 1994:452.

Hudak BB, Jones MD: Meconium aspiration. In: *Current Therapy in Neonatal-Perinatal Medicine—2.* Nelson NM (editor). Philadelphia: Decker, 1990.

Jepson HA, Talashek ML, Tichy AM: The Apgar score: Evolution, limitations, and scoring guidelines. *Birth* 1991; 18(2):83.

Kerwin ME, Osborne M, Eicher PS: Effect of position and support on oral-motor skills of a child with bronchopulmonary dysplasia. *Clin Pediatr* January 1994:8.

Knoppert DC, Mackanjee HR: Current strategies in the management of bronchopulmonary dysplasia: The role of corticosteroids. *Neonatal Network* 1994; 13(3):53.

Krause K, Younger V: Nursing diagnoses as guidelines in the care of the neonatal ECMO patient. *JOGNN* 1992; 21(3):169.

Lapido M: Respiratory distress revisited. *Neonatal Network* 1989; 8(3):9.

Lott JW: *Neonatal Infection: Assessment, Diagnosis, and Management.* Petaluma, CA: NICU Ink, 1994.

Mag-akat Angeles D: Pathophysiology and nursing management of pulmonary hypertension of the newborn. *MCN* 1992; 17:314.

Maisels MJ: Jaundice. In: *Neonatology: Pathophysiology and Management of the Newborn*, 4th ed. Avery GB et al (editors). Philadelphia: Lippincott, 1994.

Merenstein GB, Gardner SL: *Handbook of Neonatal Intensive Care*, 3rd ed. St Louis: Mosby, 1993.

Miller E, Armstrong C: Surfactant replacement therapy: Innovative care for the preterm infant. *JOGNN* 1990; 19(1):14.

Moya FR, Gross I: Combined hormonal therapy for the prevention of respiratory distress syndrome and its consequences. *Semin Perinatol* 1993; 17(4):267.

Newman TB, Maisels MJ: Evaluation and treatment of jaundice in the full term newborn: A kind, gentle approach. *Pediatrics* 1992; 89(5):809.

NRP Instructor Update. Elk Grove Village, IL: American Academy of Pediatrics and American Heart Association, 1993; 2(1).

Nugent J: *Acute Respiratory Care of the Neonate.* Petaluma, CA: Neonatal Network, 1991.

Osborne SE, Kassity NA: Neonatal resuscitation program update. *Neonatal Intensive Care* 1993; 6(7):32.

Payne NR, Schilling CG, Steinberg S: Selecting antibiotics for nosocomial bacterial infections in patients requiring neonatal intensive care. *Neonatal Network* 1994; 13(3):41.

Rozycki HJ, Kirkpatrick BV: New developments in bronchopulmonary dysplasia. *Pediatr Annals* 1993; 22(9):532.

Shapiro SM: Brainstem auditory evoked potentials in an experimental model of bilirubin neurotoxicity. *Clin Pediatr* August 1994:460.

Sunnehag A, Gustafsson, Ewald U: Very immature infants (< 30 wk) respond to glucose infusion with incomplete suppression of glucose production. *Pediatr Res* 1994; 36(4):550.

Tan KL: Comparison of the efficacy of fiberoptic and conventional phototherapy for neonatal hyperbilirubinemia. *J Pediatr* 1994; 125(4):607.

PART SEVEN

POSTPARTUM

CHAPTER 33

POSTPARTAL ADAPTATION AND NURSING ASSESSMENT

I had heard about the negatives—the fatigue, the loneliness, loss of self. But nobody told me about the wonderful parts: holding my baby close to me, seeing her first smile, watching her grow and become more responsive day by day. How can I describe the way I felt when she stroked my breast while nursing, or looked into my eyes or arched her eyebrows like an opera singer? This was the deepest connection I'd felt to anybody. Sometimes the intensity almost frightened me. For the first time I cared about somebody else more than myself, and I would do anything to nurture and protect her.

~ THE NEW OUR BODIES, OURSELVES ~

KEY TERMS

Afterpains

Boggy uterus

Diastasis recti abdominis

Fourth trimester

Fundus

Involution

Lochia

Lochia alba

Lochia rubra

Lochia serosa

Maternal role attainment

Postpartum blues

Puerperium

Subinvolution

OBJECTIVES

Describe the basic physiologic changes that occur in the postpartal period as a woman's body returns to its prepregnant state.

Discuss the physiologic adjustments that normally occur during the postpartal period.

Delineate a normal postpartal assessment.

Discuss the physical and developmental tasks that the mother must accomplish during the postpartal period.

The **puerperium,** or postpartal period, is the period during which the woman adjusts, physically and psychologically, to pregnancy and birth. It begins immediately after birth and continues for approximately 6 weeks or until the body has returned to a near prepregnant state. The puerperium is often referred to as the **fourth trimester.** Although the time span is less than 3 months, this term demonstrates the idea of continuity.

This chapter describes the physiologic and psychologic changes and adaptations that occur postpartally and the basic aspects of a thorough postpartal assessment.

POSTPARTAL PHYSICAL ADAPTATIONS

Comprehensive nursing assessment is based on a sound understanding of the normal anatomic and physiologic processes of the puerperium. These processes involve the reproductive organs and other major body systems.

Reproductive System

Involution of the Uterus

The term **involution** is used to describe the rapid reduction in size of the uterus and its return to a condition similar to its prepregnant state, although it remains slightly larger than it was before the first pregnancy.

Following separation of the placenta, the decidua of the uterus is irregular, jagged, and varied in thickness. With the dramatic decrease in the levels of circulating estrogen and progesterone following placental separation the uterine cells atrophy, and the hyperplasia of pregnancy begins to reverse. The process is one in which the size of the cells decreases markedly, rather than a decrease in cell numbers (Cunningham et al 1993). Proteolytic enzymes are released, and macrophages migrate to the uterus to promote autolysis (self-digestion). Protein material in the uterine wall is broken down and absorbed. The spongy layer of the decidua is cast off as lochia, and the basal layer of the decidua remains in the uterus to become differentiated into two layers within the first 48 to 72 hours after birth. The outermost layer becomes necrotic and is sloughed off in the lochia. The layer closest to the myometrium contains the fundi of the uterine endometrial glands, and these glands lay the foundation for the new endometrium. Except at the placental site this process is completed in approximately 3 weeks.

Involution of the placental site is a similar process but takes up to 6 weeks for completion. Following separation, the placental site contracts to an area 8 to 9 cm in diameter that appears raised and irregular. Bleeding from the larger uterine vessels is controlled by compression of the retracted uterine muscle fibers. The placental site consists of multiple thrombosed vascular sinusoids that are treated by the body as any other vascular clot. Some of these vessels are eventually destroyed and replaced by new vessels with smaller lumens.

Rather than forming a fibrous scar in the decidua, the placental site heals by a process of exfoliation. The placental site is undermined by the growth of the endometrial tissue both from the margins of the site and from the fundi of the endometrial glands left in the basal layer of the site. The infarcted superficial tissue then becomes necrotic and is sloughed off. *Exfoliation* is one of the most important aspects of involution. If the healing of the placental site left a fibrous scar, the area available for further implantation would be limited, as would the number of possible pregnancies.

Factors that retard uterine involution and their rationales are listed in Table 33–1. Some factors that enhance involution include an uncomplicated labor and birth, complete expulsion of the amniotic membranes and the placenta, breastfeeding, and early ambulation.

Changes in Fundal Position

Immediately following the explusion of the placenta, the uterus contracts firmly to the size of a large grapefruit. The **fundus** (top portion of the uterus) is situated in the midline, one-half to two-thirds of the way between the symphysis pubis and the umbilicus (Figure 33–1). The walls of the contracted uterus, each about 4 to 5 cm thick, are close together, and the uterine blood vessels are firmly compressed by the myometrium. Within 6–12 hours after birth the fundus of the uterus rises to the level of the umbilicus because of blood and clots that remain within the

TABLE 33–1	Factors That Retard Uterine Involution

Factor	Rationale
Prolonged labor	Muscles relax due to prolonged time of contraction during labor.
Anesthesia	Muscles relax.
Difficult birth	The uterus is manipulated excessively.
Grandmultiparity	Repeated distention of uterus during pregnancy and labor leads to muscle stretching, diminished tone, and muscle relaxation.
Full bladder	As the uterus is pushed up and to the right, pressure on it interferes with effective uterine contraction.
Incomplete expulsion of placenta and/or membranes	The presence of even small amounts of tissue interferes with ability of uterus to remain firmly contracted.
Infection	Inflammation interferes with uterine muscle's ability to contract effectively.

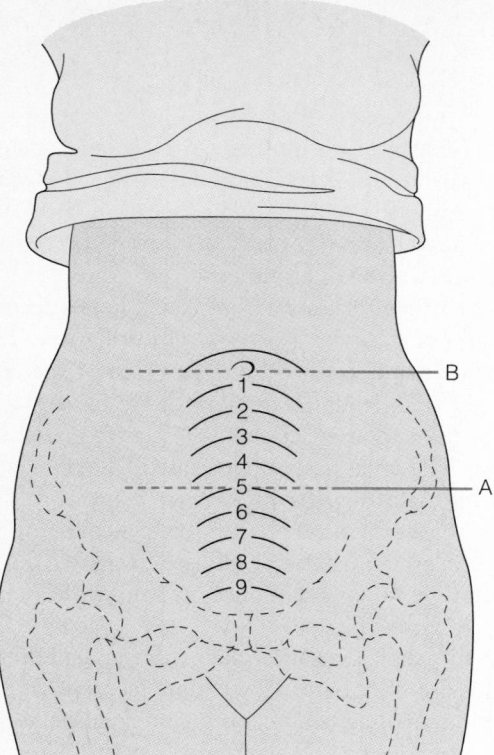

FIGURE 33-1 Involution of the uterus. Immediately after delivery of the placenta the top of the fundus is in the midline and approximately halfway between the symphysis pubis and the umbilicus. About 6–12 hours after birth the fundus is at the level of the umbilicus. The height of the fundus then decreases about one fingerbreadth (approximately 1 cm) each day.

uterus and changes in support of the uterus by the ligaments (Zlatnik 1994). A fundus that is above the umbilicus and boggy (feels soft and spongy rather than firm and well contracted), is associated with excessive uterine bleeding. As blood collects and forms clots within the uterus, the fundus rises; firm contractions of the uterine muscle are interrupted, causing a **boggy uterus.** When the fundus is higher than expected and deviated from the midline (usually to the right), bladder distention should be suspected. Because the uterine ligaments are still stretched, a full bladder can move the uterus.

After birth the top of the fundus remains at the level of the umbilicus for about half a day. On the first postpartum day the top of the fundus is located about 1 cm below the umbilicus. The top of the fundus descends approximately one fingerbreadth per day until it descends into the pelvis on about the tenth day (Blackburn & Loper 1992).

If the mother is breastfeeding, the release of endogenous oxytocin from the posterior pituitary in response to suckling hastens this process. Barring complications, such as infection or retained placental fragments, the uterus approaches its prepregnant size and location by 5–6

weeks (Cunningham et al 1993). If infection is present, the uterine fundus descends much more slowly. This slowing of descent is called **subinvolution** (for further discussion of subinvolution see Chapter 36).

Lochia

One of the unique capabilities of the uterus is its ability to rid itself of the debris remaining after birth. This discharge, termed **lochia,** is classified according to its appearance and contents. **Lochia rubra** is dark red in color. This discharge occurs for the first 2 to 3 days and contains epithelial cells, erythrocytes, leukocytes, shreds of the decidua, and occasionally fetal meconium, lanugo, and vernix caseosa. Lochia should not contain large clots; if it does, the cause should be discovered without delay. A few small clots (no larger than a nickel) are considered normal. **Lochia serosa** follows from about the third until the tenth day. It is a pinkish to brownish color and is composed of serous exudate (hence the name), shreds of degenerating decidua, erythrocytes, leukocytes, cervical mucus, and numerous microorganisms.

The blood cell component decreases gradually, and a creamy or yellowish discharge persists for an additional week or two. This final discharge, termed **lochia alba,** is composed primarily of leukocytes, decidual cells, epithelial cells, fat, cervical mucus, cholesterol crystals, and bacteria. When the lochia stops, the cervix is considered closed, and chances of infection ascending from the vagina to the uterus decrease.

Like menstrual discharge, lochia has a musty, stale odor that is not offensive. Microorganisms are always present in the vaginal lochia, and by the second day following birth the uterus is contaminated with the vaginal bacteria. Researchers speculate that infection does not develop because the organisms involved are relatively nonvirulent. In addition, by the time the bacteria reach the raw, exposed surface of the uterus, the process of granulation has begun, forming a protective barrier. Any foul smell to the lochia or used peri-pad suggests infection and the need for prompt additional assessment, such as white blood cell count and differential, and assessment for uterine tenderness and fever.

The total volume of lochia is approximately 240 to 270 mL (8 to 9 oz), and the daily volume decreases gradually. Discharge is heavier in the morning than at night because lochia tends to pool in the vagina and uterus when the woman is recumbent and is discharged when she arises, because of gravity. The amount of lochia may also be increased by exertion or breastfeeding.

Evaluation of lochia is necessary not only to determine the presence of hemorrhage but also to assess uterine involution. The type, amount, and consistency of lochia determine the state of healing of the placental site, and a progressive change from bright red at birth to dark red to pink to white/clear discharge should be observed. Persistent discharge of lochia rubra or a return to lochia rubra indicates subinvolution or late postpartal hemorrhage (see Chapter 36).

Caution should be exercised in the evaluation of bleeding immediately after birth. The continuous seepage of blood is more consistent with cervical or vaginal lacerations and may be effectively diagnosed when the bleeding is evaluated in conjunction with the consistency of the uterus. Lacerations should be suspected if the uterus is firm, of expected size, and if no clots can be expressed.

Cervical Changes

Immediately following birth the cervix is spongy, flabby, and formless and may appear bruised. However, the original form of the cervix is regained within a few hours (Zlatnik 1994). The external os is markedly irregular and closes slowly. It admits two fingers for a few days following birth, but by the end of the first week only a fingertip opening remains.

The shape of the external os is permanently changed following the first vaginal birth. The characteristic dimplelike os of the nullipara changes to the lateral slit (smile) os of the multipara. After significant cervical laceration or several lacerations, the cervix may appear lopsided. After the slight change in the size of the cervix, a diaphragm or cervical cap will need to be refitted if the woman is using one of these methods of contraception.

Vaginal Changes

Following birth the vagina appears edematous and may be bruised. Small superficial lacerations may be evident, and the rugae have been obliterated. The apparent bruising of the vagina is due to pelvic congestion and will quickly disappear. The hymen, torn and jagged, heals irregularly, leaving small tags called the *carunculae myrtiformes*.

The size of the vagina decreases, and vaginal rugae begin to return by 3 weeks. This facilitates the gradual return to smaller, although not nulliparous, dimensions. By 6 weeks the nonlactating woman's vagina usually appears normal. The lactating woman is in a hypoestrogenic state because of ovarian suppression, and her vaginal mucosa may be pale and without rugae. This may lead to dyspareunia (painful intercourse) (Zlatnik 1994). Tone and contractibility of the vaginal opening may be improved by perineal tightening exercises (Kegel's exercises, discussed in Chapter 15), which may begin soon after birth. The labia majora and labia minora are flabbier in the woman who has borne a child than in the nullipara.

Perineal Changes

During the early postpartal period the soft tissue in and around the perineum may appear edematous (Figure 33–2). If an episiotomy or laceration is present, the edges

CRITICAL THINKING IN PRACTICE

You have completed your assessment of Patty Clark, a 24-year-old, G2P2, woman who is 24 hours past birth. The fundus is just above the umbilicus, and slightly to the right. Lochia rubra is present, and a pad is soaked every 2 hours. What would you do?

Answers can be found in Appendix I.

should be approximated. Occasionally, ecchymosis occurs, and this may delay healing.

Recurrence of Ovulation and Menstruation

The return of menstruation and ovulation varies for each postpartal woman. Menstruation generally returns in nonnursing mothers between 6 and 10 weeks after birth, and 50% of the first cycles are anovulatory (Blackburn & Loper 1992). Overall, 40% of nonnursing mothers resume menstruation by 6 weeks, and 90% resume within 24 weeks after birth.

The return of menstruation and ovulation in nursing mothers is usually prolonged and is associated with the length of time the woman breastfeeds and whether formula supplements are used. If a nursing mother breastfeeds for less than 1 month, the return of menstruation and ovulation is similar to the nonnursing mother. In women who continue to breastfeed, the average time for the return of menstruation is 30–36 weeks, and 17–28 weeks for the return of ovulation (Blackburn & Loper 1992).

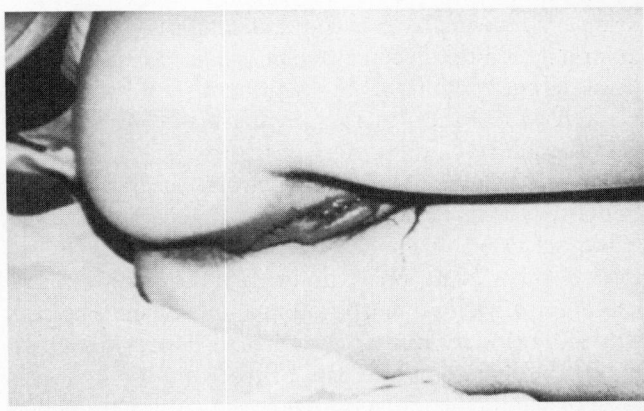

FIGURE 33-2   Bruising and edema of the vulva and perineum in a primipara 3 days after a forceps delivery. SOURCE: Bennett VR, Brown LK: *Myles Textbook for Midwives,* 11th ed. Edinburgh: Churchill-Livingstone, 1989, p 235.

Abdomen

The uterine ligaments (notably the round and broad ligaments) are stretched and require time to recover. The abdominal wall itself has also been stretched and will appear loose and somewhat flabby for a time. With exercise abdominal muscle tone will improve greatly within 2 to 3 months. In the grandmultipara, in the woman in whom overdistention of the abdomen has occurred, or in the woman with poor muscle tone before pregnancy the abdomen may fail to regain good tone and may remain flabby. **Diastasis recti abdominis,** a separation of the rectus abdominis muscles, may occur with pregnancy, especially in women with poor abdominal muscle tone. If diastasis occurs, part of the abdominal wall has no muscular support but is formed only by skin, subcutaneous fat, fascia, and peritoneum. Improvement depends on the physical condition of the mother, the total number of pregnancies, and the type and amount of physical exercise. If rectus muscle tone is not regained, support may be inadequate during future pregnancies. This may result in a pendulous abdomen and increased maternal backache. Fortunately, diastasis responds well to exercise, and abdominal muscle tone can improve significantly.

The striae (stretch marks), which occurred as a result of stretching and rupture of the elastic fibers of the skin, take on different colors based on the mother's skin color. The striae of caucasian mothers are red to purple at the time of birth and gradually fade to silver or white. The striae of mothers with darker skin are darker than the surrounding skin and remain darker.

Lactation

During pregnancy, breast development in preparation for lactation results from the influence of both estrogen and progesterone. After birth the interplay of maternal hormones leads to the establishment of milk production.

Gastrointestinal System

Hunger following birth is common, and the mother may enjoy a light meal. Frequently, she is quite thirsty and will drink large amounts of fluid. Drinking fluids helps replace fluid lost during labor, in the urine, and through perspiration.

The bowels tend to be sluggish after birth due to the lingering effects of progesterone and decreased abdominal muscle tone. The practice of omitting solid food during labor may cause a delay in the first bowel movement.

The pain from an episiotomy, any lacerations, and hemorrhoids may lead the woman to delay elimination for fear of increasing the pain or tearing her stitches. In most instances the initial bowel movement is not uncomfortable. However, refusing or delaying the bowel movement may cause constipation and more discomfort when elimination finally occurs.

Fluids and solid foods are delayed for the woman who has had a cesarean birth until bowel sounds return.

Clear liquids are generally begun by the day after surgery (first postoperative day), and the diet is quickly advanced to solid food once bowel sounds return. The woman may experience some discomfort from flatulence initially. This is relieved by early ambulation and use of antiflatulent medications. It may take a few days for the bowel to regain its tone. The woman who has had a cesarean or a difficult birth may benefit from stool softeners. In some cases it may be necessary to administer an enema or suppository to promote elimination.

Urinary Tract

Increased bladder capacity, swelling and bruising of the tissues around the urethra, decreased sensitivity to fluid pressure, decreased sensation of bladder filling, and inability to void in the recumbent position put the puerperal woman at risk for overdistention, incomplete emptying, and buildup of residual urine. In addition women who have had a regional anesthetic block have inhibited neural functioning of the bladder and are more susceptible to urinary retention.

Urinary output increases during the early postpartal period (first 12 to 24 hours) due to *puerperal diuresis.* The kidneys must eliminate an estimated 2000 to 3000 mL of extracellular fluid with a normal pregnancy. With pregnancy-induced hypertension (PIH), chronic hypertension, and diabetes, even greater fluid retention is experienced, and postpartal diuresis is increased accordingly.

Bladder elimination presents an immediate problem. If stasis exists, chances increase for urinary tract infection because of bacteriuria and the presence of dilated ureters and renal pelves, which persist for about 6 weeks after birth. A full bladder may also increase the tendency of the uterus to relax by displacing the uterus and interfering with its contractility, leading to hemorrhage.

Hematuria, resulting from bladder trauma, may occasionally occur after birth, but the presence of lochia may mask this sign. If hematuria occurs in the second or third postpartal week, there may be a bladder infection. Acetone may be present in the urine of women with diabetes or of women with prolonged labor and dehydration. Slight (1+) proteinuria may occur during the first week following birth. However, proteinuria may be associated with an infectious process (cystitis, pyelitis), so it should be further evaluated. A urine specimen contaminated with lochia may be the cause of proteinuria, so any specimen should be obtained as a midstream or a catheterized specimen.

Vital Signs

During the postpartal period, with the exception of the first 24 hours, the woman should be afebrile. A temperature of up to 38 C (100.4 F) may occur after birth as a result of the exertion and dehydration of labor. Infection must be considered in the woman with a temperature of 38 C or above after the first 24 hours.

Blood pressure readings should remain stable and within normal range following the birth. A decrease may indicate physiologic readjustment to decreased intrapelvic pressure, or it may be related to uterine hemorrhage. Blood pressure elevations, especially when accompanied by headache, suggest PIH, and the woman should be evaluated further.

Puerperal bradycardia with rates of 50 to 70 beats per minute commonly occurs during the first 6 to 10 days of the postpartal period. It may be related to decreased cardiac strain, the decreased blood volume following placental separation, contraction of the uterus, and increased stroke volume. Tachycardia occurs less frequently and is related to increased blood loss or difficult, prolonged labor and birth.

Blood Values

The blood values should return to the prepregnant state by the end of the postpartal period. Pregnancy-associated activation of coagulation factors may continue for variable amounts of time. This condition, in conjunction with trauma, immobility, or sepsis, predisposes the woman to development of thromboembolism. Plasma fibrinogen is maintained at pregnancy levels for a week, accounting for the higher sedimentation rate observed in the early postpartum period.

Leukocytosis with white blood cell counts of 15,000 to 20,000 per μL persists in the early postpartal days. The leukocytosis cannot be relied upon to indicate infection. Other clinical signs of infection (elevation of temperature, redness, swelling, and pain) must be evaluated.

Blood loss averages 200 to 500 mL with a vaginal birth and 700 to 1000 mL with cesarean birth. Hemoglobin and erythrocyte values vary during the early puerperium, but they should approximate or exceed prelabor values within 2 to 6 weeks. As extracellular fluid is excreted, hemoconcentration occurs, with a concomitant rise in hematocrit. A drop in values indicates an abnormal blood loss. The following is a convenient rule of thumb: a 2-point drop in hematocrit equals a blood loss of 500 mL (Varney 1987).

Weight Loss

An initial weight loss of 10 to 12 lb occurs as a result of the birth of infant, placenta, and amniotic fluid. Puerperal diuresis accounts for the loss of an additional 5 lb during the early puerperium. By the sixth to eighth week after birth many women have returned to approximately prepregnant weight if they gained the average 25 to 30 lb. For others a return to prepregnant weight takes longer.

Postpartal Chill

Frequently, the mother experiences a shaking chill immediately after birth, which may be related to a neurologic response or to vasomotor changes. If not followed by fever, it is not of clinical concern, but it is uncomfortable for the woman. Covering the woman with warmed bath blankets will help alleviate the chill and increase her comfort. The mother may also find a warm beverage helpful. Chills and fever later in the puerperium indicate infection and require further evaluation.

Postpartal Diaphoresis

The elimination of excess fluid and waste products via the skin during the puerperium greatly increases perspiration. Diaphoretic episodes frequently occur at night, and the woman may awaken drenched with perspiration. This perspiration is not significant clinically, but the mother should be protected from chilling.

Afterpains

Afterpains occur more commonly in multiparas than in primiparas and are caused by intermittent uterine contractions. Although the uterus of the primipara usually remains consistently contracted, the lost tone of the uterus of the multipara results in alternate contraction and relaxation. This phenomenon also occurs if the uterus has been markedly distended, as with multiple pregnancies or hydramnios, or if clots or placental fragments were retained. These afterpains may cause the mother severe discomfort for 2 to 3 days following birth. The administration of oxytocic agents (IV infusion with Pitocin or PO Methergine) stimulates uterine contraction and increases the discomfort of the afterpains. Because oxytocin is released when the infant suckles, breastfeeding also increases the severity of the afterpains. The nursing mother may find it helpful to take a mild analgesic approximately 1 hour before feeding her infant. The nurse can assure the nursing mother that the prescribed analgesics are not harmful to the newborn and help improve the quality of the breastfeeding experience. An analgesic is also helpful at bedtime if the afterpains interfere with the mother's rest.

POSTPARTAL PSYCHOLOGIC ADAPTATIONS

The postpartal period is a time of readjustment and adaptation for the entire childbearing family, but especially for the mother. The woman experiences a variety of responses as she adjusts to a new family member, postpartum discomforts, changes in her body image, and the reality that she is no longer pregnant. One young mother described her responses well:

> I feel like it's the day after Christmas. I'm relieved that everything went well and I have a fine baby, but I feel so let down. I had an image of what my delivery would be like, and everything was a little different. I figured that as soon as I delivered, I would feel fine. Why didn't someone tell me I would

still be sore; the pain didn't magically disappear! When I was pregnant, everyone treated me as though I was a little fragile. Now when people call or visit, all they talk about is the baby. I don't think I'm really jealous, but I do miss the attention. During this past day I've started to realize that my life will never, ever be the same again. I've always wanted to be a mother, but I'm not really sure how to do it. Isn't that strange?

During the first day or two following birth the woman tends to be passive and somewhat dependent. The new mother follows suggestions, is hesitant about making decisions, and is still rather preoccupied with her needs. She may have a great need to talk about her perceptions of her labor and birth. This helps her work through the process, sort out the reality from her fantasized experience, and clarify anything that she did not understand.

During this time food and sleep are major focuses for her. The woman is talkative but passive. In her early work Rubin (1961) labeled this the *taking-in* period.

By the second or third day after birth the new mother has had time to relive her experience, adjust to her new life, rest, and recover from childbirth. She is then ready to resume control of her life. The new mother may be concerned about controlling bodily functions such as elimination. If she is breastfeeding, she may worry about the quality of her milk and her ability to nurse her baby. She requires assurance that she is doing well as a mother. If her baby spits up following feeding, she may view it as a personal failure. She may also feel demoralized by the fact that the nurse handles her baby proficiently while she feels unsure and tentative. Rubin (1961) labeled this phase as *taking-hold*.

Today's mothers seem to be more independent and to adjust more rapidly. Ament (1990) found that women did exhibit behavior characteristic of "taking-in" and "taking-hold" but found that the time frames were shorter than those cited by Rubin. Ament found that taking-in occurred only during the first 24 hours after childbirth. It will be interesting to see what further study brings to this subject.

Postpartally, the woman must adjust to a changed body image. Often women, especially primiparas, are surprised and rather dismayed to discover that they do not return to their prepregnant weight and shape as soon as the baby is born. Women often express dissatisfaction about their appearance and concern about the return of their weight and figure to normal. Multiparas tend to be more positive about their appearance postpartally than primiparas. This may be because the multipara's previous experience has prepared her for the fact that the body does not immediately return to a prepregnant state.

The psychologic outcomes of the postpartal period are far more positive when the parents have access to a support network. Women and their partners may find that family relationships become increasingly important,

and the attention that their infant receives from family members is a source of satisfaction to the new parents. In many cases the ties to the woman's family become especially good. Fathers may report that their relationships with their in-laws become far more positive and supportive. But the increased family interaction can be a source

RESEARCH IN PRACTICE

Sandra Ferketich and Ramona Mercer identified predictors of paternal role competence based on the risk status of the partner's pregnancy. Fathers were classified according to whether their partners had experienced a low-risk pregnancy (LRM) or had had an antenatal hospitalization for a high-risk condition (HRM). In this longitudinal study, the authors explored paternal competence, self-esteem, sense of mastery of infant care-giving skills, partner relationship, family functioning, depression, anxiety, support, feelings about labor and delivery, infant's health status, relationship with their own parents, negative life events stress, and paternal attachment. The fathers were tested during their partner's pregnancy at 24–34 weeks' gestation, during the postpartal hospitalization, and after the birth at 1, 4, and 8 months.

The hypothesis that HRM fathers would report significantly less paternal competence than the LRM group was not validated by the study. However, the second hypothesis, that a significant relationship exists between paternal competence and paternal attachment, was supported with Pearson r correlations ranging from 0.46 to 0.62 for all testing times and both groups. For HRM fathers, the major predictor of paternal competence was level of state anxiety, which explained from 15% to 24% of the variance. Other important predictors, tested at specific times, included the variables of family function and educational level (during hospitalization) and labor and delivery experience (at 8 months postpartum). For the LRM fathers, mastery was the major variable, with predictive ranges of 26% to 29%. Depression also correlated negatively with paternal competence and predicted from 5% to 31% of the variance.

Clinical Application of Study

Nurses can assess the anxiety level of those fathers whose partners have a high-risk pregnancy and assist these men in dealing with this problem if necessary. Labor and delivery nurses especially should remember that the labor and delivery experiences of these HRM fathers impact paternal competence several months after the birth.

For the fathers whose partners had a low-risk pregnancy, the nurse should assess for depression and help the father find assistance. Also, the nurse should focus on assisting these fathers to gain mastery in caring for their child because this factor significantly impacts feelings of paternal competence.

SOURCE: Ferketich S, Mercer R: Predictors of paternal role competence by risk status. *Nurs Res* 1994; 43 (2):80.

of stress, especially for the new mother, who tends to have more contact with the families.

Childbearing couples often change their social network somewhat following the birth of their child. Once the new parents have made the transition to parenthood, they both tend to have more contact with other parents of small children. For the woman, interaction with co-workers often declines postpartally, but contact with friends increases. Thus the woman maintains the size of her support group but alters it to meet the changes that have occurred in her life-style.

Perhaps the greatest concern involves women and their partners who have no family available and no friends to form a social network. Isolation when the woman feels an increased need for support can result in tremendous stress and is often a contributing factor in situations of child neglect or abuse.

A prime focus of research in recent years has been maternal role attainment. **Maternal role attainment** is the process by which a woman learns mothering behaviors and becomes comfortable with her identity as a mother. The formation of a maternal identity indicates that the woman has attained the maternal role. Formation of a maternal identity occurs with each child a woman bears. As the mother grows to know this child and forms a relationship with her or him, the mother's maternal identity gradually, systematically evolves, and she "binds in" to the infant (Rubin 1984).

Maternal role attainment occurs in four stages (Mercer 1985). (The formal and informal stages of maternal role attainment correspond with the taking-in and taking-hold stages previously identified by Rubin [1961]):

1. The *anticipatory stage* occurs during pregnancy. The woman looks to role models, especially her own mother, for examples of how to mother.
2. The *formal stage* begins when the child is born. The woman is still influenced by the guidance of others and tries to act as she believes others expect her to act.
3. The *informal stage* begins when the mother begins to make her own choices about mothering. The woman begins to develop her own style of mothering and finds ways of functioning that work well for her.
4. The *personal stage* is the final stage of maternal role attainment. When the woman reaches this stage, she is comfortable with the notion of herself as "mother."

In most cases maternal role attainment occurs within 3 to 10 months following birth. Social support, the woman's age and personality traits, the temperament of her infant, and the family's socioeconomic status all influence the woman's success in attaining the maternal role.

Mothers, whether primiparas or multiparas, have a variety of concerns following childbirth related to their own physiologic changes, newborn care, and methods to manage recovery from childbirth. One example of how nurses can help new mothers with such concerns is a Maternal Concerns Questionnaire developed by Sheil et al (1995) that helps the mother identify the degree of concern she has regarding her own and the baby's needs, concerns related to her partner and family, and concerns related to the community. For each area the mother is able to note specific needs and rate them as no concern, little concern, moderate concern, or much concern. After the mother completes the questionnaire, the nurse can identify her individual concerns and informational needs and address them in individualized nursing care planning and teaching.

Postpartum Blues

The **postpartum blues** consist of a transient period of depression that occurs during the first week or two after birth in most women. It may be manifested by mood swings, anger, weepiness, anorexia, difficulty sleeping, and a feeling of letdown. Because of the practice of early postpartum discharge, the depression often occurs at home. Psychologic adjustments and hormonal changes are thought to be the main cause, although fatigue, discomfort, and overstimulation may play a part. The postpartum blues usually resolve naturally, especially if the woman receives understanding and support. If symptoms persist or intensify, the woman may need evaluation for postpartum depression (see Chapter 36).

Cultural Influences in the Postpartal Period

The new mother's beliefs about her postpartal care are influenced by her culture and personal values. Her expectations regarding food, fluids, rest, hygiene, medications and relief measures, support and counsel, as well as other aspects of her life, will be influenced by the beliefs and values of her family and cultural group. Sometimes a new mother's wishes will differ from what the physician and/or nurse expects.

Nurses also belong to a particular culture, as well as to the health care cultural group. As a part of the health care cultural group nurses may take on some practices that support the general beliefs, such as offering food in the recovery period following birth, providing iced fluids, expecting the woman to ambulate as soon as possible, and assuming the woman will want to shower and perhaps wash her hair soon after birth. It is important for nurses to recognize that they are approaching their client's care from the own perspective, but in order to individualize care for each mother individual choices need to be assessed, offered, and supported.

Although listing particular practices of differing cultural groups always involves some generalization, it is helpful for nurses to understand some of the possible differences in beliefs and practices. For example, a woman of

European heritage may expect to eat a full meal and have large amount of iced fluids following the birth, in the belief that the food restores energy and the fluids help replace fluid lost during the labor. She may want to ambulate shortly after the birth and shower, wash her hair, and put on a fresh gown. She may expect a short stay in the hospital and may or may not be interested in educational classes.

Many cultures emphasize certain postpartal routines or rituals for mother and baby that are designed to restore the harmony, or the hot-cold balance, of the body. Some women of Mexican, African, and Asian cultures may avoid cold after birth. This prohibition includes cold air, wind, and all water (even if heated). Dietary changes also reflect the need to avoid cold foods and restore the balance between hot and cold (Andrew & Boyle 1995; Spector 1991). For instance a traditional Mexican woman may avoid eating "hot" foods such as pork just after the birth of her baby (considered a "hot" experience). It is important to note that each individual may define hot and cold conditions as well as hot and cold foods differently. Therefore the nurse should ask each woman what she can eat and what foods she thinks would be helpful for healing (Andrew & Boyle 1995; Spector 1991). The nurse may encourage family members to bring preferred food and drink for the mother.

In many cultures the extended family frequently plays an essential role during the puerperium. The grandmother is often the primary helper to the mother and newborn. She brings wisdom and experience, allowing the new mother time to rest as well as giving her ready access to someone who can help with problems and concerns as they arise. It is important to assure access of all family members during the postpartal period. Visiting rules may be waived to allow family members or authority figures access to the mother and newborn. These practices show respect and foster a blending of old and new behaviors to meet the goals of all concerned. It is always important to remember that the parent retains "ownership" of what care is appropriate and desired.

Development of Parent-Infant Attachment

During the postpartal period the parents continue to strengthen the bonds with their baby that were established in the prenatal period. This process of attachment has been the focus of significant research in recent years. It is described in depth in Chapter 35.

POSTPARTAL NURSING ASSESSMENT

Comprehensive care is based on a thorough assessment, with identification of individual needs or potential problems. (See the accompanying Postpartal Assessment Guide: First Week After Birth on page 1051.)

TABLE 33–2	Postpartal High-Risk Factors
Factor	**Maternal Implication**
PIH	↑ Blood pressure ↑ CNS irritability ↑ Need for bed rest → ↑ risk thrombophlebitis
Diabetes	Need for insulin regulation Episodes of hypoglycemia or hyperglycemia ↓ Healing
Cardiac disease	↑ Maternal exhaustion
Cesarean birth	↑ Healing needs ↑ Pain from incision ↑ Risk of infection ↑ Length of hospitalization
Overdistention of uterus (multiple gestation, hydramnios)	↑ Risk of hemorrhage ↑ Risk of anemia ↑ Stretching of abdominal muscles ↑ Incidence and severity of afterpains
Abruptio placentae, placenta previa	Hemorrhage → anemia ↓ Uterine contractility after birth → ↑ infection risk
Precipitous labor (<3 hours)	↑ Risk of lacerations to birth canal → hemorrhage
Prolonged labor (>24 hours)	Exhaustion ↑ Risk of hemorrhage Nutritional and fluid depletion ↑ Bladder atony and/or trauma
Difficult birth	Exhaustion ↑ Risk of perineal lacerations ↑ Risk of hematomas ↑ Risk of hemorrhage → anemia
Extended period of time in stirrups at birth	↑ Risk of thrombophlebitis
Retained placenta	↑ Risk of hemorrhage ↑ Risk of infection

Risk Factors

The emphasis on ongoing assessment and education during the puerperium is designed to meet the needs of the childbearing family and to detect and treat possible complications. Table 33–2 identifies factors that may place the new mother at risk during the postpartal period. The nurse uses this knowledge during the assessment and is particularly alert for possible complications that may occur in an individual because of identified risk factors.

Critical Thinking Question

Using your knowledge of general physical assessment, plan a logical approach to postpartum physical assessment.

Physical Assessment

Several principles should be remembered in preparing for and completing the assessment of the postpartal woman:

- Select the time that will provide the most accurate data. Palpating the fundus when the woman has a

Text continues on page 1054

First Week After Birth

Physical Assessment/ Normal Findings	Alterations and Possible Causes*	Nursing Responses to Data†
Vital Signs		
Blood pressure (BP): Should remain consistent with baseline BP during pregnancy.	High BP (PIH, essential hypertension, renal disease, anxiety). Drop in BP (may be normal; uterine hemorrhage).	Evaluate history of preexisting disorders and check for other signs of PIH (edema, proteinuria). Assess for other signs of hemorrhage (↑ pulse, cool clammy skin).
Pulse: 50–90 beats/minute. May be bradycardia of 50–70 beats/minute. Respirations: 16–24/minute. Temperature: 36.2–38 C (98–100.4 F).	Tachycardia (difficult labor and birth, hemorrhage). Marked tachypnea (respiratory disease). After first 24 hours temperature of 38 C (100.4 F) or above suggests infection.	Evaluate for other signs of hemorrhage (↓ BP, cool clammy skin). Assess for other signs of respiratory disease. Assess for other signs of infection; notify physician/certified nurse-midwife.
Breasts		
General appearance: Smooth, even pigmentation, changes of pregnancy still apparent; one may appear larger.	Reddened area (mastitis).	Assess further for signs of infection.
Palpation: Depending on postpartal day, may be soft, filling, full, or engorged.	Palpable mass (caked breast, mastitis). Engorgement (venous stasis). Tenderness, heat, edema (engorgement, caked breast, mastitis).	Assess for other signs of infection: If blocked duct, consider heat, massage, position change for breastfeeding. Assess for further signs. Report mastitis to physician/certified nurse-midwife.
Nipples: Supple, pigmented, intact; become erect when stimulated.	Fissures, cracks, soreness (problems with breastfeeding), not erectile with stimulation (inverted nipples).	Reassess technique; recommend appropriate interventions.
Abdomen		
Musculature: Abdomen may be soft, have a "doughy" texture; rectus muscle intact.	Separation in musculature (diastasis recti abdominis).	Evaluate size of diastasis; teach appropriate exercises for decreasing the separation.
Fundus: Firm, midline; following expected schedule of involution.	Boggy (full bladder, uterine bleeding).	Massage until firm; assess bladder and have woman void if needed; attempt to express clots when firm. If bogginess remains or recurs, report to physician/certified nurse-midwife.
May be tender when palpated.	Constant tenderness (infection).	Assess for evidence of endometritis.
Lochia		
Scant to moderate amount, earthy odor; no clots.	Large amount, clots (hemorrhage). Foul-smelling lochia (infection).	Assess for firmness, express additional clots; begin peri-pad count. Assess for other signs of infection; report to physician/certified nurse-midwife.

*Possible causes of alterations are placed in parentheses.

†This column provides guidelines for further assessment and initial nursing actions.

FIRST WEEK AFTER BIRTH continued

Physical Assessment/ Normal Findings	Alterations and Possible Causes*	Nursing Responses to Data[†]
Normal progression: First 1–3 days: rubra. Days 3–10: serosa (alba seldom seen in hospital).	Failure to progress normally or return to rubra from serosa (subinvolution).	Report to physician/certified nurse-midwife.
Perineum Slight edema and bruising in intact perineum.	Marked fullness, bruising, pain (vulvar hematoma).	Assess size; apply ice glove or ice pack; report to physician/certified nurse-midwife.
Episiotomy: No redness, edema, ecchymosis, or discharge; edges well approximated.	Redness, edema, ecchymosis, discharge, or gaping stitches (infection).	Encourage sitz baths; review perineal care, appropriate wiping techniques.
Hemorrhoids: None present; if present, should be small and nontender.	Full, tender, inflamed hemorrhoids.	Encourage sitz baths, side-lying position; tucks pads, anesthetic ointments, manual replacement of hemorrhoids, stool softeners, increased fluid intake.
Costo-Vertebral Angle (CVA) Tenderness None.	Present (kidney infection).	Assess for other symptoms of urinary tract infection (UTI); obtain clean-catch urine; report to physician/certified nurse-midwife.
Lower Extremities No pain with palpation; negative Homan's sign.	Positive findings (thrombophlebitis).	Report to physician/certified nurse-midwife.
Elimination Urinary output: Voiding in sufficient quantities at least every 4–6 hours; bladder not palpable.	Inability to void (urinary retention). Symptoms of urgency, frequency, dysuria (UTI).	Employ nursing interventions to promote voiding; if not successful, obtain order for catheterization. Report symptoms of UTI to physician/certified nurse-midwife.
Bowel elimination: Should have normal bowel movement by second or third day after birth.	Inability to pass feces (constipation due to fear of pain from episiotomy, hemorrhoids, perineal trauma).	Encourage fluids, ambulation, roughage in diet; sitz baths to promote healing of perineum; obtain order for stool softener.

Cultural Assessment[‡]	Variations to Consider	Nursing Responses to Data[†]
Determine customs and practices regarding postpartum care. Ask the mother if she would like fluids, and ask what temperature she prefers. Ask the mother what foods or fluids she would like.	Individual preference may include: Receiving room temperature or warmed fluids rather than iced drinks. Inclusion of special foods or fluids to hasten healing after childbirth.	Provide for specific request if possible. If woman is unable to provide specific information, the nurse may draw from general information regarding cultural variation. Mexican women may want food and fluids that restore hot-cold balance to the body. Women of European background may ask for iced fluids.

*Possible causes of alterations are placed in parentheses.

[†]This column provides guidelines for further assessment and initial nursing actions.

[‡]These are only a few suggestions. It is not our intent to imply this is a comprehensive cultural assessment.

FIRST WEEK AFTER BIRTH continued

Cultural Assessment[‡]	Variations to Consider	Nursing Responses to Data[†]
Ask the mother if she would prefer to be alone during breastfeeding.	Some women may be hesitant to have someone with them when their breast is exposed.	

Psychosocial Assessment/ Normal Findings	Variations to Consider	Nursing Responses to Data
Psychologic Adaptation		
During first 24 hours: Passive; preoccupied with own needs; may talk about her labor and birth experience; may be talkative, elated, or very quiet.	Very quiet and passive; sleeps frequently (fatigue from long labor; feelings of disappointment about some aspect of the experience; may be following cultural expectation).	Provide opportunities for adequate rest; provide nutritious meals and snacks that are consistent with what the woman desires to eat and drink; provide opportunities to discuss birth experience in nonjudgmental atmosphere if the woman desires to do so.
By 24–48 hours: Beginning to assume responsibility; some women eager to learn; easily feels overwhelmed.	Excessive weepiness, mood swings, pronounced irritability (postpartum blues, feelings of inadequacy; culturally prescribed behavior).	Explain postpartum blues; provide supportive atmosphere; determine support available for mother; consider referral for evidence of profound depression.
Attachment		
En face position; holds baby close; cuddles and soothes; calls by name; identifies characteristics of family members in infant; may be awkward in providing care.	Continued expressions of disappointment in sex, appearance of infant; refusal to care for infant; derogatory comments; lack of bonding behaviors (difficulty in attachment, following expectations of cultural/ethnic group).	Provide reinforcement and support for infant caretaking behaviors; maintain nonjudgmental approach and gather more information if caretaking behaviors are not evident.
Initially may express disappointment over sex or appearance of infant but within 1–2 days demonstrates attachment behaviors.		
Client Education		
Has basic understanding of self-care activities and infant care needs; can identify signs of complications that should be reported.	Unable to demonstrate basic self-care and infant care activities (knowledge deficit; postpartum blues; following prescribed cultural behavior and will be cared for by grandmother or other family member).	Determine whether woman understands English and provide interpreter if needed; provide reinforcement of information through conversation and through written material (remember that some women and their families may not be able to understand written materials due to language difficulties or inability to read); provide information regarding infant care skills that are culturally consistent; give woman opportunity to express her feelings; consider social service home referral for women who have no family or other support, are unable to take in information about self-care and infant care, and demonstrate no caretaking activities.

[†]This column provides guidelines for further assessment and initial nursing actions.

[‡]These are only a few suggestions. It is not our intent to imply this is a comprehensive cultural assessment.

full bladder, for example, may give false information about the progress of involution.

- An explanation of the purpose of regular assessment should be given to the woman.
- The woman should be relaxed, and the procedures should be done as gently as possible to avoid unnecessary discomfort.
- The data obtained should be recorded and reported as clearly as possible.
- The nurse should take care to protect herself from exposure to bodily fluids. (See Essential Precautions in Practice: During Postpartal Assessment.)

While the nurse is performing the physical assessment, she or he should also be teaching the woman. For example, when the nurse is assessing the breasts of a nursing woman, breast milk production, the letdown reflex, and breast self-examination can be discussed. Mothers may be very receptive to instruction on postpartal abdominal tightening exercises when the nurse assesses the woman's fundal height and diastasis. The assessment also provides an excellent time to provide information about the body's postpartal physical and anatomic changes as well as danger signs to report. Because the time the woman spends in the postpartum unit is often limited, nurses should use every available opportunity for client education regarding self-care. One of the best opportunities comes during the normal postpartal assessment. To assist nurses in recognizing these opportunities, examples of client teaching during the assessment have been provided throughout the following discussion.

Vital Signs

The nurse may choose to organize the physical assessment in a variety of ways. Many nurses choose to begin by assessing vital signs because the findings will be more accurate when they are obtained with the woman at rest. In addition, establishing whether the vital signs are within the expected normal range will assist the nurse in determining other assessments that might be needed. For instance, if the temperature is elevated, the nurse considers the time since birth and begins to gather information regarding whether the woman may be dehydrated or if an infection may be present.

Alterations in vital signs may indicate complications, so they are assessed at regular intervals. The blood pressure should remain stable. The pulse often shows a characteristic slowness that is no cause for alarm. Pulse rates return to prepregnant norms very quickly unless complications arise.

Temperature elevations (less than 38 C [100.4 F]) due to normal processes should last for only a few days and should not be associated with other clinical signs of infection. Any elevation should be evaluated in light of other signs and symptoms. The woman's history should also be carefully reviewed to identify other factors, such as premature rupture of membranes (PROM) or prolonged labor, which might increase the incidence of infection in the genital tract.

The nurse informs the woman of the results of the vital signs assessment. Information regarding the normal changes in blood pressure and pulse can be provided. This may be an opportunity to assess whether the mother knows how to assess her own and her infant's temperatures and how to read a thermometer.

Auscultation of Lungs

The breath sounds should be clear. Women who have been treated for preterm labor or PIH are especially at risk for pulmonary edema (see Chapter 18).

Breasts

The nurse can first assess the fit and support provided by the woman's bra. The nurse provides information about how to select a supportive bra. A properly fitting bra provides support to the breasts and helps maintain breast shape by limiting stretching of supporting ligaments and connective tissue. If the mother is breastfeeding, the straps of the bra should be cloth, not elastic (because cloth has less stretch and provides more support) and easily adjustable. The back should be wide and have at least three rows of hooks to adjust for fit. Traditional nursing bras have a fixed inner cup and a separate half-cup that can be unhooked for breastfeeding while continuing to support the breast. Purchasing a nursing bra one size too large during pregnancy will usually result in a good fit because the breasts increase in size with milk production.

The bra is then removed so the breasts can be examined. The nurse notes the size and shape of the breasts and any abnormalities, reddened areas, or engorgement. The breasts are also lightly palpated for softness, slight firmness associated with filling, firmness associated with engorgement, warmth, or tenderness. The nipples are assessed for fissures, cracks, soreness, or inversion. The nurse teaches the woman the characteristics of the breast and explains how to recognize problems such as fissures or cracks.

The nonnursing mother is assessed for evidence of breast discomfort, and relief measures are taken if necessary. (See discussion of lactation suppression in the nonnursing mother in Chapter 34.) Breast assessment findings for a nonnursing woman may be recorded as follows: Breasts soft, filling, no evidence of nipple tenderness or cracking.

Abdomen and Fundus

Before examination of the abdomen the woman should void. This practice assures that a full bladder is not causing displacement of the uterus or any uterine atony; if atony is present, other causes (such as uterine relaxation associated with a regional block, overstretched uterus, or distended bladder) must be investigated.

The nurse determines the relationship of the fundus to the umbilicus and also assesses the firmness of the fundus. The nurse notes whether the fundus is in the midline or displaced to either side of the abdomen. The most common cause of displacement to the side is a full bladder; thus this finding requires further assessment. If the fundus is in the midline but higher than expected, it is usually associated with clots within the uterus. The results of the assessment should then be recorded. (See Procedure 33–1 on page 1056.)

While completing the assessment, the nurse teaches the woman about fundal position and how to determine firmness. The mother can be assisted in gently massaging her fundus if it is not firm.

A well-contracted uterus feels as firm as the uterus does during a strong labor contraction. If handled gently, the uterus should not be overly tender. Excessive pain in the uterus during postpartal examination should alert the nurse to possible uterine infection. If the uterus is not

firm, the nurse should gently massage the fundus with the fingertips of the examining hand, then assess the results. If the uterus becomes firm, the chart should read "Uterus: boggy → firm c̄ light massage." A good habit for the nurse to develop during the postpartal examination is to have the woman lie flat on her back with her head on a pillow and legs flexed. Then the nurse can release the perineal pad to observe the results of uterine massage based on the amount of expelled blood. Occasionally, oxytocic agents such as IV Pitocin and methylergonovine maleate (Methergine) are administered postpartally to maintain uterine contraction and prevent hemorrhage (see Drug Guide: Methylergonovine Maleate [Methergine] in Chapter 34).

The boggy uterus that does not contract with light, gentle massage may need more vigorous massage. The amount and character of any expelled blood obtained while massaging the fundus is assessed. When a woman has postpartal uterine atony, the nurse should do the following:

1. Reevaluate for full bladder; if the bladder is full, have the woman void.

2. Question the woman on her bleeding history since the birth or last examination. How heavy does her flow seem? Has she passed any clots? How frequently has she changed pads? Were the pads saturated?

3. For the nursing mother, put the newborn to the mother's breast to stimulate oxytocin production.

4. Reassess the fundus; if the fundus is still boggy, alert the certified nurse-midwife or physician, because further intervention is now needed.

Following the uterine assessment and before assessing the lochia, the nurse examines for diastasis recti. The separation in the rectus muscle is evaluated according to its length and width. The separation is palpated first just

Nursing Action	**Rationale**

Objective: Prepare woman.

Explain procedure; have the woman void; position woman flat in bed with head comfortable on a pillow; if the procedure is uncomfortable, woman may flex legs.

Having the woman void assures that a full bladder is not causing any uterine atony.
Having woman flat prevents falsely high assessment of fundal height. Flexing the legs relaxes the abdominal muscles. The uterus may be tender if frequent massage has been necessary.

Objective: Determine uterine firmness.

Gently place one hand on the lower segment of the uterus; using the side of the other hand, palpate the abdomen until the top of the fundus is located. Determine whether the fundus is firm. If it is not firm, massage lightly until firm.

Provides support for uterus.
Provides a larger surface for palpation and is less uncomfortable for the woman. A firm fundus indicates that the muscles are contracted and bleeding will not occur.

Objective: Determine the height of the fundus.

Measure the height of the top of the fundus in fingerbreadths above, below, or at the umbilicus (Figure 33–3).

Fundal height gives information about the progress of involution.

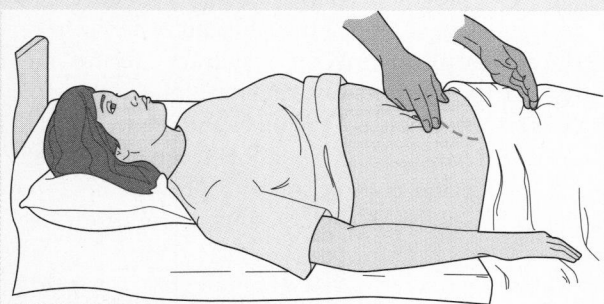

FIGURE 33-3   Measurement of descent of fundus. The fundus is located two fingerbreadths below the umbilicus

Objective: Ascertain position.

Determine whether fundus is deviated from the midline. If not in midline, locate position. Evaluate bladder for distention. Ascertain voiding pattern; use measuring device to measure urine output for next few hours (until normal elimination status is established).

Fundus may be deviated when bladder is full.

Objective: Correlate uterine status with lochia.

Observe lochia for amount, presence of clots, color, and odor.

As normal involution occurs, the lochia decreases in amount and changes from rubra to serosa. Increased amounts of lochia may be associated with uterine relaxation; failure to progress to next type of lochia may indicate uterine relaxation or infection.

Objective: Record findings.

Fundal height is recorded in fingerbreadths; for example the chart should read "2 FB ↓ U; 1 FB ↑ U."

If massage had been necessary, the chart could read "Uterus: Boggy → firm c̄ light massage."

Allows for consistency of reporting among care givers.

below the umbilicus, and the width is ascertained. Then the separation is palpated for length toward the symphysis pubis and toward the xiphoid process. If palpation is difficult due to abdominal relaxation, the woman is asked to lift her head unassisted by the nurse. This action contracts the rectus muscles and more clearly defines their edges.

Methods of charting these results vary from institution to institution. Some prefer to record the diastasis measured from the umbilicus down and then from the umbilicus up, so the chart should read "Diastasis: U ↓ 4 cm by 1 cm, U ↑ 2 cm by 1 cm." Others prefer recording the entire length, so the chart should read "Diastasis: 6 cm by 1 cm." Either method is acceptable.

In the woman who has had a cesarean birth the abdominal incision should be inspected for signs of healing, such as approximation and minimal redness, and for any signs of infection, including drainage, foul odor, or redness. During the assessment the nurse teaches the woman about her incision. Characteristics of normal healing may be reviewed and signs of infection discussed.

Lochia

The next aspect to be evaluated is the lochia, which is assessed for character, amount, odor, and the presence of clots. Disposable gloves must be worn when assessing the perineum and lochia. Nurses may put on the gloves before beginning the assessment, just before assessing the abdomen and fundus, or when they are ready to assess the perineum and lochia. (See Essential Precautions in Practice: During Postpartal Assessment on page 1054.) During the first 1–3 days the lochia should be rubra. A few small clots are normal and occur as a result of blood pooling in the vagina. However, the passage of numerous or large clots is abnormal, and the cause should be investigated immediately. After 2–3 days the lochia becomes serosa.

Lochia should never exceed a moderate amount, such as four to eight partially saturated peri-pads daily, with an average of six. However, because this is influenced by an individual woman's pad-changing practices, she should be questioned about the length of time the current pad has been in use, whether the amount is normal, and whether any clots were passed prior to this examination, such as during voiding. If heavy bleeding is reported but not seen, the woman is asked to put on a clean perineal pad and is then reassessed in 1 hour (Figure 33–4). Clots and heavy bleeding may be caused by uterine relaxation (atony) or retained placental fragments, and they require further assessment. Because of the evacuation of the uterine cavity during cesarean birth, women with such surgery usually have less lochia after the first 24 hours than mothers who give birth vaginally. Therefore amounts of lochia that would be normal in women who had vaginal births are suspect in women who have undergone cesarean birth. Research suggests that estimations of blood loss are influenced by the brand of peri-pad used

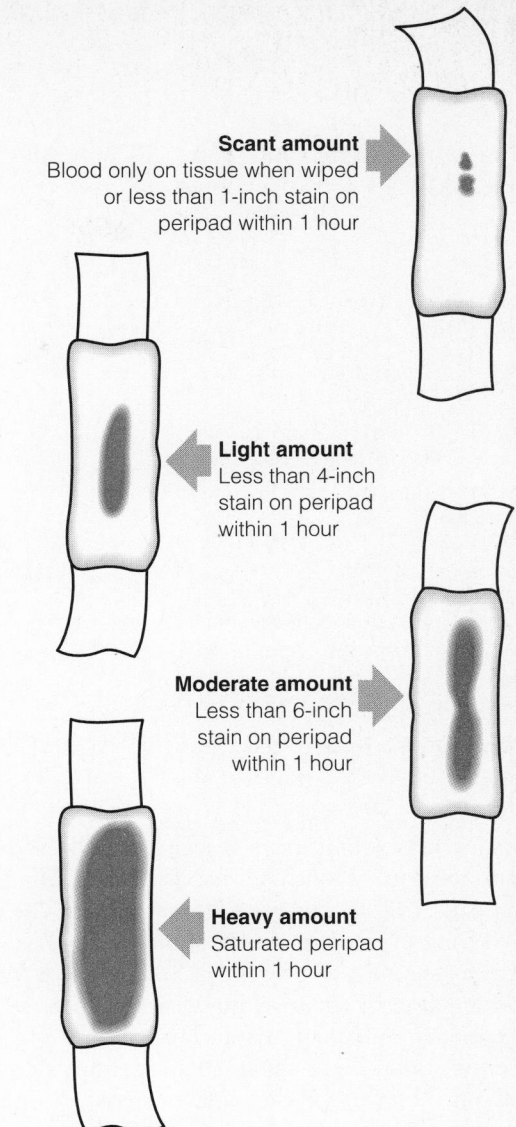

FIGURE 33-4 Suggested guidelines for assessing lochia volume. SOURCE: Jacobson H: A standard for assessing lochia volume. *Am J Mat Child Nurs* May/June 1985; 10:175.

Luegenbiehl et al 1990). Consequently, if standards for estimating blood loss are established in a clinical facility, they should be brand specific. When a more accurate assessment of blood loss is needed, the perineal pads can be weighed. When pads are weighed, 1 g is considered equivalent to 1 mL blood.

If the woman is at increased risk for bleeding or is actually experiencing heavy flow of lochia rubra, the physician may order methylergonovine maleate (Methergine).

The odor of the lochia is nonoffensive and never foul. If foul odor is present, so is an infection.

The amount of lochia is charted first, followed by character; for example "Lochia: moderate rubra."

Client teaching that may be addressed during assessment of the lochia may center on normal changes that can be expected in the amount and color of the flow. Hygienic

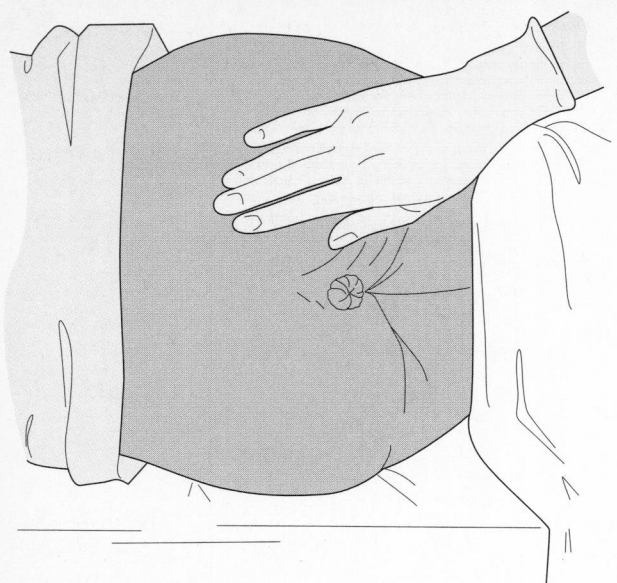

FIGURE 33-5 Intact perineum with hemorrhoids. Note how the examiner's hand raises the upper buttocks to fully expose the anal area.

measures, such as wiping from front to back on the perineum and the need to wash her hands after toileting and changing pads, may be reviewed if appropriate. The timing of teaching hygienic practices should be approached delicately, as should the content to be included. When the nurse approaches the teaching with the goals of promoting comfort, enhancing tissue healing, and preventing infection, value-laden statements regarding personal beliefs about the need for cleanliness or control of body odor are avoided.

Perineum

The perineum is inspected with the woman lying in a Sims's position. The buttock is lifted to expose the perineum and anus.

If an episiotomy was done or a laceration required suturing, the wound is assessed. The state of healing is evaluated by observing for redness, edema, ecchymosis, discharge, and approximation. After 24 hours some edema may still be present, but the skin edges should be "glued" together (well approximated) so that gentle pressure does not separate them. Gentle palpation should elicit minimal tenderness, and there should be no hardened areas suggesting infection. Ecchymosis interferes with normal healing, as does infection.

Foul odors associated with drainage indicate infection. Further observation of the incision for warmth, tenderness, edema, and separation should also be made.

The nurse next assesses whether hemorrhoids are present around the anus. If present, they are assessed for size, number, and pain or tenderness (Figure 33–5).

During the assessment the nurse talks with the woman to determine the effectiveness of comfort measures that have been used. The nurse provides teaching about the episiotomy. Some women do not thoroughly understand what an episiotomy is and where it is and may believe that the stitches must be removed, as with other types of surgery. Frequently, when women fear that the stitches must be removed manually, they are afraid to ask about them. As the nurse explains the findings of the assessment, information about the episiotomy, its location, and signs that are being assessed can be addressed. In addition the nurse can casually add that the sutures are special and that they dissolve slowly over the next few weeks as the tissues heal. By the time the sutures are dissolved, the tissues are strong, and the incision edges will not separate. This is also an opportunity to teach comfort measures that may be used (see Chapter 34).

An example of charting a perineal assessment might read "Midline episiotomy; no edema, tenderness, or ecchymosis present. Skin edges well approximated. Patient reports pain relief measures are controlling discomfort."

Lower Extremities

If thrombophlebitis occurs, the most likely site will be in the woman's legs. To assess for this condition, her legs should be stretched out, with the knees slightly flexed, and should be relaxed. The foot is then grasped and sharply dorsiflexed. No discomfort or pain should be present. If pain is elicited, the nurse-midwife or physician is notified that the woman has a positive Homan's sign (see Figure 36–2). The pain is caused by inflammation of a vessel. The legs are also evaluated for edema. This may be done by comparing both legs because usually only one leg is involved. Any areas of redness, tenderness, and increased skin temperature should be noted.

Early ambulation is an important aspect of the prevention of thrombophlebitis. Most women are able to get up shortly after birth. The cesarean birth client requires passive range of motion exercises until she is ambulating more freely.

Client teaching associated with assessment of the lower extremities focuses on the signs and symptoms of thrombophlebitis. In addition the nurse may review self-care measures to promote circulation and measures to prevent thrombophlebitis, such as leg exercises that may be accomplished in bed and dorsiflexion on an hourly basis, ambulation, avoiding pressure behind the knees, avoiding use of the knee gatch on the bed, and avoiding crossing the legs.

Results of the assessment are usually contained in a summary nursing note. If tenderness and warmth have been noted, they might be recorded as follows: "Tenderness, warmth, and slight redness noted on posterior aspect of left calf—positive Homan's. Woman advised to avoid pressure to this area; lower leg elevated and moist heat applied per agency protocol. Call placed to Dr Smith to report findings."

Elimination

During the hours after birth the nurse carefully monitors a new mother's bladder status. A displaced uterus, palpable bladder, or boggy uterus are signs of bladder distention and require nursing intervention.

The postpartal woman should be encouraged to void every 4–6 hours. The bladder should be assessed for distention until the woman demonstrates complete emptying of the bladder with each voiding. The nurse may employ techniques to facilitate voiding, such as helping the woman out of bed to void or pouring warm water on the perineum. Catheterization is required when the bladder is distended and the woman cannot void or when she is voiding small amounts (< 100 mL) frequently. Although many physicians/CNMs write orders stating the woman can be catheterized in 8 hours if no voiding has occurred, the nurse needs to assess the bladder and any voiding pattern rather than a time interval. The cesarean birth mother may have an indwelling catheter inserted prophylactically. The same assessments should be made in evaluating bladder emptying once the catheter is removed.

During the physical assessment the nurse elicits information from the woman regarding the adequacy of her fluid intake, whether she feels she is emptying her bladder completely when she voids, and any signs of urinary tract infection (UTI) she may be experiencing.

In the same way the nurse obtains information about the new mother's intestinal elimination and any concerns she may have about it. Many mothers fear that the first bowel movement will be painful and possibly even damaging if an episiotomy has been done. Stool softeners may be ordered to increase bulk and moisture in the fecal material and to allow more comfortable and complete evacuation. Constipation is avoided to prevent pressures on sutures that may increase discomfort. Encouraging ambulation, forcing fluids (up to 2000 mL/day or more), and providing fresh fruits and roughage in the diet enhance bowel elimination and assist the woman in reestablishing her normal bowel pattern.

During the assessment the nurse may provide information regarding postpartum diuresis and why the woman may be emptying her bladder so frequently. The need for additional fluid intake with suggestions of specific amounts may be helpful. The woman should drink at least eight 8-oz glasses of water or juice in addition to other fluids. Signs of retention and overflow voiding are discussed, and symptoms of UTI may be reviewed with the mother at this time if it seems an appropriate moment for teaching. Methods of assisting bowel elimination may be reviewed, and opportunities for the woman to ask questions are provided.

Rest and Sleep Status

As part of the postpartal assessment the nurse evaluates the amount of rest a new mother is getting. If the woman reports difficulty sleeping at night, the nurse should try to determine the cause. If it is simply the strange environment, a warm drink, backrub, or mild sedative may prove helpful. Appropriate nursing measures are indicated if the woman is bothered by normal postpartal discomforts such as afterpains, diaphoresis, or episiotomy or hemorrhoidal pain.

A daily rest period should be encouraged, and hospital activities should be scheduled to allow time for napping. The nurse can also provide information about the fatigue a new mother experiences and the impact it can have on her emotions and sense of being in control.

Nutritional Status

Determination of postpartal nutritional status is based primarily on information provided by the mother and on direct assessment. During pregnancy the daily recommended dietary allowances call for increases in calories, proteins, and most vitamins and minerals. After birth the nonnursing mother's dietary requirements return to prepregnancy levels.

Visiting the mothers during mealtime provides an opportunity for unobtrusive nutritional assessment and counseling. The nonnursing mother should be advised about the need to reduce her caloric intake by about 300 kcal and to return to prepregnancy levels for other nutrients. The nursing mother should increase her caloric intake by about 200 kcal over the pregnancy requirements, or a total of 500 kcal over the nonpregnant requirement. Basic discussion will prove helpful, followed by referral as needed. In all cases literature on nutrition should be provided so that the woman will have a source of information following discharge.

The dietitian should be informed of any mother who is a vegetarian or whose cultural or religious beliefs require specific foods. Appropriate meals can then be prepared for her. Many women, especially those who gained more than the recommended number of pounds, are interested in losing weight after birth. The dietitian can design weight-reduction diets to meet nutritional needs and food preferences. The nurse may also refer women with unusual eating habits or numerous questions about good nutrition to the dietitian.

New mothers are also advised that it is common practice to prescribe iron supplements for 4–6 weeks after birth. The hematocrit is then checked at the postpartal visit to detect any anemia.

As a part of the nutritional assessment the nurse can provide teaching about the nutritional needs of the woman during the postpartal period. See Table 33–3 as well as the discussion in Chapter 17.

Critical Thinking Question

What techniques might you use to accurately assess the new mother's psychologic status?

2–3 servings of milk, yogurt, and cheese group

2–3 servings of meat or protein group

3–5 servings of vegetable group

4 servings of whole grain

2–4 servings of fruit group

6–11 servings of bread, cereal, rice, and pasta group

Fats, oils, and sweets sparingly

Psychologic Assessment

Adequate assessment of the mother's psychologic adjustment is an integral part of postpartal evaluation. This assessment focuses on the mother's general attitude, feelings of competence, available support systems, and caregiving skills. It also evaluates her fatigue level, sense of satisfaction, and ability to accomplish her developmental tasks.

Fatigue is often a highly significant factor in a new mother's apparent disinterest in her newborn. Frequently, the woman is so tired from a long labor and birth that everything seems to be an effort. To avoid inadvertently classifying a very tired mother as one with a potential attachment problem, the nurse should do the psychologic assessment on more than one occasion. After a nap the new mother is often far more receptive to her baby and her surroundings.

Some new mothers have little or no experience with newborns and may feel totally overwhelmed. They may show these feelings by asking questions and reading all available material or by becoming passive and quiet because they simply cannot deal with their feelings of inadequacy. Unless a nurse questions the woman about her plans and previous experience in a supportive, nonjudgmental way, one might conclude that the woman was disinterested, withdrawn, or depressed. Problem clues might include excessive continued fatigue, marked depression, excessive preoccupation with physical status and/or discomfort, evidence of low self-esteem, lack of support systems, marital problems, inability to care for or nurture the newborn, and current family crises (such as illness or unemployment). These characteristics frequently indicate a potential for maladaptive parenting, which may lead to child abuse or neglect (physical, emotional, intellectual) and cannot be ignored. Referrals to public health nurses or other available community resources may provide greatly needed assistance and alleviate potentially dangerous situations.

Assessment of Early Attachment

Attachment is a desired outcome of maternal-newborn interactions during the postpartal period. The nurse in the postpartum setting can periodically observe and note progress toward attachment. This content is discussed in detail in Chapter 35.

DATABASE: THE FOURTH TRIMESTER

The first several postpartal weeks have been termed the fourth trimester to stress the idea of continuity as the family adjusts to having a new member and as the woman's body returns to a prepregnant state. During this period the woman must accomplish certain physical and developmental tasks:

- Restoring physical condition
- Developing competence in caring for and meeting the needs of her infant
- Establishing a relationship with her new child
- Adapting to altered life-styles and family structure resulting from the addition of a new member

The new mother and her family may have an inadequate or incorrect understanding of what to expect during the early postpartal weeks. She may be concerned with restoring her figure and surprised because of continuing physical discomfort from sore breasts, episiotomy, or hemorrhoids. Fatigue is perhaps her greatest, yet most underestimated, problem during the early weeks. This may be aggravated if she has no extended family support or if there are other young children at home.

Developing skill and confidence in caring for an infant may be especially anxiety provoking for a new mother. As she struggles to establish a mutually acceptable pattern with her baby, small unanticipated concerns may seem monumental. The woman may begin to feel inadequate and, if she lacks support systems, isolated.

Nurses have been in the forefront of health care providers attempting to improve the care given during the postpartal period. Many obstetricians, certified nurse-midwives, and nurse practitioners now routinely see all postpartal women 1 to 2 weeks after birth in addition to the routine 6-week checkup. These visits provide opportunities for physical assessment as well as assessment of the mother's psychologic and informational needs and needs of the family.

Assessment at Two and Six Weeks After Birth

The routine physical assessment, which can be made rapidly, focuses on the woman's general appearance, breasts, reproductive tract, bladder and bowel elimination, and any specific problems or complaints. (See the accompanying Postpartal Assessment Guide: Two Weeks and Six Weeks After Birth.) In addition the nurse should talk with the mother about her diet, fatigue level, family adjustment, and psychologic status. The nurse explores any problems with child care and refers the mother to a

Text continues on page 1065

Two Weeks and Six Weeks After Birth

Physical Assessment/ Normal Findings	Alterations and Possible Causes*	Nursing Responses to Data†
Vital Signs		
Blood pressure: Return to normal prepregnant level.	Elevated blood pressure (anxiety, essential hypertension, renal disease).	Review history, evaluate normal baseline; refer to physician/certified nurse-midwife if necessary.
Pulse: 60–90 beats/minute (or prepregnant normal rate).	Increased pulse rate (excitement, anxiety, cardiac disorders).	Count pulse for full minute, note irregularities; marked tachycardia or beat irregularities require additional assessment and possible physician/certified nurse-midwife referral.
Respirations: 16–24/minute.	Marked tachypnea or abnormal patterns (respiratory disorders).	Evaluate for respiratory disease; refer to physician/certified nurse-midwife if necessary.
Temperature: 36.2 C–37.6 C (98 F–99.6 F).	Increased temperature (infection).	Assess for signs and symptoms of infection or disease state.
Weight		
2 weeks: Probable weight loss of 14–20+ lb.	Little or no weight loss (fluid retention, subinvolution, excessive caloric intake).	Evaluate dietary habits and nutritional state; review blood pressure to evaluate fluid retention or blood losses.
6 weeks: Returning to normal prepregnant weight.	Retained weight (excessive caloric intake).	Determine amount of daily exercise. Provide dietary teaching. Refer to dietitian if necessary for additional dietary counseling.
	Extreme weight loss (excessive dieting, inadequate caloric intake).	Discuss appropriate diets; refer to dietitian for additional counseling if necessary.
Breasts		
Nonnursing: 2 weeks: May have mild tenderness; small amount of milk may be expressed; breasts returning to prepregnant size. 6 weeks: Soft, with no tenderness; return to prepregnant size.	Some engorgement (incomplete suppression of lactation). Redness; marked tenderness (mastitis). Palpable mass (tumor).	Engorgement usually seen when no medication has been given to suppress lactation or may occur after lactation suppression medication is stopped. Advise client to wear a supportive, well-fitted bra and avoid hot showers; evaluate for signs and symptoms of mastitis (rare in nonnursing mothers).
Nursing: Full, with prominent nipples; lactation established.	Cracked, fissured nipples (feeding problems). Redness, marked tenderness, or even abscess formation (mastitis). Palpable mass (full milk duct, tumor).	Counsel about nipple care. Evaluate client condition, evidence of fever; refer to physician/certified nurse-midwife for initiation of antibiotic therapy, if indicated. Opinion varies as to value of breast examination for nursing mothers; some feel a nursing mother should examine her breasts monthly, after feeding, when breasts are empty; if palpable mass is felt, refer to physician for further evaluation.

*Possible causes of alterations are placed in parentheses.

†This column provides guidelines for further assessment and initial nursing interventions.

TWO WEEKS AND SIX WEEKS AFTER BIRTH *continued*

Physical Assessment/ Normal Findings	Alterations and Possible Causes*	Nursing Responses to Data†
Breasts *continued*		For breast inflammation instruct the mother to 1. Keep breast empty by frequent feeding. 2. Rest when possible. 3. Take aspirin for pain. 4. Force fluids. If symptoms persist for more than 24 hours, instruct her to call her physician/certified nurse-midwife.
Abdominal Musculature		
2 weeks: Improved firmness, although "bread dough" consistency is not unusual, especially in multipara. Striae pink and obvious.	Marked diastasis recti (relaxation of muscles).	Evaluate exercise level; provide information on appropriate exercise program.
Cesarean incision healing.	Drainage, redness, tenderness, pain, edema (infection).	Evaluate for infection; refer to physician/ certified nurse-midwife if necessary.
6 weeks: Muscle tone continues to improve; striae may be beginning to fade, may not achieve a silvery appearance for several more weeks; linea nigra fading.		
Elimination Pattern		
Urinary tract: Return to prepregnant urinary elimination routine.	Urinary incontinence, especially when lifting, coughing, laughing, and so on (urethral trauma, cystocele).	Assess for cystocele; instruct in appropriate muscle tightening exercises; refer to physician/certified nurse-midwife.
	Pain or burning when voiding, urgency and/or frequency, pus or white blood cells (WBC) in urine, pathogenic organisms in culture (urinary tract infection).	Evaluate for urinary tract infection; obtain clean-catch urine; refer to physician/certified nurse-midwife for treatment if indicated.
Routine urinalysis within normal limits (proteinuria disappeared).	Sugar or ketone in urine—may be some lactose present in urine of breastfeeding mothers (diabetes).	Evaluate diet; assess for signs and symptoms of diabetes; refer to physician/certified nurse-midwife.
Bowel habits: 2 weeks: May still be some discomfort with defecation, especially if client had severe hemorrhoids or third- or fourth-degree extension.	Severe constipation or pain when defecating (trauma or hemorrhoids).	Discuss dietary patterns; encourage fluid, adequate roughage. Continue use of stool softener if necessary to prevent pain associated with straining; continue sitz baths, periods of rest for severe hemorrhoids; assess healing of episiotomy and/or lacerations; severe constipation may require administration of laxatives, stool softeners, and an enema.
6 weeks: Return to normal prepregnancy bowel elimination.	Marked constipation.	See above.

*Possible causes of alterations are placed in parentheses.

†This column provides guidelines for further assessment and initial nursing interventions.

TWO WEEKS AND SIX WEEKS AFTER BIRTH continued

Physical Assessment/ Normal Findings	Alterations and Possible Causes*	Nursing Responses to Data†
Elimination Pattern continued		
Bowel habits continued	Fecal incontinence or constipation (rectocele).	Assess for evidence of rectocele; instruct in muscle tightening exercises; refer to physician/certified nurse-midwife.
Reproductive Tract		
Lochia: 2 weeks: Lochia alba, scant amounts, fleshy odor.	Foul odor, excessive in amounts (infection). Return to lochia rubra or persistence of lochia rubra or serosa (subinvolution, infection).	Assess for evidence of infection and/or subinvolution; culture lochia; refer to physician/certified nurse-midwife.
6 weeks: No lochia, or return to normal menstruation pattern.	See above.	See above.
Fundus and perineum: 2 weeks: Uterus no longer palpable abdominally; uterine muscles still somewhat lax and uterus may be displaced; introitus of vagina still lacking tone—gapes when intra-abdominal pressure is increased by coughing or straining.	Uterus not decreasing in size appropriately (subinvolution, infection).	Assess for evidence of subinvolution and/or infection; refer to physician/certified nurse-midwife if indicated.
Episiotomy and/or lacerations healing; no signs of infection.	Evidence of redness, tenderness, poor tissue approximation in episiotomy and/or laceration (wound infection).	
6 weeks: Uterus almost returned to prepregnant size with almost completely restored muscle tone.	Continued flow of lochia, failure to decrease appropriately in size (subinvolution).	Assess for evidence of subinvolution and/or infection; refer to physician for further evaluation and for dilatation and curettage if necessary.
Hemoglobin and Hematocrit Levels		
6 weeks: Hb 12 g/dL. Hct 37% ± 5%.	Hb < 12 g/dL. Hct 32% (anemia).	Assess nutritional status, begin (or continue) supplemental iron; for marked anemia (Hb ≤ 9 g/dL) additional assessment and/or physician/certified nurse-midwife referral may be necessary.

Psychosocial Assessment/ Normal Findings	Alterations and Possible Causes*	Nursing Responses to Data†
Attachment		
Bonding process demonstrated by soothing, cuddling, and talking to infant; appropriate feeding techniques; eye-to-eye contact;	Failure to bond demonstrated by lack of behaviors associated with bonding process, calling infant by nickname that promotes	Provide counseling; talk with the woman about her feelings regarding the infant; provide support for the caretaking activities

*Possible causes of alterations are placed in parentheses.

†This column provides guidelines for further assessment and initial nursing interventions.

TWO WEEKS AND SIX WEEKS AFTER BIRTH *continued*

Psychosocial Assessment/ Normal Findings	Alterations and Possible Causes*	Nursing Responses to Data†
Attachment *continued*		
calling infant by name.	ridicule, inadequate infant weight gain, infant is dirty, hygienic measures are not being maintained, severe diaper rash, failure to obtain adequate supplies to provide infant care (malattachment).	that are being performed; refer to public health nurse for continued home visits.
Parent interacts with infant and provides soothing, caretaking activities.	Parent is unable to respond to infant needs (inability to recognize needs, inadequate education and support, fear, family stress).	Provide support for caretaking activities observed; provide information regarding caretaking activities, such as responding to infant cry; methods of wrapping infant; methods of soothing the infant such as swaddling, rocking, increasing stimuli by singing to the infant or decreasing stimuli by putting infant to rest in quiet room; methods of holding the infant; differences in the cry. Identify support system such as friends, neighbors; provide information regarding community resources and support groups.
Parents express feelings of comfort and success with the parent role.	Evidence of stress and anxiety (difficulty moving into or dealing with the parent role).	Provide support and encouragement; provide information regarding progression into parent role and assist parents in talking through their feelings; refer to community resources and support groups.
Woman is in the informal or personal stage of maternal role attainment.	Woman is still greatly influenced by others, has not developed an image or style of her own (woman remains in the anticipatory stage).	Provide role modeling for the woman in working through problem solving with the infant; provide encouragement as she thinks through decisions and develops her sense of problem solving; encourage her to make decisions regarding infant care.
Adjustment to Parental Role		
Parents are coping with new roles in terms of division of labor, financial status, communication, readjustment of sexual relations, and adjusting to new daily tasks.	Inability to adjust to new roles (immaturity, inadequate education and preparation, ineffective communication patterns, inadequate support, current family crisis).	Provide counseling; refer to parent groups.
Education		
Mother understands self-care measures.	Inadequate knowledge of self-care (inadequate education).	Provide education and counseling.
Parents are knowledgeable regarding infant care.	Inadequate knowledge of infant care (inadequate education).	
Siblings are adjusting to new baby.	Excessive sibling rivalry.	
Parents have a method of contraception.	Birth control method not chosen.	

*Possible causes of alterations are placed in parentheses.

†This column provides guidelines for further assessment and initial nursing interventions.

pediatric nurse practitioner or pediatrician if needed. Available community resources, including public health department follow-up visits, are mentioned when appropriate. If not already discussed, teaching about family planning is appropriate at this time, and information regarding birth control methods is provided.

In ideal situations a family approach involving the father, infant, and possibly other siblings permits a total evaluation and provides an opportunity for all family members to ask questions and express concerns. In addition disturbed family patterns can sometimes be more readily diagnosed and therapy can be suggested or even instituted to prevent future problems of neglect or abuse.

The fourth trimester is the several weeks following birth during which the woman's physical condition returns to a nonpregnant state and she gains competence and confidence in herself as a parent.

KEY CONCEPTS

The uterus involutes rapidly, primarily through a reduction in cell size.

Involution is assessed by measuring fundal height. The fundus is at the level of the umbilicus within a few hours after birth and should decrease by approximately one fingerbreadth per day.

The placental site heals by a process of exfoliation, so no scar formation occurs.

Lochia progresses from rubra to serosa to alba and is assessed in terms of type, quantity, and characteristics.

The abdomen may have decreased muscle tone (flabby consistency) initially. Diastasis recti abdominis should be measured.

Constipation may develop postpartally due to decreased tone, limited diet, and denial of the urge to defecate due to fear of pain.

Decreased bladder sensitivity, increased capacity, and postpartal diuresis may lead to problems with bladder elimination. Frequent assessment and prompt intervention are indicated. A fundus that is boggy but does not respond to massage, is higher than expected, or deviates to the side usually indicates a full bladder.

Postpartally, a healthy woman should be normotensive and afebrile. Bradycardia is common.

Postpartally the WBC is often elevated. Activation of clotting factors predisposes the woman to thrombus formation.

Psychologic adaptations are traditionally described as taking-in and taking-hold.

In consideration of the client's background, cultural variations and individual preferences should be recognized and respected.

Postpartal assessment should be completed in a systematic way, usually cephalocaudally. It provides a tremendous opportunity for informal client teaching.

REFERENCES

Ament LA: Maternal tasks of the puerperium reidentified. *JOGNN* July/August 1990; 19:330.

Andrew MA, Boyle JS: *Transcultural Concepts in Nursing Care.* Philadelphia: Lippincott, 1995.

Belsky J, Rovine M: Social-network contact, family support, and the transition to parenthood. *J Marriage Fam* 1984; 46:455.

Blackburn ST, Loper DL: *Maternal, Fetal and Neonatal Physiology.* Philadelphia: Saunders, 1992.

Cunningham FG et al: *Williams Obstetrics,* 19th ed. Norwalk, CT: Appleton & Lange, 1993.

Food and Nutrition Board, National Academy of Sciences—National Research Council: *Recommended Dietary Allowances,* 10th ed. Washington, DC: 1989.

Jacobson H: A standard for assessing lochia volume. *MCN* May/June 1985; 10:174.

Karch A, Boyd E: *Handbook of Drugs.* Philadelphia: Lippincott, 1989.

LaDu EB: Childbirth care for Hmong families. *MCN* November/December 1985; 10:382.

Luegenbiehl DL et al: Standardized assessment of blood loss. *MCN* July/August 1990; 15:241.

Mercer RT: The process of maternal role attainment over the first year. *Nurs Res* July/August 1985; 34:198.

Rubin R: *Maternal Identity and the Maternal Experience.* New York: Springer, 1984.

Rubin R: Puerperal change. *Nurs Outlook* 1961; 9:753.

Sheil EP et al: Concerns of childbearing women: A maternal concerns questionnaire as an assessment tool. *JOGNN* 1995; 24(2):149.

Spector RE: *Cultural Diversity in Health and Illness.* Norwalk, CT: Appleton & Lange, 1991.

Varney H: *Nurse Midwifery,* 2nd ed. Boston: Blackwell Scientific Publications, 1987.

Zlatnik: FJ: The puerperium: Normal and abnormal. In: *Danforth's Obstetrics and Gynecology,* 7th ed. Scott JB et al (editors). Philadelphia: Lippincott, 1994.

CHAPTER 34

THE POSTPARTAL FAMILY: NEEDS AND CARE

T he word "family" to me has always had very meaningful and positive thoughts and experiences associated with it. I vividly remember growing up being the oldest of six children. With constant love, affection, and support from my parents, I always thought, "How can they do it? How can they nurture and raise so many kids and yet still make every one of us feel so special and important?" I truly believed that I would never be able to accomplish the successful parenting they so consistently provided to all of us, and I was actually scared and fearful to begin a family of my own.

My husband and I now laugh about these thoughts I shared with him 4½ years ago as our family continues to grow quite rapidly. Trying to raise a 4-year-old, a 2-year-old, and a 10-week-old is extremely challenging, but it is the most rewarding experience in my life.

In addition to parenting three very small children I have balanced a full-time position as a nurse-manager, and I completed my master's degree this spring. All of this has demanded an enormous amount of energy, motivation, and self-control. I realize now that my uneasiness and hesitation to begin our family was merely a time in my life in which I lacked the self-esteem and self-confidence to be a successful parent.

OBJECTIVES

Relate the use of nursing diagnoses to the findings of the "normal" postpartum assessment and analysis.

Delineate nursing responsibilities for client education during the early post-partum period.

Discuss appropriate nursing interventions to meet identified nursing goals for the childbearing family.

Compare the nursing needs of a woman who experienced a cesarean birth with

the needs of a woman who gave birth vaginally.

Summarize the nursing needs of the childbearing adolescent during the post-partum period.

Describe possible approaches to follow-up nursing care for the childbearing family.

Determine the nurse's responsibilities related to early postpartum discharge.

$\mathcal{C}$ertain premises form the basis of effective nursing care during the postpartal period.

- The best postpartal care is family centered and disrupts the family unit as little as possible. This approach uses the family's resources to support an early and smooth adjustment to the newborn by all family members.

- Knowledge of the range of normal physiologic and psychologic adaptations occurring during the postpartal period allows the nurse to recognize alterations and initiate interventions early. Communicating information about postpartal adaptations to the family facilitates their adjustment to their situation.

- Nursing care is aimed at accomplishing specific goals that ultimately meet individual needs. These goals are formulated after careful assessment and consideration of factors that could influence the outcome of care.

Chapter 33 provided a thorough discussion of postpartal assessment. This chapter describes how the nurse can use the remaining steps of the nursing process effectively to plan and provide care. Specific nursing responses to the mother's physical needs and the family's psychosocial needs are described at length. See also the Postpartal Critical Pathway.

NURSING DIAGNOSIS DURING THE POSTPARTUM PERIOD

For most postpartal women physical recovery goes smoothly and is considered a healthy process. Because of this perception, it is all too common for care givers to think that the woman and her family have no "real" needs and thus that no care plan is needed. Nothing could be further from the truth. Every member of the family has needs, although they may not be obvious, especially if they are psychologic or educational.

The postpartal family's needs, which should be identified during assessment, are the basis for developing nursing diagnoses. Once a nursing diagnosis is made and recorded, systematic action, as delineated in a nursing care plan, can be taken to meet the identified need.

Many nurses have suggested that nursing diagnoses are difficult to make in a wellness setting because of their emphasis on "problems." Nurses involved in the effort to formulate standardized diagnoses recognize this difficulty and are working to develop diagnoses that are more useful in wellness settings.

Many agencies that use nursing diagnoses prefer to use only the NANDA list. Consequently, physiologic al-

terations form the basis of many postpartal diagnoses. Examples of such diagnoses include the following:

- Altered patterns of urinary elimination related to dysuria and/or urinary retention
- Self-care deficit: bathing/hygiene related to fatigue
- Constipation related to fear of tearing stitches and/or pain
- Pain related to perineal edema from birth, episiotomy, and generalized muscular discomfort
- Risk for infection related to episiotomy
- Sleep pattern disturbance related to frequent interruption of rest for newborn care

Diagnoses related to family coping or instructional needs are also used frequently. Examples of these diagnoses include the following:

- Knowledge deficit related to lack of knowledge regarding newborn care, self-care, infant feeding, and infant growth and development
- Family coping: Potential for growth related to successful adjustment to new baby

After completing the assessment and diagnosis steps of the nursing process, the nurse identifies expected outcomes and selects nursing interventions that will enable the expected outcomes to be met.

NURSING PLAN AND IMPLEMENTATION DURING THE POSTPARTAL PERIOD

Many women remain on a postpartum unit for only a short time, so it is often possible to assign a woman's care to the same nurse. However, for consistency of care it is essential to develop a specific plan of care. Implementation of the plan by all personnel caring for the postpartal woman promotes consistency, progress in client education, and more effective ongoing assessment and evaluation. The nursing care plan is individualized for the postpartum woman and the infant, even if a separate staff in the nursery is caring for the newborn. The plan of care needs to consider the newborn's schedule of activities during the day, such as feeding times, because the mother's day is frequently determined by the infant's activities. An important component of nursing care is client teaching. Sophisticated, detailed forms and guidelines are often available to assist in health teaching. Such tools are a useful adjunct but cannot take the place of the nurse's client-specific plan. As part of the teaching that occurs, desired patient outcomes or goals should be discussed with the mother as soon as possible upon arrival in the postpartum unit. Examples of these desired client outcomes (adapted from the Rose Women's Center, Denver, Colorado) are the following:

- Maintains health for self and baby
- Reviews educational resources for self and baby care
- Demonstrates care for self and baby
- Displays appropriate interaction between parent and baby
- Practices principles of infant safety
- Demonstrates proper breastfeeding and breast care or describes formula preparation for bottle feeding, feeding techniques, and breast care

Additional outcomes for the cesarean birth mother include the following:

- States in own words the reason for the cesarean birth
- Maintains desired pain control
- Maintains moderate mobility level

All components of the nursing process culminate in reaching the desired outcomes identified for the woman and her family. The Postpartal Critical Pathway on page 1070 describes the normal progression of a mother during the early postpartal period and notes critical points that should be attained to assure normal recovery from the pregnancy and birth.

Promotion of Maternal Physical Well-Being

Maternal physical well-being is promoted by monitoring the status of the uterus, monitoring vital signs on a regular schedule, and providing medications as needed for women with problems involving the Rh factor, women who are not rubella immune, and women with some degree of anemia following childbirth.

Monitoring Uterine Status

The nurse completes an assessment of the uterus as discussed in Chapter 33. The assessment interval is every 15 minutes for the first hour after childbirth, every 30 minutes for the next hour, and then hourly for approximately 2 hours. After that the nurse monitors uterine status every 8 hours or more frequently if problems such as bogginess (softening of the uterus due to inadequate contraction of the muscle tissue), positioning out of midline, heavy lochia flow, or the presence of clots arise (Table 34–1).

The amount, consistency, color, and odor of the lochia are monitored on an ongoing basis. Changes in lochia that need to be assessed further, documented, and

| TABLE 34–1 | Key Facts To Remember About Monitoring Postpartal Uterine Status |

Position of the Uterine Fundus Following Birth

Immediately after birth: The top of the fundus is in the midline about midway between the symphysis pubis and umbilicus.

Six to 12 hours after birth: The top of the fundus is in the midline and at the level of the umbilicus.

One day after birth: The top of the fundus is in the midline and one finger-breadth below the umbilicus.

Second day after birth and thereafter: The top of the fundus remains in the midline and descends about one fingerbreadth per day.

Normal Characteristics of Lochia

Lochia rubra is red and is present for the first 2–3 days.

Lochia serosa is pinkish red and is presented from day 3–day 10.

Lochia alba is creamy white and is present from day 11 to about day 21.

reported to the physician/certified nurse-midwife are presented in Table 34–2.

The physician may order medication such as methylergonovine maleate (Methergine) to promote uterine contractions. In some cases an IV with Pitocin may be ordered if the uterus does not remain firm and uterine bleeding is excessive. See Drug Guide: Methylergonovine Maleate (Methergine) in this chapter and Drug Guide: Pitocin in Chapter 26.

Teaching for Home Care The woman may be taught to assess her fundus for firmness and position and to gently massage the fundus to promote uterine muscle contraction. In addition she needs to monitor the amount and color of the lochia flow to determine if normal progression is occurring. Being aware of normal involutional changes will help the woman identify problems and know when to contact her health care provider once she is discharged.

Rubella Vaccine

Women who have a rubella titer of less than 1:10 or are ELISA antibody-negative are usually given rubella vaccine in the postpartal period (Scott et al 1994). Because

CRITICAL THINKING IN PRACTICE

Ellen Baker is 24 hours past birth. She tells you that she is passing clots and asks you if this is normal. What will you tell her?

Answers can be found in Appendix I.

TABLE 34-2   Changes in Lochia That Cause Concern

Change	Possible Problem	Nursing Action
Presence of clots	Inadequate uterine contractions that allow bleeding from vessels at the placental site.	Assess location and firmness of fundus. Assess voiding pattern. Record and report findings.
Persistent lochia rubra	Inadequate uterine contractions; retained placental fragments; infection	Assess location and firmness of fundus. Assess activity pattern. Assess for signs of infection. Record and report findings.

the vaccine needs to be given when the woman is not pregnant, administering the injection just after childbirth has the advantage of targeting a time period that the woman is definitely not pregnant and in most cases does not want another pregnancy in the next 3 months. If the woman is not rubella immune and is also Rh negative and receives RhoGAM, the RhoGAM will interfere with the production of antibodies to rubella (Varney 1987). In this case most physicians/certified nurse-midwives continue to order rubella vaccine and repeat the rubella titer in a few weeks to determine immunity (see Table 34–3 on page 1072).

Teaching for Self-Care The nurse needs to ensure that the woman understands the purpose of the vaccine and that she must avoid becoming pregnant in the next 3 months. To ensure that the woman understands, an informed consent is usually signed prior to administration. Because the avoidance of pregnancy is so important, counseling regarding contraception is suggested.

Text continues on page 1073

DRUG GUIDE

METHYLERGONOVINE MALEATE (METHERGINE)

Overview of Action

Methylergonovine maleate is an ergot alkaloid that stimulates smooth muscle tissue. Because the smooth muscle of the uterus is especially sensitive to this drug, it is used postpartally to stimulate the uterus to contract in order to decrease blood loss by clamping off uterine blood vessels and to promote the involution process. In addition the drug has a vasoconstrictive effect on all blood vessels, especially the larger arteries. This may result in hypertension, particularly in a woman whose blood pressure is already elevated.

Route, Dosage, and Frequency

Methergine has a rapid onset of action and may be given intramuscularly, orally, or intravenously.

Usual IM dose: 0.2 mg following delivery of the placenta. The dose may be repeated every 2–4 hours if necessary.

Usual oral dose: 0.2 mg every 4 hours (six doses).

Usual IV dose: Because the adverse effects of Methergine are far more severe with IV administration, this route is seldom used.

Maternal Contraindications

Pregnancy, hepatic or renal disease, cardiac disease, and hypertension contraindicate this drug's use.

Maternal Side Effects

Hypertension (particularly when administered IV), nausea, vomiting, headache, bradycardia, dizziness, tinnitus, abdominal cramps, palpitations, dyspnea, chest pain, and allergic reactions may be noted.

Effects on Fetus or Neonate

Because Methergine has a long duration of action and can thus produce tetanic contractions, it **should never be used during pregnancy or in labor,** when it may result in fetal trauma or death.

Nursing Considerations

1. Monitor fundal height and consistency and the amount and character of the lochia.

2. Assess the blood pressure before and routinely throughout drug administration.

3. Observe for adverse effects or symptoms of ergot toxicity.

POSTPARTAL CRITICAL PATHWAY

Category	1–4 Hours Postpartum	4–8 Hours Postpartum	8–24 Hours Postpartum
Referral	Report from labor nurse if not continuing in an LDR room	Lactation consultation if needed	Home nursing referral if indicated
Assessments	Postpartum assessments q$\frac{1}{2}$h × 2, q1h × 2, then q4h. Includes: • Fundus firm, in midline, at or below umbilicus • Lochia rubra < 1 pad/h; no free flow or passage of clots with massage • Bladder: voids large amts urine spontaneously; bladder not palpable following voiding • Perineum: sutures intact; no bulging or marked swelling; no c/o severe pain. Minimal bruising may be present. If hemorrhoids present, no tenseness or marked engorgement; < 2 cm diameter • Breasts: Soft, colostrum present Vital signs: • BP WNL; no hypotension; not > 30 mm systolic or 15 mm diastolic over baseline • Temperature: < 38 C (100.4 F) • Pulse: Bradycardia normal; consistent with baseline • Respirations: 12–20/min; quiet; easy Comfort level: < 3 on scale of 1 to 10	Continue postpartum assessment q4h × 2, then q8h Breasts: Evaluate nipple status; should be no evidence of cracks or bruising Observe feeding technique with newborn Vital signs assessment q8h: all WNL; report temperature >38 C (100.4 F) Continue assessment of comfort level	Continue postpartum assessment q8h Breasts: nipples should remain free of cracks, fissures, bruising Feeding technique with newborn: should be good or improving Vital signs assessment q8h: all WNL; report temperature > 38 C (100.4 F) Continue assessment of comfort level
Comfort	Institute comfort measures: • Perineal discomfort: peri-care, sitz baths, topical analgesics • Hemorrhoids: sitz baths, topical analgesics, digital replacement of external hemorrhoids, side-lying or prone position • Afterpains: prone with sm. pillow under abdomen; warm shower or sitz baths; ambulation • Administer pain medication _____	Continue with pain management techniques	Continue with pain management techniques
Teaching/ psychosocial	Explain postpartum assessments Teach self-massage of fundus & expected findings Instruct to call for assistance first time OOB and prn Demonstrate peri-care, surgigator, sitz bath prn Explain comfort measures Begin newborn teaching: bulb suctioning, positioning, feeding, diaper change, cord care Orient to room if transferred from LDR room Provide information on early postpartum period	Discuss psychologic changes of postpartum period Stress need for frequent rest periods Continue newborn teaching: soothing/ comforting techniques, swaddling; return demonstrations indicate woman's understanding Provide opportunities for questions and review; reinforce previous teaching Breastfeeding: Nipple care: air-drying, lanolin; proper latch-on technique; tea bags Bottle feeding: supportive bra, ice bags, breast binder	Reinforce previous teaching; answer questions Discuss involution; anticipated physical changes in first 2 weeks postpartum; postpartum exercises; need to limit visitors Discuss postpartum nutrition: balanced diet, nutritionally rich Breastfeeding: • Increase calories by 500 kcal over nonpregnant state (200 kcal over pregnant intake) • Explain milk production, let-down reflex, use of supplements, breast pumping, and milk storage Bottle feeding: • Return to normal caloric intake for nonpregnant state • Explain formula preparation and storage Discuss sibling rivalry. Mother should have plan for supporting siblings at home. Teaching evaulation completed.

Category	1–4 Hours Postpartum *continued*	4–8 Hours Postpartum *continued*	8–24 Hours Postpartum *continued*
Therapeutic nursing interventions and reports	Ice pack to perineum to ↓ swelling & ↑ comfort Straight cath. prn × 1 if distended or voiding small amts If continues unable to void or voiding sm. amts, insert Foley catheter and notify CNM/physician	Sitz baths prn If woman Rh⁻ and infant Rh⁺, RhoGAM work up; obtain consent; complete teaching Obtain consent for rubella vaccine if indicated; explain purpose, procedure, implications Obtain hematocrit Determine rubella status	Continue sitz baths prn May shower if ambulating s̄ difficulty D/C buffalo cap if present
Activity	Assistance when OOB first time, then prn Ambulate ad lib Rests comfortably between checks	Encourage rest periods Ambulate ad lib; may leave birthing unit	Up ad lib
Nutrition	Regular diet Fluid intake ≥ 2000 mL/day	Continue diet and fluids	Continue diet and fluids
Elimination	Voiding large amts straw-colored urine	Voiding large quantities May have bowel movement	Same
Medications	Methergine 0.2 mg q4h prn if ordered Stool softener _____ Tucks pads prn	Continue meds Lanolin to nipples PRN; tea bags to nipples if tender; heparin flush to buffalo cap (if present) q8h or as ordered	Continue medications May take own prenatal vitamins RhoGAM administered if indicated Rubella vaccine administered if indicated
Discharge planning/ home care	Evaluate knowledge of normal postpartum, newborn care Evaluate support systems	Discuss typical newborn schedule; plan for periods of rest Birth certificate paperwork completed Evaluate plans for transporting newborn; car seat available	Review discharge instruction sheet and checklist Describe postpartum warning signs and when to call CNM/physician Provide prescriptions. Gift pack given to woman Arrangements made for baby pictures if desired Postpartum visit scheduled Newborn check scheduled
Family involvement	Identify available support persons Assess family perceptions of birth experience Parenting: demonstrates culturally expected early parenting behaviors	Involve support persons in care, teaching; answer questions Evidence of parental bonding behaviors apparent	Continue to involve support persons in teaching Evidence of parental bonding behaviors present Plans made for providing support to mother following discharge. Support persons verbalize understanding of need for woman to rest, eat nutritionally, recover

| TABLE 34-3 | Essential Information for Common Postpartum Drugs |

EMPIRIN #3 (325 mg aspirin and 30 mg codeine)

Drug Class: Narcotic analgesic

Dose/Route: Usual adult dose: 1–2 tablets PO every 4 hours PRN

Indication: For relief of mild to moderate pain

Adverse Effects: Aspirin: Nausea, dyspepsia, epigastric discomfort, dizziness
Codeine: Respiratory depression, apnea, light-headedness, dizziness, nausea, sweating, dry mouth, constipation, facial flushing, suppression of cough reflex, ureteral spasm, urinary retention, pruritis

Nursing Implications: Determine if woman is sensitive to aspirin or codeine; has history of impaired hepatic or renal function.
Observe woman carefully for respiratory depression.
Monitor bowel sounds, urine output.
Administer with food or after meals if GI upset occurs; encourage woman to drink one full glass (240 mL) with the tablet to reduce the risk of the tablet lodging in the esophagus.

Client Teaching: Inform client about name of drug, expected action, possible side effects, that it is secreted in breast milk (Note: Some physicians/certified nurse-midwives may avoid ordering the medication for nursing mothers), and review safety measures (assess for dizziness, use side rails, call for assistance when getting out of bed and ambulating, report to nurse any signs of adverse effects); ask if she has any questions.

Nursing Diagnoses Related to Drug Therapy: Knowledge deficit related to lack of information about drug therapy.

Risk for injury related to dizziness secondary to effect of drug.

PERCOSET (325 mg acetaminophen and 5 mg oxycodone)

Drug Class: Narcotic analgesic

Dose/Route: 1–2 tablets PO every 4 hours PRN

Indication: For moderate to moderately severe pain; can be used in aspirin-sensitive women

Adverse Effects: Acetaminophen: Hepatotoxicity, headache, rash, hypoglycemia
Oxycodone: Respiratory depression, apnea, circulatory depression, euphoria, facial flushing, constipation, suppression of cough reflex, ureteral spasm, urinary retention

Nursing Implications: Determine if woman is sensitive to acetaminophen or codeine; has bronchial asthma, respiratory depression, convulsive disorder.
Observe woman carefully for respiratory depression. Consider that post–cesarean birth woman may have depressed cough reflex, so teaching and encouragement to deep breathe and cough are needed.
Monitor bowel sounds, urine and bowel elimination.

Client Teaching: Teaching should include name of drug, expected effect, possible adverse effects, that drug is secreted in the breast milk, encouragement to report any signs of adverse effects immediately.

Nursing Diagnoses Related to Drug Therapy: Ineffective breathing patterns related to depression.

Constipation related to slowed gastrointestinal activity.

RUBELLA VIRUS VACCINE, Live (Meruvax 2)

Dose/Route: Single-dose vial, inject subcutaneously in outer aspect of the upper arm

Indication: Stimulate active immunity against rubella virus

Adverse Effects: Burning or stinging at the injection site; about 2–4 weeks later may have rash, malaise, sore throat, or headache.

Nursing Implications: Determine if woman has sensitivity to neomycin (vaccine contains neomycin); is immunosuppressed, or has received blood transfusions (not to be administered within 3 months of blood transfusion, plasma transfusion, or serum immune globulin). Note: If a woman is to receive both RhoGAM and rubella, there is a possibility that the formation of antibodies to rubella may be suppressed by the RhoGAM injection. Most physicians will go ahead and order both injections and retest for maternal rubella immune status in about 3 months (Varney 1987).

Client Teaching: Name of drug, expected effect, possible adverse effects, possible comfort measures to use if adverse effects occur; rubella titer will be assessed in about 3 months. Instruct woman to AVOID PREGNANCY FOR 3 MONTHS following vaccination. Provide information regarding contraceptives and their use.

Nursing Diagnoses Related to Drug Therapy   Knowledge deficit related to lack of information about drug therapy. Knowledge deficit related to lack of information about types and use of contraceptives.

RhoGAM (Rh immune globulin specific for D antigen)

Dose/Route: Postpartum: One vial IM within 72 hours of birth
Antepartal: One vial microdose RhoGAM IM at 28 weeks in Rh negative women; after amniocentesis, spontaneous or therapeutic abortion, or ectopic pregnancy

Indication: Prevention of sensitization to the Rh factor in Rh negative women and to prevent hemolytic disease in the newborn in subsequent pregnancies. Mother must be Rh negative, not previously sensitized to Rh factor. Infant must be Rh positive, direct antiglobulin negative.

Adverse Effects: Soreness at injection site

Nursing Implications: Confirm criteria for administration are present. Assure correct vial is used for the client (each vial is cross-matched to the specific woman and must be carefully checked).
Inject entire contents of vial.

Client Teaching: Name of drug, expected action, possible side effects; report soreness at injection site to nurse; woman should carry information regarding Rh status and dates of RhoGAM injections with her at all times; explain use of RhoGAM with subsequent pregnancies.

Nursing Diagnoses Related to Drug Therapy: Knowledge deficit related to lack of information about the need for RhoGAM and future implications.

Pain related to soreness at injection site.

| TABLE 34-3 | *continued* |

SECONAL SODIUM (secobarbital sodium)

Drug Class: Sedative, short-acting barbiturate

Dose/Route: 100 mg PO at bedtime

Indication: Promote sleep

Adverse Effects: Somnolence, confusion, ataxia, vertigo, nightmares, hypoventilation, bradycardia, hypotension, nausea, vomiting, rashes

Nursing Implications: Determine if woman has sensitivity to barbiturates or respiratory distress. Monitor respirations, blood pressure, pulse. Modify environment to increase relaxation and promote sleep.
Monitor for drug interaction if woman also is taking tranquilizers or TACE.

Client Teaching: Name of drug, expected effect, possible adverse effects, safety measures (side rails, use call bell, ask for assistance when out of bed); medication is secreted in breast milk.

Nursing Diagnoses Related to Drug Therapy: Risk for injury related to possible ataxia or vertigo.
Altered thought processes related to drug-induced confusion.
Knowledge deficit related to lack of information about drug therapy.

RhIgG (RhoGAM)

All Rh negative women who meet specific criteria should receive RhIgG (RhoGAM) within 72 hours after childbirth to prevent sensitization from the fetomaternal transfusion of the Rh positive fetal red blood cells. To prevent sensitization, the dosage is usually 300 μg of $Rh_0(D)$ immune globulin. See discussion of criteria in Procedure 19–2.

Teaching for Self-Care   The Rh negative woman needs to understand the implications of her Rh negative status in future pregnancies. (See Chapter 18 for a detailed discussion.) The nurse provides opportunities for questions during teaching.

Promotion of Comfort and Relief of Pain

Discomfort may be present to varying degrees in the postpartal woman. Potential sources of discomfort include an edematous perineum; a distended bladder; an episiotomy, perineal laceration, or extension; a vaginal hematoma; engorged hemorrhoids; engorged breasts; or sore nipples.

TEACHING MOMENT

You may be surprised by how quickly the postpartum woman shows signs of bladder distention, possibly as soon as 1 to 2 hours after childbirth. This is because of the normal postpartum diuresis. You can help prevent overdistention by palpating the woman's bladder frequently and encouraging her to void. If she is unable to void and catheterization becomes necessary, be prepared for difficulty in visualizing the urethra because of localized swelling and discomfort and tenderness in the area.

Relief of Perineal Discomfort

There are many nursing interventions available for the relief of perineal discomfort. Before selecting a method, the nurse needs to have assessed the perineum to determine the degree of edema and such. It is also important to ask the woman if there are special measures that she feels will be particularly effective or to offer her choices when possible. It is important for the nurse to use disposable gloves while applying all relief measures and to complete a hand washing before and after using the gloves. (See Essential Precautions in Practice: During Postpartal Care on page 1074.)

At all times it is important to remember hygienic practices such as moving from the front (area of the symphysis pubis) to the back (area around the anus) of the perineum. This is important to remember while placing ice packs, placing perineal pads, and applying topical anesthetics or pain relief products. Avoiding contamination between the anal area and the urethral/vaginal area is important to prevent infection.

Ice Pack   If an episiotomy is done at the time of birth, an ice pack is generally applied to reduce edema and provide numbing of the tissues, which promotes comfort. In some agencies chemical ice bags are used. These are usually activated by folding both ends toward the middle. Inexpensive ice bags may be made by filling a disposable glove with ice chips or crushed ice and then taping the top of the glove. To protect the perineum from burns caused by contact with the ice pack, the disposable glove needs to first be rinsed under running water to remove any powder that may be present and then wrapped in an absorbent towel or washcloth before placing it against the perineum. To attain the maximum effect of this cold treatment, the ice pack should remain in place approximately 20 minutes and then be removed for about 10 minutes before replacing it. Ice packs may be continued for as long as necessary. Usually, they are needed for the first 24 hours.

Teaching for Home Care   The nurse provides information regarding the purpose of the ice pack, anticipated effects, benefits, and possible problems and how to prepare an ice pack for home use if edema is present and early discharge is planned.

Sitz Bath   The warmth of the water in the sitz bath provides comfort, decreases pain, and promotes circulation to the tissues, which promotes healing and reduces the incidence of infection. Sitz baths may be ordered TID and PRN. The nurse prepares the sitz bath by cleansing the sitz tub or portable sitz. Water at 102–105 F is added. The woman is instructed to remain in the sitz for 20 minutes. Care needs to be taken during the first sitz bath because the warm moist heat and warm environment may cause the woman to faint. Placing a call bell well within reach and checking on the woman at frequent intervals will increase her comfort and maintain safety. The woman needs to be observed at frequent intervals for signs that she may faint, such as dizziness, a floaty or spacy feeling, or difficulty hearing. It is important for the woman to have a clean unused towel to pat dry her perineum after the sitz bath and to have a clean perineal pad ready to apply.

Recently, cool sitz baths have gained popularity because they are effective in reducing perineal edema. Until definite research supports one temperature (warm or cold) as more effective, it may be best to offer the woman a choice.

Teaching for Home Care   The nurse provides information regarding the purpose and use of the sitz bath, anticipated effects, benefits and possible problems, and safety measures to prevent injury from fainting, slipping, or excessive water temperature. Home use of sitz baths may be recommended for the woman with an extensive episiotomy, and the woman may use a portable sitz or her bathtub. It is important for the nurse to emphasize that in using a bathtub only 4–6 in water is drawn, the temperature of the water needs to be assessed, and the water is used only for the sitz and not for bathing. If a tub bath is taken, the water should be released, the tub cleaned, and new water drawn prior to the sitz to prevent infection.

The popularity of hot tubs among the general population has led many institutions to install hot tubs or jet hydrotherapy tubs instead of traditional sitz tubs. Because of the intense competition for obstetric patients, newer facilities often feature these tubs in each room (Rhode & Barger 1990).

Topical Agents   Topical anesthetics such as Dermoplast aerosol spray or Americain spray may be used to relieve perineal discomfort. The woman is advised to apply the anesthetic following a sitz bath or perineal care. Because of the danger of tissue burns, she must be cautioned not to apply anesthetic before using a heat lamp.

Witch hazel compresses may be used to relieve perineal discomfort and edema. Nupercainal ointment or TUCKS may be ordered for relief of hemorrhoidal pain. It is important for the nurse to emphasize the need for the woman to wash her hands before and after using the topical treatments.

Teaching for Self-Care   The nurse provides information regarding the anesthetic spray or topical agent. The woman needs to understand the purpose, use, anticipated effects, benefits, and possible problems associated with the product. Demonstration of application by the nurse can be combined with explanation. A return demonstration is a useful method of evaluating the woman's understanding.

Perineal Care   Perineal care after each elimination cleanses the perineum and helps promote comfort. Many agencies provide "peri bottles" that the woman can use to squirt warm tap water over her perineum following elimination. To cleanse her perineum, the woman may use a Surgigator, moist antiseptic towelettes, or toilet paper in a blotting (patting) motion and should be taught to start at the front (area just under the symphysis pubis) and proceed toward the back (area around the anus) to prevent contamination from the anal area. In addition, to prevent contamination, the perineal pad should be applied from front to back, placing the front portion against the perineum first.

Teaching for Self-Care The nurse demonstrates how to cleanse the perineum and assists the woman as necessary. Additional information regarding the use of perineal pads may be offered. The pads need to be placed snugly against the perineum but should not produce pressure. If the pad is worn too loosely, it may rub back and forth, irritating perineal tissues and causing contamination between the anal and vaginal areas. Many women have never used a perineal pad or belt and will need additional assistance in using them during the postpartal period. (See Teaching Guide: Care of an Episiotomy on page 1076.)

Relief of Hemorrhoidal Discomfort

Some mothers experience hemorrhoidal pain after giving birth. Relief measures include the use of sitz baths, anesthetic ointments, rectal suppositories, or witch hazel pads applied directly to the anal area. The woman may be taught to digitally replace external hemorrhoids in her rectum. She may also find it helpful to maintain a side-lying position when possible or to tighten her buttocks when sitting down to reduce contact of the perineum with the seat and to avoid prolonged sitting. The mother is encouraged to maintain an adequate fluid intake, and stool softeners are administered to ensure greater comfort with bowel movements. The hemorrhoids usually disappear a few weeks after birth if the woman did not have them prior to her pregnancy.

Relief of Afterpains

Afterpains are the result of intermittent uterine contractions. A primipara may not notice afterpains because her uterus is able to maintain a contracted state. Multiparous women and those who have had an overdistended uterus (due to multiple gestation or hydramnios) frequently experience discomfort from afterpains as the uterus intermittently contracts more vigorously. Breastfeeding women are also more likely to experience afterpains than bottle-feeding women because of the release of oxytocin when the infant suckles. The nurse can suggest the woman lie prone with a small pillow under the lower abdomen. The woman needs to be told that the discomfort may feel intensified for about 5 minutes but then will diminish greatly if not completely. The prone position applies pressure to the uterus and therefore stimulates contractions. When the uterus maintains a constant contraction, the afterpains cease. Additional nursing interventions may be to encourage a sitz bath (for warmth), positioning, ambulation, or administration of an analgesic agent such as Motrin, Tylenol, or Percoset. When administering an analgesic, the nurse must make a clinical judgment about the type, dosage, and frequency based on the medication ordered. The mother's description of the type and severity of her pain is usually the most reliable method of determining which analgesic would provide her the comfort she desires, therefore encouraging self-care activities and beginning to learn how to take care of her infant. Many women have concerns about the effects on the infant if they are breastfeeding. For breastfeeding mothers a mild analgesic administered an hour before feeding will promote comfort and enhance maternal-infant interactions.

Teaching for Self-Care The nurse provides information about the cause of afterpains and methods to decrease discomfort. Any medications that are ordered are explained, along with expected effect, benefits, possible side effects, and any special considerations such as the possibility of dizziness or sleepiness with particular medications.

Relief of Discomfort from Immobility

Discomfort may also be caused by immobility. The woman who pushed for a long time during labor may experience muscular aches. It is not unusual for women to experience joint pains and discomfort in both arms and legs. Early ambulation is encouraged to help reduce the incidence of complications such as constipation and thrombophlebitis. It also helps promote a feeling of general well-being.

TEACHING MOMENT

It is not unusual for the postpartum mother to feel faint the first few times she gets up. Be alert for signs of faintness such as loss of color in her lips or face; complaints of feeling warm, dizzy, or having buzzing in her ears; and difficulty hearing. If any of these signs are noted, immediately support her body so she doesn't fall. Then help her sit with her head between her knees or lie down.

The nurse assists the woman the first few times she gets up during the postpartal period. Fatigue, effects of medications, loss of blood, and possibly even lack of food intake may result in feelings of dizziness or faintness when the woman stands up. Because this may be a problem during the woman's first shower, the nurse should remain in the room, check the woman frequently, and have a chair close by in case she becomes faint. Dizziness may be aggravated by standing still and by the warmth of the water, so it is best to keep the first shower somewhat brief. On many postpartal units ammonia inhalants are taped to the bathroom door for use in case of fainting. During this first shower the nurse instructs the woman in the use of the emergency call button in the bathroom; if she becomes faint during a future shower, she can call for assistance.

Teaching for Self-Care The nurse provides information about ambulation and the importance of monitoring any signs of dizziness or weakness.

CARE OF AN EPISIOTOMY

Assessment   During the time following labor and birth the nurse assesses the woman's understanding of the purpose of the episiotomy, factors that contribute to wound healing, and comfort measures available if the woman experiences discomfort. The woman's level of knowledge may be influenced by several factors, including, for example, childbirth preparation activities and previous childbirth experience.

Nursing Diagnosis   The key nursing diagnosis will probably be: Knowledge deficit related to lack of information about self-care measures to promote episiotomy healing and personal comfort.

Nursing Plan and Implementation   The teaching will focus on the process of healing, factors that increase the risk of infection, and steps the woman can take to promote healing and increase her personal comfort.

Client Goals   At the completion of the teaching the woman will be able to do the following:

1. Identify factors that promote and those that interfere with wound healing.

2. Summarize self-care activities to promote healing and increase personal comfort.

3. Demonstrate the correct procedure for taking a sitz bath.

4. Discuss the judicious use of prescribed analgesics as needed.

Teaching Plan

Content   Describe the process of wound healing, including the value of healing by first intention as opposed to a jagged tear. Discuss the risk of contamination of the episiotomy by bacteria from the anal area.

Explain techniques that are used to keep the episiotomy clean and promote healing such as the following:

*   Sitz bath

*   Use of peri-bottle or surgigator following each voiding or defecation

*   Pad change following each elimination and at regular intervals

Describe comfort measures:

*   Ice pack or glove immediately following birth

*   Sitz bath

*   Judicious use of analgesics or topical anesthetics

*   Tightening buttocks before sitting

Identify signs of episiotomy infection. Advise the woman to contact care giver if infection develops.

Evaluation   At the end of the teaching session the woman will be able to verbalize principles of wound healing and episiotomy care. She also will be able to demonstrate self-care measures such as peri-care and taking a sitz bath.

Teaching Method   *Many women fail to consider the episiotomy a surgical incision. Discussion helps them understand the importance of good wound care.*

Discussion and demonstration as indicated. Demonstration may be necessary for sitz bath or Surgigator.

Discussion and opportunity for questions.

Discussion and printed handouts. Some of this content may also be covered during a small postpartum class.

Relief of Discomfort from Excessive Perspiration

Postpartal diaphoresis may cause discomfort for new mothers. The nurse can offer a fresh dry gown and bed linens to enhance comfort. Some women may feel refreshed by a shower. It is important to consider cultural practices and realize that some women of Mexican or Asian cultural background may prefer not to shower in the first few days following birth. Because diaphoresis also may lead to increased thirst, the nurse can offer fluids as the woman desires. Again, cultural practices are important to consider. Women of Western European background may prefer iced water; Asian women may prefer water at room temperature. It is important for the nurse to ascertain the woman's wishes rather than operate solely from the nurse's own value/cultural belief system.

Teaching for Self-Care The nurse provides information regarding the normal physiologic occurrence of the diaphoresis and methods to increase comfort.

Suppression of Lactation in the Nonnursing Mother

Lactation may be suppressed through drug therapy and mechanical inhibition. The drugs used are hormones that inhibit the secretion of prolactin. However, because many of these drugs, such as chlorotrianisene (TACE), are estrogen-based medications and are associated with an increased incidence of thromboembolic disease, most practitioners prescribe them much less frequently than formerly.

Because medication used to suppress lactation is not always completely successful, mechanical methods of lactation suppression are becoming increasingly popular. Although signs of engorgement do not usually occur until the second or third postpartum day, prevention of engorgement is best accomplished by beginning mechanical (nonpharmaceutical) methods of lactation suppression as soon as possible after birth. Ideally, this involves having the woman begin wearing a supportive, well-fitting bra within 6 hours after birth. The bra is worn continuously until lactation is suppressed (usually about 5 days) and is removed only for showers. The bra provides support and eases the discomfort that can occur with tension on the breasts because of fullness. A snug breast binder may be used if the woman does not have a bra available or if she finds the binder more comfortable. Ice packs should be applied over the axillary area of each breast for 20 minutes four times daily. This, too, should be begun soon after birth. Ice is also useful in relieving discomfort if engorgement occurs.

Teaching for Home Care

The mother is advised to avoid any stimulation of her breasts by her baby, herself, breast pumps, or her sexual partner until the sensation of fullness has passed (usually about 1 week). Such stimulation will increase milk production and delay the suppression process. Heat is to be avoided for the same reason, and the mother is encouraged to let shower water flow over her back rather than her breasts. Suppression takes only a few days in most cases, but small amounts of milk may be produced up to a month after birth.

Promotion of Rest and Graded Activity

Following birth most women feel exhausted and in need of rest. Other women are euphoric and full of psychic energy, ready to retell their experience of birth repeatedly. The nurse evaluates individual needs, always with the goal of providing opportunities for rest. The nurse can provide time for the excited, euphoric woman to air her feelings and then can encourage a period of rest. The nurse may also help the family limit visitors and provide a comfortable sleep chair or bed for the father.

Physical fatigue often influences many other adjustments and functions with the new mother. It may also reduce milk flow, thereby increasing problems with breastfeeding. The mother requires energy to make the psychologic adjustments to a new infant and to assume new roles. She makes these adjustments more smoothly when she gets adequate rest.

The nurse may encourage rest by organizing activities to avoid frequent interruptions for the woman. If the new mother chooses, rest times may be arranged by having the newborn remain in the holding nursery for a period of time, or the mother can rest or sleep when the baby is sleeping in her room.

Postpartal Exercises

The woman is encouraged to begin simple exercises and continue them at home. She is advised that increased lochia or pain means she should reevaluate her activity and make necessary alterations. Most agencies provide a booklet describing suggested postpartal activities. (Exercise routines vary for women undergoing tubal ligation following birth or for cesarean birth clients.) See Figure 34–1 on page 1078 for some common exercises.

Resumption of Activities

Activity may be increased gradually after discharge. The new mother should avoid heavy lifting, excessive stair climbing, and strenuous activity. One or two daily naps are essential and are most easily achieved if the mother sleeps when her baby does.

By the second week at home, light housekeeping may be resumed. Although it is customary to delay returning to work for 6 weeks, most women are physically able to resume practically all activities by 4 to 5 weeks. Delaying returning to work until after the final postpartal examination will minimize the possibility of problems.

Promotion of Maternal Psychologic Well-Being

The birth of a child, with the role changes and increased responsibilities it produces, is a time of emotional stress for the new mother. This stress is increased by the tremendous physiologic changes as her body adjusts to a nonpregnant state. During the early postpartal days mood swings and tearfulness are common.

At first the mother may repeatedly discuss her experiences in labor and birth. This allows her to integrate her experiences. If she feels that she did not cope well with labor, she may have feelings of inadequacy and may benefit from reassurance that she did well.

Open discussion of feelings is possible only if the postpartum nurse has established a warm, supportive

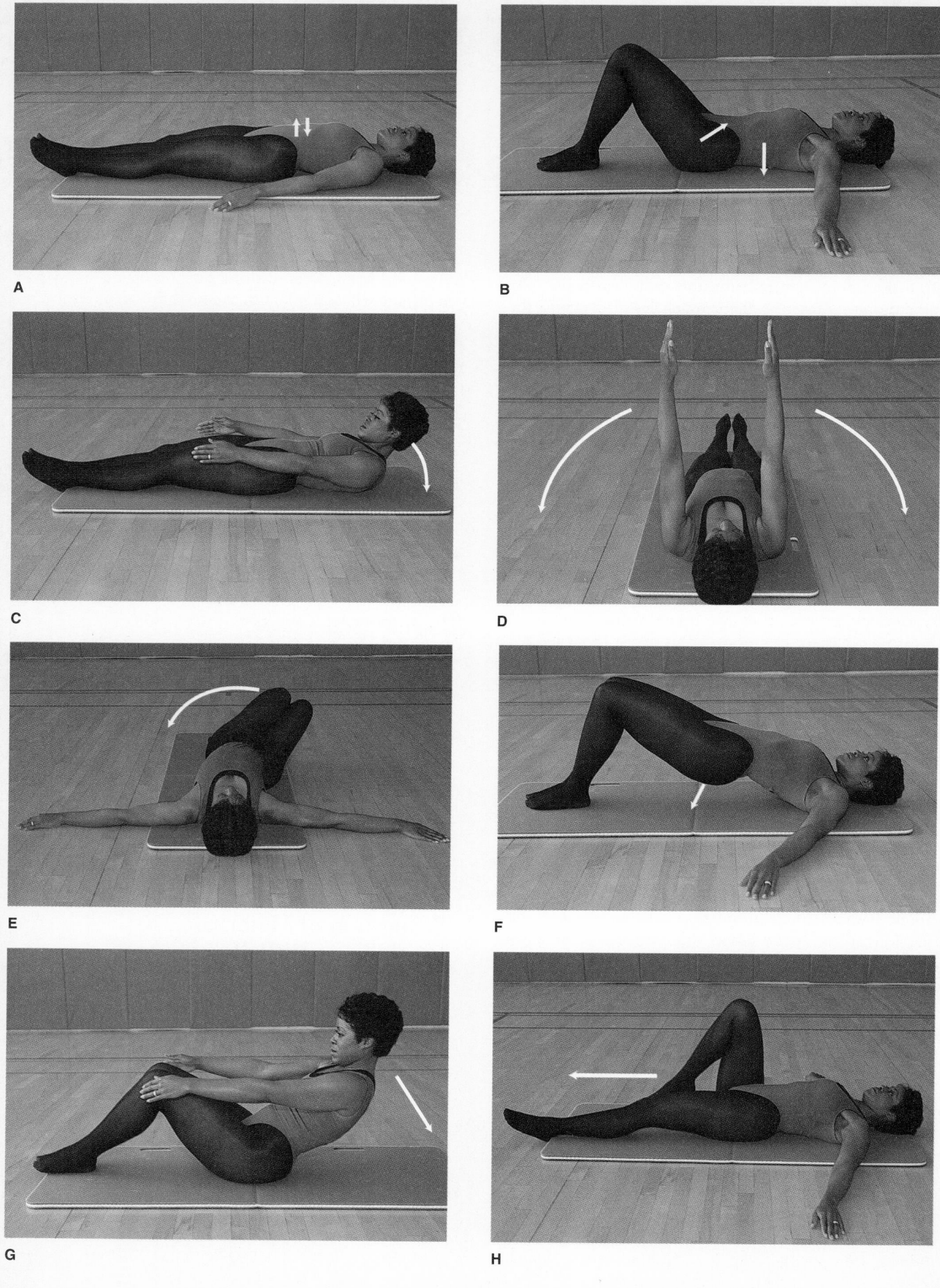

A

B

C

D

E

F

G

H

relationship with the woman. Follow-up visits from the nurse who assisted her in labor and birth provide additional opportunities for the mother to relive her experiences and come to terms with them.

During the postpartal period the mother must adjust to the loss of her fantasized child and accept the child she has borne. This may be more difficult if the child is not of the desired sex or if she or he has birth defects.

Immediately following the birth (the *taking-in* period) the mother is focused on bodily concerns, and teaching other than for self-care may not be totally effective. Because early discharge is common, however, classes and information should be offered and printed handouts provided for reference as questions arise at home.

Following the initial dependent period, the mother becomes very concerned about her ability to be a successful parent (the *taking-hold* period). Skillful intervention by the nurse, with continual reassurance that the woman is a successful mother, is vital. During this time the mother is most receptive to teaching, and tactful instruction and demonstration assist her in mothering effectively. The nurse must carefully avoid "taking over" the infant. By functioning as an adviser and allowing the mother to perform the actual care, the nurse demonstrates confidence in the mother's skill and ability, which in turn increases the mother's self-confidence about her effectiveness as a parent. Recognition and praise of her success increase the mother's feeling of control and competence in her ability to take care of her infant. Feelings of self-esteem in the mother are greatly increased through positive feedback.

The depression, weepiness, and "let down feeling" that characterize the postpartum blues are often a surprise for the new mother. She and her family may require reassurance that these feelings are normal and an explanation about why they occur. It is vital to provide a supportive environment that permits the mother to cry without feeling guilty.

After our baby was born, I felt so lost. Here was the little one we had waited for, and we were so happy; yet it seemed that I couldn't do anything right. I had watched my friends diaper their babies, and yet I couldn't get the diaper on without a struggle. How could those little legs move around so quickly, and just at the wrong moment? Our baby cried each time I tried to change her T-shirt, and she always got her hands caught in the sleeves. I wondered if I would ever learn how to care for this little one.

Our nurse was so wonderful. She was just always there at the right time, and even though she could see that I was having trouble, she spoke so gently and helped me feel that I could learn this. She showed me all kinds of little tricks about getting that diaper on while keeping our baby's legs quiet, and really showed me how to care for our baby. The nurse did everything so smoothly; yet her gentle, supportive encouragement as she helped me gave me the courage to keep trying. By the time we went home, I had mastered dressing our baby, and I felt that I could do what I would need to do. I could really be the mother that I wanted to be. It seemed like such a little thing in my nurse's busy day, when I think of all the work that she had to do, but I will always remember her. She showed that she cared for all of us, and she quietly changed our lives. I hope our nurse knows that.

Promotion of Effective Parent Education

Meeting the educational needs of the new mother and her family is one of the primary challenges facing the postpartum nurse. Effective education provides the childbearing family with sufficient knowledge to meet many of their own health needs and to seek assistance if necessary.

Educational assessment may be accomplished through observation, sensitivity to nonverbal clues, and tactfully phrased questions. For example, asking "What plans have you made for handling things when you get

◄ FIGURE 34-1 Postpartal exercises. Begin with five repetitions two or three times daily, and gradually increase to ten repetitions. First day: *A* Abdominal breathing. Lying supine, inhale deeply, using the abdominal muscles. The abdomen should expand. Then exhale slowly through pursed lips, tightening the abdominal muscles. *B* Pelvic rocking. Lying supine with arms at sides, knees bent, and feet flat, tighten abdomen and buttocks, and attempt to flatten back on floor. Hold for a count of ten; then arch the back, causing the pelvis to "rock." On the second day add: *C* Chin to chest. Lying supine with legs straight, raise head and attempt to touch chin to chest. Slowly lower head. *D* Arm raises. Lying supine, arms extended at a 90-degree angle from body, raise arms so they are perpendicular and hands touch. Lower slowly. On fourth day add: *E* Knee rolls. Lying supine with knees bent, feet flat, arms extended to the side, roll knees slowly to one side, keeping shoulders flat. Return to original position, and roll to opposite side. *F* Buttocks lift. Lying supine, arms at sides, knees bent, feet flat, slowly raise the buttocks, and arch the back. Return slowly to starting position. On sixth day add: *G* Abdominal tighteners. Lying supine, knees bent, feet flat, slowly raise head toward knees. Arms should extend along either side of legs. Return slowly to original position. *H* Knee to abdomen. Lying supine, arms at sides, bend one knee and thigh until foot touches buttocks. Straighten leg and lower it slowly. Repeat with other leg. After 2–3 weeks more strenuous exercises such as sit-ups and side leg raises may be added as tolerated. Kegel exercises, begun antepartally, should be done many times daily during postpartum to restore vaginal and perineal tone.

Family functioning changes when any mother brings a new infant home. When the new mother is an adolescent, even more family adaptations may be required. Kathryn Records tested an adolescent family assessment model by examining adolescent mothers' caregiving knowledge and behavior, approval from family and friends, and family functioning. In this study care giving was defined as meeting the infant's needs by performing an activity. Approval involved receiving acceptance or positive affirmation for one's actions from either the peer group or the family. Family functioning was examined in both the young mother's original family and, if applicable, the new family of the adolescent mother and infant.

The sample for this study consisted of 134 adolescent mothers who lived in the same household as their infants. The sample included White (37%), Mexican American (48%), Native American (12%), and Black (3%) mothers. The typical participant relied on her baby's grandparents as secondary care givers, had participated in a teen parent program for 7 months, and had no experience babysitting prior to her pregnancy. Data were collected using several methods, including family and peer approval instruments, an infant care-giving inventory, a family function assessment, and an interpersonal relationship inventory. Psychometric properties of all instruments were analyzed and discussed, and the author did not find satisfactory stability with either the care-giving inventory or the peer approval instrument.

Results showed that the young mothers had a moderate level of care-giving knowledge and moderately high levels of peer and family approval. The mothers described a moderate level of family functioning in new families as well as in families of origin. Multiple regression revealed that White ethnicity and the age of the first child accounted for 15% of the variance for care-giving behavior. Native American ethnicity and age of first child explained 10% of family functioning. In other words, as the child grew older, care-giving behavior decreased for White mothers and family functioning decreased for Native American mothers. Care-giving knowledge and family approval did not contribute to the model of family functioning.

Clinical Application of Study

As the author notes, these results need to be interpreted with caution due to the unsatisfactory stability of two of the instruments. However, the observed decrease in family functioning as the child ages could negatively affect both mother and child. Nurses need to be alert for this possibility in families with adolescent mothers and should develop intervention strategies as needed.

SOURCE: Records K: Adolescent mothers: Caregiving, approval, and family functioning. *JOGNN* 1994; 23(9):791.

home?" will elicit a more detailed response than, "Will someone be available to help you at home?"

To assess learning needs, some agencies provide a client handout listing the most frequently identified areas of concern for new mothers. The mother checks those that apply to her or writes in concerns not included.

In many educational settings, planning primarily involves the development of objectives that clarify what is to be taught and describe how the learner will demonstrate achievement of each objective. In planned postpartal classes, objectives are predetermined and generalized to meet the needs of most participants. Even in nonstructured, individualized situations, however, objectives can be identified by the nurse—"Mrs Warren, when we are finished, you will be able to show how to manually express your breast milk and explain how to properly store it."

The educational method chosen to implement the objectives varies. Agencies with many clients and limited staff may rely heavily on structured classes. Smaller units may provide individualized instruction through the use of videotapes. Because more effective learning occurs when there is sensory involvement and active participation, television and movies (sight and hearing) are more helpful than lecture (hearing only), and demonstration–return demonstration (sight, touch, hearing, and possibly smell and taste) is even more effective.

Postpartal units use a variety of approaches—scheduled classes or demonstrations, handouts, group discussions, movies, videotapes, and individual interaction. Some agencies have access to a television channel and can show instructional films at scheduled times during the day. Women should have pencils and paper provided to jot down questions that arise as they view the material. Afterward nurses are available to clarify material or answer any questions about the content.

Timing is important in implementing educational activities. The new mother is more receptive to teaching after the first 24 to 48 hours, when she is ready to assume responsibility for her own care and that of her newborn. However, many women are discharged in the early, dependent phase. Because of this, teaching should be done, and handouts should be provided for future reference. Some clinicians suggest that client education in early postpartum discharge programs is most effective if based on comprehensive assessment, home follow-ups, and individualized teaching (Harrison 1990; Sheil et al 1995).

Timing is also important for new fathers, who are more likely to attend sessions planned for them if they are scheduled in the evening after visiting hours. If material is planned for siblings, late afternoon teaching after school or naps might be most effective.

Demonstration–return demonstration techniques offer opportunities for an individual to practice in a supervised situation. Emphasizing understanding of principles rather than simply mimicking of techniques facilitates transfer of the learning to the home situation.

Teaching should not be limited to "how to" activities, however. Anticipatory guidance is essential in assisting the family to cope with role changes and the realities of a new baby. Small group discussions provide a chance for the new parents to talk about fears and expectations. Questions may arise regarding sexuality, contraception, child care, and even the grief associated with giving up the fantasized infant in order to accept the actual one.

Information is also essential for individuals with specialized educational needs—the mother who had a cesarean birth, the adolescent mother, the parents of an infant with congenital anomalies, and so on. They may feel overwhelmed, have difficult feelings to work through, and not even realize what it is they need to know. Nurses who are attuned to these individual problems can begin providing guidance as soon as possible.

Methods for evaluating learning vary according to the objectives and teaching methods. Return demonstrations, question-and-answer sessions, and even programed instruction are opportunities for evaluating learning, as are formal evaluation tools.

Evaluation of attitudinal or less concrete learning is more difficult. For example, a mother's ability to express her frustrations over an unanticipated cesarean birth or a new mother's decision to delay for several weeks a family dinner originally scheduled for the first weekend after she arrives home may be the nurse's only clues that learning has occurred. Follow-up phone calls after discharge may provide additional evaluative information and continue the helping process as the nurse assesses the family's current educational status and begins planning accordingly.

Promotion of Family Wellness

A satisfactory maternity experience may have a positive impact on the entire family. The new or expanding family that receives appropriate information and has adequate time to interact with its newest member in a supportive environment will feel more comfortable and secure at home.

Mother-Baby Units

In the past newborns were typically separated from their parents immediately after birth. Today most facilities encourage parents to spend time with their infants. Some facilities offer the option of mother-baby units (also called mother-baby primary nursing, mother-infant nursing, combined care, and family-centered maternity care). This concept works very well when combined with the practice of single-room maternity care (LDRP, ie, labor, delivery, recovery, postpartum; or LDR). A mother-baby unit is based on the concept that mother and infant will both benefit from time spent together, so the infant remains at the mother's bedside, and both are cared for by the same nurse. Some agencies call this option *rooming-in*. In other facilities the rooming-in policy varies slightly in that nursery personnel remain responsible for the child at the mother's bedside while postpartum staff care for the mother.

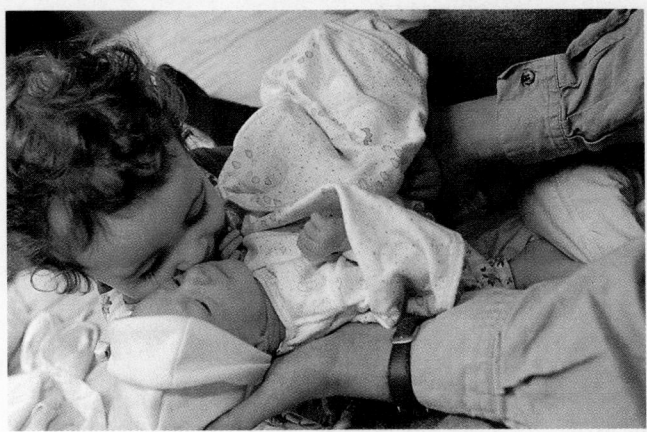

FIGURE 34-2 The sister of this newborn becomes acquainted with the new family member during a nursing assessment.

In a mother-baby unit the newborn's crib is placed near the mother's bed, where she can see her baby easily. The crib should be a self-contained unit stocked with items the mother might require in providing care. A bulb syringe for suctioning the mouth or nares should always be accessible, and the mother and father/partner should be familiar with its use.

Mothers are frequently very tired after birth, so the responsibility for providing total infant care could be overwhelming. The mother-baby policy must be flexible enough to permit the mother to return the baby to the nursery if she finds it necessary because of fatigue or physical discomfort.

The mother-baby unit is conducive to a self-demand feeding schedule for both breastfeeding and bottle-feeding infants. The lactating mother may find it especially beneficial to be able to nurse her child every 1½ to 3 hours as desired.

Many agencies have unlimited visiting hours for the father or significant others of the mother's choice. Fathers, after washing their hands, are able to care for their infant in a mother-baby unit. These opportunities to hold and care for the child promote paternal self-confidence and foster paternal attachment.

Sibling Visitation

Sibling visitation helps meet the needs of both the siblings and their mother. A visit to the hospital reassures children that their mother is well and still loves them. It also provides an opportunity for the children to become familiar with the new baby. For the mother the pangs of separation are lessened as she interacts with her children and introduces them to the newest family member.

Most agencies now recognize the importance of providing siblings with opportunities to see their mother and meet the infant during the early postpartal period (Figure 34–2). Approaches to this issue vary from specified visiting hours for siblings to unlimited visiting privileges.

Teaching for Home Care Although the parents have prepared the child for the presence of a new brother or sister, the actual arrival of the infant requires some adjustments. If the woman gives birth in a birthing center, her children may be present for the birth. They then have an opportunity to spend time with their new sibling and their parents. They may even remain throughout the woman's hospitalization, especially if it is brief, and all go home as a family.

For the mother who is returning home to small children it is often helpful to have the father carry the new baby inside. This practice keeps the mother's arms free to hug and hold her older children. She thereby reaffirms her love for them before introducing them to their new sibling. Many mothers have found that bringing a doll home with them for the older child is helpful. The child cares for the doll alongside his or her parents, thereby identifying with the parent. This identification helps decrease anger and the need to regress to get attention.

Often older children enjoy working with the parents to care for the newborn. Involvement in care helps the older child develop a sense of closeness to the baby. It also helps the child learn acceptable behavior toward the newborn, feel a sense of accomplishment, and develop tenderness and caring. With constant supervision and assistance as necessary, even very young children can hold the baby or a bottle during feeding. Breastfeeding mothers may allow siblings to help give the new infant an occasional bottle of water.

Regression is a common occurrence even when siblings have been well prepared. The nurse can provide anticipatory guidance so that parents do not become overly upset if their previously toilet-trained child begins to have accidents or requests a bottle to feed from.

Regardless of age, an older sibling needs reassurance that he or she is still special to the parents, a truly loved and valued family member. Words of love and praise coupled with hugs and kisses are very important. So, too, is special parent-child time. Both parents should spend quality time in a one-to-one experience with each of their older children. This may require some careful planning, but its worth cannot be overestimated. It confirms the parents' love for the child and often helps the child accept the new baby.

The child, especially one of the opposite sex from the newborn, may raise queries about the appearance of the genitals as compared to his or her own. A simple explanation, such as, "That's what little girls (boys) look like," is often sufficient.

Resumption of Sexual Activity

Nursing interventions in the postpartal period acknowledge that the parent is also a sexual being. Couples were formerly discouraged from engaging in sexual intercourse until 6 weeks postpartum. Currently, the couple is advised to abstain from intercourse until the episiotomy is healed and the lochial flow has stopped (usually by the end of the third week). Because the vaginal vault is still "dry" (hormone-poor), some form of lubrication, such as K-Y jelly, may be necessary during intercourse. The female-superior or side-by-side positions for coitus may be preferable because they enable the woman to control the depth of penile penetration.

Breastfeeding couples should be forewarned that during orgasm, milk may spout from the nipples due to the release of oxytocin. Some couples find this pleasurable or amusing; other couples choose to have the woman wear a bra during sex. Nursing the baby prior to lovemaking may reduce the chance of milk release.

Other factors may inhibit satisfactory sexual experience: The baby's crying may "spoil the mood"; the woman's changed body may be unattractive to her or to her partner; and maternal sleep deprivation may interfere with a mutually satisfying experience. Couples may also be frustrated if there is decreased libido or other changes in the woman's physiologic response to sexual stimulation. These changes are due to hormonal changes and may persist for several months. Many couples report that even 4 months following childbirth they continue to experience a decline in sexual activity due to the woman's lingering discomfort (often related to episiotomy pain), fatigue, decreased physical strength and dissatisfaction with personal appearance (Fishman et al 1986).

Teaching for Home Care Anticipatory guidance during the prenatal and postnatal periods can forewarn the couple of these eventualities and of their temporary nature. See Teaching Guide: Resumption of Sexual Activity After Childbirth.

Couples can be encouraged to express their affection and love through kissing, holding, and talking. Because the man's level of desire does not show the same decrease as the woman's, he requires forewarning that he may experience a decrease in sexual intercourse for up to a year following childbirth (Fishman et al 1986).

Contraception

Because many couples resume sexual activity before the postpartal examination, family-planning information should be made available before discharge. A couple's decision to use a contraceptive is often motivated by a desire to gain control over the number of children they will conceive or to determine the spacing of future children. In choosing a specific method, consistency of use outweighs the absolute reliability of a given method. Risk factors and contraindications of the various methods must be identified by the nurse to help the couple select a contraceptive method that has practical application and is compatible with the couple's health and physical needs.

Often different methods of contraception are appropriate at different times in the couple's life. Thus they should have a clear understanding of all of the methods

RESUMPTION OF SEXUAL ACTIVITY AFTER CHILDBIRTH

Assessment The nurse recognizes that couples, especially if they have become parents for the first time, may have questions about resuming sexual activity. Although the woman may initiate this discussion, often the nurse can best assess the woman's (and her partner's) understanding by providing some general information followed by some tactful questions.

Nursing Diagnosis The key nursing diagnosis will probably be: Knowledge deficit related to lack of information about changes in sexual activity that commonly occur postpartally.

Nursing Plan and Implementation For the teaching plan to be effective the nurse must first establish rapport with the couple and should promote an environment that is conducive to teaching and discussion. It is helpful to provide privacy during the session so that the couple feels free to ask questions without fear of interruption. The format is generally a question and answer or discussion approach.

Client Goals At the completion of the teaching the couple will be able to do the following:

1. Discuss the changes in the woman's body that affect sexual activity.

2. Formulate alternative approaches to sexual activity based on an understanding of these changes.

3. Identify the length of time it is advisable to wait before resuming sexual activity.

4. Discuss information needed to make contraceptive choices.

Teaching Plan

Content Present information about changes that may affect sexual activity, including the following:

- Tenderness of the vagina and perineum
- Presence of lochia and the healing process
- Dryness of the vagina
- Breast engorgement and tenderness
- Escape of milk during sexual activity

The nurse discusses healing at the placental site and stresses that the presence of lochia indicates that healing is not yet complete. The nurse points out that because the vagina is "hormone-poor" postpartally, vaginal dryness may be problematic. This can be avoided by using a water-soluble lubricant. Escape of milk during sexual activity can be minimized by having the breastfeeding mother nurse immediately beforehand.

Discuss the importance of contraception even during the early postpartal period. Provide information on the advantages and disadvantages of different methods. The woman's body needs adequate time to heal and recover from the stress of pregnancy and childbirth. Couples who are opposed to contraception may choose abstinence at this time.

Discuss impact of fatigue and the new baby's schedule on the woman's feelings of desire. Refer to physician/certified nurse-midwife for additional information if needed.

Evaluation The nurse determines the couple's learning by providing time for discussion and questions. If the couple indicates that they plan to use a particular contraceptive method, the nurse may ask them about aspects of the method to ascertain that they have correct and complete information.

Teaching Method *Discussion is a logical approach. It may be useful to make a universal statement and link it with a question to determine a couple's initial level of knowledge. For example, "Many women experience vaginal dryness when they resume intercourse for the first several weeks after childbirth. Are you familiar with this change and the cause for it?"*
Use the information gained during this discussion to determine the depth to which to cover the material.

Provide printed information to clarify content and serve as a resource for the couple following discharge.

Have samples of different types of contraceptives available.
Provide literature on specific contraceptive methods.

Many couples are unprepared for the impact of fatigue and the baby on lovemaking. Information enables the couple to anticipate this impact.

available to them so that they can make an appropriate choice. The currently available contraceptive methods are discussed in detail in Chapter 9.

Nursing Plan and Implementation for Cesarean Birth

After a cesarean birth the new mother has postpartal needs similar to those of women who gave birth vaginally. Because she has undergone major abdominal surgery, however, the woman who has had a cesarean also has nursing care needs similar to those of other surgical clients. The anticipated course of recovery is presented in the Cesarean Birth Critical Pathway on page 1086.

Promotion of Maternal Physical Well-Being

The chances of pulmonary infection are increased due to immobility after the use of narcotics and sedatives and because of the altered immune response in postoperative clients. For this reason the woman is encouraged to cough and deep breathe and to use incentive spirometry every 2 to 4 hours while awake for the first few days following cesarean birth.

Leg exercises are done every 15 minutes in conjunction with the postpartal check in the recovery room. The exercises should be continued every 2 hours until the woman is ambulatory. The leg exercises increase circulation, help prevent thrombophlebitis, and aid in the improvement of abdominal motility by tightening abdominal muscles.

Monitoring and managment of the woman's pain experience are carried out during the postpartum period. Sources of pain include incisional pain, gas pain, referred shoulder pain, periodic uterine contractions (afterbirth pains), and pain from voiding, defecation, or constipation.

Nursing interventions are oriented toward preventing or alleviating pain or helping the woman cope with pain. The nurse should undertake the following measures:

- Administer analgesics as needed, especially during the first 24 to 72 hours. Their use will relieve the woman's pain and enable her to be more mobile and active.

- Offer comfort through proper positioning, back rubs, oral care, and the reduction of noxious stimuli such as noise and unpleasant odors.

- Encourage the presence of significant others, including the newborn. This practice provides distraction from the painful sensations and helps reduce the woman's fear and anxiety.

- Encourage the use of breathing, relaxation, and distraction techniques (for example, stimulation of cutaneous tissue) taught in childbirth preparation class.

The use of patient-controlled analgesia (PCA) following cesarean birth is becoming increasingly popular. With this approach the woman is given a bolus of analgesia, usually morphine or meperidine, at the beginning of therapy. Using an IV pump system, the woman presses a button to self-administer small doses of the medication as needed. For safety the pump is preset with a time lockout so that the woman cannot deliver another dose before a specified time has elapsed. Women using PCA feel less anxious, have a greater sense of control with less dependence on the nursing staff, experience rapid pain relief without grogginess and a drugged feeling, sleep better, and avoid the discomfort of injections (Bucknell & Sikorski 1989). Other agencies report good pain relief using epidural morphine (Inturrisi et al 1988) or transcutaneous electrical nerve stimulation therapy (TENS).

Critical Thinking Question

Can you identify any disadvantages to patient-controlled analgesia (PCA)?

The accumulation of gas in the intestines may produce discomfort for the woman during the first postpartal days. Measures to prevent or minimize gas pains include leg exercises, abdominal tightening, ambulation, avoiding carbonated or very hot or cold beverages, avoiding the use of straws, and providing a high-protein liquid diet for the first 24 to 48 hours.

The woman may find it helpful to lie prone or on her left side. Lying on the left side allows gas to rise from the descending colon to the sigmoid colon so that it can be expelled more readily. Other women report that a rocking chair helps them obtain relief. Medical interventions for gas pain include the use of antiflatulents (such as Mylicon), suppositories, and enemas.

Preventive measures to avoid pain secondary to constipation include encouraging fluids and administering a stool softener or mild cathartic.

The nurse can minimize discomfort and promote satisfaction as the mother assumes the activities of her new role. Instruction and assistance in assuming comfortable positions when holding and/or breastfeeding the infant will do much to increase her sense of competence and comfort. Sitting in a chair or tailor fashion in bed, leaning slightly forward with the infant propped on a pillow in her lap will prevent irritation to the incision. Another preferred position for breastfeeding during the first postoperative days is lying on the side with the newborn positioned along the mother's body.

By the first or second day after the cesarean birth, the mother is usually receptive to learning how to care for herself and her infant. Special emphasis should be given to home management. She should be encouraged to let others assume responsibility for housekeeping and cooking. Fatigue not only prolongs recovery but also interferes with breastfeeding and mother-infant interaction. Demonstration of proper body mechanics in getting out of bed without the use of a side rail and ways of caring for the infant that prevent strain and torsion on the incision are also indicated.

The cesarean birth woman usually does extremely well postoperatively. If birth was accompanied by spinal anesthesia, the side effects of general anesthesia are avoided. Even after general anesthesia, however, most women are ambulating by the day after the surgery. Usually by the second or third postpartal day the woman can shower, which seems to provide a mental as well as physical lift. If staples have been used, the incision is sometimes left open to the air, and showering is permitted without covering it. Most women are discharged on the third postoperative day.

Promotion of Parent-Infant Interaction After Cesarean Birth

Many factors associated with cesarean birth may hinder successful and frequent maternal-infant interaction. These include the physical condition of the mother and newborn and maternal reactions to stress, anesthesia, and medications. The mother and her infant may be separated after birth because of hospital routines, prematurity, or neonatal complications. A healthy infant born by an uncomplicated cesarean birth is no more fragile than an infant born vaginally. Many agencies are beginning to provide time for the family together in the operating room if the mother's and infant's conditions permit, but some agencies still automatically place cesarean birth newborns in a high-risk nursery for a time.

Signs of depression, anger, or withdrawal in the cesarean birth mother may indicate a grief response to the loss of the fantasized vaginal birth experience. Fathers as well as mothers may experience feelings of "missing out," guilt that the surgery was the result of something they did "wrong," and even jealousy toward another couple who had a vaginal birth. The couple may also feel guilty that they are considering their personal needs and not simply the welfare of the infant.

The nurse can support the parents in a variety of ways. Initially, nurses must work through their own feelings about cesarean birth. The nurse who considers a vaginal birth "normal" and refers to it as such indicates that a cesarean birth is therefore "abnormal" rather than simply an alternative method. Thus language and terminology, though seemingly insignificant, can convey to the couple negative messages about their cesarean birth experience.

The nurse should offer positive support to the couple. The cesarean birth couple needs the opportunity to tell their story repeatedly to work through their feelings. The nurse can provide factual information about their situation and support the couple's effective coping behaviors. The nurse should provide the parents with choices by allowing them to participate in decision making about the options available to them.

The perception of and reactions to a cesarean birth experience depend on how the woman defines that experience. Her reality is what she perceives it to be. If the woman's attitude is more positive than negative, successful resolution of subsequent stressful events is more likely. Because the definition of events is transitory in nature, the possibility of change and growth is present. Often the mothering role is perceived as an extension of the childbearing role, and inability to fulfill expected childbearing behavior (vaginal birth) may lead to parental feelings of role failure and frustration. The nurse can help families alter their negative definitions of cesarean birth and bolster and encourage positive perceptions.

NURSING PLAN AND IMPLEMENTATION FOR THE POSTPARTAL ADOLESCENT

Currently, more than 90% of teen mothers who give birth keep their infants. These adolescent mothers are at a greater risk for sexually transmitted diseases, reduced socioeconomic status, and rehospitalization. Infants born to adolescent mothers are at increased risk for low birth weight, prematurity, sudden infant death syndrome (SIDS), minor acute infections, and death (Stevens-Simon & McAnarney 1991). Adolescent mothers exhibit fewer maternal attachment behaviors than older mothers in the first 3 days postpartum (Norr & Roberts 1991). The attainment of the maternal role and the quality and quantity of parent-child interactions may be limited for adolescents due partly to lack of knowledge combined with egocentric thinking (Strauss & Clark 1992). In addition to their exposures to the risks of pregnancy, complications, and poor birth outcome, they are likely to experience a subsequent pregnancy while still in their teens. One study suggests that all teen mothers of normal birth weight infants require additional education to prevent rehospitalization of their infants (Wilson et al 1990).

The adolescent may have special postpartal needs, depending on her level of maturity, support systems, and cultural background. The nurse needs to assess maternal-infant interaction, roles of support people, plans for discharge, knowledge of childrearing, and plans for follow-up care. It is imperative to have a community health service be in touch with the young woman shortly after discharge.

Contraception counseling is an important part of teaching. Often the young woman tells the nurse that she

Text continues on page 1088

Cesarean Birth Critical Pathway

Category	Day of Surgery	Postoperative Day #1	Postoperative Day #2
Referral	Report from OR nurse	Lactation consultation if needed	Home nursing referral if indicated
Assessments	Assessments q15 min × 4, then q$\frac{1}{2}$h × 2, then q4h if stable Vital signs: • BP WNL; no hypotension; no ↑ >30 mm systolic or 15 mm diastolic over baseline • Pulse: bradycardia normal; consistent with baseline • Respirations: 12–20/min; quiet, easy • Temperature 36.2–37.6 C (98–99.6 F); check initially; if WNL then q4h Pulse oxymetry: monitor first 2h; >90% Auscultate breath sounds: lungs clear, no adventitious sounds Breasts: soft, colostrum present Lochia: scant initially; rubra; no free flow or passage of clots Assess top of fundus (or sides depending on incision location) for firmness Dressings: clean & dry Comfort ≤5 on scale of 1 to 10 Auscultate for bowel sounds Check Homan's sign q shift: negative	Continue postpartum/postoperative assessments q4h until 24h postop, then q8h Vital signs assessment: all WNL; report temperature >38 C (100.4 F) Fundal height, location and firmness: normally firm, in the midline, at umbilicus Lochia—type, amount, odor; normally rubra, scant to moderate, earthy odor Lung sounds Bowel sounds checked until return of bowel sounds Assess abdomen for distention; should be soft, nondistended Dressings Homan's sign Breasts: Evaluate nipple status; should be no evidence of cracking or bruising Observe feeding technique with newborn Continue assessment of comfort level	Continue postpartum and postoperative assessments as described q8h Vital signs assessment q8h; all WNL; report temperature >38 C (100.4 F) Breasts: full; nipples should remain free of cracks, fissures, bruising Feeding technique with newborn: should be good or improving Incision: clean, dry; no redness, edema, drainage
Comfort	Institute comfort measures: position of comfort, adequate warmth Pain medication _____ by IV, PCA, or IM as ordered Epidural or intrathecal narcotic analgesia: follow analgesia orders from anesth. × 24h	Continue with pain management techniques Pain medication _____ as ordered PO once IV d/c'd Stool softener as ordered	Continue with pain management techniques
Teaching/ psychosocial	Orient to room if transferred from OR or delivery room Explain comfort measures, pain relief options Teach self-massage of fundus and expected findings If sufficiently alert, provide assistance with breastfeeding or bottle feeding Begin initial newborn teaching for woman or support person: bulb suctioning, positioning, diaper change, cord care Teach pericare	Provide information on early postpartum period Discuss postpartum psychologic changes Continue newborn teaching: soothing/comforting techniques, swaddling; return demonstrations indicate woman's understanding Provide opportunities for question and review; reinforce previous teaching Breastfeeding: nipple care; air-drying, lanolin, proper latch-on technique; tea bags Breast pumping if newborn in NICU Bottle feeding: supportive bra, ice bags, breast binder	Discuss incisional care Discuss involution, anticipated physical changes first two weeks postpartum, postpartum exercises, need to limit visitors Discuss postpartum nutrition: balanced diet, high protein and vitamin C to encourage wound healing Breastfeeding: • Increase calories by 500 kcal over nonpregnant state (200 kcal over pregnant intake) • Explain milk production, let-down reflex, use of supplements, breast pumping, and milk storage; answer questions Bottle feeding: • Return to normal caloric intake for nonpregnant state • Explain formula preparation and storage Discuss sibling rivalry: mother should have plan for supporting siblings at home Teaching evaluation completed

Category	Day of Surgery *continued*	Postoperative Day #1 *continued*	Postoperative Day #2 *continued*
Therapeutic nursing interventions and reports	Monitor level of conciousness if general anesthesia given Should rouse easily, respond to questions Monitor return of motor ability and sensation if regional block given If receiving epidural or intrathecal narcotics, report any of the following: decreased respiratory effort; respirations < 11; changes in respiratory pattern; signs of airway obstruction; pin-point pupils; excessive drowsiness or signs of sedation; c/o severe itching, excessive nausea, vomiting, urinary retention If receiving intrathecal narcotics: assess resp q30min × 12; then q1h for 12 hours Change peripad as needed; weigh pads if lochia flow >1 saturated pad/h; presence of boggy uterus and clots Massage uterus until firm Turn, cough, deep breathe q2h Reinforce dressings if necessary	If woman Rh⁻ and infant Rh⁺, RhoGAM work up; consent obtained; teaching completed Administer RhoGAM if indicated Obtain consent for rubella vaccine if indicated; explain purpose, procedure, implications Obtain CBC D/C Foley	D/C buffalo cap Administer rubella vaccine if indicated Remove staples before discharge
Activity	Bed rest; position of comfort Siderails up for safety Maintain flat in bed if spinal anesthesia given May dangle p8h c̄ assistance (12h p spinal)	Encourage leg exercises when in bed Progressive ambulation with assistance then independently as tolerated May shower with assistance p24h	Up ad lib as tolerated; encourage ambulation May shower independently
Nutrition	NPO until bowel sounds present, then begin clear liquids I&O q8h	Advance diet as tolerated once passing flatus Encourage fluids (2000 mL/day) D/C I&O when IV out and fluid intake adequate	Soft—regular if passing flatus Encourage fluid intake
Elimination	Foley catheter; catheter care q4–8h	D/C Foley Voiding large amt straw-colored urine Straight cath if bladder distended or unable to void	Same May have bowel movement; ask woman to report it to nurse
Medications	Continue pitocin infusion as ordered IV antibiotics as ordered Antiemetics prn as ordered If epidural or intrathecal narcotic analgesia used: • Naloxone 0.2 mg IV for respirations < 8/min or signs of resp distress • Diphenhydramine 25 mg IV or IM q2h prn itching	Buffalo cap IV when fluid intake adequate Heparin flush to BC per agency policy Antiflatulents PRN Stool softener _____	Continue medications May take own prenatal vitamins
Discharge planning/ home care	Evaluate knowledge of post cesarean recovery, newborn care	Discuss typical newborn schedule; stress need to plan for periods of rest Birth certificate paperwork completed Evaluate plans for transporting newborn; car seat available Arrangements made for baby pictures if desired	Review discharge instruction sheet and checklist Describe postpartum warning signs and when to call CNM/physician Provide prescriptions; gift pack to woman Newborn check schedule Postoperative/postpartum visit schedule
Family involvement	Evaluate support system Provide opportunities for woman and support persons to watch newborn assessments Recognize possible impact of culture on responses	Involve support persons in care, teaching; answer questions Evidence of parental bonding behaviors present Demonstrates culturally expected early parenting behaviors Contact social services if indicated	Plans made for care and support of mother following discharge Support person verbalizes understanding of need for woman to rest, eat nutrionally, recover, avoid overexertion Evidence of parental bonding behaviors clearly present

does not plan on engaging in sex again. This denial mechanism is unrealistic, and the nurse must help the young woman realize this. The nurse should make sure that the woman has some method of birth control available to her and that she understands ovulation and fertility in relation to her menstrual cycle. This is an excellent opportunity for sex education.

Promotion of Parenting Skills

The nurse has many opportunities for teaching the adolescent about the newborn in the postpartal unit. Because the nurse serves as a role model, the manner in which she handles the baby greatly influences the young mother. The father should be included in as much of the teaching as possible.

A newborn physical exam done at the bedside gives the adolescent immediate feedback about the newborn's health and shows her the proper methods of handling an infant. The nurse can teach as the examination progresses, giving the new mother information about the fontanelles, cradle cap, shampooing the newborn's hair, and so on. The nurse might also use this time to teach the young mother about infant stimulation techniques. Because adolescent mothers tend to concentrate their interactions in the physical domain, they need to comprehend the importance of verbal, visual, and auditory stimulation for newborns as well.

Performing an examination at the bedside also gives the adolescent permission to explore her baby, while she may have been hesitant to do. A Brazelton neonatal assessment (Chapter 28) will help the mother understand the newborn's response to stimuli, a key factor in the adolescent's response to the individuality of her newborn once she goes home. Parents who have some idea of what to expect from their infants will be less frustrated with the newborn's behavior.

The adolescent mother appreciates positive feedback about her fine newborn and her developing maternal responses. This praise and encouragement will increase her confidence and self-esteem.

Group classes for adolescent mothers should include infant care skills, information about growth and development, infant feeding, well-baby care, and danger signals in the ill newborn. If classes are offered in the hospital during the postpartum stay, the adolescent mother should be strongly encouraged to attend. If the child's father is involved, he should also be encouraged to attend and participate. The nurse can correct misconceptions and unrealistic expectations about growth and development. The nurse should also make a thorough assessment of the support systems and resources already in place for the mother and additional resources from the hospital or the community that may be appropriate for the situation.

Ideally, teenage mothers should visit adolescent clinics where mother and baby are assessed for several years after birth. In this way classes on parenting, vocational guidance, and school attendance can be followed closely. School systems' classes for young mothers are an excellent way of helping adolescents finish school and learn how to parent at the same time.

NURSING PLAN AND IMPLEMENTATION FOR THE WOMAN WHO RELINQUISHES HER INFANT

Sometimes a pregnancy is unwanted. The expectant woman may be an adolescent, unmarried, or economically restricted. She may dislike children or the idea of being a mother. She may feel that she is not emotionally ready for the responsibilities of parenthood. Her partner may disapprove of the pregnancy. These and many other reasons may cause the woman to continue to reject the idea of her pregnancy. An emotional crisis arises as she attempts to resolve the problem. She may choose to have an abortion, to carry the fetus to term and keep the baby, or to have the baby and relinquish it for adoption.

Many mothers who choose to give their infants up for adoption are young and/or unmarried. More young women choose to keep the child than to give it up, however. Approximately two-thirds of children born to single women are raised by their mothers alone.

The decision of a mother to relinquish her infant is an extremely difficult one. There are social pressures against giving up one's child. Some women may want to prove to themselves that they can manage on their own by keeping their infants.

The mother who chooses to let her child be adopted usually experiences intense ambivalence. These feelings may heighten just before birth and upon seeing her baby. After childbirth the mother will need to complete a grieving process to work through her loss.

Critical Thinking Question

How have attitudes toward single mothers and their children changed over the years? What impact do you think these changes have had on relinquishment as an option?

Provision of Support to the Woman Relinquishing Her Infant

The mother who decides to relinquish her child usually has made considerable adjustments in her life-style to give birth to this child. She may not have told friends and relatives about the pregnancy and so lacks an extended support system. During the prenatal period the nurse can help her by encouraging her to express her grief, loneliness, guilt, and other feelings. It is often helpful to encourage the mother to visit the hospital prior to birth.

She may be given a tour of the labor and delivery area as well as the postpartum area. Accomplishment of this requires good communication from the physician and/or the adoption agency. Often many of the fears, anxieties, and questions can be resolved prior to the arrival at the hospital.

When the relinquishing mother is admitted to the maternity unit, the staff should be informed about the mother's decision to relinquish the infant. Any special requests regarding the birth should be respected, and the woman should be encouraged to express her emotions.

After the birth the mother should be able to decide whether she wants to see the newborn. Seeing the newborn often facilitates the grieving process. When the mother sees her baby, she may feel strong attachment and love. The nurse needs to assure the woman that these feelings do not mean that her decision to relinquish the child is a wrong one; relinquishment is often a painful act of love (Arms 1990). Postpartal nursing management also includes arranging ongoing care for the relinquishing mother.

Promotion of Acceptance When a Woman Denies Pregnancy

Initial denial of pregnancy by women usually progresses to acceptance of the pregnant state. Occasionally, however, a nurse may encounter a woman who denies she is pregnant even as she is admitted to the maternity unit. It may seem impossible to the nurse that a woman who is so obviously pregnant could maintain this delusion. Because of this denial, the woman has not sought prenatal care. Preparation for the birth experience may be incomplete, and the mother and infant may be at risk.

The nurse must establish a trusting relationship with this woman. While building rapport with the woman, the nurse should gently guide her to accept reality.

Promotion of Family Wellness

In the event that a woman decides to keep an unwanted child, the nurse should be aware of the potential for parenting problems. Families with unwanted children are more prone to crisis than others, although in many cases parents grow to love their child after attachment occurs. The nurse should be ready to initiate crisis management strategies or make appropriate referrals as the need arises.

NURSING PLAN AND IMPLEMENTATION REGARDING DISCHARGE INFORMATION

The postpartum stay allowed by most third-party payers has decreased dramatically in recent years. Hospital stays that were measured in weeks in the 1940s are now mea-

sured in hours. Postpartum nursing care that has traditionally included a strong focus on the adjustments of the mother, newborn, and family is very difficult to accomplish because of the brief length of stay. Mothers and newborns are being discharged before many of their important postbirth health care needs can be addressed. These include establishing breastfeeding, ruling out infections, supporting infant-family bonding, and patient education. Home health services are increasingly being recognized as a cost-effective means of meeting the postbirth needs of mothers and newborns. Postpartum nursing care has been advocated as a national priority of maternal-child nursing (Williams & Cooper 1993).

Ideally, preparation for discharge begins the moment a woman enters the birthing unit to give birth. Nursing efforts should be directed toward assessing the couple's knowledge, expectations, and beliefs and then providing anticipatory guidance and teaching accordingly (Table 34–4). Because teaching is one of the primary responsibilities of the postpartum nurse, many agencies have elaborate teaching programs and classes. Before the actual discharge, however, the nurse should spend time with the couple to determine if they have any last-minute questions. In general, discharge teaching should include at least the following information:

1. The woman should contact her care giver if she develops any of the signs of possible complications:
   a. Sudden persistent or spiking fever
   b. Change in the character of the lochia—foul smell, return to bright red bleeding, excessive amount
   c. Evidence of mastitis, such as breast tenderness, reddened areas, malaise
   d. Evidence of thrombophlebitis, such as calf pain, tenderness, redness
   e. Evidence of urinary tract infection, such as urgency, frequency, burning on urination
   f. Evidence of infection in an incision (either episiotomy or cesarean), such as redness, edema, bruising, discharge, or lack of approximation
   g. Continued severe or incapacitating postpartal depression

2. The woman should review the literature she has received that explains recommended postpartum exercises, the need for adequate rest, the need to avoid overexertion initially, and the recommendation to abstain from sexual intercourse until lochia has ceased. The woman may take a shower and may continue sitz baths at home if she desires.

3. The woman should be given the phone numbers of the postpartum unit and nursery and encouraged to call if she has any questions, no matter how simple.

Text continues on page 1092

TABLE 34-4   Areas to Include in Postpartal Teaching

Knowledge and Skills To Be Taught	Teaching Method			
	Video	**Verbal Only**	**Verbally Reinforced**	**Demonstration**
Care of the Mother				
Breast care				
Breast feeding or lactation suppression				
Possible problems and care				
Involutional changes				
Position of fundus				
Aftercontractions				
Changes in lochia				
Signs of possible problems				
Bladder function				
Fluid needs				
Signs of possible problems				
Bowel function				
Normal patterns				
Dietary assistance				
Perineal care				
Expected healing changes in episiotomy				
Comfort measures (rinsing with warm water, use of analgesic/anesthetic spray, sitz bath), home care				
Signs of possible problems				
Rest and activity				
Scheduling rest periods, handling fatigue				
Ambulation				
Watching for circulatory problems in legs				
Emotional changes				
Changes in mood, crying, depression				
Care of the Father/Partner				
Emotional changes				
Emotional changes and challenges that may occur				
Encouragement to seek support as needed				
Physiologic and psychologic changes that may occur in the mother and newborn				
Infant care concerns				
Possible supportive measures for the new family				
Care of the Baby				
Observing the baby				
General appearance				
Senses				
Visual				
Hearing				
Touch				
Smell				
Taste				
Vital signs				
Normal parameters				
How to take a temperature				
Skin				
Coloring				
Normal sign rashes				
Diaper care				
Stool cycle				
Normal characteristics				
Signs of diarrhea and treatment				
Signs of constipation and treatment				

TABLE 34-4 *continued*

Knowledge and Skills To Be Taught	Teaching Method			
	Video	Verbal Only	Verbally Reinforced	Demonstration
Care of the Baby *continued*				
Observing the baby *continued*				
Emotional and comforting needs				
Protective reflexes				
Blinking				
Sneezing				
Swallowing				
Normal reflexes				
Moro				
Fencing				
Head lag				
Stepping				
Feeding the baby				
Schedule				
Breastfeeding				
Positioning, initiating and ending feeding				
Infant cues for feeding				
Identifying problem areas and possible solutions				
Breast care				
Bottle-feeding				
Positioning				
Preparation of bottles and formula				
Burping or bubbling the baby				
Holding, wrapping and diapering the baby				
Various holds (cradle, football)				
Securing baby in blanket to provide warmth				
Diapering				
Comparison of reusable (cloth) and single use (paper)				
Methods of diapering and care of soiled diapers				
Perineal skin care				
Positioning the baby for sleep				
Bathing the baby				
Supplies				
Method				
Safety				
Use of bulb syringe and care if choking				
Positioning				
Car seat				
Health promotion				
When to call health care provider				
Temp				
Diarrhea				
Eating problems				
Malaise				
Protecting baby from infections				
Immunization schedule				
Aspects of Parenting				
Interaction with newborn				
Newborn cues and capacity for interaction				
Parenting needs				
Acquaintance with individual characteristics of their newborn and possible techniques to use				
Resources available				

4. The woman should receive information on local agencies and/or support groups, such as La Leche League and Mothers of Twins, that might be of particular assistance to her.

5. Both breastfeeding and bottle-feeding mothers should receive information geared to their specific nutritional needs. They should also be told to continue their vitamin and iron supplements until their postpartal examination.

6. The woman should have a scheduled appointment for her postpartal examination and for her infant's first well-baby examination before they are discharged.

7. The mother should clearly understand the correct procedure for obtaining copies of her infant's birth certificate.

8. The new parents should be able to provide home care for their infants and should know when to anticipate that the cord will fall off, when the infant can have a tub bath, when the infant will need his or her first immunizations, and so on. They should also be comfortable feeding and handling the baby and should be aware of basic safety considerations, including the need to use a car seat whenever the infant is in a car.

9. The parents should be aware of signs and symptoms in the infant that indicate possible problems and who they should contact about them.

The nurse can also use this final period to reassure the couple of their ability to be successful parents. She can stress the infant's need to feel loved and secure. She can also urge parents to talk to each other and work together to solve any problems that may arise.

Follow-up visits are mentioned when appropriate. If not already discussed, teaching about family planning is appropriate at this time, and information regarding birth control methods is provided.

In ideal situations a family approach involving the father, infant, and possibly other siblings would permit a total evaluation and provide an opportunity for all family members to ask questions and express concerns. In addition disturbed family patterns might be more readily diagnosed and therapy instituted to prevent future problems of neglect or abuse.

EVALUATION

Anticipated outcomes of nursing care include:

- The mother has learned pain relief measures and has increased comfort.

- The mother will be rested and will understand how to increase her activities over the next few days and weeks.

- The mother verbalizes support measures that will enhance her physiologic and psychologic well-being.

- The mother verbalizes her understanding of self-care measures.

- The new parents demonstrate how to care for their baby.

- The new parents have had opportunities to form attachment with their baby.

KEY CONCEPTS

Nursing diagnoses can be used effectively in caring for women postpartally.

Postpartum discomfort may be due to a variety of factors, including engorged breasts, an edematous perineum, an episiotomy or extension, engorged hemorrhoids, or hematoma formation. Various self-care approaches are helpful in promoting comfort.

Lactation suppression may be accomplished by mechanical techniques or by administering medication.

The new mother requires opportunities to discuss her childbirth experience with an empathetic listener.

The first day or two following birth are marked by maternal behaviors that are more dependent and comfort oriented. Then the woman becomes more independent and ready to assume responsibility.

Rooming-in provides the childbearing family with opportunities to interact with their new member during the first hours and days of life. This enables the family to develop some confidence and skill in a "safe" environment.

Sexual intercourse may resume once the episiotomy has healed and lochia has stopped. Couples should be forewarned of possible changes; for example, the vagina may be "dry," the level of desire may be influenced by fatigue, or the woman's breasts may leak milk during orgasm.

Following cesarean birth, a woman has the nursing care needs of a surgical client in addition to her needs as a postpartum client. She may also require assistance in working through her feelings if the cesarean birth was unexpected.

Postpartally, the nurse evaluates the adolescent mother in terms of her level of maturity, available support systems, cultural background, and existing knowledge and then plans care accordingly.

The mother who decides to relinquish her baby needs emotional support. She should be able to decide whether to see and hold her baby and should have any special requests regarding the birth honored.

Prior to discharge the couple should be given any information necessary for the woman to provide appropriate self-care. They should have a beginning skill in caring for their newborn and should be familiar with warning signs of possible complications for mother or baby. Printed information is valuable in helping couples deal with questions that may arise at home.

Because of the trend toward early discharge, follow-up care is more important than ever. Many approaches are used, especially home visits and telephone follow-up.

REFERENCES

Arms S: *Adoption: A Handful of Hope.* Berkeley, CA: Celestial Arts, 1990.

Bucknell S, Sikorski K: Putting patient-controlled analgesia to the test. *MCN* January/February 1989; 14:37.

Fishman SH et al: Changes in sexual relations in postpartum couples. *JOGNN* January/February 1986; 15:58.

Foster S: Bromocriptine: Suppressing lactation. *MCN* March/April 1982; 7:99.

Gosha J, Brucker MC: A self-help group for new mothers: An evaluation. *MCN* January/February 1986; 11:20.

Harrison LL: Patient education in early postpartum discharge programs. *MCN* January/February 1990; 15:39.

Inturrisi M et al: Epidural morphine for relief of postpartum, postsurgical pain. *JOGNN* July/August 1988; 17:238.

Jansson P: Early postpartum discharge. *AJN* May 1985; 85:547.

LaFoy J, Geden EA: Postepisiotomy pain: Warm versus cold sitz bath. *JOGNN* September/October 1989; 18:399.

Norr KF, Roberts JE: Early maternal attachment behaviors of adolescents and adult mothers. *J Nurse-Midwifery* 1991; 36(6):334.

Nursing '91. *Drug Handbook*, Springhouse, PA.

Peters F et al: Inhibition of lactation by long-acting bromocriptine. *Obstet Gynecol* 1986; 67:82.

Ramler D, Roberts : A comparison of cold and warm sitz baths for relief of postpartum perineal pain. *JOGNN* November/December 1986; 15:471.

Rhode MN, Barger MK: Perineal care then and now. *J Nurse-Midwifery* July/August 1990; 35(4):220.

Scott JR et al: *Danforth's Obstetrics and Gynecology*, 7th ed. Philadelphia: Lippincott, 1994.

Sheil EP et al: Concerns of childbearing women: A maternal concerns questionnaire as an assessment tool. *JOGNN* 1995; 24(2):149.

Stevens-Simon C, McAnarney ER: Adolescent maternal weight gain and low birth weight: A multifactorial model. *Am J Clin Nutr* 1991; 47:948.

Strauss SS, Clark BA: Decision-making patterns in adolescent mothers. *Image* 1992; 24(1):69.

Varney H: *Nurse Midwifery*, 2nd ed. Boston: Blackwell Scientific Publications, 1987.

Williams LR, Cooper MK: Nurse-managed postpartum home care. *JOGNN* 1993; 22(1):25.

Wilson MD, Duggan AK, Joffe A: Rehospitalization of infants born to adolescent mothers. *J Adol Health Care* 1990; 11(6):510.

Wong S, Stepp-Gilbert E: Lactation suppression: Nonpharmaceutical versus pharmaceutical method. *JOGNN* July/August 1985; 14:302.

CHAPTER 35

ATTACHMENT

*I*t's one of those "grass-is-greener" things—I envied, sometimes even hated Sam when he went out to work. I don't know what I was imagining—that he hung around talking, went out to lunch, did interesting things. One time he was watching me bathe Annie in the sink. He asked if he could do it—he stood there, soaping her back over and over like he couldn't get enough of it, and he talked about how he hated to leave us in the morning and how he worried he would be closed out, left looking in at what she and I had together.

~ THE NEW OUR BODIES, OURSELVES ~

KEY TERMS

Attachment

Bonding

En face

Engrossment

Entrainment

Reciprocity

OBJECTIVES

Describe the attachment process, including the phases of maternal-infant interaction.

Identify the factors influencing the first maternal-infant interaction.

Explore the factors affecting other family members' interactions with the infant.

Explain the types of questions and observations used for evaluating the maternal-infant relationship.

Describe methods the nurse can use to facilitate a positive attachment process.

Identify complications that can affect the maternal-infant attachment process.

There has been a great deal of research on attachment in recent years. The goals of the research have been to describe, operationally define, and relate attachment to cognitive and social outcomes; to support or refute psychologic theories; and to determine public child care policy.

The early literature on attachment related primarily to the infant's tie to her or his mother, which was understood to develop in the second half of the first year of life when the infant was capable of recognizing the mother. This literature was derived in part from experience with maternally deprived infants. More recently, researchers have investigated the attachment the mother develops with the fetus and that of the infant with other significant family members. The importance of the attachment between fathers and infants has gained attention, and sibling attachment continues to be studied.

This chapter begins by exploring the nature and operation of attachment. Having established this knowledge base, the chapter concludes by discussing nursing assessment and interventions related to attachment.

NATURE OF ATTACHMENT

An **attachment** is an enduring two-way bond or relationship of affection between persons. Affectional ties exist in families between parents, between parents and their children, and between siblings.

Attachment originally referred to a child's tie to his or her mother, although it was recognized that the tie was actually to any mother figure, a primary care giver, who was usually, although not necessarily, the biologic mother. Attachment may now refer to an infant's tie to a parent or a parent's tie to the child. The essence of an infant's attachment to a parent is organization and patterning of behavior that results in feelings of closeness to the attachment figure. Elements of this attachment behavior are clinging, crying, smiling, sucking, following, and eye-to-eye contact.

Bonding is considered a process of parent-infant attachment that occurs at or soon after birth, but it is only one brief phase in the development of the enduring reciprocal emotional relationship between parent and child called attachment (Taylor 1990).

PERSPECTIVES ON ATTACHMENT

Attachment is viewed from three major perspectives: psychoanalytic, ethologic, and social learning theory.

From a psychoanalytic perspective attachment is explained by instinctual responses and object relations. Attachment is innate, an instinctual drive. The mother is the object of the drive. Fathers are important as support for the mother, but initial attachment with anyone other than the mother is thought to interfere with and be detrimental to the child's development. Other attachments will follow once attachment to the mother is assured. The quality of later attachment depends on the quality of attachment to the mother.

Within an ethologic framework attachment consists of species-specific behavior. Examples of such behaviors are ducklings imprinting on the first moving object seen after hatching, monkeys clinging to parents when alarmed, and cats licking newborn kittens to stimulate respiratory and gastrointestinal functioning.

According to social learning theory framework, attachment is formed through secondary drives. The mother meets her infant's needs, and the infant associates need satisfaction, comfort, and love with the mother.

Concepts of the origin of attachment, behaviors denoting attachment, and interventions to promote attachment may differ, depending on the theoretical perspective taken.

WHAT THE MOTHER BRINGS TO THE FIRST INTERACTION

Prenatal Influences

A mother has a specific genetic makeup of intelligence, personality and temperament, body structure, physical health, and biochemical/hormonal status. Each of these factors influences the environment the mother can provide for the fetus and newborn and affects her ability to relate well to her child. Her cultural and ethnic background will influence her attitudes, behaviors, and practices related to pregnancy and childbirth. Her experiences in infancy and childhood, the mothering she received, and her exposure to appropriate role models will shape her own mothering practices. New mothers do a lot of "trying on for size" of the mothering behaviors that they see in others (their own mothers, sisters, or friends), using the coping mechanisms of introjection and projection. They then adopt those behaviors that they feel most comfortable with.

The mother's current developmental level and relationships with significant others will provide the foundation for the developing relationship with her fetus and the newborn. Often she will "rework" the relationship with her own mother at this time and develop a closer relationship to her mother as a result (Zachariah 1994).

Family readiness for pregnancy is crucial for providing an environment in which attachment to the fetus and newborn can occur. The optimum environment is created when the baby is planned and wanted and the family has the necessary resources to provide for the infant.

Present Pregnancy

Each mother brings to her first visual contact with her newborn her reactions to that particular pregnancy, from conception through birth. A variety of factors may influence her response to the pregnancy and the baby: whether the pregnancy was planned and a baby wanted (Brazelton & Cramer 1990), complications she experienced in pregnancy, and the support she received from family and friends. Life events essentially unrelated to her pregnant condition may have enhanced a woman's response to pregnancy or depleted the energy reserves and coping ability necessary to pregnancy adjustments. Stress during pregnancy can interfere with attachment, but support from family and others can offset some of the adverse effects of such stress (Fuller et al 1993).

By the time of birth each mother has developed an emotional orientation of some kind toward the fetus. This attachment is based on a tactile-kinesthetic awareness combined with fantasy images and perceptions. For many women an emotional bond to the fetus develops soon after conception and deepens during pregnancy.

By the third trimester, significant attachment has occurred, as evidenced by nesting behaviors such as preparing the baby's room; expectations about the baby's gender, appearance, and temperament; and selection of names (Taylor 1990). In preparation for birth and postnatal attachment, the pregnant woman needs to complete the developmental task of gaining a sense of the fetus's separate presence. Stainton (1990) described four distinct phases in the attainment of this sense: incorporating the fetus into one's body- and self-image, differentiating the fetus from self, gaining a sense of the fetus, and becoming attached to the fetus. Fathers, too, become attached to the fetus. Stainton (1990) noted that parents infrequently use the term "fetus" when referring to the newborn infant. Instead, parents state that they feel the presence of the infant motivates words such as "he" or "she," regardless of whether the gender was known.

Events such as hearing the fetal heart or visualizing the fetus on a screen through sonography affect the mother's perception of her fetus and appear to increase her feelings of attachment. Counting fetal movements using a fetal activity diary (FAD) may hasten the pregnant woman's sense of attachment to the fetus (Mikhail et al 1991). Research also indicates that knowledge of whether the fetus is male or female does not seem to affect attachment. The prenatal attachment process is a unique combination of maternal-paternal-fetal interaction styles involving intimacy, assigning meanings, and reading cues. The parents' relationship with their fetus is contained within the context of their life situation, personal histories, and the whole experience of pregnancy.

Pascoe and French (1989) found that women who did not plan to become pregnant or who conceived for reasons of status or security were frequently among those who had minimal feelings of closeness to the fetus throughout the pregnancy. Those who felt well adjusted in their marriage and emotionally ready to have a baby were able to develop strong affectionate feelings.

WHAT THE NEWBORN BRINGS TO THE FIRST INTERACTION

Each partner in an interpersonal interaction contributes in some way to the process. In years past, the newborn's influence on the beginning mother-infant relationship was ignored. More recently, research on the capacities of newborns has shown that they are indeed active partners in the exchange and take part, shaping their own human environment from the moment of birth. Newborns do this by virtue of who they are and what they do—their appearance and behavior.

Appearance

At the moment of birth, certain information about the newborn's external appearance is available. Each characteristic may have a special meaning for the parents as it relates to their hopes, fears, and expectations. The relatively obvious things are usually noted first: sex, size, shape, color, and presence or absence of abnormality or injury. The eyes are a particularly important feature.

Behaviors

The newborn has, and may demonstrate at birth, certain functional behaviors, such as crying, sucking, eliminating, looking, listening, and startling. In the first days of life, the infant selectively attends to the human face, prefers the human voice over other sounds, and becomes quiet and alert when picked up and held over the shoulder.

In addition to having behaviors in common with other neonates, each newborn, like the parent, is already a unique combination of genetic potential and life experience. The newborn's life experience is shorter and more limited in scope, of course, but it can have a powerful effect on behavior. The past history and present personality of each mother and father combine with the characteristics and behavior of their infant to influence the quality and direction of the parent-infant relationship.

THE SETTING

The physical environment, human environment, and condition of the mother and newborn at first contact may influence the opportunities for interaction.

Critical Thinking Question

What can the nurse do with an expectant couple to facilitate attachment with the fetus?

Physical Environment

Childbirth may occur in a variety of settings. The most frequent setting by far is a maternity unit in a hospital. The physical surroundings are usually relatively strange to the woman as she moves from the admitting area to the labor room, birthing area, recovery area, and her room in the postpartal unit.

She may encounter a variety of unfamiliar equipment and procedures. Noise levels are often high. Food is usually withheld until after the birth. The stress of accommodating to the physical environment can interfere with the progress of labor and birth and with the comfort of mother-infant interaction. In addition the parents may be separated from the newborn. Agency policy and practices that limit interaction, such as strict adherence to specific time frames for feedings, discouraging the mother from unwrapping and looking at her newborn, or prolonged separation, although far less common today, may create a problem for some mothers.

Consumer and professional efforts to increase the comfort of hospital births while decreasing the risks sometimes associated with home birth have produced an intermediate type of setting: hospital-independent birth centers or hospital birthing rooms. These facilities are more homelike in appearance and do not require moves from one area to another during the progression from labor through early recovery. The newborn remains with the parents in this setting, and the arrangement provides the environment for facilitating early parent-infant contact and flexible rooming-in.

The first early discharge programs were offered to families with support at home (Taylor 1990). Programs that provide postdischarge nursing assessment and counseling in the home have historically been associated with health maintenance organizations. Now many institutions have early discharge requirements regardless of the support system at home; this has had a significant impact on the traditional nursing methods of providing newborn care instructions and facilitating attachment between parents and newborn (Weinberg 1994). Using home visits, postpartum telephone follow-up, or postpartum visits to the birthing center, nurses can continue the health care instructions started earlier, and parents can describe how the family is managing at home and integrating the newborn into the family.

Human Environment

Labor and birth usually occur in a social setting. Very few women express the wish to be alone during childbirth; most respond with distress to the idea of abandonment at such a time. Birthing centers generally provide for fairly constant nursing supervision of women in active labor, in the course of the birth, and in the early postpartum period. Often, however, there is a different caretaker present in each phase of the childbearing activities. This requires the woman to relate to a variety of nurses—each with advice, expectations, and attitudes—at a very vulnerable time.

The care giver's philosophy can greatly influence the progress of the attachment process. For example, in any birthing setting, if the care givers are supportive, lights can be dimmed and skin-to-skin contact, if desired, can be initiated immediately after birth. But care givers in the same setting may actually reduce opportunities for attachment by having the baby in an admitting room warmer for an unnecessarily long time so that the mother must wait to view or hold her baby.

In almost all settings the laboring woman is able to have any support person she desires with her during labor and birth. This practice increases the possibility that a woman will have the support of one trusted person for the whole childbirth experience. The quality of support available from professionals or laypersons varies considerably according to their clinical and psychosocial skills. There are indications that a woman's perceptions of her physical care and emotional support can influence her mothering responses.

Condition of the Interactors

When the postbirth conditions are optimal, mother and newborn are ready to relate effectively to each other and to benefit from the interaction. The mother is emotionally high and alert, primed for maternal responsiveness by her hormonal state. The newborn is in a quiet alert state, capable of attending to the mother's face and voice. However, several common conditions diminish or divert the mother's physical and psychologic energies. Fatigue, pain, cold, chills and shaking, hunger, and thirst are frequent after childbirth. The mother may also have received drugs for relaxation and pain relief and may be encumbered in her movements by intravenous tubing.

Certain conditions may also lower the newborn's potential for human interaction. In addition to the physiologic adaptations necessary for extrauterine existence, physical maturity, nutritional adequacy, neurologic intactness, bodily discomfort, suctioning, extremes of temperature, and levels of analgesic and anesthetic agents have all been related to the infant's behavioral responses in the first hours of life—as well as later. Prophylactic eye treatments interfere with newborns' ability to keep their eyes open and focused on the mother's face. Generally speaking, any situation, condition, or stimulus that detracts from the energy either partner can use to attend to the other diminishes the probability of optimal interaction between the two.

MOTHER-INFANT INTERACTION

Introductory Phase

After the baby's birth, the mother seeks to establish a realistic image of her infant and integrate the infant into her self-perception and her social systems through an

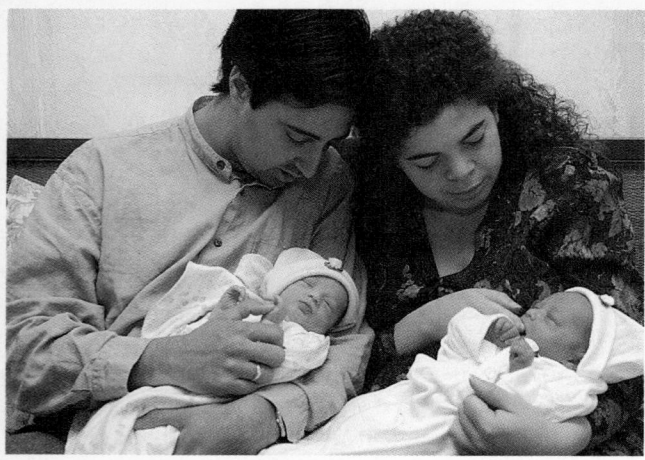

FIGURE 35-1   The new parents interact with their infants.

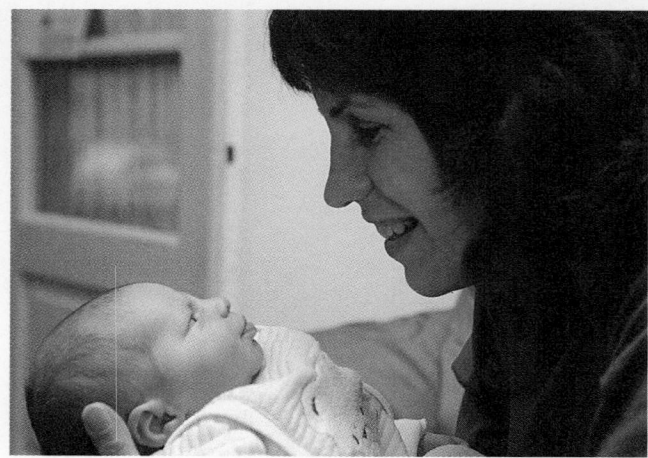

FIGURE 35-2   En face position.

acquaintance-attachment process (Beal 1991). Observers of very early mother-newborn interactions in birthing settings have presented evidence that a fairly regular pattern of maternal behaviors is exhibited at first contact with the normal newborn (Klaus & Kennell 1982; Rubin 1984). In a progression of touching activities, the mother proceeds from fingertip exploration of the newborn's extremities toward palmar contact with the larger body areas and finally to enfolding the infant with the whole hand and arms. The time taken to accomplish these steps varies from minutes to days, depending, it appears, on the timing of the first contact, the clothing barriers present, and the physical condition of the baby. There also may be ethnic or cultural differences in patterns of interaction. Maternal excitement and elation tend to increase during the time of the initial meeting (Figure 35–1).

The mother also increases the proportion of time spent in the **en face** position (Figure 35–2). That is, she arranges herself or the newborn so that her face and eyes and the infant's meet in the same vertical plane of rotation. The majority of women cradle their infant in their left arm, which is probably related to hand dominance. There is an intense interest in having the infant's eyes open. When the eyes are open, the mother characteristically greets the baby and talks in high-pitched tones to her or him.

Clinical observations indicate that behaviors differ somewhat in unconventional birth situations. Home and Leboyer births seem to speed up the behaviors described. Often after a home birth the mother turns almost immediately to pick up and hold the newborn and to rub the infant's cheek with her fingertip. The newborn is often offered the breast before the placenta is expelled. In a birth patterned after the Leboyer method the mother, and sometimes the father, is encouraged to gently massage the infant's whole body while waiting for the placenta to be expelled. Production of prolactin during breastfeeding enhances attachment by creating calm, relaxed feelings in the mother.

In most instances the mother relies heavily on her senses of sight, touch, and hearing in getting to know what her baby is really like. She responds verbally to any sounds emitted by the newborn, such as cries, coughs, sneezes, and grunts. Mothers are able to distinguish their infant's odor, and the sense of smell may be involved in the acquaintance process.

While interacting with the newborn, the mother is undergoing her own emotional reactions to the labor and birth and to the baby. Sometimes direct comments and nonverbal cues clearly reflect her emotions; sometimes the mother reports only later on her feelings at the time. An expression of "I can't believe it" and a feeling of emotional distance from the newborn are quite common: "I felt he was a stranger." Feelings of connectedness between the newborn and the rest of the family can be expressed in positive or negative terms: "He's got your cute nose, Daddy" or "Oh, no! She looks just like the first one, and she was an impossible baby." A mother's facial expressions or the frequency and content of her questions may demonstrate concerns about the infant's general condition or normality, especially if her pregnancy was complicated or if a previous baby was not normal.

During the initial mother-newborn interaction the neonate, too, is continuously communicating. Elements of the newborn's appearance and behavior may be perceived by the mother as if they represented intentionality and interpersonal dialogue, and they do influence her responses. The newborn's size says to the mother, "You nourished me well—you did a good job." Individual features say, "I am a part of you or of my father. I belong with you." Even the time of birth can be read as a message: "I'm cooperative—or uncooperative." The intensity, timing, configuration, and other elements of the newborn's observable activity, however reflexive, are regularly responded to as a very personal communication from the baby to the mother.

When newborns no longer need to concentrate most of their energy in physical and physiologic response to the immediate crisis of birth, they are able to lie quietly with their eyes open, looking about, moving occasionally, making sucking motions, possibly attempting to get hand to mouth. Placed in appropriate proximity to the mother, the baby appears to focus briefly on her face and to attend to her voice repeatedly in the first moments. When their mother is talking and they are attending, babies are likely to move arms, legs, fingers, or eyelids in an exact synchrony with their mother's minute voice changes.

During the introductory contact after birth, the mother gathers a certain amount of information about her baby. This learning about the partner is the first step in any interpersonal acquaintance. From the remarks, questions, and activities of a new mother in the earliest postpartal days, it is apparent that she is applying herself to the task of getting acquainted with her newborn. She wants to know what kind of baby she is taking into her family system and what the infant's reaction to her is. She is also consciously involved in clarifying the nature of her own developing feelings toward the newborn. In part she is becoming acquainted with herself as the mother of this particular infant. Gottlieb (1978) described a discovery process in which a mother *identifies* the infant as her own, pointing out what the infant looks like and what the baby can do. Next she *relates* the behavior or appearance to someone or something familiar: "Her nose is just like her daddy's." A third step in the process is *interpreting* or giving meaning to the infant's behavior or appearance: "Look at that face; he's going to be a feisty one!"

The degree to which a mother develops feelings of affectionate closeness or attachment to the fetus before birth is highly correlated with the course of maternal feelings and interactions toward the baby immediately after the birth and in the acquaintance phase as assessed by the maternal-fetal attachment scale (Fuller 1990). Muller's (1993) prenatal attachment inventory, which is based on the attachment model, may also be helpful in developing strategies to enhance positive attachment for pregnant women. Minimal closeness before birth seems to lead to less enjoyment of the newborn, less responsiveness to needs, and less empathy when the infant is in distress. Women who feel an intense attachment and interaction before birth appear to pick up the relationship at that level after birth and to develop increased feelings of closeness in the acquaintance phase. They eagerly respond to the newborn's needs and are gratified by the baby's apparent well-being. In addition they are likely to be more successful at initiating and maintaining breastfeeding than are minimally attached mothers. Liking the infant at the start apparently contributes to the woman's understanding of her newborn as an individual with unique needs and adds to her willingness to respond to those needs. The positive orientation at the beginning of contact probably also influences the woman to believe that her baby appreciates her.

The newborn plays an important part in determining the outcome of the mother-infant relationship. If infants respond in an organized way to the usual caretaking stimuli and are regular in biologic rhythms, they tend to be easy to understand. If infants give clear behavioral cues about needs, their responses to mothering will be predictable. Such predictability makes a mother feel effective and competent. If the newborn responds to the mother's care with a predominantly positive mood rather than with irritability, and if the baby has relatively long periods of being quietly awake and attentive, the infant is pleasant to be near and to interact with. Other behaviors that make an infant more attractive to caretakers are smiling, grasping a finger, nursing eagerly, cuddling, and being easy to console.

The newborn is also becoming acquainted with his or her mother. Newborns gather what information they can about their new world. They attend to sights, sounds, tastes, and smells and experience different tactile and kinesthetic sensations. Within a few days after birth, infants show signs of recognizing recurrent situations and responding to changes in routine.

Critical Thinking Question

How might the baby's temperament influence the bonding or attachment process with the parents?

Phase of Mutual Regulation

In performing the necessary tasks of newborn care, such as feeding, bathing, and comforting, the new mother develops awareness that there is some discrepancy between her wishes and needs and her baby's needs and desires. This awareness ushers in a phase of mutual regulation of behaviors in which mother and baby modify their relationship in an attempt to make it as enjoyable as possible for both. The relative amounts of control to be exerted by the mother and baby in the interpersonal adjustment are an issue in the early postpartal weeks. Maternal goals in resolving this issue of control are, of course, variable, both among different mothers and in the same mother at different times. In some mother-infant pairs, the maternal goal is primarily to change the infant to meet the mother's needs. In other pairs it is quite apparent that the mother's intent is primarily to interpret correctly and to gratify completely all of her baby's needs. Either of those approaches is likely to result in relational disturbances, the degree of distress and tension depending to a large extent on the newborn's reactions to the maternal behaviors used to reach the goal. For example, the mother who wishes her baby to adjust rather than she adjusting to her baby will have a smoother postnatal course if she is blessed with a highly adaptive infant who is positive in mood. The mother who is intent on meeting every need of her child at the same moment it arises will meet with failure very quickly if the newborn is unpredictable, is irregular in daily rhythms, and presents behavioral cues that are difficult to interpret.

The ideal solution to the control issue would be somewhere between the two extremes. A mother who realizes that she is a person with her own needs will be less vulnerable to the buildup of anger, frustration, anxiety, and guilt. In all but the most ideal situations, each partner must undergo disappointments, and each must at some time subordinate his or her own needs to the needs of the other. The most important consideration is that each should obtain a good measure of enjoyment from the ongoing interactions.

Generally speaking, enjoyment is enhanced during the early months if the infant can make clear her or his needs behaviorally and if the mother's personality allows her to let the infant lead the interaction. Mutual maternal-infant regulation is never instantaneous; it is a process that continues throughout infancy and childhood. Fortunately, there appears to be a tendency toward improved organization of behavior in the newborn period and an increasing ability to nurture in the mother during the same time.

It is during the mutual adjustment phase that negative maternal feelings are likely to surface or intensify. Because "everyone knows that mothers love their babies," these negative feelings often go unexpressed and are allowed to build up. If they are expressed, the response of friends, relatives, or health care personnel is often to deny the feeling to the mother: "You don't mean that"; "You can't feel that way"; "Your baby is not ugly; he is beautiful." Some negative feelings are normal in the first few days following birth, and the nurse should be supportive when the mother vocalizes these feelings.

Reciprocity

Reciprocity within a mother-infant system may be described as a series of simultaneous behaviors and responses between the mother and infant (Barnard 1978; Brazelton & Cramer 1990). A high degree of reciprocity characterizes successful mutual regulation between a mother and baby. Reciprocity involves mutual cuing behaviors, expectancy, rhythmicity, and synchrony. There are intimations of reciprocity in the early hours of life. The mother and her infant respond to each other's cues. They develop rhythms in interaction that form the basis for communication. During several weeks of interaction, they establish a pattern of behavior in which they mesh with each other. When this meshing or synchrony is attained, the mother and infant perform a reciprocal process of cyclic attention and nonattention. The significant behavior cues and factors that influence both mother and infant are illustrated in Figure 35–3.

Brazelton and his colleagues (1974) studied this reciprocal process in the laboratory and carefully analyzed the component parts. They described five phases of the cycle: (1) initiation, (2) orientation, (3) acceleration, (4) deceleration, and (5) turning away. The first two phases establish the partners' expectations regarding the interaction. Both mother and infant use clusters of behaviors as the interaction develops. Feedback between partners enables them to modulate their behaviors. Sensitivity and adjustment by the mother allow the infant to maintain a physiologically homeostatic state and to develop a longer attention cycle. The infant may begin to develop recognizable patterns of behavior by about 2 weeks of age, and patterns are often well established by 6 weeks.

If the observer is aware of what to look for, the segments of an interactional cycle can be described as they are observed. The following is a hypothetical example of an interactional period as it is likely to appear when things are going well:

Initiation: The infant is held on the mother's knee, facing her. He looks toward her with a relaxed expression and makes slow movements with his arms and hands.

Orientation: As the infant makes eye contact with his mother, his eyes brighten and become alert, and he turns his whole body toward her, extending arms and legs in her direction. He reaches toward the mother.

State of attention: The mother smiles and talks to the infant, and he responds by smiling, moving his arms and legs in pedaling motions, cooing, and making other sounds. The eyes alternately become alert and dull as he responds to the smiles and words of his mother. The limbs move rhythmically, in time with the mother's voice. There is a constant, slow, smooth reaching and circular movement occurring as the tension within the infant's body rises and falls. The infant assumes the look of expectancy.

Acceleration: The infant continues to move, to wave his hands and feet about, and to increase his smiling activity. His eyes are bright and alert. He strains toward his mother in the intensity of the interaction, all the time watching her and cuing to her smile. For the most part the body movement is smooth, but there may be occasional jerkiness.

Peak of excitement: As the infant becomes wholly involved in the interaction, his movements may become jerky and intense. He brings his hand to his mouth and tries to insert his thumb while still smiling and cooing. The other hand clutches his thigh and he leans forward to his mother as she continues to smile at him. As he endeavors to reach forward, his back arches and his body tends to twist toward one side.

Deceleration: The excitement begins to pass, and the infant's movements slow. There is a gradual decrease in body movement, the bright look dims, the eyes become dull, and the lids appear to droop. The smiles fade, and vocalization decreases. Suddenly,

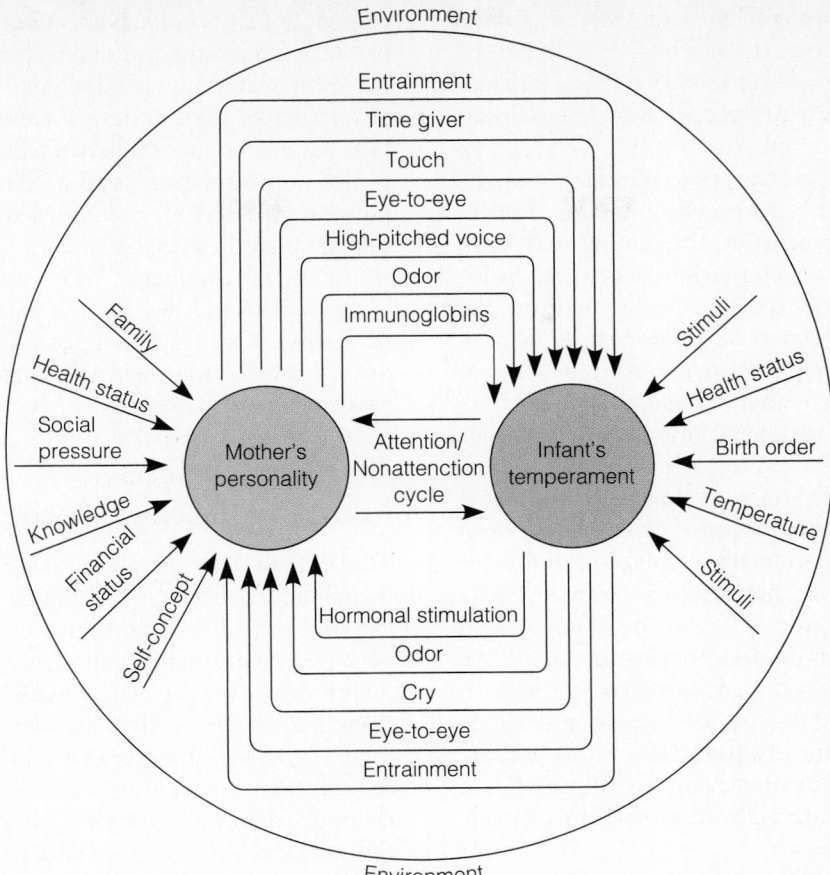

FIGURE 35-3   Factors and behavioral cues that influence maternal-infant interaction.

the infant yawns and begins to suck his thumb as he leans away from his mother. His hands drop to his lap with the fingers widespread, and he appears to be relaxing.

Withdrawal or turning away: The infant's activity slows down almost completely. He slumps against his mother's hands with his body half turned away from her. His eyes are dull and focused in the direction of an object to the side. There is a faint smile on his face. The mother stops smiling and talking to the infant. She just sits holding him quietly, waiting for his next cue. The mother briefly raises her head and glances beyond the infant. This prompts a reaction in the infant. He looks toward his mother, smiles briefly, and looks away again, then turns back to the mother, ready to resume another period of interaction.

The responsibility for monitoring cues and for sensitively initiating or maintaining the interaction rests primarily with the mother. The infant uses the nonattention time to recover from the tension of interaction, to organize behavior, and to process what has been taken in during the attentive periods.

The development of reciprocity between a mother and her infant is evidence of the bond or attachment that has formed between them. It enables the mother to let go of the infant she knew as a fetus during pregnancy. A new relationship now develops with an individual who has a unique character and who evokes a response entirely different from the fantasy response of pregnancy. When reciprocity is synchronous, the interaction between mother and infant is mutually gratifying and is sought and initiated by both partners. Pleasure and delight develop in each other's company, and there is mutual development of love and growth.

Reciprocity may take weeks to develop, and it usually requires sensitive stimuli from both partners. As infants become more organized in their behavior and as senses develop, they are able to give positive feedback to their mothers. As they transmit the appearance of listening, they follow voice and movements and respond with intentionality to the mother as an individual whom they recognize and with whom they seek to communicate; this is called **entrainment.** Entrainment demonstrates the synchronization of the baby's movements with the pattern and rhythms of the parent's speech. When there is a change in the mother's speech pattern, such as a pause or accented syllable, the baby's behavior changes subtly. When either the mother or the newborn is sick and the initial acquaintance is delayed, a delay in the development of reciprocity is also likely to develop over time (Cusson 1993).

Overstimulation or inappropriate stimulation by the mother may interfere with the synchrony of the interaction. In the resultant asynchrony, the mother may be in the attention phase of the reciprocal process when the infant is in the nonattention phase. This asynchrony can lead to frustration on the part of either partner or both and may lead to a disharmonious relationship as both become established in their interactional patterns. In extreme instances mother and infant may cease to communicate with each other.

Infants vary in their strategies for dealing with an overload of stimulation. Four types of reaction have been described in infants responding to unpleasant and inappropriately timed stimuli (Brazelton & Cramer 1990): (1) active physical withdrawal, (2) rejection, (3) decreased sensitivity, and (4) communication of distress. An infant can move away from the source of stimulation, can push the stimulus away, can lapse into drowsiness or sleep, or can fuss and cry. Some of these strategies, if they become characteristic of an infant's behavior, are easier to live with than others; they interact with a mother's expectations and her personality.

The nurse may have the opportunity to observe reciprocity developing between a mother and her newborn in the early weeks of life. If nurses recognize the appearance of asynchrony, they may be able to initiate intervention before the asynchronous behaviors become firmly established.

Attachment Behaviors

Attachment is a bond of affection. Behavioral cues must be observed to detect indications of the presence or absence of the bond. Researchers have used a variety of behaviors as indicators of attachment. In the immediate newborn period important behaviors include smiling at the infant; addressing him or her by name or in affectionate terms; kissing, touching, and enfolding the infant close to the body; cradling the infant and assuming the *en face* position; making positive comments about the appearance and behavior of the infant; finding family resemblances; and expressing positive feelings to the spouse. Breastfeeding can enhance attachment by providing the opportunity for frequent skin contact between the newborn and mother. The tactile stimulation associated with breastfeeding can communicate warmth, closeness, and comfort. The increased closeness of breastfeeding provides both newborn and mother with the opportunity to learn each other's cues and needs. Later, expression of enjoying caring for the infant, feeling the infant belongs to the parents, thinking about the infant when away from him or her, making warm comments about the infant, and

responding appropriately to infant cues indicate that the parent has developed a bond with the infant.

The maternal role includes both emotional and physical tasks. The emotional component includes qualities that enable the mother to feel warmth, affection, attachment, protectiveness, and devotion to the child. The physical tasks include the knowledge and skill to provide care for the infant, that is, to feed, diaper, bathe, and provide a safe environment.

Whether and how soon a parent displays behaviors indicating attachment depend on many factors; the process is believed to be facilitated by a warm, supportive environment.

Attachment Behaviors in the Adolescent Mother

Adolescents demonstrate attachment behaviors toward their infants, although differences in attachment behaviors between adolescent mothers and older mothers have been observed. Pregnant adolescents show attachment to their fetus during pregnancy, as do adult pregnant women (Kemp et al 1990). However, later, when dealing with their newborns, these young mothers tend to be more anxious, have lower attachment scores, and interact less favorably than older mothers. The younger the adolescent, the less likely she is to display typical adult maternal behaviors of touching, synchrony with her newborn, vocalization, and proximity of mother and newborn (Porter & Sobong 1990). It also appears that the most important areas of interaction in the early postpartal period for the adolescent are physical and motor. These mothers appear to be more attuned to these behaviors than to auditory and visual interaction.

Strong ego functioning, as demonstrated by the mother's ability to adapt to pregnancy and to plan for her future, appears to affect the mother's interaction with her newborn. The response of the newborn is also critical. Infants who are healthy are more likely to affect the relationship positively. Adolescents may have problems with parenting because they tend to have less realistic expectations of what an infant can do at a given age. Nurses need to assess the adolescent's perception of what life will be like with her infant and provide anticipatory guidance regarding common problems and how to solve them. This promotes the development of a repertoire of "mothering knowledge and skill" that may positively influence her perception of her capability to care for her infant. In addition, cognitively immature adolescents may not foresee the consequences of their actions. Neglectful parenting may become a problem. However, many adolescent mothers live with their mothers, who provide support during pregnancy and provide a significant proportion of the care of the infant.

With these considerations in mind the nurse must be attentive to the early maternal-infant interaction, use appropriate modeling and teaching techniques, include the adolescent's mother when appropriate, and refer adolescent mothers for follow-up care and early intervention programs when indicated.

FATHER-INFANT INTERACTION

The father has traditionally been seen only as a source of support for the pregnant woman. He contributed to the growth and development of his newborn indirectly by nurturing and supporting his partner through the pregnancy and the early postpartal weeks. As fathers have become more involved in the pregnancy and birth experience, researchers have begun to study their experiences and feelings about the fetus and newborn. When fathers are involved in pregnancy through a close couple's relationship, they have a more positive report of the birth and new baby.

The majority of fathers demonstrate attachment behaviors toward the fetus during pregnancy; that is, they talk to the fetus, refer to it by name, enjoy watching their partner's abdomen move as the fetus moves, think about the baby, and show other similar behaviors (Longobucco & Freston 1989). Fathers who identify with the pregnancy by having physical symptoms similar to pregnancy symptoms have higher attachment scores. A positive birth experience also leads to greater levels of attachment in fathers.

A father experiences feelings toward his newborn that are similar to the mother's feelings of attachment (Graham 1993). In the past the significance of any psychologic response called fatherliness was minimized. It was implied that, because the man did not have deep physiologic roots of fatherliness, his feelings were somehow less important than the mother's and were weaker and longer in developing. Evidence now shows that a father does have a strong attraction to his newborn and highly positive emotional reactions to first contact. The first hours after birth appear to be significant in the development of the father-mother-infant bond.

Greenberg and Morris (1974) noted the reactions of first-time fathers to early contact with their newborns. They used the term **engrossment** to label characteristics of the effect of the newborn on the father—his sense of absorption, preoccupation, and interest in the infant.

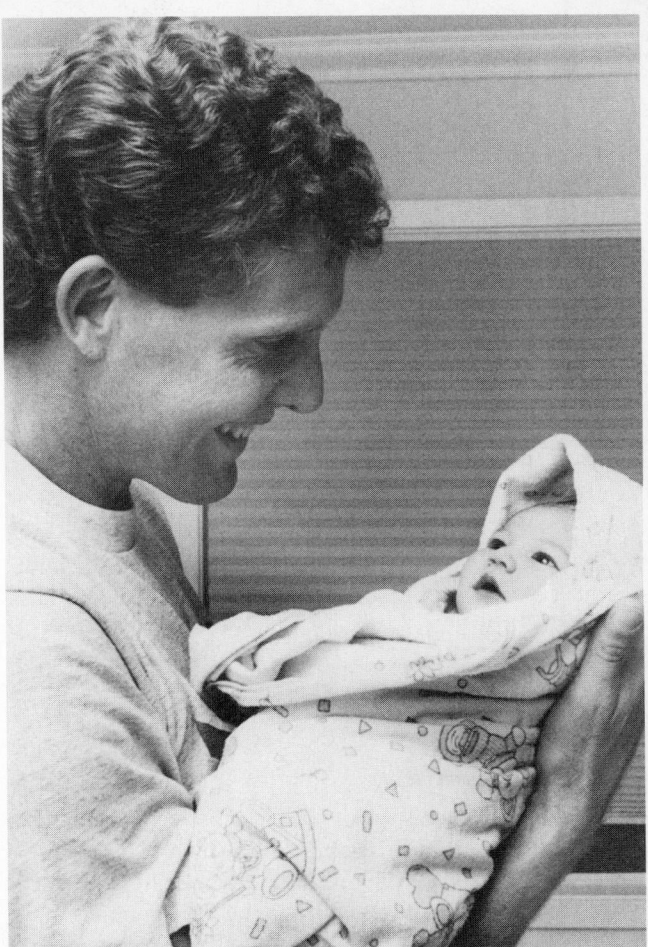

FIGURE 35-4   A bond develops between father and infant as they interact en face.

Critical Thinking Question

At times men may feel funny talking to their newborns. How can the nurse encourage the father to vocalize with his baby?

The father's emotional reaction to the first sight of the baby and to later contacts tends to be very positive. The intensity of his feelings may come as a surprise to him. The new father's involvement with his newborn can draw time and energy away from the ongoing couple relationship. The man who has been encouraged to support his partner in her new mothering role may feel some guilt about preoccupation with the baby, and the woman may feel ignored or excluded from a significant relationship. It seems likely that couples who shared experiences, relationships, and material things before the birth will also be able to share their infant's attention and the responsibilities of parenting.

When the new father initiates interaction, the newborn responds (Figure 35–4). As with the mother-newborn interaction, the baby contributes his or her part. The infant cries and moves, indicating alertness and well-being. Spontaneous and reflexive movements and grimaces are emitted, and the father responds by voice and touch. From the beginning the father's interactive behaviors are different from the mother's, and these variations are perceptible to the infant. A father's odor, voice pitch, appearance, and touch qualities all differ from a mother's. In a face-to-face "play situation" a mother tends to use her hands to enfold and enclose her baby's body and limbs with gentle molding and smoothing motions. The father punctuates his conversation with finger pokes and more exaggerated changes in facial expression, which act to increase the baby's excitement level. Observers have noted differences in an infant's responses to interaction with mother or father as early as 2 weeks after birth.

Mothers, too, appear to notice a difference. Often in the early weeks, when asked if they play with the baby, mothers say, "No, but my husband does" (Graham 1993). An outcome of father-infant interaction is to further acquaint the mother with her baby's range of possible behaviors in the context of a shared relationship.

The following are some components of positive father-infant interaction that can be assessed:

Tactile contact: Does he touch the baby with his fingertips and whole hand? Does he hold, kiss, or rock the baby?

Inspection: Does he assume an en face position, smile at the baby, and identify distinct characteristics of the infant?

Verbalization: Does the father talk to the baby, call the baby by name, and use affectionate terms?

Caretaking: Does the father respond to the baby's cues and demands for attention? Does he burp, clean, diaper, or feed the infant when possible?

Even with early discharge births, the nurse can assess how the father interacts and how involved he is with his newborn soon after birth. During the follow-up home or return postpartum visit, the nurse assesses the infant's state of activity. For example, is the baby active and alert or inactive and passive? Is the father involved with the baby only during periods of sleep or crying? How does the father behave when he is alone with the infant? Is there a change when mother, infant, and father are together (Novak & Novak 1990)?

It might be helpful if, during the pregnancy, nurses explain the potential for engrossment of the father after birth. If both parents are aware that each has needs at this time, they may be better able to support each other's growing relationship to this new family member. To make nursing goals appropriate and intervention effective, more knowledge is needed about the long-term effects of different levels of direct paternal involvement on the quality of the father-child relationship and other family relationships.

SIBLINGS AND OTHERS

Most parents try to prepare their children for the arrival of a new baby. Many birthing units have expanded their services to allow children's participation at the sibling's birth, help children learn about newborns in special classes, and encourage sibling contact with the infant on the postpartum unit and sibling visits in the intensive care nursery. These opportunities help children become involved in the socialization of the new baby into the family (Murphy 1993). The type and extent of the siblings' preparation may depend on the age of the children and the type of relationships that exist in the home. If the new baby is seen as nonthreatening to the relationships the children have with their parents, there will probably be less disruption, and the new baby will be accepted without serious problems.

Research has found that children's reactions to the birth of a sibling are varied, but may include imitating the mother's caretaking activities. However, sometimes other types of alterations in sibling behavior are seen, such as changes in toileting and sleep habits or increased attention-seeking activities. These may represent the child's attempt to "try on" baby behavior (Murphy 1993). Gullick and Crase (1993) used the older child's expectations and observation inventories to study the reaction of firstborn children to the birth of a sibling. They found that firstborn children tend to show more positive responses to the sibling birth than their parents expected.

Murphy (1992) described a behavior pattern called sibling mutuality in which children demonstrate sensitivity in reading the infant's cues and responding appropriately. Children who develop sibling mutuality usually have had many opportunities for uncensored, uninterrupted interaction with their infant brother or sister. The postpartum activities that have been reported to facilitate acquaintance with the newborn sibling include inviting the child to touch the baby, pointing out features of the newborn, and having infant capabilities explained during the newborn's exam (Murphy 1993).

Other research has shown that, during initial contact with the new baby, girl siblings tend to position themselves closer than boys to the baby (Faller & Ratcliffe 1993). Anderberg (1988) found the following factors to be associated with the frequency of sibling attachment and acquaintance behaviors: previous experience with loss, the siblings' prenatal relationship with the newborn, and the parents' parenting style. The birth of the new baby initiates the relationship between the siblings, so activities that promote positive feelings and attachment to the baby are important to that relationship. The initial birthing experience can be a positive activity for siblings if the period of separation from the mother is short and the need for competition for mom's attention is reduced (Faller & Ratcliffe 1993).

Recent work with infants has shown that they are capable of maintaining a number of attachments. These attachments may include siblings, grandparents, aunts, and uncles. Some infants were found to be capable of forming attachments with five or more people simultaneously without loss of quality. The social setting and personalities of the individuals appear to be significant factors in permitting the development of multiple attachments. In addition the advent of open visiting hours and rooming-in facilitates participation of siblings and grandparents in the attachment process.

ATTACHMENT WITH ADOPTED CHILDREN

Attachment with adopted children occurs even though many factors thought to be important in the attachment process, such as early contact, may not be possible. Factors that aid the attachment process for adoptive parents include physical contact with the child, such as touching, kissing, or feeding, and shared activities. More problems seem to occur when the child is over the age of 4 years when the placement occurs. Factors that interfere are the child's negative behavior and rejection by the older child. Some mothers indicate that attachment is hindered by lack of energy and resources and by conflicts in roles, factors that also affect biologic mothers. As with biologic mothers, the support system of partner, relatives, and friends is very important.

The quality of attachment in adoptive mother-infant pairs is no different from that in nonadoptive situations, at least in middle-class families (Koepke et al 1991). A warm, supportive environment with competent and confident parents promotes the formation of affectionate bonds. Adoptive parents who miss their infant's birth still form emotional bonds with their infants and should not be made to feel that they have missed something crucial. Adoptive parents have identified the need for education on infant care when they receive the infant. Indeed, education about physical contact and infant care have been shown to foster the attachment process (Koepke et al 1991). Parental education policies should be an integral part of institutions dealing with adoption (Lobar & Phillips 1994).

In some situations adoptive parents are permitted to be present at the birth and to experience early contact and provide initial care. Some hospitals are allowing adoptive parents to room-in and receive instruction and practice in infant care under supervision of hospital staff. In other situations the child may be older and may have developed a relationship with another care giver. In these situations the adoptive parents need assistance and support to allow time for the acquaintance process to occur, to become sensitive to each other's cues, and to develop reciprocity. With appropriate adjustments for time of placement, similar assessments of attachment and interventions to promote attachment can be used in adoptive and biologic families. Adoption support groups provide opportunities for older adopted children to interact with other adopted children to discuss issues and decrease their feelings of being "different" (Lobar & Phillips 1994).

ATTACHMENT WITH SEVERELY HANDICAPPED CHILDREN

An anomaly in the infant may affect the attachment process. Because reciprocity is an important part of the process of attachment, the process may be at risk when one of the interactors is unable to perform her or his role. When a mother interacts with a nonhandicapped child, the more the child smiles, looks, or vocalizes, the more responsive the mother becomes. When the child is blind, deaf, or mentally retarded, the mother must adapt her interactive behaviors. However, she may not know how to compensate for the child's deficits and may need instruction and role modeling (Landry & Chapieski 1989).

Many handicapped children *do* exhibit attachment behaviors. Quinn's (1991) study of Down syndrome parents found that characteristics of Down children such as being mild mannered, easy to handle, and having the ability to give clear cues, signals, and responses to their parents facilitate high attachment scores for these families, regardless of the child's degree of mental retardation.

The nurse can promote attachment in families with handicapped children in a variety of ways, such as enhancing the parent's sensitivity to subtle cues. For example, a head turn or ceasing self-stimulatory behavior may be the child's way of recognizing the mother or father. Parents may be either positively or negatively unrealistic about the child's capabilities. Parents can be helped to think realistically about the child's abilities and to respond to the child's signals. Because attachment does occur with severely handicapped children, the implications of separation must be considered when recommending placement of such children. When neither parental attachment nor ability of the child to form an attachment exists, placement of the child outside the home is more likely to be an acceptable and appropriate option. When the parents choose to keep the child at home, professionals should help foster attachment.

NURSE'S ROLE

Nurses come into professional contact with women and their families at any point in the maternity cycle in public health offices, hospitals, doctor's offices, child protection centers, or childbirth education classes. Facilitating a mother-infant relationship is usually only one of a number of concurrently operating goals of health care. Much can be done during the performance of other nursing tasks to support the development of maternal attachment.

Usually, a maternity or public health nurse is concerned with the care of a specific woman and her baby at a given point in time. The nurse can draw on general knowledge of norms, averages, and risk factors, but must apply what is pertinent from that store of information to a mother with a specific history and personality, in a relationship with a specific infant, and within a specific environment. Individuals classified as high risk are sometimes able to cope effectively with whatever risks are involved and to relate affectionately to a particular newborn. It also happens that what appears to be a perfect image of a potential mother can be shattered by unpredictable events occurring after the image was created.

Effective evaluation of a mother-infant relationship requires a broad understanding of a mother and newborn pair as it exists within a family and a wider social setting. How the nurse evaluates a mother-newborn relationship can be concurrently diagnostic, preventive, and therapeutic. While interacting with a maternity client, the nurse can assess the woman's ability to trust people and to enjoy relationships, her skills in communication, and her feeling tone. At the same time the nurse can work to develop a mutually trusting relationship and an increase in maternal self-esteem and self-confidence.

Through direct interaction the nurse can also model appropriate behaviors, such as nurturing, communicating, and problem solving, that can be unconsciously picked up and imitated or consciously studied and tested by the mother. When feelings are expressed, the nurse can accept them nonjudgmentally. This practice enables the client to accept her feelings and perhaps to examine and understand them. It also encourages the further expression of feelings.

As the nurse reaches tentative conclusions in the evaluation of a mother-infant relationship, it is often appropriate to share ideas with the mother, both because the mother is a source of validation of the nurse's observation and because being included in the process of assessment can be ego-enhancing for the mother. Some mothers can be very accurate in predicting their own postpartal adjustment and the quality of their support network. Nurses should critically evaluate the use of broad-based parent-infant relationship assessment tools. These tools should include father's as well as mother's perspectives, verbal and nonverbal behaviors, cultural differences, and interchange in the parent-infant relationship (Coffman 1992).

Critical Thinking Question

How can the nurse positively influence the bonding or attachment process in this era of short birthing stays?

Assessment of Early Attachment

If attachment is accepted as a desired outcome of nursing care, a nurse in any of the various postpartal settings can periodically observe and note progress toward this goal. The mother's behavior toward her infant reflects where she is in Rubin's (1984) phases of maternal role development. The following questions can be addressed in the course of nurse-client interactions:

1. *Is the mother attracted to her newborn?* Does she seek face-to-face contact and eye contact? Is she actively reaching out or only passively holding her newborn? Has she progressed from fingertip touch to palmar contact to enfolding the infant close to her body? Is attraction increasing or decreasing? If the mother does not exhibit increasing attraction, why not? Do the reasons lie primarily within her, the baby, or the environment?

2. *Is the mother inclined to nurture her infant?* Is she progressing in her interactions with her infant? Has she selected a rooming-in arrangement if it is available?

3. *Does the mother act consistently?* Is she developing a consistent and predictable approach to the care of her infant? Does she tend to respond to the same situation in the same way each time? If not, is the source of unpredictability within her or her infant?

4. *Does the mother seek information as needed?* Does she seek information and evaluate it objectively? Does she develop solutions based on adequate knowledge of valid data? How did she prepare herself for the parenting role? Does she evaluate the effectiveness of her maternal care and make appropriate adjustment?

5. *Is she sensitive to the newborn's needs as they arise?* How quickly does she interpret her infant's behavior and react to cues? Does she respond when the baby cries or fusses? Does she seem happy and satisfied with the infant's responses to her efforts? Is she pleased with feeding behaviors? How much of this ability and willingness to respond is related to the baby's nature and how much to her own?

6. *Does she seem pleased with her baby's appearance and sex?* Is she experiencing pleasure in interaction with her infant? What times are the most and least enjoyable? What interferes with the enjoyment? Does she speak to the baby frequently and affectionately? Does she call him or her by name? Does she point out family traits or characteristics she sees in the newborn?

7. *Are there any cultural factors that might modify the mother's response?* For instance, is it customary for the grandmother to assume most of the child care responsibilities while the mother recovers from childbirth?

8. *Are there other factors that might modify the mother's response?* For example, her prior experience with mothering and her physical condition may influence her ability to attach to her baby.

When these questions are addressed and the facts have been assembled by the nurse, the nurse's intuitive feelings and formal background of knowledge should combine to answer three more questions: Is there a problem in attachment? What is the problem? What is its source? Each nurse can then devise a creative approach to the problem in the context of a unique developing mother-infant relationship.

Assessment of attachment behaviors has become increasingly important in light of current theories that correlate malattachment with an increased incidence of parenting problems, failure to thrive, and child neglect or abuse. When assessing attachment behaviors, the nurse should be careful not to generalize or give too much importance to any one factor. Adaptive behavior may vary from one situation to the next. Cultural factors such as decreased eye contact should also be considered. All cultures may not recognize or value the same behaviors that are valued by Western culture.

Assessment of the mother-infant (or father-infant) interaction should be made on various occasions to avoid attaching too much significance to one behavior on a given occasion. Some behaviors that may indicate a maladaptive attachment process include refusal by the mother to see her newborn, failure in normal progression of touching when holding or exploring the infant, making no attempt to establish eye-to-eye contact, inability to choose a name, or choosing a name that is so unusual that it implies hostility or ridicule (such as "Jim Beam," "Spirits," "Tornado," or the like).

An attachment assessment form is reproduced in Figure 35–5. It provides for recording observations during the prenatal period through 6 weeks of life. Those involved in care of the family can use such a form to become aware of potential problems and provide interventions to enhance attachment.

Guidelines for Intervention

Nursing actions that minimize the parents' mental distress and physical discomfort or maximize feelings of well-being and pleasure have the potential of enhancing the quality of mother-infant interaction. Following are some suggested objectives and ways of achieving them:

1. Determine the childbearing and childrearing goals of the infant's mother and father, and use them wherever possible in planning nursing care for the family. This includes giving the parents choices about their labor and birth experience and their initial time with their new infant.

2. Arrange the health care setting so that individual nurse-client professional relationships can be developed and maintained throughout a pregnancy and during the first months of mother-infant adaptation. A consistent care giver during the mother's prenatal experience allows a comfortable, trusting relationship to develop in which the mother feels free to express concerns, ask questions, and explore choices. In the hospital, a primary nurse can develop rapport and assess the mother's strengths and needs.

3. Enhance the couple's relationship and increase their communication capacity during the pregnancy. A feeling of closeness and personal satisfaction often results when the father plays an active role in the labor and birth process by acting as the woman's coach and support person. Comfort with such a role will develop most easily if the parents attend prenatal classes. As they learn about pregnancy and birth, anxiety decreases.

4. Use anticipatory guidance from conception through the postpartal period to prepare the parents for expected problems of adjustment. Prenatal classes often focus on possible problems a new family might encounter. In addition, literature on a variety of concerns, from feeding to sibling rivalry to infant stimulation, helps the new parents cope. If such information is available in the hospital and at the office or clinic, parents can choose according to their need.

5. Include parents in any nursing intervention planning and evaluation. Give choices whenever possible.

6. Remove barriers to voluntary contact among family members and the infant. This may be accomplished by providing time in the first hour after birth for the new family to become acquainted with as much privacy as possible. Warmth may be maintained by placing the infant against the mother's bare chest and covering both with a warmed blanket. When the father is holding his new daughter or son, the baby may be wrapped in two or three warmed blankets. Postponing eye prophylaxis facilitates eye contact between parents and their newborn. Sibling attendance at the birth or sibling visits also play a role in integrating the newest family member.

7. Initiate and support measures to alleviate parental fatigue.

8. Help parents identify, understand, and accept both positive and negative feelings related to the overall parental experience.

9. Support and assist parents in determining the personality and unique needs of their infant. Whenever possible, rooming-in should be available. This practice gives the mother a chance to learn her infant's normal patterns and develop confidence in caring for him or her. It also allows the father more uninterrupted time with his infant in the first days of life. If the mother and baby are doing well and if help is available for the mother at home, early discharge permits the family to begin establishing their life together.

The following are specific strategies to promote the role of the father in pregnancy and childbirth:

1. Include the father in all prenatal visits.

2. Encourage his participation in prenatal and parenting classes.

3. Provide educational material depicting active, involved fathers.

4. Address concerns of fathers related to childbirth and infant care.

Name _____ Age _____ Marital status: Single _____ Married _____ Separated _____

Gravida _____ Para _____ AB _____ Date of birth _____

Expected date of confinement _____ Method of feeding _____

Summary of labor and birth (anesthesia, complications, presence of a supportive person):

_____

Directions: This form is provided to systematically assess and record the components of the attachment process based on information obtained from available records, observations, and interviews with the parent(s) and other health care providers.

Prenatal Period

	Yes	No
Planned the pregnancy	_____	_____
Comments _____		
Confirmed the pregnancy	_____	_____
Comments _____		
Accepted the pregnancy	_____	_____
Comments _____		
Received early prenatal care	_____	_____
Comments _____		
Described fetal movement	_____	_____
Comments _____		
Personalized the fetus	_____	_____
Comments _____		
Asked what the fetus was like in utero	_____	_____
Comments _____		
Attended prenatal classes	_____	_____
Comments _____		
Planned for infant's needs	_____	_____
Comments _____		
Thought of possible names	_____	_____
Comments _____		
Client in good health	_____	_____
Comments _____		
Father of infant involved	_____	_____
Comments _____		
Areas of concern _____		

First Postpartum Day *(from birth through first day)*

	Yes	No
Calls infant by name	_____	_____
Comments _____		
Describes infant in affectionate terms	_____	_____
Comments _____		
Offers positive comments about infant's physical appearance	_____	_____
Comments _____		
Finds family resemblances	_____	_____
Comments _____		
Looks and reaches out to infant	_____	_____
Comments _____		
Hugs and touches infant	_____	_____
Comments _____		
Kisses infant	_____	_____
Comments _____		
Smiles at infant	_____	_____
Comments _____		
Expresses positive emotional feelings to infant's father or significant other	_____	_____
Comments _____		
Experiences average discomfort	_____	_____
Comments _____		
Welcomes visitors	_____	_____
Comments _____		
Areas of concern _____		

Delivery Period *(birth through 4 hours)*

	Yes	No
Accepts sex of infant	_____	_____
Comments _____		
Calls infant by name	_____	_____
Comments _____		
Calls infant by affectionate terms	_____	_____
Comments _____		
Comments on beauty of infant	_____	_____
Comments _____		
Realistically appraises the physical appearance of infant	_____	_____
Comments _____		
Looks and reaches out to infant	_____	_____
Comments _____		
Touches infant	_____	_____
Comments _____		
Smiles at infant	_____	_____
Comments _____		
Areas of concern _____		

Postpostpartum Period *(from second day to 6 weeks)*

	Yes	No
Wants to be near infant	_____	_____
Comments _____		
Enjoys caring for infant	_____	_____
Comments _____		
Holds infant close	_____	_____
Comments _____		
Feels infant belongs to her	_____	_____
Comments _____		
Feels infant notices her	_____	_____
Comments _____		
When away, thinks about infant	_____	_____
Comments _____		
Verbalizes warm comments about infant	_____	_____
Comments _____		
Recuperates with little difficulty	_____	_____
Comments _____		
Responds sensitively and appropriately to infant	_____	_____
Comments _____		
Areas of concern _____		

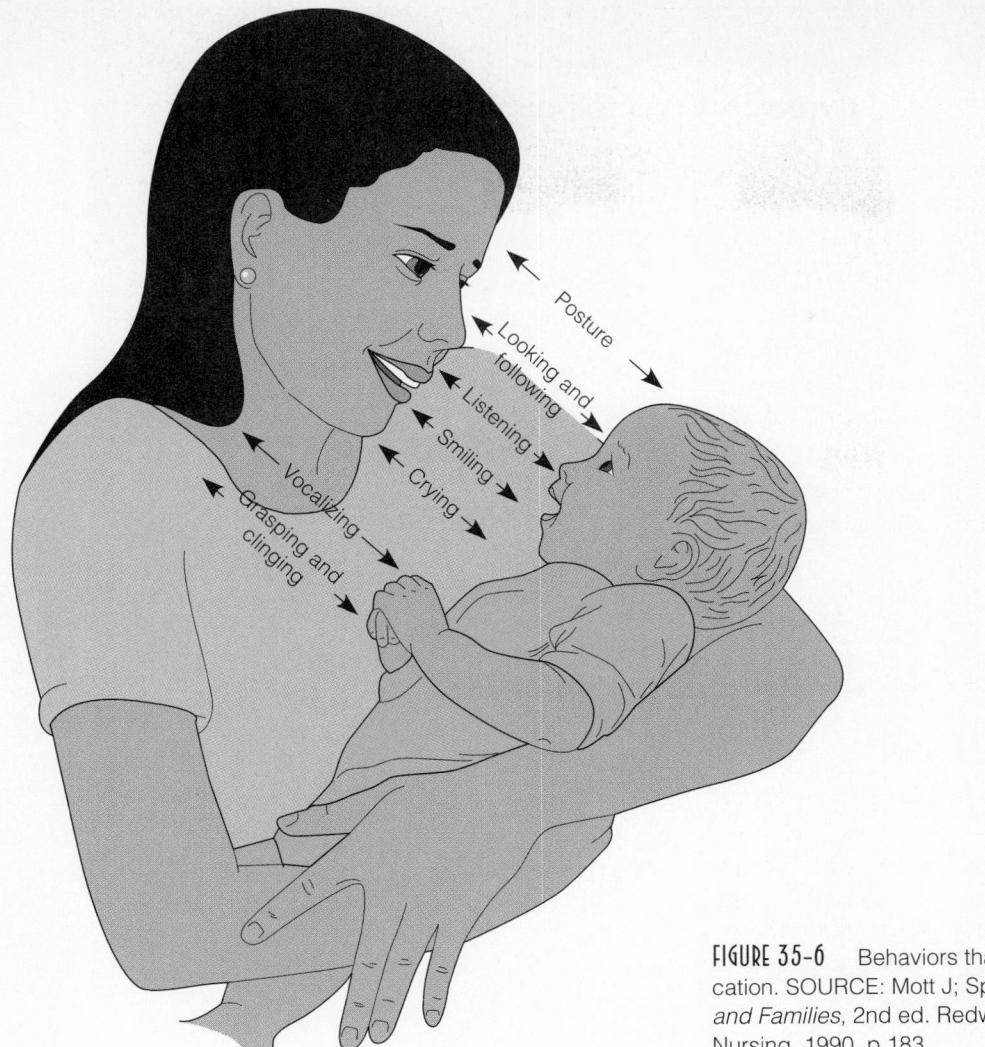

FIGURE 35-6 Behaviors that enhance parent-infant communication. SOURCE: Mott J; Sperhac A: *Nursing Care of Children and Families,* 2nd ed. Redwood City, CA: Addison-Wesley Nursing, 1990, p 183.

5. Have a prenatal session for fathers only, with involved fathers as discussion leaders.

6. Encourage discussion of changes in role and parenting issues.

7. Facilitate the father's presence at labor and birth, and provide support for the role he wishes.

8. Encourage the father to hold his newborn.

9. Allow the parents to have time alone with their infant after birth.

10. Give the father the opportunity to room-in with the mother.

11. Encourage the father's participation in feeding, holding, and diapering the infant.

◀ **FIGURE 35-5** Attachment assessment form with provision for continuity from the prenatal period through delivery and the first postpartum day to 6 weeks postpartum. SOURCE: *Early Parent-Infant Relationships.* White Plains, NY: National Foundation/March of Dimes, 1978, p 74.

12. Include the father in well-baby checks.

13. Provide postpartum classes that include both parents.

14. Facilitate discussion of difficulties in sharing responsibilities for infant care.

15. Encourage formation of parent support groups.

The importance of attachment is widely recognized, as are the adverse effects that may result when attachment does not occur. Formation of the attachment bond depends on numerous factors (Figure 35–6), and the bond may be enhanced by the sensitive approach of a health care provider in a humanistic environment in which parental preferences are given primary consideration. See Teaching Guide: Enhancing Attachment on page 1110.

Facilitating Attachment During Maternal-Newborn Complications

The mother who experienced a high-risk labor and birth or who has complications in the immediate postpartal period has an increased risk of encountering difficulties in

ENHANCING ATTACHMENT

Assessment   The nurse provides maximum opportunity for parents to interact with their infant immediately after birth and while in the birthing unit. Observation and documentation of these interactions will assist the nurse in determining family's needs for teaching, support, or interventions.

Nursing Diagnosis   The nursing diagnoses will probably be: Altered family processes related to addition of a new baby to the family or Knowledge deficit related to lack of information about emotional needs of newborn.

Nursing Plan and Implementation   The teaching plan includes information about the infant's physical status and normal characteristics, comforting techniques, and the baby's emotional needs immediately after birth and during the newborn period. Parents are encouraged to maintain continuous contact through rooming-in.

Parent Goals   At the completion of the teaching the parents will be able to do the following:

1. Demonstrate appropriate nurturing behaviors such as touching, bonding, talking to, kissing, and holding their baby.

2. Discuss normal characteristics and emotional needs of the newborn.

3. List at least three comforting techniques.

Teaching Plan

Content   Present information on periods of reactivity and expected newborn responses.

Describe normal physical characteristics of newborn.

Explain the bonding process, its gradual development, and the reciprocal interactive nature of the process.

Discuss infant's capabilities for interaction, such as nonverbal communication abilities. The nonverbal communications include movement, gaze, touch, facial expressions, and vocalizations—including crying. Emphasize that eye contact is considered one of the cardinal factors in developing infant-parent attachment and will be integrated with touching and vocal behaviors.

Discuss that touching, including stroking, patting, massaging, and kissing, will progress to interactive touch between parent and infant; discuss need to assimilate these behaviors into daily routine with baby.

Describe and demonstrate comforting techniques, including use of sound, swaddling, rocking, and stroking.

Discuss progression of the infant's behaviors as infant matures and importance of parents' consistent response to infant's cues and needs.

Provide information about available pamphlets, videos, and support groups in the community.

Evaluation   The nurse may evaluate the learning by providing time for discussion, questions, and return demonstrations in the birthing unit, during postpartal return visit or home visit. Continued observation of parent's positive interaction with their baby during remainder of stay in birthing unit provides a beginning means of evaluating learning.

Teaching Method   Discussion

Discussion and presentation of slides showing newborn characteristics

Show video on interactive capabilities of newborns

Discussion, demonstration, and handouts

Demonstration and return demonstration

Discussion, time for questions

attachment. She is more likely to have had medications, analgesia, or anesthesia during the intrapartal period, which may influence early interaction with her newborn. In the immediate postpartal period, she may be more likely to receive medications or analgesics or to face problems that limit her energy. Complications involving the mother or infant may necessitate separation during the early stages of attachment. Although these are only a few of the factors that may be present, they may be significant if they interfere with the bonding or attachment process.

See Chapters 19 and 31 for more in-depth discussion of the attachment process with maternal-newborn complications.

When the Newborn Is Hospitalized

Problems in attachment are more likely after the parents and baby have been separated due to prolonged hospitalization of the infant. In addition, Mercer (1993) found that an infant's gestational age at birth is a critical factor in the attachment process because a woman's progression through the tasks of pregnancy influences her perceptions of her infant as measured by the Maternal-Fetal Attachment tool. Therefore maternal-infant attachment is at particular risk in the case of prematurity because of both gestational age and the potential need for hospitalization (Haut, Peddicord and O'Brien, 1994). Fortunately, however, most mothers and fathers develop a closeness to their infants and nurture them in a normal, adaptive way, despite separation. When problems do occur, the mother's affective state and the father's role are critical components (Weingarten et al 1990). It is possible that when a mother is separated from her infant, she needs extra nurturing in order to provide the necessary nurturing for the infant. Thus an important role for the father may be to nurture his partner so that she can nurture the infant.

When infants require lengthy intensive care, special efforts by the nurse may facilitate attachment. It is important that parents believe that the child "belongs" to them rather than to the medical team. Parents are encouraged to participate in care and to give suggestions about care. A care plan that includes specific nursing diagnoses such as "Family coping: potential for growth" or "Altered role performance" provides for nursing interventions that are established according to the stages of parenting behaviors outlined in Figure 31–20. For example, if the mother entered the nursery, lowered the crib rail, and established an en face position while talking to the infant, she would be ready to move into stage II. In this case, if there is a specific problem, with the feeding schedule or technique, for example, the parents might be encouraged to work with the nurses to help establish the care plan.

Jenkins and Tock (1986, p 34) describe sending an informative letter to the parents "from the baby" on a weekly basis to promote proximity. The letter describes the competencies of the infant and behaviors such as "I like to open my eyes when I eat, but I get so tired that I soon close them." Davis and Truesdale (1993) described the development of "keepsake momentos" to promote parent-infant bonding and attachment. These momentos included the following:

- *First bottle.* This momento signifies a milestone because parents of ill or premature newborns may wait weeks or months for their infant's first bottle feeding.

RESEARCH IN PRACTICE

Mothers of full-term infants acquire and modify their maternal role and identify through constant caretaking interactions with their babies beginning at birth. However, mothers of preterm infants have limited initial access to their children and thus may have difficulty establishing maternal identity. Mary Zabielski designed a study to identify how preterm mothers acquire their maternal role and to determine whether qualitative differences exist between mothers of preterm and full-term babies in terms of maternal role attainment.

The sample included 42 first-time mothers, half of whom had recently delivered full-term babies and half of whom had preterm infants. All of the mothers had a singleton birth, were 19 years of age or older, and were 10 to 15 months postdelivery at the time of the study. The investigator identified preterm mothers first and then matched the full-term mothers using demographic variables. Quantitative data collection instruments consisted of a demographic data sheet, neonatal morbidity scale, family inventory of life events, and three other instruments designed to categorize maternal role and identity. The psychometric properties of all instruments were presented. A semi-structured interview provided qualitative data.

Data analysis showed no statistically significant differences between the preterm and full-term mothers' perceptions of support or amount of family stress. Furthermore, the preterm and full-term mothers demonstrated no statistically significant differences in either timing of maternal identity recognition or maternal role satisfaction.

Content analysis of the qualitative data resulted in the identification of eight common themes: role expectations, acknowledgement, qualities, actions, readiness, partner interactions, change, and self-continuity. The main theme of role expectations included maternal role anticipation, role rights or privileges, and role obligations. Although many of the participants experienced fulfillment of maternal role expectations, certain preterm mothers identified not meeting role expectations, such as taking their baby home from the hospital with them. One preterm mother still did not feel like a mother at the time of the interview. Several qualitative differences arose between the preterm and full-term mothers even though common themes were identified. Preterm mothers focused on role partner interaction, and full-term mothers emphasized role qualities.

Clinical Application of Study

As the author notes, neonatal nurses need to empower preterm mothers to have all forms of contact with their infants, including caretaking activities. Mothers can be encouraged to make decisions about their child's care to increase their feelings of having met maternal role expectations.

SOURCE: Zabielski M: Recognition of maternal identity in preterm and fullterm mothers. *Mat Child Nurs J* 1994; 22(1):2.

- *First haircut.* Even though shaving part of the infant's head may be necessary, it can be very disturbing for the parents. The hair is given to the parents in a heart-shaped window envelope after explaining the need for the haircut and that as little as possible was cut.

- *Personalized letter.* Decorated individually for each infant, this momento identifies that baby's special needs, such as feeding and positioning hints, physical and occupational therapy needs, and favorite music and play activities.

During the postpartal period, continued family interaction should be encouraged through supportive staff, liberal visiting policies, and educational offerings for both father and mother. Staff should be trained in assessment techniques and alert for evidence of malattachment so that appropriate interventions may be initiated. If necessary, referrals to the community health nurse or social services may provide the ongoing assistance needed. Telephone hotlines may provide a useful resource for a frustrated or worried parent, as may classes or parents' groups during the early weeks after birth.

Malattachment

The most common element in the lives of parents who neglect or abuse their children is a "lack of empathic mothering" in their own lives. This phrase describes inadequate responses of the caretaker to the infant, frequently beginning in the perinatal period and related to poorly developed maternal-infant attachment or insufficient bonding (Helfer & Kempe 1988). This finding has added to the attention given to promoting adequate parent-infant bonding. Factors that may contribute to malattachment include an abnormal pregnancy, an abnormal labor or birth, neonatal separation, other separation in the first 6 months, illnesses in the infant during the first year of life, illnesses in the mother during the first year of the baby's life, lack of social support, physical condition (ie, fatigue or altered sleep patterns), and inadequate problem-solving and stress reduction skills.

In the prenatal period, warning signs that may indicate lack of acceptance of the pregnancy and a potential for malattachment include negative maternal self-perception, excessive mood swings or emotional withdrawal, failure to respond to quickening, excessive maternal preoccupation with appearance, numerous physical complaints, and failure to prepare for the infant during the last trimester (Helfer & Kempe 1988).

Signs of maladaptive responses at birth may include lack of interest in seeing the newborn; withdrawal, sadness, or disappointment; negative comments such as "She's such an ugly thing"; or expressions of marked disappointment when told the infant's sex. When shown the infant, the mother may avoid looking at the child or may regard the child without expression. She may decline to hold the infant, or if she does agree to do so, she may not touch or stroke the infant's face or extremities. The mother may also avoid asking questions or talking to the infant and may suddenly decide she does not want to breastfeed.

During the early postpartal period, evidence of maladaptive mothering may include limited handling of or smiling at the infant; lack of preparation or questions about infant needs and care; and a failure to exhibit close, gentle, physical contact with the infant (for example, holding the infant away from her body, playing rough, or avoiding eye contact and the en face position). The mother may also describe her infant negatively or use animal characteristics in a hostile manner when referring to the infant: "He looks just like a withered old monkey to me!"

The father, too, may exhibit signs of malattachment to his infant. Examples of maladaptive paternal behaviors include inattentiveness and indifference toward the child; rough, unrelaxed handling; and tense, rigid posture. The father may also choose inappropriate types of play and exhibit no protective behavior toward his child.

When maladaptive behaviors are identified, various interventions can be used. A team approach involving all nursing shifts is advised. Any positive behaviors are communicated so that each staff member can continue to offer support and stimulate further development of such strengths.

The mother needs a supportive, understanding person she can interact with as she works through her feelings about her baby. Personal or telephone contact may be maintained after discharge so that the mother can continue to have contact with a supportive person with whom she is already acquainted. The mother should be encouraged to call the postpartal unit or newborn nursery if she has questions.

KEY CONCEPTS

The three major perspectives on attachment are psychoanalytic, ethologic, and social learning theories.

A mother's genetic makeup and background influence the environment she can provide for the fetus and newborn.

Attachment to the fetus develops during pregnancy.

The infant is a significant partner in the attachment interaction.

The childbirth setting is important in creating an environment for early parent-infant interaction.

Mother-infant interaction proceeds through phases: introductory, acquaintance, mutual regulation, reciprocity and rhythmicity, and attachment.

Attachment behaviors may differ in adolescent mothers.

Fathers, siblings, and others also become attached to the fetus and newborn.

Attachment occurs with adopted children and with handicapped children.

Attachment can be systematically assessed.

Interventions can facilitate attachment.

Complications in parent-infant attachment can occur because of maternal illness or hospitalization of the infant.

REFERENCES

Anderberg GL: Initial acquaintance and attachment behavior of siblings with the newborn. *JOGNN* 1988; 17(1):49.

Barnard K: *Nursing Child Assessment Satellite Training Scale.* Seattle: Univ of Washington, 1978.

Beal J: Methodological issues in conducting research on parent-infant attachment. *J Pediatr Nurs* 1991; 6(1):11.

Brazelton TB, Cramer BG: *The Earliest Relationship.* Reading, MA: Addison-Wesley, 1990.

Brazelton TB et al: The origins of reciprocity: The early mother-infant interaction. In: *The Effect of the Infant on Its Caregiver.* Lewis M, Rosenblum LA (editors). New York: Wiley, 1974.

Coffman S: Parent and infant attachment: Review of nursing research 1981–1990. *Pediatr Nurs* 1992; 18(4):421.

Cusson RM: Instruments in neonatal research: Measuring attachment behavior. *Neonatal Network* 1993; 12(4):69.

Davis R, Truesdale M: Creative approaches to promoting parent-infant bonding. *J Pediatr Nurs* 1993; 8(3):201.

Faller HS, Ratcliffe L: Sibling visitation: How far should the pendulum swing? *J Pediatr Nurs* 1993; 8(24):92.

Fuller JR: Early patterns of maternal attachment. *Health Care Women Int* 1990; 11:433.

Fuller SG, Moore LR, Lester JW: Influence of family functioning on maternal-fetal attachment. *J Perinatol* 1993; 13(6):453.

Gottlieb L: Maternal attachment in primiparas. *JOGNN* 1978; 7:39.

Graham MV: Parental sensitivity to infant cues: Similarities and differences between mothers and fathers. *J Pediatr Nurs* 1993; 8(6):376.

Greenberg M, Morris N: Engrossment: The newborn's impact upon the father. *Am J Orthopsychiat* 1974; 44:520.

Gullicks JN, Crase SJ: Sibling behavior with a newborn: Parents' expectations and observations. *JOGNN* 1993; 22(5):438.

Haut C, Peddicord K, O'Brien E: Supporting parental bonding in the NICU: A care plan for nurses. *Neonatal Network* 1994; 13(8):19.

Helfer RE, Kemps RS: *The Battered Child.* Chicago: Univ of Chicago Press, 1988.

Jenkins RL, Tock MKS: Helping parents bond to their premature infant. *MCN* 1986; 11:32.

Kemp VH, Sibley DE, Pond EF: A comparison of adolescent and adult mothers on factors affecting maternal role attainment. *Mat Child Nurs J* 1990; 19(1):63.

Klaus M, Kennell J: *Parent Infant Bonding.* St Louis: Mosby, 1982.

Koepke JE et al: Becoming parents: Feelings of adoptive mothers. *Pediatr Nurs* 1991; 17(4):333.

Landry SH, Chapieski ML: Joint attention and infant toy exploration: Effects of Down syndrome and prematurity. *Child Dev* 1989; 60:103.

Lobar SL, Phillips S: The couple choosing private infant adoption. *Pediatr Nurs* 1994; 20(2):141.

Longobucco DC, Freston MS: Relation of somatic symptoms to degree of paternal-role preparation to first-time expectant fathers. *JOGNN* 1989; 18(6):482.

Mercer RT: Commentary: Development of the prenatal attachment inventory. *West J Nurs Res* 1993; 15:211.

Mikhail MS et al: The effect of fetal movement counting on maternal attachment to fetus. *Am J Obstet Gynecol* 1991; 165:988.

Muller ME: Development of the prenatal attachment inventory. *West J Nurs Res* 1993; 15:199.

Murphy SO: Using multiple forms of family data: Identifying pattern and meaning in sibling-infant relationships. In: *Qualitative Methods in Family Research.* Gilgun J, Daly K, Handel G (editors). Newbury Park, CA: Sage, 1992.

Murphy SO: Siblings and the new baby: Changing perspectives. *J Pediatr Nurs* 1993; 8(5):277.

Novak J, Novak R: Facilitating fathering. In: *Nursing Interventions for Infants and Children.* Craft M, Denehy J (editors). Philadelphia: WB Saunders, 1990.

Pascoe JM, French J: Development of positive feelings in primiparous mothers toward their normal newborns. *Clin Pediatr* 1989; 28(1):452.

Porter LS, Sobong LC: Differences in maternal perception of the newborn among adolescents. *Pediatr Nurs* January/February 1990; 16:101.

Quinn MM: Attachment between mothers and their Down syndrome infants. *West J Nurs Res* 1991; 13(3):382.

Rubin R: *Maternal Identity and the Maternal Experience.* New York: Springer, 1984.

Stainton MC: Parents' awareness of their unborn infant in the third trimester. *Birth* 1990; 17(2):92.

Taylor PM: Bonding and attachment. In: *Current Therapy in Neonatal-Perinatal Medicine-2.* Nelson NM (editor). Philadelphia: Decker, 1990.

Weinberg SH: An alternative to meet the needs of early discharge: The tender beginnings postpartum visit. *MCN* 1994; 19(6):339.

Weingarten CT et al: Married mothers' perceptions of their premature or term infants and the quality of their relationships with their husbands. *JOGNN* 1990; 19(1):64.

Zachariah R: Maternal-fetal attachment: Influence of mother-daughter and husband-wife relationships. *Res Nurs* 1994; 17:37.

CHAPTER 36

THE POSTPARTAL FAMILY AT RISK

*W*e are surviving. Just. Why don't they give Croix de Guerre to people who can go without more than two hours total daily sleep for five weeks? I thought babies ate at six-ten-two-six-ten-two—mine does. He also eats at five-seven-nine-eleven and four-eight-twelve. I am getting rather used to going around with my breasts hanging out. They are either drying from the last feed or getting ready for the next one. But the love—I never knew, never imagined that I would love him like this. This incredible feeling of boundless, endless love—a wish to protect his innocence from ever being hurt or wounded or scratched. And that awful, horrible, mad feeling in the first week that you'll never be able to keep anything so precious and so vulnerable alive.

~ THE NEW OUR BODIES, OURSELVES ~

KEY TERMS

Early postpartal hemorrhage

Endometritis

Late postpartal hemorrhage

Mastitis

Oophoritis

Pelvic cellulitis (parametritis)

Peritonitis

Puerperal morbidity

Pulmonary embolism

Salpingitis

Subinvolution

Thrombophlebitis

Uterine atony

OBJECTIVES

Describe assessment of the postpartum woman for predisposing factors, signs, and symptoms of various postpartum complications to facilitate early and effective management of complications.

Incorporate preventive measures for various complications of the postpartum period into nursing care of the postpartum woman.

List the causes of and appropriate nursing interventions for hemorrhage during the postpartal period.

Develop a nursing care plan that reflects a knowledge of etiology, pathophysiol-

ogy, and current medical management for the woman experiencing postpartum hemorrhage, reproductive tract infection, thromboembolic disease, urinary tract infection, mastitis, or a postpartal psychiatric disorder.

Evaluate the mother's knowledge of self-care measures, signs of complications to be reported to the primary care provider, and measures to prevent recurrence of complications.

Describe the role of telephone follow-up and home visits in the extended care of postpartum families at risk.

The postpartal period is often seen as a smooth, uneventful time that follows the anticipation of pregnancy and the excitement and work of labor and birth—and often it is. However, it is important for the nurse to be aware of problems that may develop postpartally and their implications for the childbearing family. This chapter discusses several serious complications of the postpartal period and describes their care on the postpartum unit as well as the home care that may apply.

CARE OF AT-RISK WOMEN ON THE POSTPARTUM UNIT

When providing care to the childbearing woman during the postpartal period, the nurse continues to apply the nursing process to make ongoing assessments, institute preventive measures, and detect, as early as possible, the development of any complications. If a complication does develop, assessment remains important to determine the effectiveness of therapy and to detect any signs that the problem is worsening.

HOME CARE OF POSTPARTUM WOMEN

Early postpartum discharge, occurring within 24 to 48 hours of the birth, is becoming increasingly common. Health care outreach services can be especially valuable for clients at risk for postpartum complications, sometimes enabling the family to remain at home together rather than being separated by the mother's readmission to the hospital.

Comprehensive nursing assessment of postpartum clients assumes particular importance when early discharge is anticipated. Systematic data collection allows the nurse to note the normality of findings and to identify early signs of complications that would necessitate a longer hospital stay. Data collected prior to hospital discharge represent baseline findings against which subsequent data, collected by telephone or home visits, may be judged.

Signs and symptoms of many postpartum complications (late hemorrhage, mastitis, thromboembolic disease, and major depression) typically occur only *after* the woman has returned home, despite the fact that she met criteria for early discharge. Telephone or home visit follow-up may allow early recognition of such complications and help the mother get earlier intervention from her primary provider.

Telephone or home visit follow-up care by a professional nurse may also be initiated or extended in response to referral from a physician who has diagnosed a postpartal complication. In either event the nurse will continue systematic assessment and will plan and implement strategies in collaboration with the physician and family.

Postpartum Assessment by Telephone or During Home Visit

Because 92% of all American homes are accessible by telephone, this outreach method is reasonable for extending services to the postpartum family (Donaldson 1988). The telephone follow-up option is explained to families prior to discharge from the hospital, and a mutually agreeable time is set for the call, usually within 3 to 7 days after discharge or earlier if desired. Calls typically last about 20 minutes and are preplanned and goal directed. The initial goal is assessment, albeit indirect, of the woman's perception of her current circumstances, her recovery from childbirth, her and her partner's adjustment to parenthood, the newborn's condition, family-newborn bonding, and any problems or concerns that have arisen since homecoming.

The following areas are specifically assessed to determine the existence of postpartum complications: (1) progression of lochia, amount of flow, presence of foul odor or large clots; (2) fever; (3) dysuria or difficulty voiding; (4) pain in the pelvis or perineum; (5) painful, reddened hot spots or shooting pains in the breasts during or between feedings; and (6) areas of edema, redness, tenderness, or warmth in the legs. Assessment of the woman's emotional status, affect, comfort level, problems eating or sleeping, fatigue, reactions to the baby, and adaptation to new role demands may alert the nurse to postpartum mood disorders. To perform an effective telephone assessment, the nurse must be able to listen skillfully, use open-ended questions and wait for answers, and extend warm positive regard so that the mother feels comfortable talking candidly to a faceless caller.

A home visit has the advantage of allowing direct assessment to identify postpartum families at risk. The initial visit, planned in collaboration with the family, is usually made within the first 24 to 72 hours after discharge. The visiting nurse performs a systematic assessment of mother and newborn, family members' adjustment to their new life situation and its inherent role changes, maternal self-care, and newborn care. When the father and other children are present, the nurse has an excellent opportunity to assess the family dynamics among all members within the security of their home. The nurse is also able to assess the residence for adequacy of resources and evidence of safety hazards and to plan interventions accordingly.

Postpartal Nursing Diagnosis, Plan, and Implementation by Telephone or During Home Visit

The nurse formulates nursing diagnoses based on analysis of the assessment data elicited during the telephone call or home visit. If, for example, the woman reports that she has not had a bowel movement since delivery 2 days ago, the nurse would elicit additional data. The nurse learns that the woman is taking a narcotic several times daily for afterbirth contractions and perineal pain. Further, the woman is concerned that defecation will "hurt the stitches." When asked to recall what she has eaten for the last 24 hours, the client reveals that her intake is deficient in roughage and fluids. Analysis of this data justifies the nursing diagnosis: Risk for constipation related to decreased intestinal mobility from narcotic, fear of painful defecation, and inadequate dietary intake of fluids and roughage.

The plan of care developed during a telephone conversation is limited to supportive counseling, teaching, and referral. In the case of the woman with risk for constipation several nursing measures would be appropriate: (1) advising her to respond immediately to an urge to defecate, (2) reassuring her that defecation will not be painful if the stool is soft, (3) encouraging her to decrease strain on her sutures and perineum by propping her feet on a small footstool during defecation, (4) advising her to increase her intake of fluids and dietary fiber, and (5) referring her to the physician for a stool softener or laxative, if necessary.

When nursing assessment reveals signs of an initial or recurring postpartum complication, immediate referral to the primary provider is advisable because complications require dependent nursing measures that the physician prescribes.

Postpartal Evaluation by Telephone or During Home Visit

In postpartum outreach services, subsequent telephone calls or home visits provide an opportunity to determine whether the goals of care resulting from the first postpartal contact have been met or whether the plan needs revision. For example, in the preceding situation the woman was able to report during the telephone conversation with the nurse the next morning that she had a soft formed bowel movement without undue discomfort and found the suggested measures particularly helpful. She reports that she used a large dictionary as a "footstool" and found eating whole grain cereal with fruit, followed by coffee, a helpful measure and one she will continue to prevent constipation. The nurse can conclude that the plan has been effective. Moreover, because the mother's concerns were taken seriously and handled in a timely manner, a more serious problem was averted, and the mother is likely to feel more comfortable interacting with this concerned nurse in the future.

CARE OF THE WOMAN WITH POSTPARTAL HEMORRHAGE

Hemorrhage in the postpartal period is described as either early or late postpartal hemorrhage. **Early postpartal hemorrhage** (or immediate postpartal hemorrhage) occurs in the first 24 hours after birth. **Late postpartal hemorrhage** (delayed postpartal hemorrhage) occurs after the first 24 hours. Postpartal hemorrhage has traditionally been defined as loss of greater than 500 mL of blood after the end of the third stage of labor. That definition is being questioned in light of recent quantitative studies indicating that blood loss during normal birth is 500 to 600 mL. Furthermore, blood loss during both vaginal and cesarean births is commonly underestimated by half (Gant & Cunningham 1993). As the amount of blood loss increases, as in the case of hemorrhage, estimates are likely to be even less accurate (Newton 1966).

Early Postpartal Hemorrhage

The main causes of early postpartal hemorrhage are uterine atony (relaxation of the uterus), laceration of the genital tract, retained placental fragments, and blood coagulation problems. Certain factors predispose women to hemorrhage:

- Overdistention of the uterus due to hydramnios, a large infant, or multiple gestation
- Grand multiparity
- Use of anesthetic agents (especially halothane) to relax the uterus
- Trauma due to obstetric procedures such as midforceps delivery, intrauterine manipulation, or forceps rotation
- A prolonged or very rapid labor
- Use of oxytocin to induce or augment labor
- Uterine infection
- Maternal malnutrition, anemia, pregnancy-induced hypertension (PIH), history of hemorrhage, or history of blood coagulation problems

Uterine Atony

The most common cause of early postpartum hemorrhage is **uterine atony,** the relaxation of the uterus following birth. It can frequently be anticipated in the presence of:

- Overdistention of the uterus
- Dysfunctional labor that has already indicated the uterus is contracting abnormally
- Oxytocin use during labor
- Use of anesthesia or other drugs like magnesium sulfate that produce uterine relaxation

Hemorrhage from uterine atony may be slow and steady or sudden and massive. The blood may escape the

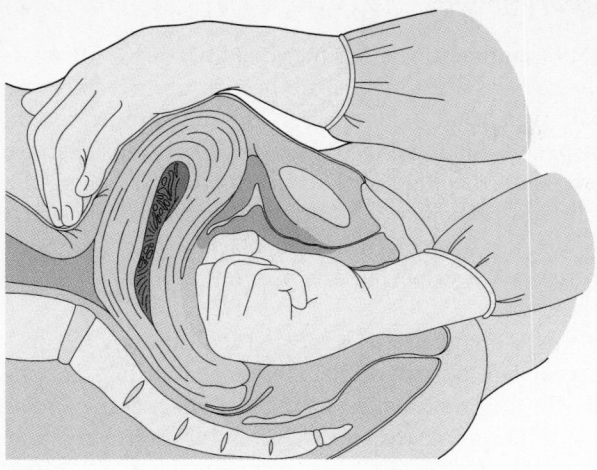

A

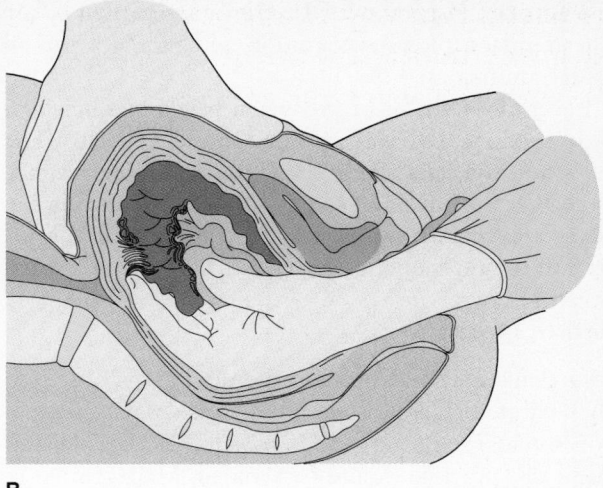

B

FIGURE 36-1 *A* Manual compression of the uterus and massage with the abdominal hand usually will effectively control hemorrhage from uterine atony. *B* Manual removal of placenta. The fingers are alternately abducted, adducted, and advanced until the placenta is completely detached. Both procedures are performed only by the medical clinician. SOURCE: Adapted from Cunningham FG, MacDonald PC, Gant NF [editors]: *Williams Obstetrics,* 18th ed. Norwalk, CT: Appleton & Lange, 1989, pp 417–418.

vagina or collect in the uterus, evident as large clots. Changes in maternal blood pressure and pulse may not occur until blood loss has been significant because of the increased blood volume associated with pregnancy.

In most cases the clinician can predict when a woman is at risk for hemorrhage. The key to successful management is prevention, beginning with adequate nutrition, good prenatal care, early diagnosis, and management of complications that may arise. Traumatic procedures should be avoided, and the birth should take place in a facility that has blood immediately available. Any woman at risk should be typed and cross-matched for blood and have intravenous lines in place. Excellent labor management and childbirth technique are imperative.

After expulsion of the placenta the fundus should be palpated to ensure that it is firm and well contracted. If it is not firm (if it is boggy), fundal massage should be performed until the uterus contracts. If bleeding is excessive, the physician undertakes bimanual uterine compression (Figure 36–1*A*) while ordering the administration of intravenous oxytocin (Pitocin) at a rapid rate. (An undiluted bolus of oxytocin *should not* be given because it can cause hypotension). Because of longer-lasting effects, methylergonovine maleate (Methergine) may be ordered for the immediate management of uterine atony. (See Drug Guide: Methylergonovine Maleate [Methergine] in Chapter 34.) Oxygen is also administered by mask. The combination of bimanual compression and oxytocin is usually effective in treating uterine atony.

If bleeding persists, the cervix and vagina should be inspected for lacerations. The physician may manually examine the uterine cavity for retained placental fragments or may perform a curettage. If the atony does not respond to these measures, 250 μg of 15-methyl prostaglandin F_2 (Prostin 15M) may be administered in-tramuscularly (Zlatnik 1994). The dose may be repeated at 15- to 90-minute intervals, if necessary. The side effects, such as nausea, vomiting, and diarrhea, are unpleasant and are often treated with medication. Other side effects include fever, flushing, and elevated diastolic blood pressure.

In a small-scale study, prostaglandin E was injected directly into the uterine cavity, causing rapid, sustained uterine contractions and cessation of hemorrhage within minutes. Side effects are minimized because a minute amount is needed and systemic circulation is bypassed (Peyser & Kupferminic 1990).

If the hemorrhage is not severe, the need for blood transfusion will be determined after blood values have been obtained and the true extent of the hemorrhage determined. Severe, uncontrolled hemorrhage, in addition to the previously described measures, may require immediate blood transfusion, inspection for uterine rupture, blood coagulation studies, curettage, bilateral internal iliac artery ligation, angiographic embolization, or hysterectomy (Mitty et al 1993).

Lacerations of the Reproductive Tract

Early postpartum hemorrhage is associated with lacerations of the perineum, vagina, or cervix in 20% of cases (Kapernick 1991). Several factors predispose women to higher risk of reproductive tract lacerations:

- Nulliparity
- Epidural anesthesia
- Precipitous birth
- Forceps-assisted birth
- Macrosomia

Thorough inspection of the reproductive tract by the birth attendant allows recognition and timely repair of most lacerations.

Lacerations are suspected when bright red bleeding persists in the presence of a firmly contracted uterus. The nurse who suspects a laceration on the basis of these findings notifies the physician so that immediate suturing can be used to control the hemorrhage and repair the integrity of the reproductive tract.

Retained Placenta

Hemorrhage may also occur if the placenta is only partially separated. The most common cause of partial separation is massage of the fundus *prior* to placental separation, so this practice should be avoided. Management of hemorrhage due to a partial separation, once it has occurred, includes uterine massage and manual removal of the placenta (Figure 36–1*B*). After expulsion of the placenta the consistency of the fundus is assessed. Rarely, placenta accreta, an abnormal adherence of the placenta to the uterine wall, is the cause of the hemorrhage and may require curettage or emergency hysterectomy.

Late Postpartal Hemorrhage

Late postpartum hemorrhage generally occurs 1 to 2 weeks after delivery and is most often the result of abnormal involution of the placental site or retained placental fragments. In the case of retained placenta, fragments may become necrosed, and fibrin may be deposited, forming a *placental polyp*.

Medical Therapy

Careful examination of the placenta after birth for missing pieces or cotyledons is the best preventive measure for late postpartal hemorrhage. The membranes should be inspected for missing sections or for vessels that are transverse to the edge of the placenta outward along the membranes, which may indicate succenturiate placenta and a retained lobe. If retained placental fragments or membranes are suspected, the uterine cavity may also be checked.

Often a boggy uterus is the first indication of the possibility of late postpartal hemorrhage. Bleeding is controlled by intravenous oxytocin, methylergonovinemaleate (Methergine), (usual dosage is 0.2 mg every four hours for six doses), ergotrate, or prostaglandins. Antibiotics are also used to prevent infection. Volume expanders and/or blood products are used if large amounts of blood are lost. Sonography is used to determine the presence of retained placental fragments. Curettage, formerly standard treatment, is now thought by some to traumatize the implantation site and thereby increase bleeding (Cunningham et al 1993).

APPLYING THE NURSING PROCESS

Nursing Assessment

Careful and ongoing assessment of the woman during labor and birth and evaluation of her prenatal history, will help identify factors that put her at risk for postpartal hemorrhage. Following birth, periodic assessment for evidence of bleeding is a major nursing responsibility. Careful observation and documentation of vaginal bleeding are important to determine if further medical intervention is needed. This assessment can be done visually, by pad counts, or by weighing the perineal pads. See Essential Precautions in Practice: During Postpartal Hemorrhage.

Nursing Diagnosis

Nursing diagnoses that may apply when a woman experiences postpartal hemorrhage include the following:

- Knowledge deficit related to lack of information about signs of delayed postpartal hemorrhage

- Fluid volume deficit related to blood loss secondary to uterine atony, lacerations, or retained placental fragments

Nursing Plan and Implementation

Regular and frequent assessment of fundal height and evidence of uterine tone or contractility will alert the nurse to the possible development or recurrence of hemorrhage. A soft, boggy uterus is massaged until firm. If the uterus is not contracting well and appears larger than anticipated, the nurse may express clots during fundal massage. Once clots are removed, the uterus tends to contract more effectively.

If the woman seems to have a slow, steady, free flow of blood, the nurse begins weighing the perineal pads (approximately 500 mL fluid weighs 1 lb or 454 g and monitors the woman's vital signs at least every 15 minutes—more frequently if indicated. If the fundus is displaced upward or to one side due to a full bladder, the nurse encourages the woman to empty her bladder—or catheterizes her if she is unable to void—to allow for efficient uterine contractions.

TEACHING MOMENT

As you know, bogginess indicates that the uterus is not contracting well, which results in increased uterine bleeding. This blood may remain in the uterus and form clots or may result in increased flow. In assessing the amount of blood loss, you must first massage the uterus until it is firm and then express clots. Don't be misled by the fact that a woman has a firm uterus. Significant bleeding can occur from causes other than uterine atony. To accurately determine the amount of blood loss, it is not sufficient to assess only the peri-pad. You should also ask the woman to turn on her side so you can assess the Chux pad for pooling of blood.

The nurse assesses the woman for signs of anemia, such as fatigue, pallor, headache, thirst, and orthostatic changes in pulse or blood pressure, and reviews the results of all hematocrit determinations. All medical interventions, intravenous infusions, blood transfusions, oxygen therapy, and medications such as methylergonovine maleate are monitored and evaluated for effectiveness. Urinary output should be monitored to determine adequacy of fluid replacement and renal perfusion. The nurse also encourages the woman to obtain adequate rest and helps her plan activities so that rest is possible.

The woman who is experiencing anemia and fatigue related to hemorrhage may need assistance with self-care and progressive ambulation for several days. When she is able to be out of bed to shower, use of a shower chair can enable independence while providing a measure of safety, should she experience weakness or dizziness. The emergency call light should be easily accessible.

The mother may find it difficult to care for her baby because of the fatigue associated with blood loss. The nurse can often find ways to promote attachment while still recognizing the health needs of the mother. The mother may require additional assistance in caring for her infant. If she has intravenous lines in place, even carrying the newborn may be awkward. For the mother who feels compelled to do as much as possible, the nurse may also need to "give permission" to the mother to return her infant to the nursery so she can have adequate periods of uninterrupted rest.

Involving the father in the plan of care is a productive strategy. He can support the mother's recovery by helping to meet her physical needs while encouraging her to rest. The mother is likely to feel less concern over her limited opportunities for newborn care if she can witness the father's interactions with and care for the newborn. The couple may wish for arrangements to be made for the father to stay in the hospital room, sleeping on a cot and eating with the mother so that limited rooming-in with the newborn is still an option. In that way, even if the mother is too fatigued to assume an infant care role, she can enjoy the infant's presence and experience bonding. The extent to which the father becomes involved with care of the mother and baby must be carefully balanced with his need to be rested for extra responsibilities he will assume when his partner and newborn child are discharged from the hospital.

Teaching for Self-Care

Because of current trends toward early discharge, the healthy mother may be sent home as soon as 4 hours after birth. She and her family or other support persons should receive clear, preferably written, explanations of the normal postpartal course, including changes in the lochia and fundus and signs of abnormal bleeding. Instructions for the prevention of bleeding should include fundal massage, ways to assess the fundal height and consistency, and inspection of the episiotomy and lacerations, if present. The woman should receive instruction in perineal care. The woman and her family are advised to contact their care giver if any of the following occur: excessive or bright red bleeding (saturation of more than one pad per hour), a boggy fundus that does not respond to massage, abnormal clots, leukorrhea, high temperature, or any unusual pelvic or rectal discomfort or backache. If iron supplementation is ordered, instructions for proper dosage should be provided in order to enhance absorption and avoid constipation and stomach upset. The nurse stresses the importance of reexamination of uterine size in 2 weeks. See Table 36–1.

Home Care

For most postpartum women, routine discharge instructions include advice such as: "You take care of the baby and let someone else care for you, the family, and the household." Because of her fatigue and weakened condition, the woman who experienced postpartum hemorrhage may be unable even to care for her newborn unassisted. The care givers at home need clear, concise explanations of her condition and needs for recovery. For example, all should understand the woman's need to rest and to be allotted extra time for a rest period following any necessary activity.

The woman may continue to need help with self-care for a time. She should be advised to rise slowly to minimize the likelihood of orthostatic hypotension. Until she

TABLE 36-1   Signs of Postpartal Hemorrhage

Excessive or bright red bleeding

A boggy fundus that does not respond to massage

Abnormal clots

Any unusual pelvic discomfort or backache

Persistent bleeding in the presence of a firmly contracted uterus

Rise in the level of the fundus of the uterus

Increased pulse or decreased BP

Hematoma formation or bulging/shiny skin in the perineal area

Decreased level of consciousness

regains strength, the mother should be seated when holding the newborn.

The person who will assume responsibility for grocery shopping and meal preparation will need advice about the importance of including foods high in iron in the daily menus. Enlisting the client's selection of preferences from a list of such foods will facilitate compliance with the diet. The nurse also explains the rationale for continuing medications containing iron.

The woman should continue to count perineal pads for several days so she will recognize any recurring problem with excessive blood loss. The debilitated condition and anemia associated with hemorrhage increase the woman's risk of puerperal infection. She and her care givers should use good hand washing and minimize exposure to infection in the home. They should be given a list of signs of infection and an appreciation of the importance of alerting the physician immediately should signs occur.

A sense of emergency often exists in the event of late postpartum hemorrhage. Because it commonly occurs 1 to 2 weeks after delivery, the couple is at home, involved in the day-to-day activities demanded by their new roles, when the unexpected, excessive bleeding begins. Quick decisions about child care arrangements must often be made so that the mother may be returned to the hospital. Both mother and father are likely to be alarmed by the excessive bleeding and concerned about her prognosis. There will be additional worries about separation from the newborn, especially when the mother is breastfeeding. The father may be in the unenviable position of being torn between the needs of the mother and the newborn. Ideally, arrangements can be made to minimize separation of the family members.

In addition to meeting the woman's physical needs, which may include those related to recovery from emergency D&C, the nurse will assess both members of the couple for impending crisis by addressing these factors: (1) What is their perception of the current situation, and is the perception realistic? (2) What coping strategies

have been helpful in previous difficult circumstances? Are they in use at this time, and are they effective? (3) What degree of support do they have from significant others? Do they have necessary resources? Providing realistic information, offering to call those in their support network, and exploring effective coping strategies can be of immeasurable value as they try to maintain a sense of balance in this difficult situation.

Evaluation

Anticipated outcomes of nursing care include:

- Signs of postpartal hemorrhage are detected quickly and managed effectively.
- Maternal-infant attachment is maintained successfully.
- The woman is able to identify abnormal changes that might occur following discharge and understands the importance of notifying her care giver if they develop.

Hematomas

Hematomas occur as a result of injury to a blood vessel, often without noticeable trauma to the superficial tissue. The soft tissue in the area offers no resistance, and hematomas containing 250 to 500 mL of blood may develop rapidly. Predisposing factors include the increased vascularity and pelvic congestion of pregnancy, PIH, genital varicosities, use of pudendal and epidural regional anesthesia, primigravidity, precipitous labor, prolonged second stage of labor, infant size greater than 4000 g, blood dyscrasias, and forceps-assisted birth. Hematomas may be vulvar, vaginal (especially in the area of the ischial spines), or subperitonial. Signs and symptoms vary somewhat with the type of hematoma.

Medical Therapy

Small vulvar hematomas may be treated with the application of ice packs and continued observation. Large hematomas or those increasing in size require surgical intervention to evacuate the clot and achieve hemostasis by ligating the bleeding point. Antibiotics, replacement of blood and coagulation factors, and vaginal packing may also be indicated. When large amounts of vaginal packing are necessary, voiding may be difficult, if not impossible, because of pressure on the urethra. An indwelling catheter is often necessary until the vaginal packing is removed. Infrequently, a pelvic hematoma that is extensive or difficult to control may require angiographic embolization or additional surgery (Zlatnik 1994).

Nursing Assessment

Often the first clue that a hematoma is forming is the woman's complaints of severe vulvar pain (pain that seems out of proportion or excessive), usually from her "stitches," or of severe rectal pressure. On examination, the large hematoma appears as a unilateral tense, fluctuant, bulging mass at the introitus or within the labia majora. With smaller hematomas the nurse checks for unilateral bluish or reddish discoloration of skin of the perineum and buttocks. The area feels firm and is painful to the touch. The nurse should estimate the size of the hematoma carefully with the first assessment to better identify increases in size and the potential blood loss. Frequent visualization of the perineum in women who are still under the effect of regional anesthesia is especially important.

Hematomas that develop in the upper portion of the vagina may cause difficulty voiding because of pressure on the urethra or meatus. Diagnosis is confirmed through careful vaginal examination.

Hematomas that occur upward into the broad ligament may be more difficult to detect. The woman may complain of severe lateral uterine pain, flank pain, or abdominal distention. Occasionally, the hematoma can be discovered with high rectal examination or with abdominal palpation, although these procedures may be quite uncomfortable for the woman. Signs and symptoms of shock in the presence of a well-contracted uterus and no visible vaginal blood loss should alert the nurse to the possibility of a hematoma.

Continuous assessment of vaginal bleeding after surgery to control a hematoma is required to detect a recurrence.

Critical Thinking Question

If hypovolemic shock is present, what signs might you see?

Nursing Diagnosis

Nursing diagnoses that may apply when a woman develops a hematoma postpartally include the following:

- Risk for injury related to tissue damage secondary to prolonged pressure from a large vaginal hematoma
- Pain related to tissue trauma secondary to hematoma formation

Nursing Plan and Implementation

If birth required the use of forceps or a vacuum extractor, or if it was traumatic because of the infant's size or position, the postpartal nurse can promote comfort and de-crease the possibility of hematoma formation by applying an ice pack to the woman's perineum during the first hour after birth and intermittently thereafter for the next 8–12 hours.

The discomfort experienced by a woman who develops a hematoma cannot be overlooked. If a hematoma develops despite preventive measures, a sitz bath after the first 24 hours will aid fluid absorption once the bleeding has stopped and will promote comfort, as will the judicious use of analgesics.

Evaluation

Anticipated outcomes of nursing care include:

- Hematoma formation is detected quickly and managed successfully.
- The woman's discomfort is relieved effectively.
- Tissue damage is avoided or minimized.

Subinvolution

Subinvolution of the uterus occurs when the uterus fails to follow the normal pattern of involution but instead remains enlarged. Deficiency of immunologic factors has been implicated in lack of involution of uteroplacental arteries, however, retained placental fragments or infection are the most frequent causes of subinvolution. With subinvolution the fundus is higher in the abdomen than expected. In addition, lochia often fails to progress from rubra to serosa to alba. Lochia rubra that persists longer than 2 weeks postpartum is highly suggestive of subinvolution (Cunningham et al 1993). Leukorrhea and backache may occur if infection is the cause. Subinvolution is most commonly diagnosed during the routine postpartal examination at 4 to 6 weeks. The woman may relate a history of irregular or excessive bleeding or describe the symptoms listed previously. An enlarged, softer than normal uterus when palpated with bimanual examination indicates subinvolution. Treatment involves oral administration of methylergonovine maleate (Methergine) 0.2 mg orally every 3 to 4 hours for 24 to 48 hours. When metritis is present, antibiotics are also administered. If this treatment is not effective, or if the cause is believed to be retained placental fragments, curettage may be indicated (Cunningham et al 1993).

CARE OF THE WOMAN WITH A REPRODUCTIVE TRACT INFECTION

Puerperal infection is an infection of the reproductive tract associated with childbirth that can occur any time from birth to 6 weeks postpartum. The most common infection is metritis/endometritis and is limited to the uterine cavity. However, infection can spread by way of the lymphatics and blood vessels to become a progressive disease resulting in peritonitis or pelvic cellulitis. The woman's prognosis is directly related to the stage of the disease at the time of diagnosis, the invading organism, and the woman's state of health and ability to resist the disease state.

The standard definition of **puerperal morbidity** established in the 1930s by the Joint Committee on Maternal Welfare is a temperature of 38 C (100.4 F) or higher with the temperature occurring on any 2 of the first 10 postpartum days, exclusive of the first 24 hours, and when taken by mouth by a standard technique at least four times a day. However, serious infections can occur in the first 24 hours or may cause only persistent low-grade temperatures. Therefore careful assessment of all postpartum women with elevated temperatures is essential.

Antibiotic therapy alone has not caused the decrease in postpartum morbidity and mortality that is seen today. Aseptic technique, fewer traumatic operative births, a better understanding of labor dystocia, improved surgical intervention, and a population that is generally at less risk from malnutrition and chronic debilitative disease have also contributed to this reduction. Postpartum sepsis will accounts for up to 16% of maternal mortality (Monga & Oshiro 1993).

Causative Factors

The vagina and cervix of approximately 70% of all healthy pregnant women contain pathogenic bacteria that, alone or in combination, are sufficiently virulent to cause extensive infections. Why the organisms do not cause infection during pregnancy is not altogether clear; however, recent studies indicate that more than the presence of a pathogen in the woman's reproductive tract is necessary for infection to begin.

Although the uterus is considered a sterile cavity prior to rupture of the fetal membranes, bacterial contamination of amniotic fluid with the membranes will intact at term is more common than previously believed and may contribute to premature labor. Following rupture of the membranes and during labor, contamination of the uterine cavity by vaginal or cervical bacteria can easily occur. Chorioamnionitis and cesarean birth after the onset of labor are the most significant factors in the development of postpartal uterine infection (Monga & Oshiro 1993). The relationships between puerperal infection and duration of ruptured membranes, multiple vaginal examinations, and internal fetal monitoring are not well documented and remain controversial. Poor nutritional status; anemia; vaginal infection with group B streptococcus; endocervical infections with *Chlamydia trachomatis* and *Mycoplasma hominis*; underlying disease, such as diabetes; and lacerations of the reproductive tract increase the risk of puerperal infection. Most infections are polymicrobial (caused by more than one organism) and include both aerobes and anaerobes.

Infectious Agents

The most common aerobic bacteria found in women with postpartal infection are group B B-hemolytic streptococci, other streptococci, and *Gardenerella vaginalis*. Other aerobic bacteria implicated in puerperal infections include *Escherichia coli* and *Staphylococcus aureus* (associated with an increasing number of cases of postpartum toxic shock). *E coli* may be introduced as a result of contamination of the vulva or reproductive tract from feces during labor and birth. Group A B-hemolytic streptococci, a less common cause (Nathan et al 1993), may be transmitted from the skin or nasopharynx of the woman herself or more probably from an external source such as personnel and equipment. Thus aseptic technique is essential.

Anaerobic bacteria most frequently isolated from women with postpartal infection include *Bacteroides* species, *Peptostreptococcus* species, and occasionally, *Clostridium perfringens*.

Genital mycoplasmas, *Ureaplasma urealyticum* and *Mycoplasma hominis*, are found in as many as 69% of women with postpartal endometritis, but their role in the infection is unclear because the endometritis responds to antibiotics that are not effective against these particular organisms (Monga & Oshiro 1993).

Late-onset postpartal endometritis is most commonly associated with the genital mycoplasmas and *Chlamydia trachomatis*. *C trachomatis* has a longer replication time and latency period than other bacteria and is not consistently eradicated by antibiotics used for early postpartum infections.

Types of Infections
Localized Infections

Localized infections of the episiotomy or of lacerations to the perineum, vagina, or vulva are usually not severe. However, necrotizing fasciitis, an infection of the superficial fascia and subcutaneous tissue arising in an episiotomy site, is an uncommon but rapidly developing, life-threatening infection. Early signs are erythema, edema, and induration at the episiotomy site with later development of skin discoloration and systemic shock. Treatment includes intravenous and oral antibiotics and aggressive surgical debridement (Monga & Oshiro 1993).

Wound infection of the abdominal incision site following cesarean birth is also possible. The skin edges become reddened, edematous, firm, and tender. The skin edges then separate, and purulent material, sometimes mixed with bloody liquid, drains from the wound. The woman may complain of localized pain and dysuria and may have a low-grade fever (less than 38.3 C or 101 F). If the wound abscesses or is unable to drain, high temperature and chills may result.

Endometritis (Metritis)

Endometritis, an inflammation of the endometrium, may occur postpartally. After expulsion of the placenta, the placental site provides an excellent culture medium for bacterial growth. The site (in the contracted uterus) is a 4 cm round, dark red, elevated area with a nodular surface composed of numerous veins, many of which become occluded due to clot formation. The remaining portion of the decidua is also susceptible to infection because of its thinness (approximately 2 mm) and its large blood supply. The cervix may also present a bacterial breeding ground due to the multiple small lacerations attending normal labor and spontaneous birth. Pathogenic bacteria deposited at the cervix during vaginal examination and those already present infect the decidua and eventually involve the entire mucosa. If the infection is confined to the surface of the mucosa, this area will become necrotic and be sloughed off within 3 to 5 days.

In mild cases of endometritis the woman will generally have discharge that may be scant or profuse, bloody, and foul smelling. In more severe cases symptoms may include uterine tenderness and jagged, irregular temperature elevation, usually between 38.3 C (101 F) and 40 C (104 F). Tachycardia, chills, and evidence of subinvolution may be noted. Foul-smelling lochia generally is cited as a classic sign of endometritis, but in the case of infection with β-hemolytic streptococcus the lochia may be scant and odorless (Cunningham et al 1993).

Salpingitis and Oophoritis

Occasionally, bacteria may spread into the lumen of the fallopian tubes, producing infection in the tubes known as **salpingitis** and ovaries known as **oophoritis.** Such infections are most often caused by a gonorrheal infection, *Chlamydia trachomatis*, anerobic baccilli and cocci, and gram-negative aerobes. Symptoms include bilateral (or unilateral) lower abdominal and pelvic pain, fever, chills, possible adnexal mass (if abscess develops), and tachycardia. Approximately 50–60% of women with salpingitis severe enough to cause infertility from tubal obstruction have never had a recognized episode of salpingitis (Eschenbach 1994). If tubal closure results, sterility may ensue.

Pelvic Cellulitis (Parametritis) and Peritonitis

Pelvic cellulitis (parametritis) refers to infection involving connective tissue of the broad ligament and, in more severe forms, the connective tissue of all the pelvic structures. It is generally spread by way of the lymphatics in the uterine wall but may also occur if pathogenic organisms invade a cervical laceration that extends upward into the connective tissue of the broad ligament. This laceration then serves as a direct pathway that allows the pathogens already in the cervix to spread into the pelvis. **Peritonitis** refers to infection involving the peritoneum.

A pelvic abscess may form in the case of postpartal peritonitis and most commonly is found in the uterine ligaments, cul-de-sac of Douglas, and the subdiaphragmatic space. Pelvic cellulitis may be a secondary result of pelvic vein thrombophlebitis. This condition occurs when the clot, usually in the right ovarian vein, becomes infected, and the wall of the vein breaks down from necrosis, spilling the infection into the connective tissues of the pelvis.

As the course of pelvic cellulitis advances, a mass of exudate develops along the base of the broad ligament that may push the uterus toward the opposite wall (if the infection is unilateral), where it will become fixed. If the exudate spreads into the rectocervical septum, a firm mass develops behind the cervix instead. The abscess that results should be drained or resolved through appropriate antibiotic therapy to avoid rupture of the abscess into the peritoneal cavity and development of a possibly fatal peritonitis.

A woman suffering from parametritis may demonstrate a variety of symptoms, including marked high temperature (38.9–40 C or 102–104 F), chills, malaise, lethargy, abdominal pain, subinvolution of the uterus, tachycardia, and local and referred rebound tenderness. If peritonitis develops, the woman will be acutely ill with severe pain; marked anxiety; high fever; rapid, shallow respirations; pronounced tachycardia; excessive thirst; abdominal distention; nausea; and vomiting.

Medical Therapy

Diagnosis of the infection site and causative organism is accomplished by careful history and complete physical examination, blood tests, aerobic and anaerobic endometrial cultures (although this may be of limited value because multiple organisms are usually present), and urinalysis to rule out urinary tract infection. When a localized infection develops, it is treated with antibiotics, sitz baths, and analgesics as necessary for pain relief. If an abscess has developed or a stitch site is infected, the suture is removed, and the area is allowed to drain. Research indicates that treating the mother with prophylactic antibiotics (cephalosporin or ampicillin) after clamping the umbilical cord decreases the incidence of reproductive tract infection by about 50% (Monga & Oshiro 1993).

Endometritis (metritis) is treated by the administration of antibiotics. The route and dosage are determined by the severity of the infection. Careful monitoring is also necessary to prevent the development of a more serious infection.

Parametritis and peritonitis are treated with intravenous antibiotics. Broad-spectrum antibiotics effective against the most commonly occurring causative organisms are chosen initially until the results of culture and sensitivity reports are available. If multiple organisms are present, the approach to antibiotic therapy is continued unless no improvement is observed; then the antibiotic is changed.

An abscess is frequently manifested by the development of a palpable mass and may be confirmed with ultrasound. An abscess usually requires incision and drainage to avoid rupture into the peritoneal cavity and the possible development of peritonitis. Following drainage of the abscess, the cavity may be packed with iodoform gauze to promote drainage and facilitate healing.

The woman with a severe systemic infection is acutely ill and may require care in an intensive care unit. Supportive therapy includes maintenance of adequate hydration with intravenous fluids, analgesics, ongoing assessment of the infection, and possibly continuous nasogastric suctioning if paralytic ileus develops.

APPLYING THE NURSING PROCESS

Nursing Assessment

The woman's perineum should be inspected every 8–12 hours for signs of early infection. The REEDA scale helps the nurse remember to consider redness, edema, ecchymosis, discharge, and approximation. Any degree of induration (hardening) should be immediately reported to the clinician.

Fever, malaise, abdominal pain, foul-smelling lochia, larger than expected uterus, tachycardia, and other signs of infection should be noted and reported immediately so that treatment can begin.

Nursing Diagnosis

For nursing diagnoses that might apply see the Nursing Care Plan: Puerperal Infection.

Nursing Plan and Implementation

Careful attention to asceptic technique during labor, birth, and the postpartum period is essential.

The nurse caring for a woman during the postpartal period is responsible for teaching the woman self-care measures that are helpful in preventing infection. The woman should understand the importance of good perineal care, hygiene practices to prevent contamination of the perineum (such as wiping from front to back, changing the perineal pad after voiding), and thorough hand washing. Once edema and perineal pain are under control, the nurse can also encourage sitz baths, which are cleansing and promote healing. Adequate fluid intake coupled with a diet high in protein and vitamin C, which are necessary to promote wound healing, also helps prevent infection.

If the woman has a draining wound or purulent lochia, it is especially important that those in contact with soiled items and linens practice good hand washing. Clear, concise instructions about wound care and how to appropriately discard soiled dressings must be provided to safeguard the woman and her care givers.

If the woman is seriously ill, ongoing assessment of urine specific gravity and intake and output is necessary. The nurse also carefully administers antibiotics as ordered and regulates the intravenous fluids. Ongoing as-

sessment of the woman's condition is vital to detect subtle changes in her health status. The nurse also recognizes the woman's comfort needs related to hygiene, positioning, oral hygiene, and pain relief.

Promoting maternal-infant attachment can be difficult with the acutely ill woman. The nurse may provide pictures of the infant and keep the mother informed of the infant's well-being. If she feels up to it, the new mother will also benefit from brief visits with her infant.

For the woman who wishes to breastfeed when her condition allows, maintenance of lactation by pumping the breasts can be a positive nursing action. Knowing that the promise of a special mothering opportunity is simply delayed, not eliminated, by the infectious process may improve the woman's morale (Coates & Riordan 1992).

The partner of a seriously ill woman has particular needs. He will be concerned about her condition and torn between spending time with her and with the newborn. Because maternal-infant bonding may be compromised, father-newborn bonding can be especially important. Mementos, such as a footprint, a note "written" by the baby to the mother, or a videotape of the baby can be comforting to the mother during their separation.

Home Care

The woman with a puerperal infection needs assistance when she is discharged from the hospital. If the family cannot provide this home assistance, a referral to home care services is needed. Home care services should be contacted as soon as puerperal infection is diagnosed so that the nurse can meet with the woman for a family and home assessment and development of a home care plan.

The family needs instruction in the care of a newborn, including feeding, bathing, cord care, immunizations, and significant observations that should be reported. A well-baby appointment should be scheduled. Breastfeeding mothers should be instructed to inspect the infant's mouth for signs of thrush and to report the finding to their physician.

The mother should be instructed regarding activity, rest, medications, diet, and signs and symptoms of complications, and she should be scheduled for a return medical visit. She needs to know the importance of taking the entire course of prescribed antibiotics even though she may begin to feel better before the bottle is empty. She also needs to be informed about the importance of pelvic rest. That is, she should not use tampons or douches nor have intercourse until she has been examined by the physician and told it is safe to resume those activities.

Evaluation

Anticipated outcomes of nursing care include:

- The infection is quickly identified and treated successfully without further complications.

Text continues on page 1128

PUERPERAL INFECTION

Nursing Assessment

Nursing History

1. Predisposing health factors: malnutrition, anemia, and debilitated condition
2. Predisposing factors associated with labor and birth: prolonged labor, hemorrhage, premature and/or prolonged rupture of membranes, soft tissue trauma, invasive techniques (eg, internal monitoring, frequent vaginal exams), operative procedures, maternal exhaustion

Physical Examination

1. Localized episiotomy infections may demonstrate:
   a. Complaints of unusual degree of discomfort, localized pain
   b. Reddened edematous lesion
   c. Purulent drainage, sanguineous drainage
   d. Failure of skin edges to approximate
   e. Fever (generally below 38.3 C or 101 F)
   f. Dysuria
2. Endometritis: Mild case may be asymptomatic or characterized only by low-grade fever, anorexia, and malaise. More severe cases may demonstrate:
   a. Fever of 38.3–39.4 C (101–103+ F)
   b. Anorexia, extreme lethargy
   c. Chills
   d. Rapid pulse (tachycardia)
   e. Lower abdominal pain or uterine tenderness
   f. Lochia: Appearance varies, depending on causative organism. May appear normal, be profuse, bloody, and foul smelling; may be scant and serosanguineous to brownish and foul smelling.
   g. Severe afterpains

h. Vomiting, diarrhea
i. Uterine subinvolution

3. Pelvic cellulitis (parametritis) may demonstrate:
   a. Signs and symptoms of severe infection (see previous discussion of endometritis)
   b. Severe abdominal pain, usually lateral to the uterus on one or both sides and apparent with both abdominal palpation and pelvic examination
   c. Possible abscess formation; dependent on location; may be palpated vaginally, rectally, or abdominally

4. Puerperal peritonitis may demonstrate:
   a. Symptoms just described plus severe abdominal pain
   b. Abdominal rigidity, guarding, rebound tenderness
   c. Possible vomiting and diarrhea
   d. Tachycardia, shallow respirations, anxiety, restlessness
   e. Marked bowel distention if paralytic ileus develops, absent bowel sounds

Diagnostic Studies

1. Elevated WBC, although it may be within normal puerperal limits (15,000–30,000/mm^3)
2. Culture of intrauterine material to reveal causative organism
3. Urine culture to rule out an asymptomatic urinary tract infection (should be normal)
4. Elevated sedimentation rate
5. Bimanual examination
6. Ultrasonography

NURSING DIAGNOSIS: Risk for injury related to the spread of infection

EXPECTED OUTCOME: Women will be free of infection.

Nursing Interventions

Evaluate history for factors that would contribute to a possible infection or retard wound health.

Employ principles of medical asepsis in hand washing and disposal of contaminated material by client and care giver. Promote normal wound healing by:

1. Sitz baths two to four times daily for 10–15 minutes or surgigator
2. Peri-care following elimination
3. Wiping front to back after voiding
4. Frequent changing of peri-pads
5. Applying pads front to back
6. Early ambulation
7. Diet high in protein, vitamin C, iron
8. Fluid intake to 2000 mL/day

Evaluate degree of healing using the REEDA scale. Report signs and symptoms of wound infection, including redness, edema, excessive pain, inadequate approximation of wound edges, purulent drainage, fever, anorexia, or malaise.

Obtain culture from wound site and administer antibiotics per physician order.

Increase wound drainage by:

1. Assisting physician in opening wound for drainage when indicated
2. Anticipating packing of a cavity greater than 2–3 cm with iodoform gauze

Rationale

Careful evaluation of client history enables the nurse to identify those women who are at risk for infection and for delayed wound healing.

Infection may be spread through direct contact with bacteria on hands, contaminated material, and so forth. Warm water is cleansing, promotes healing through increased vascular flow to affected area, and is soothing to woman. Peri-care promotes removal of urine and fecal contaminants from perineum. Wiping front to back and applying pads front to back prevent introduction of fecal material, including E coli, to episiotomy and reproductive tract. Changing pads frequently decreases the media for bacterial growth. Ambulation promotes drainage of lochia. Protein, vitamin C, and iron are essential for wound healing.

REEDA scale provides consistent, objective tool for evaluation of wound healing. Wound infection produces characteristic signs and symptoms that reflect the body's response to the invading organism.

Antibiotic therapy based on knowledge of causative organism is treatment of choice for localized infection.

Abscesses may develop when infected material accumulates in closed body cavity.

Iodoform packing maintains patency of opening so drainage can continue.

PUERPERAL INFECTION continued

Nursing Interventions	Rationale
Report signs of progressive infection, such as uterine subinvolution, foul-smelling lochia, uterine tenderness, severe lower abdominal pain, fever, elevated WBC, malaise, chills, lethargy, tachycardia, nausea and vomiting, abdominal rigidity.	More severe infections, such as endometritis, pelvic cellulitis, or peritonitis, can develop and produce characteristic signs as the body responds systemically to the invading pathogens.
Administer IV fluids and antibiotics as ordered.	IV fluids maintain adequate hydration; antibiotics are the treatment of choice to combat the infection.
Maintain semi-Fowler's position.	Promotes comfort and helps prevent spread of infection.
Encourage adequate rest.	Reduces metabolic demands, thereby providing adequate oxygen and nutrients to the affected area to facilitate healing.
Monitor vital signs, especially temperature, every 4 hours and more frequently if they are significantly abnormal. Note temperature trends.	Tachycardia and fever occur because the body's metabolic rate increases in response to its efforts to combat infection. A profound systemic infection can produce septic shock with decreased blood pressure and increased respirations.
Monitor I&O, urine specific gravity, and level of hydration as ordered.	Vigorous fluid and electrolyte therapy is necessary not only because of vomiting and diarrhea, but also because both fluid and electrolytes become sequestered in lumen and wall of bowel.
Maintain continuous nasogastric suction per physician order, and assess bowel sounds.	Continuous nasogastric suction is used to decompress the bowel when paralytic ileus complicates the course and results in cessation of gastrointestinal (GI) motility.
Transfer woman to intensive care if indicated by her condition.	Woman with peritonitis is in critical condition, and quality of nursing care this patient receives may determine the difference between recovery and demise.

OUTCOME MET IF:

- Woman's temperature is 97–99 F (36.1–37.2 C).
- Woman's WBC $<30,000$ mm^3.
- Woman has no uterine tenderness per palpation.
- Woman's lochia is not foul smelling.
- Woman's incision or episiotomy show no signs of redness, edema, purulent discharge, or inadequate approximation.
- Woman has no nausea and vomiting.

NURSING DIAGNOSIS: Pain related to the presence of infection

EXPECTED OUTCOME: Woman will obtain relief of pain.

Nursing Interventions	Rationale
Promote comfort by:	Comfort is essential to enable the woman to rest and recover.
1. Ensuring adequate periods of rest	
2. Minimizing disturbing environmental stimuli	External environmental stimuli may increase pain perceptions. Plan rest periods to increase client's emotional reserve.
3. Judicious use of analgesics and antipyretics	
4. Providing emotional support	
5. Using supportive nursing measures, such as back rubs, instruction in relaxation techniques, maintenance of cleanliness, provision of diversional activities	Relaxation and cleanliness promote comfort and decrease pain.

OUTCOME MET IF:

- Pain level ≤5 at all times on a 10-point pain scale.

NURSING DIAGNOSIS: Risk for altered parenting related to delayed parent-infant attachment secondary to woman's malaise and other symptoms of infection

EXPECTED OUTCOME: Woman will bond with her infant.

PUERPERAL INFECTION *continued*

Nursing Interventions	**Rationale**

Provide and maintain mother-infant interaction:

1. Provide opportunities for the mother to see and hold her infant

2. Encourage the mother to feed the infant if she feels able. Assist the mother with feeding when IV is in place.

3. If breastfeeding mother is unable to nurse, assits her in pumping her breasts to maintain milk production.

4. Encourage partner or support person to discuss infant with woman and to become involved in infant's care if the woman is not able to do do.

5. Provide pictures or video of the infant for the mother.

6. Encourage verbalization of anxieties, fears, and concerns.

Assess breastfeeding infant's mouth for signs of thrush, a common side effect of antibiotics taken by the mother. Treatment should be initiated, but breastfeeding need not be stopped.

Critically ill woman may become very depressed not only from disease process but also because her anticipated postpartal course is now denied her, and she may interpret this as a failure of her ability to mother her infant.

Success at infant feeding generally enhances the woman's outlook and encourages mother-infant interaction.

Assists woman to feel involved with her infant and reassures her that her baby is receiving care and love.

Promotes attachment

Reduces the woman's anxiety

Thrush, a monilial infection caused by Candida albicans, *often occurs when normal oral flora are destroyed by antibiotic therapy.*

OUTCOME MET IF:

- Woman/family demonstrates two or more of the following physical interactions: good eye contact, touching baby, holding baby close, attempting to comfort baby, and kissing baby.

- Woman/family demonstrates two or more of the following social interactions: calling baby by name, making positive comments about baby, asking questions about baby, and talking to baby.

NURSING DIAGNOSIS: Knowledge deficit related to lack of information about the condition and its treatment

EXPECTED OUTCOME: Woman will be able to discuss her condition, its treatment, and her care needs following discharge.

Nursing Interventions	**Rationale**

Provide information regarding predisposing factors, signs and symptoms, and treatment. Discuss the value of a nutritious diet in promoting healing.

Review hygiene practice, such as correct wiping after voiding, and hand washing, to prevent the spread of infection.

Discuss home care routines to be used following postpartal infection.

Women have the right and responsibility to be actively involved in their own health care to the extent that they are able. To be an active participant, the woman needs appropriate information.

OUTCOME MET IF:

- Woman/family verbalizes understanding of signs and symptoms to report to health care provider, hygiene practices that prevent the spread of infection, and value of appropriate diet and foods that meet this need.

Essential Nursing Activities to Achieve Outcomes

Nursing Assessments

1. Assess predisposing health and labor/birth factors.

2. Take vital signs (BP, P, R, T) every 4 hours or more frequently if abnormal finding. A temperature of 100 F or higher on 2 of the first 10 postpartum days, exclusive of the first 24 hours, may indicate an infection.

3. Record I&O.

4. Note WBC: should be <30,000 mm^3.

5. Inspect incision/episiotomy for redness, approximation, and drainage.

6. Assess the uterus for tenderness to palpation, enlargement, and rigidity.

7. Assess lochia for color, odor, amount.

8. Assess pain level every 3–4 hours.

9. Monitor for nausea and vomiting.

10. Assess the knowledge level of the woman and family.

11. Monitor parent-infant interaction.

Nursing Interventions/Prevention

1. Obtain accurate history.

2. Instruct woman on:
   a. Peri-care after each voiding
   b. Wiping front to back after voiding
   c. Applying pads front to back
   d. Frequent changing of pads
   e. Need for early ambulation
   f. Proper diet
   g. Increasing fluid intake
   h. Sitz bath two to three times/day

3. Evaluate woman/family's understanding of all information.

4. Obtain blood cultures per physician order with elevated temperatures.

5. Document accurately all assessment information.

6. Report all abnormal findings to appropriate health care provider.

7. Instruct woman on signs and symptoms of infection that need to be reported to health care provider.

- The woman understands the infection and the purpose of therapy; she carries out any ongoing antibiotic therapy if indicated following discharge.
- Maternal-infant attachment is maintained.

CARE OF THE WOMAN WITH THROMBOEMBOLIC DISEASE

Thromboembolic disease may occur antepartally, but it is generally considered a postpartal complication. *Venous thrombosis* refers to thrombus formation in a superficial or deep vein with the accompanying risk that a portion of the clot might break off and result in pulmonary embolism. When the thrombus is formed in response to inflammation in the vein wall, it is termed **thrombophlebitis.** In this type of thrombosis the clot tends to be more firmly attached and therefore is less likely to result in embolism. In *noninflammatory venous thrombosis* (also called phlebothrombosis) the clot tends to be more loosely attached, and the risk of embolism is greater. The primary factor responsible for noninflammatory deep vein thrombosis is venous stasis (Cunningham et al 1993).

Factors contributing directly to the development of thromboembolic disease postpartally include (1) increased amounts of certain blood clotting factors; (2) postpartal thrombocystosis (increased quantity of circulating platelets) and their increased adhesiveness; (3) release of thromboplastin substances from the tissue of the decidua, placenta, and fetal membranes; and (4) increased amounts of fibrinolysis inhibitors. Predisposing factors are (1) obesity, increased maternal age, and high parity; (2) anesthesia and surgery with possible vessel trauma and venous stasis due to prolonged inactivity; (3) previous history of venous thrombosis; (4) maternal anemia, hypothermia, or heart disease; (5) use of estrogen for suppression of lactation; (6) endometritis (metritis); and (7) varicosities.

Superficial Leg Vein Disease

Superficial thrombophlebitis is far more common postpartum than during pregnancy. Often the clot involves the saphenous veins. This disorder is more common in women with preexisting varices (enlarged veins), although it is not limited to these women. Symptoms usually become apparent about the third or fourth postpartal day: tenderness in a portion of the vein, some local heat and redness, absent or low-grade fever, and occasionally slight elevation of the pulse. Treatment involves application of local heat, elevation of the affected limb, bed rest and analgesics, and the use of elastic support hose. Anticoagulants are usually not necessary unless complications develop. Pulmonary embolism is extremely rare. Occasionally, the involved veins have incompetent valves, and as a result the problem may spread to the deeper leg veins, such as the femoral vein.

Deep Vein Thrombosis (DVT)

Deep venous thrombosis/thrombophlebitis is more frequently seen in women with a history of thrombosis. Certain obstetric complications such as hydramnios, PIH, and operative birth are associated with an increased incidence.

Clinical manifestations may include edema of the ankle and leg and an initial low-grade fever often followed by high temperature and chills. Depending on the vein involved, the woman may complain of pain in the popliteal and lateral tibial areas (popliteal vein), entire lower leg and foot (anterior and posterior tibial veins), inguinal tenderness (femoral vein), or pain in the lower abdomen (iliofemoral vein). Homan's sign (Figure 36–2) may or may not be positive, but pain often results from calf pressure. Because of reflex arterial spasm, sometimes the limb is cool to the touch—the so-called milk leg or *phlegmasia alba dolens*—and peripheral pulses may be decreased.

Septic pelvic thrombophlebitis may develop in conjunction with infections of the reproductive tract and is more common in women who have had a cesarean birth. The classic sign is fever of unknown origin. However, when the ovarian vein is involved, lower abdominal pain also occurs. If untreated, tachycardia, nausea, ileus, and elevated white count usually develop.

Medical Therapy

Because cases are seldom clear-cut, diagnosis involves a variety of approaches, such as client history and physical examination, occlusive cuff impedence plethysmography (IPG), Doppler ultrasonography, and contrast venography. In questionable cases, contrast venography provides the most accurate diagnosis of deep vein thrombosis. Unfortunately, venography is not practical for multiple examinations or prospective screening and may itself induce phlebitis.

Treatment involves the administration of intravenous heparin, using an infusion pump to permit continuous, accurate infusion of medication. Strict bed rest and elevation of the legs are required, and analgesics are given as necessary to relieve discomfort. If fever is present, deep thrombophlebitis is suspected, and the woman is also given antibiotic therapy. In most cases thrombectomy is not necessary.

Once the symptoms have subsided (usually in several days), the woman may begin walking while wearing elastic support stockings. Intravenous heparin is continued, and treatment with sodium warfarin (Coumadin) is begun. Osteoporosis may occur with prolonged heparin therapy (Cosico et al 1993). When prothrombin time

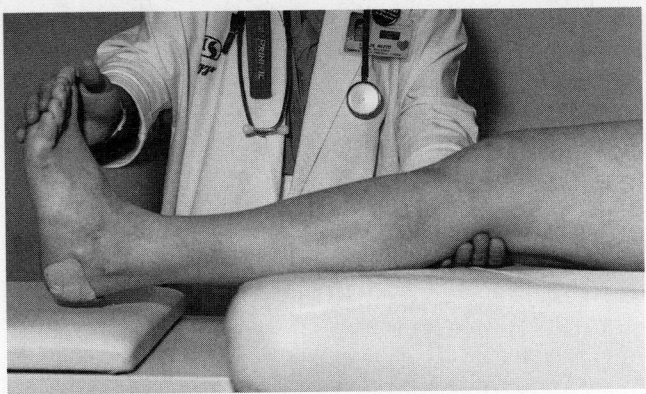

FIGURE 36-2 Homan's sign. With the client's knee flexed to decrease the risk of embolization, the nurse dorsiflexes the client's foot. Pain in the foot or leg is a positive Homan's sign.

reaches 1.5 to 1.7, the heparin is discontinued. The woman will continue on Coumadin for 2 to 6 months at home. While on warfarin, prothrombin times are assessed periodically to maintain correct dosage levels.

APPLYING THE NURSING PROCESS

Nursing Assessment

The nurse carefully assesses the woman's history for factors predisposing to development of thrombosis and/or thrombophlebitis. In addition, as part of regular postpartal assessment, the nurse is alert to any client complaints of pain in the leg, inguinal area, or lower abdomen because such pain may indicate deep venous thrombosis. The nurse also assesses the woman's legs for evidence of edema, temperature change, or pain with palpation. Measurement of the affected portion of the leg using a nonstretchable tape measure helps quantify the amount of edema.

Nursing Diagnosis

Nursing diagnoses that may apply to a postpartal woman with thromboembolic disease are found in the Nursing Care Plan: Thromboembolic Disease on page 1130.

Nursing Plan and Implementation

Women with varicosities should be evaluated for the need for support hose during labor and the postpartum period. Adequate fluid intake is necessary during labor to avoid dehydration. Because trauma is often a factor in the development of thrombophlebitis, the nurse avoids keeping the woman's legs elevated in stirrups for prolonged periods. If stirrups are used, they should be comfortably padded and adjusted to provide correct support and prevent pressure on popliteal vessels. In addition early ambulation is encouraged following birth, and the use of the knee gatch on the bed should be avoided. Women confined to bed following a cesarean birth are encouraged to do regular leg exercises to promote venous return.

Once the diagnosis of deep venous thrombosis is made, the nurse maintains the heparin therapy, provides for appropriate comfort measures, and monitors the woman closely for signs of pulmonary embolism. The nurse also assesses for evidence of bleeding related to heparin and keeps the antagonist for heparin, protamine sulfate, readily available.

Teaching for Self-Care

The nurse instructs the woman to avoid prolonged standing or sitting because these positions contribute to venous stasis. She is also instructed to avoid crossing her legs because of the pressure it causes. The nurse also advises her to take frequent breaks such as when taking car trips or if she has a job where she sits most of the day. Walking is acceptable because it promotes venous return. The woman is reminded to identify her history of thrombosis/thrombophlebitis to her physician during subsequent pregnancies so that preventive measures may be instituted early.

Women who are discharged on warfarin must understand the purpose of the medication and be alert to signs of hemorrhage such as bleeding gums, epistaxis, petechiae or ecchymosis, or evidence of blood in the urine or stool. Because careful monitoring is important, the woman should clearly understand the need to keep scheduled appointments for prothrombin time assessment. Certain medications such as aspirin and nonsteroidal anti-inflammatory drugs increase anticoagulant activity, so they should be avoided. In fact the woman should check for possible medication interaction before taking any medication while on warfarin. A woman may choose to carry a MedicAlert card in case of emergency and should inform all medical care providers, including

Text continues on page 1133

CRITICAL THINKING IN PRACTICE

Lei Chang, G1P1, had a cesarean birth after a prolonged labor and failure to progress. You notice that, as she is walking in the hallway with her husband, Lei is limping slightly, and you comment on that observation. Lei responds that she is having pain in her right lower leg. She says, "Maybe I pulled a muscle during labor." What would you do?

Answers can be found in Appendix I.

THROMBOEMBOLIC DISEASE

Nursing Assessment

Nursing History

1. Predisposing factors, including the following:
   a. Increased maternal age
   b. Obesity
   c. Increased parity
   d. Prolonged labor with associated pressure of the fetal head on the pelvic veins
   e. PIH
   f. Heart disease
   g. Hypercoagulability of the early puerperium
   h. Anemia
   i. Immobility
   j. Hemorrhage
   k. Previous history of venous thrombosis
   l. Varicose veins

2. Initiating factors, including the following:
   a. Trauma to deep leg veins due to faulty positioning for birth
   b. Operative birth, including cesarean birth
   c. Abortion
   d. Postpartal pelvic cellulitis

Physical Examination

1. Superficial thrombophlebitis:
   a. Tenderness along the involved vein
   b. Areas of palpable thrombosis
   c. Warmth and redness in the involved area

2. Deep venous thrombosis (DVT):
   a. Positive Homan's sign (pain occurs when foot is dorsiflexed while leg is extended)
   b. Tenderness and pain in affected area
   c. Fever (initially low, followed by high fever and chills)
   d. Edema in affected extremity
   e. Pallor and coolness in affected limb
   f. Diminished peripheral pulses
   g. Increased potential for pulmonary embolus

Diagnostic Studies

1. Doppler ultrasonography demonstrates increased circumference of affected extremity.
2. Occlusive cuff IPG
3. Venography confirms diagnosis.
4. Computerized axial tomography or MRI may be used for confirmation.

NURSING DIAGNOSIS: Altered tissue perfusion in periphery related to obstructed venous return

EXPECTED OUTCOME: Tissue perfusion is adequate in extremities.

Nursing Interventions	Rationale

Report signs and symptoms of developing thrombophlebitis (see client assessment section of nursing care plan).

Early detection of developing thrombophlebitis permits prompt treatment. As the thrombus increases in size, signs of obstruction also increase.

Maintain bed rest and warm, moist soaks as ordered, with legs elevated.

Bed rest is ordered to decrease possibility that portion of clot will dislodge and cause pulmonary embolism. Warmth promotes blood flow to affected area. Elevation of legs decreases edema and prevents venous stasis.

For DVT administer intravenous heparin as ordered, by continuous intravenous drip, heparin lock, or subcutaneously, including the following:

1. Monitor IV or heparin lock site for signs of infiltration.
2. Obtain Lee-White clotting times or partial thromboplastin time (PTT) per physician order, and review prior to administering heparin.
3. Observe for signs of anticoagulant overdose with resultant bleeding, including the following: hematuria, epistaxis, ecchymosis, and bleeding gums.
4. Provide protamine sulfate per physician order to combat bleeding problems related to heparin overdosage.

Heparin does not dissolve clot but is administered to prevent further clotting. It is safe for breastfeeding mothers because heparin is not secreted in mother's milk.

Protamine sulfate is heparin antagonist, given intravenously, which is almost immediately effective in counteracting bleeding complications caused by heparin overdose.

Immediately report the development of any signs of pulmonary embolism, including the following:

1. Sudden onset of severe chest pain, often located substernally
2. Apprehension and sense of impending catastrophe
3. Cough (may be accompanied by hemoptysis)
4. Tachycardia
5. Fever
6. Hypotension
7. Diaphoresis, pallor, weakness
8. Shortness of breath
9. Neck engorgement
10. Friction rub and evidence of atelectasis upon auscultation

Pulmonary embolism is major complication of deep venous thrombosis/thrombophlebitis. Signs and symptoms may occur suddenly and require immediate emergency treatment; prognosis is related to size and location of embolism.

THROMBOEMBOLIC DISEASE *continued*

Nursing Interventions	Rationale
Initiate or support any emergency treatment. Initiate progressive ambulation following the acute phase; provide properly fitting elastic stockings prior to ambulation for management of superficial thrombophlebitis and DVT. For DVT obtain prothrombin time (PT) and review prior to beginning warfarin. Repeat periodically per physician order.	Elastic stockings or "TEDs" help prevent pooling of venous blood in lower extremities. PT is the test most commonly used to monitor the blood of clients receiving warfarin. Warfarin sodium (Coumadin) inhibits Vitamin K–dependent activation of clotting factors II, VII, IX, and X. Goal of treatment is to maintain prothrombin time (PT) at 1.5 to 2 times normal.

OUTCOME MET IF:
- Woman has absence of pain and edema in extremity.
- Woman's pulses are palpable.
- Woman's skin is warm and normal color for race.

NURSING DIAGNOSIS: Pain related to tissue hypoxia and edema secondary to vascular obstruction

EXPECTED OUTCOME: Woman will obtain relief of pain.

Nursing Interventions	Rationale
Administer analgesics as ordered for relief of pain. Provide supportive nursing comfort measures, such as back rubs, provision of quiet time for sleep, diversional activities. Maintain limb in elevated position.	Analgesics are to relieve pain and enable the woman to rest. Aspirin or ibuprofen products are contraindicated because they inhibit platelet adhesiveness. Acetaminophen may be ordered by the physician. Elevation of affected limb promotes venous return and helps decrease edema.

OUTCOME MET IF:
- Woman's pain level ≤5 at all times.

NURSING DIAGNOSIS: Risk for altered parenting related to decreased maternal-infant interaction secondary to bed rest and IVs

EXPECTED OUTCOME: Woman will demonstrate evidence of positive physical and social interaction with newborn.

Nursing Interventions	Rationale
Maintain mother-infant attachment when mother is on bed rest. Provide frequent contacts for mother and infant; modified rooming-in is possible if the crib is placed close to the mother's bed and nurse checks often to help mother lift or move infant.	Maternal-infant attachment is enhanced by frequent contact and opportunities to interact.

OUTCOME MET IF:
- Parents will demonstrate two or more of the following physical interactions: good eye contact, touching baby, holding baby close, attempting to comfort baby, kissing baby.
- Parents will demonstrate two or more of the following social interactions: calling baby by name, making positive comments about baby, asking questions about baby, asking questions about baby care, and talking to baby.

NURSING DIAGNOSIS: Altered family processes related to illness of family member

EXPECTED OUTCOME: Woman and her family will cope effectively with her illness.

Nursing Interventions	Rationale
Encourage woman to express her concerns to her partner. Assist couple in planning ways to manage while woman is hospitalized and after her discharge.	Illness of any family member impacts the entire family. This is especially true when the family situation is such that the mother is the primary nurturer and she is absent. Family members attempt to continue their own roles while also assuming the tasks of the missing mother. This can result in crisis.

THROMBOEMBOLIC DISEASE continued

Nursing Interventions	Rationale

Encourage partner or support person to bring other children to hospital to visit mother and meet new sibling.

Encourage partner or support person to bring in family pictures. Encourage phone calls.

Contact social services if indicated to obtain additional assistance for family if needed.

OUTCOME MET IF:
- Family visits woman frequently.
- Woman and family verbalize plan for division of family tasks while the woman is hospitalized and understanding of potential needs of woman once released from hospital.

NURSING DIAGNOSIS: Knowledge deficit related to lack of information about the DVT/thrombophlebitis, its treatment, preventive measures, and the medication, warfarin

EXPECTED OUTCOME: Woman will understand her condition, its treatment, and long-term implications.

Nursing Interventions	Rationale

Discuss ways of avoiding circulatory stasis such as avoiding prolonged standing, sitting and crossing legs.

Review need to wear support stockings and to plan for rest periods with legs elevated.

In the presence of DVT, discuss the following:

1. The use of warfarin, its side effects, possible interactions with other medications, and need to have dosage assessed through periodic checks of the prothrombin time

2. Signs of bleeding, which may be associated with warfarin sodium and which need to be reported immediately, including the following: hematuria, epistaxis, ecchymosis, bleeding gums, and rectal bleeding

3. Monitor menstrual flow: bleeding may be heavier.

4. Review need for woman to eat a consistent amount of leafy green vegetables (lettuce, cabbage, brussels sprouts, broccoli) every day.

5. Instruct the woman to report *any* bleeding that continues more than 10 minutes.

6. Instruct the woman to do the following:
   - Routinely inspect the body for bruising.
   - Carry MedicAlert card indicating she is on anticoagulant therapy.
   - Use electric razor to avoid scratching skin.
   - Use soft bristle toothbrush.
   - Avoid alcohol intake or keep intake at minimum.
   - Avoid taking any other drugs without checking with the physician.
   - Note that stools may change color to pink, red, or black as a result of anticoagulant use.
   - Advise all health providers, including dentists, that she is taking anticoagulants.

Such discussion is essential to help the woman understand the condition, her medication, and its implications. She must have a clear understanding to be able to provide effective self-care.

These foods are high in vitamin K and will affect balance between dose of warfarin and PT.

OUTCOME MET IF:
- Woman verbalizes understanding of ways to avoid circulatory stasis, need to wear supportive stockings, medication dosage and side effects, and the importance of a balanced diet high in vitamin K.
- Woman verbalizes understanding of signs and symptoms of bleeding that need to be reported to health care provider.

Essential Nursing Activities to Achieve Outcomes

1. Assess for the following:
   a. Homan's sign
   b. Pain or tenderness in extremity
   c. Edema in extremity
   d. Skin color
   e. Peripheral pulses
   f. Temperature
   g. Side effects of medication: hematuria, epistaxis, ecchymosis, bleeding gums
   h. Sudden chest pain
   i. Apprehension
   j. Cough
   k. Tachycardia
   l. Shortness of breath
   m. Diaphoresis
2. Ensure the woman has bed rest as ordered.

3. Elevate affected extremity.
4. Apply warm, moist packs.
5. Administer medications as ordered.
6. Promptly report/treat any signs or symptoms of bleeding or pulmonary embolism.
7. Answer any questions the woman or her family may have regarding treatment or medications.
8. Provide discharge teaching regarding:
   a. Ways to avoid circulatory stasis
   b. Medications
   c. Support stockings
   d. Rest periods with legs elevated
   e. Importance of complying with prescribed medical plan
   f. Signs/symptoms to report to health care provider
9. Provide list or make appropriate referrals to available community resources.

dentists, that she is taking anticoagulants. She should also have vitamin K available in case bleeding occurs. Warfarin is excreted in the breast milk and thus may present problems for breastfeeding mothers. Women who wish to continue nursing may be maintained at home on low doses of subcutaneous heparin, because heparin is not excreted in breast milk.

Home Care

Because the mother with postpartum thromboembolic disease will depend on others for much of her initial home care, it is helpful for the father to be involved in preparations for discharge. Ample opportunities should be provided for questions to be answered and instructions clarified, verbally and in writing. The nurse will evaluate the extent to which both mother and father have understood instructions regarding the plan of care. It is especially important before discharge to assess the couple's plans in order to assure complete bed rest for the mother. They might explore ways for her to maintain bed rest and still spend quality time with her newborn and any other children. For example, young children can sit on the bed for storytelling or play quiet games, and the newborn's crib can be placed adjacent to the mother's bed.

Many concerns will not surface until the couple actually returns home and fully comprehends the reality of their situation. For that reason it is valuable to provide them with an accessible resource person and to plan telephone or home visit follow-up care.

The father may be assuming multiple roles in the circumstances—household manager, parent, worker, and care giver. Fatigue is inevitable. There may be financial concerns as a result of prolonged health care and/or his extended time away from work to care for the family. The couple must keep their communication lines open and spend quality time together. Referral to social services and assessment of the presence and use of a continued support system and coping strategies are necessary to avert potential crises.

Signs of postpartum thrombophlebitis may not occur until after discharge from the hospital. Consequently, all couples must be taught about the signs and symptoms and to appreciate the importance of reporting them immediately and of not massaging the affected leg. Should signs and symptoms occur after discharge from the postpartum unit, a short readmission might be required. Every effort is made in that case to allow mother, father, and newborn to remain together.

Evaluation

Anticipated outcomes of nursing care include:

- If thrombosis/thrombophlebitis develops, it is detected quickly and managed successfully without further complications.

- At discharge the woman is able to explain the purpose, dosage regimen, and necessary precautions associated with any prescribed medications such as anticoagulants.

- The woman can discuss self-care measures and ongoing therapies (such as the use of elastic stockings) that are indicated.

- The woman has bonded successfully with her newborn and is able to care for the baby effectively.

Pulmonary Embolism

A sudden onset of dyspnea accompanied by sweating, pallor, cyanosis, confusion, systemic hypotension, cough (with or without hemoptysis), tachycardia, shortness of breath, fever, and increased jugular pressure may indicate **pulmonary embolism,** a blockage of the pulmonary artery. Chest pain that mimics heart attack, coupled with the woman's verbalized fear of imminent death and complaint of pressure in the bowel and rectum, should alert the nurse to the extensive size of the embolus. A friction rub and evidence of atelectasis may be noted upon auscultation. A gallop (heart) rhythm may be present even if respiratory inspiration is normal, although smaller emboli may present with only transient syncope, tightness of the chest, or unexplained pyrexia.

Even x-ray films and EKG changes and laboratory data are not always reliable. If a case of pulmonary embolism is suspected, prompt treatment should begin even in the absence of corroborative data. If the embolism is small and heparin therapy is begun quickly, the chance of survival is excellent. However, when a large thrombus occludes a major pulmonary vessel, death may occur before therapy can even begin.

Therapy involves the administration of a variety of intravenous medications, such as meperidine hydrochloride to relieve the pain, lidocaine to correct any arrhythmias, and drugs such as papaverine hydrochloride and aminophylline to reduce spasms of the bronchi and coronary and pulmonary vessels. Oxygen is administered, and heparin infusion is begun. In severe cases an embolectomy may be necessary, although fibrinolytic therapy with medications (such as streptokinase) that lyse clots may be tried first.

CARE OF THE WOMAN WITH A URINARY TRACT INFECTION (UTI)

The postpartal woman is at increased risk of developing urinary tract problems due to the normal postpartal diuresis, increased bladder capacity, decreased bladder sensitivity from stretching and/or trauma, and possible inhibited neural control of the bladder following the use of general or regional anesthesia and contamination from catheterization.

Emptying the bladder is vital. Women who have not sufficiently recovered from the effects of anesthesia cannot void spontaneously, and catheterization is necessary.

Retention of residual urine, bacteria introduced at the time of catheterization, and a bladder traumatized by childbirth combine to provide an excellent environment for the development of cystitis.

Overdistention of the Bladder

Overdistention occurs postpartally when the woman is unable to empty her bladder as a result of the predisposing factors previously identified.

Medical Therapy

Overdistention in the early postpartal period is often managed by draining the bladder with a straight catheter as a one-time measure. If the overdistention recurs or is diagnosed later in the postpartal period, an indwelling catheter is generally ordered for 24 hours.

APPLYING THE NURSING PROCESS

Nursing Assessment

The overdistended bladder appears as a large mass, reaching sometimes to the umbilicus and displacing the uterine fundus upward. There is increased vaginal bleeding, the fundus is boggy, and the woman may complain of cramping as the uterus attempts to contract. Some women also experience backache and restlessness.

Nursing Diagnosis

Nursing diagnoses that may apply when a woman has difficulties due to overdistention include the following:

- Risk for infection related to urinary stasis secondary to overdistention
- Urinary retention related to decreased bladder sensitivity and normal postpartal diuresis

Nursing Plan and Implementation

Diligent monitoring of the bladder during the recovery period and preventive health measures greatly reduce the chance for overdistention of the bladder. Encouraging the mother to void spontaneously and helping her use the toilet, if possible, or the bedpan if she has received conductive anesthesia, prevent overdistention in most cases. The nurse assists the woman to a normal position for voiding (ie, sitting with the legs and feet lower than the trunk) and provides privacy to encourage voiding. The woman should be medicated for whatever pain she may be having before attempting to void because pain may cause a reflex spasm of the urethra. Ice packs applied to the perineum immediately postpartum will minimize any edema, which may interfere with voiding. Pouring warm water over the perineum or having the woman void in a sitz bath may also help.

If catheterization becomes necessary, careful, meticulous, aseptic technique should be employed during catheter insertion. The vagina and vulva are traumatized to some degree by vaginal birth, and edema is common. This edema may obscure the urinary meatus; therefore the nurse needs to be extremely careful in cleansing the vulva and inserting the catheter. It is imperative to discard a catheter that has inadvertently been introduced into the vagina and thus contaminated. Because catheterization is an uncomfortable procedure due to the postpartal trauma and edema of the tissue, the nurse should be careful and gentle not only in inserting the catheter but also in handling and cleaning the perineal area.

If the amount of urine drained from the bladder reaches 900–1000 mL, the catheter should be clamped and taped firmly to the woman's leg. The procedure, including taking the woman's vital signs before and after the procedure and noting her responses, should be carefully charted. After an hour the catheter may be unclamped and removed or, in the case of an indwelling catheter, placed on gravity drainage. This technique protects the bladder and avoids rapid intra-abdominal decompression. When the indwelling catheter is removed, a urine specimen is often sent to the laboratory. The tip of the catheter may also be removed and sent for culture.

Evaluation

Anticipated outcomes of nursing care include:

- The woman voids adequately to meet the demands of the increased fluid shifts during the postpartal period.
- The woman doesn't develop infection due to stasis of urine.
- The woman actively incorporates self-care measures to decrease bladder overdistention.

Cystitis (Lower Urinary Tract Infection)

E coli has been demonstrated to be the causative agent in most cases of postpartal cystitis and pyelonephritis (in both lower and upper UTI). In most cases the infection ascends the urinary tract from the urethra to the bladder and then to the kidneys because vesiculoureteral reflux forces contaminated urine into the renal pelvis.

Medical Therapy

When cystitis is suspected, a clean-catch midstream urine sample is obtained for microscopic examination, culture, and sensitivity tests. The specimen may require collection by the nurse with the woman on a bedpan because few postpartal women can collect a true midstream, clean-catch specimen without contaminating the specimen with lochia. A catheterized specimen is avoided when possible because of the increased risk of infection. When the bacterial concentration is greater than 100,000 colonies of the same organism per milliliter of fresh urine, infection is generally present. Counts between 10,000 and 100,000 suggest infection, particularly if clinical symptoms are noted.

Treatment is theoretically delayed until urine culture and sensitivity reports are available. In the clinical setting, however, antibiotic therapy is often initiated using one of the short-acting sulfonamides, nitrofurantoin (Macrodantin), or, in the case of sulfa allergy, ampicillin. The antibiotic is begun immediately and then can be changed if indicated by the results of the sensitivity report (Cunningham et al 1993). Antispasmodics may be given to relieve discomfort.

Pyelonephritis (Upper Urinary Tract Infection)

Pyelonephritis is an inflammation of the renal pelvis that is usually the result of infection. In most cases the infection has ascended from the lower urinary tract. It occurs more commonly on the right, although both kidneys may be affected. If untreated, the renal cortex may be damaged and kidney function impaired.

Medical Therapy

When pyelonephritis is diagnosed, antibiotic therapy is begun immediately. If sensitivity reports so indicate, the antibiotic can be changed later. Bed rest and careful monitoring of intake and output are necessary to detect the development of bacterial shock. Fluids are encouraged; if nausea and vomiting are severe, however, fluids are administered intravenously. Antispasmodics, analgesics, and antipyretics are given to relieve discomfort. The woman usually continues to take antibiotics for 2 to 4 weeks after clinical and bacteriologic response. A clean-catch urine culture should be obtained 2 weeks after completion of therapy and then periodically for the next 2 years. An intravenous pyelogram may be ordered in 2 to 4 months to identify any residual renal damage.

Continuation of breastfeeding during therapy is limited only by the degree of the mother's malaise and clinical discomfort. For the breastfeeding mother the antibiotic should be selected carefully to avoid problems for the infant via the milk.

APPLYING THE NURSING PROCESS

Nursing Assessment

Symptoms of cystitis often appear 2 to 3 days after birth. The initial symptoms of cystitis may include frequency, urgency, dysuria, and nocturia. Hematuria and suprapubic pain may also be present. A slightly elevated temperature may occur, but systemic symptoms are often absent.

When a urinary tract infection progresses to pyelonephritis, systemic symptoms usually occur, and the woman becomes acutely ill. Symptoms include chills, high fever, flank pain (unilateral or bilateral), nausea, and vomiting, in addition to all the signs of lower UTI. Costovertebral pain also may be present. The nurse obtains a urine culture so that sensitivity tests can identify the causative organism.

Nursing Diagnosis

Nursing diagnoses that may apply if a woman develops a UTI postpartally include the following:

- Knowledge deficit related to lack of information about long-term effects of pyelonephritis
- Knowledge deficit related to lack of information about self-care measures to prevent UTI

Nursing Plan and Implementation

As with other conditions, the nurse plays an important role in preventing the development of UTI. Screening for asymptomatic bacteriuria in pregnancy should be routine. Frequent emptying of the bladder during labor and the postpartum period should be encouraged to prevent overdistention and trauma to the bladder. Catheterization technique and nursing actions to prevent overdistention were previously discussed and also apply. The woman with pyelonephritis must understand the importance of follow-up care after discharge to prevent recurrence or further complications.

Teaching for Self-Care

The postpartal woman should be advised to continue good perineal hygiene following discharge. She is also advised to maintain a good fluid intake and to empty her bladder whenever she feels the urge to void, but at least every 2 to 4 hours while awake. The new mother should void before sexual intercourse (to prevent bladder trauma) and following intercourse (to wash contaminants from the vicinity of the urinary meatus). Wearing cotton crotch underwear to facilitate air circulation also reduces the risk of urinary tract infection.

Evaluation

Anticipated outcomes of nursing care include:

- Signs of urinary tract infection are detected quickly, and the condition is treated successfully.
- The woman incorporates self-care measures to prevent the recurrence of UTI as part of her personal hygiene routine.
- The woman continues with any long-term therapy or follow-up.
- Maternal-infant attachment is maintained, and the woman is able to care for her newborn effectively.

CARE OF THE WOMAN WITH MASTITIS

Mastitis is an inflammation of the breast generally caused by *Staphylococcus aureus* and primarily seen in breastfeeding mothers. Symptoms seldom occur before the second to fourth week postpartum, so birthing center nurses often are not fully aware of how uncomfortable and acutely ill the woman may be. The most common source of the bacteria is the infant's nose and throat, although other sources include the hands of the mother or of hospital personnel or the woman's circulating blood.

Poor drainage of milk, presence of a pathogenic organism, lowered maternal defenses due to fatigue or stress, poor hygiene practices, or nipple tissue damage make the woman susceptible to mastitis. Tight clothing, missed feedings, poor support of pendulous breasts, lack of regular breast pumping when away from the baby, or a baby who suddenly begins to sleep through the night can all result in milk stasis, which is a milder inflammatory condition.

Thomsen and associates (1984) has suggested a classification of inflammatory symptoms of the breast based on leukocytes and bacterial counts per milliliter of breast milk: (1) milk stasis, (2) noninfectious inflammation of the breast, and (3) infectious mastitis. Milk stasis is a relatively mild, short-lived condition, usually without fever and not requiring antibiotics. Noninfectious inflammation of the breast presents with more severe inflammatory symptoms that last for several days. Infectious mastitis is a more serious infection with fever, headache, flulike symptoms, and a warm, reddened, painful area of the breast (Figure 36–3).

In other cases *Candida albicans* is the causative organism of mastitis, entering the breast through a small fissure or abrasion on the nipple. Signs include late-onset nipple pain, followed by shooting pain during and between feedings. Eventually, the skin of the affected breast will become pink, flaking, and pruritic.

Medical Therapy

Diagnosis is usually based on symptoms and physical examination, even while waiting for laboratory results. The need for culture and antibody sensitivity of the breast milk remains controversial, although most experts agree on the need for cultures if there is a recurrence of the mastitis. Treatment involves bed rest, increased fluid intake, a supportive bra, feeding the baby frequently, local application of heat, and analgesics for discomfort. Early treatment may prevent the progression of milk stasis and noninfectious inflammation to mastitis. Treatment of mastitis includes all of the measures mentioned previously plus a 10-day course of antibiotics (usually a penicillinase-resistant penicillin). Improved outcome, a decreased duration of symptoms, and decreased incidence of breast abscess result if the breasts continue to be emptied by either nursing or pumping. Whether to continue nursing or not has been controversial in the past, but most experts now recommend continued nursing in most cases. The woman should be contacted within 24 hours of initiation of treatment to ensure that symptoms are subsiding (Lawrence 1994).

Occasionally, the process of mastitis may continue, and a frank abscess develops. The mother's milk and any drainage from the nipple should be cultured and antibiotic therapy instituted. In addition it is usually necessary to incise surgically and drain the abscessed area. If multiple abscesses are present, multiple incisions will be necessary, usually under general anesthesia. After incision and drainage, the area is packed with sterile gauze. The packing is gradually decreased to permit proper healing.

Often the breast is covered with a sterile surgical dressing, and access to the breast is temporarily inhibited, making breastfeeding impossible. If possible, the dressing should be applied so that the woman can continue to pump her breast, thereby avoiding engorgement and maintaining lactation. A recent study recommended ultrasonically guided percutaneous treatment for acute puerperal breast abscesses (Karstrup et al 1993). This method allows continued breastfeeding.

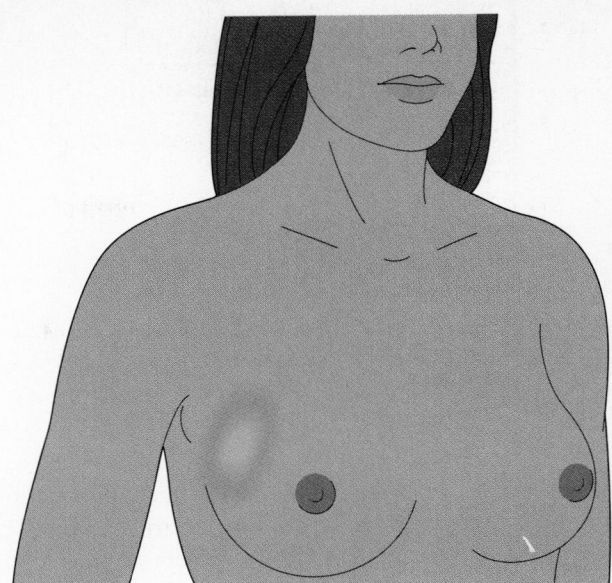

FIGURE 36-3 Mastitis. Erythemia and swelling are present in the upper outer quadrant of the breast. Axillary lymph nodes are enlarged and tender.

APPLYING THE NURSING PROCESS

Nursing Assessment

Daily assessment of breast consistency, skin color, surface temperature, nipple condition, and presence of pain is essential to detect early signs of problems that may predispose to mastitis. The mother should be observed nursing her baby to ensure use of proper breastfeeding technique.

If an infection has developed, the nurse should assess for contributing factors such as cracked nipples, poor hygiene, engorgement, supplemental feedings, change in routine or infant feeding pattern, abrupt weaning, or lack of proper breast support so that these factors may be corrected as part of the treatment plan.

Nursing Diagnosis

Nursing diagnoses that may apply to the woman with mastitis include the following:

- Knowledge deficit related to lack of information about appropriate breastfeeding practices
- Ineffective breastfeeding related to pain secondary to development of mastitis

Nursing Plan and Implementation

Prevention of mastitis is far simpler than therapy. Ideally, mothers should be instructed in proper breastfeeding technique prenatally. If not, instruction should begin as soon as possible in the postpartal period. The nurse should help the mother breastfeed soon after birth and should review correct technique. All women, even those not breastfeeding, are encouraged to wear a good supportive bra at all times to avoid milk stasis, especially in the lower lobes.

Meticulous hand washing by all personnel is the primary measure for preventing epidemic nursery infections and subsequent maternal mastitis. Prompt attention to mothers who have blocked milk ducts eliminates stagnant milk as a growth medium for bacteria. If the mother finds that one area of her breast feels distended, she can rotate the position of her infant for nursing, manually express milk remaining in the breast after nursing (usually only necessary if the infant is not sucking well), or massage the caked area toward the nipple as the infant nurses. Early identification of and intervention for sore nipples are also essential, as is prompt assessment of the nursing mother's breasts when thrush is discovered in her newborn's mouth.

Teaching for Self-Care

The nurse stresses to the breastfeeding woman the importance of adequate breast and nipple care to prevent the development of cracks and fissures, a common portal for bacterial entry. For a detailed discussion of breastfeeding see Chapter 30.

The woman should be aware of the importance of regular, complete emptying of the breasts to prevent engorgement and stasis. She should also understand the role of let-down in successful breastfeeding and the principle of supply and demand. Breastfeeding mothers who will

TABLE 36-2   Comparison of Findings of Engorgement, Plugged Duct, and Mastitis

Characteristics	Engorgement	Plugged Duct	Mastitis
Onset	Gradual, immediately postpartum	Gradual, after feedings	Sudden, after 10 days
Site	Bilateral	Unilateral	Usually unilateral
Swelling and heat	Generalized	May shift, little or no heat	Localized, red, hot, and swollen
Pain	Generalized	Mild but localized	Intense but localized
Body temperature	<38.4 C	<38.4 C	>38.4 C
Systemic symptoms	Feels well	Feels well	Flulike symptoms

SOURCE: Lawrence RA: *Breastfeeding—A Guide for the Medical Profession.* St Louis: Mosby, 1994, p 261.

be returning to work outside the home need information on how to do so successfully. Because mastitis tends to develop following discharge, it is important to include information about signs and symptoms in the discharge teaching (Table 36–2). All flulike symptoms should be considered a sign of mastitis until proved otherwise. If symptoms develop, the woman should contact her care giver immediately because prompt treatment helps to avoid abscess formation.

Home Care

The home care nurse who suspects mastitis on the basis of assessment findings refers the woman to the physician. The nurse may be asked to obtain a sample of breast milk to be cultured for identification of the causative organism.

The woman who develops mastitis may need to temporarily discontinue breastfeeding. In that case she will need to learn techniques for bottle-feeding and formula preparation, including sterilization, if necessary. The home care nurse can help the mother obtain an appropriate breast pump to help her maintain lactation and can provide opportunities for demonstration and return demonstration of pumping.

News that one must discontinue breastfeeding, even temporarily, is generally met with feelings of disappointment. Some mothers experience a sense of failure. Helping the mother deal with such feelings is an important component of care. Referral to a lactation consultant or to La Leche League can be invaluable to the woman's physical and emotional adjustment to mastitis.

Evaluation

Anticipated outcomes of nursing care include:

- The woman is aware of the signs and symptoms of mastitis.
- The woman's mastitis is detected early and treated successfully.
- The woman can continue breastfeeding if she chooses.

- The woman understands self-care measures she can employ to prevent the recurrence of the mastitis.

CARE OF THE WOMAN WITH A POSTPARTAL PSYCHIATRIC DISORDER

Many types of psychiatric problems may occur in the postpartum period. The classification of postpartum psychiatric disorders is a subject of some controversy. The *Diagnostic and Statistical Manual of Mental Disorders*, 4th edition (DSM-IV), has added a postpartum onset specifier to the mood disorder diagnostic category of psychiatric disorders. Inwood (1989) proposes that postpartum psychiatric disorders be considered one diagnosable syndrome with three subclasses: (1) adjustment reaction with depressed mood, (2) postpartum psychosis, and (3) postpartum major mood disorder. The incidence, etiology, symptoms, treatment, and prognosis vary with each subclass.

Adjustment reaction with depressed mood is also known as postpartum, maternal, or "baby" blues. It occurs in as many as 75% of mothers and is characterized by mild depression interspersed with happier feelings. Postpartum blues typically occurs within a few days after the baby's birth and is self-limiting, lasting from a few hours to 2 weeks. It is more severe in primiparas and seems related to the rapid alteration of estrogen, progesterone, and prolactin levels after birth. New mothers experiencing postpartum blues commonly report feeling overwhelmed, unable to cope, fatigued, anxious, irritable, and oversensitive. A key feature is episodic tearfulness, often without an identifiable reason.

Validating the existence of this phenomenon, labeling it as a real but normal adjustment reaction, and providing reassurance can offer a measure of relief. Assistance with self and infant care, information, and family support is helpful to recovery. The partner should be encouraged to watch for and report signs that the new mother is not returning to a more normal mood but is instead slipping into a deeper depression.

Postpartum psychosis, which has an incidence of 1 to 2 per 1000, usually becomes evident within the first 3 months postpartum. Though rare, this phenomenon receives considerable publicity because of the tragic 10% rate of suicide or infanticide associated with it (Inwood 1989).

Symptoms include agitation, hyperactivity, insomnia, mood lability, confusion, irrationality, difficulty remembering or concentrating, poor judgment, delusions, and hallucinations. Recovery is usually good unless schizophrenia is diagnosed. There is a 10% to 25% recurrence rate in subsequent pregnancies. Risk factors include (1) previous puerperal psychosis; (2) manic-depressive history; (3) prenatal stressors, such as lack of social support, lack of a partner, and low socioeconomic status; (4) obsessive personality; and (5) a family history of a mood disorder. Treatment may include hospitalization, antipsychotics, sedatives, electroconvulsive therapy, removal of the infant, social support, and psychotherapy.

Postpartum major mood disorder, also known as postpartum depression, develops in about 10% of all postpartum women. Although it may occur at any time during the first postpartum year, the greatest risks occur around the fourth week, just prior to the initiation of menses, and upon weaning.

Many of the symptoms of this major depression are indistinguishable from serious depression at other times: sadness, frequent crying, insomnia, appetite change, difficulty concentrating and making decisions, feelings of worthlessness, obsessive thoughts of inadequacy as a person and parent, lack of interest in usual activities (including sexual relations), and lack of concern about personal appearance. Persistent anxiety further contributes to the woman's feeling out of control. Irritability and hostility toward others, including the newborn, may be evident. Beck (1993) describes these debilitating symptoms as "teetering on the edge" between sanity and insanity. Women participating in Beck's qualitative research on postpartum depression described a sense of living their daily life in a sort of fog, from which they believed they would never emerge. Once they improved, they often grieved over the time lost with their newborns while in this "fog."

Risk factors for postpartum depression include:

- Primiparity
- Ambivalence about maintaining the pregnancy
- History of postpartum depression or bipolar illness
- Lack of social support
- Lack of a stable relationship with parents or partner
- The woman's dissatisfaction with herself
- Lack of a supportive relationship with her parents, especially her father, as a child (Inwood 1989)

RESEARCH IN PRACTICE

Cheryl Beck used grounded theory methodology to discover the underlying social-psychologic problem of postpartum depression and to examine the processes used by participants to resolve this fundamental problem. The sample for this study consisted of 12 white, postpartum, married women who had attended a postpartum depression support group. The time period since the women had delivered ranged from 6 weeks to 3 years. Data collection incorporated in-depth interviews and field notes from the support group meetings.

The author used a constant comparative method to analyze the data. Analysis revealed the basic social-psychologic problem of postpartum depression to be loss of control. As described by the author, the basic social-psychologic process unfolded as "teetering on the edge" or walking the fine line between being sane and insane.

Teetering on the edge consists of four stages or constructs: encountering terror, dying of self, struggling to survive, and regaining control. Each stage contains several categories. Encountering terror, or stage one, encompasses the three conditions of horrifying anxiety attacks, enveloping fogginess, and relentless obsessive thinking. As a consequence of the conditions in stage one, stage two resulted as a perceived dying of the mother's normal self. This stage includes alarming feelings of unrealness, isolating of self, and contemplating and attempting self-destruction. In "alarming unrealness" the participants said they did not feel real, and even their husbands asked where their wives had gone. Stage three, struggling to survive, incorporated the strategies of battling the system, praying for relief, and seeking solace in a support group. Mothers described having to battle the health care system to get appropriate referrals, listen to patronizing advice from physicians, and find financial resources to cover their psychiatric care. The final stage of teetering on the edge entails regaining control. This stage is characterized by unpredictable transitioning, mourning lost time, and guarded recovery.

Clinical Application of Study

When a nurse interacts with a client who displays or describes symptoms of postpartum depression, the nurse can assess the woman's stage of "teetering on the edge" and help both the mother and her partner recognize the potential for movement through that process. The nurse could also discuss this study with the client as a means of helping the mother identify effective coping strategies and seeing that other women were able to resolve the basic psychologic problem of loss of control.

SOURCE: Beck C: Teetering on the edge: A substantive theory of postpartum depression. *Nurs Res* 1993; 42(1):42.

Certain other factors that have been highly correlated with postpartum depression may be assessed via screening questions for the disorder: (1) history of infertility, (2) early menarche (before age 11), (3) unrealistic expectations of parenthood, and (4) adverse emotional reactions (irritability or depression) resulting from earlier use of oral contraceptives (LaGrone 1992).

Medication, individual or group psychotherapy, and practical assistance with child care and other demands of daily life are common treatment measures. Support groups have proven to be successful adjuncts to such treatment. Within a support group of postpartal women and their partners, a couple may feel consolation that they are not alone in their experience. Moreover, it provides a forum for gaining information about postpartum depression, learning stress reduction measures, and experiencing renewed self-esteem and support (Berchtold & Burroughs 1990).

APPLYING THE NURSING PROCESS

Nursing Assessment

Assessment for factors predisposing a client to postpartum depression or psychosis should begin prenatally. Questions designed to detect problems can be included as part of the routine prenatal history interview or questionnaire. Women with a personal or family history of psychiatric disease, particularly postpartum depression or psychosis, need prenatal instructions on the signs and symptoms of depression and may need additional emotional support. If not done previously, the woman is assessed for predisposing factors during her labor and postpartum stay.

In providing daily care the nurse observes the woman for signs of depression: anxiety, irritability, poor concentration, forgetfulness, sleeping difficulties, appetite change, fatigue, tearfulness, and statements indicating feelings of failure and self-accusation. Severity and duration of symptoms should be noted. Behavior and verbalization that are bizarre or seem to indicate a potential for violence against herself or others, including the infant, are reported as soon as possible for further evaluation.

The nurse needs to be aware that many normal physiologic changes of the puerperium are similar to symptoms of depression (lack of sexual interest, appetite change, and fatigue). It is essential that observations be as specific and as objective as possible and that they be carefully documented.

Nursing Diagnosis

Possible nursing diagnoses that may apply to a woman with a postpartum psychiatric disorder include:

- Ineffective individual coping related to postpartum depression
- Risk for altered parenting related to postpartal mental illness

Nursing Plan and Implementation

Nurses working in antepartal settings or teaching childbirth classes play indispensable roles in helping prospective parents appreciate the life-style changes and role demands associated with parenthood. Offering realistic information and anticipatory guidance and debunking myths about the perfect mother or perfect newborn may help prevent postpartum depression.

The nurse should alert the mother, spouse, and other family members to the possibility of postpartum blues in the early days after birth and reassure them of the short-term nature of the condition. Symptoms of postpartum depression should be described and the mother encouraged to call her health care provider if symptoms become severe, if they fail to subside quickly, or if at any time she feels she is unable to function. Encouraging the mother to plan how she will manage at home and providing concrete suggestions on how to cope will aid in her adjustment to motherhood. Telephone follow-up at 3 weeks postpartum to ask if the mother is experiencing difficulties is also helpful (Inwood 1989). Home visits, especially for early discharge families, are essential to fostering positive adjustments for the new family constellation.

Women with a history of depression or postpartum psychosis should be referred to a mental health professional for counseling and biweekly visits between the second and sixth weeks postpartum for evaluation of depression. Medication, social support, and assistance with child care may also be necessary.

In all women the presence of three symptoms or one symptom for 3 days may signal serious depression. Referral to a mental health professional should be made immediately. Immediate referral should also be made if rejection of the infant or threatened or actual aggression against the infant has occurred. In such cases the newborn is never left unattended with the mother.

Home Care

A diagnosis of postpartum depression or other psychiatric disorder will pose major problems for the family, especially the father. The symptoms of these disorders are difficult to witness and may be harder to understand than physical problems like hemorrhage or infection. The father may feel hurt by his partner's hostility and may worry that she is becoming insane, or be baffled by her mood swings and lack of concern about herself, the newborn, or household responsibilities. He may be troubled by their lack of intimacy or deteriorating communication. Certainly, he has cause for concern about how the newborn and any other children are being affected. There may be very real practical matters to handle—running the household; managing the children, including the totally dependent newborn; and caring for the mother—added to his usual routines and work responsibilities. It is not surprising that even in the most supportive families relationships may suffer in response to these circumstances. It is often a family member who in desperation makes contact with the health care agency. This is especially difficult when the mother is reluctant to admit she is suffering emotional difficulty or is too ill to recognize her own needs.

Information, emotional support, and assistance in providing or obtaining care for the infant may be needed. The nurse can assist family members by identifying community resources and making referrals to public health nursing services and social services. Postpartum follow-up (home visits, group support, and telephone follow-up), which all postpartum women need, is especially important for the woman at risk for or experiencing postpartum depression (Hampson 1989).

Evaluation

Anticipated outcomes of nursing care include:

- Signs of potential postpartal disorders are detected quickly, and therapy is implemented.
- The newborn is cared for effectively by the father or another support person until the mother is able to do so.

KEY CONCEPTS

Nursing assessment and intervention play large roles in preventing postpartum complications.

The main causes of early postpartal hemorrhage are uterine atony, lacerations of the vagina and cervix, and retained placental fragments.

The most common postpartal infection is endometritis, which is limited to the uterine cavity.

Thromboembolic disease originating in the veins of the leg, thigh, or pelvis may occur in the antepartum or postpartum periods and carries with it the potential for creating a pulmonary embolus.

A postpartal woman is at increased risk for developing urinary tract problems due to normal postpartal diuresis, increased bladder capacity, decreased bladder sensitivity from stretching and/or trauma, and, possibly, inhibited neural control of the bladder following the use of anesthetic agents.

Mastitis is an inflammation of the breast often caused by *Staphylococcus aureus* and is primarily seen in breastfeeding women. Symptoms seldom occur before the second to fourth postpartal week.

Although many different types of psychiatric problems may be encountered in the postpartal period, depression is the most common. Episodes occur frequently in the week after birth and are typically transient.

Telephone calls and home visits are effective measures for extending comprehensive care into the home setting of the postpartum family at risk.

REFERENCES

Andrew A et al: Subinvolution of the uteroplacental arteries: An immunohistochemical study. *Int J Gynecol Pathol* 1993; 12(1):28.

Beck CT: Teetering on the edge: A substantive theory of postpartum depression. *Nurs Res* 1993; 42(1):42.

Berchtold N, Burroughs M: Reaching out: Depression after delivery support group network. *NAACOG's Clin Issues Perinatal Women Health Nurs* 1990; 1(3):385.

Coates M, Riordan J: Breastfeeding during maternal or infant illness. *NAACOG's Clin Issues Perinatal Women Health Nurs* 1992; 3(4):683.

Cosico JN et al: Indications, management and patient education for anticoagulation therapy during pregnancy. *MCN* 1993; 17(3):130.

Cunningham FG, MacDonald PC, Gant NF (editors): *Williams Obstetrics*, 19th ed. Norwalk, CT: Appleton & Lange, 1993.

Diagnostic and Statistical Manual of Mental Disorders: DSM IV, 4th ed. Washington DC: American Psychiatric Association, 1994.

Donaldson NE: Effect of telephone postpartum follow-up: A clinical trial. *Diss Abstr Int* 49:2567B. University Microfilms International DA8809495, 1988.

Eschenbach DA: Pelvic infections and sexually transmitted diseases. In: *Danforth's Obstetrics and Gynecology*, 7th ed. Scott JR et al (editors). Philadelphia: Lippincott, 1994.

Gant NF, Cunningham FG: *Basic Gynecology and Obstetrics*. Norwalk, CT: Appleton & Lange, 1993.

Hampson SJ: Nursing interventions for the first three postpartum months. *JOGNN* March/April 1989; 18:116.

Inwood DG: Postpartum psychiatric disorders. In: *Comprehensive Textbook of Psychiatry*, 5th ed, vol 1. Kaplan HI, Sadock BJ (editors). Baltimore: Williams & Wilkins, 1989.

Kapernick PS: Postpartum hemorrhage and the abnormal puerperium. In: *Current Obstetric and Gynecologic Diagnosis and Treatment*. Pernoll ML (editor). Norwalk, CT: Appleton & Lange, 1991.

Karstrup S et al: Acute puerperal breast abscesses: US-guided drainage. *Radiology* 1993; 188(3):807.

LaGrone D: Postpartum depression: Challenges in obstetric, gynecologic, and neonatal nursing. Paper presented at the Medical Center of Central Georgia, Macon, July 16, 1992.

Lawrence RA: *Breastfeeding: A Guide for the Medical Profession*, 4th ed. St Louis: Mosby, 1994.

Mitty HA et al: Obstetric hemorrhage: Prophylactic and emergency arterial catheterization and embolotherapy. *Radiology* 1993; 188(1):183.

Monga M, Oshiro BT: Puerperal infections. *Semin Perinatol* 1993; 17(6):426.

Nathan L et al: The return of life-threatening puerperal sepsis caused by group A streptococci. *Am J Obstet Gynecol* 1993; 169(3):571.

Newton M: Postpartum hemorrhage. *Am J Obstet Gynecol* 1966; 94:711.

Peyser MR, Kuperminic MJ: Management of severe postpartum hemorrhage by intrauterine irrigation with prostaglandin E_2. *Am J Obstet Gynecol* 1990; 162:694.

Thomsen AC, Esperson T, Maiggard S: Course and treatment of milk stasis, noninfectious inflammation of the breast, and infectious mastitis in nursing women. *Am J Obstet Gynecol* 1984; 149(5):492.

Zlatnik FJ: The normal and abnormal puerperium. In: *Danforth's Obstetrics and Gynecology*, 7th ed. Scott JR et al (editors). Philadelphia: Lippincott, 1994.

APPENDICES

COMMON ABBREVIATIONS IN MATERNAL-NEWBORN AND WOMEN'S HEALTH NURSING

accel	Acceleration of fetal heart rate	EDC	Estimated date of confinement
AC	Abdominal circumference	EDD	Estimated date of delivery
AFAFP	Amniotic fluid α-fetoprotein	EFM	Electronic fetal monitoring
AFP	α-fetoprotein	EFW	Estimated fetal weight
AFV	Amniotic fluid volume	EIA	Enzyme immunoassay
AGA	Average for gestational age	ELF	Elective low forceps
AID or AIH	Artificial insemination donor (H designates mate is donor)	ELISA	Enzyme-linked immunosorbent assay
		epis	Episiotomy
ARBOW	Artificial rupture of bag of waters	ERT	Estrogen replacement therapy
AROM	Artificial rupture of membranes	FAD	Fetal activity diary
BAT	Brown adipose tissue (brown fat)	FAE	Fetal alcohol effects
BBT	Basal body temperature	FAS	Fetal alcohol syndrome
BL	Baseline (fetal heart rate baseline)	FBD	Fibrocystic breast disease
BOW	Bag of waters	FBM	Fetal breathing movements
BPD	Biparietal diameter *or* Bronchopulmonary dysplasia	FBS	Fetal blood sample *or* Fasting blood sugar test
BPP	Biophysical profile	FECG	Fetal electrocardiogram
BSE	Breast self-examination	FHR	Fetal heart rate
BSST	Breast self-stimulation test	FHT	Fetal heart tones
CC	Chest circumference *or* Cord compression	FL	Femur length
C–H	Crown-to-heel length	FM	Fetal movement
CID	Cytomegalic inclusion disease	FPG	Fasting plasma glucose test
CMV	Cytomegalovirus	FSH	Follicle-stimulating hormone
CNM	Certified nurse-midwife	FSHRH	Follicle-stimulating hormone–releasing hormone
CNS	Clinical nurse specialist		
CPAP	Continuous positive airway pressure	G or grav	Gravida
CPD	Cephalopelvic disproportion *or* Citrate-phosphate-dextrose	GDM	Gestational diabetes mellitus
		GIFT	Gamete intrafallopian transfer
CRL	Crown-rump length	GnRF	Gonadotropin-releasing factor
C/S	Cesarean section (or C-section)	GnRH	Gonadotropin-releasing hormone
CST	Contraction stress test	GTD	Gestational trophoblastic disease
CVA	Costovertebral angle	GTPAL	Gravida, term, preterm, abortion, living children; a system of recording maternity history
CVS	Chorionic villus sampling		
D & C	Dilatation and curettage		
decels	Deceleration of fetal heart rate	HA	Head-abdominal ratio
DFMR	Daily fetal movement response	HAI	Hemagglutination-inhibition test
dil	Dilatation	HC	Head compression
DRG	Diagnostic related groups	hCG	Human chorionic gonadotropin
DTR	Deep tendon reflexes	hCS	Human chorionic somatomammotropin (same as hPL)
ECMO	Extracorporal membrane oxygenator		
EDB	Estimated date of birth	HMD	Hyaline membrane disease

hMG	Human menopausal gonadotropin	Pap smear	Papanicolaou smear
hPL	Human placental lactogen	PDA	Patent ductus arteriosus
HPV	Human papilloma virus	PEEP	Positive end-expiratory pressure
HVH	Herpesvirus hominis	PG	Phosphatidylglycerol *or* Prostaglandin
IDM	Infant of a diabetic mother	PI	Phosphatidylinositol
IPG	Impedance phlebography	PID	Pelvic inflammatory disease
IU	International units	PIH	Pregnancy-induced hypertension
IUD	Intrauterine device	Pit	Pitocin
IUFD	Intrauterine fetal death	PKU	Phenylketonuria
IUGR	Intrauterine growth restriction	PMS	Premenstrual syndrome
IVF	In vitro fertilization	PPHN	Persistent pulmonary hypertension
LADA	Left-acromion-dorsal-anterior	Preemie	Premature infant
LADP	Left-acromion-dorsal-posterior	primip	Primapara
LBW	Low birth weight	PROM	Premature rupture of membranes
LDR	Labor, delivery, and recovery room	PSI	Prostaglandin synthesis inhibitor
LGA	Large for gestational age	PUBS	Percutaneous umbilical blood sampling
LH	Luteinizing hormone	RADA	Right-acromion-dorsal-anterior
LHRH	Luteinizing hormone–releasing hormone	RADP	Right-acromion-dorsal-posterior
LMA	Left-mentum-anterior	RDS	Respiratory distress syndrome
LML	Left mediolateral (episiotomy)	REM	Rapid eye movements
LMP	Last menstrual period *or* Left-mentum-posterior	RIA	Radioimmunoassay
		RLF	Retrolental fibroplasia
LMT	Left-mentum-transverse	RMA	Right-mentum-anterior
LOA	Left-occiput-anterior	RMP	Right-mentum-posterior
LOF	Low outlet forceps	RMT	Right-mentum-transverse
LOP	Left-occiput-posterior	ROA	Right-occiput-anterior
LOT	Left-occiput-transverse	ROM	Rupture of membranes
L/S	Lecithin/sphingomyelin ratio	ROP	Right-occiput-posterior *or* Retinopathy of prematurity
LSA	Left-sacrum-anterior		
LSP	Left-sacrum-posterior	ROT	Right-occiput-transverse
LST	Left-sacrum-transverse	RRA	Radioreceptor assay
MAS	Meconium aspiration syndrome	RSA	Right-sacrum-anterior
mec	Meconium	RSP	Right-sacrum-posterior
mec st	Meconium stain	RST	Right-sacrum-transverse
ML	Midline (episiotomy)	SET	Surrogate embryo transfer
MRI	Magnetic resonance imaging	SFD	Small for dates
MSAFP	Maternal serum α-fetoprotein	SGA	Small for gestational age
MUGB	4-methylumbelliferyl quanidinobenzoate	SIDS	Sudden infant death syndrome
multip	Multipara	SMB	Submentobregmatic diameter
NEC	Necrotizing enterocolitis	SOB	Suboccipitobregmatic diameter
NGU	Nongonococcal urethritis	SPA	Sperm penetration assay
NP	Nurse practitioner	SRBOW	Spontaneous rupture of the bag of waters
NSCST	Nipple stimulation contraction stress test	SROM	Spontaneous rupture of membranes
NST	Nonstress test *or* Nonshivering thermo-genesis	STI	Sexually transmitted infection
		STH	Somatotropic hormone
NSVD	Normal sterile vaginal delivery	STS	Serologic test for syphilis
NTD	Neural tube defects	SVE	Sterile vaginal exam
OA	Occiput anterior	TC	Thoracic circumference
OC	Oral contraceptives	TCM	Transcutaneous monitoring
OCT	Oxytocin challenge test	TDI	Therapeutic Donor Insemination
OF	Occipito-frontal diameter of fetal head	TNZ	Thermal neutral zone
OFC	Occipito-frontal circumference	TOL	Trail of labor
OGTT	Oral glucose tolerance test	TORCH	Toxoplasmosis, rubella, cytomegalovirus, herpesvirus hominis type 2
OM	Occipitomental (diameter)		
OP	Occiput posterior	TSS	Toxic shock syndrome
p	Para	$\overline{u}$	Umbilicus

UA	Uterine activity	VBAC	Vaginal birth after cesarean
UAC	Umbilical artery catheter	VDRL	Venereal Disease Research Laboratories
UAU	Uterine activity units	VLBW	Very low birth weight
UC	Uterine contraction	WIC	Supplemental food program for Women, Infants, and Children
UPI	Uteroplacental insufficiency		
US	Ultrasound	ZIFT	Zygote intrafallopian transfer

THE PREGNANT PATIENT'S BILL OF RIGHTS*

The Pregnant Patient has the right to participate in decisions involving her well-being and that of her unborn child, unless there is a clearcut medical emergency that prevents her participation. In addition to the rights set forth in the American Hospital Association's "Patient's Bill of Rights," the Pregnant Patient, because she represents *two* patients rather than one, should be recognized as having the additional rights listed below.

1. *The Pregnant Patient has the right*, prior to the administration of any drug or procedure, to be informed by the health professional caring for her of any potential direct or indirect effects, risks or hazards to herself or her unborn or newborn infant which may result from the use of a drug or procedure prescribed for or administered to her during pregnancy, labor, birth or lactation.

2. *The Pregnant Patient has the right*, prior to the proposed therapy, to be informed, not only of the benefits, risks and hazards of the proposed therapy but also of known alternative therapy, such as available childbirth education classes which could help to prepare the Pregnant Patient physically and mentally to cope with the discomfort or stress of pregnancy and the experience of childbirth, thereby reducing or eliminating her need for drugs and obstetric intervention. She should be offered such information early in her pregnancy in order that she may make a reasoned decision.

3. *The Pregnant Patient has the right*, prior to the administration of any drug, to be informed by the health professional who is prescribing or administering the drug to her that any drug which she receives during pregnancy, labor and birth, no matter how or when the drug is taken or administered, may adversely affect her unborn baby, directly or indirectly, and that there is no drug or chemical which has been proven safe for the unborn child.

4. *The Pregnant Patient has the right*, if cesarean birth is anticipated, to be informed prior to the administration of any drug, and preferably prior to her hospitalization, that minimizing her and, in turn, her baby's intake of nonessential preoperative medicine will benefit her baby.

5. *The Pregnant Patient has the right*, prior to the administration of a drug or procedure, to be informed of the areas of uncertainty if there is NO properly controlled follow-up research which has established the safety of the drug or procedure with regard to its direct and/or indirect effects on the physiological, mental and neurological development of the child exposed, via the mother, to the drug or procedure during pregnancy, labor, birth or lactation—(this would apply to virtually all drugs and the vast majority of obstetric procedures).

6. *The Pregnant Patient has the right*, prior to the administration of any drug, to be informed of the brand name and generic name of the drug in order that she may advise the health professional of any past adverse reaction to the drug.

7. *The Pregnant Patient has the right* to determine for herself, without pressure from her attendant, whether she will accept the risks inherent in the proposed therapy or refuse a drug or procedure.

8. *The Pregnant Patient has the right* to know the name and qualifications of the individual administering a medication or procedure to her during labor or birth.

9. *The Pregnant Patient has the right* to be informed, prior to the administration of any procedure, whether that procedure is being administered to her for her or her baby's benefit (medically indicated) or as an elective procedure (for convenience, teaching purposes or research).

10. *The Pregnant Patient has the right* to be accompanied during the stress of labor and birth by someone she cares for, and to whom she looks for emotional comfort and encouragement.

11. *The Pregnant Patient has the right*, after appropriate medical consultation, to choose a position for labor and for birth which is least stressful to her baby and to herself.

12. *The Obstetric Patient has the right* to have her baby cared for at her bedside if her baby is normal, and to feed her baby according to her baby's needs rather than according to the hospital regimen.

*Prepared by Doris Haire, Chair, Committee on Health Law and Regulation, International Childbirth Education Association, Inc, Rochester, NY.

13. *The Obstetric Patient has the right* to be informed in writing of the name of the person who actually delivered her baby and the professional qualifications of that person. This information should also be on the birth certificate.

14. *The Obstetric Patient has the right* to be informed if there is any known or indicated aspect of her or her baby's care or condition which may cause her or her baby later difficulty or problems.

15. *The Obstetric Patient has the right* to have her and her baby's hospital medical records complete, accurate and legible and have their records, including Nurses' Notes, retained by the hospital until the child reaches at least the age of majority, or to have the records offered to her before they are destroyed.

16. *The Obstetric Patient, both during and after her hospital stay, has the right* to have access to her complete hospital medical records, including Nurses' Notes, and to receive a copy upon payment of a reasonable fee and without incurring the expense of retaining an attorney.

It is the Obstetric Patient and her baby, not the health professional, who must sustain any trauma or injury resulting from the use of a drug or obstetric procedure. The observation of the rights listed above will not only permit the Obstetric Patient to participate in the decisions involving her and her baby's health care, but will help to protect the health professional and the hospital against litigation arising from resentment or misunderstanding on the part of the mother.

NAACOG'S STANDARDS FOR THE NURSING CARE OF WOMEN AND NEWBORNS*

STANDARD I: NURSING PRACTICE

Comprehensive nursing care for women and newborns focuses on helping individuals, families, and communities achieve their optimum health potential. This is best achieved within the framework of the nursing process.

The nurse is responsible for decisions and actions within the domain of nursing practice, which may include

- integration of the nursing process components of assessment, planning, implementation, and evaluation in all areas of nursing practice;

- individualization and prioritization of nursing care to meet the physical, psychological, spiritual, and social needs of patients;

- collaboration with the individual, family, and other members of the health-care team;

- promotion of a safe and therapeutic environment for both the recipients and providers of nursing care;

- demonstration and validation of competence in nursing practice;

- acquisition of specialized knowledge and skills and additional formal education to provide specialized care; and

- provision for complete and accurate documentation of care.

The written or computerized patient record is the documented means of communication among all members of the health-care team. It also promotes continuity of care and provides a mechanism for evaluating care. The record should contain accurate and complete recordings of the patient's history and physical examination as well as the nursing plan of care, including goals, interventions, health education, and evaluation of patient and family responses. Additional documentation may include planned follow-up and appropriate referrals. All information contained in the patient record and related to the care of the patient and family is confidential and should be released only according to institutional policy. **Note: To apply this universal standard to a specific area of gynecologic, obstetric, or neonatal nursing practice, refer directly to the specialty-specific nursing practice standards section.**

STANDARD II: HEALTH EDUCATION AND COUNSELING

Health education for the individual, family, and community is an integral part of comprehensive nursing care. Such education encourages participation in, and shared responsibility for, health promotion, maintenance, and restoration.

Comprehensive health education includes

- identification of the needs and abilities of the learner;

- collaboration with the patient and other health-care providers in design, content, and follow-up of the educational plan;

- provision of accurate and current information;

- provision of information based on educationally sound principles of teaching and learning;

- recognition of patient rights, responsibilities, and alternative choices;

- utilization of available educational resources to provide health education information to individuals/families in the community; and

- documentation and evaluation of health education including patient response.

The nurse participates in and/or coordinates the health education and counseling process. It begins with the initial patient contact or admission to the unit or service and is an ongoing, continuous process. **Note: To apply this universal standard to a specific area of gynecologic, obstetric, or neonatal nursing practice, refer directly to the specialty-specific nursing practice standards section.**

*From *NAACOG Standards for the Nursing Care of Women and Newborns*, 4th ed, Washington, DC: NAACOG, 1991. NAACOG is now known as AWHONN (Association of Women's Health, Obstetric, and Neonatal Nurses).

STANDARD III: POLICIES, PROCEDURES, AND PROTOCOLS

Written policies, procedures, and protocols clarify the scope of nursing practice and delineate the qualifications of personnel authorized to provide care to women and newborns within the health-care setting.

The components of policies, procedures, and protocols are based on

- recognition of the organization's philosophy;
- recognition of the unit's philosophy;
- coordination with the overall mission of the organization;
- assessment of the practice setting and determination of types of services to be provided;
- incorporation of a multidisciplinary approach in their development;
- identification of specific areas of practice to be addressed;
- reflection of current practice, standards, and local regulations; and
- anticipated use as references for health-care providers, orientation of new personnel and students, quality assurance activities, and/or guiding nursing actions in emergency situations.

The development of policies, procedures, and protocols should include consideration of staff availability, skill, and licensure; the physical plant and equipment; effects on other departments; and fiscal impact. Policies, procedures, and protocols should be reviewed and revised at least on an annual basis or more frequently as science/technology changes.
Note: To apply this universal standard to a specific area of gynecologic, obstetric, or neonatal nursing practice, refer directly to the specialty-specific nursing practice standards section.

STANDARD IV: PROFESSIONAL RESPONSIBILITY AND ACCOUNTABILITY

Comprehensive nursing care for women and newborns is provided by nurses who are clinically competent and accountable for professional actions and legal responsibilities inherent in the nursing role.

Responsibility and accountability for knowledge and competence in nursing practice for women and newborns include

- awareness of changing practices and professional and ethical issues;
- knowledge and clinical skills gained through in-service education, professional continuing education, research data, and professional literature;
- implementation of newly acquired knowledge and skills;
- collaboration through networking and sharing with other professionals;
- participation in the development of standards and policies, procedures, and protocols;
- participation with professional committees within the institution;
- participation in periodic peer- and self-evaluations; and
- recognition of certification as one mechanism for the demonstration of special knowledge within a specialty area of practice.

Legal accountability extends to the

- nurse practice acts;
- parameters of professional practice established by professional organizations;
- institutional standards;
- legislative changes that affect practice; and
- policies, procedures, and protocols within the practice environment.

STANDARD V: UTILIZATION OF NURSING PERSONNEL

Nursing care for women and newborns is conducted in practice settings that have qualified nursing staff in sufficient numbers to meet patient-care needs.

Each practice setting should have sufficient nursing personnel to meet patient-care requirements. Nursing staff who provide direct care to women and newborns should be supervised by registered nurses who are clinically proficient in the specialty area of practice. The patient-care unit or service is managed by a professional nurse who is prepared educationally and clinically to assume a leadership position. In all practice settings, the nurse may practice independently or collaboratively with other health-care team members. It is essential that nurses know both the responsibilities and the limitations of professional nursing practice specific to the practice setting.

Many variables are considered in determining both the number and type of nursing staff needed for a practice setting. Among these variables are those related to the patient, practice, organization, and personnel. Patient-related variables may include

- patient demographics and acuity of patients served;
- length of stay;
- educational needs;
- cultural factors and level of comprehension;
- communication barriers; and

- discharge or home-care needs.

Practice-related variables may include

- difference in educational and experiential level of nursing staff;
- nursing philosophy;
- type of nursing-care delivery system;
- use of assistive personnel;
- use of nurses in expanded roles; and
- participation in teaching programs.

Organizational variables may include

- scope of services provided;
- availability of support services;
- patient volume;
- mission or philosophy of the organization;
- risk-management concerns;
- quality assurance programs;
- policies, procedures, and protocols;
- physical plant;
- marketing strategies; and
- fiscal considerations.

Personnel variables relate to the type and number of professional and nonprofessional staff and may include

- education, skill, and experience of the nursing leadership;
- educational preparation, skill, and experience of staff;
- types and mix of nursing staff;
- availability of qualified alternative staff to deal with emergencies or unanticipated volumes;
- distribution of staff, eg, temporary reassignment, floating, on-call, cross-training, and supplemental staffing;
- responsibilities for orientation, precepting, or students;
- turnover rates; and
- clerical and technical support.

Competency-based job descriptions should be available for each level of nursing staff. Orientation for all personnel should include a general overview of the organization and specific information about the individual practice setting. Performance evaluations for all personnel should be conducted, documented, and discussed on a regular basis with input from the individual, colleagues, and supervisory staff.

STANDARD VI: ETHICS

Ethical principles guide the process of decision making for nurses caring for women and newborns at all times and especially when personal or professional values conflict with those of the patient, family, colleagues, or practice setting.

The nurse should have the opportunity to participate in the ethical decision-making process. To participate actively, nurses should

- clarify their own personal and professional values;
- recognize the difficulty in selecting a course of action that is morally and ethically acceptable to all parties;
- communicate openly and assertively;
- identify options; and
- seek consultations.

Nurses must carefully examine their own value systems since values influence the decision-making process. Opportunities should be provided in the practice setting for discussion of potential ethical issues. Each practice setting should have a framework for decision making regarding bioethical dilemmas. Ethical dilemmas generally arise when there is a conflict between loyalties, rights, duties, or values.

For nurses, most ethical dilemmas occur when there is a real or perceived requirement to act in a manner contrary to personal values or when care ordered or provided does not seem compatible with the best interest of the patient. Common areas of concern may include

- nursing autonomy and decision making;
- maternal interests versus fetal interests;
- issues of duty, obligation, and loyalty (for example, employer to employee, professional to public, professional to professional);
- patients' rights to resources, privacy, confidentiality, information, participation in decision making, and refusal of therapy;
- the right to live or die;
- life cycle concerns, including contraception, sterilization, pregnancy termination, genetic manipulation, infanticide, sexuality and choices of life style, and euthanasia;
- fetal or neonatal conditions incompatible with life;
- fetal tissue use; and
- biomedical intervention.

The bioethics literature can provide nurses with strategies to cope with or resolve decisions in situations when conflicts of values occur. For ethical decision-making frameworks to be applied to practice situations, working relationships must be established in which individuals may express their own points of view. All persons potentially affected by an ethical decision have the right to participate in the decision-making process.

Standard VII: Research

Nurses caring for women and newborns utilize research findings, conduct nursing research, and evaluate nursing practice to improve the outcomes of care.

Knowledge of the research process and participation in scientific inquiry are necessary to

- conduct or participate in the conduct of research according to ethical guidelines;

- use research findings to provide appropriate and safe nursing care;

- use research findings as a basis for validating standards of nursing care;

- evaluate the relevance and application of research findings from nursing and related disciplines; and

- validate the effect of nursing practice on patient outcomes.

Standard VIII: Quality Assurance

Quality and appropriateness of patient care are evaluated through a planned assessment program using specific, identified clinical indicators.

Each unit or service should have a written quality assurance plan that reflects a philosophy that is coordinated with the organization's mission and overall quality assurance program. Objectives of the unit-based or service-based quality assurance plan should include

- assurance of consistent quality patient outcomes;

- identification and correction of potential nursing practice deficiencies;

- promotion of professional nursing practice based on appropriate nursing standards; and

- education and participation of staff in quality assurance activities.

The unit nurse manager is responsible for developing and implementing the unit-based quality assurance plan. The plan should include

- responsibilities of all personnel in the quality assurance process;

- the scope of service provided;

- important aspects of care or service involving high-risk, high-volume, and problem-prone patients or activities;

- clinical indicators or measurable standards that affect the aspects of care and service that have been identified as important;

- specific criteria and thresholds for use in monitoring clinical indicators;

- methods for the collection and analysis of data, including reference to collection tools, sample size, time frame, and staff responsibility;

- determination of appropriate corrective action, when indicated, that will fall into one of three categories: educational, organizational, or behavioral change;

- follow-up assessment of identified problems;

- documentation of all aspects of the quality assurance program, including results; and

- a process for communication related to quality assurance activities within the total organization.

CLINICAL ESTIMATION OF GESTATIONAL AGE

► **Examination First Hours**

CLINICAL ESTIMATION OF GESTATIONAL AGE
An Approximation Based on Published Data*

PHYSICAL FINDINGS		WEEKS GESTATION 20–48
VERNIX		APPEARS (21) · COVERS BODY, THICK LAYER · ON BACK, SCALP, IN CREASES (38–39) · SCANT, IN CREASES (40–41) · NO VERNIX (42–48)
BREAST TISSUE AND AREOLA		AREOLA & NIPPLE BARELY VISIBLE, NO PALPABLE BREAST TISSUE (20–35) · AREOLA RAISED (36–37) · 1-2 MM NODULE (38–39) · 3-5 MM (38) · 5-6 MM (39) · 7-10 MM (40–43) · ?12 MM (44–48)
EAR	FORM	FLAT, SHAPELESS (20–35) · BEGINNING INCURVING SUPERIOR (36–37) · INCURVING UPPER 2/3 PINNAE (38–39) · WELL-DEFINED INCURVING TO LOBE (40–48)
	CARTILAGE	PINNA SOFT, STAYS FOLDED (20–35) · CARTILAGE SCANT RETURNS SLOWLY FROM FOLDING (36–37) · THIN CARTILAGE SPRINGS BACK FROM FOLDING (38–39) · PINNA FIRM, REMAINS ERECT FROM HEAD (40–48)
SOLE CREASES		SMOOTH SOLES ₹ CREASES (20–33) · 1-2 ANTERIOR CREASES (34–35) · 2-3 ANTERIOR CREASES (36–37) · CREASES ANTERIOR 2/3 SOLE (38–39) · CREASES INVOLVING HEEL (40–41) · DEEPER CREASES OVER ENTIRE SOLE (42–48)
SKIN	THICKNESS & APPEARANCE	THIN, TRANSLUCENT SKIN, PLETHORIC, VENULES OVER ABDOMEN EDEMA (20–33) · SMOOTH THICKER NO EDEMA (34–37) · PINK (38–39) · FEW VESSELS (40–41) · SOME DESQUAMATION PALE PINK (42) · THICK, PALE, DESQUAMATION OVER ENTIRE BODY (43–48)
	NAIL PLATES	APPEAR (20–21) · NAILS TO FINGER TIPS (22–41) · NAILS EXTEND WELL BEYOND FINGER TIPS (42–48)
HAIR		APPEARS ON HEAD (20–22) · EYE BROWS & LASHES (23–27) · FINE, WOOLLY, BUNCHES OUT FROM HEAD (28–37) · SILKY, SINGLE STRANDS LAYS FLAT (38–41) · ?RECEDING HAIRLINE OR LOSS OF BABY HAIR SHORT, FINE UNDERNEATH (42–48)
LANUGO		APPEARS (20–21) · COVERS ENTIRE BODY (22–33) · VANISHES FROM FACE (34–37) · PRESENT ON SHOULDERS (38–41) · NO LANUGO (42–48)
GENITALIA	TESTES	TESTES PALPABLE IN INGUINAL CANAL (30–37) · IN UPPER SCROTUM (38–41) · IN LOWER SCROTUM (42–48)
	SCROTUM	FEW RUGAE (30–37) · RUGAE, ANTERIOR PORTION (38–39) · RUGAE COVER (40–41) · PENDULOUS (42–48)
	LABIA & CLITORIS	PROMINENT CLITORIS, LABIA MAJORA SMALL WIDELY SEPARATED (32–37) · LABIA MAJORA LARGER NEARLY COVERED CLITORIS (38–41) · LABIA MINORA & CLITORIS COVERED (42–48)
SKULL FIRMNESS		BONES ARE SOFT (20–29) · SOFT TO 1" FROM ANTERIOR FONTANELLE (30–33) · SPONGY AT EDGES OF FONTANELLE CENTER FIRM (34–37) · BONES HARD SUTURES EASILY DISPLACED (38–41) · BONES HARD, CANNOT BE DISPLACED (42–48)
POSTURE	RESTING	HYPOTONIC LATERAL DECUBITUS (20–26) · HYPOTONIC (27–29) · BEGINNING FLEXION THIGH (30–31) · STRONGER HIP FLEXION (32–33) · FROG-LIKE (34–35) · FLEXION ALL LIMBS (36–37) · HYPERTONIC (38–41) · VERY HYPERTONIC (42–48)
	RECOIL - LEG	NO RECOIL (24–29) · PARTIAL RECOIL (34–37) · PROMPT RECOIL (42–48)
	ARM	NO RECOIL (27–33) · BEGIN FLEXION NO RECOIL (34–35) · PROMPT RECOIL MAY BE INHIBITED (36–37) · PROMPT RECOIL AFTER 30" INHIBITION (40–48)

*Brazie JV and Lubchenco LO. The estimation of gestational age chart. In Kempe, Silver and O'Brien. Current Pediatric Diagnosis and Treatment, ed 3. Los Altos, Calif. Lange Medical Publications, 1974, ch 4.
Form courtesy of Mead Johnson Laboratories, Evansville, IN.

ACTIONS AND EFFECTS OF SELECTED DRUGS DURING BREASTFEEDING*

aAnticholinergics

Atropine: May cause hyperthermia in the newborn; may decrease maternal milk supply

Anticoagulants

Coumarin derivatives (Warfarin): Only small amount in breast milk; check PTT

Heparin: Relatively safe to use; check PTT

Phenindione (Hedulin): Passes easily into breast milk; neonate may have increased prothrombin time and PTT

Anticonvulsants

Phenytoin (Dilantin), phenobarbital: Generally considered safe; if high doses of phenobarbital are ingested, may cause drowsiness; short-acting pheno-barbiturates (secobarbital) preferred, as they appear in lower concentration in milk

Antihistamines

Diphenhydramine (Benadryl), pheniramine (Dimetane), Coricidin, Drixoral: May cause decreased milk supply; infant may become drowsy, irritable, or have tachy-cardia

Antimetabolites

Unknown, probably long-term anti-DNA effect on the infant; potentially very toxic

Antimicrobials

Aminoglycosides: May cause ototoxicity or nephro-toxicity if given for more than 2 weeks

Ampicillin: Skin rash, candidiasis; diarrhea

Chloramphenicol: Possible bone marrow suppression; Gray syndrome; refusal of breast

Methacycline: Possible inhibition of bone growth; may cause discoloration of the teeth; use should be avoided

Metronidazole (Flagyl): Possible neurologic disorders or blood dyscrasias; delay breastfeeding for 12 hours after dose

Penicillin: Possible allergic response; candidiasis

Quinolones (synthetic antibiotics): Can cause arthro-pathies

Sulfonamides: May cause hyperbilirubinemia; use contraindicated until infant over 1 month old

Tetracycline: Long-term use and large doses should be avoided; may cause tooth staining or inhibition of bone growth

Antithyroids

Thiouracil: Contraindicated during lactation; may cause goiter or agranulocytosis

Barbiturates

May produce sedation

Phenothiazines: May produce sedation

Bronchodilators

Aminophylline: May cause insomnia or irritability in the infant

Ephedrine, cromolyn (Intal): Relatively safe

Caffeine

Excessive consumption may cause jitteriness

Cardiovascular

Methyldopa: Increase in milk volume

Propranolol (Inderal): May cause hypoglycemia; possibility of other blocking effects, especially if infant has renal or liver dysfunction

Quinidine: May cause arrhythmias in infant

Reserpine (Serpasil): Nasal stuffiness, lethargy, or diarrhea in infant

Corticosteroids

Adrenal suppression may occur with long-term administration of doses greater than 10 mg/day

Diuretics

Furosemide (Lasix): Not excreted in breast milk

Thiazide diuretics (Esidrix, Hydrodiuril, Oretic): Safe but can cause dehydration, reduce milk production

Heavy metals

Gold: Potentially toxic

Mercury: Excreted in the milk and hazardous to infant

Hormones

Androgens: Suppress lactation

Thyroid hormones: May mask hypothyroidism

Laxatives

Cascara: May cause diarrhea in infant

Milk of magnesia: Relatively safe

Phenolphthalein: May cause diarrhea in infant

Narcotic analgesics

Codeine: Accumulation may lead to neonatal depression

*Based on data from Kacew S: Adverse effects of drugs and chemicals in breast milk on the nursing infant. *J Clin Pharmacol* 1993;33:213–221; Riordan J, Auerbach KG: *Breastfeeding and Human Lactation.* Boston: Jones and Bartlett, 1993, pp 135–166.

Meperidine: May lead to neonatal depression

Morphine: Long-term use may cause newborn addiction

Nonnarcotic analgesics, NSAIDs

Acetaminophen (Tylenol):   Relatively safe for short-term analgesia

Ibuprofen (Motrin):   Safe

Propoxyphene (Darvon):   May cause sleepiness and poor nursing in infant

Salicylates (aspirin):   Safe after first week of life; monitor protime

Oral contraceptives

Combined estrogen/progestin pills: Significantly decrease milk supply; may alter milk composition; may cause gynecomastia in male infants

Progestin only: Safe if started after lactation is established

Radioactive materials for testing

Gallium citrate (^{67}G):   Insignificant amount excreted in breast milk; no nursing for 2 weeks

Iodine: Contraindicated; may affect infant's thyroid gland

^{125}I: Discontinue nursing for 48 hours

^{131}I: Nursing should be discontinued until excretion is no longer significant; after a test dose, nursing may be resumed after 24 to 36 hours; after a treatment dose, nursing may be resumed after 2 to 3 weeks

Technetium-99m: Discontinue nursing for 3 days (half-life = 6 hours)

Sedatives/Tranquilizers

Diazepam (Valium):   May accumulate to high levels; may increase neonatal jaundice; may cause lethargy

Lithium carbonate: Controversial; may cause neonatal flaccidity and hypotonia

Substance Abuse

Alcohol: Potential motor developmental delay; mild sedative effect

Amphetamines: Controversial; may cause irritability, poor sleeping

Cocaine, crack: Extreme irritability, tachycardia, vomiting, apnea

Marijuana: Drowsiness

SELECTED MATERNAL-NEWBORN LABORATORY VALUES

NORMAL MATERNAL LABORATORY VALUES

Test	Non-Pregnant Values	Pregnant Values
Hematocrit	37%–47%	32%–42%
Hemoglobin	12–16 g/dL*	10–14 g/dL*
Platelets	150,000–350,000/mm^3	Significant increase 3–5 days after birth (predisposes to thrombosis)
Partial thromboplastin time (PTT)	12–14 seconds	Slight decrease in pregnancy and again in labor (placental site clotting)
Fibrinogen	250 mg/dL	400 mg/dL
Serum Glucose:		
Fasting	70–80 mg/dL	65 mg/dL
2-hour postprandial	60–110 mg/dL	Less than 140 mg/dL
Total protein	6.7–8.3 g/dL	5.5–7.5 g/dL
White blood cell total	4500–10,000/mm^3	5000–15,000/mm^3
Polymorphonuclear cells	54%–62%	60%–85%
Lymphocytes	38%–46%	15%–40%

NORMAL NEONATAL LABORATORY VALUES

Test	Normal Values
Hematocrit	51%–56%
Hemoglobin	16.5 g/dL (cord blood)
Platelets	150,000–400,000/mm^3
White blood cell total	18,000/mm^3
White blood cell differential:	
Bands	1600/mm^3 (9%)
Polymorphonuclear (segs)	9400/mm^3 (52%)
Eosinophils	400/mm^3 (2.2%)
Basophils	100/mm^3 (0.6%)
Lymphocytes	5500/mm^3 (31%)
Monocytes	1050/mm^3 (5.8%)
Serum glucose	40–80 mg/dL
Serum electrolytes:	
Sodium	135–147 mEq/L
Potassium	4–6 mEq/L
Chloride	90–114 mEq/L
Carbon dioxide	15–25 mEq/L
Bicarbonate	18–23 mEq/L
Calcium	7–10 mg/dL

*at sea level

Source: *Essentials Handbook.*

1995–1996 NANDA-APPROVED NURSING DIAGNOSES

Activity intolerance
Activity intolerance, risk for
Adjustment, impaired
Airway clearance, ineffective
Anxiety
Aspiration, risk for
Body image disturbance
Body temperature, risk for altered
Breastfeeding, effective
Breastfeeding, ineffective
Breastfeeding, interrupted
Breathing pattern, ineffective
Cardiac output, decreased
Caregiver role strain
Caregiver role strain, risk for
Constipation
Constipation, colonic
Constipation, perceived
Coping (family), ineffective: compromised
Coping (family), ineffective: disabling
Coping (family), potential for growth
Coping (individual), ineffective
Coping, defensive
Decisional conflict
Denial, ineffective
Diarrhea
Disuse syndrome, risk for
Diversional activity deficit
Dysreflexia
Family processes, altered
Fatigue
Fear
Fluid volume deficit
Fluid volume deficit, risk for
Fluid volume excess
Gas exchange, impaired
Grieving, anticipatory
Grieving, dysfunctional
Growth and development, altered
Health seeking behaviors (specify)

Health maintenance, altered
Home maintenance management, impaired
Hopelessness
Hyperthermia
Hypothermia
Incontinence, bowel
Incontinence, functional (urinary)
Incontinence, reflex (urinary)
Incontinence, stress (urinary)
Incontinence, total (urinary)
Incontinence, urge (urinary)
Infant feeding pattern, ineffective
Infection, risk for
Injury, risk for
Knowledge deficit (specify)
Management of therapeutic regimen, ineffective
Mobility, impaired physical
Noncompliance (specify)
Nutrition, altered: less than body requirements
Nutrition, altered: more than body requirements
Nutrition, altered: potential for more than body requirements
Oral mucous membrane, altered
Pain
Pain, chronic
Parental role conflict
Parenting, altered
Parenting, risk for altered
Peripheral neurovascular dysfunction, risk for
Personal identity disturbance
Poisoning, risk for
Post-trauma response
Powerlessness
Protection, altered
Rape-trauma syndrome
Rape-trauma syndrome: compound reaction

Rape-trauma syndrome: silent reaction
Relocation stress syndrome
Role performance, altered
Self care deficit: bathing/hygiene
Self care deficit: dressing/grooming
Self care deficit: feeding
Self care deficit: toileting
Self esteem disturbance
Self esteem, chronic low
Self esteem, situational low
Self-mutilation, risk for
Sensory/perceptual alterations (specify)
Sexual dysfunction
Sexuality patterns, altered
Skin integrity, impaired
Skin integrity, risk for impaired
Sleep pattern disturbance
Social interaction, impaired
Social isolation
Spiritual distress (distress of the human spirit)
Spontaneous ventilation: inability to sustain
Suffocation, risk for
Swallowing, impaired
Thermoregulation, ineffective
Thought processes, altered
Tissue integrity, impaired
Tissue perfusion, altered: peripheral
Tissue perfusion, altered: renal, cerebral, cardiopulmonary, gastrointestinal (specify type)
Trauma, risk for
Unilateral neglect
Urinary elimination, altered
Urinary retention
Ventilatory weaning response, dysfunctional
Verbal communication, impaired
Violence, risk for: self-directed or directed at others

SOURCE: Wilkinson J.M.: *Nursing Diagnosis and Intervention Pocket Guide*, 6th ed. Redwood City, CA: Addison-Wesley Nursing, 1995.

PROJECTED RECOMMENDATIONS FOR ISOLATION PRECAUTIONS (CDC 1995)

The guidelines established by the Centers for Disease Control and Prevention (CDC) in 1995 have two levels of prevention—standard precautions, designed to be used with all clients, and transmission-based precautions, designed to be used with clients with suspected or confirmed infections with epidemiologically important organisms transmitted by airborne or droplet route or by direct contact with contaminated surfaces or dry skin. Section A of this Appendix describes the projected 1995 CDC guidelines, and section B summarizes the 1991 OSHA Bloodborne Pathogen Standard, which are an integral part of the Standard Precautions (CDC, 1995).

SECTION A   PROJECTED RECOMMENDATIONS FOR ISOLATION PRECAUTIONS (CDC 1995)

Type Precaution	Handwashing	Gloves	Gown	Mask, Eye Protection, Face Shield	Room Assignment of Client
Standard Precautions *To be used with all clients	Between all client contacts; immediately after removing gloves; after any contact with bodily fluids or secretions; or after any contact with contaminated items.	Nonsterile gloves worn when coming in contact with any bodily substances (saliva, urine, feces, blood, etc), mucous membranes, or nonintact skin.	Nonsterile, clean gown used during procedures in which splashing of bodily fluids is anticipated. Gown is discarded after tasks are finished.	Mask and eye protection or face shield worn whenever splashing or spraying of bodily fluids is probable.	Private room preferred if client is unable to maintain own hygiene or environmental control of room; otherwise room with multiple clients is acceptable.
Transmission-based precautions: Droplet *To be used for clients with known or suspected infections with microorganisms > 5 microns known to be transmitted by droplets from sneezing, talking, coughing, etc.	Same as above.	Same as above.	Same as above.	A mask is worn when working within three feet of the client.	Private room preferred if possible; if not possible a spatial separation of at least three feet must be maintained between client and other individuals such as other clients, visitors, etc.
Transmission-based precautions: Airborne *To be used for clients with known or suspected infection with microorganisms (≤ 5 microns) that can remain in the air or be dispersed widely by air currents.	Same as above.	Same as above.	Same as above.	A special mask (particulate respirator) is recommended for entering the rooms of clients with tuberculosis. Individuals who have never had varicella or rubeola should not enter the rooms of clients diagnosed with or suspected of having these infections.	Client room should have the following: • monitored negative air pressure • at least 6 air exchanges per hour • appropriate discharge of air from room. In addition, the door to room should be kept closed at all times. Client may be in a semi-private room with another client who has the same diagnosis.

Transmission-based precautions: Contact	Same as above.	Use nonsterile, clean gloves in providing direct client care or during contact with potentially contaminated items.	Clean, nonsterile gown is recommended if contact with bodily substances, equipment, or surfaces is anticipated.	Same as for standard precautions.	Private room if possible.

*To be used for clients with known or suspected infection with epidemiologically important microorganisms that can be transmitted by direct contact with the client or by indirect contact (for example, by touching objects or equipment in the client's room).

Note: CDC Guidelines are extrapolated from: Draft guideline for isolation precautions in hospitals: notice of comment period. *Federal Register* 59(214):55552-55570. November 7, 1994. The final version of the guidelines may differ. Reviewed by Marguerite McMillan Jackson RN, Doctoral Candidate, CIC, FAAN. Administrative Director Medical Center Epidemiology Unit, University of California San Diego.

SECTION B OCCUPATIONAL SAFETY AND HEALTH ADMINISTRATION (OSHA) BLOODBORNE PATHOGENS STANDARD (1991)

The Bloodborne Pathogens Standard (1991) will be an integral part of the Standard Precautions (CDC 1995). This standard is to be used to prevent contact with blood or other materials that are potentially infectious. If the circumstance arises that body fluids are difficult to differentiate, all body fluids are considered potentially infectious. The essential elements of the Bloodborne Pathogens Standard are as follows:

- Handwashing guidelines should include:
  - Washing hands with soap and water prior to and immediately after contact with all clients and/or any contaminated items.
  - Hands are to be washed immediately after removing gloves.
  - Handwashing materials are to be made readily available in each work setting.
- Nonsterile, disposable gloves are to be worn whenever contact with blood or other potentially infectious body fluids may be anticipated. Gloves should be replaced if they are punctured or torn. Disposable gloves are to be used only once.
- Masks, eye protection, and face shields are to be worn whenever potentially contaminated material may be splashed, sprayed or spattered on the face, eyes, nose or mouth.
- Special care is to be taken when using or discarding sharp instruments (needles, scalpels or other sharp devices).
  - Needles are never to be recapped using two hands.
  - If the needle needs to be recapped, a one-handed 'scoop' technique may be used, or a special device for recapping may be used.
  - Used needles should not be removed from the syringe by hand.
  - Needles should not be manipulated, twisted or broken by hand.
  - All sharps (needles, scalpels, and sharp disposable instruments) should be placed in an appropriate puncture-resistant container. The container should be clearly marked and/or color-coded, be leakproof on the sides and bottom, be located as close to the client as possible, be maintained in an upright position, and have a lid so spillage is not possible.
- During resuscitation, special disposable devices should be used as an alternative to the direct mouth-to-mouth method.

From: Department of Labor, Occupational Safety and Health Administration: *Federal Register* 56:64003-64182, Dec 6, 1991. Reviewed by Marguerite McMillan Jackson RN, Doctoral Candidate, CIC, FAAN. Administrative Director Medical Center, University of California San Diego.

ANSWERS TO CRITICAL THINKING IN PRACTICE

Chapter 3

After an infant is born, a primary concern of the nurse is to assess the couple's ability to meet the needs of their newborn. Assessment of the family's structural traits (form, roles, culture, values, communication patterns, power structure, and social network), functional traits (affective, socialization, reproductive, coping, economic, physical care, and health care functions), and developmental tasks is needed. In this case, the nurse must elicit more detailed information from the couple concerning these issues. A nurse also assumes the role of teacher and counselor when discussing the needs of the infant and demonstrating care to the parents. A supportive, caring approach with young couples can often allay their fears. The nurse must provide education about the current and ongoing health care needs of the infant.

Chapter 9

Rita has described a normal menstrual cycle. While it is variable in frequency, it is not outside the range of what is acceptable in a teenager. The flow that she thinks is heavy is really quite normal and the fact that she has cramps indicates that she is having ovulatory cycles.

It is important to reassure Rita that there is nothing wrong with her menstrual cycle. It would be appropriate to suggest an anti-prostaglandin such as ibuprofen for the relief of dysmenorrhea. Of utmost importance is to follow up on her request for birth control pills. It may be that she is considering becoming sexually active and needs contraception. Sometimes teenagers have a difficult time asking for what they really want and this is an ideal situation in which to bring up issues of sexuality with a young woman.

Chapter 10

The use of feminine hygiene products can result in vaginitis and actually promote sexually transmitted diseases, especially PID. Feminine hygiene products, especially douches, alter the acid-base balance of the vagina, allowing opportunistic organisms to replicate. Also, douching washes out the protective normal flora of the vagina, and the altered acid-base vaginal environment prevents the protective bacteria from growing. The action of douching can propel pathogenic organisms up-

ward and promote an ascending infection such as PID. CW should be told that douching is seldom necessary, and that cleansing daily with soap and water are adequate hygienic measures (Rosenberg and Phillips, 1992).

CW should be told that she is at increased risk for PID because she has multiple sexual partners, uses an IUD, and douches. She should be counselled to consider other forms of contraceptives that are more protective against STDs and to consider limiting her sexual activity to a monogamous relationship.

Chapter 11

Marsha's story of how she got her injury is not consistent with the type of injury she has. Injuries that are accidental are usually to the extremities and not the trunk. Also, the bruising and edema suggest that the injury happened several hours ago. You should suspect that Marsha received her injuries from physical abuse, probably by Fred. The type of injury and the delay in coming for treatment are possible indicators of abuse. Also the fact that she looks to Fred to agree with her statements is suspicious. You should make every attempt to separate Marsha from Fred, so that she can speak more openly if she chooses. It is likely that if Fred is in the room she will deny the abuse for fear of further abuse. You do not want to put her in danger. You may need to be creative in separating Fred from Marsha, since often the abuser does not want to leave.

Chapter 13

At this point it would be important to realize that this is this couple's first exposure to the health care system of the United States and that the goal should be to make their first experience a positive one, as this may greatly influence their utilization of the system in the future. Take a moment to critically examine your own cultural values. Perhaps reflect upon your value of the importance of seeking early prenatal care and realize that for the Southeast Asian individual, seeking health care is usually related to a crisis and relief of symptoms. Pregnancy is not viewed as an illness, and therefore this couple would not usually be entering the health care system. What has brought them here today? Is Mrs Nguyen experiencing any problems with her pregnancy?

While reflecting upon questions such as these, one of the first things you can do to make this a positive experience for them is to immediately arrange for an interpreter. Once the interpreter is available, you will be able to obtain a more thorough history of Mrs Nguyen's pregnancy. Include a cultural assessment as part of your history. What are their expectations of the health care system? Are they using any traditional healing practices? Based upon the information provided, you will be able to provide prenatal education and care with consideration for their cultural values and beliefs.

Chapter 14

Certainly Karen should continue with her exercising, including light weight lifting. She also can continue to use the heated pool. Current recommendations, however, suggest nonuse of hot tubs during pregnancy. There is a potential for hot tub (and sauna) hyperthermia in early pregnancy to induce fetal damage. Temperatures in hot tubs have the potential to raise core body temperatures after 10 to 15 minutes of use. The central nervous system is especially vulnerable to heat exposure in the developing fetus (Milunsky et al, 1992).

Chapter 15

Competing in the marathon is not recommended. Even though Constance is in excellent shape, we do not know what impact prolonged participation in such a strenuous event might have on her fetus. Uterine blood flow is decreased during exercise as blood is shunted to the muscles, and the normal fetus seems able to withstand this. We don't know, however, whether this decreased blood flow to the fetus interferes with the fetus's ability to dissipate heat, especially since the fetus is not able to decrease temperature via perspiration or respiration (Fishbein & Phillips, 1990). With this in mind, ACOG guidelines recommend that, during pregnancy, competitive athletes avoid competition, and all women exercise for shorter intervals (no longer than 15 minutes at a time).

Chapter 16

Cindy has only recently turned 15. She may not be aware of good nutrition, and probably has minimal knowledge about how her nutritional habits impact the growing fetus. The nurse can begin by showing Cindy and her boyfriend pictures of the uterus, placenta, and umbilical cord, and discussing how the fetus is nourished. She then needs to help Cindy understand good nutritional habits and which of her favorite foods in the different food groups will also be healthy for her fetus. The use of audiovisual aids is important in teaching young teenagers. The nurse needs to determine food practices in Cindy's home. Who is cooking and preparing the food? How much control does Cindy have? If the mother prepares the food, the nurse and Cindy can discuss ways of sharing information about good nutrition with Cindy's mother. Evaluation of nutritional habits and reinforcement for positive changes throughout her pregnancy will be important. Since this was a planned pregnancy with a supportive boyfriend, compliance in health behaviors to produce a healthy baby is likely.

Expected weight gain in pregnancy also needs to be discussed. Body image is a concern in the teen years. Knowing a specific amount of weight that needs to be gained each trimester for normal growth of a healthy fetus, and that this weight will be lost after pregnancy, will be important for both Cindy and her boyfriend.

Chapter 17

Although Jane's intake is supporting an appropriate weight gain, her diet is not nutritionally adequate. Comparing her diet to the Food Guide Pyramid shows that she lacks servings from the grain and dairy groups and that she has a high intake from the meat group.

Grain group	Jane should not restrict her intake from this group. Breads, pasta, and other grain products will not cause weight gain unless they are prepared with large amounts of fat or eaten in excessive quantities.
Meat group	The number of servings from this group exceeds the recommended intake. This contributes to Jane's fat and calorie intake even though she may be selecting lean cuts of meat. The number of servings should be decreased and each portion size should be about 2–3 ounces.
Dairy group	A restricted dairy intake has decreased Jane's calcium intake. The items she does consume from this group tend to have a high fat content. She could use dairy products that have a reduced fat content in order to limit her calorie intake but maintain the calcium level in her diet.
Vegetable group	Broccoli and green leafy vegetables such as beet greens, collards, and kale will provide calcium to the diet but must be consumed in amounts greater than usual serving sizes in order to obtain adequate calcium (Table 17-5). Most salad greens contain very little calcium.
Beverages	The total amount of fluid consumed is adequate. The consumption of soda should be limited because it would increase the calorie intake without contributing to the nutrient content of the diet.

Chapter 18

It is not unusual for women to be upset and frustrated with news that they may have newly diagnosed glucose intolerance during pregnancy. It has been described that women with gestational diabetes approach the new diagnosis as a crisis or anxiety-provoking situation. These women may experience more difficulty with coping and learning than do women with chronic diabetes who become pregnant (Keohane 1991).

It is important for the nurse to first assess the woman's knowledge about gestational diabetes before attempting to provide any teaching. The woman will benefit most from discussions that build on her current knowledge level. It will usually take several sessions to ensure that the new information is accurately understood and retained.

The nurse can reassure Mrs Chang that the baby should be fine, and can stress the importance of keeping her glucose levels in a normal range. Women with gestational diabetes usually require treatment with diet therapy alone, but occasionally may need insulin administration to control hyperglycemia.

It is felt that gestational diabetes does not cause birth defects because it occurs later in pregnancy, after the baby's organs are formed. The two most common risks to the baby are macrosomia, potentially causing a problem in labor and birth, and hypoglycemia.

Chapter 19

This approach is not appropriate for Rachel. While it is unusual for a nonpregnant woman to develop pyelonephritis from a bladder infection, 25% to 65% of pregnant women with bacteriuria develop pyelonephritis unless their bladder infection is treated (Shortliffe 1992). This is related to the anatomic and physiologic changes of pregnancy, including decreased ureteral peristalsis, ureteral dilation, and increased bladder capacity. Since Rachel is 6 months pregnant, she is probably being seen monthly for prenatal care. Because prompt treatment is essential, you should urge her to call her care giver and discuss her symptoms.

Chapter 24

We hope you would encourage her to take medication if she felt she needed it. There are many types of analgesic agents and many types of regional blocks that can help her if she decides she needs them. Sometimes, giving permission for someone to ask relieves her anxiety and decreases the need for intervention.

Chapter 25

The pattern described is within normal limits. No further action is needed because the pattern is reassuring.

Chapter 26

Once uterine contractions reach the desired characteristics (frequency of every 2–3 minutes, duration of 40–60 seconds, and moderate to strong intensity), and cervical dilitation is 5–6 cm, the infusion rate can be decreased by increments similar to those by which it was increased. In this case you should decrease the rate to the step it was just prior to 6 mU/min (36 mL/hr).

Chapter 27

The twin at greatest risk of developing tissue hypoxia is David. Hypoxia develops when there is inadequate delivery of oxygen to the tissues. This occurs when there is inadequate circulation to the tissues or, as in this case, the blood delivered to the tissues has a decreased oxygen-carrying capacity. The oxygen-carrying capacity of blood is calculated as: 1.26 mL O_2/gram of hemoglobin (the O_2-carrying capacity of fetal hemoglobin) multiplied by the grams of hemoglobin in the sample. Thus, the oxygen vols% and the oxygen-carrying capacity of David's blood is $1.26 \times 11 = 13.86$ vols%. Therefore, David is at greater risk of developing tissue hypoxia than is his brother.

Caution should be exercised when using oxygen saturation monitors to assess hypoxia. The monitors determine the amount of oxygenated versus deoxygenated hemoglobin in the blood and report this value as a percentage; for example, "94% saturated" means 94 percent of the hemoglobin has bound to oxygen molecules. The monitors do not evaluate the amount of hemoglobin present in the blood, nor the actual oxygen-carrying capacity. In this case, David is at greater risk of developing tissue hypoxia despite his oxygen saturation of 100% because he has a lower oxygen-carrying capacity and his tissues are receiving less oxygen per volume of blood.

Chapter 28

The unique behavioral and temperament characteristics of newborn infants should be discussed. Additionally, aspects of the Brazelton exam may be helpful to show Mrs Reyes how her infant changes state with different stimuli and intervention. Teaching her how to console her newborn may also be helpful.

Chapter 29

Reassure mother that you will help her baby as you carry out the following activities:

- Position the infant with her head lowered and to the side.
- Bulb suction the nares and mouth repeatedly until the airway is cleared.
- Hold and comfort the infant when normal respirations are restored.
- Reassure the mother, and review this procedure with her.

Note: If bulb suctioning alone does not clear the airway, use DeLee wall suction and administer oxygen as needed to restore normal respirations.

Chapter 29

We hope you would first examine the infant's genitalia and wipe between the labia to verify the source of bleeding. If there were no external lacerations, you would explain to the mother that a small amount of bleeding, called pseudomenstruation, sometimes occurs in newborn girls because of maternal hormone levels. This is considered normal and generally resolves in a few days. The tissue she observes is a vaginal skin tag, also a normal finding. It usually disappears in a few weeks.

Chapter 30

Acknowledge Ann's frustration and pain. Tell her you are glad she called and ask how you may be of help. Let her ventilate about how she feels. Explain that her breasts are engorged, which is a problem that many women encounter. It is not unusual for infants to refuse to nurse when the breast is hard and the nipple difficult to grasp.

Identify methods to relieve the engorgement.

a. Warm or cool soaks, whichever she prefers, for comfort and to stimulate let-down.

b. Express a small amount of milk.

c. Put the baby to breast after stimulating let-down and expressing a little milk. (The breast will be softer and it will be easier to grasp the nipple.)

d. Use analgesics. (If taken immediately before nursing, less medication will go to the baby.)

Explain to Ann that her emotional upheaval is probably the "baby blues" or "postpartum blues" and that they usually subside in 24–72 hours. Instruct her to call her physician if the blues do not subside, or if she develops symptoms of depression.

Ask why she started supplemental feedings. Upon questioning, Ann tells you that she had started supplementing her baby with formula after each feeding because her mother-in-law told her that the baby was nursing too frequently (every 1–3 hours, sometimes clustering 3–4 feedings in one 2–3 hour period). She told Ann that the baby was obviously not getting enough breast milk. After receiving supplemental feedings, the baby began feeding once every 3–5 hours.

Tactfully explain that although Ann's mother-in-law meant well, her comments indicate a lack of information about breastfeeding; that is,

a. Breast milk digests faster than formula, so breastfeeding babies feed more frequently.

b. On average, babies nurse 8–12 times in 24 hours.

c. After lactation is well established, the baby will nurse less frequently. During growth spurts, however, all babies nurse more frequently for a few days.

Explain that Ann may still breastfeed successfully, and if she desires to continue breastfeeding, she should stop supplementing with formula.

Chapter 31

We hope that you would tell her that nurses always wear gloves during the initial assessment of a newborn, during all admission procedures until the newborn has its first bath, and sometimes during diaper changes. You should also tell her that her baby will not be isolated from the other babies when in the nursery, and that her baby can remain with her if she wishes. It is important to recognize the concern that Mrs Corrigan may have about people knowing that her baby may have HIV, and to assess her own feelings of social isolation.

Chapter 32

It is important to give this mother clear, factual information regarding the type, cause, and usual course of the baby's respiratory problem. You see that Linn's laboratory tests, chest x-ray, and clinical course so far are indicative of transient tachypnea of the newborn. Respiratory distress syndrome is probably not the problem since Linn is not premature and didn't have any asphyxia at birth. You recognize that prior experience with a premature newborn with respiratory distress and prolonged hospitalization will add to this mother's fear and anxiety regarding her new baby. Therefore, in addition to giving factual information regarding the baby's condition, it is important for you to see whether the mother can be brought to the nursery to see her baby, or to have the mother receive a picture of the baby for reassurance. Before the mother visits the baby, clearly describe the oxygen and monitoring equipment that is helping Linn so that the mother will not be alarmed upon seeing her daughter.

Chapter 33

These findings are not within the normal range. At 24 hours past birth the fundus should be approximately one finger-breadth below the umbilicus and located in the midline. A uterus that is deviated to the right may indicate that the bladder is full and the woman needs to urinate. You should determine whether she is having difficulty urinating and emptying her bladder; if so, you can try some nursing measures to help her void. The lochia will still be rubra, but the amount is excessive and may be related to a boggy uterus.

Chapter 34

Clots are a sign of a problem in any postpartal woman. You will need to obtain further information regarding the size of the clots, obtain the mother's vital signs, assess the uterus for position and firmness, and assess the amount of lochial flow. The clot may be associated with uterine relaxation and fundal massage may be needed. It is important to first obtain more information.

Chapter 36

You should have Lei return to her room via wheelchair. Assess her leg for warmth, edema, redness, tenderness, and Homan's sign. Discuss with Lei that she should not massage her leg or get out of bed until you consult with the primary provider concerning your findings. Notify her primary health care provider and document your assessment findings.

RESOURCE DIRECTORY

This Resource Directory lists associations, support groups, and other organizations that can provide information or other assistance to maternal-newborn nurses and their clients. The resources are organized by topic, usually with brief descriptions of their services. Because many of these organizations have branches or chapters throughout North America, we recommend that you refer to your telephone directory for the location of the local branch.

GENERAL INFORMATION RESOURCES

National Center for Health Statistics (NCHS)
(produces vital and health statistics for the United States)
Scientific and Technical Information Branch
Department of Health and Human Services
6525 Belcrest Road, Room 1064
Hyattsville, MD 20782
(301) 436-8500

National Health Information Center
(provides information on health organizations and publications; selected diseases; Medicare, Medicaid, and other insurances)
working through The Office of Disease
Prevention and Health Promotion
P.O. Box 1133
Washington, DC 10013-1133
(301) 565-4167; (800) 336-4797

National Institute of Child Health and Human Development (NICHD)
National Institutes of Health
9000 Rockville Pike
Bldg. 31A, Room 2A32
Bethesda, MD 20892
(301) 496-5133

National Library of Medicine (NLM)
(collects and disseminates biomedical information; publishes indexes of journal and research literature related to biomedical fields)
Public Information Office
8600 Rockville Pike
Bethesda, MD 20894
(301) 496-6308; (800) 272-4787

National Maternal and Child Health Clearinghouse
(provides information and publications regarding maternal/child health, nutrition, pregnancy, etc)
2070 Chain Bridge Road, Suite 450
Vienna, VA 22182
(703) 625-8410

National Technical Information Service (NTIS)
(source of specialized social, scientific, business, and economic information, mostly originated or sponsored by federal agencies)
Department of Commerce
5285 Port Royal Road
Springfield, VA 22161
(703) 487-4600

Office of Research for Women's Health
National Institute of Health
9000 Rockville Pike
Bldg. 1, Room 201
Bethesda, MD 20892
(301) 402-1770

ONLINE COMPUTER SERVICES

Knight-Ridder Information, Inc.
2440 El Camino Real
Mountain View, CA 94040
(415) 254-7000; (800) 334-2564

National Library of Medicine
MEDLARS Management Section
Bldg. 38A, Room 4N-421
8600 Rockville Pike
Bethesda, MD 20894
(800) 638-8480

Ovid Technologies
5650 S. Green Street
Murray, UT 84123
(801) 281-3884; (800) 289-4277

RESOURCES BY TOPIC

ABORTION

National Abortion Federation
(provides information and referrals for abortion services)
1436 U Street, NW, Suite 103
Washington, DC 20009
(202) 667-5881; (800) 772-9100

National Abortion Rights Action League
(pro-choice political action group)
1156 15th Street NW, Suite 700
Washington, DC 20005
(202) 828-9300

National Right to Life Committee
(pro-life political action group)

Planned Parenthood Federation of America
810 Seventh Avenue
New York, NY 10019
(212) 541-7800; (800) 829-7732
See also Family Planning

ADOPTION

AASK (Adopt a Special Kid)
(provides assistance to families who adopt older and handicapped children)
2201 Broadway, Suite 702
Oakland, CA 94612
(510) 451-1748; FAX (510) 451-2023

Adoptees' Liberty Movement Association (ALMA) Society
(provides assistance for adopted children to locate natural parents and for natural parents to locate relinquished children)
P.O. Box 727
Radio City Station
New York, NY 10101-0727
(212) 581-1568

Child Welfare Administration
(provides information on adoption, foster care, and child abuse)
80 Lafayette
New York, NY 10013
(718) 291-1900

Child Welfare League of America
(provides information about adoption, especially of children with special needs)
Four 41st Street NW, Suite 310
Washington, DC 20001-2085
(202) 638-2952

AIDS (ACQUIRED IMMUNE DEFICIENCY SYNDROME)

American Foundation for AIDS Research (AmFar)
(provides funding for scientific research, education, and clinical trials. Does not provide general information)
733 3rd Ave., 12th Floor
New York, NY 10017
(212) 682-7440

American Social Health Association
Home Office
P.O. Box 13827
RTP, NC 27709

AIDS INFORMATION HOTLINE
(800) 342-AIDS

SIDA Hotline
(provides AIDS information in Spanish)
(800) 344-7432

TTY/TTD Hotline
(provides AIDS information for the deaf)
(800) 243-7889

Community Health Education Core
(conducts research and maintains an extensive research library on women's health and HIV prevention)
Columbia University School of Public Health
722 W. 168th Street, Box 29
New York, NY 10032
(212) 740-7292

National AIDS Clearinghouse
(provides treatment directory)
P.O. Box 6003
Rockville, MD 20849-6003
(800) 458-5231
for information regarding clinical trials:
(800) TRIALS-A

Shanti Project
(provides counseling and assistance to individuals with AIDS)
1546 Market Street
San Francisco, CA 94102
(415) 864-2273

ALCOHOL ABUSE

Al-Anon/Alateen
P.O. Box 862
Midtown Station
New York, NY 10018-0862
(212) 302-7240; (800) 344-2666

Alcoholics Anonymous
475 Riverside Drive
New York, NY 10115
(212) 870-3400

National Clearinghouse for Alcohol and Drug Information
P.O. Box 2345
Rockville, MD 20847
(301) 468-2600; (800) 729-6686

Victim Outreach Program
Mothers Against Drunk Drivers (MADD)
(operates Victim Outreach Program to aid victims through the court process. Conducts research)
1341 W. Mockingbird Lane, #240W
Dallas, TX 75247
(214) 744-6233

Women for Sobriety, Inc.
(support group for women with drinking problems)
P.O. Box 618
Quakertown, PA 18951
(215) 536-8026; (800) 333-1606

BIRTH CONTROL

See Family Planning

BIRTH DEFECTS

American Cleft Palate Association
(provides information about cleft palates and cleft palate centers and parent support groups)
1218 Grandview Ave.
Pittsburgh, PA 15211
(412) 481-1376

Cystic Fibrosis Foundation
2250 N. Druid Hills Rd., Suite 275
Atlanta, GA 30329
(404) 325-6973; (800) 476-4483

Institutes for the Achievement of Human Potential
(resource for parents with brain-injured children)
8801 Stenton Avenue
Philadelphia, PA 19118
(215) 233-2050

March of Dimes Birth Defects Foundation
Public Health Education Foundation
1275 Mamaroneck Avenue
White Plains, NY 10605
(914) 428-7100

Spina Bifida Association of America
(provides information and support to parents of infants with neural tube defects)
4590 McArthur Blvd., NW, Suite 250
Washington, DC 20007-4226
(800) 621-3141
See also Down Syndrome; Genetic Disorders; Sickle Cell Anemia

BREAST CANCER

Reach to Recovery
(support program for women who have undergone mastectomies as a result of breast cancer)
American Cancer Society
19 W. 56th St.
New York, NY 10019
(212) 586-8700
See also Cancer

BREASTFEEDING

Human Lactation Center
(limited to research on international infant/maternal feeding practices. No information provided)
666 Sturges Highway
Westport, CT 06880
(203) 259-5995

La Leche League International
(provides information about breastfeeding and support for breastfeeding mothers)
1400 N. Meachen Rd.
Chalmburg, IL 60173
(708) 519-7730
(800) 525-3243 (800 LaLeche)

Lact-Aid
(provides services, literature, and supplies to promote breastfeeding)
P.O. Box 1066
Athens, TN 37371-1066
(615) 744-9090
See also Childbirth; Infant Health

Lactation Consultants Association, Ltd. (ILCA)
P.O. Box 4031
University of Virginia Station
Charlottesville, VA 22903

CANCER

American Cancer Society National Office
1599 Clifton Rd. NE
Atlanta, GA 30329-4251
(404) 320-3333; (800) 227-2345

Cancer Information Service, Cancer Inquiries
(provides cancer information for the general public)
National Cancer Institute
900 Wisconsin Ave.
Bethesda, MD 20814
(301) 496-5583
(to access regional offices for cancer information in English or Spanish)
(800) 4-CANCER
See also Breast Cancer; DES Exposure; Smoking

CESAREAN BIRTH

C/SEC, Inc. (Cesarean/Support Education and Concern)
(provides information about cesarean birth)
22 Forest Road
Framingham, MA 01701
(508) 877-8266

VBAC (Vaginal Birth After Cesarean)
10 Great Plain Terrace
Needham, MA 01292

CHILD ABUSE

C. Henry Kempe National Center for Prevention and Treatment of Child Abuse and Neglect
(publishes a newsletter with information on prevention and treatment of child abuse)
University of Colorado Medical Center
Department of Pediatrics
1205 Oneida Street
Denver, CO 80220
(303) 321-3963

Clearinghouse on Child Abuse and Neglect Information
Office of Child Development
P.O. Box 1182
Washington, DC 20013
(703) 714-6120 FAX

National Committee for Prevention of Child Abuse (NCPCA)
(provides literature on child abuse prevention programs)
332 South Michigan Avenue, Suite 1600
Chicago, IL 60604
(312) 663-3520

CHILD HEALTH AND DEVELOPMENT

Canadian Institute of Child Health
885 Meadowlands Drive East, Suite 512
Ottawa, Ontario K2C 3N2
(613) 224-4144

National Center for Education in Maternal and Child Health
38th and R Streets, NW
Washington, DC 20057
(202) 625-8400

National Institute of Child Health and Human Development (NICHD)
9000 Rockville Pike
Bldg. 31, Room 2A32
Bethesda, MD 20892
(301) 496-4000

4 Parents Helpline
(provides non-medical support, information and referrals to parents and care givers)
Work and Family Resources of the Community College of Denver
1391 N. Speer Blvd.
Denver, CO 80204
(303) 620-4444

CHILDBIRTH

American Foundation for Maternal and Child Health, Inc.
(clearinghouse for scientific information on obstetric care)
439 E. 51st Street
New York, NY 10002
(212) 759-5510

Birth: Issues in Prenatal Care and Education
(quarterly journal)
(publisher also provides directory of instructional materials for childbirth educators)
Blackwell Scientific Publications, Inc.
3 Cambridge Center, Suite 208
Cambridge, MA 02142
(617) 876-7000

International Childbirth Education Association
(provides information to educators and consumers on childbirth education)
P.O. Box 20048
Minneapolis, MN 55420
(612) 854-8660

Maternity Center Association
(freestanding birth center that provides information and advocacy functions)
48 East 92nd Street
New York, NY 10128
(212) 369-7300

National Association of Childbearing Centers
(organization that provides information and suggests guidelines for birth centers)
3123 Gottschall Road
Perkiomenville, PA 18074
(215) 234-8068

4 Parents Helpline
(provides non-medical support, information and referrals to parents and care givers)
Work and Family Resources of the Community College of Denver
1391 N. Speer Blvd.
Denver, CO 80204
(303) 620-4444

CHILDBIRTH EDUCATION/PREPARATION

American Academy of Husband-Coached Childbirth
(provides information on the Bradley method of childbirth)
P.O. Box 5224
Sherman Oaks, CA 91413
(818) 788-6662;
(800) 42-BIRTH within CA
(800) 423-2397 outside CA

American Society for Psychoprophylaxis in Obstetrics
(provides information about the Lamaze method of childbirth)
1200 19th Street NW, Suite 300
Washington, DC 20036-2412
(202) 857-1128; (800) 368-4404

Childbirth Graphics, Ltd.
(provides audiovisual and other types of teaching aids for childbirth education)
P.O. Box 20540
Rochester, NY 14602-0540
(716) 272-0300; FAX (716) 272-0716

Read Natural Childbirth Foundation, Inc.
(provides information about the Dick-Read method of childbirth)
P.O. Box 956
San Rafael, CA 94915
(415) 456-8462
See also Cesarean Birth; Childbirth

CIRCUMCISION

American Academy of Pediatrics
(report on circumcision available for a minimal fee)
141 Northwest Point Blvd.
Elk Grove, IL 60007-0927
(708) 228-5005

Childbirth Education Foundation
(Eastern area contact for No-CIRC; promotes reform in childbirth practices, especially in the treatment of the newborn)
P.O. Box 5
Richboro, PA 18954
(610) 828-0131

National Organization of Circumcision Information Resource Center (No-CIRC)
(western area contact)
P.O. Box 2512
San Anselmo, CA 94960
(415) 488-9883

CONGENITAL DISORDERS/DEFECTS

See Birth Defects; Genetic Disorders

CONTRACEPTION

See Family Planning

COUNSELING SERVICES

Family Service America
(organization of local family counseling agencies throughout North America)
11700 Westlake Park Drive
Milwaukee, WI 53224
(414) 359-1040

Women in Transition (WIT)
(provides counseling information and referrals for women in distress and transition because of divorce, widowhood, and separation)
215 12th Street, 6th Floor
Philadelphia, PA 19107-3606
(215) 751-1111

DES (DIETHYLSTILBESTROL) EXPOSURE

Cancer Information Service, Cancer Inquiries
(provides information to DES mothers and daughters)
National Cancer Institute
900 Wisconsin Ave.
Bethesda, MD 20814
(301) 496-5583
(to access regional offices for cancer information in English or Spanish)
(800) 4-CANCER

DES Action
(provides information on DES and the DES cancer network)
1615 Broadway, Suite 510
Oakland, CA 94612
(510) 465-4011

DOWN SYNDROME

National Association for Down's Syndrome (NADS)
(provides information about Down syndrome)
1605 Chantilly Drive, #250
Atlanta, GA 30324
(404) 633-1555;
(800) 232-6372

National Down's Syndrome Society Hotline
666 Broadway
New York, NY 10012
(800) 221-4602; in New York (212) 460-9330
See also Birth Defects; Genetic Disorders

FAMILY

Displaced Homemakers Network
(national advocacy group for women over 35 who have lost their primary means of support through death, divorce, or disabling of spouse)
1625 K Street NW, #300
Washington, DC 20006
(202) 467-6346

Fathers for Equal Rights
P.O. Box 010847
Flagler Station
Miami, FL 33101
(305) 895-6351

Family Service America
(provides counseling and assistance to families)
11700 Westlake Park Drive
Milwaukee, WI 53223
(414) 359-1040

Parents Without Partners
(support group for single parents)
8807 Colesville Road
Silver Spring, MD 20910
(800) 637-7974

Step Family Foundation
333 West End Ave.
New York, NY 10023
(212) 877-3244

FAMILY PLANNING

Association of Voluntary Sterilization, Inc. (AVS)
(provides information on sterilization and referral service)
79 Madison Ave.
New York, NY 10168
(212) 561-8000

Couple to Couple League International, Inc. (CCL)
(teaches natural family planning techniques; publishes manual on the symptothermal method, The Art of Natural Family Planning)
P.O. Box 111184
Cincinnati, OH 45211
(513) 471-2000

Planned Parenthood Federation of America
810 Seventh Avenue
New York, NY 10019
(212) 541-7800; (800) 829-7732

Family Life Information Exchange
P.O. Box 30686
Bethesda, MD 20814
(301) 654-6190

FOOD AND NUTRITION

See Nutrition

GENETIC DISORDERS

National Center for Education in Maternal and Child Health
(provides educational services and technical assistance to organizations, agencies, and individuals with interests in maternal and child health issues)
38th & R Streets, NW
Washington, DC 20057
(202) 625-8400

HEARING-IMPAIRED CHILDREN

American Society for Deaf Children
(provides education and support to parents of hearing-impaired children)
2848 Arden Way, Suite 210
Sacramento, CA 95825-1373
(916) 482-0120
(800) 942-ASDC

International Organization for the Education of the Hearing Impaired
(provides information on speech and oralism in newborns and information regarding "at risk" infants. Grants financial assistance for the funding of hearing aids, speech therapy, etc. for parents of hearing-impaired children under 5 years)
c/o Alexander Graham Bell Association for the Deaf
3417 Volta Pl., NW
Washington, DC 20007-2778
(202) 337-5220

INFANT DEATH

Compassionate Friends
(self-help organization offering friendship and understanding to bereaved parents and siblings due to the death of a child of any age for any reason)
P.O. Box 3696
Oak Brook, IL 60522-3696
(708) 990-0010

SHARE (Source of Help in Airing and Resolving Experiences)
(support group for parents who have suffered loss of newborn baby)
c/o St. John's Hospital
800 E. Carpenter Street
Springfield, IL 62769
(217) 525-5675
See also Sudden Infant Death Syndrome

INFANT HEALTH

American Foundation for Maternal and Child Health
(clearinghouse for research on the perinatal period)
439 E. 51st St.
New York, NY 10022
(212) 759-5510

American Red Cross
(offers classes to prepare expectant parents for care and nurturing of infant)
431 18th St., NW
Washington, DC 20006
(202) 737-8300

National Center for Clinical Infant Programs
(promotes optimum development and mental health for infants and their families)
2000 14th St., N., Suite 380
Arlington, VA 22201-2500
(703) 528-4300
See also Child Health and Development

INFERTILITY

Fertility Research Foundation (FRF)
(provides medical and consultation services for infertile couples; publishes journals, Fertility Review *and* Infertility*)*
875 Park Avenue
New York, NY 10021
(212) 744-5500

Resolve, Inc.
1310 Broadway
Somerville, MA 02144-1731
(617) 643-2424

Test-Tube Fertilization
Eastern Virginia Medical School
Norfolk General Hospital
The Howard and Georgeanna Jones Institute for Reproductive Medicine
601 Colley Avenue
Norfolk, VA 23507
(804) 446-8948

INTRAUTERINE PROCEDURES

National Institute for Child Health and Human Development (NICHD)
9000 Rockville Pike
Bldg. 31, Room 2A32
Bethesda, MD 20892
(301) 496-4000

LEGAL CONCERNS

National Center on Women and Family Law
(collects information on battered women, child support, and custody)
799 Broadway, Room 402
New York, NY 10003
(212) 674-8200

Reproductive Freedom Project (ACLU)
American Civil Liberties Union
132 West 43rd Street
New York, NY 10036
(212) 944-9800

MEDICAL ORGANIZATIONS

American Academy of Family Physicians
8880 Ward Parkway
Kansas City, MO 64114
(816) 333-9700

American Academy of Pediatrics
141 Northwest Point Blvd.
Elk Grove Village, IL 60007
(312) 569-2025; (800) 433-9016

American College of Obstetricians and Gynecologists
409 12th St., SW
Washington, DC 20024
(202) 638-5577

American Medical Association
515 N. State St.
Chicago, IL 60610
(312) 464-5000

Society of Obstetricians and Gynaecologists of Canada
774 Echo Drive
Ottawa, Ontario K1S 5N8
(613) 730-4192

MEDICATIONS (PRESCRIPTION AND OVER-THE-COUNTER)

Food and Drug Administration (FDA)
Office of Consumer Affairs
Public Inquiries
5600 Fishers Lane (HFE-2)
Rockville, MD 20857
(301) 443-5006

MIDWIFERY

The Farm
(offers lay midwifery program, published midwifery handouts and Spiritual Midwifery; *publishes periodical* The Birth Gazette*)*
P.O. Box 34, The Farm
Summertown, TN 38483
(615) 964-3574
See also Nurse-Midwifery

MULTIPLE BIRTH

Center for the Study of Multiple Birth
333 East Superior Street, Suite 464
Chicago, IL 60611
(312) 266-9093

National Organization of Mothers of Twins Club
P.O. Box 23188
Albuquerque, NM 87192
(505) 275-0955

NURSE-MIDWIFERY

American College of Nurse Midwives
1 Dupont Circle NW
Washington, DC 20036-1120

Journal of Nurse-Midwifery
(periodical)
Elsevier Science Publishing Co., Inc.
655 Ave. of the Americas
New York, NY 10010
(212) 989-5800

NURSING ORGANIZATIONS

American Association of Nurse Anesthetists (AANA)
222 S. Prospect Avenue
Park Ridge, IL 60068-4001
(708) 692-7050

American Nurses Association and Foundation
600 Maryland Ave., SW, Suite 100 West
Washington, DC 20024
(202) 651-7000

Canadian Nurses Association
50 The Driveway
Ottawa, Ontario 4
Canada
(613) 237-2133

Association of Women's Health, Obstetric and Neonatal Nurses (AWHONN)
700 14th St., NW #600
Washington, DC 20005
(202) 662-1600

National League for Nursing (NLN)
350 Hudson St.
New York, NY 10014
(212) 989-9393
See also Nurse-Midwifery

NUTRITION

American Institute of Nutrition
9650 Rockville Pike
Bethesda, MD 20814
(301) 530-7050

Food and Drug Administration (FDA)
Office of Consumer Affairs
Public Inquiries
5600 Fishers Lane (HFE-88)
Rockville, MD 20857
(301) 443-5006

OBESITY

See Nutrition; Weight Control

OCCUPATIONAL HEALTH

Clearinghouse for Occupational Safety and Health Information
National Institute for Occupational Safety and Health
4676 Columbia Parkway
Cincinnati, OH 45226
(513) 533-8236

PREGNANCY

COPE (Coping with the Overall Pregnancy/ Parenting Experience)
530 Tremont Street
Boston, MA 02116
See also Childbirth; Family Planning; Women's Health

PREMENSTRUAL SYNDROME

See Women's Health

RAPE

See telephone directory for local Rape Centers

Women Against Rape
P.O. Box 02084
Columbus, OH 43202
(614) 291-9751
See also Sexual Abuse and Assault

SEX EDUCATION

Advocacy for Youth
(develops programs and material to educate teenagers on sex and sexual responsibility)
1025 Vermont Ave., NW, Suite 200
Washington, DC 20005
(202) 347-5700; FAX (202) 347-2263

Planned Parenthood Federation of America
810 Seventh Avenue
New York, NY 10019
(212) 541-7800; (800) 829-7732
See also Family Planning

SEXUAL ABUSE AND ASSAULT

Child Assault Prevention (CAP) Project
Women Against Rape
P.O. Box 02084
Columbus, OH 43202
(614) 291-9751

National Committee for Prevention of Child Abuse
332 S. Michigan Avenue, Suite 1600
Chicago, IL 60604
(312) 663-3520

Voices in Action, Inc.
(provides a communication and peer support network for victims of incest and those affected by it)
P.O. Box 148309
Chicago, IL 60614
(312) 327-1500

SEXUALLY TRANSMITTED INFECTIONS

Center for Prevention Services
(Conducts research. Provides information to physicans)
Centers for Disease Control
1600 Clifton Road, NE
Atlanta, GA 30333
Physicians ONLY call: (404) 639-3311
STD Hotline: (800) 227-8922

V.D. National Hotline
(800) 227-8922
See also AIDS; Sex Education

SICKLE CELL ANEMIA

Center for Sickle Cell Disease
2121 Georgia Avenue, NW
Washington, DC 20059
(202) 806-7930

SMOKING

The following organizations provide information about the effects of smoking as well as how to quit smoking. See the white pages of your telephone directory for local chapters.

American Cancer Society
19 W. 56th St.
New York, NY 10019
(212) 586-8700

American Heart Association
7272 Greenville Avenue
Dallas, TX 75231
(214) 373-6300

American Lung Association
1740 Broadway
New York, NY 10019
(212) 315-8700

SUDDEN INFANT DEATH SYNDROME (SIDS)

Loyola University
(maintains scientific research center for the investigation of SIDS)
2160 S. 1st Ave.
Maywood, IL 60153
(708) 216-9000

National Sudden Infant Death Syndrome Clearinghouse (NSIDSC)
8201 Greensboro Dr., Suite 600
McLean, VA 22102
(703) 821-8955, ext. 361
See also Infant Death

WEIGHT CONTROL

The following groups provide information about weight control and support for their members. See the white pages of your telephone directory for local chapters.

Overeaters Anonymous
P.O. Box 44620
Rio Rancho, NM 87174-4020
(505) 891-2664

TOPS (Take Off Pounds Sensibly)
P.O. Box 07360
4575 S. Fifth Street
Milwaukee, WI 53207-0360
(414) 482-4620

Weight Watchers International, Inc.
Jericho Atrium
500 North Broadway
Jericho, NY 11753-2196
(516) 939-0400
See also Nutrition

WOMEN'S HEALTH

Boston Women's Health Book Collective
(publishes Our Bodies, Ourselves, *a well-known book on women's health)*
240 Elm St.
Summerville, MA 02144-2935
(617) 625-0271

Coalition for Homelessness
(Advocates for the rights of the homeless. Provides education regarding homelessness)
126 Hyde
San Francisco, CA 94102
(415) 346-3740

Community Health Education Core
(conducts research and maintains an extensive research library on women's health, as well as HIV prevention)
Columbia University School of Public Health
722 W. 168th Street, Box 29
New York, NY 10032
(212) 740-7292

Office of Research for Women's Health
National Institute of Health
9000 Rockville Pike
Bldg. 1, Room 201
Bethesda, MD 20892-0161
(301) 402-1770

National Women's Health Network
(provides information about and is involved in legislative action for women's health issues)
514 10th, NW, Suite 400
Washington, DC 20004
(202) 347-1140

Women's Sports Foundation
(provides information about women's sports, physical fitness, and related topics)
Eisenhower Park
East Meadow, NY 11554
(800) 227-3988
See also Childbirth; Family Planning; Occupational Health

CREDITS

PHOTOGRAPHY CREDITS

Special thanks to Wendy Harle, Development and Public Affairs, Massachusetts General Hospital, Boston, MA; Laurie Miller, Womencare, Arlington, MA; Teresa Corrigan, Perinatal Education and Lactation Center, California Pacific Medical Center, San Francisco, CA; Sequoia Hospital, Redwood City, CA; and Boston Regional Medical Center, Stoneham, MA.

Part Openers   I: William Gage/Custom Medical Stock Photography. II: Philip Matson/Tony Stone Images, Inc. III: Mark Segal/Tony Stone Worldwide, Ltd. IV: David Young Wolff/Tony Stone Worldwide, Ltd. V: S. I. U./Science Source/Photo Researchers, Inc. VI: Terry Vine/Tony Stone Images, Inc. VII: John Fortunato/Tony Stone Worldwide, Ltd.

Chapter 1   1-1, 3: Richard Tauber. 1-2: Amy Snyder.

Chapter 3   3-1 (clockwise, starting upper left): Alain McLaughlin, Elena Dorfman, Robert Brenner/Photo Edit, Elena Dorfman, © Joseph Sohm/Photo Researchers, Inc. 3-3: Amy Snyder.

Chapter 4   4-1: Richard Tauber.

Chapter 5   5-22, 23: Courtesy of Dr. E. S. E. Hafez, Wayne State University, Detroit, MI.

Chapter 6   6-5b, 22, 23, 24: © Lennart Nilsson, *A Child is Born*, Dell, New York, NY © 1990. 6-18, 19, 20, 21: © Petit Format/Nestle/Science Source/Photo Researchers, Inc.

Chapter 7   7-4b: Courtesy of Lovena L. Porter. 7-4c: from Speroff, L. et al., *Clinical Gynecological Endocrinology and Infertility* 4th ed. 1989, p. 520 © 1989 Williams & Wilkins Co., Baltimore, MD. 7-6, 7: Courtesy of Jane Cangleton and Reproductive Genetics Center. 7-8, 9: Courtesy of Dr. Arthur Robinson, National Jewish Hospital and Research Center. 7-10, 11, 12: from Smith's *Recognizable Patterns of Human Malformations*. Philadelphia: Saunders. 7-14, 15: from Thompson, J. S., Thompson, M. W., *Genetics in Medicine* 4th ed. 1986, Saunders, Philadelphia.

Chapter 8   8-1: © Mark Ludak/Impact Visuals. 8-2: Courtesy of Edward Zieserl, MD. 8-3: Richard Tauber.

Chapter 9   9-4a, 5a, 7, 9 (top): Kathleen Cameron. 9-9 (bottom): Alain McLaughlin.

Chapter 10   10-4, 5: Center for Disease Control. 10-6: © Visuals Unlimited. 10-7: © Kenneth Greer/Visuals Unlimited.

Chapter 12   12-3a, 4: Anne Dowie. 12-3b, 3c: Stella Johnson, 1995. 12-3d: Custom Medical Stock Photography. 12-5: Richard Tauber.

Chapter 14   14-3: Suzanne Arms. 14-5: Amy Snyder.

Chapter 15   15-1, 2, 9: Richard Tauber. 15-3: Stella Johnson, 1995. 15-7, 8: Elena Dorfman. 15-10: Suzanne Arms.

Chapter 16   16-1: Amy Snyder. 16-2: H. Gans/The Image Works. 16-3: Stella Johnson, 1995.

Chapter 17   17-2: Michael Newman/PhotoEdit.

Chapter 18   18-1: Stella Johnson, 1995.

Chapter 19   19-4: Courtesy of Tokos Medical Corporation. 19-7, 8: Amy Snyder.

Chapter 20   20-1: Richard Tauber. 20-2, 16: Amy Snyder. 20-3: Courtesy of Diane Roth. 20-4: Callen: *Ultrasonography and Obstetrics and Gynecology*, 2nd ed. 1988, Fig. 4-1, pg. 49. Saunders, Philadelphia. 20-5: Callen: *Ultrasonography and Obstetrics and Gynecology*, 2nd ed. 1988, Fig. 4-2, pg. 50. Saunders, Philadelphia. 20-6: Callen: *Ultrasonography and Obstetrics and Gynecology*, 2nd ed. 1988, Fig. 4-3, pg. 51. Saunders, Philadelphia. 20-7: Callen: *Ultrasonography and Obstetrics and Gynecology*, 2nd ed. 1988, Fig. 4-5, pg. 55. Saunders, Philadelphia. 20-8: Callen: *Ultrasonography and Obstetrics and Gynecology*, 2nd ed. 1988, Fig. 4-4, pg. 53. Saunders, Philadelphia. 20-9: Callen: *Ultrasonography and Obstetrics and Gynecology*, 2nd ed. 1988, Fig. 4-8, pg. 58. Saunders, Philadelphia. 20-10: Callen: *Ultrasonography and Obstetrics and Gynecology*, 2nd ed. 1988, Fig. 4-7, pg. 57. Saunders, Philadelphia. 20-12, 13: "Umbilical Artery Doppler Flow Studies during Pregnancy"; by Jayme L. Cundiff, Kathleen Haubrich and Nancy G. Hinzman. *JOGNN*, Vol. 19, No. 6, pp. 475–481. 20-20: © John Watney/Photo Researchers, Inc.

Chapter 21　21-12: Stella Johnson, 1995.

Chapter 22　22-4, 9: Stella Johnson, 1995. 22-5: Courtesy of Medical Systems, Inc., Wallingford, CT. 22-7: Courtesy of Utah Medical Products, Inc., Midvale, UT.

Chapter 23　23-1, 3, 6, 9, 10: Stella Johnson, 1995. 23-2, 4, 5, 7: Suzanne Arms.

Chapter 25　25-20: Courtesy of Dr. Dan Farine, University of Toronto.

Chapter 27　27-13, 14: Elizabeth Elkin.

Chapter 28　28-2, 3b, 3c, 4a, 4b, 5a, 5b, 6a, 7, 8, 9, 10: Reprinted by permission of V. Dubowitz, M. D., Hammersmith Hospital, London, England. 28-3a: Barbara Corey, RNC, MSN, MNP. 28-4c, 5c, 6b, 31: Suzanne Arms. 28-13, 16, 32: Elizabeth Elkin. 28-23, 30: from Korones S. B.: *High Risk Newborn Infants* 4th ed. St. Louis: Mosby, 1986. 28-24, 33: Reproduced with permission from Potter, E. L., Craig, J. M.: *Pathology of the Fetus and Infant* 3rd ed. © 1975 by Year Book Medical Publishers, Chicago. 28-25, 27, 29, 35a: Courtesy of Mead Johnson & Company, Evansville, IN. 28-26: Courtesy of Dr. Ralph Platow, from Potter, E. L., Craig, J. M.: *Pathology of the Fetus and Infant* 3rd ed. © 1975 by Year Book Medical Publishers, Chicago. 28-28, 35b, 36, 37, 38, 39, 40: Stella Johnson, 1995.

Chapter 29　29-1, 5, 7, 8, 9: Stella Johnson, 1995. 29-2, 4: Elizabeth Elkin.

Chapter 30　30-1, 5, 6b, 10, 11, 12: Stella Johnson, 1995. 30-14: © Suzanne Arms Wimberly from Renfrow, Arms, Fisher: *Breastfeeding: Getting Breastfeeding Right for You.* Berkeley, CA: Celestial Arts, 1990.

Chapter 31　31-4, 6, 8, 16: Stella Johnson, 1995. 31-5: From Dubowitz L, Dubowitz V: *Gestational Age of the Newborn.* Menlo Park, CA: Addison-Wesley. 31-12: Courtesy of Kadlac Medical Center/Carol Thompson. 31-13: Courtesy of Theresa Kledyck. Table 31-4: Courtesy of Dr. Paul Winchester.

Chapter 32　32-1, 5, 7, 10, 15, 16: Stella Johnson, 1995. 32-12: Elizabeth Elkin.

Chapter 33　33-2: from Myles *Textbook for Midwives*, 11th ed by Bennett and Brown. Churchill Livingstone, 1989, pg. 235, Fig. 16-2.

Chapter 34　34-1: Anne Dowie. 34-2: Stella Johnson, 1995.

Chapter 35　35-1, 2: Stella Johnson, 1995. 35-4: Elizabeth Elkin.

Chapter 36　36-2: Amy Snyder.

One Family's Story photos by Richard Tauber.

ART CREDITS

Chapter 2　2-1: Nea Hanscomb.

Chapter 3　3-2, 4: Nea Hanscomb.

Chapter 5　5-1, 6, 11, 12, 15, 16, 18, 20, 26: Kristin N. Mount. 5-2, 3, 4, 10, 17, 19, 21, 24: Nea Hanscomb. 5-5, 9, 25: Wendy Hiller Gee/Biomed Arts/Nea Hanscomb. 5-7, 8, 13, 14: Joanne Bales/Precision Graphics.

Chapter 6　6-1, 2, 3, 4, 14: Nea Hanscomb. 6-5a, 7, 8, 9, 10, 15, 16: Kristin N. Mount. 6-6, 11, 17: Joanne Bales/Precision Graphics.

Chapter 7　7-1, 2, 5, 13: Nea Hanscomb. 7-3: The Left Coast Production Group. 7-4a, 16, 17, 18, 20, 21: Joanne Bales/Precision Graphics. 7-19: Kristin N. Mount.

Chapter 9　9-1, 2, 3, 8: Nea Hanscomb. 9-4b, 5b, 5c, 5d, 6: Joanne Bales/Precision Graphics.

Chapter 10　10-1, 2: Joanne Bales/Precision Graphics. 10-3: Kristin N. Mount.

Chapter 12　12-1: Nea Hanscomb. 12-2: The Left Coast Production Group. 12-6: Joanne Bales/Precision Graphics.

Chapter 13　13-1, 3, 4, 6: Kristin N. Mount. 13-5: Joanne Bales/Precision Graphics.

Chapter 14　14-1: Nea Hanscomb. 14-2: The Left Coast Production Group. 14-4, 6, 7, 8, 9: Kristin N. Mount.

Chapter 15　15-4: The Left Coast Production Group. 15-5: Nea Hanscomb. 15-6, 11: Kristin N. Mount.

Chapter 17　17-1: Robert Vioghts. 17-3: The Left Coast Production Group.

Chapter 19　19-1, 3, 6: Joanne Bales/Precision Graphics. 19-2, 9: Kristin N. Mount. 19-5: Nea Hanscomb.

Chapter 20　20-11, 14, 15, 17, 18: Nea Hanscomb. 20-19: Kristin N. Mount.

Chapter 21　21-1, 2, 3: Kristin N. Mount. 21-4, 5, 6, 7, 8, 11, 13, 15, 16, 17, 18: Joanne Bales/Precision Graphics. 21-9: Nea Hanscomb. 21-10: Nea Hanscomb. 21-13, 14: Kristin N. Mount.

Chapter 22 22-1, 8: Kristin N. Mount. 22-2, 3, 6, 10, 11, 12, 27: Joanne Bales/Precision Graphics. 22-13, 14, 15, 16, 17, 18, 19, 20, 21, 22, 23, 24, 25, 26: Nea Hanscomb.

Chapter 23 Table 23-3 (top, middle-top, middle-bottom, bottom): Nea Hanscomb. Table 23-3 (middle): Kristin N. Mount. 23-8, 12, 13: Joanne Bales/Precision Graphics.

Chapter 24 24-1, 3a, 3c: Joanne Bales/Precision Graphics. 24-2, 3b, 3d, 4, 5, 6, 7, 8, 9: Kristin N. Mount.

Chapter 25 25-1, 6, 16, 18, 21, 22, 24: Nea Hanscomb. 25-2: The Left Coast Production Group. 25-3, 4, 5, 7, 8, 9, 10, 11, 12, 13, 14, 17, 19, 23: Joanne Bales/Precision Graphics. 25-15: Kristin N. Mount.

Chapter 26 26-1, 2, 5, 6: Joanne Bales/Precision Graphics. 26-3: Wendy Hiller Gee/Biomed Arts/Nea Hanscomb. 26-4, 7: Nea Hanscomb.

Chapter 27 27-1, 3, 4, 7, 11: Nea Hanscomb. 27-2, 5, 6, 8: Kristin N. Mount. 27-9, 10: Joanne Bales/Precision Graphics.

Chapter 28 28-1, 12: The Left Coast Production Group. 28-11: Nea Hanscomb. 28-14, 15: Joanne Bales/Precision Graphics. 28-24, 28-25, 34: Kristin N. Mount.

Chapter 29 29-3: Kristin N. Mount. 29-6, 10, 11, 12, 13, 15: Joanne Bales/Precision Graphics. 29-14, 16: The Left Coast Production Group.

Chapter 30 30-2, 6a, 7, 8, 13: Joanne Bales/Precision Graphics. 30-3: Nea Hanscomb. 30-4: Kristin N. Mount. 30-9: The Left Coast Production Group.

Chapter 31 Table 31-4: Kristin N. Mount. 31-1, 2, 7, 11, 14, 15: Nea Hanscomb. 31-9, 10: Joanne Bales/Precision Graphics.

Chapter 32 32-2, 3, 9: Joanne Bales/Precision Graphics. 32-4, 6, 8, 11, 13, 14: Nea Hanscomb.

Chapter 33 33-1: Kristin N. Mount. 33-3, 5: Joanne Bales/Precision Graphics. 33-4: Nea Hanscomb.

Chapter 35 35-3: Nea Hanscomb. 35-5: The Left Coast Production Group. 35-6: Joanne Bales/Precision Graphics.

Chapter 36 36-1, 3: Kristin N. Mount.

Abdominal effleurage Gentle stroking used in massage.

Abortion Loss of pregnancy before the fetus is viable outside the uterus; miscarriage.

Abruptio placentae Partial or total premature separation of a normally implanted placenta.

Abstinence Refraining voluntarily, especially from indulgence in food, alcoholic beverages, or sexual intercourse.

Acceleration Periodic increase in the baseline fetal heart rate.

Acini cells Secretory cells in the human breast that create milk from nutrients in the bloodstream.

Acme Peak or highest point; time of greatest intensity (of a uterine contraction).

Acrocyanosis Cyanosis of the extremities.

Acrosomal reaction Break–down of the hyaluronic acid in the corona radiata by enzymes from the heads of sperm; allows one spermatozoon to penetrate the ovum zona pellucida.

Active acquired immunity Formation of antibodies by the pregnant woman in response to illness or immunization.

Acute grief The most severe stage of the grief response; usually resolved within 1 to 2 months and followed by a gradual return to the pre-loss level of functioning.

Adnexa Adjoining or accessory parts of a structure, such as the uterine adnexa: the ovaries and fallopian tubes.

Adolescence Period of human development initiated by puberty and ending with the attainment of young adulthood.

Afterbirth Placenta and membranes expelled after the birth of the infant, during the third stage of labor. Also called secundines.

Afterpains Cramplike pains due to contractions of the uterus that occur after childbirth. They are more common in multiparas, tend to be most severe during nursing, and last 2 to 3 days.

AIDS (Acquired immune deficiency syndrome) A sexually transmitted viral disease that so far has proved fatal in 100% of cases.

Allele One of a series of alternative genes at the same locus; one form of a gene.

Alveoli Small units of the breast tissue in which milk is synthesized by the alveolar secretory epithelium.

Amenorrhea Suppression or absence of menstruation.

Amniocentesis Removal of amniotic fluid by insertion of a needle into the amniotic sac; amniotic fluid is used to assess fetal health or maturity.

Amnion The inner of the two membranes that form the sac containing the fetus and the amniotic fluid.

Amnionitis Infection of the amniotic fluid.

Amniotic fluid The liquid surrounding the fetus in utero. It absorbs shocks, permits fetal movement, and prevents heat loss.

Amniotic fluid embolism Amniotic fluid that has leaked into the chorionic plate and entered the maternal circulation.

Amniotomy The artificial rupturing of the amniotic membrane.

Ampulla The outer two-thirds of the fallopian tube; fertilization of the ovum by a spermatozoon usually occurs here.

Androgen Substance producing male characteristics, such as the male hormone testosterone.

Android pelvis Male-type pelvis.

Antepartum Time between conception and the onset of labor; usually used to describe the period during which a woman is pregnant.

Anterior fontanelle Diamond-shaped area between the two frontal and two parietal bones just above the newborn's forehead.

Anthropoid pelvis Pelvis in which the anteroposterior diameter is equal to or greater than the transverse diameter.

Apgar score A scoring system used to evaluate newborns at 1 minute and 5 minutes after birth. The total score is achieved by assessing five signs: heart rate, respiratory effort, muscle tone, reflex irritability, and color. Each of the signs is assigned a score of 0, 1, or 2. The highest possible score is 10.

Apnea A condition that occurs when respirations cease for more than 20 seconds, with generalized cyanosis.

Areola Pigmented ring surrounding the nipple of the breast.

Artificial rupture of membranes (AROM) Use of a device such as an amnihook or allis forceps to rupture the amniotic membranes.

Artificial insemination Introduction of viable semen into the vagina by artificial means for the purpose of impregnation.

Assisted reproductive technology (ART) Term used to describe the highly technologic approaches used to produce pregnancy.

Attachment Enduring bonds or relationship of affection between persons.

Attitude Attitude of the fetus refers to the relationship of the fetal parts to each other.

Autosome A chromosome that is not a sex chromosome.

Babinski reflex Reflex found normally in infants under 6 months of age in which the great toe dorsiflexes when the sole of the foot is stimulated.

Bacterial vaginosis A bacterial infection of the vagina, formerly called *Gardnerella vaginalis* or *Hemophilus vaginalis*, characterized by a foul-smelling, grayish vaginal discharge that exhibits a characteristic fishy odor when 10% potassium hydroxide (KOH) is added. Microscopic examination of a vaginal wet prep reveals the presence of "clue cells" (vaginal epithelial cells coated with gram-negative organisms).

Bag of waters (BOW) The membrane containing the amniotic fluid and the fetus.

Ballottement A technique of palpation to detect or examine a floating object in the body. In obstetrics, the fetus, when pushed, floats away and then returns to touch the examiner's fingers.

Barr body Deeply staining chromatin mass located against the inner surface of the cell nucleus. It is found only in normal females. Also called sex chromatin.

Basal body temperature (BBT) The lowest waking temperature.

Baseline rate The average fetal heart rate observed during a 10-minute period of monitoring.

Baseline variability Changes in the fetal heart rate that result from the interplay between the sympathetic and the parasympathetic nervous systems.

Battledore placenta Placenta in which the umbilical cord is inserted on the periphery rather than centrally.

Bimanual palpation Examination of the pelvic organs by placing one hand on the abdomen and one or two fingers of the other hand into the vagina.

Biophysical profile Assessment of five variables in the fetus that help to evaluate fetal risk: breathing movement, body movement, tone, amniotic fluid volume, and fetal heart rate reactivity.

Birth center A setting for labor and birth that emphasizes a family-centered approach rather than obstetric technology and treatment.

Birth plan Decisions made by the expectant couple about aspects of the childbearing experience that are most important to them.

Birth rate Number of live births per 1000 population.

Birthing room A room for labor and birth with a relaxed atmosphere.

Bishop score A prelabor scoring system to assist in predicting whether an induction of labor may be successful. The total score is achieved by assessing five components: cervical dilatation, cervical effacement, cervical consistency, cervical position, and fetal station. Each of the components is assigned a score of 0 to 3, and the highest possible score is 13.

Blastocyst The inner solid mass of cells within the morula.

Blended family Families established through remarriage; may include children from previous marriages of each spouse as well as children of the current marriage.

Bloody show Pink-tinged mucous secretions resulting from rupture of small capillaries as the cervix effaces and dilates.

Body stalk Future umbilical cord; structure that attaches the embryo to the yolk sac and contains blood vessels that extend into the chorionic villi.

Boggy uterus A term used to describe the uterine fundus when it is not firmly contracted after the birth of the baby and in the early postpartum period; excessive bleeding occurs from the placental site and maternal hemorrhage may occur.

Bonding Process of parent-infant attachment occurring at or soon after birth.

Brachial palsy Partial or complete paralysis of portions of the arm resulting from trauma to the brachial plexus during a difficult birth.

Bradley method Partner-coached natural childbirth.

Bradycardia Slow heart rate.

Braxton Hicks contractions Intermittent painless contractions of the uterus that may occur every 10 to 20 minutes. They occur more frequently toward the end of pregnancy and are sometimes mistaken for true labor signs.

Brazleton's neonatal behavioral assessment A brief examination used to identify the infant's behavioral states and responses.

Breasts Mammary glands.

Breast self-examination Recommended monthly procedure by which women may detect changes or abnormalities in their breasts.

Breech presentation A birth in which the buttocks and/or feet are presented instead of the head.

Broad ligament The ligament extending from the lateral margins of the uterus to the pelvic wall; keeps uterus centrally placed and provides stability within the pelvic cavity.

Bronchopulmonary dysplasia (BPD) Chronic pulmonary disease of multifactorial etiology characterized initially by alveolar and bronchial necrosis, which results in bronchial metaplasia and interstitial fibrosis. Appears in x-ray films as generalized small, radiolucent cysts within the lungs.

Brown adipose tissue (BAT) Fat deposits in neonates that provide greater heat-generating activity than ordinary fat. Found around the kidneys, adrenals, and neck; between the scapulas; and behind the sternum. Also called brown fat.

Calorie Amount of heat required to raise the temperature of 1 kg of water 1 degree Celsius.

Capacitation Removal of the plasma membrane overlying the spermatozoa's acrosomal area with the loss of seminal plasma proteins and the glycoprotein coat. If the glycoprotein coat is not removed, the sperm will not be able to penetrate the ovum.

Caput succedaneum Swelling or edema occurring in or under the fetal scalp during labor.

Cardinal ligaments The chief uterine supports, suspending the uterus from the side walls of the true pelvis.

Cardinal movements of labor The positional changes of the fetus as it moves through the birth canal during labor and birth. The positional changes are descent, flexion, internal rotation, extension, restitution, and external rotation.

Cardiopulmonary adaptation Adaptation of the neonate's cardiovascular and respiratory systems to life outside the womb.

Cephalhematoma Subcutaneous swelling containing blood found on the head of an infant several days after birth, which usually disappears within a few weeks to 2 months.

Cephalic presentation Birth in which the fetal head is presenting against the cervix.

Cephalopelvic disproportion (CPD) A condition in which the fetal head is of such a shape or size, or in such a position, that it cannot pass through the maternal pelvis.

Certified nurse-midwife (CNM) An RN who has received special training and education in the care of the family during childbearing and the prenatal, labor and birth, and postpartal periods. After a period of formal education, the nurse-midwife takes a certification test to become a CNM.

Cervical cap A cup-shaped device placed over the cervix to prevent pregnancy.

Cervical dilatation Process in which the cervical os and the cervical canal widen from less than a centimeter to approximately 10 cm, allowing birth of the fetus.

Cervix The "neck" between the external os and the body of the uterus. The lower end of the cervix extends into the vagina.

Cesarean birth Birth of the fetus by means of an incision into the abdominal wall and the uterus.

Chadwick's sign Violet bluish color of the vaginal mucous membrane caused by increased vascularity; visible from about the fourth week of pregnancy.

Chemical conjunctivitis Irritation of the mucus membrane lining of the eyelid; may be due to instillation of silver nitrate ophthalmic drops.

Child abuse Nonaccidental physical or threatened harm, including mental or emotional injury, sexual abuse, and sexual exploitation.

Child neglect Failure by parents or other custodians to meet the medical, emotional, physical, or supervisory needs of a child.

Chloasma Brownish pigmentation over the bridge of the nose and the cheeks during pregnancy and in some women who are taking oral contraceptives. Also called mask of pregnancy.

Chorioamnionitis An inflammation of the amniotic membranes stimulated by organisms in the amniotic fluid, which then becomes infiltrated with polymorphonuclear leukocytes.

Chorion The fetal membrane closest to the intrauterine wall that gives rise to the placenta and continues as the outer membrane surrounding the amnion.

Chorionic villus sampling Procedure in which a specimen of the chorionic villi is obtained from the edge of the developing placenta at about 8 weeks' gestation. The sample can be used for chromosomal, enzyme, and DNA tests.

Chromosomes The threadlike structures within the nucleus of a cell that carry the genes.

Chronic grief Grief response involving a denial of the reality of the loss, which prevents any resolution.

Circumcision Surgical removal of the prepuce (foreskin) of the penis.

Circumoral cyanosis Bluish appearance around the mouth.

Circumvallate placenta A placenta with a thick white fibrous ring around the edge.

Cleavage Rapid mitotic division of the zygote; cells produced are called blastomeres.

Client advocacy An approach to client care in which the nurse educates and supports the client and protects the client's rights.

Climacteric The period of time that marks the cessation of a woman's reproductive function; the "change of life" or menopause.

Clitoris Female organ homologous to the male penis; a small oval body of erectile tissue situated at the anterior junction of the vulva.

Coitus Sexual intercourse between a male and female.

Coitus interruptus Method of contraception in which the male withdraws his penis from the vagina prior to ejaculation.

Cold stress Excessive heat loss resulting in compensatory mechanisms (increased respirations and nonshivering thermogenesis) to maintain core body temperature.

Colostrum Secretion from the breast before the onset of true lactation; contains mainly serum and white blood corpuscles. It has a high protein content, provides some immune properties, and cleanses the neonate's intestinal tract of mucus and meconium.

Colposcopy The use of an instrument inserted into the vagina to examine the cervical and vaginal tissues by means of a magnifying lens.

Conception Union of male sperm and female ovum; fertilization.

Conceptional age The number of complete weeks since the moment of conception. Because the moment of conception is almost impossible to determine, conceptional age is estimated at 2 weeks less than gestational age.

Condom A rubber sheath that covers the penis to prevent conception or disease.

Conduction Loss of heat to a cooler surface by direct skin contact.

Condyloma Wartlike growth of skin, usually seen on the external genitals or anus. There are two types, a pointed variety and a broad, flat form usually found with syphilis.

Conjugate Important diameter of the pelvis, measured from the center of the promontory of the sacrum to the back of the symphysis pubis. The diagonal conjugate is measured and the true conjugate is estimated.

Conjugate vera The true conjugate, which extends from the middle of the sacral promontory to the middle of the pubic crest.

Contraception The prevention of conception or impregnation.

Contraction Tightening and shortening of the uterine muscles during labor, causing effacement and dilatation of the cervix; contributes to the downward and outward descent of the fetus.

Contraction stress test A method of assessing the reaction of the fetus to the stress of uterine contractions. This test may be utilized when contractions are occurring spontaneously or when contractions are artificially induced by OCT (oxytocin challenge test) or BSST (breast self-stimulation test).

Convection Loss of heat from the warm body surface to cooler air currents.

Coombs' test A test for antiglobulins in the red cells. The indirect test determines the presence of Rh-positive antibodies in maternal blood; the direct test determines the presence of maternal Rh-positive antibodies in fetal cord blood.

Cornua The elongated portions of the uterus where the fallopian tubes open.

Corpus The upper two-thirds of the uterus.

Corpus luteum A small yellow body that develops within a ruptured ovarian follicle; it secretes progesterone in the second half of the menstrual cycle and atrophies about 3 days before the beginning of menstrual flow. If pregnancy occurs, the corpus luteum continues to produce progesterone until the placenta takes over this function.

Cotyledon One of the rounded portions into which the placenta's uterine surface is divided, consisting of a mass of villi, fetal vessels, and an intervillous space.

Couvade In some cultures, the male's observance of certain rituals and taboos to signify the transition to fatherhood.

Crack A form of free base cocaine that is smoked.

Crisis Any naturally occurring turning point, such as courtship, marriage, pregnancy, parenthood, or death.

Crisis intervention Actions taken by the nurse to help the client deal with an impending, potentially overwhelming crisis, regain his or her equilibrium, grow from the experience, and improve coping skills.

Critical thinking Intellectual processes that include separating fact from opinion, identifying prejudices and stereotypes that may influence interpretation of information, exploring differing ideas and views, and arriving at conclusions or insights.

Crowning Appearance of the presenting fetal part at the vaginal orifice during labor.

Deceleration Periodic decrease in the baseline fetal heart rate.

Decidua Endometrium or mucous membrane lining of the uterus in pregnancy that is shed after childbirth.

Decidua basalis The part of the decidua that unites with the chorion to form the placenta. It is shed in lochial discharge after childbirth.

Decidua capsularis The part of the decidua surrounding the chorionic sac.

Decidua vera (parietalis) Nonplacental decidua lining the uterus.

Decrement Decrease or stage of decline, as of a contraction.

Depo-Provera A long acting, injectable progestin contraceptive.

Descriptive statistics Statistics that describe or summarize a set of data.

Desquamation Shedding of the epithelial cells of the epidermis.

Developmental framework Focuses on the family over time as it progresses through predictable stages of the life cycle.

Diagonal conjugate Distance from the lower posterior border of the symphysis pubis to the sacral promontory; may be obtained by manual measurement.

Diaphragm A flexible disk that covers the cervix to prevent pregnancy.

Diastasis recti abdominis Separation of the recti abdominis muscles along the median line. In women, it is seen with repeated childbirths or multiple gestations. In the newborn, it is usually caused by incomplete development.

Dilatation and curettage (D and C) Stretching of the cervical canal to permit passage of a curette, which is used to scrape the endometrium to empty the uterine contents or to obtain tissue for examination.

Dilatation of the cervix Expansion of the external os from an opening a few millimeters in size to an opening large enough to allow the passage of the infant.

Diploid number of chromosomes Containing a set of maternal and a set of paternal chromosomes; in humans, the diploid number of chromosomes is 46.

Dissociation relaxation A pattern of active relaxation in which the woman learns to tighten one area of the body and then relax other areas simultaneously. This relaxation pattern is very effective for some women during labor.

Doula A supportive companion who accompanies a laboring woman to provide emotional, physical, and informational support and acts as an advocate for the woman and her family.

Down syndrome An abnormality resulting from the presence of an extra chromosome number 21 (trisomy 21); characteristics include mental retardation and altered physical appearance. Formerly called mongolism.

Drug-dependent infant The newborn of an alcoholic or drug-addicted woman.

Ductus arteriosus A communication channel between the main pulmonary artery and the aorta of the fetus. It is obliterated after birth by rising PO_2 and changes in intravascular pressure in the presence of normal pulmonary functioning. It normally becomes a ligament after birth but sometimes remains patent (patent ductus arteriosus, a treatable condition).

Ductus venosus A fetal blood vessel that carries oxygenated blood between the umbilical vein and the inferior vena cava, bypassing the liver; it becomes a ligament after birth.

Duncan's mechanism Occurs when the maternal surface of the placenta presents upon delivery rather than the shiny fetal surface.

Duration The time length of each contraction, measured from the beginning of the increment to the completion of the decrement.

Dysmenorrhea Painful menstruation.

Dyspareunia Painful intercourse.

Dystocia Difficult labor due to mechanical factors produced by the fetus or the maternal pelvis, or due to inadequate uterine or other muscular activity.

Early adolescence 14 years of age and under.

Early decelerations Periodic change in fetal heart rate pattern caused by head compression; deceleration has a uniform appearance and early onset in relation to maternal contraction.

Early postpartal hemorrhage See *Postpartal hemorrhage.*

Eclampsia A major complication of pregnancy. Its cause is unknown; it occurs more often in the primigravida and is accompanied by elevated blood pressure, albuminuria, oliguria, tonic and clonic convulsions, and coma. It may occur during pregnancy (usually after the 20th week of gestation) or within 48 hours after childbirth.

Ectoderm Outer layer of cells in the developing embryo that gives rise to the skin, nails, and hair.

Ectopic pregnancy Implantation of the fertilized ovum outside the uterine cavity; common sites are the abdomen, fallopian tubes, and ovaries. Also called oocyesis.

Effacement Thinning and shortening of the cervix that occurs late in pregnancy or during labor.

Effleurage A light stroking movement of the fingertips over the abdominal area during labor; used to provide distraction during labor contractions.

Ejaculation Expulsion of the seminal fluids from the penis.

Emancipated minor An adolescent who has the right to live as an adult because she or he is self-supporting, living away from home, married, pregnant, a parent, or in the military.

Embryo The early stage of development of the young of any organism. In humans the embryonic period is from about 2 to 8 weeks of gestation, and is characterized by cellular differentiation and predominantly hyperplastic growth.

Embryonic membranes The amnion and chorion.

Endoderm The inner layer of cells in the developing embryo that give rise to internal organs such as the intestines.

Endometriosis Ectopic endometrium located outside the uterus in the pelvic cavity. Symptoms may include pelvic pain or pressure, dysmenorrhea, dispareunia, abnormal bleeding from the uterus or rectum, and sterility.

Endometritis Infection of the endometrium.

Endometrium The mucous membrane that lines the inner surface of the uterus.

En face An assumed position in which one person looks at another and maintains his or her face in the same vertical plane as that of the other.

Engagement The entrance of the fetal presenting part into the superior pelvic strait and the beginning of the descent through the pelvic canal.

Engorgement Vascular congestion or distention. In obstetrics, the swelling of breast tissue brought about by an increase in blood and lymph supply to the breast, preceding true lactation.

Engrossment Characteristic sense of absorption, preoccupation, and interest in the infant demonstrated by fathers during early contact with their infants.

Entrainment Phenomenon in which a newborn moves in rhythm to adult speech.

Epidural block Regional anesthesia effective through the first and second stages of labor.

Episiotomy Incision of the perineum to facilitate birth and to avoid laceration of the perineum.

Epstein's pearls Small, white blebs found along the gum margins and at the junction of the hard and soft palates; commonly seen in the newborn as a normal manifestation.

Erb-Duchenne palsy Paralysis of the arm and chest wall as a result of a birth injury to the brachial plexus or a subsequent injury to the fifth and sixth cervical nerves.

Erythema toxicum Innocuous pink papular rash of unknown cause with superimposed vesicles; it appears within 24 to 48 hours after birth and resolves spontaneously within a few days.

Erythroblastosis fetalis Hemolytic disease of the newborn characterized by anemia, jaundice, enlargement of the liver and spleen, and generalized edema. Caused by isoimmunization due to Rh incompatibility or ABO incompatibility.

Estimated date of birth (EDB) During a pregnancy, the approximate date when childbirth will occur; the "due date."

Estrogen replacement therapy (ERT) Use of estrogen and a progestin to decrease the symptoms of menopause and to help prevent osteoporosis.

Estrogens The hormones estradiol and estrone, produced by the ovary.

Ethnocentrism An individual's belief that the values and practices of his or her own culture are the best ones.

Evaporation Loss of heat incurred when water on the skin surface is converted to a vapor.

Exchange transfusion The replacement of 70% to 80% of circulating blood by withdrawing the recipient's blood and injecting a donor's blood in equal amounts, for the purpose of preventing the accumulation of bilirubin or other by-products of hemolysis in the blood.

External os The opening between the cervix and the vagina.

External (cephalic) version Procedure involving external manipulation of the maternal abdomen to change the presentation of the fetus from breech to cephalic.

Fallopian tubes Tubes that extend from the lateral angle of the uterus and terminate near the ovary; they serve as a passageway for the ovum from the ovary to the uterus and for the spermatozoa from the uterus toward the ovary. Also called oviducts and uterine tubes.

False labor Contractions of the uterus, regular or irregular, that may be strong enough to be interpreted as true labor but that do not dilate the cervix.

False pelvis The portion of the pelvis above the linea terminalis; its primary function is to support the weight of the enlarged pregnant uterus.

Family-centered care An approach to health care based on the concept that a hospital can provide professional services to mothers, fathers, and infants in a homelike environment that would

enhance the integrity of the family unit.

Family structure The organization of the family unit, the manner in which members are arranged, and how members relate to each other.

Family systems framework Focuses on the interaction of various family members rather than solely describing their functions.

Female condom A thin, disposable polyurethane sheath with a flexible ring at each end which is placed inside the vagina and serves to prevent sperm from entering the cervix, thus preventing conception.

Female partner abuse Violence against a female by her husband or partner in an ongoing domestic relationship.

Female reproductive cycle (FRC) The monthly rhythmic changes in sexually mature women.

Ferning Formation of a palm-leaf pattern by the crystallization of cervical mucus as it dries at mid-menstrual cycle. Helpful in determining time of ovulation. Observed via microscopic examination of a thin layer of cervical mucus on a glass slide. This pattern is also observed when amniotic fluid is allowed to air dry on a slide and is a useful and quick test to determine whether amniotic membranes have ruptured.

Fertility awareness methods Natural family planning.

Fertility rate Number of births per 1000 women aged 15 to 44 in a given population per year.

Fertilization Impregnation of an ovum by a spermatozoon; conception.

Fetal acoustic stimulation test (FAST) A fetal assessment test that uses sound from a speaker, bell, or artificial larynx to stimulate acceleration of the fetal heart; may be used in conjunction with the nonstress test.

Fetal activity diary (FAD) A method for tracking fetal activity taught to pregnant women.

Fetal alcohol effects (FAE) The less severe fetal manifestations of maternal alcohol ingestion, including mild to moderate cognitive problems and physical growth retardation.

Fetal alcohol syndrome (FAS) Syndrome caused by maternal alcohol ingestion and characterized by microcephaly, intrauterine growth retardation, short palpebral fissures, and maxillary hypoplasia.

Fetal attitude Relationship of the fetal parts to one another. Normal fetal attitude is one of moderate flexion of the arms onto the chest and flexion of the legs onto the abdomen.

Fetal blood sampling Blood sample drawn from the fetal scalp (or from the fetus in breech position) to evaluate the acid-base status of the fetus.

Fetal bradycardia A fetal heart rate less than 120 beats per minute during a 10-minute period of continuous monitoring.

Fetal death Death of the developing fetus after 20 weeks' gestation. Also called fetal demise.

Fetal distress Evidence that the fetus is in jeopardy, such as a change in fetal activity or heart rate.

Fetal heart rate (FHR) The number of times the fetal heart beats per minute; normal range is 120 to 160.

Fetal lie Relationship of the cephalocaudal axis (spinal column) of the fetus to the cephalocaudal axis (spinal column) of the woman. The fetus may be in a longitudinal or transverse lie.

Fetal movement record See *Fetal activity diary.*

Fetal position Relationship of the landmark on the presenting fetal part to the front, sides, or back of the maternal pelvis.

Fetal presentation The fetal body part that enters the maternal pelvis first. The three possible presentations are cephalic, shoulder, or breech.

Fetal tachycardia A fetal heart rate of 160 beats per minute or more during a 10-minute period of continuous monitoring.

Fetoscope An adaptation of a stethoscope that facilitates auscultation of the fetal heart rate.

Fetoscopy A technique for directly observing the fetus and obtaining a sample of fetal blood or skin.

Fetus The child in utero from about the seventh to ninth week of gestation until birth.

Fibrocystic breast disease Benign breast disorder characterized by a thickening of normal breast tissue and the formation of cysts.

Fimbria Any structure resembling a fringe; the fringelike extremity of the fallopian tubes.

Folic acid An important vitamin directly related to the outcome of pregnancy and to maternal and fetal health.

Follicle-stimulating hormone (FSH) Hormone produced by the anterior pituitary during the first half of the menstrual cycle, stimulating development of the graafian follicle.

Fontanelle In the fetus, an unossified space or soft spot consisting of a strong band of connective tissue lying between the cranial bones of the skull.

Foramen ovale Special opening between the atria of the fetal heart. Normally, the opening closes shortly after birth; if it remains open, it can be repaired surgically.

Forceps Obstetric instrument occasionally used to aid in childbirth.

Foremilk Breast milk obtained at the beginning of the breastfeeding episode.

Fourth trimester First several postpartal weeks during which the woman returns to an essentially prepregnant state and becomes competent in caring for her newborn.

Frequency The time between the beginning of one contraction and the beginning of the next contraction.

Fundus The upper portion of the uterus between the fallopian tubes.

Galactorrhea Nipple discharge.

Gamete Female or male germ cell; contains a haploid number of chromosomes.

Gamete intrafallopian transfer (GIFT) Retrieval of oocytes by laparoscopy; immediately combining oocytes with washed, motile sperm in a catheter; and placement of the gametes into the frimbriated end of the fallopian tube.

Gametogenesis The process by which germ cells are produced.

Genotype The genetic composition of an individual.

Gestation Period of intrauterine development from conception through birth; pregnancy.

Gestational age The number of complete weeks of fetal development, calculated from the first day of the last normal menstrual cycle.

Gestational age assessment tools Systems used to evaluate the newborn's external physical characteristics and neurologic and/or neuromuscular development to accurately determine gestational age. These replace or supplement the traditional calculation from the woman's last menstrual period.

Gestational diabetes mellitus A form of diabetes of variable severity with onset or first recognition during pregnancy.

Gestational trophoblastic disease (GTD) Disorder classified into two types: benign (hydatidiform mole) and malignant.

Gonadotropin-releasing hormone (GnRH) A hormone secreted by the hypothalamus that stimulates the anterior pituitary to secrete FSH and LH.

Goodell's sign Softening of the cervix that occurs during the second month of pregnancy.

Graafian follicle The ovarian cyst containing the ripe ovum; it secretes estrogens.

Grasping reflex Normal newborn reflex elicited by stimulating the palm with a finger or object, resulting in newborn firmly holding on to the finger or object.

Gravida A pregnant woman.

Grief work The inner process of working through or managing the bereavement.

Gynecoid pelvis Typical female pelvis in which the inlet is round instead of oval.

Habituation Infant's ability to diminish innate responses to specific repeated stimuli.

Haploid number of chromosomes Half the diploid number of chromosomes. In humans there are 23 chromosomes, the haploid number, in each germ cell.

Harlequin sign A rare color change that occurs between the longitudinal halves of the newborn's body, such that the dependent half is noticeably pinker than the superior half when the newborn is placed on one side; it is of no pathologic significance.

Hegar's sign A softening of the lower uterine segment found upon palpation in the second or third month of pregnancy.

HELLP syndrome A cluster of changes including hemolysis, elevated liver enzymes, and low platelet count; sometimes associated with severe preeclampsia.

Hemolytic disease of the newborn *Hyperbilirubinemia* secondary to Rh incompatibility.

Heterozygous A genotypic situation in which two different alleles occur at a given locus on a pair of homologous chromosomes.

Hindmilk Breast milk released after initial letdown reflex; high in fat content.

Homozygous A genotypic situation in which two similar genes occur at a given locus on homologous chromosomes.

Hormone replacement therapy (HRT) Administration of hormones, usually estrogen and a progestin, to alleviate the symptoms of menopause.

Hot flashes Vasomotor changes related to menopause that result in sensations of heat, flushing, or sweating.

Huhner test Postcoital examination to evaluate sperm and cervical mucus.

Human chorionic gonadotropin (hCG) A hormone produced by the chorionic villi and found in the urine of pregnant women. Also called prolan.

Human placental lactogen (hPL) A hormone synthesized by the syncytiotrophoblast that functions as an insulin antagonist and promotes lipolysis to increase the amounts of circulating free fatty acids available for maternal metabolic use.

Hydatidiform mole Degenerative process in chorionic villi, giving rise to multiple cysts and rapid growth of the uterus with hemorrhage.

Hydramnios An excess of amniotic fluid, leading to overdistention of the uterus. Frequently seen in diabetic pregnant women, even if there is no coexisting fetal anomaly. Also called polyhydramnios.

Hydrops fetalis See *Erythroblastosis fetalis.*

Hyperbilirubinemia Excessive amount of bilirubin in the blood; indicative of hemolytic processes due to blood incompatibility, intrauterine infection, septicemia, neonatal renal infection, and other disorders.

Hyperemesis gravidarum Excessive vomiting during pregnancy, leading to dehydration and starvation.

Hyperventilation A pattern of breathing in labor in which the woman breathes rapidly during the uterine contractions. Characterized by a feeling of not being able to "catch" a breath and a tingling of the lips, face, and fingertips; progresses to carpal-pedal spasms if not relieved.

Hypnoreflexogenous method A combination of hypnosis and conditioned reflexes used during childbirth.

Hypocalcemia Abnormally low level of serum calcium.

Hypoglycemia Abnormally low level of sugar in the blood.

Hysterectomy Surgical removal of the uterus.

Hysterosalpingogram Result of testing by instillation of radiopaque substance into the uterine cavity to visualize the uterus and fallopian tubes.

Hysteroscopy Use of a special endoscope to examine the uterus.

In vitro fertilization (IVF) Procedure during which oocytes are removed from the ovary, mixed with spermatozoa, fertilized, and incubated in a glass petri dish; then up to four viable embryos are placed in the woman's uterus.

Inborn error of metabolism A hereditary deficiency of a specific enzyme needed for normal metabolism of specific chemicals.

Incompetent (dysfunctional) cervix The premature dilatation of the cervix, usually in the second trimester of pregnancy.

Increment Increase or addition; to build up, as of a contraction.

Induction of labor The process of causing or initiating labor by use of medication or surgical rupture of membranes.

Infant A child under 1 year of age.

Infant mortality rate Number of deaths of infants under 1 year of age per 1000 live births in a given population per year.

Infant of a diabetic mother (IDM) At-risk infant born to a woman previously diagnosed as diabetic, or who develops symptoms of diabetes during pregnancy.

Inferential statistics Statistics that allow an investigator to draw conclusions about what is happening between two or more variables in a population and to suggest or refute casual relationships between them.

Infertility Diminished ability to conceive.

Informed consent A legal concept that protects a person's rights to autonomy and self-determination by specifying that no action may be taken without that person's prior understanding and freely given consent.

Infundibulopelvic ligament Ligament that suspends and supports the ovaries.

Innominate bone The hip bone, ilium, ischium, and pubis.

Intensity The strength of a uterine contraction during acme.

Interactional framework Focuses on the family members' subjective views of the situation, emphasizing internal family dynamics.

Internal os An inside mouth or opening; the opening between the cervix and the uterus.

Internal version Procedure used to vaginally deliver a second twin. The obstetrician inserts a hand into the uterus, grasps the feet of the fetus, and changes the fetus from a transverse to a breech presentation.

Intrapartum The time from the onset of true labor until the birth of the infant and delivery of the placenta.

Intrauterine catheter A catheter that can be placed through the cervix into the uterus to measure uterine pressure during labor. Some types of catheters may be inserted for the purpose of infusing warmed saline to add additional intrauterine fluid when oligohydramnios is present.

Intrauterine device (IUD) Small metal or plastic form that is placed in the uterus to prevent implantation of a fertilized ovum.

Intrauterine fetal surgery Surgery performed on a fetus to correct anatomic lesions that are not compatible with life if left untreated.

Intrauterine growth restriction (IUGR) Fetal undergrowth due to any etiology, such as intrauterine infection, deficient nutrient supply, or congenital malformation. Formerly called intrauterine growth retardation.

Introitus Opening or entrance into a cavity or canal such as the vagina.

Involution Rolling or turning inward; the reduction in size of the uterus following childbirth.

Ischial spines Prominences that arise near the junction of the ilium and ischium and jut into the pelvic cavity; used as a reference point during labor to evaluate the descent of the fetal head into the birth canal.

Isthmus The straight, narrow part of the fallopian tube with a thick muscular wall and an opening (lumen) 2–3 mm in diameter; the site of tubal ligation. Also a constriction in the uterus that is located above the cervix and below the corpus.

Jaundice Yellow pigmentation of body tissues caused by the presence of bile pigments. See also *Physiologic jaundice*.

Karyotype The set of chromosomes arranged in a standard order.

Kegel's exercises Perineal muscle tightening that strengthens the pubococcygeus muscle and increases its tone.

Kernicterus An encephalopathy caused by deposition of unconjugated bilirubin in brain cells; may result in impaired brain function or death.

Kilocalorie (kcal) Equivalent to 1000 calories, it is the unit used to express the energy value of food.

Klinefelter syndrome A chromosomal abnormality caused by the presence of an extra X chromosome in the male; characteristics include tall stature, sparse pubic and facial hair, gynecomastia, small firm testes, and absence of spermatogenesis.

Labor The process by which the fetus is expelled from the maternal uterus. Also called childbirth, confinement, or parturition.

Lactase deficiency See *Lactose intolerance*.

Lactation The process of producing and supplying breast milk.

Lacto-ovovegetarians Vegetarians who include milk, dairy products, and eggs in their diets, and occasionally fish, poultry, and liver.

Lactose intolerance A condition in which an individual has difficulty digesting milk and milk products.

Lactovegetarians Vegetarians who include dairy products but no eggs in their diets.

La Leche League Organization that provides information on and assistance with breastfeeding.

Lamaze method A method of childbirth preparation. See also *psychoprophylaxis*.

Lanugo Fine, downy hair found on all body parts of the fetus, with the exception of the palms of the hands and the soles of the feet, after 20 weeks' gestation.

Laparoscopy Procedure that enables direct visualization of pelvic organs.

Large for gestational age (LGA) Excessive growth of a fetus in relation to the gestational time period.

Last menstrual period (LMP) The last normal menstrual period experienced by the woman prior to pregnancy; sometimes used to calculate the infant's gestational age.

Late adolescence Between 18 and 19 years of age.

Late decelerations Periodic change in fetal heart rate pattern caused by uteroplacental insufficiency; deceleration has a uniform shape and late onset in relation to maternal contraction.

Late postpartal hemorrhage See *Postpartal hemorrhage*.

Leboyer method Birthing technique that eases the newborn's transition to extrauterine life wherein lights in the birthing room are dimmed and noise is kept to a minimum.

Lecithin/sphingomyelin (L/S) ratio Lecithin and sphingomyelin are phospholipid components of surfactant; their ratio changes during gestation. When the L/S ratio reaches 2:1, the fetal lungs are thought to be mature and the fetus will have a low risk of respiratory distress syndrome if born at that time.

Leiomyoma A benign tumor of the uterus, composed primarily of smooth muscle and connective tissue. Also referred to as a myoma or a fibroid.

Leopold's maneuvers A series of four maneuvers designed to provide a systematic approach whereby the examiner may determine fetal presentation and position.

Letdown reflex Pattern of stimulation, hormone release, and resulting muscle contraction that forces milk into the lactiferous ducts, making it available to the infant. Also called milk ejection reflex.

Leukorrhea Mucous discharge from the vagina or cervical canal that may be normal or pathologic, as in the presence of infection.

Lie Relationship of the long axis of the fetus and the long axis of the pregnant woman. The fetal lie may be longitudinal, transverse, or oblique.

Lightening Moving of the fetus and uterus downward into the pelvic cavity.

Linea nigra The line of darker pigmentation extending from the umbilicus to the pubis noted in some women during the later months of pregnancy.

Local anesthesia Injection of an anesthetic agent into the subcutaneous tissue in a fanlike pattern.

Lochia Maternal discharge of blood, mucus, and tissue from the uterus; may last for several weeks after birth.

Lochia alba White vaginal discharge that follows lochia serosa and that lasts from about the 10th to the 21st day after birth.

Lochia rubra Red, blood-tinged vaginal discharge that occurs following birth and lasts 2 to 4 days.

Lochia serosa Pink, serous, and blood-tinged vaginal discharge that follows lochia rubra and lasts until the seventh to tenth day after birth.

Long-term variability (LTV) Large rhythmic fluctuations of the FHR that occur from two to six times per minute.

L/S ratio See *Lecithin/sphingomyelin ratio*.

Luteinizing hormone (LH) Anterior pituitary hormone responsible for stimulating ovulation and for development of the corpus luteum.

Macrosomia A condition seen in neonates of large body size and high birth weight, as those born of prediabetic and diabetic mothers.

Malposition An abnormal position of the fetus in the birth canal.

Malpresentation A presentation of the fetus into the birth canal that is not "normal," that is, brow, face, shoulder, or breech presentation.

Mammogram A soft tissue radiograph of the breast without the injection of a contrast medium.

Mastitis Inflammation of the breast.

Maternal mortality The number of maternal deaths from any cause during the pregnancy cycle per 100,000 live births.

Mature milk Breast milk that contains 10% solids for energy and growth.

McDonald's sign A probable sign of pregnancy characterized by an ease in flexing the body of the uterus against the cervix.

Meconium Dark green or black material present in the large intestine of a full-term infant; the first stools passed by the newborn.

Meconium aspiration syndrome (MAS) Respiratory disease of term, postterm, and SGA newborns caused by inhalation of meconium or meconium-stained amniotic fluid into the lungs; characterized by mild to severe respiratory distress, hyperexpansion of the chest, hyperinflated alveoli, and secondary atelectasis.

Meiosis The process of cell division that occurs in the maturation of sperm and ova that decreases their number of chromosomes by one-half.

Menarche Beginning of menstrual and reproductive function in the female.

Mendelian inheritance A major category of inheritance whereby a trait is determined by a pair of genes on homologous chromosomes. Also called single gene inheritance.

Menopause The permanent cessation of menses.

Menorrhagia Excessive or profuse menstrual flow.

Menstrual cycle Cyclic buildup of the uterine lining, ovulation, and sloughing of the lining occurring approximately every 28 days in non-pregnant females.

Mentum The chin.

Mesoderm The intermediate layer of germ cells in the embryo that gives rise to connective tissue, bone marrow, muscles, blood, lymphoid tissue, and epithelial tissue.

Metrorrhagia Abnormal uterine bleeding occurring at irregular intervals.

Middle adolescence Between 15 and 17 years of age.

Mifepristone (RU 486) Experimental postcoital contraceptive.

Milia Tiny white papules appearing on the face of a neonate as a result of unopened sebaceous glands; they disappear spontaneously within a few weeks.

Milk/plasma ratio Comparison of the concentration of substances in the breast milk and the maternal blood serum.

Miscarriage See *Spontaneous abortion.*

Mitosis Process of cell division whereby both daughter cells have the same number and pattern of chromosomes as the original cell.

Molding Shaping of the fetal head by overlapping of the cranial bones to facilitate movement through the birth canal during labor.

Mongolian spot Dark, flat pigmentation of the lower back and buttocks noted at birth in some infants; usually disappears by the time the child reaches school age.

Moniliasis Yeastlike fungal infection caused by *Candida albicans.*

Monosomy Chromosome disorder in which one chromosome of a pair is missing.

Mons pubis Mound of subcutaneous fatty tissue covering the anterior portion of the symphysis pubis.

Moro reflex Flexion of the newborn's thighs and knees accompanied by fingers that fan, then clench, as the arms are simultaneously thrown out and then brought together, as though embracing something. This reflex can be elicited by startling the newborn with a sudden noise or movement. Also called the startle reflex.

Morula Developmental stage of the fertilized ovum in which there is a solid mass of cells.

Mosaicism Condition of an individual who has at least two cell lines with differing karotypes.

Mottling Discoloration of the skin in irregular areas; may be seen with chilling, poor perfusion, or hypoxia.

Mucous plug A collection of thick mucus that blocks the cervical canal during pregnancy. Also called operculum.

Multigravida Woman who has been pregnant more than once.

Multipara Woman who has had more than one pregnancy in which the fetus was viable.

Multiple pregnancy More than one fetus in the uterus at the same time.

Myometrium Uterine muscular structure.

Nägele's rule A method of determining the estimated date of birth (EDB): after obtaining the first day of the last menstrual period, subtract 3 months and add 7 days.

Natural childbirth Prepared childbirth, in which the couple attends a prenatal education program and learns exercises and breathing patterns that are used during labor and childbirth.

Neonatal mortality rate Number of deaths of infants in the first 28 days of life per 1000 live births.

Neonatal mortality risk The chance of death within the newborn period.

Neonatal transition The first few hours of life in which the newborn stabilizes its respiratory and circulatory functions.

Neonate Infant from birth through the first 28 days of life.

Neonatology The specialty that focuses on the management of high-risk conditions of the newborn.

Nevus flammeus Large port-wine stain.

Nevus vasculosus "Strawberry mark": raised, clearly delineated, dark red, rough-surfaced birth mark commonly found in the head region.

Newborn screening tests Tests that detect inborn errors of metabolism that, if left untreated, cause mental retardation and physical handicaps.

Nidation Implantation of a fertilized ovum in the endometrium.

Nipple A protrusion about 0.5 to 1.3 cm in diameter in the center of each mature breast.

Nipple preparation Prenatal activities designed to toughen the nipple in preparation for breastfeeding.

Non-Mendelian (multifactorial) inheritance The occurrence of congenital disorders that result from an interaction of multiple genetic and environmental factors.

Nonstress test (NST) An assessment method by which the reaction (or response) of the fetal heart rate to fetal movement is evaluated.

Norplant A subdermal progestin contraceptive which is implanted in a woman's arm and provides contraceptive protection for up to 5 years.

Nuchal cord Term used to describe the umbilical cord when it is wrapped around the neck of the fetus.

Nuclear family A configuration usually referring to a husband, wife, and all minor children living together in a single household, separate from the family of origin.

Nulligravida A woman who has never been pregnant.

Nullipara A woman who has not delivered a viable fetus.

Obstetric conjugate Distance from the middle of the sacral promontory to an area approximately 1 cm below the pubic crest.

Older adolescent Between 18 and 19 years of age.

Oligohydramnios Decreased amount of amniotic fluid, which may indicate a fetal urinary tract defect.

Oocyte Early primitive ovum before it has completely developed.

Oogenesis Process during fetal life whereby the ovary produces oogenia, cells that become primitive ovarian eggs.

Oophoritis Infection of the ovaries.

Ophthalmia neonatorum Purulent infection of the eyes or conjunctiva of the newborn, usually caused by gonococci.

Oral contraceptives "Birth control pills" that work by inhibiting the release of an ovum and by maintaining a type of mucus that is hostile to sperm.

Orgasm Climax of the sexual experience.

Orientation Infant's ability to respond to auditory and visual stimuli in the environment.

Ortolani's maneuver A manual procedure performed to rule out the possibility of congenital hip dysplasia.

Ovarian ligaments Ligaments that anchor the lower pole of the ovary to the cornua of the uterus.

Ovary Female sex gland in which the ova are formed and in which estrogen and progesterone are produced. Nor-

mally there are two ovaries, located in the lower abdomen on each side of uterus.

Ovulation Normal process of discharging a mature ovum from an ovary approximately 14 days prior to the onset of menses.

Ovum Female reproductive cell; egg.

Oxygen toxicity Excessive levels of oxygen therapy that result in pathologic changes in tissue.

Oxytocin Hormone normally produced by the posterior pituitary, responsible for stimulation of uterine contractions and the release of milk into the lactiferous ducts.

Oxytocin challenge test (OCT) See *Contraction stress test (CST)*.

Papanicolaou (Pap) smear Procedure to detect the presence of cancer of the uterus by microscopic examination of cells gently scraped from the cervix.

Para A woman who has borne offspring who reached the age of viability.

Paracervical block A local anesthetic agent injected transvaginally adjacent to the outer rim of the cervix.

Parametritis Inflammation of the parametrial layer of the uterus.

Parent-newborn attachment Close affectional ties that develop between parent and child. See also *Attachment*.

Passive acquired immunity Transfer of antibodies (IgG) from the mother to the fetus in utero.

Pedigree Graphic representation of a family tree.

Pelvic cavity Bony portion of the birth passages; a curved canal with a longer posterior than anterior wall.

Pelvic cellulitis Infection involving the connective tissue of the broad ligament or, in severe cases, the connective tissue of all the pelvic structures.

Pelvic diaphragm Part of the pelvic floor composed of deep fascia and the levator ani and the coccygeal muscles.

Pelvic floor Muscles and tissue that act as a buttress to the pelvic outlet.

Pelvic inflammatory disease (PID) An infection of the fallopian tubes that may or may not be accompanied by a pelvic abscess; may cause infertility secondary to tubal damage.

Pelvic inlet Upper border of the true pelvis.

Pelvic outlet Lower border of the true pelvis.

Pelvic tilt Also called pelvic rocking; exercise designed to reduce back strain and strengthen abdominal muscle tone.

Penis The male organ of copulation and reproduction.

Percutaneous umbilical blood sampling (PUBS) A technique used to obtain pure fetal blood from the umbilical cord while the fetus is in utero. Also called cordocentesis.

Perimetrium The outermost layer of the corpus of the uterus. Also known as the serosal layer.

Perinatal mortality rate The number of neonatal and fetal deaths per 1000 live births.

Perinatology The medical specialty concerned with the diagnosis and treatment of high-risk conditions of the pregnant woman and her fetus.

Perineal body Wedge-shaped mass of fibromuscular tissue found between the lower part of the vagina and the anal canal.

Perineum The area of tissue between the anus and scrotum in a man or between the anus and vagina in a woman.

Periodic breathing Sporadic episodes of apnea, not associated with cyanosis, that last for about 10 seconds and commonly occur in preterm infants.

Periods of reactivity Predictable patterns of neonate behavior during the first several hours after birth.

Peritonitis Infection involving the peritoneum.

Persistant occiput posterior position Malposition of the fetus in which the fetal occiput is posterior in the maternal pelvis.

Persistent pulmonary hypertension of the newborn (PPHN) Respiratory disease resulting from right-to-left shunting of blood away from the lungs and through the ductus arteriosus and patent foramen ovale.

Phenotype The whole physical, biochemical, and physiologic makeup of an individual as determined both genetically and environmentally.

Phenylketonuria A common metabolic disease caused by an inborn error in the metabolism of the amino acid phenylalanine.

Phosphatidylglycerol (PG) A phospholipid present in fetal surfactant after about 35 weeks' gestation.

Phototherapy The treatment of jaundice by exposure to light.

Physiologic anemia of infancy A harmless condition in which the hemoglobin level drops in the first 6 to 12 weeks after birth, then reverts to normal levels.

Physiologic anemia of pregnancy Apparent anemia that results because during pregnancy the plasma volume increases more than the erythrocyte increase.

Physiologic jaundice A harmless condition caused by the normal reduction of red blood cells, occurring 48 or more hours after birth, peaking at the fifth to seventh day, and disappearing between the seventh to tenth day.

Pica The eating of substances not ordinarily considered edible or to have nutritive value.

Placenta Specialized disk-shaped organ that connects the fetus to the uterine wall for gas and nutrient exchange. Also called afterbirth.

Placenta accreta Partial or complete absence of the decidua basalis and abnormal adherence of the placenta to the uterine wall.

Placenta previa Abnormal implantation of the placenta in the lower uterine segment. Classification of type is based on proximity to the cervical os: *total*—completely covers the os; *partial*—covers a portion of the os; *marginal*—is in close proximity to the os.

Platypelloid pelvis An unusually wide pelvis, having a flattened oval transverse shape and a shortened anteroposterior diameter.

Pneumothorax The accumulation of air in the thoracic cavity between the parietal and visceral pleura.

Polar body A small cell resulting from the meiotic division of the mature oocyte.

Polycythemia An abnormal increase in the number of total red blood cells in the body's circulation.

Polydactyly A developmental anomaly characterized by more than five digits on the hands or feet.

Positive signs of pregnancy Indications that confirm the presence of pregnancy.

Postconception age periods Period of time in embryonic/fetal development calculated from the time of fertilization of the ovum.

Postmature newborn See *Postterm newborn.*

Postpartal hemorrhage A loss of blood of greater than 500 mL following birth. The hemorrhage is classified as *early* or *immediate* if it occurs within the first 24 hours and *late* or *delayed* after the first 24 hours.

Postpartum After childbirth or delivery.

Postpartum blues A maternal adjustment reaction occurring in the first few postpartal days, characterized by mild depression, tearfulness, anxiety, headache, and irritability.

Postterm newborn Any infant born after 42 weeks' gestation.

Postterm labor Labor that occurs after 42 weeks of gestation.

Postterm pregnancy Pregnancy that lasts beyond 42 weeks' gestation.

Precipitous birth (1) Unduly rapid progression of labor. (2) A birth in which no physician is in attendance.

Precipitous labor Labor lasting less than 3 hours.

Preeclampsia Toxemia of pregnancy, characterized by hypertension, albuminuria, and edema. See also *Eclampsia.*

Pregnancy-induced hypertension (PIH) A hypertensive disorder including preeclampsia and eclampsia as conditions, characterized by the three cardinal signs of hypertension, edema, and proteinuria.

Premature infant See *Preterm infant.*

Premature rupture of the membranes (PROM) See *Rupture of membranes.*

Premenstrual syndrome (PMS) Cluster of symptoms experienced by some women, typically occurring from a few days up to 2 weeks prior to the onset of menses.

Prenatal education Programs offered to expectant families, adolescents, women, or partners to provide education regarding the pregnancy, labor, and birth experience.

Prep Shaving of the pubic area.

Presentation The fetal body part that enters the maternal pelvis first. The three possible presentations are cephalic, shoulder, or breech.

Presenting part The fetal part present in or on the cervical os.

Presumptive signs of pregnancy Symptoms that suggest but do not confirm pregnancy, such as cessation of menses, quickening, Chadwick's sign, and morning sickness.

Preterm infant Any infant born before 38 weeks' gestation.

Preterm labor Labor occurring between 20 and 38 weeks of pregnancy. Also called premature labor.

Primigravida A woman who is pregnant for the first time.

Primipara A woman who has given birth to her first child (past the point of viability), whether or not that child is living or was alive at birth.

Probable signs of pregnancy Manifestations that strongly suggest the likelihood of pregnancy, such as a positive pregnancy test, enlarging abdomen, and positive Goodell's, Hegar's, and Braxton Hicks signs.

Progesterone A hormone produced by the corpus luteum, adrenal cortex, and placenta whose function is to stimulate proliferation of the endometrium to facilitate growth of the embryo.

Progressive relaxation A relaxation technique that involves relaxing first one portion of the body and then another portion, until total body relaxation is achieved; may be used during labor.

Prolactin A hormone secreted by the anterior pituitary that stimulates and sustains lactation in mammals.

Prolapsed cord Umbilical cord that becomes trapped in the vagina before the fetus is born.

Prolonged labor Labor lasting more than 24 hours.

Prostaglandins Complex lipid compounds synthesized by many cells in the body.

Pseudomenstruation Blood-tinged mucus from the vagina in the newborn female infant; caused by withdrawal of maternal hormones that were present during pregnancy.

Psychoprophylaxis (Lamaze) Psychophysical training aimed at preparing the expectant parents to cope with the processes of labor and to avoid concentration on the discomforts associated with childbirth.

Ptyalism Excessive salivation.

Puberty Developmental stage early in adolescence when reproductive ability begins and secondary sex characteristics develop.

Pubic Pertaining to the pubes or pubis.

Pudendal block Injection of an anesthetizing agent at the pudendal nerve to produce numbness of the external genitals and the lower one third of the vagina, to facilitate childbirth and permit episiotomy if necessary.

Puerperal morbidity A maternal temperature of 100.4 F (38 C) or higher on any 2 of the first 10 postpartal days, excluding the first 24 hours. The temperature is to be taken by mouth at least 4 times per day.

Puerperium The period after completion of the third stage of labor until involution of the uterus is complete, usually 6 weeks.

Quickening The first fetal movements felt by the pregnant woman, usually between 16 to 18 weeks' gestation.

Radiation Heat loss incurred when heat transfers to cooler surfaces and objects not in direct contact with the body.

Rape Sexual activity, often intercourse, against the will of the victim.

Read method Natural childbirth preparation centered on eliminating the fear-tension-pain syndrome.

Reciprocal inhibition The principle that it is impossible to feel relaxed and tense at the same time; the basis for relaxation techniques.

Reciprocity Process in which a newborn gives cues and the parent or other caregiver interprets, then responds to the cues.

Recommended dietary allowances (RDA) Government-recommended allowances of various vitamins, minerals, and other nutrients.

Regional anesthesia Injection of local anesthetic agents so that they come into direct contact with nervous tissue.

Relaxin A water-soluble protein secreted by the corpus luteum that causes relaxation of the symphysis and cervical dilatation.

Respiratory distress syndrome (RDS) Respiratory disease of the newborn characterized by interference with ventilation at the alveolar level, thought to be caused by the presence of fibrinoid deposits lining the alveolar ducts. Formerly called hyaline membrane disease.

Retinopathy of prematurity Formation of fibrotic tissue behind the lens; associated with retinal detachment and arrested eye growth, seen with hypoxemia in preterm infants.

Rh factor Antigens present on the surface of blood cells that make the blood cell incompatible with blood cells that do not have the antigen.

RhoGAM An anti-Rh (D) gamma-globulin given after delivery to an Rh-negative mother of an Rh-positive fetus or child. Prevents the development of permanent active immunity to the Rh antigen.

Rhythm method The timing of sexual intercourse to avoid the fertile time associated with ovulation.

Risk factors Any findings that suggest the pregnancy may have a negative outcome, either for the woman or her unborn child.

Rooming-in unit A hospital unit where the infant can reside in the same room with the mother after birth and during their postpartal stay.

Rooting reflex An infant's tendency to turn the head and open the lips to suck when one side of the mouth or cheek is touched.

Round ligaments Ligaments that arise from the side of the uterus near the fallopian tube insertion to help the broad ligament keep the uterus in place.

Rugae Transverse ridges of mucous membranes lining the vagina, which allow the vagina to stretch during the descent of the fetal head.

Rupture of membranes (ROM) Rupture may be PROM (premature), SROM (spontaneous), or AROM (artificial). Some clinicians may use the abbreviation RBOW (rupture of bag of water).

Sacral promontory A projection into the pelvic cavity on the anterior upper portion of the sacrum; serves as an obstetric guide in determining pelvic measurements.

Salpingitis Infection of the fallopian tubes.

Saltatory pattern A fetal heart rate pattern of marked or excessive variability.

Scalp stimulation test (SST) A test used during labor to assess fetal well-being by pressing a fingertip on the fetal scalp. A fetus not under excessive stress will respond to the digital stimulation with heart rate accelerations.

Scarf sign The position of the elbow when the hand of a supine infant is drawn across to the other shoulder until it meets resistance.

Schultze's mechanism Delivery of the placenta with the shiny or fetal surface presenting first.

Self-quieting activity Infant's ability to use personal resources to quiet and console him- or herself.

Semen Thick whitish fluid ejaculated by the male during orgasm and containing the spermatozoa and their nutrients.

Sepsis neonatorum Infections experienced by a neonate during the first month of life.

Sex chromosomes The X and Y chromosomes, which are responsible for sex determination.

Sexually transmitted infection (STI) Refers to infections ordinarily transmitted by direct sexual contact with an infected individual. Also called sexually transmitted disease.

Short-term variability (STV) Refers to the differences between successive heart beats as measured by the R–R wave interval of the QRS cardiac cycle. Measured only by internal electronic fetal monitoring.

Show A pinkish mucous discharge from the vagina that may occur a few hours to a few days prior to the onset of labor.

Simian line A single palmar crease frequently found in children with Down syndrome.

Sinusoidal pattern A wave form of fetal heart rate where long-term variability is present but there is no short-term variability.

Situational contraceptives Contraceptive methods that involve no prior preparation, for instance, abstinence or coitus interruptus.

Skin turgor Elasticity of skin; provides information on hydration status.

Small for gestational age (SGA) Inadequate weight or growth for gestational age; birth weight below the tenth percentile.

Spermatogenesis The process by which mature spermatozoa are formed, during which the number of chromosomes is halved.

Spermatozoa Mature sperm cells of the male animal, produced by the testes.

Spermicides A variety of creams, foams, jellies, and suppositories that, when inserted into the vagina prior to intercourse, destroy sperm or neutralize any vaginal secretions and thereby immobilize sperm.

Spinal block Injection of a local anesthetic agent directly into the spinal fluid in the spinal canal to provide anesthesia for vaginal and cesarean births.

Spinnbarkeit The elasticity of the cervical mucus that is present at ovulation.

Spontaneous abortion Abortion that occurs naturally. Also called miscarriage.

Station Relationship of the presenting fetal part to an imaginary line drawn between the pelvic ischial spines.

Sterility Inability to conceive or to produce offspring.

Stillbirth The delivery of a dead infant.

Striae gravidarum Stretch marks; shiny reddish lines that appear on the abdomen, breasts, thighs, and buttocks of pregnant women as a result of stretching the skin.

Structural-functional framework Defines the family as a social system.

Subconjunctival hemorrhage Hemorrhage on the sclera of a newborn's eye usually caused by changes in vascular tension during birth.

Subdermal implants (Norplant) Silastic capsules containing levonorgestrel; when 6 are implanted in a woman's upper arm, they act as a contraceptive for up to 5 years.

Subinvolution Failure of a part to return to its normal size after functional enlargement, such as failure of the uterus to return to normal size after pregnancy.

Sucking reflex Normal newborn reflex elicited by inserting a finger or nipple in the newborn's mouth, resulting in forceful, rhythmic sucking.

Surfactant A surface-active mixture of lipoproteins secreted in the alveoli and air passages that reduces surface tension of pulmonary fluids and contributes to the elasticity of pulmonary tissue.

Suture (1) Fibrous connection of opposed joint surfaces, as in the skull. (2) The uniting of edges of a wound.

Symphysis pubis Fibrocartilaginous joint between the pelvic bones in the midline.

Syndactyly Malformation of the fingers or toes in which there may be webbing or complete fusion of two or more digits.

Telangiectatic nevi (stork bites) Small clusters of pink-red spots appearing on the nape of the neck and around the eyes of infants; localized areas of capillary dilatation.

Teratogens Nongenetic factors that can produce malformations of the fetus.

Term The normal duration of pregnancy.

Testes The male gonads, in which sperm and testosterone are produced.

Testosterone The male hormone; responsible for the development of secondary male characteristics.

Therapeutic abortion Medically induced termination of pregnancy when a malformed fetus is suspected or when the woman's health is in jeopardy.

Thermal neutral zone (TNZ) An environment that provides for minimal heat loss or expenditure.

Thrombophlebitis Inflammation of a vein wall resulting in thrombus.

Thrush A fungal infection of the oral mucous membranes caused by *Candida albicans*. Most often seen in infants; characterized by white plaques in the mouth.

Tocolysis Use of medications to arrest preterm labor.

Tonic neck reflex Postural reflex seen in the newborn. When the supine infant's head is turned to one side, the arm and leg on that side extend while the extremities on the opposite side flex. Also called the fencing position.

TORCH An acronym used to describe a group of infections that represent potentially severe problems during pregnancy. TO = toxoplasmosis, R = rubella, C = cytomegalovirus, H = herpesvirus.

Total serum bilirubin Sum of conjugated (direct) and unconjugated (indirect) bilirubin.

Touch relaxation A relaxation technique that involves relaxing an area of body as another person provides a "touch" cue to that specific area. Touch relaxation is very effective during labor contractions.

Toxic shock syndrome Infection caused by *Staphylococcus aureaus*, found primarily in women of reproductive age.

Transitional milk Breast milk produced from the end of colostrum production until about 2 weeks postpartum.

Transverse diameter The largest diameter of the pelvic inlet; helps determine the shape of the inlet.

Transverse lie A lie in which the fetus is positioned crosswise in the uterus.

Trichomonas vaginalis A parasitic protozoan that may cause inflammation of the vagina, characterized by itching and burning of vulvar tissue and by white, frothy discharge.

Trimester Three months, or one-third of the gestational time for pregnancy.

Trisomy The presence of three homologous chromosomes rather than the normal two.

Trophoblast The outer layer of the blastoderm that will eventually establish the nutrient relationship with the uterine endometrium.

True pelvis The portion that lies below the linea terminalis, made up of the inlet, cavity, and outlet.

Trunk incurvation (Galant reflex) Normal newborn reflex elicited when newborn is prone and the spine is stroked, causing the pelvis to turn to the stimulated side.

Tubal ligation Sterilization of a woman accomplished by transecting or occluding the fallopian tubes.

Turner syndrome A number of anomalies that occur when a woman has only one X chromosome; characteristics include short stature, little sexual differentiation, webbing of the neck with a low posterior hairline, and congenital cardiac anomalies.

Ultrasound High-frequency sound waves that may be directed, through the use of a transducer, into the maternal abdomen. The ultrasonic sound waves reflected by the underlying structures of varying densities allow various maternal and fetal tissues, bones, and fluids to be identified.

Umbilical cord The structure connecting the placenta to the umbilicus of the fetus and through which nutrients from the woman are exchanged for wastes from the fetus.

Uterine atony Relaxation of uterine muscle tone following birth.

Uterine inversion Prolapse of the uterine fundus through the cervix into the vagina; may occur just prior to or during delivery of the placenta; associated with massive hemorrhage requiring emergency treatment.

Uterosacral ligaments Ligaments that provide support for the uterus and cervix at the level of the ischial spines.

Uterus The hollow muscular organ in which the fertilized ovum is implanted and in which the developing fetus is nourished until birth.

Vagina The musculomembranous tube or passageway located between the external genitals and the uterus of a woman.

Vaginal birth after cesarean (VBAC) Practice of permitting a trial of labor and possible vaginal birth for women following a previous cesarean birth for nonrecurring causes such as fetal distress or placenta previa.

Variable deceleration Periodic change in fetal heart rate caused by umbilical cord compression; decelerations vary in onset, occurrence, and waveform.

Vasectomy Surgical removal of a portion of the vas deferens (ductus deferens) to produce infertility.

Vegan A "pure" vegetarian; one who consumes no food from animal sources.

Vena caval syndrome Symptoms of dizziness, pallor, and clamminess that result from lowered blood pressure when a pregnant woman lies supine and the enlarged uterus presses on the vena cava. Also known as supine hypotensive syndrome.

Vernix caseosa A protective cheese-like whitish substance made up of sebum and desquamated epithelial cells that is present on the fetal skin.

Version Turning of the fetus in utero.

Vertex The top or crown of the head.

Vulva The external structure of the female genitals, lying below the mons veneris.

Vulvovaginal candidiasis (VVC) See *Moniliasis.*

Weaning The process of discontinuing breastfeeding and accustoming an infant to another feeding method.

Wharton's jelly Yellow-white gelatinous material surrounding the vessels of the umbilical cord.

Young adolescent Less than 14 years of age.

Zona pellucida Transparent inner layer surrounding an ovum.

Zygote A fertilized egg.

Zygote intrafallopian transfer (ZIFT) Retrieval of oocytes under ultrasound guidance followed by in vitro fertilization and laparoscopic replacement of fertilized eggs into fimbriated end of the fallopian tube.

Assisted reproductive technology (ART), 17, 147–148. *See also* Infertility

Association of Women's Health, Obstetric, and Neonatal Nurses (AWHONN), NAACOG Standards of Nursing Care, 25, 1149

Asthenospermia, 146

Atony, uterine, 667–668, 1044, 1055, 1057, 1117–1119
  defined, 1116

Atresia
  choanal, congenital, 824, 830, *965t*
  rectal, 835

Atrial septal defect (ASD), *968t*

Attachment
  adolescent mothers and, 1085, 1088
  with adopted children, 1105
  assessment of, 50, 820, 1060, 1104, 1106–1108
    form for, *1108f*
  at-risk newborns and, 973–981, *975f, 978f,* 1036–1039, 1105
    preterm, 945–946, *947f,* 950–951, *951f*
  behaviors, 1096, 1109, *1109f*
  cesarean birth and, 1085
  defined, 1095
  en face position and, 1098, *1098f*
  engrossment in, 1103
  entrainment in, 1101–1102
  environment for, 1096–1097
  facilitating, 664–665, 868, 870–871, 1096–2097, 1105–1106
  fathers and, 1103–1104
  intervention guidelines, 1107, 1109, *1109f*
  malattachment warning signs, 1112
  maternal-fetal, 1095–1096, 1124
  maternal-newborn, 1049, 1097–1103
    initial, 664–665
    postpartal complications and, 1109–1112
  newborn influence on, 664–665, 1096, 1098–1099, 1104
  parent-newborn, 811, 820, 865, 868, 870, 977–979
  prenatal influences on, 1095–1096, 1099
  reciprocity process in, 1100–1102, *1101f,* 1105
  siblings and, 1104
  teaching guide to enhance, 1110

Attention/nonattention cycle, 1100–1102, *1101f*

Attitudes. *See also* Beliefs
  about pregnancy, 327–328
  of the family, 39–40
  sexual, 193–194

Auditory capacity, newborn, 808, 831, 847, 946, 1105

Autosomal inheritance
  dominant, 156–157, *157f*
  nondisjunction, 106
  recessive, 157–158, *158f*

Autosomes, defined, 151

AWHONN (Association of Women's Health, Obstetric, and Neonatal Nurses), NAACOG Standards of nursing care, 25, 1149

Azoospermia, 146

AZT (zidovudine), 457, 960

Babinski reflex, 838, *839t,* 854

Backache, *369t,* 373–374

Bacterial vaginosis (BV), 200, *238f,* 239, *241t, 523t*

Bactrim, *389t*

BAER (brain stem auditory evoked response) test, 946

Bag of waters (BOW), 113

Balanced translocation, 161
  carrier, 154, *155f*

Ballard score, 811–820, *812f, 814f–821f*

Ballottement, *317t,* 318

Barbiturates, *389t, 462t*
  for labor discomfort, 678

Barlow's maneuver, *836f,* 837

Barr body, 155–156

Barrier contraceptives, 205–208, *207f, 208f,* 211

Bartter's syndrome, 114

Basal body temperature (BBT), 136–137, *137f,* 203, *204f*

Basal metabolic rate (BMR), in pregnancy, 315

Baseline rate, 617–619

Baseline variability, 619–621, *619f, 620f*

BAT (brown adipose tissue), 798–799, *798f,* 935, 1012–1013

Bathing
  cultural practices and, 1076
  during pregnancy, 380
  postpartal, 1074, 1075
  sitz, 1074

Bathing newborns
  at admission, 863
  circumcision care, 875, 877
  sponge baths, 874–877

supplies for, *875t*
tub baths, 877, *877f*
umbilical cord care during, teaching guide, 876

Battered women
  characteristics of, 268–270
  cycle of violence and, 270–271
  management of, 272–278
    nursing care plan, 275
  signs of, 272–273
  trauma to, during pregnancy, 518

Battledore placenta, 744–745, *744f*

BBT (basal body temperature), 136–137, *137f,* 203, *204f*

Beckwith-Wiedemann syndrome, 929

Beginning families, defined, 35, *42t,* 43

Behavior
  attachment, 1096–1103
  change, learning theories and, 59–62
  entrainment, 1101–1102
  feeding, 896–897, *897t*
  newborn, 806–808
    assessment of, 855–856
    drug-dependent, 955–956
    preterm, 952
  states
    fetal, 589
    newborn, 807–808, 837

Beliefs
  about food, 424, 425–426, *426f*
  about labor, 644–646
  about menstruation, 197–198
  about pregnancy, 58, *58t,* 77, 365, *365t*
  about sexuality, 193–194
  family, 45–46
  health, 56–58, *57t, 58t,* 327–328

Benzedrine, *462t*

Beta blockers, 388

Beta-adrenergic agonists, 488

Betamethasone (Celestone Solupan), 484–485
  drug guide, 485

Betamimetics, 488, 760

Bilateral salpingo-oophorectomy (BSO), 253, 254

Bilirubin, 799–802, *800f, 802t,* 937, 1019
  encephalopathy (kernicterus), 1019

Bill of rights, pregnant patient's, 1147

Billings contraception method, 204

Biocept-G test, for pregnancy, 319

Biophysical profile, 445, 458, 539–541, *540t, 541t*

and ovulatory function, 138
in placental functions, 120, 315
Ethics
    AIDS patients and, 456
    dilemmas of, 15–18
    principles of, 13–14
    standards of care and, 11–12
Ethnic identity, family and, 45–46
Ethnocentrism, 329
Evaporation heat loss, defined, 797
Exchange transfusion, 1022, *1022t*, 1027–1029
    procedure for, 1028–1029
Exenteration, pelvic, 258–259
Exercises
    childbirth, 374, 382–384, *383f*, *384f*
    during pregnancy, *365t*, 381–384, *383f*, *384f*
    Hoffman's, 378–379, *379f*
    Kegel's, 263, 304, 383, *384f*, 1045
    pelvic tilt, 374, 382, *383f*
    perineal, prenatal, 383, *384f*
    postpartal, 1077, *1078f*, 1079
    preconception, 293
Exosurf (artificial surfactant), 993
Expectant family, 363–368
    adolescent, 394–407
    over age 35, 407–411
Extended family, 37
External (cephalic) version, 758–760, *758f*
Extracorporeal membrane oxygenation (ECMO), 993, 1002
Extremities, newborn assessment, 835–837, *835f*, *836f*, *837f*, 851–853
Eyes, newborn
    assessment, 829–830, *830f*, 844–846
    movements of, 806, 837, 844–845
    preventing infection in, 866–867, *867f*, 868

Fabry disease, 162
Face
    newborn assessment, 828–831, *830f*, *831f*, 843–844
    paralysis in, 826, 828, *829f*
Face presentation, 566, *566t*, *567f*, 716–717, *716f*, *717f*
Factrel, *145t*
FAD (Family Assessment Device), 50
FAD (fetal activity diary), 378
FAE (fetal alcohol effects), 953–955
Failure to progress, in labor, *595t*
Faintness, *370t*, 374–375
    postpartal, 1074–1075

Fallopian tubes. *See also* Ectopic pregnancy
    artificial insemination, 17, 146–147
    blood supply to, *78f*
    fertilization location in, *112f*
    functions of, 82
    structure of, 80–81, *81f*
False labor, 576–577, *577t*, 678
False pelvis, 85–88, *86f*
Family
    adjustments, to newborn illness, 973–981, *975f*, *978f*
    assessment of, *39t*, 48–51, *49f*, *50t*, *51t*
    as client, 47–48
    defined, 35
    female-headed, 37, 45–46, 173, 175
    functions of, 38–40
        factors affecting, 45–47
    genetic counseling and, 165–168, *168t*
    grief work of, 477, 732, 974, 1036–1038, 1085, 1088–1089
    homelessness and, 175–176
    nutrition counseling and, 433
    postpartal period, 1048–1050
    stages of, 35, 42–45, *42t*, *44t*
    structure of, 35–38
        factors affecting, 45–47
    theoretical frameworks for, 40–45
Family APGAR test, 50
Family Assessment Device (FAD), 50
Family Environment Scale, 50
Family and Medical Leave Act, 179
Family planning, natural, 202–205, *204f*
Family systems framework, defined, 41–42
Family violence. *See* Violence
Family-centered nursing, 4, 34, 47–52
FAS (fetal alcohol syndrome), 390, 463, 953–955
FAST (fetal acoustic stimulation test), 546, *546f*
Fat (dietary), in pregnancy, 314, 419
Fathers, 4, 335, 364
    adolescent, 398–400, 1088
    cesarean birth and, 1085
    postpartal period and, 1048, 1080, 1081
    reactions to pregnancy, 324–326
    strategies to promote role of, 1107, 1109, *1109f*
Fatigue, 316, *369t*, 370–371
    postpartal, 1059, 1060, 1077, 1119
FBD (fibrocystic breast disease), 219–221, *225t*

FBM (Fetal breathing movements), 539–540, *540t*
Fear, as labor complication, 700–703, *702f*
Feeding. *See also* Bottle feeding; Breastfeeding
    behavior cues, 896–897, *897t*
    first, of newborn, 807, 867–868, 938–943
    gavage, 931, 940–943, 950
    total parenteral nutrition, 940
    transpyloric, 940, 950
Feet, newborn assessment, 814, *815f*, 837, *837f*, 853
Feetman Family Functioning Scale, 50
Female condom, 205–206, *206*
Female partner abuse. *See* Battered women
Feminization of poverty, 173–176
Femur length, fetal, 535, *536f*
Fentanyl, 680, 970, 993, 1004
Ferning capacity, 95, 138–139, *139f*
Fertility
    components of normal, 132–133, *133t*
    cycle of, summary, *97t*, *98t*, *136t*, *195t*
Fertility awareness contraception methods, 202–205, *204f*
Fertilization, 101, *106f*, 108–110
    age, of fetus, 123
    location of, in fallopian tube, *112f*
    moment of, 109–110
Fetal acoustic stimulation test (FAST), 546, *546f*
Fetal activity diary (FAD), 378
Fetal activity monitoring
    electronic
        external, 615, *616f*, *618t*
        indications for, 615, *615t*
        internal, 615–617, *616f*, *617f*, *618t*
        maternal psychologic reactions to, 628–629
        nursing procedure for, 614
        relative merits of, *618t*, 629
    maternal, 542–543
        Cardiff Count-to-Ten scoring card, *377f*, 543
        diaries/movement records, 378
        teaching guide for, 376–377
Fetal alcohol effects (FAE), 953–955
Fetal alcohol syndrome (FAS), 390, 463, 953–955
Fetal attitude, 565, *565f*
Fetal breathing movements (FBM), 539–540, *540t*

early discharge from, 4, 55
  maternity units, 296, *297f*
Hot flashes, 215
Hot tubs, 1074
  hazards of, 129, 380
hPL (human placental lactogen), 119,
  120, 315
HSG (hysterosalpingography),
  142–143
HSV (herpes simplex virus), 164,
  205, 210
  fetal-neonatal risks, 521–523
Huhner's test, 139, 141
Human chorionic gonadotropin
  (hCG), 95, 119, *145t*, 315,
  368
Human development, stages of,
  124–128, *124–127f*
Human Genome Project, 17–18
Human immunodeficiency virus. *See*
  HIV infection
Human menopausal gonadotropin
  (hMG), 144, *145t*
Human placental lactogen (hPL),
  119, 120, 315
Human reproduction, 69–170
Hunter syndrome, 162
Huntington's chorea, 157
Hurler disease, 162
Hyaline membrane disease (HMD).
  See Respiratory distress syn-
  drome
Hydatidiform mole, 480–481, *480f*
Hydramnios, 115, 442, 530, 749–750
  risk factors, *595t, 1050t,* 1128
Hydrocele, 835
Hydrocephalus, congenital, 946,
  965t
Hydrochlorothiazide, 388
Hydromorphone, 680
Hydrops fetalis, 511, 1020
Hyperbilirubinemia, 443, 515, 771
  in IDM newborn, 930
  pathophysiology of, 1019–1020
Hypercalcemia, 422
Hyperemesis gravidarum, 474–475
Hyperglycemia, in preterm newborn,
  936
Hypermenorrhea, 202
Hyperoxia-hyperventilation test, 1004
Hyperphenylalaninemia, *469t*
Hypertension
  chronic, *338t,* 509
  inherited, 160
  pregnancy-induced. *See* Pregnancy-
    induced hypertension
Hyperthermia, 129, 799
Hyperthyroidism, risk factors, *338t,*
  469t

Hypertonic labor patterns, 703–706,
  704f
Hyperventilation, in labor, 650–651
Hyperviscosity, in LGA newborn,
  929
Hypnosis, for childbirth, 302–303,
  303t
Hypocalcemia, 443, 837
  care of, 1017–1018
  in IDM newborn, 930
  in SGA newborn, 924
Hypoglycemia, 447, 837
  care of, 1013, *1014f, 1015f,*
    1016–1017
  glucose chemstrip test (procedure),
    1014–1016
  in IDM newborn, 930
  in LGA newborn, 929
  in postmaturity syndrome,
    932
  in SGA newborn, 924
Hypoglycemics, oral, 444
Hypomenorrhea, 202
Hypoplastic left heart syndrome,
  969t
Hypospadias, 146, 835
Hypothermia, newborn. *See* Cold
  stress
Hypothyroidism, 138, 165, 885
  congenital, 971, 972
  risk factors, *338t, 469t*
Hypotonic labor patterns, *704f,*
  706–707, 713, 714
Hypovolemia, 824, 1030
Hypoxemia, 935
Hypoxia, 992
  fetal, 674, 728
HypRho-D. *See* Rh immune globulin
Hysterectomy
  abdominal, 251, 253–256
  postoperative care, 257
  vaginal, 255, 256
Hysterogram, 142–143
Hysterosalpingography (HSG),
  142–143
Hysteroscopy, 143

Identical twins, 110, *111f*
Identification bands, 664, 728
Idiopathic respiratory distress syn-
  drome. *See* Respiratory dis-
  tress syndrome
IDMs (infants of diabetic mothers),
  813–814, 930–932, *930f*
IgA immunoglobins, 805, 892
IGT (impaired glucose tolerance),
  440t
Ileococcygeus muscle, *84t,* 85, *85t*

Ilotycin Ophthalmic (erythromycin
  ophthalmic)
  drug guide, 866
  instillation of (procedure), 867,
    867f
Imminent abortion, 476, *477f*
Immune response, in HIV infection,
  456–462
Immunity
  active acquired, 805
  passive acquired, 805, 892
  in preterm newborn, 937
Immunizations
  during pregnancy, 385, *387t,* 457
  of newborns, 884–886, 1068–1069,
    1072t
Immunoassays, to diagnose pregnancy, 318–319
Immunoglobins, 805
Immunologic system
  in HIV infection, 456–462
  neonatal transition period, 805
  in preterm newborn, 937
Impaired glucose tolerance (IGT),
  440t
Imperforate anus, 835
Imperforate anus, congenital, *967t*
Implantation (nidation), 96, 111–112,
  112f, 113f
  blastocyst, *97f*
In vitro fertilization (IVF), 17,
  146–147, 149
Inborn errors of metabolism, 158,
  162, 164–165, 971–973
Incompetent cervix, 483
Incomplete abortion, 476, *477f*
Inderal (propranolol hydrochloride),
  437
Indomethacin (Indocin), 489, 944,
  945
Induction of labor
  elective, 762
  indications for, 762
  nursing care plan, 766–768
  oxytocin for, drug guide, 763–765
  predictors of inducibility, *763t*
  risk factors, *595t*
Infants
  birth weight (statistics), 27, *28f*
  of diabetic mothers (IDMs), *815f,*
    930–932, *930f*
    maturity rating and, 813–814
  mortality rate (statistics), 27–29,
    29t, 457
  of substance-abusing mothers
    (ISAMs)
    complications of, 955–956
    fetal alcohol syndrome, 953–955
    home care for, 960

MAS (meconium aspiration
syndrome), 932, 955,
1000–1003
Mastectomy, 229
Mastitis
chronic cystic, 219–221, *225t*
plasma cell, 225–226, *225t*
postpartal, 1136–1138, *1137f,*
1138t
Mastodynia, 219
Maternal age, 26, *27t, 28f*
adolescent, 393–407
risk factors, *337t, 395t*
age-related risks, *163t,* 396–397
chromosomal abnormalities, risk
factors, *162t*
genetic testing and, 160–162, *163t*
35 and over, *337t,* 407–411
Maternal Attachment Assessment
Strategy, 50
Maternal Concerns Questionnaire,
1049
Maternal mortality rate, defined, 29,
29t
Maternal nutrition, 413–434
adolescent pregnancy and,
427–429
assessing, 416, 427, 430–433
diet histories, 428–429, 431
questionnaire for, *432f*
breastfeeding and, *414t, 415t,* 420,
430, 1059, *1060t*
calcium, 314, 419–420, *420t,* 430
calories, 417
teaching guide for increasing,
418–419
carbohydrates, 314, 417
daily food plan for, *415t*
deficiencies in, 129
for diabetic pregnancy, 444
eating disorders and, 428
factors influencing, 414–415,
424–427, *426f*
fats, 314, 419
fluid intake, 314, 423–424, 430
Food Guide Pyramid, 416, *417f*
lactose intolerance and, 424–425
minerals, 314, *414f,* 419–421,
420t, 428, 429, 430
pica, 425
postpartal, 429–430, 1059, *1060t*
pregnancy outcome and, 414, 416,
420–424, 427
protein, 417, 419, *419t,* 424, 430
psychosocial factors, 426–427
recommended dietary allowances,
414–417, *414t,* 428
requirements for, 418–424
vegetarianism, 419, 424

vitamins, 314, 421–423
weight gain, optimal, 314, 416,
416t, 424, 428, 429
Maternal role attainment, defined,
1049
Maternal serum alpha-fetoprotein
(MSAFP) testing, 163–164,
553
Maternity leaves, 179
Mature milk, defined, 892
Maturity assessment
fetal, 553–554
newborn, 811–820, *812f, 814–821f*
by weight/gestational age,
819–820, *820f, 821f*
preterm, 934–935, *935f*
Measles, German. *See* Rubella
Measurements, newborn, 822–823,
822f, 823t, 841, 862, *862f*
Mechanisms of labor (cardinal movements), 579, *581f*
Meconium
defined, 803
stools, 803, *803f, 803t,* 835
Meconium aspiration syndrome
(MAS), 932, 955, 1000–1003
Meconium staining of amniotic fluid,
554, 653, 709
amnioinfusion to treat, 769
risk factors, *595t*
Medical diagnosis, *versus* nursing
diagnosis, 22
Medical records, confidentiality of,
13
Medications. *See also specific medication*
breastfeeding and, 439, 894, 907,
909, 1135, 1154
effects on fetus, 388–389, *389t,*
462t
postpartal, commonly used,
1072–1073t
tocolytic, 487–489
Mediterranean ethnicity, thalassemias
and, *163t,* 167, 455–456
Medroxyprogesterone acetate, 145
Megaloblastic anemia, 423
Meiosis, 93–94, 105–110, *107f*
compared with mitosis, *105f*
Menadione (vitamin K), 422
Menarche
adaptation to, 198
defined, 73, 95
Mendelian (single-gene) inheritance,
156–159
Meningomyelocele, 423
Menopause, 82, 214–216
Menorrhagia, 202
Menotropins, 144, *145t*
Menstruation

amenorrhea, 201–202
beliefs about, 197–198
cycle of
anovulatory cycles, 202
blood supply during, *94f*
comfort issues with, 77,
199–200
normal, 198
phases of, 95–96, *95t, 97t, 136t*
variations in, 201–202
defined, 95
dysmenorrhea, 80, 201
menarche, 73, 95, 198
premenstrual syndrome, 200–201
recurrence of, postpartal, 1045
teaching about, 198–202
toxic shock syndrome and, 199
Meperidine hydrochloride (Demerol),
676, 799, 1084, 1134
drug guide, 677
Mepivacaine hydrochloride (Carbocaine), 680, 693, 694
Mesoderm, 112, *113t*
Metabolic acidosis, 992, *992f*
Metabolic disorders
genetic counseling for, 166
inborn errors, 158, 162, 164–165,
971–973
screening for, in newborn,
884–885
Metabolism, in pregnancy, 314
Metachromatic leukodystrophy, 162
Metaphase stage, chromosomal, 106,
151f
Methadone, *462t,* 465, 955, 956
Methergine (methylergonovine
maleate), 666, 1047, 1055,
1057, 1068, 1117, 1118, 1121
drug guide, 1069
Methicillin, *1035t*
Methotrexate, *389t,* 479
Methylergonovine maleate
(Methergine), 666, 1047,
1055, 1057, 1068, 1117, 1118,
1121
drug guide, 1069
Methylmalonic aciduria, 162
Metritis, 1121–1123
Metrodin, *145t*
Metronidazole (Flagyl), 239–240,
523t
drug guide, 240
Metrorrhagia, 202
Mexican Americans, *57t,* 424–425
MgSO₄ (magnesium sulfate), 488,
499, 708, 760
drug guide, 490
Microangiopathic hemolytic anemia,
496–497

CERVICAL DILATATION ASSESSMENT AID

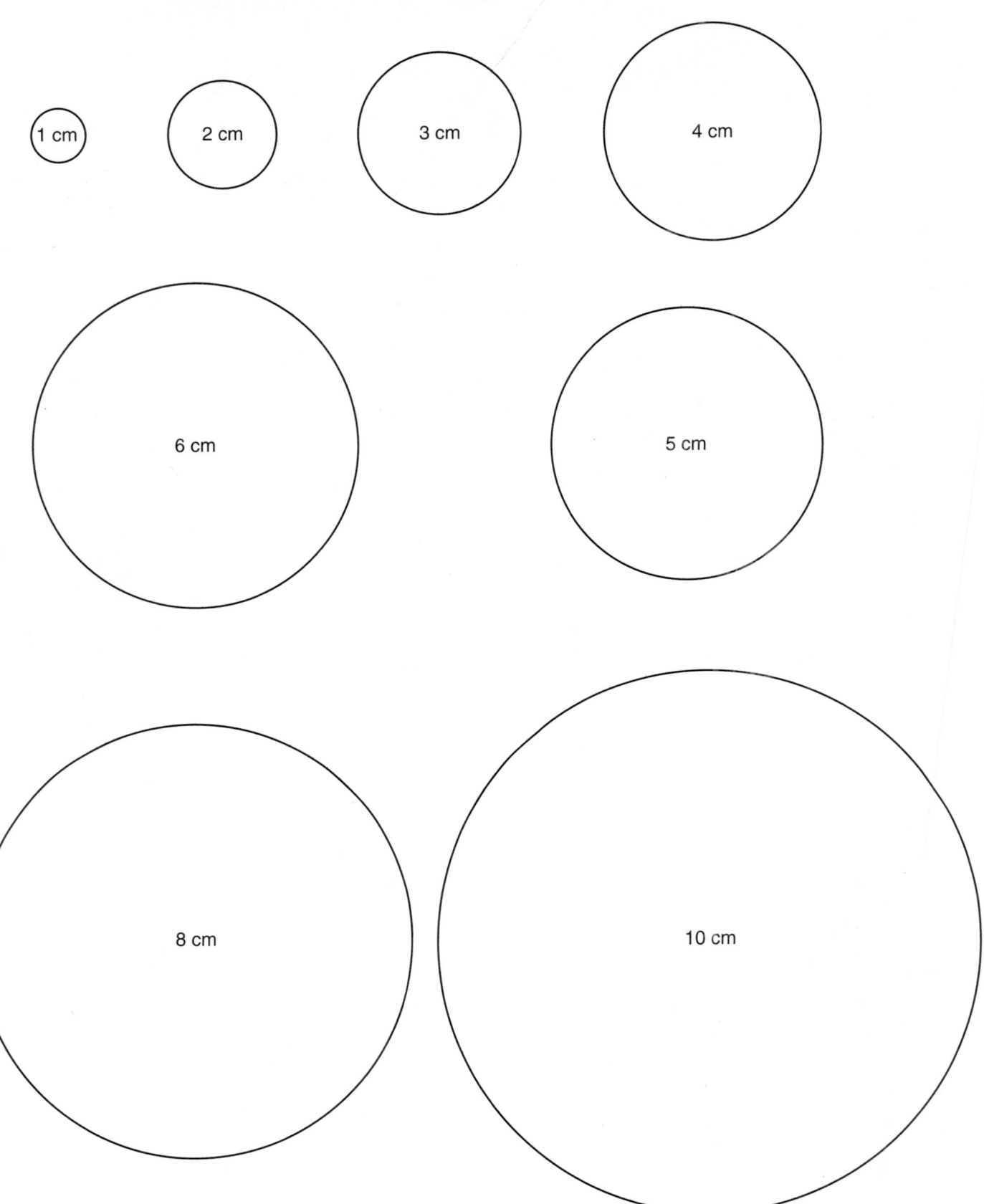